Compliments of

AstraZeneca

A research-based pharmaceutical

company committed

to bringing you innovative

cardiovascular medications.

160189 6/99

Hypertension:
A Companion to Brenner and Rector's
The Kidney

Hypertension:
A Companion to Brenner and Rector's
The Kidney

Suzanne Oparil, M.D.

Director, Vascular Biology and Hypertension Program
Division of Cardiovascular Disease

Professor of Medicine
University of Alabama at Birmingham School of Medicine
Birmingham, Alabama

Michael A. Weber, M.D.

Chair, Department of Medicine
Brookdale University Hospital and Medical Center

Professor of Medicine and Clinical Associate Dean
State University of New York Health Science Center at Brooklyn
Brooklyn, New York

W.B. Saunders Company

A Harcourt Health Sciences Company
St. Louis   Philadelphia   London   Sydney   Toronto

W.B. SAUNDERS COMPANY
A *Harcourt Health Sciences Company*

The Curtis Center
Independence Square West
Philadelphia, Pennsylvania 19106

Library of Congress Cataloging-in-Publication Data

Hypertension: a companion to Brenner & Rector's the kidney / [edited by] Suzanne Oparil, Michael A. Weber.

p.   cm.

Companion v. to: Brenner & Rector's the kidney / edited by Barry M. Brenner. 5th ed. c 1996.

ISBN 0–7216–7764–9

1. Hypertension.   I. Oparil, Suzanne.   II. Weber, Michael A.   III. Brenner & Rector's the kidney. [DNLM: 1. Hypertension—therapy.
2. Hypertension—physiopathology.   3. Hypertension—complications.
4. Life Style.   5. Antihypertensive Agents—therapeutic use.
WG 340 H99426 1999]

RC685.H8H76783 1999   616.1'32—dc21

DNLM/DLC   98–47451

HYPERTENSION: A Companion to Brenner and Rector's *The Kidney*   ISBN 0–7216–7764–9

Printed in the United States of America.

Last digit is the print number: 9   8   7   6   5   4   3   2   1

*We dedicate this volume to our families
and to the mentors, collaborators, and associates
who have made our work in hypertension possible.
In particular, we express appreciation
to Harriet Dustan and John Laragh
for their pivotal contributions to our field
and to our personal careers.*

Contributors

Koshy Abraham, M.D.
Clinical Instructor
University of Florida
Clinical Instructor
University of Florida Shands Teaching
  Hospital
Gainesville, Florida
  Hypertension in the Elderly

Ayub Akbari, M.D.
Fellow, Department of Nephrology
University of Ottawa
Ottawa, Canada
  Hypertension in Pregnant Women

Michael H. Alderman, M.D.
Department of Epidemiology and Social
  Medicine
Albert Einstein College of Medicine
Bronx, New York
  Total Risk

Syed S. Ali, M.D.
Fellow, Endocrinology
Wayne State University School of
  Medicine
Detroit, Michigan
  *Metabolic Abnormalities in
  Hypertension*

Phyllis August, M.D.
Professor of Medicine
Chief, Hypertension Division
Weill Medical College of Cornell
  University
Attending Physician
New York Presbyterian Hospital
New York, New York
  Hypertension in Women

George L. Bakris, M.D.
Associate Professor of Preventive and
  Internal Medicine
Vice-Chairman, Department of Preventive
  Medicine
Director, Hypertension/Clinical Research
  Center
Rush Medical College
Chicago, Illinois
  *Diabetes and Syndrome X: Focus on
  Reduction of Cardiovascular and Renal
  Events*

John H. Bauer, M.D.
Professor of Medicine
University of Missouri
Nephrology Consultant
Harry S. Truman Memorial Veterans
  Hospital
Columbia, Missouri
  *Hypertension in Patients on Renal
  Replacement Therapy*

Henry R. Black, M.D.
Charles J. and Margaret Roberts Professor
  and Chairman of Preventive Medicine
Professor of Internal Medicine
Senior Attending Physician
Rush Medical College of Rush University
Rush–Presbyterian–St. Luke's Medical
  Center
Chicago, Illinois
  *Benefits of Treating Hypertension—
  Lessons From Clinical Trials*

George L. Blackburn, M.D., Ph.D.
Associate Professor of Surgery
S. Daniel Abraham Chair in Nutrition
  Medicine
Harvard Medical School
Director, Center for the Study of
  Nutrition Medicine
Beth Israel Deaconess Medical Center
Boston, Massachusetts
  Diet—Calories

Lee R. Bone, R.N., M.P.H.
Associate Scientist
Johns Hopkins University School of
  Hygiene and Public Health
Baltimore, Maryland
  Community Outreach

Emmanuel L. Bravo, M.D.
Staff, Department of Nephrology and
  Hypertension
Department of Molecular Cardiology
  (Research Institute)
Cleveland Clinic
Cleveland, Ohio
  Adrenal Cortex

Robert Brook, M.D.
Fellow, Division of Hypertension
University of Michigan Health System
Ann Arbor, Michigan
  *Mild Hypertension: An Important
  Frontier in Therapy of Hypertension*

Gillian R. Bullock, B.Sc., Ph.D.
Guest Professor and Head, Molecular
  Pathology Laboratory
Department of Pathology
University Hospital
Ghent, Belgium
  The AT_1 and AT_2 Angiotensin Receptors

Julie E. Buring, Sc.D.
Professor, Department of Ambulatory
  Care and Prevention
Harvard Medical School
Deputy Director, Division of Preventive
  Medicine
Brigham and Women's Hospital
Boston, Massachusetts
  *Calcium Channel Blockers in the
  Treatment of Hypertension*

John C. Burnett, Jr., M.D.
Cardiorenal Research Laboratory
Mayo Foundation
Rochester, Minnesota
  Endothelin in Hypertension

David A. Calhoun, M.D.
Assistant Professor of Medicine, Vascular
  Biology and Hypertension Program
Division of Cardiovascular Diseases
University of Alabama at Birmingham
Birmingham, Alabama
  Hypertensive Crisis; Drug Tables

Vito M. Campese, M.D.
Professor of Medicine and Interim Chief,
  Division of Nephrology
University of Southern California, Los
  Angeles, Medical Center
Los Angeles, California
  Natriuretic Peptides

**J. Jaime Caro, M.D.C.M., F.R.C.P.C.,
F.A.C.P.**
Adjunct Professor of Medicine
McGill University
Montreal, Québec, Canada
  Current Prescribing Practices

Daniel F. Catanzaro, Ph.D.
Associate Professor of Physiology in
  Medicine
Weill Medical College
Cornell University
New York, New York
  Angiotensinogen: Physiology,
  Molecular Biology, and Relevance to
  Hypertension

Hal L. Chadow, M.D.
State University of New York Health
  Science Center at Brooklyn
The Brookdale University Hospital and
  Medical Center
Brooklyn, New York
  Ischemic Heart Disease

Samuel Chan, M.D.
Fellow
Harvard Medical School
Fellow, Nutrition and Metabolism
Beth Israel Deaconess Medical Center
Boston, Massachusetts
  Diet—Calories

William C. Cushman, B.A., M.D.
Professor of Preventive Medicine and
  Medicine
University of Tennessee College of
  Medicine
Chief, Preventive Medicine Section
Veterans Affairs Medical Center
Memphis, Tennessee
  Alcohol Consumption and the
  Management of Hypertension

Björn Dahlöf, M.D., Ph.D.
Associate Professor
University of Göteborg
Consultant, Department of Internal
  Medicine
Sahlgrenska Hospital/Östra
Göteborg, Sweden
  The Losartan Intervention for Endpoint
  (LIFE) Reduction in Hypertension
  Study: Rationale, Design, and
  Characteristics of 9194 Patients With
  Left Ventricular Hypertrophy

Marc de Gasparo, M.D.
Valsartan Preclinical Leader
Novartis Pharma AG
Basel, Switzerland
  The AT_1 and AT_2 Angiotensin Receptors

J. Deinum, M.D.
Internist, Staff Member
University Hospital Dykzigt
Rotterdam, The Netherlands
  Renin and Prorenin

Paul E. de Jong, M.D., Ph.D.,
F.R.C.P.Edin.
Professor of Nephrology
Gröningen School of Medicine
Head, Renal Division
Department of Medicine
University Hospital
Gröningen, The Netherlands
  Renal Disease

Carolina Delgado, M.D.
Research Fellow
Division of Hypertension
Department of Internal Medicine
University of Michigan
Ann Arbor, Michigan
  Pathophysiology of Hypertension

Dick De Zeeuw, M.D., Ph.D.
Professor of Clinical Pharmacology
Director, Department of Clinical
  Pharmacology
Director, Gröningen Kidney Center
Gröningen School of Medicine
Gröningen, The Netherlands
  Renal Disease

Joseph A. Diamond, M.D.
Assistant Professor of Medicine
Mount Sinai School of Medicine
Assistant Attending of Medicine
Zena and Michael Wiener Cardiovascular
  Institute
Mount Sinai Medical Center
New York, New York
  Left Ventricular Hypertrophy,
  Congestive Heart Failure, and
  Coronary Flow Reserve Abnormalities
  in Hypertension

Diem T. Dinh, B.Sc.(Hons.)
Postgraduate Research Scholar
Department of Medicine
University of Melbourne
Melbourne, Victoria, Australia
  Angiotensin-Converting Enzyme: Basic
  Properties, Distribution, and
  Functional Role

Donald J. DiPette, M.D.
Professor of Medicine
Vice-Chair for In-Patient Affairs
Director, Division of General Internal
  Medicine
University of Texas Medical Branch
Galveston, Texas
  Calcitonin Gene–Related Peptide and
  Hypertension

Karen A. Duggan, B.Sc.(Hons.),
M.B.B.S., M.D., F.R.A.C.P.
Associate Professor of Medicine
Faculty of Medicine
University of New South Wales
Director, Hypertension Service
Bankstown-Lidcombe Hospital
Sydney, New South Wales, Australia
  Comorbid Conditions

Harriet P. Dustan, B.S., M.D.
(deceased)
Visiting Professor, Department of
  Pharmacology and Medicine
University of Vermont College of
  Medicine
Burlington, Vermont
  History of Clinical Hypertension: From
  1827 to 1970

William J. Elliott, M.D., Ph.D.
Associate Professor of Preventive
  Medicine, Rush Medical College of
  Rush University at Rush–Presbyterian–
  St. Luke's Medical Center
Attending Physician
Rush–Presbyterian–St. Luke's Medical
  Center
Chicago, Illinois
  Benefits of Treating Hypertension—
  Lessons From Clinical Trials; Cost-
  Effectiveness in Treating Hypertension

Maurice E. Fabiani, B.Sc.(Hons.), Ph.D.
Senior Research Fellow
Department of Medicine
University of Melbourne
Melbourne, Victoria, Australia
  Angiotensin-Converting Enzyme: Basic
  Properties, Distribution, and
  Functional Role

Pierre F. Faubert, M.D.
Associate Professor of Medicine
State University of New York Health
  Science Center at Brooklyn
Attending Physician, Division of
  Nephrology and Hypertension,
  Department of Medicine
The Brookdale University Hospital and
  Medical Center
Brooklyn, New York
  Chronic Renal Insufficiency: Slowing
  Its Progression

Alan Feit, M.D.
Cardiac Catheterization Center
State University of New York Health
  Science Center at Brooklyn
Brooklyn, New York
  Ischemic Heart Disease

Robert R. Fenichel, M.D., Ph.D.
Deputy Division Director, Division of
  CardioRenal Drug Products
United States Food and Drug
  Administration
Rockville, Maryland
  How Hypertensive Drugs Get Approved
  in the United States

John M. Flack, M.D., M.P.H.
Professor of Medicine and Community
  Medicine
Associate Chairman, Department of
  Medicine
Wayne State University Medical School
Chief of Medicine, Detroit Medical
  Center, Central Region Hospitals
Director, Cardiovascular Epidemiology
  and Clinical Applications Program
Wayne State University
Detroit, Michigan
  Hypertension in Blacks

Stanley S. Franklin, M.D.
Clinical Professor of Medicine
Associate Medical Director
UCI Heart Disease Prevention Program
College of Medicine, Department of
    Medicine
University of California, Irvine
Irvine, California
    New Interpretations of Blood Pressure:
    The Importance of Pulse Pressure

William H. Frishman, M.D.
Professor of Medicine and Pharmacology
Chairman, Department of Medicine
New York Medical College
Chief of Medicine
Westchester Medical Center
Valhalla, New York
    β-Adrenergic Blockers

Edward D. Frohlich, M.D.
Professor, Department of Medicine and
    Department of Physiology
Louisiana State University
Clinical Professor of Medicine and
    Adjunct Professor of Pharmacology
Tulane University
Vice President for Academic Affairs
Alton Ochsner Medical Foundation
New Orleans, Louisiana
    Other Adrenergic Inhibitors and the
    Direct-Acting Smooth Muscle
    Vasodilators

Todd W. B. Gehr, M.D.
Professor of Medicine, Division of
    Nephrology
Medical College of Virginia Hospitals of
    Virginia Commonwealth University
Richmond, Virginia
    Dose-Response Relationships in
    Antihypertensive Treatment;
    Angiotensin-Converting Enzyme
    Inhibitors

Robert J. Glynn, Sc.D.
Associate Professor of Medicine
    (Biostatistics)
Harvard Medical School
Statistician, Division of Preventive
    Medicine
Brigham and Women's Hospital
Boston, Massachusetts
    Calcium Channel Blockers in the
    Treatment of Hypertension

James Gould, M.D.
Associate in the Department of
    Anesthesia, Division of Cardiothoracic
    Anesthesia
Duke University Medical Center
Durham, North Carolina
    Anesthesia and Hypertension

Lennart Hansson, M.D.
Professor, University of Uppsala
Department of Geriatrics
Uppsala, Sweden
    Epidemiology of Hypertension

Stephen B. Harrap, M.B.B.S.,
F.R.A.C.P., Ph.D.
Professor and Head, Department of
    Physiology
University of Melbourne
Parkville
Consultant Physician, Royal Melbourne
    Hospital
Victoria, Australia
    Genetics

Christopher S. Hayward, B.Med.Sc.,
M.B.B.S., F.R.A.C.P.
Postdoctoral Research Fellow, National
    Heart and Lung Institute
Department of Cardiac Medicine
Imperial College School of Medicine
London, United Kingdom
    Arterial Stiffness

Charles H. Hennekens, M.D., Dr.P.H.
Eugene Braunwald Professor of Medicine
Professor of Ambulatory Care and
    Prevention
Harvard Medical School
Chief, Division of Preventive Medicine
Brigham and Women's Hospital
Boston, Massachusetts
    Calcium Channel Blockers in the
    Treatment of Hypertension

Angel H. Herrera, M.D.
Fellow in Geriatric Medicine
University of Florida
Fellow in Geriatric Medicine
Veterans Affairs Medical Center
Gainesville, Florida
    Exercise and Hypertension

Martha N. Hill, R.N., Ph.D.
Professor, Johns Hopkins University
    School of Nursing
Baltimore, Maryland
    Nursing Clinics in the Management of
    Hypertension; Community Outreach

Norman K. Hollenberg, M.D., Ph.D.
Professor, Department of Medicine
Harvard Medical School
Director of Physiologic Research
    Radiology
Brigham and Women's Hospital
Boston, Massachusetts
    Renin Inhibitors

Howard G. Hutchinson, M.D.,
F.A.C.C.
Senior Medical Director
Zeneca Pharmaceuticals
Wilmington, Delaware
    Obesity-Hypertension: Effects on the
    Cardiovascular and Renal
    Systems—The Therapeutic Approach

Joseph L. Izzo, Jr., M.D.
Professor of Medicine and Pharmacology
Chief, Clinical Pharmacology
State University of New York at Buffalo
Staff
Kaleida Health
Millard Fillmore Hospital
Buffalo, New York
    Sympathetic Nervous System in Acute
    and Chronic Blood Pressure Elevation

Colin I. Johnston, M.B.B.S., F.R.A.C.P.
Baker Medical Research Institute
Melbourne, Victoria, Australia
    Angiotensin-Converting Enzyme: Basic
    Properties, Distribution, and
    Functional Role

Ulrich Jorde, M.D.
Fellow in Cardiovascular Medicine
Albert Einstein College of Medicine
Staff
Montefiore Medical Center/Jacobi
    Hospital Center
Bronx, New York
    β-Adrenergic Blockers

Stevo Julius, M.D., Sc.D.
Professor of Internal Medicine and
    Physiology
University of Michigan
Frederick G. L. Huetwell Professor of
    Hypertension
Chief, Division of Hypertension
University of Michigan Health System
Ann Arbor, Michigan
    Mild Hypertension: An Important
    Frontier in Therapy of Hypertension

Douglas M. Kahn, D.O.
Teaching Fellow in Pulmonary and
    Critical Care Medicine
Brown University School of Medicine
Providence, Rhode Island
    Obstructive Sleep Apnea

W. B. Kannel, M.D., M.P.H.
Professor of Medicine and Public Health
Boston University School of Medicine
Boston, Massachusetts
Head, Visiting Scientist Program
Framingham Heart Study
Framingham, Massachusetts
    Coronary Atherosclerotic Sequelae of
    Hypertension

Norman M. Kaplan, M.D.
Clinical Professor of Medicine
University of Texas Southwestern
    Medical Center
Dallas, Texas
    Changing Approaches to Diagnosis
    and Treatment of Hypertension

Lena Kilander, M.D., Ph.D.
Department of Geriatrics
University of Uppsala
Uppsala, Sweden
    Epidemiology of Hypertension

Sverre E. Kjeldsen, M.D., Ph.D.
Associate Professor
University of Oslo
Chief of Section, Division of Cardiology
Department of Internal Medicine
Ullevaal Hospital
Oslo, Norway
*The Losartan Intervention for Endpoint
(LIFE) Reduction in Hypertension
Study: Rationale, Design, and
Characteristics of 9194 Patients With
Left Ventricular Hypertrophy*

Arthur L. Klatsky, M.D.
Senior Consultant in Cardiology
Senior Investigator, Division of Research
Kaiser Permanente Medical Center
Oakland, California
Alcohol and Hypertension

John B. Kostis, M.D.
John G. Detwiler Professor of Cardiology
Professor of Medicine and Pharmacology
Chairman, Department of Medicine
Robert Wood Johnson Medical School
Chief, Medical Staff
Robert Wood Johnson University Hospital
New Brunswick, New Jersey
Angiotensin II Receptor Antagonists

Lawrence R. Krakoff, M.D.
Professor of Medicine
Mount Sinai School of Medicine
New York, New York
Chief of Medicine
Englewood Hospital and Medical Center
Englewood, New Jersey
Initial Evaluation and Follow-Up

Lewis Landsberg, M.D.
Irving S. Cutter Professor and Chairman,
Department of Medicine
Northwestern University Medical School
Physician-in-Chief
Northwestern Memorial Hospital
Chicago, Illinois
*Obesity-Related Hypertension as a
Metabolic Disorder*

Eldon D. Lehmann, M.B., B.S., B.Sc.
Ph.D. Student, Department of Imaging
Imperial College, National Heart and
Lung Institute
Royal Brompton Hospital
Specialist Registrar, Academic
Department of Radiology
St. Bartholomew's Hospital
London, United Kingdom
Arterial Stiffness

Melvin A. Lester, M.D., P.C.
Staff, Internal Medicine
Vascular Medicine Clinic
Southfield, Michigan
*Metabolic Abnormalities in
Hypertension*

David M. Levine, M.D., Sc.D., M.P.H.
Professor
Johns Hopkins University School of
Medicine
Baltimore, Maryland
Community Outreach

Paul D. Levinson, M.D.
Associate Professor of Medicine
Brown University School of Medicine
Providence, Rhode Island
Chief, Endocrinology Division
Memorial Hospital of Rhode Island
Pawtucket, Rhode Island
Obstructive Sleep Apnea

Kathleen C. Light, Ph.D.
Professor of Psychology, Departments of
Psychiatry, Psychology and Physiology
Director, Stress and Health Research
Program
University of North Carolina School of
Medicine
Chapel Hill, North Carolina
*Environmental and Psychosocial Stress
in Hypertension Onset and Progression*

Marshall D. Lindheimer, M.D.
Professor of Medicine, Obstetrics and
Gynecology, and Clinical
Pharmacology
University of Chicago, Division of
Biological Sciences
Attending
University of Chicago Hospitals and
Clinics
Chicago, Illinois
Hypertension in Pregnant Women

David T. Lowenthal, M.D., Ph.D.
Professor of Medicine, Pharmacology and
Exercise Science
University of Florida
Gainesville, Florida
Director of Geriatric Research, Education,
and Clinical Center
Veterans Affairs Medical Center
Staff
University of Florida Shands Teaching
Hospital
Gainesville, Florida
*Exercise and Hypertension;
Hypertension in the Elderly*

George A. Mansoor, M.D.
Assistant Professor, University of
Connecticut School of Medicine
Attending Physician
John Dempsey Hospital
University of Connecticut Health Center
Farmington, Connecticut
White-Coat Hypertension

Harry S. Margolius, M.D., Ph.D.
Professor and Chairman, Department of
Pharmacology
Professor of Medicine
Medical University of South Carolina
Attending Physician
Medical University of South Carolina
Hospital
Ralph H. Johnson Veterans Hospital
Charleston Memorial Hospital
Charleston, South Carolina
Kallikrein-Kinin Systems

David A. McCarron, M.D.
Professor of Medicine, Division of
Nephrology
Oregon Health Sciences University
Portland, Oregon
Diet—Micronutrients

Karen C. McCowen, M.B., M.R.C.P.I.
Fellow
Harvard Medical School
Fellow, Endocrinology, Nutrition, and
Metabolism
Beth Israel Deaconess Medical Center
Boston, Massachusetts
Diet—Calories

John C. McGiff, M.D.
Professor and Chairman, Department of
Pharmacology
New York Medical College
Valhalla, New York
Eicosanoids: Do They Matter?

Nancy Houston Miller, R.N., B.S.N.
Adjunct Assistant Clinical Professor,
Department of Physiological Nursing
University of California, San Francisco
San Francisco
Associate Director, Stanford Cardiac
Rehabilitation Program
Stanford University School of Medicine
Palo Alto, California
*Nursing Clinics in the Management of
Hypertension*

Richard P. Millman, M.D.
Professor of Medicine
Brown University School of Medicine
Director, Sleep Disorders Center of
Lifespan Hospitals
Providence, Rhode Island
Obstructive Sleep Apnea

**Madhukar Misra, M.D.,
M.R.C.P.(U.K.)**
Senior Fellow in Nephrology
University of Missouri
Senior Fellow in Nephrology
Harry S. Truman Memorial Veterans
Hospital
Columbia, Missouri
*Hypertension in Patients on Renal
Replacement Therapy*

Michael J. Mulvany, Ph.D.
Professor, Department of Pharmacology
University of Aarhus
Aarhus, Denmark
Remodeling of Resistance Vessels in Essential Hypertension

Labrini Nassis, B.Sc.(Hons.)
Postgraduate Research Scholar
Department of Medicine
University of Melbourne
Melbourne, Victoria, Australia
Angiotensin-Converting Enzyme: Basic Properties, Distribution, and Functional Role

Gerjan Navis, M.D., Ph.D.
Assistant Professor of Nephrology and Clinical Pharmacology
Gröningen School of Medicine
Staff Physician, Renal Division
Department of Medicine
University Hospital
Gröningen, The Netherlands
Renal Disease

Shawna D. Nesbitt, M.D.
Assistant Professor of Internal Medicine
University of Michigan
Physician-in-Charge, Hypertension/ Hyperlipidemia Clinics
University of Michigan Health System
Ann Arbor, Michigan
Mild Hypertension: An Important Frontier in Therapy of Hypertension

Joel M. Neutel, M.D.
Assistant Professor of Medicine
University of California, Irvine
Irvine
Chief of Hypertension and Clinical Pharmacology
Veterans Affairs Medical Center
Long Beach, California
Chronotherapeutics in the Treatment of Hypertension

Margareta Öhrvall, M.D., Ph.D.
Department of Geriatrics
University of Uppsala
Uppsala, Sweden
Epidemiology of Hypertension

Suzanne Oparil, M.D.
Director, Vascular Biology and Hypertension Program
Division of Cardiovascular Disease
Professor of Medicine
University of Alabama at Birmingham School of Medicine
Birmingham, Alabama
Diet—Micronutrients—Special Foods; Hypertension in Women

Michael F. O'Rourke, M.D., D.Sc.
Professor of Medicine (Personal Chair)
University of New South Wales School of Medicine
Cardiologist, Medical Professorial Unit
St. Vincent's Hospital
Sydney, New South Wales, Australia
Arterial Stiffness

Adebayo Oyekan, Ph.D.
Assistant Professor, Department of Pharmacology
New York Medical College
Valhalla, New York
Eicosanoids: Do They Matter?

Julio A. Panza, M.D.
Senior Investigator and Head, Section on Echocardiography
Cardiology Branch, National Heart, Lung, and Blood Institute
National Institutes of Health
Bethesda, Maryland
Nitric Oxide in Hypertension

Vasilios Papademetriou, M.D., F.A.C.C., F.A.C.P.
Associate Professor of Medicine (Cardiology)
Georgetown University School of Medicine
Chief, Hypertension, Staff Cardiologist
Veterans Affairs Medical Center
Washington, District of Columbia
The Antihypertensive and Lipid Lowering to Prevent Heart Attack Trial

Mark Phillips, M.D.
Duke University Medical Center
Durham, North Carolina
Anesthesia and Hypertension

Robert A. Phillips, M.D., Ph.D.
Associate Professor of Medicine
Mount Sinai School of Medicine
Associate Attending of Medicine
Zena and Michael Wiener Cardiovascular Institute
Mount Sinai Medical Center
New York, New York
Left Ventricular Hypertrophy, Congestive Heart Failure, and Coronary Flow Reserve Abnormalities in Hypertension

Thomas G. Pickering, M.D., D.Phil.
Professor of Medicine
Weill Medical College of Cornell University
Attending Physician
New York Presbyterian Hospital
New York, New York
Blood Pressure Measurement Issues

Bojan Pohar, M.D.
Assistant Professor of Medicine
Assistant Professor of Physiology
Specialist of Internal Medicine
Center for Intensive Internal Medicine
University Medical Center Ljubljana
Ljubljana, Slovenia
Orthostatic Hypotension

James L. Pool, M.D.
Professor of Medicine and Pharmacology
Baylor College of Medicine
Houston, Texas
α-Adrenoceptor Blockers

Jerome G. Porush, M.D.
Professor of Medicine
State University of New York Health Science Center at Brooklyn
Director, Division of Nephrology and Hypertension, Department of Medicine
The Brookdale University Hospital and Medical Center
Brooklyn, New York
Chronic Renal Insufficiency: Slowing Its Progression

Jules B. Puschett, M.D.
Professor and Chairman, Department of Medicine
Tulane University School of Medicine
New Orleans, Louisiana
Diuretics

John Quilley, Ph.D.
Associate Professor, Department of Cell Biology
University of Medicine and Dentistry of New Jersey School of Medicine
Stratford, New Jersey
Eicosanoids: Do They Matter?

Paul Radensky, M.D., J.D.
Partner, Health Law Department
McDermott, Will, and Emory, Attorneys-at-Law
Miami, Florida
Outcomes in Treating Hypertension

Shahrokh Rafii, M.D.
The Brookdale University Hospital and Medical Center
Brooklyn, New York
Ischemic Heart Disease

C. Venkata S. Ram, M.D.
Clinical Professor of Medicine
University of Texas Southwestern Medical Center
Medical Director, Texas Blood Pressure Institute
Dallas, Texas
Changing Approaches to Diagnosis and Treatment of Hypertension

Garry P. Reams, M.D.
Associate Professor of Medicine
University of Missouri
Columbia, Missouri
*Hypertension in Patients on Renal
Replacement Therapy*

Ira W. Reiser
Assistant Professor, Department of
Medicine
State University of New York Health
Science Center at Brooklyn
Attending Physician, Division of
Nephrology and Hypertension,
Department of Medicine
The Brookdale University Hospital and
Medical Center
Brooklyn, New York
*Renovascular Hypertension: Diagnosis
and Treatment*

Efrain Reisin, M.D., F.A.C.C.
Professor of Medicine
Louisiana State University School of
Medicine
Chief of the Nephrology Section
Medical Center of Louisiana at New
Orleans
New Orleans, Louisiana
*Obesity-Hypertension: Effects on the
Cardiovascular and Renal
Systems—The Therapeutic Approach*

Molly E. Reusser, B.A.
Research Associate, Department of
Nephrology
Oregon Health Sciences University
Portland, Oregon
Diet—Micronutrients

J. G. Reves, M.D.
Professor and Chairman, Department of
Anesthesiology
Duke University Medical Center
Durham, North Carolina
Anesthesia and Hypertension

Elizabeth Ripley, M.D.
Assistant Professor of Medicine, Division
of Nephrology
Medical College of Virginia of Virginia
Commonwealth University
Richmond, Virginia
*Low-Dose Fixed-Combination
Antihypertensive Therapy*

David Robertson, M.D.
Elton Yates Professor of Medicine,
Pharmacology and Neurology
Director, General Clinical Research
Center
Vanderbilt University
Nashville, Tennessee
Orthostatic Hypotension

Peter Rudd, M.D., F.A.C.P.
Chief, Division of General Internal
Medicine
Stanford University School of Medicine
Stanford
Director, On-Site Primary Care Services
UCSF Stanford Health Care, South
Campus
Palo Alto, California
*Medication Compliance for
Antihypertensive Therapy*

Michael C. Ruddy, M.D.
Associate Professor of Medicine
Chief, Section of Hypertension
University of Medicine and Dentistry of
New Jersey
Robert Wood Johnson Medical School
Attending Physician
Chief, Division of Hypertension
Robert Wood Johnson University Hospital
New Brunswick, New Jersey
Angiotensin II Receptor Antagonists

Ravi K. Saini, D.V.M., Ph.D.
Director, Cardiovascular Clinical
Research
Bristol-Myers Squibb Company
Princeton, New Jersey
*Vasopeptide Inhibitors: A New Class of
Cardiovascular Agents*

M. A. D. H. Schalekamp, M.D.
Professor of Medicine
Erasmus University
Internist, Head of the Department of
Internal Medicine
University Hospital Dykzigt
Rotterdam, The Netherlands
Renin and Prorenin

Ernesto L. Schiffrin, M.D., Ph.D.,
F.R.C.P.C.
Professor of Medicine
Director, Multidisciplinary Research
Group on Hypertension
Clinical Research Institute of Montreal
University of Montreal
Staff, Division of Internal Medicine
University of Montreal Hospital Center
(CHUM, Hôtel-Dieu Campus)
Montreal, Québec, Canada
Endothelin Antagonists

Domenic A. Sica, M.D.
Professor of Medicine and Pharmacology
Chairman, Clinical Pharmacology and
Hypertension
Medical College of Virginia Hospitals of
Virginia Commonwealth University
Richmond, Virginia
*Dose-Response Relationships in
Antihypertensive Treatment; Low-Dose
Fixed-Combination Antihypertensive
Therapy; Angiotensin-Converting
Enzyme Inhibitors*

David H. G. Smith, M.D.
Assistant Professor of Medicine
University of California, Irvine
Irvine
Director, Hypertension Center
Veterans Affairs Medical Center
Long Beach, California
*Chronotherapeutics in the Treatment of
Hypertension*

James R. Sowers, M.D.
Professor of Medicine and Physiology
Director, Division of Endocrinology,
Metabolism and Hypertension
Wayne State University School of
Medicine
Detroit, Michigan
*Metabolic Abnormalities in
Hypertension*

Jeanne L. Speckman, M.Sc.
Staff
Caro Research
Concord, Massachusetts
Current Prescribing Practices

J. David Spence, B.A., M.D., M.B.A.
Professor of Neurology, Internal Medicine
and Pharmacology
University of Western Ontario
Active Staff, Stroke Service
Department of Clinical Neurological
Sciences
London Health Sciences Centre
London, Ontario, Canada
Stroke and Hypertension

Samuel Spitalewitz, M.D.
Assistant Professor, Department of
Medicine
State University of New York Health
Science Center at Brooklyn
Attending Physician, Division of
Nephrology and Hypertension,
Department of Medicine
Physician-in-Charge, The Renal and
Hypertension Clinics
The Brookdale University Hospital and
Medical Center
Brooklyn, New York
*Chronic Renal Insufficiency: Slowing
Its Progression; Renovascular
Hypertension: Diagnosis and Treatment*

Jan A. Staessen, M.D., Ph.D.
Lecturer, Hypertension and Cardiac
Rehabilitation Unit
Department of Molecular and
Cardiovascular Research
University of Leuven
University Hospital Gasthuisberg
Leuven, Belgium
*Characteristics of Published, Ongoing,
and Planned Outcome Trials in
Hypertension*

Beth A. Staffileno, D.N.Sc., R.N.
Assistant Professor, Department of
  Internal Medicine
Cardiovascular Epidemiology and Clinical
  Applications Program
Wayne State University
Detroit, Michigan
  Hypertension in Blacks

Gordon S. Stokes, M.B.B.S.(Sydney),
M.D.(N.S.W.)
Clinical Professor (Medicine)
Northern Clinical School
University of Sydney
Senior Staff Specialist
Royal North Shore Hospital
St. Leonard's, Sydney
New South Wales, Australia
  Comorbid Conditions

Scott C. Supowit, Ph.D.
Associate Professor
Department of Human Biological
  Chemistry and Genetics and
  Department of Internal Medicine
University of Texas Medical Branch
Galveston, Texas
  *Calcitonin Gene–Related Peptide and
  Hypertension*

John D. Swales, M.D.
Professor of Medicine
University of Leicester
Honorary Consultant Physician
Leicester Royal Infirmary
Leicester, United Kingdom
  *Critical Assessment of Hypertension
  Guidelines*

Nick C. Trippodo, Ph.D.
Senior Principal Scientist
Bristol-Myers Squibb Pharmaceutical
  Research Institute
Princeton, New Jersey
  *Vasopeptide Inhibitors: A New Class of
  Cardiovascular Agents*

Donald G. Vidt, M.D., M.Sc.
Professor of Medicine
Ohio State University College of
  Medicine and Public Health
Columbus
Consultant, Department of Nephrology
  and Hypertension
Cleveland Clinic Foundation
Cleveland, Ohio
  Resistant Hypertension

Imelda P. Villarosa, M.D.
Instructor in Preventive Medicine
Rush Medical College
Chicago, Illinois
  *Diabetes and Syndrome X: Focus on
  Reduction of Cardiovascular and Renal
  Events*

Ji G. Wang, M.D.
Hypertension and Cardiac Rehabilitation
  Unit
Department of Molecular and
  Cardiovascular Research
University of Leuven
University Hospital Gasthuisberg
Leuven, Belgium
  *Characteristics of Published, Ongoing,
  and Planned Outcome Trials in
  Hypertension*

Michael A. Weber, M.D.
Chair, Department of Medicine
The Brookdale University Hospital and
  Medical Center
Professor of Medicine and Clinical
  Associate Dean
State University of New York Health
  Science Center at Brooklyn
Brooklyn, New York
  *Outcomes in Treating Hypertension;
  Cost-Effectiveness in Treating
  Hypertension*

Alan B. Weder, M.D.
Professor of Medicine
University of Michigan School of
  Medicine
Assistant Division Chief, Division of
  Hypertension
Department of Internal Medicine
University of Michigan
Ann Arbor, Michigan
  Pathophysiology of Hypertension

Matthew R. Weir, M.D.
Professor of Medicine
Director, Division of Nephrology and
  Clinical Research Unit
University of Maryland School of
  Medicine
Baltimore, Maryland
  *Initial Choices in the Treatment of
  Hypertension*

William B. White, M.D.
Professor of Medicine
University of Connecticut School of
  Medicine
Chief, Section of Hypertension and
  Clinical Pharmacology
Attending Physician
University of Connecticut Health Center
Farmington, Connecticut
  White-Coat Hypertension

Arie L. M. Widerhorn
Division of Nephrology
University of Southern California, Los
  Angeles Medical Center
Los Angeles, California
  Natriuretic Peptides

William F. Young, Jr., M.D.
Associate Professor of Medicine
Mayo Medical School
Consultant, Divisions of Hypertension,
  Endocrinology and Metabolism,
  Internal Medicine
Mayo Clinic
Rochester, Minnesota
  Pheochromocytoma

Kelly B. Zarnke, M.Sc., M.D.
Assistant Professor of Internal Medicine,
  Epidemiology, and Biostatistics
University of Western Ontario
Acting Staff, Division of Clinical
  Pharmacology
Department of Internal Medicine
London Health Sciences Centre
London, Ontario, Canada
  Stroke and Hypertension

P. A. van Zwieten, M.D., Ph.D.
Professor and Chairman, Department of
  Pharmacotherapy
Academic Medical Centre
Consultant for Clinical Pharmacology,
  Departments of Cardiology and
  Cardiothoracic Surgery
University of Amsterdam
Amsterdam, The Netherlands
  *Calcium Antagonists as
  Antihypertensives*

Preface

Results of recent population surveys have underscored the enormity of the health problem posed by elevated blood pressure. With a prevalence of 20% of the adult population worldwide, high blood pressure increases the cardiovascular risk of billions of people. Careful analyses of cohort data have shown that this increased risk pertains not only to persons with frank hypertension by traditional definitions but also to those with blood pressures at the higher end of the "normal" range. The risk of cardiovascular disease is directly and linearly related to both systolic and diastolic blood pressure, although the slope of this relationship is steeper for systolic than for diastolic pressure. Recent analyses have shown that elevated pulse pressure may carry the worst prognosis of all, particularly among the elderly.

The risk of elevated blood pressure is clearly modifiable with appropriate and aggressive antihypertensive treatment. Results of recent randomized clinical trials have reinforced the concept that lowering blood pressure can prevent morbidity and mortality due to cardiovascular diseases, including stroke, congestive heart failure, myocardial infarction, and end-stage renal disease. Further, these studies have shown that lowering blood pressure to more aggressive target levels confers relatively greater benefit in those persons at highest risk, including diabetics and persons with renal insufficiency accompanied by proteinuria.

Despite the impressive successes of controlled clinical trials in preventing hypertension-related cardiovascular events, the incidence of heart failure and end-stage renal disease has increased dramatically since the early 1980s. A major contributor to this trend is inadequate control of blood pressure in the population. Hypertension control rates are disappointing (only 27% in the United States and much lower in other industrialized countries, for example, 6% in the United Kingdom) and have declined in recent years.

The challenge to the practicing physician, then, is to translate the promising results of clinical trials into everyday practice. Impediments to this effort include nonadherence to prescribed medical regimens by patients, failure to communicate the need for treatment by providers, the cost of care, failure to prescribe medications in adequate doses, and the requirement for multidrug regimens to achieve adequate control in most patients. Hope for the future lies in innovative health care delivery systems that utilize nurses, pharmacists, and other nonphysician providers, increased emphasis on adherence-enhancing measures, and reliance on referral to hypertension specialists for the care of complex and resistant patients. The team approach to care of hypertensive patients also facilitates implementation of lifestyle modification measures, including novel dietary programs, that can reduce blood pressure.

Broader recognition by health care providers of the need to treat to lower goal blood pressures and by the health care delivery system of the importance of successful antihypertensive treatment should yield immediate benefit. Results of randomized controlled trials currently in progress will yield insights into whether specific antihypertensive drugs are more—or less—effective than others in preventing morbid and mortal cardiovascular events. These studies should provide definitive answers to the question of whether blood pressure reduction per se fully accounts for the benefits of antihypertensive treatment or whether the mechanism of action of antihypertensive drugs also has a bearing on outcomes.

Interesting questions and controversies remain. High blood pressure rarely exists as a solitary abnormality. Metabolic changes such as lipid disorders and insulin resistance, often associated with obesity, are common in hypertensive patients. In addition, cardiovascular findings, including changes in the structure and function of the left ventricle or stiffening of the arteries, as well as evidence for renal hyperfiltration, are also part of this syndrome. Since these findings can be detected in the apparently normotensive offspring of patients with hypertension, the issue of how and when to best evaluate those at risk of hypertension and its consequences becomes important. Another ongoing question: although randomized clinical trials with hard endpoints are critical to hypertension guideline writers and policy makers, how can practicing physicians best judge the true effectiveness of treatment in their own individual patients? Can surrogate endpoints like regression of left ventricular hypertrophy, improvement in arterial compliance, or reduction in proteinuria be regarded as legitimate guideposts in patient management?

The science of vascular biology has become a critical part of hypertension. Changes in the endothelium and in the structure and function of the arterial wall are critical in determining the cardiovascular prognosis of patients with this condition. The renin-angiotensin-aldosterone system, together with the many other vasoactive peptides and substances with which it interacts, has become an important therapeutic target as well as a subject of basic scientific interest. There is now an active ongoing search for links between these vascular and clinical findings and the underlying genetic variations and abnormalities that are responsible for them.

It could be anticipated that application of knowledge

gained from the human genome project and other studies of the inheritance of high blood pressure and related comorbid conditions will lead to better understanding of the pathophysiology of essential hypertension and to the selection of more effective, targeted antihypertensive therapy based on the genotype of the patient.

This entirely new book is intended to be a useful reference for clinicians who provide care for hypertensive patients, for scientists who are studying the pathobiology of blood pressure control and hypertension-related target organ disease, and for health care planners from academia, industry, and government. The volume begins with a brief history of clinical hypertension and an overview of the epidemiology of hypertension worldwide. Sections 2 and 3 emphasize contemporary issues in the pathophysiology of blood pressure elevation and its cardiovascular complications and target organ damage, as well as common comorbid conditions, such as obesity and insulin resistance. A particularly novel aspect of these sections is the discussion of primary arterial pathology and arterial stiffness in the pathogenesis of hypertension, providing a mechanistic basis for the recent emphasis on pulse pressure as a predictor of cardiovascular morbidity and mortality in hypertensive subjects. Consideration of target organ damage and cardiovascular complications, as well as blood pressure level per se, as components of total cardiovascular risk is presented as a critical factor in deciding when and how aggressively to treat the patient with elevated blood pressure.

Section 4 on diagnosis emphasizes the importance of accurate blood pressure measurement, including the role of ambulatory and self-measurement of blood pressure in guiding antihypertensive therapy, as well as the complex issue of white-coat hypertension. Section 5 on general considerations in antihypertensive treatment focuses on a number of contemporary issues, including use of outcome data from recent clinical trials in making therapeutic decisions. A critical assessment of hypertension treatment guidelines and their impact on office practice is presented. Current prescribing practices, as well as the cost-effectiveness of antihypertensive therapy in a managed care setting, are discussed. Novel systems for delivering antihypertensive therapy, including nursing clinics and community outreach programs, and for optimizing compliance with antihypertensive medication occupy prominent positions in this section.

Section 6 deals with lifestyle modification in the prevention and treatment of hypertension. It discusses the value of a balanced diet rich in fruits, vegetables, and low-fat dairy products, e.g., the Dietary Approaches to Stop Hypertension (DASH) diet, as well as weight reduction, increased physical activity, and moderation of alcohol consumption as primary or adjunctive therapy in hypertensive patients.

Section 7 outlines general considerations for the initial choice of antihypertensive drug treatment, including low-dose fixed-combination therapy, and the role of chronotherapeutics in treatment decisions. Special considerations in the treatment of hypertensive patients with comorbid conditions, particularly insulin resistance, diabetes, ischemic heart disease, and renal disease, as well as in special patient groups, including women, the elderly, and blacks, are discussed in Section 8. Chapters on resistant hypertension and orthostatic hypotension round out this section.

The process of antihypertensive drug registration in the United States is described in Section 9, which also includes detailed consideration of antihypertensive drug actions by class. New antihypertensive drug classes, including endothelin antagonists, renin inhibitors, and the vasopeptidases, which combine neutral endopeptidase and angiotensin-converting enzyme–inhibiting properties, as well as the established classes, are discussed here.

Section 10 emphasizes recent advances in the diagnosis and treatment of secondary hypertension. Obstructive sleep apnea, a recently recognized and important cause of hypertension, is highlighted. Anesthesia in the hypertensive patient and the treatment of hypertensive emergencies, specialized areas that often baffle clinicians, are discussed in this section. The volume ends with a set of tables listing the antihypertensive drugs currently available in the United States.

We thank the contributing authors for their scholarly and extremely contemporary treatment of important topics in hypertension pathophysiology, diagnosis, and therapy. We also express our appreciation to Richard Zorab, Jennifer Shreiner, and the production staff at W.B. Saunders Company for their expertise and diligent attention to detail in the preparation of this text.

SUZANNE OPARIL, M.D.
MICHAEL A. WEBER, M.D.

Contents

SECTION 1

BACKGROUND AND HISTORICAL ASPECTS 1

CHAPTER 1

History of Clinical Hypertension: From 1827 to 1970   1
Harriet P. Dustan

CHAPTER 2

Epidemiology of Hypertension   4
Lennart Hansson, Lena Kilander, and Margareta Öhrvall

SECTION 2

PATHOPHYSIOLOGY 21

CHAPTER 3

Pathophysiology of Hypertension   21
Carolina Delgado and Alan B. Weder

CHAPTER 4

Genetics   29
Stephen B. Harrap

CHAPTER 5

Sympathetic Nervous System in Acute and Chronic Blood Pressure Elevation   42
Joseph L. Izzo, Jr.

CHAPTER 6

Environmental and Psychosocial Stress in Hypertension Onset and Progression   59
Kathleen C. Light

CHAPTER 7

Renin and Prorenin   70
J. Deinum and M. A. D. H. Schalekamp

CHAPTER 8

Angiotensinogen: Physiology, Molecular Biology, and Relevance to Hypertension   77
Daniel F. Catanzaro

CHAPTER 9

Angiotensin-Converting Enzyme: Basic Properties, Distribution, and Functional Role   90
Maurice E. Fabiani, Diem T. Dinh, Labrini Nassis, and Colin I. Johnston

CHAPTER 10

The AT_1 and AT_2 Angiotensin Receptors   100
Marc de Gasparo and Gillian R. Bullock

CHAPTER 11

Metabolic Abnormalities in Hypertension   110
Syed S. Ali, Melvin A. Lester, and James R. Sowers

CHAPTER 12

Obesity-Related Hypertension as a Metabolic Disorder   118
Lewis Landsberg

CHAPTER 13

Remodeling of Resistance Vessels in Essential Hypertension   125
Michael J. Mulvany

CHAPTER 14

Arterial Stiffness   134
Michael F. O'Rourke, Christopher S. Hayward, and Eldon D. Lehmann

CHAPTER 15

Endothelin in Hypertension   152
John C. Burnett, Jr.

CHAPTER 16

Nitric Oxide in Hypertension   158
Julio A. Panza

CHAPTER 17

Natriuretic Peptides   165
Vito M. Campese and Arie L. M. Widerhorn

CHAPTER 18

Eicosanoids: Do They Matter?   176
Adebayo Oyekan, John C. McGiff, and John Quilley

CHAPTER 19

Calcitonin Gene–Related Peptide and Hypertension   182
Donald J. DiPette and Scott C. Supowit

CHAPTER 20

Kallikrein-Kinin Systems   190
Harry S. Margolius

Diet—Nutrition

CHAPTER 21

Diet—Micronutrients   202
David A. McCarron and Molly E. Reusser

CHAPTER 22

Obesity-Hypertension: Effects on the Cardiovascular and Renal Systems—The Therapeutic Approach   206
Efrain Reisin and Howard G. Hutchinson

CHAPTER 23

Alcohol and Hypertension   211
Arthur L. Klatsky

SECTION 3

TARGET ORGAN DAMAGE/ CARDIOVASCULAR COMPLICATIONS 221

CHAPTER 24

Total Risk   221
Michael H. Alderman

CHAPTER 25

New Interpretations of Blood Pressure: The Importance of Pulse Pressure   227
Stanley S. Franklin

CHAPTER 26

Coronary Atherosclerotic Sequelae of Hypertension   235
W. B. Kannel

CHAPTER 27

Left Ventricular Hypertrophy, Congestive Heart Failure, and Coronary Flow Reserve Abnormalities in Hypertension   244
Robert A. Phillips and Joseph A. Diamond

CHAPTER 28

Stroke and Hypertension   277
J. David Spence and Kelly B. Zarnke

CHAPTER 29

Chronic Renal Insufficiency: Slowing Its Progression   286
Samuel Spitalewitz, Pierre F. Faubert, and Jerome G. Porush

SECTION 4

DIAGNOSIS 297

CHAPTER 30

Initial Evaluation and Follow-Up   297
Lawrence R. Krakoff

CHAPTER 31

Blood Pressure Measurement Issues   306
Thomas G. Pickering

CHAPTER 32

White-Coat Hypertension   314
George A. Mansoor and William B. White

SECTION 5

TREATMENT—GENERAL CONSIDERATIONS 323

CHAPTER 33

Outcomes in Treating Hypertension   323
Michael A. Weber and Paul Radensky

CHAPTER 34

Benefits of Treating Hypertension—Lessons From Clinical Trials   331
William J. Elliott and Henry R. Black

CHAPTER 35

Characteristics of Published, Ongoing, and Planned Outcome Trials in Hypertension   341
Jan A. Staessen and Ji G. Wang

CHAPTER 36

The Antihypertensive and Lipid-Lowering to Prevent Heart Attack Trial   360
Vasilios Papademetriou

CHAPTER 37

The Losartan Intervention For Endpoint (LIFE) Reduction in Hypertension Study: Rationale, Design, and Characteristics of 9194 Patients With Left Ventricular Hypertrophy   366
Sverre E. Kjeldsen and Björn Dahlöf

CHAPTER 38

Changing Approaches to Diagnosis and Treatment of Hypertension 371
Norman M. Kaplan and C. Venkata S. Ram

CHAPTER 39

Critical Assessment of Hypertension Guidelines 375
John D. Swales

CHAPTER 40

Current Prescribing Practices 383
J. Jaime Caro and Jeanne L. Speckman

CHAPTER 41

Calcium Channel Blockers in the Treatment of Hypertension 389
Julie E. Buring, Robert J. Glynn, and Charles H. Hennekens

CHAPTER 42

Mild Hypertension: An Important Frontier in Therapy of Hypertension 398
Stevo Julius, Shawna D. Nesbitt, and Robert Brook

CHAPTER 43

Cost-Effectiveness in Treating Hypertension 405
Michael A. Weber and William J. Elliott

CHAPTER 44

Nursing Clinics in the Management of Hypertension 409
Nancy Houston Miller and Martha N. Hill

CHAPTER 45

Community Outreach 415
Martha N. Hill, Lee R. Bone, and David M. Levine

CHAPTER 46

Medication Compliance for Antihypertensive Therapy 419
Peter Rudd

SECTION 6

LIFESTYLE MODIFICATION 433

CHAPTER 47

Diet—Micronutrients—Special Foods 433
Suzanne Oparil

CHAPTER 48

Diet—Calories 460
Karen C. McCowen, Samuel Chan, and George L. Blackburn

CHAPTER 49

Alcohol Consumption and the Management of Hypertension 466
William C. Cushman

CHAPTER 50

Exercise and Hypertension 470
Angel H. Herrera and David T. Lowenthal

SECTION 7

PHARMACOLOGICAL TREATMENT 479

CHAPTER 51

Initial Choices in the Treatment of Hypertension 479
Matthew R. Weir

CHAPTER 52

Dose-Response Relationships in Antihypertensive Treatment 492
Todd W. B. Gehr and Domenic A. Sica

CHAPTER 53

Low-Dose Fixed-Combination Antihypertensive Therapy 497
Domenic A. Sica and Elizabeth Ripley

CHAPTER 54

Chronotherapeutics in the Treatment of Hypertension 504
Joel M. Neutel and David H. G. Smith

SECTION 8

COMORBID CONDITIONS—SPECIAL CONSIDERATIONS 509

CHAPTER 55

Comorbid Conditions 509
Gordon S. Stokes and Karen A. Duggan

CHAPTER 56

Diabetes and Syndrome X: Focus on Reduction of Cardiovascular and Renal Events 518
Imelda P. Villarosa and George L. Bakris

CHAPTER 57

Renal Disease 524
Gerjan Navis, Paul E. de Jong, and Dick de Zeeuw

CHAPTER 58

Hypertension in Patients on Renal Replacement Therapy 531
Madhukar Misra, Garry P. Reams, and John H. Bauer

CHAPTER 59

Ischemic Heart Disease 539
Hal L. Chadow, Alan Feit, and Shahrokh Rafii

CHAPTER 60

Hypertension in Women 546
Phyllis August and Suzanne Oparil

CHAPTER 61

Hypertension in the Elderly 551
Koshy Abraham and David T. Lowenthal

CHAPTER 62

Hypertension in Blacks 558
John M. Flack and Beth A. Staffileno

CHAPTER 63

Resistant Hypertension 564
Donald G. Vidt

CHAPTER 64

Orthostatic Hypotension 572
Bojan Pohar and David Robertson

SECTION 9

INDIVIDUAL DRUG CLASSES 579

CHAPTER 65

How Hypertensive Drugs Get Approved in the United
States 579
Robert R. Fenichel

CHAPTER 66

Diuretics 584
Jules B. Puschett

CHAPTER 67

β-Adrenergic Blockers 590
William H. Frishman and Ulrich Jorde

CHAPTER 68

α-Adrenoceptor Blockers 595
James L. Pool

CHAPTER 69

Angiotensin-Converting Enzyme Inhibitors 599
Domenic A. Sica and Todd W. B. Gehr

CHAPTER 70

Calcium Antagonists as Antihypertensives 609
P. A. van Zwieten

CHAPTER 71

Angiotensin II Receptor Antagonists 621
Michael C. Ruddy and John B. Kostis

CHAPTER 72

Other Adrenergic Inhibitors and the Direct-Acting Smooth
Muscle Vasodilators 637
Edward D. Frohlich

New Classes

CHAPTER 73

Endothelin Antagonists 643
Ernesto L. Schiffrin

CHAPTER 74

Renin Inhibitors 646
Norman K. Hollenberg

CHAPTER 75

Vasopeptide Inhibitors: A New Class of Cardiovascular
Agents 651
Nick C. Trippodo and Ravi K. Saini

SECTION 10

SECONDARY HYPERTENSION 657

CHAPTER 76

Obstructive Sleep Apnea 657
*Douglas M. Kahn, Paul D. Levinson, and
Richard P. Millman*

CHAPTER 77

Renovascular Hypertension: Diagnosis and
Treatment 662
Samuel Spitalewitz and Ira W. Reiser

CHAPTER 78

Adrenal Cortex 674
Emmanuel L. Bravo

CHAPTER 79

Pheochromocytoma 685
William F. Young, Jr.

CHAPTER 80

Hypertension in Pregnant Women 688
Marshall D. Lindheimer and Ayub Akbari

CHAPTER 81

Anesthesia and Hypertension 702
James Gould, J. G. Reves, and Mark Phillips

CHAPTER 82

Hypertensive Crisis 715
David A. Calhoun

APPENDIX

Drug Tables 719
David A. Calhoun

Index 723

Background and Historical Aspects

CHAPTER 1

History of Clinical Hypertension: From 1827 to 1970
Harriet P. Dustan

Nineteen ninety-six was the 100th anniversary of Riva-Rocci's description of an inflatable cuff that allowed measurement of brachial systolic pressure. In 1904, Korotkov reported the auscultatory method that allowed measurement of diastolic pressure as well. These developments opened the way for recognizing hypertension as abnormal and for the eventual acceptance by physicians, many decades later, of the public health threat posed by its related vascular diseases.

NINETEENTH CENTURY BEGINNINGS

The ability to measure blood pressure answered many of the questions that had arisen after Bright's 1827 and 1836 observations of diseased kidneys and associated cardiovascular abnormalities. These early investigations are admirably summarized in Ruskin's *Classics in Arterial Hypertension.*[1] For example, Johnson (1852) described medial hypertrophy of the renal afferent arterioles, which he took as a response to increased intravascular pressure. Traube (1856) concluded that left ventricular hypertrophy was caused by "high arterial tension." Gull and Sutton (1872) were struck by the finding of generalized vascular disease with varying degrees of renal involvement and thought that "this morbid change" could have its beginnings in organs other than the kidney. Mahomed (1874) had estimated intraarterial pressure by measurement of pulse tension with a sphygmograph and concluded that arteriolar disease could be caused by elevated blood pressure. Potain (1875), who had an instrument for estimating systolic pressure by pulse compression, concluded that left ventricular hypertrophy resulted from high intraarterial pressure. Gowers (1876) first used the ophthalmoscope to describe retinal arteriolar constriction, which he found to be associated with high blood pressure as estimated by the relative incompressibility of the radial pulse. And finally, Albutt (1896) recognized that raised arterial pressure could occur without evidence of renal disease, and when found in the elderly, he called it *senile plethora.*

Albutt used the term *hyperpiesia* to indicate raised intraarterial pressure. It is a correct term of Greek derivation, but was never widely used. Instead, Frank's 1911 *essentielle Hypertonie* was given an English cast and became *essential hypertension.* This term is now used to indicate hypertension of unknown cause.

ESTABLISHING HYPERTENSION AS A THREAT TO HEALTH

Not much time passed between the demonstration of blood pressure measurement and the report that people so affected could suffer a variety of lethal consequences. In 1913, Janeway reported on the deaths of 212 hypertensive patients; 33% from heart disease (probably mostly cardiac failure), 24% from stroke, and 23% from uremia.[2]

However, most physicians were not impressed by high blood pressure and, when it occurred in elderly people, attributed it to aging. Not so with insurance companies, because in 1925, the Society of Actuaries summarized their experience with 560,000 insured men (at that time, not enough women were insured for an adequate assessment).[3] Thus, for the first time, it became known that when a large group of men was considered, the presence of hypertension was a direct threat to long life. Fifteen years later, another Society of Actuaries report showed that even hypertension of mild degree shortened life span.[4]

Since there were no generally successful treatments available, most physicians paid little attention. This was influenced not only by the lack of available treatment but also by the novelty of predicting clinical outcomes from large groups. Evidence-based medicine was many decades in the future.

By the mid 1920s, it had become obvious to physicians who did measure blood pressure that the severity of hypertension varied widely. Some people had only mild pressure elevations and lived to old age, whereas others had very high systolic and diastolic pressures with markedly shortened life spans. Physicians at the Mayo Clinic attempted to bring some guidance to their colleagues as to what their patients faced in terms of morbidity and mortality.[5, 6] First, they described malignant hypertension, so-called because 79% of patients were dead within a year of diagnosis.[5] These patients had very high pressures, both systolic and diastolic; severe retinal arteriolar vasoconstriction and sclerosis; papilledema; and very often, hemorrhages and exudates. In addition, most had other evidence of target organ damage, i.e., hypertensive heart disease or nephrosclerosis. Papilledema was the hallmark, and so it has remained for over 70 years, although the lethal nature of the vascular disease can usually be eliminated now by good blood pressure control.

Eleven years later, using retinal findings and evidence of target organ damage, the Mayo Clinic physicians presented a classification of essential hypertension.[6] This did not include severity of hypertension. They divided hypertensive subjects into four groups and showed that the more severe the retinal vascular disease and the greater the target organ damage, the shorter the life span. No blood pressure data were given, so they escaped making the conclusion, shown amply later, that the higher the pressure, the more severe the vascular disease and the greater the mortality and morbidity.

Lack of treatment did not completely suppress interest in hypertension, and in the 1930s and 1940s, physicians began long-term follow-up programs to determine the natural history of hypertension. These were published mostly in the 1950s, before the favorable impact of antihypertensive drug therapy had become obvious.[7-9] These three programs followed a total of 1781 men and women for periods ranging from 10 to 32 years. Their conclusions were relatively uniform:

1. Hypertensive men died earlier than hypertensive women.
2. Hypertension in young people carried a poor prognosis, but if a hypertensive patient lived beyond 60 years, life expectancy was little diminished.
3. "Labile" rather than "fixed diastolic" hypertension had a better prognosis.
4. Generally speaking, the higher the pressure, the shorter the life span, but occasionally, patients with systolic pressure as high as 200 mm Hg lived into old age.
5. Hypertension plus target organ damage carried a poorer prognosis than hypertension alone.

THE FRAMINGHAM HEART STUDY

These natural history studies showed us the varied clinical course that hypertension could take but taught us nothing about the multifactorial nature of vascular disease. That information came from the Framingham Study, which began in 1948 as a longitudinal survey of the population of one small city in the United States with regard to the prevalence, incidence, morbidity, and mortality of vascular diseases. It has been funded by the National Institutes of Health for over 50 years. The knowledge gleaned from it has formed the basis for much of cardiovascular disease prevention. It was this study that first described the combined importance of hypertension, hypercholesterolemia, glucose intolerance, and cigarette smoking in the genesis of coronary heart disease.[10] This was the study that finally convinced physicians that elevated systolic pressure is as damaging to blood vessels as high diastolic pressure is, if not more so.[11] The value of information gained from the Framingham Heart Study has been, and will continue to be, enormous.

DISCOVERY OF SECONDARY HYPERTENSIONS

Bright's observations originally identified the kidney as the source of elevated intravascular pressure, but later studies in the 19th century refuted that interpretation. This left open the possibility of other causes. That possibility was bolstered by laboratory investigations of the 1930s and 1940s that clearly established the multifactorial nature of blood pressure control and, therefore, the likelihood of several origins of hypertension.

We now recognize a number of so-called secondary hypertensions, most of which have been discovered through the serendipitous study of hypertensive patients with signs or symptoms inappropriate for essential hypertension.

By 1970, five major secondary causes had been described: pheochromocytoma (1922),[12] Cushing's syndrome (1932),[13] aortic coarctation (1947),[14] renal arterial disease (1954),[15] and primary aldosteronism (1955).[16]

TREATMENTS FOR HYPERTENSION

Even before Riva-Rocci's and Korotkov's methods for measuring arterial pressure were available, attempts were made to lower values as determined by pulse compressibility equipment. These attempts included electrotherapy with high-frequency currents that, unlike low-frequency currents, did not "produce the phenomenon of tetany."[17] For the patient, this therapy had the added advantage of being applied in a cage, so that he or she really felt that something important was being done.

Another treatment at the time that supposedly addressed a basic fault was irradiation of the adrenals. One of its promoters was Cottenot, who stated that "modern concepts tell us how important this adrenal hyperplasia is in vascular pathology. Many people believe it to be the essential factor in vascular hypertension and atheroma."[18] This approach, which began around 1910, continued into the 1930s, but fortunately, it was not widely used.

In the 1920s through 1940s, as the longitudinal natural history studies were going on, some physicians were attempting to lower the arterial pressure of severely hypertensive patients to see what effect, if any, this would have on the already-known poor prognosis. These attempts were based on what little was known of the pathophysiology of hypertension. There was concern, however, because of the widespread belief that elevated pressure was "essential" for organ perfusion and that lowering it would result in organ failure.

The first of these treatments (and the only one still used today) was a sodium-restricted diet. A low-chloride diet for treatment of heart failure in hypertension had been instituted by the Paris physicians Ambard and Beaujard in 1904 (they had no method for measuring sodium).[19] It was adopted by Allen in the United States and was probably the genesis of Kempner's very low sodium, rice-fruit diet.[20] Kempner thought that the low-protein component of the diet was as important in blood pressure control as sodium restriction was, but Grollman and colleagues, who used dialyzed milk as a major protein source, were able to show that a normal-protein, but restricted-salt, diet had an antihypertensive effect equivalent to that of the rice-fruit diet.[21]

Medicines of those days included thiocyanate for hypertensive headaches and veratrum viride. The latter was a strikingly successful antihypertensive drug, but it was almost impossible to take because the margin between good blood pressure control and incapacitating vomiting was so narrow as to preclude its wide use.[22]

Between 1935 and 1950, the most widely used treatment was probably sympathectomy. A variety of operations were devised, including total, lumbodorsal, supradiaphragmatic, and infradiaphragmatic sympathectomy. The operation helped some people but, when effective drugs became available, was quickly abandoned.

Other treatments of limited usefulness and relatively short life were kidney extract injections[23] and pyrogen therapy.[24] Pentaquine, the first ganglion blocker to be tried, also lowered pressure, but its side effects were considered prohibitive.[25]

THE MODERN ERA OF TREATMENT

Around 1950, treatment of hypertension changed for the better. Two drugs, hydralazine, a vasodilator, and hexamethonium, a ganglion blocker, became available.[26, 27] They were orally active and of long-term effectiveness. The side effects could be troublesome and sometimes dangerous, but doctors accustomed to their use could often achieve benefit for their patients. Another drug introduced a bit later was reserpine.[28] Using these three agents to treat malignant hypertension showed that lowering blood pressure cleared retinopathy, improved cardiac performance, and stabilized renal function.[29, 30]

The next advance in therapy was the introduction of an orally active, nonmercurial diuretic, chlorothiazide. Not only could this agent return pressure responsiveness in patients whose pressures had become tolerant to ganglion blockers, but it was also often effective in treating mild to moderate hypertension.

HYPERTENSION AS A CAUSE OF VASCULAR DISEASE

At long last, physicians had the ability to establish the relationship between elevated pressure and vascular disease—one that had been suspected for over 100 years. Two possibilities were considered: that hypertension and vascular disease were manifestations of an underlying fault, but not causally related, and that hypertension caused vascular disease. The task of investigating these two hypotheses was undertaken by the Veterans Administration Cooperative Study Group headed by Freis.

The first Veterans Administration report appeared in 1967.[31] It evaluated 143 men with diastolic pressures of 115 to 129 mm Hg in a randomized, placebo-controlled trial. Seventy-three men received active treatment with hydrochlorothiazide, hydralazine, and reserpine as needed to reduce blood pressure, and 70 men were given placebo. In the treated group, strokes were markedly lessened, and heart failure and accelerated hypertension were not seen. However, coronary heart disease events were practically unchanged by treatment. In 1970, results from the study of men with diastolic pressures of 90 to 114 mm Hg were

reported.[32] Again, treatment greatly lessened stroke and abolished heart failure and accelerated hypertension without affecting the incidence of coronary heart disease syndromes.

THE END OF THIS TALE

These Veterans Administration study results were the basis for Mary Lasker's insistence that something positive be done about the public health threat of hypertension, which led to the establishment by the National Heart, Lung, and Blood Institute of the National High Blood Pressure Education Program. Its intensive efforts to train physicians and patients about the dangers of hypertension have led to marked decreases in deaths from stroke and heart attack.

References

1. Ruskin A. Classics in Arterial Hypertension. Springfield, IL, Charles C Thomas, 1956; pp 164–272.
2. Janeway TC. A clinical study of hypertensive cardiovascular disease. Arch Intern Med 12:755, 1913.
3. Society of Actuaries. Blood Pressure: Report of the Joint Committee on Mortality of the Association of Life Insurance Medical Directors and the Actuarial Society of America. New York, Society of Actuaries, 1925.
4. Society of Actuaries. Blood Pressure Study 1939, New York, NY. New York, Society of Actuaries and Association of Life Insurance Medical Directors, 1940.
5. Keith NM, Wagener HP, Kernohan JW. The syndrome of malignant hypertension. Arch Intern Med 41:44, 1928.
6. Keith NM, Wagener HP, Barker NW. Some different types of essential hypertension: Their course and prognosis. Am J Med Sci 197:132, 1939.
7. Bachgaard P, Kopp H, Neilson J. One thousand hypertensive patients followed from 16–22 years. Acta Med Scand 154 (suppl 312):175, 1956.
8. Mathisen HS. The prognosis in essential hypertension. Acta Med Scand 154 (suppl 312):154:185, 1956.
9. Palmer RS. Treatment of hypertension. J Chronic Dis 10:500, 1959.
10. Kannel WB, Sorlie P. Hypertension in Framingham. *In* Paul O (ed). Epidemiology and Control of Hypertension. New York, Stratton Intercontinental Medical Book Corporation, 1975; p 553.
11. Kannel WB, Gordon T, Schwartz MJ. Systolic vs diastolic blood pressure and risk of coronary heart disease: The Framingham Study. Am J Cardiol 27:335, 1971.
12. L'Abbe M, Tinel J, Doumer E. Crises solaires et hypertension paroxystique en rapport avec une tumeur surrenale. Bull Soc Med Hop 46:982, 1922.
13. Cushing H. The basophil adenomas of the pituitary body and their clinical manifestations (pituitary basophilism). Bull Johns Hopkins Hosp 50:137, 1932.
14. Reifenstein GH, Levine SA, Gross RE. Coarctation of the aorta: A review of 104 autopsied cases of the "adult type," 2 years of age or older. Am Heart J 33:146, 1947.
15. Howard JE, Berthrong M, Gould BM. Hypertension resulting from unilateral renal vascular disease and its relief by nephrectomy. Bull Johns Hopkins Hosp 94:51, 1954.
16. Conn JW. Presidential address. Part II: Primary aldosteronism, a new clinical syndrome. J Lab Clin Med 45:6, 1955.
17. Postal-Vinay N. Treating hypertension. *In* A Century of Arterial Hypertension, 1896–1996. Chichester, Eng, John Wiley & Sons, 1996; p 105.
18. Postal-Vinay N. Treating hypertension. *In* A Century of Arterial Hypertension, 1896–1996. Chichester, Eng, John Wiley & Sons, 1996; p 111.
19. Ambard L, Beaujard E. Causes de hypertension arterielle. Arch Gen Med 1:520, 1904.

20. Kempner W. Treatment of hypertensive vascular disease with rice diet. Am J Med 4:545, 1948.
21. Grollman A, Harrison TR, Mason MF. Sodium restriction in the diet for hypertension. JAMA 129:533, 1945.
22. Wilkins RW. Recent experiences with the pharmacologic treatment of hypertension. In Bell ET (ed). Hypertension. Minneapolis, University of Minnesota Press, p 492, 1951.
23. Page IH, Helmer OM, Kohlstaedt KG, et al. The blood pressure reducing property of extracts of kidneys in hypertensive patients and animals. Ann Intern Med 15:347, 1941.
24. Page IH, Taylor RD. Pyrogens in the treatment of malignant hypertension. Mod Concepts Cardiovasc Dis 18:51, 1949.
25. Freis ED, Wilkins R. Effects of pentaguine in patients with hypertension. Proc Soc Exp Biol Med 64:731, 1947.
26. Schroeder HA. The effect of 1-hydrazinophalazine in hypertension. Circulation 5:28, 1952.
27. Freis ED, Finnerty FA, Schnaper HW, Johnson RL. The treatment of hypertension with hexamethonium. Circulation 5:20, 1952.
28. Wilkins RW, Judson WE. Use of Rauwolfia serpentina in hypertensive patients. N Engl J Med 248:48, 1953.
29. Perry HM Jr, Schroeder HA. The effect of treatment on mortality ratio in severe hypertension. Arch Intern Med 102:418, 1958.
30. Dustan HP, Schneckloth RE, Corcoran AC, et al. The effectiveness of the long term treatment of malignant hypertension. Circulation 18:644, 1958.
31. Veterans Administration Cooperative Study Group on Antihypertensive Agents. Effect of treatment on morbidity in hypertension. I: Results in patients with diastolic blood pressure averaging 115 through 129 mm Hg. JAMA 202:1028, 1967.
32. Veterans Administration Cooperative Study Group on Antihypertensive Agents. Effects of treatment on morbidity in hypertension. II: Results in patients with diastolic blood pressure averaging 90 through 114 mm Hg. JAMA 213:1143, 1970.

CHAPTER 2

Epidemiology of Hypertension

Lennart Hansson, Lena Kilander, and Margareta Öhrvall

There is an abundance of epidemiological information about blood pressure and hypertension. Arterial pressure has been measured in numerous populations worldwide. Usually this has been in the form of observational surveys, such as the Framingham Heart Study, which over the years has provided a unique database on the relationship between arterial pressure and various cardiovascular disorders.[1-13] Many other important observational studies have contributed to our understanding of the distribution of blood pressure in the population and of the links between blood pressure and cardiovascular disease, e.g., the Bergen study,[14, 15] the Taiwan population screening,[16] the Tecumseh study,[17] the study of men born in 1913,[18-21] the South Wales population survey,[22, 23] the Solomon Islands survey,[24] the Yanomano Indian study,[25] the Uppsala study of middle-aged men,[26] the Kenya urban and tribal study,[27] the U.S. Community Hypertension Evaluation Clinic (CHEC) Program,[28] and the long-term blood pressure survey in Japan,[29] to mention just a few.

Much important information on blood pressure epidemiology has also been obtained from screening examinations of individuals in which the aim has been to recruit subjects for various intervention projects, such as the Multiple Risk Factor Intervention Trial (MRFIT)[30] or the Hypertension Detection and Evaluation Program.[31] The ongoing multinational Monitoring of Trends and Determinants of Cardiovascular Disease (MONICA) project under the auspices of the World Health Organization[32] has already produced important information on the epidemiology of hypertension, and many further contributions can be expected from this important undertaking. Similarly, the National Health and Nutrition Examination Survey (NHANES) in the United States, with its repeated investigation of representative population samples, has yielded large amounts of reliable data on blood pressure (Table 2–1).[33, 34] Finally, much has been learned from life insurance data, particularly in

the United States.[35, 36] Even minor elevations of systolic or diastolic blood pressure have been found to be associated with marked reductions in longevity.[35, 36]

Virtually all of the epidemiological information on blood pressure has been obtained with classic noninvasive methodology using a cuff with a sphygmomanometer and a stethoscope. However, Sokolow's group has presented long-term data on cardiovascular risk in relation to ambulatory blood pressure,[37] and more data are emerging in which (noninvasive) ambulatory measurements have been obtained in relatively large populations, such as the Pressioni Arteriose Monitorate e Loro Associazioni (PAMELA) study in Italy,[38] as well as population-based reference values in men aged 50 years from Uppsala, Sweden.[39] Data on 50-year-old women are now available from the Uppsala study, and there are no significant differences between

Table 2–1. Prevalence (%) of Hypertension in the Second NHANES Study 1976–1980*

Age (yr)	Males		Females	
	White	Black	White	Black
18–24	2.9	2.4	0.9	3.2
25–34	8.9	13.3	3.7	7.3
35–44	12.1	23.8	8.9	26.9
45–54	26.2	26.0	21.6	58.3
55–64	31.3	46.4	34.4	60.1
65–74	37.5	42.9	48.3	72.8

From Drizd T, Danneberg AL, Engel A. Blood pressure levels in persons 18–74 years of age in 1976–1980, and trends in blood pressure from 1960 to 1980 in the United States. Vital and Health Statistics, Series 11, 234, DHHS publ No. (PHS) 86-1684. Washington, DC, U.S. Government Printing Office, 1986.
Abbreviation: NHANES, National Health and Nutrition Examination Survey.
* The second NHANES defined hypertension as >160/95 mm Hg on three measurements on one occasion (or current antihypertensive treatment).

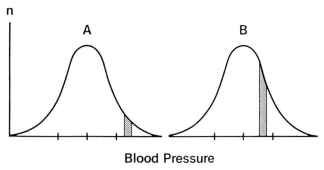

Figure 2–1. Schematic illustration of the distribution of blood pressure in a population. The part of the curve to the right of the *hatched dividing zone* represents "hypertension." The prevalence of "normotension" and "hypertension" depends on where the dividing line is drawn, as illustrated by the identical curves A and B.

Table 2–2. 1993 WHO/International Society of Hypertension Definitions of Hypertension

	Systolic BP (mm Hg)		Diastolic BP (mm Hg)
Normotension	<140	and	<90
Mild hypertension	140–180	and/or	90–105
Subgroup borderline hypertension	140–160	and/or	90–95
Moderate/severe hypertension	>180	and/or	>105
ISH	>160	and	<90
Subgroup borderline ISH	140–160	and	<90

From Zanchetti A, Chalmers J, Arakawa K, et al. The 1993 guidelines for the management of mild hypertension: Memorandum from a WHO/ISH meeting. Blood Pressure 2:86–100, 1993.
Abbreviations: WHO, World Health Organization; BP, blood pressure; ISH, isolated systolic hypertension.

men and women in 24-hour ambulatory blood pressures (Schwan Å, unpublished, 1999).

It is easy to understand why such a massive amount of data has been compiled on this topic. The link between blood pressure and cardiovascular disease has been well established for decades, and the methodology for measuring blood pressure, based on Riva-Rocci's technique,[40, 41] with Korotkoff's modification,[42] is simple and inexpensive to use. Moreover, the treatment of hypertension with antihypertensive drugs has proved to be one of the medical success stories of the 20th century.[43] Undoubtedly, this has had a stimulating effect on attempts to detect hypertensive individuals.

It is not easy to draw a line between hypertension and normotension that is universally accepted. Not long ago, there were strong arguments in favor of distinguishing hypertension and normotension as two separate entities, a view advocated by Sir Robert Platt.[44] His main adversary in this classic debate, Sir George Pickering, on the other hand, claimed that arterial pressure is a normally distributed variable and that any distinction between normal and elevated blood pressure therefore must depend on a chosen line of separation.[45] As it turned out, Pickering's opinion was correct and represents the prevailing view today. The fact that blood pressure in a population is distributed as a nearly gaussian curve means that the prevalence of hyper-

tension is directly dependent on where the line of separation between hypertension and normotension is drawn. In other words, the definition of hypertension will determine its prevalence (Fig. 2–1). It should be noted, though, that the distribution of blood pressure is somewhat skewed to the right, particularly in elderly populations. This means that by using the same definition of hypertension in young and old subjects, the prevalence will be greater in the old population (Fig. 2–2). A number of international and national hypertension societies and expert groups have published their views on the definitions of hypertension. The most recent definitions by the World Health Organization (WHO) and the International Society of Hypertension (ISH) are given in Table 2–2,[46] and those of the sixth report of the Joint National Committee for the Prevention, Detection, Evaluation, and Treatment of High Blood Pressure (JNC VI) are given in Table 2–3.[47]

The huge amount of data available makes it necessary to be highly selective when attempting to review the epidemiology of hypertension. Realistically, no text on a topic of this magnitude can ever be expected to cover every aspect of the field. It is the aim of this chapter to provide brief information on the "classic" epidemiological aspects of hypertension and to discuss some new findings, such as the importance of birth weight for adult hypertension and the links between arterial hypertension and dementia or cognitive impairment.

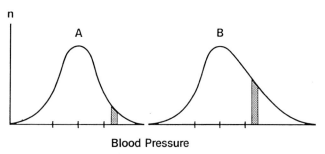

Figure 2–2. Schematic illustration of the distribution of blood pressure in two populations. The part of the curve to the right of the *hatched dividing zone* represents "hypertension." The prevalence of "normotension" and "hypertension" depends on the shape of the curves, even if the dividing line is drawn at the identical level of blood pressure as in curves A and B. Skewing to the right is typical of the distribution of blood pressure in an elderly population.

Table 2–3. Classification of Blood Pressure for Adults Aged 18 Years and Older

Category	Systolic (mm Hg)		Diastolic (mm Hg)
Optimal	<120	and	<80
Normal	<130	and	<85
High-normal	130–139	or	85–89
Hypertension			
Stage 1	140–159	or	90–99
Stage 2	160–179	or	100–109
Stage 3	≥180	or	≥110

Data from Joint National Committee on Prevention, Detection, Evaluation, and Treatment of High Blood Pressure. The Sixth Report. Arch Intern Med 157:2413–2446, 1997.

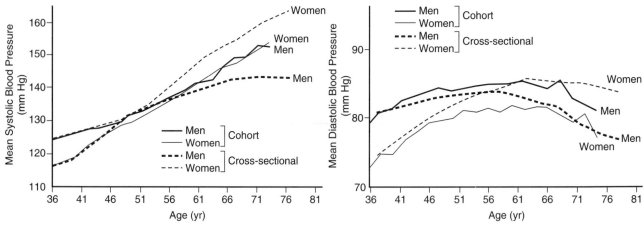

Figure 2–3. Average age trends in systolic *(left)* and diastolic *(right)* blood pressure levels for cross-sectional and cohort data. (From Kannel WB, Wolf PA, McGee DL, et al. Systolic blood pressure, arterial rigidity, and risk of stroke. JAMA 245:1225–1229, 1981.)

BLOOD PRESSURE IN INDUSTRIALIZED POPULATIONS

Blood pressure in industrialized or Westernized populations, with few exceptions, rises with age.[4, 8, 13, 14, 17, 20, 22] This is different from some nonindustrialized populations in which blood pressure remains virtually unchanged with increasing age.[25, 27, 48] The reason for this is not entirely clear, although it was suggested in the multinational Intersalt survey that the rise in blood pressure with age is not seen in populations with a low salt intake.[49] The rise in blood pressure with age is exemplified by the data from the Framingham Heart Study (Fig. 2–3).[6] Systolic blood pressure rises continuously in both men and women during adult life, whereas the rise in diastolic blood pressure levels off and even declines after about age 60 years. The rise in blood pressure is present from birth and continues during childhood and adolescence (Fig. 2–4). Young men have slightly higher blood pressures than women of the same age and not until about age 50 years does the blood pressure in women rise above that of men (Fig. 2–3). As shown in the South Wales population survey, the rise in blood pressure over a 10-year period is greatest in the subjects with the highest initial levels of blood pressure (Fig. 2–5).[23]

Even within countries with apparently homogeneous populations, differences in blood pressure have been reported between different regions.[50] In Great Britain, marked differences in the rate of cardiovascular disease exist, with the lowest rates seen in the southeast and East Anglia and the highest rates in northern England and Scotland.[51] There is a corresponding difference in blood pressure as well. As shown in the British Heart Study[52, 53] and the Nine Towns Study,[54] the highest levels of blood pressure were observed in the regions with the highest prevalence of cardiovascular disease.

The reasons for these differences in blood pressure within a country such as Great Britain, with a relatively homogeneous population, are not entirely clear. Genetic differences seem unlikely. When the genetic influence was assessed in terms of blood group, no association between the ABO blood group and blood pressure was found.[55] There are strong associations between socioeconomic status and blood pressure. Lower blood pressure has been reported in individuals with nonmanual work tasks.[52, 56] A link also exists between social class and heavy drinking: The highest rate of drunk behavior reported to the Temperance Board was in the lowest social class in Tibblin's

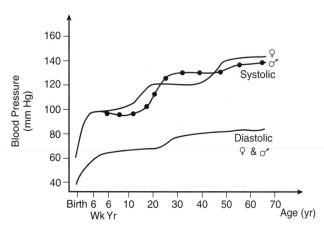

Figure 2–4. Schematic illustration of blood pressure in relation to age.

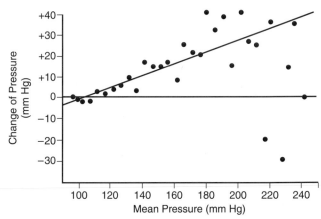

Figure 2–5. Mean change in systolic blood pressure over 10 years in relation to initial mean systolic blood pressure in women aged 15 to 74 years. (This figure was first published in the BMJ, from Miall WE, Lovell HG. Relation between change of blood pressure and age. BMJ 1967; 2:660–664, and is reproduced by permission of the BMJ.)

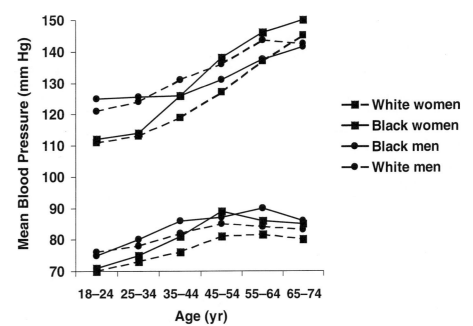

Figure 2–6. Mean systolic *(top)* and diastolic *(bottom)* blood pressures for white and black men and women during the years 1976 to 1980. (From Rowland M, Roberts J. NCHC Advance Data, No. 84, Vital and Health Statistics of the National Center for Health Statistics, October 8, 1982.)

epidemiological survey of men born in 1913.[18] Alcohol intake could be a plausible explanation of the relationship between socioeconomic class and blood pressure, since in the British Heart Study and the Nine Towns Study, the intake of alcohol was strongly linked to the level of blood pressure.[54, 57]

Another potentially contributing factor is body build. Body mass index is strongly associated with blood pressure.[52, 56] Differences in sodium or potassium intake are apparently of minor importance, as judged from the large multinational Intersalt study.[49] Poor living conditions in childhood and adolescence have been suggested as an important risk factor for adult atherosclerotic heart disease.[58] The importance of low birth weight in this context has attracted much attention in recent years. This topic is discussed later.

Race is an important determinant of blood pressure in many populations, e.g., the United States. Adult black individuals have higher blood pressure, and more hypertension, than white individuals in the United States[28, 31] (Figs. 2–6 and 2–7).[59] However, black individuals in the United Kingdom have blood pressure levels similar to those of the white population.[60] This may be attributed to the fact that both racial groups in the British study were from the same social class. The higher levels of blood pressure in American black individuals have been ascribed to a variety of possible differences in psychological, biological,[61] biochemical, and endocrine factors.[62] It is likely that a combination of factors is of importance in this context. It should be noted that hypertension is not unduly common in Africa. In fact, several rural populations in Africa have low blood pressure that does not rise with age, as is discussed later. The fact that black individuals in the United States have an excess prevalence of high blood pressure compared with white individuals, as well as higher rates of mortality from stroke and hypertensive heart disease,[63] might therefore be due to factors other than race, e.g., psychosocial factors or selective migration.

It can be concluded that in most industrialized populations:

1. Blood pressure rises with age.
2. Initially, the rise in blood pressure is steeper in men than in women, but after the menopause, women show a greater rise and reach levels of blood pressure that are higher than in men.
3. There are geographical variations in blood pressure even within seemingly homogeneous populations that can not be explained by simple genetic markers, such as the ABO blood groups or sodium and potassium intake.

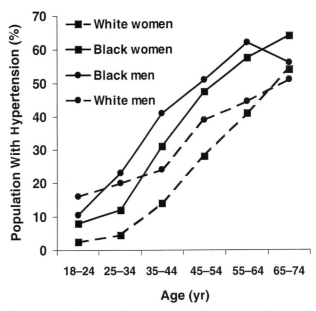

Figure 2–7. Prevalence of hypertension (>140 mm Hg systolic or >90 mm Hg diastolic) in white and black men and women in the United States, 1976 to 1980. (From Rowland M, Roberts J. NCHC Advance Data, No. 84, Vital and Health Statistics of the National Center for Health Statistics, October 8, 1982.)

4. Alcohol intake, body mass index, and social class all appear to be of importance in this context, and to some extent, all three variables are linked.
5. In some industrialized countries, notably the United States, race plays an important role, blood pressure being higher in black individuals. In other countries, black and white subjects have similar levels of blood pressure.

BLOOD PRESSURE IN NONINDUSTRIALIZED POPULATIONS

Much information is available about blood pressure in nonindustrialized populations. An unchanged level of blood pressure during adult, life is not uncommon, but with urbanization or migration from rural to urban settings, rapid changes (increases) in blood pressure may occur. Regretfully, there is virtually no information about the effects on blood pressure of movement from an urban to a rural setting, simply because such changes have yet to occur on a large scale.

Many nonindustrialized populations, such as the Yanomamo Indians in the Amazon, are characterized by low blood pressure.[25] However, low blood pressure is by no means a uniform finding in nonindustrialized or rural populations. Thus, Langford and coworkers found higher blood pressures in a rural black population in the United States compared with an urban black U.S. population.[64] Similar observations have been made in rural and urban Zaire.[65] There is obviously no automatic protection against high blood pressure conferred by living in a rural setting. Differences in blood pressure between rural and urban populations are often rather small. In fact, greater differences in blood pressure have been observed within countries with a relatively homogeneous population, such as in Great Britain. In the British Heart Study, an age-adjusted range of systolic blood pressure of 9 mm Hg was found in middle-aged men in the 24 towns examined.[53] This is a greater difference than is usually found in comparisons between urban and rural populations of the same ethnic background.

The low and stable blood pressure with aging in the Yanomamo Indians has already been mentioned.[25] Similar observations have been made in Bushmen from Kalahari and Botswana in the southern part of Africa.[66, 67] Blood pressure actually tended to fall with age in the Botswana bushmen.[67] In the Xhosa people of South Africa, living in the rural parts of Transkei, blood pressure has been reported to be low and to show little rise with aging.[27] Early observations from East Africa are in agreement with the findings in the nonindustrialized populations in South Africa briefly reviewed here. Thus, in Kenya, a report based on 1000 hospital records in 1929 pointed out that not a single case of hypertension was found and that blood pressure fell with age.[68] In the study by Page and colleagues of the inhabitants of six Solomon Island societies, there was little or no hypertension.[24] Blood pressure remained unchanged or decreased with increasing age in the three least acculturated populations (Baegu, Aita, and Kwaio), whereas blood pressure in women increased with age in the three most acculturated populations (Nasioi, Nagovisi, and Lau).[24] These differences are not easy to explain. It has been suggested that some of these populations, in particular the Lau society, which lives near the coast and makes its livelihood from fishing and therefore also has the greatest salt intake, may show a rise in blood pressure because of its free access to salt.[69] This may be so, but the Intersalt study that recorded sodium excretion and blood pressure in more than 50 populations worldwide found, after exclusion of four extreme populations, no significant relationship between salt intake (assessed as sodium excretion in the urine) and blood pressure.[49] Only the rise in blood pressure with age was associated with salt intake.[49]

Comparisons between geographically distinct populations are of certain interest because they may provide information on blood pressure that integrates the effects of ethnicity, culturization, and diet. A survey of 1100 subjects aged 22 to 89 years in three different parts of the world can be used as an example. In each of the three areas of investigation, Africa (Tanzania and Uganda), the Amazon region of Brazil, and northern Italy, 370 subjects were studied.[70] Each group comprised 111 men and 259 women. As expected, there were a number of differences in the general characteristics of the three groups (Table 2–4).[70] Systolic blood pressure was significantly lower in the Africans: 8% lower than in the Brazilians and 11% lower than in the Italians.[70] Similarly, diastolic blood pressure was significantly lower (by 13%) in the Africans versus the other two groups.[70] There was no rise in blood pressure with age in the African group (if anything there was a trend toward a fall in blood pressure), whereas there was the expected rise with age in the other two groups (Fig. 2–8). The lack of rise in blood pressure with age is in agreement with previous observations in African populations[66, 67] and also in isolated "no-salt" cultures.[25] Whether the lack of rise in blood pressure with age in the African group can be ascribed to low salt intake is not clear. The Africans did in fact use less salt than the other

Table 2–4. General Characteristics of the Three Populations*

Variance	Africa	Brazil	Italy	Significance by Analysis of p Value
Whites:blacks ratio	0:370	234:136	370:0	
Systolic blood pressure (mm Hg)	144	155†	160†‡	<.0001
Diastolic blood pressure (mm Hg)	83	95†	95†	<.0001
Body mass index (kg/m²)	20.4	26.1†	26.8†‡	<.0001
Serum cholesterol (mg/dl)	160	186†	227†	<.001
Serum glucose (mg/dl)	91	108†	103†	<.0001
Ethanol consumption (g/day)	43	10†	39§	<.0001
Smoking (cigarettes/day)	0.2	1.4†	2.3†‖	<.0001

Modified from Pavan L, Casiglia E, Pauletto P, et al. Blood pressure, serum cholesterol and nutritional state in Tanzania and the Amazon: Comparison with an Italian population. J Hypertens 15(10):1083–1090, 1997.
Mean values: †$p < .0001$ versus Africa;‡$p < .05$; §$p < .0001$ versus Brazil; †‖$p < .01$.
* Subjects aged 57.3 + 11.0 yr; $n = 370$, 111 men and 259 women in each sample.

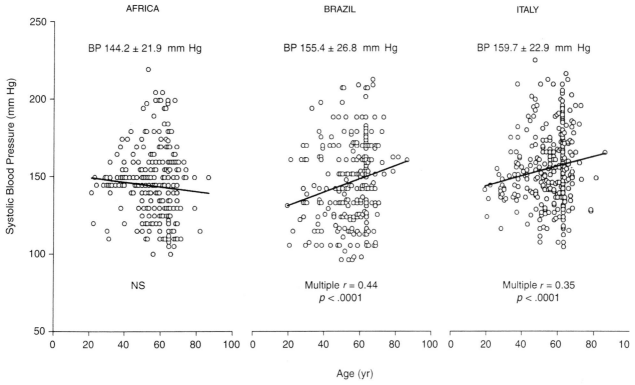

Figure 2–8. Correlations between systolic blood pressure (BP) and age for the populations from Africa, Brazil, and Italy. NS, not significant. (From Pavan L, Casiglia E, Pauletto P, et al. Blood pressure, serum cholesterol and nutritional state in Tanzania and the Amazon: Comparison with an Italian population. J Hypertens 15[10]:1083–1090, 1997.)

two groups, 4 g/day versus 10 g/day in the Brazilians and 11 g/day in the Italians.[70] The finding is in agreement with the results of the Intersalt study, which found that low-salt populations did not show a rise in blood pressure with age.[49] There are, however, a number of other differences between the groups that could be of importance in this context.

It can be concluded that in most nonindustrialized populations:

1. Blood pressure is lower than in industrialized populations.
2. The rise in blood pressure with age is by no means an obligatory finding. On the contrary, a stable level of blood pressure during adult life is common.
3. The reasons behind the differences in blood pressure observed between industrialized and nonindustrialized populations are complex and not fully understood. Dietary factors as well as a number of psychosocial variables appear to be of importance.
4. The rise in blood pressure associated with migration from rural to urban habitants provides an interesting illustration of the effects on blood pressure of a change in lifestyle and is discussed next.

EFFECT OF MIGRATION

Much information on the epidemiology of blood pressure and hypertension can be derived from migration studies. Migration so far has been unidirectional—from rural to

urban settings. This is obviously a complex issue: Who are the individuals who break out from their original place of habitation to seek new fortunes in an urban setting? Most likely they are different in a number of ways from those left behind. Moreover, what are the changes that these migrants meet? Most likely more "stress," but also greater access to tobacco, alcohol, and a Westernized diet with more salt, calories, animal fat, and animal protein. An increase in blood pressure is virtually always found in populations that have migrated from rural to urban living. This can be exemplified by the observations in a Pacific island population that migrated from the Tokelau Island to New Zealand to take up living in an urban and industrialized society.[71] A marked rise in blood pressure was observed, as well as an age-dependent rise in blood pressure that had not been a characteristic feature of this population as long as it remained on its Pacific atolls.[71] Similar observations have been made in China on the Yi people who moved from a very primitive rural life to a somewhat more cultured lifestyle,[72] as well as in several studies from Africa.[27, 65, 73] In particular, Poulter and associates contributed significantly to this field.[69, 74–76] They pointed out that the differences in blood pressure between migrants and those who remain in their original habitat are not due to selective migration.[75] Migration from a rural to an urban setting usually means that a number of factors of importance for blood pressure undergo change. These include dietary habits, usually leading to a higher intake of calories, salt, animal protein, simple carbohydrates, saturated fat, and processed foods.[69] Often there is an increase in the amount of alcohol consumed as well. In addition, a number of sociocultural factors change.

PSYCHOSOCIAL FACTORS

Numerous sociocultural or psychosocial factors play a role in determining the level of blood pressure and the development of hypertension, although these are considerably more difficult to measure and quantify than dietary practices. Noise exposure is an example. Exposure to loud industrial noise (>90 dB) has been shown to raise blood pressure and "stress" hormones acutely.[77, 78] Long-term exposure to industrial noise in car factory workers is associated with higher levels of blood pressure and a higher prevalence of hypertension.[79] Increased levels of blood pressure have also been reported in Iranian weavers working with industrialized carpet production[80] and in Germans living on streets with heavy traffic.[81]

Another recent example of the influence of psychosocial factors on blood pressure is the report of a 30-year follow-up on an isolated order of nuns in Umbria, Italy, and a matched control group of laywomen.[82] In spite of having the same genetic background, the women who lived in secluded cloisters did not show the remarkable rise in blood pressure with age seen in a well-matched group of women leading a normal Italian life. The 30-year data on 144 nuns and 138 laywomen show no significant difference at baseline in blood pressure, family history of hypertension, sodium excretion in the urine, or body mass index. However, with time, there was an increasing difference in blood pressure between the two groups. Although there was almost no change in blood pressure in the group of nuns, the laywomen showed the expected rise with aging (Fig. 2–9).[82] The explanation of this difference is complex, but it likely involves marked differences in psychosocial factors. The nuns did not use birth control pills, but neither did any of the laywomen. There were no smokers in either group. Alcohol intake was 189 g/wk in the nuns and 196

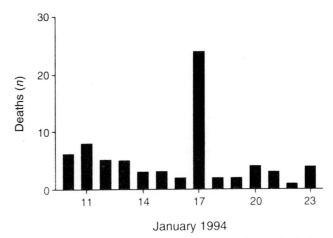

Figure 2–10. The number of sudden cardiovascular deaths in Los Angeles in January 1994. The earthquake took place on the 17th. (From Leor J, Poole WK, Kloner RA. Sudden cardiac death triggered by an earthquake. N Engl J Med 334:413–419, 1996. Copyright © 1996 Massachusetts Medical Society. All rights reserved.)

g/wk in the laywomen, which corresponds to about two bottles of wine weekly. Based on the urinary excretion of sodium at the 30-year follow-up, the two groups had the same salt intake, but the nuns now showed significantly higher levels of serum cholesterol and triglycerides.[82] It is worth noting that the difference in blood pressure was associated with a marked and statistically significant difference in cardiovascular risk as well. Thus, there were 10 versus 21 fatal and 21 versus 48 nonfatal strokes and myocardial infarctions in the nuns compared with the laywomen over the 30-year observation period.[82]

Perhaps the most striking illustration of the powerful associations between psychosocial factors and cardiovascular risk was provided by the earthquake in Los Angeles in January 1994. The number of sudden deaths related to atherosclerotic cardiovascular disease was considerably higher on that date compared with other days of that month (Fig. 2–10).[83]

In summary, numerous variables are altered when people migrate from a rural to an urbanized habitat. It is obvious from migration studies that sociocultural factors, including dietary habits, play an important role in the cause of hypertension.

BLOOD PRESSURE AND BIRTH WEIGHT

There is accumulating evidence that impaired growth in fetal life is related to higher levels of cardiovascular risk factors, such as high blood pressure, impaired glucose tolerance, and possibly even higher fibrinogen and total low-density lipoprotein-cholesterol levels. An association between birth weight and syndrome X, including type 2 diabetes mellitus, hypertension, and hyperlipidemia, has been described. In addition to low birth weight, small head circumference and low ponderal index were seen at birth in subjects with this syndrome.[84–89] Similar negative associations between size at birth and blood pressure have been repeatedly observed in studies of adult men and women. The findings of an association between maternal physique and health, poor fetal growth, and high death rates from

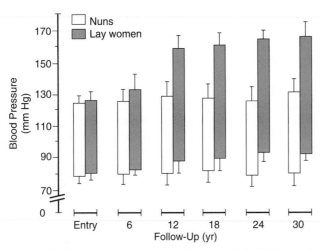

Figure 2–9. Blood pressure in 144 nuns living in secluded cloisers and 138 matched lay women during a 30-year follow-up. (From Timio M, Lippi G, Venanzi S, et al. Blood pressure trend and cardiovascular events in nuns in a secluded order: 30-year follow-up study. Blood Press 6:81–87, 1997.)

Table 2–5. Mean Systolic Blood Pressure (mm Hg) at Age 50 Years by Birth Weight and Gestation Age

Gestation Age (wk)	Birth Weight (g)				p Value for Trend
	<3250	3250–3749	3750–4249	≥4250	
≤37	132.5	141.2	158.3	162.5	<.01
38–41	136.7	135.8	132.9	128.6	.02
≥42	125.5	137.4	133.4	142.5	.23

Data from Leon DA, Koupilova I, Lithell HO, et al. Failure to realise growth potential in utero and adult obesity in relation to blood pressure in 50 year old Swedish men. BMJ 312:401–406, 1996.

cardiovascular disease have led to studies of the relation between intrauterine growth and blood pressure. These studies have reported an inverse relationship between birth weight and adult blood pressure. In a study by Barker and coworkers, the intrauterine environment has been said to have an important effect on blood pressure and hypertension in adults.[90–94]

In an investigation of the associations of fetal growth with blood pressure and mortality from circulatory diseases in adult life, a cohort of 1335 men in Uppsala, Sweden, born 1920 to 1924, was examined. Birth weights for 577 of these men collected from obstetrical records showed a negative association with systolic blood pressure at age 50 years. This association was strongest in men who were born at term (Table 2–5) and in those who had high body mass index at age 50 years (Table 2–6). Birth weight was also negatively associated with hypertension at 50, 60, and 70 years of age in men with high growth potential.[95] A failure to express one's growth potential in utero is related to high blood pressure in middle age.[96] Men who had a low birth weight but grew to above median height are those whose fetal growth was impaired in that they failed to realize their growth potential in utero. Further, these men had low-weight placentas and may have suffered from placental insufficiency, possibly reflecting fetal undernutrition. The birth weight varied appreciably in relation to the social class of the infants' families. Infants born to women of high social class and with high educational level had the highest birth weight. At age 50 years, systolic blood pressure was strongly negatively associated with education. None of the associations between birth weight and adult

Table 2–6. Mean Systolic Blood Pressure (mm Hg) at Age 50 Years by Birth Weight and Body Mass Index

BMI (kg/m²)	Birth Weight (g)				p Value for Trend
	<3250	3250–3749	3750–4249	≥4250	
<23.5	128.5	131.3	127.7	125.4	.51
23.5–25.9	134.5	132.7	130.0	129.1	.02
≥26.0	141.7	140.3	136.2	137.8	.02

Data from Leon DA, Koupilova I, Lithell HO, et al. Failure to realise growth potential in utero and adult obesity in relation to blood pressure in 50 year old Swedish men. BMJ 312:401–406, 1996.
Abbreviation: BMI, body mass index.

blood pressure was materially affected by adjustment for these sociodemographic characteristics.[97]

It has been suggested that differences in blood pressure are established in utero and progressively amplified throughout life. Hemodynamic changes in utero or persisting changes in growth factor concentrations may be linked to increased left ventricular mass, which may explain the association with cardiovascular disease.[98] Studies have also reported relationships between size at birth and the function of the hypothalamopituitaryadrenal axis in childhood,[99] size at birth, and plasma insulin-like growth factor-1 concentration in childhood,[100] and size at birth and arterial compliance in adults.[94] Since variance in birth weight is explained by various environmental and genetic fetal and maternal factors, there may be some common genetic influences first causing impaired fetal growth and later being related to the occurrence of cardiovascular disease in adult life.

BLOOD PRESSURE AND DEMENTIA

Cerebral target organ damage in hypertension has previously been regarded as restricted to stroke. However, in recent years, there has been an increasing interest in hypertension as a potential risk factor also for cognitive decline and dementia. *Dementia* denotes a persistent deterioration of memory and other cognitive functions, severe enough to interfere with daily activities. Advanced dementia causes severe functional deficits and a major decline in quality of life for the patient and his or her family. Its economic impact for society is enormous and is expected to rise, since an increasing proportion of the population is reaching very advanced ages.

There are two major subgroups of dementia disorders: neurodegenerative dementia, including Alzheimer's disease (AD), and vascular dementia (VaD), i.e., dementia caused by cerebrovascular disease. Interest in vascular causes of dementia is increasing owing to the recognition that VaD is common in old age and to the prospect of preventive treatment.[101] In Japan, VaD is responsible for more than half of all dementia cases.[102] The same distribution has been reported from a population-based study of 85-year-olds in Gothenburg, Sweden.[103] Still, there is no consensus concerning criteria for dementia[104] nor for VaD.[105] It is, therefore, difficult to estimate the true prevalence in a general population.

Changing Concepts Over Time

The story of modern dementia research starts in the middle of the 1970s, when dementia in old patients was recognized as a disease entity, and not merely as a nonspecific aging phenomenon. At that time, AD was recognized to be no longer a rare condition, affecting only subjects younger than 65 years, but a "major killer."[106, 107] In 1974, Hachinski and colleagues introduced the term *multiinfarct dementia* (MID), meaning dementia due to cerebrovascular disease and accompanied by multiple infarcts—large or small.[108] In the 1980s, *MID without multiple infarcts* was increasingly recognized, and the wider term *vascular de-*

mentia (VaD), dementia resulting from any type of cerebrovascular disease, was introduced.[109]

At present, evidence suggests that late-onset AD and VaD have common pathways.[110] Vascular lesions may contribute to the clinical manifestation of dementia/AD.[111] An interaction between cerebrovascular disease/atherosclerosis and apolipoprotein E4 allele has been suggested in cognitive decline[112] and in dementia.[113] β-Amyloid seems to interact with endothelial cells,[114] and microvascular factors such as blood-brain barrier and carrier dysfunction may be important in some cases of AD.[115–117] Even in nondemented subjects, there is an association between hypertension and a higher density of neurofibrillary tangles in brain.[118]

High Blood Pressure and Dementia

Stroke and neuroradiological findings of cerebrovascular disease are among the diagnostic criteria of VaD,[105] but they have also been associated with AD and unspecified dementia.[103, 119] In a recent 15-year follow-up of a Swedish population, high blood pressure in 70-year-olds predicted later development of AD as well as of VaD.[110] In the Canadian Study of Health and Aging, observed risk factors for VaD included hypertension, heart disease, and alcohol abuse.[120] In a prospective Japanese study, high systolic blood pressure and stroke were identified as risk factors for VaD.[102]

High Blood Pressure and Early Cognitive Decline

Cognitive functions are distributed along a continuum. The borderlines between "healthy," "forgetful," and "demented" are not clear-cut. Dementia research is now focusing on the identification of risk factors for early cognitive decline, in which prevention or postponement of further deterioration might be possible[121] (Fig. 2–11). Several investigations point to an association between hypertension and impaired cognitive function in nondemented subjects.

Cognitive functions have been followed longitudinally in a few studies only. In a study published in 1971—"Intelligence and Blood Pressure in the Aged"—diastolic blood pressure above 105 mm Hg at baseline predicted

cognitive deterioration at a follow-up after 10 years (n = 87).[122] The authors suggested that "the basis for the cognitive decline associated with aging should be considered secondary to some pathological processes, and not merely as a 'normal aging process.'" In another prospective study, 103 middle-aged persons were followed up for 11 years. High diastolic blood pressure at baseline and at follow-up, and initiation of antihypertensive treatment, were related to impaired performance in one single cognitive test.[123] In a 15-month follow-up of 58 young hypertensive patients, cognitive performance was restored in the treated patients but not in those without treatment.[124]

In the following studies, cognitive functions were measured at one occasion only. Hence, the outcome measurement is "low cognitive function" rather than "cognitive impairment." The most widely used cognitive test is the Mini-Mental State Examination (MMSE).[125] It is a screening instrument for cognitive disturbances that focuses on orientation, short-term verbal memory, calculation, figure copying, praxis, and language functions, with a maximal score of 30 points.

Three population-based studies have shown a relation between high blood pressure at baseline and low cognitive function 10 to 25 years later. In Framingham, blood pressure was measured five times every second year in 1702 stroke-free subjects, and cognitive functions were assessed by a composite score of eight standard psychometric tests 10 to 15 years later.[126] Untreated subjects with hypertension at all five occasions performed 0.25 SD lower than normotensives. Performance in a test of logical memory was most discriminating. In the Honolulu-Asia study, there was a weak inverse relation between systolic blood pressure at baseline and results in the MMSE 25 years later (n = 3735).[127] When men with a previous stroke were excluded, the relation just reached statistical significance. In the Uppsala longitudinal study on adult men without stroke, diastolic, but not systolic, blood pressure at 50 years of age was inversely related to cognitive functions 20 years later, independent of socioeconomic factors.[128] The mean cognitive score in men with diastolic blood pressure of 70 mm Hg or less was 0.5 SD higher than in men with diastolic blood pressure of 105 mm Hg or higher at baseline (Fig. 2–12). Cognition was assessed by a composite score of the MMSE and the Trail Making Tests,[129] which measure subcorticofrontal functions such as psychomotor speed, attention, and flexibility.

Results from cross-sectional studies are not unanimous. In one of the first studies of a stroke-free population (n = 2433), diastolic blood pressure of 90 mm Hg or more was related to low cognitive function.[130] In a study from southern Italy (n = 1339), those with low results in the MMSE (<24, 30% of the population) had higher diastolic blood pressure. The relationship was significant in treated subjects only.[131] Similarly, low cognitive function has been related to high systolic blood pressure (n = 598, Edinburgh);[132] to high diastolic blood pressure (n = 921, Britain);[133] and to hypertension (n = 1927, Austria).[134] Other studies found no relation between blood pressure and cognitive function[135–137] or even a positive association,[138] possibly due to recall biases, since hypertension was defined by self-reported medical history.

In the Uppsala cohort, cross-sectional relations between 24-hour ambulatory blood pressure measurements and cog-

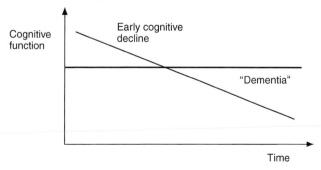

Figure 2–11. Schematic illustration of the development of dementia. Dementia denotes a persistent and severe deterioration of cognitive functions. The "dementia threshold" is arbitrarily defined. Intervention in the early stages of cognitive decline may hypothetically prevent or postpone manifest dementia.

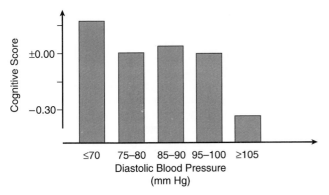

Figure 2–12. Relations between diastolic blood pressure at age 50 years and measurements of cognitive function 20 years later in 929 stroke-free 70-year-old men in the Uppsala cohort. Test for trend, adjusted for education and occupation: $p = .0040$. (Courtesy of L. Kilander, 1998.)

nitive functions were studied.[128] High 24-hour blood pressure, but not high office blood pressure, was related to low cognitive function. The relationship held in both treated and untreated subjects (Fig. 2–13). Further, a nondipping nocturnal blood pressure pattern and diabetes, respectively, were related to low performance, independently of blood pressure levels.

These results support the hypothesis that hypertension is causally related to cognitive impairment, possibly through silent cerebrovascular lesions. However, other interpretations must also be considered. Since cognitive functions were measured on only one occasion, factors linked to low cognitive function at baseline may provide alternative explanations. There is a strong relationship between educational level and other measures of socioeconomic status, and performance on cognitive tests. Another interpretation is that causation might be reverse, i.e., alterations in blood pressure regulation and cognitive impairment may both be

secondary to lesions in cerebral blood pressure regulatory centres. High nocturnal blood pressure has been found to be related, primarily or secondarily, to white matter lesions in hypertensive subjects.[139] However, cerebral lesions more commonly cause a decrease in blood pressure as discussed later.

Low Blood Pressure and Dementia and Cognitive Decline

Low blood pressure and orthostatic hypotension are common features in manifest dementia, irrespective of its cause.[140–144] On the basis of cross-sectional data, it has been suggested that low blood pressure or orthostatic hypotension may be a risk factor for dementia.[141, 142, 145–147] In a study of a very old Swedish population, aged 75 to 101 years, including subjects with dementia ($n = 1736$), blood pressure was positively related to results of the MMSE.[148] In a recent study of ordinary clinical practice, one third of the responding Swedish geriatricians believed that demented patients would benefit from a higher blood pressure.[149] However, there is no evidence from longitudinal studies that low blood pressure or orthostatic hypotension[150] is an independent predictor of cognitive decline. Low blood pressure or a resolution of hypertension seems to be secondary to late stages of dementia, with advanced neuronal damage.[144, 145] In the Uppsala cohort, neither low blood pressure on treatment nor extreme nocturnal dipping was related to lower cognitive function.[128] In the Gothenburg longitudinal study, dementia in 85-year-olds was accompanied by low blood pressure, but was preceded by high blood pressure 15 years earlier[110] (Fig. 2–14). Low blood pressure may be caused by cerebral lesions with reduced sympathetic outflow from brain, by sensory deprivation, or by weight loss.[144, 151] A neuropathological study suggested that blood pressure alteration in AD is due to degeneration

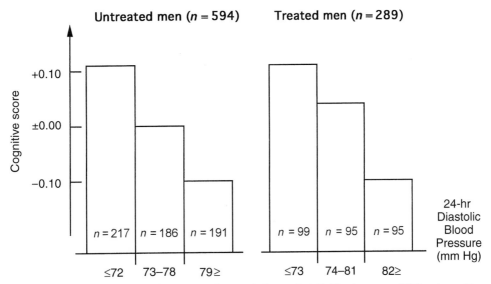

Figure 2–13. An inverse relation between 24-hour ambulatory diastolic blood pressure (DBP) and cognitive score at age 70 years in stroke-free men in the Uppsala cohort, similar in treated and untreated subjects. Mean cognitive score did not differ between the groups, in spite of higher 24-hour DBP in the treated men. Test for trend, adjusted for education, occupation, and insulin sensitivity index: $p = .014$ in untreated men; $p = .272$ in treated men. (Courtesy of L. Kilander, 1998.)

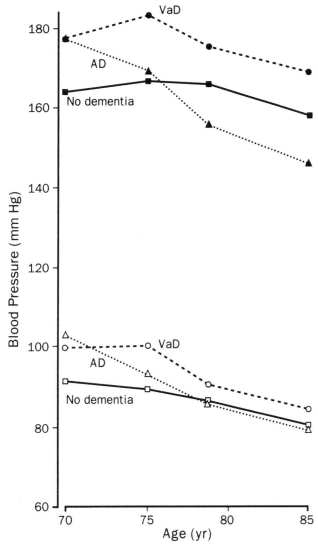

Figure 2–14. Longitudinally measured blood pressure from ages 70 to 85 years in relation to type of dementia with onset at ages 79–85 years. AD, Alzheimer's disease; VaD, vascular dementia. (From Skoog I, Lernfelt B, Landahl S, et al. 15-year longitudinal study of blood pressure and dementia. Lancet 347[9009]:1141–1145, 1996, © by The Lancet Ltd, 1996.)

of central nervous blood pressure regulatory pathways (the C-1 nucleus).[152] The relationship between severity of dementia and low blood pressure may also be a result of greater longevity in patients with a lower risk of vascular disease.

Randomized Clinical Trials

Possible positive or negative effects of antihypertensive treatment on cognitive function and quality of life have been investigated in several clinical trials. To summarize, there is no evidence that blood pressure–lowering, or antihypertensive, agents (diuretics, β-blockers, calcium channel blockers, and angiotensin-converting enzyme inhibitors) have short-term adverse effects on cerebral function or quality of life in elderly patients.[153–156] Some studies reported improved psychomotor performance and quality

of life after treatment.[157] The Hypertensive Old People in Edinburgh (HOPE) Study included untreated elderly patients with mild or moderate hypertension.[158] Cognitive tests were performed at baseline and after 6 months of treatment ($n = 69$). Those patients with the greatest reductions in diastolic blood pressure (≥ 19 mm Hg) had improved scores in some tests compared with those with the least blood pressure lowering. There were no differences between type of treatment (captopril or bendrofluazide).

In larger trials including the Department of Veterans Affairs Cooperative Study,[159] the Systolic Hypertension in the Elderly Project (SHEP) (5 years' follow-up),[160] and the MRC trial of hypertension in older adults (4.5 years' follow-up)[161]—no clear differences in cognitive function between placebo and active treatment were shown. Drop-outs had lower baseline cognitive performance, i.e., were at higher risk of cognitive decline.

The ongoing placebo-controlled Study on Cognition and Prognosis in the Elderly (SCOPE) investigates possible effects of antihypertensive treatment on cognition in very old patients with blood pressure in the "gray zone." A substudy of the Systolic Hypertension in Europe (SYST-EUR) trial is addressing the same question,[162] while the Perindopril Protection Against Recurrent Stroke (PROGRESS) study is examining possible beneficial effects of treatment in stroke patients with normal or high blood pressure.[163]

The most plausible interpretations of these findings is that high blood pressure contributes to impaired cognitive function, and low blood pressure in established dementia is an effect, rather than a cause, of the dementia process. Pathophysiological mechanisms may be multifactorial, including ischemia, dysfunction of the blood-brain barrier, and hemodynamic dysfunction. There is evidence of links between hypertension, impaired cognitive function, white matter lesions, cerebral atrophy, and reduced regional cerebral glucose metabolism.[164–166] Subjects with extensive white matter lesions had higher systolic blood pressure, decreased regional cerebral glucose metabolism, and poorer performance in cognitive tests measuring subcorticofrontal functions.[167] However, many questions concerning causality in the complex of vascular risk factors, white matter lesions, and cognitive impairment still remain.[168] Since a linkage with vascular risk factors has been established, it is urgent to investigate whether cognitive decline can be postponed by more intensive risk factor reduction, including antihypertensive treatment. The hypothesis that antihypertensive treatment prevents cognitive decline and dementia remains to be proved. Participants in clinical trials are highly selected with regard to compliance and, thus, also with regard to high baseline cognitive functions. Trials including patients at high risk of developing dementia are needed to provide a rigorous test of treatment effects on cognitive decline.

RISKS ASSOCIATED WITH HYPERTENSION

The level of blood pressure is directly linked to mortality or the remaining life span. The first major set of data on this topic included the follow-up observations of some 4

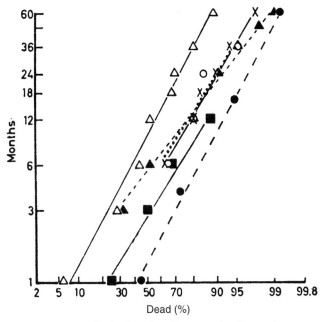

Figure 2–15. Mortality in six series of untreated malignant hypertension. (From Pickering GW, Cranston WI, Pears MA. The Treatment of Hypertension. Springfield, IL, Charles C Thomas, 1961.)

cardiovascular morbidity are clearly linked to the level of blood pressure. In a classic meta-analysis of seven epidemiological studies of the association between blood pressure and the risk of stroke, MacMahon and colleagues showed a steep linear relationship between blood pressure and risk (Fig. 2–16).[170] The observations in these seven studies were based on 843 strokes.[170] The same authors also analyzed the relationship between blood pressure and the risk of coronary heart disease morbidity and mortality in nine observational studies (Fig. 2–17).[171] In this analysis, the result was based on 4856 coronary heart disease events.[170] Risk of both of these major cardiovascular events is clearly linked to the level of blood pressure, at least down to a diastolic blood pressure of 76 mm Hg. In an update of this analysis, which included estimates from later remeasurements of blood pressure in the Framingham Heart Study, the straight linear relationship between diastolic blood pressure and the risk of coronary heart disease was demonstrable down to a diastolic blood pressure of 73 mm Hg.[86] In other words, a J-shaped relationship between blood pressure and risk was not seen in this extensive analysis of observational data.[84] Even if a J-shaped relationship between blood pressure and cardiovascular risk exists, the lowest point of the J-curve is found at a relatively low diastolic blood pressure in population surveys. Thus, only in the diastolic blood pressure range of 20 to 74 mm Hg is there a suggestion of higher coronary heart disease mortality compared with the higher blood pressure brackets in the 30-year follow-up of the Framingham Heart Study (Table 2–7).[8]

Numerous cardiovascular disease manifestations in addition to stroke[2, 6, 169] and coronary heart disease,[1, 7, 169] including congestive heart failure,[3, 8, 11] intermittent claudication,[8] and angina pectoris,[7, 8, 170] are linked to the level of blood pressure. These are dealt with separately in other chapters of this book.

million life insurance policy holders in the study of the Society of Actuaries in 1959.[35] Sir George Pickering and associates, in a mini–meta-analysis, drew attention to the horrendous mortality of untreated malignant hypertension at about the same time (Fig. 2–15). Further, the risks of

Stroke and usual DBP
(in 5 categories defined by baseline DBP)
7 prospective observational studies: 843 events

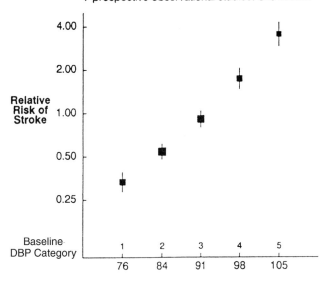

Figure 2–16. Relationship between diastolic blood pressure (DBP) and stroke in seven prospective observational studies. DBP, diastolic blood pressure. (From MacMahon S, Peto R, Cutler J, et al. Blood pressure, stroke, and coronary heart disease. Part 1: Prolonged differences in blood pressure: Prospective observational studies corrected for the regression dilution bias. Lancet 335[8692]:765–774, 1990, © by The Lancet Ltd, 1990.)

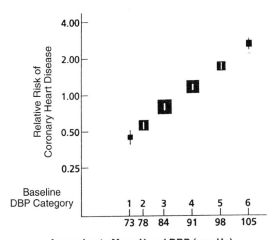

Approximate Mean Usual DBP (mm Hg)
(estimated from later remeasurements in the Framingham Study)

Figure 2–17. Relationship between diastolic blood pressure (DBP) and coronary heart disease in nine prospective observational studies. (From MacMahon S, Peto R, Cutler J, et al. Blood pressure, stroke, and coronary heart disease. Part 1: Prolonged differences in blood pressure: Prospective observational studies corrected for the regression dilution bias. Lancet 335[8692]:765–774, 1990, © by The Lancet Ltd, 1990.)

Table 2–7. Fatal Coronary Heart Disease in Relation to Diastolic Blood Pressure in Men and Women Aged 35 to 74 Years—30-Year Follow-Up Data From the Framingham Heart Study

Diastolic Blood Pressure (mm Hg)	n	Annual Incidence/1000
20–74	16,174	26
75–84	18,091	23
85–94	14,659	28
95–104	6419	48
105–160	2824	64

From Stokes J III, Kannel WB, Wolf PA, et al. The relative importance of selected risk factors for various manifestations of cardiovascular disease among men and women from 35 to 64 years old: 30 years of follow-up in the Framingham Study. Circulation 75(suppl V):65–73, 1987.

References

1. Kannel WB, Schwartz MJ, McNamara PM. Blood pressure and risk of coronary heart disease: The Framingham Study. Dis Chest 56:43–52, 1969.
2. Kannel WB, Wolf PA, Verter J, McNamara PM. Epidemiologic assessment of the role of blood pressure in stroke. The Framingham Study. JAMA 214:301–310, 1970.
3. Kannel WB, Castelli WP, McNamara PM, et al. Role of blood pressure in the development of congestive heart failure. The Framingham Study. N Engl J Med 287:781–787, 1972.
4. Kannel WB. Role of blood pressure in cardiovascular morbidity and mortality. Prog Cardiovasc Dis 7:5–24, 1974.
5. Kannel WB, Gordon T. Elevation of cardiovascular risk in the elderly: The Framingham study. Bull N Y Acad Med 54:573–583, 1978.
6. Kannel WB, Wolf PA, McGee DL, et al. Systolic blood pressure, arterial rigidity, and risk of stroke. JAMA 245:1225–1229, 1981.
7. Wilson P, Castelli W, Kannel W. Coronary risk prediction in adults (The Framingham Heart Study). Am J Cardiol 59:91–94, 1987.
8. Stokes J III, Kannel WB, Wolf PA, et al. The relative importance of selected risk factors for various manifestations of cardiovascular disease among men and women from 35 to 64 years old: 30 years of follow-up in the Framingham Study. Circulation 75(suppl V):65–73, 1987.
9. Dannenberg AL, Garrison RJ, Kannel WB. Incidence of hypertension in the Framingham Study. Am J Publ Health 78:676–679, 1988.
10. Levy D, Garrison RJ, Sagae DD, et al. Prognostic implications of echocardiographically determined left ventricular mass in the Framingham Heart Study. N Engl J Med 322:1561–1566, 1990.
11. Kannel WB, Belanger AJ. The epidemiology of heart failure. Am Heart J 121:951–957, 1991.
12. Sytkowski PA, D'Agostino RB, Belanger AJ, Kannel WB. Secular trends in long-term sustained hypertension, long-term treatment, and cardiovascular mortality. The Framingham Heart Study 1950 to 1990. Circulation 93:697–703, 1996.
13. Franklin SS, Gustin W IV, Wong ND, et al. Hemodynamic patterns of age-related changes in blood pressure. The Framingham Heart Study. Circulation 96:308–315, 1997.
14. Bøe J, Humerfelt S, Wedervang F. The blood pressure in a population, blood pressure readings and height and weight determinations in the adult population of the city of Bergen. Acta Med Scand Suppl 321:1–270, 1957.
15. Lund-Johansen P. Hemodynamics in early essential hypertension. Acta Med Scand 181(suppl 482):1–101, 1967.
16. Lin TY, Hung TP, Chen CM, et al. A study of normal and elevated blood pressure in a Chinese urban population in Taiwan (Formosa). Clin Sci 18:301–312, 1959.
17. Epstein FH, Francis T, Hayner NS, et al. Prevalence of chronic diseases and distribution of selected physiologic variables in a total community, Tecumseh, Michigan. Am J Epidemiol 81:307–322, 1965.
18. Tibblin G. High blood pressure in men aged 50. A population study of men born in 1913. Acta Med Scand Suppl 453, 1967.
19. Svärdsudd K. High blood pressure. Thesis, University of Göteborg, Sweden, 1978, pp 1–43.
20. Svärdsudd K, Tibblin G. A longitudinal blood pressure study. Change of blood pressure during 10 years in relation to initial values: The study of men born in 1913. J Chron Dis 33:627–636, 1980.
21. Ribacke M, Tibblin G, Rosengren A, Eriksson H. Is hypertension changing? Blood pressure development in cohorts of 50-year old men between 1963 and 1993. Blood Press 5:133–137, 1996.
22. Miall WE, Chinn S. Blood pressure and aging: Results of a 15–17 year follow-up study in South Wales. Clin Sci Mol Med 45(suppl 1):23–33, 1973.
23. Miall WE, Lovell HG. Relation between change of blood pressure and age. BMJ 2:660–664, 1967.
24. Page LB, Damon A, Moellering RC Jr. Antecedents of cardiovascular disease in six Solomon Island societies. Circulation 49:1132, 1974.
25. Oliver WJ, Cohen EL, Neel JV. Blood pressure, sodium intake, and sodium related hormones in the Yanomamo Indians, a "no-salt" culture. Circulation 52:146–151, 1975.
26. Hedstrand H, Åberg H. Detection and characterization of middle-aged men with hypertension. Acta Med Scand 199:273–280, 1976.
27. Sever PS, Peart WS, Gordon D, Beighton P. Blood pressure and its correlates in urban and tribal Africa. Lancet 2:60–64, 1980.
28. Stamler J, Stamler R, Riedlinger WF, et al. Hypertension screening of 1 million Americans: Community Hypertension Evaluation Clinic (CHEC) Program, 1973–1975. JAMA 235:2299–2306, 1976.
29. Ueshima H, Tatara K, Asakura S, Okamoto M. Declining trends in blood pressure level and the prevalence of hypertension, and changes in related factors in Japan 1956–1980. J Chron Dis 40:137–147, 1987.
30. Stamler J, Wentworth D, Neaton JD. Is the relationship between serum cholesterol and risk of premature death from coronary heart disease continuous and graded? Findings in 35,222 primary screenees of the Multiple Risk Factor Intervention Trial (MRFIT). JAMA 256:2823–2828, 1986.
31. Hypertension Detection and Follow-Up Program Cooperative Group. Blood pressure studies in 14 communities: A two-stage screen for hypertension. JAMA 237:2385–2391, 1977.
32. The WHO Monica Project. Geographical variation in the major risk factors of coronary heart disease in men and women aged 35–64 years. World Health Stat Q 41:115–129, 1988.
33. Drizd T, Danneberg AL, Engel A. Blood pressure levels in persons 18–74 years of age in 1976–1980, and trends in blood pressure from 1960 to 1980 in the United States. Vital and Health Statistics, Series 11, 234, DHHS publ No. (PHS) 86-1684. Washington, DC, U.S. Government Printing Office, 1986.
34. Burt VL, Whelton PK, Roccella EJ, et al. Prevalence of hypertension in the US adult population: Results from the Third National Health and Nutrition Examination Survey, 1988–1991. Hypertension 25:305–313, 1995.
35. Build and Blood Pressure Study. Vols 1 and 2. Chicago, Society of Actuaries, 1959.
36. Lew EA. High blood pressure, other risk factors and longevity: The insurance viewpoint. Am J Med 55:281–294, 1973.
37. Perloff D, Sokolow M. Ambulatory blood pressure: Mortality and morbidity. J Hypertens 9(suppl 8):S31–S33, 1991.
38. Mancia G, Sega R, Bravi C, et al. Ambulatory blood pressure normality: Results from the PAMELA Study. J Hypertens 13:1377–1390, 1995.
39. Schwan Å. Reference values for 24-hour non-invasive ambulatory blood pressure: A population study of men aged 50. Scand J Prim Health Care 11:21–25, 1993.
40. Riva-Rocci S. Un sfigomanometro nuovo. Gaz Med Torino 47:981–996, 1896.
41. Riva-Rocci S. Un sfigomanometro nuovo. Gaz Med Torino 47:1001–1017, 1896.
42. Korotkoff NS. K voprusu o metodoach eezldovania krovyoanovo-davlenia. Izv Imperatoor Vorenno Med Akad 11:365–367, 1905.
43. Hansson L. What are we really achieving with long-term drug therapy? Am J Hypertens 1:414–420, 1988.
44. Platt R. The nature of essential hypertension. Lancet 2:55–57, 1959.
45. Pickering GW. The Nature of Essential Hypertension. London, J & A Churchill, 1961.
46. Zanchetti A, Chalmers J, Arakawa K, et al. The 1993 guidelines for

the management of mild hypertension: Memorandum from a WHO/ISH meeting. Blood Press 2:86–100, 1993.

47. Joint National Committee on Prevention, Detection, Evaluation, and Treatment of High Blood Pressure. The Sixth Report. Arch Intern Med 157:2413–2446, 1997.

48. Sinnet PF, Whyte HM. Epidemiology studies in total Highland population in New Guinea: Environment, culture and health status. Hum Ecol 1:245, 1973.

49. Intersalt Co-operative Research Group. Intersalt: An international study of electrolyte excretion and blood pressure. Results for 24 hour urinary sodium and potassium excretion. BMJ 297:319–328, 1988.

50. Marmot MG. Geography of blood pressure and hypertension. Br Med Bull 40:380–386, 1984.

51. Office of Population, Censuses and Surveys. Mortality and geography. A review in the mid-1980s. The Registrar General's Decennial Supplement for England and Wales. Series DS, no. 9. London, Her Majesty's Stationery Office, 1990.

52. Shaper AG, Pocock SJ, Walker M, et al. British Regional Heart Study: Cardiovascular risk factors in middle-aged men in 24 towns. BMJ 283:179–186, 1981.

53. Shaper AG, Ashby D, Pocock SJ. Blood pressure and hypertension in middle-aged British men. J Hypertens 6:367–374, 1988.

54. Bruce NG, Cook DG, Shaper AG, Thompson AG. Geographical variation in blood pressure in British men and women. J Clin Epidemiol 43:385–398, 1990.

55. Whincup PH, Cook DG, Phillips AN, Shaper AG. ABO blood group and ischaemic heart disease in British men. BMJ 300:1679–1682, 1990.

56. Bruce N, Wannamethee G, Shaper AG. Life style factors associated with geographic blood pressure variations among men and women in the UK. J Hum Hypertens 7:229–238, 1993.

57. Shaper AG, Wannamethee G, Whincup PH. Alcohol and blood pressure in middle-aged British men. J Hum Hypertens 2:71–78, 1988.

58. Forsdahl A. Are poor living conditions in childhood and adolescense an important risk factor for arteriosclerotic heart disease? Br J Prev Soc Med 31:91–95, 1977.

59. Rowland M, Roberts J. NCHC Advance Data, No. 84, Vital and Health Statistics of the National Center for Health Statistics, October 8, 1982.

60. Cruickshank JK, Jackson SHD, Beevers DG, et al. Similarity of blood pressure in blacks, whites and Asians in England: The Birmingham Factory Study. J Hypertens 3:365–371, 1985.

61. Anderson NB, Myers HF, Pickering T, Jackson JS. Hypertension in blacks: Psychosocial and biological perspectives. [Editorial review] J Hypertens 7:161–172, 1989.

62. Falkner B. Differences in blacks and whites with essential hypertension: Biochemistry and endocrine. Hypertension 15:681–686, 1990.

63. Freis ED. Age, race, sex and other indices of risk in hypertension. Am J Med 55:275–280, 1973.

64. Langford HG, Watson RL, Douglas BH. Factors affecting blood pressure in population groups. Trans Assoc Am Phys 81:135–146, 1969.

65. M'Buyamba-Kabangu J-R, Fagard R, Staessen J, et al. Correlates of blood pressure in rural and urban Zaire. J Hypertens 5:371–375, 1987.

66. Kaminer B, Lutz WPW. Blood pressure in bushmen of the Kalahari Desert. Circulation 22:289–295, 1960.

67. Truswell AS, Kenelly BM, Hansen JDL, Lee RB. Blood pressure of !Kung bushmen in northern Botswana. Am Heart J 84:5–12, 1972.

68. Donnison CP. Blood pressure in the African native. Lancet 1:6–7, 1929.

69. Poulter NR, Sever PS. Blood pressure in other populations. *In* Swales JD (ed). Textbook of Hypertension. Oxford, Blackwell, 1994; pp 22–36.

70. Pavan L, Casiglia E, Pauletto P, et al. Blood pressure, serum cholesterol and nutritional state in Tanzania and the Amazon: Comparison with an Italian population. J Hypertens 15:1083–1090, 1997.

71. Beaglehole R, Salmond CE, Hooper A, et al. Blood pressure and social interaction in Tokelau and migrants in New Zealand. J Chron Dis 30:803–812, 1977.

72. He J, Tell GS, Tang Y-C, et al. Effect of migration on blood pressure: The Yi People Study. Epidemiology 2:88–97, 1991.

73. Scotch NA. Sociocultural factors in the epidemiology of Zulu hypertension. Am J Public Health 53:1205–1213, 1963.

74. Poulter NR, Khaw KT, Hopwood BEC, et al. Blood pressure and its correlates in an African tribe in urban and rural environments. J Epidemiol Community Health 38:181–186, 1984.

75. Poulter NR, Khaw KT, Sever PS. Higher BPs of urban migrants from an African low BP population are not due to selective migration. Am J Hypertens 1:143S–145S, 1988.

76. Poulter NR, Khaw KT, Hopwood BEC, et al. The Kenyan Luo migration study: Observations on the initiation of a rise in blood pressure. BMJ 300:967–972, 1990.

77. Andrén L, Hansson L, Björkman M, Jonsson A. Noise as a contributory factor in the development of elevated arterial pressure in man. Acta Med Scand 207:493–498, 1981.

78. Andrén L, Lindstedt G, Björkman M, et al. Effect of noise on blood pressure and "stress" hormones. Clin Sci 62:141, 1982.

79. Jonsson A, Hansson L. Prolonged exposure to a stressful stimulus (noise) as a cause of raised blood pressure in man. Lancet 1:86–87, 1977.

80. Parvizpoor D. Noise exposure and prevalence of high blood pressure among weavers in Iran. J Occup Med 18:730–731, 1976.

81. von Eiff AW, Neus H. Verkehrslärm und Hypertonie-Risiko. 1. Mitteilung. Münch Med Wochenschr 122:894–896, 1980.

82. Timio M, Lippi G, Venanzi S, et al. Blood pressure trend and cardiovascular events in nuns in a secluded order: 30-year follow-up study. Blood Press 6:81–87, 1997.

83. Leor J, Poole WK, Kloner RA. Sudden cardiac death triggered by an earthquake. N Engl J Med 334:413–419, 1996.

84. Barker DJP, Osmond C, Golding J, et al. Growth in utero, blood pressure in childhood and adult life, and mortality from cardiovascular disease. BMJ 298:564–567, 1989.

85. Law CM, Shiell AW. Is blood pressure inversely related to birth weight: Strength of evidence from systematic review of the literature. J Hypertens 14:935–941, 1996.

86. Hales CN, Barker DJP, Clark PMS, et al. Fetal and infant growth and impaired glucose tolerance at age 64. BMJ 303:1019–1022, 1991.

87. Lithell HO, McKeigue PM, Berglund L, et al. Relationship of birth weight and ponderal index to non–insulin-dependent diabetes and insulin response to glucose challenge in men aged 50–60 years. BMJ 312:406–410, 1996.

88. Martyn CN, Meade TW, Stirling Y, Barker DJ. Plasma concentrations of fibrinogen and factor VII in adult life and their relation to intra-uterine growth. Br J Haematol 89:142–146, 1995.

89. Barker DJP, Hales CN, Fall CHD, et al. Type 2 (non insulin dependent) diabetes mellitus, hypertension and hyperlipidemia (syndrome X) relation to foetal groth. Diabetologia 36:62–67, 1993.

90. Wadsworth MEJ, Cripps HA, Midwinter RE, Colley JRT. Blood pressure in a national birth cohort at the age of 36 related to social and familiar factors, smoking and body mass. BMJ 291:1534–1538, 1985.

91. Gennser G, Rymark P, Isberg PE. Low birth weight and risk of high blood pressure in adulthood. BMJ 296:1498–1500, 1988.

92. Barker DJP, Bull AR, Osmond C, Simmonds SJ. Fetal and placental size and risk of hypertension in adult life. BMJ 301:259–262, 1990.

93. Barker DJP, Godfrey KM, Osmond C, Bull A. The relation of fetal length, ponderal index and head circumference to blood pressure and the risk of hypertension in adult life. Paediatr Perinat Epidemiol 6:35–44, 1992.

94. Martyn CN, Barker DJP, Jespersen S, et al. Growth in utero, adult blood pressure, and arterial compliance. Br Heart J 73:116–121, 1995.

95. Koupilova I, Leon DA, Lithell HO, Berglund L. Size at birth and hypertension in longitudinally followed 50–70 year old men. Blood Press 6:223–228, 1997.

96. Leon DA, Koupilova I, Lithell HO, et al. Failure to realise growth potential in utero and adult obesity in relation to blood pressure in 50 year old Swedish men. BMJ 312:401–406, 1996.

97. Koupilova I, Leon DA, Vågerö D. Can confounding by socio-demographic and behavioral factors explain the association between size at birth and blood pressure at age 50 in Sweden? J Epidemiol Community Health 51:14–18, 1997.

98. Vijayakumar M, Fall CH, Osmond C, Barker DJ. Birth weight, weight at one year, and left ventricular mass in adult life. Br Heart J 73:363–367, 1995.

99. Clark PH, Hindmarsh PC, Shiell AW, et al. Size at birth and adrenocortical function in childhood. Clin Endocrinol (Oxf) 45:721–726, 1996.

100. Fall CH, Pandit AN, Law CM, et al. Size at birth and plasma insulin-like growth factor-1 concentrations. Arch Dis Child 73:287–297, 1995.
101. Hachinski V. Preventable senility: A call for action against the vascular dementias. Lancet 340:645–648, 1992.
102. Yoshitake T, Kiyohara Y, Kato I, et al. Incidence and risk factors of vascular dementia and Alzheimer's disease in a defined elderly Japanese population. Neurology 45:1161–1168, 1995.
103. Skoog I, Nilsson L, Palmertz B, et al. A population-based study of dementia in 85-year-olds. N Engl J Med 328:153–158, 1993.
104. Erkinjuntti T, Østbye T, Steenhuis R, Hachinski V. The effect of different diagnostic criteria on the prevalence of dementia. N Engl J Med 337:1667–1674, 1997.
105. Wetterling T, Kanitz R-D, Borgis K-J. Comparison of different diagnostic criteria for vascular dementia (ADDTC, DSM-IV, ICD-10, NINDS-AIREN). Stroke 27:30–36, 1996.
106. Katzman R. The prevalence and malignancy of Alzheimer disease. A major killer. [Editorial] Arch Neurol 33:217–218, 1976.
107. Blessed G, Tomlinson BE, Roth M. The association between quantitative measures of dementia and of senile changes in the cerebral gray matter of elderly subjects. Br J Psychiatry 114:797–811, 1968.
108. Hachinski VC, Lassen NA, Marshall J. Multi-infarct dementia. A cause of mental deterioration in the elderly. Lancet 27:207–210, 1974.
109. Scheinberg P. Dementia due to vascular disease: A multifactorial disorder. Stroke 19:1291–1299, 1988.
110. Skoog I, Lernfelt B, Landahl S, et al. 15-year longitudinal study of blood pressure and dementia. Lancet 347:1141–1145, 1996.
111. Martyn C. Blood pressure and dementia. Lancet 347:1130–1131, 1996.
112. Kalmijn S, Feskens EJM, Launer LJ, Kromhout D. Cerebrovascular disease, the apolipoprotein e4 allele, and cognitive decline in a community-based study of elderly men. Stroke 27:2230–2235, 1996.
113. Hofman A, Ott A, Breteler M, et al. Atherosclerosis, apolipoprotein E, and prevalence of dementia and Alzheimer's disease in the Rotterdam study. Lancet 349:151–154, 1997.
114. Thomas T, Thomas G, McLendon C, et al. β-Amyloid–mediated vasoactivity and vascular endothelial damage. Nature 380:168–171, 1996.
115. Scheltens PH, Barkhof F, Valk J, et al. White matter lesions on magnetic resonance imaging in clinically diagnosed Alzheimer's disease. Brain 115:735–748, 1992.
116. Scheibel AB, Duong T, Jacobs R. Alzheimer's disease as a capillary dementia. Ann Med 21:103–107, 1989.
117. Kalaria RN, Hedera P. Beta-amyloid vasoactivity in Alzheimer's disease. [Letter] Lancet 347:1492–1493, 1996.
118. Sparks DL, Scheff SW, Liu H, et al. Increased incidence of neurofibrillary tangles in non-demented individuals with hypertension. J Neurol Sci 131:162–169, 1995.
119. Loeb C, Gandolfo C, Croce R, Conti M. Dementia associated with lacunar infarction. Stroke 23:1225–1229, 1992.
120. Lindsay J, Hébert R, Rockwood K. The Canadian study of health and aging: Risk factors for vascular dementia. Stroke 28:526–530, 1997.
121. Lancet conference 1996. The challenge of the dementias. Lancet 347:1303–1307, 1996.
122. Wilkie F, Eisdorfer C. Intelligence and blood pressure in the aged. Science 172:959–962, 1971.
123. Prouty Sands L, Meredith W. Blood pressure and intellectual functioning in late midlife. J Gerontol 47:P81–P84, 1992.
124. Miller RE, Shapiro AP, King HE, et al. Effect of antihypertensive treatment on the behavioral consequences of elevated blood pressure. Hypertension 6:202–208, 1984.
125. Folstein MF, Folstein SE, McHugh PR. "Mini-Mental State": A practical method for grading the cognitive state of patients for the clinician. J Psychiatr Res 12:189–198, 1975.
126. Elias MF, Wolf PA, D'Agostino RB, et al. Untreated blood pressure level is inversely related to cognitive functioning: The Framingham Study. Am J Epidemiol 138:353–364, 1993.
127. Launer L, Masaki K, Petrovitch H, et al. The association between midlife blood pressure levels and late-life cognitive function. The Honolulu-Asia Aging Study. JAMA 274:1846–1851, 1995.
128. Kilander L, Nyman H, Hansson L, et al. Hypertension and associated metabolic disturbances are related to cognitive impairment. A 20-year follow-up of 999 men. Hypertension 31:780–786, 1998.

129. Lezak M. Neuropsychological Assessment, 3rd ed. New York, Oxford University Press, 1995.
130. Wallace RB, Lemke JH, Morris MC, et al. Relationship of free-recall memory to hypertension in the elderly. The Iowa 65 + Rural Health Study. J Chronic Dis 38:475–481, 1985.
131. Cacciatore F, Abete A, Ferrara N, et al. The role of blood pressure in cognitive impairment in an elderly population. J Hypertens 15:135–142, 1997.
132. Starr JM, Whalley LJ, Inch S, Shering A. Blood pressure and cognitive function in healthy old people. J Am Geriatr Soc 753–756, 1993.
133. Gale CR, Martyn CN, Cooper C. Cognitive impairment and mortality in a cohort of elderly people. BMJ 312:608–611, 1996.
134. Freidl W, Schmidt R, Stronegger W-J, Reinhart B. The impact of sociodemographic, environmental, and behavioral factors, and cerebrovascular risk factors as potential predictors of the Mattis Dementia Rating Scale. J Gerontol 52A:M111–M116, 1997.
135. Scherr P, Hebert L, Smith L. Evans D. Relation of blood pressure to cognitive function in the elderly. Am J Epidemiol 134:1303–1315, 1991.
136. Woo J, Ho SC, Lau S, et al. Prevalence of cognitive impairment and associated factors among elderly Hong Kong Chinese aged 70 years and older. Neuroepidemiology 13:50–58, 1994.
137. van Boxtel M, Gaillard C, Houx P, et al. Can the blood pressure predict cognitive task performance in a healthy population sample? J Hypertens 15:1069–1076, 1997.
138. Launer L, Dinkgreve M, Jonker C, et al. Are age and education independent correlates of the Mini-Mental State Exam performance of community-dwelling elderly? J Gerontol 48:P271–P277, 1993.
139. Kario K, Matsuo T, Kobayashi H, et al. Nocturnal fall of blood pressure and silent cerebrovascular damage in elderly hypertensive patients. Hypertension 27:130–135, 1996.
140. Kilander L, Boberg M, Lithell H. Peripheral glucose metabolism and insulin sensitivity in Alzheimer's disease. Acta Neurol Scand 87:294–298, 1993.
141. Landin K, Blennow K, Wallin A, Gottfries C-G. Low blood pressure and blood glucose levels in Alzheimer's disease. Evidence for a hypometabolic disorder? J Intern Med 233:357–363, 1993.
142. Passant U, Warkentin S, Karlson S, et al. Orthostatic hypotension in organic dementia: Relationship between blood pressure, cortical blood flow and symptoms. Clin Auton Res 6:29–36, 1996.
143. Hogan DB, Ebly EM, Rockwood K. Weight, blood pressure, osmolarity, and glucose levels across various stages of Alzheimer's disease and vascular dementia. Dement Geriatr Cogn Disord 8:147–151, 1997.
144. Guo Z, Viitanen M, Fratiglioni L, Winblad B. Low blood pressure and dementia in elderly people: The Kungsholmen project. BMJ 312:805–808, 1996.
145. Desmond DW, Moroney JT, Sano M, Stern Y. Recovery of cognitive function after stroke. Stroke 27:1798–1803, 1996.
146. Perlmuter LC, Greenberg JJ. Do you mind standing? Cognitive changes in orthostasis. Exp Aging Res 22:325–341, 1996.
147. Elmståhl S, Rosén I. Postural hypotension and EEG variables predict cognitive decline: Results from a 5-year follow-up of healthy elderly women. Dement Geriatr Cogn Disord 8:180–187, 1997.
148. Guo Z, Fratiglioni L, Winblad B, Viitanen M. Blood pressure and performance on the Mini-Mental State Examination in the very old. Am J Epidemiol 145:1106–1113, 1997.
149. Kilander L, Boberg M, Lithell H. How do we treat, or not treat, high blood pressure in the oldest old? A practice study in Swedish geriatricians. Blood Press 6:372–376, 1997.
150. Rutan GH, Hermanson B, Bild DE, et al. Orthostatic hypotension in older adults. The Cardiovascular Health Study. Hypertension 19:508–519, 1992.
151. Cronin-Stubbs D, Beckett LA, Scherr PA, et al. Weight loss in people with Alzheimer's disease: A prospective population based analysis. BMJ 314:178–179, 1997.
152. Burke WJ, Coronado PG, Schmitt CA, et al. Blood pressure regulation in Alzheimer's disease. J Auton Nerv Syst 48:65–71, 1994.
153. Croog S, Elias M, Colton T, et al. Effects of antihypertensive medications on quality of life in elderly hypertensive women. Am J Hypertens 7:329–339, 1994.
154. Neutel JM, Smith DHG, Lefkowitz MP, et al. Hypertension in the elderly: 24 h ambulatory blood pressure results from a placebo-controlled trial. J Hum Hypertens 9:723–727, 1995.

155. Beto JA, Bansal VK. Quality of life in treatment of hypertension. A metaanalysis of clinical trials. Am J Hypertens 5:125–133, 1992.

156. Muldoon MF, Waldstein SR, Jennings JR. Neuropsychological consequences of antihypertensive medication use. Exp Aging Res 21:353–368, 1995.

157. Croog S, Levine S, Testa M, et al. The effects of antihypertensive therapy on the quality of life. N Engl J Med 314:1657–1664, 1986.

158. Starr JM, Whalley LJ, Deary IJ. The effects of antihypertensive treatment on cognitive function: Results from the HOPE study. J Am Geriatr Soc 44:411–415, 1996.

159. Goldstein G, Materson BJ, Cushman WC, et al. Treatment of hypertension in the elderly. II: Cognitive and behavioral function. Hypertension 15:361–369, 1990.

160. Applegate WB, Pressel S, Wittes J, et al. Impact of the treatment of isolated systolic hypertension on behavioral variables. Arch Intern Med 154:2154–2160, 1994.

161. Prince MJ, Bird AS, Blizard RA, Mann AH. Is the cognitive function of older patients affected by antihypertensive treatment? Results from 54 months of the Medical Research Council's treatment trial of hypertension in older adults. BMJ 312:801–805, 1996.

162. Slovick DI, Amery A, Birkenhager W, et al. SYST-EUR multicentre trial on the treatment of isolated systolic hypertension in the elderly: First interim report. J Hum Hypertens 7:201–203, 1993.

163. Whitlock G, MacMahon S, Anderson C, et al. Blood pressure lowering for the prevention of cognitive decline in patients with cerebrovascular disease. Clin Exp Hypertens 19:843–855, 1997.

164. van Swieten JC, Geyskes GG, Derix MMA, et al. Hypertension in the elderly is associated with white matter lesions and cognitive decline. Ann Neurol 30:825–830, 1991.

165. Schmidt R, Fazekas F, Koch M, et al. Magnetic resonance imaging cerebral abnormalities and neuropsychologic test performance in elderly hypertensive subjects. Arch Neurol 52:905–910, 1995.

166. Salerno J, Grady C, Mentis M, et al. Brain metabolic function in older men with chronic essential hypertension. J Gerontol 50A:M147–M154, 1995.

167. DeCarli C, Murphy DGM, Tranh M, et al: The effect of white matter hyperintensity volume on brain structure, cognitive performance, and cerebral metabolism of glucose in 51 healthy adults. Neurology 45:2077–2084, 1995.

168. Longstreth WT, Manolio TA, Arnold A, et al: Clinical correlates of white matter findings on cranial magnetic resonance imaging of 3301 elderly people: The Cardiovascular Health Study. Stroke 27:1274–1282, 1996.

169. Pickering GW, Cranston WI, Pears MA. The Treatment of Hypertension. Springfield, IL, Charles C Thomas, 1961.

170. MacMahon S, Peto R, Cutler J, et al. Blood pressure, stroke, and coronary heart disease. Part 1: Prolonged differences in blood pressure: Prospective observational studies corrected for the regression dilution bias. Lancet 335:765–774, 1990.

171. MacMahon S. Blood pressure and the risks of cardiovascular disease. *In* Swales JD (ed). Textbook of Hypertension. Oxford, Blackwell, 1994; pp 46–57.

SECTION 2

Pathophysiology

CHAPTER 3

Pathophysiology of Hypertension

Carolina Delgado and Alan B. Weder

Regulation of blood pressure is one of the most complex of physiologic functions, dependent on the integrated actions of cardiovascular, renal, neural, and endocrine systems. Hypertension is a disorder of the average level about which blood pressure is regulated, and although it is of clinical importance because chronically elevated blood pressure damages the heart, blood vessels, and kidneys, at least in its early stages hypertension does not cause obvious disturbances of cardiovascular function. Most of the functional cardiovascular derangements of hypertension arise from the compensatory mechanisms elevated blood pressure provokes, e.g., vascular and ventricular hypertrophy, or from its contribution to vascular damage, e.g., atherosclerosis and nephrosclerosis. Investigating the pathophysiology of hypertension therefore means understanding the mechanisms of normal blood pressure control and seeking evidence of subtle abnormalities that precede (or at least coincide with) the rise of blood pressure to hypertensive levels.

Because hypertension represents a quantitative dysfunction of the highly interactive elements of the cardiovascular system, traditional reductionist research modes are unlikely to yield more than fragments of the answer to the question of what causes hypertension.[1–3] Pathophysiologic thinking is one such reductionist approach. Essentially mechanistic and concerned largely with the immediate or proximate causes of disease, such research seeks to identify the structures and functions that result in elevated blood pressure. Pathophysiologic studies have been of great value in describing the underlying causes of differences between hypertensives and normotensives but less successful in identifying root causes of hypertension. To address causality, findings gathered in the physiologic investigation of cardiovascular control systems will need to be integrated into broader frameworks: the value of evolutionary research for organizing the findings derived from pathophysiologic research has been pointed out before.[4] The goal of evolutionary thinking is to understand how heritable traits affect fitness, i.e., reproductive success, and ultimately to describe not only the fundamental genetic complement underpinning hypertension but also the environmental factors necessary for expression of the phenotype and the physiologic processes mediating the interaction of genes and environment. Each such complement of genes, each set of environmental exposures, and each history of their interaction will be unique, so that a truly comprehensive description of the pathophysiology of hypertension will probably never be possible. But by integrating broad frames such as evolution into our pathophysiologic thinking, we are likely to get a better understanding of ultimate causation.

This introduction attempts to lay out some of the broad principles of cardiovascular regulation that are relevant to a consideration of the pathophysiology of essential hypertension. We do not aim to summarize the mechanisms to be explored in detail by experts in the succeeding chapters of this volume but rather to demonstrate how complex the task of formulating an integrated pathophysiologic picture of hypertension is likely to be. We begin by emphasizing three fundamental features of blood pressure control:

1. Blood pressure regulation is flexible and responsive to local organ perfusion requirements.
2. Blood pressure regulation is integrated into overall cardiovascular-renal function to serve total-body homeostasis.
3. The level at which blood pressure is regulated changes throughout life history.

BLOOD PRESSURE CONTROL AND LOCAL NEEDS

At its most basic level, blood pressure provides the driving force that moves blood through the vascular system. Because maintenance of this function is absolutely critical to life, it is not surprising that natural selection has favored organisms that have evolved mechanisms that contribute to blood pressure stability. Nor is it unexpected that such mechanisms are powerful and highly redundant, providing ample "backup" to cope with changes in environmental factors, including electrolyte intake, physical activity, threats, and trauma. Indeed, it would be remarkable if the situation were otherwise.

All mammals have fundamentally the same circulatory system, so blood pressure control systems are likely to be highly evolutionarily conserved across species, and it may therefore not seem surprising that mean arterial blood pressure in the aortic root is essentially constant in mammals, about 100 mm Hg.[5] This constancy is in contrast to many anatomic features, e.g., heart weight, and physiologic functions, e.g., heart rate, that are scaled to average body mass across a wide range of species sizes.[6] In many cases, unscaled variables, i.e., those not related to body size, are constrained by fundamental and invariant physical or chemical features important to life, such as diffusion distances. Since several other critical aspects of circulatory function are similarly unscaled, notably capillary and red blood cell diameters, it seems plausible to assume that blood pressure is part of a system finely adapted in many ways to ensure optimal delivery of metabolic substrates at the tissue level. That the level of blood pressure characteristic of mammals is an adaptation of their particular body plan is evidenced by the differing average blood pressure levels found in other animals. Birds, e.g., operate at a higher average blood pressure level than do mammals, and the reasons for the difference are not clear.[6]

Whereas the constancy of blood pressure in mammals might seem to imply rigidity of function, nothing could be further from the truth. The only example of naturally elevated blood pressure in a nonhuman mammalian species is instructive in demonstrating how flexible blood pressure regulation can be. Giraffes have evolved to occupy an ecologic niche of arboreal feeding by means of selection for an extreme elongation of the neck. Although closely related to the other ruminants, where blood pressure averages the expected value of about 100 mm Hg mean, giraffes demonstrate extraordinarily high blood pressures at the level of the heart, with estimates of resting blood pressure of 180 mm Hg[7] to over 300 mm Hg.[8]

Elevated blood pressure in these animals serves to maintain blood flow to the brain, so that blood pressure level at the base of the skull is about 100 mm Hg. The cardiovascular system has accommodated the particular structural adaptations of giraffe anatomy by altering force generation at the left ventricle and thus aortic root pressure to provide precisely the energy necessary to drive blood to the brain. It is theoretically possible for natural selection to have altered the structural plan of the giraffe body to one in which the brain migrated to a more central body location and therefore could operate at a "normal" systemic blood pressure. However, such an adaptation would involve wrenching changes in the established body plan and ontologic course of vertebrate development that would undoubtedly be difficult to fashion. Nature usually shapes its adaptations conservatively. The giraffe's neck, for instance, although markedly different in appearance from that of the taxonomically related cow, nonetheless contains the same seven cervical vertebrae. In meeting the cardiovascular demand imposed by its anatomic adaptation, rather than redesigning the system, how much more efficient to draw on built-in features of the cardiovascular repertoire—notably the ability to regulate average blood pressure level—and to use those features to match the specific circulatory demands imposed by neck elongation. Thus although generally fixed within a narrow range in mammals, when necessary, blood pressure can be maintained indefinitely at a markedly increased level when critical local needs require it.

The giraffe illustrates an important principle of blood pressure control: Blood pressure level is flexible and responsive to important physiologic needs, e.g., brain perfusion. From the viewpoint of the fitness of the organism in terms of natural selection, this functional trade-off of high blood pressure for optimal brain perfusion is perfectly reasonable, even if some adverse consequences flow from the compromise. The adaptationist paradigm holds that, in general, natural selection favors any individual or suite of novel features (in the case of the giraffe, a long neck and the attendant elevated blood pressure) when the net impact of such changes is favorable in terms of reproductive success of the affected individual's genes. Importantly, not every preserved element need be in itself adaptive. Thus, whereas employing high blood pressure as a way of matching circulatory function to an unusual anatomic situation is an elegant solution to an adaptive challenge, it does not imply that giraffes do not pay a price for maintaining high aortic root pressures. They evidence a large number of pathologic effects of high blood pressure, including massive left ventricular hypertrophy and extraordinary arterial vascular smooth muscle hypertrophy in the limbs.[9, 10] It seems likely that such cardiovascular adaptations are potentially deleterious, but any such adverse consequences are more than balanced by the advantages of a long neck on overall fitness.

BLOOD PRESSURE CONTROL AND INTEGRATED CARDIOVASCULAR-RENAL FUNCTION

In addition to providing perfusion to critical organs such as the brain, blood pressure plays a key role in the optimization of other organ and whole-body functions. Starling recognized as long ago as 1909 that total-body sodium and water balance is regulated in part by renal arterial perfusion pressure.[11] This concept was further characterized by subsequent investigators, most notably by Guyton and associates, who proposed that blood pressure and sodium homeostasis are related through the mechanism of pressure natriuresis: When perfusion pressure increases, renal sodium output increases and extracellular fluid and blood volumes contract by an amount sufficient to return arterial blood pressure to its baseline.[12, 13] Guyton[13] characterized the relationship between natriuresis and mean arterial blood pressure by a pressure-natriuresis curve characteristic of each individual, which is shifted to a higher value on the pressure axis when hypertension is chronically sustained.

The fundamental phenomena central to this theory have been confirmed in both experimental and clinical studies, and more recent evidence suggests that the renal medulla may be the anatomic site of critical importance in pressure natriuresis in rats.[14] Unlike renal cortical blood flow and glomerular filtration rate, which are autoregulated and therefore essentially constant over a wide range of perfusion pressures in experimental models, rat renal medullary blood flow increases by 5 to 10% as mean perfusion pressure rises from 80 to 160 mm Hg.[15] Vasa recta capillary pressure also rises as perfusion pressure increases, resulting in increased renal interstitial pressure, which shifts nephron function toward a natriuretic mode. Evidence that the renal medulla is a possible cause of hypertension was provided by Roman, who used laser Doppler flowmetry to measure medullary blood flow in prehypertensive 3- to 5-week-old spontaneously hypertensive rats (SHR).[16] Medullary blood flow was decreased in these animals before blood pressure rose, compatible with a role for the medullary microvasculature in the genesis of hypertension. Others have demonstrated that cross-transplantation of kidneys from genetically hypertensive to genetically normotensive rats results in a rise in blood pressure and, conversely, that transplantation of a kidney from a normotensive rat lowers blood pressure in hypertensive strains.[17–19] Therefore, a structural renal characteristic, such as might be encoded in the medullary vasculature, is an attractive candidate mechanism of hypertension in such animals. Other structural renal abnormalities may also be important, as proposed by Norrelund and colleagues, who showed that afferent renal arteriolar diameter cosegregates with blood pressure in F2 animals derived from an SHR × WKY cross.[20] Since increased afferent arteriolar resistance could restrict renal medullary flow, these two vascular systems could reinforce each other. Functional disorders of the renal medullary circulation may also be important, as evidenced by studies demonstrating that inhibition of nitric oxide synthase can restore medullary autoregulation.[21] Other factors, such as vasoactive hormones, can also affect medullary flow and resistance. Thus, medullary vascular mechanisms may be affected by many of the substances that alter renal sodium handling.

Others working with dog models concluded that renal medullary blood flow is well autoregulated,[22, 23] and thus the renal medullary circulation may not be a critical determinant of pressure natriuresis in all species. Clearly the importance of such abnormalities cannot be confirmed directly in humans. Whether or not theories of the cause of essential hypertension predicated on vascular abnormalities in the kidney are correct in detail, the underlying principle is important: Blood pressure is regulated as part of overall cardiovascular-renal homeostasis to serve the needs of the total organism. Regulation of blood pressure cannot be otherwise if the model of Guyton and associates is correct, as deviations from that determined by the overall functioning of the integrated system would result in cardiovascular disaster.[13] In characterizing the pathophysiologic basis of hypertension, it will be important to include integrated physiologic thinking as well as detailed mechanistic descriptions. Hierarchically organized complex systems such as those governing cardiovascular functions are generally characterized by emergent properties, such as pressure natriuresis, that are present only at higher functional levels and cannot be understood by examination of their individual components.[24, 25] This message is directed toward proponents of molecular biologic approaches to hypertension pathogenesis, who sometimes appear to be so fascinated with their search for ultimate, i.e., genetic, causes of disease that they lose sight of the infinitely complex hierarchies of function and control that characterize organisms.[1]

CHANGING THE SET POINT: GROWTH, DEVELOPMENT, AND HYPERTENSION

As pointed out in 1978 by Sir George Pickering, *hypertension* is defined by an arbitrary division in the continuous blood pressure distribution.[26] Two sets of definitions are commonly used, one for adults and one for children and adolescents. Adult levels exceeding a threshold, usually 140 mm Hg systolic or 90 mm Hg diastolic in the United States, are defined as being *hypertensive*. Such cutpoints are based largely on tradition rather than on any biological significance of the values. In childhood, hypertension is defined as a blood pressure exceeding the 95th percentile

for age,[27] another arbitrary division that results in a constantly changing threshold for hypertension during development. Such definitions are of heuristic value in identifying individuals on whom medical attention should be focused. But perhaps the real message of the different definitions is that they acknowledge an important feature of blood pressure during postnatal development: Blood pressure rises with age. Long ignored, the significance of the childhood, and indeed even prenatal, antecedents of hypertension are receiving increasing attention.[4, 28]

The rise of blood pressure during childhood and adolescence follows a very stereotypical course, with a rapid increase during the first few weeks of life, a gradual increase throughout childhood, and a dramatic rise during puberty.[27] Blood pressure then remains relatively constant in most individuals throughout the remainder of the second and well into third decade, after which it again begins to rise.[4] It is during this period that most diastolic hypertension develops, i.e., blood pressures finally exceed 90 mm Hg diastolic. However, it has long been recognized that adult blood pressures are related to adolescent levels: Serial measures of blood pressure within individuals are correlated, and the coefficient of correlation becomes increasingly strong with aging.[28] As a consequence, adolescents with the highest relative rank of blood pressure have the highest risk of future hypertension. So where does hypertension begin? Is it when the blood pressure is established in the upper rank, as certainly can be determined during adolescence? Or alternatively, must we wait until middle age to diagnose hypertension? Because the pattern of high blood pressure is established early in life, hypertension may have its roots in early developmental events, and events contributing to high blood pressure in youth may result in pathophysiologic changes that cannot be subsequently reprogrammed or that set the stage so that events affecting blood pressure later in life have an enhanced hypertension-promoting effect.

Although the precise mechanisms affected early in development are unknown, several schema incorporating the general principle of early events conditioning later responses have been proposed:

1. *Vascular remodeling.* Observations by Folkow[29] and Sivertsson[30] that hypertensive vessels undergo adaptation by structural remodeling, which increases the wall:lumen ratio, identified an important mechanism that maintains chronically increased vascular resistance in established hypertension. Although partially reversible by long-term antihypertensive therapy, this structural adaptation persists to a degree even in effectively treated patients and progresses in uncontrolled hypertension.[31] Since structural changes are present even in borderline hypertension, it is likely that this adaptation begins early in the course of the blood pressure rise, probably before the hypertensive range is reached.[32, 33]

2. *Hyperkinetic borderline hypertension.* Julius and coworkers described serial changes in cardiovascular function that result in a transition in the hemodynamics of blood pressure control from a state of increased cardiac output, largely sustained by the autonomic nervous system, to one of a sustained elevation of blood pressure dependent on increased vascular resistance and unre-

lated to increased autonomic tone.[34, 35] The initiating factor for the early hyperkinetic circulatory state, increased sympathetic and decreased parasympathetic tone, is postulated to cause β_1-receptor downregulation in the heart that, perhaps in concert with changes in myocardial function,[36] results in a regression of cardiac output to normal values. At the same time, structural enhancement of vascular resistance (increased wall:lumen ratio), induced by high blood pressure and sympathetic overactivity, results in a progressive increase in vascular tone even as sympathetic drive falls. The net effect of these adaptations is a transition from a state of increased cardiac output to one of increased vascular resistance.[37, 38] Because the transition occurs over decades, serial longitudinal hemodynamic studies have been difficult to organize, but Lund-Johansen and Omvik documented the transition in a small group of subjects who presented with hyperkinetic borderline hypertension in youth and ended with typical high-resistance essential hypertension 20 years later.[39]

3. *Allometric dysfunction.* Weder and Schork proposed a schema in which the coordinated programs matching somatic and renal growth could be disrupted by an excessively vigorous growth pattern in youth and adolescence.[4] They postulated that the vigorous growth associated with modern childhood and adolescence, coupled with compression of the period of active growth by earlier puberty, might result in a fixed mismatch of some critical growth-related renal function and somatic metabolic demands. Such a mismatch might be compensated for by increased blood pressure, and since the fundamental defect could not be corrected after the cessation of growth at puberty, this fixed defect could promote hypertension throughout life. Although the precise nature of the renal defect leading to such a situation is unknown, possible candidates are underdevelopment of the medullary microcirculation or cortical afferent arterioles, which, as noted previously, appear to be important aspects of renal structure affecting sodium handling. Aspects of this schema are pertinent to the subsequent discussion of how modernity causes hypertension.

4. *Synchronicity.* Schork and associates noted that in inbred animal strains, there is a temporal coupling of growth and blood pressure such that growth spurts regularly precede rises in blood pressure.[40] Similar findings have been reported for humans when serial changes in body size and blood pressure have been examined.[41] The vigor of the rise in blood pressure after a growth spurt appeared to be greater in genetically hypertensive rats compared with a genetically normotensive strain, suggesting that genetic programs controlling the coupling function could be responsible for initiating states of increasing blood pressure initially triggered by normal growth processes.

5. *Telomere shortening.* Aviv and Aviv proposed the interesting hypothesis that telomere shortening, a phenomenon accompanying normal aging, might contribute to hypertension.[42] If true, an early acceleration of telomeric loss—or alternatively, congenitally short telomeres or a deficiency in telomerase, the enzyme that repairs damaged telomeres—could condition a later acceleration of hypertension.

6. *Birth weight and hypertension.* Largely through the work of Barker, a relationship between low birth weight, increased placental weight, and increased risk of adult hypertension has been established.[43, 44] These observations suggest that in utero events can condition, or in Barker's terminology, program, an infant to a phenotype characterized by insulin resistance and a tendency toward the development of hypertension and diabetes.[43] Barker argues that in utero growth retardation sets the stage for a thrifty phenotype that manifests itself as disease late in life.

The mechanism of such programming has been further investigated by Seckl, who has provided evidence that placental 11β-hydroxysteroid dehydrogenase activity may play a key role in such programming.[45] This enzyme converts physiologic glucocorticoids such as cortisol to inactive metabolites, thus decreasing the transfer of maternal steroids to the fetus. Experimental studies show that steroid exposure inhibits fetal growth but increases placental weight, the pattern identified by Barker as predisposing to hypertension.[43] Seckl demonstrated that in rats, in utero exposure to steroids increases the blood pressure of offspring,[46] suggesting that factors that control fetal steroid exposure, especially 11β-hydroxysteroid dehydrogenase activity, could play a role in promoting hypertension.

All these mechanisms share a common theme: Events at one point in development have consequences for the blood pressure level at a later stage. In searching for causal events, then, we would be well advised to look at the times at which such events are operative.

HYPERTENSION: PROXIMATE AND ULTIMATE CAUSATION

Having stressed the importance to research in hypertension of the essential functions of the circulatory system, the integrated nature of cardiovascular-renal homeostasis and the importance of the temporal evolution of the level of blood pressure, let us turn to a consideration of why humans get hypertension.

No one can say with absolute certainty when hypertension first appeared in human history, but it is generally accepted to be a relatively modern disease of civilization. The emphasis on the importance of the acculturated environment somewhat undervalues the role of genes, and the term *syndrome of impaired genetic homeostasis* has been suggested as a better characterization of the problem.[47] The strongest support for the view that hypertension results from a fundamental mismatch between our ancient genes and our modern environment comes from observations of blood pressure in populations of modern-day hunter-gatherers.[48] Individuals in many of these societies pursue a lifestyle probably quite like that of the Neolithic period and do not develop hypertension or the progressive rise in systolic and mean blood pressure that is universally observed in individuals living in Westernized societies. Since adult hunter-gatherers have typical mammalian blood pressures, i.e., mean arterial blood pressures of about 100 mm Hg, elevated blood pressures in Westernized societies may reflect a response to some physiologic need imposed by our acculturation. Although we do not have an adaptive problem as obvious as the giraffe's long neck, modern environmental novelty apparently activates the flexible, powerful, highly evolutionarily preserved systems that alter the set point of blood pressure control to a higher level in some individuals. Unlike the giraffe, we do not seem to "need" high blood pressure, for in general, there is no obvious physiologic dysfunction induced by lowering blood pressure through antihypertensive treatment. Further, clinical trials show that the adverse consequences of sustained high blood pressure are ameliorated by such treatment.

Yet the indisputable fact that genes contribute to human hypertension implies an adaptive role for those genes.[49] We are unaware of any data suggesting an adaptive advantage or disadvantage for hypertension itself. Except for the relatively rare event of fatal malignant hypertension in youth, which could obviously affect reproductive potential, diseases arising from or aggravated by essential hypertension generally occur during postreproductive years. Thus, when considering high blood pressure in an evolutionary context, it is important to focus on issues other than high blood pressure, since that is not a trait likely to be related to reproductive success. It is reasonable to view hypertension as a pleiotropic effect of a genetic suite that subserves some important function other than blood pressure regulation.[1, 40] The keys to hypertension are likely to reside in genetic-environmental interactions, with the genes involved those of our ancient hunter-gatherer–adapted genome and the environment that of our new human-created world: Hypertension is a response to environmental novelty.

What is it that Westernized society does to our bodies that causes high blood pressure? The increased dietary sodium intake of acculturated societies has been extensively studied, and the Intersalt trial has provided good evidence that in populations with minimal sodium intake, the prevalence of hypertension is very low.[50] However, other factors may also be important, as exemplified by the Kuna of Panama, some of whom follow a traditional lifestyle yet consume sodium at levels typical of Westernized societies and do not evidence hypertension.[51] Others have suggested that the ratio of sodium:potassium intake may be critical and have identified the weight gain associated with migration from rural to urban settings as a factor associated with the development of hypertension.[52] The most obvious features of Westernized lifestyle are calorie intake in excess of need and calorie expenditure far below that of our early ancestors. Hunting and gathering involved nomadic foraging and persistent pursuit of game, both of which required vigorous physical exertion. Even as agriculture arose, life remained strenuous, and not until industrialization did humans begin to escape a lifestyle of obligatory physical activity. Such a lifestyle required considerable energy throughput, and the estimated daily energy expenditure of adult members of hunter-gatherer and traditional (nonmechanized) agricultural societies was on the order of 3000 kcal/day,[53, 54] whereas individuals in our modern industrialized societies expend about 2000 kcal/day or less.

This shift is almost entirely the result of mechanization, as illustrated by estimates of the effect of mechanized farming in Japan, which reduced daily work expenditure for the average farmer by over 50%.[55] The shift from a balanced energy throughput, characterized by high intake but equally high expenditure, to one of intake in excess of expenditure resulted in an altered body habitus with an increase in body fat and a loss of muscle mass.[56, 57] Even recently studied hunter-gatherers, who have already been somewhat affected by the modern world, have skinfold thicknesses half those of Westernized North Americans.[58] The experience of the Inuit of the Northwestern Territories of Canada during the period when hunting by dog sled and kayak was superseded by travel on snowmobiles, all-terrain vehicles, and power boats is particularly powerful and instructive, as the effect of modernization occurred quickly and resulted in dramatic changes in body composition within a generation.[59] Eaton noted that for 20- to 29-year-old males, lean body mass declined 10.1% and body fat (estimated from skinfold thicknesses) increased 88.7% over one 20-year period; for women in the same age category, lean body mass fell 12.1% while body fat rose 40.1%.[60] Along with the observed changes in body habitus, which seem to inevitably follow Westernization, comes hypertension. It is reasonable to think that the effects on body habitus and blood pressure are related: The question is, how?

The most logical place to search for the causes of hypertension is in normal blood pressure regulatory systems, and the optimal time is before blood pressure rises to pathological levels. In order to carry out such studies, we need to examine further how blood pressure changes during normal growth and development. Blood pressure rises in several reasonably stereotypical spurts, most notably during adolescence. This adolescent spurt is probably part of our fundamental human biology, as it appears in hunter-gatherer adolescents as well as in Westernized individuals.[61] However, hunter-gatherers do not go on to develop hypertension later in life, whereas we do. Most interest has traditionally focused on the period during which hypertension actually develops—adulthood. However, increasing attention is being paid to childhood and adolescence as evidence accumulates that the forces driving the blood pressure up may already be in play by that time. An alteration in the natural history of the adolescent growth spurt may be important in the pathophysiology of adult hypertension.

Schork and associates observed that the rise in blood pressure in young rats that corresponds to the adolescent blood pressure spurt in humans is coupled to a growth spurt: Rapid growth precedes a rise in blood pressure in a regular manner.[40] More recently, longitudinal observations in humans demonstrated the same sequence with the adolescent blood pressure spurt trailing the onset of the growth spurt by about 1 to 2 years.[41] The appearance of this sequence in both humans and rats suggests that blood pressure rises to serve some need imposed by growth, presumably as part of maintenance of overall homeostasis.[40] In humans, secular trends in growth and development suggest that the overall program of maturation may be greatly accelerated by modern life.[62] Interestingly, evidence suggests that human ancestors were quite tall, probably on average as tall as the upper 15% of the modern population,[63, 64] so the amount of linear growth itself may not be the problem.

Historical data show a progressive compression of the period of active growth and development in children and adolescents,[65] such that the growth of contemporary adolescents is probably near its biological limits for both the final height achieved and the rate at which linear growth proceeds.[66] Coupled with vigorous linear growth is a tendency to adiposity that results in a high average body mass index in the tallest adolescents. In addition, sexual maturity is now probably achieved almost as early as biologically possible,[62] and the relative obesity of adolescents may again play an important role. It has been suggested that a critical fat mass is a trigger of menarche (perhaps mediated by increasing leptin levels[67]), presumably because sufficient fat accumulation increases the potential for successful pregnancy and childbearing.[68] The earlier and greater accumulation of body fat by acculturated children may be part of the reason that sexual development is now much more rapid than in earlier times. We have previously proposed that this compression of growth and development has affected growth programs preserved during evolution and adapted for a more leisurely pace, resulting in mismatches between structure and function, perhaps at the level of the kidney.[4] If this hypothesis is correct, a rise in blood pressure to high levels in adolescents who grow rapidly to a large size and mature early is simply a mechanism by which the body maintains overall homeostasis. Since those adolescents who are driven by rapid and vigorous growth to develop high blood pressure are predisposed to adult hypertension, it may be that the effects of modern civilization are mediated in part by a disruption of normal, i.e., Paleolithic, growth patterns.

An important distinction between hunter-gatherers and us is lack of an adult rise in blood pressure in non-Westernized people. It is during this adult phase that hypertension actually develops. Hypertension has at least two developmental phases, an early phase (childhood and adolescence), during which the stage is set for future hypertension, and a later phase, during which progressively rising blood pressure finally achieves hypertensive levels. It seems likely that the later phase of hypertension development is a product of the same environmental influences that affected early growth and development, but in adulthood, where linear growth is no longer possible, the result of caloric excess is progressive adiposity, which ultimately promotes a rise in blood pressure and the development of hypertension. Some support for this view comes from an intriguing observation reported in the Framingham cohort that lean young hypertensives go on to develop obesity in adulthood, suggesting that factors that promote hypertension in youth may predispose to adiposity in adults.[69] As described previously, Barker and coworkers suggested that this tendency toward hypertension and obesity may actually be set during in utero development.[70] A pathophysiologic schema by which obesity may promote hypertension has been proposed by Landsberg[71] and is presented in Chapter 12, Obesity-Related Hypertension as a Metabolic Disorder.

Our Paleolithic genes are affected by modern lifestyle factors with the result that we achieve less than optimal muscularity and a considerable excess of body fat, yet we grow linearly at an accelerated rate and achieve sexual maturity at a young age. These alterations in human natural history appear to provoke a rise in blood pressure through mechanisms not yet well described: Physiologists still have much to contribute to reveal the detailed mechanisms by which the set point of blood pressure regulation is altered.

GENETICS OF HYPERTENSION

The ultimate goal of reductionist biology is to uncover the genes causing hypertension. The speculations we have put forward previously raised several important issues for investigators of the genetics of hypertension, which are now coming to attract increasing attention in hypertension research.

First, we must consider how to look. The model most commonly applied to genetic studies of complex diseases such as hypertension, which has been termed the *Baconian-Cartesian-Newtonian-Darwinian-Comtean research paradigm,* may be misguided.[2] Such an approach presupposes that agents causing disease can be isolated without altering their fundamental nature, that such agents do not change as the result of being measured, and that interference with the action of such agents does not alter the effects of other factors influencing the phenomenon of interest. Yet the factors promoting hypertension are a tightly integrated web of environmental-genetic interactions played out in subtle alterations of complex developmental schema. As has been emphasized by Sing and associates, individual disease susceptibility genes are likely to have small effects on final phenotypes, and the majority of prevalent cases of disease most likely result from what has been termed *context-dependent effects of allelic variations.*[2] Although the consequences of such factors in some cases may converge on a critical biologic measure, e.g., renal medullary resistance, reducing that factor to its genetic basis does not mean searching for a gene for small medullary capillaries.

Second, when to look? Since the development of hypertension begins in youth, it would be appropriate to direct considerable attention to that phase if one is interested in understanding what causes hypertension in later life. Relatively little attention has been paid to the precursors of hypertension, probably because it is difficult to identify "prehypertensives" with precision, and because such studies would require extensive longitudinal follow-up. Perhaps most promising at present are studies in the genetic hypertension models, where the important observations of Harrap and colleagues suggest that events early in life mediated through the renin-angiotensin system are critical to the full expression of hypertension in adulthood.[72] Although studies in humans are far more difficult and less conclusive than those in animal models, some progress has been possible, as best typified by the work of Barker on possible in utero effects on the subsequent evolution of hypertension.[43] If deterministic genetic processes are active only during critical developmental phases, identification of causal genes may require that studies be conducted while such genes are expressed. We have recently demonstrated that inbred rats show a time-dependent linkage between a genetic marker and blood pressure and that detection of the linkage may be possible only within a critical temporal window.[73]

Third, where to look? The search for genes contributing to hypertension must be framed in the context of a developmental disorder or regulation. Many of the advances in molecular genetics have begun with studies of mendelian variants of disease, and hypertension is no exception. The elucidation of the molecular bases of such diseases as glucocorticoid-remediable aldosteronism,[74] the syndrome of apparent mineralocorticoid excess,[75] and Liddle's syndrome[76] have been exciting, and work on other rare phenotypes, such as the hypertension-brachydactyly syndrome,[77] continues. However, it seems unlikely that such diseases will lead directly to an understanding of the genes underpinning essential hypertension. Whereas a traditional linkage approach to hypertension has discovered one allelic variant contributing to hypertension—the $A(-6)$ mutation in the promoter sequence of the angiotensinogen gene[78]—and whereas continued efforts employing linkage-based as well as candidate gene approaches are being pursued vigorously, complementary strategies will have to be developed to address at least two important issues. If gene-environment interactions are critical to the promotion of hypertension, more attention will need to be given to environmental covariates in genetic analyses. At present, most studies are focused on the hypertensive state (defined by blood pressure level or the prescription of antihypertensive drugs) or intermediate phenotypes, such as the often-associated insulin-resistant state. A better understanding of what factors in the environment are critical promoters of hypertension will be required before a reasonably complete model of hypertension can be developed. Further, geneticists have treated hypertension as if it results from the continued action of causal genes, i.e., genes whose role can be uncovered by studies undertaken at the time the blood pressure has reached hypertensive levels. However, experimental work and epidemiologic observations suggest that early events are important, perhaps crucial, for the development of hypertension, and such early influences may not be evident by the time blood pressure rises.

There are a huge number of additional issues to be addressed at every organizational level to answer the question of what causes hypertension. How we ask those questions frames the answer we will get. Let us hope that we are clever enough to ask the right questions.

References

1. Strohman RC. Ancient genomes, wise bodies, unhealthy people: Limits of a genetic paradigm in biology and medicine. Perspect Biol Med 37:112, 1993.
2. Sing C, Havilland MB, Reilly SL. Genetic architecture of common multifactorial disease. *In* Chadwick D, Cardew G (eds). Variation in the Human Genome. Ciba Foundation Symposium 197. Chichester, United Kingdom, John Wiley & Sons, 1996; pp 211–232.
3. Schork NJ. Genetically complex cardiovascular traits. Origins, problems, and potential solutions. Hypertension 29:145, 1997.
4. Weder AB, Schork NJ. Adaptation, allometry, and hypertension. Hypertension 24:145, 1994.
5. Patterson JL, Goetz RH, Doyle JT, et al. Cardiorespiratory dynamics in the ox and giraffe, with comparative observations on man and other mammals. N Y Acad Sci 127:393, 1965.
6. Calder WA III. Scaling of physiological processes in homeothermic animals. Annu Rev Physiol 43:301, 1981.
7. Van Critters RL, Franklin DL, Vatner SF, et al. Cerebral hemodynamics in the giraffe. Trans Assoc Am Physicians 82:293, 1969.
8. Goetz RH, Warren JV, Gauer OH, et al. Circulation of the giraffe. Circ Res 8:1049, 1960.
9. Goetz RH. Preliminary observations on the circulation in the giraffe. Trans Am Coll Cardiol 5:239, 1955.
10. Dagg AI, Foster JB. The Giraffe. Its Biology, Behavior, and Ecology. New York, Van Nostrand Reinhold, 1976.
11. Starling EH. The Fluids of the Body. London, Constable, 1909; pp 104–133.
12. Guyton AC, Coleman TG, Cowley AV Jr, et al. Arterial pressure regulation. Overriding dominance of the kidneys in long-term regulation and in hypertension. Am J Med 52:584, 1972.
13. Guyton AC. Long-term arterial pressure control: An analysis from animal experiments and computer and graphic models. Am J Physiol 259:R685, 1990.
14. Cowley AW. Role of the renal medulla in volume and arterial pressure regulation. Am J Physiol 273:R1, 1997.
15. Mattson DL, Lu S, Roman RJ, Cowley AW. Relationship between renal perfusion pressure and blood flow in different regions of the kidney. Am J Physiol 264:R578, 1993.
16. Roman RJ. Altered pressure natriuresis relationship in young spontaneously hypertensive rats. Hypertension 9:III-131, 1987.
17. Churchill PC. Kidney cross transplant in Dahl salt-sensitive and salt-resistant rats. Am J Physiol 262:H809, 1992.
18. Fox U. The primary role of the kidney in causing blood pressure difference between Milan hypertensive strain (MHS) and normotensive rats. Clin Exp Pharmacol Suppl 3:71, 1976.
19. Knoft DW. Source of the kidney determines blood pressure in young renal transplanted rats. Am J Physiol, 265:F104, 1993.
20. Norrelund H, Christensen KL, Samani NJ, et al. Early narrowed afferent arteriole is a contributor to the development of hypertension. Hypertension 24:301, 1994.
21. Fenoy FJ, Ferrer P, Carbonell L, et al. Role of nitric oxide on papillary blood flow and pressure natriuresis. Hypertension 25:408, 1995.
22. Majid DS, Navar LG. Medullary blood flow responses to changes in arterial pressure in canine kidney. Am J Physiol 270:F833–838, 1996.
23. Majid DSA, Godfrey M, Navar LG. Pressure natriuresis and renal medullary blood flow in dogs. Hypertension 29:1051, 1997.
24. Mayr E. Toward a New Philosophy of Biology. Cambridge, MA, Harvard University Press, 1988; pp 44–48.
25. Folkow B. Increasing importance of integrative physiology in the era of molecular biology. News Physiol 9:93, 1994.
26. Pickering G. Normotension and hypertension: The mysterious viability of the false. Am J Med 65:561, 1978.
27. Horan JM, Falkner B, Kimin SYS, et al. Report of the Second National Heart, Lung, and Blood Institute Task Force on Blood Pressure Control in Children—1987. Pediatrics 79:1, 1987.
28. Lever AV, Harrap SB. Essential hypertension: A disorder of growth with origins in childhood? J Hypertens 10:101, 1992.
29. Folkow B. Cardiovascular structural adaptation: Its role in the initiation and maintenance of primary hypertension. Clin Sci Mol Med 55:3, 1978.
30. Sivertsson R. The hemodynamic importance of structural vascular changes in essential hypertension. Acta Physiol Scand 79:3, 1970.
31. Schachter M. Drug-induced modification of vascular structure: Effects of antihypertensive drugs. Am Heart J 122:316, 1991.
32. Takeshita A, Mark AL. Decreased vasodilator capacity of forearm resistance vessels in borderline hypertension. Hypertension 2:610, 1980.
33. Zweifler AJ, Nicholls MG. Diminished finger volume pulse in borderline hypertension: Evidence for early structural vascular abnormality. Am Heart J 104:812, 1982.
34. Julius S, Quadir H, Gajendragadkar S. Hyperkinetic state: A precursor of hypertension? A longitudinal study of borderline hypertension. *In* Gross F, Strasser T (eds). Mild Hypertension: Natural History and Management. London, Pittman, 1979; pp 116–126.
35. Julius S, Schork NJ, Schork MA. Sympathetic hyperactivity in early stages of hypertension: The Ann Arbor data set. J Cardiovasc Pharmacol 12:121, 1988.
36. Julius S, Randall OS, Esler MD, et al. Altered cardiac responsiveness and regulation in the normal cardiac output type of borderline hypertension. Circ Res 36–37(suppl I):I-199–I-207, 1975.
37. Julius S. Editorial review: The blood pressure seeking properties of the central nervous system. J Hypertens 6:177–185, 1988.
38. Julius S. Changing role of the autonomic nervous system in human hypertension. J Hypertens 8:S59–S65, 1990.
39. Lund-Johansen P, Omvik P. Hemodynamic patterns of untreated hypertensive disease. *In* Laragh JH, Brenner BM (eds). Hypertension: Pathophysiology, Diagnosis, and Management. New York, Raven, 1990; pp 305–327.

40. Schork NJ, Jokelainen P, Grant EJ, et al. Relationship of growth and blood pressure in inbred rats. Am J Physiol 266:R702, 1994.

41. Akahoshi M, Soda M, Carter R, et al. Correlation between systolic blood pressure and physical development in adolescents. Am J Epidemiol 144:51, 1996.

42. Aviv A, Aviv H. Reflections on telomeres, growth, aging, and essential hypertension. Hypertension 29:1067, 1997.

43. Barker DJP (ed). Fetal and Infant Origins of Adult Disease. London, BMJ, 1993.

44. Law CM, Shiell AW. Is blood pressure related to birth weight? The strength of evidence from a systematic review of the literature. J Hypertens 14:935, 1996.

45. Seckl JR. Glucocorticoids, feto-placental 11β-hydroxysteroid dehydrogenase type 2, and the early life origins of adult disease. Steroids 62:89, 1997.

46. Benediktsson R, Lindsay RS, Noble J, et al. Glucocorticoid exposure in utero: New model for adult hypertension. Lancet 341:339, 1993.

47. Neel JV, Weder AB, Julius S. Type II diabetes, essential hypertension, and obesity as "syndromes of impaired genetic homeostasis": The "thrifty genotype" hypothesis enters the 21st century. Perspect Biol Med 42:44–74, 1998.

48. James GD, Baker PT. Human population biology and blood pressure: Evolutionary and ecological considerations and interpretations of population studies. *In* Hypertension: Pathophysiology, Diagnosis, and Management, 2nd ed. Laragh JH Brenner BM (eds). New York, Raven, 1995; pp 115–126.

49. Ward R. Familial aggregation and genetic epidemiology of blood pressure. *In* Laragh JH Brenner BM (eds). Hypertension: Pathophysiology, Diagnosis, and Management, 2nd ed. New York, Raven, 1995; pp 67–88.

50. Intersalt Cooperative Research Group. Intersalt: An international study of electrolyte excretion and blood pressure. Results for 24 hour urinary sodium and potassium excretion. BMJ 297:319, 1988.

51. Hollenberg NK, Martinez G, McCullough M, et al. Aging, acculturation, salt intake, and hypertension in the Kuna of Panama. Hypertension 29:171, 1997.

52. Poulter NR, Hopwood BEC, Mugambi M, et al. The Kenyan Luo migration study: Observations on the initiation of a rise in blood pressure. BMJ 300:967, 1990.

53. Hill K, Hawkes K, Hurtado M, Kaplan H. Seasonal variance in the diet of Ache hunter-gatherers in eastern Paraguay. Hum Ecol 12:101, 1984.

54. Heini AF, Mingholli G, Diaz E, et al. Free-living energy expenditure assessed by two different methods in lean rural Gambian farmers. Am J Clin Nutr 61:893, 1995.

55. Shimamoto T, Komachi Y, Inada H, et al. Trends for coronary heart disease and stroke and their risk factors in Japan. Circulation 79:503, 1989.

56. Larsen CS. Functional implications of post cranial size reduction on the prehistoric Georgia coast, USA. J Hum Evol 10:489, 1981.

57. Smith P, Bloom RA, Berkowitz J. Diachronic trends in human cortical thickness of Near Eastern populations. J Hum Evol 131:603, 1984.

58. Eaton SB, Konner M, Shostak M. Stone agers in the fast lane: Chronic degenerative diseases in evolutionary perspective. Am J Med 84:739, 1988.

59. Rode A, Shepard RJ. Physiological consequences of acculturation: A 20-year study of fitness in an Inuit community. Eur J Appl Physiol 69:516, 1994.

60. Eaton SB. Where's the beef? Evolution, body composition, and insulin resistance. In preparation.

61. Oliver WJ, Cohen EL, Neel JV. Blood pressure, sodium intake, and sodium related hormones in the Yanomamo Indians, a no-salt culture. Circulation 52:146, 1975.

62. Tanner JM. Earlier maturation in man. Sci Am 218:21, 1968.

63. Roberts MB, Stringer CB, Parfitt BP. A hominid tibia from middle Pleistocene sediments at Boxgrove, UK. Nature 369:311, 1994.

64. Walker A. Perspectives on the Nariokotome discovery. *In* Walker A, Leakey R (eds). The Nariokotome Homo erectus skeleton. Cambridge, MA, Harvard University Press, 1993; pp 411–430.

65. Tanner JM. Growth as a measure of the nutritional and hygienic status of a population. Horm Res 38(suppl 1):106–115, 1992.

66. Stini WA. Adaptive strategies of human populations under nutritional stress. *In* Watts ES, Johnston FE, Lasker GW (eds). Biosocial Interrelations in Population Adaptation. The Hague, The Netherlands, Mouton, 1975; pp 19–41.

67. Chehab FF, Mounzih K, Lu R, Lim ME. Early onset reproductive function in normal female mice treated with leptin. Science 275:88, 1997.

68. Frisch RE. Body fat, puberty and fertility. Biol Rev 59:161, 1984.

69. Kannel WB, Brand N, Skinner JJ, et al. The relation of adiposity to blood pressure and development of hypertension. Ann Intern Med 67:48, 1967.

70. Barker DJP, Bull AR, Osmond C, Simmonds S. Fetal and placental size and risk of hypertension in adult life. BMJ 301:259–262, 1990.

71. Kreiger DR, Landsberg L. Obesity and hypertension. *In* Laragh JH, Brenner BM (eds). Hypertension: Pathophysiology, Diagnosis, and Management, 2nd ed. New York, Raven, 1995; p 2367.

72. Harrap SB, Van der Merwe WM, Griffin SA, et al. Brief angiotensin converting enzyme inhibitor treatment in young spontaneously hypertensive rats reduces blood pressure long-term. Hypertension 16:603, 1990.

73. Iyengar S, Schork NJ, Jokelainen P, et al. The function of growth in the regulation of blood pressure: Model organisms as a paradigm for human disease. Am J Human Genet Suppl 61:A280, 1997.

74. Lifton RP, Dluhy RG, Powers M, et al. A chimaeric 11β-hydroxylase/aldosterone synthase gene causes glucocorticoid-remediable aldosteronism and human hypertension. Nature 355:262–265, 1992.

75. Stewart PM, Krozowski ZS, Gupta A, et al. Hypertension in the syndrome of apparent mineralocorticoid excess due to mutation of the 11β-hydroxysteroid dehydrogenase type 2 gene. Lancet 347:88–91, 1996.

76. Shimkets RA, Warnock DG, Bostis CM, et al. Liddle's syndrome: Heritable human hypertension caused by mutations in the β subunit of the epithelial sodium channel. Cell 79:407–414, 1994.

77. Schuster H, Wienker TF, Bahring S, et al. Severe autosomal dominant hypertension and brachydactyly in a unique Turkish kindred maps to human chromosome 12. Nat Genet 13:98–100, 1996.

78. Inoue I, Nakajima T, Williams CS, et al. A nucleotide substitution in the promoter of human angiotensinogen is associated with essential hypertension and affects basal transcription in vitro. J Clin Invest 99:1786, 1997.

4 Genetics

Stephen B. Harrap

Attempts to understand and explain the genetic basis of blood pressure levels have encompassed studies of blood pressure correlations among relatives,[1–3] associations between blood pressure and genetically determined traits such as blood group[4–6] and human leukocyte antigen (HLA) antigens[7, 8] and, recently, direct analysis of DNA sequence and mutations. Beyond scientific curiosity, the impetus behind the research is the establishment of fundamental understanding as the basis for new methods of detecting, preventing, and treating high blood pressure and allied cardiovascular disease. However, the task is difficult. Some of the complexities, such as the variability of the blood pressure phenotype and the interaction with environmental factors, were apparent early. The discovery of the molecular basis of rare, familial Mendelian diseases that affect blood pressure diseases[9] engendered optimism about genetic discoveries related to more common conditions such as clinical essential hypertension. However, the common conditions have proved much more difficult to understand than was expected, and recurring inconsistencies have dashed early hopes for quick answers.

ASSUMPTIONS AND MODELS

Before one addresses the issues concerning genetics it is important to have a clear understanding of the epidemiological characteristics and relevance of blood pressure. In particular, the clinical concept of hypertension and the relationship between hypertension and cardiovascular disease deserve scrutiny. Certain assumptions underpin many existing approaches to the genetics of blood pressure, and they have important implications for the applicability of molecular research.

Blood Pressure and Cardiovascular Disease

The Genetics of Higher Blood Pressure, Not Just of Hypertension, Is Important

Much interest in the genetics of blood pressure has focused on hypertension, but the rationale for this focus owes more to clinical medicine than it does to cardiovascular endpoints and their burden on the entire population.

HYPERTENSION IS AN ARBITRARILY DEFINED RISK FACTOR, NOT A DISEASE. The importance of high blood pressure rests in its contribution to increased risk of cardiac and vascular conditions such as stroke and ischemic heart disease that cause disability and death.[10] The greatest relative cardiovascular risk is associated with the highest blood pressures. This correlation justifies the medical approach of screening blood pressure and treating hypertensive subjects so as to reduce individual risk. However, the distribution of blood pressure levels in the population is unimodal (Fig. 4–1), and the definition of hypertension is arbitrary and operational.[11, 12] Classifications such as *hypertensive* and *normotensive* do not necessarily differentiate individuals in a meaningful biological or genetic context and are not, therefore, necessarily appropriate as the basis for genetic analyses.

THERE IS A CONTINUOUS RELATIONSHIP BETWEEN BLOOD PRESSURE AND CARDIOVASCULAR RISK. Epidemiological analyses indicate that the relationship between blood pressure and risk of cardiovascular disease is continuous.[10] In other words, across the entire population, each increment in pressure is associated with higher risk. This phenomenon is obvious when the relationship between blood pressure and cardiovascular disease is displayed as relative risk (Fig. 4–2). However, such representations obscure the real impact of blood pressure in a population.

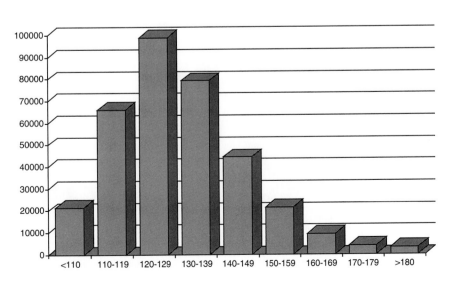

Figure 4–1. Systolic blood pressure distribution in 347,987 men aged 35 to 57 years in the Multiple Risk Factor Intervention Trial. These data show a unimodal distribution with a skew toward upper values. (Data from Stamler J, Stamler R, Neaton JD. Blood pressure, systolic and diastolic, and cardiovascular risks. U.S. population data. Arch Intern Med 153:598–615, 1993. Copyright 1993, American Medical Association.)

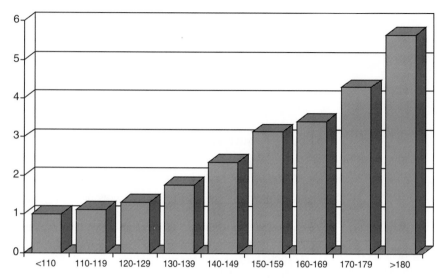

Figure 4–2. Rate of deaths from coronary heart disease (adjusted for age, race, serum cholesterol, cigarettes per day, diabetes, and income) relative to the group with the lowest systolic blood pressure in 347,987 men aged 35 to 57 years in the Multiple Risk Factor Intervention Trial. These data show a stepwise increase in relative risk for each increment in systolic blood pressure. (Data from Stamler J, Stamler R, Neaton JD. Blood pressure, systolic and diastolic, and cardiovascular risks. U.S. population data. Arch Intern Med 153:598–615, 1993. Copyright 1993, American Medical Association.)

MUCH CARDIOVASCULAR DISEASE ATTRIBUTABLE TO BLOOD PRESSURE OCCURS IN "NORMOTENSIVES." When the number of people exposed to a certain level of blood pressure is multiplied by the relevant relative risk, a different picture emerges.[13] The absolute number of people affected indicates that blood pressure–related cardiovascular disease is a problem among the population in general, and is found in people without hypertension.[14] Using estimates of relative risk and the data concerning prevalence, it is possible to calculate risk of blood pressure–related disease among a population. Results provide an indication of the cardiovascular disease that can be attributed to blood pressure at every level of pressure, using the rate of cardiovascular disease at the lowest blood pressure as a baseline. Such an analysis was undertaken in the Multiple Risk Factor Intervention Trial (MRFIT) of 347,987 men (aged 35 to 57 years) in which "excess deaths" from coronary heart disease were estimated in relation to systolic blood pressure levels.[14] The excess deaths (Fig. 4–3) were those that were attributable to the systolic blood pressure after taking into account other cardiovascular risk factors.[14] These figures were derived by first calculating expected numbers of deaths within deciles of a risk score based on age, race, serum cholesterol, cigarettes per day, use of medication for diabetes, and income, and then summing these estimates across risk score deciles within each blood pressure category and subtracting this number from the observed number of deaths. After taking into account other risk factors in this way, the findings showed that 31.9% of coronary heart disease deaths attributable to systolic blood pressure occurred in men with a systolic pressure of less than 140 mm Hg, compared with 24.1% of excess coronary heart disease deaths attributable to systolic blood pressure in subjects with pressures greater than 160 mm Hg.

The MRFIT data demonstrate an important general principle of preventive medicine: Many people exposed to a modest risk (average blood pressure) may generate more cases than do a small number exposed to a conspicuous risk (hypertension).[13] Genetic studies that focus only on hypertension (particularly "extreme" hypertension) are uncovering evidence relevant to only a portion of blood pressure–related cardiovascular morbidity and mortality. In contrast, genetic analyses of physiological variation in blood pressure offer insights into the molecular basis of

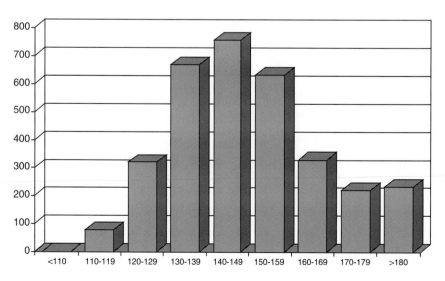

Figure 4–3. Number of "excess deaths" from coronary heart disease attributable to systolic blood pressure relative to the group with the lowest systolic blood pressure in 347,987 men aged 35 to 57 years in the Multiple Risk Factor Intervention Trial. See text for details. These data show that a large number of people exposed to a modest risk (average blood pressure) account for many cases of cardiovascular death in a population. (Data from Stamler J, Stamler R, Neaton JD. Blood pressure, systolic and diastolic, and cardiovascular risks. U.S. population data. Arch Intern Med 153:598–615, 1993. Copyright 1993, American Medical Association.)

blood pressure levels to which the majority of cardiovascular disease can be ascribed. The determinants of higher blood pressure, not just of hypertension, should be the goal of genetic research.

Blood Pressure Is Only One Component of Multifactorial Cardiovascular Risk

The second issue relevant to genetics touches on the place of blood pressure in the multifactorial etiology of cardiovascular disease. Blood pressure is only one of a number of cardiovascular risk factors. Others, such as body weight, cholesterol, diabetes, and fibrinogen, show familial aggregation and are presumed to be determined by a number of genes.[15, 16]

GENETIC COMPLEXITY. If the genes controlling each cardiovascular risk phenotype are independent, then the number of genes contributing to cardiovascular disease is potentially quite large, as it is the product of the number of risk factors and the number of genes controlling each risk factor. By inference, the predictive power and impact on cardiovascular risk of any single gene would be relatively small. In this case, individual cardiovascular phenotypes could be studied in isolation, but large numbers of subjects would be required to reliably detect such effects.

GENETIC SIMPLICITY. The epidemiological associations and correlations among individual cardiovascular phenotypes suggest that each is a component of an underlying metabolic syndrome.[17, 18] If this is the case, it is possible that the component phenotypes are determined by a limited number of genes that control pivotal metabolic physiology. The discovery of such genes would be of fundamental importance to predicting and preventing cardiovascular disease. The identification of genes of fundamental cardiovascular metabolic relevance is predicated on a multifactorial approach in which blood pressure as well as other relevant phenotypes are measured and analyzed concurrently. In this way, among the genes that affect blood pressure, those that also affect body weight and cholesterol could be identified and the metabolic syndrome might be understood at a molecular level.

Appropriate and Informative Research Design

Considerations of the genetics of hypertension must be based on achieving useful and meaningful benefits in the prevention and treatment of stroke and heart attack. Hypertensive subjects are only a very small part of the cardiovascular disease picture. Research design must take into account the epidemiological imperatives. There is a need to consider more inclusive designs that derive information from individuals with all levels of blood pressure, not just hypertension, and from other cardiovascular risk factors, not just blood pressure. Under ideal circumstances, these priorities could be met by representative population sampling and multifactorial cardiovascular risk assessment. The time and resources for such research are not readily available and demand careful planning. Nevertheless, judged against the remarkable investment in molecular DNA technologies, questions worth answering about the genetics of cardiovascular disease deserve similar resources to ensure appropriate and informative research design.

GENES VERSUS ENVIRONMENT

What is the evidence that in humans, genes affect blood pressure, and how can such effects be understood in relation to the influences of the environment?

Biometric Analyses

Before it was possible to track genes, biometric analyses were used to model the aggregation of traits within families and postulate explanations based on genetic or environmental causation.[1–3] In general, the closer the genetic relatedness, the closer the blood pressures. For example, the correlation coefficient for blood pressure between monozygotic twins is approximately 0.75, whereas blood pressures of nontwin siblings show correlation coefficients of about 0.25. At face value, this would indicate a potent influence of genes on blood pressure. However, other factors are involved. For relatives with the same degree of genetic relatedness, significant differences in blood pressure correlation exist. For example, the correlation coefficient between dizygotic twins is usually significantly greater than that between nontwin siblings, yet the genetic similarity is 50% in both instances. Similarly, the correlation between parents and offspring who also share 50% of their genetic material is usually significantly less than that between siblings. These differences can be ascribed to nongenetic,—that is, environmental—influences.

Family Environments

The identification and specification of environmental factors are difficult. Nevertheless, certain familial patterns emerge. In particular, generational effects can be inferred from the closer correlation between siblings than between parents and offspring. Presumably, behavior and lifestyles are shared more closely by brothers and sisters than by children and parents.

The timing and the ages at which environmental exposure is shared are also relevant. Adopted and unrelated siblings show significant blood pressure correlations,[1] presumably as a result of living as children in the same household. However, parents who also share the same household environment show significantly less correlation than do adopted siblings. This contrast suggests either that young people are more prone to experiencing environmental effects on blood pressure or that adopted siblings share lifestyles and behavioral characteristics more similar to each others' than to those of their parents.

Different degrees of environmental similarity are also important within generations. The greater correlation between dizygotic twins than between nontwin siblings is evidence of such processes. In the case of twins, the relevant environmental exposure may be the same pregnancy. It has been argued that there are critical periods for setting the course of physiology and pathophysiology in later life. The intrauterine environment may be important in this regard.[19] However, twins also grow up together, and susceptibility to environmental influence during infancy and childhood is also important.[20, 21]

In adulthood, the influence of shared environment is less apparent. The blood pressure correlation coefficient between parents is often of the order of 0.10 and is barely statistically significant.[22–25] In part, this reflects the attraction of partners who share similar characteristics—so-called assortive mating. In this process, partners are more likely to share genes that determine characteristics such as height and body build and, therefore, blood pressure. It has been shown that the correlation between spouses does not increase significantly as the period of shared environment increases.[22]

Separating Genes and Environment

Difficulty arises when attempts are made to partition variation in blood pressure into genetic and environmental compartments. Although often quoted, statements maintaining that blood pressure is 40% determined by genes are misleading and counterintuitive. It makes little sense to infer from a blood pressure of 160 mm Hg that 64 mm Hg are genetic and 96 mm Hg environmental.

Biometric analyses are attempts to test how well certain mathematical models explain blood pressure variation within families. Even the most comprehensive and best-fitting models are unlikely to mirror biological truths such as the extraordinarily complex dynamics affecting gene expression and gene environment interaction.

Population Environments

The concept of *environment* encompasses economic, social, psychological, and biological elements. The vagaries and variability of environmental components have made difficult any meaningful characterization of the environment to which an individual is exposed.[26] However, indisputable evidence of environmental effects comes from studies of large numbers of people who migrate or who remain geographically stable but whose environment changes with time.

Migration

There are a number of well-documented studies in which blood pressure changed significantly after migration.[27–30] Such changes must be due to alterations in the environment, because genes remain unchanged. These changes in blood pressure are often associated with increases in body weight. However, attempts to define the exact constituents of the environment that explain these effects have been inconclusive.

Secular Trends

Along with a decline in the coronary epidemic, average blood pressures in Western societies have been falling.[31–34] In the absence of major changes in the genetic substrate, such effects reflect the influence of the environment on the population as a whole.

Comparisons among populations have been used to identify correlates of blood pressure differences. However, the magnitude of these differences is rather small and is confounded by intercorrelated environmental characteristics.[35] It is important to note that the influence of such factors among individuals within populations is difficult to demonstrate.

Population Environment Affects the Population Mean

Of particular relevance is the observation that environmental change appears to shift the population average blood pressure such that there are changes at every level of the distribution.[36] Therefore, a population's mean pressures are indicative of the prevailing social, economic, and biological components of the environment.

Population Genetics

The apparent absence of environmental factors as explanations for substantial differences among individuals focuses attention on genetic differences. On average, individuals differ at 1 in every 1000 base pairs, which amounts to about 3 million differences in DNA coding between any two people. Although most of these differences are of no consequence, some define unique characteristics.

Shared physical features within families are accepted as being genetic. It is not unreasonable to presume that the effects of genes are more than superficial and that physiology is, to a significant extent, inherited. The biometric studies of family blood pressures are consistent with this concept.

Polygenes

The nature of the genetic determinants of blood pressure remains to be determined. However, there is general agreement that a number of genes are involved. Some evidence for a polygenic model is based on the unimodal distribution of pressures, which contrasts with the expectation that a major gene causing hypertension would result in a clear delineation between affected and unaffected individuals, that is, a bimodal distribution. However, the shape of the distribution of pressures is not a reliable guide to underlying genetic patterns, as the clarity of genetic effects may be blurred by other factors (Fig. 4–4A).

The most important evidence supporting blood pressure polygenes comes from biometric studies that indicate that the blood pressure correlation among relatives is seen across the blood pressure range. In other words, parents with low blood pressure tend to have children with low blood pressure with the same likelihood that parents with average or high pressure have children with average or high blood pressure, respectively. Such a continuous relationship could not be explained by a single major gene. Instead, there has emerged the concept of a number of polygenes, each with an incremental effect on blood pressure. For example, a population's blood pressure range of 100 mm Hg could be explained by the presence of 10 polygenes, each contributing an additive effect of 10 mm Hg, or by the presence of 5 polygenes, each contributing individual effects of 20 mm Hg, and so on (see Fig. 4–4B). The effect of gene dose has been demonstrated clearly in animal studies.[37]

Explaining Individual Blood Pressure

Individual blood pressure can be understood as the result of two underlying influences.[38] One, the dose of polygenes, would determine rank within the population distribution. The other, population environment, would determine the mean for the population. Therefore, the actual blood pressure of an individual would be defined by ranking in relation to the population mean, and in this way would show dependence on both genes and environment (Fig. 4–5).

Gene Environment Interaction

It is possible that certain genotypes predispose to larger changes in blood pressure for a given change in the population environment. This phenomenon might explain the skewed distribution of blood pressure in Western societies. Migration studies have identified subgroups of individuals who appear to have exaggerated blood pressure responses to migration.[39] These clusters are often familial, although they are not explained by simple genetic inheritance.[39]

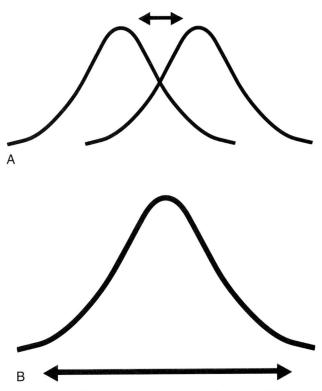

Figure 4–5. A. Changes in the population environment with migration tend to shift the distribution of blood pressure levels as a whole. **B.** Blood pressure differences within a population are likely to be explained by genetic differences among individuals.

GENETIC RESEARCH

The limelight in genetic research has fallen on the molecular biological laboratory and statistical genetic analysis. However, the most modern technology and sophisticated mathematics cannot overcome fundamental weaknesses in sampling and experimental design. What are the factors that determine whether sampling for genetic research will be informative and appropriate?

Linkage and Association Studies

Given the fundamental aim of identifying genetic mutations that affect blood pressure, two basic approaches are used. In linkage studies, families form the research substrate in which coinheritance of blood pressure and molecular markers is tested. For this purpose, the minimum family unit comprises two relatives, often a pair of siblings.[40, 41] Chromosomal regions or genes influencing blood pressure are defined as those in which molecular identity between siblings is associated with similarity in blood pressure; greater than would be expected by chance. Similarity can be judged qualitatively, as in the case of affected sibling pair studies, or quantitatively, as a derivative of the numeric difference in blood pressure between sibling pairs. Statistical methods are available for both approaches.[42, 43]

Association studies are essentially case-control studies in which the research substrate is the population. If a particular genetic marker evolved at the same time and is physically very close to a mutation affecting blood pres-

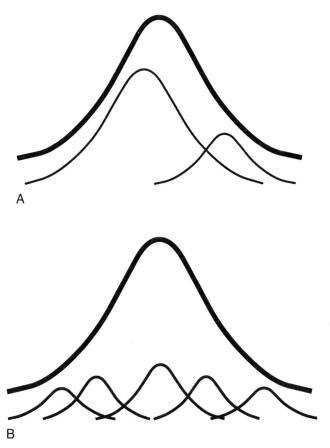

Figure 4–4. A. The unimodal population distribution of blood pressure could be explained by two genetically distinct subpopulations defined by one major gene. **B.** The unimodal population distribution of blood pressure could be explained by many genetically distinct subpopulations defined by a number of polygenes.

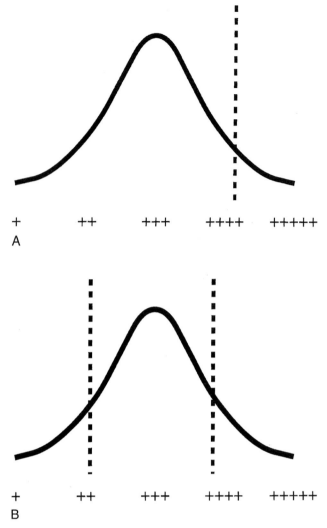

+   ++   +++   ++++   +++++

A

+   ++   +++   ++++   +++++

B

Figure 4–6. A. Assuming that blood pressure rank is the result of the individual "dose" of polygenes, the genetic contrast between hypertensive people (to the right of the *dashed line*) and normotensive people (to the left of the *dashed line*) is not particularly great. **B.** Assuming that blood pressure rank is the result of the individual "dose" of polygenes, the genetic contrast between subjects with high (to the right of the *right dashed line*) and low (to the left of the *left dashed line*) blood pressure is greater than the dichotomous strategy.

sure, then the frequency of the marker should differ significantly between cases and controls. The definition of cases and controls can be qualitative (hypertensive versus normotensive) or quantitative (high versus low blood pressure). In blood pressure genetics, it has been proposed that the power of association studies will be superior to the power of linkage studies if the effect of individual polygenes is relatively small.[44, 45] New methods combine features of linkage and association studies. The transmission disequilibrium test is a means of defining the linkage of markers that have shown positive association with a particular trait.[46, 47]

Phenotypes

Whether using linkage or association approaches, phenotyping is a critical issue. The variation of blood pressure

with the seasons, diurnal rhythms, and posture are but a few of the explanations for the biological variability of blood pressure. Such variability can be minimized by careful standardization of technique and training of observers. Repeated measurements or 24-hour recordings can further reduce variation.[48, 49] However, given the intercorrelation between single measurements and continuous recordings, it has yet to be demonstrated in a genetic analysis that the additional investment of comprehensive measurement approaches is worthwhile, especially as more stringent criteria for defining statistical significance are demanding larger numbers of study subjects.[50]

Intermediate Phenotypes

It has been suggested that as blood pressure represents an integrated phenotype resulting from the interaction of numerous physiological control systems, blood pressure should be subgrouped according to underlying physiology. The clinical parallel is the concept that hypertension is a composite syndrome that can be differentiated according to underlying mechanisms.[51, 52] The implication is that subgrouping blood pressure or hypertension according to intermediate phenotypes might concentrate specific polygenes that operate through particular mechanisms. Although conceptually appealing, there are difficulties with this approach, not the least of which are the additional expense, time, and effort required to define subsidiary phenotypes. Furthermore, there is no guarantee that the phenotypes represent any more than a patterned, physiological, compensatory response to blood pressure variation or a complication of high blood pressure per se, rather than a clue to a genetically determined causative mechanism. There has been limited published success in using the combined blood pressure–intermediate phenotype approach.[53]

Sampling Bias

Bias is a particular problem in association studies, in which the frequency of certain genetic variants is compared in cases and controls. Typically, the cases have been subjects with clinical hypertension and the controls have been those with normal blood pressure. Herein lies the potential for bias unless cases and controls are matched carefully. Examples of bias exist in which the racial characteristics of cases and controls differ.[54] However, the causes of bias can be far more subtle and difficult to identify.

The best controls are those of similar age and sex who have experienced similar exposure to environmental factors and share a common genetic background. Performing association studies within families[55] is one approach, and dizygous twins would best fulfill these criteria. However, association studies require phenotypic contrast between cases and controls, and the high correlation of blood pressures between twins makes the coincidence of high and low blood pressure in a pair of twins an uncommon event. Relatively large numbers of twins must be screened to identify such combinations. Nevertheless, the effort may well be worthwhile.

Genetic Contrast

The issue of contrast deserves comment, as the usual comparison in association studies is between hypertensive and normotensive subjects. These groups sit on either side of an arbitrary line drawn in the population distribution (Fig. 4–6A). According to the polygenic model applied to population blood pressures, the hypertensive normotensive comparison provides less genetic contrast than does a comparison between the upper and lower ends of the population distribution (Fig. 4–6B). Theoretically, genetic contrast can be enhanced by selecting families from the top and bottom of the distribution. This approach has been developed in the settings of both linkage and association studies. In linkage approaches, the selection of siblings with discordant phenotypes has been proposed.[56, 57] In association studies, the Four Corners Approach devised by Watt selects from the upper and lower ends of the blood pressure distribution to ensure phenotypic contrast.[58–60] Importantly, however, Watt's method uses information from two generations by taking into account the measured pressures of each subject and of both the subject's parents. A subject with high blood pressure for his or her age and sex who also has parents with high blood pressure for their ages and genders is the most likely to be carrying genetic determinants of high blood pressure, and subjects with low personal and parental pressures are least likely to be carrying genetic determinants of high blood pressure.

Avoiding Extremes

Contrast, however, should not be taken to extremes. Although there may be a theoretical argument for selecting from the extremes of the blood pressure distribution to increase statistical power,[57, 61] there are dangers in this approach. Pickering showed that familial correlation appeared to decline at very high levels of pressure and interpreted this as the result of inclusion of nonfamilial, secondary forms of hypertension.[62] Even if secondary, nongenetic forms of hypertension are excluded, selection for extremes leaves doubts regarding the general applicability of results. For example, extremely discordant sibling pairs (one in the top 10% and the other in the bottom 10% of the blood pressure distribution) may offer statistical power,[57] but they are most unusual. A balance between contrast and representativeness is needed; to achieve it, the Four Corners Approach derives genetic information from groups representing approximately the upper and lower thirds of the blood pressure distribution.

GENETIC DISEASE AND BLOOD PRESSURE

Among the triumphs of molecular biology stand the definitions of genetic causes of rare Mendelian forms of blood pressure deviation.[9, 63, 64] Table 4–1 lists the known major genetic causes of hypertension and low blood pressure and the genes implicated.

Molecular and Genetic Heterogeneity

The molecular definitions of these rare diseases have revealed as much to concern as to reassure geneticists interested in clinical hypertension. They have shown that syn-

Table 4–1 Genetic Causes of Hypertension and the Genes Implicated

Disease	Phenotype	Genetic Cause
Glucocorticoid remediable hyperaldosteronism[65]	Autosomal dominant, hypertension, variable hyperaldosteronism	Chimeric 11β-hydroxylase/aldosterone synthase gene
Syndrome of apparent mineralocorticoid excess[66]	Autosomal recessive, volume expansion, hypokalemia, low renin and aldosterone	Mutations in the 11β-hydroxysteroid dehydrogenase gene
Liddle's syndrome[67, 68]	Autosomal dominant, hypertension, volume expansion, hypokalemia, low renin and aldosterone	Mutations in subunits of the epithelial sodium channel SCNN1B and SCNN1G genes
Pseudohypoaldosteronism type II (Gordon's syndrome)[69]	Autosomal dominant, hypertension, hyperkalemia, volume expansion, normal glomerular filtration rate	Linkage to chromosomes 1q31–q42 and 17p11–q21
Gitelman's syndrome[70]	Autosomal recessive, low blood pressure, hypokalemic alkalosis, hypocalciuria	Mutations in the Na-Cl cotransporter NCCT gene
Bartter's syndrome[71, 72]	Autosomal recessive, low blood pressure, hypokalemic alkalosis, hypercalciuria	Mutations in the Na-K-2Cl cotransporter NKCC2 gene or mutations in the K channel ROMK gene
Bartter's syndrome type III[73]	Autosomal recessive, low blood pressure, hypokalemic alkalosis, hypercaliuria without nephrocalcinosis	Mutations in the chloride channel CLCNKB gene
Pseudohypoaldosteronism type 1, severe[74]	Autosomal recessive, low blood pressure, renal salt wasting, hyperkalemia and metabolic acidosis, elevated aldosterone levels	Mutations in subunits of the epithelial sodium channel SCNN1B and SCNN1G genes
Pseudohypoaldosteronism type 1, mild[75]	Autosomal dominant, low blood pressure, renal salt wasting, hyperkalemia and metabolic acidosis, elevated aldosterone levels that remit with age	Mutations in mineralocorticoid receptor gene
Polycystic kidney disease[76]	Autosomal dominant, renal cysts, hypertension, renal failure, liver cysts, cerebral aneurysms, valvular heart disease	Mutations in the PKD1 and PKD2 genes
Multiple endocrine neoplasia type 2A[77]	Autosomal dominant, medullary thyroid carcinoma, pheochromocytoma, hyperparathyroidism	Mutations in the RET proto-oncogene

dromes that are clinically indistinguishable are frequently heterogeneous at a molecular level.[67, 68, 72, 74] Large varieties of mutations in particular genes or even mutations in other genes can result in the same clinical picture. Phenotypic similarity is usually the result of convergence at an early stage in the pathway from DNA to blood pressure. Common effects on cellular transmembrane transport, signaling, or enzymatic activity can result from diverse DNA mutations. The inferences are clear: No simple test of an individual mutation is useful in population screening for the clinical syndrome. Furthermore, the subgrouping of clinical hypertension according to intermediate phenotypes may not be as powerful as anticipated in leading back to a particular mutation or even to a particular gene.

Phenotypic Heterogeneity

Studies of major genes within families have also revealed considerable variation in phenotype associated with inheritance of the same mutation.[78] Within a family, phenotypes of mutation-positive individuals may range from normal to severely affected. Differences in environmental exposure are not likely to be sufficiently large or potent to explain such discrepancies. The likely explanation is differences among family members in other genes. Such genes might affect blood pressure per se or might affect the ability of the physiological control systems to counter the effects of the hypertension mutation.

If relatively limited genetic variation within families can have such profound effects on the phenotypic consequences of major genes, then it is certainly possible that more marked genetic variation within populations could obscure the phenotypic effects of single polygenes. These considerations have important implications for the potential to associate or link genes and blood pressure and for the individual predictive reliability of genetic mutations or markers defined from large group analyses. Polygenetic effects defined under closely controlled research conditions may be submerged by the diverse genetic background of a population unless such effects are robust.

Phenotypic Clues

The Mendelian conditions previously discussed not only illustrate that genetic mutation can cause variation in blood pressure above and below the population mean but also provide potentially important clues to the physiological systems involved in blood pressure control. Prominent among these is the action of mineralocorticoids and the renal handling of salt and water.[79] Of the large number of physiological possibilities, it seems that perturbations of sodium reabsorption, particularly in the distal nephron segments, are sufficiently robust to overcome physiological adaptive responses that might return blood pressure to normal. It is possible that less severe mutations in genes that control sodium handling could explain variations in blood pressure within a population and individual sensitivity of blood pressure to changes in dietary sodium.

GENETICS AND HIGH BLOOD PRESSURE

Candidate Genes

Many of the genetic discoveries in rare Mendelian diseases resulted from targeted searches based on known physiological explanations. A similar approach based on physiological plausibility can be applied to identify candidate genes in the population as a whole. The priority of candidates depends on the weight of favorable evidence and on a number of extenuating circumstances.

Candidacy Based on Rare Mendelian Diseases

The epithelial sodium channel subunit genes[67, 80, 81] and the 11β-hydroxysteroid dehydrogenase gene have been tested in hypertensive subjects from the population.[82] These studies have yielded largely negative results in relation to the presence of major genetic mutations in the general population or the linkage of these genetic loci with clinical hypertension. However, a recent study indicates that the SCNN1B and SCNN1G genes encoding the β- and γ-subunits of the epithelial sodium channel may have important effects in determining systolic blood pressure in the general population.[83] In quantitative sibling pair linkage analyses, significant linkage was observed between markers in and around SCNN1B and SCNN1G. When sibling pairs were genetically identical at these loci, their average difference in systolic blood pressure was about half that of sibling pairs who were not identical at these loci ($p = .001$). Although the causative mutation(s) have yet to be identified, these findings illustrate the potential relevance of rare syndromes in defining candidates for genetic analyses. Other genetic loci from Table 4–1 are also worthy candidates.

Candidacy Based on Physiological Plausibility

Careful physiological study of blood pressure and, in particular, the predisposition to high blood pressure provides important clues to genes worthy of investigation. In contrast to the rare Mendelian syndromes, the pathophysiology is not predominantly renal and includes other neuronal and metabolic abnormalities.[84–89]

Candidacy Based on Positional Mapping

In addition to justification based on functional relevance, candidates can command greater attention if they fall within chromosomal regions that are linked with blood pressure in chromosomal or genome-wide mapping studies.

The list of candidates that might be derived from pathophysiological evidence or positional mapping is potentially enormous. To date, a handful of candidate genes have captured the attention of genetic researchers. Some of the candidates that have been linked to or associated with high blood pressure are shown in Table 4–2.

Mapping Methods

Mapping of quantitative trait loci has become a relatively common method of identifying chromosomal regions that

Table 4–2 Genes Implicated in High Blood Pressure
6-Phosphogluconate dehydrogenase[40]
ACE[90, 91]
Angiotensinogen[92]
Glucocorticoid receptor[93]
Insulin receptor[94]
Complement C3F[95]
β_2-Adrenergic receptor[96, 97]
Lipoprotein lipase[98]
Type 1A dopamine receptor[99]
α_{1B}-Adrenergic receptor[99]
α-Adducin[100]
Endothelial nitric oxide synthase[101]
Pancreatic phospholipase[102]
α_2-Adrenergic receptor[103]
SA gene[104]
Angiotensin II type 1 receptor[105]
G-protein $\beta3$ subunit[106]
Prostacyclin synthase[107]
Growth hormone[108]

Abbreviations: ACE, angiotensin-converting enzyme.

contribute to variation in phenotypes related to complex and common diseases.[109–116] One advantage of mapping is the possibility of discovering new and unexpected genes and pathophysiological mechanisms. However, the implicated regions are often very large and may harbor hundreds of candidate genes. Nevertheless, the mapping approaches help to narrow the field of interest and the resolution of maps, and the sophistication of measurement and analysis is improving rapidly.

MICROSATELLITE MAPS. The development and continued refinement of comprehensive genetic maps allows a reasonably thorough search across the 22 autosomal chromosomes and the X chromosome. The maps make use of DNA sequence differences to characterize individuals. At many points along the genome, individuals vary widely in the number of repeats of small sequences of DNA known as *microsatellites;* for example, the $(CA)_n$ repeats. About 450 such points make up a map of reasonable resolution.

SINGLE NUCLEOTIDE POLYMORPHISM MAPS. Alternatively, larger numbers of less polymorphic markers such as the single nucleotide polymorphisms can be used.[117–119] They make up approximately 80% of all known DNA polymorphisms, and their potential strengths are their abundance and mutational stability. Instead of being highly polymorphic at each point, they usually have only two variants (alleles), making them amenable to simple plus/minus–style assays that take advantage of the parallel development in DNA microarray chip technology.[120]

GENOMIC MISMATCH SCREENING. New techniques are being developed for linkage mapping that potentially obviate the need for genotyping or sequencing. Genomic mismatch screening is a new method of genetic mapping that attempts to purify and map the regions of identity in two complex genomes in a single test based on their ability to form extensive mismatch-free hybrid molecules.[121–124] This approach is also able to utilize microarray technology to find relevant chromosomal regions.[125]

Functional Mutations

Particular candidates assume greater importance if particular markers are associated with significant differences in biochemical or physiological phenotypes. Major genetic mutations that cause large changes in gene expression or performance of the resultant polypeptide or protein are obviously relevant to Mendelian diseases. However, in the general population, more common mutations that cause less extreme derangement are likely to be of greater relevance. For example, the simple I/D polymorphism of the angiotensin-converting enzyme gene has been associated in some studies with differences in enzyme activity[126, 127] and in responsiveness to angiotensin II.[128] Other studies do not support these particular findings.[129, 130] Variants of the angiotensinogen gene have been shown to be associated with differences in plasma angiotensinogen levels.[92] A common polymorphism of the glucocorticoid receptor gene[93] has been related to tissue-specific differences in steroid sensitivity.[131]

Inconsistency

A recurring observation in genetic analyses has been the inconsistency among various reports using the same genetic markers. Almost every published positive result has been followed by a negative result.[129, 132–142] The discrepancies among studies using the same gene and genetic markers have caused great disappointment, heightened by the enormous promise and early excitement about the molecular revolution. Explanations for the inconsistencies are not obvious. The combination of chance and editorial bias[143] explains some of the positive results that have not stood the test of time. However, comparable studies with careful design and satisfactory statistical power have also been unable to agree. Differences among the study populations are likely to be relevant in this regard.

Environmental Differences

Environmental differences may be such that the effects of a susceptibility gene may not be expressed in one population whereas the gene may be associated with high blood pressure in another population. Such hypotheses are difficult to test without controlling for environmental differences, for example, in the context of a migration study.

Genetic Differences

There may be significant differences in average genetic background among various populations that contribute to discrepancies among studies. These differences may operate in two ways: (1) the effect of a functional mutation found in two populations may be suppressed in one population by the effect of other genes that are prevalent in that population only, or (2) the genetic marker that is informative in one population may be uninformative in another because, through evolutionary diversion, it no longer reliably reflects the presence of a functional mutation.

Reproducibility

Whatever the explanation, the implication is that until proved otherwise, genetic results should not be generalized to all populations. Even within the same population, it is important to replicate genetic analyses using independent samples before declaring the case proven.

Statistical Issues

The question of what proves a genetic case has been argued largely in terms of levels of statistical significance and statistical power. The concern is in relation to both false-positive (type I) and false-negative (type 2) errors.

The likelihood of false-positive results is increased when particular genetic hypotheses are tested by a large number of investigators and when large numbers of genetic markers are tested in a particular investigation. With automated molecular machinery, such situations become more commonplace. These issues have been addressed in recent guidelines that suggest that all genetic analyses, even those of single candidate genes, should be judged as if they were part of a genome-wide scan in which chance positive results are most likely.[50] These theoretically determined acceptable significance levels are far more stringent than previous standards and have been challenged by empirical observations.[144] The most effective means of detection of false-positive results is failure of replication. First reports should be considered hypothesis-generating and incomplete without subsequent formal hypothesis-testing.

The issue of false-negative results is far more difficult. The calculations of statistical power and sample sizes that provide confidence in negative results are extraordinarily complex and are based on numerous unproven and untestable assumptions. Matters such as the phenotypic effect of the proposed mutation, its linkage with the markers under examination, the mode of inheritance, and the degree of gene-gene and gene-environment interaction are all relevant. If it is not possible to be confident of a negative result, what should be done? Such findings often fall victim to the editorial desire for positive studies. Rather than losing data of questionable power, there may be good reasons to create a repository with an accessible database that would allow other investigators to assess whether it would be worthwhile to readdress certain issues using their own resources.

THE FUTURE

There is still a long distance to travel before research into genetic mutations of significance to blood pressure have an impact on the general population. What are the likely outcomes of genetic research in relation to blood pressure? If genetic discovery provides insights into the fundamental mechanisms controlling blood pressure, the possibilities include the identification of individual predisposition to high blood pressure through DNA testing, the development of novel pharmacological treatments and gene therapy, and even public health measures.

New Tests

Defining predisposition is predicated on the availability of reliable DNA tests to detect tangible and meaningful increases in risk. However, DNA tests should be informative for all common mutations that affect the function of the gene in question, and should also take into account the influence of relevant components of the genetic background known to modulate the phenotypic consequences of the functional mutation. In this regard, the new DNA microarray chip technologies might provide rapid and comprehensive screening. However, before such tests can be recommended widely it will be necessary to demonstrate distinct advantages of potentially expensive and invasive molecular diagnostics over simple measurements with a sphygmomanometer.

Despite widespread public misconception, genetic tests in the context of complex human multifactorial disease provide an indication of predisposition, not predestination. Because genetic tests can be performed when a person is young, it will be especially important to avoid the creation of unnecessary lifelong anxiety as the result of a positive laboratory result.

New Therapies

Tailored Treatments

For hypertensive individuals who need treatment to lower blood pressure, genetic discovery may lead to the development of novel pharmaceutical approaches based on genetically determined mechanisms. The implication is also that before treatment, hypertensive subjects will be screened for the particular mutations responsible for such pathophysiological mechanisms. In this way, treatment can be tailored through the use of genetic information to select the most appropriate and efficacious class or combinations of therapies.

Gene Therapy

Beyond genetic assistance in deciding on pharmacotherapy for hypertension, the possibility of gene therapy has been raised.[145–150] Some approaches are simply clever means of offering "symptomatic" treatment to achieve physiological changes that can otherwise be achieved by pharmacological treatment. Other approaches might attempt to modulate a fundamental genetic defect. But as long as uncertainty exists about the identity of the gene or genes responsible and about the size of the expected benefit, gene therapy to remedy an underlying abnormality seems an unlikely option to pursue.

The arguments against using gene therapy include that it is specialized, expensive, and technically demanding and that hypertension is not a purely genetic condition. Furthermore, other effective, safe, and cheap therapies exist. Safety also remains a significant concern. For a common condition such as hypertension, even a small risk may outweigh the potential benefits of any new approach. Human gene therapy is in its infancy and there remain doubts about the stability of viruses used to transfect DNA into host cells. Unforeseen complications may not become evident for many years, and evidence of the long-term safety of gene therapy in serious genetic disease will be required before the treatment of less serious disease should be considered. Finally, treatment of hypertension benefits only some of the individuals who will experience cardiovascular disease as a result of blood pressure.

Public Health Strategies

It is possible that the investment in molecular technology may be repaid in the currency of prevention. Chromosomal mapping may reveal hitherto unknown genes that code for novel peptides or proteins that confer genetic susceptibility. Specific lifestyle or behavioral factors may be revealed as triggers of such genetic predisposition. If the consequences of such genes can be interrupted and countered effectively by cheap and acceptable changes in personal behavior, the entire population stands to gain. Such an outcome may be the greatest contribution geneticists might hope to make to the field of blood pressure and cardiovascular disease.

References

1. Mongeau JG, Biron P, Sing CF. The influence of genetics and household environment upon the variability of normal blood pressure: The Montreal Adoption Survey. Clin Exp Hypertens A 8:653–660, 1986.
2. Longini IM Jr, Higgins MW, Hinton PC, et al. Environmental and genetic sources of familial aggregation of blood pressure in Tecumseh, Michigan. Am J Epidemiol 120:131–144, 1984.
3. Tambs K, Moum T, Holmen J, et al. Genetic and environmental effects on blood pressure in a Norwegian sample. Genet Epidemiol 9:11–26, 1992.
4. Heise ER, Moore MA, Reid QB, Goodman HO. Possible association of MN locus haplotypes with essential hypertension. Hypertension 9:634–640, 1987.
5. Miller JZ, Grim CE, Conneally PM, Weinberger MH. Association of blood groups with essential and secondary hypertension. A possible association of the MNS system. Hypertension 1:493–497, 1979.
6. Nance WE, Krieger H, Azevedo E, Mi MP. Human blood pressure and the ABO blood group system: An apparent association. Hum Biol 37:238–244, 1965.
7. Gerbase DeLima M, DeLima JJ, Persoli LB, et al. Essential hypertension and histocompatibility antigens. A linkage study. Hypertension 14:604–609, 1989.
8. Gerbase DeLima M, Ladalardo MA, DeLima JJ, et al. Essential hypertension and histocompatibility antigens. An association study. Hypertension 19:400–402, 1992.
9. Lifton RP. Genetic determinants of human hypertension. Proc Natl Acad Sci U S A 92:8545–8551, 1995.
10. MacMahon S, Peto R, Cutler J, et al. Blood pressure, stroke, and coronary heart disease. Part I: Prolonged differences in blood pressure: Prospective observational studies corrected for the regression dilution bias. Lancet 335:765–774, 1990.
11. Pickering G. Normotension and hypertension: The mysterious viability of the false. Am J Med 65:561–563, 1978.
12. Pickering G. Hypertension: Definitions, natural histories and consequences. Am J Med 52:570–583, 1972.
13. Rose G. Strategy of prevention: Lessons from cardiovascular disease. BMJ Clin Res Ed 282:1847–1851, 1981.
14. Stamler J, Stamler R, Neaton JD. Blood pressure, systolic and diastolic, and cardiovascular risks. U.S. population data. Arch Intern Med 153:598–615, 1993.
15. Deutscher S, Epstein FH, Kjelsberg MO. Familial aggregation of factors associated with coronary heart disease. Circulation 33:911–924, 1966.
16. Meade TW, Mellows S, Brozovic M, et al. Haemostatic function and ischaemic heart disease: Principal results of the Northwick Park Heart Study. Lancet 2:533–537, 1986.
17. Kesaniemi YA, Lilja M, Kervinen K, Rantala A. Multiple metabolic syndrome: Aspects of genetic epidemiology and molecular genetics. Ann Med 24:461–464, 1992.
18. Hjermann I. The metabolic cardiovascular syndrome: Syndrome X, Reaven's syndrome, insulin resistance syndrome, atherothrombogenic syndrome. J Cardiovasc Pharmacol 20:S5–S10, 1992.
19. Barker DJ, Bull AR, Osmond C, Simmonds SJ. Fetal and placental size and risk of hypertension in adult life. BMJ 301:259–262, 1990.
20. Langley Evans SC, Welham SJ, Sherman RC, Jackson AA. Weanling rats exposed to maternal low-protein diets during discrete periods of gestation exhibit differing severity of hypertension. Clin Sci 91:607–615, 1996.
21. Harrap SB, Van der Merwe WM, Griffin SA, et al. Brief angiotensin converting enzyme inhibitor treatment in young spontaneously hypertensive rats reduces blood pressure long-term. Hypertension 16:603–614, 1990.
22. Knuiman MW, Divitini ML, Bartholomew HC, Welborn TA. Spouse correlations in cardiovascular risk factors and the effect of marriage duration. Am J Epidemiol 143:48–53, 1996.
23. Sackett DL, Anderson GD, Milner R, et al. Concordance for coronary risk factors among spouses. Circulation 52:589–595, 1975.
24. Speers MA, Kasl SV, Freeman DH Jr, Ostfeld AM. Blood pressure concordance between spouses. Am J Epidemiol 123:818–829, 1986.
25. Speers MA, Kasl SV, Ostfeld AM. Marital correlates of blood pressure. Am J Epidemiol 129:956–972, 1989.
26. Rose G, Marmot MG. Social class and coronary heart disease. Br Heart J 45:13–19, 1981.
27. Salmond CE, Prior IA, Wessen AF. Blood pressure patterns and migration: A 14-year cohort study of adult Tokelauans. Am J Epidemiol 130:37–52, 1989.
28. Sever PS, Poulter NR. A hypothesis for the pathogenesis of essential hypertension: The initiating factors. J Hypertens Suppl 7:S9–S12, 1989.
29. Ward RH, Chin PG, Prior IA. Tokelau Island Migrant Study. Effect of migration on the familial aggregation of blood pressure. Hypertension 2:43–54, 1980.
30. Winkelstein W Jr, Kagan A, Kato H, Sacks ST. Epidemiologic studies of coronary heart disease and stroke in Japanese men living in Japan, Hawaii and California: Blood pressure distributions. Am J Epidemiol 102:502–513, 1975.
31. Wilhelmsen L. ESC Population Studies Lecture 1996. Cardiovascular monitoring of a city over 30 years. Eur Heart J 18:1220–1230, 1997.
32. Epstein FH. International trends in coronary heart disease epidemiology. Ann Clin Res 3:293–299, 1971.
33. Sarti C, Vartiainen E, Torppa J, et al. Trends in cerebrovascular mortality and its risk factors in Finland during the last 20 years. Health Rep 6:196–206, 1994.
34. Wietlisbach V, Paccaud F, Rickenbach M, Gutzwiller F. Trends in cardiovascular risk factors (1984–1993) in a Swiss region: Results of three population surveys. Prev Med 26:523–533, 1997.
35. INTERSALT Cooperative Research Group. Intersalt: An international study of electrolyte excretion and blood pressure. Results for 24-hour urinary sodium and potassium excretion. BMJ 297:319–328, 1988.
36. Rose G, Day S. The population mean predicts the number of deviant individuals. BMJ 301:1031–1034, 1990.
37. Kim HS, Krege JH, Kluckman KD, et al. Genetic control of blood pressure and the angiotensinogen locus. Proc Natl Acad Sci U S A 92:2735–2739, 1995.
38. Harrap SB. Hypertension: Genes versus environment. Lancet 344:169–171, 1994.
39. Ward RH. Genetic and sociocultural components of high blood pressure. Am J Phys Anthropol 62:91–105, 1983.
40. Wilson AF, Elston RC, Tran LD, Siervogel RM. Use of the robust sib-pair method to screen for single-locus, multiple-locus, and pleiotropic effects: Application to traits related to hypertension. Am J Hum Genet 48:862–872, 1991.
41. McCarthy MI, Kruglyak L, Lander ES. Sib-pair collection strategies for complex diseases. Genet Epidemiol 15:317–340, 1998.
42. Kruglyak L, Lander ES. Complete multipoint sib-pair analysis of qualitative and quantitative traits. Am J Hum Genet 57:439–454, 1995.
43. Amos CI, Elston RC, Wilson AF, Bailey Wilson JE. A more powerful robust sib-pair test of linkage for quantitative traits. Genet Epidemiol 6:435–449, 1989.

44. Risch N, Merikangas K. The future of genetic studies of complex human diseases. Science 273:1516–1517, 1996.

45. Jones HB. The relative power of linkage and association studies for the detection of genes involved in hypertension. Kidney Int 53:1446–1448, 1998.

46. Spielman RS, Ewens WJ. The TDT and other family-based tests for linkage disequilibrium and association. Am J Hum Genet 59:983–989, 1996.

47. Spielman RS, Ewens WJ. A sibship test for linkage in the presence of association: The sib transmission/disequilibrium test. Am J Hum Genet 62:450–458, 1998.

48. Mancia G, Omboni S, Parati G. Lessons to be learned from 24-hour ambulatory blood pressure monitoring. Kidney Int Suppl 55:563–568, 1996.

49. Ravogli A, Trazzi S, Villani A, et al. Early 24-hour blood pressure elevation in normotensive subjects with parental hypertension. Hypertension 16:491–497, 1990.

50. Lander E, Kruglyak L. Genetic dissection of complex traits: Guidelines for interpreting and reporting linkage results. Nat Genet 11:241–247, 1995.

51. Williams RR, Hunt SC, Hasstedt SJ, et al. Multigenic human hypertension: Evidence for subtypes and hope for haplotypes. J Hypertens Suppl 8:S39–S46, 1990.

52. Drayer JI, Weber MA, Laragh JH, Sealey JE. Renin subgroups in essential hypertension. Clin Exp Hypertens A 4:1817–1834, 1982.

53. Hopkins PN, Lifton RP, Hollenberg NK, et al. Blunted renal vascular response to angiotensin II is associated with a common variant of the angiotensinogen gene and obesity. J Hypertens 14:199–207, 1996.

54. Barley J, Carter ND, Cruickshank JK, et al. Renin and atrial natriuretic peptide restriction fragment length polymorphisms: Association with ethnicity and blood pressure. J Hypertens 9:993–996, 1991.

55. Thomson G. Mapping disease genes: Family-based association studies. Am J Hum Genet 57:487–498, 1995.

56. Risch NJ, Zhang H. Mapping quantitative trait loci with extreme discordant sib pairs: Sampling considerations. Am J Hum Genet 58:836–843, 1996.

57. Risch N, Zhang H. Extreme discordant sib pairs for mapping quantitative trait loci in humans. Science 268:1584–1589, 1995.

58. Watt G. Design and interpretation of studies comparing individuals with and without a family history of high blood pressure. J Hypertens 4:1–7, 1986.

59. Watt GC. Strengths and weaknesses of family studies of high blood pressure. J Hum Hypertens 8:327–328, 1994.

60. Watt GC, Foy CJ, Holton DW, Edwards HE. Prediction of high blood pressure in young people: The limited usefulness of parental blood pressure data. J Hypertens 9:55–58, 1991.

61. Zhang H, Risch N. Mapping quantitative-trait loci in humans by use of extreme concordant sib pairs: Selected sampling by parental phenotypes [published erratum appears in Am J Hum Genet 60:748–749, 1997]. Am J Hum Genet 59:951–957, 1996.

62. Pickering GW. The nature of essential hypertension. Lancet 1:1027–1028, 1959.

63. Lifton RP. Molecular genetics of human blood pressure variation. Science 272:676–680, 1996.

64. Karet FE, Lifton RP. Mutations contributing to human blood pressure variation. Recent Prog Horm Res 52:263–276, 1997.

65. Lifton RP, Dluhy RG, Powers M, et al. A chimaeric 11 beta-hydroxylase/aldosterone synthase gene causes glucocorticoid-remediable aldosteronism and human hypertension. Nature 355:262–265, 1992.

66. Mune T, Rogerson FM, Nikkila H, et al. Human hypertension caused by mutations in the kidney isozyme of 11 beta-hydroxysteroid dehydrogenase. Nat Genet 10:394–399, 1995.

67. Shimkets RA, Warnock DG, Bositis CM, et al. Liddle's syndrome: Heritable human hypertension caused by mutations in the beta subunit of the epithelial sodium channel. Cell 79:407–414, 1994.

68. Hansson JH, Nelson Williams C, Suzuki H, et al. Hypertension caused by a truncated epithelial sodium channel gamma subunit: Genetic heterogeneity of Liddle syndrome. Nat Genet 11:76–82, 1995.

69. Mansfield TA, Simon DB, Farfel Z, et al. Multilocus linkage of familial hyperkalaemia and hypertension, pseudohypoaldosteronism type II, to chromosomes 1q31–42 and 17p11–q21. Nat Genet 16:202–205, 1997.

70. Simon DB, Nelson Williams C, Bia MJ, et al. Gitelman's variant of Bartter's syndrome, inherited hypokalaemic alkalosis, is caused by mutations in the thiazide-sensitive Na-Cl cotransporter. Nat Genet 12:24–30, 1996.

71. Simon DB, Karet FE, Hamdan JM, et al. Bartter's syndrome, hypokalaemic alkalosis with hypercalciuria, is caused by mutations in the Na-K-2Cl cotransporter NKCC2. Nat Genet 13:183–188, 1996.

72. Simon DB, Karet FE, Rodriguez Soriano J, et al. Genetic heterogeneity of Bartter's syndrome revealed by mutations in the K+ channel, ROMK. Nat Genet 14:152–156, 1996.

73. Simon DB, Bindra RS, Mansfield TA, et al. Mutations in the chloride channel gene, CLCNKB, cause Bartter's syndrome type III. Nat Genet 17:171–178, 1997.

74. Strautnieks SS, Thompson RJ, Gardiner RM, Chung E. A novel splice-site mutation in the gamma subunit of the epithelial sodium channel gene in three pseudohypoaldosteronism type 1 families. Nat Genet 13:248–250, 1996.

75. Geller DS, Rodriguez Soriano J, Vallo Boado A, et al. Mutations in the mineralocorticoid receptor gene cause autosomal dominant pseudohypoaldosteronism type I. Nat Genet 19:279–281, 1998.

76. Bacallao RL, Carone FA. Recent advances in the understanding of polycystic kidney disease. Curr Opin Nephrol Hypertens 6:377–383, 1997.

77. Cirafici AM, Salvatore G, De Vita G, et al. Only the substitution of methionine 918 with a threonine and not with other residues activates RET transforming potential. Endocrinology 138:1450–1455, 1997.

78. Gates LJ, MacConnachie AA, Lifton RP, et al. Variation of phenotype in patients with glucocorticoid remediable aldosteronism. J Med Genet 33:25–28, 1996.

79. White PC. Inherited forms of mineralocorticoid hypertension. Hypertension 28:927–936, 1996.

80. Chang H, Fujita T. Lack of mutations in epithelial sodium channel beta-subunit gene in human subjects with hypertension. J Hypertens 14:1417–1419, 1996.

81. Munroe PB, Strautnieks SS, Farrall M, et al. Absence of linkage of the epithelial sodium channel to hypertension in black Caribbeans. Am J Hypertens 11:942–945, 1991.

82. Brand E, Kato N, Chatelain N, et al. Structural analysis and evaluation of the 11β-hydroxysteroid dehydrogenase type 2 (11β-HSD2) gene in human essential hypertension. J Hypertens 16:1627–1634, 1998.

83. Wong ZYH, Stebbing M, Ellis JA, et al. Genetic linkage of the β- and γ- subunits of the epithelial sodium channel with systolic blood pressure in the general population. Lancet 353:1222–1225, 1999.

84. Esler M, Jennings G, Lambert G. Noradrenaline release and the pathophysiology of primary human hypertension. Am J Hypertens 2:140S–146S, 1989.

85. Esler M, Jennings G, Biviano B, et al. Mechanism of elevated plasma noradrenaline in the course of essential hypertension. J Cardiovasc Pharmacol 8:S39–S43, 1986.

86. Ferrier C, Cox H, Esler M. Elevated total body noradrenaline spillover in normotensive members of hypertensive families. Clin Sci 84:225–230, 1993.

87. Floras JS. Epinephrine and the genesis of hypertension. Hypertension 19:1–18, 1992.

88. Harrap SB, Fraser R, Inglis GC, et al. Abnormal epinephrine release in young adults with high personal and high parental blood pressures. Circulation 96:556–561, 1997.

89. Ferrannini E, Buzzigoli G, Bonadonna R, et al. Insulin resistance in essential hypertension. N Engl J Med 317:350–357, 1987.

90. Fornage M, Amos CI, Kardia S, et al. Variation in the region of the angiotensin-converting enzyme gene influences interindividual differences in blood pressure levels in young white males. Circulation 97:1773–1779, 1991.

91. O'Donnell CJ, Lindpaintner K, Larson MG, et al. Evidence for association and genetic linkage of the angiotensin-converting enzyme locus with hypertension and blood pressure in men but not women in the Framingham Heart Study. Circulation 97:1766–1772, 1998.

92. Jeunemaitre X, Soubrier F, Kotelevtsev YV, et al. Molecular basis of human hypertension: Role of angiotensinogen. Cell 71:169–180, 1992.

93. Watt GC, Harrap SB, Foy CJ, et al. Abnormalities of glucocorticoid metabolism and the renin-angiotensin system: A Four Corners Approach to the identification of genetic determinants of blood pressure. J Hypertens 10:473–482, 1992.

94. Ying LH, Zee RY, Griffiths LR, Morris BJ. Association of a RFLP for the insulin receptor gene, but not insulin, with essential hypertension. Biochem Biophys Res Commun 181:486–492, 1991.

95. Schaadt O, Sorensen H, Krogsgaard AR. Association between the C3F-gene and essential hypertension. Clin Sci 61:363S–365S, 1981.

96. Timmermann B, Mo R, Luft FC, et al. Beta-2 adrenoceptor genetic variation is associated with genetic predisposition to essential hypertension: The Bergen Blood Pressure Study. Kidney Int 53:1455–1460, 1998.

97. Kotanko P, Binder A, Tasker J, et al. Essential hypertension in African Caribbean associates with a variant of the beta adrenoceptor. Hypertension 30:773–776, 1997.

98. Wu DA, Bu X, Warden CH, et al. Quantitative trait locus mapping of human blood pressure to a genetic region at or near the lipoprotein lipase gene locus on chromosome 8p22. J Clin Invest 97:2111–2118, 1996.

99. Krushkal J, Xiong M, Ferrell R, et al. Linkage and association of adrenergic and dopamine receptor genes in the distal portion of the long arm of chromosome 5 with systolic blood pressure variation. Hum Mol Genet 7:1379–1383, 1991.

100. Casari G, Barlassina C, Cusi D, et al. Association of the alpha-adducin locus with essential hypertension. Hypertension 25:320–326, 1995.

101. Miyamoto Y, Saito Y, Kajiyama N, et al. Endothelial nitric oxide synthase gene is positively associated with essential hypertension. Hypertension 32:3–8, 1998.

102. Frossard PM, Lestringant GG. Association between a dimorphic site on chromosome 12 and clinical diagnosis of hypertension in three independent populations. Clin Genet 48:284–287, 1995.

103. Lockette W, Ghosh S, Farrow S, et al. Alpha$_2$ adrenergic receptor gene polymorphism and hypertension in blacks. Am J Hypertens 4:390–394, 1995.

104. Iwai N, Ohmichi N, Hanai K, et al. Human SA gene locus as a candidate locus for essential hypertension. Hypertension 23:375–380, 1994.

105. Bonnardeaux A, Davies E, Jeunemaitre X, et al. Angiotensin II type 1 receptor gene polymorphisms in human essential hypertension. Hypertension 24:63–69, 1994.

106. Siffert W, Rosskopf D, Siffert G, et al. Association of a human G-protein beta$_3$ subunit variant with hypertension. Nat Genet 18:45–48, 1998.

107. Nakayama T, Soma M, Kanmatsuse K. Organization of the human prostacyclin synthase gene and association analysis of a novel CA repeat in essential hypertension. Adv Exp Med Biol 433:127–130, 1997.

108. Julier C, Delepine M, Keavney B, et al. Genetic susceptibility for human familial essential hypertension in a region of homology with blood pressure linkage on rat chromosome 10. Hum Mol Genet 6:2077–2085, 1997.

109. Luo DF, Buzzetti R, Rotter JI, et al. Confirmation of three susceptibility genes to insulin-dependent diabetes mellitus: IDDM4, IDDM5, and IDDM8. Hum Mol Genet 5:693–698, 1996.

110. Blouin JL, Dombroski BA, Nath SK, et al. Schizophrenia susceptibility loci on chromosomes 13q32 and 8p21. Nat Genet 20:70–73, 1998.

111. Ober C, Cox NJ, Abney M, et al. Genome-wide search for asthma susceptibility loci in a founder population. The Collaborative Study on the Genetics of Asthma. Hum Mol Genet 7:1393–1398, 1998.

112. Cloninger CR, Van Eerdewegh P, Goate A, et al. Anxiety proneness linked to epistatic loci in genome scan of human personality traits. Am J Med Genet 81:313–317, 1998.

113. Smith JR, Freije D, Carpten JD, et al. Major susceptibility locus for prostate cancer on chromosome 1 suggested by a genome-wide search. Science 274:1371–1374, 1996.

114. Satsangi J, Parkes M, Louis E, et al. Two-stage genome-wide search in inflammatory bowel disease provides evidence for susceptibility loci on chromosomes 3, 7 and 12. Nat Genet 14:199–202, 1996.

115. Daniels SE, Bhattacharrya S, James A, et al. A genome-wide search for quantitative trait loci underlying asthma. Nature 383:247–250, 1996.

116. Comuzzie AG, Hixson JE, Almasy L, et al. A major quantitative trait locus determining serum leptin levels and fat mass is located on human chromosome 2. Nat Genet 15:273–276, 1997.

117. Kruglyak L. The use of a genetic map of biallelic markers in linkage studies. Nat Genet 17:21–24, 1997.

118. Zhao LP, Aragaki C, Hsu L, Quiaoit F. Mapping of complex traits by single-nucleotide polymorphisms. Am J Hum Genet 63:225–240, 1998.

119. Wang DG, Fan JB, Siao CJ, et al. Large-scale identification, mapping, and genotyping of single-nucleotide polymorphisms in the human genome. Science 280:1077–1082, 1998.

120. Chee M, Yang R, Hubbell E, et al. Accessing genetic information with high-density DNA arrays. Science 274:610–614, 1996.

121. McAllister L, Penland L, Brown PO. Enrichment for loci identical-by-descent between pairs of mouse or human genomes by genomic mismatch scanning. Genomics 47:7–11, 1998.

122. Mirzayans F, Mears AJ, Guo SW, et al. Identification of the human chromosomal region containing the iridogoniodysgenesis anomaly locus by genomic-mismatch scanning. Am J Hum Genet 61:111–119, 1997.

123. Nelson SF. Genomic mismatch scanning: Current progress and potential applications. Electrophoresis 16:279–285, 1995.

124. Cheung VG, Nelson SF. Genomic mismatch scanning identifies human genomic DNA shared identical by descent. Genomics 47:1–6, 1998.

125. Cheung VG, Gregg JP, Gogolin Ewens KJ, et al. Linkage-disequilibrium mapping without genotyping. Nat Genet 18:225–230, 1998.

126. Rigat B, Hubert C, Alhenc Gelas F, et al. An insertion/deletion polymorphism in the angiotensin I converting enzyme gene accounting for half the variance of serum enzyme levels. J Clin Invest 86:1343–1346, 1990.

127. Costerousse O, Allegrini J, Lopez M, Alhenc Gelas F. Angiotensin I converting enzyme in human circulating mononuclear cells: Genetic polymorphism of expression in T-lymphocytes. Biochem J 291:33–40, 1993.

128. Ueda S, Elliott HL, Morton JJ, Connell JM. Enhanced pressor response to angiotensin I in normotensive men with the deletion genotype (DD) for angiotensin converting enzyme. Hypertension 25:1266–1269, 1995.

129. Harrap SB, Davidson HR, Connor JM, et al. The angiotensin I converting enzyme gene and predisposition to high blood pressure. Hypertension 21:455–460, 1993.

130. Lachurie ML, Azizi M, Guyene TT, et al. Angiotensin converting enzyme gene polymorphism has no influence on the circulating renin-angiotensin-aldosterone system or blood pressure in normotensive subjects. Circulation 91:2933–2942, 1995.

131. Panarelli M, Holloway CD, Fraser R, et al. Glucocorticoid receptor polymorphism, skin vasoconstriction, and other metabolic intermediate phenotypes in normal human subjects. J Clin Endocrinol Metab 83:1846–1852, 1998.

132. Brand E, Chatelain N, Keavney B, et al. Evaluation of the angiotensinogen locus in human essential hypertension: A European study. Hypertension 31:725–729, 1998.

133. Rotimi C, Morrison L, Cooper R, et al. Angiotensinogen gene in human hypertension. Lack of an association of the 235T allele among African Americans. Hypertension 24:591–594, 1994.

134. Nabika T, Bonnardeaux A, James M, et al. Evaluation of the SA locus in human hypertension. Hypertension 25:6–13, 1995.

135. Harrap SB, Samani NJ, Lodwick D, et al. The SA gene: Predisposition to hypertension and renal function in man. Clin Sci 88:665–670, 1995.

136. Jeunemaitre X, Lifton RP, Hunt SC, et al. Absence of linkage between the angiotensin converting enzyme locus and human essential hypertension. Nat Genet 1:72–75, 1992.

137. Hunt SC, Williams CS, Sharma AM, et al. Lack of linkage between the endothelial nitric oxide synthase gene and hypertension. J Hum Hypertens 10:27–30, 1996.

138. Berge KE, Berg K. No effect of TaqI polymorphism at the human renal kallikrein (KLK1) locus on normal blood pressure level or variability. Clin Genet 44:196–202, 1993.

139. Kamitani A, Wong ZY, Fraser R, et al. Human alpha-adducin gene, blood pressure, and sodium metabolism. Hypertension 32:138–143, 1998.

140. Kreutz R, Hubner N, Ganten D, Lindpaintner K. Genetic linkage of the ACE gene to plasma angiotensin converting enzyme activity but not to blood pressure. A quantitative trait locus confers identical complex phenotypes in human and rat hypertension. Circulation 92:2381–2384, 1995.

141. Bonnardeaux A, Nadaud S, Charru A, et al. Lack of evidence for

linkage of the endothelial cell nitric oxide synthase gene to essential hypertension. Circulation 91:96–102, 1995.

142. Fornage M, Turner ST, Sing CF, Boerwinkle E. Variation at the M235T locus of the angiotensinogen gene and essential hypertension: A population-based case-control study from Rochester, Minnesota. Hum Genet 96:295–300, 1995.

143. Dickersin K. The existence of publication bias and risk factors for its occurrence. JAMA 263:1385–1389, 1990.

144. Sawcer S, Jones HB, Judge D, et al. Empirical genomewide significance levels established by whole genome simulations. Genet Epidemiol 14:223–229, 1997.

145. Kurtz TW, Gardner DG. Transcription-modulating drugs: A new frontier in the treatment of essential hypertension. Hypertension 32:380–386, 1998.

146. Jin L, Zhang JJ, Chao L, Chao J. Gene therapy in hypertension: Adenovirus-mediated kallikrein gene delivery in hypertensive rats. Hum Gene Ther 8:1753–1761, 1997.

147. Phillips MI. Antisense inhibition and adeno-associated viral vector delivery for reducing hypertension. Hypertension 29:177–187, 1997.

148. Lin KF, Chao J, Chao L. Human atrial natriuretic peptide gene delivery reduces blood pressure in hypertensive rats. Hypertension 26:847–853, 1995.

149. Lin KF, Chao L, Chao J. Prolonged reduction of high blood pressure with human nitric oxide synthase gene delivery. Hypertension 30:307–313, 1997.

150. Martens JR, Reaves PY, Lu D, et al. Prevention of renovascular and cardiac pathophysiological changes in hypertension by angiotensin II type 1 receptor antisense gene therapy. Proc Natl Acad Sci U S A 95:2664–2669, 1998.

CHAPTER 5

Sympathetic Nervous System in Acute and Chronic Blood Pressure Elevation

Joseph L. Izzo, Jr.

The sympathetic nervous system (SNS) is unique in its capacity for both momentary (seconds to minutes) and sustained (days to years) regulation of blood pressure.[1, 2] Recognition of the interactive role of the SNS in various hypertensive syndromes has been hindered by the system's complexity, the cumbersome and expensive techniques required to study it, and our current tendency to focus on isolated biological processes at the expense of integrative physiology. The SNS is widely distributed throughout the body and participates in virtually all major physiological processes. As it becomes clearer that both primary and secondary hypertension are multisystem processes with linked neural, circulatory, and metabolic abnormalities, a logical question is whether the SNS may play a permissive or causal role in these processes. This chapter discusses how inappropriately increased SNS activity occurs in both primary and secondary hypertension and how it contributes to the multifaceted age-related abnormalities of the syndrome of essential hypertension, including increased blood pressure, obesity, insulin resistance, premature structural change, target organ damage, and premature death. Emphasis is placed on recent clinical investigation.

ORGANIZATION AND FUNCTION OF THE SNS

For the purposes of this discussion, the SNS is considered to include the vasomotor control centers within the central nervous system (CNS), the peripheral afferent and efferent sympathetic nerves, and the adrenal medulla. The multilayered cross-linked organization of the central and peripheral SNS provides numerous mechanisms by which the SNS can affect blood pressure and contribute to the pathogenesis of hypertension.

Central Control of SNS Outflow

Elegant studies in the laboratories of Reis and others[3, 4] have identified the functional role of several CNS nuclei in acute and chronic blood pressure regulation (Fig. 5–1). Reflex and behavioral control of arterial pressure are integrated in the rostral ventrolateral (RVL) nucleus of the medulla oblongata, which is sometimes called the *vasomotor control center*.[3, 5] Cell bodies of efferent SNS cardiovascular stimulatory neurons lie in the C_1 subregion, which also receives and sends neural projections to and from many other CNS centers.[4] The most critical RVL input comes from the adjacent nucleus tractus solitarius (NTS), which receives afferent fibers from stretch-sensitive mechanoreceptors in the carotid sinus and aortic arch (aortocarotid baroreflexes) and the cardiac atria and ventricles (cardiopulmonary baroreflexes).[6, 7] Signals from the NTS *inhibit* RVL sympathetic outflow and tend to buffer acute blood pressure changes.[8, 9] The NTS integrates a variety of signals from stimulatory and inhibitory centers in the brain stem, basal ganglia, and cortex, including the overlying area postrema located in the floor of the fourth ventricle.[10] The area postrema, which does not have a blood-brain barrier, is stimulated by circulating angiotensin II (Ang II). Area postrema stimulation cancels the inhibitory effect of the NTS and *increases* RVL sympathetic outflow.[11–14] The NTS-RVL complex also receives input from peripheral chemoreceptor afferent neurons in the kidneys and skeletal muscle that are *excitatory* to RVL sympathetic outflow.[6, 15]

Brain Stem in Hypertensive Models

CNS centers that control SNS outflow clearly affect acute and chronic blood pressure levels in animal models of hypertension. Brain stem regions in particular seem to

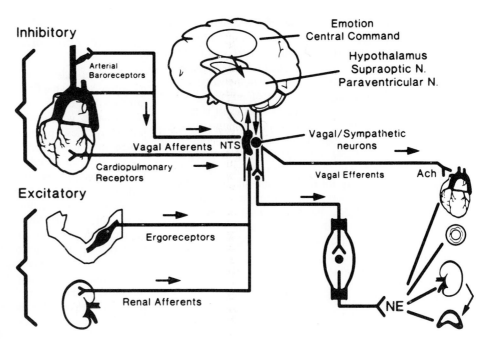

Figure 5–1. Central nervous system control of sympathetic outflow. Efferent sympathetic nervous system (SNS) output is the result of integrated actions of several central nervous system centers. The cerebral cortex and peripheral chemoreceptors are usually stimulatory, whereas baroreflexes in the aorta and carotic sinus (arterial baroreflexes) and the heart and lungs (cardiopulmonary baroreflexes) inhibit SNS outflow. The hypothalamus integrates behavioral input, and the nucleus tractus solitarius (NTS) is the principal controller of brain stem SNS outflow. Ach, acetylcholine. (From Abboud FM. The sympathetic system in hypertension. Hypertension 4[suppl II]:208–225, 1982.)

participate in all forms of experimental hypertension. Ablation of the NTS in normotensive rats causes increased SNS outflow and either severe blood pressure lability[8] or severe chronic hypertension,[7] which can be abolished by simultaneous lesions of the RVL.[16] In contrast, lesions in the area postrema lower blood pressure in rats with genetic[14] and steroid-induced hypertension.[13, 17] Stimulation of the area postrema by Ang II is believed to be a major sustaining mechanism in genetic and steroid-induced hypertension.[11, 13, 14, 17]

Hypothalamus, Behavioral Integration, and Cardiovascular Responses

Stress, emotions, and drugs affect SNS function through a variety of CNS centers. The hypothalamus is the principal brain region that integrates and differentiates environmental and behavioral input signals that, in turn, modify RVL output. The posterolateral hypothalamus mediates defense reactions, such as the "fight-or-flight" response, which includes RVL activation, increased heart rate and blood pressure, and vasodilatation in skeletal muscle.[18, 19] Various other integrated CNS response patterns are also necessary to meet different emotional and physiological demands. These responses appear to involve different patterns of cortical and hypothalamic stimulation. For example, an individual can experience different patterns of hemodynamic stimulation that are dependent on the individual's state of mind. Stimuli perceived as challenging or manageable are characterized by SNS-mediated increases in cardiac output, whereas stimuli perceived as threatening or outside the individual's range of control are associated with systemic vasoconstriction.[20, 21] These differential hemodynamic responses are not genetically determined because they are not predicted by family history of hypertension and because both "threat" and "challenge" patterns can be seen within the same individual.[20] In extreme situations

such as "vagal syncope," bradycardia is the result of a general parasympathetic "override" of SNS outflow that involves the nucleus ambiguus and other hypothalamic centers. Brody and colleagues found that the anteroventral third ventricular region is capable of modulating baroreflex function and SNS outflow in a complex pattern.[22–24] The median preoptic nucleus in this region serves to integrate water balance and thirst-sensing mechanisms with cardiovascular signals and may mediate organ-specific responses, such as skeletal muscle vasodilatation.[24] Thus, an interplay of CNS influences affects SNS outflow, and these may be involved in the heterogeneous syndrome of human essential hypertension. Many other CNS nuclei also modulate SNS outflow, but a full discussion is beyond the scope of this chapter. For example, epinephrine release during exercise is blunted by benzodiazepine therapy,[25] suggesting a role for locus ceruleus γ-aminobutyric acid (GABA) neurons in the process.

Hypothalamus in Hypertensive Models

In addition to acute changes in blood pressure, the hypothalamus may affect long-term blood pressure control. Ablation of the posterior hypothalamus reduces blood pressure in steroid-induced, genetic, and renal hypertension.[26] Lesions of the anterior hypothalamus dramatically increase blood pressure via massive adrenomedullary stimulation in normotensive rats, whereas electrical stimulation of this region causes hypotension.[27, 28] Ablation of the paraventricular nucleus prevents the development of hypertension in the spontaneously hypertensive rat (SHR).[29]

Spinal Cord and Peripheral Neurons

SNS efferent neuronal impulses are generated principally by cell bodies in the RVL-C$_1$ region, which project axons through the intermediolateral columns of the spinal cord to the sympathetic ganglia. Neuronal arborization within the SNS allows an extremely small number of RVL cell bodies to control an extremely diverse system of linked organ-specific responses. SNS signal amplification also occurs as a result of arborization at the level of postganglionic sympathetic nerves. Each axon contains a series of varicosities arranged like a string of beads that contain storage granules that release norepinephrine (NE) in response to antegrade axonal electrical impulses. Collateral synapses of C_1 axons on noradrenergic cell bodies in the spinal cord offer the opportunity for regional modulation of SNS responses.[5] The most important of these regional modulating influences is probably the "reno-renal reflex" that modifies contralateral renal hemodynamics in response to changes in ipsilateral renal blood flow and renal function.[30] The interlinked arborized organization of the SNS allows a spectrum of graded hemodynamic responses that range from subtle changes in regional blood flow to massive stimulation during fight-or-flight responses or major stimuli such as severe hemorrhage, hypotension, hypoglycemia, or hypothermia.

Peripheral Hyperinnervation in Hypertensive Models

A series of studies suggests that the SHR is anatomically hyperinnervated, as reflected in the increased number,[31] axonal volume,[32] and granular NE content[33] of peripheral sympathetic nerves in these animals. In addition, the amount of mRNA for nerve growth factor in caudal and mesenteric arteries and kidney is increased during development in these rats.[34, 35] Early treatment with antibody to nerve growth factor prevents the hyperinnervation and the accompanying vascular hypertrophy and lowers blood pressure.[33] A pattern of accelerated growth of renal sympathetic innervation has also been described in the SHR.[36]

Intrasynaptic Neurotransmitter Metabolism

The release of NE from storage granules in peripheral sympathetic varicosities is an exocytotic process dependent on intracellular calcium release.[37] Neuronally released NE faces one of three fates within the synapse: reuptake (uptake 1) into the presynaptic noradrenergic varicosity removes about 80% of the NE released into the synapse; uptake and metabolism by postsynaptic cells (uptake 2) releases O-methylated metabolites in urine or plasma; or diffusion (spillover) from the synaptic cleft releases NE into the extracellular fluid.[38] Because of potential differences among these three processes in individuals with differing physiological or pathological states, NE spillover has been recommended by some investigators as a more accurate index of SNS activity than plasma NE concentrations.[39, 40] Careful review of the literature reveals few if any meaningful conditions or circumstances in which an elevation of plasma NE does not provide a highly specific indicator of increased SNS activity.[41]

Intrasynaptic Modulation: Presynaptic Receptors and Cotransmitters

A variety of substances acts at specific receptors on post-ganglionic presynaptic membranes to modify local neurotransmission, either reducing or augmenting the amount of NE released with each nerve impulse.[42, 43] The most important of these presynaptic receptors is the α_2-receptor, which is usually occupied by NE. α_2-Receptors act as conservators of peripheral neurotransmission by signaling the noradrenergic neuron that NE is already present in the synaptic cleft and that subsequent nerve impulses need not release the same amount of NE as the immediately previous ones. This system thus provides a "check and balance" to excessive SNS discharge. Presynaptic α_2-receptors are probably the main site of action of central sympatholytics such as clonidine, guanfacine, guanadrel, methyldopa, and rilmenidine, which compete with NE at α_2- or imidazoline receptors to exert their effects. In direct opposition to these inhibitory presynaptic receptors are stimulatory presynaptic receptors such as β_2-receptors and Ang II receptors[42, 44] that augment the amount of NE released per nerve impulse. Rand and Majewski[43] first postulated that epinephrine facilitates SNS neurotransmission by functioning as a "cotransmitter" with NE. Under chronic stress, epinephrine initially released from the adrenal medulla is subsequently taken up into postganglionic neurons in parallel with NE. Subsequent SNS nerve impulses cause the release of both epinephrine and NE from noradrenergic nerve terminals. If stress is protracted, the stimulatory effect of intrasynaptic epinephrine on presynaptic β_2-receptors counterbalances the inhibitory effects of intrasynaptic NE on α_2-receptors. The clinical importance of this mechanism is not yet clear with respect to chronic hypertension, but studies suggest that the antihypertensive actions of nonselective β-blockers include blockade of intrasynaptic β_2-receptors.[45–47]

Interactions of the SNS and Renin-Angiotensin System

The body's two main blood pressure defense mechanisms, the SNS and the renin-angiotensin system, have a unique set of mutually reinforcing actions that combine to raise blood pressure acutely and chronically. A major consequence of SNS activation is β_1-receptor–mediated release of renin from the kidney, which in turn increases circulating Ang II, which acts at four or more levels to enhance further SNS outflow. First, circulating Ang II acts on CNS nuclei such as the area postrema, which does not have a blood-brain barrier, to enhance sympathetic outflow.[48, 49] Second, Ang II acts on stimulatory presynaptic receptors in CNS and peripheral synapses to enhance the amount of NE (or epinephrine) released by each nerve impulse,[49] similar to the function of presynaptic β-receptors. Third, Ang II facilitates the effects of NE via its inositide-dependent potentiation of calcium influx.[50] Fourth, Ang II appears to blunt baroreflex suppression of SNS outflow, although there is some controversy in this regard.[51–54] In parallel, Ang II has potent direct vasoconstrictor effects, principally via stimulation of angiotensin-1 (AT_1) receptors.[50] In addition to its effects on the SNS, Ang II stimulates other physiological responses that indirectly raise blood pressure, including increased thirst, secretion of aldosterone from the adrenal cortex, and secretion of vasopressin (antidiuretic hormone) from the posterior pituitary. Ang II acts together with catecholamines to promote structural changes such as hypertrophy of cardiac and vascular smooth muscle[55] (see Fig. 5–3) and interacts with both catecholamines and renal nerves to favor salt and water retention.[56, 57]

Other Neurotransmitters and Neuromodulators in Hypertensive Models

Various substances modify neurotransmission by direct action on neural membranes. Nitric oxide (NO) has significant neuroinhibitory features, as demonstrated by increased SNS nerve traffic after NO synthase blockade.[58, 59] Either neuronal NO deficiency or baroreflex desensitization[59] secondary to reduced NO availability has been postulated to contribute to chronic hypertension. GABA is another neurodepressant, as evidenced by the ability of valproate or muscimol to lower blood pressure in hypertensive rats.[60] Calcitonin gene–related peptide suppresses NE release from the brain stem in normal rats but not in SHRs.[61] The CNS effects of opiates,[62, 63] atriopeptins,[64] and other substances are complex and dependent on the individual nucleus affected. Endogenous neurostimulatory substances also exist. SHRs demonstrate augmented SNS responses due to activation of glutamate-sensitive neurons in the RVL.[65] Ouabain mediates increased RVL SNS outflow via an Ang II–dependent mechanism: The hypertensive effects of ouabain are abolished by AT_1-receptor blockade.[66, 67] Ouabain–Ang II interactions may also affect cardiopulmonary baroreflex sensitivity.[68]

Postsynaptic Adrenergic Receptors

Careful binding studies using specific ligands have differentiated two major adrenergic receptor types (α and β), each of which has several subtypes with different patterns of tissue localization and activation.[69] Although α-receptors respond to both NE and epinephrine, the NE effect tends to predominate. α_1-Receptors tend to be found within adrenergic synapses, particularly on postsynaptic membranes on the adventitial side of the smooth muscle layer of blood vessels. Their stimulation causes vasoconstriction. α_2-Receptors are found on endothelium, platelets, white blood cells, and fibroblasts, as well as on presynaptic neural membranes. β_1-Receptors are found predominantly on the heart and kidneys, whereas β_2-receptors are found in smooth muscle, endothelium, formed blood elements, and presynaptic neural membranes. β-Receptors are preferentially stimulated by epinephrine, which tends to increase cardiac output.

Role of Circulating Catecholamines

Contrary to their relatively weak effects on metabolic parameters,[70] physiological range elevations of circulating NE can increase plasma renin activity and diastolic blood pressure.[71, 72] Thus, circulating NE functions as a "cardiovascular hormone." Other effects of physiological increases in circulating catecholamines include increased platelet and leukocyte number[73] and increased platelet aggregation.[74] Hypertensives have greater platelet aggregability than normotensives.[75]

Cardiac Chromaffin Cells

The mammalian heart possesses unique perivascular catecholamine-producing cells that are not innervated by postganglionic sympathetic neurons and do not respond to SNS activation.[76] These cells have the potential to regulate a variety of physiological processes, including growth and development,[77] but their clinical significance is unknown.

INTEGRATED CARDIOVASCULAR AND METABOLIC REGULATION

Homeostasis Versus Acute Stress Responses

It has been almost 150 years since Claude Bernard proposed the concept of "sympathetic function," by which he meant an organized patterned response of the organism to its external environment. In his vision, vasomotor nerves helped preserve the "internal milieu" in an overall normative process later called *homeostasis*. A wide spectrum of stimuli affect SNS outflow. These range from mild to severe and from acute to chronic. A small transient decrease in blood pressure or blood sugar is a much less potent stimulus than severe hypotension, so the SNS response must be appropriately graded. Since there is basal activity of the SNS at all times, it is logical to assume that the SNS plays a role in basal regulation as well, particularly for those vital functions that affect metabolism, body temperature, and the delivery of oxygen and substrates to tissues. These overlapping SNS regulatory functions affect the circulation, extracellular fluid volume, intermediary metabolism, and thermoregulation.

Acute Blood Pressure Control

The basic physical equation describing blood pressure (the product of cardiac output and systemic vascular resistance) is shown in Figure 5–2, along with the "proximal" neurohumoral and receptor-mediated efferent factors that control blood pressure acutely.[2] It can be seen from this diagram that the SNS directly and indirectly affects many different parameters of blood pressure control.

High-Pressure (Aortocarotid) and Low-Pressure (Cardiopulmonary) Baroreceptors

Two inhibitory baroreflex sensor systems control SNS outflow: One responds to changes in arterial pressure (aortocarotid baroreflexes), the other to changes in cardiac filling

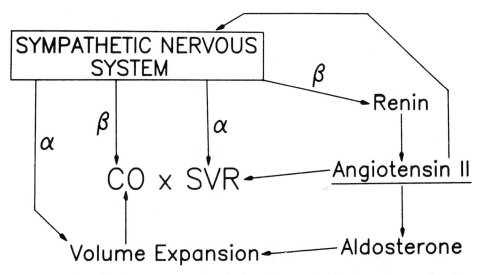

Figure 5–2. Acute blood pressure control mechanisms. Changes in blood pressure are affected by increases in cardiac output (CO) or systemic vascular resistance (SVR). Increased CO is the result of actions such as increased cardiac filling pressure or "preload," which, in turn, is the result of centralization of blood volume caused by α_1-receptor–mediated venoconstriction and renal afferent arteriolar constriction, which reduces salt and water excretion. These antinatriuretic effects are reinforced by β_1-receptor–mediated increases in renin, angiotensin II, and aldosterone and α_2-receptor–mediated effects on the renal tubular sodium transport. Concomitant stimulation of β_1-receptors increases cardiac rate and contractility and releases renin. Subsequent angiotensin II generation exerts *positive* feedback on sympathetic nervous system outflow and augments the increases in SVR that result directly from the effects of catecholamines on vascular α_1- and α_2-receptors. (Reprinted by permission of Elsevier Science from Izzo JL Jr. Sympathoadrenal activity, catecholamines, and the pathogenesis of vasculopathic hypertensive target-organ damage. Am J Hypertens 2:305S–312S, copyright 1989 by American Journal of Hypertension Ltd.)

(cardiopulmonary baroreflexes). In general, these two systems work in tandem to defend central blood volume and pressure. In response to a sudden fall in arterial pressure, the carotid sinus is "unloaded" and afferent signals are sent to the NTS to disinhibit (activate) the SNS, thereby resulting in increased heart rate, myocardial contractility, and constriction of vascular smooth muscle.[48] The arterial baroreflex system also partially inhibits the SNS during acute rises in systolic pressure and can respond to metabolic signals generated by the carotid sinus endothelium. The baroreceptors are also sensitized by prostanoids[78] and respond to other factors that alter cellular ion transport.[79, 80] Operating in tandem with the arterial system are low-pressure stretch receptors in the heart and great veins (cardiopulmonary baroreflexes) that sense changes in central blood volume. Decreases in central blood volume (cardiac "preload") or salt depletion lead to SNS activation, whereas salt loading or extracellular volume expansion suppresses SNS activity.[81, 82] The cardiopulmonary baroreflex system often supersedes the aortocarotid system in controlling SNS and renin-angiotensin activity, especially during postural adaptation or other conditions that affect central blood volume.[83–87] Guo and Thames demonstrated that renal sympathetic nerve traffic was normally suppressed by volume loading even after ablation of afferent aortocarotid nerves.[85] These results reveal the intimate relationship between cardiac filling and renal nerve activity.[85] In humans, cardiopulmonary baroreflexes can be stimulated separately by lower-body negative pressure, which increases muscle sympathetic nerve activity, renal vascular resistance, renal overflow of NE, glomerular filtration rate, plasma renin activity, and plasma Ang II, while reducing forearm and splanchnic blood flow.[88–90] As in dogs, these integrated physiological responses can occur independent of any changes in aortocarotid baroreflex activity.[91] It is also clear that the two systems have extensive interactions.[92, 93] Postural adaptation studies in humans also reveal the close relationship between cardiac filling and SNS activity: Across both supine and upright postures, plasma NE correlates more strongly with reduced cardiac stroke volume than with reduced central arterial pressure.[83]

Baroreflex Resetting and Hypertension

Arterial baroreceptors exert an important permissive influence in chronic hypertension because of their intrinsic inability to respond to chronic changes in blood pressure, a phenomenon known as *baroreflex resetting*.[94] Reset baroreceptors are still able to respond to acute changes in pressure but are not capable of returning blood pressure to normal. Thus, the SNS is never completely suppressed, even if blood pressure is high.[94–98] Although an inverse correlation remains between resting plasma NE and arterial baroreflex sensitivity in chronic hypertension,[99] SNS outflow is inappropriately high for the level of blood pressure. Chronic arterial baroreflex blunting has been linked with aging,[94] increased basal activity of the SNS,[99, 100] and increased Ang II effect.[52, 101] Altered sensitivity of cardiopulmonary baroreflexes may also play a significant role in permitting chronic increases in SNS activity and blood pressure.[102] When cardiac filling is reduced equally, borderline hypertensives exhibit augmented muscle sympathetic nerve activation compared with normotensives.[87, 91, 103, 104]

In contrast, in volume-loading experiments[85, 105] in dogs with renal failure and hypertension, blunting of both cardiopulmonary and aortocarotid baroreflexes was found.[84] Hajduczok and coworkers demonstrated that impaired cardiopulmonary baroreflexes contribute to the age-related increase in SNS activity.[102] These results are not inconsistent because they suggest a slope change in the baroreflex curve (blunting during volume loading and sensitization during unloading). CNS ouabain and Ang II[66] may play a role in cardiopulmonary baroreflex resetting because the slope of the curve in hypertensives is normalized by digitalis.[68]

Caloric Load, Glucoregulation, and Thermoregulation

Closely related to issues of perfusion of peripheral tissues is the regulation of body temperature. Sufficient cold exposure creates the need for SNS activation to constrict blood flow to the extremities and the skin, reducing convective heat loss. Parallel catabolic influences of catecholamines on adipose tissue cause simultaneous increases in caloric availability, which leads to compensatory heat generation. In rodents, the metabolism of brown adipose tissue is regulated directly by catecholamines and adrenergic receptors.[106, 107] The role of the SNS in the regulation of body temperature in humans is somewhat less clear. Peripheral vasoconstriction and vascular sensitivity to NE are increased by free fatty acids, which are liberated by the action of catecholamines on adipose tissue.[107] Landsberg and Young demonstrated that sucrose overfeeding increases SNS activity, as manifested by increased cardiac NE turnover in rats.[108] In contrast, starvation decreases SNS activity in rats and humans.[108-110] The conceptual breakthrough that excess caloric intake causes SNS activation may have important implications in the pathogenesis of hypertension associated with obesity. The SNS also plays a major role in glucose homeostasis, providing an early line of defense against hypoglycemia.[108] Both NE and epinephrine have "diabetogenic" properties, and infusion of catecholamines causes a rise in blood glucose similar to that found in pheochromocytoma. Increased SNS activity promotes hyperglycemia by a variety of mechanisms, including epinephrine-induced glucose biosynthesis from lactate and amino acids,[108, 111] and β-receptor–mediated decreases in glycogen synthase activity. The effects of NE in vivo on insulin and glucagon release are complicated by the influences of glucose, potassium, calcium, and growth hormone.[112] Stimulation of α-adrenergic receptors by catecholamines inhibits insulin secretion by pancreatic cells.[113] In contrast, pancreatic islet cells pretreated with NE show enhanced glucose-mediated secretion of insulin.[108]

Microcirculatory Protective Effects of Sympathetic Nerves

Although excessive SNS activity may be globally harmful, catecholamines and sympathetic nerves also have organ-protective effects. Reflex precapillary arteriolar constriction is necessary to protect the brain from surges in systolic blood pressure. This "baroprotective" role of sympathetic nerves was uncovered by Heistad and associates, who unilaterally denervated the cerebral vasculature in stroke-prone rats.[114-116] In these animals, fatal stroke occurred rapidly on the side from which the sympathetic nerves had been removed. In the syndrome of malignant hypertension, cerebral edema is worsened by sympathectomy, which permits increased blood flow.[116] In rats made acutely hypertensive by stellate ganglion stimulation, local sympathectomy caused abnormal brain hyperemia and local sympathetic nerve stimulation prevented the hyperemic response.[117] Renal nerves exhibit similar protective properties. In the SHR kidney, chemical sympathectomy or peripheral α-β-blockade can prevent hyperfiltration and parenchymal damage even if blood pressure is unaffected.[36]

GENETIC-ENVIRONMENTAL INTERACTIONS

Integrated Stress-Response Theories

Cannon[36a] described an integrated role of the SNS in the fight-or-flight response to external stimulation, in which stimuli such as pain, bleeding, or exposure to cold caused increases in SNS traffic and secretion of epinephrine and NE into the bloodstream. These surges in catecholamines were found to increase the delivery of oxygen and substrates to the CNS and to cardiac and skeletal muscle. As "defensive hormones," catecholamines were felt to enhance our ability to withstand hostile challenges at the expense of short-term increases in blood pressure. Selye[36b] first described the *general adaptation syndrome,* in which environmental stress elicits a sequential response pattern in the organism. An initial "alarm reaction," characterized by an immediate SNS discharge, is followed during ongoing stress by a subsequent "stage of resistance," which is characterized by chronic activation of the hypothalamic-pituitary-adrenocortical axis. Continued stress finally causes a stage of "exhaustion," with evidence of organ damage, including adrenal hypertrophy, gastrointestinal ulceration, and lymphoid shrinkage.

Acute Stress and Blood Pressure

The frequent SNS stimulation that occurs repeatedly throughout the day as a result of mental stress and activity causes transitory increases in NE production and blood pressure. Among the most important of these stimuli is physical activity. Although exercise raises blood pressure, physical conditioning overrides this stimulatory effect and leads to effective reduction in basal and stimulated SNS activity and blood pressures[118, 119] as well as cardiovascular risk.[120] Another important SNS stimulant is cigarette smoking.[121] Even though the effects of smoking are transient and blood pressure is increased only for a short time, the repetitive nature of smoking may cause an increase in average daily blood pressure. Major stressors that cause acute hypertension are burns, brain injuries, surgical interventions such as cardiopulmonary bypass, and general anesthesia, each of which results in marked SNS activation.

Exposure to cold or withdrawal from drugs such as opiates or central sympatholytics may also acutely activate the SNS. Such episodes are transient, however, and are not associated with chronic hypertension.

Chronic Stress, Personality Traits, and Blood Pressure

Blood pressures are lower in primitive societies than in complex societies; in contrast, people in lower socioeconomic groups within complex societies—who lead more stressful lives—have increased rates of hypertension.[122] Because of the difficulty in quantitating stress, however, large trials have generally ignored stress as a cardiovascular risk factor. When diary recordings have been combined with ambulatory blood pressure monitoring, correlations have been found among stressful daily events, increased blood pressure,[123–126] and increased left ventricular mass.[127, 128] A major component of workplace blood pressure elevation is stressful interpersonal relationships, particularly with one's immediate supervisor.[128] Specific personality subtypes also appear to predispose to hypertension and cardiovascular disease, but the original description that anxiety-prone individuals with "type A" personalities are at increased risk is no longer generally accepted. Rather, a personality pattern of suppressed hostility or "anger-in,"[129] with controlled, guilt-prone, and submissive characteristics, has been found to be associated with hypertension. This personality pattern correlates with elevated plasma NE, increased plasma renin activity,[130] and increased cardiovascular morbidity and mortality.[131]

Stress, Renal Sympathetic Nerves, and Hypertension

Abnormally high renal sympathetic nerve tone appears to be an important part of the pathogenesis of essential hypertension. Exaggerated stress-induced systemic and renal vasoconstriction contribute to increased systemic vascular resistance, reduced renal blood flow, and blunted natriuresis. DiBona and colleagues used an air jet stress paradigm to study renal nerves and salt and water excretion in rats. SHRs exhibit exaggerated renal vasoconstriction and excess salt and water retention during stress.[132] In humans, Hollenberg and coworkers[133] found that renal blood flow increased during mental stress in normotensives without parental history of hypertension but not in normotensives with parental history of hypertension. In borderline hypertensives, renal blood flow decreases with mental stress.[133, 134] The physiological importance of the renal nerves is further demonstrated by the observation that experimental denervation of the kidney leads to a salt-wasting state.[135] Relative salt wasting also occurs in humans after pharmacological sympathectomy with guanethidine[136] and in autonomic insufficiency.[137] Renal salt wasting is a major reason why individuals with autonomic insufficiency have abnormally low blood volume and orthostatic hypotension. Renal nerves also mediate the hypertension caused by NO synthase inhibition in rats. Renal denervation prevents the blood pressure increases that occur under this experimental condition.[138]

Circadian and Seasonal Variation in SNS Activity

The circadian rhythm of blood pressure follows the circadian rhythm of the SNS, which decreases during sleep and then peaks in the morning hours in parallel with plasma renin activity, blood volume, cortisol secretion, cardiac output, body temperature, and other variables. Panza and associates used plethysmographic techniques to demonstrate that the basal vasomotor tone of the peripheral vasculature has a diurnal rhythm that is dependent on α-receptor stimulation.[139] SNS activity decreases at night or during sleep, along with blood pressure, heart rate, cardiac output, and plasma catecholamines.[140] Superimposed on this circadian pattern are other daily SNS stimuli. Daytime blood pressure is determined principally by daily activities rather than diurnal rhythms,[141–143] as shown most clearly in shift workers.[142] In addition to these high-frequency and circadian patterns, seasonal and other long-term variations in SNS activity have also been reported. During winter months, plasma and urinary catecholamine levels are increased,[144–146] and there is increased systemic vasoconstriction, decreased blood volume and cardiac output, and in some cases, seasonal hypertension.[145] Morbidity and mortality patterns also follow the patterns of SNS activation. The morning peaks of myocardial infarction and sudden cardiac death[147, 148] or stroke[149] parallel the morning peaks of SNS activity and platelet aggregability. This diurnal pattern is abolished by β-blockers.[147] A seasonal influence on coronary and cerebrovascular disease also exists, with higher incidence of angina, heart failure, and mortality rates during winter months.[150–153]

Genetic Markers

At present, there are no genetic markers for increased SNS activity in humans. In SHRs, the Y chromosome confers higher blood pressure and SNS activity but not increased pressor responses during physical or social stress.[154] The mechanism for this effect is not known, but it may be related to the stimulatory effects of testosterone on the rate-limiting catecholamine synthetic enzyme tyrosine hydroxylase.[155] Another catecholamine synthetic enzyme, dopamine β-hydroxylase, and its regulatory genes have been found to be deficient in certain patients with autonomic failure.[156]

Family History Studies

Family history studies consistently reveal weak correlations between genetics and various indices of SNS overactivity. In a cross-sectional study of 557 Japanese, high plasma NE was found to predict future hypertension but was not related to family history of hypertension.[157] These investigators also found that family history of hypertension correlated with supranormal responses of NE and insulin to glucose loading.[158] In two smaller American studies, no relationship was found between family history of hypertension and plasma NE, urinary NE,[159] or plasma chromogranin A[160] at rest or after mental stress. A Swedish study, on the other hand, found that family history of hypertension predicted exaggerated responses of urinary catecholamines and heart rate to mental stress.[161] Similar findings, including an association with exaggerated blood pressure responses, were reported in an Italian study of children with hypertensive parents.[162] An Australian study found that normotensives with a parental history of hypertension had elevated plasma NE and increased NE spillover.[163] In a small Swiss study[164] and in African Americans,[165] family history of hypertension was associated with exaggerated responses of muscle sympathetic nerve activity to environmental stress. A Canadian study demonstrated that the abnormal heart rate and forearm blood flow responses to mental stress in normotensives with a family history of hypertension could be abolished by α-β-blockade.[166] A related phenomenon, arterial baroreflex sensitivity, is inherited separately from hypertension in humans.[167] In these studies, the overlap between those with and those without a family history of hypertension was substantial and the presence of a positive family history explained no more than 20 to 30% of the intergroup differences. Thus, increased SNS activity and hypertension appear to be related more to environmental or acquired characteristics than genetic predetermination.

SNS HYPERACTIVITY IN EARLY HYPERTENSION

General Considerations

The foregoing discussion underscores the central position of the SNS in physiological blood pressure regulation and leads to the hypothesis that the SNS plays a major pathogenetic role in human essential hypertension. At least five major questions have arisen in considering the role of the SNS in essential hypertension:

1. Is the SNS is a trigger mechanism or sustaining influence in hypertension?
2. What level of SNS activity is "normal" in the setting of chronic blood pressure increases? It can be argued that appropriate testing of pressure-dependent SNS outflow requires that hypertensive and normotensive populations be investigated at the same blood pressure levels, both low and high.
3. If the SNS regulates so many cardiovascular and metabolic signals, can these influences be identified and controlled? Assessment of SNS activation ideally requires control of time of day, body temperature, central blood volume, blood glucose, degree of emotional excitation, posture, and degree of physical activity.
4. What are the effects of aging and target organ damage on SNS outflow?
5. Are current study techniques adequate?

It may not be realistic to expect to resolve all of these uncertainties, yet an appreciation of the scope of the dilemma helps improve our understanding of the limits of existing studies.

Physiological and Pharmacological Studies

The first clinical evidence of SNS overactivity in "prehypertensives" was the observation that military recruits who later developed hypertension exhibited initially higher heart rates than those who remained normotensive.[168] Julius and colleagues concluded that because elevated cardiac output values in borderline hypertensives were not normalized by β-blockade without atropine, the elevation in cardiac output seen in borderline hypertensive subjects was due to a combination of sympathetic hyperactivity and parasympathetic dysfunction.[169, 170] Goldstein and Keiser used yohimbine to increase SNS outflow and plasma NE by blocking central α₂-receptors.[171] Increased yohimbine-dependent stimulation of plasma NE in early hypertensives suggested that baroreflex suppression of SNS outflow had partially suppressed increased SNS activity. In SHRs, sympathectomy prevents the development of hypertension.[172]

Plasma Catecholamines and Other Plasma Markers

Goldstein reviewed 78 studies published by 1982 and concluded that the majority demonstrated elevated plasma NE values in young borderline hypertensives.[173] More recently, a prospective 10-year follow-up study in initially normotensive Japanese found higher initial plasma NE values in those whose blood pressures subsequently increased than in those who remained normotensive,[157, 174] clearly suggesting a role for the SNS in the initiation of hypertension. In the Tecumseh Study, 37% of "borderline" hypertensives were found to have elevated plasma NE along with increased heart rate, cardiac index, and forearm blood flow.[175] This pattern persisted from age 5 to 23 years and was associated with a parental history of hypertension. Plasma epinephrine values have been reported to be elevated in early essential hypertensives.[176] By a cotransmitter effect, epinephrine could "prime the pump" for sustained elevation of SNS outflow. Another SNS biochemical marker, plasma chromogranin A, is elevated in hypertension.[177] Urinary catecholamines have been less consistently elevated in early hypertension.[178–180]

Kinetic and Microneurographic Studies

In the hope of improving on the relatively low sensitivity of plasma NE for detecting small changes in SNS activity, Esler and coworkers pioneered the use of steady-state radiolabeled NE infusion techniques to measure NE spillover.[40, 181] Increased whole-body NE spillover in early hypertension has been found in several studies.[182, 183] Subsequent modifications of the technique have revealed increased organ-specific NE spillover from the heart, kidney, and brain of hypertensive subjects.[181, 184] Despite the intuitive appeal of this kinetic approach, there are some discrepancies with data derived from direct muscle sympathetic nerve recordings. For example, kinetic techniques do not reveal increased skeletal muscle SNS traffic in hypertension, a finding consistently demonstrated by venous plasma NE values and by muscle sympathetic nerve recordings.[185–188] Curiously, muscle sympathetic nerve activity has been reported to correlate with renal NE spillover[189] and jugular vein NE spillover[190] but not muscle NE spillover. Furthermore, obese individuals demonstrate reduced cardiac and increased renal NE spillover,[191] data that seem at odds with studies showing increased muscle sympathetic nerve activity in obesity.[192, 193] Taken together, these observations cast some doubt on the validity of the kinetic techniques.

SNS, Obesity, and Insulin Resistance

Obesity, insulin resistance, hypertension, dyslipidemia, and atherosclerosis often coexist as *metabolic syndrome X*.[194, 195] Which of these linked abnormalities is causal is an interesting question. It is attractive to speculate that each may be caused by a more basic cellular abnormality and that certain of these linked abnormalities can lead to the others. Obesity and hypertension are strongly positively correlated at all ages, regardless of gender or race.[196–198] Increased muscle sympathetic nerve activity has been found in obese individuals,[192, 193] and there is growing realization of the potential pathogenic role of the SNS in obesity-related hypertension.[195, 199–201] Not only does increased SNS activity cause insulin resistance, but hyperinsulinemia clearly increases SNS activity.[202, 203] Thus, the vicious circle of increased SNS activity–hyperinsulinemia–insulin resistance may be a major pathophysiological link between obesity and hypertension. Insulin-sensitizing drugs such as metformin[204] decrease SNS activity and blood pressure, and insulin therapy increases appetite in diabetics, thereby contributing to obesity. The hypothesis that increased SNS activity causes insulin resistance[111] is consistent with studies showing that when the SNS is activated by lower body negative pressure, forearm insulin resistance is induced.[205] Similarly, treatment with the central sympatholytic drug clonidine lowers SNS output and plasma catecholamines and increases insulin sensitivity.[206]

α-Adrenergic Hyperresponsiveness

The importance of peripheral vascular α-adrenergic tone in the maintenance of hypertension was demonstrated by Egan and associates, who found increased basal forearm vascular resistance in established hypertensives that could be normalized by α-blockade.[207] Philipp and colleagues[208] and Kiowski and coworkers[209] examined the relative contributions of increased plasma NE and increased α-adrenergic vascular responsiveness in established hypertension. After stratification for blood pressure, a series of hyperbolic relationships between plasma NE concentration and α-adrenergic responsiveness were found.[208] Those with high plasma NE had low α-adrenergic responsiveness, whereas those with low plasma NE had high α-adrenergic responsiveness. Thus, the impact of the SNS on blood pressure is a combined effect of the amount of agonist and the tissue sensitivity to that agonist. Racial differences in α-adrenergic responsiveness have been described as well: African Americans have greater blood pressure increases during cold and mental stress, and a study of African American children revealed lower urinary catecholamines despite higher blood pressures than their white counterparts.[210] Egan and coworkers reported that α-adrenergic hyperresponsiveness is caused by increased endothelial fatty acid uptake, suggesting another link between metabolism and hypertension.[211]

Associated Renin-Angiotensin and Renal Flow Abnormalities

Given the close relationship between SNS and renin-angiotensin activity, it would be logical to examine their interactions in essential hypertension. In early studies, Esler found higher heart rates and cardiac indices among the high-renin hypotensives who also had isolated systolichypertension.[213] In contrast, the normal-renin hypertensive group had normal heart rates and cardiac indices but elevated peripheral resistance. In addition, blood pressure lowering after β-blockade was significant only in the high-renin subgroup, suggesting that these individuals had "neurogenic hypertension." Later studies demonstrated a direct correlation between plasma renin activity and plasma NE in these younger individuals.[212, 213] In essential hypertensives, Schmieder and associates found that mental stress caused abnormal increases in glomerular filtration and plasma Ang II, which were fully blocked by ACE inhibition.[214]

AGING, SNS HYPERACTIVITY, AND CHRONIC HYPERTENSION

The presence of multiple confounders in assessing the appropriateness of SNS outflow has already been emphasized. Perhaps the most important of these confounders in chronic hypertension is the close interrelationship among aging, increased SNS activity, and hypertension. Current data strongly suggest that increased SNS activity remains a major pathogenetic component of essential hypertension at all ages and during all stages of the disorder. Similar to the linkage between obesity and hypertension, the tendency for plasma NE to increase with age may be the critical link explaining the age-related increase in blood pressure. What remains to be identified is the mechanism of the age-related increase in SNS activity.

Antihypertensive Therapy and SNS Activity in Sustained Hypertension

In the early 20th century, the notion that vasomotor nerves contributed to vasoconstriction led to the variably successful practice of surgical sympathectomy of the lower extremities to treat hypertension. The same logic led to pioneering work by Freis in the development of ganglionic blocking drugs.[215] A hallmark effect of these drugs was orthostatic hypotension caused by interruption of sympathetically mediated postural adaptation. Louis and coworkers demonstrated in the late 1960s that ganglionic-blocking drugs caused proportional falls in blood pressure and plasma NE in established hypertensives, many of whom had severe, long-standing hypertension.[216] Izzo and colleagues found that when blood pressure was lowered equally by α_1-blockade or nonspecific vasodilators, plasma NE doubled in hypertensive subjects.[217] In contrast, equal pressure-lowering with angiotensin-converting enzyme inhibitors had no effect on plasma NE,[217] suggesting that baroreflex suppression of SNS outflow persists in chronic hypertension and that the renin-angiotensin system plays a role in baroreflex blunting. Central sympatholytic drugs, such as clonidine, have been used to probe the role of the CNS and peripheral nervous system in hypertension. Goldstein and associates found that essential hypertensives with high resting plasma NE values exhibited a proportional fall in both blood pressure and plasma NE after clonidine administration,[218] confirming earlier results.[216] General clinical experience confirms the utility of the central sympatholytic agents in all forms of hypertension, a finding that supports the concept of inappropriate SNS activity in all forms of the disorder.

Aging and Increased SNS Activity

The prevalent view about the effects of aging on catecholamines has been that age adjustment eliminates differences in plasma NE between hypertensives and normotensives. On closer scrutiny, however, this dogma seems incorrect. Messerli and coworkers[219] and Izzo and colleagues[220] found a significant correlation among advancing age, increased plasma NE, and increased blood pressure in hypertensives. After adjustment for age, a strong residual correlation between plasma NE and systemic vascular resistance remained.[220] It seems likely that increased vascular resistance contributes to the decrease in cardiac inotropy that occurs with age, a phenomenon that may be related to the age-related decrease in β-receptors.[221, 222] In the Normative Aging Study, one of the strongest residual relationships among the various parameters tested as determinants of blood pressure was the age-independent relationship between urinary NE excretion and blood pressure.[223] Plasma epinephrine has also been reported to remain elevated in hypertensives beyond age 60 years, suggesting a continuing role in sustaining inappropriate SNS activity.[224] The discovery of age-related decreases in NE clearance suggested to some investigators that increases in plasma NE with age were artifactual. An early report by Esler and associates suggested that neither whole-body nor organ-specific NE spillover increased with age.[225, 226] Closer scrutiny of the data reveals that the magnitude of the observed age-related difference in NE clearance was relatively small and that NE spillover was increased by about the same proportion. Furthermore, whether increased NE comes from increased neuronal release or decreased clearance, the total amount of catecholamine at the postsynaptic membranes is increased. The finding of clear-cut age-related increases in directly recorded muscle SNS activity in hypertensives[102] adds further evidence that NE spillover data are not always

consistent with plasma catecholamines or muscle nerve traffic data. Given the concordance between plasma NE and muscle sympathetic nerve traffic[185, 186] techniques, it appears that essential hypertension is characterized by inappropriately elevated whole-body and muscle sympathetic nerve activity and increased chronic "burden" of catecholamines.

SNS HYPERACTIVITY IN SECONDARY HYPERTENSION

It addition to clear evidence that primary (essential) hypertension includes a component of inappropriate SNS activation, there is equally clear evidence that inappropriate SNS activity occurs in all forms of secondary hypertension.

Steroid-Induced Hypertension

A significant misconception exists that steroid-induced hypertension is simply "volume-dependent" hypertension. Substantial evidence in animals and humans suggests that steroid-induced hypertension is more "neurogenic" in nature and is most clearly understood as a disturbance of the equilibrium between "volume" and SNS-mediated vasoconstriction. Normally, volume loading leads to a suppression of SNS outflow.[81, 129] In steroid-induced hypertension, there is elevated or unsuppressible SNS outflow. Although rats implanted with deoxycorticosterone acetate (DOCA) develop hypertension with minimal elevations of catecholamines, their SNS outflow is accentuated by hemorrhage,[227] and pharmacological interruption of neurotransmission normalizes blood pressure.[228] Zambraski and coworkers demonstrated that miniature swine implanted with DOCA, which do not require additional salt loading to manifest hypertension, exhibit increased plasma catecholamines and normalization of blood pressures with pharmacological sympathectomy.[229, 230] In DOCA-salt rats, adrenalectomy significantly lowers blood pressure and blunts NE release by a reduced cotransmitter effect on presynaptic β-receptors.[231] Although the mechanisms by which steroid excess engenders increased SNS outflow are not fully known, Saavedra demonstrated that brain stem epinephrine synthesis increases during chronic steroid administration through induction of the epinephrine-synthesizing enzyme phenylethanolamine-N-methyl transferase.[232] Local epinephrine exerts an excitatory effect on the RVL to increase SNS outflow and may interact with impaired cardiopulmonary baroreflexes[233] to sustain the hypertension.

Renovascular Hypertension

Given the tight interrelationship between the SNS and the renin-angiotensin system, a permissive role of the SNS in renovascular hypertension should be expected. Renal nerves participate in the maintenance of hypertension in two-kidney and one-kidney renovascular hypertension in the rat, as evidenced by the observation that renal denervation substantially lowers blood pressure in these animals.[234, 235] In the one-kidney renovascular model, it has been shown that renal denervation reduced abnormal hypothalamic NE metabolism[236] and corrected SNS overactivity.[236–238] In these animals, the development of hypertension can be prevented by posterior hypothalamic lesions,[26] chemical sympathectomy,[239] or thoracolumbar dorsal rhizotomy, which selectively ablates afferent renal nerves.[240] Wyss and associates subsequently demonstrated that thoracolumbar dorsal rhizotomy performed after the blood pressure elevation was sustained could improve but not cure the hypertension.[241] Thus, renal afferent nerves are important promoters of SNS overactivity, which contributes to the genesis and maintenance of renovascular hypertension.

Renal Parenchymal Hypertension

Plasma catecholamines are elevated in chronic renal failure[242–244] in parallel with elevations in blood pressure. In uremic humans, the accompanying hypertension is associated with increased NE turnover[243] and increased muscle sympathetic nerve traffic.[245] Central sympatholytic drugs such as clonidine are extremely effective in uremic hypertension, causing proportional falls in plasma NE and blood pressure.[242, 244] Combined α-β-blockers are also extremely effective in these patients. The mechanisms of increased sympathetic discharge in uremia include cardiopulmonary baroreflex failure[84, 85] and abnormal afferent signals from renal nerves that chronically activate brain stem SNS outflow.[246]

Pheochromocytoma

The paradigm of catecholamine hypertension is pheochromocytoma. In this situation, excessive production of catecholamines directly causes hypertension and the removal of the autonomous catecholamine-secreting tissue cures the hypertension. In pheochromocytoma, plasma catecholamine levels are generally much higher than those observed in essential hypertension.[247] This argument has been used in the past to indicate that catecholamines play no role in essential hypertension. Because about 80% of NE released is immediately taken up into the nerve terminal from which it was released, however, the concentration of NE at the postsynaptic membrane in essential hypertension may be similar to that observed in pheochromocytoma.

Preeclampsia

Recent microneurographic studies have demonstrated that the syndrome of preeclampsia is associated with marked increases in SNS activity, which return to normal as blood pressure normalizes after delivery.[248] Although this syndrome has features similar to those of profound volume depletion, the degree of SNS activation is higher than would be expected from a compensatory response to hypovolemia.

SNS HYPERACTIVITY, STRUCTURAL CHANGE, AND TARGET ORGAN DAMAGE

The classical teaching that cardiac and vascular target organ damage is simply the result of mechanical trauma from long-standing hypertension is no longer accepted. A rapidly growing body of information has identified a causal relationship between excessive "neurohumoral activation" (increased SNS activity, catecholamines, and renin-angiotensin activity) and cardiovascular target organ damage (Fig. 5–3). These target organ changes can be found early in hypertension, in some cases before a sustained rise in blood pressure occurs.[2, 249] Vascular and cardiac hypertrophy and decreased arterial compliance impair the baroreflexes, thereby sustaining inappropriate SNS activity and chronic hypertension.[250] These structural changes are at least partially reversible with appropriate therapy.

Cellular Hypertrophy and the SNS

Cardiac and vascular hypertrophy are principally caused by volume or pressure overload, but it is also clear that the

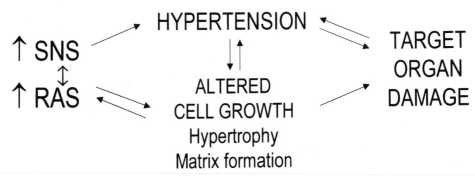

Figure 5–3. Mechanisms of chronic hypertension. The sympathetic nervous system (SNS) and renin-angiotensin system (RAS) continue to exert chronic pressor effects on the heart and vasculature, as shown in Figure 5–2. In addition, continued overactivity of the SNS-RAS axis induces further functional and structural change in the cardiovascular system. Cardiac and vascular hypertrophy, which result from mechanical and direct neurohumoral actions, tend to blunt arterial and cardiopulmonary baroreflexes, thus sustaining chronic increases in SNS-RAS outflow, which continue to promote higher blood pressure and further degeneration.

SNS and renin-angiotensin system exert direct "neurohumoral" influences on the hypertrophic process. In tissue culture, both Ang II and NE strongly promote the synthesis and release of trophic substances such as insulin-like growth factor, fibroblast growth factor, and transforming growth factor-β.[55] These substances then cause cardiac and vascular hypertrophy and favor increased deposition of collagen and other structural proteins in the extracellular matrix.[55] Korner and associates correlated tissue and adrenal NE concentrations with the degree of cardiac and vascular hypertrophy in a variety of selectively crossbred rat strains.[251] They found that hypertrophy could be prevented only when α-blockade was combined with sympathectomy and stressed the importance of α_1-receptors in the hypertrophic process.[251] Sympathectomy also has been shown to attenuate the hypertrophy of the muscularis of cerebral arterioles in SHRs.[252]

Arteriosclerosis and Decreased Vascular Compliance

Vascular stiffness or its inverse, vascular compliance, has both functional and structural components. Decreased aortic compliance causes systolic hypertension and a widening of the pulse pressure, a major predictor of heart disease and stroke. Catecholamine-dependent aortic sclerosis and loss of compliance of large and small blood vessels may depend on catecholamine-dependent protein synthesis and amino acid uptake into vascular smooth muscle, which can be blocked by sympatholytic drugs.[253] Grassi and coworkers have shown that either local phenylephrine infusion or cigarette smoking causes reversible decreases in radial arterial compliance, which is inversely related to plasma NE.[254] Reduced compliance of the carotid sinus is believed to play a significant role in the blunting of the arterial baroreflex that occurs with age, which in turn permits inappropriate SNS outflow to continue.

Cardiac Hypertrophy and Failure

In dogs, periodic blood pressure elevation can cause ventricular hypertrophy in the absence of sustained hypertension.[255] Cardiac hypertrophy reduces the ability of cardiac mechanoreceptors to respond to volume overload and blunts the inhibitory effect of cardiopulmonary baroreflexes, fostering continued inappropriate SNS outflow and chronic hypertension. Some studies have shown a positive correlation between plasma epinephrine and left ventricular wall thickness.[256] Abnormal cardiac NE kinetics have been found in hypertrophic cardiomyopathy,[257] and infusion of NE reproducibly causes dilated cardiomyopathy in animals.[258] The severity of the syndrome of heart failure is also related to the degree of neurohumoral stimulation present.[259, 260]

Integrated Effects of Inappropriate SNS Activity

Chronic hypertension and target organ damage are probably best viewed as a lifetime accumulation of acute and chronic activation of the SNS. Each individual SNS-mediated stress response is superimposed on an age-related increase in baseline SNS activity, which is in turn causally related to the hypertrophic and sclerotic effects of the SNS on the heart and blood vessels. In addition to its effects on blood pressure and cardiac and vascular hypertrophy, excess SNS activity contributes to premature cardiovascular death via acute and chronic vasoconstriction, platelet and leukocyte activation, thrombosis, and cardiac arrhythmias.

References

1. Izzo JL Jr. The sympathoadrenal system in the maintenance of elevated arterial pressure. J Cardiovasc Pharmacol 6:s514–s521, 1984.
2. Izzo JL Jr. Sympathoadrenal activity, catecholamines, and the pathogenesis of vasculopathic hypertensive target-organ damage. Am J Hypertens 2:305S–312S, 1989.
3. Reis DJ. The brain and hypertension: Reflections on 35 years of inquiry into the neurobiology of the circulation. Circulation 70:31–45, 1984.
4. Reis DJ, Ruggiero DA, Morrison SF. The C1 area of the rostral ventrolateral medulla oblongata. Am J Hypertens 2:363S–374S, 1989.
5. Ross CA, Ruggiero DA, Park DH, et al. Tonic vasomotor control by the rostral ventrolateral medulla: Effect of electrical or chemical stimulation of the area containing C1 adrenaline neurons on arterial pressure, heart rate and plasma catecholamines and vasopressin. J Neurosci 4:474–494, 1984.
6. Abboud FM. The sympathetic system in hypertension. Hypertension 4(suppl II):208–225, 1982.
7. Ferrario CM, Barnes KL, Bohonek S. Neurogenic hypertension produced by lesions of the nucleus tractus solitarii alone or with sinoaortic denervation in the dog. Hypertension 3:112–118, 1981.
8. Nathan MA, Reis DJ. Chronic labile hypertension produced by lesions of the nucleus tractus solitarii in the cat. Circ Res 40:72–80, 1977.
9. Laubie M, Schmitt H. Destruction of the nucleus tractus solitarii in the dog: Comparison with sinoaortic denervation. Am J Physiol 5:736–743, 1979.
10. Ciriello J, Calaresu FR. Projections from buffer nerves to the nucleus of the solitary tract: An anatomical and electrophysiological study in the cat. J Auton Nerv Syst 3:299–310, 1981.
11. Fink GD, Haywood JR, Bryan WJ, et al. Central site for pressor action of blood-borne angiotensin in rat. Am J Physiol 239:R358–R361, 1980.
12. Shapiro RE, Miselis RR. The central neural connections of the area postrema of the rat. J Comp Neurol 234:344–364, 1985.
13. Fink GD, Bruner CA, Mangiapane ML. Area postrema is critical for angiotensin-induced hypertension in rats. Hypertension 9:355–361, 1987.
14. Mangiapane ML, Skoog KM, Rittenhouse P, et al. Lesion of the area postrema region attenuates hypertension in spontaneously hypertensive rats. Circ Res 64:129–135, 1989.
15. Walker JL, Abboud FM, Mark AL, Thames MD. Interaction of cardiopulmonary and somatic reflexes in humans. J Clin Invest 65:1491–1497, 1980.
16. Granata AR, Ruggiero DA, Park DH, et al. Brain stem area with C1 epinephrine neurons mediates baroreflex vasodepressor responses. Am J Physiol 248:H547–H567, 1985.
17. Bruner CA, Mangiapane ML, Fink GD, Webb RC. Area postrema ablation and vascular reactivity in deoxycorticosterone-salt–treated rats. Hypertension 11:668–673, 1988.
18. Juskevich JC, Robinson DS, Whitehorn D. Effect of hypothalamic stimulation in spontaneously hypertensive and Wistar-Kyoto rats. Eur J Pharmacol 51:429–439, 1978.
19. Takeda K, Bunag RD. Sympathetic hyperactivity during hypothalamic stimulation in spontaneously hypertensive rats. J Clin Invest 62:642–648, 1978.
20. Allen K, Shykoff BE, Izzo JL Jr. Cognitive appraisal of threat or challenge predicts hemodynamic responses to mental arithmetic and speech tasks. Am J Hypertens 11:134A, 1998.
21. Shykoff BE, Allen K, Izzo JL Jr. Interactions of social support and

family history in blood pressure reactivity to psychological stressors. Am J Hypertens 11:134A, 1998.

22. Knuepfer MM, Johnson AK, Brody MJ. Vasomotor projections from the anteroventral third ventricle (AV3V). Am J Physiol 247:139–145, 1984.

23. Knuepfer MM, Johnson AK, Brody MJ. Identification of brain stem projections mediating hemodynamic responses to stimulation of the anteroventral third ventricle (AV3V) region. Brain Res 294:305–314, 1984.

24. Mangiapane ML, Brody MJ. Vasoconstrictor and vasodilator sites within anteroventral third ventricle region. Am J Physiol 253:827–831, 1987.

25. Stratton JR, Halter JB. Effect of a benzodiazepine (alprazolam) on plasma epinephrine and norepinephrine levels during exercise stress. Am J Cardiol 56:136–139, 1985.

26. Bunag RD, Eferakeya AD. Immediate hypotensive after effects of posterior hypothalamic lesions in awake rats with spontaneous, renal, or DOCA hypertension. Cardiovasc Res 10:663–671, 1976.

27. Folkow B, Johansson B, Oberg B. A hypothalamic structure with marked inhibitory effect on tonic sympathetic activity. Acta Physiol Scand 47:262–270, 1959.

28. Nathan MA, Reis DJ. Fulminating arterial hypertension with pulmonary edema from release of adrenomedullary catecholamines after lesions of the anterior hypothalamus in the rat. Circ Res 37:226–235, 1975.

29. Takeda K, Nakata T, Takesako T, et al. Sympathetic inhibition and attenuation of spontaneous hypertension by PVN lesions in rats. Brain Res 543:296–300, 1991.

30. DiBona GF. Role of the renal nerves in hypertension. Semin Nephrol 11:503–511, 1991.

31. Mangiarua EI, Lee RM. Increased sympathetic innervation in the cerebral and mesenteric arteries of hypertensive rats. Can J Physiol Pharmacol 68:492–499, 1990.

32. Albert V, Campbell GR. Relationship between the sympathetic nervous system and vascular smooth muscle: A morphometric study of adult and juvenile spontaneously hypertensive rat/Wistar-Kyoto rat caudal artery. Heart Vessels 5:129–139, 1990.

33. Brock JA, Van Helden DF, Dosen P, Rush RA. Prevention of high blood pressure by reducing sympathetic innervation in the spontaneously hypertensive rat. J Auton Nerv Syst 61:97–102, 1996.

34. Antonaccio MJ, Robson RD, Burrell R. The effects of L-dopa and alpha-methyldopa on reflexes and sympathetic nerve function. Eur J Pharmacol 25:9–18, 1974.

35. Falckh PH, Harkin LA, Head RJ. Nerve growth factor mRNA content parallels altered sympathetic innervation in the spontaneously hypertensive rat. Clin Exp Pharmacol Physiol 19:541–545, 1992.

36. Gattone VH 2d, Evan AP, Overhage JM, Severs WB. Developing renal innervation in the spontaneously hypertensive rat: Evidence for a role of the sympathetic nervous system in renal damage. J Hypertens 8:423–428, 1990.

36a. Cannon WB. Stresses and strains of homeostasis. Am J Med Sci 189:1–14, 1935.

36b. Selye H. Forty years of stress research: Principal remaining problems and misconceptions. Can Med Assoc J 115:53–56, 1976.

37. Rubin RP. The role of calcium in the release of neurotransmitter substances and hormones. Pharmacol Rev 22:389–428, 1970.

38. Iverson LL. Catecholamine uptake process. Br Med Bull 29:130–135, 1973.

39. Goldstein DS, Eisenhofer G, Garty M, et al. Implications of plasma levels of catechols in the evaluation of sympathoadrenomedullary function. Am J Hypertens 2:133S–139S, 1989.

40. Eisenhofer G, Esler MD, Goldstein DS, Kopin IJ. Neuronal uptake, metabolism, and release of tritium-labeled norepinephrine during assessment of its plasma kinetics. Am J Physiol 261:E505–E515, 1991.

41. Izzo JL Jr. Biochemical assessment of sympathetic activity. In Robertson D, Low PA, Polinsky RJ (eds). Primer on the Autonomic Nervous System. San Diego, Academic, 1996; pp 116–122.

42. Langer SZ. Pre-synaptic regulation of the release of catecholamines. Pharmacol Rev 32:337–362, 1980.

43. Rand MJ, Majewski H. Adrenaline mediates a positive feedback loop in noradrenergic neurotransmission: Its possible role in development of hypertension. Clin Exp Hypertens A6:347–370, 1984.

44. Floras JS, Aylward PE, Victor RG, et al. Epinephrine facilitates

neurogenic vasoconstriction in humans. J Clin Invest 81:1265–1274, 1988.

45. Dixon WR, Mosimann WF, Weiner N. The role of presynaptic feedback mechanisms in regulation of norepinephrine release by nerve stimulation. J Pharmacol Exp Ther 209:196–204, 1979.

46. Chang PC, Kriek E, van Brummelen P. Sympathetic activity and presynaptic adrenoceptor function in patients with long-standing essential hypertension. J Hypertens 12:179–190, 1994.

47. Draper AJ, Meghji S, Redfern PH. Enhanced presynaptic facilitation of vascular adrenergic neurotransmission in spontaneously hypertensive rats. J Auton Pharmacol 9:103–111, 1989.

48. Zimmerman BG. Evaluation of peripheral and central components of action of angiotensin on the sympathetic nervous system. J Pharmacol Exp Ther 158:1–10, 1967.

49. Zimmerman BG. Adrenergic facilitation by angiotensin: Does it serve a physiological function? Clin Sci 60:343–348, 1981.

50. Marsden PA, Brenner BM, Ballerman BJ. Mechanisms of angiotensin action on vascular smooth muscle, the adrenal, and the kidney. In Laragh JH, Brenner BM (eds). Hypertension: Pathophysiology, Diagnosis, and Treatment. New York, Raven, 1990; pp 1247–1272.

51. Scroop GC, Lowe RD. Efferent pathways of the cardiovascular response to vertebral artery infusions of angiotensin in the dog. Clin Sci 37:605–619, 1969.

52. Guo GB, Abboud FM. Angiotensin II attenuates baroreflex control of heart rate and sympathetic activity. Am J Physiol 246:H80–H89, 1984.

53. Lee WB, Lumbers ER. Angiotensin and the cardiac baroreflex response to phenylephrine. Clin Exp Pharmacol Physiol 8:109–117, 1981.

54. McCubbin JW, Page IH, Bumpus FM. Effect of synthetic angiotonin on the carotid sinus. Circ Res 5:458–460, 1957.

55. Griffin SA, Brown WCB, MacPherson F, et al. Angiotensin II causes vascular hypertrophy in part by a non-pressor mechanism. Hypertension 17:626–635, 1991.

56. Gavras I, Mulinari R, Gavras H. Renin-angiotensin and vasopressin in the development of salt-induced hypertension. J Hypertens 6:999–1002, 1988.

57. Ichihara A, Inscho EW, Imig JD, et al. Role of renal nerves in afferent arteriolar reactivity in angiotensin-induced hypertension. Hypertension 29:442–449, 1997.

58. Sander M, Hansen J, Victor RG. The sympathetic nervous system is involved in the maintenance but not initiation of the hypertension induced by N(omega)-nitro-L-arginine methyl ester. Hypertension 30:64–70, 1997.

59. Zanzinger J, Czachurski J, Seller H. Inhibition of sympathetic vasoconstriction is a major principle of vasodilation by nitric oxide in vivo. Circ Res 75:1073–1077, 1994.

60. Sasaki S, Nakata T, Kawasaki S, et al. Chronic central GABAergic stimulation attenuates hypothalamic hyperactivity and development of spontaneous hypertension in rats. J Cardiovasc Pharmacol 15:706–713, 1990.

61. Tsuda K, Tsuda S, Goldstein M, Masuyama Y. Effects of calcitonin gene–related peptide on [3H]norepinephrine release in medulla oblongata of spontaneously hypertensive rats. Eur J Pharmacol 191:101–105, 1990.

62. Feuerstein G, Siren AL, Goldstein DS, et al. Effect of morphine on the hemodynamic and neuroendocrine responses to hemorrhage in conscious rats. Circ Shock 27:219–235, 1989.

63. May CN, Whitehead CJ, Heslop KE, Mathias CJ. Evidence that intravenous morphine stimulates central opiate receptors to increase sympatho-adrenal outflow and cause hypertension in conscious rabbits. Clin Sci 76:431–437, 1989.

64. Shirakami G, Nakao K, Yamada T, et al. Inhibitory effect of brain natriuretic peptide on central angiotensin II–stimulated pressor response in conscious rats. Neurosci Lett 91:77–83, 1988.

65. Tsuchihashi T, Abe I, Fujishima M. Role of metabotropic glutamate receptors in ventrolateral medulla of hypertensive rats. Hypertension 24:648–652, 1994.

66. Budzikowski AS, Huang BS, Leenen FH. Brain "ouabain," a neurosteroid, mediates sympathetic hyperactivity in salt-sensitive hypertension. Clin Exp Hypertens 20:119–140, 1998.

67. Huang BS, Veerasingham SJ, Leenen FH. Brain "ouabain," ANG II, and sympathoexcitation by chronic central sodium loading in rats. Am J Physiol 274:H1269–H1276, 1998.

68. Lembo G, Rendina V, Iaccarino G, et al. Digitalis restores the

68. forearm sympathetic response to cardiopulmonary receptor unloading in hypertensive patients with left ventricular hypertrophy. J Hypertens 11:1395–1402, 1993.

69. Insel PA. Seminars in medicine of the Beth Israel Hospital, Boston. Adrenergic receptors—Evolving concepts and clinical implications. N Engl J Med 334:580–585, 1996.

70. Silverberg AB, Shah SD, Haymond MW, Cryer PE. Norepinephrine: Hormone and neurotransmitter in man. Am J Physiol 234:E252–E256, 1978.

71. Izzo JL Jr. Cardiovascular hormonal effects of circulating norepinephrine. Hypertension 5:787–789, 1983.

72. Licht MR, Izzo JL Jr. Humoral effect of norepinephrine on renin release in humans. Am J Hypertens 2:788–791, 1989.

73. Sloand JA, Hooper M, Izzo JL Jr. Effects of circulating norepinephrine on platelets, leukocytes, and RBC counts by alpha-1 adrenergic stimulation. Am J Cardiol 63:1140–1142, 1989.

74. Clayton S, Cross MJ. The aggregation of blood platelets by catecholamines and by thrombin. J Physiol (Lond) 169:82P–83P, 1963.

75. Vlachakis ND, Aledort L. Hypertension and propranolol therapy: Effect on blood pressure, plasma catecholamines, and platelet aggregation. Am J Cardiol 45:321–325, 1980.

76. Huang MH, Friend DS, Sunday ME, et al. An intrinsic adrenergic system in mammalian heart. J Clin Invest 98:1298–1303, 1996.

77. Abboud FM. An intrinsic cardiac adrenergic system can regulate cardiac development and function. J Clin Invest 98:1275–1276, 1996.

78. Chapleau MW, Hajduczok G, Abboud FM. Paracrine role of prostanoids in activation of arterial baroreceptors: An overview. Clin Exp Hypertens A Theory Pract 13:817–824, 1991.

79. Sharma RV, Chapleau MW, Hajduczok G, et al. Mechanical stimulation increases intracellular calcium concentration in nodose sensory neurons. Neuroscience 66:433–441, 1995.

80. Chapleau MW, Lu J, Hajduczok G, Abboud FM. Mechanism of baroreceptor adaptation in dogs: Attenuation of adaptation by the K+ channel blocker 4-aminopyridine. J Physiol 462:291–306, 1993.

81. Luft FC, Rankin LI, Henry DP, et al. Plasma and urinary norepinephrine at extremes of sodium intake in normal man. Hypertension 1:261–266, 1979.

82. Romoff MS, Kreusch G, Campese VM, et al. Effect of sodium intake on plasma catecholamines in normal subjects. J Clin Endocrinol Metab 48:26–31, 1979.

83. Izzo JL Jr, Sander E, Larrabee PS. Effect of postural stimulation on systemic hemodynamics and sympathetic nervous activity in systemic hypertension. Am J Cardiol 65:339–342, 1990.

84. Thames MD, Johnson LN. Impaired cardiopulmonary baroreflex control of renal nerves in renal hypertension. Circ Res 57:741–747, 1985.

85. Guo GB, Thames MD. Abnormal baroreflex control in renal hypertension is due to abnormal baroreceptors. Am J Physiol 245:420–428, 1983.

86. Thames MD, Miller BD, Abboud FM. Baroreflex regulation of renal nerve activity during volume expansion. Am J Physiol 243:810–814, 1982.

87. Simon AC, Safar ME, Weiss YA, et al. Baroreflex sensitivity and cardiopulmonary blood volume in normotensive and hypertensive patients. Br Heart J 39:799–805, 1977.

88. Tidgren B, Hjemdahl P, Theodorsson E, Nussberger J. Renal responses to lower body negative pressure in humans. Am J Physiol 259:F573–F579, 1990.

89. Schmedtje JF Jr, Varghese A, Gutkowska J, Taylor AA. Correlation of plasma norepinephrine and plasma atrial natriuretic factor during lower body negative pressure. Aviat Space Environ Med 61:555–558, 1990.

90. Joyner MJ, Shepherd JT, Seals DR. Sustained increases in sympathetic outflow during prolonged lower body negative pressure in humans. J Appl Physiol 68:1004–1009, 1990.

91. Westheim A, Os I, Kjeldsen SE, et al. Renal haemodynamic and sympathetic responses to head-up tilt in essential hypertension. Scand J Clin Lab Invest 50:815–822, 1990.

92. Eckberg DL, Abboud FM, Mark AL. Modulation of carotid baroreflex responsiveness in man: Effects of posture and propanolol. J Appl Physiol 41:383–387, 1976.

93. Thames MD, Schmid PG. Interaction between carotid and cardiopulmonary baroreflexes in control of plasma ADH. Am J Physiol 241:431–434, 1981.

94. Gribbin B, Pickering TG, Sleight P, Peto R. Effect of age and high blood pressure on baroreflex sensitivity in man. Circ Res 29:424–430, 1971.

95. Sleight P. Importance of cardiovascular reflexes in disease. Am J Med 84(suppl 3A):92–96, 1988.

96. Randall OS, Esler MD, Bulloch EG, et al. Relationship of age and blood pressure to baroreflex sensitivity and arterial compliance in man. Clin Sci Mol Med 51:357s–360s, 1976.

97. Olshan AR, O'Connor DT, Cohen IM, et al. Baroreflex dysfunction in patients with adult-onset diabetes and hypertension. Am J Med 74:233–242, 1983.

98. Matsukawa T, Gotoh E, Hasegawa O, et al. Reduced baroreflex changes in muscle sympathetic nerve activity during blood pressure elevation in essential hypertension. J Hypertens 9:537–542, 1991.

99. Goldstein DS. Arterial baroreflex sensitivity, plasma catecholamines, and pressor responsiveness in essential hypertension. Circulation 68:234–240, 1983.

100. Sanders JS, Ferguson DW, Mark AL. Arterial baroreflex control of sympathetic nerve activity during elevation of blood pressure in normal man: Dominance of aortic baroreflexes. Circulation 77:279–288, 1988.

101. Ismay JJA, Lumbers ER, Stevens AD. The action of angiotensin II on the baroreflex response of the conscious ewe and the conscious fetus. J Physiol 288:467–479, 1979.

102. Hajduczok C, Chapleau MW, Abboud FM. Increase in sympathetic activity with age. II: Role of impairment of cardiopulmonary baroreflexes. Am J Physiol 260:H1121–H1127, 1991.

103. Mark AL, Kerber RE. Augmentation of cardiopulmonary baroreflex control of forearm vascular resistance in borderline hypertension. Hypertension 4:39–46, 1982.

104. Rea RF, Hamdan M. Baroreflex control of muscle sympathetic nerve activity in borderline hypertension. Circulation 82:856–862, 1990.

105. Thames MD, Miller BD, Abboud FM. Sensitization of vagal cardiopulmonary baroreflex by chronic digoxin. Am J Physiol 243:815–818, 1982.

106. Saito M, Minokoshi Y, Shimazu T. Metabolic and sympathetic nerve activities of brown adipose tissue in tube-fed rats. Am J Physiol 257:E374–E378, 1989.

107. Rothwell NJ, Stock MJ. A role for brown adipose tissue in diet-induced thermogenesis. Obes Res 5:650–656, 1997.

108. Landsberg L, Young JB. Catecholamines and the adrenal medulla. In Wilson JD, Foster DW (eds). Textbook of Endocrinology, 7th ed. Philadelphia, WB Saunders, 1985; pp 891–965.

109. Kushiro T, Kobayashi F, Osada H, et al. Role of sympathetic activity in blood pressure reduction with low calorie regimen. Hypertension 17:965–968, 1991.

110. Andersson B, Elam M, Wallin BG, et al. Effect of energy-restricted diet on sympathetic muscle nerve activity in obese women. Hypertension 18:783–789, 1991.

111. Izzo JL Jr, Swislocki ALM. Symposium on insulin and cardiovascular disease. Workshop III—Insulin resistance: Is it truly the link? Am J Med 90(suppl 2A):26S–31S, 1991.

112. Bravo EL. Metabolic factors and the sympathetic nervous system. Am J Hypertens 2:339S–344S, 1989.

113. Kjeldsen SE, Rostrup M, Moan A, et al. The sympathetic nervous system may modulate the metabolic cardiovascular syndrome in essential hypertension. J Cardiovasc Pharmacol 20(suppl 8):S32–S39, 1992.

114. McKenzie ET, McCulloch J, O'Keane M, et al. Cerebral circulation and norepinephrine: Relevance of the blood-brain barrier. Am J Physiol 231:483–488, 1976.

115. Sadoshima S, Busjia D, Brody MJ, et al. Sympathetic nerves protect against stroke in stroke-prone hypertensive rats. Hypertension 3:124–127, 1981.

116. Sadoshima S, Thames M, Heistad DD. Cerebral blood flow during elevation of intracranial pressure: Role of sympathetic nerves. Am J Physiol 241:78–84, 1981.

117. Tuor UI. Acute hypertension and sympathetic stimulation: Local heterogeneous changes in cerebral blood flow. Am J Physiol 263:H511–H518, 1992.

118. Winder WW, Hickson RC, Hagberg JM, et al. Training-induced changes in hormonal and metabolic responses to submaximal exercise. J Appl Physiol 46:766–771, 1979.

119. Winder WW, Hagberg JM, Hickson RC, et al. Time course of sympathoadrenal adaptation to endurance exercise training in man. J Appl Physiol 45:370–374, 1978.

120. Paffenbarger RS Jr, Hyde RT, Wing AL, Hsieh C. Physical activity, all-cause mortality, and longevity of college alumni. N Engl J Med 314:605–613, 1986.

121. Cryer PE, Haymond MW, Shah SD, Santiago JV. Norepinephrine and epinephrine release and adrenergic medication of smoking-associated hemodynamic and metabolic effects. N Engl J Med 295:573–577, 1976.

122. Harburg E, Erfurt JC, Chape C, et al. Socioecological stressor areas and black-white blood pressure. Detroit J Chronic Dis 26:595–611, 1973.

123. Sokolow M, Werdegar D, Kain HK, Hinman AT. Relationship between level of blood pressure measured casually and by portable recorders and severity of complications in essential hypertension. Circulation 34:279–298, 1964.

124. Perloff D, Sokolow M, Cowan R. The prognostic value of ambulatory blood pressures. JAMA 249:2792–2798, 1983.

125. Pickering TG, Harshfield GA, Blank S, et al. Behavioral determinants of 24-hour blood pressure patterns in borderline hypertension. J Cardiovasc Pharmacol 8:89–92, 1986.

126. Clark LA, Denby L, Pregibon D, et al. A quantitative analysis of the effects of activity and time of day on the diurnal variations of blood pressure. J Chronic Dis 40:671–681, 1987.

127. Devereux RB, Pickering TG, Harshfield GA, et al. Left ventricular hypertrophy in patients with hypertension: Importance of blood pressure response to regularly recurring stress. Circulation 3:470–476, 1983.

128. Schnall PL, Pieper C, Schwartz JE, et al. The relationship between "job strain," workplace diastolic blood pressure, and left ventricular mass index. JAMA 263:1929–1935, 1990.

129. Schneider RH, Egan BM, Johnson EH, et al. Anger and anxiety in borderline hypertension. Psychosom Med 48:242–248, 1986.

130. Julius S, Petrin J. Autonomic nervous and behavioral factors in hypertension. In Laragh JH, Brenner BM (eds). Hypertension: Pathophysiology, Diagnosis, and Management. New York, Raven, 1990; pp 2083–2090.

131. Alderman MH, Madhaven S, Ooi WL, et al. Association of the renin-sodium profile with the risk of myocardial infarction in patients with hypertension. N Engl J Med 324:1098–1104, 1991.

132. Kapusta DR, Knardahl S, Koepke JP, et al. Selective central alpha-2 adrenoceptor control of regional haemodynamic responses to air jet stress in conscious spontaneously hypertensive rats. J Hypertens 7:189–194, 1989.

133. Hollenberg NK, Williams GH, Adams DF. Essential hypertension: Abnormal renal vascular and endocrine responses to a mild psychological stimulus. Hypertension 3:11–17, 1981.

134. Schmieder RE, Ruddel H, Schachinger H, et al. Renal hemodynamics and cardiovascular reactivity in the prehypertensive stage. Behav Med 19:5–12, 1993.

135. Kamm DE, Levinsky NG. The mechanism of denervation natriuresis. J Clin Invest 44:93, 1965.

136. Gill JR Jr, Mason DT, Bartter FC. Adrenergic nervous system in sodium metabolism: Effects of guanethidine and sodium-retaining steroids in normal man. J Clin Invest 43:177, 1964.

137. Wagner HN Jr. The influence of autonomic vasoregulatory reflexes on the rate of sodium and water excretion in man. J Clin Invest 36:1319, 1956.

138. Matsuoka H, Nishida H, Nomura G, et al. Hypertension induced by nitric oxide synthesis inhibition is renal nerve dependent. Hypertension 23:971–975, 1994.

139. Panza JA, Epstein SE, Quyyumi AA. Circadian variation in vascular tone and its relation to alpha-sympathetic vasoconstrictor activity. N Engl J Med 325:986–1039, 1991.

140. Watson RDS, Hamilton CA, Reid JL, Littler WA. Changes in plasma norepinephrine, blood pressure and heart rate during physical activity in hypertensive man. Hypertension 1:341–346, 1979.

141. Floras JS, Hassan O, Vann Jones J, et al. Factors influencing blood pressure and heart rate variability in hypertensive humans. Hypertension 11:273–281, 1988.

142. Sundberg S, Kohvakka A, Gordin A. Rapid reversal of circadian blood pressure rhythm in shift workers. J Hypertens 6:394–396, 1988.

143. Floras JS, Jones JV, Johnston JA, et al. Arousal and the circadian rhythm of blood pressure. Clin Sci Mol Med 55:395s–397s, 1978.

144. Feller RP, Hale HB. Human sympatho-adrenal responsiveness in autumn, winter and spring. Technical document, Rep. SAM-TDR-63-46. Brooks Air Force Base, TX, USAF School of Aerospace Medicine, 1963.

145. Izzo JL Jr, Larrabee PS, Sander E, Lillis LM. Hemodynamics of seasonal adaptation. Am J Hypertens 3:405–407, 1990.

146. Hata T, Ogihara T, Maruyama A, et al. The seasonal variation of blood pressure in patients with essential hypertension. Clin Exp Hypertens 3:341–354, 1982.

147. Muller JE, Stone PH, Turi ZG, et al. Circadian variation in the frequency of onset of acute myocardial infarction. N Engl J Med 313:1315–1322,1985.

148. Tofler GH, Brezinski D, Schafer AI, et al. Concurrent morning increase in platelet aggregability and the risk of myocardial infarction and sudden cardiac death. N Engl J Med 316:1514–1518, 1987.

149. Argentino C, Toni D, Rasura M, et al. Circadian variation in the frequency of ischemic stroke. Stroke 21:387–389, 1990.

150. Anderson T, Le Riche W. Cold weather and myocardial infarction. Lancet 1:291–296, 1970.

151. Protos A, Caracta A, Gross L. The seasonal susceptibility to myocardial infarction. J Am Geriatr Soc 19:526–535, 1971.

152. Mann GV, Garrett HL, Farhi A, et al. Exercise to prevent coronary heart disease. An experimental study of the effects of training on risk factors for coronary disease in men. Am J Med 46:12–27, 1969.

153. Bean WB, Mills CA. Coronary occlusion, heart failure and environmental temperatures. Am Heart J 16:701–713, 1938.

154. Ely D, Caplea A, Dunphy G, et al. Spontaneously hypertensive rat Y chromosome increases indexes of sympathetic nervous system activity. Hypertension 29:613–618, 1997.

155. Kumai T, Tanaka M, Watanabe M, et al. Possible involvement of androgen in increased norepinephrine synthesis in blood vessels of spontaneously hypertensive rats. Jpn J Pharmacol 66:439–444, 1994.

156. Robertson D, Goldberg MR, Onrot J, et al. Isolated failure of autonomic neurotransmission. Evidence for impaired beta-hydroxylation of dopamine. N Engl J Med 314:1494–1497, 1986.

157. Masuo K, Mikami H, Ogihara T, Tuck ML. Familial hypertension, insulin, sympathetic activity, and blood pressure elevation. Hypertension 32:96–100, 1998.

158. Masuo K, Mikami H, Ogihara T, Tuck ML. Differences in insulin and sympathetic responses to glucose ingestion due to family history of hypertension. Am J Hypertens 9:739–745, 1996.

159. Manuck SB, Polefrone JM, Terrell DF, et al. Absence of enhanced sympathoadrenal activity and behaviorally evoked cardiovascular reactivity among offspring of hypertensives. Am J Hypertens 9:248–255, 1996.

160. Takiyyuddin MA, Parmer RJ, Kailasam MT, et al. Chromogranin A in human hypertension. Influence of heredity. Hypertension 26:213–220, 1995.

161. Fredrickson M, Tuomisto M, Bergman-Losman B. Neuroendocrine and cardiovascular stress reactivity in middle-aged normotensive adults with parental history of cardiovascular disease. Psychophysiology 28:656–664, 1991.

162. Ferrara LA, Moscato TS, Pisanti N, et al. Is the sympathetic nervous system altered in children with familial history of arterial hypertension? Cardiology 75:200–205, 1988.

163. Ferrier C, Cox H, Esler M. Elevated total body noradrenaline spillover in normotensive members of hypertensive families. Clin Sci 84:225–230, 1993.

164. Noll G, Wenzel RR, Schneider M, et al. Increased activation of sympathetic nervous system and endothelin by mental stress in normotensive offspring of hypertensive parents. Circulation 93:866–869, 1996.

165. Calhoun DA, Mutinga ML. Race, family history of hypertension, and sympathetic response to cold pressor testing. Blood Press 6:209–213, 1997.

166. Miller SB, Ditto B. Exaggerated sympathetic nervous system response to extended psychological stress in offspring of hypertensives. Psychophysiology 28:103–113, 1991.

167. Parmer RJ, Cervenka JH, Stone RA. Baroreflex sensitivity and heredity in essential hypertension. Circulation 85:497–503, 1992.

168. Levy RL, White PD, Stroud WD, Hillman CC. Transient tachycardia: Prognostic significance alone and in association with transient hypertension. JAMA 129:585–588, 1945.

169. Nicholls MG, Julius S, Zweifler AJ. Withdrawal of endogenous sympathetic drive lowers blood pressure in primary aldosteronism. Clin Endocrinol (Oxf) 15:253–258, 1981.

170. Simon G, Kiowski W, Julius S. Effect of beta adrenoceptor antagonists on baroreceptor reflex sensitivity in hypertension. Clin Pharmacol Ther 22:293–298, 1977.

171. Goldstein DS, Keiser HR. Neural circulatory control in the hyperdynamic circulation syndrome. Am Heart J 109:387–390, 1985.

172. Lee RM, Borkowski KR, Leenen FH, et al. Interaction between sympathetic nervous system and adrenal medulla in the control of cardiovascular changes in hypertension. J Cardiovasc Pharmacol 17(suppl 2):S114–S116, 1991.

173. Goldstein DS. Plasma catecholamines and essential hypertension: An analytical review. Hypertension 5:86–99, 1983.

174. Masuo K, Mikami H, Ogihara T, Tuck ML. Sympathetic nerve hyperactivity precedes hyperinsulinemia and blood pressure elevation in a young, nonobese Japanese population. Am J Hypertens 10:77–83, 1997.

175. Julius S, Krause L, Schork NJ, et al. Hyperkinetic borderline hypertension in Tecumseh, Michigan. J Hypertens 9:77–84, 1991.

176. Hofman A, Boomsma F, Schalekamp MADH, Valkenburg HA. Raised blood pressure and plasma noradrenaline concentrations in teenagers and young adults selected from an open population. BMJ 1:1536–1538, 1979.

177. Takiyyuddin MA, Cervenka JH, Hsaio RJ, et al. Chromogranin A. Storage and release in hypertension. Hypertension 15:237–246, 1990.

178. Januszewicz W, Wocial B. Urinary excretion of catecholamines and their metabolites in patients with renovascular hypertension. Jpn Heart J 19:468–478, 1978.

179. Saito I, Takeshita E, Hayashi S, et al. Comparison of clinic and home blood pressure levels and the role of the sympathetic nervous system in clinic-home differences. Am J Hypertens 3:219–224, 1990.

180. Horky K, Kopecka J, Greogorova I, Dvorakova J. Relationship between plasma renin activity and urinary catecholamines in various types of hypertension. Endokrinologie 67:331–342, 1976.

181. Esler MD, Jennings GL, Johns J, et al. Estimation of "total" renal, cardiac and splanchnic sympathetic nervous tone in essential hypertension from measurements of noradrenaline release. J Hypertens Suppl 2:S123–S125, 1984.

182. Esler M, Ferrier C, Lambert G, et al. Biochemical evidence of sympathetic hyperactivity in human hypertension. Hypertension 17(suppl III):III-29–III-35, 1991.

183. Esler M, Lambert G, Jennings GL. Increased regional sympathetic nervous activity in human hypertension: Causes and consequences. J Hypertens 8:553–557, 1990.

184. Ferrier C, Esler MD, Eisenhofer G, et al. Increased norepinephrine spillover into the jugular veins in essential hypertension. Hypertension 19:62–69, 1992.

185. Morlin C, Wallin BG, Eriksson BM. Muscle sympathetic activity and plasma noradrenaline in normotensive and hypertensive man. Acta Physiol Scand 119:117–121, 1983.

186. Wallin BG, Morlin C, Hjemdahl P. Muscle sympathetic activity and venous plasma noradrenaline concentrations during static exercise in normotensive and hypertensive subjects. Acta Physiol Scand 129:489–497, 1987.

187. Anderson EA, Sinkey CA, Lawton WJ, Mark AL. Elevated sympathetic nerve activity in borderline hypertensive humans. Evidence from direct intraneural recordings. Hypertension 14:177–183, 1989.

188. Floras JS, Hara K. Sympathoneural and haemodynamic characteristics of young subjects with mild essential hypertension. J Hypertens 11:647–655, 1993.

189. Wallin BG, Thompson JM, Jennings GL, Esler MD. Renal noradrenaline spillover correlates with muscle sympathetic activity in humans. J Physiol 491:881–887, 1996.

190. Hajduczok G, Chapleau MW, Abboud FM. Rapid adaptation of central pathways explains the suppressed baroreflex with aging. Neurobiol Aging 12:601–604, 1991.

191. Vaz M, Jennings G, Turner A, et al. Regional sympathetic nervous activity and oxygen consumption in obese normotensive human subjects. Circulation 96:3423–3429, 1997.

192. Grassi G, Seravalle G, Cattaneo BM, et al. Sympathetic activation in obese normotensive subjects. Hypertension 25:560–563, 1995.

193. Gudbjornsdottir S, Lonnroth P, Sverrisdottir YB, et al. Sympathetic nerve activity and insulin in obese normotensive and hypertensive men [published erratum appears in Hypertension 27:1030, 1996]. Hypertension 27:276–280, 1996.

194. Ferrannini E, DeFronzo RA. The association of hypertension, diabetes, and obesity: A review. J Nephrol 1:3–15, 1989.

195. DeFronzo RA, Ferrannini E. Insulin resistance: A multifaceted syndrome responsible for NIDDM, obesity, hypertension, dyslipidemia, and atherosclerotic cardiovascular disease. Diabetes Care 14:173–194, 1991.

196. Court JM, Hill GJ. Hypertension in childhood obesity. Aust Paediatr J 10:296–300, 1974.

197. Kannel WB, Brand N, Skinner JJ, MacNamera P. The relation of adiposity to blood pressure and development of hypertension: The Framingham study. Ann Intern Med 67:48–49, 1976.

198. Stamler R, Stamler J, Riedlinger WF, et al. Weight and blood pressure findings in hypertension screening of 1 million Americans. JAMA 240:1607–1610, 1978.

199. Sowers JR, Whitfield LA, Catania RA, et al. Role of the sympathetic nervous system in blood pressure maintenance in obesity. J Clin Endocrinol Metab 54:1181–1186, 1982.

200. Daly PA, Landsberg L. Hypertension in obesity and NIDDM. Role of insulin and sympathetic nervous system. Diabetes Care 14:240–248, 1991.

201. Facchini FS, Stoohs RA, Reaven GM. Enhanced sympathetic nervous system activity. The linchpin between insulin resistance, hyperinsulinemia, and heart rate. Am J Hypertens 9:1013–1017, 1996.

202. Rowe JW, Young JB, Minaker KL, et al. Effect of insulin and glucose infusions on sympathetic nervous system activity in normal man. Diabetes 30:219–225, 1981.

203. Reaven GM, Lithell H, Landsberg L. Hypertension and associated metabolic abnormalities—The role of insulin resistance and the sympathoadrenal system. N Engl J Med 334:374–381, 1996.

204. Petersen JS, DiBona GF. Acute sympathoinhibitory actions of metformin in spontaneously hypertensive rats. Hypertension 27:619–625, 1996.

205. Jamerson K, Smith SD, Amerena J, et al. Vasoconstriction with norepinephrine causes less forearm insulin resistance than a reflex sympathetic vasoconstriction. Hypertension 23:1006–1011, 1994.

206. Rocchini AP, Mao HZ, Babu K, Rocchini AJ. Clonidine prevents insulin resistance and hypertension in obese dogs. Hypertension 32:592, 1998.

207. Egan B, Panis R, Hinderliter A, et al. Mechanism of increased alpha adrenergic vasoconstriction in human essential hypertension. J Clin Invest 80:812–817, 1987.

208. Philipp T, Distler A, Cordes U. Sympathetic nervous system and blood pressure control in essential hypertension. Lancet 2:959–963, 1978.

209. Kiowski W, van Brummelen P, Buhler FR. Plasma noradrenaline correlates with alpha-adrenoceptor–mediated vasoconstriction and blood pressure in patients with essential hypertension. Clin Sci 57:177S–180S, 1979.

210. Pratt JH, Manatunga AK, Bowsher RR, Henry DP. The interaction of norepinephrine excretion with blood pressure and race in children. J Hypertens 10:93–96, 1992.

211. Stepniakowski KT, Lu G, Miller GD, Egan BM. Fatty acids, not insulin, modulate alpha1-adrenergic reactivity in dorsal hand veins. Hypertension 30:1150–1155, 1997.

212. DeQuattro V, Campese V, Miura Y, Meijer D. Increased plasma catecholamines in high renin hypertension. Am J Cardiol 38:801–804, 1976.

213. Esler M, Julius S, Zweifler A, et al. Mild high-renin essential hypertension: Neurogenic human hypertension? N Engl J Med 296:405–411, 1977.

214. Schmieder RE, Veelken R, Schobel H, et al. Glomerular hyperfiltration during sympathetic nervous system activation in early essential hypertension. J Am Soc Nephrol; 8:893–900, 1997.

215. Freis ED. Origins and development of antihypertensive treatment. In Laragh JH, Brenner BM (eds). Hypertension: Pathophysiology, Diagnosis, and Management. New York, Raven, 1990; pp 2093–2105.

216. Louis WJ, Doyle AE, Anavekar S. Plasma norepinephrine levels in essential hypertension. N Engl J Med 288:599–601, 1973.

217. Izzo JL Jr, Licht MR, Smith RJ, et al. Chronic effects of direct vasodilation (Pinacidil), alpha-adrenergic blockade (Prazosin) and angiotensin-converting enzyme inhibition (Captopril) in systemic hypertension. Am J Cardiol 60:303–308, 1987.

218. Goldstein DS, Levinson PD, Zimlichman R, et al. Clonidine suppression testing in essential hypertension. Ann Intern Med 102:42–48, 1985.

219. Messerli FH, Frohlich ED, Suarez DH, et al. Borderline hypertension: Relationship between age, hemodynamics and circulating catecholamines. Circulation 64:760–764, 1981.

220. Izzo JL Jr, Smith RJ, Larrabee PS, Kallay MC. Plasma norepinephrine and age as determinants of systemic hemodynamics in men with established essential hypertension. Hypertension 9:415–419, 1987.

221. Izzo JL Jr. Hypertension in the elderly: A pathophysiologic approach to therapy. J Am Geriatr Soc 30:352–359, 1982.

222. O'Malley K, Docherty JR, Kelly JG. Adrenoceptor status and cardiovascular function in ageing. J Hypertens Suppl 6:S59–S62, 1988.

223. Ward KD, Sparrow D, Landsberg L, et al. Influence of insulin, sympathetic nervous system activity, and obesity on blood pressure: The Normative Aging Study. J Hypertens 14:301–308, 1996.

224. Cerasola G, Cottone S, D'Ignoto G, et al. Sympathetic activity in borderline and established hypertension in the elderly. J Hypertens Suppl 6:S55–S58, 1988.

225. Esler M, Skews H, Leonard P, et al. Age-dependence of noradrenaline kinetics in normal subjects. Clin Sci 60:217–219, 1981.

226. Esler MD, Turner AG, Kaye DM, et al. Aging effects on human sympathetic neuronal function. Am J Physiol 268:R278–R285, 1995.

227. Drolet G, Bouvier M, de Champlain J. Enhanced sympathoadrenal reactivity to haemorrhagic stress in DOCA-salt hypertensive rats. J Hypertens 7:237–242, 1989.

228. Chen Y, Nagahama S, Winternitz SR, Oparil S. Hyperresponsiveness of monoaminergic mechanisms in DOCA/NaCl hypertensive rats. Am J Physiol 249:H71–H79, 1985.

229. Zambraski EJ, Ciccone CD, Izzo JL Jr. The role of the sympathetic nervous system in 2-kidney DOCA-hypertensive Yucatan miniature swine. Clin Exp Hypertens A Theory Pract 8:411–424, 1986.

230. Thomas GD, O'Hagan KP, Zambraski EJ. Chemical sympathectomy alters the development of hypertension in miniature swine. Hypertension 17:357–362, 1991.

231. Moreau P, Drolet G, Yamaguchi N, de Champlain J. Role of presynaptic beta 2-adrenergic facilitation in the development and maintenance of DOCA-salt hypertension. Am J Hypertens 6:1016–1024, 1993.

232. Saavedra JM. Brain catecholamines during development of DOCA-salt hypertension in rats. Brain Res 179:121–127, 1979.

233. Veelken R, Hilgers KF, Ditting T, et al. Impaired cardiovascular reflexes precede deoxycorticosterone acetate–salt hypertension. Hypertension 24:564–570, 1994.

234. Katholi RE, Winternitz SR, Oparil S. Role of the renal nerves in the pathogenesis of one-kidney renal hypertension in the rat. Hypertension 3:404–409, 1981.

235. Katholi RE, Whitlow PL, Winternitz SR, Oparil S. Importance of the renal nerves in established two-kidney, one-clip Goldblatt hypertension in the rat. Hypertension 4:166–174, 1982.

236. Winternitz SR, Katholi RE, Oparil S. Decrease in hypothalamic norepinephrine content following renal denervation in the one-kidney one-clip Goldblatt hypertensive rat. Hypertension 4:369–373, 1982.

237. Katholi RE, Winternitz SR, Oparil S. Decrease in peripheral sympathetic nervous system activity following renal denervation or unclipping in the one-kidney one-clip Goldblatt hypertensive rat. J Clin Invest 69:55–62, 1982.

238. Winternitz SR, Oparil S. Importance of the renal nerves in the pathogenesis of experimental hypertension. Hypertension 5:108–114, 1982.

239. Dargie HL, Franklin SS, Reid JL. The sympathetic nervous system in renovascular hypertension in the rat. Br J Pharmacol 56:365–374, 1976.

240. Wyss JM, Aboukarsh N, Oparil S. Sensory denervation of the kidney attenuates renovascular hypertension in the rat. Am J Physiol 250:H82–H86, 1986.

241. Wyss JM, Aboukarsh N, Oparil S. Selective lesion of the renal afferents transiently lowers blood pressure in established 1 kidney, 1 clip Goldblatt hypertension. Circulation 70:429–435, 1984.

242. Campese VM, Romoff MS, Levitan D, et al. Mechanisms of autonomic nervous system dysfunction in uremia. Kidney Int 20:246–253, 1981.

243. Izzo JL Jr, Sterns RH. Abnormal norepinephrine release in uremia. Kidney Int 24(suppl 16):s221–s223, 1983.

244. Izzo JL Jr, Santarosa RP, Larrabee PS, et al. Increased plasma norepinephrine and sympathetic nervous activity in essential hypertensive and uremic humans: Effects of clonidine. J Cardiovasc Pharmacol 10(suppl 12):S225–S229, 1987.

245. Converse RL Jr, Jacobsen TN, Toto RD, et al. Sympathetic overactivity in patients with chronic renal failure. N Engl J Med 327:1912–1918, 1992.

246. Campese VM. Neurogenic factors and hypertension in chronic renal failure. J Nephrol 10:184–187, 1997.

247. Bravo EL, Tarazi RC, Fouad FM, et al. Clonidine-suppression test: A useful aid in the diagnosis of pheochromocytoma. N Engl J Med 305:623–626, 1981.

248. Schobel HP, Fischer T, Heuszer K, et al. Preeclampsia—A state of sympathetic overactivity. N Engl J Med 335:1480–1485, 1996.

249. Mancia G, Di Rienzo M, Parati G, Grassi G. Sympathetic activity, blood pressure variability and end organ damage in hypertension. J Hum Hypertens 11(suppl 1):S3–S8, 1997.

250. Korner PI, Jennings GL, Esler MD, Broughton A. Role of cardiac and vascular amplifiers in the maintenance of hypertension and the effect of reversal of cardiovascular hypertrophy. Clin Exp Pharmacol Physiol 12:205–209, 1985.

251. Korner P, Bobik A, Oddie C, Friberg P. Sympathoadrenal system is critical for structural changes in genetic hypertension. Hypertension 22:243–252, 1993.

252. Mangiarua EI, Lee RM. Morphometric study of cerebral arteries from spontaneously hypertensive and stroke-prone spontaneously hypertensive rats. J Hypertens 10:1183–1190, 1992.

253. Yamori Y, Nakada T, Lovenberg W. Effect of antihypertensive therapy on lysine incorporation into vascular protein of the spontaneously hypertensive rat. Eur J Pharmacol 38:349–355, 1976.

254. Grassi G, Giannattasio C, Failla M, et al. Sympathetic modulation of radial artery compliance in congestive heart failure. Hypertension 26:348–354, 1995.

255. Julius S, Li Y, Brant D, et al. Neurogenic pressor episodes fail to cause hypertension, but do induce cardiac hypertrophy. Hypertension 13:422–429, 1989.

256. Fujita T, Noda H, Ito Y, et al. Increased sympathoadrenomedullary activity and left ventricular hypertrophy in young patients with borderline hypertension. J Mol Cell Cardiol 21(suppl 5):31–38, 1989.

257. Brush JE Jr, Eisenhofer G, Garty M, et al. Cardiac norepinephrine kinetics in hypertrophic cardiomyopathy. Circulation 79:836–844, 1989.

258. Moss AJ, Schenk EA. Cardiovascular effects of sustained norepinephrine infusions in dogs. IV: Previous treatment with adrenergic blocking agents. Circ Res 27:1013–1022, 1970.

259. Levine TB, Francis GS, Goldsmith SR, et al. Activity of the sympathetic nervous system and renin-angiotensin system assessed by plasma hormone levels and their relation to hemodynamic abnormalities in congestive heart failure. Am J Cardiol 49:1659–1666, 1982.

260. Cohn JN, Levine TB, Olivari MT, et al. Plasma norepinephrine as a guide to prognosis in patients with chronic congestive heart failure. N Engl J Med 311:819–823, 1984.

CHAPTER

6 Environmental and Psychosocial Stress in Hypertension Onset and Progression

Kathleen C. Light

Life events that evoke negative emotions like anger, fear, and sadness have long been known to produce temporary elevations in blood pressure (BP).[1, 2] Since the application of standardized laboratory experimental methods has become widely used to assess cardiovascular and neuroendocrine responses (psychophysiological stress testing), a large body of evidence has shown that many other experiences also lead to short-term pressor responses. These experiences range from cognitive to physical challenges and positive as well as negative emotional states. These laboratory studies have also shown that different adrenergic and hemodynamic patterns are involved during different types of stressors. Challenging tasks involving active coping and mental effort typically elicit a state involving increased β-adrenergic receptor activity characterized by increased heart rate, cardiac output, cardiac contractile force (frequently indicated by decreased preejection period) and vasodilatation in skeletal muscle.[3–5] This state is similar to the pattern originally identified through studies in animal models as "preparation for fight or flight" or the defense reaction, which is characterized by enhanced activity of the sympathetic adrenomedullary system.[6, 7] Events that incorporate aspects of frustration, passive coping, loss of control, or helplessness tend to evoke less β-adrenergic activity and less cardiac activation but instead result in greater vasoconstriction, presumably owing to α-adrenergic activity.[3–5] This pattern resembles the "defeat reaction" of animal models, which is characterized by overactivity of the hypothalamic-pituitary-adrenocortical (HPAC) system.[6, 7]

These psychophysiological stress studies have also shown that even when the stressors themselves are highly standardized, individuals differ greatly in the magnitude of BP increase evoked.[3] Those individuals who demonstrate BP increases that place them in the top 25% of those studied are often labeled *high stress reactors*. An active hypothesis guiding considerable research has focused on these hyperresponsive persons as a group that may be at increased risk of developing hypertension.[8] Studies have also shown that healthy normotensive men and women differ in their stress responses, with men showing greater systolic BP increases, greater vasodilatation during stressors evoking β-adrenergic activation, and greater vasoconstriction during stressors evoking α-adrenergic activation.[5, 9] Men also show slower return of BP to prestress levels (slow recovery) after the stressful event has ended.[9] These gender differences are enhanced when women are tested in the phase of their menstrual cycle when female reproductive hormones, particularly estrogen and progesterone, are higher than when these are low. Estrogen has vasodilator effects, which may underlie both this observation and other findings suggesting that postmenopausal

women have enhanced stress-induced BP increases compared with premenopausal women.[10, 11] Ethnic differences in cardiovascular stress responses have also been shown in both normotensive and hypertensive adults, with African Americans demonstrating greater vasoconstriction during stress and sometimes greater BP increases than European Americans.[4, 12, 13] African Americans more frequently demonstrate another potentially maladaptive response to short-term stress exposure—increased sodium retention. This response, like exaggerated BP increases during stress, has been shown to occur more frequently in persons with risk factors for hypertension, including borderline hypertension and positive family history of hypertension.[14–16]

Laboratory stress studies in normotensive and hypertensive humans can be very informative about patterns of cardiovascular responses. They can also document the stability of high and low reactivity in a variety of cardiovascular measures. Stability at acceptable levels has been documented over periods ranging from weeks to months to as long as 10 years.[3, 8, 17] However, such studies cannot establish the long-term predictive significance of stress or of stress reactivity in the onset or progression of hypertension. This critical issue has been addressed in several other ways. This review summarizes recent findings in the following areas: (1) animal models involving stress showing progression to hypertension; (2) human studies showing relationship of environmental factors or personality or behavioral patterns to the development of hypertension; (3) prospective long-term follow-up studies of normotensive individuals characterized as high and low stress reactors; and (4) evidence that stress buffers and stress-management interventions are related to lower BP.

ANIMAL MODELS OF STRESS-RELATED HYPERTENSION

One of the most influential leaders in the field of stress exposure, patterns of response, and health consequences was James P. Henry.[7] His model of stress-related hypertension in mice induced by social environments that increase territorial confrontations provided some of the strongest evidence to date that chronic stress exposure can indeed be a key precipitating factor in the pathogenesis of hypertension. The development of sustained hypertension was evident in dominant males (mean BP levels of 145 mm Hg) and was worsened in subdominant males (those just below the dominant ones in social status; mean levels of 160 mm Hg) but not in the truly subordinate males (mean levels of 125 mm Hg). The elevation was greater when the colony members were changed frequently versus when stable dominance hierarchies were allowed to remain intact. According to the interpretation of Henry and Stephens, dominant males showed a classic defense reaction with sympathetic activation as they exerted themselves but maintained control. Subdominant animals showed a more extreme defense reaction associated with striving but incomplete control. Subordinate animals showed a defeat reaction with enhanced corticosterone and HPAC activity.[18] In keeping with this as the era of genetic and molecular biology, it is important to emphasize that even in this model of social environmental hypertension, genetic influences are critical.

When Henry extended his work on social stress from mice to rats, he compared chronic social stress effects in rat strains that normally do not develop hypertension in standard laboratory environments.[7, 19] Wistar-Kyoto hyperactive rats, classified as very peaceable, showed no BP rise with chronic unstable social environments, whereas the moderately peaceable Sprague-Dawley animals showed some rise in BP, and the aggressive Long-Evans rats showed much larger increases in BP, with rise in BP positively correlated with number of scars from aggressive encounters. This research has recently been extended by Mormede, who reports that among six rat strains, both behavioral and adrenal and heart weight evidence can be used to identify those strains more vulnerable to social stress.[20] However, even strains showing high social stress sensitivity must also have related target organ vulnerability (renal, cardiac, or vascular) before the excess sympathetic adrenomedullary activity evoked by chronic social instability results in sustained BP increases.[20, 21]

A second prominent model of stress-related hypertension is the borderline hypertensive rat (BHR) as developed and studied by Lawler and colleagues.[22–26] This first-generation backcross of a spontaneously hypertensive rat (SHR) with a normotensive Wistar Kyoto rat typically develops only high-normal or borderline hypertension in the usual laboratory environment. With daily exposure to a brief period of a shock avoidance conflict task for 16 weeks, the BHRs develop hypertension with target organ damage that persists even if the stress exposure is terminated. This stress-induced hypertension is blunted if the animals receive daily swimming exercise as well as the conflict task (Fig. 6–1).[25] Hypertension also develops in BHRs if they are placed on a high intake of salt, and the combination of high salt and stress leads to greater adverse cardiovascular effects than either environmental factor individually.

A primary role for renal involvement in the hypertension resulting from either high stress or high salt is suggested by the observation that renal denervation delays onset of the rise in pressure. Work by DiBona and associates has shown that stress induces greater increases in sodium retention in SHRs and BHRs than in normotensive rat strains, and that this effect of stress can be prevented by renal denervation or reduction in central sympathetic outflow owing to administration of sympathetically active agents into the ventricles of the brain.[27–29] Lawler and colleagues have reported that in the early period of stress exposure plus high salt, norepinephrine content decreases in nuclei of the hypothalamus that are known to be involved in the classic defense reaction.[24]

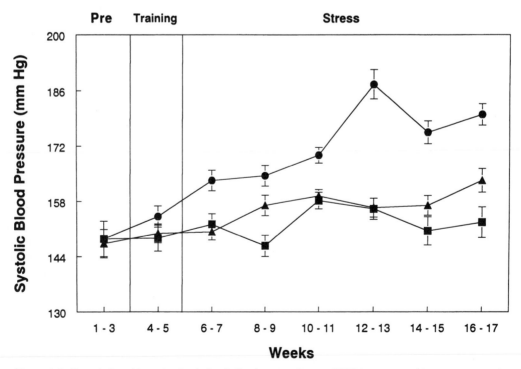

Figure 6–1. Stress-induced hypertension in borderline hypertensive rats (BHR) is attenuated by concurrent swim training. Mean (±SEM) tail cuff systolic blood pressure for each 2-week period before the stress manipulations (Pre), during the 2 weeks when the stress was being progressively lengthened (Training), and during the 12 weeks of daily swim or tail shock, or both (Stress), in rats exposed to daily shock plus swim training *(triangles)*, shock only *(circles)*, or neither intervention *(squares)*. (From Cox RH, Hubbard JW, Lawler JE, et al. Exercise training attenuates stress-induced hypertension in the rat. Hypertension 7:747–751, 1985.)

A third animal model of stress-related hypertension described by Anderson and coworkers is the mongrel dog exposed to daily shock avoidance while on increased salt and low potassium intake.[30-32] This model requires both stress exposure and high salt intake to induce hypertension; neither factor alone is sufficient. The reversible hypertension that results involves retention of sodium, and either renal denervation or potassium supplementation is sufficient to prevent or reverse hypertension in this model. Thus, even in animals lacking clear genetic predisposition, a reversible form of hypertension may arise when three adverse environmental factors are present: excessive salt, potassium deficiency, and regular stress exposure.

These animal models provide the most definitive evidence to date that chronic life stress exposure can contribute to the development of hypertension in individuals with genetic susceptibility and/or when combined with other adverse environmental factors such as a high-salt/low-potassium diet. These observations lay the foundation for studies of environmental stress in humans, which cannot provide such direct and definitive evidence but do show important associations with parallels to the animal models.

ENVIRONMENTAL STRESS EXPOSURE: CHRONIC JOB OR HOME LIFE STRESS AND ACUTE TRAUMATIC STRESS

Observations of people who move from stable, rural, traditional societies to unstable, urban, Westernized environments have indicated that contemporary urban conditions contribute to increases in BP over the life span.[33] For example, the nomadic Samburo warriors of Kenya show no BP increase with age in their traditional environment, yet when they join the Kenyan military, they show BP increases similar to those of recruits from more urban areas.[34, 35] The principal factors that change with such a move and are believed to contribute to the pressure rise include: (1) diet, (2) physical activity, (3) increased obesity, (4) reduction of supportive ties to the family and larger community, and (5) increased mental effort and active coping to perform work and home life activities under time pressure and competition. Waldron and colleagues, after examining BP data from 84 different cultures and social groups, concluded that BP increases were independent of changes in salt intake and obesity (in men), and that the remaining factors, particularly economic competition and loss of family ties, appear to be the more universal contributing causes.[36]

Among Westernized societies, both urban and rural, people with less education, lower-status occupations, less total household income, and generally lower socioeconomic status (SES) have higher BP.[37] Although African Americans have on average fewer educational and economic resources and higher BP than age-matched European Americans, ethnic differences do not account for these differences in BP between lower and higher SES groups. Clear BP differences are seen between lower and higher SES African Americans, as between lower and higher SES whites and members of other ethnic minorities. Sources of these group differences have been reviewed by Anderson and associates.[38, 39] All explanations involve multiple contributing factors, including *chronic stress,* defined as increased frequency of threats to the well-being of the individual and her or his close family and friends. This definition of chronic stress is so general that it leaves completely open which specific elements that differ between SES groups are most critical in their impact on BP. However, its generality is also one of its strengths in that it spans both the objective and the more individualized subjective perception of actual and anticipated life experiences as components of the stress exposure. Thus, it leaves room for individual differences in response to the same experience and for multiple models focusing on specific dimensions of low SES, such as economic insecurity or lack of control at work or at home.

One specific model that grew from the observed SES differences in BP is Dressler's model of lifestyle incongruity.[40] This model associates increased chronic stress and sympathetic nervous system activity with the extent to which the individual's material acquisitions are higher than average for his or her occupation and income level (i.e., living beyond one's means). High lifestyle incongruity has been associated with increased BP levels. Dressler's current model also addresses incongruity in regard to noneconomic issues that are related to expectations about behavior and multiple roles or status within the family and community. Both economic and social incongruity appear to act, in part, through another important factor—reduction in social support from family and other sources.

Low occupational status and low control within the workplace are associated with lower SES, and both have been associated with increased job stress. Ever since early work by Rose and coworkers on air traffic controllers,[41] the hypothesis that daily stress exposure on the job may contribute to hypertension has been gaining support. Karasek and colleagues' model of "job strain" was developed to formalize the study of stress on the job across a variety of occupations.[42] Job strain focuses on two dimensions of work stress: (1) psychological demands, i.e., how hard and how fast the worker perceives she or he must work, and (2) job decision latitude, i.e., the level of control over the nature and pace of the work. *Job strain* is defined as occurring when high psychological demand occurs together with low decision latitude.

Research on job strain as a contributing stress exposure factor in the onset and exacerbation of elevated BP has included over 14 studies since the late 1980s. As summarized by Pickering, the method of BP assessment is critical.[33] Clinic assessments of BP are more time-efficient, but ambulatory BP obtained at intervals of every few minutes throughout a normal weekday spent at work and at home has distinct advantages for assessing response to daily work life demands at work and as they spill over to influence responses after work. Of 7 studies using clinic assessments only, none has found a relationship between job strain and increased BP. Of another 7 studies that employed ambulatory monitoring, all but 1 have observed a positive relationship for men. The most definitive work has come from Schnall and associates, who have shown that job strain is related to higher BP at work and also at home and during sleep, to increased left ventricular mass, and to hypertensive status in a case-control study in 196 men.[43, 44] They have also reported that job strain interacts with age such that the increase in BP with age is greater for high–job strain men, and that the combination of high job strain and increased alcohol use is related to greater increases in BP. Further, in a 3-year follow-up study, this research team found that increases in pressure over time are greater for high–job strain than low–job strain men, controlling for BP at study entry.

High work demand and low control on the job have been related to increased urinary epinephrine but not cortisol,[45] suggesting that enhanced adrenergic receptor activity may contribute to the BP increase in high–job strain individuals. It is worth noting that research reported by Pickering[33] and another study by Light and coworkers[46] have observed no increase in work BP in women reporting job strain, although men in the same study showed the predicted relationship. This observation is consistent with recent work by Lundberg[47] and by Luecken and colleagues[48] suggesting that stress related to child care and other family duties is a greater influence than job-related stress on the mental and physical well-being of working women.

PERSONALITY AND BEHAVIORAL PATTERNS ASSOCIATED WITH ELEVATED BLOOD PRESSURE

A number of psychological characteristics have been related to higher BP levels and/or increased prevalence of hypertension. Several of these traits are of relevance because they are presumed to act, in part, by increasing the individual's exposure to stress or perception of stress (e.g., cynical hostility) or because they themselves may be a consequence and thus a marker of excessive stress exposure (e.g., hopelessness and depressive symptoms).

Type A or the coronary-prone behavior pattern is associated with increased risk of atherosclerosis and coronary morbidity.[49] This pattern includes three semiindependent component traits: hostile outlook, competitiveness, and time urgency.[50] Of these traits, hostile outlook was the primary predictive factor in most studies that examined relationships of the individual factors. Additional research on hostility by Barefoot and others has confirmed that this trait is stable over time and predicts both cardiovascular and all-cause mortality, in part through its relationship to increased BP.[50–53] Hostile outlook, described as a combination of angerability and cynical mistrust, leads to increased BP, vasoconstriction, and plasma cortisol and testosterone responses to laboratory stressors, as well as higher 24-hour urinary cortisol and ambulatory BP levels in normotensive and hypertensive individuals.[54–57] Some experts have interpreted such findings as evidence that hostile individuals demonstrate greater and more frequent stress reactions in daily life because they perceive more situations as threatening and because they provoke more conflicts and negative interpersonal interactions. Some studies have found no excessive BP responses to stress in high-hostility men and women during purely cognitive tasks like mental arithmetic or the Stroop color-word task;[58, 59] but other investigations in which the stressors involved interpersonal interactions, including efforts to control or dominate others or harassment and frustration by others, have consistently found greater pressor responses in high-hostility persons.[60] High-hostile young men reporting greater frequency and longer

duration of angry episodes in their lives also demonstrate adrenergic receptor downregulation, suggesting greater chronic sympathetic nervous system activity.[57]

Some studies have reported an apparently paradoxical association between low rather than high self-reports of hostility and higher BP. Work by Shapiro, Jamner, and coworkers has suggested that these persons are not truly low in hostility, but instead they employ a defensive coping style, characterized by reluctance to admit to anger, anxiety, or other socially undesirable thoughts or feelings.[61, 62] Defensive copers among paramedics and nurses showed higher ambulatory BP on the job, particularly under more stressful conditions. Defensive coping, like hostility, is more consistently related to high stress responsivity in men than in women, possibly because of differences in social expectations about expression of emotion between genders.[63, 64] These observations indicate that it is not appropriate to conclude that there is a simple, unidirectional relationship between high scores on a hostility scale and risk of hypertension. Further, several large-scale investigations have found that hostility scores decrease with increasing education and income.[65, 66] Thus, it is important to separate the effects of social class from hostility by matching groups for education and economic resources or controlling statistically for group differences in these variables.

Anger-arousing experiences have long been known to raise BP and increase vasoconstriction.[1, 2] One way hostile outlook may influence cardiovascular risk is through frequent bouts of anger. Three patterns of anger coping—high anger-out (hair trigger and explosive verbal and physical expression of anger), low anger-out (inability or unwillingness to show or express anger even when appropriate and justified), and high anger-in (denial of angry feelings toward others with unjustified self-blame)—have been hypothesized to lead to increased BP reactivity to stress and to hypertension.[67, 68] The original research by Harburg and colleagues on African Americans living in high-crime areas of Detroit suggested that anger suppression or low anger-out was directly related to elevated BP in these stress-vulnerable people.[69] This pattern has been related to increased BP and heart rate during role play of conflicts and harassment in the laboratory, as well as to increased BP in wives after discussion of conflicts with their husbands.[53, 70–74] Anger suppression, like hostility with its association of high-anger expression, has been related to downregulation of β-adrenergic receptors, suggesting a stable pattern of sympathetic overactivity.[57, 76, 77] Engebretson and associates originally suggested that high cardiovascular reactivity was more frequent in both high–anger-in and high–anger-out persons if the stressor involved some provocation of angry feelings.[71] A recent prospective analysis of middle-aged men from the Kuopio, Finland, study indicated that subjects who were at the extreme ends of the distribution for either anger-in or anger-out had a significantly higher risk of developing hypertension over the next 5 years.[75] These results confirm that extremes in either expressing or suppressing angry feelings are maladaptive and that moderation is the lowest-risk solution.

Another psychological factor related to increased BP is the desire to dominate and impress others, termed *power motivation*. McClelland found that inhibited power motivation in men predicted hypertension-related pathology in a 20-year study,[78] but few studies have confirmed an association between power motivation and either high reactivity or increased BP levels. Further, a number of negative studies exist. The parallel of this pattern to Henry and colleagues' psychosocial model of hypertension in rats and mice[7, 18] is compelling and may provide a basis for integrating the contradictory results. Dominant and subdominant rats develop hypertension only if they are members of a strain that is vulnerable to stress-induced hypertension, and the BP increase occurs when aggressive contacts are high. In the truly dominant males, this occurs only when the social group members change, so that frequent bouts of aggression are required to assert dominance. In humans, the appropriate parallel might be that inhibited power motivation may lead to hypertension only when the individual's work and home environments are also unstable and the individual's social dominance is repeatedly threatened.

A related characteristic is the preference for active coping, or John Henryism.[79–84] This trait is defined by the belief in individual control and that hard work and persistence despite obstacles will lead to future success. The theory regarding the active coping behavior pattern states specifically that it will not be related to increased sympathetic activity and BP if the environment is supportive and has adequate resources. Only if the individual's environment is deficient in some way, thus leading to excessive effort and sympathetic overactivity, will hypertension develop. James and associates showed that high John Henryism was associated with increased BP in lower–social class rural African Americans, whose environment offered little opportunity for success.[79, 80] African American and white adolescents with the combination of high John Henryism and lower social class had increased BP and higher vascular resistance.[84] In another study in which the sample was limited to well-educated and employed African American and white adults, Light and coworkers observed that ambulatory BP at work was increased in women and African Americans with high-status professional and managerial jobs who scored high in this preference for active coping.[83] This effect was not seen among white male professionals and managers, and this was interpreted as evidence that this role is more threatening and less supportive for women and African Americans because of lack of peers in these jobs.

Attention has also focused on depressive symptoms and their relation to hypertension and cardiovascular risk.[85, 86] Depression is different from previous psychological factors because it is assumed to be an impermanent mood state (characterized by sadness and loss of interest in work, hobbies, family, and friends) rather than a stable trait. However, longitudinal studies indicate that depressive states tend to recur and that past history of depression is a primary predictor of subsequent depressive states. Although fewer reports have supported a relationship of depression to hypertension versus depression to cardiovascular and total mortality, the overall consistency of the pattern is compelling. Depression (as well as its correlated measure of distress, anxiety) is linked prospectively to onset of hypertension in both men and women, and in African American as well as white samples.[87] In elderly patients with established hypertension, men and women with higher depression scores show greater hypertension-related disease progression and increased incidence of stroke.[88, 89] Depressive symptoms are predictive of more severe cardiac

events. In patients with confirmed coronary heart disease, depressive symptoms are linked to increased MI, stroke, surgical intervention, and cardiac death, to decreased heart rate variability, and to increased cardiac activation and myocardial ischemia during Holter monitoring or mental stress in the laboratory.[85, 90–94]

Depression can develop in susceptible persons as a reaction pattern to life stress, including stresses associated with health crises such as MI and other serious cardiovascular diagnoses.[90, 91] In young healthy women, depressive symptoms were related to increased cardiac adrenergic tone and enhanced norepinephrine increases during a speech stressor.[95] Thus, stressful life events may contribute to worsening of depressive symptoms, and depression may in turn worsen sympathetic and cardiovascular responses to stress, producing a vicious circle effect. Frasure-Smith and coworkers have confirmed that in patients with a recent MI, depression predicts premature death due to recurrent MI, arrhythmic events, and congestive heart failure at 6, 12, and 18 months' follow-up; risk was further increased in those whose post-MI depression was not their first depressive episode.[85, 90, 91] The effects of depression are strongest in the subgroup with premature ventricular complexes, a group especially vulnerable to arrhythmia and sudden death associated with alterations in cardiac autonomic activity, such as may be induced by severe acute life stress.

Hopelessness and pessimism are common among depressed and vitally exhausted individuals, but these can also occur without the severe sadness or loss of interest in life that are the true hallmarks of depression.[96] Unlike depression, which is more common in women than in men and less common in African Americans than in other ethnic groups, hopelessness is reported equally in both genders, and it may be equally or more common in minorities and those from lower social classes.[97] In the Kuopio Ischemic Heart Disease Study, men with moderate to high hopelessness at baseline were 2.5 to 4 times more likely than men with lower levels of hopelessness to die of cardiovascular causes over a 6-year follow-up period, even after controlling for baseline BP, smoking, and other traditional cardiovascular risk factors.[98] Hopelessness also predicted all-cause mortality in this group of 2428 middle-aged men and carotid atherosclerotic lesion progression in the 942 men showing some carotid plaque at initial testing.[98, 99] The effect of persistent hopelessness was equivalent to that of smoking 2.5 packs of cigarettes daily. Pessimism before coronary bypass surgery is also linked to increased likelihood of having a perioperative MI.[100, 101] Less research has focused on the linkage of hopelessness and pessimism to hypertension, but the few studies reported to date support this relationship.[102] For example, in postmenopausal women, those who both had low SES and used a stable pessimistic attributional style (believing that bad events are permanent and cannot be controlled or improved) had increased ambulatory BP.[103] Helplessness and pessimism, like depression, are seen as both consequences of previous life stress and states that enhance the adverse cardiovascular effects of subsequent stress exposure.[104] Additional work on these important factors, which appear to parallel the defeat and helplessness state in animal models,[6, 7] is currently in progress.

Altogether, there is substantial and growing evidence to

support the association of hypertension and cardiac events with a number of psychological factors that involve stress as a causal factor in initiating the psychological condition or in contributing to its adverse cardiovascular consequences. Psychological states like hostility, depression, and hopelessness are thus ripe for serving as risk identifiers and as focal points for behavioral or pharmacological interventions to reduce risk. Ongoing clinical trials, such as the Sadheart Trial of pharmacotherapy for depressive symptoms and the Enhanced Recovery in Coronary Heart Disease (ENRICHD) Trial of cognitive-behavioral therapy for clinical depression and/or social isolation in patients with recent MI are assessing the potential importance of these approaches to help develop and refine treatment based on psychological risk factors.[102]

HIGH CARDIOVASCULAR RESPONSE TO STRESS IN PREDICTION OF LATER BLOOD PRESSURE ELEVATION

The hypothesis that those individuals who show exaggerated BP, heart rate, or other cardiovascular responses to behavioral stressors have increased risk of becoming hypertensive has generated considerable research and much debate since the late 1970s.[8, 105] Indirect evidence supporting this hypothesis included observations that persons with borderline hypertension or those with hypertensive parents showed increased BP responses to stress in many studies, although not in all. Other evidence indicated that high response to stress was a stable characteristic of certain people, documented by highly correlated response levels when compared across stressors or on retesting after intervals as long as 1 to 10 years. Notably, response levels showed greater stability than did reactivity scores (calculated as increases from resting baseline levels).[3, 17] More direct support for this hypothesis has been derived from several longitudinal studies. A number of these have employed a single stressor, often the cold pressor test, which elicits a BP increase via α-adrenergically mediated vasoconstriction. These investigations have not always yielded positive findings,[105] but the two largest investigations with the longest follow-up interval have supported the reactivity hypothesis by showing that individuals with the greatest BP increases to painful cold later developed hypertension at a higher rate than those with lesser BP increases.[106, 107]

Several smaller-scale studies, particularly those focusing on young borderline-hypertensive individuals, have shown that high reactivity to active coping stressors like mental arithmetic that evoke BP increases through β-adrenergic activity and increased heart rate and cardiac output is predictive of later sustained hypertension.[108, 109] Similar studies with active coping stressors using normotensive subjects have generated both positive and negative findings after partialling out effects related to higher prestress BP, which is associated with high stress reactivity and later hypertension.[110–112] BP increases during *anticipation of upcoming physical or mental stress* and during *recovery after stress* are added effects of stress reactivity; increases in these measures are strongly predictive of later hypertension.[108, 109, 113] Figure 6–2 shows the relationship of BP responses during anticipation of an exercise stress test to hypertension incidence 4 years later.[113]

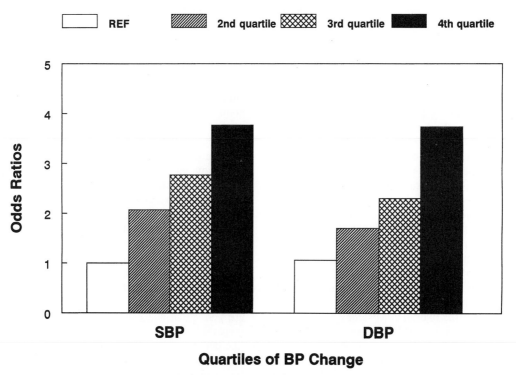

Figure 6–2. Association between systolic blood pressure (SBP) and diastolic blood pressure (DBP) responses in anticipation of exercise and 4-year incidence of high blood pressure (BP). REF, reference category in logistic regression models. (From Everson SA, Kaplan GA, Goldberg DE, Salonen JT. Anticipatory blood pressure response to exercise predicts future high blood pressure in middle-aged men. Hypertension 27:1059–1064, 1996.)

Two prospective studies that included women as well as men in the sample have examined responses to multiple stressors. In the study by Matthews and colleagues involving parents and their children, high pressor reactivity to active coping stressors was related to increased BP after 6.5 years; the effects were more consistent for men and boys than for women and girls.[114] In the much larger Coronary Artery Risk Development in Young Adults (CARDIA) study involving over 3300 African American and white young adults,[115] results after 5 years of follow-up indicated that high systolic BP reactivity to the active coping task, but not to the passive cold pressor test, was predictive of greater BP elevations and increased incidence of hypertension in African American and white men, even after controlling for baseline BP levels and other key covariates. In women regardless of race, neither task was effective in predicting later BP (Table 6–1).[115] The gender difference seen in the latter studies may have been related, in part, to the fact that women tend to develop hypertension at a later age, perhaps related to protective effects of female reproductive hormones during the ages under study. Another possibility is that video games may differentially engage higher active coping effort in men than in women.

Prior work by our group has supported the interpretation by the CARDIA investigators that individuals showing enhanced cardiac responses due to β-adrenergic activity during active coping stressors have a greater likelihood of demonstrating BP increases as young adults. In our investigation, the sample under study was small, but the follow-up testing involved over 60 measures of BP from each subject obtained through ambulatory monitoring on a regular workday, providing greater confidence in the outcome measures.[110] Both high heart rate reactors and high BP responders to an active coping reaction time task demonstrated increased BP at work and at home as well as in the clinic 10 years later. The predictive effect of high heart rate reactivity most directly points to mediation via β-adrenergic activity, since our laboratory has confirmed through use of β-antagonists that heart rate and systolic BP elevations in response to active coping reaction time tasks primarily reflect such activity.[4, 5]

More recently, our group has completed a second 10-year follow-up study using ambulatory BP monitoring.[116] This study reconfirmed that initially normotensive young men who were high heart rate and systolic BP responders to stress showed greater BP increases and a high incidence of borderline hypertension 10 years later. The results also showed that prediction of later development of borderline hypertension was strongest for the men who had hypertensive parents as well as high stress responsivity. Finally, the study indicated that the stress exposure and stress buffers in the person's home and work environments could influence the predictive effect of high cardiovascular responsivity to stress. Clinic pressure was higher in high stress responders who reported high scores on the Daily Stress Inventory, but not for those reporting low daily stress. Similarly, ambulatory pressure at work was greater in high stress responders reporting low support from their work supervisor and greater during leisure at home from those reporting low overall social support, but not in high responders who had greater support in their lives. These findings encourage reconsideration of the reactivity hypoth-

Table 6–1. Odds Ratios of Having Significant Blood Pressure Increase (8 mm Hg) Over 5-Year Follow-Up Function of Gender and Systolic Reactivity to Video Game: The CARDIA Study*

	Systolic Reactivity to Video Game (mm Hg)†	OR (95% CI)
Men	5	0.8 (0.77, 0.92)
	10	1
	20	1.4 (1.19, 1.69)
	30	2.0 (1.41, 2.86)
Women	5	1.0 (0.89, 1.05)
	10	1
	20	1.1 (0.91, 1.07)
	30	1.1 (0.83, 1.59)

From Markovitz JH, Raczynski JM, Wallace D, et al. Cardiovascular reactivity to video game predicts subsequent blood pressure increases in young men: The CARDIA study. Psychosom Med 60:186–191, 1998.
Abbreviations: OR, odds ratio; 95% CI, 95% confidence interval; BP, blood pressure.
*n = 889 with BP increase; n = 2722 without BP increase.
†Reference group = 10 mm Hg.

esis, expanding it to take into account genetic factors (e.g., parental hypertension); differences across individuals in chronic stress exposure, which affects expression of the predisposition to high heart rate and BP responses; and differences in exposure to stress buffers like social support.

In sum, these investigations provide cautious encouragement for continued research addressing high reactivity to stress as a potential risk factor for hypertension. Future research should avoid some of the oversimplified approaches of the past and utilize available opportunities to examine stress-response patterns in association with information about family history and factors relating to chronic stress level.

STRESS BUFFERS AND STRESS-REDUCTION INTERVENTIONS

As one of the spokesmen for models of stress and disease in humans, Cohen has incorporated a category of factors labeled *stress buffers* in his model.[117] Stress buffers include any factor that reduces perceived level of distress in individuals exposed to stress, that limits exposure to stressors, or that decreases adverse physiological reactions to stress. The best-documented stress buffer is social support. Social isolation has been associated with high rates of premature death from cardiovascular disease and all causes combined.[118–121] In patients with MI, increased emotional social support was related to decreased mortality, even after controlling for age, Killip class, and other cardiovascular risk factors.[121] Laboratory studies have shown that BP and other cardiovascular responses to mental challenges are less when a supportive and nonevaluative person is present.[122–124] Similarly, even support from a pet dog or cat has been shown to reduce stress responses.[125] In contrast, when the supportive person may be evaluating the test subject based on her or his performance, or when support may increase the intensity of effort (such as arguing against racial discrimination in the presence of another person advocating the same position), cardiovascular responses can actually be increased rather than decreased when the supporter is present.[124–126]

In several studies involving ambulatory BP monitoring, high perceived support was related to lower BP.[127, 128] Brownley and associates reported that high social support did not act by itself to lower BP in 129 healthy African American and white men and women, but it did interact with hostility. In this sample, high-hostile persons lacking support had higher ambulatory BP, whereas high-hostile persons with social support showed no BP increase relative to low-hostile persons (Fig. 6–3).[128] A similar interaction was seen in a prospective study of Swedish men, in which type A men lacking social support had increased mortality but other type A men reporting more support had no increase in risk relative to type B men.[129] Additional work addressing the potential stress-buffering effect of social support is needed, however. In particular, interactions of

support with anger-coping styles and other psychological factors, with high stress reactivity, and with environmental stressors like job strain have clear potential to reveal important relationships.

Another potential stress buffer is aerobic exercise. A number of studies have compared cardiovascular responses to stress after a period of exercise versus those following a control condition.[130–135] Some of these studies showed no differences, whereas others supported the hypothesis that stress responses are reduced after exercise.[135] Two factors that may influence the outcome of such studies are whether the subject is a high reactor to stress and whether his or her BP is elevated. Research in our laboratory has suggested that moderate aerobic exercise for only 20 to 30 minutes can evoke a reduction in vascular resistance in most individuals, but that BP will not decrease in all subjects.[131, 134] BP responses during stress appear to be blunted after exercise in high stress reactors. This makes sense, since it is hard to reduce a response that is already minimal. Also, ambulatory BP levels have been shown to be reduced at work for up to 5 or more hours after exercise in borderline-hypertensive persons, whereas normotensive subjects typically show no reduction in BP, although they do show potentially beneficially decreases in total vascular resistance.[134, 136] This appears to be related to homeostatic influences, such as baroreceptor activity, that elicit compensatory adjustments in circulatory control systems to prevent a fall in BP in normotensive individuals. Other research has indicated that reduced efferent sympathetic nerve activity and lower circulating catecholamine levels contribute to the lower vascular resistance in the postexercise period.[137, 138]

These studies addressed the effects of only a single bout of exercise on responses during the postexercise period. Other investigations have examined the effects of increased aerobic fitness level due to weeks of physical training on stress responses. These studies have similarly suggested that stress responses are reduced after aerobic training in some but not all persons, with hypertensive individuals being most likely to benefit. More rapid recovery of cardiovascular responses after stress has been observed as a more general benefit of training.[135] For this reason, regular exercise is strongly recommended both as adjunctive treatment and as a preventive intervention for hypertension.[102, 138–140]

Stress-reduction interventions, including biofeedback, relaxation training, and cognitive behavioral therapies, have been extensively studied as potential ways to lower BP, with mixed success.[141–144] McGrady and Higgins attempted to develop a profile of hypertensive patients most likely to lower their BP through biofeedback. They found that young women with higher anxiety and tension levels and higher initial heart rates are the most successful in using this method.[142] Other studies have indicated that relaxation therapy is more effective with individuals whose daytime ambulatory BP is elevated versus those with lower daytime pressures.[141] Although some studies employing a "habituation control phase" have observed no changes with stress-reduction treatment,[144] falls in BP during both habituation and treatment have been seen in other well-designed investigations.[143]

There has been substantial rekindling of interest in

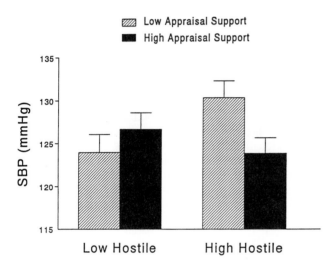

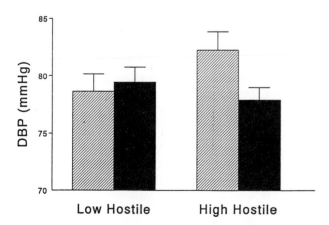

Figure 6–3. Unadjusted mean (SE) systolic blood pressure (SBP; *top*) and diastolic blood pressure (DBP; *bottom*) levels in low and high hostile subjects as a function of low- versus high-appraisal social support; *n* = 34 (high-support–high-hostile); *n* = 31 (low-support–high-hostile); *n* = 38 (high-support–low-hostile), and *n* = 26 (low-support–low-hostile). (From Brownley KA, Light KC, Anderson NB. Social support and hostility interact to influence clinic, work and home blood pressure in black and white men and women. Psychophysiology 33:434–445, 1996. Reprinted with the permission of Cambridge University Press.)

stress-reduction interventions after the reports by Ornish and colleagues[145] and by Blumenthal and coworkers[146] that stress management can be part of a lifestyle intervention program that can reduce risk and even partially reverse vascular pathology in coronary heart disease patients. The former study employed stress management only in combination with other established methods, such as low-fat diet, exercise, and weight reduction, whereas the latter used stress management as a solitary intervention and compared its benefits with an exercise training group as well as to a usual care group. Patients given a combination of relaxation, biofeedback, and cognitive therapies to help them recognize and manage stress, anger, and depression demonstrated greater reduction in risk of subsequent cardiac events or interventions compared with patients given exercise training or usual care.[146] Although more studies are clearly needed, the overall pattern suggests that stress-management techniques are effective in reducing cardiovascular risks in some individuals. Benefits are more likely with interventions using cognitive therapy as well as simpler relaxation or biofeedback approaches and in patient groups with more cardiovascular and psychological risk factors. It is expected that more research on this topic will be forthcoming soon.

SUMMARY AND INTEGRATION

The preponderance of animal and human research shows that environmental and psychosocial stress have a clear impact on BP levels over the short term, and these may have a role in the onset and progression of hypertension in individuals with genetic or environmentally enhanced susceptibility (such as a high-salt, low-potassium diet). Increased sympathetic nervous system activity is a mediator of the effect of stress on BP, although other factors are also involved. Certain personality and behavioral patterns are associated with high stress responses and greater risk of hypertension and cardiovascular disease, and certain environmentally stressful conditions (ranging from the broadest, such as low SES, to the more specific, such as high job strain) are potential risk factors for hypertension. Buffers available to reduce the adverse effects of stress on BP include social support, exercise, and stress-management therapies. Since modern life in Western societies appears to make stress exposure unavoidable, more research on strategies to reduce the effects of stress exposure is needed.

References

1. Schacter J. Pain, fear and anger in hypertensives and normotensives. Psychosom Med 19:17–29, 1957.
2. Sinha R, Lovallo WR, Parsons OA. Cardiovascular differentiation of emotions. Psychosom Med 54:422–435, 1992.
3. Sherwood A, Turner JR. A conceptual and methodological overview of cardiovascular reactivity research. *In* Turner JR, Sherwood A, Light KC (eds). Individual Differences in Cardiovascular Response to Stress. New York, Plenum, 1992; pp 3–32.
4. Light KC, Sherwood A. Race, borderline hypertension and hemodynamic responses to behavioral stress before and after beta-adrenergic blockade. Health Psychol 8:577–595, 1990.
5. Girdler SS, Hinderliter AL, Light KC. Peripheral adrenergic receptor contributions to cardiovascular reactivity: Influence of race and gender. J Psychosom Res 37:177–193, 1993.
6. Henry JP, Grim CE. Psychosocial mechanisms of primary hypertension. [Editorial review] J Hypertens 8:783–793, 1990.
7. Henry JP, Liu J, Meehan WP. Psychosocial stress and experimental hypertension. *In* Laragh JM, Brenner BM (eds). Hypertension. Pathophysiology, Diagnosis and Management. New York, Raven, 1995; pp 905–921.
8. Manuck SB. Cardiovascular reactivity in cardiovascular disease: "Once more unto the breach." Int J Behav Med 1:4–31, 1994.
9. Light KC, Girdler SS, West S, Brownley KA. Blood pressure responses to occupational challenges and laboratory stress in women. *In* Orth-Gomer K, Chesney MA, Wenger N (eds). Women, Stress and Heart Disease. Mahwah, NJ, Lawrence Erlbaum, 1998; pp 237–261.
10. Sudhir K, Jennings GL, Funder JW, Komesaroff PA. Estrogen enhances basal nitric oxide release in the forearm vasculature in perimenopausal women. Hypertension 28:330–334, 1996.
11. Owens JF, Stoney CM, Matthews KA. Menopausal status influences ambulatory blood pressure levels and blood pressure changes during mental stress. Circulation 88:2794–2802, 1993.
12. Light KC, Turner JR, Hinderliter AL, et al. Race and gender comparisons. I: Hemodynamic responses to a series of stressors. Health Psychol 12:354–365, 1993.
13. Sherwood A, May CW, Siegel WC, et al. Ethnic differences in hemodynamic responses to stress in hypertensive men and women. Am J Hypertens 8:552–557, 1995.
14. Light KC, Koepke JP, Obrist PA, et al. Psychological stress induces sodium and fluid retention in men at risk for hypertension. Science 220:429–431, 1983.
15. Light KC, Turner JR. Stress-induced changes in the rate of sodium excretion in healthy black and white men. J Psychosom Res 36:497–508, 1992.
16. Harshfield GA, Pulliam DA, Alpert BS. Patterns of sodium excretion during sympathetic nervous system arousal. Hypertension 17:1156–1170, 1992.
17. Sherwood A, Girdler SS, Bragdon EE, et al. Ten-year stability of cardiovascular responses to laboratory stressors. Psychophysiology 34:185–191, 1997.
18. Henry JP, Stephens PM. Stress, Health and the Social Environment: A Sociobiologic Appproach to Medicine. New York, Springer-Verlag, 1977.
19. Folkow B. Physiological aspects of the "defense" and "defeat" reactions. Acta Physiol Scand 161(suppl 640):34–37, 1997.
20. Mormede P. Genetic influences on the responses to psychosocial challenges in rats. Acta Physiol Scand 161(suppl 640):65–68, 1997.
21. Ely D, Caplea A, Dunphy G, et al. Physiological and neuroendocrine correlates of social position in normotensive and hypertensive rat colonies. Acta Physiol Scand 161(suppl 640):92–95, 1997.
22. Lawler JE, Barker GF, Hubbard JW, et al. Effect of stress on blood pressure and cardiac pathology in rats with borderline hypertension. Hypertension 3:496–501, 1981.
23. Sanders BJ, Cox RH, Lawler JE. Cardiovascular and renal responses to stress in borderline hypertensive rat. Am J Physiol 255:R431–R438, 1988.
24. Lawler JE, Zheng G, Li S, et al. Norepinephrine levels in discrete brain nuclei in borderline hypertensive rats exposed to compound stressors. Brain Res Bull 41:87–92, 1996.
25. Cox RH, Hubbard JW, Lawler JE, et al. Exercise training attenuates stress-induced hypertension in the rat. Hypertension 7:747–751, 1985.
26. Sanders BJ, Lawler JE. The borderline hypertensive rat (BHR) as a model for environmentally induced hypertension: A review and update. Neurosci Biobeh Rev 16:207–217, 1992.
27. DiBona GF, Jones SY. Renal manifestations of NaCl sensitivity in borderline hypertensive rats. Hypertension 17:44–53, 1991.
28. Koepke JP, Jones SY, DiBona GF. Sodium responsiveness of central alpha-adrenergic receptors in spontaneously hypertensive rats. Hypertension 11:326–333, 1988.
29. Koepke JP, DiBona GF. Central adrenergic receptor control of renal function in conscious hypertensive rats. Hypertension 8:133–141, 1986.
30. Anderson DE, Kearns WD, Better WE. Progressive hypertension in dogs by avoidance conditioning and saline infusion. Hypertension 5:286–291, 1983.
31. Anderson DE, Kearns WD, Worden TJ. Potassium infusion attenuates avoidance-saline hypertension in dogs. Hypertension 5:415–420, 1983.

32. Anderson DA, Dietz JR, Murphy P. Behavioral hypertension in sodium-loaded dogs is accompanied by sustained sodium retention. J Hypertens 5:99–105, 1987.

33. Pickering TG. The effects of environmental and lifestyle factors on blood pressure and the intermediary role of the sympathetic nervous system. J Hum Hypertens 11(suppl 1):S9–S18, 1997.

34. Shaper AG. Cardiovascular studies in the Samburo tribe of northern Kenya. Am Heart J 63:437–442, 1962.

35. Shaper AG, Leonard PJ, Jones KW, et al. Environmental effects on the body build, blood pressure and blood chemistry of nomadic warriors serving in the army in Kenya. East Afr Med J 46:282–289, 1969.

36. Waldron I, Nowotarski M, Freimer M, et al. Cross-cultural variation in blood pressure: A quantitative analysis of the relationship of blood pressure to cultural characteristics, salt consumption and body weight. Soc Sci Med 16:419–430, 1982.

37. Kaplan GA, Keil JE. Socioeconomic factors and coronary heart disease: A review of the literature. Circulation 88:1978–1998, 1993.

38. Anderson NB, Myers H, Pickering T, et al. Hypertension in blacks: Psychosocial and biological perspectives. J Hypertens 7:161–172, 1989.

39. Anderson NB, McNeilly M, Myers H. Toward understanding race difference in autonomic reactivity. In Turner JR, Sherwood A, Light KC (eds). Individual Differences in Cardiovascular Response to Stress. New York, Plenum, 1992; pp 125–145.

40. Dressler WW. Social support, lifestyle incongruity, and arterial blood pressure in a southern black community. Psychsom Med 53:608–620, 1991.

41. Rose RM, Jenkins CD, Hurst MW. Health change in air traffic controllers: A prospective study. I: Background and description. Psychosom Med 40:142–165, 1978.

42. Karasek RA, Baker D, Marxer F, et al. Job decision latitude, job demands and cardiovascular disease: A prospective study in Swedish men. Am J Pub Health 75:694–705, 1981.

43. Schnall PL, Pieper C, Schwartz JE, et al. The relationship between "job strain," workplace diastolic blood pressure and left ventricular mass index. JAMA 263:1929–1935, 1990; also see Correction, JAMA 267:1209, 1992.

44. Schnall PL, Schwartz JE, Landsbergis PA, et al. Relation between job strain, alcohol and ambulatory blood pressure. Hypertension 19:488–494, 1992.

45. Pollard TM, Ungpakorn G, Harrison GA, et al. Epinephrine and cortisol responses to work: A test of the models of Frankenhaeuser and Karasek. Ann Behav Med 18:229–237, 1996.

46. Light KC, Turner JR, Hinderliter AL. Job strain and ambulatory work blood pressure in healthy young men and women. Hypertension 20:214–218, 1992.

47. Lundberg U. Work and stress in women. In Orth-Gomer K, Chesney MA, Wenger NK (eds). Women, Stress and Heart Disease. Mahwah, NJ, Lawrence Erlbaum, 1998; pp 41–56.

48. Luecken LJ, Suarez EC, Kuhn CM, et al. Stress in employed women: Impact of marital status and children at home on neurohormone output and home strain. Psychosom Med 59:352–359, 1997.

49. Rosenman RH, Brand RJ, Scholtz RI, et al. Multivariate prediction of coronary heart disease during the 8.5 year follow-up in the Western Collaborative Group Study. Am J Cardiol 37:903–912, 1976.

50. Houston BK, Chesney MA, Black GW, et al. Behavioral clusters and coronary heart disease risk. Psychosom Med 54:447–461, 1992.

51. Barefoot JC, Dahlstrom WG, Williams RB Jr. Hostility, CHD incidence and total mortality: A 25-year follow-up study of 255 physicians. Psychosom Med 45:59–63, 1983.

52. Dembroski TM, MacDougall JM, Costa PT, et al. Components of hostility as predictors of sudden death and myocardial infarction in the Multiple Risk Factor Intervention Trial. Psychosom Med 51:514–522, 1989.

53. Smith TW. Hostility and health: Current status of a psychosomatic hypothesis. Health Psychol 11:139–150, 1992.

54. Weidner G, Friend R, Ficarotto TJ, et al. Hostility and cardiovascular reactivity to stress in women and men. Psychosom Med 51:36–45, 1990.

55. Girdler SS, Jamner LD, Shapiro D. Hostility, testosterone and vascular reactivity to stress: Effects of gender. Int J Behav Med 4:242–263, 1998.

56. Jamner LD, Shapiro D, Hui KK, et al. Hostility and differences between clinic, self-determined and ambulatory blood pressure. Psychosom Med 55:203–211, 1993.

57. Suarez EC, Shiller AD, Kuhn CM, et al. The relationship between hostility and beta-adrenergic receptor physiology in healthy young males. Psychosom Med 59:481–487, 1997.

58. Sallis JF, Johnson CC, Trevorrow TR, et al. The relationship between cynical hostility and blood pressure reactivity. J Psychosom Res 31:111–116, 1987.

59. Smith MA, Houston BK. Hostility, anger expression, cardiovascular responsivity and social support. Biol Psychol 24:39–48, 1987.

60. Everson SA, McKey BS, Lovallo WR. Effect of trait hostility on cardiovascular responses to harassment in young men. Int J Behav Med 2:172–191, 1995.

61. Jamner LD, Shapiro D, Goldstein IB, et al. Ambulatory blood pressure and heart rate in paramedics: Effects of cynical hostility and defensiveness. Psychosom Med 53:393–406, 1992.

62. Shapiro D, Goldstein IB, Jamner LD. Effect of cynical hostility, anger out, anxiety and defensiveness on ambulatory blood pressure in black and white college students. Psychosom Med 58:354–364, 1996.

63. Helmers KF, Krantz DS. Defensive hostility, gender and cardiovascular levels and responses to stress. Ann Behav Med 18:246–254, 1996.

64. King AC, Taylor CB, Albright CA, et al. The relationship between repressive and defensive coping styles and blood pressure responses in healthy middle-aged men and women. J Psychosom Res 34:461–471, 1990.

65. Scherwitz L, Perkins L, Chesney M, et al. Cook-Medley Hostility Scale and subsets: Relationships to demographic and psychosocial characteristics in young adults in the CARDIA Study. Psychosom Med 53:36–49, 1991.

66. Barefoot JC, Peterson BL, Dahlstrom WG, et al. Hostility patterns and health implications: Correlates of Cook-Medley Hostility Scale scores in a national survey. Health Psychol 10:18–24, 1991.

67. Manuck SB, Morrison RL, Bellack AS, et al. Behavioral factors in hypertension: Cardiovascular responsivity, anger and social competence. In Chesney MA, Rosenman RM (eds). Anger and Hostility in Cardiovascular and Behavioral Disorders. Washington, DC, Hemisphere, 1985; pp 149–172.

68. Houston BK. Personality characteristics, reactivity, and cardiovascular disease. In Turner JR, Sherwood A, Light KC (eds). Individual Differences in Cardiovascular Response to Stress. New York, Plenum, 1992; pp. 103–123.

69. Harburg E, Erfurt J, Hauenstein L, et al. Socio-ecological stress, suppressed hostility, skin color and Black-White male blood pressure: Detroit. Psychosom Med 35:276–296, 1973.

70. Durel LA, Carver CS, Spitzer SB, et al. Associations of blood pressure with self-report measures of anger and hostility among black and white men and women. Health Psychol 8:557–575, 1989.

71. Engebretson TO, Matthews KA, Scheier MF. Relations between anger expression and cardiovascular reactivity: Reconciling inconsistent findings through a matching hypothesis. J Pers Soc Psychol 58:844–854, 1989.

72. Powch IG, Houston BK. Hostility, anger-in and cardiovascular reactivity in white women. Health Psychol 15:200–208, 1996.

73. Houston BK. Anger, hostility and psychophysiological reactivity. In Siegman AW, Smith TW (eds). Anger, Hostility and the Heart. Hillsdale, NJ, Lawrence Erlbaum, 1996; pp 97–115.

74. Dimsdale JE, Pierce C, Schoenfeld D, et al. Suppressed anger and blood pressure: The effects of race, sex, social class, obesity and age. Psychosom Med 48:430–436, 1986.

75. Everson SA, Goldberg DE, Kaplan GA, et al. Anger expression and incident hypertension. Psychosom Med 60:730–735, 1998.

76. Mills PJ, Dimsdale JE. Anger suppression: Its relationship to beta-adrenergic receptor sensitivity and stress-induced changes in blood pressure. Psychol Med 23:673–678, 1993.

77. Julius S, Amerena J, Smith S, et al. Autonomic and behavioral factors in hypertension. In Laragh JH, Brenner BM (eds). Hypertension: Pathophysiology, Diagnosis and Management. New York, Raven, 1995; pp 2557–2570.

78. McClelland DC. Inhibited power motivation and high blood pressure in men. J Abnorm Psychol 8:182–190, 1979.

79. James SA, Harnett SA, Kalsbeek WD. John Henryism and blood pressure differences among black men. J Behav Med 6:259–278, 1983.

80. James SA, Keenan NL, Strogatz DS, et al. Socioeconomic status, John Henryism and blood pressure in black adults: The Pitt County Study. Am J Epidemiol 135:59–67, 1992.

81. Duijkers TJ, Drijver M, Kromhout D, et al. John Henryism and blood pressure in a Dutch population. Psychosom Med 50:353–359, 1988.

82. James SA. John Henryism and the health of African Americans. Cult Med Psychiatry 18:163–182, 1994.

83. Light KC, Brownley KA, Turner JR, et al. Job status and high-effort coping influence work blood pressure in women and blacks. Hypertension 25:554–559, 1995.

84. Wright LB, Treiber FA, Davis H, et al. Relationship of John Henryism to cardiovascular functioning at rest and during stress in youth. Ann Behav Med 18:146–150, 1996.

85. Frasure-Smith N, Lesperance F, Talajic M. Depression and 18-month prognosis after myocardial infarction. Circulation 91:999–1005, 1995.

86. Barefoot JC, Schroll M. Symptoms of depression, acute myocardial infarction and total mortality in a community sample. Circulation 93:1976–1980, 1996.

87. Jonas BS, Franks P, Ingram DD. Are symptoms of anxiety and depression risk factors for hypertension? Longitudinal evidence from the NHANES I Epidemiologic Follow-up Study. Arch Fam Med 6:43–49, 1997.

88. Wassertheil-Smoller S, Applegate WB, Berge K, et al. Change in depression as a precursor of cardiovascular events. SHEP Cooperative Research Group (Systolic Hypertension in the Elderly). Arch Intern Med 156:553–561, 1996.

89. Simonsick EM, Wallace RB, Balzer DG, et al. Depressive symptomatology and hypertension-associated morbidity and mortality in older adults. Psychosom Med 57:427–435, 1995.

90. Lesperance F, Frasure-Smith N, Talajic M. Major depression before and after myocardial infarction: Its nature and consequences. Psychosom Med 58:1–9, 1996.

91. Frasure-Smith N, Lesperance F, Talajic M. The impact of negative emotions on prognosis following myocardial infarction: Is it more than depression? Health Psychol 14:388–398, 1995.

92. Carney RM, Rich MW, Freedland KE, et al. Major depressive disorder predicts cardiac events in patients with coronary artery disease. Psychosom Med 50:627–633, 1988.

93. Carney RM, Saunders RD, Freedland KE, et al. Association of depression with reduced heart rate variability in patients with coronary artery disease. Am J Cardiol 76:562–564, 1995.

94. Krittayaphong R, Cascio WE, Light KC, et al. Heart rate variability in patients with coronary artery disease: Differences in patients with higher and lower depression scores. Psychom Med 59:231–235, 1997.

95. Light KC, Kothandapani RV, Allen MT. Enhanced cardiovascular and catecholamine responses in women with depressive symptoms. Int J Psychophysiol 28:157–166, 1998.

96. Dua JK. Health, affect and attributional style. J Clin Psychol 51:507–518, 1995.

97. Greene SM. Levels of measured hopelessness in the general population. Br J Clin Psychol 20:11–14, 1981.

98. Everson SA, Goldberg DE, Kaplan GA, et al. Hopelessness and risk of mortality and incidence of myocardial infarction and cancer. Psychosom Med 58:113–121, 1996.

99. Everson SA, Kaplan GA, Goldberg DE, et al. Hopelessness and 4-year progression of carotid atherosclerosis. The Kuopio Ischemic Heart Disease Risk Factor Study. Arterioscler Thromb Vasc Biol 17:2–7, 1997.

100. Scheier MF, Matthews KA, Owens J, et al. Dispositional optimism and recovery from coronary artery bypass surgery: The beneficial effects on physical and psychological well-being. J Pers Soc Psychol 57:1024–1040, 1989.

101. Buchanan GM. Explanatory style and coronary heart disease. *In* Buchanon GM, Seligman MEP (eds). Explanatory Style. Hillsdale, NJ, Lawrence Erlbaum, 1995; pp 225–232.

102. Horan MJ, Lenfant C. Epidemiology of blood pressure and predictors of hypertension. Hypertension 15(suppl I):I20–I24, 1990.

103. Grewen K, Girdler SS, West SG, et al. Pessimistic attributional style and low social class are linked to higher ambulatory blood pressure in postmenopausal women. Manuscript in preparation, 1998, available by request.

104. Forest KB, Moen P, Dempster-McClain D. The effects of childhood family stress on women's depressive symptoms: A life course approach. Psychol Women Q 20:81–100, 1996.

105. Pickering TG, Gerin W. Cardiovascular reactivity in the laboratory and the role of behavioral factors in hypertension: A critical review. Ann Behav Med 12:3–16, 1990.

106. Menkes MS, Matthews KA, Krantz DS, et al. Cardiovascular reactivity to the cold pressor as a predictor of hypertension. Hypertension 14:524–530, 1989.

107. Kasagi F, Akahoshi M, Shimaoki K. Relation between cold pressor test and development of hypertension based on 28-year follow-up. Hypertension 25:71–76, 1995.

108. Falkner B, Onesti G, Hamstra B. Stress response characteristics of adolescents with high genetic risk for essential hypertension. Clin Exp Hypertens 3:583–591, 1981.

109. Borghi C, Costa FV, Boschi S, et al. Predictors of stable hypertension in young borderline hypertensive subjects: A five-year follow-up study. J Cardiovasc Pharmacol 8(suppl 5):S138–S141, 1986.

110. Light KC, Dolan CA, Davis MR, et al. Cardiovascular responses to an active coping challenge as predictors of blood pressure patterns 10 to 15 years later. Psychosom Med 54:217–238, 1992.

111. Murphy JK, Alpert BS, Walker SS. Ethnicity, pressor reactivity and children's blood pressure: Five years of observations. Hypertension 20:327–332, 1992.

112. Carroll D, Smith GD, Sheffield D, et al. Pressor reactions to psychological stress and prediction of future blood pressure: Data from the Whitehall II Study. BMJ 310:771–776, 1995.

113. Everson SA, Kaplan GA, Goldberg DE, et al. Anticipatory blood pressure response to exercise predicts future high blood pressure in middle-aged men. Hypertension 27:1059–1064, 1996.

114. Matthews KA, Woodall KL, Allen MT. Cardiovascular reactivity to stress predicts future blood pressure status. Hypertension 22:479–485, 1993.

115. Markovitz JH, Raczynski JM, Wallace D, et al. Cardiovascular reactivity to video game predicts subsequent blood pressure increases in young men: The CARDIA Study. Psychosom Med 60:186–191, 1998.

116. Light KC. Psychosocial mechanisms and cardiovascular reactivity in borderline hypertension. Paper presented at the International Symposium on Borderline Hypertension: Detection and Management, Bologna, Italy, June 11, 1997.

117. Cohen S. Psychosocial models of the role of social support in the etiology of physical disease. Health Psychol 7:269–297, 1988.

118. House JS, Robbins C, Metzner HL. The association of social relationships and activities to mortality: Prospective evidence from Tecumseh Community Health Study. Am J Epidemiol 116:123–140, 1982.

119. Berkman L, Syme SL. Social networks, host resistance and mortality: A nine-year follow-up of Alameda County residents. Am J Epidemiol 109:186–204, 1979.

120. Williams RB, Barefoot JC, Califf RM, et al. Prognostic importance of social and economic resources among medically treated patients with angiographically documented coronary artery disease. JAMA 267:520–524, 1992.

121. Berkman LF, Leo-Summers L, Horwitz RI. Emotional support and survival after myocardial infarction. Ann Intern Med 117:1003–1009, 1992.

122. Gerin W, Milner D, Chawla S. Social support as a moderator of cardiovascular reactivity: A test of the direct and buffering hypotheses. Psychosom Med 57:16–22, 1995.

123. Lepore SJ, Allen KA, Evans GW. Social support lowers cardiovascular reactivity to an acute stressor. Psychosom Med 55:518–524, 1993.

124. Kamarck TW, Annunciato B, Amateau LM. Affiliation moderates the effects of social threat on stress-related cardiovascular responses: Boundary conditions for a laboratory model of social support. Psychosom Med 57:183–194, 1995.

125. Allen K, Blascovich J, Tomaka J, et al. Presence of human friends and pet dogs as moderators of autonomic responses to stress in women. J Pers Soc Psychol 61:582–589, 1991.

126. McNeilly MD, Robinson EL, Anderson NB, et al. Effects of racist provocation and social support on cardiovascular reactivity in African American women. Int J Behav Med 2:321–338, 1995.

127. Linden W, Chambers L, Maurice J, et al. Sex differences in social support, self-deception, hostility and ambulatory cardiovascular activity. Health Psychol 12:376–380, 1993.

128. Brownley KA, Light KC, Anderson NB. Social support and hostility interact to influence clinic, work and home blood pressure in black and white men and women. Psychophysiology 33:434–445, 1996.

129. Orth-Gomer K, Unden A. Type A behavior, social support and coronary risk: Interaction and significance for mortality in cardiac patients. Psychosom Med 55:37–43, 1990.

130. Roskies E, Seraganian P, Oseasohn R, et al. The Montreal Type A Intervention Project: Major findings. Health Psychol 5:45–69, 1986.

131. Sherwood A, Light KC, Blumenthal JA. Effects of aerobic exercise on hemodynamic responses during psychosocial stress in normotensive and borderline hypertensive Type A men: A preliminary report. Psychosom Med 23:89–104, 1989.

132. Boone JB, Probst MM, Rogers MW, et al. Postexercise hypotension reduces cardiovascular responses to stress. J Hypertens 11:449–453, 1993.

133. Steptoe A, Kearsley N, Walters N. Cardiovascular activity during mental stress following vigorous exercise in sportsmen and inactive men. Psychophysiology 30:245–252, 1993.

134. West SG, Brownley KA, Light KC. Postexercise vasodilation reduces diastolic blood pressure responses to stress. Ann Behav Med 20:77–83, 1998.

135. Fillingim RB, Blumenthal JA. Does aerobic exercise reduce stress responses? In Turner JR, Sherwood A, Light KC (eds). Individual Differences in Cardiovascular Response to Stress. New York, Plenum, 1992; pp. 203–217.

136. Brownley KA, West SG, Hinderliter AL, et al. Acute aerobic exercise reduces ambulatory blood pressure in borderline hypertensive men and women. Am J Hypertens 9:200–206, 1996.

137. Floras JS, Sinkey CA, Aylward PE, et al. Postexercise hypotension and sympathoinhibition in borderline hypertensive men. Hypertension 14:28–35, 1989.

138. Piepoli M, Coats AJS, Adamopoulos S, et al. Persistant peripheral vasodilation and sympathetic activity in hypotension after maximal exercise. J Appl Physiol 75:1807–1814, 1993.

139. World Hypertension League. Physical exercise in the management of hypertension: A consensus statement by the World Hypertension League. J Hypertens 9:283–287, 1991.

140. Gifford RW Jr, Committee Members. The Fifth Report of the Joint National Committee on Detection, Evaluation and Treatment of High Blood Pressure. Pub no. 93-1088. Bethesda, MD, National Institutes of Health, 1993; pp 11–15.

141. Van Montfrans GA, Karemaker JM, Weiling W, et al. Relaxation therapy and continuous ambulatory blood pressure in mild hypertension: A controlled study. BMJ 300:1368–1372, 1990.

142. McGrady A, Higgins JT Jr. Prediction of response to biofeedback-assisted relaxation in hypertensives: Development of a hypertensive predictor profile (HYPP). Psychosom Med 51:277–284, 1989.

143. Goebel M, Viol GW, Orebaugh C. An incremental model to isolate specific effects of behavioral treatments in essential hypertension. Biofeed Self-Regul 18:255–280, 1993.

144. Johnston DW, Gold A, Kentish J, et al. Effect of stress management on blood pressure in mild primary hypertension. BMJ 306:963–966, 1993.

145. Ornish D, Brown SE, Scherwitz LW, et al. Can lifestyle changes reverse coronary heart disease? Lancet 336:129–133, 1990.

146. Blumenthal JA, Jiang W, Babyak MA, et al. Stress management and exercise training in cardiac patients with myocardial ischemia: Effects on prognosis and evaluation of mechanisms. Arch Intern Med 157:2213–2223, 1997.

CHAPTER 7

Renin and Prorenin

J. Deinum and M. A. D. H. Schalekamp

A century ago, Tigerstedt and Bergmann[1] coined the name *renin* for a hypertensive factor in rabbit kidney.[1] They showed that this factor was present in the renal cortex and was secreted into renal venous blood. It was retained by dialysis membranes and sensitive to heat, which suggested its protein nature. After these initial observations, renin sank into oblivion for some decades until interest flared up after the experiments by Goldblatt and coworkers,[2] who showed that clamping of a renal artery in the dog caused hypertension. They believed that the hypertensive principle was a humoral factor. This was shown to be renin by Pickering and colleagues.[3] From then on, the unraveling of the structure of the renin-angiotensin system (RAS) made steady progress, culminating in the cloning of the genes of its constituents (for a thorough review of the history of renin, see ref. 4).

The RAS is a proteolytic cascade (Fig. 7–1), connected to a signal-transduction system, in which renin cleaves the decapeptide angiotensin I (AI) from the N-terminal domain of angiotensinogen. AI is proteolytically converted to angiotensin II (AII) by angiotensin-converting enzyme (ACE). AII acts through at least two kinds of receptors, the AT_1 and AT_2 receptors (AT1R and AT2R). Most of the physiological effects of AII are mediated through the AT1R. The AT2R is mainly expressed during ontogeny, and although no functions have been elucidated yet, it may be associated with cell differentiation and regeneration.[5, 6] Other angiotensin receptor subtypes have been proposed by some, but these are not fully characterized or generally accepted by the scientific community (see Chap. 10, AT_1 and AT_2 Angiotensin Receptors). Not shown in Figure 7–1 is prorenin, the enzymatically inactive biosynthetic precursor of renin. Prorenin circulates in the blood, in concentrations nine times that of active renin. Plasma prorenin can acquire enzymatic activity in vitro by proteolytic as well as by nonproteolytic activation processes, but it has not been established whether these occur in vivo.

SYNTHESIS AND BIOCHEMISTRY OF RENIN AND PRORENIN

The renin gene, spanning 12 kb, is located on chromosome 1 and consists of 10 exons with a coding sequence of 1218 bases. The initial translation product of the renin gene is preprorenin, consisting of 406 amino acids. The "pre"sequence of 23 amino acids is cleaved on entering the rough endoplasmic reticulum. Prorenin (M_r 47,000) enters either a regulated or a constitutive secretory pathway.[7] In the regulated pathway, which in humans has only been demonstrated in the juxtaglomerular cells of afferent arterioles in the kidney, prorenin is converted to renin (M_r 40,000). This

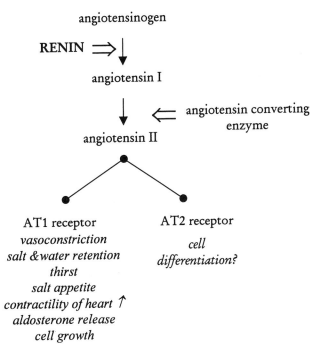

angiotensinogen

RENIN $\Rightarrow$

angiotensin I

angiotensin converting enzyme

angiotensin II

AT1 receptor
vasoconstriction
salt & water retention
thirst
salt appetite
contractility of heart ↑
aldosterone release
cell growth

AT2 receptor
cell
differentiation?

Figure 7–1. Schematic outline of the renin-angiotensin system. *Large arrows* denote proteolytic steps. ●——● denotes binding steps.

process takes place in dense secretory granules where a processing enzyme cleaves the 43 amino acid N-terminal prosegment. Release of stored renin from these secretory granules occurs after appropriate stimuli (see later). In the constitutive pathway, which is present in the kidney as well as in extrarenal sites of renin gene expression, there is a continuous flow of prorenin to the cell membrane and the extracellular space.[7]

Renin and prorenin are glycoproteins and belong to the class of aspartic proteases, which are characterized by two aspartic residues in their active center, located in a cleft between two homologous lobes.[8] Aspartic proteases are secreted as zymogens, which have an N-terminal propeptide obstructing the active site-cleft, thereby inhibiting enzymatic activity. Well-known examples of aspartic proteases are pepsin, cathepsin D, chymosin, and human immunodeficiency virus protease. Activation of pepsinogen occurs at low pH both proteolytically and nonproteolytically. Nonproteolytic activation involves a conformational change of the molecule by which the propeptide moves away from the cleft. The proteolytic autoactivation of pepsinogen involves intra- and intermolecular reactions, resulting in cleavage of the propeptide from the pepsin part of the molecule. Aspartic proteases have low substrate specificity, are inhibited by the statin-containing peptide pepstatin, and usually have low pH optima. Hence, they are active only in acidic environments such as the stomach and, intracellularly, the lysosomes. Although renin has the typical structure of aspartic proteases, its higher pH optimum and its absolute specificity for angiotensinogen set it apart.

Proteolysis of angiotensinogen by renin is a first-order, one-substrate reaction. Angiotensinogen concentration in human plasma is approximately 1500 nM,[9] which is near

the Michaelis constant. This means that AI generation in plasma is determined by both the renin concentration and the angiotensinogen concentration.

Prorenin is proteolytically converted to renin in vitro by the addition of proteases such as trypsin or plasmin. In plasma, the conversion is caused by endogenous kallikrein that is generated from prekallikrein after destruction of the natural inhibitors of contact activation of the coagulation cascade by exposure to low pH or low temperature.[10] This highly interesting in vitro connection between the coagulation system and the RAS has not been demonstrated to operate in vivo, although patients with prekallikrein deficiency have an increased prorenin:renin ratio in their plasma. Purified prorenin from either amniotic fluid or plasma or recombinant prorenin can also be activated nonproteolytically by exposure to low pH (acid activation) or cold (cryoactivation). In this case, the activation is nonproteolytic and is rapidly reversible during incubation at neutral pH and 37°C.[11] It is generally assumed that this activation is comparable to the nonproteolytic activation of pepsinogen at low pH and is caused by a conformational change of the molecule in which the propeptide moves out of the enzymatic cleft, thus permitting entry of the scissile bond of angiotensinogen into the catalytic center.

Another interesting phenomenon is that incubation of prorenin with an active site–directed renin inhibitor induces a slowly developing change in the conformation of prorenin, which is recognized by a monoclonal antibody that is specific for renin and does not react with native prorenin. Apparently, the inactive conformation of prorenin is not stable but is in equilibrium with an intermediary form that allows access of the renin inhibitor to the active center. Binding of the inhibitor then causes further destabilization of this intermediary, inactive conformation of prorenin until the renin epitope is fully exposed. This process is likely to involve the same conformational changes that occur during the nonproteolytic cryoactivation and acid activation of prorenin, although the complex with renin inhibitor lacks enzymatic activity.[12] Figure 7–2 depicts a scheme of the pathways leading to active prorenin.

CIRCULATING AND LOCAL RENIN

Classically, the RAS is considered an endocrine system. Circulating renin splices AI from angiotensinogen and AI is converted by ACE to AII in the pulmonary circulation. AII is then transported to its target sites. Although in the strictest sense renin is not a hormone, it can be considered as such because it is rate determining in AII generation and subject to tight control. Hence, according to this concept, the level of renin in plasma is believed to be an adequate measure of RAS activity.

It has become clear that this is an oversimplified view of the system. First, the view that AT1Rs are activated by AII that is formed in the lungs and then transported to the tissues via the circulation needs to be qualified because AI to AII conversion is not restricted to the vascular endothelium in the lungs.[13] Second, AI is found not only in the circulation but also in extrarenal tissues, generated locally by blood-derived renin that is produced by the kidney or by renin that is produced in situ. The essence of this new

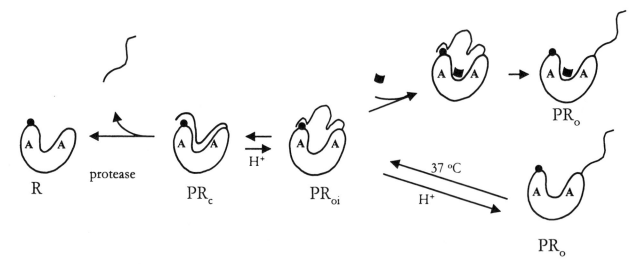

Figure 7–2. Mechanisms of prorenin activation. PR_c, native (closed) prorenin: The enzymatic cleft is closed by the propeptide and the renin epitope is covered. PR_{oi}, intermediary form of prorenin in which the propeptide has changed its conformation. A renin inhibitor, but not angiotensinogen, can bind to the active center, and the renin epitope is still covered. PR_o, prorenin in active conformation. The renin epitope is exposed. If no inhibitor is present, the molecule is enzymatically active. R, renin; A, aspartyl residue in active center. ◣ indicates renin inhibitor; ● indicates epitope, specific for renin-like conformation.

concept is that the RAS acts in a paracrine or even an autocrine way. For this concept, the term *local* RAS, as opposed to *circulating* RAS, has been coined. We propose to restrict the term *local* RAS to those tissues where (1) on the peptide level, all of the components of the RAS are present and (2) renin gene expression has been demonstrated on both the mRNA and the protein levels. This applies to the kidney and probably also to brain, adrenal gland, gonads, and eye.[14, 15] It may not apply to vascular tissue and the heart.

Local AI and AII production has been demonstrated in the vascular beds of the limbs and in cardiac tissue.[16–19] In fact, most cardiac AII appears to originate from AI produced in situ. At least under normal conditions, this production depends on blood-derived renin.[20] The same is true for AII generation in other vascular beds. The kidney is the only source of active renin in blood, whereas prorenin in the circulation originates from kidney as well as from extrarenal tissues with a local RAS. Uptake of renin from plasma may occur through renin-binding proteins[21] or mannose 6-phosphate receptors.[22] The latter, which are expressed on cardiac cells, bind and internalize renin as well as prorenin. It is not known whether angiotensinogen is also internalized. The observation that renin can be taken up from the circulation by cells raises the question whether intracellular AI generation may occur and, hence, whether an intracrine RAS exists in addition to the generally accepted endocrine, paracrine, and autocrine systems. Interestingly, prorenin is activated in the course of its internalization. The intracellular activation of prorenin might finally provide us with a long-sought function for prorenin other than its role as the precursor for renin in the kidney.

Cellular binding and intracellular activation of prorenin seem at odds with the finding that infusion of recombinant prorenin in cynomolgus monkeys did not result in an increase in blood pressure.[23] On the other hand, the interesting model of Mullins and associates[24] provides evidence of a role for the tissue RAS in blood pressure regulation.

They inserted the murine *Ren* 2-renin gene in the genome of a rat strain. Transgenic rats developed an AII-dependent hypertension with grossly elevated plasma prorenin levels and near-normal renin levels. The renin gene was overexpressed in adrenals, but not in kidney. Although the mechanism by which renin causes hypertension in these rats is still elusive, the model shows that the RAS may well cause hypertension without evidence of increased activity of the system in the circulation. A scheme of how circulating and local RASs may function is depicted in Figure 7–3. It may be clear, however, from the sometimes conflicting observations mentioned previously that a vast field of research on the workings of the RAS lies ahead.

REGULATION OF RENIN AND PRORENIN

Renin secretion by the kidney is regulated by a number of factors. First, a baroreceptor mechanism in the afferent arteriole stimulates renin secretion from juxtaglomerular cells during low perfusion pressure. Second, the delivery of sodium chloride to the distal tubule is sensed in the macula densa—low levels stimulate renin secretion; high levels inhibit. The third factor is β_1-adrenoreceptor–mediated—stimulation causes renin release; inhibition decreases renin output. Humoral factors may also influence renin secretion. The most important is AII itself, which inhibits renin secretion. A summary of various clinical conditions and pharmacological interventions that may change renin secretion can be found in Table 7–1. Many of these interventions cause an increase in plasma renin within minutes.

Because prorenin is not stored but is secreted continuously by the kidney, it cannot respond rapidly to stimuli. Only when a stimulus persists will prorenin levels rise. Most stimuli that acutely increase renin secretion will also increase prorenin levels in the long run, probably through increased gene transcription.[25] Figure 7–4 shows renin:total

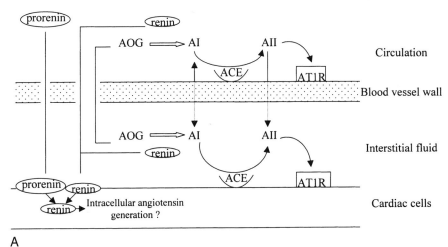

Figure 7–3. Schematic representation of concepts of the renin-angiotensin system (RAS). *A,* The endocrine concept of the RAS in which activity of the RAS is determined by blood (kidney)–derived renin. *Top,* The classical view of the RAS in which angiotensin generation occurs in the blood is depicted. *Below,* The concept of generation of angiotensins in the interstitial space by blood-derived renin and angiotensinogen is shown. In situ–generated angiotensin I (AI) is either delivered to the circulation or locally converted to angiotensin II (AII) (that does *not* reach the blood). Renin and prorenin may bind to cells *(lower left).* AOG, angiotensinogen; ACE, angiotensin-converting enzyme; AT1R, AT₁ receptor. *B,* The concept of a local RAS in which (pro)renin and angiotensinogen are produced locally and the whole system acts in a paracrine, autocrine, or maybe even intracrine way. Prorenin and possibly AI are delivered to the blood. Renin and prorenin may also bind to cells, but this is not depicted in the figure.

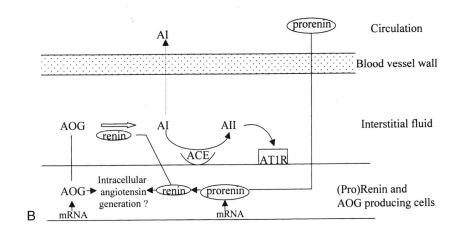

Table 7–1 Clinical Conditions Affecting Plasma Renin Levels

Regulatory Mechanism at the Level of the Juxtaglomerular Cell	Decreased Plasma Renin	Increased Plasma Renin
↑ or ↓ perfusion pressure	Salt loading Mineralocorticoid excess Liddle's syndrome Cushing's syndrome	Renovascular hypertension Malignant hypertension Cirrhosis with ascites Hemorrhage Diuretics Gastrointestinal fluid loss Upright posture Heart failure Nephrotic syndrome
↑ or ↓ salt delivery to macula densa β₁-Adrenergic stimulation or inhibition	Salt loading Autonomic dysfunction β-Blockade Adrenergic neuronal blockade	Sodium restriction Direct vasodilator therapy Pheochromocytoma Hypoglycemia Hyperthyroidism Sympathicomimetic agents
Feedback inhibition by angiotensin II		ACE Inhibitor Angiotensin II receptor antagonist
Unknown	Hyporeninemic hypoaldosteronism Low-renin hypertension	Acute glomerulonephritis High-renin hypertension

Abbreviation: ACE, angiotensin-converting enzyme.

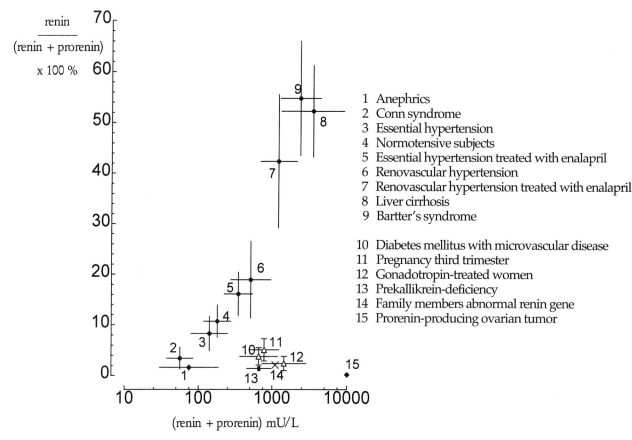

Figure 7–4. Relationship between renin:total renin (renin + prorenin) ratio and total renin (renin + prorenin) in plasma from subjects with various clinical conditions. Shown are mean ± SEM and geometric mean (95% CI), respectively.

renin (renin plus prorenin) ratios as a function of total renin in various chronic clinical conditions. It appears that total renin is determined by the underlying stimulus and that the degree of prorenin-to-renin conversion increases with rising total renin levels. There are some exceptions to the rule, e.g., pregnancy and diabetes mellitus with microvascular complications. Subjects with prekallikrein deficiency (our observation) or heterozygous for a renin gene mutation causing a premature stop codon[26] also have relatively high prorenin levels. There is no clear explanation for this phenomenon. One can hypothesize that as long as the renin and total renin levels conform to the curve in Figure 7–4, the kidney responds physiologically to a disturbance of homeostasis through one of the aforementioned regulatory mechanisms of renin and prorenin release. If the renin:total renin ratio is off the line, there may be some disturbance in the renin and prorenin synthesis machinery, possibly at the level of extrarenal renin gene transcription or intrarenal prorenin-to-renin conversion.

RENIN AND PRORENIN IN CLINICAL HYPERTENSION

Despite the pivotal role of renin in blood pressure regulation and in hypertension, measurements of renin and prorenin in plasma usually are not helpful in diagnosis or treatment. Plasma renin levels are similar in normotensive and hypertensive patients. Renin-profiling (plasma renin activity vs. 24-hour sodium excretion) in essential hypertension has been advocated as an important prognostic indicator of cardiovascular disease and a pointer to therapy.[27] Its clinical usefulness, however, is controversial. Patients with low plasma renin levels and hence a relatively inactive RAS may still respond favorably to ACE inhibitors, although this effect may be mediated by interference with systems other than the RAS.

Renin should be measured, however, in patients with hypertension and hypokalemia. In hypokalemic hypertension due to hypermineralocorticoid states such as hyperaldosteronism, apparent mineralocorticoid excess or glucocorticoid remediable hypertension, plasma renin is invariably suppressed. Patients with Liddle's syndrome (a genetic hypertensive disorder associated with hypokalemia, in which sodium reabsorption in the kidney is constitutively elevated) also have low plasma renin levels. Renin measurements may be helpful in the evaluation of renovascular hypertension. A steep increase in plasma renin after administration of captopril suggests renal artery stenosis, and an increased renal venous:arterial renin ratio of the kidney with the stenotic artery with a suppressed ratio on the other side is suggestive of renovascular hypertension.

Bartter's syndrome, characterized by hypokalemic alkalosis, without hypertension but with developmental abnormalities, is associated with high renin levels. Recently, it has become possible to make the diagnosis by genetic analysis. Hyporeninemic hypoaldosteronism, which may occur in diabetes mellitus, is confirmed by renin measurement. Effectiveness of replacement therapy in adrenal insufficiency can be readily monitored by renin measurement. Although heart failure is often accompanied by an active RAS and symptoms can be treated effectively by ACE inhibitors, measurement of renin does not add to diagnosis or management because increased plasma renin may be a reflection of the use of diuretics, ACE inhibitors or AII receptor antagonists by these patients rather than a marker of severity of heart failure.

The clinical value of measuring prorenin has not been established. It may serve, however, as a marker in Wilm's tumor.[28] In recent years, prorenin has also been advocated as a marker for microvascular disease in diabetes mellitus. Since prorenin increases before the first manifestation of nephropathy, microalbuminuria (unpublished observation and ref. 29), it may become the badly needed predictor of diabetic nephropathy. Prorenin levels, probably of ovarian origin, are very high in pregnancy, but apart from research purposes, there is no reason to measure prorenin in pregnancy.

Genetic factors undoubtedly play a role in essential hypertension, and renin is a likely "candidate gene." Renin gene variants in essential hypertension have been investigated in both association and linkage studies. None of the studies could implicate the renin gene in hypertension. Therefore, interest in the renin gene has waned. However, the heterogeneity of hypertension may have obscured a subset of hypertensive patients in whom a renin gene variant determines phenotype.

The RAS can be manipulated at various levels by pharmacological agents. Three highly successful classes of antihypertensive drugs act, in a large part, through interference with the RAS (β-blockers through suppressed renin levels, ACE inhibitors through decreased AII generation, and AT_1 receptor antagonists through blocking the actions of AII). In view of the central role of renin in the RAS, renin inhibitors are potentially attractive drugs for hypertension or heart failure, with theoretical advantages over the other three classes. They are highly selective for the RAS, whereas β-blockers and ACE inhibitors are not (ACE metabolizes numerous vasoactive peptides). In addition, AII does not increase after renin inhibition as it does after AT1R blockade, with possible untoward effects through AT2R overstimulation. Although potent nonpeptide renin inhibitors have been synthetized, development for clinical use has been hampered by the lack of orally active compounds with adequate biological availability (see Chap. 74, Renin Inhibitors). Commercial considerations may be the reason why no progress is being made in the clinical development of renin inhibitors.

METHODS FOR MEASURING RENIN AND PRORENIN

Which method to use for measuring renin has been subject to hot debates.[30] Renin is usually assayed through its enzymatic activity. In this indirect method of quantification, the renin-containing sample is incubated with renin substrate in the presence of inhibitors of AI-converting and -degrading enzymes. AI is then quantitated by radioimmunoassay. Many groups advocate the use of the so-called plasma renin activity (PRA) assay, which uses endogenous angiotensinogen as the substrate. PRA usually correlates well with the plasma renin concentration (PRC). In the PRC assay, angiotensinogen is added to the samples in order to obtain zero-order kinetics of AI generation. Only when endogenous angiotensinogen concentration is very high (e.g., in women on oral contraceptives, patients on high doses of glucocorticoids, and those with hyperthyroidism) or very low (in patients with cirrhosis) will PRA be high or low, respectively, relative to PRC.

Prorenin has no enzymatic activity, and must therefore be converted to renin by limited proteolysis. This can be achieved by the addition of trypsin or by acidification of plasma to pH 3.3. The difference in enzymatic activity before and after activation is a measure of the prorenin concentration. Direct immunoradiometric assays (IRMAs) specific for renin are available.[31] These are less time-consuming and easier to standardize than the enzyme-kinetic assays and are well suited for most clinical purposes. Prorenin can also be measured by these IRMAs after its proteolytic conversion to renin. A new way of measuring total renin is by converting native prorenin to prorenin with a renin-like conformation by the addition of a renin inhibitor to the sample. This modified prorenin can then be measured with IRMAs using monoclonal antibodies that react with renin but not with native prorenin[32] or monoclonal antibodies that react specifically with the propeptide (manuscript submitted).

CONCLUSION

New evidence suggests that the angiotensin receptors are not only activated by AII from the circulation but also by AII formed in situ and that this AII is derived not only from circulating AI but also from in situ formed AI. The kidney delivers renin to extrarenal tissues, including heart and blood vessels, to form both AI and AII in these tissues. In addition, prorenin may be taken up from the circulation and then become enzymatically active, via either proteolytical conversion to renin or a nonproteolytic conformational change. Whereas there is much detailed knowledge of the proteolytic and nonproteolytic activation of prorenin in vitro, there is no conclusive evidence that, in vivo, prorenin plays a role in physiology other than as the biosynthetic precursor of renin in the kidney. The reported extrarenal activation of endocytosed prorenin could be a step in its metabolic degradation in lysosomes rather than part of the pathway to AII formation. The presence of prorenin in plasma, in relatively high concentrations, remains therefore enigmatic.

It is now well established that prorenin is produced in a number of extrarenal tissues, but how it is activated, where AI and AII are formed, and how RAS components from the circulation contribute to local AI and AII production still have to be clarified. This is a field of potential clinical relevance in light of the growing body of evidence that the beneficial effects of ACE inhibitors and AT1R antagonists in heart failure and hypertension do not depend solely in their actions on the circulating RAS.

Clinical research on renin inhibitors has come to a standstill, but these drugs are attractive as research tools and potentially also as therapeutic agents. Renin gene variants have not been shown to influence phenotype, but intermediary phenotypes have not been studied.

In the near future, the newly developed direct IRMAs for renin and prorenin may replace the time-honored indirect radioimmunoassays that measure renin-dependent AI generation in vitro, just as the bioassay of AI was replaced by the radioimmunoassay in the late 1960s.

Acknowledgment

We are grateful to Frans Derkx for the many discussions we have had on the intricacies of renin and prorenin. He also helped with the preparation of Figure 7–4.

References

1. Tigerstedt R, Bergmann PG. Niere und kreislauf. Scand Arch Physiol 8:223–271, 1898.
2. Goldblatt H, Lynch J, Hanzal RF, et al. Studies on experimental hypertension. I: The production of persistent elevation of systolic blood pressure by means of renal ischemia. J Exp Med 59:347–379, 1934.
3. Pickering GW, Prinzmetal M. Some observations on renin, a pressor substance contained in normal kidney, together with a method for its biological assay. Clin Sci 3:211–227, 1938.
4. Peart WS. Evolution of renin. Hypertension 18(suppl III): III-100–III-108, 1991.
5. Unger T, Chung O, Csiios T, et al. Angiotensin receptors. J Hypertens Suppl 14:S95–S103, 1996.
6. Griendling K, Lassègue B, Alexander W, et al. Angiotensin receptors and their therapeutic implications. Annu Rev Pharmacol Toxicol 36:281–306, 1996.
7. Hsueh WA, Baxter JD. Human prorenin. Hypertension 17:469–479, 1991.
8. Szecsi PB. The aspartic proteases. Scand J Clin Lab Invest 52(suppl 210):5–22, 1992.
9. Derkx FHM, Stuenkel C, Schalekamp MPA, et al. Immunoreactive renin, prorenin and enzymatically active renin in plasma during pregnancy, and in women taking contraceptives. J Clin Endocrinol Metab 63:1008–1015, 1986.
10. Derkx FHM, Bouma BN, Schalekamp MADH, et al. Prorenin-renin conversion by the contact-activation system in plasma: Role of plasma protease inhibitors. J Lab Clin Med 103:560–567, 1984.
11. Derkx FHM, Schalekamp MPA, Schalekamp MADH. Prorenin-renin conversion. Isolation of an intermediary form of activated prorenin. J Biol Chem 262:2472–2477, 1987.
12. Derkx FHM, Deinum J, Lipovski M, et al. Nonproteolytic "activation" of prorenin by active site-directed renin inhibitors as demonstrated by renin-specific monoclonal antibody. J Biol Chem 267:22837–22842, 1992.
13. Danser AHJ, Koning MMG, Admiraal PJJ, et al. Metabolism of angiotensin I by different tissues in the intact animal. Am J Physiol 263:H418–H428, 1992.
14. Deschepper CF, Mellon SH, Cumin F, et al. Analysis by immunocytochemistry and in situ hybridization of renin and its mRNA in kidney, testis, adrenal and pituitary of the rat. Proc Natl Acad Sci U S A 83:7552–7556, 1986.
15. Wagner J, Danser AHJ, Derkx FHM, et al. Demonstration of renin mRNA, angiotensinogen mRNA and angiotensin converting enzyme mRNA expression in the human eye: Evidence for an intraocular renin-angiotensin system. Br J Ophthalmol 80:159–163, 1996.
16. Admiraal PJJ, Danser AHJ, Jong MS, et al. Regional angiotensin II production in essential hypertension and renal artery stenosis. Hypertension 21:173–184, 1993.
17. Hilgers KF, Kuczera M, Wilhelm MJ, et al. Angiotensin formation in the isolated rat hindlimb. J Hypertens 7:789–798, 1989.
18. Lindpaintner K, Ganten D. The cardiac renin-angiotensin system. An appraisal of present experimental and clinical evidence. Circ Res 68:905–921, 1991.
19. de Lannoy LM, Danser AHJ, Bouhuizen AMB, et al. Localization and production of angiotensin II in the isolated perfused rat heart. Hypertension 31:1111–1117, 1998.
20. Danser AHJ, van Kats JP, Admiraal PJ, et al. Cardiac renin and angiotensins. Uptake from plasma versus in situ synthesis. Hypertension 24:37–48, 1994.
21. Sealey JE, Catanzaro DF, Lavin TN, et al. Specific prorenin/renin binding (ProBP). Identification and characterization of a novel membrane site. Am J Hypertens 9:491–502, 1996.
22. van Kesteren CA, Danser AHJ, Derkx FHM, et al. Mannose 6-phosphate receptor–mediated internalization and activation of prorenin by cardiac cells. Hypertension 30:1389–1396, 1997.
23. Lenz T, Sealey JE, Maack T, et al. Half-life, hemodynamic, renal, and hormonal effects of prorenin in cynomolgus monkeys. Am J Physiol 260:R804–R810, 1991.
24. Mullins JJ, Peters J, Ganten D. Fulminant hypertension in transgenic rats harboring the mouse *Ren-2* gene. Nature 344:541–544, 1990.
25. Toffelmire EB, Skater K, Corvol P, et al. Response of plasma prorenin and active renin to chronic and acute alterations of renin secretion in normal humans. J Clin Invest 83:679–687, 1989.
26. Villard E, Lalau JD, van Hooft IS, et al. A mutant renin gene in familial elevation of prorenin. J Biol Chem 269:30307–30312, 1994.
27. Alderman MH, Ooi WL, Cohen H, et al. Plasma renin activity: Risk factor for myocardial infarction in hypertensive patients. Am J Hypertens 10:1–8. 1997.
28. Leckie BJ, Birnie G, Carachi R. Renin in Wilm's tumor: Prorenin as an indicator. J Clin Endocrinol Metab 79:1742–1746, 1994.
29. Allen TJ, Cooper MJ, Gilbert RE, et al. Serum total renin is increased before microalbuminuria in diabetes. Kidney Int 50:902–907, 1996.
30. Sealey JE, Trenkwalder P, Gahnem F, et al. Commentary: Plasma renin methodology: Inadequate sensitivity and accuracy of direct renin assay for clinical applications compared with the traditional enzymatic plasma renin activity assay. J Hypertens 13:27–30, 1995. See also J Hypertens 13:19–26, 31, 367–369, 371, 1995.
31. Ménard J, Guyenne T, Corvol P, et al. Direct immunometric assay of active renin in human plasma. J Hypertens 3(suppl 3):S275–S278), 1985.
32. Derkx FHM, De Bruin RJA, Van Gool JMG, et al. Clinical validation of renin monoclonal antibody–based sandwich assays of renin and prorenin, and use of renin inhibitor to enhance prorenin immunoreactivity. Clin Chem 42:1051–1063, 1996.

CHAPTER

8

Angiotensinogen: Physiology, Molecular Biology, and Relevance to Hypertension

Daniel F. Catanzaro

Although renin was first discovered in 1898,[1] it was not until 1939 that it was shown to be a proteolytic enzyme that generated a hypertensive factor by cleavage of a plasma protein later named *angiotensinogen*.[2] In 1957, Skeggs and coworkers[3] obtained the sequence of a tetradecapetide isolated from trypsin-treated plasma that contains the amino terminus angiotensinogen. Six years later, they purified angiotensinogen from hog plasma.[4] In the early 1980s, Tewksbury and colleagues[5–7] purified angiotensinogen from human plasma: Rat and human angiotensinogen cDNAs were cloned, and the incomplete nucleotide and amino acid sequences were deduced.[8, 9]

The availability of cloned sequences and a growing interest in the genetics of hypertension led to the initial report in 1992 of linkage and association between the angiotensinogen gene and human hypertension.[10] Since then, over 40 studies have attempted to replicate these findings, with mixed success. Analysis of the tissue distribution of angiotensinogen mRNA also fueled speculation about the role of a tissue renin angiotensin system in the pathogenesis of hypertension. Studies in transgenic animals further implicated a role for angiotensinogen in hypertension. Together, the conclusions drawn from these studies shifted the emphasis away from renin and its regulatory mechanisms and toward the angiotensinogen gene as a site for lesions in essential hypertension.

The purpose of this chapter is to review the molecular biology and genetics of angiotensinogen in relation to the biochemistry and physiology of the renin-angiotensin system. Much of the history and biochemistry of angiotensinogen have been extensively reviewed by Tewksbury.[11] There are also several excellent reviews of the molecular biology and genetics of angiotensinogen.[12–15]

BIOCHEMICAL CHARACTERISTICS OF THE REACTION BETWEEN RENIN AND ANGIOTENSINOGEN

Angiotensinogen is the only known substrate for renin. In most species, angiotensinogen circulates at a concentration close to the K_m for its cleavage by renin. Thus, varying the concentration of circulating angiotensinogen can affect the rate of angiotensin formation. However, under normal conditions, angiotensinogen concentrations remain relatively constant and only renin responds to changes in blood pressure and sodium balance to maintain blood pressure homeostasis. Moreover, even if the angiotensinogen concentration were to increase, the rise in angiotensin should result in a decrement in plasma renin to return angiotensin levels to baseline. Therefore, it seems unlikely that circulating angiotensinogen levels would have a major effect on the activity of the renin-angiotensin system, unless some defect in the mechanisms controlling renin secretion were also present.

EVIDENCE FOR A ROLE OF ANGIOTENSINOGEN IN BLOOD PRESSURE CONTROL

Relatively few studies have examined the relationship between plasma angiotensinogen levels and blood pressure. In a study of 17 patients, plasma renin substrate was 24% to 30% higher in hypertensives and their offspring than in normotensives.[16] In another study of over 500 patients, Walker and associates[17] reported a correlation of 0.39 between plasma renin substrate and recumbent diastolic blood pressure. Plasma angiotensinogen levels were elevated by 18% in hypertensive patients compared with normotensives. In a smaller study, Ito and coworkers[18] reported 18% higher plasma angiotensinogen levels in hypertensive ($n = 19$) than in normotensive ($n = 9$) patients. A four-corners approach that sampled parents and offspring with high and low blood pressure extremes reported significantly higher plasma angiotensinogen levels in the hypertensive offspring of hypertensive parents.[19] Plasma cortisol and 18-OH corticosterone levels were also elevated, which may account for the higher plasma angiotensinogen levels. In a study of patients with Cushing's syndrome, elevated plasma cortisol levels were associated with an average 50% increase in plasma angiotensinogen, whereas plasma renin concentration was suppressed by 30%, and plasma renin activity was unchanged.[20]

Angiotensinogen levels have long been known to be elevated by estrogen.[21] This effect of estrogens on plasma angiotensinogen levels has been observed in many animal and human studies.[22–24] During pregnancy, plasma angiotensinogen levels gradually rise until the 20th week of gestation to about fourfold above the postpartum level, closely following plasma estradiol levels.[25] Plasma renin activity also increases five- to sixfold, probably because of the fall in blood pressure that normally occurs during pregnancy.[25] The rise in substrate requires that plasma renin concentration rise only about two- to threefold to sustain the blood pressure.

Plasma angiotensinogen levels are also elevated in women taking oral contraceptives containing estrogens.[26, 27] In most women who remain normotensive while taking oral contraceptives, plasma renin concentration is suppressed, resulting in the maintenance of normal plasma renin activity and blood pressure. These studies also brought to light the fact that plasma angiotensinogen levels are rate-limiting for the production of angiotensin I.[27]

Therefore, it was postulated that in women who become hypertensive while taking oral contraceptives, renin secretion from the kidneys is inadequately suppressed in response to the increased angiotensin production that results from increases in plasma angiotensinogen, and hypertension develops[27–29]

Animal studies have also suggested a role for angiotensinogen in blood pressure control. Normal and salt-depleted rats injected with antiangiotensinogen antiserum or purified gamma globulin fraction showed a 30 or 40 mm Hg fall in blood pressure, respectively, that lasted about 30 minutes.[30] Similar injections of nonimmune serum had no effect on blood pressure.[30]

ANGIOTENSINOGEN IN TISSUES

Liver is the major site of angiotensinogen gene expression, but angiotensinogen mRNA is expressed in a variety of extrahepatic sites, including brain, large arteries, kidney, adipose tissues, and heart.[31, 32] Because plasma concentrations of angiotensinogen are close to K_m, any local increase brought about by local synthesis could increase angiotensin production in that tissue. It has been estimated that up to 85% of angiotensin is formed within tissues rather than in the plasma.[33] The kidney is the only known site where prorenin is converted to renin and the only source of plasma renin. Renin present in other tissues may be taken up from the circulation, perhaps through membrane-associated renin-binding sites.[34, 35] There is as yet no evidence that local synthesis of angiotensinogen affects the rate of angiotensin formation in tissues.

TRANSGENIC STUDIES

Studies in mice and rats made transgenic for renin and angiotensinogen genes of various species have been interpreted as providing evidence for a central role of angiotensinogen in blood pressure regulation. However, to fully appreciate the significance of these studies, it is necessary to understand the species-specificity and kinetics of the reaction between renin and angiotensinogen. The plasma renin concentration in mice is normally extraordinarily high (>200 ng angiotensin I/ml/hr), but angiotensinogen levels are low and limit angiotensin I production by mouse renin. In addition, the reactions between renins and angiotensinogens of different species show different kinetics. Human renin does not cleave mouse or rat angiotensinogen, and mouse or rat renin does not cleave human angiotensinogen, although rodent substrate may partly inhibit human renin.[36] Thus, transgenic mice and rats harboring either the human renin or the human angiotensinogen gene are unable to generate angiotensin I from human angiotensinogen unless mated together to yield doubly transgenic lines expressing both human genes.

Transgenic Studies With Human Renin and Angiotensinogen Genes

Doubly transgenic lines of mice and rats expressing both human renin and angiotensinogen that develop elevated blood pressures have been reported by a number of laboratories.[37–39] Hypertension in these mice most likely represents a pathological condition brought about by the inappropriate secretion of human renin from outside the kidneys. Normally, an increase in blood pressure should suppress the secretion of renin from the kidneys. Although these transgenic lines express human renin in the juxtaglomerular cells—the normal site of renin gene expression in the kidney—human renin is also expressed at unusual sites where renin secretion might not be normally regulated.[40–42]

Recently, Yan and colleagues[42] prepared transgenic lines containing a 45-kb insert spanning the human renin gene that contained much longer flanking DNA sequences than earlier models. These mice express human renin at physiologically appropriate sites and secrete active renin into the circulation only from the kidneys. Moreover, their plasma renin levels respond appropriately to a variety of physiological stimuli.[43] When these mice were infused with either rodent or human angiotensinogen, blood pressure increased, but circulating levels of both mouse and human renin decreased.[43] Furthermore, when these 45-kb hREN mice were crossed with hAGT overexpressing lines, the doubly transgenic offspring were normotensive, and both human and mouse renin concentrations were suppressed to maintain a normal plasma renin activity.[44] Thus, neither the abnormal expression of angiotensinogen in some of the tissues nor plasma levels of human angiotensinogen that were approximately fourfold higher than in normal human plasma resulted in a rise in blood pressure, because the human as well as the mouse renin responded appropriately to the elevated angiotensinogen levels.

Transgenic Studies With Renin and Angiotensinogen Genes From Rodents

In an earlier study, mice transgenic for the rat angiotensinogen gene had plasma angiotensinogen levels that were elevated 2.5- to 3-fold, yet were markedly hypertensive (mean arterial pressure 130–160 mm Hg).[45] It should be noted that mouse renin cleaves rat angiotensinogen 23 times faster than mouse angiotensinogen. Because mouse plasma renin levels are normally extraordinarily high, the required suppression of renin secretion may be out of the range of the regulatory mechanisms that control renin secretion in the mouse. The apparently low plasma angiotensinogen levels might reflect the rapid cleavage of rat substrate under these conditions. Hypertension in rats transgenic for the mouse *Ren-2* gene has also been attributed to the enhanced kinetics of the reaction between mouse renin and rat angiotensinogen.[46]

Angiotensinogen Knockouts and Gene Titration Experiments

The ability of mice with the angiotensinogen gene deleted to survive and reproduce shows that angiotensinogen is not essential for life. However, these animals are hypotensive and have renal disorders.[47] The demonstration that titration of plasma angiotensinogen levels in mice by gene targeting leads to semiproportional changes in blood pressure has also implicated a role for angiotensinogen in hypertension.[48, 49] However, the additional angiotensinogen genes that were inserted into these mice may not have all the sequences required to yield fully appropriate expression. As discussed previously, with limiting concentrations of angiotensinogen, the rate of angiotensin formation is more sensitive to changes in substrate concentration in mice than in other species. Furthermore, mice may not be able to regulate the extraordinarily high plasma renin levels sufficiently to compensate for changes in substrate concentration. Therefore, the substrate-dependence of blood pressure in these titration experiments may be a peculiarity of the mouse renin-angiotensin system.

GENETIC STUDIES

In recent years, genetic studies have promoted a role for angiotensinogen in the cause of essential hypertension. Since Jeunemaitre and associates[10] first reported linkage and association between the human angiotensinogen gene and hypertension in 1992, there have been over 40 similar studies. Most have utilized association methods; there have also been a smaller number of linkage studies. Although these studies have produced conflicting results, they have maintained a focus on angiotensinogen as a possible causative factor in essential hypertension. However, despite these numerous studies and speculations, no one has adequately addressed the mechanisms through which changes in angiotensinogen expression could cause elevations in blood pressure.

Linkage Versus Association

Linkage and *association* are terms often used interchangeably in describing inherited traits. However, they have specific definitions that refer to their unique qualities. *Linkage* in genetic terms means that two genes, or two mutations, either within the same gene or in two different genes, are on the same chromosome. By virtue of their physical proximity on the chromosome, the two genes or two mutations will more frequently occur together than would be expected by chance, unless there is recombination between the parental chromosomes. Thus, linkage methods examine whether certain alleles are transmitted within families to affected individuals.

There are many variations of linkage analysis, but the kind that has been applied most frequently to studies of the angiotensinogen gene in hypertension is the affected sib pair method. This is the simplest linkage method that makes no assumptions about the mode of inheritance and does not require genotyping of the parents. Sib pair studies examine whether a genetic marker close to the gene under examination (in this case, the angiotensinogen gene) is more frequently shared among siblings with hypertension than would be expected by chance.

Association studies examine whether a certain polymorphism occurs more frequently in subjects or individuals expressing a phenotype (in this case, hypertension) than those without it. These studies have the advantage that they are relatively simple to carry out because, unlike linkage studies, they do not require identification of hypertensive siblings. In contrast to linkage, which is a characteristic of the chromosome, association is a characteristic of a population. Association studies depend neither on a genetic model nor on knowledge of the genotypes of parents or siblings. Thus, whereas linkage and association may relate a disease to the same genetic polymorphism, linkage examines its transmission within families and association examines its distribution through populations.

Initial Reports of Linkage and Association

In their initial report, Jeunemaitre and associates[10] examined linkage between the angiotensinogen gene and hypertension in sib pairs from two independent study groups—one from Utah and the other from Paris. Despite an apparent excess of shared alleles in the Utah cohort, linkage did not reach significance in this sample. However, significant linkage was detected in the Paris cohort, and when data from the two study populations were combined, the level of significance was slightly increased. Most recently, an extended linkage analysis that included the original patient population from the Jeunemaitre and associates'[10] study found no evidence for linkage between hypertension and the angiotensinogen gene.[50] Moreover, analytical methods applied in the latter study failed to show linkage in the original data set from Jeunemaitre and associates.[10] The findings of linkage studies are summarized in Table 8–1.

Table 8–1 Linkage Studies of the Angiotensinogen Gene in Essential Hypertension

Study	Ethnicity (Country)	Study Population	Significance Level for Linkage
Jeunemaitre et al, 1992[10]	White (United States)	244 sib pairs	NS
		50 severe HT	$p < .01$
		135 sib pairs	$p < .05$
	White (France)	60 severe HT	$p < .02$
Caulfield et al, 1994[61]	White (United Kingdom)	63 families	$p < .001$
		31 severe HT	$p < .001$
Caulfield et al, 1995[71]	African (Caribbean)	63 sibships	$p = .001$
Brand et al, 1998[50]	White (Europe)	630 sib pairs	NS

Abbreviations: NS, not significant; HT, hypertension.

The study by Jeunemaitre and associates[10] also identified 15 distinct single nucleotide polymorphisms in the human angiotensinogen gene. Among them, two transversions in exon 2, a T→C substitution that results in conversion of amino acid 235 from methionine to threonine (M235T) and a C→T substitution that results in conversion of amino acid 147 from threonine to methionine (T147M), were significantly associated with hypertension in both study cohorts. In addition, 235T, but not 147M, was associated with approximately 15% higher circulating plasma angiotensinogen concentrations in homozygotes compared with heterozygotes or controls. Among the numerous studies that followed the report of Jeunemaitre and associates,[10] most have used association methods to study the distribution of angiotensinogen 235 M and T alleles among hypertensive subjects and normotensive controls. Their findings are summarized in Tables 8–2 through 8–5. Table 8–6 summarizes studies that have examined associations with specific diseases. To emphasize the differences in allele frequencies and associations that have been reported between different ethnic groups, studies are tabulated according to the ethnicity of the population.

Angiotensinogen Polymorphisms in Whites

In whites, there have been inconsistent findings of association between the angiotensinogen 235 genotype and hypertension. Among 20 studies of white populations, 9 found a positive association of T235 with blood pressure, and 11 found no association (see Table 8–2). These different findings may be accounted for, at least in part, by differences in study design. In a recent meta-analysis (see later), Kunz and coworkers[51] listed the "selection, definition, and/or characterization of cases and controls" as the main variables that could affect the outcome and/or interpretation of association studies. In addition, sample size and the frequency of angiotensinogen 235 alleles may also play a significant role. In the sections that follow, the relevance of each of these specific variables is discussed in detail.

Definition of Hypertension

The definition of hypertension varied widely among studies, ranging from relatively mild (blood pressure > 140/90 mm Hg) to more severe (diastolic blood pressure < 105 mm Hg) (see Table 8–2). Current drug treatment and onset of hypertension before a certain age (usually 50 years) were often applied as alternative criteria or in addition to specific blood pressure levels. However, mild and severe criteria for hypertension were applied approximately equally between studies that found an association between angiotensinogen 235 alleles and blood pressure and those that did not.

Matching of Case Subjects and Controls

In many studies, controls tended to be younger and less obese than case subjects. Although a number of studies failed to report age, sex, and body mass index (BMI), in most studies, there was some matching of these parameters between cases and controls.

Sample Size

One possible explanation for many negative findings is that small increases in risk associated with T235 might not reach statistical significance. This is suggested by the greater frequency of T235 in hypertensives than in controls in seven of nine studies that failed to demonstrate significant association (see Table 8–2). Moderate risk associated with 235T might not reach significance in relatively small samples but should become significant in larger samples. However, positive and negative findings were reported approximately equally in both small and large study populations, and a greater number of large studies reported no association. Jeunemaitre and colleagues[52] recently estimated that to replicate the difference in allele frequencies reported in their initial study with 80% power would require 400 or more cases and 400 or more controls. Assuming this criterion, there are only two studies, both from the Jeunemaitre group, that show association and two studies from two different groups[53, 54] that show no association.

Criteria for Selection of Case Subjects and Controls

It is noteworthy that almost all the studies that found a positive association required a family history for inclusion of hypertensive subjects, whereas only two, relatively small studies that found no evidence of association applied family history to the selection of hypertensives. A genetic factor causing hypertension would be expected to be more prevalent in individuals from families with hypertension. However, equally importantly, only a small number of studies required an absence of family history for inclusion in the control group.[55–58]

Frequency of Angiotensinogen Alleles

In their initial report, Jeunemaitre and associates[59] found a frequency of T235 of 0.44 in the Utah study cohort and 0.52 in the French cohort. Although most subsequent studies of white populations reported frequencies of T235 in control groups of approximately 0.40, this ranged from 0.31[60] to 0.49.[61] Thus, the frequency of T235 reported by Johnson and coworkers[60] in their hypertensive population was lower than the frequency of 235T among the control groups reported in other studies. Similarly, the frequencies of T235 in control groups studied by Caulfield and colleagues[61] and Kiema and associates[53] were higher than in most hypertensive groups in which no association was found.

Thus, the selection of subjects and controls is a highly important variable that can affect the outcome of a study. Most studies showed that the distribution of genotypes in controls was in Hardy-Weinberg equilibrium, suggesting that they fulfill the important criterion of representing a freely interbreeding population. However, a mixture of populations with different genetic backgrounds (see later) in the hypertensive population could result in spurious associations of genetic markers and disease. In this respect, it is noteworthy that two studies[53, 62] that examined large numbers of subjects from relatively isolated populations found no association between angiotensinogen 235 alleles and blood pressure.

Meta-Analysis of Association Studies

Meta-analysis provides a tool to compare the findings of different studies and to pool the data into a composite estimate of risk. A recent meta-analysis[51] of 12 of the studies listed in Table 8–2 (shown by *asterisks* in the Population column) indicated that T235 is associated with a 20% increased risk of hypertension (odds ratio 1.20;95% CI 1.11 to 1.29). However, the quality of a meta-analysis is limited by the quality of the data in the studies it seeks to combine.[63, 64] As the authors of the meta-analysis pointed out, there are many differences between studies as well as a number of deficiencies within the individual studies that might influence their outcome and interpretation. The authors carried out a number of sensitivity analyses in which data sets from studies that failed to adequately define parameters were deleted. When the meta-analysis was repeated with all the studies that provided data in a format that could be subjected to risk analysis, the odds ratio increased slightly to 24% (95% CI 1.17 to 1.32) (see Table 8–2).

Only five studies in the original meta-analysis required a positive family history as a mandatory criterion for inclusion as a case, and only three required a negative family history for inclusion as a control. If negative findings were due to lower sensitivity, meta-analysis might reveal a significant, albeit low risk of hypertension associated with angiotensinogen 235 alleles. When studies were segregated by a positive family history of hypertension, the risk associated with 235T increased to 42%, whereas the risk fell to an insignificant 8% increase in studies in which family history was unknown. However, it is important to note that not all studies reporting a positive family history yielded positive associations. It is also noteworthy that the two studies that considered family history, but found no association, were among the smallest studies reported. Meta-analysis of the 10 studies reporting no association revealed an odds ratio of 1.09, CI 1.00 to 1.18, suggesting that a week association may exist even in these populations.

Angiotensinogen Polymorphisms in Africans and African Americans

Hypertension in Africans and African Americans is more prevalent and severe than in whites. Although none of the 10 published studies (see Table 8–3) found an association of 235T and hypertension, a number of them reported an association with plasma angiotensinogen levels. Most studies of African peoples were relatively small. The largest study examined 220 cases and 280 controls and found no association with either hypertension or plasma angiotensinogen levels.[65] As with studies of whites, definitions of hypertension and use of family history in selecting cases and controls varied widely. Controls also tended to be younger and less obese than cases.

The frequency of 235T among Africans and African Americans is much higher than in whites, ranging from 0.73 to 0.91, which could reduce the sensitivity to detect an association with hypertension. Among Japanese, the frequency of T235 is similarly high (~0.75; see Table 8–4), but almost every study of Japanese reported a significant association with hypertension (see later). The highest frequency of 235T was found in Nigerians,[66, 67] and lower frequencies were observed in African Americans and African Caribbeans (~0.80) (see Table 8–3), consistent with their estimated 25% European admixture.[66]

Angiotensinogen Polymorphisms in Japanese

Of the eight studies that examined the association of angiotensinogen 235 with hypertension in Japanese, six found significant association, and one found association in a subpopulation less than 50 years old[68] (see Table 8–4). The one study that found no association of blood pressure with 235T found a significant association with 174M.[69] None of the studies of Japanese examined plasma angiotensinogen levels. The Japanese are probably the most heterogeneous ethnic group that has been studied, which has been suggested to account for the strength of the association detected.[14] Although most studies were relatively small and did not report age, sex, or BMI, those that did appeared to have good matching between cases and controls, and the definition of hypertension was more consistent than in other populations.

Angiotensinogen Polymorphisms in Other Ethnic Groups

The findings of two studies that examined the association of angiotensinogen 235 in a mixed ethnic group and among a large population of native Canadians are summarized in Table 8–5.

Angiotensinogen Polymorphisms in Hypertensive Subtypes

Table 8–6 summarizes the findings of studies that have investigated the association of angiotensinogen 235T with blood pressure in various hypertensive subtypes, including pregnancy-related forms of hypertension, cerebrovascular disease, and diabetes. Several studies reported positive associations, whereas others found none.

Criteria for Association Studies

As discussed by Lander and Schork,[70] a positive association between a marker and a disease can arise for one of three reasons, of which one is completely artifactual. First, the polymorphism may actually cause the disease, in which case the polymorphism should be associated with the disease in all populations. Second, a polymorphism may not actually cause the disease, but may be genetically linked to the causative mutation. The persistence of such linkage in a population depends on the distance between the two polymorphisms and the number of generations since the two polymorphisms first appeared on the chromosome. Third, a positive association may arise from population admixture. If the frequency of a polymorphism differs

Text continued on page 87

Table 8-2 Molecular Genetic Studies of Whites

Study	Population (Inclusion in Meta-analysis*) Country	Genetic or Hypertensive Status	n	T235 (%)	Assoc. With BP	Assoc. With Plasma AGT	OR (95% CI)	T174M Association With BP	Family History (Cases)	Age (yr) (m/f If Reported)	Sex (% Male)	BMI (kg/m²)	Definition of Hypertension (or BP for Continuous Measurements) and Selection of Population	Notes
Jeunemaitre et al, 1992[10]	United States*	HT	132	44	+	+	1.46 (1.03–2.06)	+	+	49.4	52	29.7	Drug treatment, age of onset < 60 yr	P
		NT	140	35							50			
Jeunemaitre et al, 1992[10]	France*	HT	83	52	+	+	1.76 (1.15–2.72)		+	42.8	48	24.9	Drug treatment, age of onset < 60 yr or DBP > 95 mm Hg	R
		NT	89	38						44.6	45	22.5		
Jeunemaitre et al, 1993[35]	France*	HT	136	44	−	+	1.41 (0.99–1.99)		+	47	47	25.0	DBP > 95 mm Hg	R (Enalapril reduced plasma AGT ~200 ng/ml irrespective of genotype)
		HT	119	49	+	+			−	53	53	23.1		
		NT	90	38						44	44			
Schmidt et al, 1995[72]	Europe*	HT	219	56	+		1.83 (1.29–2.59)		+	51	65	26.8	BP > 140/90 mm Hg and/or drugs; 24-hr BP > 145/95 mm Hg	R / R (Association evident only in hypertensives with early onset and family history)
		NT	92	41						46	65	25.0		
		NT	139	40						32	65			
Johnson et al, 1996[60]	Australia*	ISH	171	39	+		1.39 (1.12–1.72)			72	47	25.1	SBP > 160 mm Hg, DBP < 90 mm Hg, BP ≥ 160/90 mm Hg	P
		SDH	218	38	+					68	59	26.8		
		NT	366	31						69	55	25.1		
Jeunemaitre et al, 1997[56]	France*	HT	477	47	+	+	1.45 (1.19–1.76)	−	+	49	48	25.4	Age of onset < 55 yr, DBP > 95 mm Hg and/or drugs	R
		NT	364	38						46	44	23.6		
Schunkert et al, 1997[73]	Germany	MM	216		+	+				57.6	49	27.0	144/89 mm Hg; 149/92 mm Hg	P (T allele associated with 4 mm Hg SBP, 2 mm Hg DBP and number of medications)
		MT or TT	418							57.8	48	27.4		
Borecki et al, 1997[58]	United States (Framingham)	HT	129	51	+		1.63 (1.15–2.31)			61/61	56		Cases: 2 or more drugs; Controls: BP < 140/90 mm Hg, no drugs	
		NT	126	39						61/61	56			
		Random	250	43						57/57	53			
Tiret et al, In Jeunemaitre et al, 1997[52]	France	HT	802	46	+		1.27 (1.10–1.48)							Association evident in males and in females with early-onset HT (<45 yr)
		NT	658	40										

Study	Location	Comparison	N	%		OR (95% CI)			Age	%	BMI	HT definition	R/P	Comments
Bennett et al, 1993[57]	Australia*	HT / NT	92 / 94	42 / 39	− / −	1.13 (0.75–1.71)	+			52 / 46	25.7 / 25.1	Drug treatment	R	Weak association of plasma AGT with genotype
Hegele et al, 1994[62]	Hutterite Canada	Cont. Variable	741	41	−		+		37/38	45	28.1/28.2	NA	P	Association of AGT codon 174 genotype with SBP in men (p = .028)
Caulfield et al, 1994[61]	Europe*	HT / NT	63 / 64	51 / 49	−	1.08 (0.66–1.77)	+	−				Age of onset < 60 yr, DBP > 95 mm Hg and/or drug treatment	R	
Barley et al, 1994[74]	Britain*	HT / NT	65 / 74	40 / 40	−	1.00 (0.62–1.62)		−				SBP > 140 mm Hg or DBP > 90 mm Hg		
Fornage et al, 1995[75]	United States*	HT / NT	104 / 195	41 / 40	−	1.04 (0.74–1.47)		−	60/64, 61/63	43 / 43	26.5/25.6, 26.6/25.6	BP > 140/90 mm Hg and/or drug treatment	P	
Tiret et al, 1995[53]	Europe*	HT / NT	630 / 741	40 / 40	−	1.00 (0.86–1.17)		−	57 / 52	100 / 100	28.0, 26.4	DBP > 95 mm Hg and/or drugs	P	
Hingorani et al, 1996[76]	United Kingdom*	HT / NT	223 / 187	45 / 42	−	1.12 (0.86–1.49)		−	56 / 53	62 / 55	26.1, 26.9	BP > 160/90 mm Hg	P	
Kiema et al, 1996[53]	Finland*	HT / NT	508 / 523	49 / 48	−	1.04 (0.88–1.23)		−	51/52, 51/52	50 / 49	29.4/26.5, 28.7/26.2	DBP > 105 mm Hg or DBP > 95 mm Hg and high risk	P	
Beige et al, 1997[77]	Germany	HT	343	47	ND			−	55	52	26.8	SBP > 140 mm Hg or DBP > 95 mm Hg	R	Continuous distribution of BP in treated and untreated HT unrelated to genotype
Bigda et al, 1997[78]	Poland	NT	145	60	ND			−	22.8	NR	23.1	BP < 140/90	P	Ambulatory BP data analyzed in tertiles
Borecki et al, 1997[58]	United States (ARIC)	HT / NT / Random	299 / 284 / 384	43 / 39 / 43		1.18 (0.93–1.49)	+ / −		62/61, 62/61, 60/59	49 / 49 / 48		Cases: 2 or more drugs, family history; Controls: BP < 140/90 mm Hg, no drugs	P	
Mondorf et al, 1998[79]	Germany*	HT / NT	121 / 125	43 / 35	ND	1.40 (0.97–2.01)		−	46.4 / 47.3	52 / 55	25.8 / 25.1	NR; renovascular HT excluded	R	No association of AGT genotype with captopril response
Totals for risk analysis		HT / NT	4591 / 4212	45 / 40		1.24 (1.17–1.32)								

Abbreviations: BP, blood pressure; AGT, angiotensinogen; OR, odds ratio; BMI, body mass index; P, population; R, referral center; HT, hypertensive; NT, normotensive; DBP, diastolic blood pressure; ISH, isolated systolic hypertension; SDH, systolic-diastolic hypertension; SBP, systolic blood pressure; M, 235 methionine; T, 235 threonine; Cont, continuous; NA, not applicable; ND, not determined; NR, not reported.

Table 8–3 Molecular Genetic Studies of Africans and African Americans

Study	Population (Inclusion in Meta-analysis*) Country	Genetic or Hypertensive Status	n	T235 (%)	Assoc. With BP	Assoc. With Plasma AGT	T174M Association With BP	History of HT—Family—Cases; Personal—Controls	Age (yr) (m/f If Reported)	Sex (% Male)	BMI (kg/m²)	Definition of Hypertension (or BP for Continuous Measurements) and Selection of Population	Sel.	Notes
Rotimi et al, 1994[85]	African American	HT	57	82	−		−		42	28	32.3	SBP > 140 mm Hg or DBP > 90 mm Hg and/or drugs	P	
	African American	NT	130	83				−	51	41	28.7		P	
	Nigerian	ND	122	93										
Rutledge et al, 1994[86]	African American	HT	109	87				+	54	53		JNC criteria	R	Allele frequencies differ from those in whites
Barley et al, 1994[74]	Britain	HT	43	80	−							SBP > 140 mm Hg or DBP > 90 mm Hg		
		NT	15	73										
Bloem et al, 1995[87]	White	NT	148	42	−	+		−	15.0/14.9	53	21.4/21.2	NA	P	
	African American	NT	62	81	−	−		−	14.6/14.8	49	25.0/25.0			
Caulfield et al, 1995[71]	African	HT	150	86	−			+	64		26.4	DBP > 95 mm Hg or drugs	P	
	Caribbean	NT	93	84				−	54		24.9			
Forrester et al, 1996[65]	African	HT	220	81	−	−	−		54	38	27.5	BP > 160/90 mm Hg	P	Weak association of plasma AGT and BMI with BP
	Caribbean	NT	280	80					44	29	25.7			
Rotimi et al, 1996[66]	Nigerian		329	91								Not selected for HT. Equal proportions of HT and NT. Population distribution of HT	P	Nigerians have higher percentage of 235T consistent with 25% European admixture in Jamaica and United States
	Jamaican		167	81									P	
	African American		218	81									P	
Bloem et al, 1997[88]	African American	NT	76	59		+			12	47	22.2	NA		Haplotype analysis reveals associations with plasma AGT levels. Calculated by adding frequencies of haplotypes
	White	NT	139	31		+			12	58	19.8			
Rotimi et al, 1997[67]	Nigerian	HT	116	92	−	+	−		54		24.1	162/96		Sampling from extremes of BP distribution
		NT	138	90					54		22.0	118/70		
Borecki et al, 1997[58]	United States (ARIC)	HT	37	80	−			+	62/59	35		Cases: 2 or more drugs, family history		
		NT	74	77					59/59	40		Controls: BP < 140/90 mm Hg, no drugs		
		Random	160	76										

Abbreviations: BP, blood pressure; AGT, angiotensinogen; BMI, body mass index; HT, hypertensive; NT, normotensive; ND, not determined; SBP, systolic blood pressure; DBP, diastolic blood pressure; P, population; R, referral center; JNC, Joint National Committee on Prevention, Detection, Evaluation, and Treatment of High Blood Pressure; NA, not applicable.

Table 8-4 Molecular Genetic Studies of Japanese

Study	Population (Inclusion in Meta-analysis*) Country	Genetic or Hypertensive Status	n	T235 (%)	Association With BP	Association With Plasma AGT	OR (95% CI)	T174M Association With BP	History of HT Family—Cases; Personal—Controls	Age (yr) (m/f If Reported)	Sex (% Male)	BMI (kg/m²)	Definition of Hypertension (or BP for Continuous Measurements) and Selection of Population	Notes
Hata et al, 1994[80]	Japanese	HT / NT	105 / 81	89 / 75	+		2.70 (1.54–4.72)		−	61 / 34			SBP > 160 mm Hg or DBP > 95 mm Hg	R
Iwai et al, 1994[81]	Japanese	HT / NT	82 / 83	86 / 77	+		1.83 (1.04–3.25)		+	56 / 53	57 / 57	22.4 / 23.9	BP > 160/95 mm Hg	R
Kamitani et al, 1994[82]	Japanese	HT / NT	108 / 104	79 / 68	+		1.77 (1.14–2.74)							
Iwai et al, 1995[68]	Japanese	TT / TM / MM	225 / 102 / 20		−					55 / 55 / 56	52 / 55 / 60	23.1 / 23.2 / 24.5	151/87 147/85 149/86	R AGT genotype predictor of SBP and DBP in subpopulation < 50 yr
Morise et al, 1995[69]	Japanese	HT / NT	80 / 100	79 / 79	−		1.00 (0.60–1.67)	+	+ / −	49 / 52	62 / 55		Cases: BP > 160/90 mm Hg Controls: BP < 130/90 mm Hg	R
Nishiuma et al, 1995[83]	Japanese	HT / NT	64 / 149	72 / 60	+		1.71 (1.09–2.69)		+		100 / 100		SBP > 140 mm Hg or DBP > 90 mm Hg, or drugs	P
Kataoka et al, 1996[84]	Japanese	NT	131	76	+									Children
Jeunemaitre et al, 1997[59]	Japanese	HT / NT	92 / 122	91 / 76	+		3.19 (1.78–5.73)	−					SBP > 160 mm Hg and/or DBP > 90 mm Hg	Association of G-6A polymorphism
Totals for risk analysis		HT / NT	531 / 639	83 / 71			1.98 (1.63–2.44)							

Abbreviations: BP, blood pressure; AGT, angiotensinogen; OR, odds ratio; BMI, body mass index; HT, hypertension; NT, normotensive; SBP, systolic blood pressure; DBP, diastolic blood pressure; P, population; R, referral center; M, 235 methionine; T, 235 threonine.

Table 8–5 Studies of Other Ethnic Groups

Study	Population	Genetic or Hypertensive Status	n	T235 (%)	Association With BP	Age (yr) (m/f If Reported)	Sex (% Male)	BMI (kg/m²)	Definition of Hypertension (or BP for Continuous Measurements) and Selection of Population		Notes
Gharavi et al, 1997[89]	White, Hispanic, and Asian	MM	11		+	44	63	27.8	150/97 (O) 138/88 (A)	R	Ambulatory BP
		MT	22			45	59	26.1	147/95 (O) 141/89 (A)		
		TT	17			46	76	26.8	161/104 (O) 152/97 (A)		
Hegele et al, 1997[90]	Native Canadian	Cont. dist.	497	89	+	35	43	28.1	119/68		Marginal association with systolic BP (p = .037)

Abbreviations: BP, blood pressure; AGT, angiotensinogen; OR, odds ratio; BMI, body mass index; M, 235 methionine; T, 235 threonine; O, office; A, ambulatory; Cont. dist., continuous distribution.

Table 8–6 Studies of Special Disease Groups

Study	Population Country	Hypertensive Status	n	T235 (%)	Association With BP	Association With Plasma AGT
Ward et al, 1993[91]	White	PE	41	65	+	+
		PIH	108	44	+	−
		NT	93	44	+	
	Japanese	NT	478	40		
		PIH	41	90	+	
		PE	18	89	+	
		PEPG	13	88	−	
		NT	80	71		
Barley et al, 1995[92]	White	TIA	100/45		34	
		CON				
Schmidt et al, 1996[93]	Type 1 diabetics	DN+	180	44	−	
		DN−	243	45		
		DN+	310	44		
	Type 2 diabetics	DN−	353	44		
		CON	230	NS		
Tarnow et al, 1996[94]	Type 1 diabetics Denmark	DN+	195	38	−	−
		DN−	185	38		
Hopkins et al, 1996[95]		HT	34		Diminished renal plasma flow in response to Ang II in	
		NT	57		T235 homozygotes	
Kobashi, 1995[96]	Japanese	PIH	139	80–92	+	
		NT	279	56		

Abbreviations: BP, blood pressure; AGT, angiotensinogen; PE, preeclampsia; PIH, pregnancy-induced hypertension; NT, normotensive; PEPG, preeclamptic primagravida; TIA, transient ischemic attack; CON, control; DN, diabetic nephropathy (+, present; −, absent); HT, hypertension; Ang II, angiotensin II.

between two populations that also differ in the prevalence of a disease, then sampling across those two populations will show a positive association. If there is no apparent distinction between the two populations, a false-positive association between the polymorphism and the disease might be inferred.

Lander and Schork[70] recommended a number of steps to prevent spurious associations due to admixture. First, association studies should be carried out with relatively homogeneous populations. The finding of association in large mixed populations but not in homogeneous groups would suggest admixture. Second, parental DNA should be collected to provide an internal control representing the alleles not associated with the disease, the so-called affected family–based control, or haplotype relative risk method (see references in ref. 70). Third, a suspected associated allele is shown to be transmitted to affected offspring more frequently than a nonassociated allele.

CONCLUSIONS

Physiological studies suggest that, although changes in angiotensinogen can affect the rate of angiotensin formation, angiotensinogen levels vary relatively little, and these variations are compensated by changes in renin secretion that maintain a constant production of angiotensin. Although the findings of studies in transgenic and knockout animals suggest that angiotensinogen levels may play a role in blood pressure control, these findings are misleading because of their unphysiological regulation of renin. Most evidence for a role of angiotensinogen in essential hyper-

tension has come from genetic studies. However, the findings of these studies have been mixed, both within and between populations. The key question that remains unanswered is how a mutation in the angiotensinogen gene that causes a small (15%) increase in circulating angiotensinogen levels can cause hypertension. Unless there is some unidentified effect of such a mutation, the effect on blood pressure is difficult to reconcile with human and animal studies that show that angiotensinogen levels can change four- to fivefold without any effect on blood pressure, as long as renin secretion continues to be normally regulated. Nonetheless, it will be informative to determine the reason for the associations that have been reported between the angiotensinogen gene and blood pressure and why the strength of these associations differs between study populations and ethnic groups.

References

1. Tigerstedt R, Bergman PG. Niere und Kreislauf. Sc and Arch Physiol 8:223–271, 1898.
2. Munoz JM, Braun-Menendez E, Fasciolo JC, Leloir JF. Hypertensin: The substance causing renal hypertension. Nature 144:980, 1939.
3. Skeggs LT Jr, Kahn JR, Lentz K, Shumway NP. The preparation, purification, and amino acid sequence of a polypeptide renin substrate. J Exp Med 106:439–453, 1957.
4. Skeggs LT Jr, Lentz KE, Hochstrasser H, Kahn JR. The purification and partial characterization of several forms of hog renin substrate. J Exp Med 118:73–98, 1963.
5. Tewksbury DA. Angiotensinogen. Fed Proc 42:2724–2728, 1983.
6. Tewksbury DA, Dart RA, Travis J. The amino terminal amino acid sequence of human angiotensinogen. Biochem Biophys Res Commun 99:1311–1315, 1981.
7. Tewksbury DA, Frome WL, Dumas ML. Characterization of human angiotensinogen. J Biol Chem 253:3817–3820, 1978.

8. Ohkubo H, Kageyama R, Ujihara M, et al. Cloning and sequence analysis of cDNA for rat angiotensinogen. Proc Natl Acad Sci U S A 80:2196–2200, 1983.

9. Kageyama R, Ohkubo H, Nakanishi S. Primary structure of the preangiotensinogen deduced from the cloned cDNA sequence. Biochemistry 23:3603–3609, 1984.

10. Jeunemaitre X, Soubrier F, Kotelevtsev YV, et al. Molecular basis of human hypertension: Role of angiotensinogen. Cell 71:169–180, 1992.

11. Tewksbury DA. Angiotensinogen biochemistry and molecular biology. *In* Laragh JH, Brenner BM (eds). Hypertension: Pathophysiology, Diagnosis and Management, 2nd ed. New York, Raven, 1994; pp 1197–1216.

12. Lynch KR, Peach MJ. Molecular biology of angiotensinogen. Hypertension 17:263–269, 1991.

13. Corvol P, Jeunemaitre X, Charru A, et al. Role of the renin-angiotensin system in blood pressure regulation and in human hypertension: New insights from molecular genetics. Recent Prog Horm Res 50:287–308, 1995.

14. Corvol P, Jeunemaitre X. Molecular genetics of human hypertension: Role of angiotensinogen. Endocr Rev 18:662–667, 1997.

15. Brasier AR, Li J. Mechanisms for inducible control of angiotensinogen gene transcription. Hypertension 27:465–475, 1996.

16. Fasola AF, Martz BL, Helmer OM. Plasma renin activity during supine exercise in offspring of hypertensive patients. J Appl Physiol 25:410–415, 1968.

17. Walker WG, Whelton PK, Saito H, et al. Relation between blood pressure and renin, renin substrate, angiotensin II, aldosterone and urinary sodium and potassium in 574 ambulatory subjects. Hypertension 1:287–291, 1979.

18. Ito T, Eggena P, Barrett JD, et al. Studies on angiotensinogen of plasma and cerebrospinal fluid in normal and hypertensive human subjects. Hypertension 2:432–436, 1980.

19. Watt GC, Harrap SB, Foy CJ, et al. Abnormalities of glucocorticoid metabolism and the renin-angiotensin system: A four-corners approach to the identification of genetic determinants of blood pressure. J Hypertens 10:473–482, 1992.

20. Saruta T, Suzuki H, Handa M, et al. Multiple factors contribute to the pathogenesis of hypertension in Cushing's syndrome. J Clin Endocrinol Metab 62:275–279, 1986.

21. Helmer OM, Griffith RS. Effect of the administration of estrogens on renin substrate (hypertensinogen) content of rat plasma. Endocrinology 51:421, 1952.

22. Menard J, Corvol P, Foliot A, Raynaud JP. Effects of estrogens on renin substrate and uterine weights in rats. Endocrinology 93:747–751, 1973.

23. Menard J, Catt KJ. Effects of estrogen treatment on plasma renin parameters in the rat. Endocrinology 92:1382–1388, 1973.

24. Menard J, Bouhnik J, Clauser E, et al. Biochemistry and regulation of angiotensinogen. Clin Exp Hypertens [A] 5:1005–1019, 1983.

25. Wilson M, Morganti AA, Zervoudakis I, et al. Blood pressure, renin-aldosterone system and sex steroids throughout normal pregnancy. Am J Med 68:97–104, 1980.

26. Laragh JH, Sealey JE, Ledingham JG, Newton MA. Oral contraceptives. Renin, aldosterone, and high blood pressure. JAMA 201:918–922, 1967.

27. Newton MA, Sealey JE, Ledingham JG, Laragh JH. High blood pressure and oral contraceptives. Changes in plasma renin and renin substrate and in aldosterone excretion. Am J Obstet Gynecol 101:1037–1045, 1968.

28. Skinner SL, Lumbers ER, Symonds EM. Renin concentration in human fetal and maternal tissues. Am J Obstet Gynecol 101:529–533, 1968.

29. Sakura T, Saade GA, Kaplan NM. A possible mechanism for hypertension induced by oral contraceptives. Arch Intern Med 126:621–626, 1970.

30. Gardes J, Bouhnik J, Clauser E, et al. Role of angiotensinogen in blood pressure homeostasis. Hypertension 4:185–189, 1982.

31. Campbell DJ, Habener JF. Angiotensinogen gene is expressed and differentially regulated in multiple tissues of the rat. J Clin Invest 78:31–39, 1986.

32. Dzau VJ, Ellison KE, Brody T, et al. A comparative study of the distributions of renin and angiotensinogen messenger ribonucleic acids in rat and mouse tissues. Endocrinology 120:2334–2338, 1987.

33. Campbell DJ. The site of angiotensin production. J Hypertens 3:199–207, 1985.

34. Campbell WGJ, Ganhem F, Catanzaro DF, et al. Plasma and renal prorenin/renin, renin mRNA and blood pressure in Dahl S and R rats. Hypertension 27:1121–1133, 1996.

35. Sealey JE, Catanzaro DF, Lavin TN, et al. Specific prorenin/renin binding (ProBP): Identification and characterization of a novel membrane site. Am J Hypertens 9:491–502, 1996.

36. Gahnem F, Sealey JE, Atlas SA, Laragh JH. Inhibition of human renin by rat plasma. Am J Hypertens 5:495–501, 1992.

37. Bohlender J, Fukamizu A, Lippoldt A, et al. High human renin hypertension in transgenic rats. Hypertension 29:428–434, 1997.

38. Fukamizu A, Sugimura K, Takimoto E, et al. Chimeric renin-angiotensin system demonstrates sustained increase in blood pressure of transgenic mice carrying both human renin and human angiotensinogen genes. J Biol Chem 268:11617–11621, 1993.

39. Merrill DC, Thompson MW, Carney CL, et al. Chronic hypertension and altered baroreflex responses in transgenic mice containing the human renin and human angiotensinogen genes. J Clin Invest 97:1047–1055, 1996.

40. Fukamizu A, Seo MS, Hatae T, et al. Tissue-specific expression of the human renin gene in transgenic mice. Biochem Biophys Res Commun 165:826–832, 1989.

41. Sigmund CD, Jones CA, Kane CM, et al. Regulated tissue- and cell-specific expression of the human renin gene in transgenic mice. Circ Res 70:1070–1079, 1992.

42. Yan Y, Chen R, Pitarresi T, et al. Kidney is the only source of human plasma renin in 45 kb hREN transgenic mice. Circ Res 83:1279–1288, 1998.

43. Yan Y, Hu L, Chen R, et al. Appropriate regulation of human renin gene expression and secretion in 45 kb human renin transgenic mice. Hypertension 32:205–214, 1998.

44. Catanzaro DF, Chen R, Yan Y, et al. Appropriate regulation of renin and blood pressure in 45 kb human renin/human angiotensinogen transgenic mice. Hypertension 33:318–322, 1999.

45. Kimura S, Mullins JJ, Bunnemann B, et al. High blood pressure in transgenic mice carrying the rat angiotensinogen gene. EMBO J 11:821–827, 1992.

46. Tokita Y, Franco SR, Reimann EM, Mulrow PJ. Hypertension in the transgenic rat TGR(mRen-2)27 may be due to enhanced kinetics of the reaction between mouse renin and rat angiotensinogen [see comments]. Hypertension 23:422–427, 1994.

47. Tanimoto K, Sugiyama F, Goto Y, et al. Angiotensinogen-deficient mice with hypotension. J Biol Chem 269:31334–31337, 1994.

48. Smithies O, Kim HS. Targeted gene duplication and disruption for analyzing quantitative genetic traits in mice. Proc Natl Acad Sci U S A 91:3612–3615, 1994.

49. Kim HS, Krege JH, Kluckman KD, et al. Genetic control of blood pressure and the angiotensinogen locus. Proc Natl Acad Sci U S A 92:2735–2739, 1995.

50. Brand E, Chatelain N, Keavney B, et al. Evaluation of the angiotensinogen locus in human essential hypertension. Hypertension 31:725–729, 1998.

51. Kunz R, Kreutz R, Beige J, et al. Association between the angiotensinogen 235T-variant and essential hypertension in whites: A systematic review and methodological appraisal. Hypertension 30:1331–1337, 1997.

52. Jeunemaitre X, Ledru F, Battaglia S, et al. Genetic polymorphisms of the renin-angiotensin system and angiographic extent and severity of coronary artery disease: The CORGENE study. Hum Genet 99:66–73, 1997.

53. Kiema TR, Kauma H, Rantala AO, et al. Variation at the angiotensin-converting enzyme gene and angiotensinogen gene loci in relation to blood pressure. Hypertension 28:1070–1075, 1996.

54. Tiret L, Ricard S, Poirier O, et al. Genetic variation at the angiotensinogen locus in relation to high blood pressure and myocardial infarction: The ECTIM Study. J Hypertens 13:311–317, 1995.

55. Jeunemaitre X, Charru A, Chatellier G, et al. M235T variant of the human angiotensinogen gene in unselected hypertensive patients. J Hypertens Suppl S80–S81, 1993.

56. Jeunemaitre X, Inoue I, Williams C, et al. Haplotypes of angiotensinogen in essential hypertension. Am J Hum Genet 60:1448–1460, 1997.

57. Bennett CL, Schrader AP, Morris BJ. Cross-sectional analysis of Met235—The variant of angiotensinogen gene in severe, familial hypertension. Biochem Biophys Res Commun 197:833–839, 1993.

58. Borecki IB, Province MA, Ludwig EH, et al. Associations of candidate loci angiotensinogen and angiotensin-converting enzyme with severe hypertension: The NHLBI Family Heart Study. Ann Epidemiol 7:13–21, 1997.

59. Jeunemaitre X, Charru A, Rigat B, et al. Sib pair linkage analysis of

renin gene haplotypes in human essential hypertension. Hum Genet 88:301–306, 1992.

60. Johnson AG, Simons LA, Friedlander Y, et al. M235—T polymorphism of the angiotensinogen gene predicts hypertension in the elderly. J Hypertens 14:1061–1065, 1996.

61. Caulfield M, Lavender P, Farrall M, et al. Linkage of the angiotensinogen gene to essential hypertension [see comments]. N Engl J Med 330:1629–1633, 1994.

62. Hegele RA, Brunt JH, Connelly PW. A polymorphism of the angiotensinogen gene associated with variation in blood pressure in a genetic isolate. Circulation 90:2207–2212, 1994.

63. Detsky AS, Naylor CD, O'Rourke K, et al. Incorporating variations in the quality of individual randomized trials into metanalysis. J Clin Epidemiol 45:255–265, 1992.

64. Eysenck HJ. Meta-analysis and its problems. BMJ 309:789–792, 1994.

65. Forrester T, McFarlane AN, Bennet F, et al. Angiotensinogen and blood pressure among blacks: Findings from a community survey in Jamaica. J Hypertens 14:315–321, 1996.

66. Rotimi C, Puras A, Cooper R, et al. Polymorphisms of renin-angiotensin genes among Nigerians, Jamaicans, and African Americans. Hypertension 27:558–563, 1996.

67. Rotimi C, Cooper R, Ogunbiyi O, et al. Hypertension, serum angiotensinogen, and molecular variants of the angiotensinogen gene among Nigerians. Circulation 95:2348–2350, 1997.

68. Iwai N, Shimoike H, Ohmichi N, Kinoshita M. Angiotensinogen gene and blood pressure in the Japanese population. Hypertension 25:688–693, 1995.

69. Morise T, Takeuchi Y, Takeda R. Rapid detection and prevalence of the variants of the angiotensinogen gene in patients with essential hypertension. J Intern Med 237:175–180, 1995.

70. Lander ES, Schork NJ. Genetic dissection of complex traits. Science 265:2037–2048, 1994.

71. Caulfield M, Lavender P, Newell PJ, et al. Linkage of the angiotensinogen gene locus to human essential hypertension in African Caribbeans. J Clin Invest 96:687–692, 1995.

72. Schmidt S, Sharma AM, Zilch O, et al. Association of M235T variant of the angiotensinogen gene with familial hypertension of early onset. Nephrol Dial Transplant 10:1145–1148, 1995.

73. Schunkert H, Hense HW, Gimenez RA, et al. The angiotensinogen T235 variant and the use of antihypertensive drugs in a population-based cohort. Hypertension 29:628–633, 1997.

74. Barley J, Blackwood A, Sagnella G, et al. Angiotensinogen Met235–Thr polymorphism in a London normotensive and hypertensive black and white population. J Hum Hypertens 8:639–640, 1994.

75. Fornage M, Turner ST, Sing CF, Boerwinkle E. Variation at the M235T locus of the angiotensinogen gene and essential hypertension: A population-based case-control study from Rochester, Minnesota. Hum Genet 96:295–300, 1995.

76. Hingorani AD, Sharma P, Jia H, et al. Blood pressure and the M235T polymorphism of the angiotensinogen gene. Hypertension 28:907–911, 1996.

77. Beige J, Zilch O, Hohenbleicher H, et al. Genetic variants of the renin-angiotensin system and ambulatory blood pressure in essential hypertension. J Hypertens 15:503–508, 1997.

78. Bigda J, Narkiewicz K, Chrostowska M, et al. No effect of genetic variation at the angiotensinogen locus on ambulatory blood pressure level in normotensive subjects. Am J Hypertens 10:692–695, 1997.

79. Mondorf UF, Russ A, Wiesmann A, et al. Contribution of angiotensin

converting enzyme gene polymorphism and angiotensinogen gene polymorphism to blood pressure regulation in essential hypertension. Am J Hypertens 11:174–183, 1998.

80. Hata A, Namikawa C, Sasaki M, et al. Angiotensinogen as a risk factor for essential hypertension in Japan. J Clin Invest 93:1285–1287, 1994.

81. Iwai N, Ohmici N, Nakamura Y, et al. Molecular variants of the angiotensinogen gene and hypertension in a Japanese population. Hypertens Res 17:117–121, 1994.

82. Kamitani A, Rakugi H, Higaki J, et al. Association analysis of a polymorphism of the angiotensinogen gene with essential hypertension in Japanese. J Hum Hypertens 8:521–524, 1994.

83. Nishiuma S, Kario K, Kayaba K, et al. Effect of the angiotensinogen gene Met235–Thr variant on blood pressure and other cardiovascular risk factors in two Japanese populations. J Hypertens 13:717–722, 1995.

84. Kataoka S, Hashimoto N, Kakihara T, et al. Analysis of Met235 to Thr variant of the angiotensinogen gene in relation to the blood pressure and family history of essential hypertension in Japanese children. Acta Paediatr Jpn 38:312–316, 1996.

85. Rotimi C, Morrison L, Cooper R, et al. Angiotensinogen gene in human hypertension. Lack of an association of the 235T allele among African Americans. Hypertension 24:591–594, 1994.

86. Rutledge DR, Browe CS, Kubilis PS, Ross EA. Analysis of two variants of the angiotensinogen gene in essential hypertensive African-Americans. Am J Hypertens 7:651–654, 1994.

87. Bloem LJ, Manatunga AK, Tewksbury DA, Pratt JH. The serum angiotensinogen concentration and variants of the angiotensinogen gene in white and black children. J Clin Invest 95:948–953, 1995.

88. Bloem LJ, Foroud TM, Ambrosius WT, et al. Association of the angiotensinogen gene to serum angiotensinogen in blacks and whites. Hypertension 29:1078–1082, 1997.

89. Gharavi AG, Lipkowitz ML, Diamond JA, et al. Ambulatory blood pressure monitoring for detecting the relation between angiotensinogen gene polymorphism and hypertension. Am J Hypertens 10:687–691, 1997.

90. Hegele RA, Harris SB, Hanley AJ, et al. Angiotensinogen gene variation associated with variation in blood pressure in aboriginal Canadians. Hypertension 29:1073–1077, 1997.

91. Ward K, Hata A, Jeunemaitre X, et al. A molecular variant of angiotensinogen associated with preeclampsia [see comments]. Nat Genet 4:59–61, 1993.

92. Barley J, Markus H, Brown M, Carter N. Lack of association between angiotensinogen polymorphism (M235T) and cerebrovascular disease and carotid atheroma. J Hum Hypertens 9:681–683, 1995.

93. Schmidt S, Giessel R, Bergis KH, et al. Angiotensinogen gene M235T polymorphism is not associated with diabetic nephropathy. The Diabetic Nephropathy Study Group. Nephrol Dial Transplant 11:1755–1761, 1996.

94. Tarnow L, Cambien F, Rossing P, et al. Angiotensinogen gene polymorphisms in IDDM patients with diabetic nephropathy. Diabetes 45:367–369, 1996.

95. Hopkins PN, Lifton RP, Hollenberg NK, et al. Blunted renal vascular response to angiotensin II is associated with a common variant of the angiotensinogen gene and obesity. J Hypertens 14:199–207, 1996.

96. Kobashi G. [A case-control study of pregnancy-induced hypertension with a genetic predisposition: Association of a molecular variant of angiotensinogen in the Japanese women]. [Japanese] Hokkaido Igaku Zasshi 70:649–657, 1995.

CHAPTER 9

Angiotensin-Converting Enzyme: Basic Properties, Distribution, and Functional Role

Maurice E. Fabiani, Diem T. Dinh, Labrini Nassis, and Colin I. Johnston

The renin-angiotensin system (RAS) plays a key role in the regulation of blood pressure as well as in the maintenance of fluid and electrolyte balance. The biological actions of the RAS are mediated by the potent octapeptide angiotensin II via specific angiotensin receptors, namely AT_1 and AT_2. Classically, the biosynthesis of angiotensin II involves a series of catalytic steps in which the proteolytic enzyme renin, released from the juxtaglomerular cells of the kidney, cleaves the liver-derived $_2$-globulin angiotensinogen to form the decapeptide angiotensin 1, which is subsequently converted to angiotensin II by angiotensin-converting enzyme (ACE), primarily within the pulmonary circulation (Fig. 9–1). However, it is now clear that many tissues, including blood vessels, kidney, heart, and brain, are also capable of generating angiotensin II locally, which may subserve autocrine, paracrine, and intracrine functions. The presence of all the requisite components of a tissue-based RAS (i.e., renin, angiotensinogen, ACE, and angiotensin receptors) in such tissues lends further support to the existence of the tissue-based RAS, in addition to the well-described circulating hormonal RAS.

ACE is predominantly a membrane-bound ectoenzyme and an integral component of the RAS that is responsible for the production of angiotensin II from its inactive precursor angiotensin I as well as the degradation of bradykinin to inactive fragments. Although not generally considered the rate-limiting step in angiotensin II synthesis, ACE is nonetheless a major and indeed the final determinant of prevailing angiotensin II levels within the circulation and across many tissues. The remarkable success of ACE inhibitors in the treatment of hypertension and congestive heart failure highlights the importance of ACE and the RAS in the development of cardiovascular disease. This chapter focuses on the general biochemical properties, tissue localization, and distribution of ACE and on possible functional roles of tissue ACE.

BASIC PROPERTIES OF ANGIOTENSIN-CONVERTING ENZYME

Structure and Isoforms

ACE (kininase II, EC 3.4.15.1) is a ubiquitous zinc metallopeptidase that represents the final enzymatic step in the production of angiotensin II from angiotensin I.[1, 2] There are three main isoforms of ACE; they have been designated (1) somatic ACE, (2) plasma, or soluble, ACE, and (3), testicular, or germinal, ACE (Fig. 9–2). *Somatic ACE* is a 170 Kda glycoprotein that is found in a variety of tissues, including blood vessels, heart, kidney, brain, and so forth.

Somatic ACE is a bi-lobed ectoenzyme attached to the cell membrane, with a homodimeric extracellular region, a transmembrane anchoring domain, and a short intracellular carboxy tall.[3] The extracellular region consists of two homologous domains, both of which contain an active catalytic site.[4, 5] *Testicular,* or germinal, *ACE* is a 90 Kda glycoprotein that is found exclusively on germinal cells in the testes. Testicular ACE is also a membrane-bound enzyme and corresponds to the carboxy region of somatic ACE but has a unique N-terminal region.[6] Consequently, testicular ACE contains only one catalytically active site, equivalent to the C-terminal active site of the somatic isoform. However, somatic ACE and testicular ACE share the same hydrophobic transmembrane anchoring domain and hydrophilic intracellular C-terminal sequence. *Plasma,* or soluble, *ACE* is thought to be derived from post-translational proteolytic cleavage of the C-terminal region of somatic ACE from the cell membrane, but it lacks the transmembrane domain and intracellular portion.[7, 8] As such, soluble ACE corresponds to the extracellular region of somatic ACE and contains two active sites. Whether there is a specific processing enzyme that cleaves cell-bound ACE or whether it derives from senescent cells is not known. Recent studies employing molecular and gene knockout techniques have definitively established that cell-bound ACE, or somatic ACE, is the important enzyme for the production of angiotensin II.[9]

Human Angiotensin-Converting Enzyme Gene

The human gene that encodes ACE has been cloned and shown to be located on the q23 region of chromosome 17.[10, 11] The human ACE gene comprises 26 exons and 25 introns (Fig. 9–3). Both somatic and testicular ACE isoforms are derived from the same gene via two alternative promoters.[12, 13] The somatic promoter is located in the 5′ flanking region of the gene, upstream of exon 1, and initiates somatic ACE transcription. The testicular promoter is located within intron 12 of the gene and is responsible for transcription of testicular ACE.[14] Somatic ACE is encoded by an mRNA of 4.3 Kb, transcribed from exons 1 to 6 of human ACE gene, excluding exon 13. On the other hand, testicular ACE is encoded by an mRNA of 3 Kb, transcribed from exons 13 to 26, with exon 13 encoding the unique N-terminus of the testicular isoform.

A genetic polymorphism in the ACE gene has been identified and is believed to account for the high degree of interindividual variability in plasma ACE levels in the population.[15] The insertion/deletion polymorphism within intron 16 of the ACE gene is due to the presence or absence

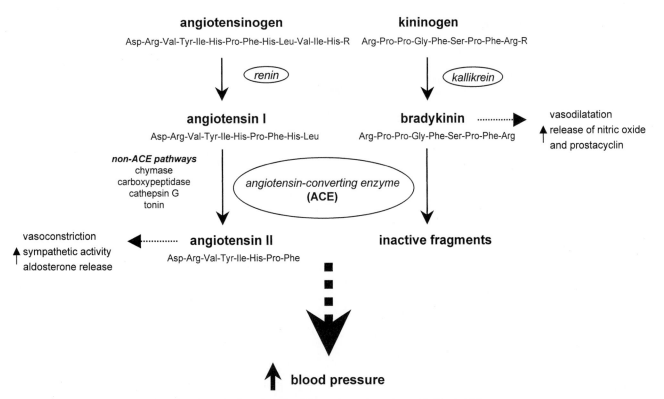

Figure 9–1. Biosynthetic pathways of the renin-angiotensin and kallikrein-kinin systems.

of a 287-base pair fragment. The D allele is associated with higher plasma ACE levels and has been linked to an increased risk of myocardial infarction and nephropathy in type I diabetics and to an increased rate of renal deterioration in glomerular diseases.[16] However, there is no association of this ACE gene polymorphism with essential hypertension in humans.[17]

Catalytic Sites

Both catalytic sites of ACE are capable of converting angiotensin I to angiotensin II.[5] However, the two active sites display different enzyme kinetics. The C-terminal site accounts for about 75% of total ACE activity, the N-terminal site accounts for only 25%.[5] Although the affinity of angiotensin I for each active site is similar, the C-terminal site is largely responsible for the conversion of angiotensin I to angiotensin II. It has been suggested that the N-terminal site is responsible mainly for the metabolism of other peptide substrates.[18]

Each active site of the ACE molecule binds one atom of zinc, which is critical for its catalytic activity.[19–21] Substitution of zinc by other divalent cations does not appear to affect substrate affinity but dramatically alters the conversion rate of peptide substrates.[20] Monovalent anions, especially chloride, enhance the ACE activity, probably by enhancing substrate binding.[22] However, the presence of chloride is not required as bradykinin and various other peptides can be hydrolyzed efficiently in the absence of

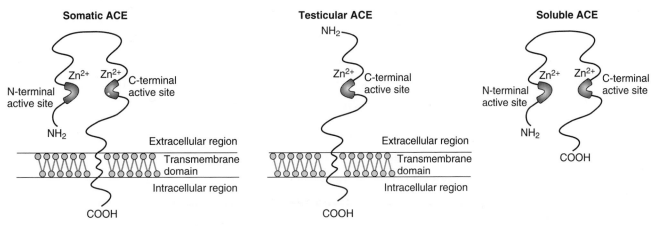

Figure 9–2. Schematic representation of the structural isoforms of angiotensin-converting enzyme (ACE).

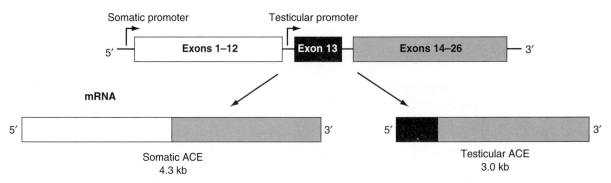

Figure 9–3. Schematic representation of the organization of the human ACE gene and transcribed mRNA for the somatic and testicular isoforms.

chloride.[22] ACE activity has an optimum pH of 7 to 8 and falls rapidly with decreasing pH (acidic environment), most likely due to protonation of the zinc-binding regions of ACE.[2]

ACE inhibitors interact differently with ACE active sites, depending on their structural configurations.[23, 24] Radioligand binding studies with [^{125}I]-351A, a *p*-hydroxy-benzamidine derivative of lisinopril, demonstrate the presence of only one binding site on both somatic and testicular ACE, suggesting that it binds only to the C-terminal active

site of ACE. In contrast, [^{125}I]-Ro31-8472, a hydroxy derivative of cilazaprilat, revealed two binding sites on somatic ACE and one binding site on testicular ACE.[4] These findings suggest that the two active sites of ACE have different conformational requirements for metabolizing peptide substrates. Accordingly, each catalytic site may selectively cleave different peptide substrates. This raises the possibility of designing specific inhibitors directed to either of these active sites to selectively block the formation or degradation or both of certain endogenous peptides.[24]

Table 9–1 Endogenous Substrates of ACE and Their Cleavage Sites

Peptide	Sequence
Angiotensin I	H-Asp-Arg-Val-Tyr-Ile-His-Pro-Phe-His-Leu-OH
Bradykinin	H-Arg-Pro-Pro-Gly-Phe-Ser-Pro-Phe-Arg-OH
Des-Arg^9 bradykinin	H-Arg-Pro-Pro-Gly-Phe-Ser-Pro-Phe-OH
β-Neoendorphin	H-Tyr-Gly-Gly-Phe-Leu-Arg-Lys-Tyr-Pro-OH
Dynorphin$^{1-8}$	H-Tyr-Gly-Gly-Phe-Leu-Arg-Arg-Ile-OH
Enkephalins	
Pentapeptide	H-Tyr-Gly-Gly-Phe-Met-OH
Heptapeptide	H-Tyr-Gly-Gly-Phe-Met-Arg-Phe-OH
Octapeptide	H-Tyr-Gly-Gly-Phe-Met-Arg-Gly-Leu-OH
Chemotactic peptide	N-formyl-Met-Leu-Phe-OH
Neurotensin	pGlu-Leu-Tyr-Glu-Asn-Lys-Pro-Arg-Arg-Pro-Tyr-Ile-Leu-OH
Substance P	H-Arg-Pro-Lys-Pro-Gln-Gln-Phe-Phe-Gly-Leu-Met-NH$_2$
Cholecystokinin-8	H-Asp-Tyr(SO$_3$H)-Met-Gly-Trp-Met-Asp-Phe-NH$_2$
Bombesin	pGlu-Gln-Arg-Leu-Gly-Asn-Gln-Trp-Ala-Val-Gly-His-Leu-Met-NH$_2$
Luteinizing hormone–releasing hormone	pGlu-His-Trp-Ser-Tyr-Gly-Leu-Arg-Pro-Gly-NH$_2$
Hematopoietic stem cell regulatory peptide	N-acetyl-Ser-Asp-Lys-Pro-OH

Abbreviation: ACE, angiotensin-converting enzyme.

Substrate Specificity

ACE is mainly a peptidyl carboxypeptidase that generates angiotensin II by cleaving the C-terminal dipeptide His-Leu from angiotensin I.[25] Similarly, ACE inactivates bradykinin by liberating the dipeptide Phe-Arg from the C-terminal end of the peptide.[25] ACE has broad substrate specificity in vitro and is capable of cleaving di- and tripeptides from the C-terminal (in some cases, from the N-terminal) region of a host of other peptides, including substance P, enkephalins, neurotensin, cholecystokinin, bombesin, and luteinizing hormone-releasing hormone.[2, 25, 26] (Table 9–1). The C-terminal active site of ACE is largely responsible for the conversion of angiotensin I to angiotensin II, whereas the N-terminal active site is responsible for cleaving other peptide substrates.[5]

ACE generally functions as a carboxy-dipeptidase against most peptide substrates. However, ACE degrades substance P by both carboxy-dipeptidase and carboxy-tripeptidase action.[27] In addition, against luteinizing hormone-releasing hormone, ACE exhibits amino-tripeptidase and carboxy-tripeptidase activity, depending on the prevailing levels of chloride.[26, 28] High chloride concentrations tend to favor the cleavage of tripeptides from the N-terminal region, whereas low chloride concentrations allow metabolism at both ends of the peptide.[28] The functional consequence and pathophysiological relevance in vivo of the broad range of peptide substrates capable of being degraded by ACE remains unknown. Recently, a specific endogenous substrate for the N-terminal catalytic site has been described. The hemoregulatory peptide N-acetyl-seryl-aspartyl-lysyl-proline has been shown to be a natural and specific substrate for the N-terminal catalytic site of human ACE.[29] Furthermore, administration of ACE inhibitors has been reported to raise the levels of this regulatory peptide in the plasma of humans.[30] This raises the interesting possibility that ACE may play a role in hemopoietic stem cell differentiation and proliferation. Moreover, ACE has been found in insects and has been shown to possess prohormone-processing activity.[31, 32]

DISTRIBUTION AND LOCALIZATION

Cardiovascular System

In vitro autoradiography and immunohistochemistry have been used extensively to map the anatomical localization of ACE in various tissues (Table 9–2). In the cardiovascular system, membrane-bound ACE is widespread on endothelial cells of the vasculature, including cerebral and coronary blood vessels.[33] In conduit blood vessels, including the aorta, pulmonary artery, mammary artery, and saphenous vein, a high level of binding of ACE has been detected in the endothelial and adventitial layers, and a low level of binding has been observed in the media. In such blood vessels, ACE binding in the adventitia is localized mainly to the vasa vasorum.[33–35]

In cardiac tissues of the rat, high-level binding sites for ACE are found on valve leaflets (pulmonary, aortic, mitral, and tricuspid) and low-level binding in the endocardium.[33, 36] In contrast, in the human heart, ACE distribution is homogeneous, with lower concentrations of ACE in cardiac valves.[37]

Central Nervous System

The localization of ACE in the brain has been studied in a variety of species, including the rat, rabbit, monkey, and human. ACE has been located in high concentrations in the cerebral vasculature of various regions of the brain (see Table 9–2).[38] High concentrations of ACE are also found in the circumventricular organs, including the subfornical organ, anterior pituitary, and vascular organ of the lamina terminalis, located outside of the blood-brain barrier.[38–40] In these regions, circulating angiotensin I may be converted to angiotensin II by ACE, which may act locally on the high density of angiotensin II receptors. Moderate to high levels of ACE are also found in other regions of the brain, such as the choroid plexus, paraventricular and supraoptic

Table 9–2 Distribution of ACE in Human Tissues and Body Fluids

Source	ACE Isoform
ENDOTHELIAL CELLS	Somatic
Arteries	
Veins	
EPITHELIAL CELLS	Somatic
Renal proximal tubules	
Gastrointestinal tract	
Submandibular gland	
Choroid plexus	
Epididymis	
Prostate gland	
CARDIOVASCULAR SYSTEM	Somatic
Heart	
Vascular adventitia	
Adrenal cortex	
BRAIN	Somatic
Basal ganglia	
Posterior pituitary	
Cerebellum	
REPRODUCTIVE SYSTEM	
Testis	Testicular
Seminiferous tubules	
Spermatozoa	
Ovary	Somatic
Corpus luteum	
Follicles	
FIBROBLASTS AND MACROPHAGES	Somatic
BODY FLUIDS	Soluble
Plasma	
Seminal fluid	
Urine	
Amniotic fluid	
Cerebrospinal fluid	
Lymph	

Abbreviation: ACE, angiotensin-converting enzyme.

hypothalamic nuclei, and dorsal vagal complex.[38, 40–43] In all of these regions, there is a good correlation between the distribution of ACE and angiotensin II receptors.

In the brain, angiotensin II is involved in stimulating drinking behavior and regulating autonomic function and in the release of pituitary hormones and monoamines.[39, 44–46] Moreover, angiotensin II is believed to act on the circumventricular organs and the paraventricular nucleus, both of which are important in mediating the central pressor and dipsogenic effects of angiotensin II.[38]

High concentrations of ACE are also present in the basal ganglia, including the caudate, putamen, globus pallidus, and substantia nigra as well as the cerebellum, hippocampus, inferior olivary nuclei, and spinal trigeminal nuclei. These sites contain very little angiotensin II and a low density of angiotensin II receptors.[38, 40] These findings suggest that, at these particular sites, ACE may be associated with the metabolism of neuropeptides such as substance P and enkephalins rather than with angiotensin II production.

Kidney and Adrenal System

In the kidney, high levels of ACE are present in epithelial cells lining the brush border of the proximal convoluted tubules.[47] Angiotensin II receptors are localized in close proximity to ACE on the basolateral and brush border membranes of the proximal convoluted tubules.[48] Angiotensin II is involved in the regulation of renal blood flow, glomerular filtration, and tubular sodium reabsorption.[48] Although it is possible that the effects of angiotensin II in the kidney are due largely to systemically delivered peptide, there is growing evidence that locally produced angiotensin II may also contribute to the renal actions of the peptide.[49]

In the rat adrenal, ACE is found in both the cortex and the medulla. In the cortex, ACE is localized to the zona glomerulosa, in the medulla, to the plasma membrane of chromaffin cells.[50, 51] Similarly, a high density of angiotensin II receptors is colocalized with ACE in these zones, suggesting a role for local production of angiotensin II.[52] Angiotensin II is a powerful stimulus for aldosterone synthesis and secretion and for catecholamine release from the adrenal medulla.[53, 54]

Reproductive System

The testicular isoform of ACE is expressed exclusively in the testis, specifically on spermatozoa and the luminal surface of seminiferous tubules (see Table 9–2).[47] In addition, somatic ACE is found in the epithelial cells of the epididymis, and high concentrations of soluble ACE are present in the seminal fluid.[55] There is stage-specific ACE expression during spermatogenesis, suggesting that ACE may play a role in sperm differentiation.[56] Other possible functions of ACE include sperm maturation and motility and processing gonadotrophins or other substrates.[57] Testicular ACE is induced by testosterone and appears during puberty.

In the human prostate, a reproductive accessory organ,

ACE has been localized to glandular epithelial structures. Moreover, ACE binding has also been demonstrated in the prostatic lumen and has been shown to be increased in prostate diseases such as benign prostatic hypertrophy (Fabiani et al., unpublished observations). It is not clear whether luminal ACE is derived from cleavage of somatic ACE from the epithelial cell membrane or active secretion into the glandular lumina.

ACE has been found in the ovary of the rat. The presence of ACE in the corpus luteum, follicles, and germinal epithelium suggests that it may be involved in follicular development (see Table 9–2).[58, 59] Evidence to support this contention is provided by the finding that the angiotensin II antagonist saralasin inhibits ovulation.[60]

Gastrointestinal Tract

In the gastrointestinal tract, high levels of ACE are found on epithelial cells lining the brush border of the small intestine (see Table 9–2).[61–63] The functional role of ACE in the gut remains obscure; however, it may digest dietary peptides into smaller fragments to facilitate absorption. ACE and angiotensin II receptors are densely distributed in the muscularis of the intestine, suggesting that locally produced angiotensin II may play a role in controlling intestinal function.[61] Moreover, in the rabbit gastric fundus, ACE has been located intracellularly in the granules of chief and neck cells. This is in stark contrast to the presence of ACE as an ectoenzyme in other tissues.[64]

FUNCTIONAL ROLE

The functional role of ACE in many tissues is still not known. Several functions of ACE have been proposed and are summarized in Table 9–3. The principal role of ACE in the circulation is the generation of angiotensin II and the degradation of bradykinin. This function of ACE is a major contribution to the regulation of blood pressure and fluid and electrolyte homeostasis (see later section). The anatomical localization of ACE in many tissues, including blood vessels, heart, kidney, brain, and reproductive organs, suggests that tissue ACE may provide an additional mechanism to control angiotensin II synthesis at a cellular level. Therefore an increase in tissue ACE activity in pathological states may lead to an increase in angiotensin II levels locally in tissues or in the circulation. Although alternative non-ACE pathways for the formation of angiotensin II, particularly cardiac chymase, have been proposed, human studies have shown that ACE inhibitors almost totally prevent the conversion of angiotensin I into angiotensin II in the intravascular compartment in vivo.[65] This suggests that ACE is the most important pathway for the formation of angiotensin II in vivo, at least in the circulation. The functional significance of non-ACE pathways remains obscure but may be of pathophysiological relevance in disease states.[66]

The wide distribution of ACE and frequent discordance with the presence of other components of the RAS suggest that the enzyme may have roles other than the synthesis of angiotensin II and the breakdown of bradykinin. For in-

Table 9-3 Proposed Functions of Tissue ACE

Site	Function

Cardiovascular system (blood vessels, heart)	Regulation of regional blood flow
	Modulation of local sympathetic activity
	Stimulation of hyperplasia and hypertrophy
	  Direct action of angiotensin II
	  Growth factors (e.g., bFGF, PDGF)
	  Activation of proto-oncogenes
	Stimulation of nitric oxide and prostacyclin from the endothelium
	Modulation of inotropic and chronotropic activity of the heart
	Inflammatory mediators

Central nervous system	Processing of neuropeptide Maintenance of fluid and electrolyte balance Regulation of systemic blood pressure Stimulation of drinking behavior Modulation of salt appetite Modulation of pituitary hormone release Modulation of sensory function Regulation of effects on learning and memory
Kidney	Regulation of fluid and electrolyte balance Regulation of renal blood flow Regulation of glomerular filtration Control of renin release
Adrenals	Stimulation of aldosterone synthesis and secretion Stimulation of catecholamine release
Reproductive organs Testis	Initiation of spermatogenesis Regulation of sperm maturation and motility Processing of gonadotrophin
Ovary	Regulation of ovulation Stimulation of estrogen
Epithelial cells	Transportation of ions Regulation of peptide metabolism
Fibroblasts and macrophages	Control of inflammation and tissue repair

Abbreviations: ACE, angiotensin-converting enzyme; bFGF, basic fibroblast growth factor; PDGF, platelet-derived growth factor.

stance, in many regions of the brain, ACE does not colocalize with angiotensin II receptors.[38, 39] It is likely that in these brain areas, ACE is involved in neuropeptide processing rather than in angiotensin II generation. Moreover, because ACE is present in high concentrations on epithelial cells of the renal proximal tubule, gastrointestinal tract, submandibular gland, choroid plexus, and placenta, it is likely that ACE is involved in ionic transport and possibly in peptide metabolism.[67]

The functional role of ACE in the male and female reproductive systems is poorly understood, but ACE may be involved in reproduction. ACE is present in high concentrations on germinal cells and spermatozoa of the testis as well as on ovarian follicles. It is possible that, in males, ACE plays a role in sperm differentiation, maturation, and motility.[57] ACE may also play a role in follicular development and ovulation in females.[58, 59]

Role in Cardiovascular Function

The functions of tissue ACE are best characterized in the cardiovascular system. The presence of all of the requisite components of the RAS in blood vessels, heart, kidney, brain, and adrenals suggests that it is intimately involved in the regulation of blood pressure and cardiovascular function and structure. ACE plays a critical role in the cardiovascular system by controlling the production of angiotensin II both systemically and locally in many tissues.

ACE may be involved in a diverse range of cardiovascular functions, such as the regulation of peripheral vascular tone and regional blood flow, modulation of local sympathetic activity, stimulation of hyperplasia and hypertrophy, release of vasoactive substances from the endothelium, and mediation of inflammation and tissue repair.[67] Angiotensin II is a potent vasoconstrictor and hence may influence peripheral vascular tone and regulate regional blood flow, including the cerebral and coronary circulations. Furthermore, ACE may modulate cardiovascular function by influencing the metabolic breakdown of bradykinin, a potent vasodilator known to liberate nitric oxide and prostacyclin from the endothelium.[68]

ACE modulates local sympathetic activity in the cardiovascular system. Angiotensin II facilitates sympathetic neuroeffector transmission in many cardiovascular tissues by several means; (1) enhancing noradrenaline release from sympathetic nerve terminals, (2) increasing the rate of synthesis of noradrenaline (3) blocking neuronal uptake of noradrenaline, and (4) amplifying the postjunctional actions of noradrenaline.[69, 70] Conversely, ACE inhibition has been demonstrated to reduce peripheral sympathetic activity and noradrenaline overflow.[71] Clinical studies have also shown that ACE inhibitors reduce plasma catecholamine levels and reduce cardiac arrhythmias in patients with congestive heart failure.[72, 73]

In the rat heart, angiotensin II receptors are present in high concentrations in the atrioventricular node, cardiac ganglia, and parasympathetic nerve bundles.[74] Thus, angiotensin II can have direct ionotropic and chronotropic effects on the heart.[54] Angiotensin II may also affect the heart by facilitating sympathetic nerve activity[75] and decreasing vagal tone.[76, 77] Conversely, ACE inhibition facilitates cardiac vagal activity.[78] Angiotensin II also interacts with the endothelium, stimulating the release of prostaglandins and nitric oxide,[79] and may be important in inflammation and tissue repair. Moreover, angiotensin II may exert growth-promoting effects, stimulating hyperplasia, hypertrophy, or both,[80] which has been implicated in pathological conditions such as hypertension, arteriosclerosis, and myocardial hypertrophy.

Angiotensin II is a powerful coronary vasoconstrictor with the ability to regulate the growth of vascular smooth muscle cells and also to induce myointimal hyperplasia after endothelial injury.[67] On the other hand, bradykinin, also a substrate for ACE, is a potent vasodilator and an antiproliferative agent. Bradykinin inhibits smooth muscle cell proliferation by stimulating the release of endothelial factors such as nitric oxide and prostacyclin. High levels of ACE may enhance the production of angiotensin II, stimulating the growth of vascular smooth cells, and may also promote bradykinin breakdown, thus losing an inhibitory pathway modulating cell proliferation. The net result is a shift of the hormonal balance in favor of enhanced cell growth in cardiovascular tissues.

PATHOPHYSIOLOGICAL ROLE

Hypertension

The RAS plays a major role in the regulation of blood pressure. The circulating RAS is responsible for the acute control of blood pressure, providing short-term hemodynamic control, whereas the local RAS is involved in the regulation of cardiovascular structure and function and hence of long-term control of blood pressure. Hyperactivity of the local RAS has been implicated in the development of hypertension, although data from animal models of hypertension are inconclusive and at times conflicting. It has been reported that vascular ACE is increased in the two-kidney, one-clip Goldblatt hypertensive rat, a high-renin model of hypertension.[82, 83] However, we could not show any increase in ACE in the spontaneously hypertensive rat (SHR) or the two-kidney, one-clip Goldblatt hypertensive rat.[84–86] On the other hand, an increase in both vascular and cardiac ACE was observed in the low-renin, one-kidney, one-clip Goldblatt hypertensive rat.[87]

It is interesting to note that brief treatment of young, prehypertensive SHRs with ACE inhibitors during a critical period of their growth has been shown to prevent or reduce the development of high blood pressure well after treatment has ceased.[88] Furthermore, it has been reported that blood pressure in SHR cosegregates with the portion of the genome that contains the ACE gene.[89, 90] However, these studies identified a large region of the genome known to contain the ACE gene, and it is possible that the hypertensive trait may be associated with an unrelated gene in close proximity to the ACE gene.

Particular attention should be drawn to the interaction of ACE with the endothelium. In hypertension there is endothelial dysfunction and impaired responses to endothelium-dependent vasodilators.[91] Treatment with ACE inhibitors appears to restore the blunted responses to these agents. The mechanism by which ACE inhibitors restore these responses is not clear but may involve bradykinin, as bradykinin can stimulate the release of vasoactive substances, particularly nitric oxide and prostaglandins, from endothelial cells.[81] ACE inhibitors may restore vasodilator responses by preventing the breakdown of bradykinin.

Cardiovascular Hypertrophy

The local RAS has been implicated in promoting cardiac and vascular cell growth and hypertrophy (see Table 9–2). Angiotensin II not only provides a hemodynamic load by means of its vasoconstrictor activity, thus increasing peripheral resistance and ventricular afterload, but may also have several nonhemodynamic effects on growth. It is a potent stimulator of hyperplasia and hypertrophy of smooth muscle cells in culture[80, 92, 93] and releases growth factors such as platelet-derived growth factor, basic fibroblast growth factor, and transforming growth factor from smooth muscle cells.[94–96] Moreover, angiotensin II activates proto-oncogenes such as c-*fos,* c-*myc,* and c-*jun,* which are known to influence cell hypertrophy and division.[95, 97, 98] As alluded to above, angiotensin II may also stimulate peripheral sympathetic activity, which is involved in growth and hypertrophy, as sympathetic denervation leads to smooth muscle atrophy.[99] ACE inhibitors promote a regression of vascular hypertrophy and an increase in vascular flow reserve.[100, 101]

In the one-kidney, one-clip Goldblatt hypertensive rat, ACE is increased in hypertrophied blood vessels and in the left ventricle, but plasma ACE remains unchanged.[102] Moreover, ACE inhibition prevents neointimal hyperplasia following the removal of the endothelium in rat carotid arteries.[103] Removal of the endothelium is characterized initially by a decrease in vascular ACE, followed by an increase in ACE in the hyperplastic blood vessel.[3, 104] ACE inhibitors inhibit tissue ACE in blood vessels, but have not proved effective in preventing re-stenosis after coronary angioplasty in humans.[105, 106]

The RAS may also be involved in cardiac hypertrophy. ACE mRNA is increased in the hypertrophied left ventricle of rats following aortic banding[107] and in the hypertrophied left ventricle of the Goldblatt hypertensive rat. The degree of left ventricular hypertrophy correlates well with cardiac angiotensin II levels.[108] ACE inhibitors, in both hypotensive and nonhypotensive doses, reduce left ventricular hypertrophy following aortic stenosis in rats.[109] By contrast, in SHRs, the ability of ACE inhibitors to promote regression of left ventricular hypertrophy seems to be related to the extent of blood pressure reduction.[110] In humans, ACE inhibitors have been reported to reverse left ventricular hypertrophy to a greater extent than other classes of antihypertensive drugs despite similar reductions in blood pressure.[111] These findings indicate that the local RAS is involved in the development of cardiovascular hypertrophy, although its precise role has not yet been fully elucidated.

Myocardial Infarction and Cardiac Remodeling

Following acute myocardial infarction induced experimentally by ligation of the left coronary artery in rats,[112] ACE concentration increases dramatically in the peri-infarct region and is associated with the development of the acute inflammatory response. When the acute inflammatory response subsides, it is followed by the formation of scar tissue which also has very high levels of ACE. The remaining viable myocardium undergoes marked hypertrophy and remodeling associated with a dramatic increase in ACE.[36] This increase in ACE in both fibrotic scar tissue and hypertrophied myocardium persists for several months. Treatment with ACE inhibitors following acute myocardial infarction has been shown to improve hemodynamics, promote regression of myocardial hypertrophy, and increase survival.[1] These favorable effects of ACE inhibitors coincide with the inhibition of cardiac ACE activity and may help to explain the beneficial effects of ACE inhibitors reported in the Cooperative New Scandinavian Enalapril Survival Study (CONSENSUS; congestive heart failure), Studies of Left Ventricular Dysfunction (SOLVD; left ventricular dysfunction), and Survival and Ventricular Enlargement (SAVE); left ventricular dysfunction after myocardial infarction) trials.[113, 114] Genetic predisposition may also play a role in myocardial infarction. The deletion polymorphism in the ACE gene is associated with an increased risk of myocardial infarction.[115]

Inflammation and Tissue Repair

The presence of ACE on macrophages and fibroblasts suggests that the enzyme may be involved in the process of inflammation and tissue repair.[116] ACE is increased in some inflammatory conditions such as sarcoidosis and after acute myocardial infarction, so the initial increase in ACE in the infarct zone is most likely associated with an influx of inflammatory cells. Furthermore, in coronary arteries, denudation of the endothelium leads to neointimal hyperplasia with infiltration of the vessel wall with inflammatory cells, proliferation of fibroblasts, and deposition of collagen associated with an increase in ACE in the hyperplastic tissue.[103]

Bradykinin, a substrate for ACE, is also a potent inflammatory mediator[26] and is known to produce hyperemia and increase vascular permeability. Substance P is also a substrate for ACE and is known to be involved in mediating pain and inflammation.[26, 118, 119] Moreover, the chemotactic peptide N-formyl-met-leu-phe is a substrate for ACE. Therefore, ACE present on macrophages may play a role in inflammation by inactivating chemotactic peptides.[25]

BLOCKADE BY ANGIOTENSIN-CONVERTING ENZYME INHIBITORS

ACE inhibitors have proved a major advance in the treatment of cardiovascular disease. These drugs were originally designed to inhibit the conversion of angiotensin I to angiotensin II by plasma ACE. Although the acute hypotensive action of ACE inhibitors correlates well with a reduction in plasma angiotensin II levels, the long-term or chronic hypotensive action of these agents cannot be ascribed solely to inhibition of plasma ACE and a decrease in circulating angiotensin II. The chronic hypotensive action of ACE inhibitors is more closely related to inhibition of tissue ACE than of plasma ACE.[120] Similarly, the ability of ACE inhibitors to reverse vascular and left ventricular hypertrophy is most likely associated with inhibition of vascular and cardiac ACE as well as with reduction of hemodynamic load by lowering blood pressure. The significant reduction in morbidity and mortality associated with ACE inhibitor therapy after myocardial infarction observed in the SOLVD[114] and SAVE[113] studies is due not only to hemodynamic improvement but also to inhibition of cardiac tissue ACE.

ACE inhibitors act by binding to the catalytic site of ACE in a stoichiometric manner[120] and restricting the accessibility of the endogenous substrate angiotensin I, hence preventing its conversion to angiotensin II. These agents inhibit ACE in a variety of tissues in a dose-dependent manner and with the same rank order of potency.[121] Given that the active site of ACE is the same in all tissues and plasma, ACE inhibitors can potentially block the enzyme at all sites. However, ACE inhibitors do not readily cross the blood-brain or blood-testis barrier. The accessibility of these compounds particularly to the brain is dependent on their lipophilicity. For example, lipophilic ACE inhibitors such as ramipril, enalapril, and perindopril gain access to the brain, whereas hydrophobic ACE inhibitors such as quinapril and lisinopril do not.[120] It is important to note however, that both classes of ACE inhibitors lower blood pressure to a similar extent, which suggests that inhibition of ACE in the brain is not necessary for the antihypertensive actions of these agents.

CONCLUSION

ACE is a ubiquitous zinc metallopeptidase that plays an important role in the regulation of blood pressure and maintenance of cardiovascular homeostasis by directly influencing the synthesis of angiotensin II as well as the degradation of bradykinin. However, ACE has wide substrate specificity and is capable of degrading a variety of other peptides, including substance P, opioid peptides, neurotensin, and luteinizing hormone-releasing hormone. ACE is predominantly a membrane-bound ectoenzyme found in a variety of tissues, including blood vessels, heart, brain, kidney, and adrenals. ACE does not always colocalize with other components of the RAS and may participate in other (noncardiovascular) biological functions, including immunity, reproduction, and neuropeptide processing. ACE inhibitors lower elevated blood pressure and promote regression of vascular and cardiac hypertrophy. The extraordinary success of ACE inhibitors in the treatment of hypertension and congestive heart failure can be attributed to inhibition of tissue as well as plasma ACE.

Acknowledgments

We gratefully acknowledge the financial support of the National Health and Medical Research Council of Australia, Commonwealth Department of Veterans' Affairs, Sir Edward Dunlop Medical Research Foundation, and Ramaciotti Medical Research Foundation.

References

1. Johnston CI. Biochemistry and pharmacology of the renin-angiotensin system. Drugs 39:21–31, 1990.
2. Skidgel RA, Erdos EG. Biochemistry of angiotensin I-converting enzyme. In Nicholls MG, Robertson JS (eds). The Renin-Angiotensin System. London, Gower Medical, 1993, pp 10.1–10.10.
3. Johnston CI. Tissue angiotensin converting enzyme in cardiac and vascular hypertrophy, repair, and remodeling. Hypertension 23:258–268, 1994.
4. Perich RB, Jackson B, Rogerson FM, et al. Two binding sites on angiotensin converting enzyme: Evidence from radioligand binding studies. Molecular Pharmacol 42:286–293, 1992.
5. Wei L, Alhenc-Gelas F, Corvol P, Clauser E. The two homologous domains of human angiotensin I-converting enzyme are both catalytically active. J Biol Chem 266:9002–9008, 1991.
6. Kumar RS, Kusari J, Roy S, et al. Structure of testicular angiotensin-

converting enzyme: A segmental isozyme. J Biol Chem 264:16754–16758, 1989.

7. Wei L, Alhenc-Gelas F, Soubrier F, et al. Expression and characterization of recombinant human angiotensin I-converting enzyme: Evidence for a C-terminal transmembrane anchor and for a proteolytic processing of the secreted recombinant and plasma enzymes. J Biol Chem 266:5540–5546, 1991.

8. Beldent V, Michaud A, Wei L, et al. Proteolytic release of human angiotensin-converting enzyme. Localization of the cleavage site. J Biol Chem 268:26428–26434, 1993.

9. Esther CR, Marino EM, Howard TE, et al. The critical role of tissue angiotensin-converting enzyme as revealed by gene targeting in mice. J Clin Invest 99:2375–2385, 1997.

10. Bernstein KE, Martin BM, Bernstein EA, et al. The isolation of angiotensin-converting enzyme cDNA. J Biol Chem 263:11021–11024, 1988.

11. Soubrier F, Alhenc-Gelas F, Hubert C, et al. Two putative active centers in human angiotensin I-converting enzyme revealed by molecular cloning. Proc Natl Acad Sci U S A 85:9386–9390, 1988.

12. Hubert C, Houot AM, Corvol P, Soubrier F. Structure of the angiotensin I-converting enzyme gene: Two alternative promoters correspond to evolutionary steps of a duplicated gene. J Biol Chem 266:15377–15383, 1991.

13. Kumar R, Thekkumkara T, Sen GC. The mRNAs encoding the two angiotensin-converting isozymes are transcribed from the same gene by a tissue-specific choice of alternative transcription initiation sites. J Biol Chem 266:3854–3862, 1991.

14. Howard TE, Shai SY, Langford KG, et al. Transcription of testicular angiotensin-converting enzyme (ACE) is initiated within the 12th intron of the somatic ACE gene. Mol Cell Biol 10:4294–4302, 1990.

15. Rigat B, Hubert C, Alhenc-Gelas F, et al. An insertion/deletion polymorphism in the angiotensin I-converting enzyme gene accounting for half the variance of serum enzyme levels. J Clin Invest 86:1343–1346, 1990.

16. Costerousse O, Danilov S, Alhenc-Gelas F. Genetics of angiotensin I-converting enzyme. Clin Exper Hyperten 19:659–669, 1997.

17. Jeunemaitre X, Lifton RP, Hunt SC, et al. Absence of linkage between the angiotensin-converting enzyme locus and human essential hypertension. Nat Gene 1:72–75, 1992.

18. Ehlers MRW, Riordan JF. Angiotensin-converting enzyme: Zinc and inhibitor binding stoichiometries of the somatic and testis isozymes. Biochemistry 30:7118–7126, 1991.

19. Bunning P. The catalytic mechanism of angiotensin-converting enzyme. Clin Exp Hypertens 5:1263–1275, 1983.

20. Bunning P, Riordan JF. The functional role of zinc in angiotensin-converting enzyme: Implications for the enzyme mechanism. J Inorg Biochem 24:183–198, 1985.

21. Schullek JR, Wilson IB. The binding of zinc to angiotensin-converting enzyme. Arch Biochem Biophys 265:346–350, 1988.

22. Bunning P, Riordan JF. Activation of angiotensin-converting enzyme by monovalent anions. Biochemistry 22:110–116, 1983.

23. Wei L, Clauser E, Alhenc-Gelas F, Corvol P. The two homologous domains of human angiotensin I-converting enzyme interact differently with competitive inhibitors. J Biol Chem 267:13398–13405, 1992.

24. Perich RB, Jackson B, Attwood MR, et al. Angiotensin-converting enzyme inhibitors act at two different binding sites on angiotensin-converting enzyme. Pharma Pharmacol Let 1:41–43, 1991.

25. Erdos EG. Angiotensin I-converting enzyme and the changes in our concepts through the years. Lewis K. Dahl memorial lecture. Hypertension 16:363–370, 1990.

26. Skidgel RA, Erdos EG. The broad substrate specificity of human angiotensin I-converting enzyme. Clin Exper Hyperten A9:243–259, 1987.

27. Skidgel RA, Engelbrecht S, Johnson AR, Erdos EG. Hydrolysis of substance P and neurotensin by converting enzyme and neutral endopeptidase. Peptides 5:769–776, 1984.

28. Skidgel RA, Erdos EG. Novel activity of human angiotensin I-converting enzyme: Release of the NH2- and COOH-terminal tripeptides from the luteinizing hormone-releasing hormone. Proc Natl Acad Sci U S A 82:1025–1029, 1985.

29. Rousseau A, Michaud A, Chauvet MT, et al. The hemoregulatory peptide N-acetyl-Ser-Asp-Lys-Pro is a natural and specific substrate of the N-terminal active site of human angiotensin-converting enzyme. J Biol Chem 270:3656–3661, 1995.

30. Azizi M, Rousseau A, Ezan E, et al. Acute angiotensin-converting enzyme inhibition increases the plasma level of the natural stem cell regulator N-acetyl-seryl-aspartyl-lysyl-proline. J Clin Invest 97:839–844, 1996.

31. Isaac RE, Schoofs L, Williams TA, et al. A novel peptide-processing activity of insect peptidyl-dipeptidase A (angiotensin I-converting enzyme): The hydrolysis of lysyl-arginine and arginyl-arginine from the C-terminus of an insect prohormone peptide. Biochem J 330:61–65, 1998.

32. Isaac RE, Schoofs L, Williams TA, et al. Toward a role for angiotensin-converting enzyme in insects. Ann N Y Acad Sci 839:288–292, 1998.

33. Yamada H, Fabris B, Allen AM, et al. Localization of angiotensin-converting enzyme in the rat heart. Circ Res 68:651–665, 1991.

34. Rogerson FM, Chai SY, Schiawe I, et al. Presence of angiotensin-converting enzyme in the adventitia of large blood vessels. J Hypertens 10:615–620, 1992.

35. Wilson SK, Lynch DR, Snyder SH. Angiotensin-converting enzyme labeled with [3H]captopril. Tissue localization and changes in different models of hypertension in the rat. J Clin Invest 80:841–851, 1987.

36. Fabris B, Jackson B, Kozuki NM, et al. Increased cardiac angiotensin-converting enzyme in rats with chronic heart failure. Clin Exper Pharmacol Physiol 17:309–314, 1990.

37. Zhuo J, Allen AM, Yamada H, et al. Localization and properties of the angiotensin-converting enzyme and angiotensin receptors in the heart. In Lindpainter K, Ganten D (eds). The cardiac renin-angiotensin system. New York, Futura, 1995.

38. Chai SY, Mendelsohn FA, Paxinos G. Angiotensin-converting enzyme in rat brain visualized by quantitative in vitro autoradiography. Neuroscience 20:615–627, 1987.

39. Mendelsohn FAO, Allen AM, Chai SY, et al. The brain angiotensin system: Insights from mapping its components. Trends Endocrinol Metabol 1:189–197, 1990.

40. Chai SY, McKenzie JS, McKineley MJ, Mendelsohn FA. Angiotensin-converting enzyme in the human basal forebrain and midbrain visualized by in vitro autoradiography. J Comp Neuro 291:179–194, 1990.

41. Lind RW, Swanson LW, Ganten D. Organization of angiotensin II immunoreactive cells and fibers in the rat central nervous system. An immunochemical study. Neuroendocrinology 40:2–24, 1985.

42. Mendelsohn FAO. Localization of angiotensin-converting enzyme in rat forebrain and other tissues by in vitro autoradiography using 125I-labeled MK351A. Clin Exper Pharmacol Physiol 11:431–435, 1984.

43. Pickel VM, Chan J, Ganten D. Dual peroxidase and colloidal gold labeling study of angiotensin-converting enzyme and angiotensin-like immunoreactivity in rat subfornical organ. J Neurosci 6:2457–2469, 1986.

44. Ganong WF. Angiotensin II in the brain and pituitary: Contrasting roles in the regulation of adenohypophyseal secretion. Horm Res 31:24–31, 1989.

45. Phillips MI. Functions of angiotensin in the central nervous system. Annu Rev Physiol 49:413–435, 1987.

46. Saavedra JM. Brain and pituitary angiotensin. Endocr Rev 13:329–380, 1992.

47. Chai SY, Johnston CI. Tissue distribution of angiotensin-converting enzyme. In Laragh JH, Brenner BM (eds). Hypertension: Pathophysiology, Diagnosis, and Management. New York, Raven 1995, pp 1683–1693.

48. Zhuo J, Mendelsohn FAO. Intrarenal angiotensin II receptors. In Robertson JIS, Nicholls MCG (eds). The Renin-Angiotensin System: Biochemistry, Physiology, Pathophysiology, and Therapeutics, Vol. 25. London, New York, Gower 1993, pp 1–25.

49. Levens NR, Peach MJ, Carey RM. Role of the intrarenal renin-angiotensin system in the control of the renal function. Circ Res 48:157–159, 1981.

50. Gonzalez-Garcia C, Keiser HR. Angiotensin II and angiotensin-converting enzyme binding in human adrenal gland and pheochromocytomas. J Hypertens 8:433–441, 1990.

51. Strittmatter SM, De Souza EB, Lynch DR, Snyder SH. Angiotensin-converting enzyme localized in the rat pituitary and adrenal glands by [3H]captopril autoradiography. Endocrinology 118:1690–1699, 1986.

52. Mendelsohn FAO. Localization and properties of angiotensin receptors. J Hypertens 3:307–316, 1985.

53. Kaplan NM. The biosynthesis of adrenal steroids: Effects of angiotensin II, adrenocorticotropin, and potassium. J Clin Invest 44:2029–2039, 1965.

54. Peach MJ. Renin-angiotensin system: Biochemistry and mechanisms of action. Physiol Rev 57:313–370, 1977.

55. El-Dorry HA, MacGregor JS, Soffer RL. Dipeptidyl carboxypeptidase from seminal fluid resembles the pulmonary rather than the testicular isoenzyme. Biochem Biophys Res Commun 115:1096–1100, 1983.

56. Sibony M, Segretain D, Gasc JM. Angiotensin-converting enzyme in murine testis: Step-specific expression of the germinal isoform during spermiogenesis. Biol Reprod 50:1015–1026, 1994.

57. Mizutani T, Schill WB. Motility of seminal plasma-free spermatozoa in the presence of several physiological compounds. Andrologia 17:150–156, 1985.

58. Daud AI, Bumpus FM, Husain A. Characterization of angiotensin I-converting enzyme (ACE)-containing follicles in the rat ovary during the estrous cycle and effects of ACE inhibitor on ovulation. Endocrinology 126:2927–2935, 1990.

59. Speth RC, Husain A. Distribution of angiotensin-converting enzyme and angiotensin II-receptor binding sites in the rat ovary. Biol Reprod 38:695–702, 1988.

60. Pellicer A, Palumbo A, DeCherney AH, Naftolin F. Blockage of ovulation by an angiotensin antagonist. Science 240:1660–1661, 1988.

61. Duggan KA, Mendelsohn FA, Levens NR. Angiotensin receptors and angiotensin I-converting enzyme in rat intestine. Am J Physiol 257:G504–G510, 1989.

62. Takada Y, Unno M, Hiwada K, Kokubu T. Immunological and immunofluorescent studies of human angiotensin-converting enzyme. Clin Sci 61 (supp 7):253S–256S, 1981.

63. Yoshioka M, Erickson RH, Woodley JF, et al. Role of rat intestinal brush-border membrane angiotensin-converting enzyme in dietary protein digestion. Am J Physiol 253:G781–G786, 1987.

64. Lallberte F, Lallberte MF, Nonotte I, et al. Angiotensin I-converting enzyme in gastric mucosa of the rabbit: Localization by autoradiography, immunofluorescence, and immunoelectron microscopy. J Histochem Cytochem 39:1519–1529, 1991.

65. Schalekamp MADH. The renin angiotensin system: New surprises ahead. J Hypertens 9(suppl 6):S10–S17, 1991.

66. Urata H, Healy B, Stewart RW, et al. Angiotensin II forming pathways in normal and failing human hearts. Circ Res 66:883–890, 1990.

67. Johnston CI, Burrell LM, Perich K, et al. The tissue renin-angiotensin system and its functional role. Clin Exper Pharmacol Physiol 19(suppl 19):1–5, 1992.

68. Regoll D, Barabe J. Pharmacology of bradykinin and related kinins. Pharmacol Rev 32:1–46, 1980.

69. Saxena PR. Interaction between the renin-angiotensin-aldosterone and sympathetic nervous systems. J Cardiovasc Pharmacol 19(suppl 6):S80–S88, 1992.

70. Story DF, Ziogas J. Interaction of angiotensin II with noradrenergic transmission. Trends Pharmacol Sci 8:269–271, 1987.

71. Taddel S, Favilla S, Duranti P, et al. Vascular renin-angiotensin system and neurotransmission in hypertensive persons. Hypertension 18:266–277, 1991.

72. Cleland JGF, Dangle HJ, Ball SG, et al. Effects of enalapril on heart failure: A double-blind study of effects on exercise performance, renal function, hormones and metabolic state. Br Heart J 54:305–312, 1985.

73. McGrath BP, Arnolda L, Mathews PG, et al. Controlled trial of enalapril in congestive cardiac failure. Br Heart J 54:405–411, 1985.

74. Allen AM, Yamada H, Mendelsohn FA. In vitro autoradiographic localization of binding to angiotensin receptors in the rat heart. Int J Cardiol 28:25–83, 1990.

75. Ziogas J, Story DF, Rand MJ. Effects of locally generated angiotensin II on noradrenergic transmission in guinea-pig isolated atria. Eur J Pharmacol 106:11–18, 1984.

76. Lumbers ER, McCloskey DI, Potter EK. Inhibition by angiotensin II of baroreceptor-evoked activity in cardiac vagal efferent nerves in the dog. J Physiol 294:69–80, 1979.

77. Potter EK. Angiotensin inhibits action of vagus nerve at the heart. Br J Pharmacol 75:9–11, 1982.

78. Rechtman M, Majewski H. A facilitatory effect of anti-angiotensin drugs on vagal bradycardia in the pithed rat and guinea-pig. Br J Pharmacol 110:289–296, 1993.

79. Mombouli JV, Nephtall M, Vanhoutte PM. Effect of the converting enzyme cilazaprilat in endothelium-dependent responses. Hypertension 18(suppl II):II22–II29, 1991.

80. Schelling P, Fischer H, Ganten D. Angiotensin and cell growth: A link to cardiovascular hypertrophy? J Hypertens 9:3–15, 1991.

81. Boulanger C, Schinin VB, Moncada S, Vanhoutte PM. Release of EDRF and exogenous nitric oxide stimulate the production of cyclic AMP in cultured endothelial cells. Br J Pharmacol 101:152–156, 1990.

82. Morshita R, Higaki J, Okunkishi H, et al. Changes in gene expression of the renin-angiotensin system in two-kidney, one-clip hypertensive rat. J Hypertens 9:187–192, 1991.

83. Okamura R, Myazaki M, Inagami T, Toda N. Vascular renin-angiotensin system in two-kidney, one-clip hypertensive rats. Hypertension 8:560–565, 1986.

84. Kohzuki M, Chen BZ, Mooser V, et al. Angiotensin-converting enzyme in the spontaneously hypertensive rat. In Sassard J (ed). Genetic Hypertension, vol. 218. Paris, Colloque INSERM, John Libbey Eurotext, 1992; pp 503–505.

85. Jandeleit K, Perich R, Jackson B, Johnston CI. Mesenteric resistance and brain microvascular angiotensin-converting enzyme in the spontaneously hypertensive rat. Clin Exper Pharmacol Physiol 19:348–352, 1992.

86. Perich R, Jackson B, Paxton D, Johnston CI. Characterization of angiotensin-converting enzyme in isolated cerebral microvessels from spontaneously hypertensive and normotensive rats. Hypertens 10:149–153, 1992.

87. Jandeleit K, Jackson B, Perich R, et al. Angiotensin-converting enzyme in macro- and microvessels of the rat. Clin Exper Pharmacol Physiol 18:353–356, 1991.

88. Harrap SB, van der Merwe WM, Griffin SA, et al. Brief angiotensin-converting enzyme inhibitor treatment in young spontaneously hypertensive rats reduces blood pressure long-term. Hypertension 16:603–614, 1990.

89. Hilbert P, Lindpaintner K, Beckmann JS, et al. Chromosomal mapping of two genetic loci associated with blood pressure regulation in hereditary hypertensive rats. Nature 353:521–529, 1991.

90. Jacob HJ, Lindpaintner K, Lincoln SE, et al. Genetic mapping of a gene causing hypertension in the stroke-prone, spontaneously hypertensive rat. Cell 67:213–224, 1991.

91. Luscher TF, Noll G. The pathogenesis of cardiovascular disease: Role of the endothelium as a target and mediator. Atherosclerosis 118(suppl):S81–S90, 1995.

92. Geisterfer AA, Peach MJ, Owens GK. Angiotensin II induces hypertrophy not hyperplasia of cultured rat aortic smooth muscle cells. Circ Res 62:485–492, 1988.

93. Weber H, Taylor DS, Molloy CJ. Angiotensin II induces delayed mitogenesis and cellular proliferation in rat aortic smooth muscle cells. J Clin Invest 93:788–798, 1994.

94. Stouffer GA, Owens GK. Angiotensin II-induced mitogenesis of spontaneously hypertensive rat-derived cultured smooth muscle cells is dependent on autocrine production of transforming growth factor-β. Circ Res 70:820–828, 1992.

95. Naftilan AJ, Pratt RE, Dzau VJ. Induction of platelet-derived growth factor and c-myc expression by angiotensin II in cultured rat vascular smooth muscle cells. J Clin Invest 83:1419–1424, 1989.

96. Itoh H, Mukoyama M, Pratt RE, et al. Multiple autocrine growth factors modulate vascular smooth muscle cell response to angiotensin II. J Clin Invest 91:2268–2274, 1993.

97. Naftilan AJ, Gilliland GK, Elderidge CS, Kraft AS. Induction of the protooncogene c-jun by angiotensin II. Mol Cell Biol 10:5536–5540, 1990.

98. Kawahara J, Sunako M, Tsuda T, et al. Angiotensin II induces expression of the c-fos gene through protein kinase C activation and calcium ion mobilization in cultured vascular smooth muscle cells. Biochem Biophys Res Commun 150:52–59, 1988.

99. McVary KT, Razzaq A, Lee C, et al. Growth of the rat prostate gland is facilitated by the autonomic nervous system. Biol Reprod 51:99–107, 1994.

100. Clozel JP, Kuhn H, Hefti F. Effects of chronic ACE inhibition on cardiac hypertrophy and coronary vascular reserve in spontaneously hypertensive rats with developed hypertension. J Hypertens 7:267–275, 1989.

101. Levy BI, Michel JB, Salzmann JL, et al. Remodeling of the heart and arteries by chronic converting enzyme inhibition in spontaneously hypertensive rats. Am J Hypertens 4(suppl):S204–S245, 1991.

102. Jandeleit K, Johnston CI, Hettiarachi M, et al. Angiotensin-converting enzyme in micro- and macrovessels. *In* MacGregor GA, Sever PS (eds). Current advances in ACE inhibition. London, Churchill Livingston, 1991; pp 230–233.

103. Powell JS, Clozel J, Muller RKM, et al. Inhibitors of angiotensin-converting enzyme prevent myointimal proliferation after vascular injury. Science 245:186–188, 1989.

104. Dzau VJ, Gibons GH. Endothelium and growth factors in vascular remodeling of hypertension. Hypertension 18(suppl II):1161–1166, 1991.

105. Bopma JJ, Califf RM, Topol EJ. Clinical trials of re-stenosis following coronary angioplasty. Circulation 84:1426–1436, 1991.

106. Serruya P, Hermans W. The new angiotensin-converting enzyme inhibitor cilazapril does not prevent re-stenosis after coronary angioplasty: Results of the MERCATOR trial. J Am Coll Cardiol 19:258A, 1992.

107. Schunkert H, Dzau VJ, Tan SS, et al. Increased rat cardiac angiotensin-converting enzyme activity and mRNA expression in pressure overload left ventricular hypertrophy: Effects on coronary resistance, contractility and relaxation. J Clin Invest 86:1913–1920, 1990.

108. Nagano M, Hyigaki J, Mikami H, et al. Converting enzyme inhibitors regressed cardiac hypertrophy and reduced tissue angiotensin II in spontaneously hypertensive rats. J Hypertens 9:595–599, 1991.

109. Linz W, Scholkens BA, Ganten D. Converting enzyme inhibition specifically prevents the development and induces regression of cardiac hypertrophy in rats. Clin Exper Hypertens 2:1325–1350, 1989.

110. Mooser V, Kotopothis A, Harrap SB, Johnston CI. Inhibition of cardiac ACE does not reduce left ventricular mass in salt-induced spontaneously hypertensive rats. *In* Sassard J (ed). General Hypertension, vol. 218. Paris, Colloque INSERM, John Libbey Eurotext, 1992, pp 253–255.

111. Dahlof B, Pennert K, Hansson L. Reversal of left ventricular hypertrophy in hypertensive patients: A meta-analysis of 109 treatment studies. Am J Hypertens 5:95–110, 1992.

112. Pfeffer MA, Pfeffer JM, Steinberg C, Finn P. Survival after an experimental myocardial infarction: Beneficial effects of long-term therapy with captopril. Circulation 72:406–412, 1985.

113. SAVE Investigators. Effects of the early administration of enalapril on mortality in patients with acute myocardial infarction: Results of the Cooperative New Scandinavian Enalapril Survival Study II (CONSENSUS II). N Engl J Med 327:678–684, 1992.

114. SOLVD Investigators. Effect of enalapril on mortality and the development of heart failure in asymptomatic patients with reduced left ventricular ejection fractions. N Engl J Med 327:685–691, 1992.

115. Camblen F, Poirler O, Lecerf L, et al. Deletion polymorphism in the gene for angiotensin-converting enzyme is a potent risk factor for myocardial infarction. Nature 359:641–644, 1992.

116. Frieland J, Setton C, Silverstein J. Induction of angiotensin-converting enzyme in human monocytes in culture. Biochem Biophys Res Commun 83:843–849, 1978.

117. Weinstock JV. The significance of angiotensin I-converting enzyme in granulomatous inflammation: Functions of ACE in granulomas. Sarcoidosis 3:19–26, 1986.

118. Ehlers MRW, Riordan JF. Angiotensin-converting enzyme: New concepts concerning its biological role. Biochemistry 28:5311–5318, 1989.

119. Shor SA, Stimler-Gerard NP, Coats SR, Drazen JM. Substance P induced broncoconstriction in the guinea pig: Enhancement by inhibitors of neutral metalloendopeptidases and angiotensin-converting enzyme. Am Rev Respir Dis 137:331–336, 1988.

120. Johnston CI. Angiotensin-converting enzyme inhibitors. *In* Nicholls MG, Robertson JIS (eds). The Renin-Angiotensin System. London, Gower, 1993; pp 87. 1–87.15.

121. Johnston CI, Fabris B, Yamada H, et al. Comparative studies of tissue inhibition by angiotensin-converting enzyme inhibitors. J Hypertens 7(suppl 5):S11–S16, 1989.

The AT$_1$ and AT$_2$ Angiotensin Receptors

CHAPTER 10

Marc de Gasparo and Gillian R. Bullock

Angiotensin II (Ang II) is an octapeptide generated in plasma by the action of true proteolytic enzymes. Essentially, kidney renin hydrolyzes liver angiotensinogen, a 14-residue peptide, to give a decapeptide, Ang I, that, in turn, is converted by lung and endothelial angiotensin-converting enzyme to the active hormone Ang II. This cascade of events is called the *renin-angiotensin system.*

Ang II has been well conserved during evolution, Leu^5 present in human and rat being replaced by Vals in ox, sheep, fowl, and reptile. Elasmobranch fish (dogfish) Ang II is teleost-like because of the Asn residue in position 1 but mammalian-like because of the Ile residue in position 5.[1] Evidence for angiotensin-like molecules has even been observed in the central nervous system of the leech.[2]

Ang II plays a central role in regulating extracellular fluid volume and systemic vascular resistance. It is a unique hormone in that it regulates blood pressure by acting on both the "container" (vessels) and its "content" (circulating fluid). Ang II, however, is not only a blood-borne hormone produced and retained in the circulation. A local tissue renin-angiotensin system exists in many tissues, such as brain, kidney, heart, and vessels, where Ang II functions as a paracrine and autocrine hormone. It induces cell growth, proliferation, and migration and controls extracellular matrix formation.

Ang II acts through a plasma membrane receptor, and with this receptor being present on so many different target cells, including vascular smooth muscle and adrenal, kidney, pituitary, and sympathetic nervous ganglion, the existence of various receptor subtypes seems highly likely.

Earlier pharmacological studies have compared the efficacy of Ang II with its precursor Ang I and its metabolite Ang III. The dose-response curves for the Ang-related peptides showed quantitative discrepancies in smooth muscle contraction and aldosterone and adrenaline release.[3] Comparison of Ang II and a large number of synthetic analogues (agonists as well as antagonists) in rat colon and uterus, in rabbit aorta, or in vagotomized and nephrectomized rat indicated marked dissimilarities between the analogues in each of the preparations,[4] suggesting differences in the structure of the receptor sites. However, it was only in the late 1980s that the existence of Ang II receptor subtypes was clearly and unequivocally proved, using new synthetic tools with selective affinity for different tissues. Thus, losartan (or similar diphenyl tetrazole derivatives) displaced radiolabeled Ang II bound to membranes pre-

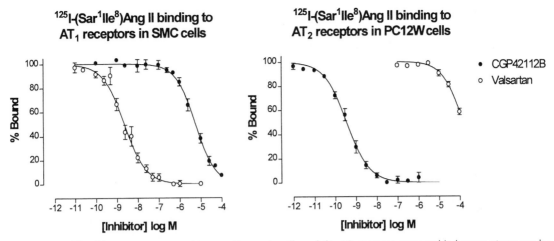

Figure 10–1. The AT₁ receptor expressed in smooth muscle cells and the AT₂ receptor expressed in human uterus can be distinguished in the binding assay with specific ligands. Valsartan *(open circles)* and CGP 42112 *(solid circles)* are specific for the AT₁ and AT₂ receptors, respectively.

pared from vascular smooth muscle cells or cortical adrenal, whereas CGP42112 and PD123177 were selective for the Ang II receptor expressed in human uterus or adrenal medulla (Fig. 10–1).[5, 6] An International Union of Pharmacology nomenclature subcommittee classified these two receptors as *AT₁* and *AT₂*.[7, 8]

Both AT₁ and AT₂ receptors have been cloned and pharmacologically characterized. Additional subtypes have been postulated but have not yet been completely characterized or cloned. For example, the fragments Ang 1-7 and Ang 3-8 (or Ang IV) have pharmacological and biochemical properties that differ from those mediated by the AT₁ and AT₂ receptors. A cytosolic binding protein as well as an Ang II–specific nuclear receptor have also been described, the function of which still remains elusive.

In this chapter, the two major Ang II receptors, AT₁ and AT₂, are reviewed and the potential beneficial effect of blockade of the AT₁ receptor is discussed.

AT₁ RECEPTOR

The cell-surface angiotensin AT₁ receptor is a member of the seven-transmembrane–spanning G-protein receptor superfamily. It has been cloned from human, rat, mouse, rabbit, pig, and dog cDNA. It is folded into a three-dimensional configuration where the seven-transmembrane–spanning helices interact with cytoplasmic and extracellular portions of the molecule to form a ligand-binding pocket. Amphibian and avian Ang II receptors have also been cloned but are pharmacologically distinct from the mammalian receptors.[9–12]

The AT₁ receptor has a molecular mass of 41 kDa and contains three consensus N-glycosylation sites and eight phosphorylation sites that are involved in receptor-effector coupling.[12] There are six cysteine residues, and the three-dimensional structure is maintained by two disulfide bridges, respectively, between the first and last extracellular domain and the second and third extracellular domain. Disruption of the disulfide bridges with dithiothreitol significantly reduced the affinity of the receptor for Ang II.[5]

Pharmacologically, the AT₁ receptor is typified by its selective affinity for biphenylimidazoles such as losartan and its insensitivity to tetrahydroimidazo-pyridine–like PD123319 or the Ang II peptidic analogue CGP 42112. The AT₁ receptor is sensitive to GTPγS, indicating that it has heterogeneous states of affinity owing to its association with G-proteins. True subtypes of the AT₁ receptor, called *AT₁ₐ* and *AT₁ᵦ*, have been characterized in rat. They are closely related but are encoded by distinct genes located on chromosomes 17 and 2, respectively. They differ in 19 amino acids, mainly in the carboxy-terminal region.[13] There are two additional phosphorylation sites in AT₁ᵦ.[14] Although AT₁ₐ and AT₁ᵦ subtypes have identical binding and functional properties, they are differentially regulated.[15] Ang II downregulates AT₁ₐ mRNA in vascular smooth muscle cells but induces upregulation of the AT₁ᵦ mRNA in rat adrenal.[16] A third subtype, AT₁c, has been described in rat placenta and has more than 80% homology to AT₁ₐ and AT₁ᵦ.[17] In humans, only one single AT₁ receptor has been reported and is encoded by a gene on chromosome 3. The properties of the rat AT₁ₐ are close to that of the human receptor. An additional and novel type of human AT₁ receptor has been cloned from a placental cDNA library. It appears pharmacologically distinct from the receptor cloned from a human heart cDNA library in its effect on calcium mobilization.[18, 19]

AT₁ Gene

The coding region of the AT₁ receptor is contained within a single exon, although the gene itself contains multiple exons.[13, 20, 21] The human gene contains five exons: exon 5 is the coding region, exon 1 enhances the protein synthesis, exon 3 is responsible for an amino-terminal extension of the AT₁ receptor.[22] The human gene promoter region contains four AP-1 protein kinase C–responsive elements, two AP-2 enhancer elements, two Sp1 GC boxes, one cyclic adenosine monophosphate (cAMP) regulatory element, one recognition site for the transcription factor polyoma virus enhances A₃ (PEA3), and a tissue-specific negative regulatory element.[20, 21, 23, 24] These are features usually associated with constitutive as well as regulated genes. Interestingly, cAMP significantly suppressed AT_1 mRNA expression in rat vascular smooth muscle cells in culture[25] and epidermal growth factor–enhanced human AT_1 promoter activity through stimulation of the PEA3 transcription factor.[26]

Distribution of the AT_1 Receptor

The anatomical distribution of the AT_1 receptor has received considerable attention using conventional binding, autoradiographic, and molecular techniques. The AT_1 receptor is expressed in somatic and brain tissues and predominates in organs and tissues involved in fluid-electrolyte balance and blood pressure regulation. It is found primarily in the adrenals, vascular smooth muscle, kidney, and heart. In the brain, it is located in specific areas implicated in the dipsogenic action of Ang II, the release of vasopressin, and the neurogenic control of blood pressure.[27, 28] This includes the circumventricular organs, the hypothalamus, the suprachiasmatic nucleus, and the nucleus of the solitary tract. The AT_{1A} and AT_{1B} are differentially expressed in the rat. The AT_{1A} subtype predominates in vascular smooth muscle, heart, and brain, whereas the AT_{1B} subtype is mainly expressed in the pituitary and adrenal gland. Marked species and tissue differences exist in both the distribution and the relative proportions of AT_1 and AT_2 receptors.

Signal Transduction of the AT_1 Receptor

Our knowledge of the AT_1 receptor signal transduction mechanism has increased considerably since the mid-1990s, and major progress has been achieved in understanding the intracellular signaling cascade.

The process of agonist binding to the receptor leads to the attachment of Gq/11 and/or Gi/0 proteins to the third cytoplasmic loop and carboxy-terminal tail of the receptor, especially the amino acids 312–314 (Tyr-Phe-Leu), and to the stimulation of various intracellular events.[29] The five classical signal transduction mechanisms of the AT_1 receptor have been extensively reviewed.[12, 28, 30, 31] Activation of phospholipase C (formation of inositol 1,4,5-triphosphate (IP_3) and diacylglycerol), voltage-dependent Ca^{2+} channels (Ca inflow); phospholipase D (cleavage of phosphatidylcholine) and phospholipase A2 (formation of prostaglandin and prostanoids); and adenylate cyclase (decrease in cAMP production) have all been demonstrated. Activation of phospholipase C and Ca mobilization from the intracellular pool, which occur within seconds, appear to be the most important steps. Activation of the two other phospholipases D and A2 and of the protein kinase C through diacylglycerol requires minutes.[32] Recently, the importance of specific kinases regulated by Ang II and leading to the phosphorylation of multiple proteins has been emphasized in vitro as well as in vivo.[32–35] The AT_1 receptor has no catalytic activity per se but is able to mimic growth factor and cytokine receptors. An analogy appears obvious. Ang II induces a rapid but transient tyrosine phosphorylation of phospholipase C-γ as observed in smooth muscle and mesangial cells. The rise in IP_3 levels that stimulate the mobilization of Ca from its intracellular pool parallels the increase in tyrosine phosphorylation of phospholipase C. Like cytokine receptors, the AT_1 receptor lacks intrinsic tyrosine kinase activity. Therefore, soluble intracellular protein tyrosine kinase should be recruited in response to the binding of Ang II to its receptor. It appears that Src kinase, especially pp60 c-src, is probably the enzyme responsible for Ang II-mediated tyrosine phosphorylation of phospholipase C-γ. In addition, binding of Ang II to the AT_1 receptor triggers a rapid tyrosine phosphorylation and activation of the intracellular kinases JAK2 and TYK2, which in turn, phosphorylate the signal transducers and activators of transcription ($STAT_1$ and $STAT_2$). Deletion analysis showed that the association with JAK2 is dependent on the AT_1 receptor motif YIPP 319–322 (Tyr-Ile-Pro-Pro).[36] Following heterodimerization and association with the protein p48, there is a translocation of STAT proteins into the nucleus, which bind to specific DNA sites and induce transcription of early growth response genes such as c-fos. Ang II also phosphorylates the cytosolic focal adhesion kinase, causing its translocation to sites of focal adhesion with the extracellular matrix. Through this mechanism, Ang II is involved in the regulation of cell morphology and movement. Ang II also causes the phosphorylation of the carboxy-terminal tail of its own receptor through the Src family. This mechanism could be involved in the sequestration and desensitization of phospholipase C and of the receptor.[33]

The mitogen-activated protein (MAP) kinase plays a central role in Ang II–induced cell growth and differentiation in vascular smooth muscle. Its activation is at least partially dependent on protein kinase C and requires prior activation of a Ca-dependent tyrosine kinase. There is a whole cascade of phosphorylation leading to MAP kinase activation, similar to the cascade of enzyme activation involved in the glycogen synthesis. Thus, MAP kinase kinase kinase (MEKKK), like raf-1, phosphorylates and activates MAP kinase kinase (MEKK), which in turn, phosphorylates MAP kinase. Activated MAP kinase phosphorylates various substrates like c-jun or myelin basic protein (MBP) involved in cell growth. Dephosphorylation and inactivation of MAP kinase occur through a MAP kinase phosphatase (MKP-1), which dephosphorylates MAP kinase on both threonine and tyrosine. This phosphatase appears to be a target for the AT_2 receptor, as discussed later.

The AT_1 receptor is involved in so-called oxidative stress. Long-term activation of the NADH/NADPH (nicotinamide adenine dinucleotide, reduced form/nicotinamide adenine dinucleotide phosphate, reduced form) oxidase pathways is implicated in AT_1-induced gene induction and cell growth. The formation of superoxide anion O_2^- and hydrogen peroxide causes endothelium dysfunction and degradation of nitric oxide. Furthermore, the altered redox state of the cell modulates the activation of cellular signaling enzymes such as protein kinase C and tyrosine kinases, alters the activity of transcription factors,[32] and appears to mediate a nonhemodynamic action of Ang II in progressive glomerular injury.[37] Clearly, the AT_1 receptor is coupled to several intracellular pathways that occur multiphasically within seconds, minutes, or hours and involves the selective activation of different pathways over time.[32] In summary, stimulation of phospholipase C and Ca mobilization occur within seconds, activation of protein kinase C and MAP kinase require minutes, and stimulation of gene transcription and NADH/NADPH oxidase activity takes hours. The relative importance of each step may be influenced by the phenotype of the cell.

AT₁ Receptor Binding Requirement

Angiotensin II

Analysis of the binding and pharmacological properties of a large number of angiotensin analogues showed that the aromatic side group of Tyr[4] and His[6] with the guanidine group of Arg[2] and the charged carboxyl-terminus are essential for the binding of Ang II to its receptor. In contrast, Tyr[4] and Phe[8] are required for the biological response.[38, 39]

Receptor Binding Site

The four cysteine residues in the extracellular domains of the AT₁ receptor maintain the three-dimensional structure of the receptor. Thus, replacing cysteine by glycine decreases the affinity of the receptor for Ang II.[40]

Binding of Ang II to the AT₁ receptor requires a sizable binding domain (Fig. 10–2) with hydrophobic and polar residues located on the extracellular loops (residues 14, 24, 27 on the N-terminal segment; residue 92 on the first extracellular loop; residues 179 and 183 on the second extracellular loop; residues 278 and 281 on the third extracellular loop) and on the superficial portion of the transmembrane helices III to VI. The terminal carboxyl group Phe[8] of Ang II binds to Lys[199] in helix V and forms a salt-linked triad with Asp[1] of Ang II. Asp[281] in the third

extracellular loop above helix VII is the docking point for the N-terminal Asp[1] of Ang II. The two major docking points Lys[199] and Asp[281] are distantly located in the receptor and probably form the intramembrane binding pocket. Efficient binding, however, requires stabilization of the octapeptide through binding to the extracellular regions of the receptor.

It appears as though the natural ligand Ang II binds to a large superficial segment of the receptor.[41, 42]

Nonpeptidic antagonists failed to bind to rabbit antibodies against Ang II. Conversely, antibodies against losartan did not bind Ang II. This suggested that Ang II receptor antagonists do not share any epitope with Ang II and suggested distinct receptor binding sites for the two molecules.[43] Chimeric mammalian-amphibian Ang II receptors and mutational studies have been used to characterize the requirement for binding of AT₁ nonpeptidic receptor antagonists. Compared with Ang II, nonpeptidic antagonists bind to distinct but overlapping areas of the receptor more deeply located within the receptor between helices III and VII. Mutation of certain amino acids, e.g., Val[108], Ala[163], Thr[198], Ser[252], Leu[300], and Phe[301], decrease binding of losartan.[44] Lys[102] and Lys[199] appear essential for the binding of both Ang II and nonpeptidic ligands. Binding of nonpeptidic antagonists is dependent on nonconserved residues located deep within the transmembrane segment VII, in particular Asn[295]. Interestingly, mutation in helix VII, especially Asn[295], had a more pronounced effect on the binding of the competitive antagonist relative to the insurmountable antagonist.[45, 46] An approximately 10-fold decrease in binding affinity was observed for competitive compared with insurmountable antagonists. This observation suggested

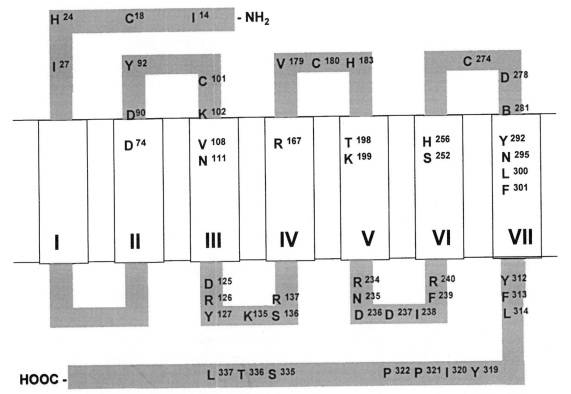

Figure 10–2. The angiotensin II (Ang II) receptors are members of the 7-transmembrane-spanning G-protein receptor superfamily. The various residues mentioned in the text are localized in this schematic representation.

that these antagonists bind distinctly to a partially overlapping site deeply buried in the spanning region. Losartan itself is a competitive antagonist in the aortic ring assay. Its metabolite EXP 3174 and other angiotensin AT_1 receptor antagonists, like valsartan, irbesartan, and CV 11974, the active metabolite of candesartan cilexetil, behave like insurmountable antagonists. They are characterized by a decrease of the maximal contraction of aortic ring following Ang II stimulation. It is not clear, however, whether this is due to specific binding requirements as suggested by Schambye and colleagues[45, 46] or whether this is linked to a slower dissociation rate from the receptor. Alternatively, the Ang II receptor may exist in two interconvertible states.[47] The insurmountable antagonist would compete with Ang II for the active receptor state with a greater affinity than for the inactive state, causing a decrease of the active receptor pool and therefore a decrease of the Ang II–induced contraction. The biological consequence of this behavior is still unknown but could be linked to the long duration of action of the insurmountable antagonists.

G-Protein Binding

Polar residues deeply buried in helices II, III, and VII and several charged residues of the second and third intracellular loops, as well as the proximal segment of the carboxy-terminal tail of the receptor, are involved in coupling the receptor to G-protein and in stimulation of IP_3 formation on exposure to Ang II.[48] Chimeric constructs of the C-terminal segment of the third intracellular loop (residues 234–240) indicate that this area plays a pivotal role in coupling selectivity and receptor signaling via G-proteins.[49] The carboxy-terminal residues Tyr^{312}-Phe^{313}-Leu^{314} are also essential for coupling and activation of Gq.[29] Other amino acids appear to be important. For example, Tyr^{292} and Asp^{74} are in spatial proximity and are necessary for the activation of the G-protein.[50, 51] Interestingly, G-protein coupling can be dissociated from internalization, as observed by mutation of Asp^{74}.[52] Truncation of the carboxy-terminal tail, especially Ser^{335}, Thr^{336}, Leu^{337}, does not change the phospholipase activity on binding of Ang II but dramatically decreases the internalization of the ligand.[53] Constitutive activation of the AT_1 receptor has been reported.[54] An interaction between Asn^{111} on the third transmembrane domain with Asp^{74} appears to exist in the nonactivated receptor.[55] Binding of Ang II would activate the receptor in allowing Tyr^{292} to interact with the conserved Asp^{74} on the second transmembrane domain. Mutation studies have been performed and an allosteric ternary complex model of ligand interaction with the AT_1 receptor has been proposed.[54]

AT_2 RECEPTOR

The AT_2 receptor was characterized by its high affinity for CGP 42112 and PD123177.[5, 6] The AT_2 receptor has a very weak affinity for the nonpeptidic antagonist losartan. Ang II does not distinguish AT_1 and AT_2 receptors. It binds to the AT_2 receptor with a similar affinity as for the AT_1 receptor, i.e., in the nanomolar range. Ang III appears to have a slightly lower affinity. Based on binding data, it was initially believed that the AT_2 receptor had a structure completely different from that of the AT_1 receptor. In

contrast to the AT_1 receptor, the AT_2 is insensitive to dithiothreitol or to $GTP\gamma S$. There is no stimulation of IP_3 formation and subsequent Ca mobilization.[56, 57] It was therefore hypothesized in 1992 that the AT_2 receptor was a member of the growth factor family coupled to some tyrosine phosphatase activity.[58]

It was a surprise when the rat AT_2 receptor was cloned simultaneously in two laboratories[59, 60] and found, like the AT_1 receptor, to have a seven-transmembrane topology with only 32% homology with the AT_1 receptor. Like the AT_1 receptor, the AT_2 receptor has a molecular mass of 41 kDa. It contains 5 N-glycosylation sites, 5 phosphorylation sites, and 14 cysteine residues, the latter making the receptor resistant to reducing agents. Lys^{102}, Arg^{167}, and Lys^{199}, which are considered to be essential for Ang II binding to the AT_1 receptor, are conserved in the AT_2 receptor. It differs more extensively from the AT_1 receptor in the carboxy-terminal tail. Unlike the AT_1 receptor, no subtypes or splice variants of the AT_2 receptor have been reported in either humans or rodents. However, Ang II binding sites have been described in rat ventral thalamic nuclei and locus coeruleus that have a high affinity for CGP 42112 and PD123177 but that differ in their sensitivity to dithiothreitol, $GTP\gamma S$, and pertussis toxin.[61] In contrast, the classic AT_2 receptor is found in the brain, e.g., in the inferior olive[62] and in neuronal cells.[63]

The AT_2 receptor cloned from mouse and human cDNA libraries has over 92% homology with the rat receptor, which was cloned first. Unlike the AT_1 receptor, the AT_2 receptor expressed in atretic ovary and in R3T3 cells does not internalize.[56, 57]

AT_2 Gene

The AT_2 gene has been mapped to the X chromosome in rat and human.[64] Interestingly, the Bp3 gene on the same chromosome, responsible for an increase in blood pressure, is unrelated to the AT_2 receptor gene.[65] The AT_2 gene is composed of three exons, and the coding sequence is found on the third exon.[66] The putative coding region is intronless.[65] The promoter region of the mouse AT_2 receptor contains several cis-acting elements, including AP-1, PEA-3, and NF-IL6.[67] It also contains interferon regulatory factors (IRF)-1 and -2. Growing R3T3 cells exhibit only IRF-2 binding, whereas confluent cells show a greater proportion of IRF-1 binding. It was speculated that the ratio of IRF-1:IRF-2 determined the AT_2 receptor expression associated with growth and/or differentiation.[68] IRF-1 upregulation following serum deprivation may be involved in enhanced Ang II–mediated apoptosis.[69]

Distribution of the AT_2 Receptor

The AT_2 receptor is developmentally regulated. AT_2 receptors are abundant in various fetal tissues, where they show a transient pattern of expression. They are found in undifferentiated mesenchyme, in connective tissues, and in mesenchyme surrounding developing cartilage, as well as in adrenal medulla, aorta, kidney, and various brain areas of the fetus.[28] In adults, the AT_2 receptor is expressed at a lower density in adrenal medulla, brain, and reproductive tissues. The proportion of AT_2 (relative to AT_1) receptors varies among species and tissues. For example, nonpregnant sheep, marmoset, and human myometrium express only the AT$_2$ receptor, whereas nonpregnant rabbit and rat myometrium express both receptor types. Also, the proportion of AT$_2$ (relative to AT$_1$) receptors in monkey varies between 10% in adrenal and a maximum of 58% in kidney cortex.[70] Most importantly, the AT$_2$ receptor is reexpressed or upregulated after vascular injury, myocardial infarction, cardiac failure, skin wound healing, and peripheral nerve injury, possibly reflecting reactivation of a fetal genetic program.[71, 72]

Signal Transduction of the AT$_2$ Receptor

Although the trisequence Asp^{125}-Arg^{126}-Tyr^{127} and the amino acid Asp^{90} involved in the G-protein activation of phospholipase C by AT$_1$ and other such receptors are retained in the AT$_2$ receptor, agonist stimulation of the AT$_2$ receptor does not induce an increase in IP$_3$ and diacylglycerol formation.[57, 73] However, like all members of the seven-transmembrane family of G-proteins, the AT$_2$ receptor is coupled to a G-protein. Using antibodies against G(α) subunits, it was demonstrated that the AT$_2$ receptor couples to pertussis toxin–sensitive proteins Giα2 and 3 in the rat fetus.[74] The intracellular third loop domain of the AT$_2$ receptor is essential for AT$_2$ function[75] and is closely linked with the cellular signaling pathway in which Gi and protein phosphatases such as MKP-1 are involved, leading to MAP kinase and JAK-STAT inactivation and to growth inhibition.[76] Recently, ceramide, which is linked to phosphatase activation, was proposed to be the second messenger.[77]

Involvement of the AT$_2$ receptor in stimulating nuclear transcription factors and matrix protein has also been described. Whereas the Ang II–induced rapid and transient increase in cytosolic calcium is blocked with an AT$_1$ receptor antagonist, the sustained rise in cytoplasmic and nuclear calcium is affected by both AT$_1$ and AT$_2$ receptor subtypes.[78] This suggests that two or more pools of calcium may exist under separate control, which may involve the AT$_2$ receptor. The biological consequence may be tissue-specific depending on the expression on one or both receptor subtypes.

FUNCTION OF THE AT$_1$ AND AT$_2$ RECEPTOR: THE YIN-YANG HYPOTHESIS

Most of the known effects of Ang II are mediated through the AT$_1$ receptor, e.g., vasoconstriction, aldosterone and vasopressin release, salt and water retention through the kidney, and sympathetic activation, as well as important autocrine and paracrine effects on cell proliferation and migration and on extracellular matrix formation.

The function of the AT$_2$ receptor has become better understood since its cloning in 1993 as a result of studies using methodological approaches such as AT$_2$ gene transfection and deletion. Thus, activation of the AT$_2$ receptor appears to stimulate intracellular mechanisms involving Tyr and Ser/Thr phosphatases and PP2-a, MKP-1, and SHP-1.[79–83] Depending on the tissue, there is an inactivation of MAP kinase, antiproliferation, promotion of apoptosis (Fig. 10–3), opening of delayed-rectifier K$^+$ channels, and closing of T-type Ca^{2+} channels in neurons, neuronal dif-

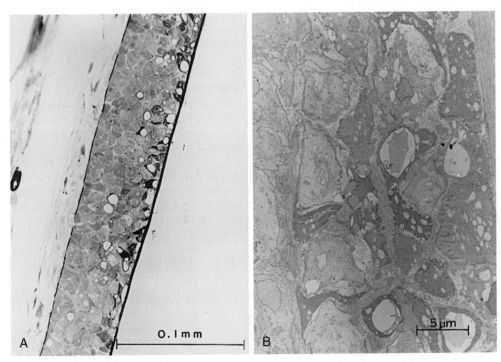

Figure 10–3. Seven-week-old spontaneously hypertensive rats were treated by gavage daily for 8 weeks with valsartan (10 mg/kg/day). The animals were perfused fixed under deep anesthesia, and rat femoral artery was collected for light and electron microscopy. **A.** In sections stained with toluidine blue, many cells appear vacuolated or with dense material, either cytoplasmic or nuclear. **B.** An adjacent section was examined by electron microscopy. The dramatic changes seen in the regions undergoing apoptosis are clearly illustrated with wholesale loss of cell structure, cytoplasmic blebbing, and condensed nuclei.

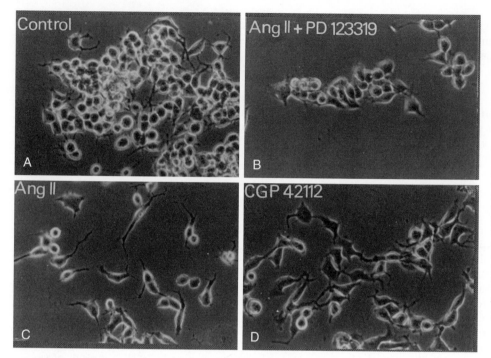

Figure 10–4. Nondifferentiated NG108-15 cells were cultured for 3 days in Dulbecco's modified Eagle's medium containing 10% fetal bovine serum in the absence (**A**) or in the presence (**B**) of 100 nM angiotensin II (Ang II); 100 nM Ang II + 10 μM PD 123319, an AT$_2$-receptor antagonist (**C**); or 100 nM CGP 42112, an AT$_2$-receptor agonist (**D**). In the presence of Ang II or CGP 42112, cells extended one or two neurite processes with a growth cone at their tip. In the presence of PD 123319, the cells kept their round appearance and formed aggregates. (**A–D,** From Laflamme L, de Gasparo M, Gallo JM, et al. Angiotensin II induction of neurite outgrowth by AT[2] receptors in NG108-15 cells—Effect counteracted by the AT[1] receptors. J Biol Chem 271:22729–22735, 1996.)

ferentiation, (Fig. 10–4) and modulation of matrix and structural proteins in endothelial and neuronal cells.[83–89]

It is hypothesized that the AT$_2$ receptor counterbalances the effect of the AT$_1$ receptor and plays a major role in development, cell differentiation, and tissue repair. Whereas Ang II promotes phosphorylation of various proteins through the AT$_1$ receptor, dephosphorylation occurs through the AT$_2$ receptor in a yin-yang manner. In cultured neonatal rat cardiac myocytes, the net growth effect of Ang II depends on the cellular AT$_1$:AT$_2$ ratio. AT$_1$ receptor–mediated proliferative effects become apparent when the AT$_2$ receptor–mediated antigrowth effects are blocked.[90] Thus, stimulation of the AT$_1$ receptor produces vasoconstriction, proliferation, and extracellular matrix formation. In contrast, stimulation of the AT$_2$ receptor causes vasodilatation and antiproliferation and modulates matrix formation. Whereas the AT$_1$ receptor is responsible for increased intracellular Ca^{2+} content, i.e., the primary signal for muscle contraction, and decreases K^+ in the cell, the AT$_2$ receptor produces the opposite. The AT$_2$ receptor is also involved in pressure natriuretic effects of Ang II in rats.[91] Reexpression of the AT$_2$ receptor in various pathological situations suggests a role of this receptor in pathophysiology. For example, there is a reciprocal relationship between AT$_1$ and AT$_2$ receptor expression in impaired ventricular function (Fig. 10–5).[92, 93] In human heart, the AT$_1$:AT$_2$ ratio correlates with right atrial pressure and left ventricular function, suggesting possible involvement of Ang II receptor subtypes in cardiac dysfunction.

Consequence of Blockade of the AT$_1$ Receptor

Blockade of the AT$_1$ receptor is accompanied by an increase in circulating levels of Ang II and its metabolites, possibly resulting in stimulation of other unblocked Ang receptors, especially the AT$_2$ receptor, which counterbalances the effects of the AT$_1$ receptor. In a model of heart failure after coronary ligature in the rat, some beneficial effects of AT$_1$ receptor blockade such as left ventricular end-systolic and end-diastolic volume and myocyte cross-sectional area were partially inhibited by an AT$_2$ antagonist, PD123319, or by a bradykinin antagonist, HOE 140.[94] Blood pressure was not affected by either AT$_2$ antagonist or bradykinin antagonist. Further, blockade of the AT$_1$ receptor in conscious sodium-depleted rats increased cyclic guanosine 3′-5′-monophosphate (cGMP) production in renal cortex microdialysates.[95, 96] A similar observation was made in rats after coronary ligature, where the aortic cGMP content was increased after treatment with losartan. This effect was blocked with the AT$_2$ antagonist PD123319.[97] It was also observed that stimulation of the AT$_2$ receptor modulates bradykinin production in the rat kidney. It is therefore postulated that the high circulating Ang II plasma level after AT$_1$ receptor blockade stimulates nitric oxide production through the AT$_2$ receptor (Fig. 10–6). This mechanism, which appears to involve a bradykinin pathway as well as a stimulation of NO synthase, may reinforce the effect of the AT$_1$ receptor blockade.

CONCLUSION

Our knowledge of the Ang II receptors has dramatically increased since the development of specific molecular tools, which permitted the characterization of at least two Ang receptor subtypes. Use of selective Ang AT$_1$ and AT$_2$ antagonists has allowed a better definition of the roles of the two best characterized Ang II receptors. Considering their coupling mechanisms and their reciprocally regulated expression, it is hypothesized that AT$_1$ and AT$_2$ receptors counterbalance each other mainly in pathological circum-

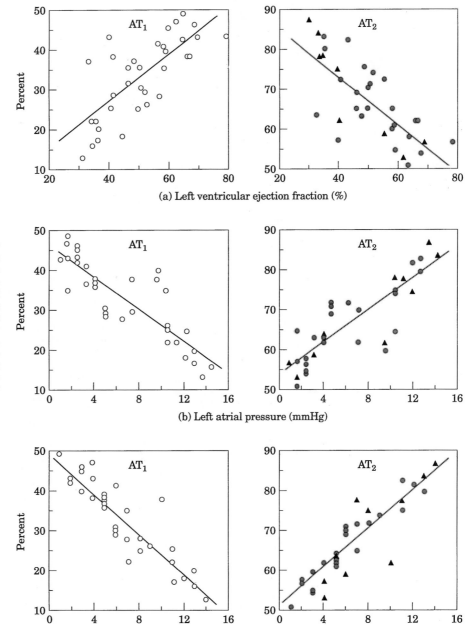

Figure 10–5. A–C. Angiotensin receptor subtypes were quantified in human atria using a binding assay. There is a correlation between the proportions of angiotensin II (Ang II) receptor subtypes and the hemodynamic parameters. The more severe the cardiac failure, the lower the amount of AT$_1$ receptor and the higher the AT$_2$ receptor. (**A–C,** From Rogg H, de Gasparo M, Graedel E, et al. Angiotensin II–receptor subtypes in human atria and evidence for alterations in patients with cardiac dysfunction. Eur Heart J 17:1112–1120, 1996.)

(a) Left ventricular ejection fraction (%)

(b) Left atrial pressure (mmHg)

(c) Right atrial pressure (mmHg)

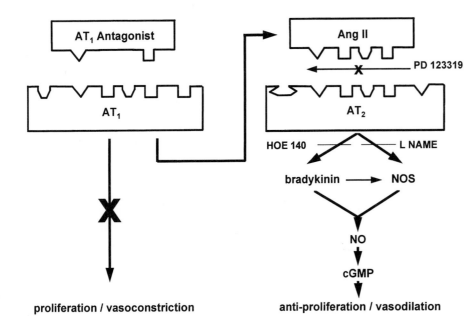

Figure 10–6. Schematic representation of a possible mechanism of action of the AT₁ receptor antagonist. Blockade of the AT₁ receptor is accompanied by increased circulating angiotensin II (Ang II) plasma levels, which stimulate the unblocked AT₂ receptor. This induces a rise in cyclic guanosine monophosphate (cGMP) formation. L-NAME, N^G-nitro-L-arginine methyl ester; NOS, nitric oxide synthase; HOE, code number of Hoechst 140, at present also known as I cantilant.

stances. Other Ang II receptor subtypes have been identified and await further characterization.

References

1. Takei Y, Hasegawa Y, Watanabe TX, et al. A novel angiotensin I isolated from an elasmobranch fish. J Endocrinol 139:281–285, 1993.
2. Salzet M, Wattez C, Baert JL, Malecha J. Biochemical evidence of angiotensin II–like peptides and proteins in the brain of the rhynchobdellid leech *Theromyzon tessulatum*. Brain Res 631:247–255, 1993.
3. Peach MJ. Renin-angiotensin system: Biochemistry and mechanisms of action. Physiol Rev 57:313–370, 1977.
4. Papadimitriou A, Worcel M. Dose-response curves for angiotensin II and synthetic analogues in three types of smooth muscle: Existence of different forms of receptor sites for angiotensin II. Br J Pharmacol 50:291–297, 1974.
5. Whitebread S, Mele M, Kamber B, de Gasparo M. Preliminary biochemical characterization of two angiotensin II receptor subtypes. Biochem Biophys Res Commun 163:284–291, 1989.
6. Chiu AT, Herblin WF, McCall DE, et al. Identification of angiotensin II receptor subtypes. Biochem Biophys Res Commun 165:196–203, 1989.
7. Bumpus FM, Catt KJ, Chiu AT, et al. Nomenclature for angiotensin receptors: A report of the Nomenclature Committee of the Council for High Blood Pressure Research. Hypertension 17:720–721, 1991.
8. de Gasparo M, Husain A, Alexander RW, et al. A proposed update of the nomenclature of angiotensin receptors. Hypertension 25:924–927, 1995.
9. Ji H, Sandberg K, Catt KJ. Novel angiotensin II antagonists distinguish amphibian from mammalian angiotensin II receptors expressed in *Xenopus laevis* oocytes. Mol Pharmacol 39:120–123, 1991.
10. Bergsma DJ, Ellis C, Nuthulaganti PR, et al. Isolation and expression of a novel angiotensin II receptor from *Xenopus laevis* heart. Mol Pharmacol 44:277–284, 1993.
11. Murphy TJ, Alexander RW, Griendling KK, et al. Isolation of a cDNA encoding the vascular type-1 angiotensin II receptor. Nature 351:233–236, 1991.
12. Sandberg K. Structural analysis and regulation of angiotensin II receptors. Trends Endocrinol Metab 5:28–35, 1994.
13. Sasamura H, Hein L, Krieger JE, et al. Cloning, characterization, and expression of two angiotensin receptor (AT-1) isoforms from the mouse genome. Biochem Biophys Res Commun 185:253–259, 1992.
14. Elton TS, Stephan CC, Taylor GR, et al. Isolation of two distinct type I angiotensin II receptor genes. Biochem Biophys Res Commun 184:1067–1073, 1992.
15. Chiu AT, Dunscomb JH, McCall DE, et al. Characterization of angio-tensin AT₁ₐ-receptor isoform by its ligand binding signature. Regul Pept 44:141–147, 1993.
16. Iwai N, Inagami T, Ohmichi N, et al. Differential regulation of rat AT₁ₐ and AT₁ᵦ receptor mRNA. Biochem Biophys Res Commun 188:298–303, 1992.
17. Hahn AWA, Jonas U, Buehler FR, Resink TJ. Identification of a 4th angiotensin-AT(1) receptor subtype in rat. Biochem Biophys Res Commun 192:1260–1265, 1993.
18. Konishi H, Kuroda S, Inada Y, Fujisawa Y. Novel subtype of human angiotensin II type 1 receptor–cDNA cloning and expression. Biochem Biophys Res Commun 199:467–474, 1994.
19. Kuroda S, Konishi H, Okishio M, Fujisawa Y. Novel subtype of human angiotensin II type 1 receptor—Analysis of signal transduction mechanism in transfected Chinese hamster ovary cells. Biochem Biophys Res Commun 199:475–481, 1994.
20. Su BG, Martin MM, Beason KB, et al. The genomic organization and functional analysis of the promoter for the human angiotensin II type 1 receptor. Biochem Biophys Res Commun 204:1039–1046, 1994.
21. Guo DF, Furuta H, Mizukoshi M, Inagami T. The genomic organization of human angiotensin II type 1 receptor. Biochem Biophys Res Commun 200:313–319, 1994.
22. Curnow KM, Pascoe L, Davies E, et al. Alternatively spliced human type 1 angiotensin II receptor mRNAs are translated at different efficiencies and encode two receptor isoforms. Mol Endocrinol 9:1250–1262, 1995.
23. Inagami T, Guo DF, Kitami Y. Molecular biology of angiotensin II receptors—An overview. J Hypertens 12:S83–S94, 1994.
24. Takayanagi R, Ohnaka K, Sakai Y, et al. Molecular cloning and characterization of the promoter for human type-1 angiotensin II receptor gene. Biochem Biophys Res Commun 200:1264–1270, 1994.
25. Makita N, Iwai N, Inagami T, Badr KF. Two distinct pathways in the down-regulation of type-1 angiotension II receptor gene in rat glomerular mesangial cells. Biochem Biophys Res Commun 185:142–146, 1992.
26. Guo DF, Inagami T. Epidermal growth factor-enhanced human angiotensin II type 1 receptor. Hypertension 23:1032–1035, 1994.
27. Steckelings U, Lebrun C, Qadri F, et al. Role of brain angiotensin in cardiovascular regulation. J Cardiovasc Pharmacol 19(suppl 6):S72–S79, 1992.
28. de Gasparo M, Bottari S, Levens NR. Characteristics of angiotensin II receptors and their role in cell and organ physiology. *In* Laragh JH, Brenner BM (eds). Hypertension: Physiology, Diagnosis, and Management. New York, Raven, 1994; pp 1695–1720.
29. Sano T, Ohyama K, Yamano Y, et al. A domain for G protein coupling in carboxyl-terminal tail of rat angiotensin II receptor type 1a. J Biol Chem 272:23631–23636, 1997.

30. Riordan JF. Angiotensin II—Biosynthesis, molecular recognition, and signal transduction. Cell Mol Neurobiol 15:637–651, 1995.

31. Griendling KK, Lassègue B, Alexander RW. Angiotensin receptors and their therapeutic implications. Annu Rev Pharmacol Toxicol 36:281–306, 1996.

32. Griendling KK, Ushiofukai M, Lassègue B, Alexander RW. Angiotensin II signaling in vascular smooth muscle—New concepts. Hypertension 29:366–373, 1997.

33. Berk BC, Corson MA. Angiotensin II signal transduction in vascular smooth muscle—Role of tyrosine kinases. [Review] Circ Res 80:607–616, 1997.

34. Schieffer B, Paxton WG, Marrero MB, Bernstein KE. Importance of tyrosine phosphorylation in angiotensin II type 1 receptor signaling. Hypertension 27:476–480, 1996.

35. Sauro MD, Sudakow R, Burns S. In vivo effects of angiotensin II on vascular smooth muscle contraction and blood pressure are mediated through a protein tyrosine kinase–dependent mechanism. J Pharmacol Exp Ther 277:1744–1750, 1996.

36. Ali MS, Sayeski PP, Dirksen LB, et al. Dependence on the motif YIPP for the physical association of jak2 kinase with the intracellular carboxyl tail of the angiotensin II AT(1) receptor. J Biol Chem 272:23382–23388, 1997.

37. Stroth U, Meffert S, Gallinat S, Unger T. Angiotensin II and NGF differentially influence microtubule proteins in PC12W cells: Role of the AT2 receptor. Mol Brain Res 53:187–195, 1998.

38. Bumpus FM. Mechanisms and sites of action of newer angiotensin agonists and antagonists in terms of activity and receptor. Fed Proc 36:2128–2132, 1977.

39. Capponi AM, Catt KJ. Angiotensin II receptors in adrenal cortex and uterus. Binding and activation properties of angiotensin analogues. J Biol Chem 254:5120–5127, 1979.

40. Yamano Y, Ohyama K, Chaki S, et al. Identification of amino acid residues of rat angiotensin II receptor for ligand binding by site directed mutagenesis. Biochem Biophys Res Commun 187:1426–1431, 1992.

41. Hunyady L, Balla T, Catt KJ. The ligand binding site of the angiotensin AT(1) receptor. [Review] Trends Pharmacol Sci 17:135–140, 1996.

42. Karnik SS, Husain A, Graham RM. Molecular determinants of peptide and non-peptide binding to the AT(1) receptor. Clin Exp Pharmacol Physiol 23:S58–S66, 1996.

43. Bensoussan M, Mitchell T, Reilly T, et al. Immunological reactivity of angiotensin-II receptor antagonists—Possible implications for receptor binding sites. Eur J Pharmacol Mol Pharmacol 247:169–175, 1993.

44. Ji H, Leung M, Zhang Y, et al. Differential structural requirements for specific binding of nonpeptide and peptide antagonists to the AT(1) angiotensin receptor—Identification of amino acid residues that determine binding of the antihypertensive drug losartan. J Biol Chem 269:16533–16536, 1994.

45. Schambye HT, Vonwijk B, Hjorth SA, et al. Mutations in transmembrane segment VII of the AT(1) receptor differentiate between closely related insurmountable and competitive angiotensin antagonists. Br J Pharmacol 113:331–333, 1994.

46. Schambye HT, Hjorth SA, Bergsma DJ, et al. Differentiation between binding sites for angiotensin II and nonpeptide antagonists on the angiotensin II type 1 receptors. Proc Natl Acad Sci U S A 91:7046–7050, 1994.

47. Robertson MJ, Dougall IG, Harper D, et al. Agonist-antagonist interaction at angiotensin receptors. Application of a two-state receptor model. Trends Pharmacol Sci 15:364–369, 1994.

48. Ohyama K, Yamano Y, Chaki S, et al. Domains for G-protein coupling in angiotensin-II receptor type-I—Studies by site-directed mutagenesis. Biochem Biophys Res Commun 189:677–683, 1992.

49. Conchon S, Barrault MB, Miserey S, et al. The C-terminal third intracellular loop of the rat AT(1a) angiotensin receptor plays a key role in G protein coupling specificity and transduction of the mitogenic signal. J Biol Chem 272:25566–25572, 1997.

50. Bihoreau C, Monnot C, Davies E, et al. Mutation of Asp(74) of the rat angiotensin-II receptor confers changes in antagonist affinities and abolishes G-protein coupling. Proc Natl Acad Sci U S A 90:5133–5137, 1993.

51. Marie J, Maigret B, Joseph MP, et al. Tyr(292) in the seventh transmembrane domain of the AT(1A) angiotensin II receptor is essential for its coupling to phospholipase C. J Biol Chem 269:20815–20818, 1994.

52. Bihoreau C, Monnot C, Davies E, et al. Mutation of Asp74 of the rat angiotensin II receptor confers changes in antagonist affinities and abolishes G-protein coupling. Proc Natl Aced Sci U S A 90:5133–5137, 1993.

53. Hunyady L, Bor M, Balla T, Catt KJ. Identification of a cytoplasmic Ser-Thr-Leu motif that determines agonist-induced internalization of the AT(1) angiotensin receptor. J Biol Chem 269:31378–31382, 1994.

54. Groblewski T, Maigret B, Larguier R, et al. Mutation of Asn(111) in the third transmembrane domain of the AT(1A) angiotensin II receptor induces its constitutive activation. J Biol Chem; 272:1822–1826,1997.

55. Balmforth AJ, Lee AJ, Warburton P, et al. The conformational change responsible for AT(1) receptor activation is dependent upon two juxtaposed asparagine residues on transmembrane helices III and VII. J Biol Chem 272:4245–4251, 1997.

56. Pucell AG, Hodges JC, Sen I, et al. Biochemical properties of the ovarian granulosa cell type 2-angiotensin II receptor. Endocrinology 128:1947–1959, 1991.

57. Dudley DT, Hubbell SE, Summerfelt RM. Characterization of angiotensin II (AT2) binding sites in R3T3 cells. Mol Pharmacol 40:360–367, 1991.

58. Bottari SP, King IN, Reichlin S, et al. The angiotensin AT2 receptor stimulates protein tyrosine phosphatase activity and mediates inhibition of particulate guanylate cyclase. Biochem Biophys Res Commun 183:206–211, 1992.

59. Mukoyama M, Nakajima M, Horiuchi M, et al. Expression cloning of type-2 angiotensin II receptor reveals a unique class of seven-transmembrane receptors. J Biol Chem 268:24539–24542, 1993.

60. Kambayashi Y, Bardhan S, Takahashi K, et al. Molecular cloning of a novel angiotensin-II receptor isoform involved in phosphotyrosine phosphatase inhibition. J Biol Chem 268:24543–24546, 1993.

61. Tsutsumi K, Saavedra JM. Heterogeneity of angiotensin AT2 receptors in the rat brain. Mol Pharmacol 41:290–297, 1992.

62. Rowe BP, Saylor DL, Speth RC. Analysis of angiotensin II receptor subtypes in individual rat brain nuclei. Neuroendocrinology 55:563–573, 1992.

63. Sumners C, Tang W, Zelezna B, Raizada MK. Angiotensin II receptor subtypes are coupled with distinct signal-transduction mechanisms in neurons and astrocytes from rat brain. Proc Natl Acad Sci U S A 88:7567–7571, 1991.

64. Koike G, Horiuchi M, Yamada T, et al. Human type 2 angiotensin II receptor gene—Cloned, mapped to the X chromosome, and its mRNA is expressed in the human lung. Biochem Biophys Res Commun 203:1842–1850, 1994.

65. Koike G, Winer ES, Horiuchi M, et al. Cloning, characterization, and genetic mapping of the rat type 2 angiotensin II receptor gene. Hypertension 26:998–1002, 1995.

66. Ichiki T, Herold CL, Kambayashi Y, et al. Cloning of the cDNA and the genomic DNA of the mouse angiotensin II type 2 receptor. Biochim Biophys Acta 1189:247–250, 1994.

67. Ichiki T, Inagami T. Expression, genomic organization, and transcription of the mouse angiotensin II type 2 receptor gene. Circ Res 76:693–700, 1995.

68. Horiuchi M, Koike G, Yamada T, et al. The growth-dependent expression of angiotensin II type 2 receptor is regulated by transcription factors interferon regulatory factor-1 and -2. J Biol Chem 270:20225–20230, 1995.

69. Horiuchi M, Yamada T, Hayashida W, Dzau VJ. Interferon regulatory factor-1 up-regulates angiotensin II type 2 receptor and induces apoptosis. J Biol Chem 272:11952–11958, 1997.

70. Chang RS, Lotti VJ. Angiotensin receptor subtypes in rat, rabbit and monkey tissues: Relative distribution and species dependency. Life Sci 49:1485–1490, 1991.

71. Dzau VJ, Horiuchi M. Differential expression of angiotensin receptor subtypes in the myocardium: A hypothesis. Eur Heart J 17:978–980, 1996.

72. Gallinat S, Yu MH, Zhu YZ, et al. Upregulation of angiotensin receptors after myocardial infarction and sciatic nerve transection: A common expression pattern. [Abstract] Hypertension 30:999, 1997.

73. Webb ML, Liu EC, Cohen RB, et al. Molecular characterization of angiotensin II type II receptors in rat pheochromocytoma cells. Peptides 13:499–508, 1992.

74. Zhang JS, Pratt RE. The AT(2) receptor selectively associates with G(1α2) and G(1α3) in the rat fetus. J Biol Chem 271:15026–15033, 1996.

75. Lehtonen JY, Hayashida W, Horiuchi M, Dzau VJ. Angiotensin II receptor subtype specific effects are mediated by intracellular third loops: Chimeric receptor approach. [Abstract] Circulation 96(suppl 1):I-478, 1997.

76. Hayashida W, Horiuchi M, Dzau VJ. Intracellular third loop domain of angiotensin II type-2 receptor—Role in mediating signal transduction and cellular function. J Biol Chem 271:21985–21992, 1996.

77. Lehtonen JY, Horiuchi M, Dzau VJ. Ceramide as a second messenger for angiotensin II type 2 receptor mediated apoptosis. [Abstract] Circulation 96(suppl 1):I-554, 1997.

78. Munzenmaier DH, Greene AS. Angiotensin II mediates a sustained rise in nuclear and cytoplasmic calcium via multiple receptor subtypes. Am J Physiol Heart Circ Physiol 38:H565–H570, 1995.

79. Nahmias C, Cazaubon SM, Briend-Sutren MM, et al. Angiotensin II AT_2 receptors are functionally coupled to protein tyrosine dephosphorylation in N 1E-115 neuroblastoma cells. Biochem J 306:87–92, 1995.

80. Nahmias C, Strosberg AD. The angiotensin AT(2) receptor—Searching for signal-transduction pathways and physiological function. Trends Pharmacol Sci 16:223–225, 1995.

81. Bedecs K, Elbaz N, Sutren M, et al. Angiotensin II type 2 receptors mediate inhibition of mitogen-activated protein kinase cascade and functional activation of SHP-1 tyrosine phosphatase. Biochem J 325:449–454, 1997.

82. Yamada T, Horiuchi M, Dzau VJ. Angiotensin II type 2 receptor mediates programmed cell death. Proc Natl Acad Sci U S A 93:156–160, 1996.

83. Kang J, Posner P, Sumners C. Angiotensin II type 2 receptor stimulation of neuronal K$^+$ currents involves an inhibitory GTP binding protein. Am J Physiol Cell Physiol 36:C1389–C1397, 1994.

84. Nakajima M, Hutchinson HG, Fujinaga M, et al. The angiotensin II type 2 (AT(2)) receptor antagonizes the growth effects of the AT(1) receptor—Gain-of-function study using gene transfer. Proc Natl Acad Sci U S A 92:10663–10667, 1995.

85. Tanaka M, Ohnishi J, Ozawa Y, et al. Characterization of angiotensin II receptor type 2 during differentiation and apoptosis of rat ovarian cultured granulosa cells. Biochem Biophys Res Commun 207:593–598, 1995.

86. Buisson B, Laflamme L, Bottari SP, et al. A G protein is involved in the angiotensin AT(2) receptor inhibition of the T-type calcium current in non-differentiated NG108-15 cells. J Biol Chem 270:1670–1674, 1995.

87. Laflamme L, de Gasparo M, Gallo JM, et al. Angiotensin II induction of neurite outgrowth by AT(2) receptors in NG108-15, cells—Effect counteracted by the AT(1) receptors. J Biol Chem 271:22729–22735, 1996.

88. Gallinat S, Csikos T, Meffert S, et al. The angiotensin AT(2) receptor down-regulates neurofilament in PC12w cells. Neurosci Lett 227:29–32, 1997.

89. Unger T, Chung O, Csikos T, et al. Angiotensin receptors. J Hypertens 14:S95–S103, 1996.

90. Vankesteren CAM, Vanheugten HAA, Lamers JMJ, et al. Angiotensin II mediated growth and antigrowth effects in cultured neonatal rat cardiac myocytes and fibroblasts. J Mol Cell Cardiol 29:2147–2157, 1997.

91. Lo M, Liu KL, Lantelme P, Sassard J. Subtype 2 of angiotensin II receptors controls pressure-natriuresis in rats. J Clin Invest 95:1394–1397, 1995.

92. Lopez JJ, Lorell BH, Ingelfinger JR, et al. Distribution and function of cardiac angiotensin AT(1)- and AT(2)-receptor subtypes in hypertrophied rat hearts. Am J Physiol 267:H844–H852, 1994.

93. Rogg H, de Gasparo M, Graedel E, et al. Angiotensin II-receptor subtypes in human atria and evidence for alterations in patients with cardiac dysfunction. Eur Heart J 17:1112–1120, 1996.

94. Liu YH, Yang XP, Sharov VG, et al. Effects of angiotensin-converting enzyme inhibitors and angiotensin II type 1 receptor antagonists in rats with heart failure—Role of kinins and angiotensin II type 2 receptors. J Clin Invest 99:1926–1935, 1997.

95. Siragy HM, Carey RM. The subtype-2 (AT(2)) angiotensin receptor regulates renal cyclic guanosine 3′,5′-monophosphate and AT(1) receptor-mediated prostaglandin E(2) production in conscious rats. J Clin Invest 97:1978–1982, 1996.

96. Siragy HM, Carey RM. The subtype 2 (AT(2)) angiotensin receptor mediates renal production of nitric oxide in conscious rats. J Clin Invest 100:264–269, 1997.

97. Gohlke P, Pees C, Unger T. AT2 receptor stimulation increases aortic cyclic GMP in SHRSP by a kinin-dependent mechanism. Hypertension 31:349–355, 1998.

CHAPTER 11

Metabolic Abnormalities in Hypertension

Syed S. Ali, Melvin A. Lester, and James R. Sowers

Essential hypertension is associated with an increased prevalence of insulin resistance and other metabolic abnormalities.[1–102] The prevalence of both essential hypertension and diabetes mellitus is increasing in industrialized cultures, such as the United States, related to such factors as aging and increasing obesity.[3, 5, 9, 91, 92] Insulin resistance, hyperinsulinemia, and hyperglycemia have been implicated as contributing factors in the pathogenesis of hypertension and atherosclerosis.[1–92] Although metabolic abnormalities, such as insulin resistance/hyperinsulinemia, often coexist with essential hypertension, the association is not uniform and the mechanisms responsible for these associations remain speculative. However, the pathophysiological significance of these observed relationships is that they predispose to premature coronary heart disease (CHD) and generalized atherosclerosis in persons with a genetic susceptibility under the influence of appropriate environmental factors. This review presents the current understanding of various metabolic disturbances associated with hypertension, the pathophysiological mechanisms involved, and the significance of the interplay between them relative to the complications of essential hypertension.

OBESITY, THE NEXUS BETWEEN HYPERTENSION AND ASSOCIATED METABOLIC ABNORMALITIES

Visceral obesity is an especially strong risk factor for hypertension, insulin resistance, dyslipidemia, type II diabetes mellitus, and increased CHD.[10–18, 88–90] Visceral fat is localized around mesenteric and omental tissues that drain directly into the portal vein. Insulin resistance in persons with visceral obesity may relate, in part, to the metabolic characteristics of visceral fat, which when compared with peripheral fat, is more resistant to the metabolic effects of insulin and more sensitive to lipolytic hormones.[11, 12] Increased release of free fatty acids into the portal system provides increased substrate for hepatic triglyceride synthesis and may impair first-pass metabolism of insulin. The increased levels of free fatty acids may, in turn, contribute to skeletal muscle insulin resistance by substrate competition between glucose and free fatty acids and the glucose–fatty acid cycle. Further, in the postabsorptive state, fatty acids account for up to 80% of substrate oxidation and, subsequently, skeletal muscle thermogenesis. Reduced fatty acid oxidation in skeletal muscle in obesity is important because it translates into a reduced rate of skeletal muscle lipoprotein lipase (LPL) activity and thermogenesis/respiration.[16] A primary (genetic) deficiency of skeletal muscle LPL activity could result in reduced fatty acid/lipid oxidation and a propensity toward increased fat distribution in visceral regions.[16, 87]

Although body mass index is a very strong determinant of blood pressure (especially systolic blood pressures),[86, 92] a visceral distribution of fat has an even greater relationship with the development of hypertension.[86, 91] The relationship between obesity and hypertension is observed in virtually all societies, ages, ethnic groups, and both genders.[86, 87, 91, 92] The risk of CHD associated with hemodynamic/metabolic abnormalities in visceral obesity was described in a report from the Quebec Cardiovascular Study, a prospective study in which over 2000 middle-aged men were followed up over a period of 5 years.[25] Two characteristic abnormalities of visceral obesity, fasting hyperinsulinemia and elevated apolipoprotein β, were the strongest independent risk factors for CHD. Another independent report indicated that the presence of small, dense, low-density lipoprotein (LDL) particles was associated with an approximately threefold increase in CHD risk and that this risk was further enhanced in the presence of elevated apolipoprotein β levels.[18] Techniques such as gradient gel electrophoresis have clearly demonstrated that the dyslipidemia characteristic of visceral obesity and related metabolic/hemodynamic abnormalities is that of increased apolipoprotein β concentrations and increases in small, dense, LDL particles (Table 11–1).[18]

LIPID ABNORMALITIES

Persons with hypertension, especially if they also manifest central obesity and insulin resistance, have the previously described lipid abnormalities, as well as elevated very low density lipoprotein (VLDL) levels (see Table 11–1).[1] Elevated levels of VLDL are due, in part, to increased portal delivery of free fatty acids to the liver, thus stimulating hepatic synthesis of these triglyceride particles. With insulin resistance, there is reduced activity of endothelium-bound LPL in skeletal muscle and adipocytes, and it is this LPL that is responsible for normal metabolism of triglyceride-rich VLDL and chylomicron particles.[17] Thus, the VLDL elevation is due to both increased production and reduced metabolism (see Table 11–1). Genetic investigations, including parent-child, large-scale family, twin, and candidate gene studies, have provided evidence for a genetic basis for the relationship between hypertension and accompanying lipid abnormalities.[1, 93–97] Indeed, there are higher heritability estimates in twins than in pedigrees for blood pressure, LDL, VLDL, and body mass index.[93] Almost 70% of adults with hypertension before 55 years of age have siblings or parents with hypertension, and 12% of all hypertensive patients have familial dyslipidemic hypertension.[93–97] Accordingly, both hypertensive and dyslipidemic states probably have a genetic basis, and both conditions have been linked to insulin resistance.

The metabolic-hypertensive syndrome consists of a combination of hypertension with either a VLDL or an LDL level above the 90th percentile or a high-density lipoprotein (HDL)–cholesterol below the 10th percentile, or both, and is present in 48% of hypertensive sibships in Utah.[93] In familial dyslipidemic hypertensives in Utah, an abnormality of HDL-cholesterol was discovered in 68%, triglycerides in 49%, and LDL-cholesterol in 27%. Elevated fasting insulin levels and increased subscapular skinfold thickness were also observed in these dyslipidemic hypertensives as well as in their twins.[94] The genetic locus associated with this atherosclerosis-predisposing metabolic disarray is closely linked to both the LDL receptor and the insulin receptor locus on the short arm of chromosome 19.[95–97] DNA sequencing has shown a point mutation for the LPL enzyme that conveys susceptibility to lipoprotein abnormalities and, possibly, hypertension.[93] In an investigation of the relationship between HDL-cholesterol and the variable region flanking the human gene, one class of alleles was associated with low HDL-cholesterol concentrations.[95] In the Bogalusa Heart Study, this allele class was associated with a family history of both diabetes and coronary artery disease.[95] In children from the Bogalusa cohort, postprandial insulin levels were positively associated with fasting serum triglycerides and pre–β-lipoprotein–cholesterol. Thus, there is considerable evidence for a genetic basis for an association of hypertension with an atherosclerotic lipid profile (high VLDL, low HDL, and small dense LDL) (see Table 11–1) as well as with insulin resistance/hyperinsulinemia.

COAGULATION/FIBRINOLYTIC ABNORMALITIES

Hypertension is often associated with coagulation abnormalities as well as lipid disturbances.[1, 5, 8, 36–46] Disturbances of the fibrinolytic system have been reported in persons with hypertension, especially those with concomitant lipid

---

Table 11–1. Lipid, Coagulation, and Fibrinolyitc Abnormalities Seen in Hypertension

Elevated plasma levels of VLDL, LDL, and Lp(a)
Decreased plasma HDL cholesterol
Increased small, dense, LDL cholesterol products
Decreased lipoprotein lipase activity
Elevated plasma levels of factors VII and VIII
Increased fibrinogen and PAI-1 levels
Elevated thrombin-antithrombin complexes
Decreased antithrombin III and protein C and S levels
Decreased plasminogen activators and fibrinolytic activity
Increased endothelial expression of adhesion molecules

Abbreviations: VLDL, very low density lipoprotein; LDL, low-density lipoprotein; Lp(a), lipoprotein(a); HDL, high-density lipoprotein; PAI-1, plasminogen activator inhibitor-1.

and glucose abnormalities and vascular disease.[1, 36–46] In order to describe these abnormalities better, it is necessary to review briefly some seminal components of the blood-clotting cascade and the plasminogen activator/plasmin system.[37–40] Generation of thrombin and the formation of a fibrin clot generally involve two components, the intrinsic and the extrinsic pathways.[37, 38] In the intrinsic pathway, monitored by the activated partial thromboplastin time, factor XII is activated during the contact phase of blood clotting. This is followed by the sequential activation of factors XI, IX, and X and prothrombin. In the extrinsic pathway, monitored by prothrombin time, a complex is formed between tissue factor and factor VI. This is followed by sequential activation of factors VII and X and prothrombin. In vivo, platelet membranes and surface membranes of endothelial cells provide a critical surface during platelet activation for initiation and propagation of the coagulation process.

Increases in several components of the coagulation cascade, including endothelium-derived von Willebrand's factor, occur in association with endothelial cell damage[1, 5, 8, 13] and macrovascular disease.[1, 13] High concentrations of factor VIII components accelerate the rate of thrombin formation and contribute to accelerated atherosclerosis. Elevated levels of fibrinogen and thrombin-antithrombin complexes increase the survival of provisional clot matrix on transformation of fibrinogen to fibrin at the site of injured endothelium.[13] Increased coagulability in association with other metabolic disorders accompanying hypertension may include deficiencies of endogenous factors (i.e., factors C and S and antithrombin C) that normally inhibit clot generation.[13, 39, 40] Plasma levels of lipoprotein(a) (Lp[a]) are often elevated in abnormal metabolic states such as diabetes mellitus.[41, 42] By inhibiting fibrinolysis, increased levels of Lp(a) potentially delay thrombolysis and contribute to plaque progression.[42] Elevated levels of plasminogen activator inhibitor-1 (PAI-1) have been reported in untreated patients with essential hypertension[37] and in men with prior myocardial infarctions and at increased risk for reinfarction.[13] Elevated PAI-1 levels are associated with abdominal obesity[11–13] and with insulin resistance/hyperinsulinemia and dyslipidemia (see Table 11–1).[3, 5, 8, 13]

PLATELET ABNORMALITIES

Platelet aggregation and adhesion are often enhanced in hypertension and associated metabolic abnormalities (Table 11–2).[3, 8, 13, 36, 45–50] These functional abnormalities are related to exaggerated elevations in platelet intracellular calcium $[Ca^{2+}]_i$ mobilization, phosphoinositide turnover, and myosin light chain phosphorylation.[36, 45–49] Both platelet $[Ca^{2+}]_i$ and relative levels of intracellular magnesium $[Mg^{2+}]_i$ have seminal roles in platelet activation. Platelet aggregation is associated with elevations in $[Ca^{2+}]_i$, a necessary first event in the aggregation process.[36] In vitro, increased $[Mg^{2+}]_i$ can inhibit platelet aggregation.[49] Additionally, magnesium infusion reduces platelet thrombus formation in a model of partial coronary and carotid occlusion.[13] There is considerable evidence that persons with essential hypertension and diabetes have elevated platelet $[Ca^{2+}]_i$ and reduced $[Mg^{2+}]_i$ (Fig. 11–1).[3, 8, 13, 36, 47] This

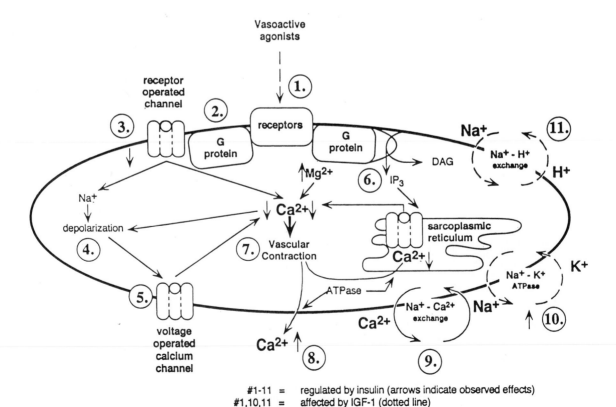

| #1-11 | = | regulated by insulin (arrows indicate observed effects) |
| #1,10,11 | = | affected by IGF-1 (dotted line) |

Figure 11–1. Mechanisms regulating divalent cation metabolism and contraction in vascular smooth muscle cells and proposed targets of insulin and insulin-like growth factor–1 (IGF-1) action. Pivotal steps in regulation of divalent cation metabolism are indicated by *circled numbers*. IP$_3$, inositol trisphosphate; DAG, diacylglycerol.

Table 11–2. Abnormalities of Platelet Function in Essential Hypertension

Increased platelet adhesiveness
Increased platelet aggregation
Decreased platelet survival
Increased platelet generation of vasoconstrictor prostanoids
Reduced platelet generation of prostacyclin and other vasodilator prostanoids
Altered platelet divalent cation homeostasis (i.e., decreased $[Mg^{2+}]_i$ and increased $[Ca^{2+}]_i$)
Increased nonenzymatic glycosylation of platelet proteins
Decreased platelet polyphosphoinositide content
Decreased platelet production of NO
Increased platelet myosin light chain phosphorylation
Increased platelet adhesion to endothelium

altered balance between relative concentrations of these divalent cations likely contributes to enhanced platelet aggregation/adhesion in persons with diabetes and associated metabolic abnormalities. Further, platelets from persons with diabetes with or without hypertension have reduced membrane fluidity thought to be related to altered membrane cholesterol:phospholipid ratios.[44] Finally, the dyslipidemia that is often associated with hypertension may contribute directly and indirectly to enhanced platelet aggregation (Table 11–2).[3, 13]

ENDOTHELIAL DYSFUNCTION

Abnormalities in the function of the vascular endothelium are thought to play a major role in the pathogenesis of accelerated atherosclerosis in persons with hypertension and associated metabolic abnormalities (Table 11–3).[55–59] Both hyperglycemia and dyslipidemia contribute to endothelial dysfunction.[56–58] Hyperglycemia results in impairment of endothelial cell nitric oxide production,[50, 56, 58] perhaps via activation of protein kinase C in endothelial cells. Activation of protein kinase C and associated reduced nitric oxide production predispose to increased synthesis of vasoconstrictor prostaglandins, endothelin, glycated proteins, endothelium adhesion molecules, and platelet and vascular growth factors, which cumulatively enhance vasomotor tone and vascular growth and remodeling.[56–59] Endothelial dysfunction is also characterized by accelerated disappearance of capillary endothelium,[58] weakening of

Table 11–3. Alterations in Vascular Endothelium Associated With Hypertension

Elevated plasma levels of von Willebrand's factor
Elevated expression, synthesis, and plasma levels of endothelin-1
Diminished prostacyclin release
Decreased release of endothelium-derived relaxing factor and reduced responsiveness to nitric oxide
Impaired fibrinolytic activity
Increased endothelial cell procoagulant activity
Increased endothelial cell surface thrombomodulin
Impaired plasmin degradation of glycosylated fibrin
Increased levels of advanced glycosylated end products
Increased superoxide anion generation
Increased expression of adhesion molecules

intercellular junctions,[57] altered protein synthesis, and expression/production of adhesion glycoproteins on endothelial cells,[56–59] promoting attachment of monocytes and leukocytes as well as their transendothelial migration.[57] Hyperglycemia enhances endothelial cell matrix production, which may contribute to basement membrane thickening,[60] and also increases the activity of enzymes involved in collagen synthesis,[60] specifically endothelial cell collagen IV and fibronectin synthesis.[60] Hyperglycemia also delays endothelial cell replication and increases cell death, in part by enhancing oxidation and glycation (glyco-oxidation).[56–60]

Insulin resistance and hyperinsulinemia are often present in persons with essential hypertension[1, 3, 5, 13] and are accompanied by abnormalities in intracellular Ca^{2+}_i metabolism, as previously described in detail (see Fig. 11–1).[3, 32, 35] Increased lipid content of skeletal muscle contributes to insulin resistance and associated hyperinsulinemia,[27, 28] akin to visceral adiposity.[29] Hyperinsulinemia promotes atherosclerosis by a number of mechanisms (Table 11–4). High levels of insulin stimulate mitogenic signaling pathways and increase DNA synthesis in vascular endothelial and smooth muscle cells.[21, 20–32] Insulin stimulates the synthesis of both endothelin and PAI-1,[21, 33] two atherogenic factors. Much of the effect of insulin on cardiovascular growth and remodeling is likely mediated through actions on an insulin-like growth factor-1 (IGF-1) receptor in endothelial/vascular smooth muscle cells (VSMC),[30–32] or indirectly by stimulating VSMC[31–33] or cardiac[33, 34] IGF-1 synthesis (Fig. 11–2). Insulin and IGF-1 are structurally related, share receptors, and have similar postreceptor signaling pathways.[32] Unlike insulin, which is not produced by cardiovascular tissue and must traverse the endothelium before acting on VSMC or cardiomyocytes, IGF-1 is synthesized by these cells and is more likely to function in an autocrine/paracrine role.[30–35, 74–76] There is increasing evidence that enhanced IGF-1 expression/synthesis plays an important role in mesangial hyperplasia and left ventricular hypertrophy, both manifestations of diabetes mellitus and hypertension.[30–35] It is likely that many of the atherosclerotic and growth effects attributed to hyperinsulinemia are mediated through an IGF-1 receptor either directly by IGF-1 or indirectly by high concentrations of insulin.[32]

Table 11–4. Abnormalities Seen in Insulin Resistance Associated With Hypertension

Elevated plasma levels of VLDL and Lp(a)
Decreased plasma HDL cholesterol
Increased lipoprotein oxidation/glycation
Increased small, dense, LDL cholesterol particles
Decreased lipoprotein lipase activity
Increased fibrinogen and PAI-1
Decreased plasminogen activator and fibrinolytic activity
Increased plasma insulin and proinsulin
Central obesity
Microalbuminuria
Increased vascular resistance
Premature atherosclerosis

Abbreviations: VLDL, very low density lipoprotein; Lp(a), lipoprotein(a); HDL, high-density lipoprotein; LDL, low-density lipoprotein; PAI-1, plasminogen activator inhibitor-1.

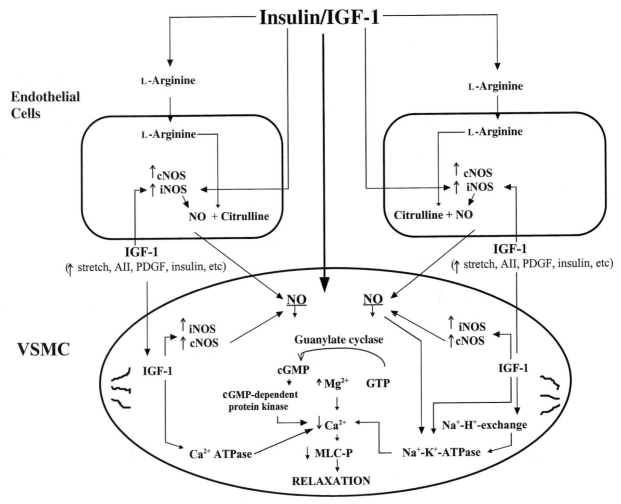

Figure 11–2. Effects of insulin and insulin-like growth factor-1 (IGF-1) on vascular smooth muscle cells (VSMC) $[Ca^{2+}]_i$ and $[Mg^{2+}]_i$ and associated VSMC contractility as mediated through modulation of both endothelial and VSMC NO production. cNOS, constitutive nitric oxide synthetase; iNOS, inducible nitric oxide synthetase; AII, angiotensin II; PDGF, platelet-derived growth factor; cGMP, cyclic guanosine monophosphate; GTP, guanosine triphosphate; ATPase, adenosine triphosphatase; MLC-P, myosin light chain phosphorylation.

GENDER AND METABOLIC ISSUES IN CORONARY HEART DISEASE

A gender-specific association between increases in blood pressure and metabolic abnormalities exists in women.[98] Hyperandrogenism may, in part, be responsible for this association. Androgen excess in women may promote insulin resistance/hyperinsulinemia,[98–101] central adiposity,[88–90] dyslipidemia, hyperuricemia,[91, 98] and hypertension.[101, 102] In particular, elevated serum levels of dehydroepiandrosterone sulfate are a risk factor for elevated blood pressure and associated metabolic risk factors in women.[98] CHD is a major health problem for American women. Cardiovascular disease is responsible for 45% of all deaths in Western society, and CHD, in particular, is responsible for one third.[8, 69] Even though CHD presents later in women than in men, it results in almost as many deaths in American women as men and is the leading cause of death among women by age 65 years.

Although CHD is less common in premenopausal women than in men, this difference begins to disappear after the onset of menopause, presumably related to the reduced production of female sex hormones (Fig. 11–3).[67, 102–106] One major risk factor for CHD, hypertension, also tracks with these age-related gender differences in CHD risk.[67, 101, 102] Men have higher blood pressure than women until ages 50 to 65 years, when systolic blood pressure in women becomes higher. The fact that the rise in blood pressure and CHD coincide with loss of ovarian function suggests that estrogen or progesterone, or both, may be protective against hypertension and CHD.[102, 103] Diabetes removes the normal gender difference in the prevalence of CHD.[8] Increased mortality in women with CHD and diabetes (mostly type II diabetes) compared with mortality in nondiabetic women was observed in an epidemiological study from California.[106] When adjusted for other ischemic heart disease risk factors, the relative risk was 2.4 for diabetic men and 3.5 for diabetic women.

High insulin levels may play a role in the absence of the usual gender-related vasoprotection in diabetic women.[61] In a 16-year follow-up of the Framingham population, long-term insulin therapy was associated with a markedly greater cardiovascular-related mortality in diabetic women compared with diabetic men.[61] It has also been observed that chronic therapy with the sulfonylurea compound glyburide, an insulin secretagogue, increased blood pressure and cardiac mass in female, but not male, stroke-prone spontaneously hypertensive rats.[68] These gender-specific increases in blood pressure produced by glyburide were accompanied by gender-specific increases in insulin levels and contractile responses to adrenergic stimulation in the presence of insulin in vitro. The investigators suggested that by chronically elevating circulating insulin levels in female rats, glyburide unmasked increases in expression of an interaction between female sex hormones and insulin that is capable of accentuating adrenergically mediated vasoconstriction and blunting vascular nitric oxide–mediated vasorelaxation.[43] These observations have important implications for therapies that render diabetic hypertensive women more hyperinsulinemic.

Treatment Considerations

Several of the newer oral hypoglycemic agents have effects on cardiovascular tissues that may ameliorate diabetic cardiovascular disease. Thiazolidinediones decrease VSMC proliferation and decrease vascular contractility.[21, 80, 81] Metformin promotes VSMC glucose uptake in conjunction with insulin and IGF-1 receptor autophosphorylation.[82] These effects can potentially overcome vascular resistance to the actions of insulin and IGF-1 in type II diabetes mellitus.[32] The thiazolidinedione troglitazone has also been shown to obviate delayed diastolic relaxation in a model of diabetic cardiomyopathy.[72] However, prospective controlled trials are needed to determine whether these agents affect CHD morbidity and mortality in diabetes.

Intriguing preliminary information suggests that therapy with angiotensin-converting enzyme (ACE) inhibitors may affect CHD and renal disease in diabetic persons. Polymorphism of the ACE gene has been associated with CHD, myocardial infarction, left ventricular hypertrophy, and diabetic nephropathy.[83–85] ACE inhibitors have a number of protective mechanisms opposing cardiovascular growth and remodeling.[86, 87] However, clinical trials will be needed to determine whether this theoretical vascular protection translates to decreased cardiovascular disease in diabetic patients. Since angiotensin II is a powerful stimulator of mesangial cell hypertrophy,[30] it is not surprising that ACE inhibition abrogates this process as well as progression of diabetic glomerulosclerosis.[86] A 5-year clinical trial of ACE inhibitor therapy administered to patients with type II diabetes in the early stages of diabetic nephropathy resulted in long-term stabilization of renal function and proteinuria, independent of blood pressure lowering.[87]

Since persons with metabolic abnormalities and hypertension generally have more atherogenic LDL particles, low HDL levels, and high triglycerides, it has been suggested that they be treated in a secondary prevention mode, lowering their LDL levels to less than 100 mg/dl.[86, 91, 92] There may also be a role for antioxidants to counteract the high oxidative stress that exists in this state. For example, probucol, an antioxidant drug, has been reported to reduce oxidation of LDL in diabetic persons.[107] Supplements of vitamin C for 4 months in older patients with type II diabetes increased glutathione and reduced LDL levels.[108] Acute infusion of vitamin C into the forearm of persons with type II diabetes resulted in an improvement in endothelium-dependent vasodilator function,[109] likely reflecting the immediate free radical–scavenging activity of vitamin C. In patients with type II diabetes, vitamin E supplementation decreased platelet aggregation and reduced the susceptibility of LDL to copper-mediated oxidation.[110] These preliminary data suggest that long-term trials of antioxidants in CHD need to be conducted. Finally, aspirin administration and discontinuation of cigarette smoking need to be emphasized in diabetics, particularly those with known CHD.[8, 9, 75] Cigarette smoking is an independent risk factor

Direct and Indirect Cardiovascular Effects of Estrogen

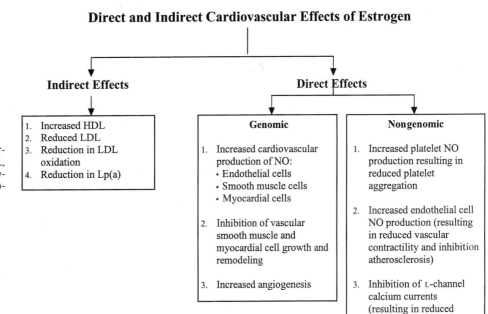

Figure 11–3. Direct and indirect cardiovascular effects of estrogen. HDL, high-density lipoprotein; LDL, low-density lipoprotein; Lp(a), lipoprotein (a).

Indirect Effects

1. Increased HDL
2. Reduced LDL
3. Reduction in LDL oxidation
4. Reduction in Lp(a)

Direct Effects

Genomic

1. Increased cardiovascular production of NO:
   • Endothelial cells
   • Smooth muscle cells
   • Myocardial cells
2. Inhibition of vascular smooth muscle and myocardial cell growth and remodeling
3. Increased angiogenesis

Nongenomic

1. Increased platelet NO production resulting in reduced platelet aggregation
2. Increased endothelial cell NO production (resulting in reduced vascular contractility and inhibition atherosclerosis)
3. Inhibition of L-channel calcium currents (resulting in reduced vascular contractility)

for death in the diabetic patient, especially women, in whom risk of cardiovascular death is doubled.[111] Future studies of the role of dietary micronutrients and macronutrients in the pathogenesis of diabetes and hypertension and related metabolic abnormalities are also needed.

Acknowledgment

The authors wish to thank Paddy McGowan for preparation of this manuscript. We also wish to acknowledge the Elliman Vascular Biology Foundation for its support.

References

1. Afonso LC, Edelson GL, Sowers JR. Metabolic abnormalities in hypertension. Curr Opin Nephrol Hypertens 6:219–223, 1997.
2. Falkner B, Hulman S, Tannenbaum J, Kushner K. Insulin resistance and blood pressure in young black males. Hypertension 16:706–711, 1990.
3. Sowers JR, Epstein M. Diabetes mellitus and associated hypertension, vascular disease, and nephropathy: An update. Hypertension 26:869–879, 1995.
4. Manolio TA, Savage PJ, Burke GL, et al. Association of fasting insulin with blood pressure and lipids in young adults: The CARDIA Study. Atherosclerosis 10:430–436, 1990.
5. Sowers JR, Standley PR, Ram JL. Hyperinsulinemia, insulin resistance, and hyperglycemia: Contributing factors in the pathogenesis of hypertension and atherosclerosis. Am J Hypertens 6:260S–270S, 1993.
6. Salomaa V, Riley W, Kaark JD, et al. Non–insulin dependent diabetes mellitus and fasting glucose and insulin concentrations are associated with arterial wall stiffness index, the ARIC study. Circulation 91:1432–1443, 1995.
7. Stein B, Weintraub WS, Gebhart S. Influence of diabetes mellitus on early and late outcome after percutaneous transluminal coronary angioplasty. Circulation 91:979–989, 1995.
8. Sowers JR. Diabetes mellitus and cardiovascular disease in women. Arch Intern Med 158:617–621, 1998.
9. The National High Blood Pressure Education Program Working Group. National High Blood Pressure Education Program Working Group report on hypertension in diabetes. Hypertension 23:145–158, 1994.
10. Haffner SM, Mykkanen LK, Laakso M. Insulin resistance, body fat distribution and sex hormones in men. Diabetes 43:212–219, 1994.
11. Landin D, Krotkiewski M, Smith U. Importance of obesity for the metabolic abnormalities associated with an abdominal fat distribution. Metabolism 38:572–576, 1989.
12. Jensen M, Haymond M, Rizza R, et al. Influence of body fat distribution on free fatty acid metabolism in obesity. J Clin Invest 83:1168–1173, 1989.
13. Walsh MF, Dominguez LJ, Sowers JR. Metabolic abnormalities in cardiac ischemia. Cardiol Clin 13:529–538, 1995.
14. Hargreaves AD, Logan RL, Elton RA, et al. Glucose tolerance, plasma insulin, HDL cholesterol and obesity: 12 year follow-up and development of coronary heart disease in Edinburgh men. Atherosclerosis 94:61–69, 1992.
15. Sowers JR. Modest weight gain and the development of diabetes: Another perspective. Ann Intern Med 122:548–549, 1995.
16. Ferraro RT, Eckel RH, Larson DE, et al. Relationship between skeletal muscle lipoprotein lipase activity and 24-hour macronutrient oxidation. J Clin Invest 92:441–445, 1993.
17. Frayn KN, Coppack SW, Fielding BA, et al. Coordinated regulation of hormone-sensitive lipase and lipoprotein lipase in human adipose tissue in vivo: Implications for the control of fat storage and fat mobilization. Adv Enzyme Regul 35:163–178, 1995.
18. Tchernof A, Lamarche M, Prud'Homme MD. The dense LDL phenotype: Association with plasma lipoprotein levels, visceral obesity, and hyperinsulinemia in men. Diabetes Care 19:629–637, 1996.
19. Fontbonne A, Charles MA, Thibut N, et al. Hyperinsulinemia as a predictor of coronary heart disease mortality in a healthy population: The Paris Prospective Study, 15-year follow-up. Diabetologia 34:356–361, 1991.
20. Ferrara LA, Mancini M, Celentano A, et al. Early changes of the arterial carotid wall in hyperinsulinemia, hypertriglyceridemia versus hypercholesterolemia. Arterioscler Thromb 13:367–370, 1993.
21. Sowers JR, Sowers PS, Peuler JD. Role of insulin resistance and hyperinsulinemia in development of hypertension and atherosclerosis. J Lab Clin Med 123:647–652, 1993.
22. Folsom AR, Eckfeldt JH, Weitzman S, et al., Atherosclerosis Risk in Communities (ARIC) Study Investigators. Relation of carotid artery wall thickness in diabetes mellitus, fasting glucose and insulin, body size, and physical activity. Stroke 25:66–73, 1994.
23. Salomaa V, Riley W, Kaark JD, et al. Non–insulin dependent diabetes mellitus and fasting glucose and insulin concentrations are associated with arterial stiffness index, the ARIC study. Circulation 91:1432–1443, 1995.
24. Agewall S, Fagerberg B, Attvall S, et al. Carotid artery wall intima-media thickness is associated with insulin-mediated glucose disposal in men at high and low coronary risk. Stroke 26:956–960, 1995.
25. Després J-P, Lamarche B, Mauriege P, et al. Hyperinsulinemia as an independent risk factor for ischemic heart disease. N Engl J Med 334:952–957, 1996.
26. Shinozaki K, Naritomi H, Shimizu T, et al. Role of insulin resistance associated with compensatory hyperinsulinemia in ischemic stroke. Stroke 27:37–43, 1996.
27. Pan DA, Lillioja S, Milner MR. Skeletal muscle membrane lipid composition is related to adiposity and insulin action. J Clin Invest 96:2802–2808, 1995.
28. Borkman M, Storlein LH, Pan DA. The relation between insulin sensitivity and the fatty acid composition of skeletal muscle phospholipids. N Engl J Med 328:238–244, 1995.
29. Poehlman ET, Toth MJ, Bunyard LB. Physiological predictors of increasing total and central adiposity in aging men and women. Arch Intern Med 155:2443–2448, 1995.
30. Bakris GL, Palant CE, Sowers JR, et al. Analogy between endothelial/mesangial cell and endothelial/vascular smooth muscle cell interactions: Role of growth factors and mechanotransduction. *In* Sowers JR (ed). Endocrinology of the Vasculature. Totowa, NJ, Humana, 1996; pp 341–355.
31. King GL, Goodman AD, Buzney S, Moses A. Receptors and insulin-like growth factors on cells from bovine retinal capillaries and aorta. J Clin Invest 75:1028–1036, 1985.
32. Sowers JR. Insulin and insulin-like growth factor in normal and pathological cardiovascular physiology. Hypertension 29:691–699, 1997.
33. Bornfeldt KE, Skottner A, Arnquist HJ. In vivo regulation of messenger RNA encoding insulin-like growth factor 1 (IGF-1) and its receptor by diabetes, insulin and IGF-1 in rat muscle. J Endocrinol 135:203–211, 1992.
34. Reiss K, Kajstura J, Capasso JM, et al. Impairment of myocyte contractility following coronary artery narrowing is associated with activation of the myocyte IGF-1 autocrine system, enhanced expression of late growth related genes, DNA synthesis, and myocyte nuclear mitotic diversion in rats. Exp Cell Res 207:348–360, 1993.
35. Sowers JR. Effects of insulin and IGF-1 on vascular smooth muscle glucose and cation metabolism. Diabetes 45:47–51, 1996.
36. Standley PR, Ali S, Bapna C, Sowers JR. Increased platelet cytosolic calcium responses to low density lipoprotein in type II diabetes with and without hypertension. Am J Hypertens 6:938–943, 1993.
37. Landin K, Tengborn L, Smith U. Elevated fibrinogen and plasminogen activator inhibitor (PAI-1) in hypertension are related to metabolic risk factors for cardiovascular disease. J Intern Med 227:273–278, 1990.
38. Furie B, Burie BC. Molecular and cellular biology of blood coagulation. N Engl J Med 326:800–806, 1992.
39. Sowers JR, Tuck ML, Sowers DK. Plasma antithrombin III and thrombin generation time: Correlation with hemoglobin A_1 and fasting serum glucose in young diabetic women. Diabetes Care 3:655–658, 1980.
40. Ceriello A, Quatraro A, Dello Russo P. Protein C deficiency in insulin dependent diabetes: A hyperglycemia-related phenomenon. Thromb Haemost 64:104–107, 1990.
41. Ramirez LC, Arauz-Pacheco C, Lackner C. Lipoprotein(a) levels in diabetes mellitus: Relationship to metabolic control. Ann Intern Med 117:42–47, 1992.
42. Stein JH, Rosenson RS. Lipoprotein Lp(a) excess and coronary heart disease. Arch Intern Med 157:1170–1176, 1997.

43. Vukovich TC, Proidl S, Knöbl P, et al. The effect of insulin treatment on the balance between tissue plasminogen activator and plasminogen activator inhibitor-1 in type 2 diabetic patients. Thromb Haemost 68:253–256, 1992.
44. Sowers JR, Lester M. Diabetes and cardiovascular disease. Diabetes Care 22(suppl 3):C14–C20, 1999.
45. Winocour PD, Bryszewska M, Watula C. Reduced membrane fluidity in platelets from diabetic patients. Diabetes 39:241–244, 1990.
46. Davi G, Catalons I, Averna M. Thromboxane biosynthesis and platelet function in type II diabetes mellitus. N Engl J Med 322:1768–1774, 1990.
47. Levy J, Gavin JR III, Sowers JR. Diabetes mellitus: A disease of abnormal cellular calcium metabolism? Am J Med 96:260–270, 1994.
48. Fakuda K, Ozaki Y, Satoh K, et al. Phosphorylation of myosin light chain in resting platelets from NIDDM patients is enhanced: Correlation with spontaneous aggregation. Diabetes 46:488–493, 1997.
49. Nadler JL, Malayan S, Luong H, et al. Evidence that intracellular free magnesium deficiency plays a key role in increased platelet reactivity in type II diabetes mellitus. Diabetes Care 15:835–841, 1992.
50. Karlet ME, Mammen EF, Sowers JR. Hyperaggregable platelets in type II diabetes with and without hypertension. [Abstract] High Blood Pressure Council 48th Annual Sessions 1994; p 76.
51. Tribe RM, Poston L. Oxidative stress and lipids in diabetes: A role in endothelial vasodilator function? Vasc Med 1:195–206, 1996.
52. McMillen DE. Development of vascular complications in diabetes. Vasc Med 2:132–142, 1997.
53. Bucala R, Makita Z, Koschinsky T, et al. Lipid advanced glycosylation: Pathway for lipid oxidation in vivo. Proc Natl Acad Sci U S A 90:6434–6438, 1993.
54. Yan SD, Schmidt AM, Anderson J. Enhanced cellular oxidant stress by the interaction of advanced glycation end products with their receptors/binding proteins. J Biol Chem 269:9989–9997, 1994.
55. Baumgartner-Parzer SM, Wagner L, Pettermann M, et al. Modulation by high glucose of adhesion molecule expression in cultured endothelial cells. Diabetologia 38:1367–1370, 1995.
56. Tesfamariam B, Brown ML, Cohen RA. Elevated glucose impaired endothelium-dependent relaxation by activating protein kinase C. J Clin Invest 87:1643–1648, 1991.
57. Rattan V, Sultana C, Shen Y. Oxidant stress-induced transendothelial migration of monocytes is linked to phosphorylation of PECAM-1. Am J Physiol 273:E453–E461, 1997.
58. Tooke JE. Microvascular function in human diabetes. Diabetes 44:721–726, 1995.
59. Paston L, Taylor PD. Endothelium-mediated vascular function in insulin-dependent diabetes mellitus. Circ Res 88:245–255, 1995.
60. Cagliero E, Roth T, Roy S. Characteristics and mechanisms of high-glucose–induced over-expression of basement membrane components in cultured human endothelial cells. Diabetes 40:102–110, 1991.
61. Garcia MJ, McNamara PM, Gordon T. Morbidity and mortality in diabetics in the Framingham population: Sixteen-year follow-up study. Diabetes Care 13:631–654, 1990.
62. Barrett-Connor E, Cohn BA, Wingard DL. Why is diabetes mellitus a stronger risk factor for fatal ischemic heart disease in women than in men? JAMA 265:627–631, 1991.
63. USRDS 1995 Annual Data Report. Incidence and causes of treated ESRD. Am J Kidney Dis 26:S39–S50, 1995.
64. Goldberg RJ, Larson M, Levy D. Factors associated with survival to 75 years of age in middle-aged men and women: The Framingham Study. Arch Intern Med 156:505–509, 1996.
65. Albert C. Sex differences in cardiac arrest survivors. Circulation 93:1170–1176, 1996.
66. Hanes DS, Weir MR, Sowers JR. Gender considerations in hypertension pathophysiology and treatment. Am J Med 101(suppl 3A):10S–21S, 1996.
67. Lissner L, Bengtsson C, Lapidus L. Fasting insulin in relation to subsequent blood pressure changes and hypertension in women. Hypertension 20:797–801, 1992.
68. Peuler JD, Johnson BAB, Sowers JR. Sex specific effects of an insulin secretagogue in stroke prone hypertensive rats. Hypertension 22:214–220, 1993.
69. Skafar DF, Ram J, Sowers JR. Female sex hormones and cardiovascular disease in women. J Clin Endocrinol Metab 82:3913–3918, 1997.
70. Bell DSH. Diabetic cardiomyopathy: A unique entity or a complication of coronary artery disease? Diabetes Care 18:708–714, 1995.
71. Ren J, Davidoff AJ. Diabetes rapidly induces contractile dysfunctions in isolated ventricular myocytes. Am J Physiol 272:H148–H158, 1997.
72. Ren J, Dominguez LJ, Sowers JR, et al. Troglitazone attenuates high-glucose–induced abnormalities in relaxation and intracellular calcium in rat ventricular myocytes. Diabetes 45:1822–1825, 1996.
73. Oswald G, Cororan S, Yudkin J. Prevalence and risks of hyperglycaemia and undiagnosed diabetes in patients with acute myocardial infarction. Lancet 1:1264–1267, 1984.
74. Standley PR, Zhang F, Sowers JR, et al. Insulin attenuates vasopressin-induced calcium transient and voltage-dependent calcium response in rat vascular smooth muscle cells. J Clin Invest 88:1230–1236, 1991.
75. Walsh MF, Dunbar JC, Sowers JR, et al. Insulin-like growth factor I diminishes in vivo and in vitro vascular contractility: Role of vascular nitric oxide. Endocrinology 137:2798–2803, 1996.
76. Ram JL, Fares MA, Standley PR, et al. Insulin inhibits vasopressin-elicited contraction of vascular smooth muscle cells. J Vasc Med Biol 4:250–254, 1993.
77. Sowers JR. Effects of ACE inhibitors and calcium channel blockers on insulin sensitivity and other components of the syndrome. Nephrol Dial Transplant 10:52–55, 1995.
78. Flack JM, Sowers JR. Epidemiologic and clinical aspects of insulin resistance and hyperinsulinemia. Am J Med 91:1S–11S, 1991.
79. Sowers JR, Epstein M. Diabetes mellitus and hypertension, emerging therapeutic perspectives. Cardiovasc Drug Rev 13:149–210, 1995.
80. Zhang F, Sowers JR, Ram JL, et al. Effects of pioglitazone on L-type calcium channels in vascular smooth muscle. Hypertension 24:170–175, 1994.
81. Song J, Walsh MF, Igwe R, et al. Troglitazone reduces contraction by inhibition of vascular smooth muscle cell Ca^{2+} currents and not endothelial nitric oxide production. Diabetes 46:659–664, 1997.
82. Dominguez LJ, Davidoff AJ, Sowers JR. Effects of metformin on tyrosine kinase activity, glucose transport, and intracellular calcium in rat vascular smooth muscle. Endocrinology 137:113–121, 1996.
83. Ruiz J, Blanche H, Cohen N. Insertion/deletion polymorphism of the angiotensin-converting enzyme gene is strongly associated with coronary heart disease in non–insulin dependent diabetes mellitus. Proc Natl Acad Sci U S A 91:3662–2665, 1994.
84. Schunkert H, Hense HW, Holmer SR. Association between deletion polymorphism of the angiotensin-converting enzyme gene and left ventricular hypertrophy. N Engl J Med 330:1634–1638, 1994.
85. Doria A, Warram JH, Krolewski AS. Genetic predisposition to diabetic nephropathy. Evidence for a role of the angiotensin I-converting enzyme gene. Diabetes 43:690–695, 1994.
86. Sowers JR. Impact of lipid and ACE inhibitor therapy on cardiovascular disease and metabolic abnormalities in the diabetic and hypertensive patient. J Hum Hypertens 11:9–16, 1997.
87. Ravid M, Savin H, Jutrin I, et al. Long-term stabilizing effect of angiotensin-converting enzyme inhibition on plasma creatinine and on proteinuria in normotensive type II diabetic patients. Ann Intern Med 118:577–581, 1993.
88. Sinagru D, Greco D, Scarpitta AM, et al. Blood pressure, insulin secretion and resistance in nonhypertensive and hypertensive obese female subjects. Int J Obes 19:610–613, 1995.
89. Colberg SG, Simoneau JA, Thaete FL, et al. Skeletal muscle utilization of FFA in women with visceral obesity. J Clin Invest 95:1846–1853, 1995.
90. Iso H, Kiyama M, Naito Y, et al. The relation of body fat distribution and body mass index with hemoglobin A$_1$C, blood pressure and blood lipids in urban Japanese men. Int J Epidemiol 20:88–94, 1991.
91. Bakris GL, Weir MR, Sowers JR. Therapeutic challenges in the obese diabetic patient with hypertension. Am J Med 101(suppl 3A):33S–46S, 1996.
92. Sowers JR, Farrow SL. Treatment of elderly hypertensive patients with diabetes, renal disease and coronary heart disease. Am J Geriatr Cardiol 6:57–70, 1996.
93. Hunt SC, Hasset SJ, Kuida H, et al. Genetic heritability and common environmental components of resting and stressed blood pressures, lipids, and body mass index in Utah pedigrees and twins. Am J Epidemiol 129:625–638, 1989.

94. Selby JV, Newman B, Quiroga J, et al. Concordance for dyslipidemic hypertension in male twins. JAMA 265:2079–2084, 1991.

95. Amos CI, Cohen JC, Srinivas SR, et al. Polymorphism in the 5′ flanking region of the insulin gene and its potential relation to cardiovascular disease risk: Observations in a biracial community. The Bogalusa Heart Study. Atherosclerosis 79:51–57, 1989.

96. Johansen K, Stolnicki A, Smith R, et al. Coronary artery disease, HDL cholesterol, and insulin-gene flanking sequences. Diabet Med 6:429–433, 1989.

97. Nishina PM, Johnson JP, Naggert JK, et al. Linkage of atherogenic lipoprotein phenotype to the low density lipoprotein receptor locus on the short arm of chromosome 19. Proc Natl Acad Sci U S A 89:708–712, 1992.

98. Mantzoros CS, Emmanuel I, Sowers JR. Relative androgenicity, blood pressure levels, and blood pressure levels of young healthy females. Am J Hypertens 8:606–614, 1995.

99. Nestler JE. Sex hormone–binding globulin: A marker for hyperinsulinemia and/or insulin resistance. [Editorial] J Clin Endocrinol Metab 76:273–274, 1993.

100. Preziosi P, Barrett-Connor E, Papoz L, et al. Interrelation between plasma sex hormone binding globulin and plasma insulin in healthy adult women: The Telecody Study. J Clin Endocrinol Metab 76:283–287, 1993.

101. Hughes GS, Mathur RS, Margolius HS. Sex steroid hormones are altered in essential hypertension. J Hypertens 7:181–187, 1989.

102. Munetta S, Murakami E, Hiwada K. Gender difference in blood pressure regulation in essential hypertension. Hypertens Res 7:71–78, 1994.

103. Stampfer MJ, Colditz GA, Willett WC, et al. Postmenopausal estrogen therapy and cardiovascular disease. Ten-year follow-up from the Nurses' Health Study. N Engl J Med 325:756–762, 1991.

104. Rossouw JE, Finnegan LP, Harlan WR, et al. The evolution of the Women's Health Initiative: Perspectives from the NIH. J Am Med Womens Assoc 50:50–55, 1995.

105. Williams JK, Adams RM, Klopfenstein HS. Estrogen modulates responses of atherosclerotic coronary arteries. Circulation 81:1680–1687, 1990.

106. Barrett-Connor E, Wingard DL. Sex differential in ischemic heart disease mortality in diabetics: A prospective population-based study. Am J Epidemiol 118:489–496, 1983.

107. Babey AV, Gebicki JM, Sullivan DR, et al. Increased oxidizability of plasma lipoproteins in diabetic patients can be prevented by probucol therapy and is not due to glycation. Biochem Pharmacol 43:995–1000, 1992.

108. Paolisso G, Balbi V, Volpe C. Metabolic benefits derived from chronic vitamin supplementation in aged non–insulin dependent diabetics. J Am Coll Nutr 14:387–392, 1995.

109. Ting HH, Timimi FK, Boles KS, et al. Vitamin C improves endothelium-dependent vasodilation in patients with non–insulin-dependent diabetes mellitus. J Clin Invest 97:22–28, 1996.

110. Reaven PD, Herold DA, Barnett J, et al. Effects of vitamin E on susceptibility of low-density lipoprotein and subfractions to oxidation and on protein glycation in NIDDM. Diabetes Care 18:807–816, 1995.

111. Scala Moy C, Laporte R, Dorman J. Insulin dependent diabetes mellitus mortality: The risks of cigarette smoking. Circulation 82:37–43, 1990.

CHAPTER

12 Obesity-Related Hypertension as a Metabolic Disorder

Lewis Landsberg

HYPERTENSION AND OBESITY

Nature of the Association

Hypertension and obesity are closely linked. Obesity predicts the subsequent development of hypertension, and less commonly recognized, hypertension increases the risk for the subsequent development of obesity.[1] Both hypertension and obesity are complex regulatory disturbances that are, from a pathophysiological standpoint, poorly understood. It is clear that trivial attributions such as cuff artifact and excessive salt intake, as well as purely hemodynamic considerations, cannot account for the association of obesity with hypertension.[2] How, then, can the fact be explained that 50% of the obese are hypertensive? The importance of this clinical question cannot be doubted: Obesity is associated with hypertension in a substantial portion of patients with increased blood pressure. Clarification of the underlying pathophysiology might suggest sound approaches to prevention and therapy.

Clues From Body Fat Distribution

It is now well established that a particular obesity phenotype is uniquely associated with the propensity to develop hypertension and other cardiovascular risk factors. In the mid-1950s, Jean Vague, a French clinician, noted that the cardiovascular and metabolic complications of obesity were most common in those individuals with the upper body fat distribution pattern.[3] Vague's observations drew little comment until the 1980s, when epidemiological surveys, particularly from Scandinavia, using the waist:hip ratio as a convenient surrogate for body fat distribution, confirmed a relationship between abdominal or upper body obesity and cardiovascular risk.[4, 5] These findings have been replicated in many different regions of the globe and are now widely accepted. Cardiovascular risk, including hypertension, thus tracks with the upper body or abdominal form of obesity.

Another series of investigations, carried out at the same time, indicated that insulin resistance and type II diabetes mellitus were also associated with the upper body fat pattern. Studies from the laboratories of Kissebah and coworkers[6] and Bjorntorp and associates[7] demonstrated that insulin resistance and hyperinsulinemia were more common in subjects with the upper body fat distribution phenotype. In addition, insulin levels began to emerge as an independent risk factor for hypertension.[8, 9] The relationship between insulin and hypertension, although strongest in the obese, was present in the nonobese as well. Insulin and hypertension, therefore, appear to be linked and related to upper body fat distribution.

Risk Factor Constellation: The Insulin Resistance Syndrome

Since the mid-1980s, (upper body) obesity, insulin resistance, hypertension, and a characteristic dyslipidemia have been noted to occur together with such frequency that this constellation has been recognized as a distinct syndrome.[10] Referred to as the *insulin resistance syndrome*, the *metabolic syndrome,* or *syndrome X,* these abnormalities impart considerable cardiovascular risk. Other abnormalities, including microalbuminuria, salt sensitivity, type II diabetes mellitus, small, dense, low-density lipoprotein (LDL), and hyperuricemia, have been noted with increased incidence in this group of patients. It is important to note that not all individuals show all manifestations of this syndrome; although insulin resistance appears to be a critical factor, the other manifestations need not all be present.

The nature of the relationship between these abnormalities has remained obscure, but the various manifestations of this syndrome may be considered to be a consequence of the metabolic adaptation to the obese state. In this formulation, insulin and the sympathoadrenal system play critical roles in the pathogenesis of the hypertension and dyslipidemia that characterize the insulin resistance syndrome.

DIET AND SYMPATHETIC NERVOUS SYSTEM ACTIVITY

Nutrient-Specific Effects

It has been known since the mid-1970s that dietary intake influences the sympathetic nervous system (SNS): fasting suppresses,[11] whereas overfeeding stimulates sympathetic activity.[12–14] It is, moreover, the carbohydrate and fat macronutrient content of the diet that stimulates the SNS;[14] protein is without effect.

Role of Insulin

The fact that diet influences the activity of the SNS implies a mechanism within the central nervous system that senses nutritional status and initiates changes in sympathetic outflow in response to nutritional signals. At least one such mechanism has been elucidated,[15, 16] and insulin plays an important role. As shown in Figure 12–1, during fasting, the small fall in plasma glucose and the larger fall in plasma insulin decrease insulin-mediated glucose metabolism in critical hypothalamic neurons sensitive to glucose and insulin.[17–21] This decrease in glucose metabolism stimulates an inhibitory pathway between the hypothalamus and the brain stem sympathetic centers, suppressing these tonically active centers and diminishing central sympathetic outflow. Conversely, during carbohydrate intake, or in the

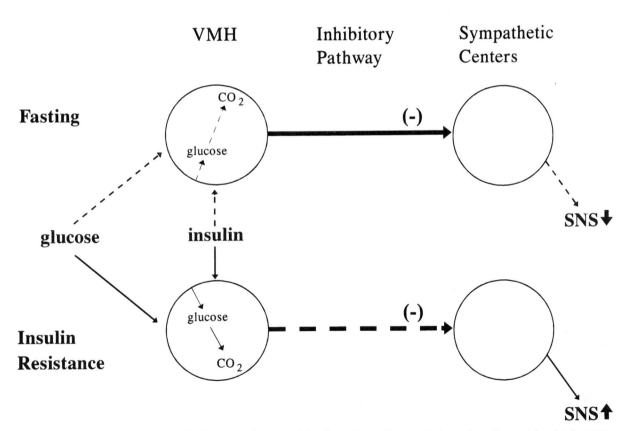

Figure 12–1. Model of the relationship between glucose and insulin and central sympathetic outflow. See text for details. VMH, ventromedial hypothalamus; SNS, sympathetic nervous system. (From Landsberg L, Young JB. The role of the sympatho-adrenal system in modulating energy expenditure. *In* James WPT [ed]. Obesity. Clin Endocrinol Metab 13:475, 1984.)

presence of insulin resistance, the small increase in glucose level, in conjunction with the larger rise in plasma insulin, stimulates insulin-mediated glucose uptake in these hypothalamic neurons. This increase in glucose metabolism suppresses the descending inhibitory pathway, thereby disinhibiting tonically active brain stem sympathetic centers, with a resultant increase in central sympathetic outflow. The experimental evidence on which this model is based has been summarized previously.[16] Interestingly, this model is based on descending inhibition, a consistent organizing principle within the central nervous system.

Dietary Thermogenesis and Energy Balance

What, then, is the physiological role of these dietary-induced changes in SNS activity? Substantial evidence now indicates that these changes in sympathetic activity provide a link between dietary intake and metabolic energy production.[15] Fasting or decreased caloric intake results in a significant decrease in resting metabolic rate. Overfeeding, conversely, increases metabolic heat production. Insulin and the SNS mediate these changes in metabolic rate, which are referred to as *dietary thermogenesis.*

The thermogenic effector organ in rodents and other small mammals is brown adipose tissue.[15] Norepinephrine, the adrenergic neurotransmitter, increases heat production by interacting with the β_3-adrenergic receptor. Although physiologically important in human neonates, the role of brown adipose tissue as a major thermogenic effector in adult humans remains uncertain. Regardless of the effector organ, however, it is clear that sympathetic stimulation increases metabolic rate in adult humans.[15]

The SNS thus mediates the phenomenon known as *dietary thermogenesis.* Suppression of sympathetically mediated thermogenesis during fasting or restricted caloric intake would increase survival by diminishing metabolic rate. The role of a mechanism evolved to dissipate calories taken in excess is intuitively less obvious. An organism faced with a subsistence diet low in protein, for example, might satisfy basic nitrogen requirements for growth and development by consuming increased quantities of the low-protein diet and, through utilization of dietary thermogenesis, burn off the excess calories as heat, thereby avoiding obesity. Such reasoning is supported by the observations that protein is without effect on the SNS and low-protein diets are markedly stimulatory.[22, 23] Whatever the teleological significance, the capacity for dietary thermogenesis provides a buffer against weight gain. It has been amply demonstrated, moreover, that individuals differ in their capacity for dietary thermogenesis and that these differences have a genetic basis.[24] As shown in Figure 12–2, the energy balance equation, a capacity for dietary thermogenesis would increase the range of energy intakes over which energy balance could be achieved.

INSULIN AND SYMPATHETIC NERVOUS SYSTEM ACTIVITY IN OBESITY-RELATED HYPERTENSION

Is there any way that the close association of obesity and hypertension can be understood in terms of the metabolic

$$\begin{matrix} \text{ENERGY} \\ \text{INTAKE} \end{matrix} = \begin{matrix} \text{ENERGY} \\ \text{OUTPUT} \end{matrix} + \text{STORAGE}$$

Dietary Calories	"Basal" Metabolism Exercise "Thermogenesis"	Fat

Figure 12–2. The energy balance equation. At equilibrium, energy intake equals energy output and there is no net storage. *Energy intake* (dietary calories) and *storage* (fat) are discrete and obvious categories. Energy output consists of several compartments. In sedentary individuals, basal metabolic rate accounts for approximately 75% of daily energy expenditure, and exercise approximately 15%. The category *thermogenesis* refers to increased heat reduction in response to dietary intake and cold exposure and represents the component that is mediated by the sympathetic nervous system. This compartment approximates 10% of total energy production. The capacity for dietary thermogenesis, therefore, increases the range of energy intake over which energy balance can be achieved.

economy of the obese state? Since sympathetically mediated thermogenesis can act as a buffer against weight gain, a hypothesis was developed (Fig. 12–3) that relates insulin resistance, and consequent sympathetic stimulation, to hypertension in the obese.[25] The formulation expressed in this hypothesis is as follows: insulin resistance is a mechanism

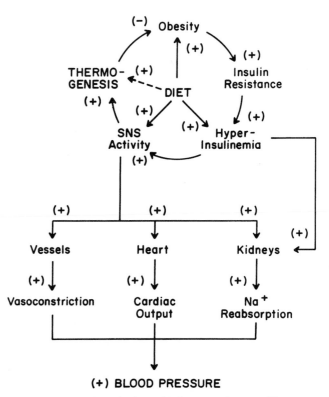

Figure 12–3. Hypothetical relationship between obesity and hypertension. This formulation, described in detail in the text, views insulin resistance as a compensatory mechanism recruited in the obese to restore energy balance and stabilize body weight. The hypertension is the inadvertent consequence of hyperinsulinemia and sympathetic stimulation. SNS, sympathetic nervous system. (From Landsberg L. Diet, obesity and hypertension: An hypothesis involving insulin, the sympathetic nervous system, and adaptive thermogenesis. Q J Med 236:1081, 1986.)

in the obese recruited to stabilize body weight and limit further weight gain; the hyperinsulinemia that results stimulates the SNS, driving thermogenic mechanisms that increase metabolic rate and stabilize body weight. The price to pay for this compensatory mechanism is hyperinsulinemia and sympathetic stimulation. Sympathetically mediated vasoconstriction and cardiac stimulation, and enhanced sodium reabsorption induced by insulin and the SNS, exert a prohypertensive effect that, in susceptible individuals, results in hypertension.

The hypothesis implicit in Figure 12–3 is testable.[26] Data have, in fact, been accumulated demonstrating that

1. The obese are not resistant to the effects of insulin on the SNS.[27]
2. Sympathetic activity is increased in the obese.[28, 29]
3. There is a relationship between insulin and glucose and sympathetic activity in the obese.[25]
4. Both insulin and sympathetic stimulation are related to hypertension.[30]

The data in Figure 12–4 are derived from a population-based cohort (the Normative Aging Study). They show the percentage of individuals with hypertension as a function of urinary norepinephrine excretion and postglucose insulin levels, markers for SNS activity and insulin resistance, respectively. Those individuals in the highest tertile of insulin resistance and sympathetic activation had a 3.5

times greater prevalence of hypertension than those in the lowest tertile of each of these variables. The interaction term in the analysis of variance, furthermore, was positive between insulin and SNS activity.[30] In addition, when hyperinsulinemia is diminished in the obese as a consequence of either diminished caloric intake[31] or acutely with somatostatin,[32, 33] both SNS activity and blood pressure fall. Available data thus support the hypothesis that insulin-mediated sympathetic stimulation contributes to hypertension in subjects with obesity.

DYSLIPIDEMIA OF THE INSULIN-RESISTANCE SYNDROME

A number of studies have shown that the insulin level itself is related to the low high-density lipoprotein (HDL)–cholesterol and high triglyceride level characteristic of the insulin resistance syndrome. This important role of insulin was confirmed in the Normative Aging Study.[34] Epinephrine appears to play a role as well.[35] In distinction to SNS activity, which increases with obesity, epinephrine excretion, a marker of adrenal medullary activity, actually diminishes.[28] The lowered epinephrine levels in obesity are related to the dyslipidemia after adjustment for the effects of insulin, body fat, and body fat distribution (Fig. 12–5).[35] Lower levels of epinephrine excretion are related to higher

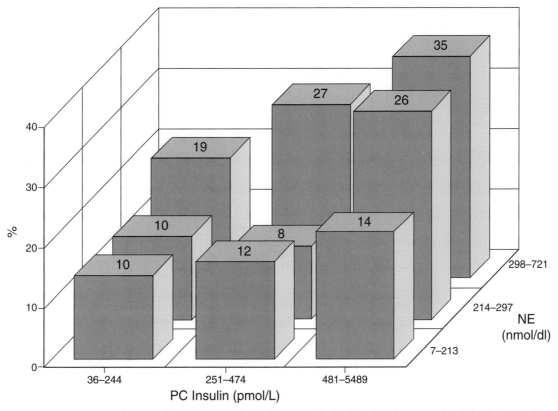

Figure 12–4. Relationship between hypertension and postglucose insulin levels and 24-hour norepinephrine (NE) excretion, from 752 subjects in the Normative Aging Study. The percentage of subjects with hypertension is shown as tertiles of postglucose insulin level and 24-hour urinary NE. The incidence of hypertension in subjects in the upper tertile in both of these categories was 35% as compared with 10% for those subjects in the lowest tertile of these variables. (From Ward KD, Sparrow D, Landsberg L, et al. Influence of insulin, sympathetic nervous system activity, and obesity on blood pressure: The Normative Aging Study. J Hypertens 14[3]:301–308, 1996.)

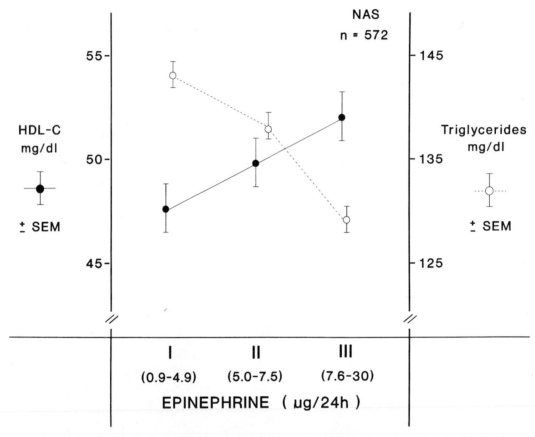

Figure 12–5. Relationship between epinephrine excretion and high-density lipoprotein cholesterol (HDL-C) and triglycerides. HDL cholesterol increases and triglycerides decrease with increasing urinary epinephrine excretion. NAS, Normative Aging Study. (From Landsberg L. Pathophysiology of obesity-related hypertension: Role of insulin and the sympathetic nervous system. J Cardiovasc Pharmacol 23[suppl 1]S1–S8, 1994.)

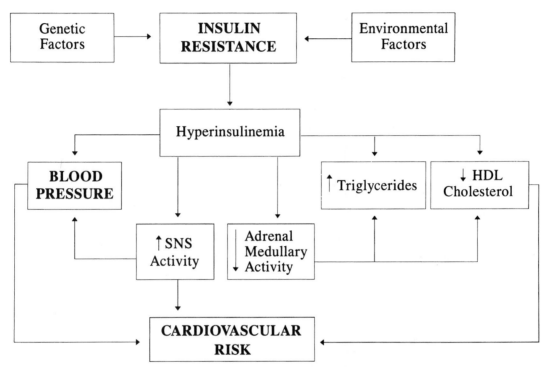

Figure 12–6. Postulated pathophysiology of the insulin-resistance syndrome. Insulin resistance, a consequence of both genetic and environmental factors, and occurring most frequently in the obese, results in hyperinsulinemia. Hyperinsulinemia contributes to hypertension both directly by effects on renal sodium excretion and, most importantly, by sympathetic stimulation. Hyperinsulinemia contributes to the characteristic dyslipidemia both directly by effects on triglycerides and high-density lipoprotein (HDL) cholesterol and indirectly by diminishing adrenal medullary activity. The hypertension and dyslipidemia together greatly increase cardiovascular risk. The sympathetic nervous system (SNS) and the adrenal medulla, therefore, act as effectors in the link between insulin, hypertension, and cardiovascular disease. (From Reaven GM, Lithell H, Landsberg L. Hypertension and associated metabolic abnormalities—The role of insulin resistance and the sympathoadrenal system. N Engl J Med 334:374–381, 1996. Copyright © 1996 Massachusetts Medical Society. All rights reserved.)

levels of triglycerides and lower levels of HDL-cholesterol, whereas, conversely, higher epinephrine excretion rates are associated with the favorable lipid pattern of high HDL-cholesterol and low triglycerides.

SUMMARY AND THERAPEUTIC IMPLICATIONS

The contribution of the sympathoadrenal system to the pathogenesis of the insulin resistance syndrome is summarized in Figure 12–6. Increased insulin and sympathetic activity contribute to the hypertension, whereas low levels of epinephrine and high levels of insulin contribute to the characteristic dyslipidemia.

The central role of insulin resistance and consequent hyperinsulinemia in the pathogenesis of the hypertension and other manifestations of the insulin resistance syndrome suggests that therapeutic strategies aimed at diminishing insulin resistance may be particularly useful. Caloric restriction, which reduces insulin resistance, diminishes both sympathetic activity and blood pressure.[31] Preliminary evidence also suggests that insulin sensitizers, such as the thiazolidinediones, may be useful therapeutically to lower blood pressure as well as insulin levels,[36] although the long-term safety of these compounds may preclude their general use.

Different classes of antihypertensive agents exert very different effects on insulin sensitivity and, therefore, on the metabolic abnormalities that constitute the insulin resistance syndrome.[37] Rational therapeutic strategies should include agents that have a beneficial, or at least neutral, effect on insulin sensitivity.

References

1. Kannel WB, Brand N, Skinner JJ, et al. The relation of adiposity to blood pressure and development of hypertension. Ann Intern Med 67:48, 1967.
2. Krieger DR, Landsberg L. Obesity and hypertension. *In* Laragh JH, Brenner BM (eds). Hypertension: Pathophysiology, Diagnosis, and Management, 2nd ed. New York, Raven, 1995; p 2367.
3. Vague J. The degree of masculine differentiation of obesities: A factor determining predisposition to diabetes, atherosclerosis, gout, and uric calculous disease. Am J Clin Nutr 4:20, 1956.
4. Lapidus L, Bengtsson C, Larsson B, et al. Distribution of adipose tissue and risk of cardiovascular disease and death: A 12 year follow up of participants in the population study of women in Gothenburg, Sweden. BMJ 289:1257, 1984.
5. Larsson B, Svardsudd K, Welin L, et al. Abdominal adipose tissue distribution, obesity, and risk of cardiovascular disease and death: 13 year follow up of participants in the study of men born in 1913. BMJ 288:1401, 1984.
6. Kissebah AH, Vydelingum N, Murray R, et al. Relation of body fat distribution to metabolic complication of obesity. J Clin Endocrinol Metab 54:254, 1982.
7. Krotkiewski M, Bjorntorp P, Sjostrom L, et al. Impact of obesity on metabolism in men and women: Importance of regional adipose tissue distribution. J Clin Invest 72:1150, 1983.
8. Modan M, Halkin H, Almog S, et al. Hyperinsulinemia: A link between hypertension, obesity and glucose intolerance. J Clin Invest 75:809, 1985.
9. Ferrannini E, Buzzigoli G, Bonadonna R, et al. Insulin resistance in essential hypertension. N Engl J Med 317:350, 1987.
10. DeFronzo RA, Ferrannini E. Insulin resistance: A multifaceted syndrome responsible for NIDDM, obesity, hypertension, dyslipidemia, and atherosclerotic cardiovascular disease. Diabetes Care 14:173, 1991.
11. Young JB, Landsberg L. Suppression of sympathetic nervous system during fasting. Science 196:1473, 1977.
12. Young JB, Landsberg L. Stimulation of the sympathetic nervous system during sucrose feeding. Nature 269:615, 1977.
13. Young JB, Saville E, Rothwell NJ, et al. Effect of diet and cold exposure on norepinephrine turnover in brown adipose tissue in the rat. J Clin Invest 69:1061, 1982.
14. Schwartz JH, Young JB, Landsberg L. Effect of dietary fat on sympathetic nervous system activity in the rat. J Clin Invest 72:361, 1983.
15. Landsberg L, Young JB. The role of the sympatho-adrenal system in modulating energy expenditure. *In* James WPT (ed). Clinics in Endocrinology and Metabolism Obesity, vol 13. London, WB Saunders, 1984; p 475.
16. Landsberg L, Young JB. Insulin-mediated glucose metabolism in the relationship between dietary intake and sympathetic nervous system activity. Int J Obes 9(suppl 2):63, 1985.
17. Rappaport EB, Young JB, Landsberg L. Effects of 2-deoxy-glucose on the cardiac sympathetic nerves and the adrenal medulla in the rat: Further evidence for a dissociation of sympathetic nervous system and adrenal medullary responses. Endocrinology 110:650, 1982.
18. Young JB. Effect of experimental hyperinsulinemia on sympathetic nervous system activity in rats. Life Sci 49:193, 1988.
19. Rowe JW, Young JB, Minaker KL, et al. Effect of insulin and glucose infusions on sympathetic nervous system activity in normal man. Diabetes 30:219, 1981.
20. Young JB, Landsberg L. Impaired suppression of sympathetic activity during fasting in the gold thioglucose-treated mouse. J Clin Invest 65:1086, 1980.
21. Hausberg M, Mark AL, Hoffman RP, et al. Dissociation of sympathoexcitatory and vasodilator actions of modestly elevated plasma insulin levels. J Hypertens 13:1015, 1995.
22. Kaufman LN, Young JB, Landsberg L. Effect of protein on sympathetic nervous system activity in the rat: Evidence for nutrient-specific responses. J Clin Invest 77:551, 1986.
23. Young JB, Kaufman LN, Saville ME, et al. Increased sympathetic nervous system activity in rats fed a low protein diet: Evidence against a role for dietary tyrosine. Am J Physiol 248:R627, 1985.
24. Bouchard C, Tremblay A, Despres JP, et al. The response to long-term overfeeding of identical twins. N Engl J Med 322:1477, 1990.
25. Landsberg L. Diet, obesity and hypertension: An hypothesis involving insulin, the sympathetic nervous system, and adaptive thermogenesis. Q J Med 236:1081, 1986.
26. Landsberg L. Pathophysiology of obesity-related hypertension: Role of insulin and the sympathetic nervous system. J Cardiovasc Pharmacol 23:S1, 1994.
27. O'Hare JA, Minaker KL, Meneilly GS, et al. Effect of insulin on plasma norepinephrine and 3,4-dihydroxyphenylalanine in obese men. Metabolism 38:322, 1989.
28. Troisi RJ, Weiss ST, Parker DR. Relation of obesity and diet to sympathetic nervous system activity. Hypertension 17:669, 1991.
29. Grassi GH, Seravalle G, Cattaneo BM, et al. Sympathetic activation in obese normotensive subjects. Hypertension 25:560, 1995.
30. Ward KD, Sparrow D, Landsberg L, et al. Influence of insulin, sympathetic nervous system activity, and obesity on blood pressure: The Normative Aging Study. J Hypertens 14:301, 1996.
31. Tuck ML. Obesity, the sympathetic nervous system, and essential hypertension. Hypertension 19:167, 1992.
32. Carretta R, Fabris B, Fischetti F, et al. Reduction of blood pressure in obese hyperinsulinemic patients during somatostatin infusion. J Hypertens 7(suppl 6):S196, 1989.
33. Elhai D, Krieger DR, Young JB, et al. Effects of somatostatin infusion on plasma norepinephrine (NE) and cardiovascular function in men. [Abstract] Clin Res 39:385A, 1991.
34. Ward KD, Sparrow D, Vokonas PS, et al. The relationships of abdominal obesity, hyperinsulinemia and saturated fat intake to serum lipid levels: The Normative Aging Study. Int J Obes 18:137–144, 1994.
35. Ward KD, Sparrow D, Landsberg L, et al. The relationship of epinephrine excretion to serum lipid levels: The Normative Aging Study. Metabolism 43:509, 1994.
36. Ogihara T, Rakugi H, Ikegami H, et al. Enhancement of insulin sensitivity by troglitazone lowers blood pressure in diabetic hypertensives. Am J Hypertens 8:316, 1995.
37. Reaven GM, Lithell H, Landsberg L. Hypertension and associated metabolic abnormalities—The role of insulin resistance and the sympathoadrenal system. N Engl J Med 334:374, 1996.

13 Remodeling of Resistance Vessels in Essential Hypertension

Michael J. Mulvany

CHAPTER

Established essential hypertension is usually associated with normal cardiac output but increased peripheral resistance (see, e.g., ref. 1). Since capillary pressure is approximately normal in essential hypertension,[2] the main increase in resistance lies in those precapillary vessels that contribute to, and control, the peripheral resistance. These vessels are known as *resistance vessels*, and evidence from animal models suggests that they consist of both the *arterioles* (arteries with not more than one layer of smooth muscle cells) and the more proximal *small arteries* (prearteriolar arteries with lumen diameters < approximately 300 μm).[3]

The reason for the increased resistance is not known, but physical considerations indicate that either the resistance vessels are narrowed or there is a decrease in the number of parallel-connected vessels, a process known as *rarefaction*. Evidence for both of these possibilities has been provided in essential hypertension. Animal studies point to both structural and functional abnormalities in the resistance vasculature,[4] although as discussed later, structural abnormalities appear to predominate in essential hypertension.

Until recently, most information about resistance vessels and hypertension was based on the many animal studies. However, it has become increasingly clear that these are not necessarily relevant to the human situation, and recent work has been directed at investigating resistance vessels in essential hypertensive patients. In particular, techniques have been developed for examination of the vessels in vitro as well as direct visualization of vessels. In this review, the evidence obtained with these techniques in essential hypertension is discussed in relation to earlier evidence from hemodynamic studies and histological examination of biopsy and autopsy material. The review supplements earlier reviews on this topic[4-6] and is primarily concerned with the structural changes in the resistance vasculature that are associated with essential hypertension.

LOCATION OF PERIPHERAL RESISTANCE

In animal models, the contribution of the various segments of the vasculature to peripheral resistance can be determined from direct measurement of the pressure in vessels from the aorta through to the capillaries to the veins. Earlier investigations in anesthetized animals showed that a substantial portion of the systemic pressure is dissipated in the small arteries and that these contribute to increased peripheral resistance in spontaneously and renal hypertensive rats (for reviews, see refs. 3 and 4). These findings in anesthetized animals have been confirmed in conscious animals.[7-9] Furthermore, it has been shown that small arteries of the rat contribute to the control of peripheral resis-

tance,[10] indicating that small arteries are indeed resistance vessels.

In humans, assessments of pressure in the peripheral vasculature are confined to measurements of capillary pressure, which is shown to be about 13 mm Hg, about 14% of systemic pressure.[2] Moreover, the capillary pressure of essential hypertensive patients is about 17% of systemic pressure,[2] similar to that in normotensive controls. This indicates that the main increase in resistance lies proximal to the capillaries, i.e., in the resistance vessels. The available evidence suggests, therefore, that studies of the causes of the increased peripheral resistance associated with essential hypertension should be concerned with the precapillary vessels, and the animal data suggest that both the arterioles and the small arteries should be investigated.

RESISTANCE VESSEL STRUCTURE

The resistance vessels exert their function through the resistance that they present to blood flow. Resistance is determined by the lumen diameter (to the fourth power according to the Poiseuille relation), and the lumen diameter is a function of the passive and active mechanical properties of the vessel. The passive properties may be described by the lumen diameter:pressure relation under conditions in which the smooth muscle cells are fully relaxed. The active properties are a function of the activation level of the individual smooth muscle cells and the quantity and arrangement of these. Assuming a given level of activation within the individual smooth muscle cells, and that these produce a given level of force per cross-sectional area, then the pressure against which the vessel can contract will (according to the Laplace relation) be proportional to the ratio of wall thickness:lumen diameter (wall:lumen ratio, or more correctly media:lumen ratio on the basis that the force-producing smooth muscle cells lie within the media).[11]

The primary structural features of the vessel are thus the diameter and the wall (or media) thickness, measured under conditions of zero smooth muscle cell activation and under a given transmural pressure. From knowledge of diameter and wall thickness, another key parameter can be determined—the wall cross-sectional area. The importance of this parameter is that it indicates the amount of material within the vascular wall and thus provides information about the biological processes that determine the vascular structure in relation to growth and/or regression. Finally, the wall:lumen ratio can be calculated. As indicated earlier, this parameter provides information about the ability of the vessels to contract against an intravascular pressure, the parameter thus having important physiological implications.

DEFINITIONS OF RESISTANCE VESSEL REMODELING

In 1989, Baumbach and Heistad[12] demonstrated that hypertension could be associated with changes in the structure of resistance vessels, such that the vessels had a decreased lumen and increased media:lumen ratio but no change in media cross-sectional area (or volume). This ability for structure to be altered without change in volume confirmed earlier results by Short[13] concerning resistance vessels in essential hypertension. Baumbach and Heistad[12] described this ability of resistance vessels to change their structure without changing their volume just as *remodeling*. For a number of years after this, the term *vascular remodeling* was used alone to describe a change in lumen associated with rearrangement of material. However, this term clashed with the way in which cardiologists, and indeed vascular biologists, used the term to describe any change in the structure of the cardiovascular system. Therefore, together with Baumbach and Heistad, a number of workers in the field (including the present author) made the new suggestion shown in Figure 13–1 for describing *remodeling* more precisely.[14]

It was proposed that the term *remodeling* be used in situations in which there is a structurally determined change in lumen diameter and that it be classified into the six changes indicated in Figure 13–1. It was suggested that remodeling should be termed *inward* or *outward* remodeling, depending on whether the process had resulted in a decrease or increase, respectively, in vessel diameter. Furthermore, since as discussed later, remodeling can result in an increase, no change, or a decrease in the amount of material, there should be a subclassification into *hypertrophic*, *eutrophic*, and *hypotrophic* remodeling, respectively. It was hoped that by providing a framework for defining the various modes of vascular remodeling, it would be easier to define the abnormalities more precisely and to provide a surer basis for discussing the mechanisms involved.

EVIDENCE FOR ALTERED RESISTANCE VESSEL STRUCTURE IN HYPERTENSION

As pointed out originally by Folkow,[15] many of the hemodynamic features associated with essential hypertension could be accounted for by alterations in the structure of the resistance vessels. In vivo hemodynamic experiments (in which forearm blood flow was measured with the vasculature fully relaxed under conditions of reactive hyperemia) showed that the relaxed peripheral resistance in essential hypertensive patients was increased and that the pressor response to maximal concentrations of agonists was increased but that the threshold concentration of agonists that caused vascular contraction was not altered. From simple physical reasoning, it was argued that these findings could be accounted for by the slight change in the structure of the resistance vessels, such that the lumen was slightly reduced, and the wall (or more correctly media) thickness was increased.[16–19]

Support for this concept was available from autopsy studies in the last century that indicated that the small

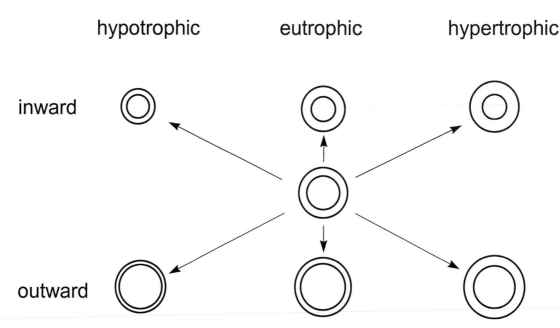

Figure 13–1. How remodeling can modify the cross-sections of blood vessels. The starting point is the vessel at the center. Remodeling can be hypertrophic (e.g., increase of cross-sectional area, vessels in *right column*), eutrophic (no change in cross-sectional area, vessels in *center column*), or hypotrophic (e.g., decrease of cross-sectional area, vessels in *left column*). These forms of remodeling can be inward i.e., reduction in lumen diameter, vessels in *top row*) or outward (i.e., increase in lumen diameter, vessels in *bottom row*). (Adapted from Mulvany MJ, Baumbach GL, Aalkjær C, et al. Vascular remodelling. [Letter to editor] Hypertension 28:505–506, 1996.)

arteries of patients with hypertension (then Bright's disease) had abnormally high wall:lumen ratios.[20, 21] However, it was not clear whether this was due to a structural change or to the vessels having contracted more strongly during the fixation process. Further support for the predictions of the hemodynamic experiments came later, when Furuyama[22] and Suwa and Takahashi[23] attempted to circumvent the problem of possible fixation-induced contraction by estimating vascular diameter from the total length of the internal elastic lamina (which corrugates during vascular contraction). These investigations also showed an increased wall:lumen ratio of vessels in autopsy material from essential hypertensives. The validity of the method is, however, dependent on the assumption that the internal elastic lamina becomes smooth at the same pressure in hypertensive and control subjects, an assumption that has been questioned.[24]

Short[13] fixed autopsy samples of mesenteric vasculature while these were being perfused under pressure and also showed that wall:lumen ratios were increased in essential hypertensives. It should be pointed out that even this elegant study had the weakness that the actual pressure in vessels at the moment of fixation could not be controlled, nor was the possibility excluded that the fixative caused contraction of the vessels. Further histological evidence for structural change in resistance vessels comes from investigations of autopsied hearts[25] and of cardiac transplant recipient hearts[26] that indicated that for a given diameter, the wall of coronary resistance vessels was thickened in hypertension.

IN VITRO DEMONSTRATION OF REMODELING OF RESISTANCE VESSEL STRUCTURE IN HYPERTENSION

Until recently, there had been few investigations of isolated small arteries in essential hypertension. However, the development of the technique of gluteal skin biopsy taken under local anesthesia, from which it is possible to dissect out small arteries for mounting on wire-myographs,[27, 28] has allowed carefully controlled investigations of small arteries in essential hypertensive patients. Such studies have provided strong support for the findings of the histological investigations.[28–32] These gluteal biopsy studies have demonstrated uniformly that essential hypertension is associated with a reduced lumen and increased media:lumen ratio in resistance vessels of essential hypertensive patients. In particular, this work has also confirmed the early finding of Short[13] that the altered morphology is not associated with an increase in the cross-sectional area of the media (measured normal to the longitudinal axis).[33] Thus, the available evidence indicates that in essential hypertension, the resistance vessels have experienced inward eutrophic remodeling (Fig. 13–2).[33] Furthermore, the size of the individual smooth muscle cells within the media is also normal,[30] whereas the functional responses of the smooth muscle are little affected.[28] In this respect, it should be noted that although the maximal response of the vessels from the essential hypertensives to agonists is increased, the increase corresponds to the increased medial thickness: The force production per unit of smooth muscle cross-section (active media stress) is normal (Fig. 13–3). These findings thus

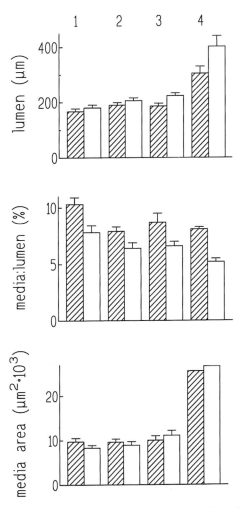

Figure 13–2. Lumen diameter, media:lumen ratio, and media cross-sectional area of resistance arteries from essential hypertensive *(hatched bars)* patients compared with resistance arteries from age- and sex-matched control subjects *(open bars)*. Summary of results from four investigations (1: ref. 28; 2: ref. 29; ; 3: ref. 55; 4: ref. 31). *Error bars* show SE. Eight to 16 subjects in each group.

support the concept that the altered hemodynamic characteristics of the resistance vasculature in essential hypertension are due mainly to a rearrangement of otherwise normal cells around a smaller diameter.

The inward eutrophic remodeling seen in essential hypertension is in contrast to other situations, in which different modes of remodeling have been noted. Thus, in human renovascular hypertension, the reduction in resistance vessel lumen diameter is accompanied by an increase in medial cross-sectional area, an inward hypertrophic response[34] (see Fig. 13–1 *top right*).

The possibility that pulse pressure could be an independent determinant of resistance vessel structure has also been investigated. Although disputed,[35] there is convincing evidence that in elderly hypertensive patients, resistance vessel media:lumen ratio is correlated with pulse pressure.[36]

It should be noted that the mode of remodeling in the resistance vessels of hypertensive individuals differs from that seen in large arteries.[37] This is likely because the functional requirements of large arteries do not include a narrowing of the lumen; their function is primarily to

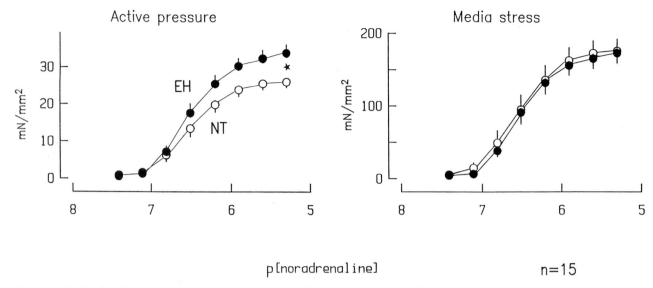

Figure 13–3. Noradrenaline concentration-response curves of isolated subcutaneous small arteries from essential hypertensive (EH) subjects *(solid circles)* and from normotensive (NT) controls *(open circles)*. Noradrenaline doses are given as p[noradrenaline] = −log(noradrenaline concentration [M]), and responses are expressed as effective active pressure (pressure against which vessel could contract, on the basis of the Laplace relation[27] *[left]*) and media stress (right). * $p < .05$. *Error bars* show SE. Fifteen subjects in each group. (From Aalkjær C, Heagerty AM, Petersen KK, et al. Evidence for increased media thickness, increased neuronal amine uptake, and depressed excitation-contraction coupling in isolated resistance vessels from essential hypertensives. Circ Res 61:181–186, 1987.)

transport blood, with the flow rate being unchanged in hypertension. Thus, an increase in media:lumen ratio of a large artery—with a normal lumen—necessarily involves an increase in the amount of material.[38]

IN VIVO VISUALIZATION

In humans, the vascular beds most suited to direct observation are in the eye and the nailfold. However, little information has been obtained by this means in essential hypertension. Vascular damage in the retina increases with the degree of hypertension, and it has been reported that this is reduced by antihypertensive treatment.[39] Studies of the branching pattern of retinal blood vessels have revealed abnormalities in hypertension.[40] Moreover, observations of the conjunctiva of essential hypertensive subjects show a rarefaction of the vasculature,[41] and similar findings are reported concerning the capillaries of the nailfold[42] and the finger dorsum,[43] in which the abnormality appears to be structural rather than functional. Thus, as in spontaneously hypertensive rats,[41, 44, 45] available evidence supports the possibility that rarefaction of the vasculature is one of the causes of the increased peripheral resistance in essential hypertension, although more work is needed to validate this.[46] It should also be pointed out that a theoretical analysis has suggested that rarefaction can account for only a minor proportion of the increased resistance in essential hypertension.[47]

REVERSAL OF RESISTANCE VESSEL REMODELING WITH ANTIHYPERTENSIVE TREATMENT

Numerous animal studies based on in vitro examination of resistance vessels have shown that reversal of hypertension

with antihypertensive drugs can lead to a normalization of resistance vessel structure.[3] Furthermore, it appears that with most classes of drugs, the degree of normalization corresponds to the degree of antihypertensive effect.[48] One reported exception was treatment of spontaneously hypertensive rats with the β-blocker metoprolol, in which a reduction in blood pressure was not accompanied by any change in resistance vessel structure.[48]

In the past few years, a number of investigators have performed comparable in vitro clinical experiments. Again, the general finding has been that normalization of blood pressure of essential hypertensive patients results in normalization of vascular structure, this being the case for treatment with angiotensin-converting enzyme (ACE) inhibitors[32, 49–51] (for a review, see ref. 52) and calcium antagonists.[53, 54] A notable exception has (as in the rat studies) been β-blocker treatment, in which atenolol therapy did not cause normalization of resistance vessel structure[32, 49] (Fig. 13–4 and Table 13–1), even when administered for up to 2 years.[55] The reason for this difference is not clear, but it may be related to the different hemodynamic profile of β-blocker treatment compared with other treatments: The antihypertensive effect of β-blockers without intrinsic sympathomimetic activity (ISA) is due primarily to reduced cardiac output rather than reduced peripheral resistance.[56] In this respect, it is established that flow is an important determinant of structure in rat resistance vessels. For example, decreased flow causes inward hypotrophic remodeling.[57]

The action of diuretics on vascular structure is not clear. An in vivo study showed that forearm resistance was little affected by hydrocholorothiazide treatment, but was reduced by ACE inhibitor treatment.[58] In contrast, in vitro experiments have suggested that hydrocholorothiazide-amiloride treatment can cause normalization of resistance artery structure.[54]

The finding that antihypertensive agents other than β-

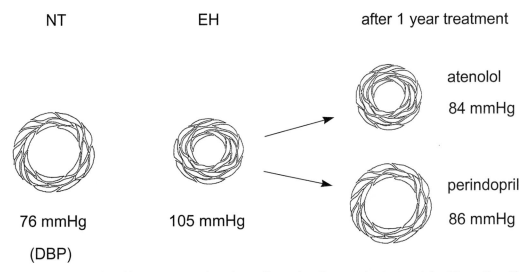

Figure 13–4. Data in Table 13–1 are used to show effects of antihypertensive treatment for 12 months with perindopril (angiotensin-converting enzyme inhibitor) or atenolol (β-blocker) on the structure of subcutaneous small arteries from patients with essential hypertension (EH). Treatment of EH with perindopril normalizes the vascular structure to that seen in normotensive controls (NT), without changing the medial cross-sectional area. Treatment with atenolol did not alter the structure of the resistance vessels. DBP, diatolic blood pressure.

blockers can cause normalization of resistance vessel structure has not been seen in all studies: One in vitro myograph study showed no effect of isradipine or spirapril.[59] The discrepancy could be related, as discussed later, to inherent difficulties in the myograph technique.

MEASUREMENT OF REMODELING

The previously discussed considerations of how remodeling of resistance vessels should be defined presupposes that accurate measurements of their dimensions can be made. Some of the pitfalls associated with that assumption are as follows.

Given the elastic nature of the vascular wall, the dimensions of a vessel depend on the conditions under which they are measured. The "structure" of a blood vessel must therefore be determined under clearly defined mechanical conditions, e.g., a particular intravascular pressure, such that its intrinsic dimensions (lumen diameter, wall thickness) will then be a function of the amount of material in the wall, the manner in which it is arranged, and the elastic moduli of the various wall components. However, the dimensions will also be a function of the degree of smooth muscle activation in the vessel wall and the magnitude of the intravascular pressure. Meaningful measurements of vascular "structure" therefore require that the intravascular pressure and state of activation be defined. For comparative purposes, it is usual for structure to be measured with the smooth muscle completely relaxed and, as far as possible, with a specific intravascular pressure, often 100 mm Hg (13.3 kPa). The figure of 100 mm Hg is used both because it is a round number and because the elastic characteristics of the vascular wall give a logarithmic lumen–intravascular pressure relation such that above 100 mm Hg, there is little increase in lumen diameter.[60]

The measurements referred to previously have generally been made under standardized conditions using myographs, either with vessels mounted on wires as ring preparations[27] or with vessels cannulated and under pressure.[61] Such in

Table 13–1 Characteristics of Subcutaneous Small Arteries Taken From Patients With Essential Hypertension Before and After Treatment With Perindopril or Atenolol

	Patients				
	Before Treatment		After Treatment		
Variable	Perindopril	Atenolol	Perindopril	Atenolol	Controls
Patients (n)	13	12	13	12	25
Lumen (μm)*	208 ± 12	222 ± 13	247 ± 12†	208 ± 12‡	237 ± 11
Media (μm)*	15.7 ± 0.9	15.1 ± 2.5	13.9 ± 0.7	13.6 ± 0.6	10.9 ± 0.8§
Media:lumen (%)*	7.94 ± 0.65	7.14 ± 0.47	5.96 ± 0.42†	6.79 ± 0.45‡	5.82 ± 0.34§
Media cross-sectional area (μm² · 10³)*	12.1 ± 1.2	12.1 ± 0.9	11.6 ± 0.8	9.8 ± 0.8†	10.9 ± 0.8

Data from Thybo NK, Stephens N, Cooper A, et al. Effect of antihypertensive treatment on small arteries of patients with previously untreated essential hypertension. Hypertension 25:474–481, 1995.
*Values are given as means ± SEM.
†$p < .05$, before vs. after, paired *t*-test.
‡$p < .05$, effect of treatment, perindopril vs. atenolol, grouped *t*-test.
§Control vs. pooled data for patients before treatment, grouped *t*-test.

vitro measurements have the advantage over histological measurements that fixation artifacts are avoided. On the other hand, in the wire-myographs, vessels are examined with zero longitudinal force, so that retraction artifacts are introduced.[60, 62] Furthermore, with the pressure-myograph, the precision of measurement of media thickness is not optimal. Nevertheless, the results of comparative studies of vessels from normotensive and hypertensive individuals can be reproduced in different laboratories,[28–32] and the wire- and pressure-myograph techniques provide qualitatively consistent results.[60, 63]

Another potential difficulty in measuring structure is the question of which vessels should be compared: Should this be on the basis of branching pattern, or on the basis of location?[3] Thus, different sampling techniques can give different results. For measurements of wall:lumen ratio or smooth muscle cell volume, this is not so serious, for these parameters are less dependent on the precise location.[64] However, lumen diameter, wall cross-sectional area, and number of smooth muscle cells per unit length are strongly dependent on the position in the vascular tree. Therefore, for these parameters, slight differences in the architecture of hypertensive and normotensive vessels can give erroneous results because of comparisons made at different levels in the vascular tree. This is particularly of concern in relation to reports of growth in the resistance vessels of hypertensive individuals, and such conclusions need to be treated with caution.[33] More sophisticated sampling techniques are called for in this setting.[13, 65]

Another point of discussion is whether the "structure" of a vessel should be determined at the intravascular pressure that it has experienced in vivo. However, the purpose of comparing vessels under identical experimental conditions is to compare their intrinsic properties, not their properties in vivo. Clearly, extrapolation of results obtained under standardized conditions to the in vivo situation must be made with caution.

Finally, an inherent disadvantage of the myograph technique is that only a few vessels can be studied per individual, and there is thus inevitably large variability between patients. For a given patient group, the interindividual coefficient of variance (SD/mean) is approximately 20% for lumen diameter and 35% for medial cross-sectional area (see, e.g., ref. 32). Accurate comparisons therefore require large numbers of subjects. Development of techniques that will allow noninvasive measurement of larger amounts of material is needed.

Nevertheless, despite all these reservations, media:lumen ratio of small arteries studied on a myograph is correlated to forearm minimal vascular resistance.[66] This suggests that the in vitro measurements do, even with the small amount of material involved, provide clinically relevant information.

FUNCTIONAL PROPERTIES OF RESISTANCE VESSELS IN HYPERTENSION

Evidence concerning the threshold sensitivity of the vasculature of essential hypertensive patients (i.e., the minimal dose that will give a response) is sparse. The vasculature in the forearm[17] and the hand[18] shows no abnormality concerning noradrenaline sensitivity. However, Robinson and coworkers[67] and Hulthen and associates[68] found that the ratio between the sensitivity of the forearm vasculature of essential hypertensives to calcium antagonists and to nitroprusside was increased, suggesting some functional abnormality. Also, in the renal vasculature, Ljungman and colleagues[69] reported a slight increase in the sensitivity to venous infusion of angiotensin II, although some central mechanism could have been involved.

The lack of evidence for substantially altered sensitivity of the resistance vasculature in essential hypertension is also seen in in vitro experiments. As mentioned previously, in subcutaneous small arteries from essential hypertensive subjects, the sensitivity to noradrenaline (see Fig. 13–3), serotonin, and vasopressin is normal.[28, 31] Other functional parameters found to be normal in small arteries from essential hypertensive subjects include intracellular pH under both resting and activated conditions, suggesting that the activity of transsarcolemmal Na,H-exchange is not altered in essential hypertension.[70] An exception to this is the response to endothelin, which is reduced in subcutaneous small arteries from patients with essential hypertension,[31] possibly due to enhanced expression of the endothelin-1 gene.[71]

ENDOTHELIUM-MEDIATED RESPONSES OF RESISTANCE VESSELS IN HYPERTENSION

In contrast to these negative results regarding vascular sensitivity to vasoconstrictors, many reports indicate that the endothelium-dependent vasodilator effect of acetylcholine infused into the forearm is reduced in essential hypertension.[72–74] The response to acetylcholine appears to be mediated through activation of nitric oxide synthase.[75] Impaired endothelium-mediated relaxation has also been seen in the heart, using intracoronary Doppler catheter and quantitative angiography. These findings are, however, controversial.[76, 77] It has also been shown, in the forearm, that the response of the vasculature to nitric oxide itself may be impaired in hypertension.[78]

In vitro investigations of endothelium-dependent vasodilatation have given equally disparate results. Thus, in some cases,[79, 80] but not in others,[81, 82] resistance arteries from essential hypertensive patients had reduced responses to acetylcholine. These conflicting results are puzzling. It has been suggested that plasma cholesterol levels may play a dominant role in the acetylcholine response[83] and that the higher cholesterol levels normally associated with hypertension could be responsible for the reduced acetylcholine response.[84, 85]

IS RESISTANCE VESSEL STRUCTURE A DETERMINANT OF BLOOD PRESSURE?

Angiotensin II causes proliferation of vascular smooth muscle cells in vitro.[86–88] Furthermore, infusion of angiotensin II into rats at subpressor doses using osmotic minipumps[89] causes increases in both the media:lumen ratio and the media cross-sectional area of mesenteric small arteries, even if rats were treated with hydralazine to prevent the rise in blood pressure. Moreover, as discussed previously, in human essential hypertension (see Fig. 13–4 and Table 13–1), treatment with an ACE inhibitor causes a greater reduction in media:lumen ratio than treatment with a β-blocker, even when both treatments have the same hypotensive effect.[32, 49] It therefore appears that the altered resistance vessel structure that is seen in hypertension is not purely a secondary response to the increased blood pressure. Thus, resistance vessel structure could play a direct role in determining the blood pressure.

The possibility that resistance vessel structure has a direct influence on blood pressure can be tested by, first, making some intervention that changes blood pressure and alters resistance vessel structure. Thereafter, one can determine whether the rate of blood pressure normalization when the intervention is removed is related to the structure of the resistance vessel before removal of the intervention. Initial work by Pickering[90] suggested that this was the case, but subsequent research has in general failed to provide much support for such a clearcut relation, as discussed previously.[91] Some examples of this follow.

First, in the angiotensin II infusion model referred to previously, as soon as the angiotensin II infusion is stopped, the blood pressure returns to normal[92] despite the changes in the resistance vessel structure.[89] Similarly, in the one-kidney, one-clip Goldblatt hypertension model, the increase in blood pressure that occurs over a few weeks, and that causes changes in the resistance vessel structure,[93] is halted as soon as the clip is removed.[94] The decrease in blood pressure is due to massive release of "medullipin," but once again, the altered resistance vessel structure is not able to sustain the hypertension. Yet another example is in human essential hypertension, where Korner and coworkers[95] have shown that when antihypertensive therapy was withdrawn from patients being treated for essential hypertension, the blood pressure returned to hypertensive levels most rapidly in those patients in whom the total peripheral resistance was lowest. Again, this suggests a dissociation between vascular structure and ability to maintain blood pressure.

In none of these examples is there any indication that resistance vessel structure has a direct effect on blood pressure. In each case, reasons can be found for why the structural effect is overridden.[96] Nevertheless, the previous analysis shows that structure does not play a dominant role in blood pressure determination.

RESISTANCE VESSEL STRUCTURE AND BLOOD PRESSURE

The previous considerations suggest that although resistance vessel structure and blood pressure are closely connected, changes in one are not automatically associated with changes in the other. Instead, the available data suggest that the resistance vessels should be considered as the effector organ of neurohumoral drive, with the altered structure merely having an amplifier effect (Fig. 13–5). As suggested by Julius,[97] the cardiovascular system apparently seeks to maintain a "required blood pressure" that is a compromise between the requirements of a number of factors, e.g., renal function. If, e.g., the pressure is too low, a signal is sent to increase the neurohumoral drive. The effect of this signal is dependent on both its strength and the resistance vessel structure (e.g., media:lumen ratio). The resulting increase in peripheral resistance increases the pressure, the process continuing until the pressure equals

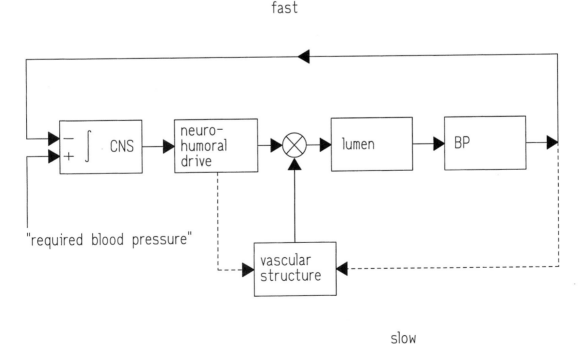

Figure 13–5. Schematic shows the proposed role for resistance vessel structure in the control of blood pressure (BP). *Solid lines* show fast processes, *dashed lines* show slow processes. The schematic embodies ideas proposed principally by Folkow,[15] but also by Lever,[100] Korner and Angus,[47] and Julius.[97] ∫, integrator; ⊗, multiplier. CNS, central nervous system.

the required pressure. This is a rapid process, a negative feedback mechanism, inherently stable, mediated through a variety of systems, not only the baroreceptors.

However, there are also slow processes for maintaining the "required blood pressure." The resistance vessel media:lumen ratio is not static but, in the long term, can be altered by (1) neurohumoral influences (as discussed earlier), and (2) the pressure (as has been shown in experiments in which a clip is placed on one femoral artery[98]). Thus, if for some reason the required pressure increases, there will initially be an increase in the neurohumoral drive, and the fast process will cause the pressure to rise. Then the slow process will ensue, with an increase in resistance vessel media:lumen ratio, due both to the increased neurohumoral drive and to the increased pressure. With the increase in resistance vessel media:lumen ratio, the neurohumoral drive necessary to maintain the increased blood pressure will be reduced. Thus, in the long run, the increased pressure will be maintained by a normal neurohumoral drive, but with an increased media:lumen ratio—the situation normally seen in essential hypertension.

The implication of these arguments is that the resistance vessels should not be considered as prime determinants of blood pressure. Rather, they should be considered as effector organs of the cardiovascular control system.

ANTIHYPERTENSIVE TREATMENT AND RESISTANCE VESSEL STRUCTURE

The previous arguments can account for the finding (see Fig. 13–4) that blood pressure can be reduced without normalizing the structure of the resistance vessels. Therefore, normalization of structure is not absolutely necessary for successful antihypertensive treatment, but reduction of blood pressure without normalization of resistance vessel structure will reduce the vascular reserve. Thus, the decreased coronary vascular reserve seen in essential hypertension will be exacerbated rather than relieved.[99] Therefore, normalization of vascular structure must, in principle, be seen as being an important goal of antihypertensive treatment. Investigations are now required to determine whether improvement of vascular reserve is dependent on normalization of resistance vessel structure and, more importantly, whether correction of vascular reserve also improves the prognosis of essential hypertensive patients.

Acknowledgments

This review was written while the author was receiving support from the Danish Medical Research Council, the Danish Heart Foundation, and the European Union (Working Party on Cellular and Molecular Mechanisms of Resistance Artery Remodelling [CAMMRAR]).

References

1. Lund-Johansson P. Haemodynamics in essential hypertension. Clin Sci 59:343–354, 1980.
2. Williams SA, Boolell M, MacGregor GA, et al. Capillary hypertension and abnormal pressure dynamics in patients with essential hypertension. Clin Sci 79:5–8, 1990.
3. Mulvany MJ, Aalkjær C. Structure and function of small arteries. Physiol Rev 70:921–961, 1990.
4. Mulvany MJ. Resistance vessels in hypertension. *In* Swales J (ed). Textbook of Hypertension. Oxford, Blackwell, 1994; pp 103–119.
5. Mulvany MJ. Structural changes in the resistance vessels in human hypertension. *In* Laragh JH, Brenner BM (eds). Hypertension: Pathophysiology, Diagnosis and Management. New York, Raven, 1995; pp 503–513.
6. Lee RM, Owens GK, Scott-Burden T, et al. Pathophysiology of smooth muscle in hypertension. Can J Physiol Pharmacol 73:574–584, 1995.
7. Christensen KL, Mulvany MJ. Mesenteric arcade arteries contribute substantially to vascular resistance in conscious rats. J Vasc Res 30:73–79, 1993.
8. Christensen KL, Mulvany MJ. Blood pressure at base of mesenteric arcades in conscious SHR and WKY rats. [Abstract] J Hypertens 11 (suppl 3):s411, 1993.
9. Fenger Gron J, Mulvany MJ, Christensen KL. Mesenteric blood pressure profile of conscious, freely moving rats. J Physiol Lond 488:753–760, 1995.
10. Fenger Gron J, Mulvany MJ, Christensen KL. Intestinal blood flow is controlled by both feed arteries and microcirculatory resistance vessels in freely moving rats. J Physiol Lond 498:215–224, 1997.
11. Mulvany MJ. Determinants of vascular hemodynamic characteristics. Hypertension 6 (suppl 3):III-13–III-18, 1984.
12. Baumbach GL, Heistad DD. Remodeling of cerebral arterioles in chronic hypertension. Hypertension 13:968–972, 1989.
13. Short D. The vascular fault in chronic hypertension with particular reference to the role of medial hypertrophy. Lancet 1:1302–1304, 1966.
14. Mulvany MJ, Baumbach GL, Aalkjær C, et al. Vascular remodelling. [Letter to editor] Hypertension 28:505–506, 1996.
15. Folkow B. Structural, myogenic, humoral and nervous factors controlling peripheral resistance. *In* Harington M (ed). Hypotensive Drugs. London, Pergamon, 1956; pp 163–174.
16. Doyle AE, Black H. Reactivity to pressor agents in hypertension. Circ Res 12:974–980, 1955.
17. Folkow B, Grimby G, Thulesius O. Adaptive structural changes of the vascular walls in hypertension and their relation to the control of the peripheral resistance. Acta Physiol Scand 44:255–272, 1958.
18. Sivertsson R. The hemodynamic importance of structural vascular changes in essential hypertension. Acta Physiol Scand Suppl 343:1–56, 1970.
19. Egan BM, Schork N, Panis R, Hinderliter A. Vascular structure enhances regional resistance responses in mild essential hypertension. J Hypertens 6:41–48, 1988.
20. Johnson G. On certain points in the anatomy of Bright's disease of the kidney. Trans R Med Chir Soc 51:57–58, 1868.
21. Gull WW, Sutton HG. Chronic Bright's disease with contracted kidney. Med Chir Trans 55:273–326, 1872.
22. Furuyama M. Histometrical investigations of arteries in reference to arterial hypertension. Tohoku J Exp Med 76:388–414, 1962.
23. Suwa N, Takahashi T. Morphological and Morphometric Analysis of Circulation in Hypertension and Ischaemic Kidney. Munich, Urban & Schwarzenberg, 1971.
24. Lee RMKW, Forrest JB, Garfield RE, Daniel EE. Comparison of blood vessel wall dimensions in normotensive and hypertensive rats by histometric and morphometric methods. Blood Vessels 20:245–254, 1983.
25. Schwartzkopff B, Motz W, Knauer S, et al. Morphometric investigation of intramyocardial arterioles in right septal endomyocardial biopsy of patients with arterial hypertension and left ventricular hypertrophy. J Cardiovasc Pharmacol 20(suppl 1):S12–S17, 1992.
26. Jenkins JT, Boyle JJ, McKay IC, et al. Vascular remodelling in intramyocardial resistance vessels in hypertensive human cardiac transplant recipients. Heart 77:353–356, 1997.
27. Mulvany MJ, Halpern W. Contractile properties of small arterial resistance vessels in spontaneously hypertensive and normotensive rats. Circ Res 41:19–26, 1977.
28. Aalkjær C, Heagerty AM, Petersen KK, et al. Evidence for increased media thickness, increased neuronal amine uptake, and depressed excitation-contraction coupling in isolated resistance vessels from essential hypertensives. Circ Res 61:181–186, 1987.
29. Izzard AS, Cragoe EJ, Heagerty AM. Intracellular pH in human resistance arteries in essential hypertension. Hypertension 17:780–786, 1991.
30. Korsgaard N, Aalkjær C, Heagerty AM, et al. Histology of subcuta-

neous small arteries from patients with essential hypertension. Hypertension 22:523–526, 1993.

31. Schiffrin EL, Deng LY, Larochelle P. Blunted effects of endothelin upon small subcutaneous resistance arteries of mild essential hypertensive patients. J Hypertens 10:437–444, 1992.
32. Thybo NK, Stephens N, Cooper A, et al. Effect of antihypertensive treatment on small arteries of patients with previously untreated essential hypertension. Hypertension 25:474–481, 1995.
33. Heagerty AM, Aalkjær C, Bund SJ, et al. Small artery structure in hypertension: Dual processes of remodelling and growth. Hypertension 21:391–397, 1993.
34. Rizzoni D, Porteri E, Castellano M, et al. Vascular hypertrophy and remodeling in secondary hypertension. Hypertension 28:785–790, 1996.
35. Cooper A, Heagerty AM. Blood pressure parameters as determinants of small artery structure in human essential hypertension. Clin Sci (Colch) 92:551–557, 1997.
36. James MA, Watt PA, Potter JF, et al. Pulse pressure and resistance artery structure in the elderly. Hypertension 26:301–306, 1995.
37. Safar ME, Frohlich ED. The arterial system in hypertension. A prospective view. Hypertension 26:10–14, 1995.
38. Schiffrin EL, Hayoz D. How to assess vascular remodelling in small and medium-sized muscular arteries in humans. J Hypertens 15:571–584, 1997.
39. Dahlöf B. Hypertensive retinal vascular changes: Relationship to left ventricular hypertrophy and arteriolar changes before and after treatment. Blood Press 1:35–44, 1992.
40. Stanton AV, Wasan B, Cerutti A, et al. Vascular network changes in the retina with age and hypertension. J Hypertens 13:1724–1728, 1995.
41. Harper RN, Moore MA, Marr MC, et al. Arteriolar rarefaction in the conjunctiva of human essential hypertensives. Microvasc Res 16:369–372, 1978.
42. Gasser P, Buhler FR. Nailfold microcirculation in normotensive and essential hypertensive subjects, as assessed by video-microscopy. J Hypertens 10:83–86, 1992.
43. Antonios TFT, Singer DRJ, Markandu ND, et al. Study of skin capillaries in essential hypertension using sodium fluorescence angiography and video-microscopy. [Abstract] Hypertension 32:789–812, 1998.
44. Sokolova IA, Manukhina EB, Blinkov SM, et al. Rarefication of the arterioles and capillary network in the brain of rats with different forms of hypertension. Microvasc Res 30:1–9, 1985.
45. le Noble JL, Tangelder GJ, Slaaf DW, et al. A functional morphometric study of the cremaster muscle microcirculation in young spontaneously hypertensive rats. J Hypertens 8:741–748, 1990.
46. Engelson ET, Schmid-Schonbein GW, Zweifach BW. The microvasculature in skeletal muscle. Microvasc Res 31:356–374, 1986.
47. Korner PI, Angus JA. Structural determinants of vascular resistance properties in hypertension. Haemodynamic and model analysis. J Vasc Res 29:293–312, 1992.
48. Christensen KL, Jespersen LT, Mulvany MJ. Development of blood pressure in spontaneously hypertensive rats after withdrawal of long-term treatment related to resistance vessel structure. J Hypertens 7:83–90, 1989.
49. Schiffrin EL, Deng LY, Larochelle P. Effects of a beta-blocker or a converting enzyme inhibitor on resistance arteries in essential hypertension. Hypertension 23:83–91, 1994.
50. Sihm I, Schroeder AP, Aalkjær C, et al. Normalization of structural cardiovascular changes during antihypertensive treatment with a regimen based on the ACE-inhibitor perindopril. Blood Press 4:241–248, 1995.
51. Rizzoni D, Muiesan ML, Porteri E, et al. Effects of long-term antihypertensive treatment with lisinopril on resistance arteries in hypertensive patients with left ventricular hypertrophy. J Hypertens 15:197–204, 1997.
52. Safar ME, van Bortel LM, Struijker Boudier HA. Resistance and conduit arteries following converting enzyme inhibition in hypertension. J Vasc Res 34:67–81, 1997.
53. Schiffrin EL, Deng LY. Structure and function of resistance arteries of hypertensive patients treated with a beta-blocker or a calcium channel antagonist. J Hypertens 14:1247–1255, 1996.
54. Sihm I, Schroeder AP, Aalkjær C, et al. Effect of antihypertensive treatment on cardiac and subcutaneous artery structure: A comparison between calcium channel blocker and thiazide-based regimens. Am J Hypertens 11:263–271, 1998.
55. Schiffrin EL, Deng LY, Larochelle P. Progressive improvement in the structure of resistance arteries of hypertensive patients after 2 years with an angiotensin I-converting enzyme inhibitor. Comparison with effects of a beta-blocker. Am J Hypertens 8:229–236, 1995.
56. Man in't Veld AJ, van der Meiracker AH. Effect of antihypertensive drugs on cardiovascular hemodynamics. In Laragh JH, Brenner BM (eds): Hypertension: Physiology, Diagnosis and Management. New York, Raven, pp 2117–2130, 1990.
57. Pourageaud F, DeMey JGR. Structural properties of rat mesenteric small arteries after 4-wk exposure to elevated or reduced blood flow. Am J Physiol 273:H1699–H1706, 1997.
58. Dahlof B, Hansson L. The influence of antihypertensive therapy on the structural arteriolar changes in essential hypertension: Different effects of enalapril and hydrochlorthiazide. J Intern Med 234:271–279, 1993.
59. Thurmann PA, Stephens N, Heagerty AM, et al. Influence of isradipine and spirapril on left ventricular hypertrophy and resistance arteries. Hypertension 28:450–456, 1996.
60. Lew MJ, Angus JA. Wall thickness to lumen diameter ratios of arteries from SHR and WKY: Comparison of pressurised and wire-mounted preparations. J Vasc Res 29:435–442, 1992.
61. Halpern W, Osol G. Blood vessel diameter measurement. Prog Appl Microcirc 8:32–39, 1985.
62. McKinnon W, Poston L, Singer DR, MacGregor GA. Resistance artery morphology in essential hypertension and in normal subjects: Some methodological considerations. J Hum Hypertens 8:623–625, 1994.
63. Falloon BJ, Heagerty AM. In vitro perfusion studies of human resistance artery function in essential hypertension. Hypertension 24:16–23, 1994.
64. Korsgaard N, Mulvany MJ. Morphological and functional properties of proximal and distal mesenteric resistance vessels. Proc Int Union Physiol Sci 17:169, 1989.
65. Gundersen HJG, Bagger P, Bendtsen TF, et al. The new stereological tools: Disector, fractionator, nucleator and point sampled intercepts and their use in pathological research and diagnosis. Acta Pathol Microbiol Immunolol Scand 96:857–881, 1988.
66. Rosei EA, Rizzoni D, Castellano M, et al. Media:lumen ratio in human small resistance arteries is related to forearm minimal vascular resistance. J Hypertens 13:341–347, 1995.
67. Robinson BF, Dobbs RJ, Bayley S. Response of forearm resistance vessels to verapamil and nitroprusside in normotensive and hypertensive men: Evidence for a functional abnormality of vascular smooth muscle in primary hypertension. Clin Sci 63:33–42, 1982.
68. Hulthen UL, Bolli P, Kiowski W, Bühler FR. Inhibition of the arteriolar smooth muscle Na$^+$=K$^+$=pump induces an enhanced vasoconstriction in borderline but not in established essential hypertension. Gen Pharmacol 14:193–196, 1983.
69. Ljungman S, Aurell M, Hartford M, et al. Effects of subpressor doses of angiotensin II on renal hemodynamics in relation to blood pressure. Hypertension 5:368–374, 1983.
70. Izzard AS, MacIver DH, Cragoe EJ, Heagerty AM. Intracellular pH in rat mesenteric resistance arteries during the development of experimental hypertension. Clin Sci 81:65–72, 1991.
71. Schiffrin EL, Deng LY, Sventek P, Day R. Enhanced expression of endothelin-1 gene in resistance arteries in severe human essential hypertension. J Hypertens 15:57–63, 1997.
72. Panza JA, Quyyumi AA, Brush JEJ, Epstein SE. Abnormal endothelium-dependent vascular relaxation in patients with essential hypertension. N Engl J Med 323:22–27, 1990.
73. Linder L, Kiowski W, Bühler FR, Lüscher TF. Indirect evidence for the release of endothelium-derived relaxing factor in human forearm circulation in vivo: Blunted response in essential hypertension. Circulation 81:1762–1767, 1990.
74. Taddei S, Virdis A, Mattei P, Salvetti A. Vasodilation to acetylcholine in primary and secondary forms of human hypertension. Hypertension 21:929–933, 1993.
75. Imaizumi T, Hirooka Y, Masaki H, et al. Effects of L-arginine on forearm vessels and responses to acetylcholine. Hypertension 20:511–517, 1992.
76. Cockcroft JR, Chowienczyk PJ, Benjamin N, Ritter JM. Preserved endothelium-dependent vasodilation in patients with essential hypertension. N Engl J Med 330:1036–1040, 1994.
77. Van Zwieten PA. Endothelial dysfunction in hypertension. A critical evaluation. Blood Press Suppl 2:67–70, 1997.
78. Preik M, Kelm M, Feelisch M, Strauer BE. Impaired effectiveness of nitric oxide-donors in resistance arteries of patients with arterial hypertension. J Hypertens 14: 903–908, 1996.

79. Deng LY, Li JS, Schiffrin EL. Endothelium-dependent relaxation of small arteries from essential hypertensive patients: Mechanisms and comparison with normotensive subjects and with responses of vessels from spontaneously hypertensive rats. Clin Sci (Colch) 88:611–622, 1995.

80. Rizzoni D, Porteri E, Castellano M, et al. Endothelial dysfunction in hypertension is independent from the etiology and from vascular structure. Hypertension 31:335–341, 1998.

81. Thybo NK, Mulvany MJ, Jastrup B, et al. Some pharmacological and elastic characteristics of isolated subcutaneous small arteries from patients with essential hypertension. J Hypertens 14:993–998, 1996.

82. James MA, Watt PA, Potter JF, et al. Endothelial function in subcutaneous resistance arteries from elderly hypertensive and normotensive subjects. Clin Sci (Colch) 92:139–145, 1997.

83. Goode GK, Garcia S, Heagerty AM. Dietary supplementation with marine fish oil improves in vitro small artery endothelial function in hypercholesterolemic patients: A double-blind placebo-controlled study. Circulation 96:2802–2807, 1997.

84. Goode GK, Miller JP, Heagerty AM. Hyperlipidaemia, hypertension, and coronary heart disease. Lancet 345:362–364, 1995.

85. Cockcroft JR, Chowienczyk PJ, Ritter JM. Hyperlipidaemia, hypertension, and coronary heart disease. Lancet 345:862–863, 1995.

86. Campbell JH, Tachas G, Black MJ, et al. Molecular biology of vascular hypertrophy. Basic Res Cardiol 86(suppl 1):3–11, 1991.

87. Stouffer GA, Owens GK. Angiotensin II–induced mitogenesis of spontaneously hypertensive rat–derived cultured smooth muscle cells is dependent on autocrine production of transforming growth factor-beta. Circ Res 70:820–828, 1992.

88. Dubey RK, Roy A, Overbeck HW. Culture of renal arteriolar smooth muscle cells. Mitogenic responses to angiotensin II. Circ Res 71:1143–1152, 1992.

89. Griffin SA, Brown WC, Macpherson F, et al. Angiotensin II causes vascular hypertrophy in part by a non-pressor mechanism. Hypertension 17:626–635, 1991.

90. Pickering GW. The role of the kidney in acute and chronic hypertension following renal artery constriction in the rabbit. Clin Sci 5:229–247, 1945.

91. Mulvany MJ. Resistance vessel growth and remodelling: Cause or consequence in cardiovascular disease. J Hum Hypertens 9:479–485, 1995.

92. Brown AJ, Casals-Stenzel J, Gofford S, et al. Comparison of fast and slow pressor effects of angiotensin II in the conscious rat. Am J Physiol 241:H381–H388, 1981.

93. Korsgaard N, Mulvany MJ. Cellular hypertrophy in mesenteric resistance vessels from renal hypertensive rats. Hypertension 12:162–167, 1988.

94. Muirhead EE, Pitcock JA, Nasjletti A, et al. The antihypertensive function of the kidney. Hypertension 7 (suppl I):I-127–I-135, 1985.

95. Korner PI, Bobik A, Jennings GL, et al. Significance of cardiovascular hypertrophy in the development and maintenance of hypertension. J Cardiovasc Pharmacol 17(suppl 2):S25–S32, 1991.

96. Folkow B. Hypertensive structural changes in systemic precapillary resistance vessels: How important are they for in vivo haemodynamics? J Hypertens 13:1546–1559, 1995.

97. Julius S. The blood pressure seeking properties of the central nervous system. J Hypertens 6:177–185, 1988.

98. Bund SJ, West KP, Heagerty AM. Effects of protection on resistance artery morphology and reactivity in spontaneously hypertensive and Wistar-Kyoto rats. Circ Res 68:1230–1240, 1991.

99. Strauer BE, Schwartzkopff B. Left ventricular hypertrophy and coronary microcirculation in hypertensive heart disease. Blood Press Suppl 2:6–12, 1997.

100. Lever AF. Slow pressor mechanisms in hypertension: A role for hypertrophy of resistance vessels? J Hypertens 4:515–524, 1986.

CHAPTER

14 Arterial Stiffness

Michael F. O'Rourke, Christopher S. Hayward, and Eldon D. Lehmann

Only in the case of young children do we find that the elasticity of arteries is so perfectly adapted to the requirements of the organism as it is in the case of the lower animals.
  C. S. ROY, 1880[1]

The amount of energy expended by the heart as measured by its oxygen consumption or CO_2 output has been shown to be proportional to the pressure developed . . . ; hence the amount of energy that the heart expends per beat, other things being equal, varies . . . with the elasticity of the arterial system.
  J. C. BRAMWELL, A. V. HILL, 1922[2]

The subject of arterial elasticity is one of the most perplexing to confront even the most astute clinician. Conceptually, the subject appears very simple. The arteries interpose between heart and peripheral arterioles, serving as a cushion as well as a conduit. Left ventricular ejection is intermittent, but flow through the arterioles is continuous. Adequate cushioning of flow pulsations, generated by the heart, depends on the elastic properties of the arterial system. The concept is simple, but complexities arise as soon as one addresses the subject in any detail. These complexities include the terms and measures used to describe and quantify arterial elastic properties (Table 14–1), the inho-

mogeneous composition of the arterial wall, the differences in elastic properties at different sites and at different distending pressures, and the differing effects of smooth muscle tone, of aging, and of hypertension on arteries at different sites. Complexities also arise because arterial elastic properties have indirect as well as direct effects on arterial hemodynamics, with these manifesting as alterations in intensity and timing of wave reflection. As the arteries stiffen with age, wave reflection returns early to the ascending aorta, boosting systolic pressure during late systole;[3] this is not necessarily apparent with conventional sphygmomanometric measurement in the arm, since an-

Table 14–1 Indices of Arterial Stiffness

Elastic modulus*	The pressure step required for (theoretical) 100% stretch from resting diameter at fixed vessel length $(\triangle P \cdot D)/\triangle D$ (mm Hg)
Arterial distensibility*	Relative diameter (or area) change for a pressure increment; the inverse of elastic modulus $\triangle D/(\triangle P \cdot D)$ (mm Hg^{-1})
Arterial compliance*	Absolute diameter (or area) change for a given pressure step at fixed vessel length $\triangle D/\triangle P$ (cm/mm Hg) (or cm²/mm Hg)
Volume elastic modulus*	Pressure step required for (theoretical) 100% increase in volume $\triangle P/(\triangle V/V)$ (mm Hg) $= \triangle P/(\triangle D/D)$ mm Hg (where there is no change in length)
Young's modulus*	Elastic modulus per unit area; the pressure step per square centimeter required for (theoretical) 100% stretch from resting length $\triangle P \cdot D/(\triangle D \cdot h)$ (mm Hg/cm)
Pulse wave velocity*	Speed of travel of the pulse along an arterial segment Distance/$\triangle t$ (cm/s)
Characteristic impedance*	Relationship between pressure change and flow velocity in the absence of wave reflections $\triangle P/\triangle v$ [(mm Hg/cm)/s]
Stiffness index	Ratio of logarithm (systolic/diastolic pressures) to (relative change in diameter) $\beta = \dfrac{\ln (P_s/P_d)}{(D_s - D_d)/D_d}$ (nondimensional)
"Capacitive compliance"	Relationship between pressure fall and volume fall in the arterial tree during the exponential component of diastolic pressure decay $\triangle V/\triangle P$ (cm³/mm Hg)
"Oscillatory compliance"	Relationship between oscillating pressure change and oscillating volume change around the exponential pressure decay during diastole $\triangle V/\triangle P$ (cm³/mm Hg)

From O'Rourke MF. Mechanical principles in arterial disease. Hypertension 26:2–9, 1995.
Abbreviations: P, pressure; D, diameter; V, volume; h, wall thickness; t, time; v, flow velocity; s, systolic; d, diastolic.
*These indices are site-specific and vary with distending pressure.

other phenomenon, caused by wave reflection, causes the peripheral pulse wave to be amplified in younger subjects, but not in the aged (Fig. 14–1, *left*).[4]

The importance of this subject has been highlighted by the attention given to isolated systolic hypertension, in which arterial stiffness is increased,[3] and where observational studies and therapeutic trials have shown a strong association with cardiovascular events and a marked reduction in these events with antihypertensive therapy.[5] The Systolic Hypertension in the Elderly Project (SHEP)[5] was the turning point, showing that reduction of elevated systolic pressure reduces all-cause mortality, including fatal strokes and cardiac events, even when diastolic pressure is in the normal range (or below). SHEP was the first major trial of antihypertensive therapy in a group of patients whose diagnosis of hypertension was not based on elevation of diastolic pressure. Leading up to this was evidence that in older persons (over 55 years), elevation of systolic pressure is a more robust indicator of cardiovascular events than is elevation of diastolic pressure. Such findings were apparent in the Framingham cohort for coronary vascular events in 1971,[6] and for cerebral vascular events in 1981.[7] Subsequent investigations consolidated the "ascendancy" of systolic pressure over diastolic pressure,[8] as well as the greater importance of systolic and pulse pressure over diastolic pressure in older subjects. Longitudinal follow-up of the Framingham cohort has shown a progressive rise in systolic pressure with age, but an even greater increase in pulse pressure, together with a decrease in diastolic pressure over age 55 years (Fig. 25–2, Chap. 25, New Interpretations of Blood Pressure: The Importance of Pulse Pressure).[9] These changes are attributable to progressive arterial stiffness with age.[3] Whereas diastolic pressure is closely related to cardiovascular events in younger subjects,[10] this association is lost or even reversed over the age of 55 years. Indeed, pulse pressure is emerging as a major risk factor for cardiovascular, and especially cardiac, events in older subjects—more robust than systolic and certainly more robust than diastolic pressure.[11-16] These findings draw attention to arterial elasticity and arterial stiffening and away from diastolic pressure, mean pressure, and peripheral resistance.

A change in focus from resistance to elasticity—from smallest resistance vessels to largest elastic vessels—is warranted because of the change in the population of patients who require treatment for hypertension. This point was made elegantly by Harriet Dustan[17] in 1989:

It is really not surprising that up until this time the focus was on diastolic hypertension. From a 1989 perspective it is hard to realize what a serious problem diastolic pressure was before the era of anti hypertensive drug therapy. This condition affected middle-aged persons at the height of their productivity. It either killed them suddenly by cerebral hemorrhage or slowly and miserably by cardiac or renal failure. No one was concerned about elderly persons with ISH (isolated systolic hypertension) particularly those who had lived longer than seventy years. However when the effectiveness of anti hypertensive drug treatment for diastolic hypertension was shown, the stage was set for a change in attitude to ISH.

Problems related to increased peripheral resistance in hypertension[18, 19] are usually easily controlled with modern drug therapy. The challenge facing clinicians is to seek equal success in dealing with problems related to increased arterial stiffness.

HISTORICAL PERSPECTIVE

Elasticity of the arterial system is a physiological concept that predates that of arteriolar resistance. It first emerged with the proof by Harvey in 1628 that arterial diastole

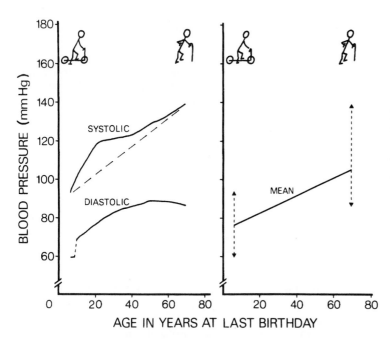

Figure 14–1. Change in brachial artery pressure with age. *Left,* Average systolic and diastolic pressures at different ages as reported in the U.S. National Health Survey (DHEW Publication No. [HRA] 78-1648, 1977). The *dotted line* indicates the probable change in aortic systolic pressure with age, allowing for substantial amplification of the peripheral pressure wave in young, fully grown adults. *Right,* Predicted change in mean pressure and brachial pulse pressure with age. (Modified from O'Rourke MF. Arterial Function in Health and Disease. Edinburgh, Churchill Livingstone, 1982.)

(dilatation) corresponds to cardiac systole and that passive stretch of the arteries contributes to forward blood flow during cardiac relaxation.[20] In his second open letter to Riolan,[21] Harvey also described the phenomenon of wave reflection. Hales,[22] the first to measure blood pressure, formulated the concept of peripheral resistance in tiny blood vessels but also likened the large arteries to the inverted air-filled dome (Windkessel) of the contemporary fire engine, which absorbed pulsations imposed by the hand (or steam)-driven pump, and permitted water to emerge from the fire hose nozzle in a continuous stream (Fig. 14–2). The simplest model of the circulation equates the Windkessel with total arterial compliance, and the fire hose nozzle with peripheral resistance. The corresponding electrical model is a resistance/capacitance (RC) circuit, with a capacitor representing total compliance and a resistor representing total resistance.

After Hales, and throughout the 19th century, fundamental studies on elasticity were conducted by physician-scientists such as Young[23] and Weber and Weber,[24] using arterial segments. During this period, the relationship between arterial elastic properties and pulse wave velocity (PWV) was established by Moens[25] and Korteweg,[26] and the equations

for blood flow in elastic tubes were derived by the mathematicians Navier[27] and Stokes.[28] At the same time, clinicians and physiologists began to focus on vascular problems. Poiseuille[29] confirmed Hales' observation that resistant properties are concentrated in the smallest arterial vessels, then established the overwhelming importance of the radius in determining resistance.[30] Bright[31] noted the relationship between high blood pressure (expressed as hardness of the pulse) and renal, cardiac, and cerebral vascular disease. His work was subsequently taken up at the same hospital (Guy's of London) by the brilliant young F. A. Mahomed. Dr. Mahomed improved on Marey's sphygmograph and then described aging change and the natural history of essential hypertension on the basis of radial pressure wave contour and augmentation of the secondary systolic wave.[32–34] Sphygmographs were widely used in clinical practice and to illustrate books and journal articles during the late 19th century, before being replaced by the cuff sphygmomanometer, which provided numbers and a veneer of scientific accuracy.

The cuff sphygmomanometer was looked on initially with healthy skepticism by influential clinicians such as Sir James Mackenzie of London[35] before being accepted

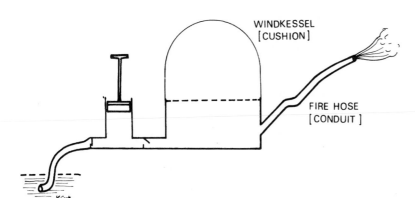

Figure 14–2. The Windkessel model of the arterial system. The arterial system is likened to an ancient fire cart, with distensible properties "lumped" in the inverted air-filled dome and peripheral resistance represented by the nozzle of the fire hose. (From O'Rourke MF. Arterial Function in Health and Disease. Edinburgh, Churchill Livingstone, 1982.)

uncritically and simplistically as by James Orr in the third edition of Mackenzie's text, which was published posthumously. This text misinterpreted the significance of systolic and diastolic pressure: "As regards the relative importance of systolic and diastolic pressure, it may be said that the systolic pressure represents the maximum force of the heart while the diastolic pressure measures the resistance the heart has to overcome."[36] This statement, in Mackenzie's name, appears to have initiated the myth that elevated systolic pressure is innocuous and that elevated diastolic pressure is the single hemodynamic manifestation of hypertensive disease. By the mid-20th century, life insurance data had clearly established elevated diastolic pressure and hypertension as the "silent killer,"[37] but similar data were available for systolic pressure as well. Data on systolic pressure were largely overlooked, and textbooks of the time, and later, concentrated on diastolic pressure and on processes causing elevation of peripheral resistance. Effective antihypertensive therapies became available in the 1950s and were shown to be capable of breaking the vicious circle of malignant hypertension.[18, 19, 38] Therapies were improved and have been responsible for the phenomenon described by Dustan[7] that has shifted attention from diastolic to systolic and pulse pressures—and so to arterial stiffness.

HYPERTENSIVE MECHANISMS WITH AGING

Most of the changes in blood pressure with age can be explained on the basis of arterial stiffening and vascular rarefaction, as also modified by the change in pressure wave amplification in the upper limb with age. Age-related changes in blood pressure are usually considered in terms of systolic and diastolic pressure (see Fig. 14–1, *left*) but would be better considered in terms of changes in mean pressure and pulse pressure.[39, 40] Cardiac output remains constant or falls with age (see Fig. 14–1, *right*), and the increases in mean pressure are attributable to increased resistance due to rarefaction of the peripheral vascular bed consequent on apoptosis of cells and atrophy of organs. Such an explanation was first offered by Mackenzie.[35] Increased pulse pressure is also attributable to arterial stiffening.[3, 9, 12–16, 39, 40] The changes in systolic and diastolic pressure with age in any individual are a consequence of relative change in resistance and stiffness. If stiffness predominates, diastolic pressure will be lower than if resistance predominates.[9, 39, 40]

A mechanism has been proposed to account for the apparent greater value of diastolic pressure over systolic pressure in predicting cardiovascular events according to actuarial data.[4, 16] Actuarial data have come mainly from young people, usually men in their 20s who obtain insurance coverage when joining the workforce. In this age group, systolic pressure in the upper limb is considerably higher than in the ascending aorta and central arteries, as a consequence of wave reflection and wave amplification, whereas diastolic pressure is similar at both sites (see Fig. 14–1, *left*).[4] With aging, the contour of the central pressure wave changes, and amplification decreases, so that values of systolic and diastolic pressure become almost identical

in central and peripheral arteries at age 80 years. If it had been possible to measure central systolic pressure or to predict it from the peripheral waveform, systolic pressure elevation in actuarial studies would likely have had the same significance at all ages, including the elderly, and as robust an association with adverse events as diastolic pressure in the young.

ELASTIC PROPERTIES OF ARTERIES

The arterial media is responsible for the elastic properties of arteries.[3, 4] Three components dominate: elastin lamellae and fibers, collagen fibers, and smooth muscle. Arteries are of three types: the large, predominantly elastic conduit arteries, including the aorta and the brachiocephalic and carotid arteries; the smaller peripheral muscular conduit arteries, such as the brachial, radial, and femoral arteries; and the smallest prearteriolar arteries, which appear to be entirely muscular. The different classes of arteries respond differently to the aging process, to elevation of blood pressure, and to drugs. In the aorta and predominantly "elastic" arteries, smooth muscle appears to have little effect on caliber or distensibility.[4, 41–44] In the large muscular arteries, change in smooth muscle tone induced by neural stimulation, endothelial mechanisms, or drugs can have a substantial effect on caliber and distensibility.[4, 44–47] Vasodilatation is often accompanied by increased distensibility, presumably because of the transfer of tension from collagenous to elastin fibers in the vessel wall.[4] In the smallest prearteriolar vessels, the effects of smooth muscle tone dominate over elastin or collagen fiber. Methods for gauging distensibility of these vessels have not been extensively investigated, but effects of change in smooth muscle tone appear striking.[48–50]

The two-phase (elastin and collagen) content of load-bearing elements in the arterial media is responsible for its behavior under stress.[3, 4, 51] At low pressures, stress is borne almost entirely by the elastin lamellae. With rise in pressure, less extensible collagenous fibers are progressively recruited, and the vessel appears stiffer. Hence, the relationship between pressure and diameter is nonlinear (Fig. 14–3). The artery is more distensible (less stiff) at low distending pressure and less distensible (stiffer) at high distending pressure. At any pressure, distensibility can be determined from the tangent to the pressure-diameter curve.

The smaller muscular peripheral conduit arteries show nonlinear elastic properties similar to those seen in the aorta and carotid arteries, but their elastic properties and caliber are more influenced by smooth muscle. The aorta is little affected by vasodilator mechanisms, and dilatation is always caused by increased distending pressure and almost always associated with increased stiffness. In contrast, the smaller arteries are under the influence of vasodilator mechanisms, and the dilated artery may be more (rather than less) distensible. An association between dilatation and increased distensibility and compliance is seen with a variety of vasodilator drugs[3, 4, 47, 52] and with physical training: The dilated femoral artery of the bicycle athlete[53] and the dilated right brachial artery of the hammer thrower[54] are more compliant than those of normal individuals. The smallest prearteriolar arteries show the relation-

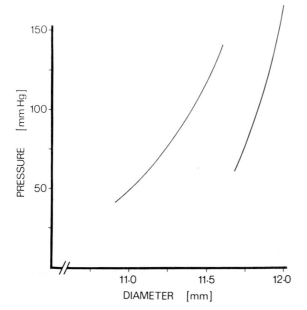

Figure 14–3. Pressure-diameter relationships shown schematically for an elastic artery of a normal subject (left curve) and for an age-matched patient with long-standing hypertension (right curve). (From Nichols WW, O'Rourke MF. McDonald's Blood Flow in Arteries, 4th ed. London, Arnold, 1998.)

ship between dilatation and increased distensibility to an even greater degree. The caliber and distensibility of these arteries are dominated by smooth muscle tone, not by distending pressure.[47–50]

INDICES OF ARTERIAL STIFFNESS

The terms that have been used to quantify arterial elastic properties are summarized in Table 14–1. All are site-specific, and values depend on the mean pressures at which they are calculated. All are affected by vasodilator influences because they are calculated from direct or indirect measures of arterial pressure, diameter, flow, and wall thickness. Ultrasonic and magnetic resonance techniques permit measurements of diameter, wall thickness, and flow to be made noninvasively in humans. Accurate measurement of pressure-diameter amplitude plots and pressure wave contour by applanation tonometry[4, 47] has also contributed. Unfortunately, there has been a profusion of terms, definitions, and units—often confusing and contradictory.[55, 56]

Arterial compliance can be determined by relating the absolute change in diameter of an artery to the imposed pressure step. *Cross-sectional compliance* relates the lumen cross-sectional area to the imposed pressure step. If length is unchanged, this is identical to the volume elastic modulus of the vessel wall. *Compliance* is an absolute term (square centimeters per millimeter of mercury [cm²/mm Hg] or cubic centimeters per millimeter of mercury [cm³/ mm Hg]) that takes into account vessel size as well as stiffness of the arterial wall. Clearly, compliance of large arteries will be greater than compliance of small arteries. Paradoxically, compliance of an abnormal artery (as in

Marfan's syndrome) may be greater than that of a normal artery.[4]

Arterial distensibility is a measure of relative arterial compliance, and it relates relative change in diameter to pressure step in units of inverse millimeters of mercury (mm Hg⁻¹). Arterial distensibility is more appropriate for comparing stiffness of different-sized arteries and of diseased arteries. The dilated aorta in Marfan's syndrome is less distensible, although more compliant, than the normal aorta.

Elastic modulus or *stiffness*[4, 55] can be considered the inverse of arterial distensibility: The greater the modulus, the less extensible (or stiffer) the artery. Young's incremental elastic modulus (E_{inc}) relates elastic modulus to arterial wall thickness and wall tension. It represents the best measure of the intrinsic composition and properties of the wall, although it assumes—incorrectly—that the wall is homogeneous. Peterson's elastic modulus (Ep) is the algebraic inverse of arterial distensibility, relating the change in pressure to a relative change in diameter.[57] Volume (bulk) elastic modulus relates the change in pressure to relative change in vessel volume.

Because all these values are pressure-dependent, attempts are usually made to express them at a given distending pressure and to make comparisons of "isobaric" values. Kawasaki and colleagues[58] and Hirai and coworkers[59] expressed pressure-diameter relationships as a logarithmic β index that behaves, at least to a degree,[55] as though it were pressure-independent.

Pulse wave velocity (PWV) (Fig. 14–4A) is an indirect measure of arterial stiffness and depends on the relationship PWV = $\sqrt{(Eh/2r\rho)}$,[4, 25, 26] where E is Young's modulus of the wall, h is wall thickness, r is vessel radius, and ρ is blood density. PWV is measured from the delay in the foot of the wave (pressure, flow, or diameter) between two sites a known distance apart in the line of pulse travel from the more proximal to the more distal artery. This is a convenient, noninvasive method for use in large arteries, but it depends on an ability to identify the wave foot accurately and on reliably estimating the arterial path length transcutaneously. PWV determinations are more accurate and reproducible when the recording sites are farther from each other.

Characteristic impedance (Z_c) is the ratio of pressure fluctuation to flow fluctuation in an artery when wave reflection is absent.[4] Characteristic impedance, as expressed in terms of flow velocity, is directly related to PWV through the formula $Z_c = \rho(PWV)$.[4] Characteristic impedance is usually determined by averaging values of input impedance at high frequencies. This usually requires invasive measurement of pressure and flow in the aorta, but it has been adapted for noninvasive determination.

The terms *capacitive compliance* and *oscillatory compliance* have been used by Cohn and associates[45, 60, 61] to describe the relationship between blood flow in an artery and the decay of pressure during diastole. These terms hark back to the concept of Grundform and Grundschwingung of the arterial pulse,[4, 62] as introduced by Frank in his analysis of arterial Windkessel behavior. They represent the most recent of many attempts to analyze the diastolic part of the arterial pressure wave to determine total arterial compliance. The practical problem in this type of analysis

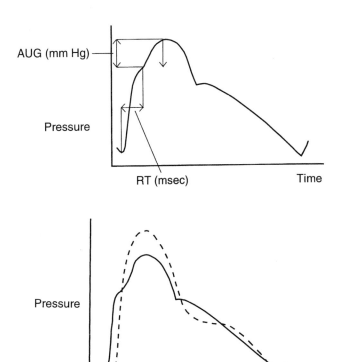

$$PWV = \frac{distance}{\Delta t}$$

Figure 14–4. Calculation of central pressure wave augmentation *(top)* and of pulse wave velocity (PWV) *(bottom)*. Augmentation (AUG) is calculated as the boost in systolic pressure from the early systolic shoulder to the peak of the wave. This may be expressed in millimeters of mercury or as a proportion of pulse pressure or amplitude from the wave foot (diastolic pressure) to the shoulder. PWV is calculated from the delay in wave foot between two sites in the line of travel of the pulse and is expressed in centimeters per second.

is to accurately separate in individual cases the residual oscillations generated by wave reflection from the exponential decline in pressure after cardiac ejection has ceased. Another approach to measurement of total arterial compliances has been described by Liu and colleagues.[63] Both this and Cohn and associates' method require accurate measurement of the arterial pulse wave, preferably in the central aorta, together with cardiac output determination.

Augmentation and *time for return of wave reflection* (see Fig. 14–4A)[4, 64] are simple measures that can be taken from the central arterial pressure wave, as recorded by high-fidelity manometry or tonometry. Both are manifestations of wave reflection. The ability to record both depends on identification of the reflected wave foot on the ascending limb of the central arterial pressure wave. Augmentation is the boost of the central systolic pressure caused by early return of wave reflection and is measured as height of the pressure wave above the systolic shoulder, expressed in millimeters of mercury or as a percentage of pulse pressure. Time for return of wave reflection is the delay between the wave foot and the appearance of this secondary wave. It is a manifestation of PWV, representing the time taken for the pulse wave to travel from the heart to peripheral sites, then to return after reflection.[4]

In the literature, there is no clear consensus on the best indices of arterial stiffness, as summarized in Table 14–1.[4, 45, 55, 56] The indices may appear to move in different directions with different interventions or with disease. In Marfan's syndrome, the diseased aorta has decreased distensibility and is stiffer than normal.[4] But if it is dilated, it may accommodate more blood per unit length for a given increase in pressure and so will appear more compliant.

Vasodilator influences may cause an artery to dilate. Even if distensibility is unchanged, this artery will have greater compliance than under control conditions, for the reason given previously.[45, 65] In hypertension, compliance of peripheral arteries may increase while compliance of central arteries decreases.[3, 66] Although studies of the effect of nitroglycerine on peripheral arteries have shown increases in distensibility, caliber, and compliance, when arterial wall thickness is considered, there may be no change in Young's incremental elastic modulus.[65]

There are other problems with measurements.[67] Pulsatile changes in diameter of an artery are very small and of the same order of magnitude as the spatial resolution of current imaging modalities (e.g., magnetic resonance imaging or B-mode ultrasound), making accurate and reproducible measurements problematic in central vessels.[67] Also, noninvasive measurements of arterial diameter may not address the vessel at right angles, so that the change in diameter of an ellipse is measured. Wall thickness is difficult to measure accurately, and it is impossible to separate the load-bearing media from the non–load-bearing intima with ultrasound. Although in a number of studies, great care has been taken to measure diameter in central vessels, pressure fluctuation has been measured in the brachial artery by sphygmomanometry, so that the effects of pulse wave amplification have been ignored, and pulse pressure has erroneously been taken as identical in all vessels. All these potential confounders must be considered in interpreting the voluminous literature on arterial stiffness. Further problems arise from the interpretation of arterial stiffness in different models of the arterial system.

MODELS OF THE ARTERIAL SYSTEM

"Lumped" Models

The simplest model of the arterial system is the Windkessel (see Fig. 14–2). This is conceptually useful for describing arterial function, but it falls down in practice because it is unrealistic—all arterial elastic properties are not lumped at the one site. The Windkessel can be used to illustrate the effects of aging or of hypertension where a decrease in arterial compliance results in higher pulse pressure for the same stroke volume (Fig. 14–5A). The characteristic feature of the Windkessel—exponential decline in pressure during diastole—is not apparent when blood pressure is normal or low (Fig. 14–5B)[68] and secondary pressure waves become apparent in diastole, indicating the presence of wave reflection. Even when blood pressure is very high, and pressure falls in a nearly exponential fashion during diastole, evidence of wave reflection is apparent as the secondary augmented pressure wave during systole and its

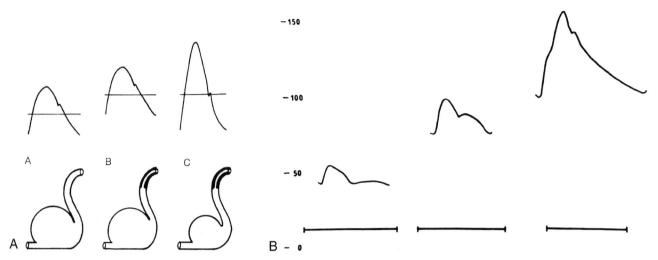

Figure 14–5. A. Effects of increased resistance and decreased compliance on arterial pressure waves (top) in three Windkessel models of the arterial system (bottom).
  A. Normal compliance, normal resistance.
  B. Normal compliance, increased resistance.
  C. Reduced compliance, increased resistance.
Mean pressure is represented by the *solid lines.* **B.** Contour of the pressure wave in the ascending aorta of a rabbit with reduction in arterial pressure (left) and increase in arterial pressure (right). The reflected wave onset normally corresponds with the cardiac incisura. During hypotension, this wave is displaced later in diastole. During hypertension, the wave moves into systole, creating an early systolic shoulder and a late systolic peak, leaving pressure to decay exponentially during diastole. (**A,** From O'Rourke MF. Arterial Function in Health and Disease. Edinburgh, Churchill Livingstone, 1982.

early appearance on the systolic upstroke of the wave (Fig. 14–5*B*).

Despite these problems, total arterial compliance has been used with some success for characterizing arterial properties in humans,[63, 69] whereas the concept of capacitive and oscillatory compliance[60, 61] effects an uneasy compromise between Windkessel and distributed models of the arterial tree. More complex Windkessel models have been described to include the effects of aortic characteristic impedance.[70] Although these can provide impedance data similar to that measured in humans under controlled conditions, they suffer the same restrictions as the simpler model because they cannot account for wave reflection and the substantial effect that wave reflection has on the systolic or diastolic part of the arterial pressure wave under different conditions (see Fig. 14–5*B*).[4]

Distributed Models

The most realistic simple model of the arterial systems is a simple elastic tube with the left ventricle at one end and lumped peripheral resistance at the other (Fig. 14–6).[71] The tube has a finite wave velocity, dependent on elastic characteristics of the wall; wave reflection occurs at the end of the tube as a result of the impedance mismatch between tube and terminal arterioles. This model is a gross simplification of the arterial system. It does not consider anatomical branching reality—especially the difference between reflecting sites in the upper and lower body—and it assumes that reflection arises from the one site. Although a simplification, this model has been very useful.[3, 4] It accounts for the contour of pressure waves in the central

aorta under control conditions and with arterial stiffening, as well as the differences between pressure and flow waves in the central aorta and lower body arteries. It also accounts for the ascending aortic impedance patterns in normal persons and with the arterial stiffening that accompanies aging and hypertension.[3, 4, 68, 71]

In this model, arterial stiffening is represented by increased wall stiffness, which results in increases in aortic characteristic impedance and PWV (Fig. 14–7).[4, 68, 71] Increased characteristic impedance causes aortic pressure to rise to a higher level at the peak of flow ejection from the heart. Increased PWV causes the reflected wave to return earlier, thus to move predominantly from diastole into systole, creating the secondary systolic wave and the discrete shoulder on the systolic upstroke of the wave, leaving pressure to decay almost exponentially during diastole.

This model well represents the whole aorta and arterial system in the trunk and lower limbs—over 80% of the body's bulk. The arterial system of head, neck, and upper limbs contributes little to the pulsatile load of the heart. Wave reflection from the head is presumed low because of the low cerebral vascular resistance.[4] Modeling studies have shown little contribution of upper limb wave reflection to pressure wave patterns in the aorta. However, the upper limb vascular system is extremely important in the measurement of blood pressure at the brachial or radial site. In contrast to the aorta, arteries in the upper limb do not show appreciable stiffening with age[72–74] or hypertension.[4, 66, 74] The upper limb arterial system can be considered as a separate single tube with constant elastic properties that makes no significant contribution to aortic reflection phenomena, aortic pressure wave patterns, or left ventricular load.[4, 47]

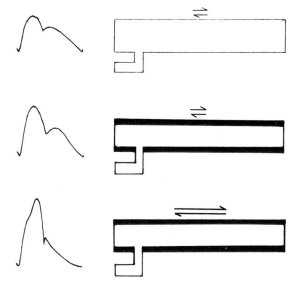

Figure 14–6. Simple tubular models of the systemic arterial system. *Top,* normal distensibility and normal pulse wave velocity. *Middle,* Decreased distensibility but normal pulse wave velocity. *Bottom,* Decreased distensibility with increased pulse wave velocity. At left are the amplitude and contour of pressure waves that would be generated at the origin of these models by the same ventricular ejection (flow) waves. Decreased distensibility per se increases pressure wave amplitude, whereas increased wave velocity causes the reflected wave to return during ventricular systole. (From O'Rourke MF, Avolio AP, Nichols WW. Left ventricular–systemic arterial coupling in humans and strategies to improve coupling in disease states. *In* Yin FCP [ed]. Vascular/Ventricular Coupling. New York, Springer-Verlag, 1987; pp 1–19.)

PATHOPHYSIOLOGICAL IMPLICATIONS OF ARTERIAL STIFFENING

Arterial stiffening increases systolic pressure, decreases diastolic pressure, and increases pulse pressure at any given mean pressure. These effects are opposite to those of arterial counterpulsation,[4] which improves cardiac function (output and metabolic requirement) by reducing systolic pressure while at the same time improving coronary perfusion by increasing pressure throughout diastole, since left ventricular perfusion occurs almost entirely during diastole. In a passive system such as the arterial tree, the best that one can hope for is a minimal rise in pressure during systole and a minimal fall during diastole.[4] An extremely compliant arterial system might be ideal, but there are other biological limitations—including the need for very large arteries and large blood volume.[75]

Studies of pulsatile pressure-flow relationships, of ascending aortic impedance, and of wave reflection provide insight into the biological compromise that has occurred in humans through evolution to achieve nearly optimal interaction between the arterial system and the pulsating heart.[4, 71, 75–77] In young adults, there is nearly optimal interaction. At the normal heart rate and blood pressure, wave reflection returns to the heart after the aortic valve shuts; the incisura (caused by the aortic valve closure) and the foot of the diastolic wave (caused by peripheral wave reflection) occur almost simultaneously. Thus, reflection does not increase left ventricular load, but it does boost

pressure during early diastole, improving coronary perfusion (see Fig. 14–5B).[4, 39] The relationship persists during the tachycardia of exercise. In young human subjects, ascending aortic impedance is extremely low over that frequency range that contains the greatest energy of the ascending aortic flow waveform—during both rest and exercise (see Fig. 14–7).[4, 39, 68]

This nearly optimal ventricular-vascular interaction is progressively distorted by arterial stiffening, as in aging and hypertension. Figure 14–8 shows changes in ascending aortic impedance modulus predicted by an increase in aortic stiffening between ages 20 and 80 years, including doubling of PWV and of aortic characteristic impedance.[4]

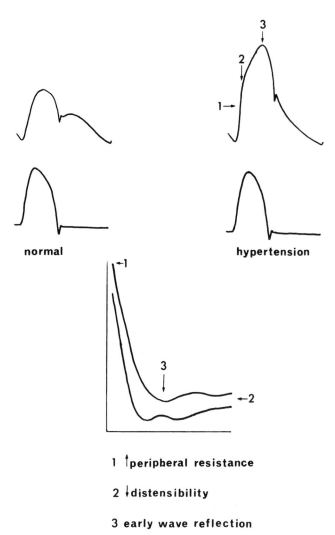

Effects of Hypertension

normal   hypertension

1 ↑peripheral resistance

2 ↓distensibility

3 early wave reflection

Figure 14–7. Effects of hypertension on aortic pressure wave contour (top) and on aortic impedance modulus (bottom). (1) Increased peripheral resistance causes increased mean pressure and an increased zero-frequency component of impedance. (2) Decreased arterial distensibility causes increased amplitude of the initial pressure peak and increased characteristic impedance. (3) Earlier return of reflected waves from arterial terminations causes the late systolic pressure peak and impedance curve to shift to the right. (From O'Rourke MF. Pulsatile arterial haemodynamics in hypertension. Aust N Z J Med 6[suppl 2]:40–48, 1976.)

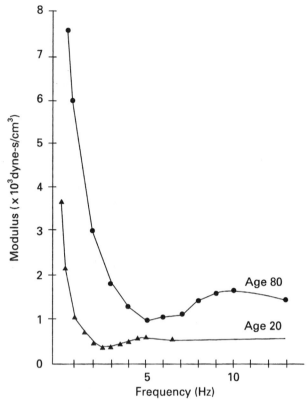

Figure 14–8. Estimated impedance modulus in a typical 20-year-old and a typical 80-year-old human subject, based on a doubling of characteristic impedance and halving of the time for wave reflection over this period. For explanation, see text. (From Nichols WW, O'Rourke MF. McDonald's Blood Flow in Arteries, 4th ed. London, Arnold, 1998.)

The twofold increase in characteristic impedance shifts the curve upward, whereas doubled wave velocity shifts the whole impedance curve to the right. The combined effect is to cause a fourfold increase of impedance at heart frequency and at the frequency of the second and third harmonics—i.e., over the frequency range that contains the greatest energy of the ventricular flow output wave. This should produce a nearly fourfold increase in pulse pressure over this age range, along with a substantial systolic augmentation of the aortic wave. In the Framingham cohort[9] (see Chap. 25, Fig. 25–2) a nearly twofold increase in brachial pulse pressure has been shown between the mid-30s and the early 80s. Allowing for changes over 15 years from ages 20 to 35, and the greater than 50% amplification of the pulse between the aorta and the upper limb arteries in young adults,[4, 16, 78] a nearly fourfold increase in aortic pulse pressure and pulsatile left ventricular load between youth and old age appears likely. Extreme examples of this process are seen in hypertensive subjects, in whom augmentation may exceed 50 mm Hg (Fig. 14–9).[79]

Ill effects of early wave reflection with arterial stiffening usually present as increased left ventricular and aortic pressure during late systole. This increases left ventricular oxygen demands and predisposes to left ventricular hypertrophy with its own multiple ill effects.[2–4] Further, increased pressure in late systole slows left ventricular relaxation[4, 80, 81] and, even in the absence of ventricular hypertrophy,

impairs left ventricular diastolic function. Arterial stiffening also impairs systolic function owing to the negative effect of early wave reflection on the aortic flow wave, tending to cause early deceleration of aortic flow (see Fig. 14–9)[79] and premature termination of ventricular ejection (Fig. 14–10).[4, 82, 83]

The predicted ill effects of arterial stiffening on coronary flow have been demonstrated in experimental animals with and without coronary stenoses and during increased inotropic stimulation.[84–86] In the presence of increased aortic stiffness, coronary occlusion has far greater ill effects on ventricular ejection and pressure generation than under control conditions.[87] Benetos and coworkers,[13] Mitchell and associates,[14] and Safar[16] pointed out the clinical implications of impaired coronary flow in persons with arterial stiffening and low diastolic pressure. The mechanism could well explain the higher cardiac mortality in persons with high pulse pressure in the recent large French and U.S. studies.[13–15] It could also explain why in trials of hypertension—in which persons most at risk of myocardial ischemia because of lower diastolic pressure were excluded—antihypertensive therapy had a greater affect on cerebrovascular than on cardiac events.[16]

ARTERIAL STIFFENING WITH AGE

Aging has a greater effect on arterial stiffening than any other process.[3, 4, 72, 73] The effects of aging are seen almost exclusively in the central elastic arteries, principally the aorta, which also dilates progressively with age.[4, 88] In a normal cohort of subjects in Sydney[88] and Beijing,[72] "aortic" PWV increased twofold between ages 15 and 70 years (Fig. 14–11). Similarity between the two populations despite wide differences in cholesterol level and prevalence of atherosclerosis suggests that this is a true aging change. Comparisons between the Beijing cohort and a cohort in the rural Guondong province of China—where salt intake and prevalence of hypertension are low—showed far less increase in aortic wave velocity in the latter group.[73] These findings suggest that high salt intake and hypertension accelerate the aging process. In a small group of normal Australian subjects, low salt intake was associated with low aortic PWV.[89] In contrast, PWV increases to a far lesser extent in the upper limb vasculature (Fig. 14–11).[72–74, 88] Studies of arterial distensibility have shown the same marked difference between central elastic and peripheral muscular arteries with age.[90]

Other manifestations of arterial stiffening associated with aging include increases in brachial pulse pressure (by 60 to 100% in the Framingham cohort between 35 and 80 years—as compared with a 3 to 10% increase in mean pressure [Fig. 25–2, Chap. 25][9]), together with increases in radial, carotid, and aortic systolic pressure augmentation.[4, 64]

Concomitant increases in diameter[91] and stiffness[72, 73, 88, 90] of elastic arteries with age suggest a common cause. Aging is associated with fracture and fragmentation of the elastin fibers or lamellae within the media.[4, 91] Other remodeling changes—including increases in collagen and glycosaminoglycans—appear to be secondary. It has been suggested that the changes in stiffness and caliber are due to fatigue and fracture of the elastin lamellae, with progres-

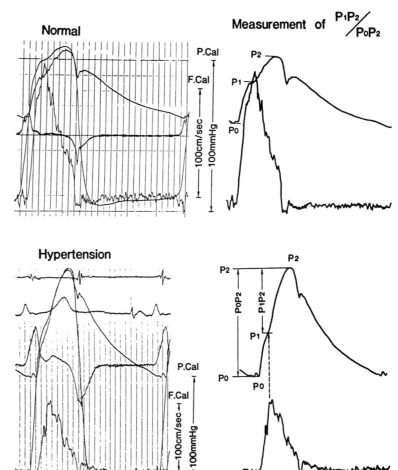

Figure 14–9. Aortic pressure and flow velocity wave shapes in patients with normal blood pressure *(top)* and hypertension *(bottom)*. Reflection wave ratio is calculated as $(P_s - P_i)/(P_s - P_d)$, where P_s = peak systolic pressure, P_i = pressure at peak flow velocity, and P_d = diastolic pressure. Recorded data at left; aortic pressure and flow redrawn at right. P.Cal, pressure calibration; F.Cal, flow calibration. (From Yaginuma T, Noda T, Tsuchiya M, et al. Interaction of left ventricular contraction and aortic input impedance in experimental and clinical studies. Jpn Circ J 49:206–214, 1985.)

sive dilatation of the aorta and recruitment of collagenous fibers within the arterial wall.[4, 39, 68] The inert elastin fibers, whose half-life is measured in decades, fracture after multiple cycles of stretch, like rubber and other elastic materials.[92] Calculations based on the properties of rubber indicate that an elastin fiber, subject to 10% stretch over 800×10^6 cycles (approximately 25 years at heart rate 70/min), will fracture, whereas elastin fibers in a peripheral artery that stretch less than 5% with each cycle will not fracture over 3000×10^6 cycles, i.e., in 100 years. This theory, which is well established in the physical sciences,[92] explains observations for the aorta and central elastic arteries and the differences between the central arteries, where distension in early life is approximately 10% with each heartbeat, and the peripheral muscular arteries, where the pulsatile change in diameter is less than 5%.[4, 90] The theory also explains how damage to the elastic lamellae may be accelerated in aortic coarctation and in some other hypertensive states in which pulsatile aortic strain is increased.[4]

HYPERTENSION

Stiffness and characteristic impedance of the aorta and large elastic arteries increase with elevation in arterial

pressure.[4, 51, 52, 69, 72, 93] In the early stage of hypertension, compliance of peripheral muscular arteries may be paradoxically increased as a result of passive arterial dilatation.[66] Changes are largely due to the physical effect of increased arterial pressure per se (increased stiffness at higher pressure) and are largely reversed by antihypertensive therapy.[4, 47, 93, 94] They are the same changes seen with aging—early return of wave reflection, greater augmentation of the central aortic and carotid pulse, and shift of ascending aortic impedance curves upward and to the right (see Fig. 14–7).[68] Increase in aortic augmentation is associated with increase in height of the secondary systolic pressure wave in the radial artery, causing it to be as high as or higher than the initial pressure peak.[4] This was recognized by Mahomed in his sphygmographic studies of hypertension in 1874 as the most consistent feature of hypertension: "The tidal wave is prolonged and too much sustained."[32]

Arterial stiffening in hypertension may be increased by the structural degeneration caused by prolonged high arterial pressure. Arterial degeneration, medial necrosis, and aneurysm formation are accelerated by hypertension. In conditions such as aortic coarctation and hyperdynamic states, this can be explained on the basis previously proposed for aging change—greater pulsatile strain over hun-

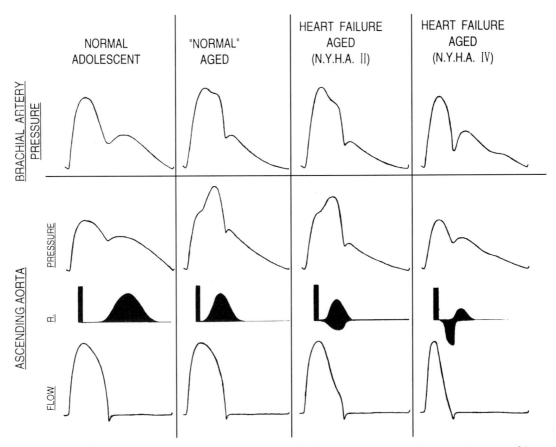

Figure 14–10. Effects of wave reflection on aortic pressure and left ventricular output with the development of heart failure in a patient with isolated systolic hypertension, all shown schematically. *From top,* Brachial artery pressure; aortic pressure; wave reflection (R) with effect on pressure shown as upward deflection and effect on flow as downward deflection; and aortic flow. N.Y.H.A., New York Heart Association. (From O'Rourke MF. Arterial hemodynamics and ventricular-vascular interaction in hypertension. Blood Press 3:33–37, 1993.)

dreds of millions of cycles.[68, 92] Inhomogeneities in the arterial wall—as at bifurcations where a muscular coat is deficient—may allow greater stretch of elastin fibers and predispose to early fracture of elastin fibers and aneurysm formation.[4]

GENDER, HEIGHT, HORMONE REPLACEMENT THERAPY, AND EXERCISE

Gender Differences

As discussed in Chapter 25, pulsatile load created by arterial characteristics is an important determinant of left ventricular mass.[3, 4] Women may therefore be expected to have lower pulsatile loads because of the beneficial vasorelaxant effect of estrogen throughout much of their adult lives. Laogun and Gosling[95] showed that arterial compliance, as determined from PWV, and arterial dimensions closely follow expected life changes, starting low in infants, rising to high levels in youth, and gradually decreasing after age 30 years (Fig. 14–12).[95] Throughout this middle age period, women have higher aortic compliance than men and approach that of men only after the age of menopause. These gender and age differences have been confirmed using a

different noninvasive technique for the distal aorta by Sonesson and coworkers.[96] In a noninvasive longitudinal study, Karpanou and colleagues found that the occurrence of menopause had a marked adverse effect on aortic root function in hypertensive women.[97]

It is surprising, therefore, that with aging, apparently healthy women have been shown to increase left ventricular mass whereas in men left ventricular mass remains unchanged.[98, 99] Both these studies demonstrated a gradual increase in left ventricular mass in women before menopause. It could therefore be argued that the estrogenic vascular effect has little benefit on ventricular-vascular coupling. The answer to this paradox may lie in the analysis of central arterial pressure waveforms. Using arterial applanation tonometry, Hayward and Kelly[100] showed that women have significantly higher augmentation of the central pulse compared with men. Like the left ventricular mass changes, these differences were apparently independent of menopause and began as early as the second decade of life (Fig. 14–13). The sex-related differences may be due, at least in part, to differences in height.

Height

The secondary peak in the central systolic pressure waveform is attributable to wave reflection (see Figs. 14–5

PWV

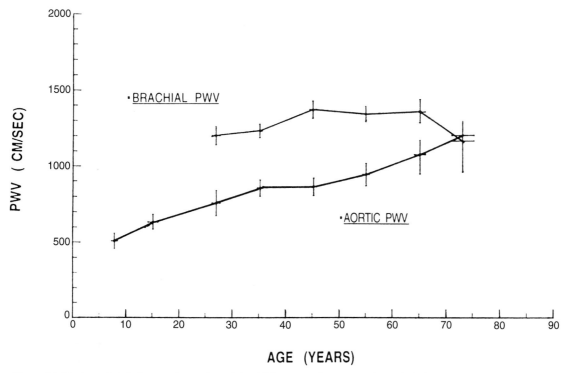

Figure 14–11. Age-related changes in aortic and brachial artery pulse wave velocity (PWV) in an Australian population. Aortic PWV increases with age, whereas brachial artery PWV does not. (From Nichols WW, O'Rourke MF. McDonald's Blood Flow in Arteries, 4th ed. London, Arnold, 1998; adapted from Ho K. Effects of Aging on Arterial Distensibility and Left Ventricular Load in an Australian Community. B.Sc.Med. Thesis, University of New South Wales, Sydney, Australia, 1982.)

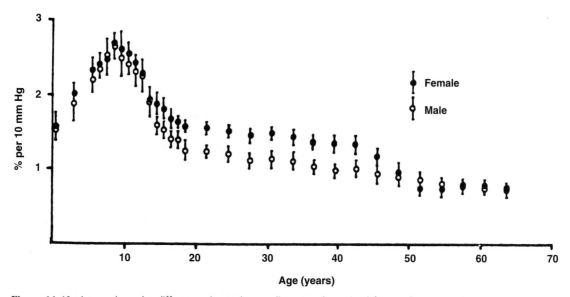

Figure 14–12. Age and gender differences in aortic compliance as determined from pulse wave velocity measured using Doppler flowmeters between the left subclavian artery and abdominal aorta in 600 healthy volunteers. The compliance is expressed per 10 mm Hg pulse pressure (± 1 SD). (From Laogun AA, Gosling RG. In vivo arterial compliance in man. Clin Phys Physiol Meas 3:201–212, 1982.)

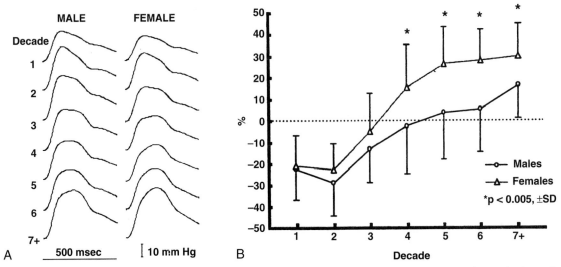

Figure 14–13. A. Calibrated average decade of life waveforms by gender (to scale). **B.** Augmentation index results for each decade of life. Males, *open circles;* females, *open triangles* (± 1 SD). (**A** and **B**, From Hayward CS, Kelly RP. Gender-related differences in the central arterial pressure waveform. Reprinted with permission from the American College of Cardiology [Journal of the American College of Cardiology, 1997, 30:1863–1871.])

through 14–10).[3, 4] A major determinant of wave reflection timing is the distance to reflecting sites. Previous investigators suggested that height is a significant inverse determinant of augmentation due to enhanced wave reflection.[101, 102] Height is significantly different between the sexes from an early age. The Cardiovascular Health Study showed that short stature is associated with concentric left ventricular remodeling, suggesting an important role for wave reflection in pulsatile load.[103] Interestingly, in the Framingham Heart Study, short stature was also associated with increased risk for myocardial infarction in women[104] and, in the second Whitehall study, for coronary events in men.[105]

Syndrome X

Gender differences in arterial function may also be important in the pathogenesis of syndrome X, which is found predominantly in women.[106] Women tend to have a lower subendocardial viability index (ratio of diastolic to systolic tension time indices),[100] which has been shown to correlate with subendocardial blood flow.[4, 13–15, 84–87] This may help to explain the regional hypoperfusion seen on nuclear cardiac scanning and electrocardiographic changes found on stress testing. Stiffening of the aorta predisposes to subendocardial hypoperfusion during increased cardiac workload or stress.[85–87]

Hormone Replacement Therapy

Since only 30% of the decrease in cardiovascular morbidity with hormone replacement after menopause can be attributed to lipid lowering,[106] much research has been directed to nonlipid vascular effects of these hormones. In hypertensive women, menopause is associated with a measurable decrease in aortic root compliance independent of associated changes in lipid status.[97] This finding is consistent with results of a study that demonstrated a measurable

change in PWV in response to hormone replacement therapy (HRT).[107] Such findings are not universal, and a number of studies failed to confirm either a change in arterial stiffness with menopause, as suggested by augmentation index,[100] or a difference between users and nonusers of HRT.[108–110]

The lack of change in arterial PWV with HRT is not inconsistent with a decrease in augmentation index. HRT causes vasodilatation and therefore may be expected to decrease wave reflection.[47] In this way, it may act similarly to other vasodilators such as nitroglycerine.[65, 93, 94] Vasodilators such as HRT that decrease the second systolic pressure peak centrally increase the disparity between central and measured peripheral systolic blood pressure.[4, 47, 111, 112] Office sphygmomanometry, which appears not to be affected by HRT,[113] may therefore underestimate a beneficial effect of HRT on cardiac afterload.

Exercise

Whereas chronic exercise has beneficial effects on arterial function,[114] acute exercise may increase wave reflection and PWV. In an invasive study of normal males,[115] arterial stiffness increased, probably related to the increase in blood pressure, but aortic characteristic impedance was unchanged during acute exercise. This apparent paradox can be explained by the exercise-induced increase in aortic diameter, which offsets the effects of increased stiffness. One effect of exercise is to increase the disparity between central and peripheral arterial pressures.[116] This may lead to an overestimation of myocardial work because the aortic systolic pressure increases far less than the brachial systolic pressure.

ARTERIAL STIFFNESS IN OTHER DISEASES

Adults with cardiovascular risk factors and with conditions such as diabetes mellitus,[117–120] familial hypercholesterolemia,[121] growth hormone deficiency,[122] renal failure,[123] ischemic heart disease[59, 124] and cerebrovascular disease[125] have stiffer arteries than normal healthy control subjects. Significant relationships have also been observed between arterial stiffness and known markers of cardiovascular risk, such as male gender, total cholesterol, low-density lipoprotein cholesterol, and high-density lipoprotein cholesterol levels. Both active and passive smoking have been shown to cause aortic stiffening.[126] Therefore, a considerable body of cohort-based observational data supports the hypothesis that noninvasive measurements of arterial biophysical properties—particularly in the aorta—may provide a marker of vascular risk. For example, patients with type 2 diabetes have stiffer aortas, corresponding to higher PWVs, than nondiabetic subjects.[117–120] The effects of chronic hyperglycemia on nonenzymatic glycosylation of matrix proteins in vivo may, in part, explain this difference. Glycosylation of collagen and elastin and accumulation of advanced glycosylation end-products have been shown to cause vessel stiffening.[127]

In animal[128] and human[129] studies, the atherosclerotic involvement of vessels at postmortem has been closely correlated with arterial stiffness assessed noninvasively just before death. In humans, Hirai and coworkers[59] also showed strong associations between aortic stiffness and the degree of coronary artery disease assessed at coronary angiography. Data support a possible role for arterial stiffness measurements as a noninvasive marker of atherosclerotic load or coronary vascular risk.[130] As highlighted earlier, aortic stiffness is an important determinant of both left ventricular function and coronary blood flow.[82–87] Whereas arterial stiffness measurements in the aorta may provide a marker of vascular change in the coronary vessels, the stiffness of the aorta is also an important determinant of coronary perfusion—becoming even more clinically significant in the presence of coronary artery disease.[84–87]

In diabetes, there appears to be a multiplicative effect of atherosclerosis and vessel stiffening.[131] Among matched groups of patients undergoing coronary artery bypass grafting, diabetic patients had stiffer aortas than did nondiabetic patients.[120] Monnier and associates[132] observed positive relationships between aortic PWV and collagen-linked fluorescence: Aortic PWV was significantly correlated with the severity of diabetic complications, suggesting that such noninvasive measurements may offer an indirect marker of long-term glycemic control. In the Bogalusa Heart Study, children with a positive parental history of diabetes also had stiffer arteries than children without such a parental history,[133] findings that have since been confirmed in healthy young adults with a positive family history of type 2 diabetes.[134]

Diabetes is a much stronger risk factor for ischemic heart disease in women than men. Ryden Ahlgren and colleagues[135] observed stiffer carotid arteries and aortas in women, but not men, with type 1 diabetes compared with gender-matched nondiabetics—results that have since been confirmed in type 2 diabetic patients.[136]

THERAPEUTIC MODIFICATION

When effects of drugs are assessed on all vascular properties, from measurement of central aortic or carotid pressure waveform, therapeutic goals can be set, observed, and achieved. An example is shown in Figure 14–14—the effect of nitroglycerine on measured ascending aortic and brachial pressure waveforms. Central pressure augmentation was reduced by the vasodilator agent to a far greater degree than was brachial systolic pressure. Changes are attributable to reduction in inappropriately early wave reflection from peripheral sites. Findings as clear-cut as this may become more common when information is sought from global, rather than local, effects of a drug.

The complexities in assessment of drug therapies arise

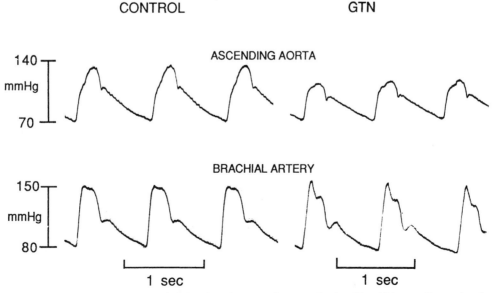

Figure 14–14. Pressure waves recorded directly in the ascending aorta (top) and brachial artery *(bottom)* under control conditions *(left)* and after sublingual nitroglycerin (GTN) 0.3 mg *(right)* in a human adult. (From Kelly RP, Gibbs HH, O'Rourke MF, et al. Nitroglycerin has more favorable effects on left ventricular afterload than apparent from measurement of pressure in a peripheral artery. Eur Heart J 11:138–144, 1990.)

from the difficulties in recording high-fidelity measures of pressure, flow, or diameter at the same or appropriate sites; the alterations in properties of an artery with changes in blood pressure or vasomotor tone; the differences in properties of arteries at different sites; and the different indices that are used for assessment of arterial stiffness, and the way that these (especially distensibility, compliance, and Young's modulus) can change in different directions with alterations in arterial caliber and wall thickness. An additional problem is the difficulty of interpreting direct and indirect effects (directly on the wall or indirectly through change in arterial pressure or vasomotor tone). Finally, many clinicians do not appreciate the subtle differences in effects of drugs on arteries at different sites and on vessels of different caliber.[4, 44, 47]

For example, nitroglycerine has a very powerful effect on muscular arteries, causing dilatation together with increases in distensibility and compliance.[4, 42, 45, 48, 65] Improvement in distensibility is attributable to unloading of collagen fibers in the wall so that the stresses are borne by elastin fibers (Fig. 14–15);[4] improvement in compliance is attributable to this and to increases in arterial caliber.[4, 45, 65] Nitroglycerine causes marked reduction in evidence of wave reflection (see Fig. 14–14) and very substantial reduction in central systolic pressure and left ventricular load. These beneficial effects have been overlooked by clinicians because of the changes that do *not* occur with nitroglycerine, including changes in peripheral resistance[4, 41] and bra-

chial systolic or diastolic pressure (as long as venous return is maintained) (see Fig. 14–14).[111, 112] Further, there is little or no change in aortic characteristic impedance or PWV[41–43] and an apparently minor change in low-frequency components of ascending aortic impedance.[41] These differences are partly due to regional effects of nitroglycerine on arterial smooth muscle—minimal in the aorta, maximal in the small muscular arteries, and minimal in the arterioles.[44, 47] Many clinicians are not aware of the effects of nitroglycerine on muscular arteries (except the coronaries) and consider the drug to be exclusively a coronary artery and venous dilator.

There is even greater confusion concerning the effects of less powerful arterial dilator drugs on arterial stiffness.[49, 94, 137–141] Other nitrates appear to have the same type of action as nitroglycerine, although nitroprusside does have a powerful effect on arterioles and reduces peripheral resistance.[94] Among other drugs, most attention has been directed to angiotensin-converting enzyme inhibitors and calcium channel antagonists.[49, 137–139] With felodipine[140] and diltiazem,[141] reduction in aortic stiffness, independent of blood pressure fall, has been described. We have not been able to confirm this[142] for felodipine. Reduction in muscular artery stiffness has been shown for a number of angiotensin-converting enzyme inhibitors and calcium channel antagonists.[94, 137–142] Studies of ascending aortic impedance have shown evidence of decreased wave reflection with nitroprusside, dobutamine, and nifedipine, as well as nitrates.[4, 47, 94, 138, 143] All vasodilator drugs that decrease stiffness of peripheral arteries also decrease wave reflection and so reduce augmentation of the central aortic left ventricular systolic pressure,[4, 41, 42, 93, 94, 138–143] usually without corresponding reduction of peripheral systolic pressure.[4, 111, 112, 142] As predicted,[83] reduction of early wave reflection in patients with cardiac failure appears to increase flow in late systole and improve stroke volume and cardiac output.[4, 79, 144–146]

SUMMARY

Although the issue of arterial stiffening with age, in hypertension, and in other conditions is very complex, a global overview provides concepts that are basically accurate and useful clinically. The arterial system is best viewed as a simple elastic tube with the left ventricle at one end pumping intermittently and the peripheral resistance at the other end perfused in a continuous fashion. The tube acts as a conduit between heart and periphery and as an elastic cushion as well. With each ventricular ejection, a pressure wave travels from the heart to the periphery, where it is reflected and returns retrogradely to the heart. Wave velocity in the tube and the timing of wave reflection depend on the elastic properties and the length of the tube.

In normal young adults, wave velocity in the aorta is sufficiently low (about 5 m/sec) that the reflected wave returns to the heart just as the aortic valve shuts. Thus, wave reflection occurs only in diastole, where it boosts coronary perfusion. With arterial stiffening, as occurs with aging and in hypertension, wave velocity is increased, so that the reflected wave moves from diastole into systole, causing a boost (augmentation) to late systolic pressure, a

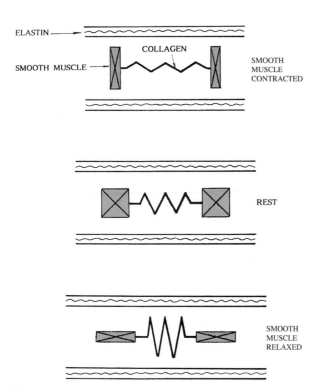

Figure 14–15. A proposed model for the arrangement of collagen, elastin, and smooth muscle in the arterial wall. The muscle is in series with the collagen elements, and both are in parallel with the elastic lamellae. Contraction of muscle transfers stress to the collagenous elements in the wall and renders the wall stiffer, whereas muscular relaxation transfers stresses to the elastic lamellae, making the wall more distensible. (From Nichols WW, O'Rourke MF. McDonald's Blood Flow in Arteries, 4th ed. London, Arnold, 1998.)

greater fall in pressure during diastole, and increased pulse pressure. Ill effects of arterial stiffening are attributable to greater systolic pressure, which increases cardiac metabolic requirements, causes hypertrophy, and predisposes to both systolic and diastolic heart failure. Ill effects are also attributable to lower pressure throughout diastole, which impairs coronary perfusion and predisposes to myocardial ischemia and coronary events.

Arterial stiffening predominantly affects the aorta and large central, elastic arteries. In contrast, most drugs have their greatest effects on peripheral, predominantly muscular arteries. Drugs may appear to have different effects at different sites and even different effects on different indices at the same site. The most important actions of drugs on arterial stiffness are indirect effects on the amplitude and timing of reflected waves. Vasodilator drugs such as nitrates increase caliber and distensibility of peripheral arteries, thus reducing wave reflection from the periphery, so that there is less effect on the heart during systole, a lesser augmentation of pressure during late systole or in heart failure (when contractility is impaired), and increased flow during late systole. Vasodilator drugs also act through reducing mean pressure and PWV, delaying return of wave reflection. Their most pronounced effect, however, is on the amplitude of wave reflection.

References

1. Roy CS. The elastic properties of the arterial wall. J Physiol 3:125–129, 1880.
2. Bramwell JC, Hill AV. Velocity of transmission of the pulse wave and elasticity of arteries. Lancet 1:891–892, 1922.
3. O'Rourke MF. Arterial stiffness, systolic blood pressure, and logical treatment of arterial hypertension. Hypertension 15:339–347, 1990.
4. Nichols WW, O'Rourke MF. McDonald's Blood Flow in Arteries, 4th ed. London, Arnold, 1998.
5. SHEP Cooperative Research Group. Prevention of stroke by antihypertensive drug treatment in older persons with isolated systolic hypertension. JAMA 265:3255–3264, 1991.
6. Kannell WB, Gordon T, Schwartz MJ. Systolic versus diastolic blood pressure and risk of coronary heart disease: The Framingham Study. Am J Cardiol 27:335–346, 1971.
7. Kannel WB, Wolf PA, McGee DL, et al. Systolic blood pressure, arterial rigidity and risk of stroke. The Framingham Study. JAMA 245:1225–1229, 1981.
8. Fisher CM. The ascendancy of diastolic blood pressure over systolic. Lancet 2:1349–1350, 1980.
9. Franklin SS, Gustin W IV, Wong ND, et al. Hemodynamic patterns of age-related change in blood pressure: The Framingham Heart Study. Circulation 96:308–315,1997.
10. MacMahon S, Peto R, Cutler J, et al. Blood pressure, stroke, and coronary heart disease. Part 1: Prolonged differences in blood pressure: Prospective observational studies corrected for the regression dilution bias. Lancet 335:765–774, 1990.
11. Darne B, Girerd X, Safar M, et al. Pulsatile versus steady state component of blood pressure: A cross-sectional analysis and a prospective analysis on cardiovascular mortality. Hypertension 13:392–400, 1989.
12. Madhavan S, Ooi WL, Cohen H, Alderman MH. Relation of pulse pressure and blood pressure reduction to the incidence of myocardial infarction. Hypertension 23:395–401, 1994.
13. Benetos A, Safar M, Rudnichi A, et al. Pulse pressure: A predictor of long-term cardiovascular mortality in a French male population. Hypertension 30:1410–1415, 1997.
14. Mitchell GF, Moye LA, Braunwald E, et al. Sphygmomanometrically determined pulse pressure is a powerful independent predictor of recurrent events after myocardial infarction in patients with impaired left ventricular function. Circulation 96:4254–4260, 1997.
15. Franklin SS, Khan SA, Wong ND, et al. The importance of pulse pressure and systolic blood pressure in predicting coronary heart disease in older adults: The Framingham Study. [Abstract] In Safar ME, London G (eds). Proceedings of the 3rd International Workshop on Structure and Function of Large Arteries. Versailles, January 1998.
16. Safar ME. Roles of systolic and pulse pressures. [Letter to the Editor] Hypertension 30:146–147, 1997.
17. Dustan HP. Isolated systolic hypertension: A long-neglected cause of cardiovascular complications. Am J Med 86:368–369, 1989.
18. Byrom FB, Dodson LF. The mechanism of the vicious circle in chronic hypertension. Clin Sci 8:1–10, 1949.
19. Ledingham JM. The vascular fault in hypertension: Byrom's work revisited. In Laragh JH, Brenner BM (eds). Hypertension: Pathophysiology, Diagnosis and Management, 2nd ed. New York, Raven, 1995; pp 37–53.
20. Harvey W. de Motu Cordis et Sanguinis in Animalibus 1628. William Fitzer Frankfurt. Translated by KJ Franklin. Oxford, Blackwell, 1957.
21. Harvey W. De Circulatione Sanguinis. Translated by KJ Franklin. Oxford: Blackwell 1957.
22. Hales S. 1733. Statical essays containing haemastaticks. History of Medicine Series. Library of New York Academy of Medicine 1964, No. 22. New York, Harper & Row, 1964.
23. Young T. Hydraulic investigations subservient to an intended Croonian lecture on the motion of the blood. Phil Trans Roy Soc (Lond) 98:164–186, 1808.
24. Weber EH, Weber WE. Wellenlehre Leipsig Fleischer, 1825.
25. Moens AI. Die Pulskurve. Leiden, 1878.
26. Korteweg DJ. Über die Fortpflanzungsgeschwindigkeit des Schalles in elastischen Rohren. Ann Physics Chem (NS) 5:52–537, 1878.
27. Navier M. Mem Acad Roy Sci 6:389, 1872. Cited by Rouse II, Ince S (eds). History of Hydraulics. Ames, IA, University of Iowa, 1980.
28. Stokes G. Trans Cambridge Phil Soc, vol 8, 1845. Cited by Rouse II, Ince S (eds). History of Hydraulics. Ames, IA, University of Iowa, 1980.
29. Poiseuille J. Recherches sur la coeur aortique. Arch Gen Med 18:550–554, 1828.
30. Poiseuille J. Recherches experimentales sur le movement des liquides dans les tubes de tres petits diametres. Compt Rend Acad Sci Paris 11:961–967, 1041–1048; 12:112–115, 1840.
31. Bright R. Selected reports of medical cases. London, Longmans, 1827.
32. Mahomed F. The aetiology of Bright's disease and the prealbuminuric stage. Med Chir Trans 57:197–228, 1874.
33. O'Rourke MF. Frederick Akbar Mahomed. Historical perspective. Hypertension 19:212–217, 1992.
34. Swales JD. Early clinical science and the investigation of hypertension: The British experience. Blood Press 5:197–200, 1996.
35. Mackenzie J. Principles of Diagnosis and Treatment of Heart Affections, 2nd ed. London, Frowde, 1917.
36. Mackenzie J. Principles of Diagnosis and Treatment of Heart Affections, 3rd ed. London, Oxford University Press, 1926.
37. Pickering G. High Blood Pressure. London, Churchill, 1968.
38. Smirk FH. High arterial pressure. Oxford, Blackwell, 1957.
39. O'Rourke MF. Arterial function in health and disease. Edinburgh, Churchill Livingstone, 1982.
40. Galarza CR, Alfie A, Waisman G, et al. Diastolic pressure underestimates age-related hemodynamic impairment. Hypertension 30:809–816, 1997.
41. Yaginuma T, Avolio AP, O'Rourke MF, et al. Effects of glyceryl trinitrate on peripheral arteries alters left ventricular hydraulic load in man. Cardiovasc Res 20:153–160, 1986.
42. Fitchett DH, Simkus GJ, Beaudry JP, Marpole DG. Reflected pressure wave in the ascending aorta: Effect of glyceryl trinitrate. Cardiovasc Res 22:494–500, 1988.
43. Carroll JD, Shroff S, Wirth P, et al. Arterial mechanical properties in dilated cardiomyopathy: Aging and the response to nitroprusside. J Clin Invest 87:1002–1009, 1991.
44. Arcaro G, Laurent S, Benetos A, et al. Heterogeneous effect of nitrates on large arteries of hypertensives. J Hypertens 9(suppl 6):S142–S143, 1991.
45. Bank AJ, Wang H, Holte JE, et al. Contribution of collagen, elastin, and smooth muscle to in vivo human brachial artery wall stress and elastic modulus. Circulation 94:3263–3270, 1996.
46. Safar ME, Bouthier JA, Levinson JA, Simon AC. Peripheral large

arteries and the response to antihypertensive treatment. Hypertension 5(suppl III):63–68, 1983.

47. O'Rourke MF, Safar ME, Dzau V (eds). Arterial Vasodilation: Mechanics and Therapy. London, Edward Arnold; Philadelphia, Lea & Febiger, 1992.

48. Westling H, Jansson L, Jonson B, Nilsén R. Vasoactive drugs and elastic properties of human arteries in vivo, with special reference to the action of nitroglycerin. Eur Heart J 5:609–616, 1984.

49. Fitchett DH. Forearm arterial compliance: A new measure of arterial compliance? Cardiovasc Res 18:651–656, 1984.

50. Kawarada A, Shimazu H, Yamakoshi K, Kamiya A. Non-invasive automatic measurement of arterial elasticity in human fingers and rabbit forelegs using photo-electric plethysmography. Med Biol Eng Comput 24:591–596, 1986.

51. Roach M, Burton AC. Reason for the shape of the distensibility curves of arteries. Can J Biochem Physiol 35:681–690, 1957.

52. Safar ME, O'Rourke MF. The Arterial System in Hypertension. Dordrecht, Kluwer, 1994.

53. Kool MJF, Struijker-Boudier HA, Wijnen JA, et al. Effects of diurnal variability and exercise training on properties of large arteries. J Hypertens 10(suppl 6):S49–S52, 1992.

54. Giannattasio C, Cattaneo BM, Mangoli A, et al. Changes in arterial compliance induced by physical training in hammer throwers. J Hypertens 10(suppl 6):S53–S56, 1992.

55. Lehmann ED, Ross JR, Gosling R. Compliance, distensibility, extensibility and "proper" definitions. J Vasc Invest 4:47–52, 1998.

56. O'Rourke MF. Mechanical principles in arterial disease. Hypertension 26:2–9, 1995.

57. Peterson LH, Jensen RE. Mechanical properties of arteries in vivo. Circ Res 8:622–639, 1960.

58. Kawasaki T, Sasayama S, Yagi S, et al. Non-invasive assessment of the age-related changes in stiffness of major branches of the human arteries. Cardiovasc Res 21:678–687, 1987.

59. Hirai T, Sasayama S, Kawasaka T, Yagi S. Stiffness of systemic arteries in patients with myocardial infarction: A noninvasive method to predict severity of coronary atherosclerosis. Circulation 80:78–86, 1989.

60. Cohn JN, Finkelstein SM. Abnormalities of vascular compliance in hypertension, aging and heart failure. J Hypertens 10(suppl):S61–S64, 1992.

61. Cohn JN, Finkelstein SM, McVeigh G, et al. Non-invasive pulse wave analysis for the early detection of vascular disease. Hypertension 26:503–508, 1995.

62. Frank O. Die Theorie der Pulswellen. Z Biol 85:91–130, 1927.

63. Liu Z, Brin KP, Yin FCP. Estimation of total arterial compliance: An improved method and evaluation of current methods. Am J Physiol 250:H588–H600, 1986.

64. Kelly RP, Hayward CS, Avolio AP, O'Rourke MF. Non-invasive determination of age-related changes in the human arterial pulse. Circulation 80:1652–1659, 1989.

65. Bank AJ, Wilson RF, Kubo SH, et al. Direct effects of smooth muscle relaxation and contraction on in vivo human brachial artery elastic properties. Circ Res 77:1008–1016, 1995.

66. Laurent S, Hayoz D, Trazzi S, et al. Isobaric compliance of the radial artery is increased in patients with essential hypertension. J Hypertens 11:89–98, 1993.

67. Lehmann ED, Gosling RG. In vivo determinants of arterial biophysical properties: Methodological considerations. Atherosclerosis 135:263–267, 1997.

68. O'Rourke MF. Pulsatile arterial haemodynamics in hypertension. Aust N Z J Med 6(suppl 2):40–48, 1976.

69. Liu Z, Ting CT, Zhu S, et al. Aortic compliance in human hypertension. Hypertension 14:129–136, 1989.

70. Westerhof NG, Elzinga G, Sipkema P. An artificial arterial system for pumping hearts. J Appl Physiol 31:776–781, 1971.

71. O'Rourke MF, Avolio AP, Nichols WW. Left ventricular–systemic arterial coupling in humans and strategies to improve coupling in disease states. In Yin FCP (ed). Vascular/Ventricular Coupling. New York, Springer-Verlag, 1987; pp 1–19.

72. Avolio AP, Chen S-G, Wang R-P, et al. Effects of aging on changing arterial compliance and left ventricular load in a northern Chinese urban community. Circulation 68:50–58, 1983.

73. Avolio AP, Deng FQ, Li W, et al. Effects of aging on arterial distensibility in populations with high and low prevalence of hypertension: Comparisons between urban and rural communities in China. Circulation 71:202–210, 1985.

74. Gallagher D. Analysis of pressure wave propagation in the human upper limb: Physical determinants and clinical applications. M.D. Thesis, University of New South Wales, Sydney, Australia, 1994.

75. Taylor MG. Wave travel in arteries and the design of the cardiovascular system. In Attinger EO (ed). Pulsatile Blood Flow. New York, McGraw-Hill, 1964; pp 343–372.

76. Milnor WR. Aortic wave length as a determinant of the relationship between heart rate and body size in mammals. Am J Physiol 237:R3–R6, 1979.

77. O'Rourke MF. Commentary on: Aortic wavelength as a determinant of the relationship between heart rate and body size in animals. Am J Physiol 240:R393–R395, 1981.

78. Kroeker EJ, Wood EH. Comparison of simultaneously recorded central and peripheral arterial pressure pulses during rest, exercise and tilted position in man. Circ Res 3:623–632, 1955.

79. Yaginuma T, Noda T, Tsuchiya M, et al. Interaction of left ventricular contraction and aortic input impedance in experimental and clinical studies. Jpn Circ J 49:206–214, 1985.

80. Hori M, Inoue M, Kitakaze M. Loading sequence is a major determinant of afterload-dependent relaxation in intact canine heart. Am J Physiol 249:H747–H754, 1985.

81. Yabe R, Takazawa K, Maeda K, et al. The influence of ascending aortic augmentation index (reflection coefficient) to left ventricular relaxation. Circulation 84:565, 1991.

82. O'Rourke MF. Arterial hemodynamics and ventricular-vascular interaction in hypertension. Blood Press 3:33–37, 1993.

83. Westerhof N, O'Rourke MF. The hemodynamic basis for the development of left ventricular failure in systolic hypertension. J Hypertens 13:943–952, 1995.

84. Buckberg GD, Fisher DE, Archie JP, Hoffman JIE. Experimental subendocardial ischemia in dogs with normal coronary arteries. Circ Res 30:67–81, 1972.

85. Ohtsuka S, Kakihana M, Watanabe H, Sugishita Y. Chronically decreased aortic distensibility causes deterioration of coronary perfusion during increased left ventricular contraction. J Am Coll Cardiol 24:1406–1414, 1994.

86. Watanabe H, Ohtsuka S, Kakihana M, Sugishita Y. Coronary circulation in dogs with an experimental decrease in aortic compliance. J Am Coll Cardiol 21:1497–1506, 1993.

87. Kass D, Saeki A, Tunin RS, Recchia FA. Adverse influence of systemic vascular stiffening on cardiac dysfunction and adaptation to acute coronary occlusion. Circulation 93:1533–1541, 1996.

88. Ho K. Effects of aging on arterial distensibility and left ventricular load in an Australian community. B.Sc.Med. Thesis, University of New South Wales, Sydney, Australia, 1982.

89. Avolio AP, Clyde KM, Beard TC, et al. Improved arterial distensibility in normotensive subjects on a low salt diet. Arteriosclerosis 6:166–169, 1986.

90. Benetos A, Laurent S, Hoeks AP, et al. Arterial alterations with aging and high blood pressure: A noninvasive study of carotid and femoral arteries. Arterioscler Thromb 13:90–97, 1993.

91. Mitchell JRA, Schwartz CJ (eds). Arterial Diseases. Oxford, Blackwell, 1965.

92. Sandor B. Fundamentals of Cyclic Stress and Strain. Madison, University of Wisconsin, 1972.

93. Merillon JP, Fontenier GH, Lerallut JF, et al. Aortic input impedance in normal man and arterial hypertension: Its modification during changes in aortic pressure. Cardiovasc Res 16:646–656, 1982.

94. Yin FCP, Guzman PA, Brin KP, et al. Effects of nitroprusside on hydraulic vascular loads on the right and left ventricles of patients with heart failure. Circulation 67:1330–1339, 1983.

95. Laogun AA, Gosling RG. In vivo arterial compliance in man. Clin Phys Physiol Meas 3:201–212, 1982.

96. Sonesson B, Hansen F, Stale H, Lanne T. Compliance and diameter in the human abdominal aorta—The influence of age and sex. Eur J Vasc Surg 7:690–697, 1993.

97. Karpanou EA, Vyssoulis GP, Papakyriakou SA, et al. Effects of menopause on aortic root function in hypertensive women. J Am Coll Cardiol 28:1562–1566, 1996.

98. Shub C, Klein AL, Zachariah PK, et al. Determination of left ventricular mass by echocardiography in a normal population: Effect of age and sex in addition to body size. Mayo Clin Proc 69:205–211, 1994.

99. Dannenberg AL, Levy D, Garrison RJ. Impact of age on echocardiographic left ventricular mass in a healthy population (The Framingham Study). Am J Cardiol 64:1066–1068, 1989.

100. Hayward CS, Kelly RP. Gender-related differences in the central arterial pressure waveform. J Am Coll Cardiol 30:1863–1871, 1997.

101. Marchais SJ, Guerin AP, Pannier BM, et al. Wave reflections and cardiac hypertrophy in chronic uremia: Influence of body size. Hypertension 22:876–883, 1993.

102. London GM, Guerin AP, Pannier B, et al. Influence of sex on arterial hemodynamics and blood pressure. Role of body height. Hypertension 26:514–519, 1995.

103. Gottdiener JS, Shemanski L, Aurigemma GP, et al. Short stature is associated with concentric LV remodelling in the elderly: The Cardiovascular Health Study. Circulation 94:1–26, 1996.

104. Kannam JP, Levy D, Larson M, Wilson PWF. Short stature and risk for cardiovascular mortality and cardiac disease events: The Framingham Heart Study. Circulation 90:2241–2247, 1994.

105. Marmot MG, Bosma H, Hemingway H, et al. Contribution of job control and other risk factors to social variations in coronary heart disease incidence. Lancet 350:235–239, 1997.

106. Kaski JC, Rosano GMC, Collins P, et al. Cardiac syndrome X: Clinical characteristics and left ventricular function. Long term follow up study. J Am Coll Cardiol 25:807–814, 1995.

107. Rajkumar C, Kingwell BA, Cameron JD, et al. Hormonal therapy increases arterial compliance in postmenopausal women. J Am Coll Cardiol 30:350–356, 1997.

108. Hayward CS, Knight DC, Wren BG, Kelly RP. Effect of hormone replacement therapy on noninvasive cardiovascular haemodynamics. J Hypertens 15:987–993, 1997.

109. Giraud GD, Morton MJ, Wilson RA, et al. Effects of estrogen and progestin on aortic size and compliance in postmenopausal women. Am J Obstet Gynecol 174:1708–1718, 1996.

110. Lehmann ED, Hopkins KD, Parker JR, et al. Aortic distensibility in postmenopausal women receiving Tibolone. Br J Radiol 67:701–705, 1994.

111. Kelly RP, Gibbs HH, O'Rourke MF, et al. Nitroglycerin has more favorable effects on left ventricular afterload than apparent from measurement of pressure in a peripheral artery. Eur Heart J 11:138–144, 1990.

112. Takazawa K, Tanaka N, Takeda K, et al. Underestimation of vasodilator effects of nitroglycerin by upper limb blood pressure. Hypertension 26:520–523, 1995.

113. Lip GYH, Beevers M, Churchill D, Beevers DG. Hormone replacement therapy and blood pressure in hypertensive women. J Hum Hypertens 8:491–494, 1994.

114. Vaitkevicius PV, Fleg JL, Engel JH, et al. Effects of age and aerobic capacity on arterial stiffness in adults. Circulation 88:1456–1462, 1993.

115. Murgo JP, Westerhof N, Giolma JP, Altobelli SA. Effects of exercise on aortic input impedance and pressure wave forms in normal humans. Circ Res 48:334–343, 1981.

116. Rowell LV, Brengelmann GL, Blackmon JR, et al. Disparities between aortic and peripheral pulse pressures induced by upright exercise and vasomotor changes in man. Circulation 37:954, 1968.

117. Lehmann ED, Gosling RG, Sönksen PH. Arterial wall compliance in diabetes. Diabet Med 9:114–119, 1992.

118. Lehmann ED, Hopkins KD, Gosling RG. Aortic compliance measurements using Doppler ultrasound: In vivo biochemical correlates. Ultrasound Med Biol 19:683–710, 1993.

119. Salomaa V, Riley W, Kark JD, et al. Non–insulin dependent diabetes mellitus and fasting glucose and insulin concentrations are associated with arterial stiffness indexes. The ARIC Study. Circulation 91:1432–1443, 1995.

120. Airaksinen KEJ, Salmela PI, Linnaluoto MK, et al. Diminished arterial elasticity in diabetes: Association with fluorescent advanced glycosylation end products in collagen. Cardiovasc Res 27:942–945, 1993.

121. Lehmann ED, Watts GF, Gosling RG. Aortic distensibility and hypercholesterolaemia. Lancet 340:1171–1172, 1992.

122. Lehmann ED, Hopkins KD, Weissberger AJ, et al. Aortic distensibility in growth hormone deficient adults. Lancet 341:309, 1993.

123. London GM, Marchais SJ, Safar ME, et al. Aortic and large artery compliance in end-stage renal failure. Kidney Int 37:137–142, 1990.

124. Bogren HG, Mohiaddin RH, Klipstein RK, et al. The function of the aorta in ischemic heart disease: A magnetic resonance and angiographic study of aortic compliance and blood flow patterns. Am Heart J 118:234–247, 1989.

125. Lehmann ED, Hopkins KD, Jones RL, et al. Aortic distensibility in patients with cerebrovascular disease. Clin Sci 89:247–253, 1995.

126. Stefanadis C, Tsiamis E, Vlachopoulos C, et al. Unfavorable effect of smoking on the elastic properties of the human aorta. Circulation 95:31–38, 1997.

127. Chappey O, Dosquet C, Wautier M-P, Wautier J-L. Advanced glycation end products, oxidant stress and vascular lesions. Eur J Clin Invest 27:97–108, 1997.

128. Farrar DJ, Bond G, Riley WA, Sawyer JK. Anatomic correlates of aortic pulse wave velocity and carotid artery elasticity during atherosclerosis progression and regression in monkeys. Circulation 83:1754–1763, 1991.

129. Wada T, Kodaira K, Fukishiro K, et al. Correlation of ultrasound-measured common carotid artery stiffness with pathological findings. Arterioscler Thromb 14:479–482, 1994.

130. Hopkins KD, Lehmann ED, Gosling RG. Aortic compliance measurements: A non-invasive indicator of atherosclerosis? Lancet 343:1447, 1994.

131. Lehmann ED, Riley WA, Clarkson P, Gosling RG. Non-invasive assessment of cardiovascular disease in diabetes mellitus. Lancet 350(suppl 1):14–19, 1997.

132. Monnier VM, Vishwanath V, Frank K, et al. Relation between complications of type 1 diabetes mellitus and collagen-linked fluorescence. N Engl J Med 314:403–408, 1986.

133. Riley WA, Freedman DS, Higgs NA, et al. Decreased arterial elasticity associated with cardiovascular disease risk factors in the young. Bogalusa Heart Study. Arteriosclerosis 6:378–386, 1986.

134. Hopkins KD, Lehmann ED, Jones RL, et al. A family history of NIDDM is associated with decreased aortic distensibility in normal healthy young adult subjects. Diabetes Care 19:501–503, 1996.

135. Ryden Ahlgren A, Länne T, Wollmer P, et al. Increased arterial stiffness in women, but not in men, with IDDM. Diabetologia 38:1082–1089, 1995.

136. Lehmann ED, Hopkins KD, Gosling RG. Increased aortic stiffness in women with NIDDM. Diabetologia 39:870–871, 1996.

137. Benetos A, Lafleche A, Asmar R, et al. Arterial stiffness, hydrochlorothiazide and converting enzyme inhibition in essential hypertension. J Hum Hypertens 10:77–82, 1996.

138. Ting CT, Chen CH, Chang MS, et al. Short- and long-term effects of antihypertensive drugs on arterial reflections, compliance, and impedance. Hypertension 26:524–530, 1995.

139. Ting CT, Chen CH, Chang MS, et al. Arterial hemodynamics in human hypertension: Effects of the calcium channel antagonist nifedipine. Hypertension 25:1326–1332, 1995.

140. Asmar RG, Benetos A, Chaouche-Teyara K, et al. Comparison of effects of felodipine versus hydrochlorothiazide on arterial diameter and pulse-wave velocity in essential hypertension. Am J Cardiol 72:794–798, 1993.

141. Stefanidis C, Dernellis J, Vlachopoulos C, et al. Aortic function in arterial hypertension determined by pressure-diameter relation: Effects of diltiazem. Circulation 96:1853–1858, 1997.

142. O'Rourke MF, Avolio AP, Lee L, Set al. Reduction of wave reflection is the principal beneficial action of felodipine in isolated systolic hypertension. Am J Hypertens 10:3–4A, 1997.

143. Binkley PF, Van Fossen DB, Nunziata E, et al. Influence of positive inotropic therapy on pulsatile hydraulic load and ventricular/vascular coupling in congestive heart failure. J Am Coll Cardiol 15:1127–1135, 1990.

144. Miyashita H, Ikeda U, Tsuruya Y, et al. Non invasive evaluation of the influence of aortic wave reflection on left ventricular ejection and auxotonic contraction. Heart Vessels 60:1–10, 1993.

145. Maruyama Y, Nishioka O, Nozaki E, et al. Effects of arterial distensibility on left ventricular ejection in the depressed contractile state. Cardiovasc Res 27:182–187, 1993.

146. Sakai T, Takazawa K, Fujita M, et al. Changes in flow velocity pattern in the left ventricular outflow tract before and after administration of nitroglycerin as assessed by Doppler echocardiography. J Cardiol 23(suppl 37):25–33, 1993.

CHAPTER

15 Endothelin in Hypertension

John C. Burnett, Jr.

Increasing evidence supports the concept that both primary and secondary forms of hypertension are linked to neurohumoral factors. The activation of neurohumoral factors can be viewed as a beneficial protective response, as in the case of the natriuretic peptides, which serve to oppose vasoconstriction and sodium retention as well as to oppose hypertrophic stimuli. In contrast, the renin-angiotensin system plays a primary role in forms of hypertension that are linked to renal etiologies. Here, angiotensin II participates in hypertension and its complications through sodium retaining (directly and via aldosterone), vasoconstricting, and growth-promoting properties. Indeed, the growing awareness of these neurohumoral systems has laid the foundation for modern pharmacological therapy in hypertension which directly antagonizes receptor-activated neurohumoral pathways or indirectly reverses adverse consequences of maladaptive humoral stimulation.

In 1988, Yanagisawa and coworkers reported the existence of a new peptide, which they called endothelin (ET) (Fig. 15–1). Three isoforms were reported (i.e., ET-1, -2, and -3); ET-1 is the most relevant to human biology and disease, as its gene and mature peptide are readily detected in humans, and it mediates diverse actions, which are discussed later.[2, 3] ET-1 exists as a 22 amino acid peptide, the product of a well-defined prohormone (proET-1) which is processed to an intermediate peptide Big ET-1 and then by a least two ET-converting enzymes to ET-1.[4, 5] The potential importance of ET-1 in cardiovascular biology and disease was suggested by its production in endothelial cells

and its potent vasoconstricting properties.[1, 6] Its importance in hypertension is supported by its plasma and tissue activation in some forms of hypertension and the ability to lower arterial pressure in human hypertension with ET receptor antagonists.[7, 8] This chapter reviews the biology of ET-1 and its receptors as well as its potential role in the pathophysiology and therapeutics of hypertension.

BIOLOGICAL ACTIONS OF ET-1

Vascular Actions

The hallmark of ET-1's actions is vasoconstriction, with an increase in arterial pressure (Fig. 15–2). In the seminal report by Yanagisawa, bolus administration of ET-1 in the rat resulted in a marked hypertensive response that was sustained.[1] In isolated porcine coronary arteries, ET-1 produced dose-dependent and sustained vasoconstriction. In other animal preparations, exogenous ET-1 produced marked increases in systemic and regional vascular resistances, often in association with decreases in cardiac output, the latter thought to be related, in part, to myocardial ischemia secondary to intense coronary vasoconstriction (Fig. 15–3).[5, 9] ET-1 was even more constricting in isolated veins compared to arteries, in part secondary to the reduced presence of nitric oxide (NO) in veins.[10]

More recently, the role of ET-1 as a vasoconstrictor and regulator of arterial pressure was elegantly demonstrated in studies in which the ET-1 gene was transferred by

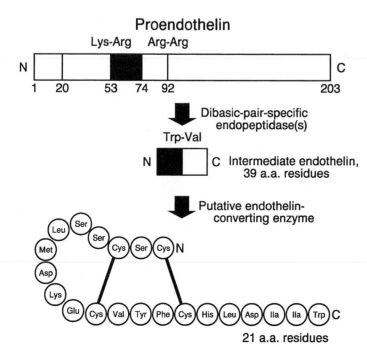

Figure 15–1. Formation of endothelin-1 (ET-1). Proendothelin (ProET) is produced from a messenger RNA template as a 203 amino acid (a.a.) protein. Initial cleavage to an intermediate peptide, Big ET-1, is then followed by cleavage to the active ET-1 by an endothelin-converting enzyme. Arg, arginine; C, carboxyl terminal; Lys, lysine; N, amino terminal; Trp, tryptophan; Val, valine. (From Yanagisawa M, Kunhara H, Kimura S, et al. A novel potent vasoconstrictor peptide produced by vascular endothelial cells. Nature 332:411–415, 1988.)

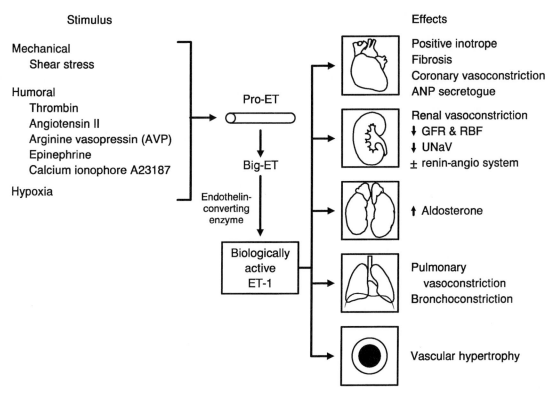

Figure 15–2. Summary of stimuli for ET-1 secretion and biological actions on specific organ systems. ANP, atrial natriuretic peptide; GFR, glomerular filtration rate; RBF, renal blood flow; UNaV, urinary sodium volume.

adenoviral gene delivery into normal rats.[11] In these studies, the transfer of the ET-1 gene resulted in an increase in arterial pressure that could be reversed by ET receptor blockade. Such vasoconstrictor responses have not been limited to animal models or tissues. Administration of ET-1 or Big ET-1 to normal humans results in potent and reversible vasoconstrictor responses. Infusion of exogenous ET-1 has been reported to produce significant coronary vasoconstriction in humans, supporting a role for ET-1 as an important potential mediator of myocardial ischemia in states of ET-1 activation, as in atherosclerosis.[12, 13] Such

vasoconstricting actions may be most important in the presence of a deficiency of counter-regulatory humoral factors such as NO, as in some forms of hypertension. Thus, the vasoconstricting action in vivo of ET-1 probably reflects not simply a direct action of ET-1 but rather the balance between ET-1 and NO. This concept has been underscored by the report that inhibition of NO in vivo markedly potentiates the coronary, renal, pulmonary, and systemic vasoconstricting and hypertensive responses to exogenous ET-1 administered at pathophysiological concentrations.[14]

Figure 15–3. Change from baseline in diastolic pressure in patients with mild to moderate hypertension assigned to receive placebo, bosentan, or enalapril. MAP, mean arterial pressure; CO, cardiac output; SVR, systemic vascular resistance. (Data from Krum H, Viskoper RJ, Lacourcière Y, et al, for the Bosentan Hypertension Investigators. The effect of an endothelin receptor antagonist, bosentan, on blood pressure in patients with essential hypertension. N Engl J Med 338:784–790, 1998.)

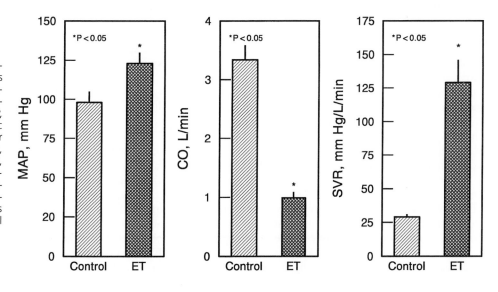

ET-1 also promotes growth of the vascular wall and has been thought to mediate vascular wall hypertrophy in states such as hypertension. This effect on vascular hypertrophy is most evident in studies in isolated vascular smooth muscle cells.[15] In such preparations, ET-1 may increase protein synthesis in vascular smooth muscle and result in cellular hypertrophy. Such actions can be reversed by ET receptor blockade or by counter-regulatory humoral factors such as atrial natriuretic peptide (ANP).

Renal Actions

The kidney has emerged as being central in the biology of ET-1. Studies have established that the renal circulation may be more sensitive than others in terms of vasoconstrictor responsiveness to ET-1.[5] ET-1 administered at concentrations that mimic those observed in pathophysiological states results in renal vasoconstriction in association with a decrease in sodium excretion.[16] These renal actions in dogs and humans appear to be mediated by the ET-A receptor (see under ET Receptors).[16, 17] More recently, in elegant studies in which ET-1 has been overexpressed locally in the kidney, glomerular sclerosis and reductions in the glomerular filtration rate, interstitial fibrosis, and cyst formation were observed,[18] suggesting a role for ET-1 in the pathogenesis of renal disease.

These studies are complemented by evidence that ET-1 administration to normal humans also produces renal vasoconstriction and sodium retention.[19] As in the animal studies, these actions of ET-1 were attenuated by ET-A receptor antagonism.[16] These renal actions have prompted studies to determine whether ET-1 has a potential role in renal disease. Such a role is supported by increased renal production of ET-1 in disease models such as acute and chronic renal failure, as well as by reports of increased urinary ET-1 in models of renal transplant rejection and contrast nephropathy.[20–23] Thus, ET-1 is an important modulator of renal function and may participate in the pathophysiology of renal diseases that are associated with elevations in arterial pressure.

Myocardial Actions

An important target for the actions of ET-1 is the heart. ET-1 has been reported to have positive inotropic actions in isolated cardiomyocytes and in the intact heart.[24, 25] Such actions may be offset by coronary vasoconstriction and myocardial ischemia, but the autocrine/paracrine action of endogenous ET-1 may be to augment myocardial contractility. In states of depressed ventricular function such as heart failure, blockade of excessive ET-1 stimulation of the heart restores the cardiac responsiveness to exogenous ET-1, but this action may be related to a greater peripheral vasodilator response rather than to a direct cardiac depressor response to the ET-1 blocker.[26–28]

ET-1 may also have growth-promoting effects on ventricular myocytes and cardiac fibroblasts. In an animal model of ventricular hypertrophy produced by pressure overload of the left ventricle, blockade of ET-1 resulted in a decrease in ventricular hypertrophy independent of any reductions in cardiac afterload.[29] In isolated cardiac fibroblasts, ET receptors are expressed and may be activated by other humoral factors such as angiotensin II.[30] Once activated, ET-1 may serve as a mediator for production of collagen and thus induce cardiac fibrosis and impair myocardial relaxation.

Humoral Actions

ET-1 has important interactions with other neurohumoral systems. Being of endothelial cell origin, ET-1 interacts importantly with NO via activation of the ET-B receptor (see later section), which is expressed in vascular endothelium. ET-1 thus releases NO, underscoring the unique balance between these two humoral pathways that mediate divergent actions on underlying vascular smooth muscle. ET-1 also releases other vasodilating humoral factors of endothelial cell origin, such as C-type natriuretic peptide (CNP) and adrenomedullin.[31, 32] In addition, the production and release of ANP are linked to ET-1.[33, 34]

An important synergism exists between angiotensin II (Ang II) and ET-1. Ang II may enhance the vascular responsiveness to a given concentration of ET-1.[35] Studies have also demonstrated that many of the myocardial actions of Ang II may occur via ET-1. Specifically, Ang II–mediated myocardial hypertrophy may involve activation of an ET receptor subtype or activation of myocardial ET-1 production or both.[36] Further, Ang II is a potent stimulus for ET-1 gene expression in isolated cultured cardiac fibroblasts.[37] It is not surprising that inhibition of Ang II generation may therefore inhibit the tissue activation of ET-1. Clavell and coworkers reported that activation of circulating and tissue ET-1 in a model of heart failure could be markedly attenuated by chronic angiotensin-converting enzyme inhibition (ACEI).[38] The latter observation supports the view that some of the actions of ACEI could occur through inhibition of ET-1 synthesis.

An additional key action of ET-1 involves stimulation of the synthesis and release of aldosterone. Studies in isolated zona glomerulosa cells have reported that ET-1 is a potent activator of aldosterone synthesis.[39] This action appears to involve activation of the ET-B receptor. The recent report that the aldosterone system coexists with ET-1 in the heart,[40] along with the known action of aldosterone on myocardial fibrosis, underscores the importance of exploring the emerging relationship between the ET-1 system and aldosterone.

ET RECEPTORS

The diverse biological actions of ET-1 are mediated by at least two receptor subtypes (Table 15–1), including the ET-A and ET-B receptors. The ET-A receptor is widely expressed and is the principal receptor for the ET system in vascular smooth muscle. The ET-A receptor possesses high affinity for ET-1 compared to ET-3. ET-A receptor activation results in vasoconstriction via activation of phospholipase C and an increase in intracellular calcium.[41] The ET-B receptor was initially thought to be expressed only in vascular endothelial cells and to release vasodilating

Table 15–1 Endothelin Receptor Characterization

Receptor	ET$_A$	ET$_B$	
Agonist potency	ET-1 > ET-2 ›› ET-3	ET-1 = ET-2 = ET-3	
Tissue	Vascular smooth muscle, cardiomyocytes	Vascular smooth muscle	Endothelium
Action	Constriction, inotropism, mitogenesis	Constriction	Dilatation
Selective agonists	None	ET-3 Sarafotoxin S6c	
Selective antagonists	BQ-123 FR-139317 ABT-167 LU-135252	BQ-788 RES-701-1	
Nonselective antagonists	Bosentan TAK-044 SB-209670 CGS-27830 PD-PD145065		

substances such as NO and prostacyclin as well as the newly identified vasodilating peptide adrenomedullin. More recent studies have demonstrated expression of the ET-B receptor in other vascular tissues, such as the aorta, pulmonary vasculature, and coronary circulation.[42] ET-B expression may be dynamic and regulated by the concentration of other humoral factors, such as Ang II and CNP.[43, 44] Further, ET-B expression may also be linked to pathophysiological states in which the endothelium is damaged.[45]

In addition to mediating vasorelaxation through the release of endogenous vasodilators, a vasoconstricting role for ET-B receptor activation has been reported in vitro, and studies suggest that ET-B receptor blockade may be necessary to reverse all of the vasoconstricting actions of ET-1.[46] Specifically, ET-A receptor antagonism with the selective ET-A receptor antagonist BQ-123 has been shown in vitro to incompletely inhibit the actions of ET-1. Furthermore, Fukuroda et al demonstrated in vitro that the combination of a selective ET-B antagonist, BQ-788, with BQ-123 produced a synergistic inhibition of ET-1–mediated vasoconstriction.[47] In vivo, Leadly et al demonstrated in normal dogs a mild vasoconstrictor response to low doses of the selective ET-B receptor agonist Sarafotoxin S6c, with increases in peripheral but not renal vascular resistance.[48] In contrast, Haynes et al reported that selective ET-B receptor activation with S6c resulted in significant vasoconstriction in the human forearm.[49]

The ET-B receptor has both direct vasoconstricting actions in isolated vessels and the ability to cause vasoconstriction indirectly by increasing endogenous ET-1 secretion, resulting in ET-A receptor activation. Specifically, in vitro studies demonstrate that the ET-B receptor upregulates the preproET-1 gene, with increased ET-1 secretion from cultured endothelial and mesangial cells and cardiac myocytes.[50, 51] Such an action could represent an essential mechanism of ET-B receptor–mediated vasoconstriction via local activation of the ET-A receptor. Rasmussen et al have recently demonstrated that ET-B receptor activation mediates systemic and pulmonary vasoconstriction, with decreases in cardiac output and SV$_{O_2}$.[52] Although selective ET-A receptor blockade attenuated the systemic vasoconstrictor action of high-dose S6c, the latter study provided

evidence that dual ET-A and ET-B receptor antagonism attenuated the potent cardiovascular actions of the ET-B receptor. The cardiopulmonary protective properties of ET-B receptor blockade may represent an important therapeutic strategy in states of ET-1 activation. Of concern, however, is the observation that the ET-B receptor may also serve as a clearance receptor and that blockade of ET-B could enhance circulating concentrations of ET-1 during dual receptor inhibition.[53] Clearly, additional studies will be required to address the role of the ET-B receptor in the presence and absence of cardiovascular disease to complement the well-documented vasoconstricting action of the ET-A receptor.

An additional concept is emerging in our understanding of the ET receptor as it relates to Ang II. In vitro studies have advanced the concept that the ET and angiotensin receptors form a common receptor family and that both peptides may be capable of dual activation or that a single dual receptor exists that may bind both peptides.[54, 55] These data may explain the difficulty in fully attenuating the deleterious actions of ET-1 or Ang II with a single receptor antagonist. The basis of the concept of a possible dual ET and Ang II receptor is a theory that predicts that binding sites of peptide hormones and binding sites of their receptors were originally encoded by complementary strands of genomic DNA. The expression of the ET-1/Ang II receptor mRNA in brain and heart tissues supports this intriguing concept.

ACTIVATION AND ROLE OF THE ET SYSTEM IN HYPERTENSION

The potent vasoconstricting and growth-promoting properties of ET-1 have suggested a potential role for ET-1 in the pathogenesis of hypertension. Circulating ET-1 is not usually increased in hypertension and any observed elevations are small and usually related to renal dysfunction.[56–60] In contrast, circulating ET-1 is markedly increased in humans with hemangioendothelioma and also in humans with severe forms of transplant-related hypertension.[61, 62] Plasma ET-1 is also increased in several models of experimental hypertension, including mineralocorticoid hypertension, the spontaneously hypertensive rat, and renovascular hypertension.[63–65] The lack of increase of plasma ET-1 in hypertension could be explained by the paracrine/autocrine function of ET-1. Such a view is supported by studies that establish that ET-1 secretion from the endothelial cell is albuminally directed, thus increasing tissue and not circulating concentrations of ET-1.[66]

As discussed above, overexpression of ET-1 by gene transfer techniques has resulted in transient increases in plasma ET-1 with associated hypertension.[11] Further, ET-1 synthesis has been shown to be increased in the vascular wall of the mineralocorticoid model of hypertension in the rat.[64] A correlation has been reported between the magnitude of vascular wall hypertrophy and ET-1 gene expression in this model of hypertension. However, this positive correlation is offset by an attenuated vascular responsiveness to exogenous ET-1, suggesting receptor downregulation.

In studies in human hypertension, the vasoconstricting responsiveness to ET-1 has been reported to be enhanced. ET-1 infusion has been shown to result in an enhanced vasoconstrictor response in the hand veins of human hypertensives.[67] This was in contrast to no difference in the response to alpha receptor stimulation and in basal plasma ET-1 concentration between hypertensive and normotensive individuals.

Hypertension in association with chronic renal disease is a common finding, and it may contribute to further renal damage as well as to an acceleration of atherosclerosis and ventricular dysfunction. Plasma and renal ET-1 have been reported to be enhanced in experimental models of chronic renal failure.[68] Further, ET receptor antagonists in experimental models of chronic renal dysfunction have resulted in a lowering of arterial pressure in association with reductions in renal glomerular sclerosis and proteinuria.

The systemic vasoconstriction that accompanies congestive heart failure (CHF), a disease state that is often the consequence of hypertension, is also linked to an activated ET-1 system. In experimental and human CHF, plasma and local tissue ET-1 are increased and correlate with the magnitude of ventricular dysfunction.[69–71] In both humans and animal models of CHF, ET receptor antagonism results in decreases in arterial pressure and systemic vascular resistance.[26, 28] Most recently, ET receptor antagonism in experimental CHF has also resulted in an improvement in survival, underscoring a recurrent theme that ET-1 plays a pathophysiological role in CHF.[29]

To date, the most convincing data to support a role for ET-1 in the pathophysiology of hypertension comes from a key investigation of the blood pressure response to chronic oral dual ETA and ETB receptor blockade in humans with essential hypertension.[8] The availability of nonpeptidergic, orally active ET receptor antagonists has permitted long-term administration and thus critical assessment of the contribution of ET-1 to cardiovascular disease states. Krum and coworkers reported the effect of the dual ET receptor antagonist bosentan on blood pressure and cardiovascular neurohumoral status in patients with essential hypertension treated with it for 4 weeks, compared to the effects of treatment with placebo or ACEI. Compared with placebo, bosentan resulted in significant reductions in diastolic pressure at doses ranging from 500

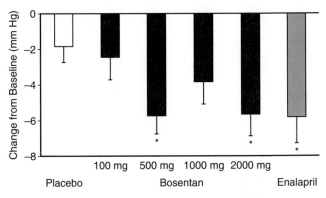

Figure 15–4. Mean ($\pm$ SE) change from baseline in diastolic pressure in patients with mild-to-moderate hypertension assigned to receive placebo, bosentan (100, 500, 1000, or 2000 mg daily), or enalapril (20 mg daily). Measurements were made while the patients were sitting upright. Asterisks denote $p < .05$ for the comparison with placebo. $p = .02$ by the trend test for the comparison of the four doses of bosentan. (Data from Krum H, Viskoper RJ, Lacourciere Y, et al. The effect of an endothelin-receptor antagonist, bosentan, on blood pressure in patients with essential hypertension. Bosentan Hypertension Investigators. N Engl J Med 338:784–790, 1998.)

to 2000 mg daily (Fig. 15–4). ET receptor blockade resulted in an absolute blood pressure decrease of 5.7 mm Hg at both the low- and the high-dose ranges, similar to the response to ACEI. No changes in heart rate were observed. Bosentan did not result in activation of the sympathetic nervous system, as determined by measurement of plasma norepinephrine, or of the renin-angiotensin system, as determined by measurement of plasma renin activity and Ang II. This report, therefore, demonstrates that long-term treatment with an ET receptor antagonist in patients with mild to moderate hypertension results in significant reductions in blood pressure compared to placebo, suggesting that ET-1 contributes to blood pressure elevation in human essential hypertension. This investigation lays the foundation for consideration of ET receptor antagonism as a potential therapeutic strategy in the treatment of human hypertension.

CONCLUSIONS

Hypertension continues to emerge as a disorder that has a genetic basis but is the result of additional primary and secondary mechanisms. The lack of adequate treatment strategies underscores our lack of understanding of the mechanisms responsible for the elevation of blood pressure and its complications, including stroke, myocardial infarction, and heart failure. A neurohumoral basis for hypertension is supported by studies of humans with hypertension, of their offspring, and of experimental models.

ET-1, a peptide primarily of endothelial origin, may play a key role. It possesses many of the properties that result not only in increased arterial pressure but also in the multiorgan complications of this disease process. The elevation of blood pressure with genetic overexpression of ET-1 by gene transfer and the lowering of blood pressure with ET receptor antagonism in humans with essential hypertension provide the rationale for aggressively examining the fundamental contribution of this peptide to this disease process.

References

1. Yanagisawa M, Kunhara H, Kimura S, et al. A novel potent vasoconstrictor peptide produced by vascular endothelial cells. Nature 332:411–415, 1988.
2. Haynes WG, Webb DJ. The endothelin family of peptides: Local hormones with diverse roles in health and disease? Clin Sci (Colch) 84:485, 1993.
3. Wei C-M, Lerman A, Rodeheffer R, et al. Endothelin in human congestive heart failure. Circulation 89:1580–1586, 1994.
4. Takahashi M, Fukuda K, Shimada K, et al. Localization of rat endothelin-converting enzyme to vascular endothelial cells and some secretory cells. Biochem J 311:657–665, 1995.
5. Grantham JA, Schirger JA, Williamson EE, et al. Enhanced endothelin-converting enzyme immunoreactivity in early atherosclerosis. J Cardiovasc Pharmacol 31:S22–S26, 1998.
6. Yokokawa K, Kohno M, Yasunari K, et al. Endothelin-3 regulates endothelin-1 production in cultured human endothelial cells. Hypertension 18:304–315, 1991.
7. Khraibi AA, Heublein DM, Knox FG, Burnett Jr JC. Increased plasma level of endothelin-1 in the Okamoto spontaneously hypertensive rat. Mayo Clin Proc 68:1–5, 1993.
8. Krum H, Viskoper RJ, Lacourcière Y, et al for the Bosentan Hypertension Investigators. The effect of an endothelin receptor antagonist, bosentan, on blood pressure in patients with essential hypertension. N Engl J Med 338:784–790, 1998.
9. Miller WL, Redfield MM, Burnett JC Jr. Integrated cardiac, renal, and endocrine actions of endothelin. J Clin Invest 83:317, 1989.
10. Moreland S, McMullen DM, Delaney CL, et al. Venous smooth muscle contains vasoconstrictor ET-B–like receptors. Biochem Biophys Res Commun 184:100–106, 1992.
11. Niranjan V, Telemaque S, deWit D, et al. Systemic hypertension induced by hepatic overexpression of human preproendothelin-1 in rats. J Clin Invest 98:2364–2372, 1996.
12. Pernow J, Kaijser J, Lennart L, et al. Comparable potent coronary constrictor effects of endothelin-1 and big endothelin-1 in humans. Circulation 94:2077–2082, 1996.
13. Lerman A, Edwards BS, Hallett JW, et al. Circulating and tissue endothelin immunoreactivity in advanced atherosclerosis. N Engl J Med 325:997–1011, 1991.
14. Lerman A, Sandok EK, Hildebrand FL Jr, Burnett JC Jr. Inhibition of endothelium-derived relaxing factor enhances endothelin-mediated vasoconstriction. Circulation 85:1894–1898, 1992.
15. Alberts GF, Peifley KA, Johns A, et al. Constitutive endothelin-1 overexpression promotes smooth muscle cell proliferation via an external autocrine loop. J Biol Chem 269:10112–10118, 1994.
16. Clavell AL, Stingo AJ, Margulies KB, et al. Role of endothelin receptor subtypes in the in vivo regulation of renal function. Am J Physiol 268:F455–F460, 1995.
17. Karet FE, Davenport AD. Endothelin and the human kidney: A potential target for new drugs. Nephrol Dial Transplant 9:465–468, 1994.
18. Hocher B, Rohmeiss P, Thone-Reineke C, et al. Endothelin 1-transgenic mice develop glomerulosclerosis, interstitial fibrosis and renal cysts, but not hypertension. J Clin Invest 99:1380–1389, 1997.
19. Rabelink TJ, Kaassjager KAH, Boer P, et al. Effects of endothelin-1 on renal function in humans: Implications for physiology and pathophysiology. Kidney Int 46:376–378, 1994.
20. Shibouta Y, Suzuki N, Shino A, et al. Pathophysiological role of endothelin in acute renal failure. Life Sci 46:1611–1618, 1990.
21. Benigni A, Zola C, Corna D, et al. Blocking both type A and B endothelin receptors in the kidney attenuates renal injury and prolongs survival in rats with remnant kidney. Am J Kidney Dis 27:416–423, 1996.
22. Textor SC, Burnett JC Jr, Romero C, et al. Urinary endothelin and renal vasoconstriction with cyclosporine or FK506 after liver transplantation. Kidney Int 47:1426–1433, 1995.
23. Margulies KB, Hildebrand FL, Heublein DM, et al. Radiocontrast increases plasma and urinary endothelin. J Am Soc Nephrol 2:1041–1045, 1991.
24. Ishikawa T, Yanagisawa M, Kimura S, et al. Positive inotropic actions of novel vasoconstrictor peptide on guinea pig atria. Am J Physiol 255:H970–H973, 1988.
25. Sakai S, Miyauchi T, Saruta T, et al. Endogenous endothelin-1 participates in the maintenance of cardiac function in rats with congestive heart failure. Circulation 93:1214–1222, 1996.
26. Borgeson DD, Grantham JA, Williamson EE, et al. Chronic oral endothelin type A receptor antagonism in experimental heart failure. Hypertension 31:755–770, 1998.
27. Spinale FG, Walker JD, Mukherjee R, et al. Concomitant endothelin receptor subtype-A blockade during progression of pacing-induced congestive heart failure in rabbits. Circulation 95:1918–1929, 1997.
28. Kiowski W, Sutsch G, Hunziker P, et al. Evidence for endothelin-1 mediated vasoconstriction in severe chronic heart failure. Lancet 346:732–736, 1995.
29. Sakai S, Miyauchi T, Kobayashi M, et al. Inhibition of myocardial endothelin pathway improves long-term survival in heart failure. Nature 384:353–355, 1996.
30. Fujisaki H, Ito H, Hirata Y, et al. Natriuretic peptides inhibit angiotensin II-induced proliferation of rat cardiac fibroblasts by blocking endothelin-1 gene expression. J Clin Invest 96:1059–1065, 1995.
31. Kullo IJ, Burnett JC Jr. C-type natriuretic peptide: The vascular component of the natriuretic peptide system. In Sowers JR (ed). Contemporary Endocrinology: Endocrinology of the Vasculature. Humana, 1996; pp 79–93.
32. Jougasaki M, Schirger JA, Simari RD, Burnett JC Jr. Autocrine role for the endothelin-B receptor in the secretion of endothelial-derived adrenomedullin. Hypertension (in press).
33. Thibault G, Doubell AF, Garcia R, et al. Endothelin-stimulated secretion of natriuretic peptides by rat atrial myocyte is mediated through endothelin-A receptors. Circ Res 74:460–474, 1994.
34. Skvorak JP, Nazian SJ, Dietz JR. Endothelin acts as a paracrine regulator of stretch-induced atrial natriuretic peptide release. Am J Physiol 269:R1093–R1098, 1995.
35. Yang Z, Richard V, von Segesser L, et al. Threshold concentrations of endothelin-1 potentiate contractions to norepinephrine and serotonin in human arteries: A new mechanism for vasospasm? Circulation 82:188–195, 1990.
36. Ito H, Hirata Y, Adachi S, et al. Endothelin-1 is an autocrine/paracrine factor in the mechanism of angiotensin II-induced hypertrophy in cultured rat cardiomyocytes. J Clin Invest 92:398–403, 1993.
37. Fareh J, Touyz RM, Schiffrin EL, Thibault G. Endothelin-1 and angiotensin II receptors in cells from rat hypertrophied heart, receptor regulation and intracellular Ca^{2+} modulation. Circ Res 78:302–311, 1996.
38. Clavell A, Mattingly M, Nir A, et al. Angiotensin-converting enzyme inhibition modulates circulating tissue endothelin in chronic canine thoracic inferior vena cava constriction. J Clin Invest 97:1286–1292, 1996.
39. Silvestre J-S, Robert V, Heymes C, et al. Myocardial production of aldosterone and corticosterone in the rat. J Biol Chem 273:4883–4891, 1998.
40. Cozza EN, Gomez-Sanchez CE, Foecking MF, et al. Endothelin binding to cultured calf adrenal glomerulosa cells and stimulation of aldosterone secretion. J Clin Invest 84:1032–1035, 1989.
41. Simonson MS, Herman WH. Protein kinase C and protein tyrosine kinase activity contribute to mitogenic signaling by endothelin-1: Cross-talk between G protein-coupled receptors and pp60^{c-src}. J Biol Chem 268:9347–9357, 1993.
42. Sumner MJ, Cannon TR, Mundin JW, et al. Endothelin ET$_A$ and ET$_B$ receptors mediate vascular smooth muscle cell contraction. Br J Pharmacol 107:858, 1992.
43. Kanno K, Hirata Y, Tsujino M, et al. Up-regulation of ET$_B$ receptor subtype mRNA by angiotensin II in rat cardiomyocytes. Biochem Biophys Res Commun 194:1282–1287, 1993.
44. Eguchi S, Hirata Y, Imai T, Marumo F. C-type natriuretic peptide upregulates vascular endothelin type B receptors. Hypertension 23:936–940, 1994.
45. Wang X, Feuerstein GZ, Ohlstein EH. Temporal expression of ECE-1, ET-1, ET-3, ET$_A$ and ET$_B$ receptor mRNAs after balloon angioplasty in the rat. J Cardiovasc Pharmacol 26:S22–S25, 1995.
46. Haynes WF, Strachan FE, Webb DJ. Endothelin ET-A and ET-B receptors mediate vasoconstriction of human resistance and capacitance vessels in vivo. Circulation 92:357–363, 1995.
47. Fukuroda T, Ozaki S, Ihara M, et al. Synergistic inhibition by BQ-123 and BQ-788 of endothelin-1-induced contractions of the rabbit pulmonary artery. Br J Pharmacol 113:336–338, 1994.
48. Leadly RJ Jr, Zhu JL, Goetz KL. Effects of endothelin-1 and Sarafotoxin S6b on regional hemodynamics in the conscious dog. Am J Physiol 260:R1210–R1217, 1991.

49. Haynes WG, Webb DJ. Endothelium-dependent modulation of responses to endothelin-1 in human veins. Clin Sci 84:427, 1993.
50. Iwasaki S, Homma T, Matsuda Y, Kon V. Endothelin receptor subtype-B mediates autoinduction of endothelin-1 in rat mesangial cells. J Biol Chem 270:6997–7003, 1995.
51. Saijonmaa O, Nyman T, Fryhrquist F. Endothelin-1 stimulates its own synthesis in human endothelial cells. Biochem Biophys Res Commun 188:286–291, 1992.
52. Rasmussen TE, Jougasaki M, Supaporn T, et al. Cardiovascular actions of ET-B activation in vivo and modulation by receptor antagonism. Am J Physiol 274:R131, 1998.
53. Fukuroda T, Fujikawa T, Ozaki S, et al. Clearance of circulating endothelin-1 by ET-B receptors in rats. Biochem Biophys Res Commun 199:1461–1465, 1994.
54. Dascal D, Nirula V, Lawus K, et al. Shared determinants of receptor binding for subtype selective, and dual endothelin-angiotensin antagonists on the AT_1 angiotensin II receptor. FEBS Lett 423:15–18, 1998.
55. Ruiz-Opazo N, Hirayama K, Akimoto K, Herrera VLM. Molecular characterization of a dual endothelin-1/angiotensin II receptor. Mol Med 4:96–108, 1998.
56. Saito Y, Nakao K, Mukoyama M, Imura H. Increased plasma endothelin level in patients with essential hypertension. N Engl J Med 322:205, 1990.
57. Kohno M, Yasunari K, Murakaw KL, et al. Plasma immunoreactive endothelin in essential hypertension. Am J Med 88:614, 1990.
58. Florijn KW, Derkx FHM, Visser W, et al. Plasma immunoreactive endothelin-1 in pregnant women with and without preeclampsia. J Cardiovasc Pharmacol 17(suppl 7):S446–S448, 1991.
59. Kohno M, Murakawa K, Horio T, et al. Plasma immunoreactive endothelin-1 in experimental malignant hypertension. Hypertension 18:93–100, 1991.
60. Cacoub P, Dorent R, Maistre G, et al. Endothelin-1 in primary pulmonary hypertension and the Eisenmenger syndrome. Am J Cardiol 72:448–450, 1993.
61. Yokokawa K, Tahara H, Kohno M, et al. Hypertension associated with endothelin secreting malignant hemangioendothelioma. Ann Int Med 114:213–215, 1991.
62. Lerman A, Click RL, Narr BJ, et al. Elevation of plasma endothelin associated with systemic hypertension in humans following orthotopic liver transplantation. Transplantation 51:646–650, 1991.
63. Schiffrin EL, Larivière R, Li J-S, et al. Deoxycorticosterone acetate plus salt induce overexpression of vascular endothelin-1 and severe vascular hypertrophy in spontaneously hypertensive rats. Hypertension 25:769–773, 1995.
64. Larivière R, Thibault G, Schiffrin EL. Increased endothelin-1 content in blood vessels of deoxycorticosterone acetate-salt hypertensive but not spontaneously hypertensive rats. Hypertension 21:294–300, 1993.
65. Fujita K, Matsumura Y, Kita S, et al. Role of endothelin-1 and the ET_A receptor in the maintenance of deoxycorticosterone acetate-salt-induced hypertension. Br J Pharmacol 114:925–930, 1995.
66. Wagner OF, Christ G, Wojta J, et al. Polar secretion of endothelin-1 by cultured endothelial cells. J Biol Chem 267:16066–16068, 1992.
67. Haynes WG, Davenport AP, Webb DJ. Endothelin: Progress in pharmacology and physiology. Trends Pharmacol Sci 14:225–228, 1993.
68. Orisio S, Benigni A, Bruzzi I, et al. Renal endothelin gene expression is increased in remnant kidney and correlates with disease progression. Kidney Int 43:354–358, 1993.
69. Rodeheffer RJ, Lerman A, Heublein D, Burnett Jr JC. Increased plasma concentrations of endothelin in congestive heart failure in humans. Mayo Clin Proc 67:719–724, 1992.
70. McMurray JJ, Ray SG, Abdullah I, et al. Plasma endothelin in chronic heart failure. Circulation 85:1374, 1992.
71. Cody RJ, Haas GJ, Binkley PF, et al. Plasma endothelin correlates with the extent of pulmonary hypertension in patients with chronic congestive heart failure. Circulation 85:504–509, 1992.

16 Nitric Oxide in Hypertension*

CHAPTER

Julio A. Panza

ENDOTHELIAL REGULATION OF VASCULAR TONE

The critical role of the vascular endothelium in modulation of the contractile state of the underlying smooth muscle was not fully realized until the publication of the seminal article by Furchgott and Zawadzki.[1] They observed that rings and strips of rabbit aorta precontracted with norepinephrine would respond with relaxation to increasing doses of acetylcholine (ACh) only if care had been taken to preserve the integrity of the endothelial lining. In contrast, when the endothelial cells were denuded by either rubbing or collagenase infusion, the response to ACh was either loss of relaxation or vasoconstriction. In the same article, Furchgott and Zawadzki[1] described their "sandwich" experiments, in which a strip of aorta without endothelium was bathed together with another strip with preserved endothelial lining. When ACh was infused in the bath, they observed that the preparation without endothelium showed relaxation similar to that of the preparation that had intact endothelial lining. These findings led to the postulation of a substance released by endothelial cells that was capable of diffusing to act on the vessel without endothelium. Although the authors could not establish the chemical structure of this substance, they coined it *endothelium-derived relaxing factor*.[1] Subsequently, agents other than ACh were shown to exert differential effects on blood vessels depending on the presence or absence of endothelium.[2] These agents, including serotonin, bradykinin, substance P, histamine, and norepinephrine, have been collectively known as *endothelial agonists*.

Although these agonists trigger endothelial release of relaxing factor(s), it is now clear that the regulatory action of the endothelium on the underlying smooth muscle is exerted through the synthesis and release of a variety of factors—some producing relaxation of the smooth muscle to cause vasodilation, others producing contraction with a corresponding increase in vascular resistance. The factors produced by the endothelium have a wide variety of chemical structures, from small molecules such as nitric oxide and oxygen free radicals, to lipid-based substances such as prostanoids and adhesion molecules, to peptides and proteins such as endothelin and growth factors. These endothelium-derived factors have contrasting effects on the contractile activity of the vascular smooth muscle and also interact with one another at different levels, producing a very complex endothelial regulation of vascular tone.[3, 4] The balance between the biological action of vasodilators

*All material in this chapter is in the public domain, with the exception of any borrowed figures or tables.

and that of vasoconstrictors determines the resulting contractile state of smooth muscle cells. The regulation of vascular tone is also importantly modified by other endothelium-independent processes, including the reactivity of vascular smooth muscle to agonists acting on its cell surface membrane, and by other systemic phenomena such as sympathetic activity, central nervous system activation, and the actions of hormones such as angiotensin II, adrenomedullin, and atrial natriuretic peptide.

VASCULAR BIOLOGY OF NITRIC OXIDE

Principal among the substances released by the endothelium to regulate vascular tone is nitric oxide, which is formed by the enzyme nitric oxide synthase (NOS) from the amino acid L-arginine.[5, 6] At least three forms of NOS have been described: neuronal NOS or NOS I existing only in the neural cells; inducible NOS (iNOS) or NOS II that can be activated by leukotrienes and cytokines to produce large amounts of nitric oxide for a relatively long period of time; and endothelial NOS (eNOS) or NOS III that produces nitric oxide constantly to maintain vascular tone. NOS III can be further stimulated by a variety of agonists. The endothelial constitutive form of NOS, in the presence of nicotinamide adenine dinucleotide phosphate, reduced form (NADPH), Ca^{2+}/calmodulin, and tetrahydrobiopterin, oxidizes L-arginine to form nitric oxide and L-citrulline.[7] This activity of NOS can be inhibited by endogenous analogues of L-arginine such as asymmetric dimethylarginine,[8] which has been shown to be increased in patients with chronic renal failure[9] and in animal models of hypercholesterolemia.[10]

Nitric oxide released by the endothelium stimulates soluble guanylate cyclase in the underlying smooth muscle. This results in elevation of intracellular levels of cyclic guanosine monophosphate with consequent vascular relaxation. The critical role of nitric oxide in the regulation of vascular tone has been shown in a variety of investigational settings. For example, mice with a knockout for the eNOS gene have increased vascular resistance with elevated systemic blood pressure.[11] Similarly, animals treated with N^G-monomethyl L-arginine (L-NMMA), an exogenous competitive inhibitor of NOS, also have elevated blood pressure.[12] In humans, it was first demonstrated by Vallance and colleagues[13] that administration of L-NMMA into the forearm circulation causes an increase in vascular resistance with consequent reduction in forearm blood flow. This observation indicates that, under normal circumstances, there is basal release of nitric oxide that is critical for the maintenance of vascular tone. Further, L-NMMA significantly blunts the response to ACh but not to nitrovasodilators in normal subjects,[13] indicating that the vasodilator effect of ACh is at least partly mediated by the stimulated release of nitric oxide.

Nitric oxide regulates vascular homeostasis by other mechanisms as well.[14] For example, nitric oxide reduces monocyte and leukocyte adhesion to endothelial cells and is an important inhibitor of platelet aggregability and platelet–vessel wall interaction. Nitric oxide decreases endothelial permeability and thus diminishes the transport of lipoproteins into the vessel wall and suppresses vascular smooth muscle proliferation and migration both in vitro and in vivo. All of these processes are important for the development of atherosclerosis, and their inhibition by nitric oxide has suggested that this molecule is one of the principal endogenous antiatherosclerotic substances produced by the cardiovascular system.

ENDOTHELIAL DYSFUNCTION IN CARDIOVASCULAR DISEASE

The significance of the endothelium in the regulation of cardiovascular homeostasis has been underscored by the discovery of impaired endothelial function in several forms of cardiovascular disease, including atherosclerosis, congestive heart failure, and pulmonary hypertension. One of the most common tests performed in clinical investigations of endothelial function is the assessment of vascular responses to ACh (an endothelium-dependent vasodilator) and sodium nitroprusside (a direct nitric oxide donor producing endothelium-independent vasodilatation). With the use of this test, impaired endothelium-dependent vascular relaxation was first demonstrated in patients with coronary atherosclerosis by Ludmer and coworkers.[15] Although assessment of endothelium-dependent and -independent vasodilatation refers only to the endothelial regulation of vascular tone, patients with atherosclerosis also have other endothelium-related abnormalities such as increased platelet aggregability, increased levels of cell adhesion molecules, and decreased fibrinolysis.

Endothelial dysfunction has also been demonstrated in conditions associated with premature development of atherosclerosis, the so-called risk factors. Hypertension,[16–20] hypercholesterolemia,[21–24] diabetes,[25, 26] smoking,[27–31] and aging[32] adversely affect endothelium-dependent vasodilation. This effect has been demonstrated at the level of both large-conductance arteries and small-resistance arterioles. Although the processes leading to endothelial dysfunction in these conditions are not known, it is plausible that the mechanisms contributing to this vascular abnormality are not the same for each condition. One could postulate the existence of a "syndrome of endothelial dysfunction" in which, regardless of the specific disease causing impaired endothelial physiology, there would be a final common consequence—the development of atherosclerosis. Thus, endothelial dysfunction could constitute a pathophysiological link between epidemiologically proven risk factors and the development of atherosclerosis.

Identification of the mechanisms of endothelial dysfunction may lead to the development of specific forms of treatment that could result in reversal of endothelial dysfunction. This, in turn, could lead to amelioration of the developing atherosclerotic process. Lipid-lowering therapy has been shown to improve endothelial vasodilator function in patients with coronary atherosclerosis.[33, 34] This could explain the beneficial effect of this treatment in patients with coronary artery disease. Similarly, the results of the Trial on Reversing Endothelial Dysfunction (TREND) study[35] suggest that enhancement of endothelial vasodilator function with the angiotensin-converting enzyme (ACE) inhibitor quinapril explains the improvement in prognosis of patients with myocardial infarction with this form of therapy. Several trials currently under way will establish the role of ACE inhibition in reversing endothelial dysfunction and improving the prognosis of patients with atherosclerosis.[36]

ENDOTHELIAL DYSFUNCTION IN HYPERTENSION

Initial studies showed impaired endothelium-dependent vasodilatation of large and small arteries in animal models of hypertension.[37–41] Subsequent investigations extended these findings to hypertensive patients. Several independent groups of investigators have demonstrated that patients with hypertension have impaired endothelium-dependent vasodilatation to ACh,[16–20] in both the peripheral and the coronary circulations. The response to the endothelium-independent agent sodium nitroprusside is not reduced, clearly demonstrating that the ability of vascular smooth muscle to respond to nitric oxide is preserved in these patients. Further, the blunted response of hypertensive patients to ACh is not related to presynaptic inhibition of norepinephrine release because α-blockade with phentolamine does not modify the response to ACh, nor does it diminish the difference in the response to endothelium-dependent vasodilatation between normotensive and hypertensive subjects.[16]

Impaired endothelium-dependent vascular relaxation has also been reported in patients with secondary hypertension.[42] A recent study assessing the vascular responses of human subcutaneous arteries in vitro has demonstrated that impaired endothelium-dependent vasodilatation is independent of the cause of hypertension.[43] There does not appear to be a relationship between the degree of alteration in vascular structure and endothelium-mediated responses.[43]

It is uncertain whether endothelial dysfunction is a primary or a secondary phenomenon in the hypertensive process. Studies have shown that elevation of blood pressure can cause endothelial dysfunction, as demonstrated by impaired responses to ACh in vessels from animals with induced coarctation of the aorta.[44] These observations suggest that endothelial dysfunction can be secondary to hypertension. On the other hand, Taddei and associates[45] showed that normotensive offspring of hypertensive parents have impaired endothelium-dependent vasodilatation to ACh compared with normotensive offspring of normotensive parents. Further, the blunted endothelium-dependent responses of offspring of hypertensive parents may be related to decreased activity of nitric oxide.[46] These findings suggest that endothelial dysfunction can precede the development of hypertension and therefore play a primary role in the hypertensive process.

The observation that induction of hypertension in animal models resulted in impaired endothelium-dependent vasodilatation led to the hypothesis that effective antihypertensive therapy may normalize or at least improve endothelial vasodilator function. In spontaneously hypertensive rats, treatment with an ACE inhibitor or a calcium channel blocker reduced blood pressure and improved endothelial dysfunction in resistance vessels,[47] whereas long-term, but not short-term, treatment with an ACE inhibitor or a calcium channel blocker improved endothelial dysfunction in a rat model of nitric oxide–deficient hypertension.[48] These studies suggested that hypertensive treatment has a beneficial effect on endothelial function. Studies of the effects of antihypertensive treatment in humans, including those studies specifically related to the use of ACE inhibitors, have yielded negative results.[49–51] One study demonstrated an acute improvement in endothelium-independent vasodilatation with ACE inhibitor treatment.[52] In this study, vasodilator responses to ACh and sodium nitroprusside were measured only 1 hour after oral administration of captopril, which may explain the discrepancy with the aforementioned studies using longer-term ACE inhibitor therapy. ACE inhibition may improve endothelial dysfunction regardless of its antihypertensive effect, as suggested in the TREND study.[35] On the other hand, studies have shown that clinically effective antihypertensive therapy does not modify the vascular response to ACh, indicating that endothelial dysfunction inhibition either is a primary phenomenon or becomes irreversible once the hypertensive process has become established.[49]

NITRIC OXIDE IN HYPERTENSION

The finding of decreased endothelium-dependent vasodilatation does not identify the mechanism leading to the defect. Endothelial regulation of vascular tone is complex, and any of the several factors released by the endothelium to produce constriction or relaxation of the underlying smooth muscle[3, 4] may affect systemic blood pressure. Given the importance of endothelium-derived nitric oxide in the regulation of basal arteriolar tone in normal humans, studies were conducted to determine whether a specific defect in the nitric oxide system might explain the reduced endothelial vasodilator function observed in hypertensive patients. The vascular effects of L-NMMA were assessed under baseline conditions and during endothelium-dependent and -independent vasodilatation. L-NMMA produced much less vasoconstriction under basal conditions in hypertensive patients than in normotensive controls[53, 54] and did not significantly modify the response to ACh in hypertensive patients.[54, 55] These reduced results demonstrate impaired activity of nitric oxide in hypertensive arteries, under baseline conditions and during stimulation with endothelium-dependent agents. The decreased response to L-NMMA cannot be ascribed to the characteristic structural changes of hypertensive arteries (i.e., increased wall:lumen ratio)[56, 57] because they predispose the vessels to a more (not a less) pronounced response to vasoconstrictor agents.[58, 59]

The finding of impaired nitric oxide activity in patients with hypertension may be critical for understanding the nature of their endothelial dysfunction. The diminished bioavailability and the associated endothelial dysfunction of hypertensive patients could be a consequence of reduced synthesis, increased breakdown, or interactions with other endothelium-derived substances that result in decreased activity of nitric oxide. These possibilities, summarized in the following paragraphs and addressed in recent investigations, provide insight into the mechanisms of endothelial dysfunction in hypertensive patients.

Decreased Production of Nitric Oxide

Nitric oxide is synthesized by endothelial cells using the amino acid L-arginine as its precursor. Previous animal[60–63] and human[23, 64] studies indicated that infusion of L-arginine can improve endothelium-dependent vasodilatation in hypercholesterolemia and atherosclerosis, suggesting that decreased availability of the substrate for NOS might be responsible for the impaired vascular responses observed in certain forms of endothelial dysfunction. If this were the case, administration of L-arginine should restore the impaired endothelium-dependent vasodilatation of hypertensive patients. However, studies undertaken to address this hypothesis gave negative results.[55, 65] In normal subjects, the endothelium-dependent vascular response to ACh was significantly potentiated by prior administration of L-arginine,[55, 65, 66] indicating that availability of substrate for nitric oxide production is a rate-limiting step in endothelium-mediated vascular relaxation. In contrast, the endothelium-dependent vascular response to ACh was not significantly modified by L-arginine in hypertensive patients.[55, 65] Thus, reduced availability of the nitric oxide precursor is not likely to account for the impaired endothelial function of hypertensive arteries.

Basal and stimulated synthesis of nitric oxide by endothelial cells involves several steps. Most endothelial agonists act on specific cell surface receptors coupled to membrane-bound G-proteins.[67] Activation of G-proteins leads to stimulation or inhibition of certain enzymes that, in turn, start the process of intracellular signal transduction leading to activation of NOS. A molecular defect at any of these steps could, therefore, lead to diminished production of nitric oxide. For example, atherosclerotic coronary arteries with abnormal responses to ACh may vasodilate normally in response to substance P,[68, 69] another endothelium-dependent vasodilator acting on different endothelial cell receptors.[2, 70] Thus, the endothelial abnormality observed in certain cardiovascular conditions may be an expression of a specific dysfunction of the muscarinic receptor stimulated by ACh. To determine whether this mechanism is operative in human hypertension, the endothelium-dependent responses of the forearm vasculature to ACh and substance P were studied in a group of hypertensive patients and normotensive controls. In this study, the endothelium-dependent vascular responses evoked by both ACh and substance P were significantly blunted in hypertensive patients compared with normal controls,[71] and there was a significant correlation between the vasodilator effects of both endothelial agonists. These findings demonstrate that the endothelial abnormality in human hypertension is not restricted to the muscarinic receptor.

In certain conditions, endothelial dysfunction may be localized to specific intracellular signal transduction pathways. Previous studies in animal models of hypercholesterolemia and endothelial regeneration showed that, early in the development of the vascular abnormalities, the responses to specific agonists are blunted selectively.[72–76] Later in the course of the disease process, all endothelium-mediated responses are depressed.[75, 76] These observations suggest that, at least in animal models, endothelial dysfunction of certain conditions progresses from an early defect of a specific intracellular signal transduction pathway to a late, more generalized abnormality of endothelial cell function.[77] To determine whether the reduced bioactivity of nitric oxide in patients with hypertension is due to a deficit at the level of a single G-protein–dependent intracellular

signal transduction pathway, the endothelium-dependent responses of the forearm vasculature to ACh and bradykinin were studied in hypertensive patients and normal controls.[78] Bradykinin is an endothelial agonist that, in contrast to ACh, acts on a pertussis toxin–insensitive G-protein to start the process leading to NOS activation. Similar to the results obtained with ACh, the increase in blood flow and decrease in vascular resistance induced by bradykinin were significantly blunted in hypertensive patients compared with normotensive controls. A significant correlation was also found between the vasodilator actions of ACh and bradykinin. These observations indicate that endothelial dysfunction in hypertension is not related to a specific defect of a single G-protein–dependent intracellular signal transduction pathway, and it differs from that observed in hypercholesterolemic patients, in whom the response to bradykinin is preserved.[79]

A more recent investigation found that the reduced nitric oxide activity in hypertensive patients is due to a defect localized more distally along the intracellular signaling pathway leading to NOS activation. Thus, hypertensive patients with blunted vasodilatation have been shown to have preserved vasodilator responses to isoproterenol,[80] a β-adrenoceptor agonist that stimulates endothelial release of nitric oxide.[81, 82] In the same study, the response to isoproterenol during nitric oxide inhibition with L-NMMA was equally blunted in controls and hypertensive patients, indicating that nitric oxide activity during isoproterenol infusion was not different between the two groups.[80] A potential explanation for these observations is that different intracellular transduction signaling pathways are used by ACh and isoproterenol to stimulate nitric oxide synthesis. In particular, endothelium-dependent relaxation to ACh is predominantly mediated through the phosphoinositide pathway, whereas β-adrenoceptor activation with isoproterenol stimulates nitric oxide synthesis using cyclic adenosine monophosphate as a second messenger. Therefore, the finding of a preserved response to isoproterenol in patients with impaired vasodilatation to ACh suggests a defect in the phosphoinositide signaling pathway as a mechanism of endothelial dysfunction in hypertensive patients.

Increased Destruction of Nitric Oxide

Studies have linked the pathogenesis of endothelial dysfunction with an increased degradation of nitric oxide. Principal among the substances involved in this process is superoxide anion, an avid scavenger of endothelium-derived nitric oxide.[83, 84] Previous studies have shown that the administration of superoxide dismutase (SOD), a scavenger of superoxide anions,[85] decreases blood pressure in hypertensive but not in normotensive rats,[86] supporting the concept that superoxide anions might trigger the development of hypertension, probably by inactivating the vasodilator effect of nitric oxide. When vascular responses to ACh were studied before and after combined administration of CuZn SOD (a form of the enzyme with poor intracellular penetrance), no significant effect was observed in endothelium-dependent vasodilatation in either normotensive controls or hypertensive patients.[87] This suggests that increased extracellular destruction of nitric oxide by superoxide anions is unlikely to play a significant role in the impaired endothelial function characteristic of hypertension. These findings do not rule out the possibility that hypertensive patients have an increased destruction of nitric oxide by superoxide anions that is not modified by administration of CuZn SOD. For example, reduced activity of nitric oxide could result from increased breakdown within the endothelial cell. The administration of CuZn SOD may not modify this abnormality, given the poor intracellular penetrance of this form of the enzyme related to its negative charge. Other forms of delivery of SOD have been used in animal studies[88] and may potentially affect vasodilator function in hypertensive patients. However, those alternative forms of SOD are not currently available for use in humans.

Superoxide anions may be generated from a variety of enzymatic and nonenzymatic sources. The xanthine oxidase system is one of the main sources of superoxide anion within and around endothelial cells, both directly and through the activation of circulating neutrophils.[89, 90] Inhibition of xanthine oxidase can be achieved by oxypurinol, which has a molecular structure similar to that of xanthine and binds to xanthine oxidase, preventing the formation of uric acid and superoxide radicals.[91] Studies have been undertaken in hypercholesterolemic and hypertensive patients to determine whether an increased breakdown of nitric oxide by xanthine oxidase–generated superoxide anions could participate in their impaired endothelium-dependent vasorelaxation. Vascular responses to the infusion of ACh and sodium nitroprusside were studied before and during the combined administration of oxypurinol.[92] In hypercholesterolemic patients, both the increase in forearm blood flow and the decrease in vascular resistance were significantly greater after the infusion of oxypurinol. In contrast, in hypertensive patients, the response to ACh was not significantly modified during the concomitant infusion of oxypurinol.[92] These results indicate that xanthine oxidase–generated superoxide anions are partly responsible for the impaired endothelial vasodilator function of patients with hypercholesterolemia; however, this mechanism does not appear to play a significant role in essential hypertension.

Other Endothelium-Derived Factors and Nitric Oxide

A mechanism that may participate in the endothelial dysfunction of hypertensive patients is related to possible interactions between nitric oxide and other endothelium-derived factors. For example, blockade of cyclooxygenase with indomethacin enhances the vasodilator effect of ACh in hypertensive but not in normotensive subjects.[42] These results suggest that vasoconstrictor prostanoids play a role in the pathophysiology of endothelial dysfunction in hypertension. More recent studies from the same group of investigators showed that the beneficial effect of indomethacin on endothelium-dependent vasodilatation was mediated by augmented availability of nitric oxide.[55] This, in turn, potentiated the response to ACh by L-arginine and attenuated the response to ACh by L-NMMA. These observations indicate that vasoconstrictor derivatives of cyclooxygenase metabolism may negatively affect the activity of nitric

oxide and thus contribute to the endothelial dysfunction of patients with hypertension.

Another potential explanation for decreased activity of nitric oxide in the hypertensive vasculature may be related to increased vascular activity of endothelin, a vasoconstrictor and mitogenic peptide produced by endothelial cells.[93] Endothelin exerts its effects through two subtypes of receptors: ET_A and ET_B.[94, 95] ET_A receptors are located mainly on vascular smooth muscle cells and mediate vasoconstriction,[96, 97] whereas ET_B receptors are located on both smooth muscle and endothelial cells. In smooth muscle cells, ET_B receptors also mediate vasoconstriction;[96, 97] however, on endothelial cells, ET_B receptors mediate stimulation of nitric oxide synthesis.[98] Nitric oxide may also inhibit the production of endothelin. Thus, there are a number of possible interactions between nitric oxide and endothelin that might lead to increased vasoconstrictor tone. Initial studies reported increased plasma levels of endothelin in patients with essential hypertension,[99–101] but other investigations showed negative results.[102–104] Because endothelin is largely released abluminally,[105] plasma levels of the peptide may not necessarily reflect the contribution of endothelin to the physiology and pathophysiology of the cardiovascular system. Finally, altered density of either ET_A or ET_B receptors may play a role in the maintenance of vascular tone even in the presence of normal release of endothelin. The development of selective antagonists of ET_A and ET_B receptors holds promise in defining the role of endothelin in mediating endothelial dysfunction in human essential hypertension and may have an impact on the therapy of this condition.[106] Studies using these agents suggest that the vascular activity of endothelin may indeed be enhanced in hypertensive patients.[107]

CONCLUSIONS

Endothelial cells play a critical role in the regulation of vascular tone and other processes related to cardiovascular homeostasis. These functions of the endothelium are mediated by many substances with different chemical structures and contrasting vascular effects. Among them, nitric oxide (a soluble gas synthesized from the amino acid L-arginine) plays a key role owing to its multiple functions, including smooth muscle relaxation, inhibition of platelet aggregability and leukocyte adhesion to the vessel wall, and prevention of oxidation of lipid molecules.

Hypertensive patients have impaired endothelium-mediated regulation of vascular tone. This abnormality is present in both patients with essential hypertension and those with secondary forms of elevated blood pressure and may be a primary mechanism leading to the hypertensive process. This form of endothelial dysfunction is largely related to decreased vascular activity of nitric oxide, which, in turn, may be related to reduced nitric oxide synthesis, increased breakdown, and interactions with endothelium-derived factors. Clinical investigations have suggested that a specific defect in the phosphoinositide pathway leading to activation of NOS may be responsible for endothelial dysfunction in essential hypertension.

Because the reduction in blood pressure accomplished by empirical forms of antihypertensive therapy or by ACE inhibition does not improve endothelial regulation of vascular tone, we must learn more about the specific mechanisms of endothelial dysfunction in hypertension in order to devise more rationalistic therapies for this condition.

References

1. Furchgott RF, Zawadzki JV. The obligatory role of endothelial cells in the relaxation of arterial smooth muscle by acetylcholine. Nature 288:373–376, 1980.
2. Furchgott RF. Role of endothelium in responses of vascular smooth muscle. Circ Res 53:557–573, 1983.
3. Bassenge E, Busse R. Endothelial modulation of coronary tone. Prog Cardiovasc Dis 30:349–380, 1988.
4. Vane JR, Änggård EE, Botting RM. Regulatory functions of the vascular endothelium. N Engl J Med 323:27–36, 1990.
5. Palmer RMJ, Ferrige AG, Moncada S. Nitric oxide release accounts for the biological activity of endothelium-derived relaxing factor. Nature 327:524–526, 1987.
6. Palmer RMJ, Ashton DS, Moncada S. Vascular endothelial cells synthesize nitric oxide from L-arginine. Nature 333:664–666, 1988.
7. Moncada S, Higgins ES. The L-arginine–nitric oxide pathway. N Engl J Med 329:2002–2012, 1993.
8. MacAllister RJ, Fickling SA, Whitley GSJ, Vallance P. Metabolism of methylarginines by human vasculature: Implications for the regulation of nitric oxide synthesis. Br J Pharmacol 112:43–48, 1994.
9. Vallance P, Leone A, Calver A, et al. Accumulation of an endogenous inhibitor of nitric oxide synthesis in chronic renal failure. Lancet 339:572–575, 1992.
10. Cooke JP, Dzau VJ. Derangements of the nitric oxide synthase pathway, L-arginine, and cardiovascular diseases. Circulation 96:379–382, 1997.
11. Huang PL, Huang Z, Mshimo H, et al. Hypertension in mice lacking the gene for endothelial nitric oxide synthase. Nature 377:239–242, 1995.
12. Ribeiro M, Antunes E, deNucci G, et al. Chronic inhibition of nitric oxide synthesis: A new model of hypertension. Hypertension 20:298–303, 1992.
13. Vallance P, Collier J, Moncada S. Effects of endothelium-derived nitric oxide on peripheral arteriolar tone in man. Lancet 2:997–1000, 1989.
14. Cooke JP, Dzau VJ. Nitric oxide synthase: Role in the genesis of vascular disease. Annu Rev Med 48:489–509, 1997.
15. Ludmer PL, Selwyn AP, Shook TL, et al. Paradoxical vasoconstriction induced by acetylcholine in atherosclerotic coronary arteries. N Engl J Med 315:1046–1051, 1986.
16. Panza JA, Quyyumi AA, Brush JE Jr, Epstein SE. Abnormal endothelium-dependent vascular relaxation in patients with essential hypertension. N Engl J Med 323:22–27, 1990.
17. Linder L, Kiowski W, Buhler FR, Luscher TF. Indirect evidence for release of endothelium-derived relaxing factor in human forearm circulation in vivo. Blunted response in essential hypertension. Circulation 81:1762–1767, 1990.
18. Yoshida M, Imaizumi T, Ando S, et al. Impaired forearm vasodilatation by acetylcholine in patients with hypertension. Heart Vessels 6:218–223, 1991.
19. Brush JE Jr, Faxon DP, Salmon S, et al. Abnormal endothelium-dependent coronary vasomotion in hypertensive patients. J Am Coll Cardiol 19:809–815, 1992.
20. Treasure CB, Manoukian SV, Klein JL, et al. Epicardial coronary artery responses to acetylcholine are impaired in hypertensive patients. Circ Res 71:776–781, 1992.
21. Creager MA, Cooke JP, Mendelson ME, et al. Impaired vasodilation of forearm resistance vessels in hypercholesterolemic humans. J Clin Invest 86:228–234, 1990.
22. Chowienczyk PJ, Watts GF, Cockcroft JR, Ritter JM. Impaired endothelium-dependent vasodilation of forearm resistance vessels in hypercholesterolaemia. Lancet 340:1430–1432, 1992.
23. Drexler H, Zeiher AM, Meinzer K, Just H. Correction of endothelial dysfunction in coronary microcirculation of hypercholesterolaemic patients by L-arginine. Lancet 338:1546–1550, 1991.
24. Casino PR, Kilcoyne CM, Quyyumi AA, et al. Role of nitric oxide in the endothelium-dependent vasodilation of hypercholesterolemic patients. Circulation 88:2541–2547, 1993.
25. McVeigh GE, Brennan GM, Johnston GD, et al. Impaired endothelium-dependent and independent vasodilation in patients with type 2 (non–insulin-dependent) diabetes mellitus. Diabetologia 35:771–776, 1992.
26. Williams SB, Cusco JA, Roddy MA, et al. Impaired nitric oxide–mediated vasodilation in patients with non–insulin-dependent diabetes mellitus. J Am Coll Cardiol 27:567–574, 1996.
27. Blache D, Bouthillier D, Davignon J. Acute influence of smoking on platelet behaviour, endothelium and plasma lipids and normalization by aspirin. Atherosclerosis 93:179–188, 1992.
28. Zeiher AM, Schachinger V, Minners J. Long-term cigarette smoking impairs endothelium-dependent coronary arterial vasodilator function. Circulation 92:1094–1100, 1995.
29. Celermajer DS, Adams MR, Clarkson P, et al. Passive smoking and impaired endothelium-dependent arterial dilatation in healthy young adults. N Engl J Med 334:150–154, 1996.
30. McVeigh GE, Lemay L, Morgan D, Cohn JN. Effects of long-term cigarette smoking on endothelium-dependent responses in humans. Am J Cardiol 78:668–672, 1996.
31. Lekakis J, Papamichael C, Vemmos C, et al. Effect of acute cigarette smoking on endothelium-dependent brachial artery dilatation in healthy individuals. Am J Cardiol 79:529–531, 1997.
32. Gerhard M, Roddy MA, Creager SJ, Creager MA. Aging progressively impairs endothelium-dependent vasodilation in forearm resistance vessels of humans. Hypertension 27:849–853, 1996.
33. Treasure CB, Klein JL, Weintraub WS, et al. Beneficial effects of cholesterol-lowering therapy on the coronary endothelium in patients with coronary artery disease. N Engl J Med 332:481–487, 1995.
34. Anderson TJ, Meredith IT, Yeung AC, et al. The effect of cholesterol-lowering and antioxidant therapy on endothelium-dependent coronary vasomotion. N Engl J Med 332:488–493, 1995.
35. Mancini GBJ, Henry GC, Macaya C, et al. Angiotensin-converting enzyme inhibition with quinapril improves endothelial vasomotor dysfunction in patients with coronary artery disease: The TREND (Trial on Reversing ENdothelial Dysfunction) study. Circulation 94:258–265, 1996.
36. Pepine CJ. Ongoing clinical trials of angiotensin-converting enzyme inhibitors for treatment of coronary artery disease in patients with preserved left ventricular function. J Am Coll Cardiol 27:1048–1052, 1996.
37. Konishi M, Su C. Role of endothelium in dilator responses of spontaneously hypertensive rat arteries. Hypertension 5:881–886, 1983.
38. Luscher TF, Vanhoutte PM. Endothelium-dependent responses to platelets and serotonin in spontaneously hypertensive rats. Hypertension 8:II-55–II-60, 1986.
39. Lockette W, Otsuka Y, Carretero O. The loss of endothelium-dependent vascular relaxation in hypertension. Hypertension 8:II-61–II-66, 1986.
40. Luscher TF, Raij L, Vanhoutte PM. Endothelium-dependent vascular responses in normotensive and hypertensive Dahl rats. Hypertension 9:157–163, 1987.
41. Luscher TF, Aarhus LL, Vanhoutte PM. Indomethacin enhances the impaired endothelium-dependent relaxations in small mesenteric arteries of the spontaneously hypertensive rat. Am J Hypertens 3:55–78, 1990.
42. Taddei S, Virdis A, Mattei P, Salvetti A. Vasodilation to acetylcholine in primary and secondary forms of human hypertension. Hypertension 21:929–933, 1993.
43. Rizzoni D, Porteri E, Castellano M, et al. Endothelial dysfunction in hypertension is independent from the etiology and from vascular structure. Hypertension 31:335–341, 1998.
44. Miller MJS, Pinto A, Mullane KM. Impaired endothelium-dependent relaxations in rabbits subjected to aortic coarctation hypertension. Hypertension 10:164–170, 1987.
45. Taddei S, Virdis A, Mattei P, et al. Endothelium-dependent forearm vasodilation is reduced in normotensive subjects with familial history of hypertension. J Cardiovasc Pharmacol 20(suppl 12):S193–S195, 1992.
46. Taddei S, Virdis A, Mattei P, et al. Defective L-arginine–nitric oxide pathway in offspring of essential hypertensive patients. Circulation 94:1298–1303, 1996.
47. Dohi Y, Criscione L, Pfeiffer K, Lüscher TF. Angiotensin blockade or calcium antagonists improve endothelial dysfunction in hypertension: Studies in perfused mesenteric resistance arteries. J Cardiovasc Pharmacol 24:372–379, 1994.

48. Takase H, Moreau P, Küng CF, et al. Antihypertensive therapy prevents endothelial dysfunction in chronic nitric oxide deficiency: Effect of verapamil and trandolapril. Hypertension 27:25–31, 1996.

49. Panza J, Quyyumi AA, Callahan TS, Epstein SE. Effect of antihypertensive treatment on endothelium-dependent vascular relaxation in patients with essential hypertension. J Am Coll Cardiol 21:1145–1151, 1993.

50. Creager MA, Roddy MA. Effect of captopril and enalapril on endothelial function in hypertensive patients. Hypertension 24:499–505, 1994.

51. Kiowski W, Linder L, Nuesch R, Martina B. Effects of cilazapril on vascular structure and function in essential hypertension. Hypertension 27:371–376, 1996.

52. Hirooka Y, Imaizumi T, Masaki H, et al. Captopril improves impaired endothelium-dependent vasodilation in hypertensive patients. Hypertension 20:175–180, 1992.

53. Calver A, Collier J, Moncada S, Vallance P. Effect of local intra-arterial N^G-monomethyl-L-arginine in patients with hypertension: The nitric oxide dilator mechanism appears abnormal. J Hypertens 10:1025–1031, 1992.

54. Panza JA, Casino PR, Kilcoyne CM, Quyyumi AA. Role of endothelium-derived nitric oxide in the abnormal endothelium-dependent vascular relaxation of patients with essential hypertension. Circulation 87:1468–1474, 1993.

55. Taddei S, Virdis A, Ghiadoni L, et al. Cyclooxygenase inhibition restores nitric oxide activity in essential hypertension. Hypertension 29:274–279, 1997.

56. Sivertsson R. The hemodynamic importance of structural vascular changes in essential hypertension. Acta Physiol Scand Suppl 343:1–56, 1970.

57. Folkow B. "Structural factor" in primary and secondary hypertension. Hypertension 16:89–101, 1990.

58. Doyle AE, Fraser JRE, Marshall RJ. Reactivity of forearm vessels to vasoconstrictor substances in hypertensive and normotensive subjects. Clin Sci 18:441–454, 1959.

59. Egan B, Panis R, Hinderliter A, et al. Mechanism of increased alpha adrenergic vasoconstriction in human essential hypertension. J Clin Invest 80:812–817, 1987.

60. Girerd XJ, Hirsch AT, Cooke JP, et al. L-Arginine augments endothelium-dependent vasodilation in cholesterol-fed rabbits. Circ Res 67:1301–1308, 1990.

61. Cooke JP, Dzau J, Creager A. Endothelial dysfunction in hypercholesterolemia is corrected by L-arginine. Basic Res Cardiol Suppl 2:173–181, 1991.

62. Rossitch E Jr, Alexander E III, Black PM, Cooke JP. L-Arginine normalizes endothelial function in cerebral vessels from hypercholesterolemic rabbits. J Clin Invest 87:1295–1299, 1991.

63. Cooke JP, Andon NA, Girerd XJ, et al. Arginine restores cholinergic relaxation of hypercholesterolemic rabbit thoracic aorta. Circulation 83:1057–1062, 1991.

64. Creager MA, Gallagher SJ, Girerd XJ, et al. L-Arginine improves endothelium-dependent vasodilation in hypercholesterolemic humans. J Clin Invest 90:1248–1253, 1992.

65. Panza JA, Casino PR, Badar DM, Quyyumi AA. Effect of increased availability of endothelium-derived nitric oxide precursor on endothelium-dependent vascular relaxation in normal subjects and in patients with essential hypertension. Circulation 87:1475–1481, 1993.

66. Imaizumi T, Hirooka Y, Masaki H, et al. Effects of L-arginine on forearm vessels and responses to acetylcholine. Hypertension 20:511–517, 1992.

67. Boulanger CM, Vanhoutte PM. G proteins and endothelium-dependent relaxations. J Vasc Res 34:175–185, 1997.

68. Egashira K, Inou T, Yamada A, et al. Heterogeneous effects of the endothelium-dependent vasodilators acetylcholine and substance P on the coronary circulation of patients with angiographically normal coronary arteries. Coron Artery Dis 3:945–952, 1992.

69. Okumura K, Yasue H, Ishizaka H, et al. Endothelium-dependent dilator response to substance P in patients with coronary spastic angina. J Am Coll Cardiol 20:838–844, 1992.

70. Saito R, Nonaka S, Konishi H, et al. Pharmacological properties of the tachykinin receptor subtype in the endothelial cell and vasodilation. Ann N Y Acad Sci 632:457–459, 1991.

71. Panza JA, Casino PR, Kilcoyne CM, Quyyumi AA. Impaired endothelium-dependent vasodilation in patients with essential hypertension: Evidence that the abnormality is not at the muscarinic receptor level. J Am Coll Cardiol 23:1610–1616, 1994.

72. Bosaller C, Habib GB, Yamamoto H, et al. Impaired muscarinic endothelium-dependent relaxation and cyclic guanosine 5'-monophosphate formation in atherosclerotic human coronary artery and rabbit aorta. J Clin Invest 79:170–174, 1987.

73. Cohen RA, Zitnay KM, Haudenschild CC, Cunningham LD. Loss of selective endothelial cell vasoactive functions caused by hypercholesterolemia in pig coronary arteries. Circ Res 63:903–910, 1988.

74. Komori K, Shimokawa H, Vanhoutte PM. Hypercholesterolemia impairs endothelium-dependent relaxations to aggregating platelets in porcine iliac arteries. J Vasc Surg 10:318–325, 1989.

75. Shimokawa H, Flavahan NA, Vanhoutte PM. Loss of endothelial pertussis toxin–sensitive G protein function in atherosclerotic porcine coronary arteries. Circulation 1983:652–660, 1991.

76. Shimokawa H, Flavahan NA, Vanhoutte PM. Natural course of the impairment of endothelium-dependent relaxations in regenerating porcine endothelial cells: Possible dysfunction of a pertussis toxin-sensitive G-protein. Circ Res 65:740–753, 1990.

77. Flavahan NA. Atherosclerotic or lipoprotein-induced endothelial dysfunction. Potential mechanisms underlying reduction in EDRF/nitric oxide activity. Circulation 85:1927–1938, 1992.

78. Panza JA, Garcia CE, Kilcoyne CM, et al. Impaired endothelium-dependent vasodilation in patients with essential hypertension. Evidence that nitric oxide abnormality is not localized to a single signal transduction pathway. Circulation 91:1732–1738, 1995.

79. Gilligan DM, Guetta V, Panza JA, et al. Selective loss of microvascular endothelial function in human hypercholesterolemia. Circulation 90:35–41, 1994.

80. Cardillo C, Kilcoyne CM, Quyyumi AA, et al. Selective defect in nitric oxide synthesis may explain the impaired endothelium-dependent vasodilation in patients with essential hypertension. Circulation 97:851–856, 1998.

81. Cardillo C, Kilcoyne CM, Quyyumi AA, et al. Decreased vasodilator response to isoproterenol during nitric oxide inhibition in humans. Hypertension 30:918–921, 1997.

82. Daves M, Chowienczyk PJ, Ritter JM. Effects of inhibition of the L-arginine/nitric oxide pathway on vasodilation caused by β-adrenergic agonists in human forearm. Circulation 95:2293–2297, 1997.

83. Rubanyi GM, Vanhoutte PM. Superoxide anions and hyperoxia inactivate endothelium-derived relaxing factor. Am J Physiol 250:H822–H827, 1986.

84. Gryglewski RJ, Palmer RM, Moncada S. Superoxide anion is involved in the breakdown of endothelium-derived vascular relaxing factor. Nature 320:454–456, 1986.

85. McCord JM, Fridovich I. Superoxide dismutase: An enzymatic function for erythrocuprein (hemocuprein). J Biol Chem 244:6049–6055, 1969.

86. Nakazono K, Watanabe N, Matsuno K, et al. Does superoxide underlie the pathogenesis of hypertension? Proc Natl Acad Sci U S A 88:10045–10048, 1991.

87. Garcia CE, Kilcoyne CM, Cardillo C, et al. Effect of copper-zinc superoxide dismutase on endothelium-dependent vasodilation of patients with essential hypertension. Hypertension 26:863–868, 1995.

88. White CW, Brock TA, Chang LY, et al. Superoxide and peroxynitrite in atherosclerosis. Proc Nat Acad Sci U S A 91:1044–1048, 1994.

89. Friedl HP, Till GO, Ryan US, Ward PA. Mediator-induced activation of xanthine oxidase in endothelial cells. FASEB J 3:2512–2518, 1989.

90. Bulkey GB. Reactive oxygen metabolites and reperfusion injury: Aberrant triggering of reticuloendothelial function. Lancet 344:934–936, 1994.

91. McKelvey G, Hollwarth E, Glanger N, et al. Mechanisms of conversion of xanthine dehydrogenase to xanthine oxidase in ischemic rat liver and kidney. Am J Physiol 27:G753–G760, 1988.

92. Cardillo C, Kilcoyne CM, Cannon RO, et al. Xanthine oxidase inhibition improves endothelium-dependent vasodilation in hypercholesterolemic but not in hypertensive patients. Hypertension 30:57–63, 1997.

93. Yanagisawa M, Kurihara H, Kimura S, et al. A novel potent vasoconstrictor peptide produced by vascular endothelial cells. Nature 332:411–415, 1988.

94. Arai H, Hori S, Aramori I, et al. Cloning and expression of cDNA encoding an endothelin receptor. Nature 348:730–732, 1990.

95. Sakurai T, Yanagisawa M, Takuwa Y, et al. Cloning of a cDNA encoding a non–isopeptide-selective subtype of the endothelin receptor. Nature 348:732–735, 1990.
96. Seo B, Oemar BS, Siebenmann R, et al. Both ET$_A$ and ET$_B$ receptors mediate contraction to endothelin-1 in human blood vessels. Circulation 89:1203–1208, 1994.
97. Haynes WG, Strachan FE, Webb DJ. Endothelin ET$_A$ and ET$_B$ receptors cause vasoconstriction of human resistance and capacitance vessels in vivo. Circulation 92:357–363, 1995.
98. De Nucci G, Thomas R, D'Orleans-Juste P, et al. Pressor effects of circulating endothelin are limited by its removal in the pulmonary circulation and by the release of prostacyclin and endothelium-derived relaxing factor. Proc Natl Acad Sci U S A 85:9797–9800, 1988.
99. Kohno M, Yasumari K, Murakawa Kl, et al. Plasma immunoreactive endothelin in essential hypertension. Am J Med 88:614–618, 1990.
100. Shichiri M, Hirata Y, Ando K, et al. Plasma endothelin levels in hypertension and chronic renal failure. Hypertension 15:493–496, 1990.

101. Saito Y, Nakao K, Mukoyama M, Imura H. Increased plasma endothelin levels in patients with essential hypertension. [Letter] N Engl J Med 322:205, 1990.
102. Davenport AP, Ashby MJ, Easton P, et al. A sensitive radioimmunoassay measuring endothelin-like immunoreactivity in human plasma: Comparison of levels in patients with essential hypertension and normotensive control subjects. Clin Sci 78:261–264, 1990.
103. Predel HG, Meyer-Lehnert H, Backer A, et al. Plasma concentrations of endothelin in patients with abnormal vascular reactivity. Effects of ergometric exercise and acute saline loading. Life Sci 47:1837–1843, 1990.
104. Schiffrin EL, Thibault G. Plasma endothelin in human essential hypertension. Am J Hypertens 4:303–308, 1991.
105. Wagner OF, Christ G, Wojta J, et al. Polar secretion of endothelin-l by cultured endothelial cells. J Biol Chem 267:16066–16068, 1992.
106. Ferro CJ, Webb DJ. The clinical potential of endothelin receptor antagonists in cardiovascular medicine. Drugs 51:12–27, 1996.
107. Cardillo C, Kilcoyne CM, Cannon RO, et al. Role of endothelin in the increased vascular tone of patients with essential hypertension. Hypertension (in press).

17 Natriuretic Peptides

CHAPTER

Vito M. Campese and Arie L. M. Widerhorn

The notion that the myocardium not only acts as a mechanical device but also exerts endocrine and paracrine functions came to the fore with the discovery by de Bold and co-workers[1] that rat atrial extracts have potent natriuretic and vasodepressor activity. This led to the discovery of atrial natriuretic peptide (ANP) and to the recognition that this hormone is important in the regulation of sodium balance and blood pressure. Subsequently, three other structurally related natriuretic peptides, brain natriuretic peptide (BNP), C-type natriuretic peptide (CNP), and urodilatin, were identified. The term *natriuretic peptides* has remained even though these peptides exert a multitude of functions other than natriuresis, including vasodilatation, antiproliferative effects, vascular remodeling, and modulation of noradrenergic transmission. CNP exerts very modest natriuretic actions, despite its name.

CHEMISTRY OF NATRIURETIC PEPTIDES

Four distinct natriuretic peptides have been recognized, and at least three are the products of separate genes and subject to independent regulation. The first to be identified was ANP, a 28-amino acid peptide synthesized and secreted by the atria.[1] ANP contains a 17-amino acid ring closed by a disulfide bond between two cysteine residues. The ANP gene in humans is located on the short arm of chromosome 1 and comprises three exons separated by two introns with regulatory elements upstream of the coding sequence.[2] ANP is stored in myocytes as a 126-amino acid prohormone (pro-ANP). When secreted, the prohormone is split into an N-terminal moiety of 98 amino acids (N-ANP) and the biologically active hormone in equimolar amounts.[3] ANP has a very short half-life (2.5 minutes), whereas N-ANP has a much longer half-life (~21 minutes) in plasma. Thus, the plasma concentration of N-ANP is approximately 50 times that of ANP. The amino acid sequence of ANP is identical in most mammals studied, with the exception of rodents and rabbits, in which isoleucine replaces methionine at position 110.

BNP is a 32-amino acid peptide, structurally similar to ANP, that retains the 17-amino acid ring structure. BNP was initially isolated from the brain of pigs[4] and dogs[5] but, despite its name, is produced predominantly by ventricular myocytes. In fact, BNP cannot be detected in the human, monkey, or rat brain but is detectable in the heart of these species. A single copy gene consisting of three exons and two introns encodes human BNP. The gene regulation of BNP is different from that of ANP: ANP is stored largely as pro-ANP, whereas BNP is stored as the mature hormone in human and rat heart and as pro-BNP in pig and sheep heart.[6]

In contrast to ANP, the structure of BNP shows marked interspecies variability. In humans, the mature circulating forms comprise a 32-amino acid residue peptide and a higher molecular-weight component, probably pro-BNP. Two precursor forms of relatively high molecular mass, prepro-BNP (134 amino acids) and pro-BNP (108 amino acids), have been identified in human cardiac tissue[7] and plasma.[8] In rats, the circulating mature form is a 45-amino acid residue peptide, whereas in pigs, two circulating forms have been identified. Because of interspecies variability in structure, it is not surprising that species-specific antisera are required for measurement of BNP in plasma, and actions of BNP differ among species. Measurements of BNP mRNA concentrations in patients with and without heart failure have demonstrated greater activity in the ventricles than in the atria, whereas ANP mRNA is virtually absent from the ventricles of normal individuals.

Two types of secretory granules have been identified in human and porcine cardiac myocytes: One contains only ANP and the other contains both ANP and BNP.[9] ANP and BNP are cosecreted,[10] and BNP can be detected by radioimmunoassay in the plasma of normal subjects at rest.[11]

CNP has little intrinsic natriuretic activity and acts more as a paracrine than as an endocrine hormone. CNP contains 22 amino acids (molecular weight 2200). Human CNP has a precursor prepro-CNP of 126 amino acids and a pro-CNP, which is then processed to form two peptides, CNP-53 and CNP-22, the only peptide with definite biological activity.[12] CNP shares the 17-amino acid ring configuration with ANP and BNP but lacks the carboxyterminal extension. Sequence analyses have revealed that there are at least two exons in the coding region for prepro-CNP, and the regulatory mechanisms for the transcription of the CNP gene appear to be different from those that regulate ANP and BNP.[13] CNP was initially isolated from porcine brain[14] and subsequently from rat and human brain extracts,[15] in which it occurs in higher concentration than either ANP or BNP. CNP is the only hormone in the heart and brain of the more primitive cartilaginous fish, and it is believed to be an ancestral molecule of the NP family.[16] The structures of CNP-22 and pro-CNP appear to be identical in all mammalian species studied.

The transcription of the CNP gene is regulated by many factors, such as tumor necrosis factor, interleukin-1, and transforming growth factor. These cytokines influence vascular cell proliferation, migration, and contraction, effects that can be modulated by CNP. In conditions characterized by widespread damage to endothelium, such as sepsis, hypoxia, and chronic renal failure, blood levels of CNP are elevated.[17] The markedly elevated plasma levels of CNP in chronic renal failure could be related in part to endothelial damage and in part to reduced clearance of the peptide. Plasma concentrations of CNP are not increased in chronic congestive heart failure, a condition associated with very high levels of ANP and BNP. Whether this reflects no increase in myocardial production or whether plasma concentrations are not necessarily a marker of tissue activation of this peptide remains to be established.

A new 32-amino acid natriuretic peptide has been isolated from human urine and termed *urodilatin*.[18] Initially, this compound was believed to be ANP excreted in the urine. However, subsequent studies have demonstrated that the structures of these two peptides are different. Compared with ANP (99 to 126 amino acids), urodilatin has 4 additional amino acids (Thr-Ala-Pro-Arg) in the NH_2 terminal. Urodilatin is synthesized exclusively in the kidney and secreted into the tubular lumen, where it binds to receptors in the inner medullary collecting duct that are coupled to guanylate cyclase. Activation of these receptors results in greater sodium excretion.[19] Immunohistochemical studies have shown urodilatin-like immunoreactivity in the distal and collecting tubules, especially in the cortical collecting duct, suggesting that urodilatin is synthesized in this part of the nephron. Urodilatin is not detectable in plasma and is presumed to be processed in the distal tubule from the same precursor as ANP.[20] However, no gene expression of urodilatin has been detected so far in the kidney.

TISSUE DISTRIBUTION OF NATRIURETIC PEPTIDES

ANP gene expression is highest in normal adult atria and much lower in ventricles. However, in pathological states, such as heart failure and ventricular hypertrophy, ANP gene expression in the ventricles may increase markedly. ANP mRNA is present in several areas of the brain, particularly in areas involved in blood pressure regulation, such as the hypothalamus and brain stem. ANP mRNA has also been found in the anterior pituitary lobe, kidney, vascular tissue, and particularly the great cardiac veins and the inferior vena cava, adrenal medulla, eye, lung, and gastrointestinal tract.[21]

BNP is produced predominantly by the ventricular myocytes. ANP mRNA is largely present in atria; BNP mRNA is located in ventricles. BNP mRNA has also been found in extracardiac tissues, including porcine and human brain, bovine adrenal medulla, and human amniotic tissue. In rats, extracardiac localization of this peptide is scant.

Immunoreactive CNP and CNP gene transcripts are found in abundance in the cerebral cortex, brain stem, cerebellum, basal ganglia, hypothalamus, and spinal cord of most species. Detectable levels of CNP have been found in a variety of peripheral tissues, including endothelium, kidney, adrenal glands, small and large bowel, thymus, uterus, and testis. Small amounts of CNP have been found in plasma and cardiac tissue.[22] CNP has been found in atrial and ventricular myocardium, suggesting that it may exert important local actions. Some have suggested that CNP in the myocardium derives from the endothelium of coronary arteries.[23] CNP has been localized in the endothelium in humans primarily as the CNP-53 amino acid precursor, suggesting that the precursor may be a storage form that is transformed into active CNP-22 when needed. CNP-53 has been detected in human plasma, suggesting a possible physiological role.[24] It is not clear, however, whether plasma concentrations of CNP provide a sensitive index of local production in the vasculature or in other tissues.

Urodilatin has been isolated only from the kidney, where it appears to play a role in the regulation of urinary sodium excretion.

NATRIURETIC PEPTIDE RECEPTORS

All natriuretic peptides exert their biological effects by interacting with specific receptors. Molecular cloning techniques have identified at least three different subtypes of natriuretic peptide receptors (NPRs) in humans—NPRa, NPRb, and NPRc. These correspond to three human chromosomes.[25] NPRa and NPRb differ from NPRc by having an extracellular ligand-binding domain, an intracellular guanylate cyclase domain, and a protein kinase–like domain that catalyzes the formation of cyclic guanosine monophosphate (cGMP) from guanosine triphosphate (GTP).[26] Intracellular cGMP targets include cGMP-dependent protein kinases, cGMP-gated ion channels, and cGMP-regulated cyclic nucleotide phosphodiesterases.[27] ANP, BNP, and urodilatin selectively activate NPRa. ANP has greater affinity for NPRa than does BNP,[28] whereas CNP has very low affinity for this receptor. By contrast, CNP binds more selectively with NPRb with an affinity three orders of magnitude greater than that of either ANP or BNP. This raises the possibility of development of specific antagonists for these receptors.

NPRc contains an extracellular ligand-binding domain and a short (37-amino acid) intracellular domain, but lacks the intracellular protein kinase–like and guanylyl cyclase regions. NPRc is thought to act through internalization and lysosomal hydrolysis of the NPR complex, followed by return to the cell surface. NPRc makes up the majority of the NPRs and is located in several tissues, including endothelium, smooth muscle cells, heart, adrenal gland, and kidney.[6] These receptors exert a clearance function for natriuretic peptides in tissues.[29, 30] Some studies suggest that NPRc acts by activating the phosphoinositol pathway[31] or inhibiting cyclic adenosine monophosphate (cAMP) production;[32] others have suggested that this receptor may mediate the antiproliferative effects of ANP, as well as the inhibitory effects of ANP on adrenergic and purinergic neurotransmission in peripheral tissues and cells.[33] The neuromodulatory effects of ANP via NPRc involve suppression of adenylyl cyclase activity via a pertussis toxin–sensitive G-protein.

The number and distribution of NPRs vary widely in different tissues. NPRa is expressed in heart, lungs, kidney, adrenal glands, adipose tissue, eye, pregnant uterus, and placenta.[34, 35] In the kidney, NPRa appears to be distributed in glomerular cells and in the inner medullary collecting ducts, consistent with the predominant role of ANP at these sites. The distribution of NPRb overlaps somewhat with that of NPRa, but this receptor is present in lower density than NPRa in large blood vessels and kidney and in higher density in the brain. The distribution of NPRb in kidney of Sprague-Dawley rats was studied by reverse transcriptase and polymerase chain reaction techniques: NPRb receptors were present in glomeruli, distal convoluted tubules, cortical and outer and inner medullary tubules, but not in the proximal convoluted tubules or in the thin or thick ascending limbs.[36] CNP mRNA was also identified in the renal cortex and medulla. These findings suggest that CNP may have paracrine or autocrine regulatory functions in rat kidney. NPRc seems to be the most abundant NPR in most tissues, such as the heart, kidney, brain, and adrenal glands, accounting for almost 90% of the total NPRs in important organs, such as the kidney.[37] The number and distribution of NPRs may vary in response to a variety of hormones, intracellular mediators, and metabolic conditions. For example, sodium depletion enhances the mRNA expression of NPRb twofold in the sheep kidney.[38]

METABOLISM OF NATRIURETIC PEPTIDES

The metabolism of ANP and BNP involves two main pathways: enzymatic degradation by neutral metalloendopeptidase (NEP) 24.11 and receptor-mediated clearance via the NPRc or clearance receptor.[35] NEP 24.11 is widely distributed throughout the body and is expressed in high concentrations in the brush border membranes in the proximal tubules of the kidney.[39]

Inhibition of NEP and NPRc produces an increase in plasma ANP concentrations, urine sodium, and volume excretion and a decrease in blood pressure.[40, 41] Coadministration of these inhibitors produces greater effects than those achieved when either of these agents is administered alone. At physiological plasma concentrations of ANP, NPRc may play a dominant role over that of NEP. In rats with heart failure, inhibition of NEP and NPRc induces a significant rise in plasma ANP with vasodilatation, natriuresis, and diuresis. Under these circumstances, the clearance receptor appears to play a lesser role than that of NEP in the metabolism of the peptide because of receptor occupancy,[42] receptor downregulation, or decreased internalization of the receptor-ligand complex.[43]

Urodilatin is not metabolized by NEP.

REGULATION OF NATRIURETIC PEPTIDE SECRETION

ANP and BNP are constitutively released from the heart. However, certain mechanical and neuroendocrine stimuli increase their rates of synthesis or secretion, or both. In response to acute stretching of the atria, there is increased secretion of ANP from atrial cardiocytes that leads to an immediate rise in plasma levels of the hormone. Release of ANP is not Ca^{2+}-dependent and derives from an acutely releasable pool that is exhausted within minutes after the initial stretch stimulus. Stretch over a 4-hour period does not alter ANP gene expression in atria but does stimulate it after 24 hours. BNP secretion and gene expression are also affected by acute stretch in some, but not other, experimental models.[44, 45] With chronic stimulation, as seen in deoxycorticosterone-salt (DOC-salt)–treated rats, both ANP and BNP mRNAs increase in atria, ventricles, and plasma.[46] ANP and BNP mRNA levels are also increased in the heart of spontaneously hypertensive rats (SHRs),[47] of dogs subjected to rapid ventricular pacing,[48] and of human subjects with congestive heart failure.[49]

Stretch of myocardial cells affects only transiently the secretion of natriuretic peptides. This suggests that chronic stimulation of ANP secretion may be under the influence of other factors, such as endothelin-1,[50] catecholamines,[51] acetylcholine, glucocorticoids, angiotensin II,[52] thyroid hormones, prostaglandins,[53] Na-K-ATPase inhibitors,[54] and vasopressin. Of these factors, endothelin-1 appears to be the most powerful stimulator of ANP, although this action is transient, probably as a result of desensitization of endothelin-1 receptor binding or downregulation of phospholipase C activity.[55] Administration of BQ123, an endothelin-a receptor antagonist, reduces stretch-induced ANP release, suggesting that endothelin-1 acts as a modulator of ANP secretion in a paracrine fashion. Endothelin-1 also stimulates BNP gene expression in cultured neonatal atrial cardiocytes[56] as well as in adult atrial tissue.

Although ANP and BNP are cosecreted, they seem to respond differently to the same stimuli. For example, unlike ANP, the plasma concentration of BNP does not change when normal subjects assume the supine position. BNP release, however, is stimulated by increases in left ventricular end-diastolic pressure, pulmonary artery pressure, and pulmonary artery wedge pressure.[57, 58] In patients with chronic renal failure, removal of fluids reduces blood levels of BNP.[59]

PHYSIOLOGICAL ACTIONS OF NATRIURETIC PEPTIDES

Natriuresis and Diuresis

ANP has diuretic, natriuretic, vasorelaxant, and antiproliferative properties.[60] In low doses, sufficient to achieve plasma levels double those of basal levels, ANP causes natriuresis but no change in blood pressure, unless the infusion is prolonged.[61, 62] ANP causes intravascular volume contraction, as documented by increases in serum albumin and hematocrit. This seems to be due in part to diuresis and in part to a shift of fluids from the capillary beds into the interstitium,[63] resulting in decreased preload and blood pressure.[64]

Qualitatively, the effects of BNP are similar to those of ANP. BNP is natriuretic in both animals and human subjects, even at doses that produce plasma levels comparable with those in heart failure. Equimolar infusions of ANP and BNP achieve similar increments in plasma concentrations, but the increase in cGMP during ANP infusion is fourfold that observed during BNP infusion. The natriuresis and contraction in plasma volume are comparable with those of the two peptides.

The mechanism of the natriuretic action of BNP and ANP is complex. ANP raises the glomerular filtration rate (GFR) in the isolated perfused rat kidney in spite of decreases in systemic arterial pressure and renal blood flow[65] and increased single-nephron GFR, measured by the micropuncture technique in the isolated rat kidney.[66] ANP also increases GFR in normal human subjects[63] and in patients with essential hypertension.[67] These findings strongly support the notion that the renal hemodynamic effects of ANP account, at least in part, for the natriuretic action of this peptide. The increase in GFR has been ascribed to constriction of the efferent glomerular arterioles, accompanied by dilatation of the afferent glomerular arterioles.[65] As opposed to ANP, and despite similar natriuretic effects, BNP does not alter GFR in humans,[68] suggesting that at least some of the natriuretic effect of natriuretic peptides must be due to mechanisms other than changes in GFR. ANP inhibits sodium transport in the proximal tubule[69] and in the inner medullary collecting duct.[70] Moreover, ANP and BNP inhibit aldosterone secretion from adrenal cells.[71] In dogs, intrarenal infusion of BNP inhibits renin secretion, probably as a result of increased sodium delivery to the macula densa. In human subjects, BNP causes a fall or no change in plasma renin activity.[72] ANP, but not BNP, inhibits the plasma aldosterone response to angiotensin II.[73]

The discovery of selective antagonists of natriuretic peptides has allowed further clarification of their physiological roles. A selective NPR antagonist, HS-142-1, was isolated from a fungal culture broth of *Aureobasidium* species. HS-142-1 selectively and reversibly blocks guanylyl cyclase–linked NPRa and NPRb and interferes with cGMP production. Studies with HS-142-1 have confirmed a role for the endogenous natriuretic peptides in the control of renal sodium excretion and in the natriuretic response

to volume expansion. This drug blocks the natriuretic and diuretic actions of ANPs in control animals as well as in animals with experimentally induced heart failure. HS-142-1 increases renal vascular resistance and renin, aldosterone, and catecholamine secretion but does not affect basal renal blood flow.[74, 75]

Urodilatin is the latest natriuretic peptide to be discovered. When injected into healthy men in doses greater than 20 ng/kg/min, urodilatin induces diuresis and natriuresis and inhibits renin secretion;[76] higher doses lower blood pressure. The natriuretic action of urodilatin is due in part to an increase in GFR and in part to direct effects on distal tubules. Urinary excretion of urodilatin increases in coincidence with renal sodium excretion, being higher during salt ingestion or after an acute saline infusion.[77] The natriuretic effect of urodilatin is stronger than that of ANP in healthy men and in experimental models of congestive heart failure.[78, 79] This has led to the suggestion that urodilatin may be more important than ANP in the regulation of sodium excretion. The mechanisms underlying the greater potency of urodilatin over ANP are not clear, but its relative resistance to NEP degradation may be a contributory factor.

Hemodynamic Effects

Sustained low-dose infusions of ANP reduce peripheral vascular resistance and blood pressure in animals and in humans,[6] whereas infusions of higher doses cause a decrease in blood pressure accompanied by a rise in peripheral vascular resistance, probably as a result of activation of counterregulatory hormones. In this instance, the hypotensive action of ANP is largely related to a shift of intravascular fluid into the interstitium, thus decreasing preload. Infusion of BNP in high doses into hypertensive rats also causes a profound and sustained fall in blood pressure.[80] However, when administered to hypertensive or normotensive human subjects in doses sufficient to raise plasma concentrations to levels comparable with those seen in heart failure, BNP causes no significant change in blood pressure or heart rate.[81] When administered in higher doses to normal human subjects, BNP causes decreases in systemic vascular resistance and blood pressure, a rise in cardiac index, and significant reductions in pulmonary capillary wedge pressure, pulmonary vascular resistance, and right atrial pressure. When administered in high doses to patients with congestive heart failure, BNP causes similar hemodynamic changes, but systemic blood pressure and pulmonary vascular resistance do not change. The vasorelaxation caused by BNP is associated with, and probably dependent on, the release of cGMP.

Cardiac myocytes contain mRNAs for NPRa and NPRb, and isolated myocytes produce cGMP when exposed to ANP or BNP.[82] This suggests that myocytes are not only a source of but also a target for natriuretic peptides. BNP causes myocardial relaxation and improves exercise hemodynamics in patients with diastolic dysfunction.[83]

ANP and BNP may attenuate the vasoconstriction caused by infusion of norepinephrine or angiotensin II. Thus, ANP and BNP may modulate changes in blood pressure caused by other neuroendocrine homeostatic mechanisms and local endothelial factors. Studies of the role of natriuretic peptides in the control of basal cardiovascular tone have been made possible by the discovery of selective antagonists. Studies have shown that HS-142-1 causes vasoconstriction of the coronary circulation in anesthetized mongrel dogs, without any significant change in systemic hemodynamics, including arterial pressure, heart rate, or cardiac filling pressure.[84] These actions were associated with a decrease in plasma cGMP; circulating ANP levels did not change. This observation suggests that ANP is an important regulator of basal coronary vascular tone.

CNP was initially considered to act principally as a neuropeptide. However, the functional significance of CNP within the central nervous system remains largely unknown. In neuronal cell lines, CNP increases cGMP production.[85] Studies in rats and sheep indicate that CNP may stimulate water drinking and reduce blood pressure and adrenocortical activity.[86] CNP may exert prejunctional inhibition of norepinephrine release.[87] The highest concentration of CNP in the body is present in the pituitary, where it may inhibit the release of luteinizing hormone via NPRa activation.[88]

CNP is also produced in blood vessels and in cultured endothelial cells[89] and acts as an endothelium-derived relaxing peptide. CNP can induce relaxation and inhibit growth of vascular smooth muscle cells[90] and has powerful venodilator effects. In vitro studies have shown that CNP dilates saphenous, femoral, and renal veins, both in the presence and in the absence of endothelium, but the venous relaxation is more potent in the absence of endothelium.[91] In addition, CNP may be an important regulator of basal coronaryvascular tone.[92] This effect may be due to receptor-mediated clearance of CNP by endothelial NPRc, CNP-mediated release of endothelium-dependent vasoconstrictors, or metabolism by endothelial neutral endopeptidase. In isolated human blood vessels in vitro, CNP also causes venous relaxation and, to a lesser degree, arterial relaxation. Arterial relaxation is less pronounced with CNP than with ANP.[92] In human gastroepiploic artery, Ikeda and colleagues[93] found that ANP raised cGMP production by one order of magnitude more than in veins. CNP stimulated cGMP production weakly and equally in these vessels. Analyzed by reverse transcription–polymerase chain reaction, expression of NPRa was four times more abundant in arteries than in veins. Expression of NPRb was approximately the same in arteries and veins.

Intravenous administration of CNP to normal rats (5 to 50 µg/kg) induces hypotension, a fall in right atrial pressure, and a small diuresis and natriuresis.[24] These responses were attenuated in SHRs.[94] In dogs, intravenous infusions of CNP cause hemodynamic effects similar to those in rats, but the natriuretic effect is less evident.[95] Intravenous injections of CNP in normal humans elicit limited biological actions. When infused intravenously in doses sufficient to achieve plasma concentrations of approximately 60 fmol/ml (circulating levels of CNP in humans are less than 10 fmol/ml), CNP has no significant biological actions.[96] When infused in doses sufficient to achieve plasma concentrations of 770 fmol/ml, CNP exerts significant natriuretic, kaliuretic, and hypotensive actions.[97] However, the natriuretic action of CNP appears to be less than that of ANP

or BNP. Whereas infusion of small doses of ANP and BNP inhibits the renin-angiotensin-aldosterone system, CNP does not appear to affect this system when infused in doses that do not affect blood pressure. Only when infused in very high doses does CNP decrease plasma concentration of aldosterone and increase plasma and urinary concentrations of cGMP.[98]

The hemodynamic actions of CNP are more pronounced than those of ANP despite lesser increases in plasma cGMP, raising the possibility that some of the actions of CNP are not mediated by cGMP. Wei and associates[91] showed that the vasorelaxant effects of CNP are inhibited by potassium chloride, but not by blockade of adrenoreceptors, nitric oxide synthase, prostaglandin synthases, or methylene blue, an inhibitor of guanylate cyclase. CNP causes potassium channel activation and membrane hyperpolarization in porcine coronary artery smooth muscle cells.

Modulation of Sympathetic Nervous System Activity

The effects of ANP on blood pressure and fluid and electrolyte balance are largely mediated via its effects on the kidney and the vasculature. However, evidence indicates that the effects of ANP on the central nervous system also contribute to fluid and electrolyte balance and hemodynamic regulation. ANP decreases sympathetic tone via an action on the brain stem.[99] In rats, injection of BNP into the ventrolateral medulla, an area of brain important in the noradrenergic control of blood pressure, causes a decrease in blood pressure and heart rate.[100] Microinjection of a monoclonal anti-ANP antibody into the anterior hypothalamus decreases blood pressure in SHRs, but not in normotensive control Wistar-Kyoto rats.[101, 102] This suggests that the activity of ANP is enhanced in the hypothalamus of SHRs as a result of either increased production of ANP in the brain or increased receptor sensitivity.[103] On the other hand, inhibition of the action of endogenous ANP in the nucleus tractus solitarius raised blood pressure, suggesting a tonic inhibitory role of this peptide in this brain region.[104] ANP synthesis in key brain nuclei that regulate the cardiovascular system is affected by changes in blood volume.[105] ANP inhibits salt appetite and water drinking, and this central action of the peptide contributes to controlling fluid and electrolyte hemeostasis.[106]

ANP and BNP are present in Purkinje's fibers of several mammals, including humans.[107–109] ANP has also been shown in the nodose ganglia of the heart, pathways that carry afferent stimuli from the cardiopulmonary area.[110] Further, ANP interferes with α_1-adrenergic receptor activation in the rat heart[111] and the human kidney.[112] The physiological relevance of these observations is not fully understood.

CNP increases catecholamine formation in the adrenal medulla via cGMP-mediated activation of tyrosine hydroxylase, a rate-limiting enzyme in the synthesis of these amines.[113] By contrast, in incubated rat hypothalamic slices, CNP inhibits spontaneous release of norepinephrine and increases its neuronal uptake and storage.[114] These studies suggest that CNP may be involved in the regulation of noradrenergic neurotransmission at the presynaptic neuronal level.

Other Actions of Natriuretic Peptides

CNP, like the other natriuretic peptides, blunts stimulated endothelin-1 production in vitro,[115] apparently via cGMP. As endothelin-1 causes vascular smooth muscle cell proliferation, CNP could locally inhibit vascular smooth muscle cell proliferation via this mechanism. CNP exerts growth inhibitory effects on human vascular smooth muscle cells and can reduce the response of these cells to growth factors.[90] In vivo, CNP infused for 14 days in rats with carotid artery injury reduced the extent of the vascular injury response.[116] CNP has been isolated from the small and large intestines of rat,[117] and administration of CNP to dogs reduced jejunal electrolyte and fluid secretion,[118] suggesting that CNP may contribute to body fluid homeostasis by modulating intestinal excretion of electrolytes. CNP has a relaxant effect on pulmonary arteries and bronchial smooth muscle cells of guinea pigs.[119] In vitro, CNP causes dose-dependent relaxation of bronchial smooth muscle and stimulates cGMP release from human respiratory epithelial cells.[120] The significance of these observations in pulmonary diseases remains to be ascertained.

INTERACTIONS AMONG NATRIURETIC PEPTIDES

Several studies have suggested that potentially important interactions among natriuretic peptides occur in vivo. Very high infusion rates (0.1 µg/kg/min) of BNP increase plasma levels of ANP in humans; much lower infusion rates of CNP (5 pmol/kg/min) increase plasma concentrations of ANP but not of BNP.[121] CNP production and release by bovine aortic endothelial cells are enhanced by ANP or BNP.[122] In the presence of background low-dose ANP infusions, coinfusion of BNP abruptly and reversibly increases plasma ANP levels by 50% and has additive physiological effects. Similarly, in the presence of background BNP infusion, coinfusion of ANP causes a reversible increase in plasma BNP concentration and results in additive physiological effects. These studies support the notion that natriuretic peptides compete for clearance by shared degradative pathways, rather than affecting each other's production rates.[121]

ATRIAL NATRIURETIC PEPTIDE IN HYPERTENSION

The role of ANP in blood pressure regulation and the pathogenesis of hypertension remains controversial.[123] A reduction of ANP secretion could result in sodium retention and salt-sensitive hypertension. This possibility is supported by studies showing that a disruption of the pro-ANP gene in mice causes salt-sensitive hypertension.[124] In NPRa knockout mice, blood pressure also increases, but this model of hypertension is not salt-sensitive.[125] By contrast,

transgenic mice overexpressing the genes for ANP or BNP have lower blood pressure than normal littermates and do not develop pulmonary hypertension when exposed to chronic hypoxia.[126, 127]

ANP levels are increased in response to salt loading in Wistar-Kyoto but not in salt-sensitive SHRs.[128] ANP infusion in a dose that achieves plasma ANP levels well within the physiological range abolishes the salt-induced exacerbation of hypertension in salt-sensitive SHRs.[129] ANP secretion in response to increased atrial pressure was impaired in prehypertensive Dahl salt-sensitive rats but exaggerated in more advanced phases when hypertension was complicated by left ventricular hypertrophy.[130] In hypertension caused by excess mineralocorticoid, the concentration of ANP increases in coincidence with the phenomenon of "escape." Administration of HS-142-1 exacerbates hypertension in this model.[131]

Measurements of plasma ANP levels in patients with essential hypertension have provided conflicting results. Some studies have shown low to normal plasma ANP levels;[132–134] others have shown increased levels.[135–137] Sagnella and coworkers[138] showed an increase in plasma ANP levels during high sodium intake in patients with essential hypertension. Kohno and colleagues[139] showed that sodium loading increased plasma ANP more in salt-sensitive than in salt-resistant patients. Nimura,[140] on the other hand, showed a blunted increase in plasma ANP in response to high dietary salt intake in salt-sensitive compared with salt-resistant patients. Ferrari and associates[141] and Weidmann and coworkers[142] observed markedly reduced plasma ANP during high sodium intake in offspring of hypertensive parents compared with offspring of normotensive parents. They suggested that relative ANP deficiency may predispose individuals to develop essential hypertension. We have demonstrated that salt-sensitive hypertensive African Americans manifest abnormal ANP secretion in response to increased dietary sodium intake. Salt-resistant patients fail to manifest the expected rise in ANP, whereas salt-sensitive patients show a paradoxical decrease in ANP. In these patients, reduced atrial secretion of ANP could be, at least in part, responsible for the reduced ability to excrete sodium and for the sodium-induced rise in blood pressure. In whites, we noticed a similar tendency for ANP to decrease during high salt intake, but the decrease did not reach statistical significance.[143] The discrepancies in the literature could be due partly to methodological differences in ANP measurements and to differences in age, dietary salt intake, left ventricular function, and genetic differences among populations studied.

ATRIAL NATRIURETIC PEPTIDE IN CONGESTIVE HEART FAILURE

In acute congestive heart failure, secretion of ANP increases in response to an acute rise in atrial filling pressure and atrial stretch. By contrast, controversy remains with regard to the acute response of BNP. In vitro studies have indicated that when isolated myocytes are subjected to acute stretch, BNP gene expression may be more immediately responsive than ANP gene expression.[144] In vivo studies, however, have indicated that acute changes in cardiac filling pressures caused by volume expansion,[145] by mitral stenosis repair in humans,[146] or by acute congestive heart failure induced by rapid left ventricular pacing in anesthetized dogs do not increase circulating BNP levels.[147] This is consistent with the observation that BNP concentrations in the normal heart are markedly less than those of ANP. In anesthetized dogs with acute congestive heart failure, an infusion of exogenous BNP sufficient to achieve circulating concentrations similar to those observed in chronic congestive heart failure resulted in markedly increased plasma and urine cGMP, reduced cardiac filling pressure, diuresis and natriuresis, attenuated release of renin, and inhibition of distal tubular sodium reabsorption.[147] This may provide a rationale for the use of BNP in the management of acute congestive heart failure. In anesthetized dogs with acute heart failure induced by rapid ventricular pacing, administration of HS-142-1, an inhibitor of NPRs, caused a decrease in GFR and an increase in distal fractional sodium reabsorption, supporting a functional role for the endogenous natriuretic peptide system in preserving sodium homeostasis and GFR in acute heart failure.[148]

In chronic heart failure, the secretion of ANP increases in proportion to the severity of the failure. Ventricular production of ANP increases, but remains lower than atrial production.[149] Plasma levels of BNP also increase in chronic heart failure and may exceed the plasma levels of ANP. Plasma BNP concentration may correlate with outcome more closely than ANP concentration.[150] BNP is considered to be a backup hormone that, in chronic congestive heart failure, is synthesized and released into the plasma to complement the actions of ANP. In contrast, the plasma concentration of CNP does not change, even though cardiac tissue content may be increased.[151] Natriuretic peptides secreted in heart failure inhibit the production of angiotensin II, aldosterone, catecholamines, and endothelins, defending the patient against sodium and water retention. The vasodilator and volume-contracting properties of these hormones reduce systemic vascular resistance, decrease ventricular filling pressure, and improve myocardial performance. Moreover, these peptides inhibit the growth of cardiac fibroblasts, thus reducing cardiac remodeling and collagen accumulation. Blocking the actions of these peptides with selective receptor antagonists results in accelerated progression of heart failure and stimulation of renin, aldosterone, catecholamines, and endothelin-1.[152]

The cGMP response to ANP in heart failure is diminished compared with that in normal subjects, probably due to downregulation of specific receptors caused by chronic exposure to high levels of the peptide. This results in further deterioration of heart failure. In contrast, the cGMP response to CNP is enhanced in patients with heart failure compared with normal subjects, suggesting receptor upregulation.[153] The significance of these changes remains obscure.

ATRIAL NATRIURETIC PEPTIDE IN CIRRHOSIS

The mechanisms of sodium retention in cirrhosis are complex and include activation of vasoconstrictors, such as angiotensin II and norepinephrine. Increased secretion of ANP compensates, at least in part, for the sodium-retaining actions of these vasoconstrictors in these patients. Plasma levels of ANP and BNP are usually increased in patients with cirrhosis,[154, 155] with the exception of patients with hyponatremia, in whom the levels may actually be decreased.[156] By contrast, urinary excretion of urodilatin is unchanged in patients with cirrhosis even in the presence of increased plasma levels of ANP,[157] suggesting that ANP and urodilatin in cirrhosis are regulated independently. Patients with well-compensated cirrhosis remain in sodium balance, presumably as a result of the natriuretic effects of these elevated levels of ANP. When cirrhosis decompensates, ANP becomes unable to offset the sodium-retaining actions of increased levels of angiotensin II and aldosterone and of increased activation of the sympathetic nervous system.[158] With the development of refractory ascites, cirrhotic patients become unresponsive to the natriuretic effects of ANP. This may be in part mediated by further increased activity of the sympathetic nervous system.[159] In a rat model of cirrhosis, the ANP response could be entirely restored by renal denervation, suggesting a key role for the sympathetic nervous system in the mediation of unresponsiveness to ANP.[160] Administration of HS-142-1 reduces renal plasma flow and GFR in cirrhotic rats with ascites, suggesting that these hormones may play a role in preservation of renal function and urine sodium excretion in this condition.[161]

ATRIAL NATRIURETIC PEPTIDE IN NEPHROTIC SYNDROME

Most,[162] although not all,[163] studies have demonstrated slightly elevated ANP levels in nephrotic patients, particularly in those with associated reduced levels of plasma renin activity. This suggests that the increase in ANP secretion may be the result of volume expansion. Bolus injection of ANP (2 μg/kg body weight) in nephrotic patients caused less natriuresis than in control subjects.[164]

ATRIAL NATRIURETIC PEPTIDE IN CHRONIC RESPIRATORY DISEASE

ANP plays an important role in the development of chronic obstructive pulmonary disease (COPD). Plasma ANP levels are elevated in chronic respiratory failure and do not change with short-term supplementary oxygen therapy.[165] BNP levels are also elevated in patients with acute hypoxic COPD and are positively correlated with the degree of hypoxia.[166] In one study, plasma levels of ANP and BNP were elevated in patients with COPD and PaO_2 less than 60 mm Hg, but not in patients with PaO_2 of 60 mm Hg or greater, and were significantly correlated with the degree of hypoxemia. Plasma CNP level was not detectable in these patients. Plasma levels of ANP and BNP were significantly decreased by long-term oxygen therapy. Moreover, plasma ANP and BNP levels were elevated in COPD patients with right ventricular hypertrophy compared with patients without right ventricular hypertrophy.[167] These data suggest that in COPD patients, the major stimulus for ANP and BNP secretion may be hypoxemia, but a rise in right ventricular pressure may also play a role.

OTHER NATRIURETIC PEPTIDES

The cardiac ventricle of rainbow trout contains a ventricular natriuretic peptide (VNP) structurally more similar to ANP than to BNP. Only VNP has been isolated from rainbow trout or from a related species, the chum salmon, *Oncorhynchus keta*. In these species, attempts to isolate ANP from atria using immunoreactivity to mammalian ANP as an assay system have been unsuccessful. Recently, a new natriuretic peptide was isolated from trout atria. However, this peptide exhibited low relaxant activity in the chick rectum and extremely low vasorelaxant activity in the rat aortic strip (only 1/400 that of human ANP). This peptide was equipotent with trout VNP and human ANP in relaxing trout epibranchial artery.[168]

Two related peptides are guanylin and uroguanylin, 15- and 16-amino acid peptides produced primarily in the gastrointestinal mucosa. These peptides act through the cGMP pathway and regulate sodium and water transport across the intestinal mucosa.[169]

CLINICAL APPLICATIONS OF NATRIURETIC PEPTIDES

Despite the potentially useful natriuretic and vasodilator actions of natriuretic peptides, these agents currently have limited if any use in clinical practice. This is in large part due to their limited effectiveness in congestive heart failure, a condition for which they originally offered the greatest promise, as well as in cirrhosis or nephrotic syndrome. Infusions of exogenous ANP in patients with heart failure are largely ineffective or increase natriuresis only transitorily. Infusion of ANP in patients with compensated cirrhosis, in doses that increased plasma concentrations to levels comparable with those observed in patients with ascites, causes decreases in left ventricular end-diastolic volume, stroke volume, cardiac output, and blood pressure, and an increase in GFR and urinary sodium excretion.[170] The hypotensive action of ANP in these patients is not associated with an appropriate increase in plasma norepinephrine.[171] Thus, the use of ANP in cirrhosis is generally limited by an intolerable drug-induced hypotension. When combined with terlipressin (a vasopressin analogue), ANP increased sodium excretion in patients with cirrhosis and refractory ascites.[172] Infusions or bolus injections of BNP still hold promise in the management of heart failure, but this requires further investigation. Infusion of urodilatin caused a significant increase in urinary sodium excretion in cirrhotic patients with or without ascites, associated with a decrease in fractional distal tubular sodium reabsorption. Urodilatin caused no changes in the renin-angiotensin-aldosterone system.[173]

ANP has also been investigated in patients with acute renal failure in a multicenter randomized trial. Dialysis-free survival did not improve in ANP-treated patients with acute renal failure, and worsened in patients with nonoliguric acute renal failure.[174]

Greater hope is provided by agents that interfere with the receptor binding or metabolism of natriuretic peptides. We have already addressed the potential usefulness of specific inhibitors of NP receptors. These agents have already helped to better define the functions of these peptides, but have not yet proved useful in the clinical arena. More promising are the inhibitors of NEP, the enzyme that degrades natriuretic peptides. Potent inhibitors of NEP have been developed and have provided useful tools to test the role of this enzyme in the inactivation of natriuretic peptides, as well as in probing the functions of these peptides. These drugs potentiate the natriuretic and hypotensive response to intravenous infusions of ANP, as well as the natriuretic response to volume expansion.[175]

NEP inhibition results in diuresis and natriuresis in congestive heart failure[176, 177] and in rats with chronic renal failure.[178] In salt-sensitive models of hypertension, such as the DOC-salt rat model, NEP inhibitors reduce blood pressure.[41] These actions occur despite minimal increases in plasma ANP levels and are associated with increased urinary excretion of cGMP, suggesting that the antihypertensive response to NEP inhibition cannot be attributed exclusively to changes in plasma concentrations of ANP and that NEP inhibitors may raise local tissue levels of ANP without increasing plasma levels. Alternatively, the actions of NEP inhibitors may be due to reduced inactivation of other vasoactive peptides, such as bradykinin.[179] This hypothesis, however, is unlikely because SCH 34826, an oral NEP inhibitor, failed to affect the depressor response to bradykinin.[41] Moreover, administration of a bradykinin antagonist failed to alter the hypotensive response to oral administration of SCH 34826 in the DOC-salt rat.

NEP inhibitors can also potentiate the renal effects of ANP, a response that is partially inhibited by bradykinin antagonists.[180] When given in combination with an inhibitor of angiotensin-converting enzyme, NEP inhibitors may further impair the degradation of bradykinin, resulting in potentiation of their beneficial effects.

References

1. de Bold AJ, Borenstein HB, Veress AT, et al. A rapid and potent natriuretic response to intravenous injection of atrial myocardial extract in rats. Life Sci 28:89–94, 1981.
2. Yandle TG. Biochemistry of natriuretic peptides. J Intern Med 235:561–576, 1994.
3. Mathisen P, Hall C, Simonsen S. Comparative study of atrial peptides ANF (1-98) and ANF (99-126) as diagnostic markers of atrial distension in patients with cardiac disease. Scand J Clin Lab Invest 53:41–49, 1991.
4. Sudoh T, Kangawa K, Minamino N, Matsuo H. A new natriuretic peptide in porcine brain. Nature 332:78–81, 1988.
5. Itoh H, Nakao K, Saito Y, et al. Radioimmunoassay for brain natriuretic peptide (BNP) detection of BNP in canine brain. Biochem Biophys Res Commun 158:120–128, 1989.
6. Espiner EA, Richards AM, Yandle TG, Nicholls G. Natriuretic hormones. Endocrinol Metab Clin North Am 24:481–509, 1995.
7. Sudoh T, Maekawa K, Kojima M, et al. Cloning and sequence analysis of cDNA encoding a precursor for human brain natriuretic peptide. Biochem Biophys Res Commun 159:1427–1434, 1989.
8. Yandle TG, Richards AM, Gilbert A, et al. Assay of brain natriuretic peptide (BNP) in human plasma: Evidence for high molecular weight BNP as a major component in heart failure. J Endocrinol Metab 76:832–838, 1993.
9. Hasegawa K, Fujiwara H, Itoh H, et al. Light and electrom microscopic localization of brain natriuretic peptide in relation to atrial

natriuretic peptide in porcine atrium: Immunohistocytochemical study using specific monoclonal antibodies. Circulation 84:1203–1209, 1991.

10. Iida T, Hirata Y, Takemura N, et al. Brain natriuretic peptide is cosecreted with atrial natriuretic peptide from porcine cardiocytes. FEBS Lett 260:98–100, 1990.

11. Togashi K, Hirata Y, Ando K, et al. Brain natriuretic peptide–like immunoreactivity is present in human plasma. FEBS Lett 250:235–237, 1989.

12. Tawaragi Y, Fuchimura K, Tanaka K, et al. Gene and precursor structures of human CNP. Biochem Biophys Res Commun 175:645–651, 1991.

13. Tawaragi Y, Fuchimura K, Nakazato H, et al. Gene and precursor structure of porcine C–type natriuretic peptide. Biochem Biophys Res Commun 172:627–632, 1990.

14. Sudoh T, Minamino N, Kangawa K, Matsuo H. C-type natriuretic peptide (CNP): A new member of natriuretic peptide family identified in porcine brain. Biochem Res Commun 168:863–870, 1990.

15. Komatsu Y, Nakao K, Suga S. CNP in rats and humans. Endocrinology 129:1104–1106, 1991.

16. Suzuki R, Togashi K, Ando K, Takei Y. Distribution and molecular forms of C-type natriuretic peptide in plasma and tissue of a dogfish, *Triakis scyllia*. Gen Comp Endocrinol 96:378–384, 1994.

17. Hama N, Itoh H, Shirakami G, et al. Detection of C-type natriuretic peptide in human circulation and marked increase of plasma CNP level in septic shock patients. Biochem Biophys Res Commun 198:1177–1182, 1994.

18. Schulz-Knappe P, Forssmann K, Herbst F, et al. Isolation and structural analysis of "urodilatin," a new peptide of the cardiodilatin-(ANP)-family, extracted from human urine. Klin Wochenschr 66:752–759, 1988.

19. Feller SM, Gangelmann M, Forssmann WG. Urodilatin: A newly described member of the ANP family. Trends Pharmacol Sci 10:93–94, 1989.

20. Greenwald JE, Needleman P, Wilkins MR, Schreiner GF. Renal synthesis of atriopeptin-like protein in physiology and pathophysiology. Am J Physiol 260:F602–F607, 1991.

21. Ruskoaho H. Atrial natriuretic peptide: Synthesis, release, and metabolism. Pharmacol Rev 44:479–602, 1992.

22. Vollmar AM, Gerbes AL, Nemer M, Sculz R. Detection of C-type natriuretic peptide (CNP) transcript in the rat heart and immune organs. Endocrinology 132:1872–1874, 1993.

23. Heublein DM, Lerman H, Clavell AL, et al. Immunohistochemical localization of C-type natriuretic peptide in human vascular and endothelial cells. J Vasc Res 29:134–171, 1992.

24. Totsune K, Takahashi K, Murakami O, et al. Elevated plasma C-type natriuretic peptide concentration in patients with chronic renal failure. Clin Sci 87:319–322, 1994.

25. Lowe DG, Klisak I, Sparkes RS, et al. Chromosomal distribution of the three members of the human natriuretic peptide receptor/guanylate cyclase gene family. Genomics 8:304–312, 1990.

26. Koller KJ, Goeddel DV. Molecular biology of the natriuretic peptides and their receptors. Circulation 86:1081–1088, 1992.

27. Lincoln TM, Cornwell TL. Intracellular cyclic GMP receptor proteins. FASEB J 7:328–338, 1993.

28. Suga S, Nakao K, Mukoyama M, et al. Receptor sensitivity of natriuretic peptide family, atrial natriuretic peptide, brain natriuretic peptide, and C type natriuretic peptide. Endocrinology 130:229–239, 1992.

29. Nuzzenzeig DR, Lewicki JA, Maack T. Cellular mechanisms of type C receptors of atrial natriuretic factor. J Biol Chem 265:20952–20958, 1990.

30. Fuller F, Porter JG, Arfsten AE, et al. Atrial natriuretic peptide clearance receptor: Complete sequence and functional expression of cDNA clones. J Biol Chem 263:9395–9401, 1988.

31. Hirata M, Chang CH, Murad F. Stimulatory effects of atrial natriuretic factor on phosphoinositide hydrolysis in cultured bovine aortic smooth muscle cells. Biochem Biophys Acta 1010:346–351, 1989.

32. Anand Srivastava MB, Sairam MR, Cartin M. Ring-deleted natriuretic analogs of atrial natriuretic factor inhibits the aldosterone response to angiotensin II in man. Clin Sci 265:8566–8572, 1986.

33. Drewett JG, Ziegler RJ, Trachte GJ. Neuromodulatory effects of atrial natriuretic peptides correlate with an inhibition of adenylate cyclase but not an activation of guanylate cyclase. J Pharmacol Exp Ther 260:689–696, 1992.

34. Itoh H, Sagawa N, Hasegawa M, et al. Expression of biologically active receptors for natriuretic peptides in the human uterus during pregnancy. Biochem Biophys Res Commun 203:602–607, 1994.

35. Nakao K, Ogawa Y, Suga S, et al. Molecular biology and biochemistry of the natriuretic peptide system. II: Natriuretic peptide receptors. J Hypertens 10:1111–1114, 1992.

36. Lohe A, Yeh I, Hyver E, et al. Natriuretic peptide B receptor and C-type natriuretic peptide in the rat kidney. J Am Soc Nephrol 6:1552–1558, 1995.

37. Maack T, Okolicany J, Koh GY, et al. Functional properties of atrial natriuretic factor receptors. Semin Nephrol 13:50–60, 1993.

38. Fraenkel MB, Aldred P, McDougall JG. Sodium status affects GC-B natriuretic peptide receptor mRNA levels but not GC-A or C receptor mRNA levels, in the sheep kidney. Clin Sci 86:517–522, 1994.

39. Seymour AA, Abboa-Offei BE, Smith PL, et al. Potentiation of natriuretic peptides by neutral endopeptidase inhibitors. Clin Exp Pharmacol Physiol 22:63–69, 1995.

40. Seymour A, Fennell SA, Swerdel JN. Potentiation of renal effects of atrial natriuretic factor (99-126) by SQ 29072. Hypertension 14:87–97, 1989.

41. Sybertz EJ, Chiu PJS, Watkins RW, Vemulapalli S. Neutral metalloendopeptidase inhibitors as ANF potentiators: Sites and mechanisms of action. Can J Physiol Pharmacol 69:1628–1635, 1991.

42. Chiu PJ, Tetzloff G, Romano MT, et al. Influence of C-ANF receptor and neutral endoperoxidase on pharmacokinetics of ANF in rats. Am J Physiol 260:R208–R216, 1991.

43. Kishimoto I, Nakao K, Suga SI, et al. Downregulation of C-receptor by natriuretic peptides via ANP-B receptor in vascular smooth muscle cells. Am J Physiol 265:H1373–H1379, 1993.

44. Mantymaa P, Vuolteenaho O, Martila M, et al. Atrial stretch induces rapid increase in brain natriuretic peptide but not in atrial natriuretic peptide gene expression in vitro. Endocrinology 133:1470–1473, 1993.

45. Kinnunen P, Vuolteenano O, Roskoaho H. Mechanisms of atrial and brain natriuretic peptide release from rat ventricular myocardium: Effect of stretching. Endocrinology 132:1961–1970, 1993.

46. de Bold AJ, Bruneau BG, de Bold MLK. Mechanical and neuroendocrine regulation of the endocrine heart. Cardiovasc Res 31:7–18, 1996.

47. Dagnino L, Lavigne JP, Nemer M. Increased transcript for B-type natriuretic peptide in spontaneously hypertensive rats. Quantitative polymerase chain reaction for atrial and brain natriuretic peptide transcripts. Hypertension 20:690–700, 1992.

48. Perrella MA, Schwab TR, O'Murchu B, et al. Cardiac atrial natriuretic factor during evolution of congestive heart failure. Am J Physiol 262:H1248–H1255, 1992.

49. Mukoyama M, Nakao K, Hosoda K, et al. Brain natriuretic peptide as a novel cardiac hormone in humans. Evidence for an exquisite dual natriuretic peptide system, atrial natriuretic peptide and brain natriuretic peptide. J Clin Invest 87:1402–1412, 1991.

50. Schiebinger RJ, Gomez-Sanchez CE. Endothelin: A potent stimulus of atrial natriuretic peptide secretion by superfused rat atria and its dependency on calcium. Endocrinology 127:119–125, 1990.

51. Schiebinger RJ, Baker MZ, Linden J. Effect of adrenergic and muscarinic cholinergic agonists on atrial natriuretic peptide secretion by isolated rat atria. Potential role of the autonomic nervous system in modulating atrial natriuretic peptide secretion. J Clin Invest 80:1687–1691, 1987.

52. Focaccio A, Volpe M, Ambrosio G, et al. Angiotensin II directly stimulates release of atrial natriuretic factor in isolated rabbit hearts. Circulation 87:192–198, 1993.

53. Gardner DG, Schultz HD. Prostaglandins regulate the synthesis and secretion of the atrial natriuretic peptide. J Clin Invest 86:52–59, 1990.

54. Bloch KD, Zamir N, Lichstein D, et al. Ouabain induces secretion of proatrial natriuretic factor by rat atrial cardiocytes. Am J Physiol 255:E383–E387, 1988.

55. Leite MF, Page E, Ambler SK. Regulation of ANP secretion by endothelin-1 in cultured atrial myocytes: Desensitization and receptor subtype. Am J Physiol 267:H2193–H2203, 1994.

56. Suzuki E, Hirata Y, Kohmoto O, et al. Cellular mechanisms for synthesis and secretion of atrial natriuretic peptide and brain natriuretic peptide in cultured rat atrial cells. Circ Res 71:1039–1048, 1992.

57. Richards AM, Crozier IG, Espiner EA, et al. Plasma brain natriuretic peptide and endopeptidase 24.11 inhibition in hypertension. Hypertension 22:231–236, 1993.

58. Kohno M, Horio T, Yokokama K, et al. Pulmonary arterial brain natriuretic peptide concentration and cardiopulmonary hemodynamics during exercise in patients with essential hypertension. Metabolism 41:1273–1275, 1992.

59. Lang CC, Choy AMJ, Henderson IS, et al. Effect of haemodialysis on plasma levels of brain natriuretic peptide in patients with chronic renal failure. Clin Sci 82:127–131, 1992.

60. Kleinert HD, Maack T, Atlas SA, et al. Atrial natriuretic factor inhibits angiotensin, norepinephrine and potassium induced vascular contractility. Hypertension 6:1–5, 1984.

61. Richards AM, Espiner EA, Ikram H, Yandle TG. Atrial natriuretic factor in hypertension: Bioactivity at normal plasma levels. Hypertension 14:261–268, 1989.

62. Janssen WMT, De Zeeuw D, van der Hem GK, De Jong PE. Antihypertensive effect of a 5-day infusion of atrial natriuretic factor in humans. Hypertension 13:640–646, 1989.

63. Weidmann P, Hasler L, Gnadinger MP, et al. Blood levels and renal effects of atrial natriuretic peptide in normal man. J Clin Invest 77:734–742, 1986.

64. Charles CJ, Espiner EA, Richards AM. Cardiovascular actions of ANF: Contributions of renal, neurohumoral, and hemodynamic factors in sheep. Am J Physiol 264:R533–R538, 1993.

65. Camargo MJF, Kleinert HD, Atlas SA, et al. Ca-dependent hemodynamic and natriuretic effects of atrial extract in isolated rat kidney. Am J Physiol 246:F447–F456, 1984.

66. Briggs JP, Steipe B, Shubert G, Schnermann J. Micropuncture studies of renal effects of atrial natriuretic substance. Pflugers Arch 395:271–276, 1982.

67. Weder AB, Sekkarie MA, Takiyyuddin M, et al. Antihypertensive and hypotensive effects of atrial natriuretic factor in men. Hypertension 10:582–589, 1987.

68. Holmes SJ, Espiner EA, Richards AM, et al. Renal, endocrine and haemodynamic effects of human brain natriuretic peptide in normal man. J Clin Endocrinol Metab 76:91–96, 1993.

69. Seymour AA, Blaine EH, Mazack EK, et al. Renal and systemic effects of synthetic atrial natriuretic factor. Life Sci 36:33–44, 1985.

70. Gunning M, Ballerman BJ, Silva P, et al. Brain natriuretic peptide: Interaction with renal ANP system. Am J Physiol F467–F472, 1990.

71. Volpe M, Odell G, Kleinert HD, et al. Effect of atrial natriuretic factor (ANF) on blood pressure renin and aldosterone in Goldblatt hypertension. Hypertension 7(suppl I):43–48, 1985.

72. McGregor A, Richards M, Expiner E, Yandle T. Brain natriuretic peptide administered to man: Actions and metabolism. J Clin Endocrinol Metab 70:1103–1107, 1990.

73. Hunt PJ, Espiner EA, Nicholls MG, et al. Differing biological effects of equimolar atrial and brain natriuretic peptide infusions in normal man. J Clin Endocrinol Metab 81:3871–3876, 1996.

74. Stevens TL, Wei C, Aarhus LL, et al. Modulation of exogenous and endogenous atrial natriuretic peptide by a receptor inhibitor. Hypertension 23:613–618, 1994.

75. Wada A, Tsutamoto T, Matsuda Y, Kinoshita M. Cardiorenal and neurohumoral effects of endogenous atrial natriuretic peptide in dogs with severe congestive heart failure using a specific antagonist for guanylate cyclase–coupled receptors. Circulation 89:2232–2240, 1994.

76. Carstens J, Jensen KT, Pedersen EB. Effect of urodilatin infusion on renal hemodynamics, tubular function and vasoactive hormones. Clin Sci 92:397–407, 1997.

77. Drummer C, Fiedler F, K'nig A, Gerzer R. Urodilatin, a kidney-derived natriuretic factor, is excreted with a circadian rhythm and is stimulated by saline infusion in man. J Am Soc Nephrol 1:1109–1113, 1991.

78. Saxenhofer H, Rashelli A, Weidmann P. Urodilatin, a natriuretic factor from kidneys, can modify renal and cardiovascular function in man. Am J Physiol 259:F832–F838, 1990.

79. Villareal D, Freeman RH, Johnson RA. Renal effects of ANF (955-126), a new atrial peptide analogue, in dogs with experimental heart failure. Am J Hypertens 4:508–515, 1991.

80. Kita T, Kida O, Yokata N, et al. Effect of brain natriuretic peptide-45, a circulating form of rat brain natriuretic peptide, in spontaneously hypertensive rats. Eur J Pharmacol 202:73–79, 1991.

81. Stephenson SL, Kenny AJ. The hydrolysis of alpha-human atrial natriuretic peptide in normal man. J Clin Endocrinol Metab 76:91–96, 1993.

82. Lin X, Hanze J, Heese F, et al. Gene expression of natriuretic peptide receptors in myocardial cells. Circ Res 77:750–758, 1995.

83. Clarkson PBM, Wheeldon NM, MacLeod C, et al. Brain natriuretic peptide: Effect on left ventricular filling patterns in healthy subjects. Clin Sci 88:159–164, 1995.

84. Supaporn T, Wennberg PW, Wei CM, et al. Role of the endogenous natriuretic peptide system in the control of basal coronary vascular tone in dogs. Clin Sci 90:357–362, 1996.

85. Toki S, Morishita Y, Sano T, Matsuda Y. HS-142-1, a novel nonpeptide ANP antagonist, blocks the cyclic GMP production elicited by natriuretic peptide in PC12 and NG 108-15 cells. Neurosci Lett 135:1117–1120, 1992.

86. Samson WK, Skala KD, Huang FLS. CNP-22 stimulates, rather than inhibits water drinking in the rat: Evidence for a unique biological action of the C-type natriuretic peptides. Brain Res 568:285–288, 1991.

87. Trachte GJ, Drewett JG. C-type natriuretic peptide neuromodulates independently of guanylyl cyclase activation. Hypertension 23:38–43, 1994.

88. Samson WK, Huang F, Fulton RJ. C-type natriuretic peptide mediates the hypothalamic actions of the natriuretic peptides to inhibit luteinizing hormone secretion. Endocrinology 132:504–509, 1993.

89. Suga S, Nakao K, Itoh H, et al. Endothelial production of C-type natriuretic peptide and its marked augmentation by transforming growth factor-β. Possible existence of "vascular natriuretic peptide system." J Clin Invest 90:1145–1149, 1992.

90. Itoh H, Pratt RE, Dzau VJ. Atrial natriuretic polypeptide inhibits hypertrophy of vascular smooth muscle cells. J Clin Invest 86:1690–1697, 1990.

91. Wei CM, Aarhus LL, Miller V, Burnett JC Jr. Actions of C-type natriuretic peptide in isolated canine arteries and veins. Am J Physiol 264:H71–H73, 1993.

92. Supaporn T, Wennberg PW, Wei CM, et al. Role of endogenous natriuretic peptide system in the control of brain coronary vascular tone in dogs. Clin Sci 90:357–362, 1996.

93. Ikeda T, Itoh H, Komatsu Y, et al. Natriuretic peptide receptors in human artery and vein and rabbit vein graft. Hypertension 27:833–837, 1996.

94. Wei CM, Kim CH, Khraibi AA, et al. Atrial natriuretic peptide and C-type natriuretic peptide in spontaneously hypertensive rats and their vasorelaxing actions in vitro. Hypertension 23(pt 2):903–907, 1994.

95. Clavell AL, Stingo AJ, Wei CM, et al. C-type natriuretic peptide: A selective cardiovascular peptide. Am J Physiol 264:R290–R295, 1993.

96. Hunt PJ, Richards A, Espiner E, et al. Bioactivity and metabolism of C-type natriuretic peptide in normal man. J Clin Endocrinol Metab 78:1428–1435, 1994.

97. Igaki T, Itoh H, Suga SI, et al. C-type natriuretic peptide in chronic renal failure and its action in humans. Kidney Int 49(suppl 55):S-144–S-147, 1996.

98. Barr CS, Rhodes P, Struthers AD. C-type natriuretic peptide. Peptides 17:1243–1251, 1996.

99. Schultz HD, Gardner DG, Deschepper CF, et al. Vagal C-fiber blockade abolishes sympathetic inhibition by atrial natriuretic factor. Am J Physiol 155:R6–R13, 1988.

100. Ermirio R, Avanzino GL, Ruggeri P, et al. Cardiovascular effects of microinjection of ANF and brain natriuretic peptide into ventrolateral medulla. Am J Physiol 259:R32–R37, 1990.

101. Yang R, Hongkui J, Chen Y, et al. Blockade of endogenous anterior hypothalamic atrial natriuretic peptide with monoclonal antibody lowers blood pressure in spontaneously hypertensive rats. J Clin Invest 86:1985–1990, 1990.

102. Oparil S, Chen YF, Peng N, Wyss JM. Anterior hypothalamic norepinephrine, atrial natriuretic peptide and hypertension. Front Neuroendocrinol 17:212–246, 1996.

103. Grove KL, Goncalves J, Picard S, et al. Comparison of ANP binding and sensitivity in brain from hypertensive and normotensive rats. Am J Physiol 272:R1344–R1353, 1997.

104. Yang RH, Jin HK, Wyss JM, et al. Pressor effect of blocking atrial natriuretic peptide in nucleus tractus solitarii. Hypertension 19:198–205, 1992.

105. Imura H, Nakao K, Itoh H, et al. The natriuretic peptide system in

the brain: Implications in the central control of cardiovascular and neuroendocrine functions. Front Neuroendocrinol 13:217–249, 1992.

106. Blackburn RE, Samson WK, Fulton RJ, et al. Central oxytocin and ANP receptors mediate osmotic inhibition of salt appetite in rats. Am J Physiol 269:R245–R251, 1995.

107. Back H, Stumpf WE, Ando E, et al. Immunocytochemical evidence for CCD/ANP-like peptides in strands of myoendocrine cells associated with the ventricular conduction system in the rat heart. Anat Embryol 175:223–226, 1986.

108. Wharton J, Andersson RH, Springall D, et al. Localization of atrial natriuretic peptide immunoreactivity in the ventricular myocardium and conduction system of the human fetal and adult heart. Br Heart J 60:267–274, 1988.

109. Hansson M, Eriksson A, Forsgren S. Natriuretic peptide immunoreactivity in nerve structures and Purkinje fibres of human, pig and sheep hearts. 29:329–336, 1997.

110. Debinski W, Gutkowska J, Kuchel O, et al. ANF-like peptides in the peripheral autonomic nervous system. Biochem Biophys Res Commun 134:279–284, 1986.

111. Atchison DJ, Ackermann U. The interaction between atrial natriuretic peptide and cardiac parasympathetic function. J Auton Nerv Syst 42:81–88, 1993.

112. Lang CC, Choy AM, Balfour DJ, Sruthers AD. Prazosin attenuates the natriuretic response to atrial natriuretic factor in man. Kidney Int 42:433–441, 1992.

113. Tsutsui M, Yanagihara N, Kouichiro M, et al. C-type natriuretic peptide stimulates catecholamine synthesis through the accumulation of cyclic GMP in cultured bovine adrenal medullary cells. J Pharmacol Exp Ther 268:584–589, 1994.

114. Vatta MS, Presas M, Bianciotti LG, et al. B and C type natriuretic peptides modulate norepinephrine uptake and release in the rat hypothalamus. Regul Pept 65:175–184, 1996.

115. Kohno M, Yasunari K, Yokokawa K, et al. Inhibition by atrial and brain natriuretic peptide of endothelin-1 secretion after stimulation with angiotensin II and thrombin of cultured hyman endothelial cells. J Clin Invest 87:1999–2004, 1991.

116. Furuya M, Aisaka K, Miyazaki T, et al. C-type natriuretic peptide inhibits intimal thickening after vascular injury. Biochem Biophys Res Commun 193:248–253, 1993.

117. Wilcox JN, Augustine A, Goeddel DV, Lowe DG. Differential regional expression of three natriuretic peptide receptor gene within primate tissues. Mol Cell Biol 11:3454–3462, 1991.

118. Morita H, Hagiike M, Horiba T, et al. Effects of brain natriuretic peptide and C-type natriuretic peptide infusion on urine flow and jejunal absorption in anesthesized dogs. J Physiol 42:349–353, 1992.

119. Takagi K, Araki N, Suzuki K, et al. Relaxant effect of CNP on guinea-pig tracheal smooth muscle. Arzneimittelforschung 42:1329–1331, 1992.

120. Geary CA, Goy MF, Boucher RC. Synthesis and vectorial export of cGMP in airway epithelium: Expression of soluble and CNP-specific guanylate cyclase. Am J Physiol 265:L598–L605, 1993.

121. Hunt PJ, Espiner EA, Richards AM, et al. Interactions of atrial and brain natriuretic peptides at pathophysiological levels in normal men. Am J Physiol 269:R1397–R1403, 1995.

122. Hu N, Levin P. Atrial and brain natriuretic peptides stimulate the production and secretion of CNP from bovine endothelial cells. J Clin Invest 95:1151–1157, 1995.

123. Oparil S. The elusive role of atrial natriuretic peptide in hypertension. [Editorial] Mayo Clin Proc 70:1015–1017, 1995.

124. John SWM, Krege JH, Oliver PM, et al. Genetic decreases in atrial natriuretic peptide and salt-sensitive hypertension. Science 267:679–681, 1995.

125. Lopez MJ, Wong SKF, Kishimoto I, et al. Salt-resistant hypertension in mice lacking guanyl cyclase-A receptor for atrial natriuretic peptide. Nature 378:65–68, 1995.

126. Ogawa Y, Itoh H, Tamura N, et al. Molecular cloning of the complementary DNA and gene that encodes mouse brain natriuretic peptide and generation of transgenic mice that overexpress the brain natriuretic peptide gene. J Clin Invest 93:1911–1921, 1994.

127. Steinhelper ME, Cochrane KL, Field LJ. Hypotension in transgenic mice expressing atrial natriuretic factor fusion genes. Hypertension 16:301–307, 1990.

128. Jin H, Chen YF, Yang RH, et al. Impaired release of atrial natriuretic factor in NaCl-loaded spontaneously hypertensive rats. Hypertension 11:739–744, 1988.

129. Jin H, Yang RH, Chen YF, Oparil S. Atrial natriuretic factor prevents NaCl-sensitive hypertension in spontaneously hypertensive rats. Hypertension 15:170–176, 1990.

130. Onwochei MO, Rapp JP. Hyposecretion of atrial natriuretic factor by prehypertensive Dahl salt-sensitive rat. Hypertension 13:440–448, 1989.

131. Yokota N, Bruneau BG, Kuroski T, et al. Atrial natriuretic factor significantly contributes to the mineralocorticoid escape phenomenon: Evidence for a guanylate cyclase–mediated pathway. J Clin Invest 94:1938–1946, 1994.

132. Schiffrin EL, St-Louis J, Essiambre R. Platelet binding sites and plasma concentrations of atrial natriuretic peptide in patients with essential hypertension. J Hypertens 6:565–572, 1988.

133. Nakaoka H, Kitahara Y, Amano M, et al. Effect of β-adrenoreceptor blockade on atrial natriuretic peptide in essential hypertension. Hypertension 10:221–225, 1987.

134. Talartschik J, Eisenhauer T, Schrader J, et al. Low atrial natriuretic peptide plasma concentrations in 100 patients with essential hypertension. Am J Hypertens 3:45–47, 1990.

135. Montorsi P, Tonolo G, Polonia J, et al. Correlates of plasma atrial natriuretic factor in health and hypertension. Hypertension 10:570–576, 1987.

136. Dessi-Fulgheri P, Palermo R, DiNoto G, et al. Plasma levels of atrial natriuretic factor in mild to moderate hypertensives without signs of left ventricular hypertrophy: Correlation with the known duration of hypertension. J Hum Hypertens 2:177–182, 1988.

137. Kohno M, Yasunari K, Toshifumi M, et al. Circulating atrial natriuretic polypeptide in essential hypertension. Am Heart J 113:1160–1163, 1987.

138. Sagnella GA, Markandu ND, Buckley MG, et al. Atrial natriuretic peptides in essential hypertension: Basal plasma levels and relationship to sodium balance. Can J Physiol Pharmacol 69:1592–1600, 1991.

139. Kohno M, Yasunari K, Murakawa K, et al. Effects of high-sodium and low-sodium intake on circulating atrial natriuretic peptides in salt-sensitive patients with essential hypertension. Am J Cardiol 59:1212–1213, 1987.

140. Nimura S. Attenuated release of atrial natriuretic factor due to sodium loading in salt-sensitive essential hypertension. Jpn Heart J 32:167–178, 1991.

141. Ferrari P, Weidmann P, Ferrier C, et al. Dysregulation of atrial natriuretic factor in hypertension-prone man. J Clin Endocrinol Metab 1:944–951, 1990.

142. Weidmann P, Ferrari P, Allemann Y, et al. Developing essential hypertension: A syndrome involving ANF deficiency? Can J Physiol Pharmacol 69:1582–1591, 1991.

143. Campese VM, Tawadrous M, Bigazzi R, et al. Salt intake and plasma natriuretic peptide and nitric oxide in hypertension. Hypertension 28:335–340, 1996.

144. Nakagawa O, Ogawa Y, Itoh H, et al. Rapid transcriptional activation of early mRNA turnover of brain natriuretic peptide in cardiocyte hypertrophy. Evidence of brain natriuretic peptide as an emergency cardiac hormone against ventricular overload. J Clin Invest 96:1280–1287, 1995.

145. Wambach G, Koch J. BNP plasma levels during acute volume expansion and chronic sodium loading in normal man. Clin Exp Hypertens 17:619–629, 1995.

146. Tharaux PL, Dussaule JC, Hubert-Brierre A, et al. Plasma atrial and brain natriuretic peptides in mitral stenosis treated by valvulotomy. Clin Sci 87:671–677, 1994.

147. Grantham JA, Borgeson DD, Burnett JC Jr. BNP: Pathophysiological and potential therapeutic roles in acute congestive heart failure. Am J Physiol 272:R1077–R1083, 1997.

148. Stevens TL, Rasmussen TE, Wei CM, et al. Renal role of the endogenous natriuretic peptide system in acute congestive heart failure. J Card Fail 2:119–125, 1996.

149. Hosoda K, Nakao K, Muroyama M, et al. Expression of brain natriuretic peptide gene in human heart. Hypertension 17:1152–1156, 1991.

150. Montwani JG, McAlpine H, Kennedy N, Struthers AD. Plasma brain natriuretic peptide as an indicator for angiotensin-converting enzyme inhibition after myocardial infarction. Lancet 341:1109–1113, 1993.

151. Wei CM, Heublein DM, Perrella MA, et al. Natriuretic peptide system in human heart failure. Circulation 88:1004–1009, 1994.

152. Stevens TL, Burnett IC Jr, Kinoshita M, et al. A functional role for

endogenous atrial natriuretic peptide in a canine model of early left ventricular dysfunction. J Clin Invest 95:1101–1108, 1995.

153. Nakamura M, Arakawa N, Funakoshi T, et al. Vasodilatory effects of C-type natriuretic peptide on forearm resistance vessels is distinct from atrial natriuretic peptide in patients with chronic heart failure. Circulation 90:1210–1214, 1994.

154. Bernardi M, Fornalé L, Di Marco C, et al. Hyperdynamic circulation of advanced cirrhosis: A reappraisal based on posture-induced changes in hemodynamics. J Hypertens 22:309–318, 1995.

155. La Villa G, Romanelli RG, Casini VR, et al. Plasma levels of brain natriuretic peptide in patients with cirrhosis. Hepatology 16:156–161, 1992.

156. Akriviadis EA, Ervin MG, Cominelli F, et al. Hyponatremia of cirrhosis: Role of vasopressin and decreased "effective" plasma volume. Scand J Gastroenterol 32:829–834, 1997.

157. Salo J, Jimenez W, Kuhn M, et al. Urinary excretion of urodilatin in patients with cirrhosis. Hepatology 24:1428–1432, 1996.

158. Wong F, Blendin L. Pathophysiology of sodium retention and ascites formation in cirrhosis: Role of atrial natriuretic factor. Semin Liver Dis 14:59–70, 1994.

159. Morali GA, Floras JS, Legault L, et al. Muscle sympathetic nerve activity and renal responsiveness to atrial natriuretic factor during the development of hepatic ascites. Am J Med 91:383–390, 1991.

160. Koepke JP, Jones S, DiBona GF. Renal nerves mediate blunted natriuresis to atrial natriuretic peptide in cirrhotic rats. Am J Physiol 252:R1019–R1023, 1987.

161. Angeli P, Jimenez W, Arroyo V, et al. Renal effects of natriuretic peptide receptor blockade in cirrhotic rats with ascites. Hepatology 20:948–954, 1994.

162. Pedersen EB, Danielsen H, Eiskjaer H, et al. Increased atrial natriuretic peptide in the nephrotic syndrome: Relationship to renal function and the renin-angiotensin-aldosterone system. Scand J Clin Lab Invest 48:141–147, 1988.

163. Rodriguez-Iturbe B, Colic D, Parra G, et al. Atrial natriuretic factor in the acute nephritic and nephrotic syndromes. Kidney Int 38:512–517, 1990.

164. Jespersen B, Eiskjaer H, Mogensen CE, et al. Reduced natriuretic effect of atrial natriuretic peptide in nephrotic syndrome: A possible role of decreased cyclic guanosine monophosphate. Nephron 71:44–53, 1995.

165. Winter RJD, Davidson AC, Treacher D, et al. Atrial natriuretic peptide concentrations in hypoxic secondary pulmonary hypertension: Relation to haemodynamic and blood gas variables and response to supplemental oxygen. Thorax 44:58–62, 1989.

166. Lang CC, Coutie WJ, Struthers AD, et al. Elevated levels of brain natriuretic peptide in acute hypoxaemic chronic obstructive pulmonary disease. Clin Sci 83:529–533, 1992.

167. Ando T, Ogawa K, Yamaki K, et al. Plasma concentrations of atrial, brain, and C-type natriuretic peptides and endothelin-1 in patients with chronic respiratory diseases. Chest 110:462–468, 1996.

168. Takei Y, Fykuzawa A, Itahara Y, et al. A new natriuretic peptide isolated from cardiac atria of trout, *Oncorhynchus mykiss*. FEBS Lett 414:377–380, 1997.

169. Greenberg RN, Hill M, Crytzer J, et al. Comparison of effects of uroguanylin, guanylin, and *Escherichia coli* heat-stable enterotoxin Sta in mouse intestine and kidney: Evidence that uroguanylin is an intestinal natriuretic hormone. J Invest Med 45:276–283, 1997.

170. La Villa G, Lazzeri C, Pascale A, et al. Cardiovascular and renal effects of low-dose atrial natriuretic peptide in compensated cirrhosis. Am J Gastroenterol 92:852–857, 1997.

171. Brenard R, Moreau R, Pussard E, et al. Hemodynamic and sympathetic responses to human atrial natriuretic peptide infusion in patients with cirrhosis. J Hepatol 14:347–356, 1992.

172. Gadano A, Moreau R, Vachiery F, et al. Natriuretic response to the combination of atrial natriuretic peptide and terlipressin in patients with cirrhosis and refractory ascites. J Hepatol 26:1229–1234, 1997.

173. Carstens J, Greisen J, Jensen AT, et al. Renal effects of a urodilatin infusion in patients with liver cirrhosis, with and without ascites. J Am Soc Nephrol 9:1489–1498, 1998.

174. Allgren RL, Marbury TC, Rahman SN, et al. Anaritide in acute tubular necrosis. N Engl J Med 336:828–834, 1997.

175. Danielewicz JC, Barclay PL, Barnish IT, et al. UK-69758, a novel inhibitor of EC 3.4.24.11 which increases ANF levels and is natriuretic and diuretic. Biochem Biophys Res Commun 164:58–65, 1989.

176. Tikkanen I, Helin K, Tikkanen T, et al. Elevation of plasma atrial natriuretic peptide in rats with chronic heart failure by SCH 39370, a neutral metalloendopeptidase inhibitor. J Pharmacol Exp Ther 254:641–645, 1990.

177. Northridge DB, Alabasterl CT, Connel J, et al. Effects of UK 69758: A novel atriopeptidase inhibitor. Lancet 2:591–593, 1989.

178. Lafferty HM, Gunning M, Silva P, et al. Enkehalinase inhibition increases plasma atrial natriuretic peptide levels, glomerular filtration rate and urinary sodium excretion in rats with reduced renal mass. Circ Res 65:640–646, 1989.

179. Gafford JT, Skidgel RA, Erdos EG, et al. Human kidney "enkephalinase." A neutral metalloendopeptidase that cleaves active peptides. Biochemistry 22:32675–32711, 1985.

180. Smits GJ, McGraw DE, Trapani AJ. Interaction of ANP and bradykinin during endopeptidase 24.11 inhibition: Renal effects. Am J Physiol 258:F1417–F1424, 1990.

18 Eicosanoids: Do They Matter?

Adebayo Oyekan, John C. McGiff, and John Quilley

Eicosanoids serve both pro- and antihypertensive mechanisms. The contribution of eicosanoids to blood pressure control resists precise definition because of the many eicosanoid products, their diverse biological effects, and transformation of products of one pathway by enzymes of a second pathway, e.g., cyclooxygenase's (COX) conversion of cytochrome P-450 monooxygenases (CYP-450)–derived mono-hydroxyeicosatetraenoic acids (16-, 18-, 19-, and 20-HETEs) to prostaglandin analogues.[1] These difficulties are evident when attempting to interpret the effects of aspirin-like drugs (nonsteroidal antiinflammatory drugs [NSAIDs]) on blood pressure regulation and renal function, changes in the latter being a principal determinant of the level of blood pressure. Inhibition of COX with an NSAID can result in either increased or decreased blood pressure in animal models of hypertension, depending on the level of participation of pro- and antihypertensive COX products in a particular hypertensive model and the experimental conditions as, e.g., salt intake, age, and sex of the animal.[2]

EICOSANOIDS ARE ESSENTIAL COMPONENTS OF DIVERSE VASCULAR MECHANISMS

Problems in interpretation of renal functional responses to NSAIDs are exemplified in the following analysis of the species of eicosanoid responsible for the effects on renal tubular and hemodynamic function produced by changes in renal perfusate chloride concentration.[3] The plasma chloride concentration may be as important to blood pressure regulation as sodium.[4]

Increasing the chloride concentration (87 mM to 117 mM) in the renal perfusate in the absence of changes in sodium concentration is associated with increased renal vascular resistance, diminished glomerular filtration rate (GFR), as well as salt and water retention.[3] Vasodilator-diuretic prostaglandins (PGE_2 and PGI_2) predominate at reduced chloride concentrations (87 mM), whereas vasoconstrictor-antidiuretic prostanoids (PGH_2 and thromboxane A_2 [TxA_2]) are elevated during hyperchloremia (117 mM).[3, 5] These findings are based on the observation that inhibition of COX prevented the renal functional response to changes in chloride in either direction.

As TxA_2 had been reported to mediate the negative effects of hyperchloremia on renal hemodynamics in the dog,[6] the failure of TxA_2 synthase inhibition to increase GFR and reverse the antinatriuresis in the rat kidney subject to hyperchloremia was unexpected and prompted a study of the prostaglandin endoperoxide, PGH_2, acting as the mediator of the negative renal functional response to hyperchloremia.[7] Since the TxA_2 receptor recognizes PGH_2, this rationale rested on firm experimental grounds. PGH_2 was, however, eliminated as a candidate for the eicosanoid mediator of hyperchloremia in that a selective antagonist of the PGH_2/TxA_2 receptor did not affect the renal functional response to elevated chloride concentration.[7]

As COX has been shown to convert CYP-450–derived arachidonate products, primarily 20-HETE and 5,6-epoxyeicosatrienoic acid (5,6-EET), to vasoconstrictor and vaso- dilator metabolites, respectively (Fig. 18–1), a vasoconstrictor transformation product of 20-HETE via COX was considered as a candidate mediator for the effects of hyperchloremia on renal function.[7] Several findings support this interpretation:

1. Hyperchloremia produced a twofold increase in 20-HETE efflux from the kidney compared with reduced chloride concentrations.
2. Inhibition of COX prevented the renal vasoconstrictor action of administered 20-HETE.[8]
3. 20-HETE is the principal eicosanoid generated by preglomerular microvessels.[9]
4. 20-HETE can be transformed to PGH_2 and TxA_2 analogues.[10]

These studies indicate that caution must be observed when a biological response is ascribed to a prostaglandin based solely on the ability of a COX inhibitor to prevent the response. Thus, one must remain cognizant of the fact that several principal CYP-450 arachidonate metabolites act via COX-derived transformation products. The importance of this caveat is strikingly evident in the cardiovascular and renal responses to inhibition of nitric oxide synthase (NOS), which elevates blood pressure in the rat through disinhibition of ω-hydroxylase activity, a mechanism in which increased formation of 20-HETE has a central role.[11] This mechanism is fully expressed only after transformation of 20-HETE by COX to an analogue of PGH_2, mediating renal vasoconstriction, and an additional step that metabolizes the 20-HETE analogue of PGH_2 to a PGE_2 analogue mediating diuresis-natriuresis (Fig. 18–2). Under these conditions, inhibition of COX attenuated the diuresis and increased renal vascular resistance produced by NOS

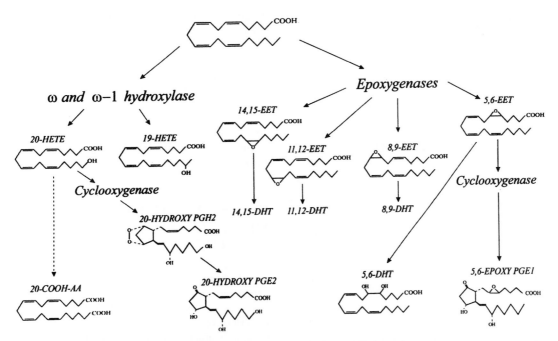

Figure 18–1. Arachidonic acid (AA) metabolism by cytochrome P450 (CYP-450)–dependent monooxygenases to ω and ω-1 hydroxyeicosatetraenoic acids (HETEs), epoxyeicosatrienoic acids (epoxides/EETS), and dihydroxyeicosatrienoic acids (diols/DHTs). For the DHTs, only the structure of 5,6-DHT is given. As 5,6-EET can be a substrate for cyclooxygenase, one of the products, the vasodilator 5,6-epoxy PGE_1, is shown. (From McGiff JC, Steinberg M, Quilley J. Missing links: Cytochrome P450 arachidonate products. Trends Cardiovasc Med 6:4, 1996.)

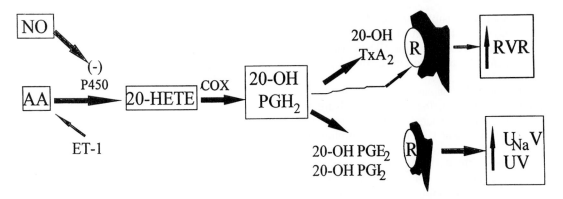

Figure 18–2. Schema showing the interrelationships among nitric oxide (NO), endothelin-1 (ET-1), and 20-hydroxyeicosatetraenoic acids (20-HETE) and the targets for interrupting 20-HETE–mediated changes in renal function. Inhibition of NO synthesis by N$^\omega$-nitro-L-arginine methyl ester (L-NAME) facilitates ET-1 stimulation of phospholipase, releasing arachidonic acid (AA), which is metabolized by ω hydroxylase cytochrome P450 (CYP450), forming 20-HETE. Transformation of 20-HETE by cyclooxygenase (COX) yields the endoperoxide analog (20-OH prostaglandin H$_2$ [PGH$_2$]), the precursor of 20-OH thromboxane A$_2$ (TxA$_2$), 20-OH prostaglandin E$_2$ (PGE$_2$), and 20-OH prostaglandin I$_2$ (PGI$_2$). These analogs can increase renal vascular resistance (RVR) through stimulation of the PGH$_2$/TxA$_2$ receptor or produce natriuresis-diuresis through stimulation of the PGE$_2$/PGI$_2$ receptors. UV, urinary volume; U$_{Na}$V, urinary volume of sodium. (From Oyekan AO, McGiff JC. Functional response of the rat kidney to inhibition of nitric oxide synthesis. Br J Pharmacol 125:1065–1073, 1998.)

inhibition. These renal functional effects required an active COX for generating the prostaglandin analogues of 20-HETE that mediate these effects, whereas blockade of the PGH$_2$/TxA$_2$ receptor prevented the increased renal vascular resistance but not the diuresis-natriuresis produced by inhibition of nitric oxide (NO) formation.[11]

The complexity of eicosanoid-dependent mechanisms is also evident when analyzing the renal functional effects of endothelin-1 (ET-1) in the anesthetized rat.[12, 13] Two critical linkages of ET-1 to eicosanoids were identified. The first was a prostaglandin-dependent mechanism that opposed the negative effect of ET-1 on GFR and renal blood flow.[13] The second was through the CYP-450 product, 20-HETE, which mediated in large part the negative renal hemodynamic effects of ET-1 as well as the seemingly paradoxical natriuretic response to the peptide. Thus, the similarity of the renal functional actions of ET-1 and 20-HETE, vasoconstriction with natriuresis, can be explained by eicosanoids acting as a second messenger for the peptide. These relationships are magnified by the abnormalities of regulatory systems that characterize hypertension, particularly deoxycorticosterone acetate–salt (DOCA-salt) hypertension, that involve ET-1 and 20-HETE.

PROHYPERTENSIVE EICOSANOIDS

In rats subjected to aortic constriction, hypertension developed with full participation of prohypertensive prostanoids in the first 2 to 3 weeks, when the renin-angiotensin system was active.[14] Blockade of PGH$_2$/TxA$_2$ receptors reduced blood pressure when carried out at this time, but not after the third week, when renin levels had returned to normal. Elevation of blood pressure in response to activation of the renin-angiotensin system is mediated, in part, by the prohypertensive prostanoids, TxA$_2$ and PGH$_2$. Nasjletti has gathered compelling evidence "that the status of the renin-angiotensin system is a major determinant of the blood pressure response to agents that inhibit thromboxane synthase or block PGH$_2$/TxA$_2$ receptors."[14] Even under these

conditions, when PGH$_2$ and TxA$_2$ contribute to elevation of blood pressure, a braking mechanism involving antihypertensive prostaglandins PGE$_2$ and PGI$_2$ can be demonstrated. In this situation, the increase in blood pressure produced by inhibition of COX eliminated the pressor effects of prostanoids by blocking the PGH$_2$/TxA$_2$ receptor.[14]

Keen and colleagues[15] demonstrated in chronically instrumented rats that a substantial component of the elevated pressor response to chronically infused angiotensin II was exerted by TxA$_2$, which potentiated the renal vasoconstrictor action of the peptide. This interaction was most in evidence at the efferent arteriole, as renal plasma flow was reduced and GFR was unaffected. Lipoxygenase products, particularly 12-hydroperoxyeicosatetraenoic acid (12-HPETE) and its peroxidase product, 12-hydroxyeicosatetraenoic acid (12-HETE), serve as second messengers for the actions of angiotensin II[16] and also suppress PGI$_2$ synthesis. Inhibition of 12-lipoxygenase will partially reverse angiotensin-dependent hypertension, an effect that in part results from disinhibition of prostacyclin synthase by eliminating 12-HPETE/12-HETE, negative modulators of the enzyme.[17]

CYP-450–RELATED ARACHIDONIC ACID METABOLISM IN THE SPONTANEOUSLY HYPERTENSIVE RAT

Arachidonate metabolites generated by CYP-450–dependent monooxygenases are increased in the spontaneously hypertensive rat (SHR) during the development of hypertension (5th to 12th weeks).[18] The distribution of CYP-450–arachidonic acid (AA) metabolic activity along the nephron is altered in the SHR and varies during the development of hypertension. Early (first 12 weeks) in the course of development of hypertension, there is a greater capacity to synthesize 20-HETE.[19] ω-Hydroxylase is overexpressed in the young SHR (approximately 5 weeks of age), resulting in increased production of 20-HETE during the period of greatest elevation in blood pressure.

Blood pressure can be normalized in the SHR if production of CYP-450–AA products is reduced by attacking the CYP-450 enzyme complex through stimulating the heme oxygenase that degrades heme-containing enzymes, including cytochromes.[20] Selective depletion of renal CYP-450 was accomplished by inducing heme oxygenase with tin, given as $SnCl_2$.[21] Heme oxygenase mRNA levels increased more than 20-fold in the rat kidney 8 hours after administration of $SnCl_2$.[22] In 7-week-old SHRs, $SnCl_2$ reduced blood pressure, increased heme oxygenase activity, reduced CYP-450 content, and decreased formation of renal AA metabolites via the CYP-450 pathway.[19] $SnCl_2$ did not affect blood pressure in Wistar-Kyoto rats or in mature 20-week-old SHRs. Induction of heme oxygenase activity also results in production of CO, which could account for some of the antihypertensive response to $SnCl_2$ in the SHR. Johnson and coworkers have shown in rats that generation of CO resulting from induction of heme oxygenase mediates a vasodepressor response.[23]

NO has been proposed to be an endogenous negative modulator of CYP-450–AA metabolism.[24] If NO tonically inhibits CYP-450 enzyme activity,[25] inhibition of NOS should increase formation of CYP-450–AA metabolites, including those mediating the renal functional response to suppression of NO. This hypothesis has been tested and confirmed.[11] Inhibition of NOS resulted in depression of renal blood flow and GFR together with a natriuresis (despite the decline in GFR) mediated by CYP-450–dependent AA metabolites. There was an associated activation of endothelin, which contributed to the stimulation of ω-hydroxylase, forming 20-HETE. This conclusion was confirmed by the ability of an Endothelin$_A$ (ET$_A$) receptor antagonist to reverse the negative renal functional response to N^G-nitro-L-arginine methyl ester (L-NAME) in a manner similar to 12,12-dibromododec-11-enoic acid, a selective inhibitor of ω-hydroxylase. The renal functional effects of both activation of ET-1 and inhibition of NO production are, therefore, best explained by increased production of 20-HETE by each stimulus. The demonstration that COX inhibition and PGH$_2$/TxA$_2$ receptor blockade antagonized the renal functional effects of L-NAME (see Fig. 18–2) provided additional evidence that 20-HETE was involved in the renal functional response to NOS inhibition. 20-HETE has been shown to be transformed via COX to biologically active prostaglandin analogues that suppress renal blood flow and GFR and promote salt excretion.[13]

Disruption of neuronal NOS (nNOS) was hypothesized to attenuate renin release, as NO can stimulate renin release and nNOS has been detected in the macula densa, the sensor site for the renin-releasing mechanism that responds to changes in tubular fluid composition/volume.[26] However, in nNOS knockout mice, a COX-2-dependent renin-releasing mechanism was activated in response to dietary salt restriction. This pathway could be blocked by a selective inhibitor of COX-2. The functional consequences of expression of COX-2 and the implications for blood pressure regulation await definition.

PREECLAMPSIA AND EICOSANOIDS

Preeclampsia is a frequent complication of pregnancy (6 to 10%) and is of placental origin, as it is terminated by delivery.[27] The activities of antipressor systems are increased in normal pregnancy: Blood pressure is not elevated and is even reduced in midgestation despite increased cardiac output and blood volume and activation of the renin-angiotensin system.[27] The pressor and vasoconstrictor responses to vasoactive hormones are blunted early in pregnancy.[28] Enhanced prostaglandin production by the placenta, as well as systemically, characterizes normal pregnancy.[29] Concomitantly with the 30- to 40-fold increase in uterine blood flow during the progression of pregnancy, PGE$_2$ concentrations in uterine venous blood of dogs increased from undetectable levels to levels approaching 1 ng/ml.[30] Inhibition of COX with indomethacin reduced uterine blood flow in late pregnancy by a mean of 80%. A deficiency in prostacyclin biosynthesis precedes the onset of hypertension in pregnancy.[31] This may be accompanied by increased production of PGH$_2$ and TxA$_2$ with progression of vascular complications, as evidenced by increasing blood pressure and proteinuria. Placental TxA$_2$ production is increased, as is platelet TxA$_2$ biosynthesis, the latter reflecting platelet activation in preeclampsia.[32]

The findings of deficient production of PGI$_2$, presumably by the endothelium, and increased thromboxane synthesis, together with platelet activation, suggested that antiplatelet treatment in the form of low-dose aspirin may reverse many of the pathological features of preeclampsia that reflect endothelial dysfunction.[33] The initial aspirin trials for treatment and prevention of preeclampsia were promising but were challenged by larger randomized studies. A multicenter, randomized, placebo-controlled trial involving almost 10,000 patients did not confirm the exuberant promises of the initial reports.[34] This study suggested that the use of low-dose aspirin prophylactically early in the second trimester was justified only in women at high risk of early-onset preeclampsia, mainly women with a history of early-onset preeclampsia. Routine prophylactic aspirin treatment was not recommended, as there was an insignificant reduction (12%) in the incidence of preeclampsia.

Ischemia/underperfusion of the uteroplacental circulation is an essential feature of preeclampsia, which appears to be primarily a disease of the endothelium.[35] Endothelial dysfunction may be the "initiating" lesion in preeclampsia: It provides a satisfactory explanation for the cardinal manifestations of preeclampsia—elevation of blood pressure, proteinuria, increased platelet activation, and microvascular alterations.[27] Ultrastructural changes signifying endothelial injury have been detected early, well before the development of the florid signs of preeclampsia, and have been suggested to result from an immunologically mediated insult to the endothelium.[36] The compromised endothelium becomes deficient in its capacity to generate "protective" mediators—primarily NO, prostacyclin, and PGE$_2$—according to current concepts.[37] However, the precise nature of the primary event remains to be defined. A case can be made for deficient NO production, which can affect gene expression and production of eicosanoids and modulate the action of pressor hormones.[11] The progression of preeclampsia to its most severe stage, eclampsia, is heralded by seizures. The therapeutic benefits of magnesium—the cornerstone for treatment of eclampsia—appear to result from effects on endothelium-related antipressor/antiaggregatory mechanisms. Magnesium may augment

PGI_2, PGE_2, and NO-dependent vascular mechanisms that oppose platelet activation and attenuate vasoconstriction mediated by pressor peptides and proaggregatory/vasoconstrictor arachidonate metabolites—TxA_2, PGH_2, and 12-HETE.[38, 39]

Estrogen-stimulated NO production has been suggested to account for the major changes in cardiovascular function during pregnancy.[40] In pregnant rats, nitrite excretion is increased, as are urinary and circulating cyclic guanosine monophosphate levels.[41] The uteroplacental complex generates NO in increasing quantity with the progression of pregnancy, the basis of a mechanism that maintains quiescence of the gravid uterus until term.[42] Increased NO production, both systemically and by the placenta and gravid uterus, contributes to refractoriness to pressor amines and peptides during pregnancy. The importance of NO in the circulatory changes of pregnancy becomes evident on chronic inhibition of NOS in pregnant rats: This produces a syndrome resembling preeclampsia.[43] However, it may be misleading to conclude that NO production is the principal mechanism underlying the circulatory adaptations to pregnancy, as there is an intimate relationship between NOS, COX, and several cytokines in this condition.[44] NO production is initiated by either interleukin-1β (IL-1β) or tumor necrosis factor-α (TNF-α) stimulation of inducible NOS (iNOS) in the gravid uterus, associated with NO-mediated enhancement of COX-2 activity. IL-1β and TNF-α can induce COX-2 gene expression in the pregnant rat uterus. COX-2 mRNA levels in rat uteri increased 3.5-fold between the 7th and the 22nd days (term) of normal pregnancy, whereas COX-1 levels were unchanged.[45] The importance of interactions between COX and NO was demonstrated by inhibiting production of NO. This maneuver diminished uterine PGE_2 production, which was restored by providing an NO donor. Further, PGE_2 is a negative modulator of IL-1 activation of NOS, i.e., PGE_2 exerts an inhibitory effect on induction of iNOS by IL-1.[44] In contrast, PGI_2 is a positive modulator of iNOS induction by the cytokine, probably through a mechanism involving increased cyclic adenosine monophosphate production.[46]

Responses of blood vessels to vasoactive agents in pregnant animals show regional variations as well as segmental differences within the vessel as, e.g., when comparing the thoracic with the abdominal aorta.[47] Enhanced endothelium-dependent relaxation of the thoracic aorta to acetylcholine in pregnant rats (compared with age-matched virgin rats) is a function primarily of increased NO production. In contrast, the relaxant response of the abdominal aorta to acetylcholine has a major CYP-450 component that is absent from the thoracic aorta of pregnant and nonpregnant rats.

CYP-450–derived arachidonate products, HETEs and EETs, are vasoactive, modulate salt and water metabolism, and have profound effects on blood pressure, as seen with respect to epoxides and blood pressure responses to salt loading.[48] Rats resistant to salt-induced elevations of blood pressure can be converted to salt-sensitive by inhibiting production of EETs, particularly the 5,6 epoxide.[49] CYP-450–dependent monooxygenase activity, in particular those isozymes that have the capacity to convert AA to vasoactive products, are affected by pregnancy, e.g., the activity of prostaglandin ω-hydroxylase of rabbit lungs is increased

100-fold during pregnancy.[50] This area of research has received little attention and promises to yield important insights into understanding the cause of preeclampsia. For example, plasma levels of ET-1 are elevated in pregnancy,[51] and as ET-1 promotes synthesis of 20-HETE, a potential mechanism exists for producing many of the features of preeclampsia.[13] A role for CYP-450–derived arachidonate metabolites in preeclampsia has been suggested, as urinary excretion of epoxides was elevated in women with preeclampsia.[52] In view of the demonstrated antipressor action of epoxides that opposes the pressor response to salt loading,[49] increased epoxide synthesis may represent a compensatory response to pressor stimuli.

DIETARY UNSATURATED FATTY ACIDS, VASCULAR REACTIVITY, AND HYPERTENSION

Ingestion of eicosapentaenoic acid and docosahexaenoic acid from marine sources has been shown to reduce the incidence of cardiovascular disease (including hypertension), reflecting, in part, decreased platelet aggregability.[53] Lahoz and associates studied the effects of dietary fats that differed in their degree of saturation on normal subjects.[54] They concluded that monounsaturated (olive oil–enriched) and polyunsaturated (bluefish-enriched) fats altered eicosanoid production, platelet aggregation, and blood pressure. The greatest effects of changes in dietary fatty acids were registered, not surprisingly, in hypertensive subjects with atherosclerotic complications, as the magnitude of response to an intervention is a function of the baseline value. A meta-analysis of 31 placebo-controlled clinical studies indicated that inclusion of fish oil in the diet produces a significant, but small, reduction in systolic and diastolic pressure in normotensive subjects.[55] The greatest reduction in blood pressure was achieved in hypertensive subjects with atherosclerotic disease.

As changes in blood pressure are a crude reflection of changes in endothelial function, the effects of fish oils on endothelial function in subjects with hypercholesterolemia were examined. Fish oils were shown to dose-dependently attenuate constriction of forearm blood vessels in healthy volunteers in response to angiotensin II and norepinephrine.[56] This effect was related to a prostaglandin mechanism, as it was abolished by indomethacin. Further, Chin and Dart demonstrated that fish oils restored altered endothelial function in subjects with hypercholesterolemia.[57] These findings were confirmed by Goode and colleagues, who obtained gluteal arteries from hypercholesterolemic patients and correlated improvement in endothelial function with increases in eicosapentaenoic acid and docosahexaenoic acid in red blood cell membranes,[58] which presumably are reliable indices of corresponding changes in endothelial membranes.

SUMMARY

Three major enzyme systems—COX, lipoxygenases, and CYP-450—generate biological mediators from AA. The arachidonate metabolites generated by CYP-450 pathways of AA metabolism have prominent effects on blood vessels and ion transport, including modulation and mediation of the actions of vasoactive hormones. The diverse properties of these AA metabolites and the wide distribution of the CYP-450 system make them prime candidates for participation in regulatory mechanisms that affect the circulation and transporting epithelia and, thereby, control of blood pressure. CYP-450–AA products are as important to renal and circulatory control as are NO and prostaglandins. The importance of renal CYP-450 arachidonate metabolites, particularly 20-HETE, to the regulation of blood pressure is underscored by the studies of Omata and coworkers[18] and Sacerdoti and associates[19] in the SHR. Treatment of young SHRs with $SnCl_2$ to deplete CYP-450 enzymes resulted in return of blood pressure to normal over a 2-day period and normalized the pressure-natriuresis relationship.[19] Moreover, chronic treatment of young SHRs with $SnCl_2$ prevented the development of hypertension.

Acknowledgments

This work is supported by National Institutes of Health Grants: HL-34300 and RO1-25394 (JCM), RO1-49275 (JQ), RO1-59884 (AO), and AHA Grant-in-Aid 9750303N (AO).

The authors wish to thank Melody Steinberg for preparation of this manuscript and editorial assistance.

References

1. McGiff JC. Cytochrome P-450 metabolism of arachidonic acid. Annu Rev Pharmacol Toxicol 31:339, 1991.
2. Quilley J, Bell-Quilley CP, McGiff JC. Eicosanoids and Hypertension. *In* Laragh JH, Brenner BM (eds). Hypertension: Pathophysiology, Diagnosis, and Management, 2nd ed, vol 2. New York, Raven, 1995; p 963.
3. Yin K, McGiff JC, Bell-Quilley CP. Role of chloride in the variable response of the kidney to cyclooxygenase inhibition. Am J Physiol 268:F561, 1995.
4. Boegehold MA, Kotchen TA. Relative contributions of dietary Na^+ and Cl^- to salt-sensitive hypertension. Hypertension 14:579, 1989.
5. Quilley CP, Lin Y-S, McGiff JC. Chloride anion concentration as a determinant of renal vascular responsiveness to vasoconstrictor agents. Br J Pharmacol 108:106, 1993.
6. Bullivant EMA, Wilcox CS, Welch WJ. Intrarenal vasoconstriction during hypochloremia: Role of thromboxane. Am J Physiol 256:F152, 1989.
7. Askari B, Bell-Quilley CP, Fulton D, et al. Analysis of eicosanoid mediation of the renal functional effects of hyperchloremia. J Pharmacol Exp Ther 282:101, 1997.
8. Carroll MA, Pilar Garcia M, Falck JR, et al. Cyclooxygenase dependency of the renovascular actions of cytochrome P450–derived arachidonate metabolites. J Pharmacol Exp Ther 260:104, 1992.
9. Kauser K, Clark JE, Masters BS, et al. Inhibitors of cytochrome P-450 attenuate the myogenic response of dog renal arcuate arteries. Circ Res 68:1154, 1991.
10. Escalante B, Sessa WC, Falck JR, et al. Vasoactivity of 20-hydroxyeicosatetraenoic acid is dependent on metabolism by cyclooxygenase. J Pharmacol Exp Ther 248:229, 1989.
11. Oyekan AO, McGiff JC. Functional response of the rat kidney to inhibition of nitric oxide synthesis: Role of cytochrome P450–derived arachidonate metabolites. Br J Pharmacol 125:1065–1073, 1998.
12. Oyekan A, Balazy M, McGiff JC. Renal oxygenases: Differential contribution to vasoconstriction induced by ET-1 and ANG II. Am J Physiol 273:R293, 1997.
13. Oyekan AO, McGiff JC. Cytochrome P-450–derived eicosanoids participate in the renal functional effects of ET-1 in the anesthetized rat. Am J Physiol 274:R52, 1998.
14. Nasjletti A. The role of eicosanoids in angiotensin-dependent hypertension. Hypertension 31:194, 1997.
15. Keen HL, Brands MW, Smith MJ, et al. Thromboxane is required for full expression of angiotensin hypertension in rats. Hypertension 29:310, 1997.
16. Stern N, Golub M, Nozawa K, et al. Selective inhibition of angiotensin II–mediated vasoconstriction by lipoxygenase blockade. Am J Physiol 257:H434, 1989.
17. Takizawa H, Dellipizzi AM, Nasjletti A. Prostaglandin I_2 contributes to the vasodepressor effect of baicalein in hypertensive rats. Hypertension 31:866, 1998.
18. Omata K, Abraham NG, Escalante B, et al. Age-related changes in renal cytochrome P-450 arachidonic acid metabolism in spontaneously hypertensive rats. Am J Physiol 262:F8, 1992.
19. Sacerdoti D, Escalante B, Abraham NG, et al. Treatment with tin prevents the development of hypertension in spontaneously hypertensive rats. Science 243:388, 1989.
20. Escalante B, Sacerdoti D, Davidian MM, et al. Chronic treatment with tin normalizes blood pressure in spontaneously hypertensive rats. Hypertension 17:776, 1991.
21. Kappas A, Maines MD. Tin: A potent inducer of heme oxygenase in kidney. Science 192:60, 1976.
22. DaSilva J-L, Tiefenthaler M, Park E, et al. Tin mediated heme oxygenase gene activation and cytochrome P450 arachidonate hydroxylase inhibition in spontaneously hypertensive rats. Am J Med Sci 307:173, 1994.
23. Johnson RA, Lavesa M, Askari B, et al. A heme oxygenase product, presumably carbon monoxide, mediates a vasodepressor function in rats. Hypertension 25:165, 1995.
24. Alonso-Galicia M, Drummond HA, Reddy KK, et al. Inhibition of 20-HETE contributes to the vascular responses to nitric oxide. Hypertension 29:320, 1997.
25. Khatsenko OG, Gross SS, Rifkind AB, et al. Nitric oxide is a mediator of the decrease in cytochrome P450–dependent metabolism caused by immunostimulants. Proc Natl Acad Sci U S A 90:11147, 1993.
26. Harding P, Sigmon DH, Alfie ME, et al. Cyclooxygenase-2 mediates increased renal renin content induced by low-sodium diet. Hypertension 29:297, 1997.
27. Barron WM, Lindheimer MD. Management of hypertension during pregnancy. *In* Laragh JH, Brenner BM (eds). Hypertension: Pathophysiology, Diagnosis, and Management, 2nd ed, vol 2. New York, Raven, 1995; p 2427.
28. Gant NF, Daley GL, Chand S, et al. A study of angiotensin II pressor response throughout primigravid pregnancy. J Clin Invest 52:2682, 1973.
29. Terragno NA, Terragno A, McGiff JC. Role of prostaglandins in blood vessels. Semin Perinatol 4:85, 1980.
30. Terragno NA, Terragno DA, Pacholczyk D, et al. Prostaglandins and the regulation of uterine blood flow in pregnancy. Nature 249:57, 1974.
31. Fitzgerald DJ, Entman SS, Mulloy K, et al. Decreased prostacyclin biosynthesis preceding the clinical manifestation of pregnancy-induced hypertension. Circulation 75:956, 1987.
32. Meagher EA, FitzGerald GA. Disordered eicosanoid formation in pregnancy-induced hypertension. Circulation 88:1324, 1993.
33. Sanchez-Ramos L, O'Sullivan MJ, Garrido-Calderon J. Effect of low-dose aspirin on angiotensin II pressor response in human pregnancy. Am J Obstet Gynecol 156:193, 1987.
34. CLASP: A randomised trial of low-dose aspirin for the prevention and treatment of pre-eclampsia among 9,364 pregnant women. Lancet 343:619, 1994.
35. Roberts JM, Taylor RN, Musci TJ, et al. Preeclampsia: An endothelial cell disorder. Am J Obstet Gynecol 161:1200, 1989.
36. Shanklin DR, Sibai BM. Ultrastructural aspects of preeclampsia. Am J Obstet Gynecol 161:735, 1989.
37. McGiff JC, Carroll MA. Eicosanoids in preeclampsia-eclampsia: The effects of magnesium. Hypertens Pregnancy 13:217, 1994.
38. Watson KV, Moldow CF, Ogburn PL, et al. Magnesium sulfate: Rationale for its use in preeclampsia. Proc Natl Acad Sci U S A 83:1075, 1986.
39. Nadler JL, Goodson S, Rude RK. Evidence that prostacyclin mediates the vascular action of magnesium in humans. Hypertension 9:379, 1987.
40. Nathan L, Cuevas J, Chaudhri G. The role of nitric oxide in the

altered vascular reactivity of pregnancy in the rat. Br J Pharmacol 114:955, 1995.

41. Conrad KP, Joffe GM, Kruszyna H, et al. Identification of increased nitric oxide biosynthesis during pregnancy in rats. FASEB J 7:566, 1993.

42. Sladek SM, Magness RR, Conrad KP. Nitric oxide and pregnancy. Am J Physiol 272:R441, 1997.

43. Baylis C, Engels K. Adverse interactions between pregnancy and a new model of systemic hypertension produced by chronic blockade of endothelial derived relaxing factor. Clin Exp Hypertens B 11:117, 1992.

44. Dong Y-L, Yallampalli C. Interaction between nitric oxide and prostaglandin E$_2$ pathways in pregnant rat uteri. Am J Physiol 270:E471, 1996.

45. Arslan A, Zingg HH. Regulation of COX-2 gene expression in rat uterus in vivo and in vitro. Prostaglandins 52:463, 1996.

46. Tetsuka T, Daphna-Iken D, Srivastava SK, et al. Cross-talk between cyclooxygenase and nitric oxide pathways: Prostaglandin E$_2$ negatively modulates induction of nitric oxide synthase by interleukin 1. Proc Natl Acad Sci U S A 91:12168, 1994.

47. Bobadilla RA, Henkel CC, Henkel EC, et al. Possible involvement of endothelium-derived hyperpolarizing factor in vascular responses of abdominal aorta from pregnant rats. Hypertension 30:596, 1997.

48. McGiff JC, Steinberg M, Quilley J. Missing links: Cytochrome P450 arachidonate products. Trends Cardiovasc Med 6:4, 1996.

49. Makita K, Takahashi K, Karara A, et al. Experimental and/or genetically controlled alterations of the renal microsomal cytochrome P450 epoxygenase induce hypertension in rats fed a high salt diet. J Clin Invest 94:2414, 1994.

50. Williams DE, Hale SE, Okita RT, et al. A prostaglandin ω-hydroxylase cytochrome P-450 (P-450$_{PG-ω}$) purified from lungs of pregnant rabbits. J Biol Chem 259:14600, 1984.

51. Clark BA, Halvorson L, Sachs B, et al. Plasma endothelin levels in preeclampsia: Elevation and correlation with uric acid levels and renal impairment. Am J Obstet Gynecol 166:962, 1992.

52. Catella F, Lawson JA, Fitzgerald DJ, et al. Endogenous biosynthesis of arachidonic acid epoxides in humans: Increased formation in pregnancy-induced hypertension. Proc Natl Acad Sci U S A 87:5893, 1990.

53. Bonaa KH, Bjerve KS, Straume B, et al. Effect of eicosapentaenoic and docosahexaenoic acids on blood pressure in hypertension. A population-based intervention trial from the Tromso Study. N Engl J Med 322:795, 1990.

54. Lahoz C, Alonso R, Ordovas JM, et al. Effects of dietary fat saturation on eicosanoid production, platelet aggregation and blood pressure. Eur J Clin Invest 27:780, 1997.

55. Morris MC, Sacks F, Rosner B. Does fish oil lower blood pressure? A meta-analysis of controlled trials. Circulation 88:523, 1993.

56. Chin JPF, Gust AP, Nestel PJ, et al. Marine oils dose-dependently inhibit vasoconstriction of forearm resistance arteries in man. Hypertension 21:22, 1993.

57. Chin JPF, Dart AM. Therapeutic restoration of endothelial function in hypercholesterolaemic subjects: The effect of fish oils. Clin Exp Pharmacol Physiol 21:749, 1994.

58. Goode GK, Garcia S, Heagerty AM. Dietary supplementation with marine fish oil improves in vitro small artery endothelial function in hypercholesterolemic patients. A double-blind placebo-controlled study. Circulation 96:2802, 1997.

CHAPTER 19

Calcitonin Gene–Related Peptide and Hypertension

Donald J. DiPette and Scott C. Supowit

Calcitonin gene–related peptide (CGRP), a potent 37–amino acid vasodilator neuropeptide, is derived from the tissue-specific alternative splicing of the primary transcript of the calcitonin/CGRP gene.[1, 2] Whereas calcitonin is produced mainly in the C cells of the thyroid, CGRP is expressed almost exclusively in specific regions of the central and peripheral nervous systems. There are two CGRP genes, which are referred to as α- and β- in the rat and I and II in humans. In the rat and in humans, the two protein sequences differ by one and three amino acids, respectively, and the biological activities of the two peptides are quite similar in most vascular beds.[3, 4] Although the emphasis of this chapter is on the role of CGRP in the pathophysiology of hypertension, CGRP has been shown to modulate multiple physiological functions, including behavioral activities, sensory neurotransmission, and motor and autonomic control in many organs. These important regulatory actions of CGRP are discussed in a number of excellent reviews.[3–10]

Within a relatively short time after the identification and cloning of the calcitonin/CGRP gene in 1982,[1] several lines of evidence indicated that CGRP had potent cardiac and vasoregulatory actions.[11–13] Since that time, a number of investigators have sought to conclusively demonstrate that CGRP is a physiologically relevant vasoactive peptide. To prove that this neuropeptide is involved in the regulation of regional organ blood flows or systemic blood pressure,

or both, certain criteria, described by Brown and Morice,[14] must be met. These criteria are

1. The peptide is synthesized or stored, or both, in specialized tissue close to the blood vessel.
2. Specific receptors for the peptide exist on the vascular smooth muscle close to the site of its release.
3. Release of the peptide is demonstrable in response to appropriate stimuli.
4. Blockade of the peptide's release or of its receptor causes changes in blood flow under some circumstances.

In this review, we show that CGRP meets all these criteria and describe its involvement in hypertension, primarily in experimental rat models where much more is known about its function than in humans.

DISTRIBUTION AND LOCALIZATION OF IMMUNOREACTIVE CGRP

Immunoreactive CGRP (iCGRP) and its receptors are widely distributed in the nervous system and the cardiovascular system.[3–9] In the peripheral nervous system, a prominent site of CGRP synthesis is the dorsal root ganglia (DRG), which contain the cell bodies of sensory nerves that terminate peripherally on blood vessels and other tissues innervated by the sensory nervous system and centrally in laminae I and II of the dorsal horn of the spinal cord.[15, 16] A dense perivascular CGRP neural network is seen in virtually all vascular beds. In these blood vessels, the CGRP-containing nerves, which are often colocalized with substance P, are found at the junction of the adventitia and the media passing into the muscle layer.[3–6, 8, 9] It is thought that circulating CGRP is largely derived from these perivascular nerve terminals and represents a spillover phenomenon related to the release of the peptide to promote vasodilatation or other functions.[4, 6, 11] The role of circulating CGRP is controversial. Receptors for CGRP have been identified in media and intima of resistance vessels.[4–6] Therefore, in accordance with the previously described criteria for a physiologically relevant vasoactive peptide, CGRP is stored in nerve fibers close to the blood vessel and its receptors are present on the vascular smooth muscle close to the site of its release.

CARDIOVASCULAR ACTIONS OF CGRP

CGRP is the most potent vasodilator discovered to date, and it also has marked positive chronotropic and inotropic effects.[4, 11–13] Its in vivo hemodynamic effects are illustrated in Figure 19–1.[13] The vasodilator effects of CGRP are much more potent and longer lasting than those of other vasodilator peptides such as substance P, bradykinin, vasointestinal peptide, and atrial natriuretic peptide.[14] CGRP

selectively dilates multiple vascular beds, with the coronary vasculature being a particularly sensitive target.[12, 13] Systemic administration of CGRP decreases blood pressure in a dose-dependent manner in normotensive animals and humans and in the spontaneously hypertensive rat (SHR).[4–6] The primary mechanism responsible for this reduction in blood pressure is peripheral arterial dilatation.[4, 5, 13] Based on pharmacological data, CGRP receptors have been classified as $CGRP_1$, and $CGRP_2$.[4] The $CGRP_1$ receptor subtype is sensitive to the CGRP antagonist $CGRP_{8–37}$, whereas the $CGRP_2$ subtype is much less sensitive. $CGRP_1$ receptors are typified by those present in heart and peripheral vessels, and $CGRP_2$ receptors are typified by those in the vas deferens.[4, 17–19] The CGRP receptors appear to be coupled to G-proteins, and in a number of tissues, including vascular smooth muscle, CGRP acts through increases in intracellular cyclic adenosine monophosphate (cAMP). CGRP is capable of activating kATP channels of vascular smooth muscle.[4, 7] The vasodilator response evoked by CGRP is also mediated, in part, by NO release, and various vascular beds differ in their degree of endothelium dependence for the dilator effects of CGRP.[4] CGRP can dilate blood vessels through NO-dependent and NO-independent mechanisms.

RELEASE OF NEUROPEPTIDES FROM SENSORY NERVE TERMINALS

CGRP (and substance P)–rich nerve fibers are components of the primary afferent nervous system, making up capsa-

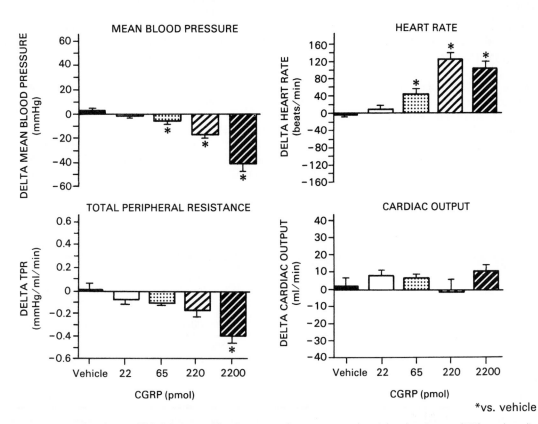

Figure 19–1. The change (delta) in mean blood pressure, heart rate, total peripheral resistance (TPR), and cardiac output in response to either vehicle or four doses of calcitonin gene–related peptide (CGRP). *Asterisk* indicates significant difference from vehicle after the Bonferroni correction of the *p* value. (From DiPette DJ, Schwarzenberger K, Kerr N, et al. Dose-dependent systemic and regional hemodynamic effects of calcitonin gene–related peptide. Am J Med Sci 297[2]:65–70, 1989.)

icin-sensitive A and C fiber afferent nerves and "type B" medium-sized neurons.[4, 20] Although these afferent nerves have traditionally been thought to "sense" stimuli in the periphery and transmit the information centrally, they also have an efferent function.[19–24] Sensory nerve terminals can release CGRP (and other neuropeptides) in response to local factors, including nerve growth factor,[25] vascular wall tension,[21, 22] bradykinin/prostaglandins,[26] endothelin,[27] and the sympathetic nervous system.[28] We and others have demonstrated that many of these factors can modulate the longer-term production and release of CGRP. Using primary cultures of adult rat DRG neurons, we have demonstrated that nerve growth factor or bradykinin/prostaglandins[29] can upregulate CGRP synthesis and release, whereas glucocorticoids[30] or α_2-adrenoreceptor agonists[31] can attenuate the stimulatory effects of nerve growth factor in CGRP. Thus, alterations in these factors, some of which are known to occur in hypertension, may mediate changes in neuronal CGRP expression. If basal CGRP synthesis is increased or decreased, these local factors could be expected to release more or less CGRP, respectively, resulting in a greater or lesser degree of vasodilatation. The release of CGRP from sensory nerve fibers can cause local vasodilatation and increased blood flow.[4] Therefore, in accordance with the previously described criteria, CGRP possesses potent vasodilator activity and is released in the vasculature in response to appropriate stimuli.

ROLE OF CGRP IN DEOXYCORTICOSTERONE-SALT AND SUBTOTAL NEPHRECTOMY–SALT–INDUCED HYPERTENSION IN THE RAT

The first evidence that CGRP plays a direct role in hypertension was provided by studies in the deoxycortisterone-salt (DOC-salt) rat, low-renin, salt-dependent model of acquired experimental hypertension. For these studies, we used DOC-salt hypertensive rats during the onset stage (4 weeks after the initiation of the experimental protocol) and four groups of normotensive rats to control for DOC-pellet implantation, uninephrectomy, or salt administration (Table

19–1). We first demonstrated that CGRP mRNA accumulation was significantly increased in DRG and, correspondingly, that iCGRP levels were elevated in laminae I and II of the spinal cord of DOC-salt hypertensive rats compared with the four groups of normotensive controls.[32] These results are in agreement with an earlier study in hypertensive humans that showed increases in circulating CGRP levels in individuals with primary aldosteronism and in salt-sensitive subjects placed on high- versus low-salt diets.[33] This increase in neuronal CGRP expression in the DOC-salt hypertensive rats was specific for the DRG; we did not observe any alterations in the brain (unpublished observations).

We originally hypothesized that CGRP expression would be markedly decreased in the hypertensive rats and that a reduction in the levels of such a potent vasodilator would, therefore, contribute to the elevated blood pressure. Because our results were the opposite of what was expected, we subsequently postulated that if CGRP was playing a role in blood pressure regulation in this setting, the stimulation of CGRP expression in DOC-salt rats was a counterregulatory vasodilator mechanism to attenuate the elevated blood pressure. To test this hypothesis, CGRP$_{8-37}$, a potent and specific CGRP receptor antagonist, was administered to identical groups of rats (see Table 19–1).[34] If the upregulation of CGRP expression in DOC-salt hypertension were a compensatory vasodilator mechanism to buffer the elevated blood pressure, CGRP$_{8-37}$ administration to the DOC-salt hypertensive rats should increase blood pressure further and have much less or no effect in normotensive controls.

For these experiments, all rats had intravenous (for drug administration) and arterial (for continuous mean arterial pressure [MAP] monitoring) catheters surgically placed and were studied in the conscious, unrestrained state. Injection of saline solution did not alter MAP in any of the five groups, and CGRP$_{8-37}$ administration did not significantly increase MAP in any of the four normotensive groups (Fig. 19–2). However, administration of the antagonist to the DOC-salt hypertensive rats rapidly (within 15 to 20 seconds after CGRP$_{8-37}$ infusion) induced, a dose-dependent increase in MAP. Because of the rapidity of the pressor response to CGRP$_{8-37}$ in the DOC-salt rat, and because the

Table 19–1 Summary of the DOC-Salt (Group A) and Normotensive Control (B–E) Groups

Treatment	A (7)	B (7)	C (5)	D (6)	E (6)
	\multicolumn{5}{c}{Group (n)}				
Surgery	NX	Sham	NX	Sham	NX
Diet	Salt	Water	Water	Salt	Salt
Implant	DOC	Placebo	Placebo	Placebo	Placebo
Final MAP (mm Hg)*	174.7 ± 5.4†	109.4 ± 4.1	125.1 ± 4.6	114.2 ± 2.7	125.4 ± 4.8

From Supowit SC, Zhao H, Hallman DM, et al. Calcitonin gene–related peptide is a depressor of deoxycorticosterone-salt hypertension in the rat. Hypertension 29(4):948, 1997.
Abbreviations: DOC, deoxycorticosterone-acetate pellet; salt, 0.9% NaCl/0.2% KCl drinking water; NX, left nephrectomy; MAP, mean arterial pressure.
*Values for MAP are reported as the mean ± SEM.
†$p < .001$, group A compared with each of the four control groups.

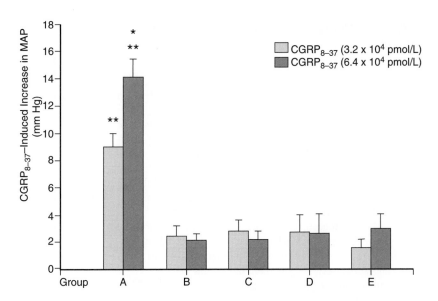

Figure 19–2. Calcitonin gene–related peptide$_{8-37}$ (CGRP$_{8-37}$) increases mean arterial pressure (MAP) in deoxycorticosterone-salt (DOC-salt) hypertensive rats but not normotensive controls. Rats were instrumented for continuous MAP recording and CGRP$_{8-37}$ administration as described in the text. With the rats fully awake and unrestrained, bolus doses of the indicated amounts of CGRP$_{8-37}$ were given. *Double asterisk, p <* .001, DOC-salt (group A) versus each of the four control groups at both CGRP$_{8-37}$ doses; *single asterisk, p < .01,* higher versus lower dose of CGRP$_{8-37}$ in DOC-salt rats. MAP values are reported as mean ± SEM. (From Supowit SC, Zhao H, Hallman DM, et al. Calcitonin gene–related peptide is a depressor of deoxycorticosterone-salt hypertension in the rat. Hypertension 29[4]:948, 1997.)

antagonist probably does not penetrate the central nervous system, the pressor activity of CGRP$_{8-37}$ seen in these experiments likely results from a direct interaction of the antagonist with peripheral vascular CGRP receptors (probably CGRP$_1$). Support for this explanation is provided by

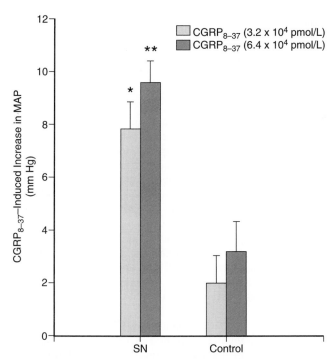

Figure 19–3. Calcitonin gene–related peptide$_{8-37}$ (CGRP$_{8-37}$) increases mean arterial pressure (MAP) in the subtotal nephrectomy (SN)–hypertensive rats but not in normotensive controls. Rats were instrumented for continuous MAP recording and CGRP$_{8-37}$ administration as described in the text. With the rats fully awake and unrestrained, bolus doses of the indicated amounts of CGRP$_{8-37}$ were given intravenously. MAP values are reported as mean ± SEM. *Single asterisk, p < .05,* SN-hypertensive rats versus control rats at the lower CGRP$_{8-37}$ dose; *double asterisk, p < .01,* SN-hypertensive rats versus control rats at the higher CGRP$_{8-37}$ dose. (From Supowit SC, Zhao H, Hallman DM, et al. Calcitonin gene–related peptide is a depressor in subtotal nephrectomy hypertension. Hypertension 11:393, 1998.)

studies that show that CGRP$_{8-37}$ is a competitive inhibitor of CGRP binding and that the CGRP$_1$ receptor subtype (present in heart and peripheral blood vessels) displays the highest sensitivity to this antagonist.[4, 17–19] Other reports demonstrate that CGRP$_{8-37}$ can inhibit the vasodilatation evoked by exogenously administered or endogenously released CGRP in vivo.[35–37] These data support the hypothesis that in DOC-salt hypertension, CGRP acts as a compensatory depressor to counteract the increase in blood pressure. They satisfy the criterion that blockade of the receptor for the peptide causes hemodynamic changes.

Because these data and other reports indicate that CGRP (and substance P)[38] may act as counterregulatory vasodilators in salt-dependent hypertension, we next examined the effect of endogenous CGRP on blood pressure in subtotal nephrectomy (SN)–salt–induced hypertension, another model of low-renin, salt-dependent hypertension.[39] SN-salt hypertensive rats (final MAP, 173 ± 5 mm Hg) and normotensive controls (final MAP, 113 ± 5 mm Hg) were instrumented and given saline solution or CGRP$_{8-37}$ as described previously. As shown in Figure 19–3, two different doses of CGRP$_{8-37}$ did not significantly alter the blood pressure in the control group. In contrast, the antagonist produced a further increase in MAP similar to that observed in the DOC-salt hypertensive rats. These results suggest that in SN-salt–induced hypertension, CGRP is also playing a compensatory depressor role.

Surprisingly, when the CGRP mRNA and peptide levels were quantified in the DRG from the SN-salt hypertensive and control rats, there were no detectable changes in CGRP expression, suggesting a second mechanism by which CGRP exerts its counterregulatory action. As opposed to increased CGRP synthesis and release, seen in DOC-salt hypertension, the mechanism of this effect may be increased vascular responsiveness to CGRP. These studies, together with those using the DOC-salt model, are consistent with the hypothesis that the ability of CGRP (and substance P) to partially counteract increased blood pressure is strongly influenced by the salt-dependence of the hypertensive state. The mechanisms by which this occurs are not known.

ROLE OF CGRP IN N^G-NITRO-L-ARGININE METHYL ESTER–INDUCED HYPERTENSION DURING PREGNANCY

Accumulating evidence suggests that CGRP is involved in the vascular adaptations that occur during normal pregnancy.[4, 40, 41] Both exogenous and endogenous CGRP have antihypertensive actions in hypertensive N^G-nitro-L-arginine methyl ester (L-NAME)–treated female rats, a non–salt-dependent model.[40, 41] Yallampalli and Garfield[42] and others have demonstrated in pregnant rats that inhibition of NO synthesis with L-NAME causes hypertension, proteinuria, fetal growth retardation, and increased fetal mortality without affecting gestational length. To examine the effects of exogenous CGRP in this setting, CGRP and L-NAME were chronically infused subcutaneously into pregnant rats, separately or together, beginning on day 17 of gestation; a control group was given saline solution.[40] As shown in Figure 19–4, L-NAME treatment significantly elevated blood pressure on days 18, 19, and 20 of pregnancy and postpartum days 1 and 2. The coadministration of CGRP with L-NAME prevented the gestational, but not the postpartum, hypertension and also significantly decreased pup mortality (not shown). Further studies revealed that this differential effect of CGRP on blood pressure during gestation, when female sex steroid hormone levels are high, and the postpartum period, when sex ste-

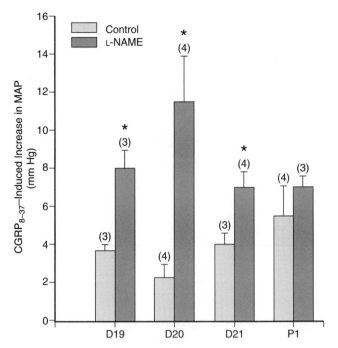

Figure 19–5. Calcitonin gene–related peptide_{8-37} (CGRP_{8-37}) increases mean arterial pressure (MAP) in the L-NAME–treated pregnant rats. Animals were instrumented for continuous MAP recording and CGRP_{8-37} administration on days 19, 20, and 21 (D19 to D21) of pregnancy and postpartum day 1 (P1). With the animals in a fully awake and unrestrained state, bolus doses of 100 μg CGRP_{8-37} were given. Changes in MAP values are reported as the mean ± SEM. Numbers in parentheses indicate number of animals in each group. *Asterisk, $p < .05$. (From Gangula PR, Supowit SC, Wimalawansa SJ. Calcitonin gene–related peptide is a depressor in L-NAME–induced preeclampsia. Hypertension 29[1]:250, 1997.)

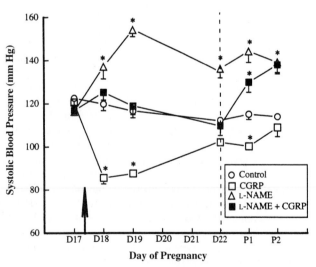

Figure 19–4. Effect of calcitonin gene–related peptide (CGRP), infused at a rate of 24 μg/day/rat either alone or in combination with 50 mg N^G-nitro-L-arginine methyl ester (L-NAME) per day, on the systolic blood pressure of pregnant rats. Agents were administered subcutaneously in osmotic minipumps dissolved in a sterile saline solution. The control group was infused with saline solution alone. Pumps were inserted on day 17 of gestation *(arrow)* after the first blood pressure measurement. Blood pressures were measured on days 17, 18, 19, and 22 of gestation (D17 to D22) and on days 1 and 2 postpartum (P1, P2). The *vertical dashed line* indicates the day of spontaneous labor. Each point represents the mean ± SEM value for five rats in each group. Values of treatment groups with *asterisks* differ significantly ($p < .05$) compared with the corresponding value of the control group (analysis of variance, Dunnett test). (From Yallampalli C, Dong YL, Wimalawansa SJ. Calcitonin gene–related peptide reverses the hypertension and significantly decreases the fetal mortality in preeclampsia rats induced by L-NAME. Hum Reprod 11:897, 1996.)

roid hormone levels are markedly reduced, is mediated by progesterone.[43] When progesterone was given along with the CGRP and L-NAME, hypertension was blocked not only in gestation but also in the postpartum period. During this latter stage, the hypotensive effects of CGRP were lost when the progesterone treatment was stopped. Similar to the findings in postpartum rats, CGRP reversed the hypertension in L-NAME–treated ovariectomized rats receiving progesterone injections. This effect of CGRP was apparent only during the progestone treatment period. These studies suggest that exogenous CGRP is antihypertensive in L-NAME–treated pregnant and nonpregnant rats and that these vasodilator effects of CGRP are modulated by progesterone.

To determine whether endogenous CGRP participates in blood pressure regulation in the L-NAME–treated pregnant rats, L-NAME–treated (starting on day 17 of gestation) and control pregnant rats were instrumented and given the CGRP antagonist as described previously.[41] Baseline blood pressure was higher in the L-NAME than the control rats on days 19, 20, and 21 of pregnancy and on postpartum day 1. As shown in Figure 19–5, CGRP_{8-37} did not change blood pressure in control groups. However, antagonist administration to the L-NAME rats further increased blood pressure on days 19, 20, and 21 of pregnancy but was without effect on postpartum day 1. CGRP mRNA and peptide levels in DRG were not different between the L-

NAME and the control rats at any time point. These data indicate that endogenous CGRP can also play a counterregulatory role in a non–salt-dependent model of hypertension. Preliminary results suggest that the sensitivity of the vasculature to CGRP is enhanced in L-NAME–induced hypertension during pregnancy and that this phenomenon is mediated, at least in part, by progesterone.

ROLE OF CGRP IN THE SHR

Although a number of studies implicate CGRP in the development and maintenance of hypertension in the SHR, conclusive results are lacking. Some investigators have reported increased levels of circulating CGRP in SHR compared with Wistar-Kyoto (WKY) controls; others have reported decreased levels.[4] Support for the latter result is provided by reports showing an age-related decrease in iCGRP and CGRP-evoked vasodilator activity in perivascular nerves associated with mesenteric vascular beds isolated from SHR compared with WKY rats.[44] In addition, we have demonstrated that CGRP mRNA levels were significantly reduced in DRG, and correspondingly, iCGRP content was lower in laminae I and II of the spinal cord of SHR compared with WKY controls.[45, 46] Studies designed to examine the role of CGRP in the maintenance of the cerebral microcirculation in SHR and WKY revealed increased responsiveness of the microvascular bed to CGRP in SHR, which was postulated to be related to decreased CGRP levels in these blood vessels.[46, 47] However, preliminary results from our laboratory show that systemic administration of CGRP$_{8-37}$ to SHR does not alter MAP, as was observed in the acquired models. Thus, CGRP is not acting as a compensatory depressor in this genetic model of hypertension. Therefore, a decrease in CGRP expression in SHR could contribute to the high blood pressure by a relative reduction of vasodilator activity.

CGRP AND HUMAN HYPERTENSION

Exogenous CGRP can markedly decrease high blood pressure in humans,[4–6] but it is not known whether endogenous CGRP participates in the pathophysiology of human hypertension. Data concerning circulating levels of iCGRP in hypertensive humans have been conflicting.[4–6, 9] These results have been attributed to several factors, including the assay itself, heterogeneity of the disease, severity and duration of the hypertensive state, the degree of end-organ damage, and the variety of antihypertensive treatment regimens used in these patients. The development of nonpeptide CGRP agonists and antagonists that can be tested in humans will enable investigators to determine whether CGRP plays a role in human hypertension. More detailed accounts of the vasoregulatory actions of CGRP in humans can be found in other reviews.[4–6, 9]

ROLE OF SUBSTANCE P IN EXPERIMENTAL HYPERTENSION

Substance P is often colocalized and coreleased with CGRP in sensory nerve terminals. This neuropeptide is a member of the tachykinin family and, like CGRP, is involved in numerous physiological activities, such as neuromodulation, smooth muscle contraction, and vasodilatation.[7, 19–23] The vasodilator activity of substance P is endothelium-dependent. This peptide participates in the regulation of blood flows of various organs. Reduced levels of substance P have been described both in stroke-prone SHR and in human essential hypertension.[38] In these settings, substance P could contribute to the elevated blood pressure through the decreased activity of a counterregulatory mechanism.

Using an experimental design similar to that used for the CGRP studies, Kohlmann and colleagues[38] employed a nonpeptide substance P receptor (NK-1) antagonist to assess the hemodynamic role of this neuropeptide in five models of experimental hypertension. In conscious unrestrained rats, the SP antagonist induced significant increases in MAP in three salt-dependent models: DOC-salt, SN-salt, and one-kidney–one-clip hypertensive rats. In contrast, the antagonist produced nonsignificant effects on MAP in two-kidney–one-clip hypertensive rats and SHR—salt-independent forms of hypertension. These data suggest that, like CGRP, substance P may act as a partial counterregulatory mechanism to counteract the blood pressure increase in models of salt-dependent hypertension. It is not known whether neuronal substance P expression is altered in any of these models or whether this peptide exerts its effects at the level of the peripheral vasculature or the central nervous system.

SUMMARY

A hypothesis regarding the role of CGRP in the hypertensive process is shown in Figure 19–6. In the three models of acquired hypertension that have been studied to date, CGRP appears to act as a compensatory vasodilator in an attempt to counteract the blood pressure increase. In the DOC-salt rat, this activity of CGRP appears to be mediated through a marked increase in the neuronal expression, and presumed release, of this peptide. The factors that cause this upregulation of CGRP have not yet been determined, but it is known that an increase in blood pressure, per se, does not enhance CGRP production.[48] The SN-salt and L-NAME models do not exhibit increases in CGRP expression, suggesting another mechanism by which this peptide could exert its antihypertensive effect. A potential second mechanism is enhanced sensitivity of the vasculature to CGRP, perhaps via the upregulation of the CGRP$_1$ receptor. It is probable that CGRP is one of several counterregulatory mechanisms that are stimulated in hypertension. Substance P has been shown to buffer the blood pressure increase in three models of salt-dependent hypertension, and compensatory antihypertensive roles have been postulated for the kallikrein-kinin system[49] and several of the natriuretic peptides.[50]

The inability of CGRP$_{8-37}$ to alter blood pressure in control rats implies that CGRP does not participate in the regulation of systemic blood pressure in the normotensive state, but this does not rule out a role for CGRP in the modulation of regional organ blood flows under normal physiological conditions. CGRP participates in the regulation of blood flow in the gut,[7] and in studies in which

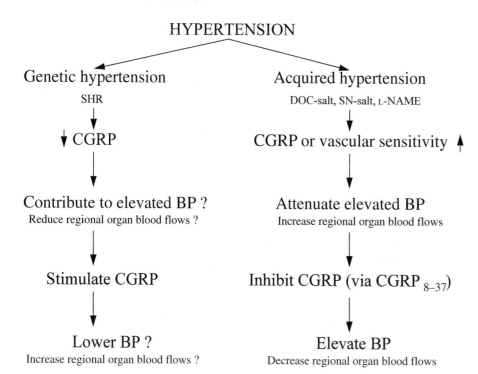

Figure 19–6. Roles of calcitonin gene–related peptide (CGRP) in experimental hypertension. SHR, spontaneously hypertensive rat; DOC-salt, deoxycorticosterone-salt; SN-salt, subtotal nephrectomy–salt; L-NAME, N^G-nitro-L-arginine methyl ester; BP, blood pressure.

CGRP$_{8-37}$ was used in normal rats, CGRP was responsible for approximately 30% of basal coronary blood flow.[51]

In genetic hypertension, as in SHR, several studies indicate that there is a marked downregulation of CGRP. Although this decrease in CGRP expression is probably not a primary cause of the hypertension in this model, the decrease in CGRP could contribute to the elevated blood pressure. Studies are currently in progress to enhance endogenous CGRP production in the SHR and to determine whether this alters blood pressure or regional organ blood flows, or both. Although a definitive role for CGRP in human hypertension has yet to be established, the weight of the evidence supports the participation of this peptide in the modulation of vasorelaxation in states of increased peripheral resistance or in an increase in blood flow to critical areas like the coronary and cerebral circulations.[6] Under these conditions, it appears that activation of perivascular sensory nerves stimulates the release of neuropeptides that, in turn, regulates vascular tone, redistributes blood flow, and perhaps modulates systemic blood pressure. CGRP has also been implicated in other cardiovascular disease states, such as congestive heart failure, as well as other pathological conditions that produce significant alterations in cardiovascular function.[4–6, 8, 9]

Acknowledgments

The authors thank Rhoda Thompson for her excellent secretarial service. We also thank Dr. Chandra Yallampalli, Dr. Pandu Gangula, Dr. Huawei Zhao, Dr. Karin Westlund-High, Dr. Sunil Wimalawansa, Diane Hallman, and Monique Christensen for their invaluable contributions to this work.

References

1. Amara SG, Jonas V, Rosenfeld MG, et al. Alternative RNA processing in calcitonin gene expression generates mRNAs encoding different polypeptide products. Nature 298:240, 1982.
2. Rosenfeld MG, Mermod JJ, Amara SG, et al. Production of a novel neuropeptide encoded by the calcitonin gene via tissue-specific RNA processing. Nature 304:129, 1983.
3. Breimer LH, MacIntyre I, Zaidi M. Peptides from the calcitonin genes: Molecular genetics, structure and function. Biochemical J 255:377, 1988.
4. Wimalawansa SJ. Calcitonin gene–related peptide and its receptors: Molecular genetics, physiology, pathophysiology, and therapeutic potentials. Endocrine Rev 17:533, 1996.
5. DiPette DJ, Wimalawansa SJ. Cardiovascular actions of calcitonin gene–related peptide. *In* Crass J, Avioli LV (eds). Calcium Regulating Hormones and Cardiovascular Function. Ann Arbor, MI, CRC, 1994; p 239.
6. Preibisz JJ. CGRP and regulation of human cardiovascular homeostatis. Am J Hypertens 6:434, 1993.
7. Dockray GJ. Physiology of enteric neuropeptides. *In* Johnson LR (ed). Physiology of the Gastrointestinal Tract. New York, Raven, 1994; p 169.
8. Zaidi M, Moonga BS, Bevis PHG, et al. The calcitonin gene peptides: Biology and clinical relevance. Crit Rev Clin Lab Sci 28:109, 1990.
9. McEwan J, Legon S, Wimalawansa SJ, et al. Calcitonin gene–related peptide: A review of its biology and relevance to the cardiovascular system. *In* Laragh JH, Brenner BN, Kaplan NM (eds). Endocrine Mechanisms in Hypertension. New York, Raven, 1989; p. 287.
10. Besson JM, Chaouch A. Peripheral and spinal mechanisms of nociception. Physiol Rev 67:67, 1987.
11. Brain SD, William TJ, Tippins JR, et al. Calcitonin gene–related peptide is a potent vasodilator. Nature 313:54, 1985.
12. Asimakis GK, DiPette DJ, Conti VR, et al. Hemodynamic action of calcitonin gene–related peptide in the isolated rat heart. Life Sci 41:597, 1987.
13. DiPette DJ, Schwarzenberger K, Kerr N, et al. Dose-dependent systemic and regional hemodynamic effects of calcitonin gene–related peptide. Am J Med Sci 297:65, 1989.
14. Brown MJ, Morice AH. Clinical pharmacology of vasodilator peptides. J Cardiovasc Pharmacol 10:582, 1987.
15. Gibson SJ, Polk JM, Bloom SR, et al. Calcitonin gene–related peptide immunoreactivity in the spinal cord of man and eight other species. J Neurosci 12:3101, 1984.
16. Marti E, Gibson SJ, Polak JM, et al. Ontogeny of peptide- and amine-containing neurones in motor, sensory, and automonic regions of rat and human spinal cord, dorsal root ganglia, and rat skin. J Comp Neurol 226:332, 1987.
17. Donoso MV, Fournier A, St. Pierre S, et al. Pharmacological charac-

terization of CGRP receptor subtype in the vascular system of the rat: Studies with hCGRP fragments and analogues. Peptides 11:885, 1990.

18. Gray GW, Marshall I, Bose C, et al. Subtypes of the calcitonin gene–related peptide (CGRP) receptor in vascular tissues. Br J Pharmacol 102:189, 1991.

19. Quirion R, Van Rossum D, Dumont Y, et al. Characterization of CGRP$_1$ and CGRP$_2$ receptor subtypes. Ann N Y Acad Sci 657:88, 1991.

20. Rang HP, Bevan SJ, Dray A. Nociceptive peripheral neurones: Cellular properties. *In* Wall PD, Melzak R (eds). Textbook of Pain. Edinburgh, Churchill Livingstone, 1994; p. 57.

21. Lembeck F, Holzer P. Substance P as neurogenic mediator of antidromic vasodilation and neurogenic plasma extravasation. Arch Pharamcol 310:175, 1979.

22. Holzer P. Local effector functions of capsaicin-sensitive sensory nerve endings: Involvement of tachykinins, calcitonin gene–related peptide and other neuropeptides. Neuroscience 24:739, 1988.

23. Yaksh TL, Bailey J, Roddy DR, et al. Peripheral release of substance P from primary afferents. *In* Dubner R, Gebhart GF, Bond MR (eds). Proceedings from the Vth World Congress on Pain. Amsterdam, Elsevier, 1988; p. 51.

24. Burnstock G, Ralevic V. New insights into the local regulation of blood flow by perivascular nerves and endothelium. Br J Plast Surg 47:527, 1994.

25. Lindsay RM, Lockett C, Sternbeg J, et al. Neuropeptide expression in cultures of adult sensory neurons: Modulation of substance P and calcitonin gene–related peptide levels by nerve growth factor. Neuroscience 33:53, 1989.

26. Vasko MR, Campbell WB, Waite KG. Prostaglandin E$_2$ enhances bradykinin stimulated release of neuropeptides from rat sensory neurons in culture. J Neurosci 14:4987, 1994.

27. Dymshitz J, Vasko MR. Endothelin-1 enhances capsaicin-induced peptide release and cGMP accumulation in cultures of rat sensory neurons. Neurosci Lett 167:128, 1994.

28. Kawasaki H, Nuki C, Saito A, et al. Adrenergic modulation of calcitonin gene–related peptide (CGRP) containing nerve-mediated vasodilation in the rat mesenteric resistance vessel. Brain Res 506:287, 1990.

29. Supowit SC, Hallman DM, Zhao H, et al. Bradykinin regulates neuronal calcitonin gene–related peptide expression and release. [Abstract] Hypertension 26:564, 1995.

30. Supowit SC, Christensen MD, Westlund KN, et al. Dexamethasone and activators of the protein kinase A and C signal transduction pathways regulate neuronal calcitonin gene–related peptide expression and release. Brain Res 686:77, 1995.

31. Supowit SC, Hallman DM, Zhao H, et al. Alpha$_2$-adrenergic receptor activation inhibits calcitonin gene–related peptide expression in cultured dorsal root ganglia neurons. Brain Res 782:184, 1998.

32. Supowit SC, Guraraj A, Ramana CV, et al. Enhanced neuronal expression of calcitonin gene–related peptide in mineralocorticoid-salt hypertension. Hypertension 25:1333, 1995.

33. Resnick LM, Preibisz JJ, Laragh JH. Calcitonin gene–related peptide–like immunoreactivity in hypertension: Relation to blood pressure, sodium and calcium metabolism. *In* Rettig R, Ganten D, Luft P (eds). Salt and Hypertension. New York, Springer-Verlag, 1989; p. 190.

34. Supowit SC, Zhao H, Hallman DM, et al. Calcitonin gene–related peptide is a depressor of deoxycorticosterone-salt hypertension in the rat. Hypertension 29:945, 1997.

35. Gardiner SM, Compton AM, Bennett T, et al. Antagonistic effects of human α-CGRP$_{8–37}$ on the in vivo regional hemodynamic action of human α-CGRP. Biochem Biophys Res Commun 171:938, 1990.

36. Gardiner SM, Compton AM, Kemp PA, et al. Human α-calcitonin gene–related peptide (CGRP)–(8–37), but not -(28–37) inhibits carotid vasodilator effects of human CGRP in vivo. Eur J Pharmacol 199:375, 1991.

37. Hughes SR, Brain SP. A calcitonin gene–related peptide (CGRP) antagonist (CGRP$_{8–37}$) inhibits microvascular response induced by CGRP and capsaicin in skin. Br J Pharmacol 104:748, 1991.

38. Kohlmann O, Cesaretti L, Ginoza M, et al. Role of substance P in blood pressure regulation in salt-dependent experimental hypertension. Hypertension 29:506, 1997.

39. Supowit SC, Zhao H, Hallman DM, et al. Calcitonin gene–related peptide is a depressor in subtotal nephrectomy hypertension. Hypertension 31:391, 1998.

40. Yallampalli C, Dong Y-L, Wimalawansa SJ. Calcitonin gene–related peptide reverses the hypertension and significantly decreases the fetal mortality in preeclampsia rats induced by N^G-nitro-L-arginine methyl ester. Hum Reprod 11:895, 1996.

41. Gangula PR, Supowit SC, Wimalawansa SJ, et al. Calcitonin gene–related peptide is a depressor in N^G-nitro-L-arginine methyl ester–induced preeclampsia. Hypertension 29:506, 1997.

42. Yallampalli C, Garfield RE. Inhibition of nitric oxide synthesis in rats during pregnancy produces symptoms identical to preeclampsia. Am J Obstet Gynecol 169:1316, 1993.

43. Gangula PR, Wimalawansa SJ, Yallampalli C. Progesterone upregulates vasodilator effects of calcitonin gene–related peptide in L-NAME–induced hypertension. Am J Obstet Gynecol 176:894, 1997.

44. Kawasaki H, Takasaki K. Age-related decrease of neurogenic release of calcitonin gene–related peptide from perivascular nerves in spontaneously hypertensive rats. Clin Exp Hypertens A14:989, 1992.

45. Westlund KN, DiPette DJ, Carson J, et al. Decreased spinal cord content of calcitonin gene–related peptide in the spontaneously hypertensive rat. Neurosci Lett 131:183, 1991.

46. Supowit SC, Ramana CV, Westlund KN, et al. Calcitonin gene–related peptide gene expression in the spontaneously hypertensive rat. Hypertension 21:1010, 1993.

47. Hong KW, Yu SS, Sin YW, et al. Decreased CGRP levels with increased sensitivity to CGRP in the pial arteries of spontaneously hypertensive rats. Life Sci 60:697, 1997.

48. Supowit SC, Zhao H, Wang DH, et al. Regulation of calcitonin gene–related peptide expression: Role of increased blood pressure. Hypertension 26:1177, 1995.

49. Nolly H, Carretero OA, Larna MC, et al. Vascular kallikrein in deoxycorticosterone acetate–salt hypertensive rats. Hypertension 23:185, 1994.

50. Lang CC, Choy AMJ, Struthers AD. Atrial and brain natruietic peptides: A dual natriuretic peptide system potentially involved in circulatory homeostasis. Clin Sci 83:519, 1992.

51. Yavita H, Sato E, Kawaguchi M, et al. Nonadrenergic noncholinergic nerves regulate basal coronary flow via release of capsaicin-sensitive neuropeptides in the rat heart. Circ Res 75:780, 1994.

20 Kallikrein-Kinin Systems

Harry S. Margolius

The kallikrein-kinin systems now occupy a more prominent position in considerations of the cause, the pathogenesis, and even the therapeutics of cardiovascular and metabolic diseases as a result of an accelerating pace of evaluation and discovery of the activities and roles of kinin system components in cardiovascular, renal, and metabolic functions and disorders. In this chapter, the structural and functional characteristics of kallikrein-kinin system components are reviewed. Some of the early observations that stimulated interest in possible connections between the systems and cardiovascular and metabolic diseases are mentioned, but most emphasis is placed on newer findings since the late 1980s that are provoking an increased level of interest in kallikrein-kinin system roles in hypertension, cardiac and renal diseases, and diabetes mellitus.[1-6]

This phylogenetically ancient system of low-molecular-weight (LMW) and high-molecular-weight (HMW) substrates, serine proteases, peptide hormones, peptidases, and inhibitors now appears to have important responsibility for the regulation of local and perhaps systemic hemodynamics, vascular permeability, the inflammatory response, activation of neuronal pathways, and the movement of electrolytes, water, and metabolic substrates across epithelia and into other tissues.[1] It is difficult to find mammalian cell types devoid of any kallikrein-kinin system components or responsiveness to kinins, suggesting that many of the regulatory roles for the systems are still undescribed.

STRUCTURE AND FUNCTION OF THE KALLIKREIN-KININ SYSTEM

Kininogens

The single human kininogen gene is localized to chromosome 3q26→qter close to two closely related genes, the α-2-HS-glycoprotein and the histidine-rich glycoprotein.[7, 8] It codes for the production of both HMW (626 amino acids, 88 to 120 kDa) and LMW (409 amino acids, 50 to 68 kDa)

kininogens via alternate splicing from 11 exons spread over a 27-kb pair span.[9] Figure 20–1 illustrates the relationships between the human kininogen gene and the mRNAs for the HMW and LMW kininogens.[10] The 9 exons upstream of the kinin sequence code for the same amino acids in both kininogens; the portion of exon 10 downstream of the kinin sequence is unique to HMW kininogen mRNA, whereas exon 11 is expressed in only LMW kininogen mRNA.

The regulation of kininogen gene expression is still incompletely characterized, but several studies have suggested that steroid hormones such as estrogens or progesterone, interleukins, acute inflammation, and dietary electrolyte changes affect the hepatic expression of kininogens.[11-13] There is an unusual pattern of kininogen gene expression in the rat, where two T kininogen genes are acute-phase genes (the expression of which is transcriptionally modified by interleukin-6 [IL-6] and glucocorticoids); there is also a K kininogen gene, which corresponds to that found in all other mammals. Although there is high homology between T and K genes (>90%), only expression of the T kininogens is increased in inflammation. This allows the study of the molecular mechanisms of regulation of gene expression in a closely related gene family. The work has shown that an evolutionary divergence of a few critical nucleotides in the promotor can markedly alter the expression of the downstream genes.[12, 13]

Another fascinating finding that indicates how much is left to learn about the regulation of kininogen gene expression is a description of the genetic basis of total kininogen deficiency in the index patient with the disorder known as *Williams' trait.*[14] In this patient, the total and lifelong absence of kininogen was not due to a major DNA deletion or insertion or any absence of kininogen gene expression, as both LMW and HMW kininogen mRNAs were detected in the patient's liver. Rather, there was a C→T mutation at nucleotide 22 in exon 5, resulting in a change from an Arg codon, CGA, to a stop codon, TGA. As this mutation occurred before the differential RNA splicing site, both

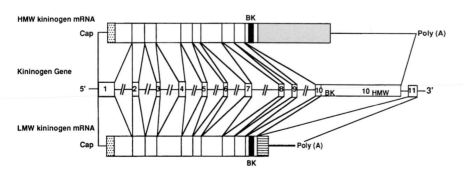

Figure 20–1. Schematic representation shows the human kininogen gene and mRNAs for high-molecular-weight (HMW) and low-molecular-weight (LMW) kininogens. Protein-coding regions are indicated by the *open boxes,* cap sites are *stippled,* and the bradykinin (BK) sequences are indicated by the *black bars.* Note that only a short segment of exons 10 and 11 is transcribed in LMW kininogen mRNA, whereas all of exon 10 but not exon 11 is transcribed in HMW kininogen mRNA. (Modified from Trends Biochem Sci, vol 11, Muller-Esterl W, Iwanaga S, Nakanishi S, Kininogens revisited, pp 336–339, Copyright 1986, with permission from Elsevier Science.)

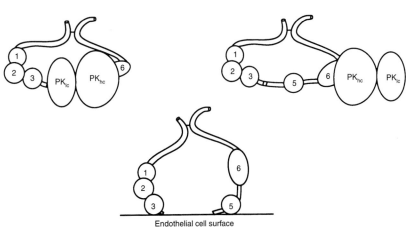

Figure 20–2. Schematic representation shows high-molecular-weight kininogen *(top)*, kininogen interacting with plasma prekallikrein (PK) *(middle)*, and changes with activation *(bottom)*. The domains are labeled as described in the text. Electron microscopic observations[16] indicate the flexibility of the prekallikrein-kininogen complexes so that the enzyme can either extend from the substrate laterally or lie on top of it, probably to cleave bradykinin. After bradykinin is cleaved, there is a conformational change that enhances binding to the endothelial cell surface. lc, light chain; hc, heavy chain. (Modified from Weisel JW, Nagasawami C, Woodhead JL, et al. The shape of high molecular weight kininogen. J Biol Chem 269:10100–10106, 1994.)

LMW and HMW mRNAs contained the stop codon. As a result, the truncated protein, if made at all, either was not secreted from the liver or was degraded.

Kininogens are single-chain glycoproteins with a common amino-terminal heavy chain and smaller, variable carboxy-terminal light chains with the kinin moiety intervening. Antibodies against the various regions are being used to define separate functions for each domain of the molecules and to mechanisms involved in prekallikrein binding to kininogen, as well as kininogen binding to vascular endothelial cells.[15, 16] The most detailed studies thus far show that HMW kininogen binds calcium via domain 1, inhibits important cysteine proteinases such as cathepsins and calpain via domains 2 and 3, binds to surfaces such as endothelium via domain 5 just downstream of bradykinin in domain 4,[17, 18] and binds plasma prekallikrein and factor XI via domain 6 of the light chain (Fig. 20–2). Work with electron microscopy of rotary shadowed preparations describes the shape changes of HMW kininogen before and after association with prekallikrein and its activation to cleave out the kinin.[16]

Additional functional properties of the two kininogens include their ability to bind platelets and neutrophils, to modulate thrombin-induced platelet activation, and to inhibit the binding of fibrinogen to platelets, while releasing kinin after their cleavage by kallikreins. This suggests that kininogens are continually and intimately involved as mediators and modulators of vascular inflammation and local injury.[19] What is not well understood is the extent of their contributions to the early (or late) phases of damage associated with hypertensive or diabetic diseases. As noted previously, the genetic abnormality responsible for the total plasma kininogen deficiency in Williams' trait has been defined, but the patients show no clinical hemostatic disorder. An animal model, the Brown Norway Katholiek rat,

which can synthesize but not secrete kininogen,[20] is being used to assess the roles of kinins in blood pressure regulation, but studies of the effects of kininogen deficiency or modification on vascular, renal, or other tissue function are still in their earliest stages.[21]

The cardiovascular system is presented with kininogens that are synthesized primarily in the liver,[22] then secreted and transported in plasma, as well as on the membranes of platelets and neutrophils, in high concentrations (HMW kininogen, 90 mg/L; LMW kininogen, 170 mg/L[19]). In addition, human vascular endothelial cells contain mRNA for HMW kininogen,[23] and kininogen is found in rat vascular smooth muscle cells grown in the absence of serum.[24]

Bradykinin upregulates the expression of kininogen-binding sites on the surface of human vascular endothelial cells.[25] More recently, the characterization of these cell surface–binding sites has generated much interest. Two groups of investigators[26, 27] have shown that the binding site for HMW kininogen on two different lines of endothelial cells is the gC1q receptor, an extrinsic membrane protein that interacts with certain domains of the complement component C1q. In addition, Colman and coworkers[28] have found that this kininogen also binds to human umbilical vein endothelial cells through zinc-dependent interactions with the urokinase receptor. They suggest this site may not represent the primary endothelial receptor for this kininogen, but that after the substrate is cleaved, it then binds with greater affinity to this second receptor. Even more recently, Hasan and colleagues[29] have identified cytokeratin 1 as a binding protein and putative kininogen receptor on the same umbilical vein endothelial cells. Interactions among kininogens and their binding sites and the ramifications of binding, subsequent proteolysis, and the influence of these events on processes such as local inflammation, cellular migration, angiogenesis, tumor metastasis, and complement or plasminogen activation[30] will become topics for intensive study in the future. Much less is known about the regulation and intravascular roles of LMW kininogen.[31]

Kallikreins and Kallikrein Inhibitors

The "true" tissue kallikrein, exemplified by renal kallikrein, is a gene product of a small gene family of 3 in the human, up to 20 in the rat, and 24 in the mouse.[1] All tissue kallikrein genes consist of five exons and four introns. The human genes are clustered on chromosome 19 at q13.2–13.4 and expressed in the epithelial or secretory cells of various ducts, including salivary, sweat, pancreatic, prostatic, intestinal, and the distal nephron. Although no human vascular wall data have established the presence of kallikrein gene expression, rat aortic smooth muscle cells in culture,[24] and rat arteries and veins express kallikrein mRNA and release enzyme into surrounding media.[32] Human neutrophils also express tissue kallikrein mRNA.[33] The assembly, trafficking, and localization of tissue kallikrein either in the sites where it has been long known to exist or in cells of the cardiovascular system are poorly understood. Given the almost ubiquitous responsiveness of these tissues and cells to kinins (and the hundreds of articles describing such responses), there is plentiful rationale for further study of the biochemical contributors to the presentation of kinins at the receptors expressed on the surfaces of these cells.

The tissue kallikreins of human and rodent are acidic glycoproteins, variably and extensively (approximately 20% molecular weight) glycosylated. The human renal enzyme is synthesized as a zymogen (prokallikrein) with an attached 17-amino acid signal peptide preceding a 7-amino acid sequence that must be cleaved to activate the enzyme. Although several proteinases are capable of activating prokallikrein in vitro, the in vivo activating enzyme is still unknown, as are the factors that regulate tissue kallikrein processing and storage. This is in contrast to knowledge available concerning the activation of plasma kallikrein, another serine proteinase different from the tissue enzyme but nevertheless carrying the same name.[1]

Once activated, human tissue kallikrein cleaves LMW kininogen to release lys-bradykinin (kallidin), whereas plasma kallikrein releases bradykinin. The two peptides are generally equipotent, and it is unknown whether this difference in peptide production is functionally significant. Several inhibitors of the tissue kallikreins exist. The most familiar are aprotinin, the bovine basic pancreatic trypsin inhibitor, a 6.5-kDa, 58-amino acid polypeptide, and another serine proteinase inhibitor (serpin), called *kallistatin*.[34] The former is commercially available and widely used experimentally (and clinically in some countries) as a tissue kallikrein inhibitor, although it is not completely specific in this regard. The latter, a 58-kDa acidic glycoprotein, slowly forms heat-stable complexes with active tissue kallikrein and other serine proteinases that can be blocked by heparin.[34] The in vivo target of kallistatin is uncertain, and it inhibits tissue kallikrein activity slowly and incompletely, but there appear to be differences in the binding of kallistatin derived from tissue extracts of spontaneously hypertensive rats (SHR) versus Wistar-Kyoto rats (WKY) to purified kallikrein.[35] In contrast, the kallikrein-binding properties of kallistatin in serum of the two strains is similar. Based on available data, it seems unlikely that this protein has a significant role in kinin system function, although further study is required. Finally, endogenous kinin generation by enzymes that are not only *not* serine proteinases, but are not of mammalian origin, has been demonstrated.[36] An extracellular cysteine proteinase of *Streptococcus pyogenes* has been shown to release biologically active kinins from HMW kininogen in vitro and from kininogens in human plasma. This could represent an important virulence mechanism in *S. pyogenes* infections.[36]

Kinins and Kinin Receptors

Kinins formed within various organs are detectable in secretory products (e.g., urine, saliva, sweat), interstitial fluid, and under some circumstances (i.e., kininase inhibition), even in venous blood. The systemic half-life of the kinins is very short (15 to 30 seconds), and concentrations of kinins in biological fluids are low—e.g., a few nanograms per liter (approximately 10^{-11} mol/L) in human plasma—but for years were overestimated by assays using inadequate inhibition of kinin-generating enzymes or nonspecific antisera that falsely elevated the estimates. These errors resulted in some faulty conclusions that, for example, seemed to eliminate the possibility of a kinin role in the effects of angiotensin-converting enzyme (ACE) inhibitors. On the other hand, the potency with which kinins exert effects on biological targets has, if anything, been underestimated, because understanding of the contributors to kinin catabolism is still incomplete.[37]

Kinin receptors are characterized as B_1, B_2, and perhaps B_3. B_1 receptors are of less functional significance than B_2. B_1 receptors were first described in rabbit vasculature,[38] especially after insult with, for example, *Escherichia coli* endotoxin or bacterial lipopolysaccharide. Under these conditions, the principal ligand for the B_1 receptor, des-Arg⁹-bradykinin, produces marked vasodilatation and hypotension, an effect not noted in normal tissue, although the peptide can also produce contraction of vascular smooth muscle. The B_1 receptor has been described in several species and cell lines; its cDNA has been cloned from a human embryonic lung fibroblast cDNA library;[39, 40] and both the murine and the human genes have been cloned and characterized.[41]

Although there are relatively few ligand-binding and second messenger studies of the B_1 receptor, it appears to be G-protein–coupled,[42] and its stimulation leads to inositol phosphate generation, transient increases in intracellular calcium, and activation of phospholipase C.[38, 39, 43] The amino acid sequence is 36% homologous with that of the B_2 receptor. The B_1 receptor is implicated in the chronic inflammatory and pain-producing responses to kinins,[44] but studies of the localization, regulation, and roles of B_1 receptors in human cells and tissues are still in early stages.[45] Such work is likely to be stimulated further by findings such as those of Bacharov and associates,[46] who found that there is a polymorphism in the putative promotor region of the human B_1 receptor gene, the prevalence of which is altered significantly in patients with renal failure and in some subgroups of uremic patients.

The B_2 receptors mediate most of the actions of kinins. Both the rodent and the human B_2 receptor genes have been cloned and expressed.[47, 48] The first rat B_2 receptor cDNA was obtained from a uterus library using *Xenopus* oocytes to assay for expression, based on bradykinin-induced ion currents.[47] The predicted protein sequence is 366 amino acids with a molecular weight of 41,696 Da and seven putative transmembrane domains. The sixth transmembrane domains of human B_1 and B_2 receptors are structurally related and contribute significantly to the ability of these receptors to distinguish between selective agonists for the subtypes.[49] Strong homology to the histamine H_2 receptor as well as to neurotensin and tachykinin receptors is evident. The potencies of bradykinin and lys-bradykinin are equal (EC_{50}, approximately 1.9 to 2.9 nmol/L), insofar as ion current responses and B_1 receptor agonists have no effect. Receptor message is widely distributed, with expression in heart, lung, brain, and testes being generally equivalent and somewhat less than in uterus.[47]

An effort to knock out the B_2 receptor has been successful[48] and has provided a valuable mouse model with which to study the roles of kinins acting via this receptor. In one of the first studies, Alfie and coworkers[50] showed that these mutant mice displayed a significantly higher blood pressure, reduced renal blood flow, and increased renal vascular resistance when maintained on a high Na^+ intake for 8 weeks, compared with knockout animals ingesting a normal Na^+ intake. Control mice showed no blood pressure differences but had a tendency to increased renal blood flow and reduced renal vascular resistance with high Na^+ intake. A subsequent study showed that these B_2 receptor knockout mice are more susceptible to myocardial ischemia or reperfusion injury (as are the Brown Norway kininogen-deficient rats)[51] providing additional evidence for the participation of an intact kininogen-kallikrein-kinin system in renal or cardiovascular homeostatic responses, at least in mice and rats.

Genomic DNA and cDNA encoding the human B_2 receptor have been isolated and the predicted amino acid sequence from each is 81% homologous to the rat smooth muscle B_2 receptor.[48, 52] Human B_2 receptor density is highest in kidney and also detectable in heart, lung, brain, uterus, and testes. The structural characterization of these receptors will be helpful for discerning kinin roles and for designing receptor antagonists or agonists for possible therapeutic use.[53, 54]

A rapidly increasing number of studies are appearing that examine the regulation of these receptors, the results of their activation after ligand binding, and their behavior in pathological circumstances.[55-62] Among the most notable is a study that shows that bradykinin can enhance exocytosis of norepinephrine from guinea pig heart sympathetic nerve endings (synaptosomes) and that the effect can be blocked by a B_2, but not B_1 receptor antagonist.[61] An ACE (kininase II) inhibitor, kininogen, or kallikrein also enhanced the release of norepinephrine from these cardiac nerve endings. This finding may have very significant implications for the possible local role of the cardiac kallikrein-kinin system in myocardial ischemic states and other pathological conditions.

Another new insight comes from recent studies by Minshall and colleagues[62] who used Chinese hamster ovary cells stably transfected with the human B_2 receptor alone or in combination with human ACE. These studies established that kinin potentiation produced by an ACE inhibitor is not simply due to inhibition of kinin breakdown, but that ACE inhibitors increased the total number of kinin-binding sites, preserved the high-affinity B_2 receptor, slowed down receptor endocytosis, and abolished receptor desensitization by ligand. These findings suggest that there is "crosstalk" between ACE and the B_2 receptor, and raise many interesting questions about the roles of both in the vascular wall and elsewhere.

A third bradykinin receptor (B_3) may exist in bovine aortic endothelial cells, the microvasculature of the guinea pig hindbrain, and cultured guinea pig tracheal smooth muscle cells.[63, 64] At these sites, variant responses to B_1 or B_2 agonists and antagonists suggest a possible interaction with another receptor. The tracheal cells appear to activate phospholipase D in response to bradykinin, and this response is not affected by either B_1 or B_2 receptor antagonists. Definitive proof awaits further cloning efforts and the development of additional receptor antagonists.

Kininases

The true half-life of kinins in biological fluids is a function of their rate of destruction. Peptidases that hydrolyze kinins are known as *kininases*, although none is known to be specific for kinins. Both aminopeptidases and carboxypeptidases can terminate biological activity, but the latter clearly predominate. The contributions of the various enzymes to kinin destruction have been studied extensively. In general, the dipeptidase kininase II (ACE) appears to be the most important within the cardiovascular system or kidney. In rat urine, another dipeptidase, neutral endopeptidase 24.11, is the major kinin-destroying enzyme.[65] Two additional carboxypeptidases, called M and N—the former concentrated in membrane fractions of various human tissues such as kidney, lung, endothelial cells, and fibroblasts and the latter in plasma and liver—are efficient kininases, cleaving the C-terminal arginine of kinins. All four of these human kininase genes have been cloned and the protein sequences established. However, it is important to note that the time sequence and extent of their contributions to the destruction of endogenous kinin are not clear. As noted by Erdös[66] the wide distribution and high affinity of carboxypeptidase M for the C-terminal arginine of kinins could suggest a ready source of substrate for the endothelial synthesis of nitric oxide.[67] This hypothesis has not been tested.

All therapeutic effects of ACE inhibitors were originally considered to result from inhibition of angiotensin II formation. It is now clear that retardation of kinin destruction (and perhaps attenuation of other enzyme actions[62]) likely plays a role in both their efficacy and their toxicity. For example, the ability of these inhibitors to reduce myocardial infarct size or attenuate postischemic reperfusion injury was shown to be abolished by blockade of kinin B_2 receptors with icatibant (HOE 140).[68] Such data, along with the corroborating plasma kinin level changes, suggest that locally produced kinins, at least in cardiac tissue, contribute to the beneficial effects of ACE inhibitors.

Controversy and uncertainty about the extent of kinin contributions to cardiovascular homeostasis persist. A case report illustrates the therapeutic rationale for more aggressive examination of this issue. Davidson and associates[69] note that anaphylactoid reactions have been described in adults undergoing low-density lipoprotein apheresis while taking ACE inhibitors. They reported a 13-year-old child with homozygous familial hypercholesterolemia and progressive ischemic cardiomyopathy who was treated with captopril who developed severe headaches, nausea, vomiting, and profound hypotension within 3 minutes of reinfusion of the cleared plasma. These adverse effects occurred even when the captopril was discontinued 72 hours before apheresis. Icatibant infused for 1 hour (200 μg/kg) before treatment and then during plasma reinfusion (100 μg/kg/h) completely prevented all symptoms and hypotension in five subsequent treatments, with captopril discontinued only 12 hours before treatment. Although the observation requires the additional support of further clinical (and/or animal) study, including measurement of the kinin level of the cleared, reinfused plasma, it reflects the pathophysiological potential of kinins, which has been generally unappreciated.

REGULATION OF THE KALLIKREIN-KININ SYSTEM

Relatively little information is currently available concerning the coordinate regulation of components of the kallikrein-kinin system in response to various biochemical, physiological, or pathological stimuli. However, such information is being gained at an increasing rate. HMW kininogen synthesis in cultured hepatocytes can be increased by glucocorticoids, and maternal estrogens are responsible for high circulating kininogen levels in neonatal rats.[22] Female rat liver kininogen mRNA levels are fourfold higher than in males. Estradiol increases, and progesterone decreases, liver kininogen mRNA, but both increase kallikrein mRNA in the kidneys of the same animals.

The assembly of components of the kallikrein-kinin system on endothelial cell surfaces and the subsequent activation of the system are dependent on heretofore unappreciated molecular interactions. For example, it was recently shown that prekallikrein activation on these cells depends on the presence of HMW kininogen, which regulates prekallikrein activation by a factor XI–dependent pathway not previously recognized.[70] More information is available about the regulation of tissue kallikrein, with renal kallikrein being the most studied. Female rat renal kallikrein mRNA is twice that of males. Various hormones including mineralocorticoids, glucocorticoids, testosterone, thyroxine, and insulin affect renal kallikrein mRNA and protein levels. Vasopressin, catecholamines, and angiotensin also affect the synthesis, activity, or release of renal kallikrein.

Thus, there is now ample opportunity to examine coordinate alterations in substrate and formative enzyme gene expression, processing, and storage or release in relation to pharmacologically induced or pathological changes in or-

gan function. This conclusion is reinforced by studies of renal kinin receptors. The first of these studies[55, 71] showed that after prolonged low sodium intake, B₂ binding site density was markedly reduced concomitant with increased renal and urinary kallikrein. This suggests that there is an inverse relation between presumptive renal kinin levels and B₂ receptor density. Subsequent studies have found that components of the renal kinin system are expressed in new sites,[72, 73] participate in heretofore unappreciated renal functions,[74–77] and are abnormal in renal disease.[78] New technology that is allowing the direct measurement of renal interstitial kinin (and other hormone) levels has shown that such levels change markedly in response to various stimuli (Fig. 20–3).[79]

INTERRELATIONS WITH OTHER REGULATORY HORMONES AND AUTACOIDS

It is clear that ACE efficiently catabolizes kinins. It has also been suggested that kallikrein can serve as a prorenin activating enzyme and that tissue kallikrein can function in an alternative pathway for the formation of angiotensin II. No definitive evidence for the latter roles exists in vivo. Nevertheless, the two systems appear likely to function in concert, at least in the kidney and the renal vasculature, to maintain blood flow and excretory capability. That is, diets low in sodium (or high in potassium) or other systemic challenges (e.g., water deprivation) stimulate renin gene expression and synthesis and concomitantly increase levels of angiotensin and aldosterone in defense of systemic and renal circulatory homeostasis, and at the same time increase renal kallikrein and kinin production in a local defense of

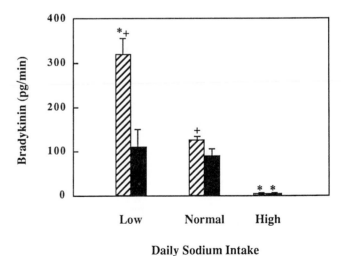

Figure 20–3. Bar graph shows renal interstitial fluid bradykinin concentration in anesthetized rats consuming a low- (0.15%), a normal (0.28%), or a high- (4.0%) sodium diet (*n* = 5 for each diet). *Hatched bars,* renal cortex; *solid bars,* renal medulla. *$p < .01$ compared with the normal diet; ⁺$p < .01$ compared with the corresponding medulla. (Modified from Siragy HM, Ibrahim MM, Jaffa AA, et al. Rat renal interstitial bradykinin, prostaglandin E₂ and cyclic guanosine 3′,5′-monophosphate: Effect of altered sodium intake. Hypertension 23:1068–1070, 1994.)

renal blood flow and glomerular filtration rate. The latter goal is accomplished by dilatation of renal cortical blood vessels, particularly afferent arterioles.

Recent evidence indicates clearly that the ACE inhibitor–induced increase in intrarenal blood flow is markedly attenuated by bradykinin B_2 receptor blockade.[80] In addition, the B_2 receptor antagonist, icatibant (HOE 140) was capable of correcting the sodium retention and reducing the levels of renin-angiotensin system activity in rats with carbon tetrachloride–induced liver cirrhosis, while also reducing the enhanced microvascular leakage seen in this model.[81] Thus, it is becoming increasingly clear that there is concerted activity between the two systems at various vascular, and probably cardiac, sites where component gene expression and receptors exist. An interesting example of this comes from a recent study that clearly showed that bradykinin prevented angiotensin II–induced hypertrophy of cardiomyocytes cocultured with endothelial cells, whereas the kinin was a hypertrophic agonist in cardiomyocytes grown alone.[82]

The reasons for the directionally opposite alterations in kallikrein-kinin and renin-angiotensin system activity, such as occur in the two-kidney, one-clip rat (with high renin and angiotensin II levels but lowered renal kallikrein), are not clearly understood. It has been suggested that the change in renal kallikrein (among the earliest observed in the kidney enzyme) in this model may be a secondary response to a more important interstitial kinin or kinin receptor change[55]—especially in the nonclipped kidney. These alterations would promote a compensatory excretory response to the contralateral insult (i.e., clipping). The availability of selective B_2 receptor antagonists and animal models with perturbed kallikrein-kinin systems (e.g., the Brown Norway rat, a mouse strain with a disrupted B_2 receptor gene[83]) will help unravel the related roles of these intertwined systems, especially in relation to vascular function in conditions such as diabetes mellitus and hypertension.

Relationships between the kallikrein-kinin system and other regulatory hormones are being uncovered at a remarkable rate. Tissue kallikrein is capable of forming atrial natriuretic peptide (ANP) from its precursors as well as catabolizing the active peptide in vitro.[84, 85] Administration of this powerful natriuretic, diuretic agent affects renal kallikrein excretion, but the significance of this effect is unclear.[86] Conversely, cardiac tissue contains a kallikrein-like enzyme that colocalizes in ANP-containing granules.[87] There also appears to be ANP synthesis in and secretion from renal cortical connecting tubule cells of the mouse and rat that also synthesize kallikrein.[88] ANP receptors, activation of which modulate renal sodium reabsorption, exist downstream in the inner medullary collecting ducts. Thus, local synthesis of ANP and kinin production appear to coexist in the same areas of the nephron. It is clear that kinins affect medullary collecting duct function,[89] but exploration of interrelations between ANP and kinin production and responsiveness at this site remains to be carried out.

Many studies have shown connections between kinins and eicosanoid synthesis,[1] but few have established a causal connection between abnormalities in components of both systems and resultant pathophysiology. The same can be said for nitric oxide, another mediator strongly implicated in kinin-induced vasodilatation and hypotension.[90] In the renal vasculature of rat and dog, kinin-induced vasodilatation depends on nitric oxide synthesis.[91] Thus, there may be a relationship between local kinin production at sites of vascular injury, acute or chronic, and nitric oxide production. This relationship is of great interest, in part because there is renal vascular hyperresponsiveness to bradykinin in the SHR, and this appears to be mediated by both nitric oxide–dependent and –independent mechanisms.[91] A full understanding of these connections might lead to new therapeutic strategies, as in the recent demonstration that suppression of epinephrine-induced arrythmias by bradykinin is a result of a kinin B_2 receptor–mediated mechanism involving the release of both nitric oxide and eicosanoids.[92]

The kallikrein-kinin system also interacts with a variety of autacoids. For example, kinins have long been known to augment blood flow through skeletal muscle and participate in skeletal muscle metabolism. Recent work has shown that bradykinin stimulates directly the translocation of GLUT4, a glucose transporter protein, from an intracellular pool to the plasma membrane of various cells, including L6 myotubules, adipocytes, and Chinese hamster ovary cells, expressing both kinin receptors and the GLUT4 transporter.[93] This may indicate that bradykinin is a local hormone responsible for exercise-stimulated glucose transport into skeletal muscle, as it is known that bradykinin is released from skeletal muscle cells during exercise.[94] Several other studies have suggested that kinins acting via B_2 receptors can stimulate norepinephrine release from either sympathetic neurons in primary cell culture or cardiac sympathetic neurons in isolated atria or whole heart.[95–97]

Finally, kinins have very interesting effects on the growth and/or mobility of various cells, most notably, vascular smooth muscle cells, mesangial cells, and fibroblasts.[98–100] The full evaluation of these effects and the determination of their physiological and pathophysiological significance are exciting areas of study.

KALLIKREINS, KININS, AND PHYSIOLOGICAL FUNCTIONS

Speculations about the roles of kallikreins and kinins in hemodynamic, excretory, and metabolic processes originated in 1909 when the hypotensive property of human urine, now known to represent excreted renal kallikrein, was discovered.[101] But insights into physiological roles were slow to appear. Study of the system was not stimulated even after two discoveries (1) of a clear reduction in kallikrein excretion in human hypertension in 1934,[102] and, (2) in the same decade, that "the average kallikrein excretion of diabetics agrees with that of healthy persons when they are treated with insulin. The situation was different in diabetics who received only a diabetic diet and no insulin: in middle-aged persons the daily excretion was then between 20 and 48 kallikrein units and hence was greatly reduced."[103] These valid clinical observations, received no attention for almost 40 years.

Some of the earliest definitive studies of kinin effects on any organ were carried out by Webster and Gilmore[104] and Gill and coworkers.[105] They established the natriuretic and diuretic capabilities of kinin in dogs and humans. This was followed by work showing that stimulation of water and electrolyte excretion was a function of increased renal blood flow. Indeed, the most consistently observed effect of kinins is to reduce vascular resistance. Unlike several other endogenous vasodilators, bradykinin can increase renal blood flow without significant changes in glomerular filtration rate or absolute proximal reabsorption but with a marked increase in fluid delivery to the distal nephron.[106] The latter effect may contribute to the increased urine volume and sodium excretion seen when exogenous kinin is administered into kidneys. It appears that natriuresis and diuresis are the result of an effect of kinins on renal papillary blood flow, which inhibits sodium reabsorption distally secondary to a washout of the medullary solute gradient, rather than on cortical blood flow, or as mentioned previously, glomerular filtration rate.[107] Support for this contention is derived from several studies using either inhibitors of renal kininases such as captopril and phosphoramidon (the latter an inhibitor of neutral endopeptidase 24.11) or long-term treatment with deoxycorticosterone, also known to raise endogenous kinin levels, followed by specific blockers of renal kinin B_2 receptors. These studies indicate that increases in papillary blood flow, urine volume, and sodium excretion induced by kininase inhibition or deoxycorticosterone can be either attenuated or abolished by kinin B_2 receptor blockade.[108]

Endogenous kinins clearly affect renal hemodynamics and excretory function. This conclusion is supported by studies of renal function in kininogen-deficient Brown Norway Katholiek rats, which show a brisk hypertensive response to a 2% NaCl diet seemingly unrelated to sodium and fluid retention.[109] Repetition of these studies in bradykinin B_2 receptor knockout mice, noted previously,[50, 51] has provided more definitive data supporting the conclusion that kinins can play an important role in preventing salt-sensitive hypertension. What is still uncertain is whether the observed natriuretic and diuretic responses are all a result of effects on renal hemodynamics in the papilla or might include a component of distal tubular inhibition of electrolyte reabsorption (or stimulation of electrolyte secretion). Some additional evidence in this regard is now available.[89] The weight of present evidence suggests that intrarenal kinins modulate renal excretory function predominantly by effects on the renal vasculature. Comparably detailed studies of tissue kallikrein-kinin system roles in the vascular beds of skeletal or cardiac muscle or in the splanchnic circulation are now appearing. Many questions are being asked about these roles in relation to organ developmental biology and blood flow regulation in physiological circumstances and specific pathological disorders.[59, 76, 110–114]

Kinin B_2 receptors are coupled to cellular systems in polarized epithelia that regulate vectorial ion and water transport.[115, 116] Many epithelia secrete anions, predominantly chloride but also bicarbonate, in voltage-clamp experiments in response to kinin; these actions are partially eicosanoid-dependent and can be blocked by Na^+-K^+-Cl^- cotransport inhibitors. However, the actions of locally generated kinins on ion, water, and substrate transport are still incompletely defined. The use of more specific system modulators such as receptor antagonists[89] or animals sub-

ject to transgenic or homologous recombination manipulations will shed light on issues of this kind.

Similarly, understanding the roles of kinins in glucose transport and metabolism requires more intensive evaluation now that extensive kallikrein-kinin system abnormalities have been identified in humans and animal models of diabetes mellitus.[117–120]

KALLIKREIN-KININ SYSTEM FUNCTION IN SYSTEMIC DISEASES

Hypertension

The notion that reduced urinary kallikrein excretion might represent a deficiency in an endogenous vasodilator system that was contributory to the hypertensive state was not enthusiastically accepted when first proposed.[102] Progress in addressing this possibility has been slow, unlike the enormous and sustained interest in the renin-angiotensin system provoked by the Goldblatt experiment. Interest in kallikrein-kinin contributions to the pathogenesis of human hypertension is now growing rapidly because of a series of provocative findings ranging from epidemiological surveys to gene-polymorphism-cosegregation analyses and studies in transgenic animals.[50, 121] Nevertheless, the case for kallikrein-kinin system involvement is still weaker than that for vasoconstrictor influences in human hypertension.

Although it is clear that patients with essential hypertension excrete less kallikrein than do normotensive subjects, there has been much overlap between groups in the population studies carried out since the early 1970s.[122] Many hypertensive subjects have normal kallikrein excretion. Black people, adults and children, excrete markedly less kallikrein than whites, regardless of blood pressure, with black hypertensive subjects generally showing the lowest measured levels.[123, 124] In recent years, studies of kallikrein and other system components in some more homogeneous human populations have begun to appear. For example, Japanese patients with low-renin hypertension show significant reductions in both active urinary kallikrein and kinin excretion.[125] They also demonstrate higher levels of a kallikrein inhibitor in urine, reduced urinary kininogen, and increased urinary kininases.[125]

Gainer and colleagues,[126] found that the wheal response to intradermal injection of bradykinin was significantly larger in African Americans than in whites. The former are known to be at increased risk of angioedema in response to ACE inhibitors, and this supersensitivity to bradykinin, along with the earlier indications of reduced tissue kallikrein levels, point to the notion of reduced kallikrein-kinin system activity playing some role in the increased incidence of hypertension in this population. On the other hand, Vajo and associates[127] failed to observe any difference in bradykinin-induced venodilatation between young, normotensive blacks and whites. Studies such as these provide a rationale and stimulus for examination of other components of the system (e.g., receptor expression, substrate or inhibitor levels, and genotypes) in relation to phenotypic characteristics of hypertensive populations.[128]

Epidemiological surveys in children stimulated interest in relationships between renal kallikrein and blood pressure.[123, 129] These efforts examined blood pressure, kallikrein, and other variables repetitively over long intervals and showed that kallikrein excretion was familially aggregated and that families of healthy children with the lowest mean kallikrein excretions showed significantly higher blood pressures than did families of children with the highest kallikrein excretions. These efforts have been extended in recent years. For example, urinary kallikrein and diastolic blood pressure are negatively correlated even in newborn infants 2 to 4 days old, and such correlations are detectable in infants up to 18 months of age.[130] Berry and coworkers[131] examined family histories of hypertension in a large population in 57 Utah pedigrees and found that individuals with a higher urinary kallikrein excretion genotype were less likely to have one or two hypertensive parents than those with a low kallikrein genotype, suggesting that the higher excretion rate genotype is associated with a reduced risk of essential hypertension. Such studies require extension and confirmation; that is, kallikrein was measured in these efforts because it became easy to measure,[132] not because it was the most likely component of the kallikrein-kinin system to demonstrate association. The most recent assessment of kallikrein gene mutations and their relevance to blood pressure regulation and cardiac disease failed to find consistent associations with either blood pressure level or myocardial infarction risk.[128] Efforts are just beginning to assess whether there might be better markers for kallikrein-kinin system abnormality in established cardiovascular disease or populations with varying levels of cardiovascular risk.

As might be expected, work in rodent or other animal forms of hypertension is proceeding more rapidly. Goldblatt hypertensive rats were the first animal models shown to have reduced urinary kallikrein excretion.[133, 134] The reduced levels occur principally in the compromised kidney of two-kidney, one-clip rats, and levels in the contralateral kidney are either normal or reduced to a lesser extent. These changes are now being studied in relation to the differential salt-handling properties of the two kidneys. Kinin B_2 receptor density, which is increased to a greater extent in the contralateral kidney than in the clipped one, is currently being examined in this model.[55] These increases could signify an augmented kinin-induced eicosanoid and/or nitric oxide production in compensatory response to the higher perfusion pressure that the contralateral kidney faces. Renal blood flow, glomerular filtration rate, and sodium excretion are greater in the contralateral than in the clipped kidney. Extensions of these studies will examine the cellular biochemical basis for the pathophysiological differences.

All genetic models of hypertension in the rat, including SHR, Dahl, Milan, New Zealand, Fawn-hooded, and Sabra strains, show kallikrein-kinin system abnormalities. However, relatively few studies have been carried out longitudinally with respect to age, and it has been generally unclear whether kallikrein-kinin system abnormalities preceded or followed the appearance of hypertension in these models. Even fewer studies have examined multiple components of the system over time. An early study in Milan rats showed significantly lower kallikrein levels in newborn pups of the hypertensive versus the control strain.[135] A more recent effort showed that renal tissue active kallikrein in SHRs

was only 53% of values in WKYs within 12 hours of birth, whereas the total enzyme level (including prokallikrein) was not different between strains.[136] The SHR-WKY difference persisted up to 12 weeks of age. This is the only evidence in a hypertensive model to suggest a possible defect in renal kallikrein synthesis rate.

A series of studies, most notably from the laboratory of El-Dahr and colleagues,[58, 59, 73, 76, 137, 138] but also from others,[74, 139] are establishing the rates of appearance and concentrations of various components of tissue kallikrein-kinin systems in the developing and maturing organs of rats and other animals. These important efforts will allow the subsequent comparisons of rates of kallikrein-kinin system development in various hypertensive strains and a determination of whether interdiction or facilitation of activity of components of the system will attenuate or possibly prevent the appearance of hypertension. Some efforts in this regard have begun and await independent confirmation.[140, 141]

More definitive connections between kinins and blood pressure regulation are appearing as long-term blockade of B_2 receptors with selective B_2 receptor antagonists in rats treated with deoxycorticosterone[142] has been shown to cause rises in blood pressure similar to those seen when kininogen-deficient Brown Norway Katholiek rats are stressed with a moderate salt intake.[109] The same increase in blood pressure after kinin B_2 receptor blockade has recently been demonstrated in SHRs in contrast to WKYs.[143] Further, chronic kinin B_2 receptor blockade in young Dahl salt-resistant rats attenuates their ability to resist a high-salt diet and blood pressure rises significantly (Fig. 20–4).[144]

Studies of kinin receptor behavior and signal transduction pathways in such models are now beginning, stimulated by these and other findings. A recent study showed that long-term blockade of kinin B_2 receptors in WKYs in both prenatal and postnatal periods resulted in significantly increased systolic blood pressure and heart rate, not to hypertensive levels but enough to suggest that endogenous kinins contribute to an "adult cardiovascular phenotype."[145] Exploration of the biochemical and cellular contributors to such phenotypes in animals and humans may provide important insights into the origins of the hypertensive diseases.

Diabetes Mellitus

The first modern study reaffirming a connection between the tissue kallikrein-kinin system and the diabetic state showed that rats with streptozotocin-induced diabetes mellitus developed significant hypertension along with altered renal kallikrein-kinin system activity.[117] Early in the course of the diabetic state, these rats, treated with insulin, show glomerular hyperfiltration along with increased synthesis, stores, and urinary excretion of renal kallikrein.[118, 119] Treatment of such rats with aprotinin or a kinin B_2 receptor antagonist reduced renal blood flow and glomerular filtration rate to levels equal to those in normal rats,[119] thus establishing a role for the kallikrein-kinin system in the renal response to the diabetic state. Similarly, patients with type 1 diabetes who had glomerular hyperfiltration showed

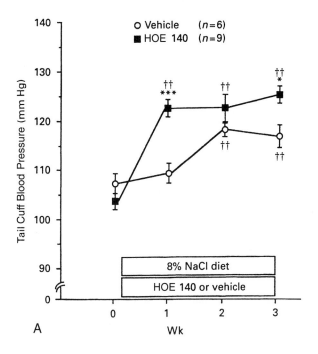

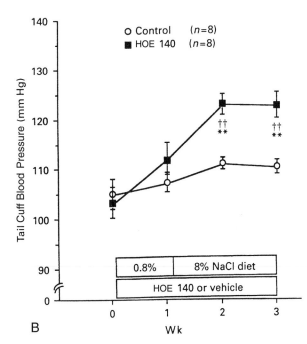

greater active kallikrein and prostaglandin E_2 excretion than patients with normal glomerular filtration rate or otherwise healthy subjects.[120] Kallikrein levels correlated directly with glomerular filtration rate and distal tubular sodium reabsorption (derived from lithium clearance). These findings in diabetic rat models and patients show that the renal kallikrein-kinin system is a contributor to the renal adaptation to diabetes and plays a role in the nephropathy. Effects of kinins on vascular proliferative responses (or inhibition of such) are preludes to an intensive examination of the role of the kallikrein-kinin system in the pathology of the human hypertensive, cardiac, and diabetic diseases.[51, 82, 98, 99, 113, 122, 146]

SUMMARY

Since the late 1960s, there have been profound advances in the understanding of the structure, localization, and regulation of components of the kallikrein-kinin system; abnormalities of this system in disease; regulation of components of the system; and most importantly, the discovery and application of specific receptor antagonists. The work summarized here has revealed enough about the contributions of the kallikrein-kinin system to cellular and organ function to allow optimism about the likelihood that new therapeutic strategies based on stimulation or interdiction of kinin actions will be important for the treatment and perhaps even the prevention of some common diseases, most notably the hypertensive disorders.

Figure 20–4. A. Systolic blood pressure of awake Dahl salt-resistant (SR/Jr) rats before and during a high (8%) NaCl diet with concomitant treatment (via osmotic minipumps) with 10 to 20 nmol d^{-1} HOE 140 or vehicle. The kinin B_2 receptor antagonist increased blood pressure after 1 week of an 8% NaCl diet. $\dagger\dagger p$ < .001 versus baseline cuff blood pressure; $**p$ < .001 versus vehicle-treated rats. **B.** Systolic blood pressure of awake Dahl salt-resistant (SR/Jr) rats fed a normal (0.8%) NaCl diet for 1 week and a high (8%) NaCl diet for 2 weeks. The rats were concomitantly treated with 20 to 40 nmol d^{-1} HOE 140 or vehicle during the 3 weeks of study. The kinin B_2 receptor antagonist increased blood pressure only after the rats were fed the high NaCl diet. $\dagger\dagger p$ < .001 versus baseline cuff blood pressure; $**p$ < .001 versus control rats. (**A** and **B,** From Mukai H, Fitzgibbon WR, Ploth DW, Margolius HS. Effect of chronic bradykinin B_2 receptor blockade on blood pressure of conscious Dahl salt-resistant rats. Br J Pharmacol 124:197–205, 1998.)

References

1. Bhoola KD, Figueroa CD, Worthy K. Bioregulation of kinins: Kallikreins, kininogens and kininases. Pharmacol Rev 44:1–80, 1992.
2. Regoli D, Calo G, Rizzi A, et al. Bradykinin receptors and receptor ligands (with special emphasis on vascular receptors). Regul Pept 65:83–89, 1996.
3. Stewart JM. Bradykinin antagonists: Development and applications. Biopolymers (Peptide Sci) 37:143–155, 1995.
4. Linz W, Wiemer G, Gohlke P, et al. Contribution of kinins to the cardiovascular actions of angiotensin-converting enzyme inhibitors. Pharmacol Rev 47:25–49, 1995.
5. Margolius HS. Kallikreins and kinins. Some unanswered questions about system characteristics and roles in human disease. Hypertension 26:221–229, 1995.
6. Katori M, Majima M. Pivotal role of renal kallikrein-kinin system in the development of hypertension and approaches to new drugs based upon this relationship. Jpn J Pharmacol 70:95–128, 1996.
7. Fong D, Smith DI, Hsieh W-T. The human kininogen gene (KNG) mapped to chromosome 3q26->qter by analysis of somatic cell hybrids using the polymerase chain reaction. Hum Genet 87:189–192, 1991.
8. Cheung PP, Cannizzaro LA, Coleman RW. Chromosomal mapping of human kininogen gene (KNG) to 3q26->qter. Cytogenet Cell Genet 59:24–26, 1992.
9. Kitamura N, Kitagawa H, Fukushima D, et al. Structural organization of the human kininogen gene and a model for its evolution. J Biol Chem 260:8610–8617, 1985.
10. Muller-Esterl W, Iwanaga S, Nakanishi S. Kininogens revisited. Trends Biochem Sci 11:336–339, 1986.
11. Chen L-M, Chung P, Chao S, et al. Differential regulation of kininogen gene expression by estrogen and progesterone in vivo. Biochim Biophys Acta 1131:145–151, 1992.
12. Chen H-M, Liao WSL. Differential acute-phase response of rat kininogen genes involves type I and type II interleukin-6 response elements. J Biol Chem 268:25311–25319, 1993.

13. Chen H-M, Liao WSL. Molecular analysis of the differential hepatic expression of rat kininogen family genes. Mol Cell Biol 13:6766–6777, 1993.

14. Cheung PP, Kunapuli SP, Scott CF, et al. Genetic basis of total kininogen deficiency in Williams' trait. J Biol Chem 268:23361–23365, 1993.

15. Tayeh MA, Olson ST, Shore JD. Surface-induced alterations in the kinetic pathway for cleavage of human high molecular weight kininogen by plasma kallikrein. J Biol Chem 269:16318–16325, 1994.

16. Weisel JW, Nagasawami C, Woodhead JL, et al. The shape of high molecular weight kininogen. J Biol Chem 269:10100–10106, 1994.

17. Hasan AAK, Cines DB, Zhang J, et al. The carboxyl terminus of bradykinin and amino terminus of the light chain of kininogens comprise an endothelial cell binding domain. J Biol Chem 269:31822–31830, 1994.

18. Hasan AAK, Cines DB, Herwald H, et al. Mapping the cell binding site on high molecular weight kininogen domain 5. J Biol Chem 271:19256–19261, 1995.

19. Colman RW, Schmaier AH. Contact system: A vascular biology modulator with anticoagulant, profibrinolytic, antiadhesive, and pro-inflammatory attributes. Blood 90:3819–3843, 1997.

20. Lattion AL, Baussant T, Ahlenc-Gelas F, et al. The high-molecular mass kininogen deficient rat expresses all kininogen mRNA species, but does not export the high-molecular mass kininogen synthesized. FEBS Lett 239:59–64, 1988.

21. Majima M, Katori M. Approaches to the development of novel antihypertensive drugs: Crucial role of the renal kallikrein-kinin system. Trends Pharmacol Sci 16:239–246, 1995.

22. Nakanishi S. Substance P precursor and kininogen: Their structures, gene organizations, and regulation. Pharmacol Rev 67:1117–1142, 1987.

23. Schmaier AH, Kuo A, Lundberg D, et al. The expression of high-molecular-weight kininogen on human umbilical vein endothelial cells. J Biol Chem 263:16327–16333, 1988.

24. Oza NB, Schwartz JH, Goud HD, et al. Rat aortic smooth muscle cells in culture express kallikrein, kininogen, and bradykininase activity. J Clin Invest 85:597–600, 1990.

25. Zini JM, Schmaier AH, Cines DB. Bradykinin regulates the expression of kininogen binding sites on endothelial cells. Blood 81:2936–2946, 1993.

26. Herwald H, Dedio J, Kellner R, et al. Isolation and characterization of the kininogen-binding protein p33 from endothelial cells. Identity with the gC1q receptor. J Biol Chem 271:13040–13047, 1996.

27. Joseph K, Ghebrehiwet B, Peerschke EIB, et al. Identification of the zinc-dependent endothelial cell binding protein for high molecular weight kininogen and factor XII: Identity with the receptor that binds to the globular "heads" of C1q (gC1q-R). Proc Natl Acad Sci U S A 93:8552–8557, 1996.

28. Colman RW, Pixley RA, Najamunnisa S, et al. Binding of high molecular weight kininogen to human endothelial cells is mediated via a site within domains 2 and 3 of the urokinase receptor. J Clin Invest 100:1481–1487, 1997.

29. Hasan AAK, Zisman T, Schmaier AH. Identification of cytokeratin 1 as a binding protein and presentation receptor for kininogens on endothelial cells. Proc Natl Acad Sci U S A 95:3615–3620, 1998.

30. Lin Y, Harris RB, Yan W, et al. High molecular weight kininogen peptides inhibit the formation of kallikrein on endothelial cell surfaces and subsequent urokinase-dependent plasmin formation. Blood 90:690–697, 1997.

31. Hasan AAK, Zhang J, Samuel M, et al. Conformational changes in low molecular weight kininogen alters its ability to bind to endothelial cells. Thromb Hemost 74:1088–1095, 1995.

32. Nolly H, Carretero OA, Scicli AG. Kallikrein release by vascular tissue. Am J Physiol 265:H1209–H1214, 1993.

33. Wu H, Venezie RD, Cohen WM, et al. Identification of tissue kallikrein mRNA in human neutrophils. Agents Actions 38:27–31, 1993.

34. Zhou GX, Chao L, Chao J. Kallistatin: A novel human tissue kallikrein inhibitor. J Biol Chem 267:25873–25880, 1992.

35. Chao J, Chao L. A major difference of kallikrein-binding protein in spontaneously hypertensive versus normotensive rats. J Hypertens 6:551–557, 1988.

36. Herwald H, Collin M, Muller-Esterl W, et al. Streptococcal cysteine proteinase releases kinins: A novel virulence mechanism. J Exp Med 184:665–673, 1996.

37. Dragovic T, Igic R, Erdös EG, et al. Metabolism of bradykinin by peptidases in the lung. Am Rev Respir Dis 147:1491–1496, 1993.

38. Schneck KA, Hess JF, Stonesifer GY, et al. Bradykinin B_1 receptors in rabbit aorta smooth muscle cells in culture. Eur J Pharmacol 266:277–282, 1994.

39. Menke JG, Borkowski JA, Bierilo KK, et al. Expression cloning of a human B_1 bradykinin receptor. J Biol Chem 269:21583–21587, 1994.

40. Webb M, McIntyre P, Phillips E. B_1 and B_2 bradykinin receptors encoded by distinct mRNAs. J Neurochem 62:1247–1253, 1994.

41. Pesquero JB, Pesquero JL, Oliveira SM, et al. Molecular cloning and functional characterization of a mouse bradykinin B_1 receptor gene. Biochem Biophys Res Commun 220:219–225, 1996.

42. Marceau F, Larrivee J-F, Saint-Jacques E, et al. The kinin B_1 receptor: An inducible G protein coupled receptor. Can J Physiol Pharmacol 75:725–730, 1997.

43. Austin CE, Faussner A, Robinson HE, et al. Stable expression of the human kinin B_1 receptor in Chinese hamster ovary cells. J Biol Chem 272:11420–11425, 1997.

44. Dray A. Kinins and their receptors in hyperalgesia. Can J Physiol Pharmacol 75:704–712, 1997.

45. Wohlfart P, Dedio J, Wirth K, et al. Different B_1 kinin receptor expression and pharmacology in endothelial cells of different origins and species. J Pharmacol Exp Ther 280:1109–1116, 1997.

46. Bacharov DR, Landry M, Pelletier I, et al. Characterization of two polymorphic sites in the human kinin B_1 receptor gene: Altered frequency of an allele in patients with a history of end-stage renal failure. J Am Soc Nephrol 9:598–604, 1998.

47. McEachern AE, Shelton ER, Bhakta S, et al. Expression cloning of a rat B_2 bradykinin receptor. Proc Natl Acad Sci U S A 88:7724–7728, 1991.

48. Borkowski JA, Ransom RW, Seabrook GR, et al. Targeted disruption of a B_2 bradykinin receptor gene in mice eliminates bradykinin action in smooth muscle and neurons. J Biol Chem 270:13706–13710, 1995.

49. Leeb T, Mathis SA, Leeb-Lundberg LMF: The sixth transmembrane domains of the human B_1 and B_2 bradykinin receptors are structurally compatible and involved in discriminating between subtype-selective agonists. J Biol Chem 272:311–317, 1997.

50. Alfie ME, Sigmon DH, Pomposiello SI, et al. Effect of high salt intake in mutant mice lacking bradykinin-B_2 receptors. Hypertension 29:483–487, 1997.

51. Yang X-P, Liu Y-H, Scicli GM, et al. Role of kinins in the cardioprotective effect of preconditioning. Study of myocardial ischemia/reperfusion injury in B_2 kinin receptor knock out mice and kininogen-deficient rats. Hypertension 30:735–740, 1997.

52. Eggerickx D, Raspe E, Bertrand D, et al. Molecular cloning, functional expression and pharmacological characterization of a human bradykinin B_2 receptor gene. Biochem Biophys Res Commun 187:1306–1313, 1992.

53. Nardone J, Hogan PG. Delineation of a region in the B_2 receptor that is essential for high-affinity agonist binding. Proc Natl Acad Sci U S A 91:4417–4421, 1994.

54. Pesquero JB, Lindsay CJ, Zeh K, et al. Molecular structure and expression of rat bradykinin B_2 receptor gene. J Biol Chem 269:26920–26925, 1994.

55. Edmond J, Bascands J-L, Rakotoarivony J, et al. Glomerular B_2 kinin-binding sites in two-kidney, one-clip hypertensive rats. Am J Physiol 260:F626–F634, 1991.

56. Hamm-Alvarez SF, Alayof BE, Himmel HM, et al. Coordinate depression of bradykinin receptor recycling and microtubule-dependent transport by taxol. Proc Natl Acad Sci U S A 85:8664–8667, 1988.

57. Tippmer S, Quitterer U, Kolm V, et al. Bradykinin induces translocation of the protein kinase C isoforms alpha, epsilon, and zeta. Eur J Biochem 229:297–304, 1994.

58. El-Dahr SS, Dipp S, Yosipiv IV, et al. Bradykinin stimulates c-fos expression, AP-1-DNA binding activity and proliferation of rat glomerular mesangial cells. Kidney Int 50:1850–1855, 1996.

59. El-Dahr SS, Yosipiv IV, Muchant DG, et al. Salt intake modulates the developmental expression of renal kallikrein and bradykinin B_2 receptors. Am J Physiol 270:F425–F431, 1996.

60. Jaffa AA, Miller BS, Rosenzweig SA, et al. Bradykinin induces tubulin phosphorylation and nuclear translocation of MAP kinase in mesangial cells. Am J Physiol 273:F916–F924, 1997.

61. Seyedi N, Win T, Lander HM, et al. Bradykinin B$_2$-receptor activation augments norepinephrine exocytosis from cardiac sympathetic nerve endings. Mediation by autocrine/paracrine mechanisms. Circ Res 81:774–784, 1997.

62. Minshall RD, Tan F, Nakamura F, et al. Potentiation of the actions of bradykinin by angiotensin-converting enzyme inhibitors. The role of expressed human bradykinin B$_2$ receptors and angiotensin-converting enzyme in CHO cells. Circ Res 81:848–856, 1997.

63. Burch RM, Kyle DJ, Stormann TM. Molecular Biology and Pharmacology of Bradykinin Receptors. Molecular Biology Intelligence Unit. Austin, TX, RG Landes, 1993; pp 1–107.

64. Pyne S, Pyne NJ. Differential effects of B$_2$ receptor antagonists upon bradykinin-stimulated phospholipase C and D in guinea-pig cultured tracheal smooth muscle. Br J Pharmacol 110:477–481, 1993.

65. Ura N, Carretero OA, Erdös EG, et al. Role of renal endopeptidase 24.11 in kinin metabolism in vitro and in vivo. Kidney Int 32:507–513, 1987.

66. Erdös EG. Some old and new ideas on kinin metabolism. J Cardiovasc Pharmacol 15(suppl 6):S20–S24, 1990.

67. Sakuma I, Stuehr DJ, Gross SS, et al. Identification of arginine as a precursor of endothelium-derived relaxing factor. Proc Natl Acad Sci U S A 85:8664–8667, 1988.

68. Linz W, Schölkens BA. Role of bradykinin in the cardiac effects of angiotensin-converting enzyme inhibitors. J Cardiovasc Pharmacol 20(suppl 9):583–590, 1992.

69. Davidson DC, Peart I, Turner S, et al. Prevention with icatibant of anaphylactoid reactions to ACE inhibitor during LDL apheresis. Lancet 343:1575, 1994.

70. Motta G, Rojkjaer R Hasan AAK, et al. High molecular weight kininogen regulates prekallikrein assembly and activation on endothelial cells: A novel mechanism for contact activation. Blood 91:516–528, 1998.

71. Bascands J-L, Pecher C, Ronaud S, et al. Evidence for the existence of two distinct bradykinin receptors on rat mesangial cells. Am J Physiol 264:F548–F556, 1993.

72. Ardaillou N, Blaise V, Costenbader K, et al. Characterization of a B$_2$-bradykinin receptor in human glomerular podocytes. Am J Physiol 271:F754–F761, 1996.

73. El-Dahr SS, Figueroa CD, Gonzalez CB, et al. Ontogeny of bradykinin B$_2$ receptors in the rat kidney: Implication for segmental nephron maturation. Kidney Int 51:739–749, 1997.

74. Toth-Heyn P, Guignard J-P. Endogenous bradykinin regulates renal function in the newborn rabbit. Biol Neonate 73:330–336, 1998.

75. Grider J, Falcone J, Kilpatrick E, et al. Effect of bradykinin on NaCl transport in the medullary thick ascending limb of the rat. Eur J Pharmacol 287:101–104, 1995.

76. El-Dahr SS, Yosipiv IV, Lewis L, et al. Role of bradykinin B$_2$ receptors in the developmental changes of renal hemodynamics in the neonatal rat. Am J Physiol 269:F786–F792, 1995.

77. Valles P, Ebner S, Manucha W, et al. Effect of glandular kallikrein on distal nephron HCO$_3^-$ secretion in MDCK cells. Am J Physiol 273:F807–F816, 1997.

78. Ouardani M, Travo P, Rakotoarivony J, et al. Decrease of bradykinin-induced glomerular contraction in diabetic rat: A new cellular interpretation. Eur J Cell Biol 73:232–239, 1997.

79. Siragy HM, Ibrahim MM, Jaffa AA, et al. Rat renal interstitial bradykinin, prostaglandin E$_2$ and cyclic guanosine 3′, 5′-monophosphate: Effect of altered sodium intake. Hypertension 23:1068–1070, 1994.

80. Endlich K, Steinhausen M. Role of kinins and angiotensin II in the vasodilating action of angiotensin converting enzyme inhibition in rat renal vessels. J Hypertens 15:633–641, 1997.

81. Wirth KJ, Bickel M, Hropot M, et al. The bradykinin B$_2$ receptor antagonist icatibant (HOE140) corrects avid Na$^+$ retention in rats with CCl$_4$-induced liver cirrhosis: Possible role of enhanced microvascular leakage. Eur J Pharmacol 337:45–53, 1997.

82. Ritchie RH, Marsh JD, Lancaster WD, et al. Bradykinin blocks angiotensin II-induced hypertrophy in the presence of endothelial cells. Hypertension 31:39–44, 1998.

83. Madeddu P, Varoni MV, Palomba D, et al. Cardiovascular phenotype of a mouse strain with disruption of bradykinin B$_2$-receptor gene. Circulation 96:3570–3578, 1997.

84. Briggs J, Marin-Grez M, Steipe B, et al. Inactivation of atrial natriuretic substance by kallikrein. Am J Physiol 247:F480–F484, 1984.

85. Currie MG, Geller DM, Chao J, et al. Kallikrein activation of a high molecular weight atrial peptide. Biochem Biophys Res Commun 120:461–466, 1984.

86. Lopez C, Jimenez W, Arroyo V, et al. Effects of atrial natriuretic peptide on urinary kallikrein excretion and renal function in rats. Eur J Pharmacol 168:1–6, 1989.

87. Simson J, Currie M, Chao L, et al. Co-localization of a kallikrein-like serine protease (arginine esterase A) and atrial natriuretic peptide in rat atrium. J Histochem Cytochem 37:1913–1917, 1989.

88. Ritter D, Chao J, Needleman P, et al. Localization, synthetic regulation, and biology of renal atriopeptin-like hormone. Am J Physiol 263:F503–F509, 1992.

89. Mukai H, Fitzgibbon WR, Bozeman G, et al. Bradykinin B$_2$ receptor antagonist increases chloride and water reabsortion in rat medullary collecting duct. Am J Physiol 271:R352–R360, 1996.

90. Fulton D, McGiff J, Quilley J. Contribution of NO and cytochrome P450 to the vasodilator effect of bradykinin in the rat kidney. Br J Pharmacol 107:722–725, 1992.

91. Cachofeiro V, Nasjletti A. Increased vascular responsiveness to bradykinin in kidneys of spontaneously hypertensive rats: Effects of N^G-nitro-L-arginine. Hypertension 18:683–689, 1991.

92. Rajani V, Hussain Y, Bolla BS, et al. Attenuation of epinephrine-induced dysrhythmias by bradykinin: Role of nitric oxide and prostaglandins. Am J Cardiol 80:153A–157, 1997.

93. Kishi K, Muromoto N, Nakaya Y, et al. Bradykinin directly triggers GLUT4 translocation via an insulin-independent pathway. Diabetes 47:550–558, 1998.

94. Stebbins CL, Carretero OA, Mindroiu T, et al. Bradykinin release from contracting skeletal muscle of the cat. J Appl Physiol 69:1225–1230, 1990.

95. Foucart S, Grondin L, Couture R, et al. Modulation of noradrenaline release by B$_1$ and B$_2$ kinin receptors during metabolic anoxia in the rat isolated atria. Can J Physiol Pharmacol 75:639–645, 1997.

96. Kurz T, Tölg R, Richardt G. Bradykinin B$_2$-receptor–mediated stimulation of exocytotic noradrenaline release from cardiac sympathetic neurons. J Mol Cell Cardiol 29:2561–2569, 1997.

97. Boehm S, Huck S. Noradrenaline release from rat sympathetic neurones triggered by activation of B$_2$ bradykinin receptors. Br J Pharmacol 122:455–462, 1997.

98. Farhy RD, Ho K-L, Carretero OA, et al. Kinins mediate the antiproliferative effect of ramipril in rat carotid artery. Biochem Biophys Res Commun 182:283–288, 1992.

99. Farhy RD, Peterson E, Scicli AG. Kinins and the events influenced by an angiotensin-converting enzyme inhibitor during neointima formation in the rat carotid artery. J Hypertens 15:421–429, 1997.

100. McAllister BS, Leeb-Lundberg F, Mellonig JT, et al. The functional interaction of EGF and PDGF with bradykinin in the proliferation of human gingival fibroblasts. J Periodontol 66:429–437, 1995.

101. Abelous J, Bardier E. Les substances hypotensives de l'urine humaine normale. Compt Rendu Soc Biol 66:511–512, 1909.

102. Elliot AH, Nuzum FR. The urinary excretion of a depressor substance (kallikrein of Frey and Kraut) in arterial hypertension. Endocrinology 18:462–474, 1934.

103. Frey EK, Kraut H, Werle E. Occurrence and routes of kallikrein in the organism. In Kallikrein (Padutin). Stuttgart, Ferdinand Enke, 1950; pp 70–96. (Translation [Everhardy WH, trans.] provided at the National Institutes of Health, Bethesda, MD, 1958.)

104. Webster ME, Gilmore J. Influence of kallidin-10 on renal function. Am J Physiol 206:714–718, 1964.

105. Gill JR Jr, Melmon KL, Gillespie L Jr, et al. Bradykinin and renal function in normal man: Effects of adrenergic blockade. Am J Physiol 209:844–848, 1965.

106. Stein J, Congbalay R, Karsh D, et al. The effect of bradykinin on proximal tubular sodium reabsorption in the dog: Evidence for functional nephron heterogeneity. J Clin Invest 51:1709–1721, 1972.

107. Roman RJ, Kaldunski M, Scicli AG, et al. Influence of kinins and angiotensin II on the regulation of papillary blood flow. Am J Physiol 255:F690–F698, 1988.

108. Fenoy FJ, Roman RJ. Effect of kinin receptor antagonists on renal hemodynamic and natriuretic responses to volume expansion. Am J Physiol 263:R1136–R1140, 1992.

109. Majima M, Yoshida O, Mihara H, et al. High sensitivity to salt in kininogen-deficient Brown Norway Katholiek rats. Hypertension 22:705–714, 1993.

110. Wall TM, Sheehy R, Hartman JC. Role of bradykinin in myocardial preconditioning. J Pharmacol Exp Ther 270:681–689, 1994.

111. Christopher TA, Ma X-L, Gauthier TW, et al. Beneficial actions of CP-0127, a novel bradykinin receptor antagonist, in murine traumatic shock. Am J Physiol 35:H867–H873, 1994.

112. Trippodo NC, Panchal, BC, Fox M. Repression of angiotensin II and potentiation of bradykinin contribute to the synergistic effects of dual metalloprotease inhibition in heart failure. J Pharmacol Exp Ther 272:619–627, 1995.

113. Parratt JR, Vegh A, Zeitlin J, et al. Bradykinin and endothelial-cardiac myocyte interactions in ischemic preconditioning. Am J Cardiol 80:124A–131A, 1997.

114. Minshall RD, Erdös EG, Vogel SLM. Angiotensin I-converting enzyme inhibitors potentiate bradykinin's inotropic effects independently of blocking its inactivation. Am J Cardiol 80:132A–136A, 1997.

115. Cuthbert A, Margolius HS. Kinins stimulate net chloride secretion by the rat colon. Br J Pharmacol 75:587–589, 1982.

116. Baird AW, Margolius HS. Bradykinin stimulates electrogenic bicarbonate secretion by the guinea pig gallbladder. J Pharmacol Exp Ther 248:268–272, 1989.

117. Mayfield RK, Namm DH, Squires J, et al. Development of hypertension in rats made diabetic with streptozotocin is associated with decreased urinary kallikrein excretion. Diabetes 34:22–28, 1985.

118. Jaffa AA, Miller DH, Bailey GS, et al. Abnormal regulation of renal kallikrein in experimental diabetes and the effects of insulin on prokallikrein synthesis, activation and excretion. J Clin Invest 80:1651–1659, 1987.

119. Harvey JN, Jaffa AA, Margolius HS, Mayfield RK. Renal kallikrein and the hemodynamic abnormalities of the diabetic kidney. Diabetes 39:299–304, 1990.

120. Harvey JN, Edmundson AW, Jaffa AA, et al. Renal excretion of kallikrein and eicosanoids in patients with type I (insulin-dependent) diabetes mellitus: Relationship to glomerular and tubular function. Diabetologia 35:857–862, 1992.

121. Pravenec M, Kren V, Kunes J, et al. Cosegregation of blood pressure with a kallikrein gene family polymorphism. Hypertension 17:242–246, 1991.

122. Katori M, Majima M. Preventative role of renal kallikrein-kinin system in the early phase of hypertension and development of new antihypertensive drugs. Adv Pharmacol 44:147–224, 1998.

123. Zinner SH, Margolius HS, Rosner B, et al. Stability of blood pressure rank and urinary kallikrein concentration in childhood. Circulation 58:908–915, 1978.

124. Levy S, Lilley J, Frigon R, et al. Urinary kallikrein and plasma renin activity as determinants of renal blood flow: The influence of race and dietary sodium intake. J Clin Invest 60:129–138, 1977.

125. Nakahashi Y, Shimamoto K, Ura N, et al. Comprehensive studies on the renal kallikrein-kinin system in essential hypertension. In Greenbaum LM, Margolius HS (eds). Kinins IV. Part B. Adv Exp Med Biol 198B:351–357, 1986.

126. Gainer JV, Nadeau JH, Ryder D, et al. Increased sensitivity to bradykinin among African Americans. J Allergy Clin Immunol 98:283–287, 1996.

127. Vajo Z, McDonald M, Takahashi B, et al. Bradykinin-induced venodilation is not different in blacks. Br J Clin Pharmacol 44:285–288, 1997.

128. Berge KE, Bakken A, Bøhn M, et al. Analyses of mutations in the human renal kallikrein (hKLK1) gene and their possible relevance to blood pressure regulation and risk of myocardial infarction. Clin Genet 52:86–95, 1997.

129. Zinner SH, Margolius HS, Rosner B, et al. Familal aggregation of urinary kallikrein in childhood. Am J Epidemiol 104:124–132, 1976.

130. McGarvey ST, Zinner SH, Margolius HS. Urinary kallikrein and blood pressure in infants and children. In Iimura O, Margolius HS (eds). Renal Function Hypertension and Kallikrein-Kinin System. Tokyo, Hokusen-Sha, 1988; pp 161–168.

131. Berry TD, Hasstedt SJ, Hunt SC, et al. A gene for high urinary kallikrein may protect against hypertension in Utah kindreds. Hypertension 13:3–8, 1989.

132. Margolius HS, Horwitz D, Geller RG, et al. Urinary kallikrein in normal subjects: Relationships to sodium intake and sodium-retaining steroids. Circ Res 35:812–819, 1974.

133. Croxatto HR, San Martin M. Kallikrein-like activity in the urine of renal hypertensive rats. Experientia 26:1216–1217, 1970.

134. Margolius HS, Geller RG, de Jong W, et al. Altered urinary kallikrein in rats with hypertension. Circ Res 30:358–362, 1972.

135. Favaro S, Barrio D, Antonello A, et al. Renal kallikrein content of spontaneously hypertensive rats. Clin Sci 49:69–71, 1975.

136. Praddaude F, Tran-Van T, Ader J-L. Renal kallikrein activity in rats developing spontaneous hypertension. Clin Sci 76:311–315, 1989.

137. El-Dahr SS. Ontogeny of the intrarenal kallikrein-kinin system: Proposed role in renal development. Microsc Res Tech 39:222–232, 1997.

138. Yosipiv IV, Dipp S, El-Dahr SS. Role of bradykinin B$_2$ receptors in neonatal kidney growth. J Am Soc Nephrol 8:920–928, 1997.

139. Velarde V, Humphreys J, Figueroa CD, Vio CP. Postnatal maturation of tissue kallikrein-producing cells (connecting tubule cells) in the rat kidney: A morphometric and immunohistochemical study. Anat Embryol 192:407–414, 1995.

140. Chao J, Zhang JJ, Lin, K-F, Chao L. Human kallikrein gene delivery attenuates hypertension, cardiac hypertrophy, and renal injury in Dahl salt-sensitive rats. Hum Gene Ther 9:21–31, 1998.

141. Chen L-M, Ma J-X, Liang Y-M, et al. Tissue kallikrein-binding protein reduces blood pressure in transgenic mice. J Biol Chem 271:27590–27594, 1996.

142. Madeddu P, Anania V, Parpaglia PP, et al. Chronic kinin receptor blockade induces hypertension in deoxycorticosterone-treated rats. Br J Pharmacol 108:651–657, 1993.

143. Braun C, Ade M, Unger T, et al. Effects of bradykinin and icatibant on renal hemodynamics in conscious spontaneously hypertensive and normotensive rats. J Cardiovasc Pharmacol 30:446–454, 1997.

144. Mukai H, Fitzgibbon WR, Ploth D, et al. Effect of chronic bradykinin B$_2$ receptor blockade on blood pressure of conscious Dahl salt-resistant rats. Br J Pharmacol 124:197–205, 1998.

145. Madeddu P, Parpaglia PP, Demonitis MP, et al. Early blockade of bradykinin B$_2$-receptors alters the adult cardiovascular phenotype in rats. Hypertension 25:453–459, 1995.

146. De Carvalho C, Sun Y, Weber KT. Wound healing following myocardial infarction in the rat: Role for bradykinin and prostaglandins. J Mol Cell Cardiol 28:1279–1285, 1996.

Diet—Nutrition

21 Diet—Micronutrients
David A. McCarron and Molly E. Reusser

SO MANY DATA, SO LITTLE CONSENSUS

Decades of research have focused on the role of specific dietary nutrients in blood pressure regulation. Sodium, potassium, calcium, and magnesium have each been examined extensively in epidemiological surveys, in clinical trials, and in laboratory investigations. And still the debates continue. Despite years of investigative effort and volumes of publications, the effects on blood pressure of these individual dietary factors remain subjects of scientific controversy and public confusion.

The most obvious example is sodium chloride, or salt, which has long been considered the foremost dietary cause of high blood pressure. This presumption received "factual" support from Dahl's epidemiological study published in 1960,[1] which included a graph with very few data points, indicating an almost perfectly linear relationship between the prevalence of hypertension and salt intake among five separate populations around the world. That often-cited study has been discounted on the basis of severe design and methodological flaws,[2] but the vast and still-expanding body of literature regarding the contribution of dietary salt to hypertension is plagued with conflicting results, and the controversy surrounding the sodium–blood pressure relationship continues to both engage and enrage nutrition and cardiovascular scientists.[3–7]

Although not of the same magnitude and intensity as sodium, studies of other micronutrients in blood pressure control are similarly equivocal and conflicting. Inadequate intakes of potassium, calcium, and magnesium have all been implicated individually in increased hypertension risk in population studies and in some but not all clinical trials. Studied in isolation, each of these micronutrients has been reported to decrease blood pressure, to increase blood pressure, and to have no effect on blood pressure. Thus, the one property that these studies share is heterogeneity; that is, modifications in nutrient intake consistently induce inconsistent responses in blood pressure.[8]

The lack of consensus regarding the blood pressure effects of these nutrients, the discrepancies in the results of the studies, and the heterogeneity of response commonly observed in clinical trials have a number of possible related explanations. It is likely that the antihypertensive effects of single nutrients are small and thus require large-scale trials for their detection. In contrast, the results of epidemiological surveys and clinical trials that include modifications of more than one nutrient may reflect larger, more easily detected additive effects. Nutrient interactions may also play a major role in the inconsistency of results in studies in which intake of one or more nutrients is manipu-

lated. Additional confounding factors in dietary studies include the degree to which baseline intake of the nutrient under study may influence individual blood pressure responses and the probability that nutrient supplements used in many studies may not have the same effect on blood pressure as nutrients present in food sources. Each of these explanations likely contributes to the unresolved questions regarding the role of specific nutrients in blood pressure regulation.

NUTRIENT INTERACTIONS

Both indirect and direct evidence support a paramount role for nutrient interactions in the prevention and treatment of high blood pressure. Early evidence came from animal and human studies of the effects of sodium on blood pressure. Kotchen and colleagues[9] first reported that the hypertensive effect of sodium chloride in Dahl salt-sensitive rats is preceded by the emergence of disturbances in calcium homeostasis. Kurtz and Morris[10] postulated that the induction of a calciuresis may signal the mechanism(s) by which sodium chloride raises blood pressure in humans. In laboratory models of salt-sensitive hypertension and cardiovascular disease, Tobian and coworkers[11, 12] demonstrated a protective effect of dietary potassium on blood pressure. These data are supported by the clinical observation of Krishna and associates[13] that short-term, severe potassium restriction induces salt sensitivity in normotensive humans and by the epidemiological data of Khaw and Barrett-Connor[14] indicating that adequate potassium intake protects against the potential adverse effects of sodium chloride on blood pressure and related target organ damage.

In the index report that characterized the calciuresis of essential hypertension, it was noted that the metabolic defect was more evident at higher levels of urinary sodium excretion.[15] This report was strikingly similar to observations reported in both the Dahl salt-sensitive rat[9] and the rat model of deoxycorticosterone acetate–salt hypertension[16] and to subsequent findings in humans.[17, 18] Subsequent studies in other laboratories have shown that reducing sodium chloride intake does not eliminate the renal defect. In the spontaneously hypertensive rat, an animal with well-characterized disturbances of calcium metabolism, including a renal calcium leak,[19] the antihypertensive effect of increasing dietary calcium has been shown to require a normal or high-normal concurrent intake of sodium chloride.[20, 21] In humans, Hamet and colleagues[22] reported that individuals consuming higher levels of sodium chloride could fall into the highest or lowest blood pressure group depending on whether they were consuming calcium in inadequate amounts or in amounts that met recommended dietary allowances, respectively.

Similar to the relationship between sodium and other nutrients, interactions among calcium, potassium, and magnesium have also been reported. However, as emphasized by Reed and coworkers[23] in their analyses of the Honolulu Heart Study, identifying these interactions is complicated by multicollinearity, which makes it inherently difficult to clearly isolate the effects of one nutrient from the effects of nutrients consumed concurrently. From the Nurses Health Study, Witteman and associates[24] observed that both dietary calcium and magnesium had strong and independent inverse associations with hypertension and that adjusting for calcium and magnesium intake eliminated the observed crude inverse association of dietary potassium and fiber with hypertension risk. It was reported in the Health Professionals Follow-Up Study that effects on blood pressure that were observed when nutrients were assessed individually were obliterated when the nutrients were considered together.[25]

Thus, numerous studies in recent years have examined relationships between nutrients and have identified some interdependencies among the major dietary electrolytes. We now recognize that nutrients participate interactively in biological functions, particularly in blood pressure regulation. Considering that nutrients are not ingested in isolation, but as combined constituents of a total diet, it is not surprising that manipulation of a single nutrient might produce inconsistent and often contradictory results in different biological settings. If one accepts the hypothesis that micronutrients express their physiological actions through integrated pathways, it is unrealistic to expect a uniform benefit in terms of blood pressure control by altering the intake of any one of them.

DIETARY NUTRIENT PATTERNS

Whenever the consumption of a single nutrient is significantly altered, a new dietary pattern is created. Nutrients occur in clusters in the typical human diet and may therefore act synergistically to alter physiological variables such as blood pressure. In a study comparing blood pressure effects of calcium carbonate supplements with increased calcium in the diet (up to 1500 mg/day), Karanja and colleagues[26] observed significant simultaneous increases in consumption of magnesium, potassium, phosphorus, riboflavin, and vitamin D in the dietary calcium group that did not occur in the calcium supplement group. In a recent review of the effect of sodium restriction on overall nutrient intake, Morris[27] found that most of the published studies did not address concomitant nutrient changes but those that did reported significant decreases in a number of essential dietary components. Although improvements were frequently observed in energy and fat intake, these were offset by reductions in calcium, potassium, fiber, and protein. Interestingly, calcium, potassium, and fiber have purported roles in blood pressure regulation, and all three are typically consumed at less than adequate levels by the general population.

COMPREHENSIVE DIETARY CLINICAL TRIALS

The Vanguard Studies

As a result of our increasing awareness of the impact and complexity of dietary interactions, nutrition research has expanded in recent years to include assessment of overall dietary patterns as they contribute to lower cardiovascular disease risk through the treatment or prevention of hypertension. The Cardiovascular Risk Reduction Dietary Intervention Trial is a 4-year series of multicenter randomized clinical studies by the Vanguard Research Group to evaluate multiple health effects of a complete nutrition program on persons at high risk of cardiovascular disease owing to established hypertension, dyslipidemia, or type 2 diabetes mellitus. Free-living adult participants in these trials were provided with their meals as a prepared meal plan that had been formulated to include levels of vitamins and minerals that meet the recommended dietary allowances of the Food and Nutrition Board of the National Research Council,[28] and the recommended micro- and macronutrient levels of national health organizations, including the American Heart Association,[29] National Cholesterol Education Program,[30] American Diabetes Association,[31] and the American Dietetics Association.[32] The clinical effects of the total nutrition plan were compared with those observed with a self-selected diet based on the exchange list system.[32]

The results of the first 10-week study, published in 1997, demonstrated significant improvements in blood pressure, lipid levels, glycemic control, homocysteine levels, weight, overall nutrient intake, and quality of life in subjects on both dietary plans. Greater improvements in most of these measures were observed with the prepared meal plan compared with a self-selected diet.[33] The second study in this series assessed the same endpoints using similar dietary interventions for 10 weeks, but reduced the amount of contact with participants to the level that would occur in actual clinical practice when dietary therapy is recommended.[34] Results from this usual-care approach were remarkably similar to those of the first study in this series. These studies demonstrate that, unlike single-nutrient alterations, consumption of a nutritionally complete and balanced dietary pattern, in which appropriate levels of nutrients are provided in combination, can improve blood pressure as well as other risk factors for cardiovascular disease, even in persons with high-normal risk profiles.

The Dietary Approaches to Stop Hypertension Trial

To specifically address the relationship between total dietary patterns and blood pressure, the National Heart, Lung, and Blood Institute initiated the multicenter, randomized, controlled Dietary Approaches to Stop Hypertension (DASH) clinical trial.[35] Published in 1997, the results of this carefully designed and executed study provide dramatic evidence of the importance of the dietary pattern of nutrients, as they occur together in food, on blood pressure regulation.[36] Three diets were assessed in the DASH study. The control diet was that considered to be a typical American diet, with 4 daily servings of fruits and vegetables and half a serving of dairy products. Potassium, calcium, and magnesium levels approximated the 25th percentile of U.S. consumption, and fiber and macronutrient levels were equivalent to the U.S. average. The second was the fruits-and-vegetables diet, which was similar to the control diet except that daily intake of fruits and vegetables was increased to 8.5 servings, which provided levels of potassium and magnesium at approximately the 75th percentile of American consumption, as well as higher dietary fiber levels. The third diet was the combination, which included 10 servings of fruits and vegetables and 2.7 servings of low-fat dairy products per day. This diet provided potassium, magnesium, and calcium at approximately the 75th percentile of consumption in the United States. Sodium content of all diets was held constant at approximately 3 g/day.

Highly significant blood pressure reductions were achieved with the combination diet compared with the control diet. With the combination diet, systolic pressure was reduced by 5 mm Hg and diastolic pressure by 3.0 mm Hg compared with the control diet. Blood pressure reductions with the fruits-and-vegetables diet compared with the control diet were also highly significant, but were only about half (2.8 mm Hg systolic and 1.1 mm Hg diastolic) of those achieved with the combination diet. The reductions with both intervention diets were observed within the first 2 weeks of study and were sustained for the remaining 6 weeks of the intervention.

Subgroup analysis did not detect any statistically significant differences in blood pressure reductions among the various subgroups of participants, including men, women; minority, nonminority; old, young. There was a between-diet difference, with greater reduction in minority than in nonminority persons; however, interaction between minority status and diet was not significant, and there was no evidence of interaction between gender and diet. The combination diet reduced blood pressure more than the fruits-and-vegetables or the control diet both in participants who met the criteria of hypertension and in those who did not. In each paired contrast, hypertensive participants had greater blood pressure reductions than those without hypertension. Interaction between hypertension status and diet was significant for systolic blood pressure and marginally significant for diastolic blood pressure.

Of high clinical significance, the blood pressure reductions observed in the hypertensive subjects on the combination compared with the control diet were 11.4 mm Hg systolic and 5.5 mm Hg diastolic; changes in hypertensive subjects on the control diet were 0.72 mm Hg systolic and 0.28 mm Hg diastolic. Blood pressure reductions in hypertensive subjects were also greater (4.1 mm Hg systolic and 2.3 mm Hg diastolic) on the combination diet than on the fruits-and-vegetables diet. The observed blood pressure reductions with the combination diet in the hypertensive subgroup were similar in magnitude to those reported in trials of antihypertensive drug treatment of mild hypertension.[37]

Other findings in the DASH study are also clinically relevant. The diet-related factors most commonly associated with blood pressure management—weight and sodium and alcohol consumption—were similar across the three diets and thus were not accountable for the blood pressure changes observed in this trial. No clinically significant adverse effects of these diet strategies were reported. Interestingly, gastrointestinal symptoms that might have been thought to be greater in the fruits-and-vegetables or combination diets were actually reported less frequently in these two diets than in the control group.

THE MORE THINGS CHANGE . . .

Our efforts to understand the blood pressure effects of micronutrients, as individual components as well as interactive constituents of the human diet, have revealed that there are no easy or uniform answers. Internationally recognized experts in the fields of nutrition and blood pressure continue to debate the merits of altering intake of one nutrient or another, and new data surface in both the medical and the lay press on a daily basis that challenge what we believed were immutable facts or that contradict the report of the previous day. Despite expansion of our knowledge with accumulated information and improved research methods and technology, our understanding of the role of micronutrients in the prevention and treatment of blood pressure abnormalities remains mired in conflicting results and scientific controversy.

This confusion is not surprising. Some of the potential sources of inconsistency among clinical studies in this area were described earlier. None of these can be simply removed from study designs. Adding to these previously noted confounders, such as heterogeneity of response, baseline intake levels, and physiological micronutrient interactions, is the enigma of hypertension itself. As the end result of an interplay between multiple, interrelated regulatory systems, each of which is itself influenced by genetic variance and environmental factors, high blood pressure is as multifaceted as the nutritional aspects of its treatment.

We do not understand the effects of single nutrients on blood pressure in every individual, and therefore it may be premature to make population-wide recommendations for specific intake levels of specific nutrients. Nevertheless, it is clear that diet does play a significant role in the control of blood pressure. We know that for many patients, appropriate dietary regimens are sufficient to manage their blood pressure, whereas for others, these regimens can be utilized to reduce antihypertensive medication requirements. Furthermore, it is clear that positive diet and lifestyle alterations offer means of preventing the development of hypertension. As stated in the Sixth Report of the Joint National Committee on Prevention, Detection, Evaluation, and Treatment of High Blood Pressure (JNC VI), lifestyle modifications—including improved nutrient intake, weight loss, and increased physical activity—"offer the potential for preventing hypertension, have been shown to be effective in lowering blood pressure, and can reduce other cardiovascular risk factors at little cost and with minimal risk."[38]

Increased awareness of the importance of comprehensive nutrient intake for hypertension prevention and treatment, combined with the growing recognition of the strong influence of multiple nutrient interactions on blood pressure control, will likely be the impetus for resolving the contradictions that pervade this field of study. In the interim, appropriate levels of all nutrients, consumed as part of a complete diet, appear to be the key to optimal blood pressure regulation for the general public. Although persons at higher risk or with established hypertension may require more aggressive management, for the population at large, micronutrient recommendations—a balanced diet and moderation in all things—have not really changed over time.

References

1. Dahl LK. Possible role of salt intake in the development of essential hypertension. *In* Bock KD, Cottier PT (eds). Essential Hypertension. Berlin, Springer-Verlag, 1960; p 53.
2. National Kidney Foundation Nonpharmacologic Management of Hypertension Organizing Committee. NKF Nonpharmacologic Management of Hypertension Program Syllabus. New York, National Kidney Foundation, 1996.
3. Intersalt Cooperative Research Group. Intersalt: An international study of electrolyte excretion and blood pressure. Results for 24-hour urinary sodium and potassium. BMJ 297:319–328, 1988.
4. Alderman MH, Anderson S, Bennett WM, et al. Scientists' statement regarding data on the sodium-hypertension relationship and sodium health claims on food labeling. Nutr Rev 55:172–175, 1997.
5. Kumanyika SK, Cutler JA. Dietary sodium reduction: Is there cause for concern? J Am Coll Nutr 16:192–203, 1997.
6. Thelle DS. Salt and blood pressure revisited. How much more evidence do we need? BMJ 312:1240–1241, 1996.
7. Luft FC, Weinberger MH. Heterogeneous responses to changes in dietary salt intake: The salt-sensitivity paradigm. Am J Clin Nutr 65:S612–S617, 1997.
8. Luft FC. Heterogeneity of hypertension: The diverse role of electrolyte intake. Annu Rev Med 42:347–355, 1991.
9. Kotchen TA, Ott CE, Whitescarver SA, et al. Calcium and calcium regulating hormones in the "prehypertensive" Dahl salt sensitive rat (calcium and salt sensitive hypertension). Am J Hypertens 2:747–753, 1989.
10. Kurtz TW, Morris RC. Dietary chloride as a determinant of "sodium-dependent" hypertension in men. N Engl J Med 317:1043–1048, 1987.
11. Tobian L. High potassium diets markedly protect against stroke deaths and kidney disease in hypertensive rats: A possible legacy from prehistoric times. Can J Physiol Pharmacol 64:840–848, 1986.
12. Tobian L, Lange J, Ulm K, et al. Potassium reduces cerebral hemorrhage and death rate in hypertensive rats, even when blood pressure is not lowered. Hypertension 7(suppl I):I-110–I-114, 1985.
13. Krishna GG, Miller E, Kapoor S. Increased blood pressure during potassium depletion in normotensive men. N Engl J Med 320:1177–1182, 1989.
14. Khaw K-T, Barrett-Connor E. Dietary potassium and stroke-associated mortality. A 12-year prospective population study. N Engl J Med 316:235–240, 1987.
15. McCarron DA, Pingree PA, Rubin RJ, et al. Enhanced parathyroid function in essential hypertension: A homeostatic response to a urinary calcium leak. Hypertension 2:162–168, 1980.
16. Kurtz TW, Morris RC Jr. Dietary chloride as a determinant of disordered calcium metabolism in salt-dependent hypertension. Life Sci 36:921–929, 1985.
17. Luft FC, Zemel MB, Sowers JR, et al. Sodium carbonate and sodium chloride: Effects on blood pressure and electrolyte homeostasis in normal and hypertensive men. J Hypertens 8:663–670, 1990.
18. Strazzullo P, Nunziata V, Cirillo M, et al. Abnormalities of calcium metabolism in essential hypertension. Clin Sci 65:137–141, 1983.
19. Young EW, Bukoski RD, McCarron DA. Calcium metabolism in essential hypertension. Proc Soc Exp Biol Med 187:123–141, 1988.
20. McCarron DA, Lucas PA, Shneidman RJ, et al. Blood pressure development of the spontaneously hypertensive rat after concurrent manipulations of dietary Ca^{2+} and Na^{+}: Relation to intestinal Ca^{2+} fluxes. J Clin Invest 76:1147–1154, 1985.
21. Hamet P, Skuherska R, Cherkaouil L, et al. Calcium levels and platelet responsiveness in spontaneously hypertensive rats on high calcium diet. [Abstract] J Hypertens 4(suppl 6):S716, 1986.
22. Hamet P, Mongeau E, Lambert J, et al. Interactions among calcium, sodium, and alcohol intake as determinants of blood pressure. Hypertension 17(suppl I):I-150–I-154, 1991.
23. Reed D, McGee D, Yano K, et al. Diet, blood pressure, and multicollinearity. Hypertension 7:405–410, 1985.
24. Witteman JCM, Willett WC, Stampfer MJ, et al. A prospective study of nutritional factors and hypertension among US women. Circulation 80:1320–1327, 1989.
25. Ascherio A, Rimm EB, Giovannucci EL, et al. A prospective study of nutritional factors and hypertension among US men. Circulation 86:1475–1484, 1992.
26. Karanja N, Morris CD, Rufolo P, et al. The impact of increasing dietary calcium intake on nutrient consumption, plasma lipids and lipoproteins in humans. Am J Clin Nutr 59:900–907, 1994.
27. Morris CD. Effect of dietary sodium restriction on overall nutrient intake. Am J Clin Nutr 65(suppl):687S–691S, 1997.
28. National Research Council (U.S.) Subcommittee on the Tenth Edition of the RDAs. Recommended Dietary Allowances. Washington, DC, National Academy Press, 1989.
29. Krauss RM, Deckelbaum RJ, Ernst N, et al. Dietary guidelines for healthy American adults: A statement for health professionals from the Nutrition Committee, American Heart Association. Circulation 94:1795–1800, 1996.
30. National Cholesterol Education Program. Report of the Expert Panel on Population Strategies for Blood Cholesterol Reduction: Executive summary. Arch Intern Med 151:1071–1084, 1991.
31. Franz MJ, Horton ES, Bantle JP, et al. Nutrition principles for the management of diabetes and related complications. [Technical Review] Diabetes Care 17:490–518, 1994.
32. American Dietetic Association and American Diabetes Association. Exchange Lists for Weight Management. Chicago, American Dietetic Association, 1989.
33. McCarron DA, Oparil S, Chait A, et al. Nutritional management of cardiovascular risk factors: A randomized clinical trial. Arch Intern Med 175:169–177, 1997.
34. Oparil S, Resnick LM, McCarron DA, et al. Effects of a comprehensive nutrition program on cardiovascular risk factors. Hypertension 28:510, 1996.
35. Sacks FM, Obarzanek E, Windhauser MM, et al. Rationale and design of the Dietary Approaches to Stop Hypertension Trial (DASH). A multicenter controlled-feeding study of dietary patterns to lower blood pressure. Ann Epidemiol 5:108–118, 1995.
36. Appel LJ, Moore TJ, Obarzanek E, et al. A clinical trial of the effects of dietary patterns on blood pressure. N Engl J Med 336:1117–1124, 1997.
37. The Treatment of Mild Hypertension Research Group. The Treatment of Mild Hypertension Study: A randomized, placebo-controlled trial of a nutritional-hygienic regimen along with various drug monotherapies. Arch Intern Med 151:1413–1423, 1991.
38. Joint National Committee on Prevention, Detection, Evaluation, and Treatment of High Blood Pressure. The Sixth Report. Arch Intern Med 157:2413–2446, 1997.

22 Obesity-Hypertension: Effects on the Cardiovascular and Renal Systems—The Therapeutic Approach

Efrain Reisin and Howard G. Hutchinson

Epidemiological studies suggest that up to 50% of obese patients have concomitant hypertension.[1, 2] The relationship between obesity and hypertension has been documented in several socioeconomic, racial, and ethnic groups.[3, 4] The relationship of weight gain to increased blood pressure is not fully understood; however, when both conditions coexist in the same patient, the hemodynamic and structural adaptations related to obesity are heightened, placing the patient at even greater risk for adverse cardiovascular and renal events.[5–7] Excess body weight is also an independent risk factor for death due to cardiovascular disease or other causes.[8]

EFFECTS OF OBESITY ON THE CARDIOVASCULAR SYSTEM

Obesity can lead to marked changes in systemic hemodynamics as well as structural adaptations in the blood vessels and heart. These adaptations can alter vascular reactivity[9] and promote cardiac hypertrophy[10] (Fig. 22–1).

Systemic Hemodynamics

High cardiac output, high plasma and total blood volume, and inappropriately normal total peripheral resistance characterize the hemodynamic profile of the obese individual.[11–13] Since heart rate usually remains unchanged, the increase in cardiac output in response to elevated metabolic requirements occurs predominantly through increased stroke volume. The increase in total blood volume occurs primarily in the cardiopulmonary area of the circulation.

The hemodynamic changes in the obese-hypertensive subject present a mixed profile owing to the interplay of the individual components of obesity and hypertension. The hemodynamic profile of the lean subject with essential hypertension is characterized by normal cardiac output and contracted intravascular volume in the presence of high total peripheral resistance. In the obese-hypertensive patient, intravascular volume, cardiac output, and total peripheral resistance are elevated compared with the lean-hypertensive subject. However, owing to the effects of the obesity component, total peripheral resistance is elevated

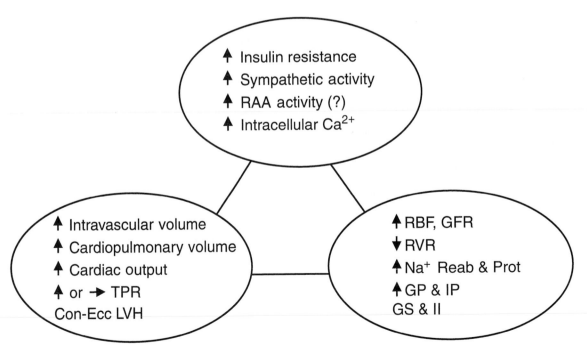

Figure 22–1. Metabolic-endocrinologic, cardiovascular, and renal damage in obesity-hypertension. RAA, renin-angiotensin-aldosterone; TPR, total peripheral resistance; Con-Ecc LVH, concentric-eccentric left ventricular hypertrophy; RBF, renal blood flow; GFR, glomerular filtration rate; RVR, renal vascular resistance; Reab, reabsorption; Prot, proteinuria; GP, intraglomerular pressure; IP, interstitial pressure; GS, glomerular sclerosis; II, interstitial infiltrate.

less than would be expected and may appear completely normal in some patients.[14, 15]

Vascular Adaptations

Cellular metabolism of cations and other components may be altered in obese subjects and may lead to changes in vascular responsiveness.[16–18] In Zucker rats, a genetically obese hyperinsulinemic model for human obesity, enhanced vascular reactivity has been observed along with a tendency toward hypertension and impaired vascular smooth muscle calcium efflux.[19] Using magnetic resonance imaging to evaluate the ascending and descending aorta of normal and hypertensive patients, Resnick and coworkers[16] showed that increased abdominal visceral fat as well as decreased intracellular magnesium and advancing age were closely associated with reduced aortic distensibility. Structural changes in resistance vessels also appear to accompany obesity;[17] however, the nature of these changes awaits clarification.[18]

Other potential effects of obesity on human blood vessels must be extrapolated from studies on red blood cells. For example, in normotensive obese subjects, cytosolic calcium in erythrocytes was increased, whereas in obese-hypertensive patients, nonobese patients with essential hypertension, and non–insulin-dependent diabetic patients with hypertension, intraerythrocyte magnesium and pH decreased.[20] If these changes were to occur in vascular smooth muscle, the result would be increased vascular tone and peripheral resistance.

Cardiac Adaptations

In response to the hemodynamic changes that occur in the obese subject, left ventricular volume and left ventricular filling pressure become elevated.[21] As demonstrated by echocardiographic studies, these alterations increase left ventricular preload, resulting in chamber dilatation and increased left ventricular wall stress. The left ventricle adapts to chamber dilatation by adding contractile elements in series. In addition, the myocardium thickens to restore wall stress to normal. The result is "eccentric" left ventricular hypertrophy, a characteristic finding in obese-normotensive subjects.[21] Earlier studies of obese subjects on autopsy that showed increased cardiac weight associated with thickened, hypertrophied ventricles corroborate these echocardiographic findings.[10] Not surprisingly, congestive heart failure has been documented as a common complication of morbid obesity, regardless of the presence of hypertension.[22, 23]

As opposed to the "eccentric" cardiac hypertrophy seen with obesity, cardiac hypertrophy in the essential hypertensive patient is "concentric," that is, the elevated total peripheral resistance results in increased ventricular afterload and increased ventricular wall stress. Contractile elements are added in parallel, resulting in the thickening of chamber walls, partially at the expense of chamber volume.[24] Cardiac dilatation is not observed during the early phases of hypertensive disease.

The coexistence of both obesity and hypertension in the same patient results in a mixed eccentric-concentric hypertrophic profile.[25] Both disorders produce an extensive rise in left ventricular stroke work as the result of the increased afterload associated with arterial hypertension and the increased preload associated with obesity. The combined hemodynamic burden of obesity and hypertension increases the risk for congestive heart failure.[24]

Obesity also appears to change the normal circadian variation of blood pressure. In a recent study, we found that up to 70% of obese-hypertensive patients failed to show an appropriate fall in systolic and diastolic blood pressure during sleep.[26] These patients have been referred to as *nondippers,* and the condition has been associated with left ventricular hypertrophy, microalbuminuria, and cerebrovascular disease.[27–29]

The hypertrophic changes that occur as a result of obesity may provide the basis for the development of cardiac arrhythmias.[30, 31] A study of obese subjects reported the presence of mononuclear cell infiltration in and around the sinoatrial node and/or its approaches, with marked fat throughout the conduction system.[32] Lipomatous hypertrophy of the interatrial septum also has been associated with obesity.[33] Such changes may explain the high rates of sudden cardiac death in morbidly obese patients.[34]

EFFECTS OF OBESITY ON THE KIDNEYS

The association of obesity and hypertension may be the cause of some renal disorders.[7] Obesity-induced hypertension, however, also may be initiated by a derangement of renal function (see Fig. 22–1). Hall and colleagues[7, 35] have studied dogs in which obesity was induced by a high-fat diet. This animal model may have characteristics similar to those of human obesity-hypertension. In these animals, investigators described sodium retention due to increased tubular sodium reabsorption at the level of the loop of Henle, a reabsorption that may cause a shift of pressure natriuresis toward higher blood pressure levels. Several mechanisms, such as insulin resistance and hyperinsulinemia, increased sympathetic activity, activation of the renin-angiotensin system, and higher renal interstitial fluid hydrostatic pressure, may generate these changes.[7, 35] This increased hydrostatic pressure may be caused by structural changes in the kidneys described in the same animal model, e.g., an increase in the number of interstitial cells and expansion of the extracellular matrix between the tubules in the renal medulla.[7] These findings led Hall and colleagues[7, 35] to believe that obesity-hypertension is associated with an abnormal relationship between arterial pressure and sodium excretion that increases tubular sodium reabsorption. They also concluded that the most important mechanisms in the pathogenesis of obesity-induced hypertension are the activation of the sympathetic nervous system and histological changes within the renal medulla.[7]

Renal Hemodynamics

In an earlier study, we showed that obese-normotensive and obese-hypertensive subjects have increased renal blood flow and reduced renal vascular resistance compared with lean matched normotensive and hypertensive patients.[36] In a more recent investigation, a similar match between lean and obese normotensive and hypertensive patients demonstrated that the glomerular filtration rate and the renal plasma flow increased in obese individuals compared with lean subjects.[37] Additionally, urinary excretion of albumin was higher in hypertensive patients compared with normotensive matched controls.[37] This increased glomerular protein traffic and heavy proteinuria are direct causes of tubular cell injury and contribute to the progression of renal disease.[38] Consequently, obese individuals will have renal hyperfiltration and hyperperfusion with increased albuminuria and increased susceptibility to the development of renal damage.[37]

Renal Damage

In a retrospective study that examined renal tissue of 180 autopsies in which groups were separated according to body mass index, 80% of the specimens from overweight patients, as opposed to only 30% of those from underweight and ideal-weight individuals, exhibited expansion of the extracellular matrix and/or an increase in the number of renomedullary interstitial cells, increased interstitial hydrostatic pressure, and increased compression of the tubules.[39] These findings may indicate that human obese-hypertensives, like the animal models discussed earlier, may have increased sodium reabsorption and hypertension.[39]

EFFECTS OF WEIGHT REDUCTION

Several studies of large numbers of patients have shown that weight reduction is an effective treatment for reducing blood pressure in obese patients with elevated blood pressure.[40, 41] In a study in which salt was not restricted, we showed that 75% of the obese-hypertensive patients returned to normal blood pressure levels after a weight loss of 10 kg, which suggests that weight loss independent of salt restriction was an effective tool in the control of blood pressure.[40] In the Dietary Intervention Study in Hypertension (DISH),[41] a large number of obese-hypertensives were offered the following management alternatives: withdrawal of antihypertensive therapy with concomitant sodium restriction or weight reduction, reinstitution of therapies, or no therapy. The average weight loss among those in the weight-reduction group was 4.5 kg after 1 year. Sixty percent remained off their medication and were still normotensive, whereas only 30% of the control subjects remained normotensive without medication. DISH investigators also reported that 46% of those patients who reduced their sodium intake remained normotensive. The authors concluded that weight reduction was the best nonpharmacological approach when antihypertensive medication was withdrawn.[41] The beneficial effects of weight reduction occurred in both sexes and in white and African American subjects alike.[41]

Systemic Hemodynamic and Cardiac Changes

In an earlier study, we showed that a weight loss of only 10 kg induced lower total circulating and cardiopulmonary blood volumes without changing total peripheral resistance.[42] These changes were related to reduced venous return and cardiac output.[42] In another study, the hemodynamic changes after weight loss were associated with reduced left ventricular internal dimension during diastole as well as decreased septal and left ventricular systolic wall thickness.[21] The hemodynamic and cardiac structural changes that accompany weight loss can significantly reduce left ventricular stroke work[43] and lead to improved cardiac function.

Renal Changes

When we studied renal hemodynamics after weight loss, we found no change in renal blood flow in obese-hypertensives.[42] To date, no other studies of the effect of weight loss on renal hemodynamics in humans have been conducted. However, animal studies have shown that calorie restriction without protein restriction in the diet of Fisher rats with only one sixth of their kidney remaining after nephrectomy[44] and of uninephrectomized spontaneously hypertensive rats[45] lowered urinary protein excretion and the glomerular filtration rate after weight loss and a drop in blood pressure. The mean glomerular injury index and the mesangial expansion index of the remaining kidney in animals treated with a low-calorie diet were significantly lower. These changes suggest that weight loss may have a beneficial effect on glomerular hyperfiltration and, consequently, may lessen proteinuria and glomerular sclerosis.[45] However, human studies are necessary to verify that these changes occur in obese-hypertensive subjects.

PHARMACOLOGICAL TREATMENT

Reasonable use of antihypertensive medications that will not enhance the preexisting metabolic abnormalities in obese-hypertensive patients should be initiated when the low-calorie diet approach fails to control blood pressure or when the patient cannot tolerate weight-control programs or is unable or unwilling to comply with them.[46]

Diuretics

Hydrochlorothiazide and chlorthalidone are effective in decreasing blood pressure in obese-hypertensives because they reduce the intravascular and extracellular fluid volume and decrease cardiac output.[46] All the studies done with obese-hypertensive patients,[47, 48] however, were short-term, and most of the patients required higher doses of diuretics to control their hypertension. The prolonged use of high dosages of diuretics may exacerbate some already existent metabolic changes in obese-hypertensive patients, e.g., dyslipidemia, increased plasma renin activity, and insulin resistance.[49]

β-Adrenergic Blocking Agents

Findings on the efficacy of these antihypertensive agents in obese-hypertensive subjects have been contradictory.[50, 51] Some studies have shown that treatment with metoprolol failed to control blood pressure,[51] but others have observed better blood pressure control with atenolol than with placebo treatment.[52] All these studies include a small number of patients with short-term follow-up, and they also have reported adverse effects on patients' lipid profiles.[52] β-Blockers may also induce reduced glucose tolerance and worsening of insulin resistance.[52] Another disadvantage to the use of these agents may be the associated risk of weight gain;[52] β-blockers prevent the action of catecholamines on fatty acid mobilization, which by decreasing the availability of fatty acids, may diminish feedback to the appetite center and induce overeating.[52]

Centrally Acting Agents

These agents control blood pressure by inhibiting the release of epinephrine and the cardiac responses to postganglionic, adrenergic nerve stimulation.[52] In a study that included a small number of obese patients, clonidine, a centrally acting agent, failed to control blood pressure in most patients using a daily dosage of up to 0.4 mg.[47] However, more large trials are necessary with a higher daily dosage to evaluate the efficacy of these agents in obese-hypertensive individuals.

α₁-Adrenergic Blocking Agents

These antihypertensives control blood pressure by inducing vasodilatation through inhibition of the postsynaptic receptors. They also may have metabolic benefits in obese-hypertensive subjects by reducing the early insulin response and increasing insulin sensitivity.[52] The α_1-adrenergic blocking agents may also lower total cholesterol and triglycerides and increase high-density lipoprotein-cholesterol levels.[52] Large studies of obese-hypertensive patients with these agents are scarce, but one study of a small number of subjects demonstrated significantly decreased systolic and diastolic blood pressure and increased insulin sensitivity.[53]

Calcium Antagonists

A highly heterogeneous group, calcium antagonists act by inhibiting the slow inward calcium channels that lead to relaxation of myocardial and smooth muscle arterial wall cells. They also may induce natriuresis by direct action on renal tubules.[52] When the dihydropyridine calcium antagonists nifedipine,[54] amlodipine,[55] nitrendipine,[56] and isradipine[57] were used in different studies with obese-hypertensive patients, they improved glucose tolerance, reduced fasting and glucose-stimulated serum insulin levels, and significantly reduced blood pressure.[54–56] However, one study on the effect of isradipine on systolic and diastolic blood pressure has shown that individual responses to treatment varied widely and that isradipine decreased diastolic blood pressure more effectively in lean-hypertensives than in obese-hypertensives.[56]

Angiotensin-Converting Enzyme Inhibitors

The use of antihypertensive medications that reduce glomerular hydrostatic pressure and glomerular hyperfiltration and may decrease proteinuria may be useful in obese-hypertensive patients.[52] In the only large prospective multicenter double-blind therapeutic trial performed in obese-hypertensive patients, we studied the efficacy and safety of the angiotensin-converting enzyme agent lisinopril compared with the diuretic hydrochlorothiazide.[48] Sixty percent of the patients treated with lisinopril had an office diastolic blood pressure less than 90 mm Hg, compared with 43% of the patients treated with hydrochlorothiazide. Plasma glucose increased significantly, and serum potassium levels decreased significantly in patients treated with hydrochlorothiazide. Most of the patients whose hypertension was controlled with hydrochlorothiazide required high doses of the medication, whereas those whose hypertension was controlled with lisinopril required low doses. We concluded that patient age and race may dictate the choice of agents. For example, lisinopril was more effective than hydrochlorothiazide in whites and in younger patients, whereas hydrochlorothiazide was more effective in African American patients.[48]

In conclusion, obesity-hypertension is characterized hemodynamically by expanded intravascular volume, which induces increased cardiac output and inappropriately normal total peripheral resistance. Obesity-hypertension is also marked by increased renal flow and glomerular filtration rate with reduced renal vascular resistance. These hemodynamic changes lead to structural changes in the heart characterized by concentric-eccentric left ventricular hypertrophy; they also generate higher renal glomerular volume and an increase in the number of interstitial cells, which may also compress the tubules and blood vessels of the renal medulla.

Weight reduction effectively controls blood pressure and improves left ventricular hypertrophy and cardiac function. Human studies of the effect of weight loss on renal hemodynamics are lacking, but animal studies suggest a benefit to kidney function and renal damage after weight loss. Angiotensin-converting enzyme inhibitors, calcium antagonists, and α_1-adrenoreceptor blocking agents also may offer an efficient antihypertensive approach in obese-hypertensive patients.

Acknowledgments

We thank Ms. Deborah Copelin for her secretarial help in the preparation of this manuscript and Ms. Anne Compliment for her editorial review.

References

1. Kannel WB, Brand N, Skinner JJ, et al. The relation of adiposity to blood pressure and development of hypertension: The Framingham Study. Ann Intern Med 67:48–49, 1967.

2. Johnson AL, Cornoni JC, Cassel JC, et al. Influence of race, sex and weight on blood pressure behavior in young adults. Am J Cardiol 35:523–530, 1975.

3. Berchtold P, Jorgens V, Finke C, et al. Epidemiology of obesity and hypertension. Int J Obes Relat Metab Disord 1:1–7, 1981.

4. Gordon T, Kannel WB. Obesity and cardiovascular disease: The Framingham Study. Baillieres Clin Endocrinol Metab 5:367–375, 1976.

5. Hubert HB, Feinleib M, McNamara PM, et al. Obesity as an independent risk factor for cardiovascular disease: A 26-year follow-up of participants in the Framingham Heart Study. Circulation 83:968–977, 1983.

6. Zamboni M, Armellini F, Sheiban I, et al. Relation of body fat distribution in men and degree of coronary narrowing in coronary artery disease. Am J Cardiol 70:1135–1138, 1992.

7. Hall JE. Renal and cardiovascular mechanisms of hypertension in obesity. Hypertension 23:381–394, 1994.

8. Stevens J, Jianwen C, Elsie R, et al. The effect of age on the association between body-mass index and mortality. N Engl J Med 338:1–7, 1997.

9. Jacobs DB, Sowers JR, Hmeidan A, et al. Effects of weight reduction on cellular cation metabolism and vascular resistance. Hypertension 21:308–314, 1993.

10. Amad KH, Brennan JC, Alexander JK. The cardiac pathology of chronic exogenous obesity. Circulation 32:740–745, 1965.

11. Frohlich ED, Messerli FH, Reisin E, et al. The problem of obesity and hypertension. Hypertension 5(suppl III):71–78, 1983.

12. Krieger DR, Landsberg L. Obesity and hypertension. In Laragh JH, Brenner BM (eds). Hypertension: Pathophysiology, Diagnosis, and Management. New York, Raven, 1990; pp 1741–1757.

13. Messerli FH, Christie B, DeCarvalho JG, et al. Obesity and essential hypertension. Hemodynamics, intravascular volume, sodium excretion, and plasma renin activity. Arch Intern Med 141:81–85, 1981.

14. Schmieder RD, Messerli FH. Does obesity influence early target organ damage in hypertensive patients? Circulation 87:1482–1488, 1993.

15. Licata G, Scaglione, Capuana G, et al. Hypertension in obese subjects: Distinct hypertensive subgroup. J Hum Hypertens 4:37–41, 1990.

16. Resnick LM, Militianu D, Cunnings AJ, et al. Direct magnetic resonance determination of aortic distensibility in essential hypertension, relation to age, abdominal visceral fat, and in situ intracellular free magnesium. Hypertension 30:654–659, 1997.

17. Rocchini AP, Moorehead C, Katch V, et al. Forearm resistance vessel abnormalities and insulin resistance in obese adolescents. Hypertension 19:615–620, 1992.

18. Boehringer K, Beretta-Piccoli C, Weidmann P, et al. Pressor factors and cardiovascular pressor responsiveness in lean and overweight normal or hypertensive subjects. Hypertension 4:697–702, 1982.

19. Ambrozy SL, Shehin SE, Chiou C-Y, et al. Effects of dietary calcium on blood pressure, vascular reactivity and vascular smooth muscle calcium efflux rate in Zucker rats. Am J Hypertens 4:592–596, 1991.

20. Resnick LM, Gupta RK, Bhargava KK, et al. Cellular ions in hypertension, diabetes, and obesity. A nuclear magnetic resonance spectroscopic study. Hypertension 17:951–957, 1991.

21. Simone G, Devereux RB, Roman MJ. Relation of obesity and gender to left ventricular hypertrophy in normotensive and hypertensive adults. Hypertension 23:600–606, 1994.

22. Messerli FH. Cardiopathy of obesity—A not-so-Victorian disease. N Engl J Med 314:378–380, 1986.

23. Drenick EJ, Bale GS, Seltzer F, et al. Excessive mortality and causes of death in morbidly obese men. JAMA 243:443–445, 1980.

24. Frohlich ED, Epstein C, Chobanian AV, et al. The heart in hypertension. N Engl J Med 327:998–1008, 1992.

25. Messerli FH, Sundgaard-Riise K, Reisin E, et al. Dimorphic cardiac adaptation to obesity and arterial hypertension. Ann Intern Med 99:757–761, 1983.

26. Weir MR, Reisin E, Falkner B, et al. Nocturnal reduction of blood pressure and the antihypertensive response to a diuretic or angiotensin converting enzyme inhibitor in obese hypertensive patients. Am J Hypertens 11:914–920, 1998.

27. Verdecchia P, Schellaci G, Boldrini F, et al. Sex, cardiac hypertrophy and diurnal blood pressure variations in essential hypertension. J Hypertens 10:683–692, 1992.

28. Bianchi S, Bigazzi R, Baldari G, et al. Diurnal variations of blood pressure and microalbuminuria in essential hypertension. Am J Hypertens 7:23–29, 1994.

29. Shimada K, Kawamoto A, Matsubayashi K, et al. Diurnal blood pressure variations and silent cerebrovascular damage in elderly patients with hypertension. J Hypertens 10:875–878, 1992.

30. Lip GYH, Gammage MD, Beevers DG. Hypertension and the heart. Br Med Bull 18:193–197, 1994.

31. De la Maza MP, Esteves A, Bunout D, et al. Ventricular mass in hypertensive obese subjects. Int J Obes Relat Metab Disord 18:193–197, 1994.

32. Bharati S, Lev M. Cardiac conduction system involvement in sudden death of obese young people. Am Heart J 129:273–281, 1995.

33. Basu S, Folliguet T, Anselmo M, et al. Lipomatous hypertrophy of the interatrial septum. Cardiovasc Surg 2:229, 1994.

34. Duflou J, Virmani R, Rabin J, et al. Sudden death as a result of heart disease in morbid obesity. Am Heart J 130:306–313, 1995.

35. Hall JE, Brands MW, Dixon WN, et al. Obesity-induced hypertension: Renal function and systemic hemodynamics. Hypertension 22:292–299, 1993.

36. Reisin E, Messerli FG, Ventura HO, et al. Renal hemodynamic studies in obesity hypertension. J Hypertens 5:397–400, 1987.

37. Ribstein J, Cailar G, Mimran A. Combined renal effects of overweight and hypertension. Hypertension 26:610–615, 1995.

38. Bruzzi I, Benigni A, Remuzzi G. Role of increased glomerular protein traffic in the progression of renal failure. Kidney Int 62:529–532, 1997.

39. Arnold MD, Brissie R, Soonz JS, et al. Obesity associated renal medullary changes. Lab Invest 70:156A, 1994.

40. Reisin E, Abel R, Modan M, et al. Effect of weight loss without salt restriction on the reduction of blood pressure in overweight hypertensive patients. N Engl J Med 298:1–6, 1978.

41. Langford HG, Blaufox MD, Oberman A, et al. Dietary therapy slows the return of hypertension after stopping prolonged medication. JAMA 253:657–669, 1985.

42. Reisin E, Frohlich ED, Messerli FH, et al. Cardiovascular changes after weight reduction in obesity hypertension. Ann Intern Med 98:315–319, 1983.

43. Backman L, Freyschuss V, Hallberg D, et al. Reversibility of cardiovascular changes in extreme obesity. Acta Med Scand 205:367–373, 1979.

44. Kovayashi S, Venkatachalam MA. Differential effects of calorie restriction on glomeruli and tubules of the remnant kidney. Kidney Int 42:710–717, 1992.

45. Reisin E, Azar S, Deboisblanc BP, et al. Low calorie unrestricted protein diet attenuates renal injury in hypertensive rats. Hypertension 21:971–974, 1993.

46. Reisin E. Treatment of obese hypertensive patients. In Izzo JL, Black HR (eds). Hypertension Primer. Dallas, American Heart Association, 1993; pp 323–325.

47. Reisin E, Weed SG. The treatment of obese hypertensive black women: A comparative study of chlorthalidone versus clonidine. J Hypertens 10:489–493, 1992.

48. Reisin E, Weir MR, Falkner B, et al. Lisinopril versus hydrochlorothiazide in obese hypertensive patients: A multi center placebo-controlled trial. Hypertension 30:140–145, 1997.

49. Mykkanen L, Kuusisto J, Pyorala K, et al. Increased risk of non-insulin dependent diabetes mellitus in elderly hypertensive subjects. J Hypertens 12:1425–1432, 1994.

50. MacMahon SW, MacDonald GJ, Bernstein L, et al. Comparison of weight reduction with metoprolol in treatment of hypertension in young overweight patients. Lancet 1:1233–1252, 1985.

51. Fagerberg B, Berglund A, Anderson OK, et al. Cardiovascular effects of weight reduction vs antihypertensive drug treatment: A comparative, randomized, 1-year study of obese men with mild hypertension. J Hypertens 9:431–439, 1991.

52. Richards RJ, Thakur V, Reisin E. Obesity related hypertension. Its physiological basis and pharmacological approaches to its treatment. J Hum Hypertens 10:559–564, 1996.

53. Pollare T, Lithell H, Selinus I, et al. Application of prazosin is associated with an increase in insulin sensitivity in obese patients with hypertension. Diabetologia 31:415–420, 1988.

54. Tuck ML, Bravo EL, Krakoff LR, et al, and the Modern Approach to the Treatment of Hypertension (MATH) Study Group. Endocrine

and renal effect of nifedipine gastrointestinal therapeutic system in patients with essential hypertension. Results of a multicenter trial. Am J Hypertens 3:S333–S341, 1990.

55. Courten M, Ferrari P, Schneider M, et al. Lack of effect of long-term amlodipine on insulin sensitivity and plasma insulin in obese patients with essential hypertension. Eur J Clin Pharmacol 44:457–462, 1993.

56. Beer NA, Jakubowitz DJ, Beer RM, et al. Effects of nitrendipine on glucose tolerance and serum insulin and dehydroepiandrosterone sulfate levels in insulin resistant obese and hypertensive men. J Clin Endocrinol Metab 76:178–183, 1992.

57. Schmieder RE, Gotzka CH, Schachunger H, et al. Obesity as a determinant for response to antihypertensive treatment. BMJ 307:537–540, 1993.

23 Alcohol and Hypertension

Arthur L. Klatsky

HISTORICAL BACKGROUND

An association between heavier alcohol consumption and hypertension (HTN) reported in World War I French servicemen[1] was apparently ignored for 60 years. Since the mid-1970s, largely because of epidemiological studies in developed countries, alcohol use has joined other correlates of HTN, such as obesity and salt intake, as a major research focus on HTN risk factors with several published reviews.[2–8] Epidemiological studies have consistently shown higher blood pressure (BP) among persons reporting usual daily intake of three drinks or more. The alcohol-HTN relationship is seen in both sexes, several ethnic groups, all adult ages, and for each of the major alcoholic beverage types (wine, beer, liquor). A clear mechanism for the association has not been established, but several aspects of the data suggest a causal relationship. Heavier drinking may be the commonest cause of reversible HTN. The data indicate that reduction of intake lowers BP and that continued intake may impair response to other forms of HTN management.

Unresolved issues include:

1. Is the relationship linear or is there a threshold dosage of alcohol for a BP effect?
2. Does alcohol interact with other dietary or behavioral factors in possible effect?
3. Is the drinking pattern (steady vs. intermittent) a major factor?
4. Is the choice of wine, liquor, or beer a factor?
5. Are there plausible mechanisms?
6. Does alcohol-associated HTN carry the same sequelae as HTN unassociated with alcohol?
7. Does reduction of alcohol intake play a role in HTN treatment or prevention?

ALCOHOL AND HYPERTENSION: EPIDEMIOLOGIC STUDIES

A review describes almost 50 cross-sectional or prospective population studies in ambulatory persons concerning the alcohol-HTN association.[8] All but two of the cross-sectional studies and all prospective studies show a link between increasing alcohol use and higher BP.

Cross-Sectional Studies

Two Kaiser Permanente cross-sectional studies remain among the largest alcohol-BP investigations; their findings are described as examples. The first study involved a diverse population of approximately 87,000 ambulatory adult subscribers to a prepaid health care plan.[9] Figure 23–1 shows the age-adjusted mean systolic and diastolic BP in each race and sex group according to the usual number of drinks per day reported on a health examination questionnaire. In both sexes, BP rose with consumption of more than 2 drinks per day. Among women of all races, consumers of 2 or fewer drinks per day had slightly lower BP than did nondrinkers. In general, the trends in systolic BP were more pronounced than those in diastolic BP. These mean differences translated into an approximately doubled HTN ($\geq$160/95) prevalence in white men and women in the 6 or more drinks per day group than in those consuming 2 or fewer drinks and the nondrinking categories. The alcohol-BP association was independent of age, sex, race, cigarette smoking, coffee use, reported past heavy drinking, and educational attainment. For example, study by adiposity tertiles (Fig. 23–2) showed that adiposity was related to BP but that alcohol use was independently related to BP within each adiposity subgroup.

One item on the examination questionnaire was: "Do you usually salt your food before tasting it?" Lacking salt excretion measurements, it was believed that those answering "yes" ingested more salt on the average than those answering "no." "Yes" answers had a strong association to alcohol intake, but among subjects subdivided by their answers to this question, the relation of alcohol intake to BP persisted (Fig. 23–3).

The second Kaiser Permanente study[10] explored several unanswered questions. Figure 23–4 shows adjusted mean BP controlled for age, adiposity, smoking, coffee use, tea use, and seven blood tests. Some other results:

1. White men reporting drinking less often than daily had no significant alcohol-BP relationship; among daily drinkers, there was a progressive rise in systolic and diastolic BP that peaked at 6 to 8 drinks per day. White women showed similar, slightly less marked, relationships.
2. African American men showed a continuous relation-

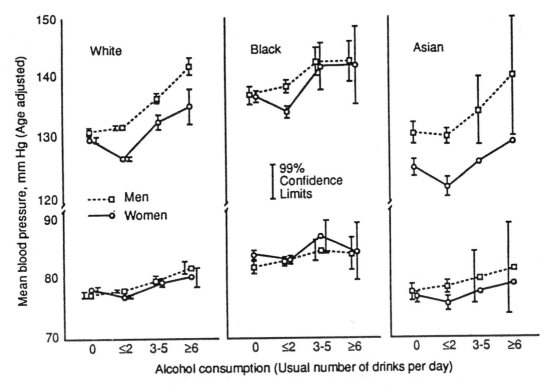

Figure 23–1. Mean systolic blood pressures *(upper graphs)* and mean diastolic blood pressures *(lower graphs)* for white, black, or Asian men and women with known drinking habits. *Small circles* represent data based on fewer than 30 persons. (From Klatsky AL, Friedman GD, Siegelaub AB, et al. Alcohol consumption and blood pressure. N Engl J Med 296:1194, 1977. Copyright © 1977 Massachusetts Medical Society. All rights reserved.)

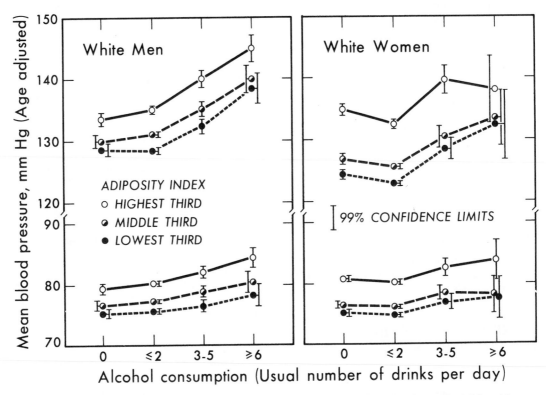

Figure 23–2. Mean systolic blood pressures *(upper graphs)* and diastolic blood pressures *(lower graphs)* for white men and women with known drinking habits according to tertiles of Quetelet's index ([wt/ht²] × 100). (From Klatsky AL, Friedman GD, Siegelaub AB, et al. Alcohol consumption and blood pressure. N Engl J Med 296:1194, 1977. Copyright © 1977 Massachusetts Medical Society. All rights reserved.)

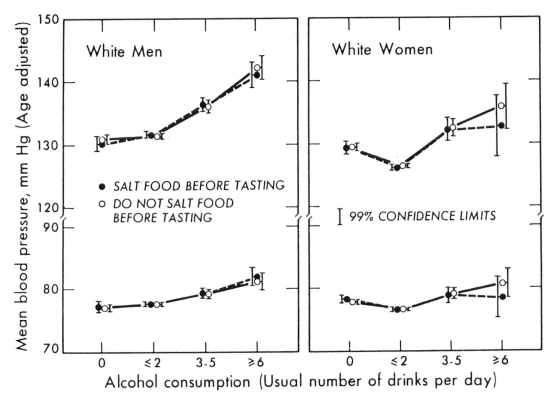

Figure 23–3. Mean systolic blood pressures *(upper graphs)* and diastolic blood pressures *(lower graphs)* for white men and women with known drinking habits according to usual salt use habit. (From Klatsky AL, Friedman GD, Siegelaub AB. Alcohol and hypertension. Compr Ther 4:60, 1978.)

ship of more drinking to higher diastolic BP, but the elevations in systolic BP leveled off at 3 to 5 drinks per day. African American women showed the least consistent alcohol-BP relationship.

3. The alcohol-BP relationship was present in all age subsets, but was slightly stronger in the oldest (≥60 years of age) persons.

4. Past drinkers did not have significantly higher BP than lifelong abstainers. Of the 651 white men who were past drinkers, 342 (52.8%) stated that their maximal drinking had been 3 or more drinks per day for at least 1 year; this subset had adjusted mean BP similar to that of lifelong abstainers. These findings suggest that HTN associated with heavier drinking regresses with abstinence.

5. Only small differences were seen in adjusted mean BP for persons indicating a clear preference for wine, liquor, or beer, suggesting that usual beverage choice was not a major factor.

6. Among white men whose usual intake was 3 or more drinks per day, those with no intake in the week before examination had substantially lower adjusted mean BP than men who reported any drinking in the past week. Those reporting 9 or more drinks in the 24 hours before examination showed no reversal of the alcohol-HTN association. These details suggest rapid regression of alcohol-associated HTN on reduction of alcohol intake.

Prospective Studies

All available data from prospective investigations show a positive association of alcohol use with BP.[8] For example, it was observed in the Framingham Study[11] in both men and women that change in alcohol consumption was positively associated with change in systolic and diastolic BP. An increase in consumption over 4 years was associated with a BP increase, whereas a decrease in consumption was associated with a BP decrease. Data from the Honolulu Heart Program Study of 8006 Japanese men showed a significant relation of alcohol intake and both systolic and diastolic BP, independent of age, body mass index, physical activity index, and intake of protein, fat, carbohydrate, milk, potassium, and calcium;[12] the relationship was clearest for systolic BP at alcohol intakes of 45 or more ounces per month. Friedman and coworkers[13] did a case-control analysis of 1031 pairs of persons over a 6-year period. Consumption of 3 or more drinks per day was predictive of HTN incidence, independent of body mass index, parental HTN history, heavy salt intake, and several other traits—more so if this intake level persisted. Other prospective studies with good control for various nutritional factors showed similar findings in 30,861 U.S. male health professionals[14] and in 58,218 female registered nurses.[15]

Studies in Hospitalized Problem Drinkers

Several early studies of hospitalized alcoholics[16–18] found BPs either lower or similar to that of the general population, leading to the suggestion that dietary deficiencies[18] or depressed myocardial function[17] was involved. Others[2] suggest that the social/medical profiles of "skid-row" alcoholics several decades ago included a larger proportion of

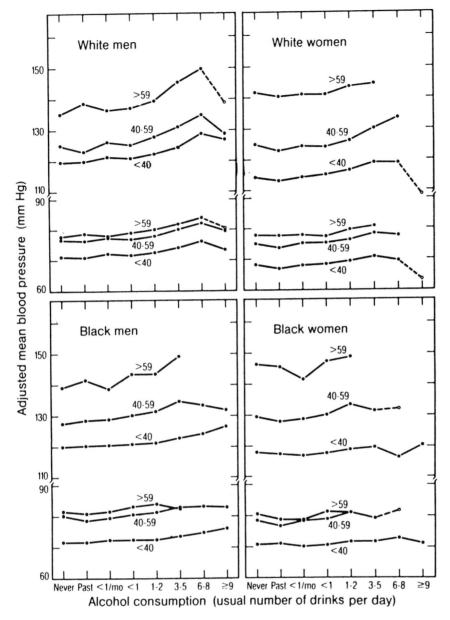

Figure 23–4. Adjusted mean systolic and diastolic blood pressures (mm Hg) according to alcohol consumption by three age groups (*top left,* white men; *lower left,* black men; *top right,* white women; *lower right,* black women). *Dashed lines* and *open circles* indicate 10 < *n* < 25. Data are omitted from the figure for categories with *n* < 11 (white women aged 40 to 59 years, nine or more drinks per day, and age over 59 years, six to eight and nine or more drinks per day; black men age over 59 years, six to eight and nine or more drinks per day; black women aged 40 to 59 years, nine or more drinks per day, and age over 59 years, three to five, six to eight, and nine or more drinks per day). (From Klatsky AL, Friedman GD, Armstrong MA. The relationship between alcoholic beverage use and other traits to blood pressure: A new Kaiser Permanente study. Circulation 73:628, 1986. By permission of the American Heart Association, Inc.)

severely ill, undernourished persons compared with a more modern experience. Other studies of alcoholics have shown higher BPs than in controls,[19–21] specifically associated in many with an alcohol withdrawal state. This aspect is discussed later.

Problems in Alcohol-Hypertension Studies

A satisfactory long-term clinical trial of alcohol, HTN, and HTN sequelae is unlikely to be performed. The closest practical alternatives are prospective observational studies and short- or intermediate-term clinical trials. Intrinsic problems in studies of alcohol and health effects are well known.[8] One of these is underreporting of heavier intake, but this is an unlikely explanation of the alcohol-HTN relation because the major effect of such underreporting would be to produce an apparent, but spurious, relationship

of HTN to *lighter* drinking. The threshold for the relationship could be higher than suggested by the epidemiological data.

The multiple traits related to alcohol drinking or to HTN make it difficult to rule out all indirect explanations, especially psychosocial stress. Properly designed intervention studies might provide evidence about indirect explanations.

INTERVENTION STUDIES IN HUMANS (CLINICAL EXPERIMENTS)

A review of HTN in heavy drinkers noted that several studies of hospitalized problem drinkers showed substantial reductions in BP within several days after admission.[22] These uncontrolled studies must be interpreted in light of the known tendency for BP to fall in hospitalized nonalcoholic patients.

To the author's knowledge, the first controlled trial of the effects of reduction of alcohol consumption on BP was the landmark clinical trial of Potter and Beevers.[23] Using a crossover design in a hospital, they studied 16 men with HTN and usual intake of approximately 4 pints of British beer. When alcohol consumption was maintained at baseline levels, BP remained high; but it fell significantly when alcohol was withdrawn for 3 to 4 days. Alcohol reintroduction produced significant BP increases. These data suggested both a pressor effect of alcohol in hypertensive men and short-term BP reductions after complete alcohol withdrawal.

The first randomized, controlled trial of alcohol restriction known to the author involved 48 normotensive men reporting approximately 4 to 5 drinks per day, studied in a 12-week crossover trial.[24] Subjects consumed 3 drinks per day for 6 weeks and 3 drinks per week for 6 weeks. Systolic BPs were significantly lower during lower alcohol consumption; changes in diastolic BP were smaller and not statistically significant. Reported changes in alcohol intake correlated well with BP changes. Further work showed similar results in hypertensives and also suggested that regular drinking might antagonize the efficacy of antihypertensive drug treatment.[25]

Several intervention studies suggest that the beneficial effects of moderation of alcohol intake supplement the effects of other nonpharmacological and drug treatments of HTN. An 18-week randomized trial of caloric restriction, 80% reduction in alcohol intake, or both, or neither, demonstrated an additive effect of weight reduction and alcohol restriction.[26] A study of exercise and alcohol restriction[27] showed that only alcohol restriction lowered BP. In a study of treated hypertensives, randomized into four groups (alcohol restriction, sodium restriction, both alcohol and sodium restriction, or neither), only alcohol restriction reduced BP.[28]

Possible interactions of alcohol with antihypertensive drugs represent an important but little studied issue. Alcohol consumers seem to respond less well to medication,[29] but it is not clear whether this is due to less compliance among drinkers or an effect on drug pharmacokinetics. One study showed that alcohol did not interfere with the hypotensive effect of a 200-mg dose of metoprolol.[30] Similar studies of other medications are needed.

Intervention studies suggest a short-term (days to weeks) pressor effect of consumption of 3 to 8 drinks per day in both hypertensive and normotensive subjects. The data show that either total abstinence from alcohol or reduction to less than 1 drink per day results in short-term BP reductions, independent of weight loss, exercise, and sodium intake. These results are compatible with a therapeutic benefit of alcohol restriction in HTN and a preventive benefit in normotensive subjects. Even without confirmation in long-term randomized controlled trials, these studies support a causal hypothesis in the alcohol-HTN relationship.

Evidence Concerning Possible Mechanisms

When reviewing physiological data concerning acute and chronic effects of alcohol on BP, we must recall the diversity of alcohol effects on various target organs that have direct or indirect roles in BP regulation. Also, experimental results may differ in health and disease. Rate, dose, and route of alcohol administration, time interval to BP measurement, and probably, psychic factors differ in reported studies. Thus, it is difficult to define the true acute effects of alcohol on BP in human subjects.

Work carried out more than six decades ago[31] showed that nonintoxicating alcohol doses produce a slight increase in heart rate and cardiac output and some increase in BP (systolic > diastolic). Later, total peripheral resistance was shown to change little; cutaneous resistance decreases, producing the familiar flushing of the skin, with compensation by visceral vasoconstriction.[32] These findings have been reported in studies of patients who consumed ethyl alcohol doses of approximately 30 to 75 ml ($\sim$2 to 5 drinks). Other acute studies of this amount of alcohol in humans showed inconsistent results: BP either increased[33] or decreased.[34–36] Larger alcohol doses, sufficient to produce respiratory depression, tend to produce hypotension, bradycardia, and asystole[37] via a combination of neural reflex mechanisms and direct myocardial effects.

An interesting recent series of Japanese studies utilized ambulatory monitoring in hypertensives to demonstrate a depressor effect of a large alcohol dose at dinner time, with persistence of lower BP for up to 8 hours.[38, 39] This work showed both pressor and depressor effects of repeated doses of 1 g/kg, with the direction of the effect dependent on time between alcohol administration and BP measurement. These changes could not be explained by measurements of plasma renin, aldosterone, insulin, cortisol, or catecholamines and were independent of the acetaldehyde-induced flushing response common among Asian Americans. These workers suggested that the BP reduction in hypertensives, which they considered to be the predominant effect of an acute alcohol load, may be associated with reduced intracellular sodium.[39] The hypertensive doses of alcohol in some clinical trials were associated with increased heart rates.[24, 25] These observations raise the possibility of impaired baroreflexes in alcohol-induced HTN.

In a randomized, balanced crossover study comparing effects of a dose of 1.3 g/kg of alcohol with an isocaloric glucose drink,[40] BP rose to a similar extent after both alcohol and the control drink, suggesting that there was no specific acute pressor effect of alcohol. Subsequently (up to 8 hours), BP fell after alcohol ingestion, but a tachycardia persisted, attributed by the investigators to a reflex response. Some animal experiments have included data concerning acute BP effects of alcohol. Intragastric administration of alcohol in dogs produced little effect,[41, 42] but intravenous administration in other studies produced a modest BP rise.[43] Several human studies of intravenous alcohol administration showed no rise in BP.[44–46]

The few chronic experimental studies in animals also had conflicting results. These studies involved feeding relatively large amounts of alcohol to rats[47] or dogs[48, 49] during a period of several months. A possible role for catecholamines in mediating the effects of alcohol on BP has been a focus in a number of investigations. Observations of an acute rise of urinary catecholamine levels after alcohol intake[50, 51] have been complemented by data showing acute rises in plasma epinephrine[52] and norepinephrine[53] after alcohol ingestion. However, the controlled study of Stott and colleagues[40] showed that the increases in norepinephrine after alcohol ingestion were similar to those following an oral glucose load. Another short-term alcohol-loading study[54] found no significant changes in catecholamines. Transient increases in catecholamine levels in the setting of alcohol consumption are due more to reduced clearance[54] or metabolism[55] than to increased secretion. Suggestions of increased renin and cortisol levels related to alcohol ingestion have not been substantiated.[55]

A few investigators have studied the possible role of these pressor substances in maintaining chronically elevated BP levels associated with alcohol use. Elevated plasma norepinephrine and renin levels have been found in alcohol-fed hypertensive rats.[56] Potter and Beevers[23] found no increases in cortisol or in renin levels during alcohol consumption in their experiments. Arkwright and associates[57] found no elevations of epinephrine, norepinephrine, renin, or cortisol in men averaging 5 drinks per day. An experiment in normal humans[58] using intraneural microelectrodes showed increased sympathetic activation in response to intravenous alcohol with a delayed (second hour) BP increase. Inhibition of these responses by dexamethasone suggested a central mechanism via corticotropin-releasing hormone. These inconsistent findings indicate a need for further studies.

Some have speculated that alcohol may directly affect peripheral vascular tone,[5, 59] perhaps via changes in calcium transport into smooth muscle cells. Using catecholamines administered locally to rat arterioles, Altura and Altura[60] found an increased constrictor response in animals fed alcohol for several weeks. However, Eisenhofer and co-workers[54] found reduced vascular reactivity to pressor substances in humans who drank. Howes and Reid[53] found in a crossover, randomized study that 7 days of alcohol ingestion reduced adrenoreceptor-mediated cardiovascular reactivity in humans.

Potter and Beevers[55] studied several factors that might predict an acute pressor response to alcohol. Only alcohol consumption in the week before study was strongly predictive of a pressor response; age, weight, baseline BP, heart rate, and serum γ-glutamyl transferase were not predictive. Yet another hypothesis has been stimulated by the observation that plasma calcium levels fell after acute alcohol loading.[54] This raised the possibility of transfer into smooth muscle cells in blood vessel walls, perhaps facilitating vasoconstriction.[57] However, a study of alcohol-fed hypertensive rats showed no major erythrocyte cell membrane changes.[61] Other (speculative) possibilities are that alcohol-induced BP increases could be related to impaired insulin sensitivity or to magnesium depletion. The latter could be related to intracellular calcium transport.

Thus, direct mechanisms that have been proposed to account for alcohol-related HTN are speculative. Firm evidence is sparse, and the physiological effects of alcohol are complex. If the alcohol-BP link proves to be causal, the mechanisms responsible will need to account for both the apparent threshold effect and the apparent lack of dose-responsiveness of BP to alcohol intake. The latter phenomenon might represent differential physiological effects of varying alcohol doses or might be due to chronic debilitating illness related to alcohol, such as cirrhosis of the liver or alcoholic cardiomyopathy.

DO ALCOHOL WITHDRAWAL REACTIONS PLAY A ROLE?

The suggestion has been repeatedly made that the alcohol-HTN association may be due to withdrawal from alcohol.[6–8, 62] The basis for this hypothesis is that temporary abstention by heavier drinkers may be presumed to be more socially presentable at a medical examination. Mild early withdrawal reactions could raise BP in a proportion of these persons. A study of 96 alcoholics admitted for detoxification showed that BP levels were related to withdrawal severity and that most hypertensives became normotensive when withdrawal cleared.[63] After discharge, BP rose only in those who resumed drinking. These investigators suggested that increased noradrenergic activity in withdrawal explained alcohol-related HTN.

The withdrawal hypothesis is not supported by the clinical trials,[23–28] which found no evidence of a BP rise on cessation of alcohol drinking in amounts less than usual intake by alcoholics. Thus, it seems unlikely that withdrawal explains the alcohol-associated HTN seen in population studies.

The withdrawal issue has two aspects. One is whether the alcohol-BP association is an artifact in that alcohol drinkers might have higher BP only when they are temporarily in a withdrawal state at medical examinations. The second is whether withdrawal is a mechanism underlying a true association. Withdrawal could raise BP both acutely, as in the detoxification ward, and chronically, in that repeated transient BP increases might lead to sustained HTN.

DOES STRESS PLAY A ROLE?

Perhaps psychological or emotional stress, which remains an unresolved confounder, could lead to both increased alcohol intake and higher BP. Increased alcohol use could be a marker for psychological problems, with no direct BP effect. Also, emotional stress could raise BP via a pharmacological effect of alcohol. There are major problems in measuring stress, but instruments are available for measuring psychological traits often considered to be influenced by stress. Australian studies showed the alcohol-BP association to be independent of a number of such psychological traits, including type A behavior, trait anxiety, recent life stress, neurosis, and extroversion or introversion.[3, 64] Reduction in BP after cessation or reduction of alcohol intake in several studies suggests that the association was not due to factors predisposing to alcohol use.[23, 24] On the other hand, one report suggests a relation of alcohol to HTN only in persons with "high-strain" jobs; these persons did not drink more than persons in normal-strain jobs, in whom no alcohol-BP relationship was seen.[65] This is a difficult area for research, and an answer about the role of stress in the alcohol-BP relationship is not likely to be seen soon.

HEALTH OUTCOMES OF ALCOHOL-ASSOCIATED HYPERTENSION

If alcohol use is one of the causes of HTN, alcohol-associated HTN should be followed by the usual health sequelae of high BP. Good data are lacking concerning alcohol use and renal failure, but two of the main complications of HTN, coronary heart disease (CHD) and stroke, are both related to alcohol use. Population studies have almost unanimously found an inverse association between lighter alcohol use and CHD;[66, 67] some studies find that heavier drinkers appear less protected than lighter drinkers (i.e., a U-shaped curve for the alcohol-CHD relationship). Increased protective high-density lipoprotein (HDL)-cholesterol levels and a possible antithrombotic effect of alcohol are plausible protective mechanisms against CHD. Since HTN is a major CHD risk factor, the role of alcohol-related HTN has been explored.[68, 69] The data suggest that approximately 50% of the observed CHD reduction was mediated by alcohol-related elevations in HDL-cholesterol levels, but a counterbalancing effect of alcohol-related HTN was also seen. It is likely that alcohol-induced HTN partially explains the upturn in the U-curve alcohol-CHD relationship at heavier drinking.

The risk factors for hemorrhagic and ischemic stroke differ somewhat, but HTN is a powerful predictor of both major stroke types. Study of relationships of alcohol drinking to stroke is made difficult by the complex relationships of alcohol to other stroke risk factors.[70, 71] For example, although HTN is a strong predictor of both hemorrhagic and ischemic stroke, cardiomyopathy, CHD, and arrhythmias are also important risk factors for ischemic stroke. To further complicate matters, anticoagulant therapy, often administered for several cardiac conditions, substantially increases risk of hemorrhagic stroke. Finally, the ability of alcohol to raise HDL-cholesterol might reduce ischemic stroke risk, while its antithrombotic action might simultaneously increase hemorrhagic stroke risk and decrease ischemic stroke risk. The relationships of alcohol to both types of stroke are less well established than for CHD, but data suggest that drinking increases risk of hemorrhagic stroke and reduces risk of ischemic stroke.[70, 71] The role of alcohol in stroke needs further study.

Thus, study of the sequelae of alcohol-associated HTN has been difficult. Follow-up data concerning hospitalizations and mortality are available from the large Kaiser Permanente study group, in which an alcohol-BP relationship was found.[8] Harmful and beneficial effects of alcohol appeared to be so balanced that it was difficult to assess the risks of alcohol-associated HTN for cardiovascular morbidity and mortality.

PROPORTION OF HYPERTENSION ATTRIBUTABLE TO ALCOHOL

Estimates of the proportion of HTN due to heavy drinking vary; the contribution of alcohol depends substantially on the drinking habits of the group under study. Considering both sexes together, published estimates are 5%[72] or 7%[3] of HTN, with attribution to alcohol of approximately 11%

of HTN in men but a much smaller proportion in women. Even these conservative estimates translate into 2 to 3 million people with alcohol-associated HTN in the United States, if one uses as the denominator 40 to 50 million hypertensives. It is probable that alcohol is the most common cause of reversible "secondary" HTN in developed countries. Published estimates of the prevalence of secondary HTN (not including alcohol) range from 5.8% in a random population sample[73] to 10% in a referral center experience.[74] In a Scottish referral center experience, 7.9% of hypertensives had an underlying cause; of these, less than one third (2.3% of all hypertensives) were considered to have a potentially reversible cause.[75]

WHAT IS THE ROLE OF ALCOHOL RESTRICTION IN HYPERTENSION MANAGEMENT?

Appropriate advise for the individual health practitioner to his or her patient about alcohol use is heavily dependent on his or her knowledge of the patient's drinking habits and his or her ability to influence the patient's behavior. What is needed is a sound assessment of the medical risk-benefit equation for the individual. The health practitioner should present the evidence clearly and allow the patient to choose a course of action. The following statements are offered as guidelines pertinent to alcohol and high BP.

1. Substantial data link heavier drinking ($\geq$3 drinks/day) to higher BP and HTN. Abstinence or restriction of intake by heavier drinkers may result in a fall in BP, either directly or by improving responsiveness to, and compliance with, other HTN treatment.[76] At lower levels of intake, up to 1 to 2 drinks per day, there is little or no biologically important effect of alcohol on BP.[8]
2. One should obtain a particularly careful history of alcohol use in subsets of hypertensive persons likely to be heavy drinkers, such as middle-aged men. From the viewpoint of therapeutic potential, young persons should be appropriately educated.
3. Lighter drinkers have lower overall mortality than either heavy drinkers or abstainers.[77, 78] Many persons should not drink at all, including those with a history of or at special risk of a drinking problem, pregnant women, and because of possible increased risk of breast cancer from alcohol,[78] young women at high risk of breast cancer. In developed countries, most adults are lighter drinkers who can control their drinking and, thus, have drinking habits that place them in a favorable risk category for cardiovascular disease. From a medical viewpoint, including management and prevention of HTN, it seems reasonable that such persons should not be advised to change their drinking behavior.[79–81]

Acknowledgments

Portions of the material in this chapter include research supported by the Alcoholic Beverage Medical Research Foundation, Inc., Baltimore, Maryland, and by the Community Service Program of Kaiser Foundation Hospitals.

References

1. Lian C. L'alcoholisme cause d'hypertension artérielle. Bull Acad Med (Paris) 74:525, 1915.
2. Gleiberman L, Harburg E. Alcohol usage and blood pressure: A review. Hum Biol 58:1, 1986.
3. MacMahon S. Alcohol consumption and hypertension. Hypertension 9:111, 1987.
4. The World Hypertension League. Alcohol and hypertension—Implications for management: A consensus statement by the World Hypertension League. J Hum Hypertens 5:227, 1991.
5. Beilin LJ, Puddy IB. Alcohol and essential hypertension. [Editorial] Alcohol 19:191, 1984.
6. Keil U, Swales JD, Grobbee DE. Alcohol intake and its relation to hypertension. *In* Verschuren PM (ed). Health Issues Related to Alcohol Consumption. Washington, DC, ILSI, 1993; p 17.
7. Klatsky AL. Alcohol use and blood pressure. *In* Izzo JL, Black HL (eds). Hypertension Primer. Dallas, American Heart Association, 1993; p 164.
8. Klatsky AL. Blood pressure and alcohol intake. *In* Laragh JH, Brenner BM (eds). Hypertension: Pathophysiology, Diagnosis, and Management, 2nd ed. New York, Raven, 1995; p 2649.
9. Klatsky AL, Friedman GD, Siegelaub AB, et al. Alcohol consumption and blood pressure. N Engl J Med 296:1194, 1977.
10. Klatsky AL, Friedman GD, Armstrong MA. The relationship between alcoholic beverage use and other traits to blood pressure: A new Kaiser Permanente study. Circulation 73:628, 1986.
11. Gordon T, Kannel WB. Drinking and its relation to smoking, BP, blood lipids, and uric acid. Arch Intern Med 143:1366, 1983.
12. Reed D, McGee D, Yano K. Biological and social correlates of blood pressure among Japanese men in Hawaii. Hypertension 4:406, 1982.
13. Friedman GD, Selby JV, Quesenberry CP, et al: Precursors of essential hypertension: The role of body weight, reported alcohol and salt use, and parental history of hypertension. Prev Med 17:387, 1988.
14. Ascherio A, Rimm EB, Giovanucci EL. A prospective study of nutritional factors and hypertension among US men. Circulation 86:1475, 1992. Stein SW, Lieber CS, Leevy CM, et al.
15. Witteman JC, Willett WC, Stampfer MJ. Relation of moderate alcohol consumption and risk of systemic hypertension in women. Am J Cardiol 65:633, 1990.
16. Wilens SL. The relationship of chronic alcoholism to atherosclerosis. JAMA 135:1136, 1947.
17. Spodick DH, Pigott VM, Chiriffe R Preclinical cardiac malfunction in alcoholism. N Engl J Med 287:677, 1972.
18. Sullivan JF, Hatch LK. Alcoholism and vascular disease. Geriatrics 19:442, 1964.
19. Mehta B, Sereny G. Cardiovascular manifestations during alcohol withdrawal. Mt Sinai J Med 46:484, 1979.
20. Saunders JB, Beevers DG, Paton A. Alcohol-induced hypertension. Lancet 2:653, 1981.
21. Bannan LT, Potter JF, Beevers DG, et al. Effect of alcohol withdrawal on blood pressure, plasma renin activity, aldosterone, cortisol and dopamine-B-hydroxylase. Clin Sci 66:659, 1984.
22. Ashley MJ, Rankin JG. Alcohol consumption and hypertension: The evidence from hazardous drinking and alcoholic populations. Aust N Z J Med 9:201, 1979.
23. Potter JF, Beevers DG. Pressor effect of alcohol in hypertension. Lancet 1:119, 1984.
24. Puddey IB, Beilin LJ, Vandongen R, et al. Evidence of a direct effect of alcohol consumption on blood pressure in normotensive men: A randomized controlled trial. Hypertension 7:707, 1985.
25. Puddey IB, Beilin LJ, Vandongen R. Regular alcohol use raises blood pressure in treated hypertensives. Lancet 1:647, 1987.
26. Puddey IB, Parker M, Beilin LJ, et al. Effects of alcohol and caloric restrictions on blood pressure and serum lipids in overweight men. Hypertension 20:533, 1992.
27. Cox KL, Puddey IB, Morton AR, et al. Controlled comparison of effects of exercise and alcohol on blood pressure and serum high density lipoprotein cholesterol in sedentary males. Clin Exp Pharmacol Physiol 17:251, 1990.
28. Parker M, Puddey IB, Beilin LJ, et al. A 2-way factorial study of alcohol and salt restriction in treated hypertensive men. Hypertension 16:398, 1990.
29. Beevers DG. Alcohol, blood pressure and antihypertensive drugs. [Editorial] J Clin Pharmacol Ther 15:395, 1990.
30. Maheswaran R, Beevers DG, Kendall MJ, et al. The interaction of alcohol and beta-blockers in arterial hypertension. J Clin Pharmacol Ther 15:405, 1990.
31. Grollman A. The action of alcohol, caffeine, and tobacco on the cardiac output (and its related functions) of normal man. J Pharmacol Exp Ther 39:313, 1930.
32. Fewings JD, Hanna MJ, Walsh JA, et al The effects of ethyl alcohol on the blood vessels of the forearm and hand in man. Br J Pharmacol Chemother 27:93, 1966.
33. Orlando J, Aronow WS, Cassidy J, et al Effect of ethanol on angina pectoris. Ann Intern Med 84:652, 1976.
34. Riff DP, Jain AC, Doyle JT. Acute hemodynamic effects of alcohol on normal human volunteers. Am Heart J 78:592, 1969.
35. Conway N. Haemodynamic effects of ethyl alcohol in patients with coronary heart disease. Br Heart J 30:638, 1968.
36. Kupari M. Drunkenness, hangover, and the heart. Acta Med Scand 213:84, 1983.
37. Eliaser M Jr, Giansiracusa FJ. The heart and alcohol. Calif Med 84:234, 1956.
38. Kawano Y, Abe H, Kojuma S, et al. Acute depressor effect of alcohol in patients with essential hypertension. Hypertension 20:219, 1992.
39. Kojima S, Kawano Y, Abe H, et al. Acute effects of alcohol on blood pressure and erythrocyte sodium concentration. J Hypertens 11:185, 1993.
40. Stott DJ, Ball SG, Inglis GC, et al. Effects of a single moderate dose of alcohol on blood pressure, heart rate, and associated endocrine and metabolic changes. Clin Sci 73:411, 1987.
41. Doekel RC, Weir EK, Looga R, et al. Potentiation of hypoxic pulmonary vasoconstriction by ethyl alcohol in dogs. J Appl Physiol 44:76, 1978.
42. Smythe CM, Heinemann HO, Bradley SE. Estimated hepatic blood flow in the dog: Effect of ethyl alcohol on it, renal blood flow, cardiac output and arterial pressure. Am J Physiol 172:737, 1953.
43. Ganz V. The acute effect of alcohol on the circulation and on the oxygen metabolism of the heart. Am Heart J 66:494, 1963.
44. Battey LL, Heyman A, Patterson JL Jr. Effects of ethyl alcohol on cerebral blood flow and metabolism. JAMA 152:6, 1953.
45. Stein SW, Lieber CS, Leevy CM, et al. The effect of ethanol upon systemic and hepatic blood flow in man. Am J Clin Nutr 13:68, 1963.
46. Miyazaki M. Circulatory effect of alcohol, with special reference to cerebral circulation. Jpn Circ J 38:381, 1974.
47. Maines JE III, Aldinger EE Myocardial depression accompanying chronic consumption of alcohol. Am Heart J 73:55, 1967.
48. Pachinger OM, Tillmanns H, Mao JC, et al. The effect of prolonged administration of alcohol on cardiac performance and metabolism in the dog. J Clin Invest 52:2690, 1973.
49. Regan TJ, Khan MI, Ettinger PO, et al. Myocardial function and lipid metabolism in the chronic alcoholic animal. J Clin Invest 54:740, 1974.
50. Greenspon AJ, Stang JM, Lewis RP, et al. Provocation of ventricular tachycardia after consumption of alcohol. N Engl J Med 301:1049, 1979.
51. Ogata M, Mendelson JH, Mello NK, et al. Adrenal function and alcoholism. II: Catecholamines. Psychosom Med 33:159, 1971.
52. Ireland MA, Vandongen R, Davidson L, et al. Acute effects of moderate alcohol consumption on blood pressure and plasma catecholamines. Clin Sci 66:643, 1984.
53. Howes LG, Reid JL. Changes in plasma free 3,4-dihydroxyphenylethylene-glycol and noradrenaline levels after acute alcohol administration. Clin Sci 69:423, 1985.
54. Eisenhofer G, Lambie DG, Johnson RH. Effects of ethanol on plasma catecholamines and norepinephrine clearance. Clin Pharmacol Ther 34:143, 1983.
55. Potter JF, Beevers DG. Factors determining the acute pressor response to alcohol. Clin Exp Hypertens Theory Pract A13:13, 1991.
56. Chan TC, Wall RA, Sutter MC. Chronic ethanol consumption, stress, and hypertension. Hypertension 7:519, 1985.
57. Arkwright PD, Beilin LJ, Vandongen R, et al. The pressor effect of alcohol consumption: A search for mechanisms. Circulation 66:60, 1982.
58. Randin D, Vollenweider P, Tappy L, et al. Suppression of alcohol-induced hypertension by dexamethasone. N Engl J Med 332:1733, 1995.
59. Knochel JP. Cardiovascular effects of alcohol. Ann Intern Med 98:849, 1983.
60. Altura BM, Altura BT. Microvascular and vascular smooth muscle actions of ethanol, acetaldehyde, and acetate. Fed Proc 41:2447, 1982.

61. Chan TC, Godin DV, Sutter MC. Erythrocyte membrane properties of the chronic alcoholic rat. Drug Alcohol Depend 12:249, 1983.

62. Wallace RB, Lynch CF, Pomrehn PR, et al. Alcohol and hypertension: Epidemiologic and experimental considerations: The Lipid Research Clinics program. Circulation 64(suppl III):III-41, 1981.

63. Spodick DH, Pigott VM, Chirife R. Preclinical cardiac malfunction in chronic alcoholism. Comparison with matched normal controls and with alcoholic cardiomyopathy. N Engl J Med 287:677–680, 1972.

64. Arkwright PD, Beilin LJ, Vandongen R, et al. Alcohol, personality, and predisposition to essential hypertension. J Hypertens 1:365, 1983.

65. Schnall C, Wiener JS. Clinical evaluation of blood pressure in alcoholics. Q J Stud Alcohol 19:432, 1958.

66. Renaud S, Criqui MH, Farchi G, et al. Alcohol drinking and coronary heart disease. *In* Verschuren PM (ed). Health Issues Related to Alcohol Consumption. Washington, DC, ILSI, 1993; p 81.

67. Klatsky AL. Epidemiology of coronary heart disease—Influence of alcohol. Alcohol Clin Exp Res 18:88, 1994.

68. Criqui MH. Alcohol and hypertension: New insights from population studies. Eur Heart J 8(suppl B):9, 1987.

69. Langer RD, Criqui MH, Reed DM. Lipoproteins and blood pressure as biologic pathways for the effect of moderate alcohol consumption on coronary heart disease. Circulation 85:910, 1992.

70. Van Gign J, Stampfer MJ, Wolfe C, et al. The association between alcohol consumption and stroke. *In* Verschuren PM (ed). Health Issues Related to Alcohol Consumption. Washington, DC, ILSI, 1993; p 43.

71. Klatsky AL. Cardiovascular effects of alcohol. Sci Am Sci Med 2:28, 1995.

72. Friedman GD, Klatsky AL, Siegelaub AB. Alcohol intake and hypertension. Ann Intern Med 98:846, 1983.

73. Berglund G, Andersson O, Wilhelmsen L. Prevalence of primary and secondary hypertension: Studies in a random population sample. BMJ 2:554, 1976.

74. Lewin A, Blaufox D, Castle H, et al Apparent prevalence of curable hypertension in the Hypertension Detection and Follow-up Program. Arch Intern Med 145:424, 1985.

75. Sinclair AM, Isles CG, Brown I, et al. Secondary hypertension in a blood pressure clinic. Arch Intern Med 147:1289, 1987.

76. Maheswaran R, Beevers M, Beevers DG. Effectiveness of advice to reduce alcohol consumption in hypertensive patients. Hypertension 19:79, 1992.

77. Klatsky AL, Armstrong MA, Friedman GD. Alcohol and mortality. Ann Intern Med 117:646, 1992.

78. Thun MJ, Peto R, Lopez AD, et al. Alcohol consumption and mortality among middle-aged and elderly U.S. adults. N Engl J Med 337:1705, 1997.

79. Friedman GD, Klatsky AL. Is alcohol good for your health? N Engl J Med 329:1882, 1993.

80. Pearson TA, Terry P. What to advise patients about drinking alcohol. JAMA 272:957, 1994.

81. National High Blood Pressure Education Program Working Group: Report on primary prevention of hypertension. Arch Intern Med 153:194, 1993.

Target Organ Damage/Cardiovascular Complications

CHAPTER 24 Total Risk
Michael H. Alderman

The purpose of blood pressure treatment is to reduce the incidence of cardiovascular disease. Efficacy and efficiency are the guiding principles by which strategies designed to achieve this goal are assessed. *Efficacy* is the extent to which a given intervention achieves disease protection. In practical terms, this is the fraction of benefit achieved by each treated person as well as the fraction of all potential beneficiaries who receive that treatment. *Efficiency,* by contrast, is the extent to which these interventions are applied only in situations where likelihood of disease and potential for prevention justify such intervention. This concept is sometimes expressed as the number needed to treat for each person benefited. The hope, of course, is that persons with trivial risk will be spared what might be lifelong medicalization.

These concepts may be straightforward, but their application is extraordinarily difficult. The appearance of orally effective and acceptable antihypertensive drugs in the late 1950s transformed the issue of who might benefit from a theoretical to an intensely practical matter. As recognition of the many factors contributing to cardiovascular disease expression expanded, and the number of tools capable of modifying these other risk factors multiplied, the complexity of responding to the challenges of managing blood pressure with efficiency and effectiveness has increased.

CLINICAL CHALLENGE

The medical management of high blood pressure depends on the answers to two fundamental questions: Whom to treat? How to treat? The difficulty, of course, is to establish the criteria by which to answer these questions. Basic to all medical treatment is to identify those persons needing and capable of responding to the intervention in question—in other words, to make a diagnosis. Usually, the condition at issue is a disease. The need is to determine its presence or absence. Detection of the tubercle bacillus initiates a definitive therapeutic process marked by rather precise milestones.

Tuberculosis is diagnosed by definitive disease-specific criteria. Regrettably, hypertension is not. It is not a disease, but rather a risk factor. Moreover, it is one, among many, that contribute to the occurrence of stroke, heart attack,

end-stage renal disease, and congestive heart failure. The relationship of blood pressure to these conditions is linear, positive, and continuous over the full range of pressures[1] (Fig. 24–1). There is no level of blood pressure, either diastolic or systolic, that distinguishes those who will from those who will not experience an event. Instead, as pressure increases, the risk of an event increases with a regular, reliable cadence. The difference in event occurrence associated with any fixed variance in pressure is, so far as is known, the same at every part of the blood pressure range.

This is *relative risk*. Thus, blood pressure level tells us what the percentage difference in event likelihood between one individual or group and another will be—as long as the two groups or individuals differ only in blood pressure level. Thus, whereas knowledge of pressure provides some information, it tells us nothing about the actual likelihood of an event for a person or the incidence in a group. The answer to that question requires that all cardiovascular disease–determining characteristics be summed. An individual's history, behavior, genetics, clinical, and laboratory measures all contribute to the *absolute risk* of disease.

In the practical world, patients and physicians are most interested in the answers to two questions: What are the chances of my experiencing a heart attack over some period of time? By what fraction would my risk of a heart attack fall if my pressure were lower? The first question relates to *absolute* and the second to *relative* risk. Most clinical decisions in management of blood pressure depend on an accurate answer to both questions.

The purpose of this chapter is to explore the use of both relative and absolute expressions of risk to address two major clinical questions. The first is whether or not to treat; the second is the nature of the treatment. The basis for answering the first question is the natural history of persons with different levels of pressure. The answer to the second question can be found through examination of treated patients.

DECISION TO TREAT

Because the relationship between blood pressure and likelihood of cardiovascular events is linear, an ideal approach to realizing the benefit of lower pressure would be univer-

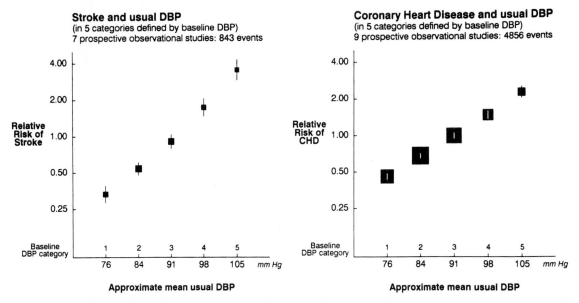

Figure 24–1. Relative risk for stroke and coronary heart disease (CHD). Estimates of the usual diastolic blood pressure (DBP) in each baseline DBP category are taken from mean DBP values 4 years after baseline in the Framingham Study. *Solid squares* represent disease risks in each category relative to risk in the whole study population; *sizes of squares* are proportional to number of events in each DBP category; and 95% confidence intervals for estimates of relative risk are denoted by *vertical lines*. (From Alderman MH. Blood pressure management: Individualized treatment based on absolute risk and the potential for benefit. Ann Intern Med 11:9:329–335, 1993.)

sal blood pressure reduction. It has been calculated that a very modest (3 to 4 mm Hg) reduction in diastolic pressure for the entire population would save more lives than successful treatment limited only to hypertensive patients. Attractive as such a public health strategy might be, the tools necessary to accomplish this goal have so far eluded medical science. The impediments to moving the population curve of blood pressure distribution to the left include absence of fully effective interventions and an inability to produce the behavior changes necessary to deliver the tools that exist. As a result, the only truly available proven safe strategy is the so-called high-risk, or medical care approach. This involves the identification and pharmacological treatment of each patient believed to be appropriate for such intervention. Since resources are limited, even though virtually everyone, whatever their pressure, might conceivably be better off with a lower pressure, only a finite number of persons can practically be treated.

The national strategy for antihypertensive therapy has been based on assignment of a level of blood pressure to distinguish those who should from those who should not be treated. The National High Blood Pressure Education Program, begun in 1972, has advocated, mostly recently, that the label of *hypertension* be applied to those whose pressures exceed either 140 mm Hg systolic or 90 mm Hg diastolic. One can hardly gainsay the value of such an approach. In fact, since 1972, stroke mortality has declined by nearly 60%, and cardiac mortality by nearly half. Although these dramatic results cannot be entirely attributed to antihypertensive therapy, there can be no doubt that the increasingly successful effort to detect, treat, and control the top 15% or so of the blood pressure distribution has yielded important health dividends.

BEYOND THE BLOOD PRESSURE THRESHOLD

Over the last few years, however, a growing consensus has emerged that recognizes a dissonance between available biomedical and epidemiological knowledge and practice.[2] No pressure threshold separates those who will from those who will not experience disease. In fact, most cardiovascular events occur below the current threshold. Moreover, with growing capacity to quantify absolute risk, the limitations of exclusive reliance on blood pressure to allocate antihypertensive resources in terms of efficacy and efficiency has become manifest. The simple strategy has led to treatment of many persons above the current threshold, despite minimal risk of an event and, therefore, trivial expectation of benefit. At the same time, many who are near but below the current threshold, despite very high risk, are arbitrarily denied therapy.

The problem is that total reliance on relative risk as defined by a particular blood pressure level is unreasonable. It is certainly true that for every 5- to 6-mm Hg increase in diastolic pressure, there is a 40% increase in stroke events. For heart attacks, a similar increase in diastolic pressure yields a 25% increase in events. This relation is a useful measure of the impact of a risk factor, in this case blood pressure, on the relative incidence of events. Moreover, the predictive value of these observational data has been confirmed through intervention trials. Repeatedly, antihypertensive drug trials have shown that a 5- to 6-mm Hg decline in diastolic pressure yields a roughly 40% fall in strokes; exactly what was predicted from observational studies. The results for heart attack have been less satisfactory: The actual benefit has been 14 to 17% in clinical trials that produced the same blood pressure difference.

Despite the remarkable precision with which relative risk can be predicted, it provides no information about either the actual likelihood of an event for an individual or the incidence for a group. This is explained by the difference between absolute and relative risk. The actual incidence (absolute risk) of events is determined by the totality of the relevant characteristics of the group or of the individual.[3] High blood pressure is not a disease, but only one of many risk factors that contribute to stroke or heart attack. For example, based on the Framingham experience, the 10-year probability of stroke may vary five- or sixfold at the same level of pressure within a group of 55-year-old white males (Fig. 24–2).[4] Thus, two patients with very "normal" systolic pressures (136 mm Hg) can have a 10-year stroke expectation indistinguishable from that of all persons that age (5.9%) or a rate more than five times that of this age cohort. Even more remarkable is that the risk for a high-risk normotensive person (A) may exceed that of another 55-year-old whose systolic blood pressure is 170 mm Hg. Clearly, blood pressure alone is a poor predictor of cardiovascular events.

Translating this expectation of disease into treatment paradigms produces several obvious anomalies. Assume that the treatment of 100 subjects matching the description of patient C would reduce the 10-year stroke incidence by 40%. In real or absolute terms, this would mean a fall from 5.4 to 3.2 events—a prevention of 2 events achieved by the treatment of 100 persons for 10 years. At the same time, a 5- to 6-mm Hg decline in diastolic pressure for 100 patients similar to subject A, assuming a similar 40% benefit, would prevent 6 times as many strokes (32.9 to 19.7) as the previous example. The estimate of benefit is based on the assumption that the difference in events associated with a given decrease in pressure is similar at all blood pressure levels. Clearly, however, no clinical trial confirms the assumption that blood pressure reduction of 5 to 6 mm Hg would generate the hoped-for benefit in persons with blood pressures below 140/90 mm Hg. However, based on the real risk of a stroke and the great potential for benefit in this situation, intervention seems justified.

A variety of instruments now define absolute risk based on the pattern of target organ disease and/or cardiovascular risk factors.[5] To one extent or another, almost all national guidelines now incorporate the need to modify the traditional blood pressure threshold, or relative risk approach.[6] Virtually all recommendations now incorporate some degree of reliance on absolute risk. At the same time, no guideline advocates that relative risk, or blood pressure thresholds, be eliminated. New Zealand has perhaps gone farthest in producing specific treatment recommendations based on absolute risk of disease after a level of pressure is reached.[7] They suggest that treatment be reserved for those with a 10-year expectation of events of 10% or greater.

WHY BOTH ABSOLUTE AND RELATIVE RISK ARE IMPORTANT

Just as dogged reliance on relative risk generates treatment decisions that are both inefficient and not optimally effective, full reliance on absolute risk would produce other problems. For example, the most important determinant of absolute risk is age. In the near-term, absolute risk, and therefore anticipated benefit, is greater in older than younger persons—even when other characteristics are similar. The fact is that a combination of relative and absolute risk provides the best strategy to decide whom to treat. Thus, it may make more sense in older persons to place greater emphasis on absolute risk, since the near-term potential for benefit is amplified at this end of the age spectrum. By contrast, for younger subjects with lower near-term absolute risk, relative risk might become more compelling. Over a longer time frame, however, the years of life added to young people might be as great as that realized by older persons who are at far-greater absolute risk. The problem is created in part because our ability to assess risk and benefit over the long-term is limited.

In sum, the wealth of available information makes one thing certain. No simple answer for all persons, in all situations, is available. Cookbook decisions incompletely apply the knowledge we have and are therefore inadequate to the needs of doctors and patients. Moreover, decisions to treat must be seen in terms of the legitimate needs of society. Cost-benefit analysis further complicates the issue

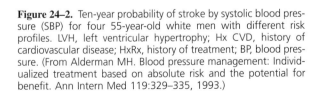

Figure 24–2. Ten-year probability of stroke by systolic blood pressure (SBP) for four 55-year-old white men with different risk profiles. LVH, left ventricular hypertrophy; Hx CVD, history of cardiovascular disease; HxRx, history of treatment; BP, blood pressure. (From Alderman MH. Blood pressure management: Individualized treatment based on absolute risk and the potential for benefit. Ann Intern Med 119:329–335, 1993.)

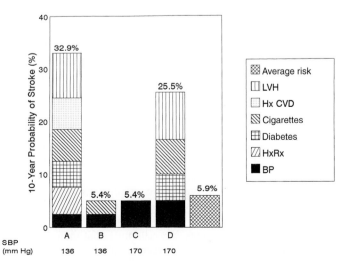

of whom to treat because resources will always be limited. As the potential for benefit recedes, the willingness to allocate scarce resources to achieve a marginal benefit evaporates.

Perhaps of more immediate concern to the physician is that individual patients differ in their desire to accept or avoid risk. The role of the physician is not to dictate the choice, but rather to ensure that his or her patient understands both the risk and the potential for benefit. To this end, the physician must understand both absolute and relative risk and be able to translate that knowledge effectively. There is good evidence that patients respond differently to therapeutic choices when they are framed in "relative" ("You can expect a 20% decline in your likelihood of an event with treatment") or a combination of "relative" and "absolute" risk calculations ("Untreated you have a 5 out of 100 chance of a stroke, treatment can reduce that by 20% to 4 out of 100").

In a sense, what is happening is a paradigm shift. Not surprisingly, such marked shifts in thinking and, in this case, practice are neither quick nor simple. Good sense and inertia combine to ensure that the change will be evolutionary rather than revolutionary.

RISK STRATIFICATION IN TREATED HYPERTENSIVE PATIENTS

The data on which the decision to treat is based derive from studies of natural history in which the value of lowering blood pressure is assessed. The model for such observational studies is the Framingham Heart Study. Begun before effective antihypertensive therapy was available, and long before its widespread use, this study examined the unmodified experience of persons at different levels of blood pressure. It thus provided a basis for estimating risk without treatment and how treatment might potentially modify that risk. This elegant, farsighted, and large-scale study has provided the basis for much of current strategy for research and practice in hypertension.

Since Framingham was initiated in the late 1940s, a variety of effective antihypertensive agents have emerged that are capable of not only lowering blood pressure but also preventing heart attacks and strokes. As a result, since the early 1970s, the detection, treatment, and control of high blood pressure—at successively lower levels—has been national policy. Although the full potential of this ambitious goal has proved elusive, more than 25 million hypertensive Americans are now receiving antihypertensive drug therapy. At least half of these, or 12 to 15 million Americans, have achieved and maintained a blood pressure less than 140/90 mm Hg. Current practice is to maintain lifelong antihypertensive therapy. Since treatment generally begins in the fifth or sixth decade of life, it can be expected to continue for as long as 40 or even 50 years. It is likely that millions of Americans have maintained "controlled blood pressure" for decades.

Effective antihypertensive treatment prevents approximately 25 to 30% of strokes and heart attacks. Therefore, 75% of events anticipated in the natural state still occur. It is unlikely that these events are randomly distributed in this newly invented cohort of "recovered" hypertensive patients. Much more likely (and, in fact, the case) is that cardiovascular risk in these treated hypertensive patients with controlled blood pressure can be predicted on the basis of identifiable characteristics—just as was the case for untreated patients. The question, of course, is what are those characteristics? Are they, for example, the same as those found so serviceable in the natural state? Answers to these questions can be found only by study of patients in this modified state, i.e., a Framingham-type study for controlled hypertensives to associate baseline characteristics with subsequent cardiovascular events that occur during the course of therapy. Identifying risk in advance provides the chance to modify therapy in the hope of further cardioprotection.

Some rigorously obtained data, following the Framingham pattern, are emerging to describe experience in long-term treatment.[8, 9] As a result, real understanding of the distribution and determinants of cardiovascular events in recovered hypertensive patients is evolving. One set of data derives from a worksite-based program of antihypertensive therapy provided primarily by nurses, with physician supervision, according to a protocol.[10] Begun in 1973, it serves several labor unions in New York City. Historical, clinical, and laboratory data were uniformly obtained and stored on computer at baseline and at each visit. All morbidity and mortality data are captured by the sponsoring unions.

The experience of 8690 hypertensive patients with an average follow-up of 5.7 years is now available. Participants who met entry blood pressure criteria included approximately 60% men, 43% whites, 30% blacks, and 24% Hispanics, with a mean age of 53 years, and a mean initial blood pressure of 152/96 mm Hg (including treated and untreated subjects). Fewer than 4% of subjects had a previous heart attack, about 2% had a stroke, and 7% of the men and nearly 9% of the women had a history of diabetes. In treatment, blood pressure averaged 140/84 mm Hg.

During 50,000 person-years of follow-up, there were 468 first cardiovascular disease events, including 282 myocardial infarctions and/or revascularization procedures, 93 strokes, 30 hospitalized first episodes of congestive heart failure, and 63 other cardiovascular deaths. These initial cardiovascular events accounted for 80% of the hospital morbidity and mortality of the group. Clearly, despite the 25% reduction in events that was expected by virtue of blood pressure reduction, cardiovascular disease remains the principal cause of morbidity and morbidity in this cohort of recovered hypertensive patients.

Of note, the pattern of events changed markedly over time (Fig. 24–3). Cardiac events were most prominent throughout, but after the first 10 years of controlled pressure, the expected age-related increase in heart attacks disappeared. Perhaps more prolonged blood pressure reduction increases the benefit of treatment. If this is true, it may partly account for the shortfall between expected and achieved cardioprotection seen in clinical trials of antihypertensive therapy. The trials may have been too short to detect the full cardioprotective effect of lowering pressure. At the same time, the incidence of congestive heart failure as a first event in these controlled hypertensive patients increased 10-fold during the study period. After 10 years in treatment, congestive heart failure replaced stroke as the second most common cardiovascular event. These data

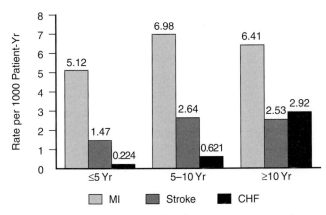

Figure 24–3. Changing patterns of cardiovascular events according to time in therapy. MI, myocardial infarction; CHF, congestive heart failure.

raise the possibility that as disease expression changes, the factors responsible for events may also change. It may ultimately be necessary to reassess risk at different time intervals to determine the factors responsible for the evolving distribution of cardiovascular events.

In this study, the goal was to identify, at entry, the patient characteristics that were associated with the development of cardiovascular morbidity and mortality over the ensuing 18 years. Based on these characteristics, criteria were identified to stratify patients into four distinct prognostic categories.

Intake characteristics assessed for their predictive value included pretreatment blood pressure. In sharp contrast to the pattern in untreated patients, diastolic blood pressure by itself was not associated with events. Systolic blood pressure had a modest positive association. However, the most powerful and only independent predictor of events was pulse pressure (Fig. 24–4). Clearly, the course of disease is predicted by different factors in patients whose environment has been altered, so that it no longer includes raised diastolic blood pressure.

The association of other historical, clinical, and laboratory factors with cardiovascular events is depicted in Figure 24–5. The bars indicate the specific hazard ratio for each characteristic. The far right bar depicts risk for those whose

only risk factor at entry was elevated blood pressure. Such patients, treated to eliminate their elevated pressure, actually had event rates below those of the Framingham subjects of comparable age and gender. Conventional risk factors, as identified in Framingham, are also predictors in these treated patients. Not surprisingly, history of stroke, heart attack, and diabetes carries the gravest prognostic threat. Most striking is the impressive increase in risk associated with a pulse pressure above 60 mm Hg. The stars in each bar indicate population-attributable risk. In a sense, this combines the severity and prevalence of a marker to estimate contribution to the group's burden of disease. Thus, whereas history of stroke or myocardial infarction conveys the greatest individual threat, the rarity of a history of these events in this relatively healthy population means that these factors contributed little to the overall incidence of events. Pulse pressure, by contrast, was of substantially greater import.

Through multivariate analysis, it was possible to identify those factors with an independent association with cardiovascular events over the next 18 years. In addition to age and gender, history of diabetes, stroke, and myocardial infarction/revascularization, and pulse pressure were each associated with a greater than 50% increase in risk. These factors, minus gender, were then used to stratify the population into four prognostic categories: low = no other risk factor; moderate = 1; high = 2; and very high subjects = 3 of these markers.

The expectation of disease events occurring over 18 years of successful antihypertensive care differed sharply among groups (Fig. 24–6). The power of this simple stratification scheme can be seen in the virtual doubling of event incidence with each increasing category. There was a nearly 10-fold difference in expectation of events between the highest and the lowest groups. It is noteworthy that although this stratification reveals impressive differences in both absolute and relative risk, the majority of events did not occur in the highest category, which included less than 10% of subjects, but in the middle categories, where the majority of subjects were found. Inclusion of markers such as left ventricular hypertrophy and plasma renin activity can substantially increase precision of the estimate of risk.

To what use can this simple stratification system be put? In different populations, determinants might differ in

Figure 24–4. Age-adjusted cardiovascular disease incidence by pretreatment blood pressure. (From Alderman MH, Cohen H, Madhavan S. Distribution and determinants of cardiovascular events during 20 years of successful antihypertensive treatment. J Hypertens 16:761–769, 1998.)

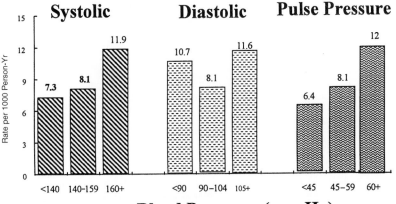

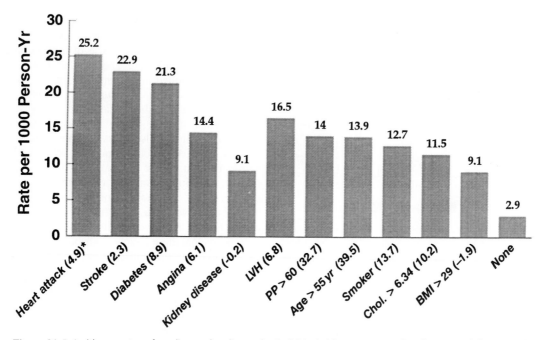

Figure 24–5. Incidence rates of cardiovascular disease by individual risk measures at baseline. LVH, left ventricular hypertrophy; PP, pulse pressure; Chol., cholesterol; BMI, body mass index. (From Alderman MH, Cohen H, Madhavan S. Distribution and determinants of cardiovascular events during 20 years of successful antihypertensive treatment. J Hypertens 16:761–769, 1998.) *Numbers in parentheses indicate population attributable risk percentage.

weight. Extrapolation from these data to groups who differ in important ways from these largely healthy, working, middle-aged persons must be made with caution. First of all, it must be clear that this scheme is of value after the decision to treat has been made. This scheme helps to predict the distribution of events during successful conventional care. Thus, risk stratification at the beginning of treatment provides some clue about where modification of conventional care might profitably be made. Just as risk in the natural state helps identify those who should receive

antihypertensive therapy, risk definition in treated patients helps identify the potential that might attend additional or varied treatment. It would be reasonable to assume that current conventional practice is sufficient for the low-risk group. For example, if current studies support the use of aspirin in hypertensive patients, this may be an intervention of sufficiently low intensity and cost to be applicable to all but perhaps the lowest-risk subjects. Since even aspirin carries some potential for adverse reaction, this might outweigh its benefit in extremely low-risk groups. Recent studies indicate a need to adjust choice of drug to particular situations. The benefit of converting-enzyme inhibitors in diabetic hypertensive patients is a case in point.

The highest-risk subjects, with an annual event rate incidence of 3.4%—higher than an average group of post–myocardial infarction patients—are clearly candidates for more vigorous intervention that could go well beyond conventional practice. Multiple therapeutic opportunities, with varying degrees of evidential support, exist. For example, treatments that have proved successful in secondary prevention of myocardial infarction, such as β-blockade, interference with the renin-angiotensin system, and reduction of low-density lipoprotein cholesterol to extremely low levels—even in patients with normal total cholesterol—should be considered.

Optimal blood pressure goals in antihypertensive treatment have generally been controversial and not evidence-based. The recently completed Hypertension Optimal Treatment (HOT) Study[11] was designed to address the question of whether treatment to a lower (<90 mm Hg diastolic) blood pressure would improve cardioprotection. Patients were randomized to three goal pressures (<90, <85, and <80 mm Hg). Although rather smaller differences between the three groups were actually achieved, the

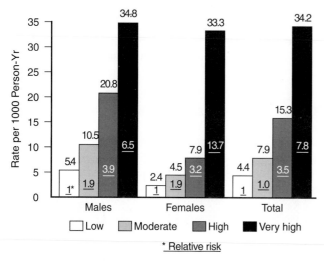

Figure 24–6. Incidence of cardiovascular disease in treated hypertensive patients by risk profile and gender. (From Alderman MH, Cohen H, Madhavan S. Distribution and determinants of cardiovascular events during 20 years of successful antihypertensive treatment. J Hypertens 16:761–769, 1998.)

authors concluded that a pressure of about 138/93 mm Hg was associated with the best outcomes. In general, further reduction of blood pressure did not provide additional cardioprotection. The single exception was for diabetic patients, who did benefit from greater blood pressure reduction.

CONCLUSIONS

The management of blood pressure in the pursuit of cardiovascular disease prevention is an inexact science. A paradigm that permits simple choices will remain elusive as long as the basis for determining risk is probabilistic. The strategy discussed here does not provide a rigid decision-tree analysis, but rather suggests an approach to the resolution of the two most important questions in blood pressure management. More refined risk assessment is the only means available to improve the basis for determining whom should be treated. Thereafter, treatment should be tailored to match the magnitude of cardiovascular risk and the potential for benefit. The optimal use of ever more effective instruments of prevention will, in large measure, depend on the wisdom by which decisions to treat high blood pressure, and the design of that treatment, are made.

References

1. MacMahon S, Peto R, Cutler J, et al. Blood pressure, stroke, and coronary heart disease. Part 1: Prolonged differences in blood pressure: Prospective observational studies corrected for the regression dilution bias. Lancet 335:765–774, 1990.
2. Menard J, Chatellier G. Mild hypertension: The mysterious viability of a faulty concept. J Hypertens 13:1071–1077, 1995.
3. Alderman MH. Blood pressure management: Individualized treatment based on absolute risk and the potential for benefit. Ann Intern Med 119:329–335, 1993.
4. Kannel WB. Hypertension and the risk of cardiovascular disease. *In* Laragh JH, Brenner BM (eds). Hypertension: Pathophysiology, Diagnosis, and Management. New York, Raven, 1990.
5. Black HR, Yi JY. A new classification scheme for hypertension based on relative and absolute risk with implications for treatment and reimbursement. Hypertension 28:719–724, 1996.
6. Joint National Committee on Prevention, Detection, Evaluation, and Treatment of High Blood Pressure. The sixth report. Arch Intern Med 157:2413–2446, 1997.
7. Jackson R, Barham P, Bills J, et al. Management of raised blood pressure in New Zealand: A discussion document. BMJ 307:107–110, 1993.
8. Bulpitt CJ, Palmer AJ, Fletcher AE, et al. Optimal blood pressure control in treated hypertensive patients. Report from the Department of Health Hypertension Care Computing Project (DHCCP). Circulation 90:225–233, 1994.
9. Samuelsson O, Pennert K, Andersson O, et al. Diabetes mellitus and raised serum triglycerides concentration in treated hypertension—Are they of prognostic importance? Observational study. BMJ 313:660–663, 1996.
10. Alderman MH, Cohen H, Madhavan S. Distribution and determinants of cardiovascular events during 20 years of successful antihypertensive treatment. J Hypertens 16:761–769, 1998.
11. Hansson L, Zanchetti A, Carruthers SG, et al. Effects of intensive blood-pressure lowering and low-dose aspirin in patients with hypertension: Principal results of the Hypertension Optimal Treatment (HOT) randomised trial. Lancet 351:1647–1649, 1998.

---

25 New Interpretations of Blood Pressure: The Importance of Pulse Pressure

Stanley S. Franklin

Hypertension as a cardiovascular risk factor continues to elude precise definition. Since the introduction of the sphygmomanometer, the chief criteria for defining high blood pressure have been peak systolic blood pressure (SBP) and end-diastolic blood pressure (DBP) as measured at the brachial artery. In contrast, *hypertension* refers to increased transmural pressure secondary to elevated arteriolar and small artery resistance; this is derived from the measurement of mean arterial pressure (MAP), utilizing the area under the curve of the pressure wave.

The principal components of blood pressure consist of both a steady-state component of resistance, represented by MAP, and a pulsatile component of impedance, represented by pulse pressure (PP).[1–5] PP is the difference between peak SBP and end DBP. At any given ventricular ejection, cardiac output, and heart rate, large artery stiffness and the influence of early wave reflection determine PP. PP, therefore, is a surrogate measurement of the cyclical influence of impedance on arterial pressure. Both arteriolar/small artery resistance and large artery impedance contribute to hypertensive cardiovascular risk. The principal question that remains to be answered is, How important is PP as a measure of this risk?

HISTORICAL PERSPECTIVE

Our understanding of the contributions of blood pressure components to cardiovascular disease risk has undergone considerable change since the introduction of the sphygmomanometer at the beginning of the 20th century. Initially, SBP was equated with the maximal force of the heart, and DBP was equated with the resistance that the heart has to overcome.[6] Drug intervention studies during the 1960s through the 1980s defined severity of hypertension solely on the basis of DBP. Since the Framingham Heart Study in 1971, more weight has been given to SBP in defining hypertensive cardiovascular risk.[7–9] Persuasive support for the benefit of treating SBP came from the 1991 landmark Systolic Hypertension in the Elderly Program (SHEP),[10] involving isolated systolic hypertension exclusively and showing significant reductions in stroke, acute myocardial infarction, and heart failure events. These findings were confirmed by the British Medical Research Council Study[11] and the Swedish Trial in Old Patients with Hypertension,[12] studies of the elderly with predominantly systolic hypertension. These population and intervention studies in elderly subjects with systolic hypertension resulted in new national[13] and international[14] guidelines in 1993: Either SBP or DBP, whichever is higher, defines hypertensive cardiovascular risk. Since the late 1980s, a body of evidence has accumulated indicating that in older hypertensive subjects, there is an inverse relation between DBP and risk of cardiovascular disease, suggesting that PP may be an important predictor of cardiovascular events.[15–26]

HEMODYNAMIC IMPLICATIONS

In elderly subjects, the hemodynamic basis for increased PP is not increased cardiac output or bradycardia, but instead, increased central artery stiffness.[1–5] The vessels affected are the elastic arteries: the thoracic aorta and its primary branches. Both increases in peripheral resistance and central artery stiffness elevate brachial artery cuff SBP. In contrast, cuff DBP rises with increases in resistance but falls with increases in stiffness; the combination of these two effects determines the final DBP.

Two clinical patterns of blood pressure elevation can be recognized. If arteriolar resistance increases greatly and there is a small increase in arterial stiffness, DBP rises to at least 90 mm Hg, a condition classified as *combined systolic/diastolic hypertension.* If arterial stiffness increases greatly and there is a small increase in resistance, DBP remains normal or decreases below normal, a condition

classified as *isolated systolic hypertension.* Both patterns are seen in the elderly, with the latter found more commonly with increasing age.

The heart is exposed to the central aortic pressure—not to the brachial artery pressure. The latter offers only a limited view of the arterial tree. To understand how information regarding large central arteries can be obtained from the peripheral brachial artery requires knowledge of arterial pulse propagation and reflection.[27–29] In normal ventricular-vascular coupling, reflected waves impact on the central arteries during diastole, resulting in improved coronary perfusion. Increases in central artery stiffness are associated with increases in pressure and velocity of the incident wave, which returns earlier and impacts the central arteries during systole rather than diastole. This increases ventricular afterload (see Chap. 14, Arterial Stiffness). The effect of early wave reflection on aortic PP can be determined by the *augmentation index,* defined as the percentage of PP from the first shoulder to the late systolic peak of the pressure wave.[28] In elderly hypertensive subjects, early wave reflection can produce increases in amplitude of SBP up to 40 to 50% in the ascending aorta.[28] These hemodynamic changes are associated with both a rise in SBP and a fall in DBP, resulting in an increase in central PP.

Normally, in young subjects with elastic arteries, wave reflection results in a progressive increase in the amplitude of PP from the central to the peripheral arteries (Fig. 25–1). This amplification phenomenon overestimates central PP when measurement is made from brachial artery cuff pressures. As a result of amplification, a young person with borderline hypertension, as measured in the brachial artery, may have a normal aortic PP. With aging, there is a change in this hemodynamic pattern. Augmentation of the central PP by early wave reflection in subjects 50 years of age or older eliminates the amplification effect found in young

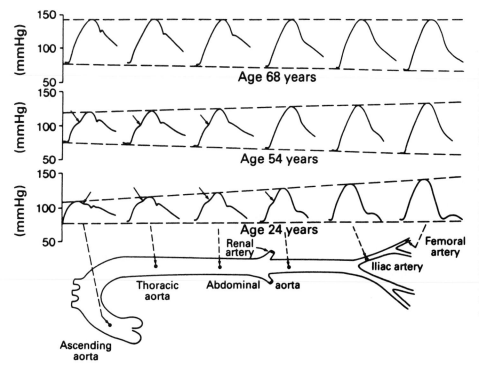

Figure 25–1. Pressure wave recorded along the arterial tree from the proximal ascending aorta to the femoral artery in three adult subjects aged 24, 54, and 68 years. In the youngest subject, amplification of the pressure wave increases approximately 60% during transmission. In contrast, the oldest subject shows minimal amplification of the pressure wave during transmission. With aging, there is a progressive increase in systolic blood pressure (SBP) and a decrease in diastolic blood pressure (DBP). (From Nichols WW, Avolio AP, Kelly RP, O'Rourke MF. Effect of age and of hypertension on wave travel and reflections. *In* O'Rourke MF, Safar ME, Dzau JV [eds]. Arterial Vasodilation: Mechanisms and Therapy. London, Edward Arnold, 1993.)

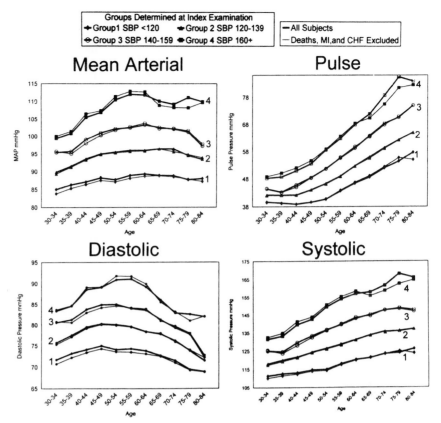

Figure 25–2. Arterial pressure components by age: Group-averaged data for all subjects and with deaths, myocardial infarction (MI), and congestive heart failure (CHF) excluded. Averaged blood pressure levels from all available data from each subject within 5-year age intervals (30 to 34 through 80 to 84) by systolic blood pressure (SBP) groupings 1 through 4. *Thick line* represents the entire study cohort (2036 subjects); *thin line* represents study cohort with deaths, nonfatal MI, and CHF excluded (1353 subjects). MAP, mean arterial pressure. (From Franklin SS, Gustin WG, Wong ND, et al. Hemodynamic patterns of age-related changes in blood pressure. The Framingham Heart Study. Circulation 96:308–315, 1997. By permission of the American Heart Association, Inc.)

subjects.[29, 30] PP in middle-aged and older subjects tends to be similar in central and peripheral arteries regardless of blood pressure values (Fig. 25–1). Therefore, brachial artery cuff measurement of PP in this age group becomes more of a surrogate measurement of central elastic artery stiffness and early pulse-wave reflection.[29, 30]

AGE-RELATED CHANGES IN BLOOD PRESSURE

Numerous studies have shown a progressive increase in blood pressure with aging in industrialized societies.[31] We reported on age-related changes in blood pressure in both normotensive and untreated hypertensive subjects in a population-based cohort from the original Framingham Heart Study[32] (Fig. 25–2). There was a linear rise in SBP from ages 30 through 84 years and a concurrent early increase in DBP and MAP. After age 60 years, DBP declined, PP rose steeply, and MAP reached an asymptote. The reduction in DBP has been attributed to "burned-out" diastolic hypertension, but this decrease in DBP was noted in both normotensive and untreated hypertensive subjects. Similarly, the concept of "selective survivorship" has been postulated as a cause of the late decline in DBP, but this was not consistent with the persistence of the late fall in DBP after removal of all deaths and patients with nonfatal myocardial infarction or heart failure from the study sample (Fig. 25–2). The most likely explanation for the fall in DBP after age 60 years, therefore, was increased large artery stiffness.[1–5, 32, 33]

The decline in DBP seen in the elderly is probably the result rather than the cause of the disease process. With age-related stiffening of the aorta, there is a decreased capacity of the elastic reservoir and a greater peripheral runoff of stroke volume during systole. With less blood remaining in the aorta at the beginning of diastole, and with diminished elastic recoil, DBP decreases with increased steepness of the diastolic decay curve.[34]

Calculated MAP from brachial blood pressure readings approximates the peripheral vascular resistance, particularly when cardiac output is not elevated.[4, 32] True vascular resistance is underestimated by the MAP equation in individuals $\geq$ age 50 years when one uses the brachial artery pressures (see Fig. 25–2). In these subjects, the area under the arterial pulse wave curve during cardiac catherization is more reliable (Fig. 25–3). The leveling off and eventual fall in DBP associated with the alteration of pulse-wave contour result in a shift of the standard form factor of 0.33 toward 0.5[35] (Fig. 25–3). Undoubtedly, after age 50 years, the MAP equation is no longer a surrogate measurement for vascular resistance.

The almost parallel increases in SBP, DBP, and MAP from ages 30 to 49 years in the Framingham Heart Study[32] support a rise in peripheral resistance. In contrast, after age 60 years, elevated large artery impedance (large artery stiffness and early pulse-wave reflection) becomes the dominant hemodynamic factor that is responsible for further elevation in SBP. Whereas measurements of cardiac output and blood pressure suggest increased vascular resistance with aging,[36] systemic vascular resistance is actually only marginally elevated in older subjects with isolated

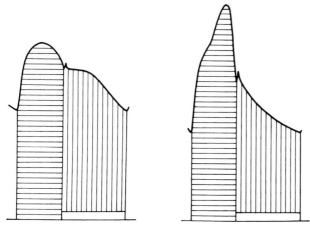

Figure 25–3. Diagrammatic representation of aortic blood pressure curve in younger *(left)* and older *(right)* subjects. The mean SBP time index is shown in the *horizontally hatched area* and the DBP time index in the *vertically hatched area*. The areas under the two curves are identical. Because cardiac periods are the same, the mean arterial pressures are identical. (From O'Rourke MF. Arterial Function in Health and Disease. Edinburgh, Churchill Livingstone, 1982.)

systolic hypertension compared with age- and sex-matched normotensive control subjects.[37, 38] Confirmatory evidence comes from catheterization studies in elderly subjects with isolated systolic hypertension in which increased impedance predominated over increased vascular resistance.[39] Antecedent untreated hypertension, moreover, was associated with an accelerated rise in SBP (and fall in DBP) after age 60 years, consistent with a greater increase in large artery impedance.[32] Higher SBP, left untreated, may accelerate large artery stiffness and thus perpetuate a vicious circle.

The age-related linear rise in SBP from ages 30 to 84 years, coupled with an early rise and late fall in DBP, suggests three hemodynamic phases. Under age 50 years, the progressive rise in DBP suggests the predominance of increased vascular resistance. The constancy of DBP during the 50s, together with the asymptotic leveling of MAP and increased slope of PP, suggests that increased vascular resistance and large artery stiffness are both increasing in a parallel manner. The fall in DBP after age 60 years signals a preponderance of large artery stiffness as the cause of further rise in SBP.

CAUSE OF LARGE ARTERY STIFFNESS

Increased arterial stiffness may be functional or structural. Young hypertensive subjects have a somewhat greater rise in SBP than in DBP. This small functional increase in PP can be explained by a "downstream" increase in resistance causing an "upstream" increase in transmural pressure, which in turn stretches large central arteries and increases their stiffness. In addition to the functional stiffening from increased transmural pressure, a variety of neurohumoral mechanisms, such as increased sympathetic tone, increased renin-angiotensin system activity, and net local vascular vasoconstrictor influences, increase large artery stiffness.[40]

With aging and hypertension, there is minimal change in

the stiffness of muscular peripheral arteries.[1, 5] In contrast, longstanding structural changes cause increased stiffness of the elastic proximal aorta. Elastin, with a half-life of 40 years, is one of the most stable proteins in the body.[41] Fatigue of elastin fibers and lamellae, however, can occur by the middle of the sixth decade of life from the accumulated cyclic stress of more than 2 billion systolic expansions of the aorta. The likely pathological explanation for the development of large artery stiffness is the thinning, fragmentation, and eventual fracturing of elastin;[42] increased collagen and calcium deposition may also play a role in this process.[42] Untreated hypertension, by increasing cyclical stress during systole, may amplify the degenerative process, leading to earlier and more severe arterial stiffening. There is evidence of gender differences in arterial stiffening, with young women having more compliant vessels than men at similar ages. With the onset of menopause, estrogen deficiency may accelerate the arterial stiffening process.[43] Other factors that have been incriminated in accelerating arterial stiffness are high dietary salt intake,[44] cigarette smoking,[45] diabetes,[19] renal failure,[46] hyperhomocysteinemia,[47] and atherosclerosis.[48]

CLINICAL RELEVANCE OF INCREASED PULSE PRESSURE

If arterial stiffness is a risk factor for cardiovascular disease, elevated PP and reduced DBP should be markers of this risk. Considerable evidence now favors the importance of PP as a predictor of a wide variety of cardiovascular diseases. Longitudinal studies in geriatric hypertensive subjects have shown that high PP and low DBP are sensitive markers for carotid artery stenosis. These include a study of eastern Finnish men,[16] the Cardiovascular Health Study,[17] the Rotterdam Elderly Study,[18] and the SHEP study.[19, 21] Patients with carotid artery stenosis detected by ultrasound are at increased risk not only for stroke events but also for coronary heart disease (CHD) and sudden death.[19] Longitudinal studies have shown that a rise in PP and a fall in DBP are associated with substantial progression of aortic atherosclerosis[20] and greater prevalence of acute myocardial infarction[22–25] and thrombotic stroke.[49] A cross-sectional study detected a similar association with hemorrhagic stroke in conjunction with thrombolytic therapy for acute myocardial infarction.[50] These clinical studies support the dominant influence of increased arterial stiffness as a risk factor for cardiovascular disease in middle-aged and geriatric hypertensive patients.

THE ELUSIVE INVERSE RELATION BETWEEN DIASTOLIC BLOOD PRESSURE AND CARDIOVASCULAR RISK

Whereas an elevated DBP was described long ago as a risk factor for cardiovascular disease,[6] the negative association of DBP with cardiovascular events[15–26] has been recognized only recently. Most early studies of blood pressure risk were based on young individuals in whom SBP and DBP tend to track together and are both strongly associated with cardiovascular risk.[32] With advancing age, however, there is a decline in DBP and in the association between DBP and cardiovascular risk.[7, 32] Thus, age is a confounding factor that limits the negative correlation between the DBP and the presence of cardiovascular disease to a middle-aged and geriatric population.[32] Furthermore, the inverse relation between DBP and cardiovascular disease is confounded by a mixed group of normotensive and hypertensive subjects. The negative association between DBP and carotid artery stenosis was noted only when elderly subjects were first stratified by the stage of systolic hypertension[21] (Fig. 25–4).

IS A LOW DIASTOLIC BLOOD PRESSURE A SUPPLEMENTARY RISK TO A HIGH PULSE PRESSURE?

Since an increased PP could be associated with a high, normal, or low DBP, there is the possibility that a very low DBP could be a risk factor for cardiovascular disease, independent of the risk of increased PP. In coronary heart disease, a decreased DBP, together with an increased PP, may contribute to reduced coronary perfusion, with resulting increased risk for acute coronary events. When DBP was added to PP in the logistic regression model, both were independent predictors of the presence of carotid stenosis in elderly subjects with isolated systolic hypertension.[21] The increased risk of carotid stenosis with low DBP was apparent when DBP values were dichotomized at 75 mm Hg and PP was greater than 75 mm Hg. These findings suggest that a marked decrease in DBP might be an addi-

tional risk marker for the presence of severe artery stiffness. Further studies are needed to confirm these results.

THE J-CURVE RELATIONSHIP BETWEEN DIASTOLIC BLOOD PRESSURE AND ACUTE CORONARY EVENTS

The finding of a J-shaped relation between DBP and the occurrence of acute myocardial infarction or sudden death has been reported in population studies. Events are fewer when the DBP is relatively low, but below critical levels (in the 70 to 80-mm Hg range), events again become more frequent.[51, 52] Several intervention trials have detected this J-curve phenomenon between the on-treatment DBP and CHD risk, suggesting to some that treatment is directly responsible for the increased CHD events.[53, 54] In contrast, a variety of randomized clinical trials have not observed a J-curve,[10–12, 55] or have observed J-curves in both the active drug– and the placebo-treated groups.[56] Moreover, further lowering of DBP (and narrowing of PP) with antihypertensive therapy in subjects in the SHEP study decreased rather than increased CHD events, perhaps by facilitating a more favorable balance between coronary perfusion and myocardial blood flow requirements.[10] Thus, elderly subjects with wide PP hypertension represent the "toe" of the J-curve, namely the members of the population for whom there is a negative correlation between DBP and the prevalence of CHD.

PATHOLOGICAL CORRELATES OF WIDE PULSE PRESSURE

Increased PP may be a surrogate marker for several possible pathological mechanisms contributing to the develop-

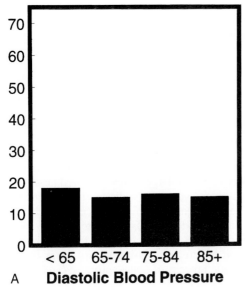
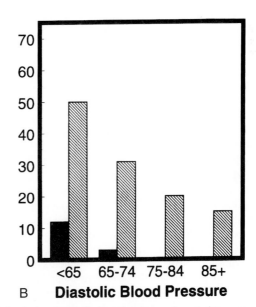

Figure 25–4. Prevalence of carotid stenosis versus DBP for isolated systolic hypertension and control groups combined and stratified by the stage of hypertension. *A,* The *solid bars* represent the entire group as a whole. There appeared to be no relation between DBP and the presence of carotid artery stenosis ($p = .960$). *B,* The *solid bars* represent the normotensive control group with SBP less than 140 mm Hg and DBP less than 90 mm Hg. The *hatched bars* represent the isolated systolic hypertension group, stages 1, 2, and 3. When the group was stratified by the stage of systolic hypertension, the inverse relationship between DBP and carotid artery stenosis was apparent ($p = .003$). (*A* and *B*, From Franklin SS, Sutton-Tyrrell K, Belle SH, et al. The importance of pulsatile components of hypertension in predicting carotid stenosis in older adults. J Hypertens 15:1143–1150, 1997.)

ment of CHD events. Increased aortic pulsatile load elevates left ventricular systolic wall stress, decreases coronary flow reserve, impairs left ventricular relaxation, and can lead to diastolic dysfunction.[57] Increased aortic pulsatile load is the major factor in the development of left ventricular hypertrophy with increased coronary blood flow requirements.[58] Simultaneously, the decrease in DBP further compromises the oxygen supply:demand ratio by reducing coronary flow.[59] Lastly, increased pulsatile shear stress leads to endothelial dysfunction with a greater propensity for coronary atherosclerosis,[60] or conversely, wide PP may simply serve as a marker for diffuse atherosclerosis.[61] Even after extensive myocardial infarction, PP remains a potent predictor of future CHD events.[26] Therefore, isolated systolic hypertension plays a dominant role in the pathogenesis of atherosclerotic disease of the large arteries and related hemorrhagic and thrombotic events,[3, 5] in vascular remodeling of the small resistance arteries,[62] and eventually, in heart failure.[63]

HEMODYNAMIC CORRELATES OF WIDE PULSE PRESSURE

The current classification of geriatric hypertension[14, 64] that uses the rise in SBP or in DBP, or both, overemphasizes small vessel resistance and underestimates the influence of large artery stiffness. This classification system fails to recognize that an increased PP and a decreased DBP are superior risk markers of cardiovascular disease because resistance and stiffness are represented fully by these blood pressure components. The emphasis on PP as a predictor of cardiovascular risk is consistent with findings from a three-component Windkessel model of the circulation.[65, 66] In this model, the cyclical stress of elastance and reflection during systole contributes more to cardiovascular risk than the steady-state stress of resistance during diastole.[33, 65, 66]

CLINICAL CORRELATES OF WIDE PULSE PRESSURE

Because of collinearity between blood pressure components, there is considerable overlap between PP and SBP in predicting cardiovascular events. At any given PP, the collinearity with SBP is maximized when DBP is high and minimized when DBP is normal or low. In young hypertensives, where SBP increases to a slightly greater extent than does DBP, SBP and PP are almost equally predictive of cardiovascular disease. In middle-aged and older hypertensives with normal or low DBP, PP is clearly superior to SBP in predicting cardiovascular risk. Thus, with equal elevation of SBP, subjects with isolated systolic hypertension are at greater risk for cardiovascular disease than those with combined systolic/diastolic hypertension. Indeed, the prevalence of hypertension in the geriatric population often exceeds 50%[67] and includes isolated systolic hypertension with large PP in approximately two thirds of cases.[68] This has important public health implications because isolated systolic hypertension is the most common type of untreated hypertension among adults over the age of 50 years.[69]

The value of a single office PP determination, shown to be predictive of cardiovascular events in large observational studies, may not be predictive in the individual subject. The white-coat effect, which frequently results in higher office than ambulatory blood pressure readings, causes a larger rise in SBP than in DBP, with a resulting increase in PP.[70] Ambulatory blood pressure readings eliminate this error. A likely explanation for this phenomenon is the transient sympathetic activation associated with the alerting reaction evoked by the visit; this may increase both the magnitude and the velocity of left ventricular emptying, with a consequent rise in PP.

ADAPTIVE AND MALADAPTIVE OVERLOAD

Increased peripheral resistance, perhaps under the influence of a hyperactive sympathetic nervous system, characterizes early hypertension, with elevations in MAP, SBP, and DBP. This results in adaptive overload with vascular smooth muscle hypertrophy of small and large arteries, early eccentric hypertrophy of the left ventricle with remodeling, normal wall stress, and perhaps intermittently increased cardiac output. The majority of large artery stiffness is extrinsic, secondary to increased transmural pressure with some vascular hypertrophy and remodeling. During this early phase of hypertension, elevated resistance is the major factor in vascular overload. Structural changes in the arteries are adaptive in that they lead to a decrease in wall stress.

In contrast, maladaptive vascular overload predominates after many years of cyclical stress. The fatiguing effect of cyclical stress on conduit arteries results in eventual fracturing of elastin molecules. This can be viewed as a vicious circle. As the elastin fibers fracture, the arterial wall dilates, thus applying more stress to the remaining elastin fibers with eventual transfer of stress to less extensible collagenous fibers.[3] The Laplace law effect contributes to this vicious circle. Arterial dilatation increases wall stress and, hence, accelerates elastin fatigue and fracturing, resulting in further elevation of SBP and PP. This maladaptive overload process begins to manifest itself in middle age and in the elderly, thereby resulting in a high absolute cardiovascular event rate.

Accelerated, malignant hypertension represents a different process. In this uncommon form of hypertension, a very rapid and large increase in peripheral resistance causes acute damage to the walls of small arteries and arterioles. The consequences of this vicious circle, in the absence of antihypertensive therapy, are rapidly increasing arterial pressure and, ultimately, organ failure. This acute syndrome must be clearly distinguished from the longstanding, chronic process of maladaptive vascular overload.

THERAPEUTIC CORRELATES OF WIDE PULSE PRESSURE

The success of therapeutic intervention trials[10–12] in reducing stroke, CHD, and heart failure events in isolated systolic hypertension confirms the potential reversibility of hemodynamic abnormalities. Most antihypertensive agents lower peripheral resistance and, secondarily, reduce central artery stiffness by decreasing transmural pressure. There is also the suggestion, at least in the short run, that certain antihypertensive drugs lower central PP by reversing early pulse-wave reflection rather than by improving central artery elasticity.[1–3, 71, 72] Angiotensin-converting enzyme inhibitors may reverse early pulse-wave reflection by means of peripheral vasodilatation and may prevent secondary stiffening from collagen deposition.[72] Furthermore, therapeutic reversal of early pulse-wave reflection may occur with little or no alteration in brachial artery cuff pressure.[42] Finally, it is invalid to assume that treatment goals have been achieved with normalization of DBP when elevated SBP and PP persist.

At the present time, we can only speculate as to the threshold level of elevated PP that requires therapeutic intervention and we have yet to establish an optimal goal of PP reduction. Further intervention studies are needed before changes can be made in current therapeutic guidelines.

FUTURE FRONTIERS: NONINVASIVE PULSE-WAVE ANALYSIS

Arterial stiffness, through its direct and indirect effects on central aortic pressure, is a key determinant of increased cardiovascular risk. Enhanced arterial stiffness may occur not only as a result of aging, with potentially irreversible degenerative changes in elastic arteries, but also as a result of reversible endothelial dysfunction. Local endothelial disturbances can occur early in the course of disease and result in increased central artery PP before there are significant increases in brachial artery cuff blood pressure. What is needed is a simple, reliable, noninvasive method for detecting early disturbances in central artery stiffness at a time when therapeutic intervention is most beneficial. This may be accomplished by using applanation tonometry to record high-fidelity pulse waveforms at various peripheral sites and to derive central waveforms by means of transfer functions.[73] Similar techniques not requiring as much operator expertise have been proposed.[74, 75] Future studies are necessary to compare various noninvasive techniques for measuring central pulse waveforms and to determine whether this information can result in earlier detection of individuals at risk for cardiovascular disease. An important question remains unanswered: Will physicians of the 21st century have a simple office method of measuring central pulse waveforms that will supplement or possibly replace the sphygmomanometer?

References

1. O'Rourke MF. Arterial Function in Health and Disease. Edinburgh, Churchill Livingstone, 1982.
2. Safar ME. Pulse pressure in essential hypertension. Clinical and therapeutic implications. J Hypertens 7:769–776, 1989.
3. Nichols WW, O'Rourke MF. McDonald's blood flow in arteries, 4th ed. London, Arnold, Hodder Headline Group, 1998.
4. Berne RM, Levy MN. Cardiovascular Physiology. St. Louis, Mosby-Year Book, 1992; pp 135–151.
5. Safar ME, Cloarec-Blauchard L, London GM. Arterial alterations in hypertension with a disproportionate increase in systolic over diastolic blood pressure. J Hypertens 14(supp 2):S103–S109, 1996.
6. Mackenzie J. Principles of diagnosis and treatment of heart affections, 3rd ed. London, Oxford University Press, 1926.
7. Kannel WB, Gordon T, Schwartz MJ. Systolic versus diastolic blood pressure and the risk of coronary heart disease. Am J Cardiol 27:335–346, 1971.
8. Stamler J, Neaton JD, Wentworth DN. Blood pressure (systolic and diastolic) and risk of fatal coronary heart disease. Hypertension 13(suppl I):I-2–I-12, 1989.
9. Rutan GH, McDonald RH, Chula LH. A historical perspective of elevated systolic vs diastolic blood pressure from an epidemiological and clinical trial viewpoint. J Clin Epidemiol 42:663–673, 1989.
10. SHEP Cooperative Research Group. Prevention of stroke by antihypertensive drug treatment in older persons with isolated systolic hypertension. JAMA 265:3255–3264, 1991.
11. Medical Research Council Working Party. MRC trial of treatment of hypertension in older adults: Principal results. BMJ 304:405–412, 1992.
12. Dahlof B, Lindholm LH, Hansson L, et al. Morbidity and mortality in the Swedish Trial in Old Patients with Hypertension (STOP-Hypertension). Lancet 338:1281–1285, 1991.
13. Joint National Committee on Prevention, Detection, Evaluation, and Treatment of High Blood Pressure. The Fifth Report (JNC V). Arch Intern Med 153:154–183, 1993.
14. World Health Organization/International Society of Hypertension. 1991 guidelines for the management of mild hypertension. [Memorandum] Hypertension 22:392–403, 1993.
15. Maarek B, Simon AC, Levenson J, et al. Heterogeneity of the atherosclerotic process in systemic hypertension poorly controlled by drug treatment. Am J Cardiol 59:414–417, 1987.
16. Salonen R, Salonen JT. Determinants of carotid intima-media thickness: A population-based ultrasonography study in eastern Finnish men. J Intern Med 229:225–231, 1991.
17. Psaty BM, Furberg CD, Kuller LH, et al. Isolated systolic hypertension and subclinical cardiovascular disease in the elderly. Initial findings from the Cardiovascular Health Study. JAMA 268:1287–1291, 1992.
18. Bots ML, Hofman A, deBruyn AM, et al. Isolated systolic hypertension and vessel wall thickness of the carotid artery. Arterioscler Thromb 13:64–69, 1993.
19. Sutton-Tyrrell K, Alcorn HG, Wolfson SK, et al. Predictors of carotid stenosis in older adults with and without isolated systolic hypertension. Stroke 24:355–361, 1993.
20. Witteman JCM, Grobbee DE, Valkenburg HA, et al. J-shaped relation between change in diastolic blood pressure and progression of aortic atherosclerosis. Lancet 343:504–507, 1994.
21. Franklin SS, Sutton-Tyrrell K, Belle SH, et al. The importance of pulsatile components of hypertension in predicting carotid stenosis in older adults. J Hypertens 15:1143–1150, 1997.
22. Darne B, Girerd X, Safar M, et al. Pulsatile versus steady component of blood pressure: A cross-sectional analysis and a prospective analysis on cardiovascular mortality. Hypertension 13:392–400, 1989.
23. Madhavan S, Ooi WL, Cohen J, Alderman MH. Relation of pulse pressure and blood pressure reduction to the incidence of myocardial infarction. Hypertension 23:395–401, 1994.
24. Fang J, Madhavan S, Cohen H, et al. Measures of blood pressure and myocardial infarction in treated hypertensive patients. J Hypertens 13:413–419, 1995.
25. Benetos A, Safar M, Rudnichi A, et al. Pulse pressure. A predictor of long-term cardiovascular mortality in a French male population. Hypertension 30:1410–1415, 1997.
26. Mitchell GF, Moye LA, Braunwald E, et al. Sphygmomanometrically determined pulse pressure is a powerful independent predictor of recurrent events after myocardial infarction in patients with impaired left ventricular function. Circulation 96:4254–4260, 1997.
27. Murgo JP, Westerhof N, Gioma JP, et al. Aortic input impedance in normal men: Relationship to pressure wave forms. Circulation 62:105–116, 1980.
28. Kelly R, Hayward C, Avolio A, et al. Noninvasive determination of age-related changes in the human arterial pulse. Circulation 80:1652–1659, 1989.
29. Benetos S, Laurent S, Hoeks AD, et al. Arterial alterations with aging and high blood pressure. Arterioscler Thromb 13:90–97, 1993.

30. Karamanoglu M, O'Rourke MF, Avolio AP, et al. An analysis of the relationship between central aortic and peripheral upper limb pressure waves in man. Eur Heart J 14:160–167, 1993.

31. Whelton PK. Blood pressure in adults and the elderly. *In* Bulpitt CJ (ed). Handbook of Hypertension, vol 6. Amsterdam, Elsevier, 1985; pp 51–69.

32. Franklin SS, Gustin WG, Wong ND, et al. Hemodynamic patterns of age-related changes in blood pressure. The Framingham Heart Study. Circulation 96:308–315, 1997.

33. Franklin SS. The concept of vascular overload in hypertension. Cardiol Clin 13:501–507, 1995.

34. Wiggers CJ. Physical and physiological aspects of arteriosclerosis and hypertension. Ann Intern Med 6:12–30, 1932.

35. Franklin SS, Weber MA. Measuring hypertensive cardiovascular risk: The vascular overload concept. Am Heart J 128:793–803, 1994.

36. Lund-Johansen P, Omvik P. Hemodynamic patterns of untreated hypertensive disease. *In* Laragh JH, Brenner BM (eds). Hypertension: Pathophysiology, Diagnosis and Management. New York, Raven, 1995; pp 323–342.

37. Terasawa F, Kuramoto K, Ying LH, et al. The study of hemodynamics in older hypertensive subjects. Acta Gerontol Jpn 56:47–52, 1972.

38. Messerli FH, Sundgaard-Risse K, Ventura HO, et al. Essential hypertension in the elderly: Haemodynamics, intravascular volume, plasma renin activity, and circulating catecholamine levels. Lancet 2:983–986, 1983.

39. Nichols WW, Nicolini FA, Pepine CJ. Determinants of isolated systolic hypertension in the elderly. J Hypertens 10(suppl 6):S73–S77, 1992.

40. O'Rourke MF, Kelly RP, Avolio AP. Wave reflection in the systemic circulation and its implications in ventricular function. J Hypertens 11:327–337, 1993.

41. Martyn CN, Greenwald SE. Impaired synthesis of elastin in wall of aorta and large conduit arteries during early development as an initiating event in pathogenesis of systemic hypertension. Lancet 350:953–955, 1997.

42. O'Rourke MF. Arterial stiffness, systolic blood pressure, and logical treatment of arterial hypertension. Hypertension 15:339–347, 1990.

43. Gangar KF, Vyas S, Whitehead M, et al. Pulsatility index in internal carotid artery in relation to transdermal oestradiol and time since menopause. Lancet 338:839–842, 1991.

44. Avolio AP, Chen SG, Wang RP, et al. Effects of aging on changing arterial compliance and left ventricular load in a northern Chinese urban community. Circulation 68:50–58, 1983.

45. Failla M, Grappiolo A, Carugo S, et al. Effects of cigarette smoking on carotid and radial artery distensibility. J Hypertens 15:1659–1664, 1997.

46. London GM, Marchais SJ, Safar ME, et al. Aortic and large artery compliance in end-stage renal failure. Kidney Int 90:2786–2796, 1990.

47. Sutton-Tyrell K, Bostom A, Selhub J, et al. High homocysteine levels are independently related to isolated systolic hypertension in older adults. Circulation 96:1745–1749, 1997.

48. Dart AM, Lacombe F, Yeoh JK, et al. Aortic distensibility in patients with isolated hypercholesterolemia, coronary artery disease, or cardiac transplant. Lancet 338:270–273, 1991.

49. Scuteri A, Cacciafesta M, Di Gernardo MG, et al. Pulsatile versus steady-state component to blood pressure in elderly females: An independent risk factor for cardiovascular disease? J Hypertens 13:185–191, 1995.

50. Selker HP, Beshansky J, Schmid CH, et al. Presenting pulse pressure predicts thrombolytic therapy-related intracranial hemorrhage. Thrombolytic Predictive Instrument (TPI) Project Results. Circulation 90:1657–1661, 1994.

51. D'Agostino RB, Belanger AJ, Kannel WB, et al. Relation of low diastolic blood pressure to coronary heart disease death in presence of myocardial infarction: The Framingham Study. BMJ 303:385–389, 1991.

52. Langer RD, Criqui MH, Barrett-Connor EL, et al. Blood pressure change and survival after age 75. Hypertension 22:551–559, 1993.

53. Cruickshank JM, Trorp JM, Zacharias FJ. Benefits and potential harm of low blood pressure. Lancet 1:581–584, 1987.

54. Weijenberg MP, Feskens EJM, Kromhout D. Blood pressure and isolated systolic hypertension and the risk of coronary heart disease and mortality in elderly men (the Zutphen Elderly Study). J Hypertens 14:1159–1166, 1996.

55. Collins R, Peto R, MacMahon S, et al. Blood pressure, stroke, and coronary heart disease, Part 2. Short-term reductions in blood pressure: Overview of randomized drug trials in their epidemiologic context. Lancet 355:827–838, 1990.

56. Staessen J, Bulpitt C, Clement D, et al. Relation between mortality and treated blood pressure in elderly patients with hypertension: Report of the European Working Party on High Blood Pressure in the Elderly. BMJ 298:1512–1516, 1989.

57. Ohtsuka S, Kakihana M, Watanabe H, et al. Alterations in left ventricular wall stress and coronary circulation in patients with isolated systolic hypertension. J Hypertens 14:1349–1355, 1996.

58. Pannier B, Brunel P, Aroussy WE, et al. Pulse pressure and echocardiographic findings in essential hypertension. J Hypertens 7:127–132, 1989.

59. Ferro G, Duilio C, Spinelli L, et al. Relation between diastolic perfusion time and coronary artery stenosis during stress-induced myocardial ischemia. Circulation 92:342–347, 1995.

60. Lyon RT, Runyon-Hass A, Davis HR, et al. Protection from atherosclerotic lesion formation by reduction of artery wall motion. J Vasc Surg 5:59–67, 1987.

61. Hirai T, Sasayama S, Kawasake T, et al. Stiffness of systemic arteries in patients with myocardial infarction: A noninvasive method to predict severity of coronary atherosclerosis. Circulation 80:78–86, 1989.

62. James MA, Watt PAC, Potter JF, et al. Pulse and resistance artery structure in the elderly. Hypertension 126:301–306, 1995.

63. Cohn JM, Finkelstein SM. Abnormalities of vascular compliance in hypertension, aging and heart failure. J Hypertens 10(suppl 6):561–564, 1992.

64. Joint National Committee on Prevention, Detection, Evaluation, and Treatment of High Blood Pressure. The Sixth Report. Arch Intern Med 157:2413–2446, 1997.

65. Elzinga G, Westerhof N. Pressure and flow generated by the left ventricle against different impedances. Circ Res 32:178–186, 1973.

66. Nichols WW, O'Rourke MF, Avolio AP, et al. Ventricular/vascular interaction in patients with mild systemic hypertension and normal peripheral resistance. Circulation 74:455–462, 1986.

67. Burt VL, Whelton P, Roccella EJ, et al. Prevalence of hypertension in the U.S. adult population. Hypertension 25:305–313, 1995.

68. Kannel WB. Blood pressure as a cardiovascular risk factor: prevention and treatment. JAMA 275:1571–1576, 1996.

69. Sagie A, Larson MG, Levy D. The natural history of borderline isolated systolic hypertension. N Engl J Med 329:1912–1917, 1993.

70. Mancia G, Bertinieri G, Grassi G, et al. Effects of blood pressure measured by the doctor on patient's blood pressure and heart rate. Lancet 2:695–698, 1983.

71. Smulyan H, Safar ME. Systolic blood pressure revisited. J Am Coll Cardiol 29:1407–1413, 1997.

72. Alvaladejo P, Bouaziz H, Duriez M, et al. Angiotensin converting enzyme inhibition prevents the increase in aortic collagen in rats. Hypertension 23:74–82, 1994.

73. Kelly R, Hayward C, Ganis J, et al. Noninvasive registration of the arterial pressure pulse waveform using high fidelity applanation tonometry. J Vasc Med Biol 1:142–149, 1989.

74. Cohn JN, Finkelstein S, McVeigh G, et al. Noninvasive pulse wave analysis for the early detection of vascular disease. Hypertension 26:503–508, 1995.

75. Brinton TJ, Kailasam MT, Wu RA, et al. Arterial compliance by cuff sphygmomanometer: Application to hypertension and early changes in subjects at genetic risk. Hypertension 28:599–603, 1996.

CHAPTER

26 Coronary Atherosclerotic Sequelae of Hypertension

W. B. Kannel

Hypertension is the most prevalent vascular disorder in the United States, as well as one of the major contributors to the leading causes of death.[1] No matter how defined, persistent inappropriate elevation of blood pressure has been shown to be a direct cause of atherosclerotic cardiovascular morbidity and mortality. Animal experiments have shown that hypertension accelerates lipid-induced atherosclerosis and that lowering the elevated blood pressure retards the pathology.[2] Also, low-pressure segments of the arterial circulation, such as the pulmonary arteries or veins, are virtually immune to atherosclerosis despite exposure to the same lipid-laden blood as the systemic arteries of the heart, brain, and limbs. Atherosclerotic disease has now replaced the fibrinoid necrosis of malignant hypertension as the major outcome of poorly controlled hypertension. However, the relation of hypertension to atherosclerosis is complex, interacting with other major risk factors that greatly influence its potential to enhance atherogenesis in the coronary arteries and elsewhere. The continuing high prevalence of hypertension in the general population, its great impact on cardiovascular morbidity and mortality rates, and our ability to treat and control it give it a high priority among measures to prevent cardiovascular disease in general and coronary disease in particular.

PREVALENCE AND INCIDENCE

Hypertension (>140/90 mm Hg) is a dangerously prevalent condition afflicting one in four American adults. About 4% of persons under age 30 years have this condition, and it increases in prevalence with age, reaching 65% in persons aged 80 years and older.[3] Each year about 2 million new hypertensive persons are added to the pool requiring evaluation and treatment. Treatment of hypertension and the cardiovascular disease it promotes accounts for a large portion of our health care expenditures.

Some 25 to 50% of the normotensive Framingham Study cohort developed hypertension over 26 years of follow-up.[4] Those with high-normal pressures developed hypertension at a two- to threefold higher rate than those with strictly normal pressures.[4, 5] The incidence of new onset of hypertension increased three- to eightfold in men and women, respectively, over the three decades from age 20 to 49 years.[5]

OPTIMAL BLOOD PRESSURE

It is difficult to specify at what blood pressure a significant excess risk of hypertensive atherosclerotic cardiovascular sequelae begins to occur. Epidemiological investigations report an excess risk of such events at blood pressures well below those designated to define *hypertension*.[6, 7] A

reasonably accurate assessment of the risk at relatively low blood pressures can be obtained from the more than 350,000 men screened for eligibility in the Multiple Risk Factor Intervention Trial (MRFIT) project.[7] An examination of 10-year mortality in relation to baseline blood pressure in that study indicates a stepwise increase from the lowest blood pressure (<110 mm Hg) on up. Compared with this lowest pressure, those patients with systolic pressures of 120 to 129 mm Hg had an 18% higher overall and 35% higher cardiovascular mortality.[7] Thus, the optimal systolic blood pressure would appear to be under 110 mm Hg because in the "normotensive" range of 110 to 139 mm Hg there occurred some 40% of all and 35% of cardiovascular deaths. On the basis of these data, it would appear that the vast majority of the population have suboptimal blood pressures, since only 6% of MRFIT screenees had pressures under 110 mm Hg. From blood pressure–related statistics, it appears that 80 to 90% of the U.S. population have suboptimal blood pressures. Because of the great prevalence in the population of persons with high-normal pressures who are at increased risk, nonpharmacological approaches to control the discretionary environmental determinants of elevated blood pressure are required.

For action by physicians using medication to control the blood pressure, somewhat higher pressures are recommended for treatment. However, it is important to recognize that the average pressure at which atherosclerotic cardiovascular events occur is quite moderate. The mean blood pressure at which men in the Framingham Study developed coronary disease was only 146/91 mm Hg, and for women this was 161/94 mm Hg (Table 26–1). This blood pressure at which cardiovascular events occurred tended to decline over the decades both in those untreated and in those under treatment. By the 1980s, half the cardiovascular events in men occurred at pressures below 135/83 mm Hg and in women at pressures below 138/80 mm Hg.

ATHEROSCLEROTIC SEQUELAE

Hypertension is clearly a major contributor to the occurrence of atherosclerotic cardiovascular disease in the general population, imposing a two- to fourfold increased risk of a major atherosclerotic cardiovascular event in persons aged 35 to 64 years (Fig. 26–1). It contributes to the risk of such events at all ages in either sex. The risk ratios are largest for heart failure and stroke, but coronary disease is the most common and lethal sequela, equaling in incidence all the other adverse outcomes combined. Although the absolute and excess risks of atherosclerotic cardiovascular disease imposed by hypertension in women are only half those in men, the relative risk is just as high in women as in men.

Table 26–1 Mean Initial Blood Pressure of Those Developing Coronary Heart Disease Versus Those Remaining Disease-Free in 14 Years in the Framingham Study

Age (yr)	Systolic Blood Pressure (mm Hg)				Diastolic Blood Pressure (mm Hg)			
	Men		Women		Men		Women	
	CHD (323)	Controls (1959)	CHD (169)	Controls (2676)	CHD	Controls	CHD	Controls
30–39	138*	132	126†	124	90*	83	83†	79
40–49	143*	135	149*	136	92*	86	91*	85
50–62	150*	141	168*	150	91*	87	97*	90
Total	146‡	135*	161‡	135	91‡	85	94‡	84

Abbreviation: CHD, coronary heart disease.
*p < .05.
†Not significant.
‡p < .01.

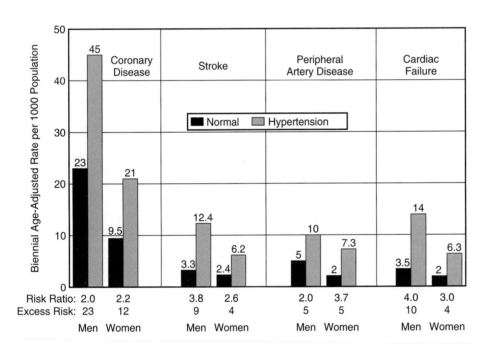

Figure 26–1. Risk of cardiovascular events by hypertensive status. Subjects aged 35 to 64 years, 36-year follow-up in the Framingham Study. (From Kannel WB. Hypertension as a risk factor for cardiac events—Epidemiologic results of long-term studies. J Cardiovasc Pharmacol 21[suppl 2]:S27–S37, 1993.)

Table 26–2 Role of Clinical Manifestations of Coronary Heart Disease by Hypertensive Status: 40-Year Follow-Up in the Framingham Study*

Clinical Manifestation	Age 35–64 Yr Age-Adjusted Annual Rate/1000				Age 65–94 Yr Age-Adjusted Annual Rate/1000			
	HBP Absent		HBP Present		HBP Absent		HBP Present	
	Men	Women	Men	Women	Men	Women	Men	Women
Myocardial infarction	4.8	0.9	9.3	2.9	11.7	3.8	20.8	8.8
Angina pectoris	4.6	2.2	9.4	5.9	6.7	4.1	9.4	7.8
Sudden death	0.74	0.20	1.95	0.55	2.6	1.1	4.8	1.8

Abbreviation: HBP, high blood pressure.
*HBP = 140/90 mm Hg or on medication.

CORONARY HAZARDS

The less than expected efficacy of antihypertensive therapy in trials to reduce the risk of coronary morbidity and mortality has led to an unjustified questioning of the role of blood pressure in the development of coronary heart disease. Hypertension has in fact been shown in prospective epidemiological studies to be a powerful independent risk factor for the development of coronary events.[8] In the Framingham Study, the risk of every clinical manifestation of coronary disease has been shown to be related to the severity of antecedent hypertension (Table 26–2). Although the coronary disease incidence rates in hypertensive women are only half that in men, the risk ratios comparing rates in hypertensives with nonhypertensives in each sex is at least as high in women as in men. Hypertension increases the risk of a myocardial infarction almost twofold in men and two- to threefold in women (Table 26–2). For reasons that are unclear, hypertension predisposes disproportionately to infarctions that go unrecognized, and the more severe the hypertension, the greater the proportion of unrecognized infarctions (Table 26–3). This association persists even after excluding persons on therapy that might mask symptoms, persons with electrocardiogram (ECG) evidence of left ventricular hypertrophy that might be confused with anterior infarctions, and persons with coexistent diabetes, who are known to be more prone to silent infarctions. Unrecognized infarctions are surprisingly common in general and particularly so in hypertensive persons. In hypertensive men, 35% of myocardial infarctions go unrecognized; in hypertensive women, 48%.

As for cardiovascular disease in general, risk of coronary events increases with the blood pressure in a continuous graded fashion with no indication of a critical value at which normal pressure leaves off and abnormal ensues (Table 26–4). It has been suggested that there is an excess risk of coronary disease at very low diastolic blood pressures. However, in the Framingham Study of healthy persons, there was no indication of a J-curve relation of diastolic blood pressure to the occurrence of coronary mortality (Fig. 26–2). Only in persons who already had a myocardial infarction was an upturn in coronary mortality seen at diastolic pressures below 75 mm Hg. The reason

for this excess of mortality at low diastolic pressures is unclear. It has been suggested that this increased coronary mortality at low diastolic blood pressures is a reflection of ill health, poor left ventricular function, or overtreatment.[9–11] Overtreatment does not appear to be a likely explanation, since the U curve has been observed in both treated and untreated subjects who have sustained a myocardial infarction in the Framingham Study and elsewhere.[10, 12] Because low diastolic pressure was associated with a poor outcome only in patients with overt coronary disease and not in those free of such disease, it is possible that the presence of a low pressure, whether induced by treatment or not, is potentially lethal in the presence of a severely compromised coronary circulation. Although the Framingham Study took into account the fall in pressure that may result from an extensive myocardial infarction and excluded subjects with heart failure, it remains possible that the low diastolic blood pressure after myocardial infarction is a surrogate of the extent of myocardial damage sustained. The data available thus far are consistent with the concept that persons with a poor coronary flow reserve are vulnerable to low coronary perfusion pressures (dia-

Table 26–4 Risk of Cardiovascular Events by Systolic Blood Pressure in Untreated Subjects: 36-Year Follow-Up in the Framingham Study

Systolic Pressure (mm Hg)	Age-Adjusted Biennial Rate/1000					
	Age 35–64 Yr			Age 65–94 Yr		
	MI	Stroke	CHF	MI	Stroke	CHF
<120	8.2	2.2	3.7	11.6	16.7	19.3
120–139	10.9	2.6	2.7	23.3	18.8	9.2
140–159	22.7	6.5	6.0	42.5	17.4	25.1
>160	22.5	12.3	15.6	51.6	36.9	33.8

Abbreviations: MI, myocardial infarction; CHF, congestive heart failure.

Table 26–3 Myocardial Infarctions Unrecognized by Hypertensive Status

Hypertensive Status	Percent of MIs Unrecognized					
	Excluding Diabetics*		Excluding Anti-HBP Rx*		Excluding LVH*	
	Men	Women	Men	Women	Men	Women
Normal	18.5	30.7	17.8	26.6	19.6	29.0
Mild	28.3	36.1	30.2	35.5	30.1	35.3
Definite	33.2	48.1	34.8	48.5	32.7	50.5

From Wilson PWF, Kannel WB. Hypertension, other risk factors and the risk of cardiovascular disease. *In* Laragh JH, Brenner BM (eds). Hypertension: Pathophysiology, Diagnosis and Management, 2nd ed, vol 1. New York, Raven, 1995; p 100.
Abbreviations: MI, myocardial infarction; HBP, high blood pressure; Rx, medication; LVH, left ventricular hypertrophy; CHD, coronary heart disease.
*Also excludes persons with CHD at examination immediately preceding MI.

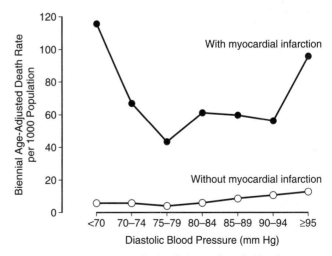

Figure 26–2. Coronary mortality in relation to diastolic blood pressure with and without myocardial infarction. (This figure was first published in the BMJ from D'Agostino RB, Belanger AJ, Kannel WB. Relation of low blood pressure to coronary heart disease in the presence of myocardial infarction. BMJ 1991; 303:385–389, and is reproduced by permission of the BMJ.)

stolic blood pressure) that are well tolerated in healthy persons.

REINFARCTION AND DEATH

Assessment of prognostic factors after myocardial infarction has been carried out extensively in relation to a wide range of clinical, demographic, and biochemical risk factors, but only a few studies have assessed the outlook beyond 5 years as the Framingham Study has done. Assessment of the influence of blood pressure on the outlook after myocardial infarction is complicated, since the blood pressure may decrease because of the infarction and may have a different association with the prognosis depending on when the blood pressure was measured with respect to the time of the infarction.[13, 14] Hypertension confers a poor prognosis after an infarction as long as the blood pressure assessment is obtained after the blood pressure stabilizes from the transient drop in pressure that often occurs immediately postinfarction.[15, 16] Patients whose blood pressures fall as a result of a myocardial infarction have a worse outlook than those whose pressures remain stable.[13, 17, 18]

In the Framingham Study, in which blood pressures were measured in survivors of myocardial infarction about 1 year after the infarction and subjects were followed for reinfarction or coronary death for up to 30 years of follow-up, both systolic and diastolic blood pressures were found to be important risk factors.[19] Mean systolic and diastolic blood pressures were higher in persons who experienced a reinfarction or coronary fatality. Adjusting for age, each 15-mm Hg increment in diastolic blood pressure increased risk of reinfarction by 40%. Each 25-mm Hg increase in systolic pressure conferred a 37% increase in risk.[19] As with reinfarction, an increase in systolic pressure of 25 mm Hg conferred a 26% increased risk of coronary mortality. These increased risks related to systolic blood pressure persisted on adjustment for other risk factors for coronary disease, including serum cholesterol, relative weight, diabetes, and male sex (Table 26–5). The strong relation of postinfarction systolic pressure with reinfarction and coronary mortality is in agreement with the findings of others who have measured blood pressures in survivors of infarction.[15, 16] In addition to postinfarction blood pressure, preinfarction blood pressure has been shown to be a risk for long-term prognosis after infarction in the Framingham Study.[19] Limited follow-up data from the Framingham Study have also shown pre- to postinfarction blood pressure reduction to be associated with a poor outlook,[13] presumably occurring in the more severe cases with major myocardial damage.

COMPONENTS OF BLOOD PRESSURE

Clinical decisions and trials concerned with the efficacy of treating hypertension have for too long emphasized the diastolic component of the blood pressure. High diastolic pressures have generally been believed to be more pathological than systolic elevations. However, there is nothing to suggest that the diastolic pressure has a greater impact than the systolic on the occurrence of cardiovascular dis-

Table 26–5 Relative Risk of Reinfarction and Coronary Mortality After Initial Myocardial Infarction by Systolic and Diastolic Blood Pressure Increments

	Reinfarction Relative Risk	Coronary Death Relative Risk
AGE-ADJUSTED RISK		
Systolic blood pressure (25 mm Hg)	1.37*	1.26*
Diastolic blood pressure (15 mm Hg)	1.40*	1.18†
AGE- AND RISK FACTOR–ADJUSTED RISK‡		
Systolic blood pressure (25 mm Hg)	1.53*‖	1.42‡

From Wong ND, Cupples LA, Ostfeld AM, Kannel WB. Risk factors for long-term prognosis after initial myocardial infarction: The Framingham Study. Am J Epidemiol 130:469–480, 1989.
*$p < .05$.
†Not significant.
‡Other risk factors: Sex, metropolitan relative weight, serum cholesterol, diabetes, heart rate, interim myocardial infarction.
‖$p < .01$.

ease in general or on coronary disease in particular.[7, 20] Comparing the impacts of the systolic and diastolic blood pressure on the rate of development of all the cardiovascular sequelae of hypertension, including coronary disease, indicates a significantly greater impact of the systolic component.[7, 20] Also, in persons in the Framingham Study with diastolic blood pressures not exceeding 90 mm Hg, the risk of cardiovascular events increased steeply with the systolic pressure at all ages in both sexes.[21]

Furthermore, in persons with an elevated systolic pressure, knowledge of the associated diastolic pressure was not helpful in estimating risk of cardiovascular events. In men in the Framingham Study, the incidence of coronary disease was substantially greater for isolated systolic than for isolated diastolic hypertension, and combined systolic and diastolic hypertension imposed only a marginally greater risk than isolated systolic hypertension.

RISK FACTOR CLUSTERING

A tendency for hypertension to cluster with other major coronary risk factors has long been noted in the Framingham Study and elsewhere, and many of the risk factors with which it tends to cluster also predict the occurrence of the hypertension.[22] It has also become increasingly apparent that the magnitude of the risk associated with any degree of blood pressure elevation is markedly influenced by the associated burden of other risk factors.[22] Only 20 to 24% of the cases of elevated blood pressure (>138 mm Hg in men and >130 mm Hg in women) that occurred in the Framingham Study did so in the absence of other risk factors (upper quintiles of total cholesterol, body mass index, triglycerides, and glucose; lower quintile of high-density lipoprotein [HDL]-cholesterol). Clusters of three or more of these additional risk factors occurred in 22% of men and 27% of women, a rate four to five times that expected by chance.

The tendency for elevated blood pressure to cluster with

other risk factors suggests that hypertension may be a reflection of some more fundamental process that accelerates atherogenesis. Abdominal obesity that promotes insulin resistance and abnormal sympathoadrenal activity has been postulated as an underlying mechanism.[23] Abnormalities of lipoprotein metabolism, insulin resistance, and glucose tolerance are commonly encountered in persons with essential hypertension or their close relatives.[24] These abnormalities do not cluster with secondary hypertension. Hyperinsulinemia, signifying insulin resistance, is found in both obese and nonobese persons with hypertension and may persist despite antihypertensive therapy.[25] However, insulin resistance and hyperinsulinemia are more severe and more closely associated with hypertension in obese than in nonobese persons. Weight gain worsens all the elements of the insulin-resistance syndrome and weight loss improves them. In the Framingham Study, the extent of risk factor clustering increased stepwise with the degree of obesity: A 5-lb increase in weight imposed a 30% increase in the extent of risk factor clustering with hypertension. Persons with elevated blood pressure characteristically have elevated triglycerides and reduced HDL-cholesterol.[25] Such persons also tend to have atherogenic small dense low-density lipoprotein particles.[26] It is not clear what percentage of hypertensive persons have the insulin-resistance syndrome, although it has been estimated that about half may have it.[24]

In the Framingham Study, the risk of developing coronary disease in hypertensive subjects increased stepwise with the extent of risk factor clustering (Table 26–6). Among persons with elevated blood pressure, it is estimated that about 40% of coronary events in men and 58% in women are attributable to clusters of two or more additional risk factors.

Whatever the cause, it is clear that risk factor clustering is to be anticipated and should be routinely screened for in persons with elevated blood pressures. Also, when two or more of the specified risk factors are found, it seems reasonable to suspect the presence of insulin resistance.

Renin

Hypertension is a heterogeneous disorder in its pathophysiology and clinical sequelae. Much research has been directed at understanding the pathophysiology of the factors that increase the risk of coronary disease in hypertension. In this connection, the role of the renin-angiotensin system has been the focus of attention for some time.[27] An activated renin-angiotensin system has been postulated to be another risk factor for coronary disease in hypertension.[28] In addition to causing vasoconstriction and sodium retention, angiotensin has been shown to shown to increase vascular smooth muscle cell growth and promote neointimal hyperplasia after vascular injury.[27] Experimentally, angiotensin-converting enzyme inhibitors have been shown to reduce myocardial ischemia, decrease atherosclerosis, prevent restenosis after arterial injury, and prevent ventricular dilatation.[27] However, it is not yet clear whether high renin plays a causal role in the risk of a myocardial infarction in hypertension or is only a marker for an activated sympathetic or neurohormonal state.[27] High renin with respect to the level of sodium excretion has been reported in case-control comparisons and a prospective epidemiological investigation to be another predictor of myocardial infarction in patients with hypertension.[28] However, several other studies have failed to confirm this claim.[29] It is possible that hypertensive patients with high renin profiles may benefit more from treatment with β-blockers or angiotensin-converting enzyme inhibitors than those with low renin with respect to avoiding coronary disease. However, this remains to be demonstrated.

Left Ventricular Hypertrophy

Left ventricular hypertrophy, whether diagnosed by ECG, chest x-ray, or echocardiogram, is an ominous manifestation of uncontrolled hypertension. Left ventricular hypertrophy by ECG criteria, particularly repolarization abnormality, is an ominous harbinger of impending coronary disease in the hypertensive patient. It further escalates the risk of all the major sequelae of elevated blood pressure, including coronary disease, its most common sequela (Fig. 26–3). Because ECG left ventricular hypertrophy carries as serious a prognosis as a myocardial infarction detected by routine ECG examination, it seems appropriate to regard hypertensive persons with this condition as if they already

Table 26–6 Sixteen-Year Coronary Heart Disease Incidence by Number of Other Risk Factors in Framingham Heart Study Offspring With Elevated Blood Pressure, Ages 30–65 Years at Baseline*

Other Risk Factors (n)	Relative Risk (95% CI)	Prevalence (%)	CHD Events n (%)	Population Attributable Risk (Multivariate)
MEN				
0	1.0 (referent)	22	10 (14)	—
1	1.33 (0.57, 3.06)	29	17 (24)	0.09
≥2	2.28 (1.09, 4.78)	49	45 (63)	0.39
Total			72 (100)	
WOMEN				
0	1.0 (referent)	18	2 (5)	—
1	2.05 (0.41, 10.18)	28	7 (18)	0.23
≥2	4.93 (1.14, 21.27)	54	31 (78)	0.68
Total			40 (100)	

Abbreviations: CI, confidence interval; CHD, coronary heart disease; SBP, systolic blood pressure; BMI, body mass index; HDL-C, high-density lipoprotein-cholesterol.
*High blood pressure is defined as SBP ≥ 138 mm Hg (men) and ≥ 130 mm Hg (women). Other risk factors included the top quintiles of other factors (total cholesterol, BMI, triglycerides, glucose) and the bottom quintile for HDL-C.

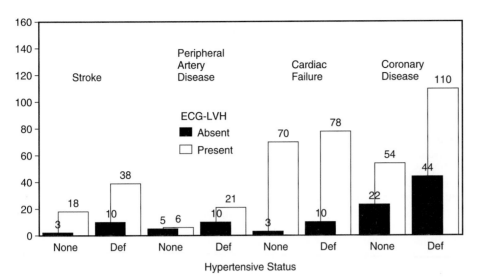

Figure 26–3. Biennial age-adjusted rate per 1000 population of cardiovascular events by hypertensive status and electrocardiogram–left ventricular hypertrophy (ECG-LVH) status. Men aged 35 to 64 years, 32-year follow-up in the Framingham Study. Def, definite. (Reprinted from Am J Cardiol, vol 77, Kannel WB. Cardioprotection and antihypertensive therapy: The key importance of addressing the associated coronary therapy, pp 6B–11B, copyright 1996 with permission from Excerpta Medica Inc.)

have coronary disease.[8] Hypertrophy on x-ray is not as ominous as the ECG version, but it adds to the risk when it accompanies the ECG hypertrophy.[8] Echocardiography is a more sensitive detector of hypertensive left ventricular hypertrophy than the ECG and has also been shown to be associated with an increased risk of developing coronary disease.[30] Risk of coronary events in the hypertensive person is related to the left ventricular mass, with no critical value that separates compensatory from pathological hypertrophy.[30]

Heart Rate

Hypertensive persons tend to have somewhat higher heart rates than normotensive people, and persons with more rapid heart rates tend to develop hypertension at a greater rate.[31] The Framingham Study observed an independent effect of the heart rate that accompanies hypertension on the rate of subsequent mortality from coronary disease (Table 26–7). The observed effect was stronger for the occurrence of fatal than for nonfatal coronary events, and

particularly for acutely fatal attacks, consistent with a direct effect of heart rate mediated through the autonomic nervous system.

THE ELDERLY

The impact of hypertension on the development of coronary disease has been perceived by many to weaken in advanced age.[11, 32] In the very old, it has been claimed that hypertension may actually be a protection against mortality.[32] This has resulted in a reluctance to treat hypertension aggressively in the aged.[11] An examination of the risk of clinical manifestations of coronary disease in hypertensive subjects in relation to age in the Framingham Study indicates a modest reduction in the risk ratio with advance in age, but this is offset by a distinctly higher absolute, excess, and attributable risk owing to the high incidence of coronary disease in the elderly, the high prevalence of hypertension, and the substantial risk ratio in this age group (Table 26–8). Because there is a disproportionate rise in systolic compared with diastolic pressure with advancing age, isolated systolic hypertension is the predominant type of hypertension in the elderly. Isolated systolic hypertension is clearly a risk for the development of coronary disease in the elderly, possibly more so than in the middle-aged (Fig. 26–4). The high systolic and pulse pressures in the hypertensive elderly appear to be a direct cause of the excess of coronary disease observed, rather than only a sign

Table 26–7 Risk of Fatal and Nonfatal Coronary Events per 40 Beat/Minute Increase in Heart Rate: Hypertensive Subjects, 30-Year Follow-Up to the Framingham Study

Event	Odds Ratio for 40 Beats/Minute Increment (BP Age-Adjusted)	
	Men	*Women*
All fatal CHD events	1.80*	1.59†
Fatal within 30 days	2.37‡	2.46§
Not fatal within 30 days	1.14†	0.82†
All fatal and nonfatal events	1.33§	0.98†

Abbreviations: BP, blood pressure; CHD, coronary heart disease.
*p < .01.
†Not significant.
‡p < .001.
§p < .05.

Table 26–8 Risk of Coronary Heart Disease Associated With Hypertension by Age in Each Sex: 40-Year Follow-Up to the Framingham Study

Age (yr)	Age-Adjusted Rate/1000		Age-Adjusted Risk Ratio		Excess Rate/1000	
	Men	*Women*	*Men*	*Women*	*Men*	*Women*
35–64	1.95	0.55	2.6	2.8	1.20	0.35
65–94	4.75	0.80	1.9	1.7	2.20	0.75

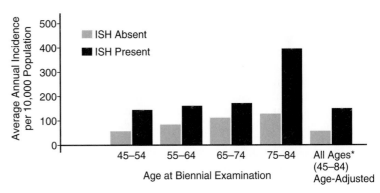

Figure 26–4. Risk of myocardial infarction with isolated systolic hypertension (ISH). Men aged 45 to 84 years, 24-year follow-up in the Framingham Study. ISH, systolic blood pressure greater than or equal to 160 mm Hg and diastolic blood pressure less than 95 mm Hg; *statistically significant $p < .01$. (Reprinted by permission of Elsevier Science from Kannel WB. Clinical heterogeneity of hypertension. Am J Hypertens, vol 4, pp 283–287, copyright 1991 by American Journal of Hypertension.)

of the diseased rigid artery, because systolic hypertension persists as a risk factor even when the associated arterial rigidity is taken into account.[33] The chief determinant of isolated systolic hypertension in the elderly appears to be an elevated blood pressure in middle age.[34] Whether predominantly systolic, diastolic, or combined, hypertension is a risk for coronary disease in the elderly. However, systolic blood pressure elevation is a more reliable predictor of coronary disease in the elderly than is diastolic pressure, and reliance on the diastolic pressure can be misleading in the elderly with systolic hypertension.[6] Although the absolute risk of developing clinical manifestations of coronary disease is lower than in men, the relative risks are higher in women than in men for all clinical events other than sudden death (Table 26–9).

PREVENTIVE IMPLICATIONS

Knowledge at midcentury about the long-term outlook of what was called *essential* hypertension was quite limited and the condition was considered benign. Physicians were unimpressed with the hazards of hypertension and, even if they were concerned, could do little about it. Since the late 1960s, we have come to recognize that this idiopathic hypertension is an insidious and, in the long-term, lethal promoter of accelerated atherogenesis and cardiovascular events. Also during this period, effective, tolerable, and safe antihypertensive medications were produced that made it possible to control elevated blood pressure, and studies were carried out to determine the efficacy of doing so.

Casual blood pressures obtained routinely in the office have been clearly shown to be related to the rate of development of cardiovascular disease in general and of coronary disease in particular, although there is some evidence that home blood pressures and 24-hour monitoring of circa-

dian blood pressure variation may be a useful refinement. Risk assessment and treatment based on the average of several office blood pressures do not appear to be ill advised. Treatment should not be initiated on the basis of a single casual office blood pressure elevation, nor should the efficacy of treatment be judged from less than the average of multiple blood pressure measurements. The lowest of a series of blood pressures obtained should not be used to determine either the need for or the efficacy of antihypertensive therapy.

In evaluating the risk of hypertension and the need to treat it, more attention needs to be given to the systolic blood pressure. For too long, there has been an overemphasis on the diastolic component of the blood pressure. Risk of coronary disease has been consistently shown to be more strongly related to the systolic than the diastolic pressure. Further, isolated systolic hypertension is not an innocuous accompaniment of advanced age. Treatment based on the systolic blood pressure and correction of isolated systolic pressure has been shown to be at least as effective as that based on the diastolic pressure.[35]

Coexistent risk factors that tend to cluster with hypertension exert a greater influence on the cardiovascular and coronary hazards of hypertension than the character of the blood pressure elevation per se. Hypertension seldom occurs in the absence of other major risk factors to which it is metabolically linked. This makes it mandatory to test for the other risk factors and to conceptualize hypertension as a component of a cardiovascular risk profile. This avoids the possibility of either overreacting to an isolated moderate blood pressure elevation or being falsely reassured by such a blood pressure elevation accompanied by multiple risk factors. When hypertension is accompanied by an elevated triglyceride, reduced HDL-cholesterol, and abdominal obesity, insulin resistance is likely to be present and treatment should be modified accordingly. Therapy of

Table 26–9 Relative Risk of Clinical Manifestations of Coronary Disease in Men Versus Women: 40-Year Follow-Up to the Framingham Study

| | Age-Adjusted Risk Ratios (High Blood Pressure/Normotension) | | | | | |
| | *Myocardial Infarction* | | *Angina Pectoris* | | *Sudden Death* | |
	35–64 yr	65–94 yr	35–64 yr	65–94 yr	35–64 yr	65–94 yr
Men	1.95	1.79	2.03	1.40	2.60	1.86
Women	3.17	2.33	2.72	1.93	2.75	1.71

hypertension to prevent coronary disease is more likely to be effective if, in addition to lowering the blood pressure, a more favorable coronary risk profile is achieved.

Not uncommonly, elderly hypertensive patients, when first encountered, may already have overt or unrecognized angina, myocardial infarction, or cardiac failure. These associated conditions must be taken into account in judging the urgency for treatment and in choosing the optimal therapeutic agents.

Antihypertensive therapy has been shown to regress left ventricular hypertrophy in hypertensive patients.[36] It is not yet established whether this induced regression results in a reduction of the formidable increase in risk imposed by the hypertrophy. However, Framingham Study data indicate that when improvements in the ECG criteria for hypertrophy occur, there is a substantially lower risk of cardiovascular sequelae compared with patients in whom there is no change or progression in these parameters (Table 26–10).[37] This suggests that therapy that eliminates or slows hypertrophy may well improve the outlook of the hypertensive patient with this dangerous condition. When left ventricular hypertrophy accompanies hypertension, there should be a greater urgency for aggressive antihypertensive therapy.

Because the heart rate increase that accompanies hypertension appears to directly influence the coronary mortality rate, antihypertensive medications that lower the heart rate may have an advantage over those that accelerate it. In an analysis of the β-blocker trials, it was found that there was a strong relationship between the reduction in heart rate achieved and the reduction in mortality.[38] Analysis of the Norwegian Multicenter Timolol Trial found that the postinfarction resting heart rate predicted later cardiac mortality and that the benefit of treatment was a result of the achieved reduction in heart rate.[39] Treatment with β-blockers has been reported to reduce silent ischemic events in relation to the heart rate reduction achieved.[39]

Because hypertension predisposes to the occurrence of silent or unrecognized myocardial infarctions, hypertensive persons should be periodically monitored by ECG examination for such an occurrence. These unrecognized infarc-

tions must be detected and dealt with because they impose a serious long-term outlook that is little different from that of clinically overt infarctions.[40]

In contrast to previous reports, a more recent meta-analysis of the efficacy of antihypertensive therapy in the elderly indicates a significant 25% decrease in coronary mortality.[41] Practitioners caring for elderly ambulatory hypertensive patients are justified in attempting to control the blood pressure, whether the hypertension is systolic, diastolic, or combined. In the very oldest and most ill and frail, treatment may be less effective, and further trials are needed before well-founded recommendations can be made. The elderly with a favorable risk profile and only mild hypertension can be managed with weight control, a moderate exercise program, salt and alcohol restriction, and counseling against smoking. These measures can help to reduce the dosage of antihypertensive medication required to control the blood pressure and to control the frequently associated risk factors. Polypharmacy may be a significant problem in managing hypertension in the elderly, who often take nonsteroidal antiinflammatory drugs for arthritis. There is much to be gained by treating hypertension in the elderly because their risk of disabling cardiovascular events is so high.

Control of hypertension to prevent coronary disease requires more than reduction of the blood pressure. Assessment of the patient should routinely include evaluation for the presence of other metabolically linked risk factors, such as dyslipidemia, glucose intolerance, abdominal obesity, and left ventricular hypertrophy. This is especially important in persons with milder hypertension where the excess risk is concentrated in those who have other risk factors or evidence of organ involvement, such as proteinuria, cardiomegaly, vascular bruits, or ECG abnormalities. Optimal preventive management should include reduced saturated fat, cholesterol, and salt intake, exercise, smoking cessation, and avoidance of excessive alcohol intake. Persuading the hypertensive cigarette smoker to quit can promptly reduce the risk of coronary disease to half that of those who continue to smoke, a risk reduction greater than that expected from blood pressure reduction.

The benefits of treating diastolic hypertension are now better appreciated, as is low-dose therapy for isolated systolic hypertension in the elderly.[35, 42] Low-dose combination therapy using antihypertensive agents with different modes of action can virtually eliminate unpleasant side effects and maintain a good quality of life in those under treatment.

SUMMARY

Since the late 1970s, the percentage of hypertensive persons who have become aware of their problem and have come under treatment has improved substantially. Concomitant with these improvements, major declines in coronary and stroke mortality have occurred. Because of the large attributable risk of hypertension as a risk factor for coronary disease and stroke, it is inferred that the improved detection and control of hypertension in the general population contributed substantially to these declines.

Epidemiological investigation has shown the importance of elevated blood pressure as a contributor to cardiovascu-

Table 26–10 Risk of Cardiovascular Events as a Function of Serial Electrocardiographic Changes in Persons with Left Ventricular Hypertrophy in the Framingham Study

	Odds Ratio	
	Men	*Women*
VOLTAGE CHANGE		
Decrease	0.46	0.56*
No change	1.00	1.00
Increase	1.86	1.61
REPOLARIZATION CHANGE		
Improved	0.45	1.19*
No change	1.00	1.00
Worsened	1.89	2.02

From Levy D, Salomon M, D'Agostino RB, et al. Prognostic implications of baseline electrocardiographic features and their serial changes in subjects with left ventricular hypertrophy. Circulation 90:1786–1793, 1994.
*Not significant.

lar morbidity and mortality. It has been demonstrated that blood pressure exerts a continuous graded influence, so the concept of an acceptable blood pressure has changed from that which is usual in an apparently healthy population to that which confers the greatest freedom from cardiovascular sequelae. Epidemiological investigation has also shown that the adverse consequences of hypertension are not primarily a result of elevation of the diastolic blood pressure and has focused more attention on the systolic component. It is now evident that hypertension seldom occurs in isolation and that high-risk hypertension is concentrated in those persons with a cluster of other metabolically linked risk factors. It is suggested that hypertension is often one component of an insulin-resistance syndrome.

Epidemiological investigation has established the continuing importance of hypertension as a risk factor for coronary disease in the elderly, and clinical trials have shown the efficacy of treating both systolic and diastolic hypertension at all ages. The ominous significance of left ventricular hypertrophy is now well documented, and the potential benefit of causing regression has been shown.

Thus, physicians now have a good deal more information to guide them in their efforts to delay or prevent the sequelae of hypertension than they had in the late 1980s. However, this increase in information has made clinical decisions and therapeutic choices in managing hypertension more complex. Evaluation and management of hypertension are no longer based solely on determining the height of the blood pressure and on lowering it to a more acceptable level. New classification schemes place more emphasis on systolic blood pressure, milder blood pressure elevations, and the presence of associated risk factors.[1] The number of available antihypertensive agents, with different modes of action, suitable for monotherapy and combined therapy, has grown. There is, however, controversy about first-choice agents and whether therapy should be tailored to take into account associated dyslipidemia, glucose intolerance, left ventricular hypertrophy, and insulin resistance.

The goal of antihypertensive therapy is to prevent cardiovascular morbidity and mortality rather than simply to bring the blood pressure under good control. Blood pressure control must be achieved in the least intrusive way, and use of low-dose combinations of agents is generally preferred over high doses of single agents to achieve goal blood pressures. Trials have clearly shown that treatment reduces stroke and heart failure events, but some question the efficacy of antihypertensive treatment, without concomitantly improving the multivariate risk profile, in reducing coronary disease. There is some interest in the possibility of cautious step-down therapy for patients whose blood pressures have been well controlled for some time. Maintaining long-term compliance with treatment remains a problem. There is continuing concern about the safety of drastic lowering of the blood pressure in hypertensive persons who have concomitant coronary disease.

References

1. Joint National Committee on Prevention, Detection, Evaluation, and Treatment of High Blood Pressure. The Sixth Report (JNC VI). Arch Intern Med 157:2413–2446, 1997.
2. Chobanian A. Adaptive and maladaptive responses of the arterial wall to hypertension. 1989 Corcoran Lecture. Hypertension 15:666–674, 1990.
3. National Heart, Lung, and Blood Institute. Chartbook on Cardiovascular, Lung and Blood Diseases. Morbidity and Mortality. Bethesda, MD, National Institutes of Health, 1996; pp 43–45.
4. Garrison RJ, Kannel WB, Stokes III, Castelli WP. Incidence and precursors of hypertension in young adults: The Framingham Offspring Study. Prev Med 16:234–251, 1987.
5. Leitschuh L, Cupples LA, Kannel WB, et al. High-normal blood pressure progression to hypertension in the Framingham Heart Study. Hypertension 17:22–27, 1991.
6. Wilson PWF, Kannel WB. Hypertension, other risk factors and the risk of cardiovascular disease. In Laragh JH, Brenner BM (eds). Hypertension: Pathophysiology, Diagnosis and Management, 2nd ed. New York, Lippincott-Raven, 1995; pp 99–114.
7. Stamler J, Stamler R, Neaton JD. Blood pressure, systolic and diastolic and cardiovascular risks. U.S. population data. Arch Intern Med 153:598–615, 1993.
8. Kannel WB. Framingham Study insights into hypertensive risk of cardiovascular disease. Hypertens Res 18:181–196, 1995.
9. Stewart IM. Relation of reduction in pressure in first myocardial infarction in patients receiving treatment for severe hypertension. Lancet 1:861–865, 1979.
10. Coope J. Hypertension: The cause of the J-curve. J Hum Hypertens 4:1–4, 1990.
11. Fletcher A, Bulpitt J. How far should blood pressure be lowered? N Engl J Med 326:251–254, 1992.
12. Staessen J, Bulpitt C, Clement D, et al. Relation between mortality and treated blood pressure in elderly patients with hypertension: Report of the European Working Party on High Blood Pressure in the Elderly. BMJ 298:1552–1556, 1989.
13. Kannel WB, Sorley P, Castelli WP, et al. Blood pressure and survival after myocardial infarction: The Framingham Study. Am J Cardiol 45:326–330, 1980.
14. Coronary Drug Project Research Group. Blood pressure in survivors of myocardial infarction. J Am Coll Cardiol 4:1135–1147, 1984.
15. Khaw K-T, Barret-Conner E. Prognostic factors for mortality in a population-based study of men and women with a history of heart disease. J Cardiopulm Rehabil 6:474–480, 1986.
16. Coronary Drug Project Research Group. Factors influencing long term prognosis after recovery from myocardial infarction—Three year findings of the Coronary Drug Project. J Chron Dis 27:267–285, 1974.
17. Coronary Drug Project Research Group. Blood pressure in survivors of myocardial infarction. J Am Coll Cardiol 6:1135–1147, 1984.
18. Norris RM, Brandt PWT, Caughey DE, et al. A new coronary prognostic index. Lancet 1:274–281, 1969.
19. Wong ND, Cupples LA, Ostfeld AM, Kannel WB. Risk factors for long term prognosis after initial myocardial infarction: The Framingham Study. Am J Epidemiol 130:469–480, 1989.
20. Kannel WB, Gordon T, Schwartz MJ. Systolic versus diastolic blood pressure and risk of coronary heart disease: The Framingham Study. Am J Cardiol 27:335–345, 1971.
21. Kannel WB. Epidemiology of essential hypertension: The Framingham Study experience. Proc R Coll Phys Edinb 21:273–287, 1991.
22. Kannel WB. Potency of vascular risk factors as the basis for antihypertensive therapy. Eur Heart J 13(suppl G):34–42, 1992.
23. Despres JP. Abdominal obesity as an important component of the insulin resistance syndrome. Nutrition 9:452–459, 1993.
24. Reaven GM, Chen YD. Insulin resistance, its consequences and coronary heart disease. [Editorial comment] Circulation 93:1780–1783, 1996.
25. Reaven GM. Insulin resistance, hyperinsulinemia, and hypertriglyceridemia in the etiology and clinical course of hypertension. Am J Med 90:7S–12S, 1991.
26. Siegal RD, Cupples LA, Schaefer EJ, Wilson PWF. Lipoproteins, apolipoproteins and low-density lipoprotein size among diabetics in the Framingham Offspring Study. Metabolism 45:1267–1272, 1996.
27. Dzau VJ. Renin and myocardial infarction in hypertension. N Engl J Med 324:1128–1130, 1991.
28. Alderman MH, Madhavan S, Ooi WL, et al. Association of the renin-sodium profile with the risk of myocardial infarction in patients with hypertension. N Engl J Med 324:1098–1104, 1991.
29. Kaplan NM. The prognostic implications of plasma renin in essential hypertension. JAMA 231:167–170, 1975.
30. Levy D, Garrison RJ, Savage DD, et al. Prognostic implications of

echocardiographically determined left ventricular mass in the Framingham Heart Study. Ann Intern Med 322:1561–1566, 1990.

31. Kannel WB. Risk factors in hypertension. J Cardiovasc Pharmacol 13(suppl):4–10, 1989.

32. Langer RD, Ganiats TG, Barrett-Conner E. Paradoxical survival in elderly men with high blood pressure. BMJ 29:1356–1358, 1989.

33. Kannel WB, Wolf PA, McGee DL, et al. Systolic blood pressure, arterial rigidity, and risk of stroke. The Framingham Study. JAMA 245:1225–1228, 1981.

34. Wilking SVP, Belanger A, Kannel WB, Steel K. Determinants of isolated systolic hypertension. JAMA 260:3451–3455, 1988.

35. SHEP Cooperative Research Group. Prevention of stroke by antihypertensive drug treatment in older persons with isolated systolic hypertension: Final results of the Systolic Hypertension in the Elderly Program (SHEP). JAMA 265:3255–3264, 1991.

36. Dahlof B, Pennert K, Hansson L. Reversal of left ventricular hypertrophy in hypertensive patients: A meta-analysis of 109 treatment studies. Am J Hypertens 5:95–110, 1992.

37. Levy D, Salomon M, D'Agostino RB, et al. Prognostic implications of baseline electrocardiographic features and their serial changes in subjects with left ventricular hypertrophy. Circulation 90:1786–1793, 1994.

38. Kjekshus JK. Beta blockers-heart rate reduction: A mechanism of action. [Comments] Eur Heart J 6(suppl):29, 1985.

39. Gunderson T, Grottum P, Pederson T, Kjekshus JK. Effect of timolol and reinfarction after acute myocardial infarction: Prognostic importance of heart rate at rest. Am J Cardiol 58:20, 1986.

40. Kannel WB, Abbott RD. Incidence and prognosis of unrecognized myocardial infarction: An update on the Framingham Study. N Engl J Med 311:1144–1147, 1984.

41. Insua JT, Sacks HS, Lau T-S, et al. Drug treatment of hypertension in the elderly. Ann Intern Med 121:355–362, 1994.

42. Collins R, Peto R, MacMahon S, et al. Blood pressure, stroke and coronary heart disease. Part 2: Short term reductions in blood pressure: Overview of randomized drug trials in their epidemiological context. Lancet 335:827–838, 1990.

CHAPTER

27 Left Ventricular Hypertrophy, Congestive Heart Failure, and Coronary Flow Reserve Abnormalities in Hypertension

Robert A. Phillips and Joseph A. Diamond

Increased left ventricular (LV) mass, diastolic dysfunction, congestive heart failure (CHF), and coronary flow abnormalities characterize hypertensive heart disease. Left ventricular hypertrophy (LVH) increases the risk of coronary heart disease, CHF, stroke, ventricular arrhythmias, and sudden death. Most antihypertensive treatments promote regression of LVH and reversal of diastolic dysfunction, which may decrease symptoms of CHF and improve survival. Adequate treatment of hypertension may prevent CHF. A variety of invasive and noninvasive techniques described herein measure LV mass, diastolic function, and coronary blood flow abnormalities. This chapter reviews the following:

- Epidemiological evidence for LVH as a risk factor for cardiovascular disease
- Structural changes in the hypertensive heart that provide the substrate for increased risk and CHF
- Cause of LVH and CHF
- Identification and treatment of LVH in clinical practice
- Diastolic dysfunction and CHF mechanisms and treatments
- Noninvasive assessment of the coronary microcirculation in patients with hypertension

DEFINITION OF HYPERTENSIVE HEART DISEASE AND EPIDEMIOLOGY OF LEFT VENTRICULAR MASS

Hypertensive heart disease occurs in association with elevated arterial blood pressure. Its manifestations include diastolic dysfunction, increased LV mass, and coronary flow abnormalities. Echocardiographically determined LVH is defined as an LV mass in the upper 2.5 to 5.0% of the adult population. It occurs in 15 to 20% of hypertensive patients.[1] Considered as a discrete, categorical variable, LVH significantly increases the risk of coronary artery disease, CHF, cerebrovascular accidents, ventricular arrhythmia, and sudden death.[2–4] LVH increases the relative risk of mortality by twofold in subjects with coronary artery disease and by fourfold in those with normal epicardial coronary arteries.[5, 6] In addition, when LV mass is considered as a continuous variable, a direct and progressive relationship exists between cardiovascular risk and the absolute amount of LV mass. During 4 years of follow-up in the Framingham Heart Study,[1] each 50 g/m^2 increase in LV mass was associated with a 1.49 increase in relative risk of cardiovascular disease for men and a 1.57 increase for women. The effect on cardiovascular mortality was even more striking, with a 1.73 relative risk for each 50 g/m^2 for men and each 2.12 g/m^2 for women (Fig. 27–1).[3]

STRUCTURE IN LEFT VENTRICULAR HYPERTROPHY

Geometric Patterns

Subjects with hypertension have different patterns of ventricular shape and geometry that are associated with markedly different risks for cardiovascular disease (Fig. 27–2). Ventricular structure is commonly categorized according to one of two ratios: (1) disproportionate septal thickening

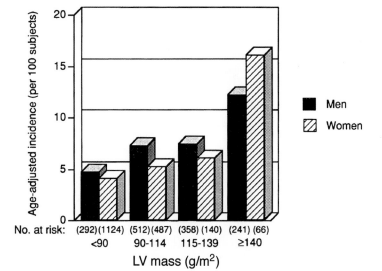

Figure 27–1. Effect of left ventricular (LV) mass on age-adjusted incidence of cardiovascular disease over a 4-year period in the Framingham Heart Study. (Adapted from Levy D, Garrison RJ, Savage DD, et al. Prognostic implications of echocardiographically determined left ventricular mass in the Framingham Heart Study. N Engl J Med 322:1561–1566, 1990. Copyright 1992 Massachusetts Medical Society. All rights reserved.)

compared with the posterior wall (ratio ≥ 1.3), a pattern that is common in persons with LV wall thickness greater than 15 mm,[7] and (2) the ratio of (2 × posterior wall thickness)/LV internal dimension, which is defined as relative wall thickness (RWT). RWT greater than or equal to 0.45 is the arbitrary cutoff often used to define concentric hypertrophy, a geometric pattern in which the LV internal dimension remains normal but LV mass increases owing to increased wall thickness. This is the pattern typically associated with pressure overload, and it results from cell thickening caused by the addition of new sarcomeres in parallel.[8] In eccentric hypertrophy, the LV internal dimension dilates, and RWT is less than 0.45. This is the pattern typically associated with volume overload; it is caused primarily by cell elongation, as sarcomeres are added at the ends of the fibers (in series).[8] Increased relative wall thickness with normal LV mass is termed *concentric remodeling.*[9]

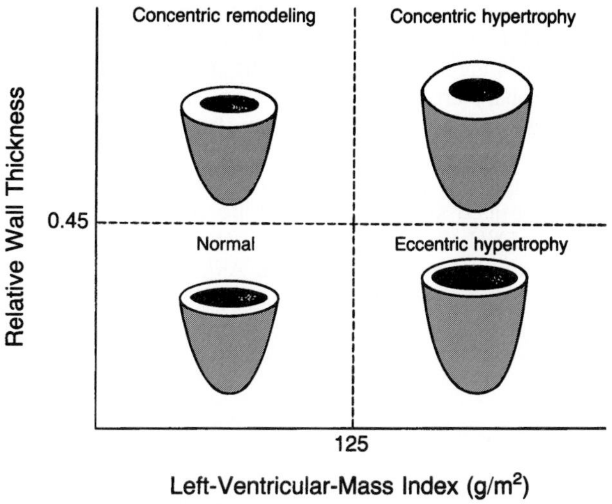

In one study of hypertensive subjects followed for 10 years, the incidence of a cardiovascular event was 30% in those with concentric LVH, 25% in those with eccentric LVH, 15% in those with concentric remodeling, and 9% in those with normal LV mass (Fig. 27–3).[10] In a study in Italy, investigators followed 694 hypertensive patients with normal LV mass (<125 g/m²) and found that concentric remodeling of the left ventricle was an important predictor of increased cardiovascular mortality, independent of conventional risk factors.[11] In the Framingham subjects without cardiovascular disease and in African Americans in Chicago (with and without coronary artery disease), those with concentric hypertrophy had the worst prognoses, followed by those with eccentric hypertrophy, concentric remodeling, and normal geometry.[12, 13] However, in the Framingham Heart Study, when conventional risk factors for coronary artery disease and ventricular muscle mass were taken into account, ventricular geometric patterns no longer provided significant prognostic information. Mortality data are not available on hypertensive subjects with disproportionate septal thickening and increased LV mass. These subjects have degrees of ventricular ectopy and depressed LV diastolic function that are similar to those of patients with concentric LVH, and they have even more atrial arrhythmias.[14]

Estimates of the prevalence of various forms of ventricular structure vary widely, depending on the hemodynamic and demographic characteristics of the population (Table 27–1). Greater severity of hypertension, advancing age, and higher peripheral resistance with normal intravascular volume increase the prevalence of concentric hypertrophy. Among subjects with LVH, eccentric hypertrophy is more common in younger subjects and those with relative volume overload.[15] The shift from an eccentric to a concentric pattern among subjects with LVH may be due to the increase in peripheral vascular resistance that occurs with aging. Compared with whites with the same level of blood pressure, blacks in both the United States and the United Kingdom tend to have increased relative wall thickness

Figure 27–2. Various forms of left ventricular (LV) geometry associated with hypertensive heart disease. Relative wall thickness is a ratio defined as: sum of septum and posterior wall/LV internal dimension, LV mass index (g/body surface area, g/m²) > 125 is approximately the 95th percentile for men. (From Frohlich ED, Apstein C, Chobanian AV, et al. Medical progress: The heart in hypertension. N Engl J Med 327:998–1008, 1992. Copyright 1992 Massachusetts Medical Society. All rights reserved.)

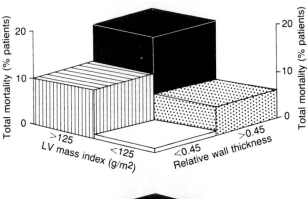

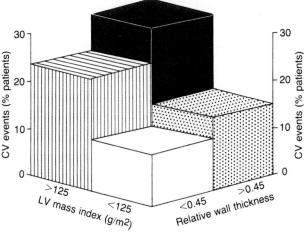

Figure 27–3. Relationship between mortality, cardiovascular (CV) events, and left ventricular (LV) geometry in hypertensive subjects followed for 10 years. The incidence of CV events and mortality was: concentric LV hypertrophy (LVH, *black bar*) > eccentric LVH *(striped bar)* > concentric remodeling *(stippled bar)* > normal LV mass and geometry *(white bar)*. (From Koren MJ, Devereux RB, Casale PN, et al. Relation of left ventricular mass and geometry to morbidity and mortality in uncomplicated essential hypertension. Ann Intern Med 114:345–352, 1991.)

and LV mass.[16–20] One explanation is the presence of a less pronounced nocturnal decline in blood pressure in blacks compared with whites.[21] Gender may also influence ventricular geometry. In the Framingham study, 31% of the men and 57% of the women with systolic hypertension had increased LV mass.[22] Hypertrophy tended to be concentric in women and eccentric in men.

There may be gender differences in the impact of hypertrophy on morbidity and mortality. In one study of 163 black men and 273 black women, after adjusting for age,

blood pressure, and ejection fraction, the relative risk for total death for individuals with LVH versus those without LVH was 2.0 (0.8–5.0, 95% CI) for men and 4.3 (1.6–11.7, 95% CI) for women. This suggests a significant gender difference in the impact of LVH on survival.[23] However, an experimental model of pressure overload by aortic banding showed an earlier transition to heart failure with onset of LV cavity dilatation, loss of concentric remodeling, increase in wall stress, and evidence of diastolic dysfunction in male weanling rats compared with females.[24]

Although it is generally accepted that obesity increases both wall thickness and LV internal dimension, whether the ultimate effect is a predominance of concentric or eccentric hypertrophy is controversial.[25–27] In an obese person, the geometric pattern of the ventricle is most likely to be determined by whether obesity-associated volume overload (leading to an eccentric pattern) predominates over afterload (leading to a concentric pattern).[28]

Myocardial Composition in Left Ventricular Hypertrophy and Congestive Heart Failure

Increases in myocyte and interstitial mass that occur as the heart hypertrophies adversely alter ventricular and vascular performance, creating a substrate for increased cardiovascular morbidity and mortality. The heart is composed of several different cell types and an extracellular matrix. Myocytes constitute approximately 75% of the heart mass (Fig. 27–4); the remaining 25% is cardiac interstitium, which is made up of the coronary vasculature, fibroblasts, macrophages, and mast cells. In hypertensive heart disease, myocytes hypertrophy and interstitial components undergo hyperplasia, hypertrophy, and remodeling.[29, 30] Excess collagen production by fibroblasts increases total interstitial and periarteriolar fibrosis. This reduces ventricular compliance. Echocardiographically derived parameters (pixel intensity, skewness, kurtosis, and the broad band of echoes about the distribution) have been shown to correlate with histologically assessed collagen volume in patients with hypertension and LVH.[31] Vascular smooth muscle cells undergo hyperplasia and hypertrophy, resulting in medial hypertrophy, coronary artery wall remodeling, and increased coronary wall to lumen ratio.[32] These structural changes decrease vasodilator capacity.

Although the precise structural changes that lead to decompensated systolic and diastolic function from compensated LVH are not currently known, myocardial fibrosis is likely to play an important role. As part of the hypertrophic response, cardiac fibroblasts undergo a phenotypic change, assuming a myofibroblast configuration. Stimu-

Table 27–1 Patterns of Heart Geometry in Hypertension

Geometric Pattern	LVH	RWT	Contributing Factors	10-year Incidence of CV Events
Normal	Absent	<0.45		9%
Concentric remodeling	Absent	>0.45	BP, TPR, race, aging, ACE genotype	15%
Concentric LVH	Present	>0.45	BP, TPR, race, ACE genotype	30%
Eccentric LVH	Present	<0.45	Obesity with volume overload	25%

From Koren MJ, Devereux RB, Casale PN, et al. Relation of left ventricular mass and geometry to morbidity and mortality in uncomplicated essential hypertension. Ann Intern Med 114:345–352, 1991.
Abbreviations: ACE, angiotensin-converting enzyme; BP, blood pressure; CV, cardiovascular; LVH, left ventricular hypertrophy; RWT, relative wall thickness; TPR, total peripheral vascular resistance.

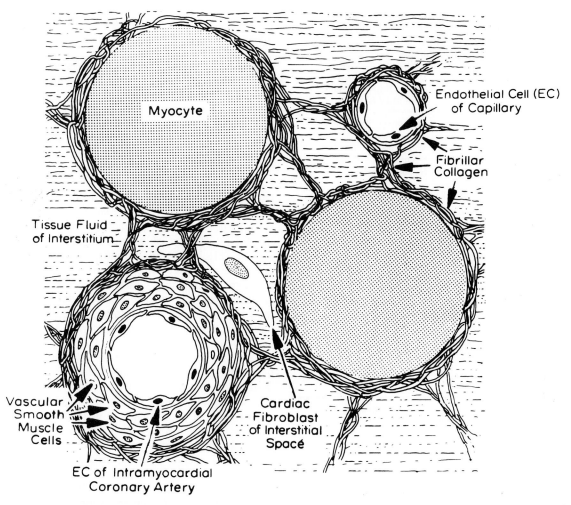

Figure 27–4. Schematic representation of the cellular composition of the myocardium. The heart is composed of several different cell types and an extracellular matrix. Monocytes constitute approximately 75% of the heart mass. The remaining 25% is the cardiac interstitium, which is composed of the coronary vasculature, fibroblasts, macrophages, and mast cells. (From Weber KT, Brilla CG. Pathological hypertrophy and cardiac interstitium. Fibrosis and renin-angiotensin-aldosterone system. Circulation 83:1849–1865, 1991.)

lated myofibroblasts proliferate and increase production of extracellular matrix proteins, including fibronectin, laminin, and collagen I and III. This results in progressive fibrosis. Many of these processes are controlled by integrins, which are cell surface receptors that mediate the cell's ability to interact with its environment.[33] Progressive fibrosis of the heart is a major component of the remodeling process in hypertensive heart disease, and it leads to left ventricular systolic dysfunction (CHF-S) through impaired myocyte contractility, oxygenation, and metabolism. Several experimental studies suggest that this process may be reversible. They include a study of hypertensive patients showed that angiotensin II type 1 (AT$_1$) receptor blockade with losartan results in decreased plasma levels of growth factors, including endothelin-1, basic fibroblast growth factor, and platelet-derived growth factor.[34] This may help to explain the positive survival impact of angiotensin-converting enzyme (ACE) inhibitors and may suggest positive benefits of AT$_1$ receptor blockers in patients with CHF-S.[35, 36]

Myocyte hypertrophy may decrease the efficiency of excitation-contraction coupling, leading to decreased efficiency of contraction and development of CHF.[37] Normally, depolarization triggers influx of calcium through dihydro-

pyridine receptors (L-type Ca^{2+} channels), leading to local cytoplasmic increases in Ca^{2+} concentration. This local increase "sparks" the release of Ca^{2+} from the sarcoplasmic reticulum through activation of ryanodine receptors. The efflux of Ca^{2+} from the sarcoplasmic reticulum causes myocyte contraction by activating the troponin-actin-myosin complex. Physical alteration of the hypertrophied myocyte in LVH increases the distance between the voltage-dependent calcium channels and the ryanodine receptors on the sarcoplasmic reticulum, resulting in failure of local Ca^{2+} to trigger sarcoplasmic Ca^{2+} release.

CAUSE OF LEFT VENTRICULAR HYPERTROPHY AND CONGESTIVE HEART FAILURE IN PATIENTS WITH HYPERTENSION

Hemodynamic Factors and Left Ventricular Hypertrophy

Because of the profound effect of LV growth on cardiovascular morbidity, it is important to determine the factors that

Table 27–2 Association Between Left Ventricular Mass and Hemodynamic and Nonhemodynamic Factors

Factor	Strength of Evidence Supporting a Causal Role in LV Mass
Blood pressure/wall stress	Very strong[29, 40–44, 50, 54]
Stroke volume	Very strong[50, 429]
Obesity	Very strong[25, 27, 71, 82, 83]
Growth hormone and IGF-1	Strong[100, 101]
Gender	Strong[24, 74, 78, 80]
Race	Strong[16, 18–20, 68]
Age	Strong (women only?)[69–73]
Intracellular [Ca^{2+}]	Strong[54, 86]
Insulin resistance	Strong[82, 103, 104]
Angiotensin II	Strong[91, 430]
Alcohol	Needs confirmation[84]
Intrinsic myocardial contractility	Needs confirmation[50]
Blood viscosity	Needs confirmation[431]
Parathyroid hormone	Needs confirmation[89]
Aldosterone (collagen synthesis)	Needs confirmation[93, 430, 432]
Sodium intake	Needs confirmation[85]
Na$^+$/H$^+$ exchanger and Na$^+$-K$^+$-Cl$^-$ cotransport system	Needs confirmation[433]
Polymorphism of the ACE gene	Controversial[62–64]
Plasma renin activity	Controversial[88–90]
Norepinephrine	Controversial[67, 88, 96, 97, 99]
Na$^+$/Li$^+$ exchanger	Controversial[433, 434]
βARK	Controversial[435, 436]

Abbreviations: ACE, angiotensin-converting enzyme; βARK, beta-adrenergic receptor kinase; IGF-1, insulin-like growth factor-1; LV, left ventricular.

initiate it. The effects on LV mass of blood pressure per se, as well as of virtually every factor known to influence blood pressure, have been investigated (Table 27–2). There is very strong evidence of a causal relationship between blood pressure and absolute LV mass. This was first reported more than 60 years ago,[29] and it led to the view that myocardial hypertrophy is an adaptive cardiac response that reduces wall stress and allows the ventricle to maintain mechanical efficiency.[38, 39] In the Framingham Heart Study, 10% of the variation in LV mass among subjects is accounted for by differences in systolic blood pressure averaged over 30 years.[40] Similarly, average blood pressure obtained during awake hours from hypertensive subjects accounts for 10 to 25% of LV mass variation,[41–43] whereas a blunted nocturnal fall in blood pressure is associated with increased LV mass.[44] Ambulatory blood pressure monitoring correlates more closely than does clinic blood pressure with LV mass and carotid artery intimal-medial thickness, and it may more accurately predict the risk for cardiovascular disease than do clinic blood pressure measurements.[42, 45–49]

In hypertensive persons, approximately 40% ($r = .66$, $p < .001$) of the variance in LV mass is accounted for by total LV load or peak meridional wall stress.[50] In normotensive persons, enhanced augmentation of systolic pressure by reflected waves, a process associated with the aging of the arterial tree, elevates wall stress and is associated with increased LV mass.[51] Other hemodynamic factors associated with increased mass are volume, which directly increases LV mass, and intrinsic contractility of the ventricle. An intrinsically hypercontractile ventricle requires less wall

thickening to overcome wall stress. Thus, an inverse relationship exists between the degree of LV mass and intrinsic myocardial contractility.[50]

The sequence of events that leads from increased wall stress to cellular hypertrophy is only beginning to be elucidated.[52] Because failure to hypertrophy in response to increased wall stress would result in a mechanical disadvantage and decreased LV function, it is likely that there are redundant systems that translate wall stress into cardiac myocyte hypertrophy. It is likely that increased wall stress activates a stretch receptor that, through a series of cellular and subcellular events, activates fetal cardiac and growth genes, such as c-*myc* and c-*jun*, to upregulate myocardial cell protein synthesis. Shear stress has been shown to activate these growth genes in endothelial cells by stimulating the production of several mitogen-activated protein kinases (Fig. 27–5).[53] The underlying molecular mechanisms that couple hypertrophic signals at the cell membrane to the reprogramming of cardiomyocyte gene expression are beginning to be elucidated. Intracellular calcium release may be an early response to myocyte stretch and other humoral stimuli, including angiotensin II, phenylephrine, and endothelin. The increase in intracellular calcium results in activation of the phosphatase calcineurin, which then dephosphorylates transcription factor NFAT3, resulting in its translocation to the nucleus. In the nucleus, AT3 interacts with another transcription factor, GATA4, to initiate transcription of genes that lead to myocyte hypertrophy,[54] such as β-myosin heavy chain and β-skeletal actin (Fig. 27–6). In the hypertrophic response, other genes are also upregulated, such as those for atrial natriuretic peptide and phospholamban.[33]

Calcineurin appears to be both necessary and sufficient to induce hypertrophy. Pharmacological inhibition of calcineurin activity with cyclosporine blocks development of hypertrophy in several circumstances: (1) in mice prone to LVH because they are genetically engineered to produce high levels of calcineurin,[54] (2) in mice genetically predisposed to develop hypertrophic cardiomyopathy,[55] and (3) in rats whose aortas were banded to produce a pressure stimulus for hypertrophy.[55] Although cyclosporine is not clinically useful in the nontransplant population, it is likely that new classes of drugs that regulate transcription will soon become available to modulate responses such as hypertrophy.

Two large community-based studies indicate that hypertension is the most common risk factor for CHF, both with and without systolic dysfunction.[56, 57] In the Framingham study, after adjusting for age and other risk factors for CHF-S in proportional hazards regression models, the risk for developing CHF in hypertensive subjects compared with normotensive subjects was nearly twofold in men and threefold in women. Hypertension was the highest risk factor for CHF-S by multivariate analysis, accounting for 39% of cases in men and 59% in women.[56] Another population-based study of CHF, in Olmsted County, Minnesota, showed similar findings. Of 216 patients studied, 52% presented with hypertension, and 137 underwent evaluation of LV systolic function. Hypertension was the underlying risk factor in 53% of subjects with left ventricular ejection fraction (LVEF) less than 50% and was present in 58% of subjects with LVEF of 50% or higher. Of note, long-term

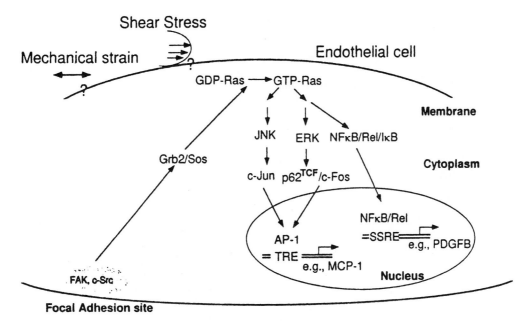

Figure 27–5. Sequential events of signaling and gene expression in endothelial cells in response to shear stress or mechanical strain. Tyrosine kinases in the focal adhesion site of endothelial cells such as FAK and c-SRC are involved in the mechanochemical transduction. Through the *Src* homology 2–containing adaptor Grb2, the small GTPase *Ras* is activated by *Sos*, a guanine nucleotide exchange factor that converts the inactive GDP-*Ras* to the activated GTP-*Ras*. As a result, JNK and ERK in the cytoplasm are activated to phosphorylate, respectively, c-*jun* and p62^{TCF}/c-*fos*, which are components of the transcription factor AP-1. In the nucleus, the action of the activated AP-1 on its target sequence, e.g., the TRE site in the promoter of the MCP-1 gene, causes an upregulation of gene expression. Concurrently, NFκB/Rel is activated by eliminating its inhibitor IκB so that genes with a shear stress–responsive element or κB site, e.g., PDGF-B, can be activated. (From Chien S, Li S, Shyy YJ. Effects of mechanical forces on signal transduction and gene expression in endothelial cells. Hypertension 31:162–169, 1998.)

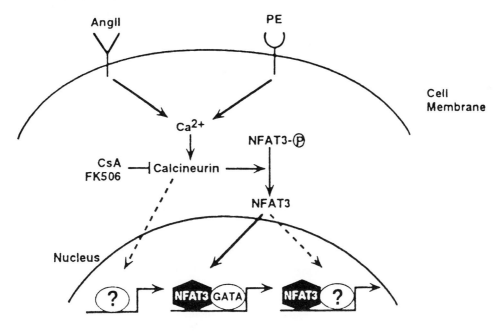

Figure 27–6. Model for the calcineurin-dependent transcriptional pathway in cardiac hypertrophy. Angiotensin II (Ang II), phenylephrine (PE), and possibly other hypertrophic stimuli acting at the cell membrane lead to elevation of intracellular Ca^{2+} and activation of calcineurin in the cytoplasm. Calcineurin dephosphorylates NFAT3, resulting in its translocation to the nucleus, where it interacts with GATA4 to synergistically activate transcription. Whether all actions of NFAT3 are mediated by its interaction with GATA4 or whether there are GATA4-independent pathways for activation of certain hypertrophic responses remains to be determined. *Solid arrows* denote pathways that are known. *Dotted lines* denote possible pathways that have not been demonstrated. (From Molkentin JD, Lu JR, Antos CL, et al. A calcineurin-dependent transcriptional pathway for cardiac hypertrophy. Cell 93:215–228, 1998.)

survival was not significantly different among subjects with normal LVEF and those with low LVEF.[57] The prognosis for hypertensive patients with newly diagnosed CHF-S was poor in both studies (≤35% survival by 5 years).

Blood pressure control effectively prevents CHF. In the Systolic Hypertension in the Elderly Program (SHEP) study, patients with isolated systolic hypertension and a prior history of myocardial infarction by electrocardiogram who were treated with diuretic-based therapy that lowered blood pressure to less than 150 mm Hg systolic had only a 2 to 3% chance of developing CHF over a 4-year period. By contrast, those patients treated with placebo had an 8 to 10% chance of developing CHF.[58] Meta-analysis of randomized, placebo-controlled antihypertensive therapy trials demonstrated that adequate blood pressure control decreases the incidence of CHF by half.[59]

Nonhemodynamic Factors and Left Ventricular Hypertrophy

A large body of data indicates that LV mass may be affected by nonhemodynamic factors (see Table 27–2). In one study, LV mass before blood pressure elevation occurred was a predictor of future blood pressure. This suggests that common factors may influence both processes.[60, 61]

There may be genetic influences on LV mass. The most studied and controversial genetic factor is an insertion/deletion polymorphism in the intron 16 (noncoding region) of the gene for angiotensin-converting enzyme (ACE). The homozygous genotype for the deletion is associated with electrocardiographic evidence of LVH.[62] The association was strongest in men who were normotensive, supporting the concept that this association is independent of hemodynamic factors. However, the Framingham study did not find a relationship between echocardiographically measured LV mass and ACE genotype. An Italian study showed that the deletion genotype was a risk factor for increased echocardiographically determined LV mass.[63] Furthermore, a study in an ethnically diverse New York City population found that the deletion genotype was associated with concentric remodeling of the left ventricle, a geometric pattern associated with increased cardiovascular risk.[64]

Epidemiological evidence for genetic influence on LV mass includes offspring studies that generally, but not uniformly, demonstrate that LV mass in children of hypertensive parents is elevated independently of blood pressure.[65, 66] However, one study, in which monozygotic twins had only minimally less intertwin variation in wall thickness than did dizygotic twins or sibling pairs, indicates that genetic influences on LV mass can be modified by environmental factors.[67]

Further evidence of genetic influence on LV mass is that race appears to be a determinant of ventricular structure. Studies made over the past 3 decades suggest that for equal levels of blood pressure, blacks have increased relative wall thickness and LV mass when compared with whites. In the Evans County, Georgia, study conducted between 1960 and 1962, the incidence of electrocardiographic evidence of LVH was two- to threefold higher in blacks at any given level of blood pressure.[68] In the early 1980s, Dunn et al., using M-mode echocardiography, showed that for the same level of blood pressure, blacks had greater LV mass.[17] Hammond et al showed that for the same blood pressure and LV mass, relative wall thickness (concentric remodeling) was greater in blacks.[18] Similarly, in the Treatment of Mild Hypertension Study (OMHS), even though blood pressure and LV mass were the same, blacks had greater wall thickness than whites.[16] Similarly, a study made in London showed that for equal levels of previously untreated blood pressure, blacks had greater LV mass and relative wall thickness than whites.[19] Hinderliter and colleagues showed that even in the absence of hypertension, young adult blacks tend to have greater relative wall thickness than whites, suggesting that differences in ventricular structure may be inherent.[20] The increase in LV mass and relative wall thickness observed in blacks may be due in part to a greater total hemodynamic burden than in whites that is related to a reduced fall in nocturnal blood pressure.[21] This altered blood pressure pattern begins in adolescence.

Gender, age, obesity, and dietary factors affect LV mass. Aging is associated with increased LV mass, and this effect may be more pronounced in women than in men.[69–73] Women have less LV mass for the same level of office-determined blood pressure,[74] but whether this difference is biological or an artifact of the method of blood pressure measurement or indexation of LV mass is controversial. For example, for similar levels of clinic blood pressure, women often have lower ambulatory blood pressures than men. This results in less hypertrophy in women for the same level of clinic pressure.[75–77] Additionally, some of the gender difference is accounted for by the presence of less lean muscle mass in women than in men.[78] When LV mass is indexed by the lean body mass (obtained by bioelectrical impedance), the gender difference in LV mass disappears.[79]

Nevertheless, some experimental data suggest that some of the gender difference may be physiologically mediated through sex hormones.[80] This is supported by data showing that LV mass is not significantly different in boys and girls during infancy and childhood, but that a difference becomes evident at puberty, when sex-specific hormonal influences occur.[81] Whether indexing for lean body mass would abolish this difference remains to be determined.

Some studies suggest that there are sex-specific determinants of LV mass. In the Tecumseh study of normotensive adults, LVH in men was associated with evidence of increased sympathetic nervous system activity and hyperinsulinemia, whereas in women, obesity was the major determinant of LVH.[82] In a study of hypertensive women by DeSimone et al, obesity was the predominant factor determining LV mass (physiological hypertrophy), whereas in men, hemodynamic factors, age, and degree of obesity all contributed.[27]

In the Framingham study, obesity increased LV mass in elderly men and women.[71] The greater incidence of hypertrophy in obese persons is accounted for by increased wall thickness and often by increased LV internal dimension.[25, 27, 83] These changes are reversible with weight loss.[83] Excessive alcohol intake is directly related to increased LV mass,[84] and excess sodium intake may be a signal for hypertrophy.[85]

Several hormones have been related to the hypertrophic process.[52, 86, 87] The role of the plasma renin-angiotensin-aldosterone axis in hypertensive end-organ pathophysiology has been extensively explored. Experimental and human studies[88, 89] have linked plasma renin activity to degree of LVH, but this is not universally accepted.[90] The product of renin activity, angiotensin I, is the substrate for ACE. Expression and regulation of the ACE gene and, thus, angiotensin II levels, may modulate development of LVH. This is supported by in vitro studies in which local release of angiotensin II in response to the mechanical stretch is a necessary permissive factor for induction of the hypertrophic growth response.[91] Although there is ample evidence that angiotensin II is involved in the hypertrophic response, it is apparently not necessary to such a response. This was shown in a study in which LVH developed in mice in response to pressure overload despite "knockout" of the angiotensin II type 1 receptor.[92] Aldosterone, the synthesis of which is partially controlled by angiotensin II appears to regulate cardiac fibroblast metabolism and growth.[93] These observations may explain why elevated plasma renin levels confer a greater risk for myocardial infarction in patients with hypertension.[94]

Several lines of evidence suggest that norepinephrine may influence LV mass. Regression of LVH in spontaneously hypertensive rats is enhanced by drugs that inhibit adrenergic stimuli.[88] Elevated plasma norepinephrine levels in the absence of hypertension cause LVH in dogs,[95] and significant increases in LV mass result from several weeks of diet-induced elevated endogenous catecholamine levels in normotensive offspring of hypertensive parents.[96] These observations may be explained by the stimulatory role of norepinephrine on the plasma renin-angiotensin-aldosterone axis and by evidence in cell culture that, through α_1-receptors, norepinephrine can activate growth-promoting oncogenes in cardiac myocytes.[97] However, the importance of adrenergic stimuli in the development of LVH has been questioned.[90] Cardiac and vascular structural changes, seen in renovascular hypertension and hyperaldosteronism, are not observed in patients with essential hypertension or pheochromocytoma.[98] Furthermore, only a minority of patients with pheochromocytoma have LVH, although pheochromocytoma is characterized by extraordinarily high levels of circulating norepinephrine.[99]

Hormones and factors that regulate cell growth may also be involved in myocardial hypertrophy. For example, marked increases in LV mass may occur in persons with acromegaly as a result of elevated levels of growth hormone and insulin-like growth factor 1;[100] the latter are higher in hypertensive patients with LVH.[101] In utero, insulin is a trophic factor that causes macrosomia.[102] Insulin levels and the degree of insulin resistance may independently modulate LV mass in normotensive and borderline hypertensive subjects.[82, 103, 104] This may be because insulin resistance leads to increased levels of intracellular calcium, possibly as a result of decreased Na^+-K^+-ATPase activity.[105] Elevated intracellular calcium may be an important stimulus for myocardial actin and myosin protein synthesis,[86] which now appears to be due to the stimulus of

calcineurin. This ionic hypothesis[106] may also explain the association between parathyroid hormone levels and LV mass in hypertensive persons.[89]

MEASUREMENT OF LEFT VENTRICULAR HYPERTROPHY AND ITS USE IN CLINICAL TRIALS AND PRACTICE

M-Mode Echocardiography

M-mode echocardiography is the most widely used, anatomically validated method of determining LV mass.[107] Most laboratories acquire M-mode tracings with two-dimensional (2-D) directed imaging.[108] To obtain a technically adequate study, the patient is imaged in the parasternal short-axis view from the highest possible interspace. This increases the likelihood of achieving an image plane orthogonal to the LV anatomic long axis, yielding a "round" LV image in the parasternal view. The M-mode cursor is then directed through the center of the 2-D parasternal short axis, just distal to the mitral valve leaflets, and the M-mode gains are adjusted to optimize endocardial and epicardial interfaces. To measure walls and prevent inclusion of right-sided and left-sided chordal echoes in the septal and posterior wall, several guidelines are helpful. The M-mode tracing should be recorded with simultaneous viewing of the 2-D image, measuring interfaces that show continuous motion throughout the cardiac cycle and discarding tracings that show abrupt posterior motion of the septum in midsystole. The latter finding reflects an incorrect angle beam from a low parasternal window. In research studies, interfaces are usually measured using the Penn convention, which excludes endocardial and epicardial surfaces from the measurement of wall thickness and includes endocardial surfaces in the measurement of LV dimension.[107] Measurements are made in diastole on the R wave of the QRS complex. LV mass is calculated according to the following formula:

$$1.04[(ivs + pwd + lvid)^3 - lvid^3] - 13.6$$

Comparable LV mass values can be obtained with measurements made according to the American Society of Echocardiography (ASE) convention, using the following formula[109]:

$$0.8 \text{ (ASE mass)} + 0.6 \text{ g}$$

ASE measurements are made at the onset of the QRS complex and are based on the leading-edge method.[110]

No uniform method is available for indexing LV mass measurements by body size or composition. The method of indexing may be irrelevant; a recent study comparing different methods of indexing LV mass suggested that prediction of mortality is similar for various indexes, including those based on height or body surface area.[111] Most published studies index mass by the subject's body surface area, expressed as g/m^2.[78] De Simone and colleagues suggested that indexing LV mass by height to the 2.7 power avoids underestimation of LVH in obese subjects.[112] Until late 1994, most publications from the Framingham Heart

Table 27–3 Partition Value for Defining Left Ventricular Hypertrophy Based on Various Indexing Methods

	LVM/Height$^{2.7}$ (g/m^2)[112]	LVM/BSA (g/m^2)[78, 437]	LVM/Height (g/m)[114, 438]	LVM/Height^2 (g/m^2)[114]
95th PERCENTILE				
Men	52	125	138	78
Women	41	100	95	58
97th PERCENTILE				
Men		134		
Women		110		
MEAN + 2 SD				
Men		143		
Women		102		

Abbreviations: BSA, body surface area; LVM, left ventricular mass, Penn convention; SD, standard deviation.

Study indexed LV mass by the subject's height in meters,[113] but that study now recommends indexing mass by the subject's height to the second power.[114] Partition values for LVH based on different indexing methods are listed in Table 27–3.

Despite careful attention to the technical points noted above, several studies indicate considerable variability in an individual measurement of LV mass.[115, 116] In the TOMHS, the width of the 95% confidence interval for a single replicate measurement of LV mass was 60 g, or approximately 35 g/m^2.[117] This raises the issue of whether 2-D–directed M-mode echocardiography should be used to guide decisions about initiation or intensity of antihypertensive therapy in the patient with borderline or stage 1 hypertension. Most of the data on reduction of cardiovascular events have been derived from trials that focused on treatment of a single risk factor. If the only risk for cardiovascular disease is diastolic blood pressure greater than 110 mm Hg, then more than 100 patients must be treated

with antihypertensive therapy to prevent one event in 5 years.[118, 119] However, patients present to the physician with varying degrees of risk, based on the absence or presence of multiple risk factors. Because of this variable, the concept is emerging that the decision of whether or not to treat and the determination of the intensity of treatment should be based on the aggregate of risk factors, that is, "absolute" risk.[118, 120] LVH is a major risk factor for future cardiovascular events, but the question that remains is how information from echocardiography should be integrated into a treatment algorithm when the measurement has such great intrinsic variability.

A statistically based resolution of the problem of inherent variability in the measurement of LV mass is needed. We derived an estimate of the probability that LVH is present for any given value of LV mass (Fig. 27–7). This calculation is based on the Z-statistic, using methodology similar to that employed to determine the probability that hypertension is present for any given level of ambulatory blood pressure.[121] If the cutoff for LVH is 125 g/m^2 (the 95th percentile for LV mass), then a subject with an LV mass index of 110 g/m^2 or greater has at least a 20% chance of having actual LVH. Because of the prognostic implications of LVH, we propose that intensive treatment for LV mass reduction begin when there is at least a 20% probability that LVH is present. Similarly, if LV mass is less than 110 g/m^2, the risk of a cardiovascular event in a patient with stage 1 hypertension is low; therefore, initiation or intensity of treatment would be determined by the presence or absence of other risk factors.

Role of Two-Dimensional Echocardiography, Magnetic Resonance Imaging, Computed Tomography, and Three-Dimensional Imaging

Two-dimensional measurements of LV mass using Simpson's rule and the area-length method have been standard-

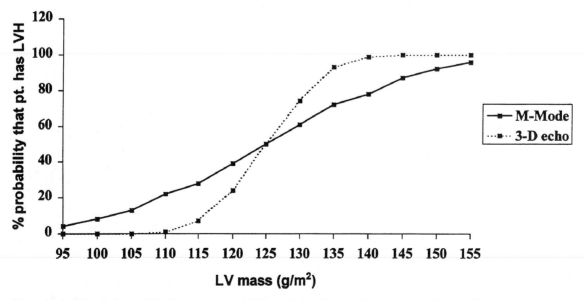

Figure 27–7. Estimated probability that an observed left ventricular (LV) mass index (LV mass/body surface area) obtained by either M-mode or three-dimensional (3-D) echocardiography is >125 g/m^2. This is based on a standard deviation for M-mode of 17.4 g/m^2 and for 3-D of 6.8 g/m^2 (assuming that body surface area is 1.7 m^2).

ized and may be reproducible.[122, 123] However, acceptance of these measurements is limited by several factors, including lack of anatomic validation of the technique, which may be a result of incorrect assumptions about ventricular geometry in unusually shaped ventricles, and technical difficulties in obtaining endocardial and epicardial interfaces, especially of the lateral wall.[109]

New techniques focus on more accurate visualization of the left ventricle. Many of them are less dependent on calculations based on geometric assumptions about the shape of the ventricle. Magnetic resonance imaging (MRI), for example, may give highly reliable and anatomically validated LV mass measurements.[124–126] Transverse slices are obtained and the endocardial and epicardial contours are determined. Computer summation of all the pixels in the circumscribed muscle area of each slice may then be determined. The multiple of slice thickness and number of slices, and the specific gravity of 1.04 g/ml, is then calculated to obtain LV mass. There are no assumptions regarding the shape of the ventricle in this method.

A similar technique may be used with ultrafast computed tomography (CT) images.[127] Although significantly more costly than echocardiography, MRI may be an effective tool for monitoring changes in LV mass for an individual patient or for groups of patients in a research protocol.[126] Less expensive and technically less demanding methods of assessing LV mass have used computer-automated algorithms with technetium-99m-sestamibi single-photon emission CT myocardial perfusion imaging.[128, 129] These techniques rely on determining counts per pixel of myocardium and thus do not depend on assumptions of the geometric shape of the ventricle. Early studies are promising; however, this technique is still in development.[130]

New techniques in echocardiography are allowing accurate, noninvasive assessments of LV mass. Three-dimensional (3-D) echocardiography eliminates the problems of geometric assumptions used in M-mode and 2-D echocardiographic techniques, allowing for more accurate assessment of LV mass. In vitro correlation of 3-D–determined LV mass and actual weight of fixed animal hearts is high, and in vivo correlation with MRI measurement in human patients is also very good over a wide range of weights.[131–135] A new generation of intravenously administered ultrasound contrast agents (microbubbles) capable of consistent and persistent detection within the LV cavity and myocardium now allow easier visualization of the endocardial and epicardial edges, permitting more accurate measurements for conventional M-mode– and 2-D–determined LV mass. In experimental studies, 3-D echocardiography performed with new echocardiographic contrast agents has been used to display myocardial mass and the mass of infarcted myocardium.[136]

REGRESSION OF LEFT VENTRICULAR MASS

Regression of LV mass with effective blood pressure reduction has been demonstrated in more than 400 clinical studies, but fewer than 10% have been double-blind and placebo-controlled.[137] Because few of these early studies were long-term, they did not determine whether regression of LVH increased survival,[138] but they hinted that it would be beneficial, as LV function was not adversely affected and diastolic function often improved.[139–144] Data indicate that regression of LV mass improves survival in hypertensive patients. In one small trial that followed hypertensive patients for more than 10 years, the cumulative incidence of nonfatal cardiovascular events was significantly higher among patients without regression of LVH in comparison to those with significant reduction of LV mass.[145] Verdecchia et al showed decreased risk of cardiac events with regression of LV mass independent of the baseline LV mass, the baseline clinic and ambulatory blood pressure, and the degree of blood pressure reduction.[146] Total cardiovascular events were also found to be fewer in the TOMHS when there was LV mass regression.[147] A mechanism that might explain these findings is that midwall fractional shortening, a sensitive measure of intrinsic myocardial systolic performance, appears to improve with regression of LV mass.[148]

Blood pressure reduction by means of all classes of antihypertensive agents, with the possible exception of pure vasodilators such as minoxidil and hydralazine reduces LV mass.[88] A meta-analysis of more than 100 studies yielded a moderately strong relationship between blood pressure reduction and LV mass regression.[149] This confirms the hemodynamic contribution to LV mass and demonstrates that greater blood pressure reduction is associated with greater regression in mass.

It is not clear, however, whether antihypertensive agents can regress LV mass independent of their effect on blood pressure. In animal studies, ACE inhibitors reduce LV mass without lowering blood pressure.[150] However, one meta-analysis of human studies suggested that for equal levels of blood pressure reduction, β-blockers, ACE inhibitors, and calcium channel blockers cause the same degree of LVH regression, whereas diuretics reduce chamber dimension but do not lead to regression of hypertrophied muscle. This conclusion has been challenged in two randomized trials that suggest that diuretics are as effective as if not more effective than other drug classes for reducing LV mass. In the TOMHS, blood pressure was reduced by a combination of weight loss and either placebo or one of five antihypertensive drug classes (a β-blocker, an α-blocker, a calcium channel blocker, an ACE inhibitor, or a diuretic).[147] At 1 and 4 years, all groups showed regression of LV mass, confirming that weight loss in conjunction with blood pressure reduction reduce LV mass. It is surprising that only the subjects receiving chlorthalidone had greater LV mass regression than did those undergoing weight loss and receiving placebo. Reduced internal dimension as well as reduced wall thickness accounted for this. The Veterans Administration (VA) Cooperative Study Group recently reported similar results: For equal levels of blood pressure reduction, hydrochlorothiazide had a greater effect on LV mass regression than did other antihypertensive agents.[151] In this trial of 493 patients who completed 1 year of maintenance antihypertensive therapy, LV mass was not reduced despite hemodynamic improvement in patients taking prazosin, clonidine, or diltiazem. In the VA trial, ACE inhibition was nearly as beneficial as diuretic-based therapy.

DIASTOLIC FUNCTION IN HYPERTENSION

Clinical Presentation and Etiology

The clinical presentation of diastolic dysfunction in hypertensive heart disease is variable, ranging from asymptomatic findings on noninvasive testing to overt CHF despite normal systolic function.[152–157] The prevalence of asymptomatic LV filling abnormalities in adults without hypertrophy and with ambulatory awake blood pressure greater than 130/85 mm Hg may be as high as 33%.[43] Once LVH or ischemia develops, these asymptomatic abnormalities may cause decreased exercise ejection fraction and blunt the expected rise in exercise cardiac output.[158] An estimated 30 to 45% of patients with CHF have normal systolic function but abnormal diastolic function (CHF-D).[157] In a large community-based study of CHF, the prognosis for patients with diastolic heart failure was poor. Survival rate at 3 months, 1 year, and 5 years was 86%, 76%, and 48%, respectively (Fig. 27–8).[57] In a cohort of patients with diastolic dysfunction and underlying coronary artery disease, 7-year cardiovascular mortality approaches 50%. Many of these patients were also hypertensive.[159] Symptoms in the presence of diastolic dysfunction are accounted

for by prolonged LV relaxation or decreased compliance, which causes shifts in the diastolic LV pressure-volume relation that result in elevated left atrial and LV filling pressures.[160]

Factors Affecting Diastolic Function

Genetic,[161] structural, metabolic, and hemodynamic factors can affect diastolic function under resting conditions and during states of increased demand or ischemia (Fig. 27–9).

Structural Factors

Reports in the late 1980s and early 1990s suggested that diastolic abnormalities occur early in the course of hypertension and precede detectable hypertrophy.[43, 153, 162–164] More recent studies challenge the notion that diastolic abnormalities are the first sign of hypertensive heart disease; they suggest that diastolic abnormalities do not precede structural changes but occur simultaneously. In general, diastolic function is inversely related to LV mass in patients with hypertension,[154, 153, 165–167] and regression of LV mass with calcium channel blockers, β-blockers, and ACE inhibitors is often,[139, 143, 144, 168–170] but not always,[171] associated with improved LV diastolic function. In the Hypertension and Ambulatory Recording Venetia Study (HARVEST), young patients with stage 1 hypertension had significantly greater LV mass and more concentric remodeling than did normotensive subjects.[172] However, there was no significant difference in Doppler mitral inflow velocity (E:A) ratio, a marker of diastolic dysfunction. Experimental data suggest that a diastolic abnormality in the absence of frank hypertrophy indicates that the heart is beginning to hypertrophy in response to hemodynamic or nonhemodynamic stimuli. For example, dogs with aortic banding simultaneously develop abnormalities of LV filling and increased LV mass.[173] This early change appears to be dependent on increased myocyte size rather than on increased fibrosis.[174] However, there is also strong evidence that abnormal filling is partially accounted for by interstitial collagen deposition that occurs with LVH and aging, leading to passive structural changes that result in increased chamber stiffness.[93, 175, 176]

Ischemia

Ischemia has pronounced effects on diastolic function, and these effects are exacerbated even in the minimally hypertrophied heart.[177] Several as yet undefined metabolic/biochemical factors that slow inactivation of the actin-myosin complex and delay relaxation are probably involved. Baseline levels of adenosine triphosphate (ATP) in the pressure-overload hypertrophied heart are similar to or slightly lower than those in control hearts.[178, 179] Although it may be normal in the resting state,[180] the rate of sarcoplasmic uptake of calcium, an energy-dependent and ATP-requiring process, is markedly reduced by hypoxia.[181] However, diastolic dysfunction in the hypertrophied ventricle may not be fully explained by depletion of high-energy phosphates. In one study, when isolated buffer-perfused rat hearts were subjected to hypoxia, significantly more ischemia devel-

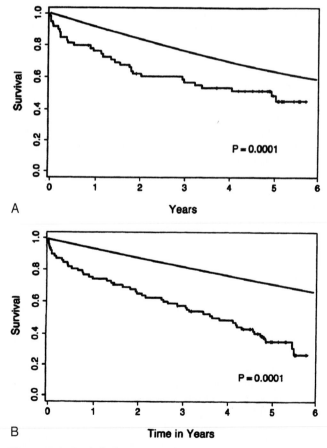

Figure 27–8. Survival of patients with an ejection fraction of ≥50% (**A**) or <50% (**B**) compared with that for age- and sex-matched population. (**A** and **B**, from Senni M, Tribouilloy CM, Rodeheffer RJ, et al. Congestive heart failure in the community. Circulation 98:2282–2289, 1998.)

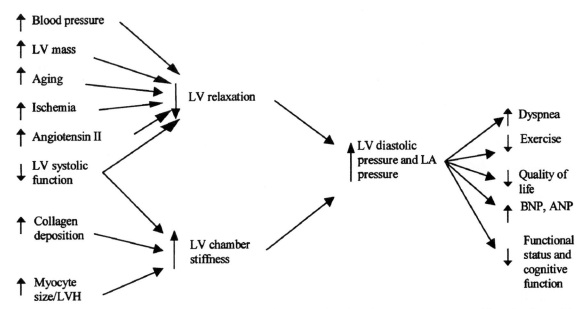

Figure 27–9. Causes of left ventricular (LV) diastolic dysfunction and its clinical consequences. ANP, atrial natriuretic peptide; BNP, brain natriuretic peptide: LA, left atrial; LV, left ventricular; LVH, left ventricular hypertrophy.

oped in hypertrophied hearts than in control hearts at equivalent rates of coronary flow and with similar rates of ATP depletion.[178] This led the authors to conclude that hypertrophy-induced alterations in calcium handling, such as changes in the calcium transients, which are abnormal even at rest,[182] might contribute to ischemia-induced diastolic dysfunction in LVH. In the intact dog, however, under conditions of increased oxygen demand, there was decreased conversion of phosphocreatinine to ATP in the hypertrophied heart,[179] suggesting that high-energy phosphate metabolism is impaired by hypertrophy. Differences in results between the isolated heart and the intact heart may be due to failure of the intact heart to deliver adequate blood flow because of decreased coronary flow reserve.

Hemodynamic Load

Increased hemodynamic load affects diastolic performance. In isolated hearts, increases in afterload early in systole impair relaxation.[183] Wall stress in untreated hypertensive persons is inversely related to diastolic function.[167] When studied with ambulatory monitoring, previously untreated borderline and mild hypertensive patients demonstrate a linear relation between blood pressure and abnormal LV filling.[43, 184] The degree to which an acute reduction in blood pressure per se improves LV diastolic performance is not known, and studies are difficult to interpret because the agents used can themselves affect performance.[185, 186]

Systolic Function

Systolic and diastolic dysfunction are closely linked. Midwall fractional shortening, a more sensitive measure of intrinsic myocardial systolic function than endocardial fractional shortening, is abnormal in a substantial portion of asymptomatic hypertensive persons.[187, 188] Schussheim et al found that depressed midwall fractional shortening and diastolic dysfunction occur simultaneously in asympto-

matic hypertensive persons with normal endocardial fractional shortening.[189] Conversely, those with normal midwall fractional shortening tend to have normal Doppler indices of mitral inflow.

Enhanced systolic performance, such as during exercise, is associated with improved diastolic function.[167, 190] Systolic function directly affects the efficiency of elastic recoil.[190] Increased recoil, in turn, augments the ability of the heart to generate negative pressure during early diastole, a "suction" phenomenon that increases LV filling. Catecholamines enhance diastolic function and improve LV filling through enhancement of myocardial restoring forces and recoil during isovolumetric relaxation.[191] OPC-18790, an experimental phosphodiesterase inhibitor, increases contractility but does not affect heart rate. During intracoronary infusion in patients with heart failure, this agent has decreased the time constant for isovolumetric relaxation (tau) without reducing afterload, reflecting enhanced active relaxation.[192] Thus, an inotropic agent may improve diastolic function.

Aging

Aging has profound effects on diastolic function, which is reflected in a reduced rate of LV relaxation and increased diastolic stiffness. This effect has been confirmed by various noninvasive measurements of diastolic function.[43, 70, 193–198] Among normal subjects in the Framingham Heart Study, age was the predominant factor affecting Doppler indices of diastolic function, with a Pearson correlation coefficient of -0.80 between age and the E:A ratio.[199] Hypertension, including isolated systolic hypertension (ISH), further depresses diastolic function in older subjects,[163, 200, 201] but this finding is controversial.[202]

The effect of exercise on age-related changes in diastolic function is also controversial. A prospectively designed exercise program in men between the ages of 60 and 82 demonstrated reversal of depressed LV diastolic function with aging.[203] However, a cross-sectional study of younger (52–76 years) male athletes demonstrated similar impairment of diastolic LV filling compared with sedentary peers.[204] In contrast, a study of healthy persons in all age ranges demonstrated improvement in diastolic function with regular modest use of alcohol or regular aerobic exercise.[205]

Hormones and Paracrine Factors

As noted earlier, catecholamines are believed to favorably affect diastolic performance by improving systolic performance. Several other studies suggest that angiotensin II adversely affects diastolic function by impairing LV relaxation and stimulating aldosterone-mediated myocardial fibrosis.[93]

Noninvasive Measurement of Diastolic Function

Diastolic function may be evaluated by several methods. The rate of isovolumetric pressure decay, early and late LV filling, and pressure-volume relations can be derived from cardiac catherization.[206–208] Although these measurements are the most accurate indexes of diastolic function, they require an invasive procedure. Inferences regarding the diastolic properties of the ventricle can be obtained noninvasively with radionuclide angiography[209] and M-mode[210] or Doppler echocardiography[211] and acoustic quantification.[212] These techniques yield information on all phases of diastole, including isovolumetric relaxation, early and late LV filling,[43, 163, 213] and temporal differences in regional filling (regional nonuniformity).[214]

Radionuclide angiography was one of the first noninvasive techniques for assessment of LV filling properties. It is based on analysis of the LV time-activity curve. The time-activity curve represents relative volume changes throughout the cardiac cycle. Several parameters of diastolic function may be computed from the time-activity curve, including the peak rate of rapid diastolic filling, the time to peak filling rate, and the relative contributions of the rapid filling to total filling volume and the time interval from end-systole to the end of rapid filling. In addition, the duration of the isovolumetric relaxation period may be computed in approximately 80% of patients. Decreased peak filling rate, increased time to peak filling rate, and decreased one-third and one-half filling fractions are reported.

Hypertensive patients with LVH and impaired diastolic filling at rest also have decreased exercise-induced augmentation in end-diastolic volume, leading to reduced stroke volume and impaired exercise ejection fraction.[215] Attention must be given to the technical details of data acquisition and analysis for evaluation of diastolic events using radionuclide angiography. In particular, the effects of cycle length variability (in gated studies), temporal resolution, temporal smoothing, and normalization parameters must be considered. For diastolic studies, high-count double-buffered, left anterior oblique 32-frame images are used.

Doppler echocardiographic evaluation of LV inflow is the most widely used noninvasive measure of diastolic function.[216] The LV diastolic flow velocity profile obtained with Doppler echocardiography correlates well with radionuclide angiographic variables in the evaluation of LV diastolic function.[209] In the setting of normal ventricular relaxation LV pressure is significantly lower than left atrial pressure immediately after mitral valve opening, and therefore the gradient between the left atrium and left ventricle is relatively high. This results in a high peak velocity of early filling (E) and significant emptying of the blood in the left atrium in early diastole. As a result, the peak velocity of the late filling wave (A) is low. If LV relaxation is prolonged, the LV pressure decline after mitral valve opening is delayed so that the gradient between the left atrium and left ventricle in early diastole is reduced, and equilibration of pressure between the two chambers may be delayed. In the setting of normal LV function, this is reflected on the Doppler recording as a reduced E and a higher A:E ratio or a prolonged deceleration time of the early filling wave or both (Figs. 27–10 and 27–11).[217–219]

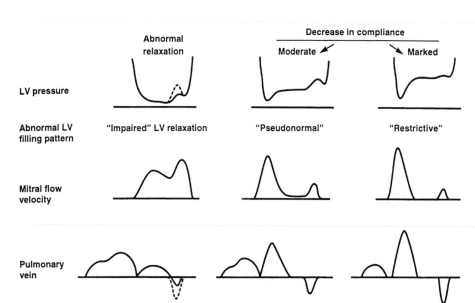

Figure 27–10. Three basic abnormal left ventricular (LV) filling (mitral flow velocity) patterns together with representative LV pressure recordings and pulmonary venous flow velocity recordings. (From Appleton CP. Left ventricular diastolic function. *In* Murphy, JG [ed]. Mayo Clinic Cardiology Review. Armonk, NY, Futura, 1997; pp 43–56. By permission of Mayo Foundation.)

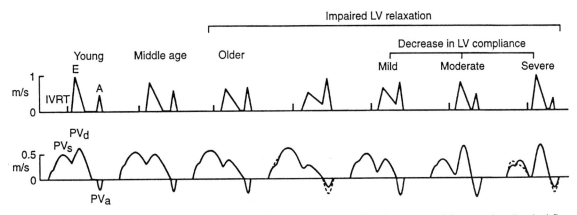

Figure 27–11. Natural history of left ventricular (LV) filling patterns. A, mitral flow velocity at atrial contraction; E, mitral flow velocity in early diastole; IVRT, isovolume relaxation time; PV_a, reverse pulmonary venous velocity at atrial contraction; PV_d, pulmonary venous flow velocity in diastole; PV_s, pulmonary venous flow velocity in systole. (From Appleton CP. Left ventricular diastolic function. *In* Murphy JG [ed]. Mayo Clinic Cardiology Review. Armonk, NY, Futura, 1997; pp 43–56.)

The enhanced A wave may be a result of two factors: (1) the LV pressure is lower than normal just before the atrial contraction due to decreased LV filling, and (2) the delayed atrial emptying causes a rise in atrial pressure. These two factors lead to a higher gradient between the left atrium and left ventricle at atrial systole and, hence, to an enhanced peak A wave.

Using Doppler echocardiography, one group studied normal subjects between the ages of 20 and 50 years (mean 35 ± 9), with heart rates 90 beats/min or fewer and no evidence of coronary artery disease. The average value peak A:E ratio was 0.67 ± 0.16; an A:E ratio of 0.99 was two standard deviations above this mean value.[43] These data have been corroborated by others, who have shown that an A:E ratio of 1 in subjects younger than 50 years of age is significantly higher than the range for normal subjects.[196] Framingham Heart Study data, however, suggest that an A:E ratio of 1 may be in the upper range of normal for a 40- to 50- year-old and is clearly abnormal only in subjects under age 40 (Fig. 27–12).[220] Studies using Doppler echocardiography show that approximately 20% of untreated borderline or mild hypertensive persons have diastolic filling abnormalities in the absence of LVH.[43, 221] In addition, there may be a threshold of average awake ambulatory blood pressure, 130/85 mm Hg, below which neither diastolic abnormalities nor LVH is detected (Fig. 27–13).[43]

Pitfalls in Interpretation of Noninvasive Measurements

Information derived from Doppler echocardiography should be interpreted in the context of the many dynamic factors that can affect Doppler variables. These include changes in afterload, systolic performance, heart rate, and cardiac filling pressures.[217, 222] For example, the peak velocity of late LV filling (peak A) is directly related to heart rate.[223] Therefore, a pharmacological intervention that simultaneously increases heart rate and the height of the A wave could be incorrectly interpreted as adversely affecting diastolic function. Conversely, a pharmacological intervention that raises LV end-diastolic pressure could be misinterpreted as being beneficial if it simultaneously lowers the A wave and raise the E wave, that is, creates "pseudonormal-

ization" of the Doppler profile. This was demonstrated in a study in which verapamil was given to patients with coronary artery disease.[224] This intervention resulted in an increased velocity of early filling (E wave) and a shortening of isovolumetric relaxation. Invasive studies, however, showed that these seemingly beneficial changes were, in fact, associated with a prolongation of the time constant of relaxation and an increase in LV end-diastolic pressure. Thus, increased LV end-diastolic pressure and left atrial filling pressures, not improved LV relaxation, caused a pattern of Doppler pseudonormalization characterized by a higher E wave, a lower A wave, and a shortened isovolumetric relaxation time.

Emerging Techniques to Measure Diastolic Function

A challenge in noninvasive evaluation of diastolic function is to devise methods by which LV end-diastolic pressure

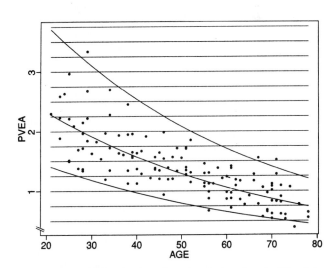

Figure 27–12. Predicted value of peak velocity of early filling:late filling (PVEA) ratio in normal subjects studied in the Framingham Heart Study. *Solid outer lines* represent the 95% confidence intervals. At approximately age 40 years, a PVEA ratio below 1 is outside of the 95% confidence interval. (Reprinted from Am J Cardiol, vol 70, Benjamin EJ, Levy D, Anderson KM, et al. Determinants of Doppler indexes of left ventricular diastolic function in normal subjects [the Framingham Heart Study], pp 508–515, Copyright 1992, with permission from Excerpta Medica Inc.)

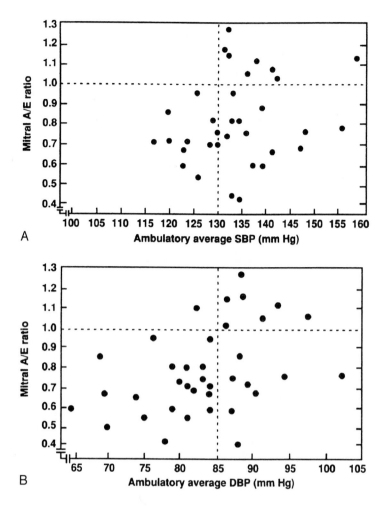

Figure 27–13. Ratio of late (A) to early (E) left ventricular inflow velocity (A:E ratio) in 37 subjects (<50 years old) plotted against average awake ambulatory systolic blood pressure (SBP) **(A)** and average ambulatory awake diastolic blood pressure (DBP) **(B)**. All subjects were untreated, had no evidence of coronary disease, and were referred for evaluation of borderline hypertension. *Horizontal hatched line* indicates that A:E ratio ≥ 1 is abnormal in this population; *vertical hatched line* indicates blood pressure above which abnormal A:E ratio was detected. **A.** Abnormal subjects had SBP > 130 mm Hg. **B.** Only 1 of 22 subjects with DBP < 85 mm Hg had abnormal A:E ratio, and this subject had SBP > 130; all other subjects with abnormal A:E ratio (7, *open circles*) had DBP > 85. (**A** and **B**, From Phillips RA, Goldman ME, Ardeljan M, et al. Determinants of abnormal left ventricular filling in early hypertension. J Am Coll Cardiol 14:979–985, 1989.)

can be serially evaluated. One group suggested that atrial natriuretic peptide (ANP), a measure of LV filling pressures, be used to interpret changes in noninvasively derived LV filling parameters.[144] Plasma ANP levels increase when the atria are stretched as a result of increased filling pressures,[225–227] and the levels fall as LV end-diastolic pressure decreases. This knowledge was exploited to interpret a Doppler evaluation of diastolic function in severely hypertensive subjects treated for 1 year with nifedipine.[144] Over the year, the Doppler early filling (E wave) increased, whereas the A wave decreased. ANP levels fell, suggesting that LV end-diastolic pressure had decreased. The investigators concluded that it was likely that the increased velocity of early filling and decreased A wave were due to improved LV relaxation.

Several new Doppler techniques are emerging that may allow for serial noninvasive interpretation of LV end-diastolic pressure. Among these is measurement of pulmonary venous inflow.[228–230] During atrial contraction, flow into the pulmonary vein reverses as the pulmonary veins become a "low-pressure sink" for the contracting atrium. Increased LV end-diastolic pressures creates more "afterload" for the atrium, leading to increased height and duration of the "reverse flow" wave. Furthermore, the difference in pulmonary venous and mitral flow velocity duration during atrial contraction is related to the increase in LV end-diastolic pressure.[229] Therefore, prolonged pulmonary ve-

nous velocity duration at atrial contraction coupled with a shortened duration of the mitral A wave suggest increasing LV end-diastolic pressure. Conversely, a shorter pulmonary venous velocity duration coupled with a lengthened transmitral A wave during atrial contraction suggest decreasing LV end-diastolic pressure (see Fig. 27–10).

Another promising Doppler technique to assess LV end-diastolic pressure rests on the observation that diastolic flow is initially directed toward the ventricular apex (transmitral A wave) and then wraps around and enters the left ventricular outflow tract just before ejection.[231, 232] This "pre-ejection wave," termed the Ar wave, can be identified on recordings of the LV outflow tract. The time from the peak of the transmitral A wave to the peak of the Ar wave (the A–Ar interval) is inversely related to LV chamber stiffness and LV end-diastolic pressure[231]—the stiffer the ventricle or the higher the LV end-diastolic pressure, the shorter the A–Ar interval.

Color M-mode assessment of LV filling expands on this concept. It is based on the interval from color M-mode peak velocity at the mitral leaflet tips to peak velocity in the apical region of the left ventricle. A first wave propagates from the left atrium to the LV apex, corresponding to early filling, and a second wave follows atrial contraction. The magnitude of these velocities is highest above the mitral tips and decreases as flow approaches the apex. The velocity at which flow propagates within the ventricle

(V_p) is given by the slope of the color wavefront. The time delay of the first wave of early filling from its appearance at the mitral leaflets to its appearance in the LV apex (TD) is also measured and is directly related to the time constant of isovolumetric relaxation. In hypertensive patients with abnormal relaxation and in patients with restrictive heart disease, there is reduced V_p and prolonged TD.[233–235] These variables may be independent of heart rate and LV end-diastolic pressure. Thus, this technique may become extremely useful in serial assessment of LV relaxation.

Doppler tissue imaging is a new ultrasound technique based on color Doppler imaging principles. It allows quantification of intramural myocardial velocities by detection of consecutive phase shifts of the ultrasound signal reflected from contracting myocardium. Large Doppler signals obtained from the ventricular wall can be selectively displayed as a color or pulsed Doppler image by eliminating small Doppler signals produced by the blood flow.[236, 237] There are significant correlations between peak early diastolic velocities in the septum, the time from the second heart sound to the peak of the early diastolic wave in the septum, and the time constant of LV pressure decay during an isovolumetric diastole (tau) as determined during cardiac catheterization.[238]

Effect of Treatment on Diastolic Congestive Heart Failure

Treatment of hypertensive patients with symptoms of CHF-D is guided by relatively few studies. Topol et al, in a landmark study, analyzed the effect of treatment on morbidity and mortality in 21 elderly hypertensive patients with marked concentric hypertrophy, supernormal LV systolic function, and depressed LV diastolic function. These patients were treated with a variety of antihypertensive and cardioactive agents because of heart failure, angina, stroke, or syncope.[156] Of the 12 patients who received vasodilators (nitrates, hydralazine, prazosin, or catopril), 6 had a severe hypotensive reaction and 1 patient died. In contrast, all 9 patients who received β-blockers or calcium antagonists improved, and 4 subjects had less dyspnea after discontinuation of digoxin and furosemide. In a more recent study of 144 patients with CHF and Doppler evidence of restrictive LV diastolic filling as measured by a shortened deceleration time of early mitral filling, cardiac mortality was assessed after 2 years of unblinded oral therapy. Various combinations of digoxin, diuretics, ACE inhibitors, nitrates and β-blockers were used. Survival was significantly better in patients with prolongation of the deceleration time over the treatment period compared with patients with no change in deceleration time.[239] The latter group used more digoxin. No other significant difference in medication use was noted. Thus, although reversing diastolic dysfunction may relieve symptoms and prolong survival, the optimal regimen is still not clear.

The few systematic studies of various agents on CHF-D are reviewed herein. The paucity of data that form the basis for conflicting recommendations by authorities on the optimal treatment of CHF-D suggests a need for a randomized trial. Drug classes whose efficacy in the treatment of CHF-D has not been proved in a clinical trial should be tested in a more rigorous fashion.

ACE Inhibitors

Two studies have evaluated the efficacy of ACE inhibitors in CHF-D. In one study, 10 subjects with hypertension, LHV, and CHF-D were treated in a nonrandomized, uncontrolled approach with the ACe inhibitor enalapril and a low-sodium diet.[170] After an average of 9 months of treatment, heart failure symptoms resolved in all subjects, without the use of diuretics. Diastolic function, as measured by Doppler echocardiography, did not change after the initial decrease in blood pressure, but improved significantly (decreased A:E ratio and deceleration time) after regression of LV mass. Another study compared treatment with enalapril to standard therapy without enalapril in 21 elderly patients with CHF-D, prior non–Q-wave myocardial infarction, and normal ejection fraction.[240] In the enalapril group, blood pressure and LV mass were significantly reduced with treatment, and this was accompanied by a significant improvement in New York Heart Association functional score (a decrease from 3.0 to 2.4, $p < .01$), increased exercise time on a treadmill, and an improvement in diastolic function as measured by Doppler echocardiography.

Calcium Channel Blockers

Two small, short-term studies have been reported in which calcium channel blockers were the mainstays of therapy for CHF. In a prospective study of 20 patients (15 of whom had hypertension), verapamil and placebo were compared in a 5-week crossover design. In comparison with baseline values, verapamil significantly improved LV filling, decreased symptoms, and improved exercise time,[241] whereas placebo had no significant effect. However, possibly because of a carryover effect of verapamil-induced improvement into the placebo phase of the crossover design, there was no difference between verapamil and placebo in LV filling. In six severely hypertensive patients followed for 4 months, of whom four received a concomitant diuretic, treatment with nifedipine was associated with symptomatic improvement.[242]

β-Blockade

To our knowledge, no study has evaluated the role of β-blockade in isolated CHF-D. A study in patients with idiopathic dilated cardiomyopathy (ejection fraction < 25%) evaluated the effect of metoprolol, up to 50 mg three times a day, on diastolic dysfunction.[243] Not only did diastolic function improve within 3 months of treatment, but the investigators suggested that better diastolic performance may have allowed for the subsequent improvement in systolic function.

Diuretics

Although no clinical trial data are available, several investigators recommend cautious use of diuretics to reduce the congested state in CHF-D.[155, 244] Diuretics reduce congestion by lowering LV preload and by reducing right ventricular filling pressure, thereby relieving pericardial restraint on the LV.[245] However, use of diuretics remains controversial because of the lack of clinical trial data and the concern that preload may be inappropriately reduced with "over-diuresis." In fact, the Fifth Report of the Joint National Committee on the Detection and Treatment of Hypertension considers diuretic therapy in diastolic dysfunction as "relatively or absolutely contraindicated" in patients with hypertensive hypertrophic cardiomyopathy with diastolic dysfunction.[246] However, diuretic-based therapy very effectively prevents the development of CHF in patients with hypertension.

Digoxin and Inotropes

Although digoxin may improve LV filling by decreasing heart rate, its ability to increase intracellular calcium may increase LV stiffness.[247] In the recent Digitalis Investigation Group trial, sponsored by the National Institutes of Health, which involved nearly 8000 patients,[248] digoxin did not appear to be deleterious in those with abnormal systolic function (CHF-S) and might have improved functional status.

OPC-18790, the experimental phosphodiesterase inhibitor described earlier, increases contractility but does not affect heart rate. During intracoronary infusion in patients with heart failure, this agent decreased the time constant for isovolumetric relaxation (tau) without reducing afterload, reflecting enhanced active relaxation.[192]

Summary of Treatment

Although 2 million Americans have CHF-D, only 71 have been enrolled in published studies that specifically evaluated the effects of drug therapy on this syndrome. Some authorities recommend that first-line treatment include β-blockers or calcium antagonists.[244, 246] However, until recently, β-blockers were contraindicated in patients with CHF. Others agree that management of symptoms in these patients often requires use of diuretics,[155] but that physicians should prescribe diuretics cautiously in this setting. Others advocate ACE inhibitors for reversal of interstitial fibrosis, which can cause diastolic dysfunction.[249] These contradictory recommendations, which are not based on evidence, underscore the urgent need for controlled clinical trials in this area.

Effect of Antihypertensive Treatment on Asymptomatic Diastolic Dysfunction

The effect of antihypertensive treatment on noninvasively detected LV filling abnormalities in asymptomatic subjects has been studied with a variety of agents. No study has reported conversion from asymptomatic to symptomatic status with treatment. Thus, analysis of therapy relies on serial measurements of noninvasively derived measures of LV filling. These studies are difficult to evaluate without data on filling pressures, which are rarely provided. For example, one 8-week study comparing verapamil and lisinopril suggested that verapamil was superior because treatment resulted in shorter time to peak LV filling, reduced

isovolumetric relaxation time, and greater first-half filling. In that study, lisinopril prolonged resting isovolumetric relaxation time.[250] An equally compelling alternative explanation is that the effect of verapamil was a result of increased filling pressures[224] and the effect of lisinopril was due to decreased filling pressures.

Calcium Channel Blockers

Many studies suggest that verapamil and dihydropyridine calcium channel blockers improve diastolic function.[139, 143, 144, 250, 251] Some of these salubrious effects are likely to be pharmacological, but some studies also suggest that improved filling is dependent on coincident LV mass regression.[139, 143, 144] Studies with diltiazem showed no significant benefit, but these were flawed by the short duration of treatment[154] or by the inclusion of patients whose LV diastolic function was nearly normal at baseline.[252]

β-Blockers

β-Blockers are routinely advocated as first-line agents in the treatment of CHF-D.[244, 253] However, the effect of β-blocker therapy on diastolic function has been variable. Some studies show improved filling (in association with, but possibly independent of, LV mass regression).[139, 168, 169] Two studies, including one in elderly hypertensive patients, failed to demonstrate LV mass regression or improvement in diastolic function.[143, 254] Because β-blockade antagonizes catecholamine-mediated LV relaxation, it has been suggested that it can improve diastolic function only if accompanied by blood pressure reduction, relief of ischemia, and prolongation of the time for LV filling.[155, 255]

ACE Inhibitors

Studies of the effect of ACE inhibitors on asymptomatic diastolic dysfunction in hypertensive patients have produced variable results. Angiotensin II has a direct negative effect on myocardial relaxation,[256] so inhibition of angiotensin II would be expected to improve LV filling. In one study in which captopril induced significant LV mass regression, Doppler indexes of LV filling did not change.[171] However, LV filling was normal at baseline; thus, it would not be expected that LV filling would improve. Both lisinopril[257] and enalapril have been shown to improve Doppler or M-mode–derived indexes of diastolic function.[141]

CORONARY MICROCIRCULATION ABNORMALITIES IN THE PATIENT WITH HYPERTENSION

In hypertensive patients with LVH, structural and functional alterations in the small coronary vessels, increasing ventricular wall stress, and alterations in the rheological properties of blood (e.g., increased viscosity) inhibit the ability of the coronary microcirculation to regulate overall coronary blood flow.[258] These abnormalities result in diminished coronary flow reserve, the increase in total coronary blood flow that occurs with maximal vasodilatation (Fig.

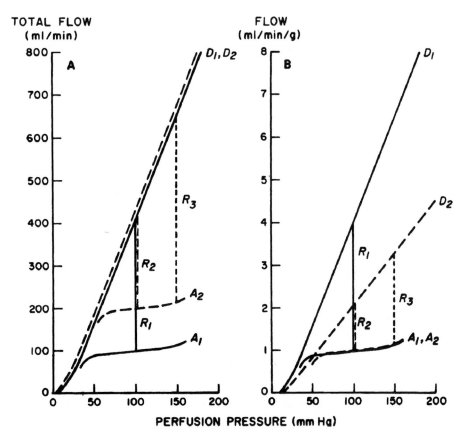

Figure 27–14. Diagram of coronary flow reserve in the presence of hypertrophy. **A.** Absolute flow is measured (ml/min). **B.** How per unit mass (ml/min/g) is measured. A, autoregulated flows; D, pressure flow line during maximal vasodilatation; R, flow reserve. Normal are A_1, D_1, R_1, and *solid lines*. Hypertrophied are A_2, D_2, R_2, R_3, and *dashed lines*. In both scenarios, coronary flow reserve is diminished. R_3 represents coronary flow reserve when perfusion pressures are elevated. (**A** and **B**, From Hoffman JI. A critical view of coronary reserve. Circulation 75[suppl I]:6–11, 1987.)

27–14). Abnormal coronary flow reserve may predispose the patient with hypertension to ischemic syndromes, which lead to heart failure, myocardial infarction, and sudden death.

Coronary Vessel Pathology in Left Ventricular Hypertrophy

Various vascular abnormalities result in a reduction in the maximal cross-sectional area of the coronary microvasculature. These abnormalities include inadequate vascular growth in response to increasing muscle mass, changes in vessel wall composition, vascular remodeling, and endothelial dysfunction.

Rarefaction of Arterioles

Morphometric studies in various animal model suggest that inadequate growth of the coronary microvascular bed limits myocardial perfusion in the presence of pressure-overload hypertrophy.[259–266] The capacity for coronary angiogenesis decreases over time. Between the ages of 9 and 14 years, heart weight in humans increases fourfold, while capillary density decreases by 28%. Capillary density in the hypertrophied heart is also age-dependent. Adults with acquired aortic stenosis have decreased capillary density, whereas children with congenital aortic stenosis maintain capillary density by increasing capillary supply in proportion to myocyte volume.[264, 267, 268] As hypertrophy progresses in the adult with hypertension, there is insufficient angiogenesis

to compensate for the increasing myocardial mass. Defective angiogenesis may be a mechanism in the inheritance of hypertension. Higher vascular resistance and lower capillary density (in the dorsum of the finger) was demonstrated in mildly hypertensive young men with hypertensive parents than in mildly hypertensive men without hypertensive parents.[269]

The mechanisms of angiogenesis are complex. Factors released with increased vascular wall tension that influence cell-to-cell interactions, extracellular matrix molecules, and the inhibition and stimulation of endothelial growth factors may be important.[270, 271] One such factor, hepatocyte growth factor, is a mesenchyme-derived pleiotropic factor that regulates cell growth, cell motility, and morphogenesis of vascular tissue (among other types of cells). Myocardial hepatocyte growth factor concentrations are low in spontaneously hypertensive rats (SHRs) and are inversely proportional to LV weight. Concentrations of cardiac and vascular angiotensin II, a suppressor of hepatocyte growth factor, are increased in SHRs. In addition, administration of an ACE inhibitor or AT_1 receptor antagonist results in a significant increase in cardiac concentration of hepatocyte growth factor.[272]

Medial Wall Thickening

Pressure overload with coronary arterial hypertension causes vascular medial hypertrophy with decreased lumen diameter and increased ratio of media thickness to lumen diameter (the media-lumen ratio).[273–276] Comparisons of coronary vascular morphology and coronary resistance in normotensive Wistar-Kyoto rats and SHRs showed a nearly twofold increase in medial thickness of the coronary arterioles of the hypertensive rats.[277] There was also a significantly increased ratio of medial thickness to vessel radius and increased minimal coronary resistance in the SHRs. The cellular basis for this increase in medial thickness is predominantly rearrangement of smooth muscle cells within the medial layers of the arterial wall, not increases in individual myocyte cell size.[278] The factors responsible for this rearrangement are slowly becoming understood. Endothelin plays a significant role, as blockade of endothelin-subtype A receptors inhibits hypertrophic vascular remodeling in salt-sensitive forms of hypertension.[279, 280] This factor and other agents important for control of smooth muscle cell hypertrophy and proliferation (endothelial growth factor, platelet-derived growth factor, angiotensin II, mechanical stretch, and fluid shear stress) induce a series of cellular kinase cascades, known collectively as the mitogen-activated protein kinase cascades, which have been implicated in vascular smooth muscle cell proliferation and hypertrophy.[281] These kinases lead to activation of the proto-oncogenes c-*fos* and c-*jun,* which are components of the nuclear transcription factor AP-1. Activation of this transcription factor results in increased gene expression for processes that initiate vascular growth and hypertrophy (see Fig 27–5).[282] The extent of vascular structural alterations may be independent from the extent of endothelial dysfunction in hypertension.[283]

Perivascular and Interstitial Fibrosis

In addition to medial hypertrophy, pressure-overload cardiac hypertrophy with hypertension causes increased vascular and perivascular deposition of collagen.[284–286] Inhibition of collage deposition in vascular and extravascular myocardial tissue in Wistar rats shows that coronary flow reserve is determined mostly by medial thickening, independent of collagen deposition. Nevertheless, collagen deposition does affect coronary blood flow, as there is greater reversal of coronary flow abnormalities after removing the pressure load on the heart (aortic banding) in rats with less collagen deposition.[286]

Increased Vascular Water Content

A 10 to 15% increase in the water content of arterial walls occurs in hypertensive patients. A high concentration of vascular water produces thickening of the vascular walls (even in the absence of hypertrophy) and may also cause a reduction in coronary flow reserve.[277]

Endothelial Dysfunction

The endothelium is an important modulator of vascular smooth muscle tone. Furchgott and Zawadzki first demonstrated that acetylcholine and other endothelial-dependent vasodilators lose their vasodilating effect when the endothelium is damaged. These vasodilators exert their effect by causing the endothelial cells to release a potent endogenous vasodilator, endothelium-derived relaxing factor, now known to be nitric oxide.[287] The nitric oxide may inhibit synthesis of extracellular matrix and inhibit mesangial cell hypertrophy and hyperplasia in the kidney. In the heart and systemic vessels, nitric oxide appears to reverse smooth muscle cell hypertrophy and hyperplasia.[288] Thus, expression of nitric oxide in hypertension may help to protect against target organ damage. Impairment of endothelial function is an early vascular abnormality that results in abnormal myocardial blood flow in patients with coronary artery disease, angina pectoris with normal coronary arteriograms, and hypertension with LVH. Most studies demonstrate a blunted response to acetycholine-stimulated endothelium-dependent vasodilation in hypertensive patients.[289–293] Imbalance between endothelium-mediated vasodilatation and vasoconstriction may be an early lesion in hypertension. In SHRs, impaired endothelium-dependent relaxation occurred before the development of overt hypertension.[294] Recent attention has focused on substance P and bradykinin, native peptides of the coronary endothelium that are extremely potent in triggering endothelium-dependent dilation of small coronary arteries. They contribute to resting coronary blood flow and partially mediate flow-dependent dilation in response to increased myocardial demand.[295, 296] A cytochrome P450 product, and not nitric oxide, may regulate production of these vasodilators.[296]

Myocardial Hypertrophy and Wall Stress

Increased wall stress (which is one factor that initiates the development of LVH in hypertensive patients) may directly moderate coronary flow reserve by causing physical compression of blood vessels. Elevated wall stress may stimulate the release of vasoactive substances that alter vascular function and growth.[277] Patients with nonhypertensive LVH without ventricular dilatation and increased wall tension (e.g., some cases of aortic stenosis and hypertrophic obstructive and hypertrophic nonobstructive cardiomyopathy with no ventricular dilatation) do not have decreased coronary flow reserve. Patients with hypertension and similar degrees of LVH and patients with aortic stenosis plus ventricular dilatation and increased LV end-diastolic pressures, however, show abnormally decreased flow reserve.[297, 298] This effect is also seen in patients with dilated cardiomyopathy[299] and in those with dilated ventricles due to aortic regurgitation.[300, 301]

Alterations of Coronary Autoregulation and Flow Reserve With Left Ventricular Hypertrophy

The coronary circulation is able to maintain relatively stable blood flow over a wide range of perfusion pressures.[302–305] This range is generally between 70 and 130 mm Hg in humans.[306] Coronary flow decreases markedly when perfusion pressure drops below the lower limit of autoregulation.

Proposed Mechanisms of Autoregulation

Both metabolic and myogenic mechanisms may product autoregulation of coronary flow. Different sites in the microvasculature may have different dominant mechanisms of control.[307] The smallest coronary arterioles are sensitive predominantly to metabolic factors, whereas larger arterioles are more reactive to myogenic stimuli. According to the metabolic theory, a decrease in coronary artery perfusion pressure results in decreased blood flow. Subsequent decreases in myocardial substrate availability or increases in production of metabolites produce vasodilatation.[308] Potential mediators include oxygen (myocardial oxygen tension), potassium and calcium ion concentrations (transmembrane potentials), osmolality, adenosine, prostaglandins, carbon dioxide, and hydrogen ion concentrations.[309–311] The endogenous vasodilator nitric oxide has been shown to inhibit coronary autoregulation.[312] Myogenic regulation is an intrinsic mechanism; application of force to vascular smooth muscle results in contraction.[313–315] In the coronary circulation, myogenic responses are difficult to demonstrate because they are closely integrated with metabolic factors.[316] These mechanisms cause both microvascular dilatation and increased recruitment of arterioles,[317] resulting in changes in intramyocardial blood volume. Myocardial contrast echocardiography can quantify autoregulatory increases in intramyocardial blood volume and thus may provide a noninvasive method for studying coronary autoregulation.[318]

Relationship Between Autoregulated Coronary Flow and Maximal Coronary Flow

Coronary flow reserve (CFR) is, for any given perfusion pressure, the decrease in coronary resistance over the resting state that occurs after maximal coronary vasodilatation. A normal human heart can increase coronary flow by a factor of 4 to 5 times above the resting state.[297] Coronary flow increases above resting autoregulated levels after transient coronary arterial occlusion (reactive hyperemia), exercise, pacing, or injection of agents like dipyridamole, adenosine, papaverine, or hyperosmolar iodinated contrast medium.[319] Loss of autoregulation occurs during these events. CFR is a dynamic value that is dependent on coronary perfusion pressure. Because there is no autoregulation during states that produce maximal coronary flow, the relationship between coronary flow and coronary perfusion pressure is linear. Relatively small changes in perfusion pressure produce large changes in CFR.

Factors That Confound the Measurement of Coronary Flow Reserve

Increased heart rate, contractility, and afterload decrease CFR and confound measurement of CFR. It is not clear whether they increase baseline flow, decrease maximal flow, or both.[320, 321] In humans, Doppler measurements of coronary blood flow during pacemaker-induced tachycardia show increased resting coronary flow velocity, but not peak velocity with papaverine administration.[321] The use of potent vasodilators to quantify CFR may result in a blunted measurement if there is any significant increase in heart rate. Body size may also influence absolute values of maximal coronary blood flow.[322]

Elevations in aortic pressure increase myocardial oxygen consumption and blood flow. Consequently, shifts in mean aortic pressure produce alterations in autoregulated (resting) blood flow. By using the relationship between mean aortic pressure, CFR, and coronary vascular resistance (coronary flow = mean aortic pressure/coronary resistance), one may calculate a coronary resistance ratio.[323] The resistance ratio may be less sensitive than the flow ratio to changes in arterial pressure.[319]

In addition to external confounding factors, there are intrinsic factors in the definition and measurement of CFR that produce confusion. CFR can be measured either as the difference between maximal and resting flow (absolute CFR) or as the ratio of maximal flow to resting flow (relative CFR). It is not clear which measurement is more clinically relevant. In hypertensive patients with LVH, it is possible to have a normal or mildly increased absolute CFR with a reduced relative CFR.[319]

Many current methods of measuring CFR are not sensitive to changes in CFR over various layers of myocardium. CFR is lower in subendocardial muscle for all perfusion pressures. Some of the newer, noninvasive techniques such as cine–computed tomography and magnetic resonance imaging may be able to measure CFR in the various layers of myocardium. However data are still very preliminary.

Effect of Hypertension and Left Ventricular Hypertrophy on Coronary Flow Reserve

CFR can be measured as absolute flow (ml/min) or as flow per unit muscle mass (ml/min/g) (see Fig. 27–14).[306] Although resting absolute coronary blood flow of the entire left ventricle increases with LVH, resting coronary blood flow per gram of myocardium is unchanged. Total maximal ventricular flow does not change significantly with acquired LVH, whereas total flow per gram of myocardium decreases. This is because of the lack of vascular growth in response to increasing muscle mass. Thus, when absolute flow is measured, resting flow is high and maximal flow is normal (see Fig. 27–14A). If flow per gram is measured, resting flow per gram myocardium is normal but maximal flow per gram myocardium is reduced (see Fig. 27–14B). Consequently, CFR is less than normal whether measured as absolute flow (ml/min) or flow per gram (ml/min/gm) of myocardium.

In the presence of hypertension, absolute CFR may be, theoretically, normal or increased, despite higher resting absolute coronary blood flow. This is because of the higher coronary perfusion pressure (shift to the right side of the curve) as shown by R_3 in Figure 27–14A. Nevertheless, in most cases of hypertensive heart disease, vascular abnormalities and increased left ventricular end diastolic pressure result in reduced maximal flow and thus in a decrease in CFR.[298, 324–326] Most[300, 325, 327] but not all[328, 329] studies show an inverse linear relationship between the extent of LVH and CFR.

Other factors (e.g., race, gender, diabetes, cigarette smoking, and prior therapies) also influence CFR.[330–334] In a recent evaluation of endothelium-dependent vasodilatation of the brachial artery, reduced flow-mediated dilation was related to age. Noticeable decline began in men after age 40 years but was preserved in women until their 50s.[335] This delay in reduction of dilatation in women may be due to protective effects of estrogen, as the decline in circulating estrogen levels appears to correlate with the onset of menopause. In a study of the coronary circulation, age and total serum cholesterol were found to be independent predictors of a blunted vasodilator response to acetylcholine.[336] Analysis of SHRs and normotensive rats showed that hypertension and aging independently result in structural alterations in the coronary resistance vasculature, with a decrease in the ratio of lumen diameter to wall thickness. Arteriolar density was not decreased by aging.[337] Racial differences were demonstrated in a study showing that blacks have decreased CFR compared with whites, independent of LVH.[330]

Hypertension may alter CFR prior to the development of LVH, as suggested by a cross-sectional analysis of hypertensive and nonhypertensive patients. Although CFR was lowest in untreated hypertensive patients with increased LV mass, patients with hypertension and normal LV mass had lower CFR than normotensive patients.[338] This finding must be viewed with caution, however, as cross-sectional studies do not allow one to analyze other factors that may influence coronary blood flow, such as duration of hypertension and prior antihypertensive therapies. Whether or not the two are linearly related, most studies suggest that LVH is strongly associated with reduced CFR. Thus, abnormalities of CFR may partially explain why patients with hypertension and LVH are at increased risk for myocardial ischemia and infarction.[339]

Effect of Blood Pressure Reduction on Autoregulated Blood Flow and Coronary Flow Reserve

Experimental and clinical studies demonstrate that blood pressure reduction in hypertensive patients with LVH may result in increased myocardial ischemia. Resting absolute coronary flow is high in these patients, and loss of autoregulated flow occurs at higher perfusion pressures (the autoregulatory curve is shifted upward and to the right). In experimentally induced LVH, although marked reductions in coronary perfusion pressure from 100 to 40 mm Hg have a minimal effect on autoregulation in the subepicardium, the ability of the subendocardium to autoregulate is reduced by more than 50%.[340] This may account for the increased size of myocardial infarctions associated with experimentally induced coronary ligation in hypertrophied hearts.[341, 342] Recovery of stunned myocardium (systolic thickening and regional myocardial blood flow) in the period immediately following transient coronary occlusion is delayed in the presence of LVH and is delayed even more when blood pressure is lowered during this early reperfusion period.[343]

In hypertensive human subjects without LVH, resting coronary blood flow does not change significantly when perfusion pressure is lowered acutely with nitroprusside from 120 to 70 mm Hg. However, when hypertrophy accompanies hypertension, there is a marked decline in flow as perfusion pressure decreases from 90 to 70 mm Hg (Fig. 27–15).[344] This suggests that a reduction of blood pressure to less than 90 mm Hg in patients with LVH could cause ischemia. This observation may in part explain the limited impact that blood pressure reduction has on reducing mortality from coronary artery disease as compared with reducing the incidence of nonfatal and fatal stroke in studies in hypertensive patients. Analysis of several large, prospective observational studies suggests that a 5 to 6 mm Hg decrease in diastolic blood pressure should cause a 20 to 25%

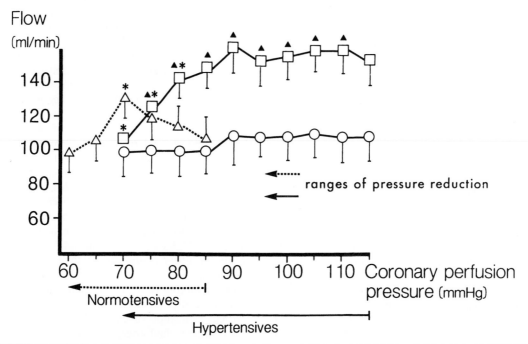

Figure 27–15. Effect of acute reduction in coronary perfusion pressure on coronary autoregulation in controls with normotension *(open triangles)*, patients with hypertension without left ventricular hypertrophy (LVH) *(circles)*, and patients with hypertension and LVH *(squares)*. The autoregulatory curve for hypertension with LVH is shifted upward and to the right. At coronary perfusion pressure < 90 mm Hg, patients with hypertension and LVH have marked loss of coronary autoregulation. *$p < .01$ difference from baseline; *solid triangles*, $p < .01$ difference from hypertensive patients without LVH *(circles)*. (From Polese A, DeCesare N, Montorsi P. Upward shift of the lower range of coronary flow autoregulation in hypertensive patients with hypertrophy of the left ventricle. Circulation 83:845–853, 1991.)

reduction in coronary events. However, this degree of reduction in blood pressure has resulted in only a 14% decrease in coronary events in clinical trials.[345, 346]

A J-curve may describe the relationship between mortality rate resulting from myocardial infarction and treated diastolic blood pressure.[347] The J-curve implies that hypertensive subjects without coronary disease benefit from decreasing their blood pressures as much as possible; however, those with ischemic disease and treated diastolic blood pressure of less than 85 to 95 mm Hg may have an upturn in coronary events. This is presumably a result of inadequate perfusion of coronary arteries. Evidence for and against the J-curve hypothesis is based on differing results and interpretations of retrospective analyses of several large treatment trials or programs.[348–352] For example, in one retrospective analysis, men with LVH or ischemic patterns on electrocardiogram had an increased incidence of myocardial infarction when treated diastolic blood pressures were below 95 mm Hg.[353] By contrast, in the SHEP trial, coronary events were decreased in subjects with evidence of LVH by electrocardiograph criteria and low, treated diastolic blood pressures.[354] Although this may argue against a J-curve, it is important to realize that these patients had low diastolic pressures prior to treatment; hence, their autoregulatory curve was already adjusted to lower pressures.

The possibility of a J-curve poses obvious treatment dilemmas for the physician. For example, although the hypertrophied heart may suffer deleterious effects from "excessively" low blood pressure, these low pressures appear to slow the rate of progression of kidney disease. This hypothesis is being tested in the African American Study of Kidney Disease and Hypertension (ASSK) (projected to be completed in 2001). Because subjects with LVH often have renal dysfunction, the point to which blood pressure is lowered may have to be a tradeoff between risk of renal complications and risk of cardiovascular complications.

Recommendations for the safest level of blood pressure reduction in patients with LVH can be only speculative at this point. In patients with isolated systolic hypertension, in whom the pretreatment diastolic blood pressure is already low, SHEP trial data indicate that further reduction of diastolic blood pressure is safe. On the other hand, patients with diastolic hypertension and LVH (without renal disease) may suffer complications of reduced coronary blood flow when blood pressure is lowered below 85 to 90 mm Hg, particularly in the presence of coronary artery disease. Whether or not lowering blood pressure below 85 to 90 mm Hg is warranted in the presence of renal disease and LVH requires further study. The presence of systolic dysfunction, particularly in patients with coronary artery disease, adds more controversial variables to this dilemma, and the therapeutic approach to such patients demands additional investigation.

Effect of Epicardial Coronary Artery Disease on Coronary Flow Reserve

Current research is focusing on the alterations in CFR that occur in the presence of coronary artery disease. At the site of coronary stenoses of up to 85% of the luminal area, autoregulation maintains normal resting flow. In more severe stenoses, there is a large pressure gradient between the aorta and the coronary artery, with a drop in coronary flow due to loss of autoregulation.[356] The ability to augment flow with maximal vasodilatation is also hampered in the presence of high-grade coronary stenoses, causing CFR to decrease.

After acute myocardial infarction, the coronary vasodilator response in the infarcted myocardial region remains severely impaired despite successful recanalization of the infarct-related artery by thrombolysis.[357] This has been attributed to dysfunction of resistance vessels in the infarcted zone. Recent studies using positron emission tomography (PET) quantification of CFR show that patients with either chronic stable angina or recent myocardial infarction have reduced CFR in regions supplied by normal arteries remote from ischemic or infarcted myocardium.[358, 359] The reasons for this are not yet clear. However, one recent PET study using [11C]hydroxyephedrine, an analogue of norepinephrine used to delineate sympathetic innervation, suggests that cardiac adrenergic signals play an important role in regulating myocardial blood flow.[360] The impairment in CFR may be a manifestation of microvascular endothelial dysfunction, an early phase of angiographically undetectable coronary atherosclerosis. These abnormalities may play a crucial role in the natural history of coronary artery disease and the ventricular remodeling that occurs after myocardial infarction.

Effect of Antihypertensive Treatment on Coronary Flow Reserve

In order to reduce the risk of coronary events in arterial hypertension, therapy should be geared to reversing the chief cardiac manifestations—LVH and coronary microcirculatory abnormalities. Studies in hypertensive rodent and canine models show that reduction of wall stress results in regression of LVH, reversal of coronary vascular abnormalities, and improved overall coronary blood flow.[386, 361–364] The effects of antihypertensive therapy on vascular pathology in humans, however, are not well understood. Heagerty et al. obtained serial skin biopsies of subcutaneous resistance arterioles in hypertensive patients. After long-term treatment with various combinations of β-blockers, calcium channel blockers, diuretics, and ACE inhibitors, the patients demonstrated partial regression of hypertrophy/hyperplasia in the medial layer of these vessels.[365] It is not known whether parallel changes occur in coronary vessels.

There are few human studies of the effects of antihypertensive therapy on CFR. Preliminary data using the gas chromatographic argon method of quantifying CFR showed improved flow reserve in hypertensive patients after 12 months of therapy with enalapril.[366] By blocking the production of angiotensin II, ACE inhibitors may be effective in improving CFR. This may be caused by reductions in perivascular and interstitial fibrosis.[367]

The effect of calcium channel blockers on CFR is even less clear. Although they produce favorable hemodynamic effects, with reversal of pressure overload and regression of LVH, several studies suggest that certain calcium channel blockers do not significantly change, or may even reduce CFR.[368-370] Theoretically, calcium channel blockers may reduce CFR by blocking the effect of endogenous vasodilators such as adenosine.[371]

Measurement of Coronary Flow Reserve

Radionuclide-Labeled Microspheres

Since the first studies using particles to study the circulation, those of Pohlman in the early 1900s, various materials (e.g., glass, ceramic, carnauba wax) have been developed as microspheres.[372, 373] Macroaggregates of albumin can be radiolabeled and can be used in humans because they can be metabolized and thus release the nuclide label for excretion. The lack of uniformity of size is a disadvantage.[374-377] Insoluble inert plastic microspheres are made in uniform spherical sizes. They are the most widely used nuclide-labeled microsphere and are considered the standard for measuring blood flow.[378] Because the microspheres are permanently lodged in tissues and are quantified by counting dissected tissue samples in a well counter, this technique is suitable only for animal research studies. The particles injected into the system circulation cannot recirculate because of capillary entrapment. The organ distribution is proportional to organ blood flow, provided that certain criteria are met: (1) An adequate number of spheres must be injected, but not so many as to produce hemodynamic alterations. (2) The spheres must be well mixed at the site of the injection. (3) All microspheres must be entrapped in the peripheral microcirculation during the first circulation. Thus, the sphere must be large enough not to pass through the organs and into the venous system.[378-381] Under these conditions, blood flow to any organ may be calculated using Heymann's formula.[378]

Noninvasive Techniques

Noninvasive imaging techniques have emerged that allow for easy and accurate quantification of CFR. These techniques include PET scans, ultrafast CT scans, contrast echocardiography, transesophageal Doppler techniques, MRI, and single-photon emission CT scans.

The most accurate noninvasive measure of regional myocardial blood flow was made possible by measurement of positron-emitting flow tracers such as [^{13}N]ammonia and rubidium-82.[382-388] Many studies have been performed using this technique to assess the impact of risk factors such as hyperlipidemia on CFR.[389, 390] In addition, serial studies may be easily performed, allowing assessment of antihypertensive, lipid-lowering therapy or smoking-cessation therapy on CFR. PET studies have also revealed early changes in CFR in young patients with borderline hypertension and in patients with family histories of coronary artery disease and hyperlipidemia but no overt evidence of epicardial coronary artery disease.[391, 392] The limitations of these tracers include the dependence of metabolism as well as perfusion on uptake; these are overcome by freely diffusible tracers such as O-15 water ($H_2{}^{15}O$) and ^{11}C-butanol.[393, 394] However, these tracers must be produced in an on-site cyclotron, and they label the myocardium and

blood pool simultaneously. Although ^{82}Rb can be produced in an inexpensive generator, the cost-effectiveness and availability of PET scanning are important issues. Other limitations include the limited resolution of positron cameras and imaging motion artifacts.

Analysis of time-video intensity curves after injection of ultrasonic contrast microbubbles allows assessment of coronary flow reserve by 2-D echocardiography.[395-398] A recent advance is the introduction for clinical use of nontoxic contrast bubbles ("second-generation microbubbles" such as sonicated 5% albumin), which may be injected intravenously.[398] The microbubbles are visualized by second-harmonic ultrasound imaging, a novel ultrasound detection method based on the nonlinear emission of harmonics by resonant microbubbles pulsating in an ultrasound field. This method allows for enhanced detection of ultrasound contrast agents within blood-containing cavities and vascularized tissue. Methods using a combination of myocardial contrast echocardiography and second-harmonic imaging have been developed to measure both CFR and myocardial blood flow reserve.[399] In vivo destruction of microbubbles by triggered imaging in which the microbubbles are exposed to ultrasound for variable periods is performed. The peak maximal videointensity at each pulsing interval is measured and plotted against the pulsing interval to generate a curve that measures absolute myocardial blood flow at baseline (Fig. 27–16). The same process may be repeated after infusion of a vasodilator to measure peak myocardial blood flow. The ratio of the two values represents the myocardial blood flow reserve ratio.

This technique has limitations. Changes in intramyocardial blood volume with coronary vasodilators affect the time-intensity curve, often resulting in underestimation of CFR. The size and type of ultrasonic contrast microbubbles also influence the time-video intensity curves. Finally, this technique requires sophisticated ultrasound systems and computer software for analysis.[399]

Transesophageal Doppler echocardiography is a relatively noninvasive method of determining CFR that does not require as much specialized technical equipment. Quantification of coronary flow by this technique has been used in the left anterior descending (LAD) coronary artery and in the coronary sinus.[400] The functional significance of stenoses of the LAD has also been successfully evaluated using this technique.[401, 402] Transesophageal Doppler echocardiography is safe and may be used for serial measurements. Adequate Doppler images are obtained in only about 70% of patients, however, and the angle between the exploring ultrasound beam and vessel direction often causes underestimation of blood flow velocities.[403]

Studies using transthoracic Doppler echocardiography to assess coronary flow velocity reserve of the LAD have also been reported. Visualization of flow in the LAD has been accomplished using a high-frequency transducer with color Doppler flow mapping,[404] and correlation with CFR as determined by intracoronary Doppler is good.[405]

Thallium-201 imaging perfusion defects are associated with depressed coronary vasodilator reserve in hypertensive patients with chest pain who do not have obstructive coronary artery disease.[406, 407] After intravenous injection, the early myocardial uptake of radionuclide imaging agents such as thallium-201 and technetium Tc-99m teboroxime

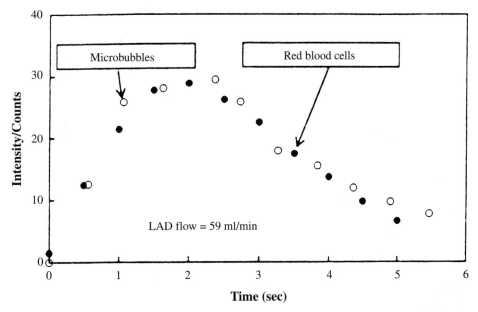

Figure 27–16. In vivo destruction of microbubbles by triggered imaging in which the microbubbles are exposed to ultrasound for variable periods. The peak maximal videointensity at each pulsing interval is measured and plotted against the pulsing interval to generate a curve that measures absolute myocardial blood flow at baseline. The same process may be repeated after infusion of a vasodilator, to measure peak myocardial blood flow. The ratio of the two values represents the myocardial blood flow reserve ratio. LAD, left anterior descending coronary artery. (From Kaul S. A glimpse of the coronary microcirculation with myocardial contrast echocardiography. [Abstract] J Invest Med 43:345–362, 1995.)

are proportional to regional myocardial blood flow over a wide range of coronary flow. With high coronary flow, however, there is a flattening of the uptake curve, which limits resolution. In the canine model, uptake of these agents significantly correlated with a wide range of regional flow as determined by the radioactive microsphere technique.[408–410] Data using this technique to quantify the effects of antihypertensive therapy on CFR are emerging.[411] This technique may provide an accessible and less costly alternative to PET scans.[412–414]

Intravenous contrast injection followed by in vivo analysis of regional contrast clearance by ultrafast CT scan quantitates blood flow and volume. There is a curvilinear relationship with microsphere measurement of coronary blood flow in the canine model.[415] A major limitation of this technique is inaccuracy of measurement at high myocardial flow rates. This may be overcome by injection of the contrast directly into the aortic root.[416] This modification, however, makes the technique invasive and thus not suited to routine clinical evaluation. Further investigation into less invasive means of administering contrast is needed.

Indirect quantification of CFR by velocity mapping of diastolic ascending aortic blood flow by MRI is under study.[417] Using this technique, retrograde flow in the ascending aorta during systole and diastole minus the antegrade flow during diastole equals the coronary diastolic flow. Phase-contrast MRI during a single breath-hold has been used in several centers.[418–421] A known magnetic gradient is applied at the area of interest. As blood flows through the gradient, its magnetic spin is altered in a manner proportional to its velocity, and thus the image encodes velocity. Flow in the LAD is quantified using this technique. After initial scout images are obtained, the location of the LAD is determined and flow-encoded images can be obtained within a single breath-hold. Multiple images are sometimes used for better localization or to determine blood flow during different parts of the cardiac cycle. Coronary flow through the artery is calculated from the velocity (obtained from the velocity-encoded MRI pictures) multiplied by the cross-sectional area of the vessel (obtained from the regular images). Direct measurement of coronary flow by MRI is hampered by the motion of the coronary arteries during cardiac contraction and respiration and the small size of the coronary arteries. New mathematical models and improved equipment are being developed to overcome these problems and allow more accurate intracoronary analysis of blood flow velocity.[422–424] MRI is a promising noninvasive technique for accurate assessment of coronary blood flow. Although it has been validated against phantom models of blood flow, comparison with invasive methods is needed.

References

1. Levy D, Anderson KM, Savage D, et al. Echocardiographically detected left ventricular hypertrophy: Prevalence and risk factors. The Framingham Heart Study. Ann Intern Med 108:7–13, 1988.
2. Casale PN, Devereux RB, Milner M, et al. Value of echocardiographic measurement of left ventricular mass in predicting cardiovascular morbid events in hypertensive men. Ann Intern Med 105:173–178, 1986.
3. Levy D, Garrison RJ, Savage DD, et al. Prognostic implications of echocardiographically determined left ventricular mass in the Framingham Heart Study. N Engl J Med 322:1561–1566, 1990.
4. Bikkina M, Larson MG, Levy D. Asymptomatic ventricular arrhythmias and mortality risk in subjects with left ventricular hypertrophy. J Am Coll Cardiol 22:1111–1116, 1993.

5. Cooper RS, Simmons BE, Castaner A, et al. Left ventricular hypertrophy is associated with worse survival independent of ventricular function and number of coronary arteries severely narrowed. Am J Cardiol 65:441–445, 1990.

6. Ghali JK, Liao Y, Simmons B, et al. The prognostic role of left ventricular hypertrophy in patients with or without coronary artery disease. Ann Intern Med 117:831–836, 1992.

7. Lewis JF, Maron BJ. Diversity of patterns of hypertrophy in patients with systemic hypertension and marked left ventricular wall thickening. Am J Cardiol 65:874–881, 1990.

8. Grossman W, Jones D, McLaurin LP. Wall stress and patterns of hypertrophy in the human left ventricle. J Clin Invest 56:56–64, 1975.

9. Ganau A, Devereux RB, Roman MJ, et al. Patterns of left ventricular hypertrophy and geometric remodeling in essential hypertension. J Am Coll Cardiol 19:1550–1558, 1992.

10. Koren MJ, Devereux RB, Casale PN, et al. Relation of left ventricular mass and geometry to morbidity and mortality in uncomplicated essential hypertension. Ann Intern Med 114:345–352, 1991.

11. Verdecchia P, Schillaci G, Borgioni C, et al. Adverse prognostic significance of concentric remodeling of the left ventricle in hypertensive patients with normal left ventricular mass. J Am Coll Cardiol 25:871–878, 1995.

12. Krumholz HM, Larson M, Levy D. Prognosis of left ventricular geometric patterns in the Framingham Heart Study. J Am Coll Cardiol 25:879–884, 1995.

13. Ghali JK, Liao Y, Cooper RS. Influence of left ventricular geometric patterns on prognosis in patients with or without coronary artery disease. J Am Coll Cardiol 31:1635–1640, 1998.

14. Nunez BD, Lavie CJ, Messerli FH, et al. Comparison of diastolic left ventricular filling and cardiac dysrythmias in hypertensive patients with and without isolated septal hypertrophy. Am J Cardiol 74:585–589, 1994.

15. Savage DD, Garrison RJ, Kannel WB, et al. The spectrum of left ventricular hypertrophy in a general population sample: The Framingham Study. Circulation 75:I26–I33, 1987.

16. Liebson PR, Grandits G, Prineas R, et al. Echocardiographic correlates of left ventricular structure among 844 mildly hypertensive men and women in the Treatment of Mild Hypertension Study (TOMHS). Circulation 87:476–486, 1993.

17. Dunn FG, Oigman W, Sungard-Rise K, et al. Racial differences in cardiac adaptation to essential hypertension determined by echocardiographic indexes. J Am Coll Cardiol 5:1348–1351, 1983.

18. Hammond IW, Alderman MH, Devereux RB, et al. Contrast in cardiac anatomy and function between black and white patients with hypertension. J Natl Med Assoc 76:247–255, 1984.

19. Mayet J, Shahi M, Foale RA, et al. Racial differences in cardiac structure and function in essential hypertension. BMJ 308:1011–1014, 1994.

20. Hinderliter AL, Light KC, Willis PW. Racial differences in left ventricular structure in healthy young adults. Am J Cardiol 69:1196–1199, 1992.

21. Harshfield GA, Alpert BS, Willey ES, et al. Race and gender influence ambulatory blood pressure patterns of adolescents. Hypertension 14:598–603, 1989.

22. Krumholz HM, Larson M, Levy D. Sex differences in cardiac adaptation to isolated systolic hypertension. Am J Cardiol 72:310–313, 1993.

23. Liao Y, Cooper RS, Mensah GA, McGee DL. Left ventricular hypertrophy has a greater impact on survival in women than in men. [Abstract] Circulation 92:805–810, 1995.

24. Douglas PS, Katz SE, Weinberg EO, et al. Hypertrophic remodeling: Gender differences in the early response to left ventricular pressure overload. J Am Coll Cardiol 32:1118–1125, 1998.

25. Lauer MS, Anderson KM, Levy D. Separate and joint influences of obesity and mild hypertension on left ventricular mass and geometry: The Framingham Heart Study. J Am Coll Card 19:130–134, 1992.

26. Schmieder RE, Messerli FH. Does obesity influence early target organ damage in hypertensive patients? Circulation 87:1482–1488, 1993.

27. De Simone G, Devereux RB, Roman MJ, et al. Relation of obesity and gender to left ventricular hypertrophy in normotensive and hypertensive adults. Hypertension 23:600–606, 1994.

28. Messerli FH. Clinical determinants and consequences of left ventricular hypertrophy. Am J Med 51–56, 1983.

29. Chantin A, Barksdale EE. Experimental renal insufficiency produced by partial nephrectomy. II. Relationship of left ventricular hypertrophy, the width of the cardiac muscle fiber and hypertension in the rat. Arch Intern Med 52:739, 1933.

30. Weber KT, Brilla CG. Pathological hypertrophy and cardiac interstitium. Fibrosis and renin-angiotensin-aldosterone system: Pathological hypertrophy and cardiac interstitium. Circulation 83:1849–1865, 1991.

31. Ciulla M, Paliotti R, Hess DB, et al. Echocardiographic patterns of myocardial fibrosis in hypertensive patients: Endomyocardial biopsy versus ultrasonic tissue characterization. J Am Soc Echocardiogr 10:657–664, 1997.

32. Schwartzkopff B, Motz W, Frenzel H, et al. Structural and functional alterations of the intramyocardial coronary arterioles in patients with arterial hypertension. Circulation 88:993–1003, 1993.

33. Hsueh WA, Law RE, Do YS. Integrins, adhesion, and cardiac remodeling. Hypertension 31:176–180, 1998.

34. Cottone S, Vadala A, Vella MC, et al. Changes of plasma endothelin and growth factor levels, and of left ventricular mass, after chronic AT1-receptor blockade in human hypertension. Am J Hypertens 11:548–553, 1998.

35. Moye LA, Pfeffer MA, Wun CC, et al. Uniformity of captopril benefit in the SAVE Study: Subgroup analysis. Survival and Ventricular Enlargement Study. Eur Heart J 15(suppl B):2–8, 1994.

36. Dahlof B, Devereux R, de-Faire U, et al. The Losartan Intervention For Endpoint Reduction (LIFE) in Hypertension study: rationale, design, and methods. The LIFE Study Group. Am J Hypertens 10:705–713, 1997.

37. Gomez AM, Valdivia HH, Cheng H, et al. Defective excitation-contraction coupling in experimental cardiac hypertrophy and heart failure. [Comments] Science 276:800–806, 1997.

38. Grossman W, Jones D, McLaurin LP. Wall stress and patterns of hypertrophy in the human left ventricle. J Clin Invest 56:56–64, 1975.

39. Badeer HS. Biological significance of cardiac hypertrophy. Am J Cardiol 14:133–137, 1964.

40. Lauer MS, Anderson KM, Levy D. Influence of contemporary versus 30-year blood pressure levels on left ventricular mass and geometry: The Framingham Heart Study. J Am Coll Card 18,5:1287–1294, 1991.

41. Rowlands DB, Glover DR, Ireland MA, et al. Assessment of left-ventricular mass and its response to antihypertensive treatment. Lancet 1:467–470, 1982.

42. Devereux RB, Pickering TG, Harshfield GA, et al. Left ventricular hypertrophy in patients with hypertension: Importance of blood pressure response to regular recurring stress. Circulation 68:470–476, 1983.

43. Phillips RA, Goldman ME, Ardeljan M, et al. Determinants of abnormal left ventricular filling in early hypertension. J Am Coll Card 14:979–985, 1989.

44. Guerrier M, Schillaci G, Verdecchia P, et al. Circadian blood pressure changes and left ventricular hypertrophy in essential hypertension. Circulation 81:528–536, 1990.

45. Devereux RB, Roman MJ, Ganau A, et al. Cardiac and arterial hypertrophy and atherosclerosis in hypertension. Hypertension 23:802–809, 1994.

46. Cavallini MC, Roman MJ, Pickering TG, et al. Is white coat hypertension associated with arterial disease or left ventricular hypertrophy? Hypertension 26:413–419, 1995.

47. Perloff D, Sokolow M, Cowan R. The prognostic value of ambulatory blood pressures. JAMA 249:2792–2798, 1983.

48. Hoegholm A, Kristensen KS, Bang LE, et al. Left ventricular mass and geometry in patients with established hypertension and white coat hypertension. Am J Hypertens 6:282–286, 1993.

49. White WB, Schulman P, McCabe EJ, Dey HM. Average daily blood pressure, not office blood pressure, determines cardiac function in patients with hypertension. JAMA 261:873–877, 1989.

50. Ganau A, Devereux RB, Pickering TG, et al. Relation of left ventricular hemodynamic load and contractile performance to left ventricular mass in hypertension. Circulation 81:25–36, 1990.

51. Saba PS, Roman MJ, Pini R, et al. Relation of carotid pressure waveform to left ventricular anatomy in normotensive subjects. J Am Coll Cardiol 22:1873–1880, 1993.

52. Morgan HE, Baker KM. Cardiac hypertrophy. Mechanical, neural and endocrine dependence. Circulation 83:13–25, 1991.

53. Schunkert H, Jahn L, Izumo S, et al. Localization and regulation of

c-fos and *c-jun* proto-oncogene induction by systolic wall stress in normal and hypertrophied rat hearts. Proc Natl Acad Sci U S A 88:11480–11484, 1991.

54. Molkentin JD, Lu JR, Antos CL, et al. A calcineurin-dependent transcriptional pathway for cardiac hypertrophy. Cell 93:215–228, 1998.

55. Sussman MA, Lim HW, Gude N, et al. Prevention of cardiac hypertrophy in mice by calcineurin inhibition. Science 281:1690–1693, 1998.

56. Levy D, Larson MG, Vasan RS, et al. The progression from hypertension to congestive heart failure. JAMA 275:1557–1562, 1996.

57. Senni M, Tribouilloy CM, Rodeheffer RJ, et al. Congestive heart failure in the community. Circulation 98:2282–2289, 1998.

58. Kostis JB, Davis BR, Cutler J, et al. Prevention of heart failure by antihypertensive drug treatment in older persons with isolated systolic hypertension. JAMA 278:212–216, 1997.

59. Moser M, Hebert PR. Prevention of disease progression, left ventricular hypertrophy and congestive heart failure in hypertension treatment trials. J Am Coll Cardiol 27:1214–1218, 1996.

60. Mahoney LT, Schieken RM, Clarke WR, Lauer RM. Left ventricular mass and exercise response predict future blood pressure: The Muscatine study. Hypertension 12:206–213, 1988.

61. De Simone G, Devereux RB, Roman MJ, et al. Echocardiographic left ventricular mass and electrolyte intake predict arterial hypertension. Ann Intern Med 114:202–209, 1991.

62. Schunkert H, Hense H-W, Holmer SR, et al. Association between a deletion polymorphism of the angiotensin-converting enzyme gene and left ventricular hypertrophy. N Engl J Med 330:1634–1638, 1994.

63. Perticone F, Ceravolo R, Cosco C, et al. Deletion polymorphism of angiotensin-converting enzyme gene and left ventricular hypertrophy in southern Italian patients. J Am Coll Cardiol 29:365–369, 1997.

64. Gharavi AG, Lipkowitz MS, Diamond JA, Jhang JS, Phillips RA. Deletion polymorphism of the angiotensin-converting enzyme gene is independently associated with left ventricular mass and geometric remodeling in systemic hypertension. Am J Cardiol 77:1315–1319, 1996.

65. Himmelmann A, Svensson A, Hansson L. Blood pressure and left ventricular mass in children with different maternal histories of hypertension: The Hypertension in Pregnancy Offspring Study. J Hypertens 11:263–268, 1993.

66. van Hooft IMS, Grobbee DE, Waal-Manning HJ, Hofman A. Hemodynamic characteristics of the early phase of primary hypertension: The Dutch Hypertension and Offspring Study. Circulation 87:1100–1106, 1993.

67. Adams TD, Yanowitz FG, Fisher AG, et al. Heritability of cardiac size: An echocardiographic and electrocardiographic study of monozygotic and dizygotic twins. Circulation 71:39–44, 1985.

68. Beaglehole R, Tyroler HA, Cassel JC, et al. An epidemiological study of left ventricular hypertrophy in the biracial population of Evans County, Georgia. J Chronic Dis 28:549–559, 1974.

69. Savage DD, Drayer JIM, Henry WL, et al. Echocardiographic assessment of cardiac anatomy and function in hypertensive patients. Circulation 59:623–632, 1979.

70. Gerstenblith G, Frederiksen J, Yin FCP, et al. Echocardiographic assessment of a normal adult aging population. Circulation 56:273–278, 1977.

71. Levy D, Garrison RJ, Savage DD, et al. Left ventricular mass and incidence of coronary heart disease in an elderly cohort: The Framingham Heart Study. Ann Intern Med 110:101–107, 1989.

72. Shub C, Klein AL, Zachariah PK, et al. Determination of left ventricular mass by echocardiography in a normal population: Effect of age and sex in addition to body size. Mayo Clin Proc 69:205–211, 1994.

73. De Simone G, Devereux RB, Roman MJ, et al. Gender differences in left ventricular anatomy, blood viscosity and volume regulatory hormones in normal adults. Am J Cardiol 68:1704–1708, 1991.

74. Hinderliter AL, Light KC, Park WWIV. Gender differences in left ventricular structure and function in young adults with normal or marginally elevated blood pressure. Am J Hypertens 5:33–36, 1992.

75. Eison H, Phillips RA, Ardeljan M, Krakoff LR. Differences in ambulatory blood pressure between men and women with mild hypertension. J Hum Hypertens 4:400–404, 1990.

76. Diamond JA, Krakoff LR, Martin K, et al. Comparison of ambulatory blood pressure and amounts of left ventricular hypertrophy in men versus women with similar levels of hypertensive clinic blood pressures. Am J Cardiol 79:505–508, 1997.

77. Verdecchia P, Porcellati C, Schillaci G, et al. Ambulatory blood pressure: An independent predictor of prognosis in essential hypertension. Hypertension 24:793–801, 1994.

78. Devereux RB, Lutas EM, Casale PN, et al. Standardization of M-mode echocardiographic left ventricular anatomic measurements. J Am Coll Cardiol 4:1222–1230, 1984.

79. Hense HW, Gneiting B, Muscholl M, et al. The associations of body size and body composition with left ventricular mass: Impacts for indexation in adults. J Am Coll Cardiol 32:451–457, 1998.

80. Cabral AM, Vasquez EC, Moyses MR, Antonio A. Sex hormone modulation of ventricular hypertrophy in sino-aortic denervated rats. Hypertension 11:93–97, 1988.

81. De Simone G, Devereux RB, Daniels SR, Meyer RA. Gender differences in left ventricular growth. Hypertension 26:979–983, 1995.

82. Marcus R, Krause L, Weder AB, et al. Sex-specific determinants of increased left ventricular mass in the Tecumseh blood pressure study. Circulation 90:928–936, 1994.

83. MacMahon SW, Wilcken DEL, MacDonald GJ. The effect of weight reduction on left ventricular mass. N Engl J Med 314:334–339, 1986.

84. Manolio TA, Levy D, Garrison RJ, et al. Relation of alcohol intake to left ventricular mass: The Framingham Study. J Am Coll Card 17,3:717–721, 1991.

85. Schmieder RE, Messerli FH, Garavaglia GE, Nunez BE. Dietary salt intake: A determinant of cardiac involvement in essential hypertension. Circulation 78:951–956, 1988.

86. Marban E, Koretsune Y. Cell calcium, oncogenes, and hypertrophy. Hypertension 15:652–658, 1990.

87. Dubus I. Origin and mechanisms of heart failure in hypertensive patients: Left ventricular remodelling in hypertensives heart disease. Eur Heart J 14:76–81, 1993.

88. Sen S, Tarazi RC, Khairallah PA, Bumpus FM. Cardiac hypertrophy in spontaneously hypertensive rats. Circ Res 35:775–781, 1974.

89. Bauwens FR, Duprez DA, De Buyzere ML, et al. Influence of the arterial blood pressure and nonhemodynamic factors on left ventricular hypertrophy in moderate essential hypertension. Am J Cardiol 68:925–929, 1991.

90. Devereux RB, Pickering TG, Cody RJ, Laragh JH. Relation of renin-angiotensin system activity to left ventricular hypertrophy and function in experimental and human hypertension. J Clin Hypertens 3:87–103, 1987.

91. Sadoshima J, Xu Y, Slayter HS, Izumo S. Autocrine release of angiotensin II mediates stretch-induced hypertrophy of cardiac myocytes in vitro. Cell 75:977–984, 1993.

92. Harada K, Komuro I, Shiojima I, et al. Pressure overload induces cardiac hypertrophy in angiotensin II type 1A receptor knockout mice. [Comments] Circulation 97:1952–1959, 1998.

93. Weber KT, Brilla CG. Pathological hypertrophy and cardiac interstitium. Fibrosis and the renin-angiotensin-aldosterone system. Circulation 83:1849–1865, 1991.

94. Alderman MH, Madhavan S, Ooi WL, et al. Association of the renin-sodium profile with the risk of myocardial infarction in patients with hypertension. N Engl J Med 324:1098–1104, 1991.

95. Laks MM, Morady F, Swan HJC. Myocardial hypertrophy produced by chronic infusion of subhypertensive doses of norepinephrine in the dog. Chest 64:75–78, 1998.

96. Trimarco B, Ricciardelli B, De Luca N, et al. Participation of endogenous catecholamines in the regulation of left ventricular mass in progeny of hypertensive parents. Circulation 72:38–46, 1985.

97. Simpson P. Role of proto-oncogenes in myocardial hypertrophy. Am J Cardiol 62:13G–19G, 1988.

98. Rizzoni D, Lorenza M, Porteri E, et al. Relations between cardiac and vascular structure in patients with primary and secondary hypertension. J Am Coll Cardiol 32:985–992, 1998.

99. Shub C, Cueto-Garcia L, Sheps S, et al. Echocardiographic findings in pheochromocytoma. Am J Cardiol 57:971–975, 1986.

100. Lim MJ, Barkan AL, Buda AJ. Rapid reduction of left ventricular hypertrophy in acromegaly after suppression of growth hormone hypersecretion. Ann Intern Med 117:719–726, 1992.

101. Andronico G, Mangano M-T, Nardi E, et al. Insulin-like growth factor 1 and sodium-lithium countertransport in essential hypertension and in hypertensive left ventricular hypertrophy. J Hypertens 11:1097–1101, 1993.

102. Geffner ME, Golde DW. Selective insulin action on skin, ovary and heart in insulin-resistant states. Diabetes Care 11:500–505, 1988.

103. Phillips RA, Krakoff LR, Ardeljan M, et al. Relation of left ventricular mass to insulin resistance and blood pressure in non-obese subjects. J Am Coll Cardiol 23:48, 1994 [Abstract].

104. Phillips RA, Krakoff LR, Dunaif A, et al. Relation among left ventricular mass, insulin resistance, and blood pressure in nonobese subjects. J Clin Endocrinol Metab 83:4284–4288, 1998.

105. Prakash TR, MacKenzie SJ, Ram JL, Sowers JR. Insulin stimulates gene transcription and activity of Na$^+$K$^+$ATPase in vascular smooth muscle cells. [Abstract] Hypertension 20:443, 1992.

106. Resnick LM. Ionic basis of hypertension, insulin resistance, vascular disease, and related disorders: The mechanism of "syndrome X." Am J Hypertens 6:123S–134S, 1993.

107. Devereux RB, Reichek N. Echocardiographic determination of left ventricular mass in man: Anatomic validation of the method. Circulation 55:613–618, 1997.

108. Feigenbaum H. The echocardiographic examination. *In* Echocardiography. Philadelphia, Lea & Febiger, 1986; pp 50–187.

109. Devereux RB, Alonso DR, Lutas EM, et al. Echocardiographic assessment of left ventricular hypertrophy: Comparison to necropsy findings. Am J Cardiol 57:450–458, 1986.

110. Sahn DJ, DeMaria A, Kisslo J, Weyman A. For the Committee on M-mode Standardization of Echocardiography. Recommendations regarding quantitation in M-mode echocardiography: Results of a survey of echocardiographic measurements. Circulation 58:1073–1078, 1978.

111. Liao Y, Cooper RS, Durazo-Arvizu R, et al. Prediction of mortality risk by different methods of indexation for left ventricular mass. J Am Coll Cardiol 29:641–647, 1998.

112. De Simone G, Daniels SR, Devereux RB, et al. Left ventricular mass and body size in normotensive children and adults: Assessment of allometric relations and impact of overweight. J Am Coll Cardiol 20:1251–1260, 1992.

113. Levy D, Anderson KM, Savage D, et al. Echocardiographically detected left ventricular hypertrophy: Prevalence and risk factors. The Framingham Heart Study. Ann Intern Med 108:7–13, 1988.

114. Lauer MS, Anderson KM, Larson M, Levy D. A new method for indexing left ventricular mass for differences in body size. Am J Cardiol 74:487–491, 1994.

115. Devereux RB. Detection of left ventricular hypertrophy by M-mode echocardiography: Anatomic validation, standardization, and comparison to other methods. Hypertension 9:II19–II26, 1987.

116. Gottdiener JS, Livengood SV, Meyer PS, Chase GA. Should echocardiography be performed to assess effects of antihypertensive therapy? Test-retest reliability of echocardiography for assessment of left ventricular mass and function. J Am Coll Cardiol 25:424–430, 1995.

117. Grandits GA, Liebson PR, Dianzumba S, Prineas RJ. Echocardiography in multicenter clinical trials: Experience from the Treatment of the Mild Hypertension Study. Control Clin Trials 15:395–410, 1994.

118. Collins R, Peto R, MacMahon S, et al. Blood pressure, stroke, and coronary heart disease. Part 2: Short-term reductions in blood pressure: Overview of randomized drug trials in their epidemiological context. Lancet 335:827–838, 1990.

119. Cook RJ, Sackett DL. The number needed to treat: A clinically useful measure of treatment effect. BMJ 310:452–454, 1995 [published erratum appears in BMJ 310:1056, 1995; see Comments].

120. Alderman MH. Blood pressure management: Individualized treatment based on absolute risk and the potential for benefit. [Comments] Ann Intern Med 119:329–335, 1993.

121. Moore CR, Krakoff LR, Phillips RA. Confirmation or exclusion of stage I hypertension by ambulatory blood pressure monitoring. Hypertension 29:1109–1113, 1997.

122. Schiller NB, Shah PM, Crawford M, et al. For the American Society of Echocardiography Committee on Standards. Recommendations for quantitation of the left ventricle by two-dimensional echocardiography. J Am Soc Echocardiogr 2:358–367, 1989.

123. Collins HW, Kronenberg MW, Byrd BF. Reproducibility of left ventricular mass measurements by two-dimensional and M-mode echocardiography. J Am Coll Cardiol 14:672–676, 1989.

124. Keller AM, Peschock RM, Malloy CR, et al. In vivo measurement of myocardial mass using nuclear magnetic resonance imaging. J Am Coll Card 8:113–117, 1986.

125. Riley-Hagan M, Peshock RM, Stray-Gundersen J, et al. Left ventricular dimensions and mass using magnetic resonance imaging in female endurance athletes. Am J Cardiol 69:1067–1074, 1992.

126. Bottini PB, Carr AA, Prisant LM, et al. Magnetic resonance imaging compared to echocardiography to assess left ventricular mass in the hypertensive patient. Am J Hypertens 8:221–228, 1995.

127. Yamaoka O, Yabe T, Okada M, Endoh S, et al. Evaluation of left ventricular mass: Comparison of ultrafast computed tomography, magnetic resonance imaging, and contrast left ventriculography. Am Heart J 126:1372–1379, 1993.

128. Wolfe CL, O'Connell JW, Sievers RE, et al. Assessment of perfused left ventricular mass in normal, ischemic, and reperfused myocardium by means of single-photon emission computed tomography of technetium-99m isonitrile. Am Heart J 126:1275–1286, 1993.

129. Williams KA, Lang RM, Reba RC, Taillon LA. Comparison of technetium-99m sestamibi-gated tomographic perfusion imaging with echocardiography and electrocardiography for determination of left ventricular mass. Am J Cardiol 77:750–755, 1996.

130. Faber TL, Folks RD, Cooke JP, et al. Left ventricular mass from ungated perfusion images: Comparison to MRI. [Abstract] J Nucl Med 38:20, 1997.

131. Gopal AS, Keller AM, Shen Z, et al. Three-dimensional echocardiography: In vitro and in vivo validation of left ventricular mass and comparison with conventional echocardiographic methods. J Am Coll Cardiol 24:504–513, 1994.

132. Gopal AS, Shen Z, Sapin PM, et al. Assessment of cardiac function by three-dimensional echocardiography compared with conventional noninvasive methods. Circulation 92:842–853, 1995.

133. Jiang L, Vazquez de Prada A, Handschumacher MD, et al. Three-dimensional echocardiography: In vivo validation for right ventricular free wall mass as an index of hypertrophy. J Am Coll Cardiol 23:1715–1722, 1994.

134. Keller AM, Gopal AS, Sapin PM, et al. Three-dimensional echocardiography: An advance in quantitative assessment of the left ventricle. Coron Artery Dis 6:42–48, 1995.

135. Rodevand O, Bjornerheim R, Kolbjornsen O, et al. Left ventricular mass assessed by three-dimensional echocardiography using rotational acquistion. Clin Cardiol 20:957–962, 1997.

136. Kaul S. New developments in ultrasound systems for contrast echocardiography. Clin Cardiol 20:27–30, 1997.

137. Schmieder RE. Reversal of left ventricular hypertrophy: Analysis of 412 published studies. [Abstract] Am J Hypertens 7:25, 1994.

138. Messerli FH, Soria F. Does a reduction in left ventricular hypertrophy reduce cardiovascular morbidity and mortality? Drugs 44(suppl 1):141–146, 1992.

139. Smith VE, White WB, Meeran MK, Karimeddini MK. Improved left ventricular filling accompanies reduced left ventricular mass during therapy of essential hypertension. J Am Coll Cardiol 8:1449–1454, 1986.

140. Schmieder RE, Messerli FH, Sturgill D, et al. Cardiac performance after reduction of myocardial hypertrophy. Am J Med 87:22–27, 1989.

141. Grandi AM, Venco A, Barzizza F, et al. Effect of enalapril on left ventricular mass and performance in essential hypertension. Am J Cardiol 63:1093–1097, 1989.

142. Trimarco B, DeLuca N, Ricciardelli B. Cardiac function in systemic hypertension before and after reversal of left ventricular hypertrophy. Am J Cardiol 62:745–750, 1988.

143. Schulman SP, Weiss JL, Becher LC, et al. The effects of antihypertensive therapy on left ventricular mass in elderly patients. N Engl J Med 322:1350–1356, 1990.

144. Phillips RA, Ardeljan M, Shimabukuro S, et al. Normalization of left ventricular mass and associated changes in neurohormones and atrial natriuretic peptide after one year of sustained nifedipine therapy for severe hypertension. J Am Coll Cardiol 17:1595–1602, 1991.

145. Muiesan ML, Salvetti M, Rizzoni D, et al. Association of change in left ventricular mass with prognosis during long-term antihypertensive treatment. J Hypertens 13:1091–1095, 1995.

146. Verdecchia P, Schillaci G, Borgioni C, et al. Prognostic significance of serial changes in left ventricular mass in essential hypertension. Circulation 97:48–54, 1998.

147. Neaton JD, Grimm RH Jr, Prineas RJ, Stamler J, et al. Treatment of Mild Hypertension Study: Final results. JAMA 270:713–724, 1993.

148. Schussheim AE, Diamond JA, Phillips RA. Midwall fractional shortening improves with regression of hypertrophy in treated hypertensives. [Abstract] Circulation 98:28, 1998.

149. Dahlof B, Pennert K, Hansson L. Reversal of left ventricular hypertrophy in hypertensive patients: A meta-analysis of 109 treatment studies. Am J Hypertens 5:95–110, 1992.

150. Linz W, Schaper J, Wiemer G, et al. Ramipril prevents left ventricular hypertrophy with myocardial fibrosis without blood pressure reduction: A one-year study in rats. Br J Pharmacol 107:970–975, 1992.

151. Gottdiener JS, Reda DJ, Massie BM, et al. for the Department of Veterans Affairs Cooperative Study Group on Antihypertensive Agents. Effect of single-drug therapy on reduction of left ventricular mass in mild to moderate hypertension: Comparison of six antihypertensive agents. [Comments] Circulation 95:2007–2014, 1997.

152. Fouad FM, Slominiski JM, Tarazi RC. Left ventricular diastolic function in hypertension: Relation to left ventricular mass and systolic function. J Am Coll Card 3:1500–1506, 1984.

153. Smith VE, Schulman P, Karimeddini M, et al. Rapid ventricular filling in left ventricular hypertrophy. II. Pathological hypertrophy. J Am Coll Cardiol 5:869–874, 1985.

154. Inouye I, Massie B, Loge D, et al. Abnormal left ventricular filling: An early finding in mild to moderate systemic hypertension. Am J Cardiol 53:120–126, 1984.

155. Bonow RO, Udelson JE. Left ventricular diastolic dysfunction as a cause of congestive heart failure: Mechanisms and management. Ann Intern Med 117:502–510, 1992.

156. Topol EJ, Traill GV, Fortuin NJ. Hypertensive cardiomyopathy of the elderly. N Engl J Med 312:277–282, 1985.

157. Soufer R, Wohlgelernter D, Vita N, et al. Intact systolic left ventricular function in clinical congestive heart failure. Am J Cardiol 55:1032–1036, 1985.

158. Cuocolo A, Sax FL, Brush JE, et al. Left ventricular hypertrophy and impaired diastolic filling in essential hypertension: Diastolic mechanisms for systolic dysfunction during exercise. Circulation 81:978–986, 1990.

159. Setaro JF, Soufer R, Remetz MS, et al. Long-term outcome in patients with congestive heart failure and intact systolic left ventricular performance. Am J Cardiol 69:1212–1216, 1992.

160. Carroll JD, Lang RM, Neumann AL, et al. The differential effects of positive inotropic and vasodilator therapy on diastolic properties in patients with congestive cardiomyopathy. Circulation 74:815–825, 1986.

161. Graettinger WF, Neutel JM, Smith DHG, Weber MA. Left ventricular diastolic filling alterations in normotensive young adults with a family history of systemic hypertension. Am J Cardiol 68:51–56, 1991.

162. Snider AR, Gidding SS, Rocchini AP, et al. Doppler evaluation of left ventricular diastolic filling in children with systemic hypertension. Am J Cardiol 56:921–926, 1985.

163. Phillips RA, Coplan NL, Krakoff LR, et al. Doppler echocardiographic analysis of left ventricular filling in treated hypertensive patients. J Am Coll Cardiol 9:317–322, 1987.

164. Dianzumba SB, DiPette DJ, Cornman C, et al. Left ventricular filling characteristics in mild untreated hypertension. Hypertension 8(suppl I):I156–I160, 1986.

165. Shapiro LM, McKenna WJ. Left ventricular hypertrophy: Relationship of structure to diastolic function in hypertension. Br Heart J 51:637–642, 1984.

166. Hartford M, Wikstrand J, Wallentin I, et al. Diastolic function of the heart in untreated primary hypertension. Hypertension 6:329–338, 1984.

167. Fouad FM, Slominski JM, Tarazi RC. Left ventricular diastolic function in hypertension: Relation to left ventricular mass and systolic function. J Am Coll Cardiol 3:1500–1506, 1984.

168. White WB, Schulman P, Karimeddini MK, Smith VE. Regression of left ventricular mass is accompanied by improvement in rapid left ventricular filling following antihypertensive therapy with metoprolol. Am Heart J 117:145–150, 1989.

169. Trimarco B, DeLuca N, Rosiello G. Improvement of diastolic function after reversal of left ventricular hypertrophy induced by long-term antihypertensive treatment with tertatolol. Am J Cardiol 64:745–751, 1989.

170. Gonzalez-Fernandez RB, Altieri PI, Diaz LM, et al. Effects of enalapril on heart failure in hypertensive patients with diastolic dysfunction. Am J Hypertens 5:480–483, 1992.

171. Shahi M, Thorn S, Poulter N, et al. Regression of hypertensive left ventricular hypertrophy and left ventricular diastolic dysfunction. Lancet 336:458–461, 1990.

172. Palatini P, Visentin P, Mormino P, et al. Structural abnormalities and not diastolic dysfunction are the earliest left ventricular changes in hypertension. HARVEST Study Group. Am J Hypertens 11:147–154, 1998.

173. Douglas PS, Berko B, Lesh M, Reichek N. Alterations in diastolic function in response to progressive left ventricular hypertrophy. J Am Coll Cardiol 13:461–467, 1989.

174. Douglas PS, Tallant B. Hypertrophy, fibrosis and diastolic dysfunction in early canine experimental hypertension. J Am Coll Cardiol 17:530–536, 1991.

175. Brilla CG, Janicki JS, Weber KT. Cardioreparative effects of lisinopril in rats with genetic hypertension and left ventricular hypertrophy. Circulation 83:1771–1779, 1991.

176. Villari B, Campbell SE, Hess OM, et al. Influence of collagen network on left ventricular systolic and diastolic function in aortic valve disease. J Am Coll Cardiol 22:1477–1484, 1993.

177. Lorell BH, Grice WN, Apstein CS. Influence of hypertension with minimal hypertrophy on diastolic function during demand ischemia. Hypertension 13:361–370, 1989.

178. Wexler LF, Lorell BH, Momomura S, et al. Enhanced sensitivity of hypoxia-induced diastolic dysfunction in pressure-overload left ventricular hypertrophy in the rat: Role of high-energy phosphate depletion. Circ Res 62:766–775, 1988.

179. Osbakken M, Douglas PS, Ivanics T, et al. Creatinine kinase kinetics studied by phosphorus-31 nuclear magnetic resonance in a canine model of chronic hypertension-induced cardiac hypertrophy. J Am Coll Card 19:233–228, 1992.

180. Ito Y, Suko J, Chidsey CA. Intracalcium and myocardial contractility. V. Calcium uptake of sarcoplasmic reticulum fractions in hypertrophied and failing rabbit hearts. J Mol Cell Cardiol 6:237–247, 1974.

181. Harding DP, Poole-Wilson PA. Calcium exchange in rabbit myocardium during and after hypoxia: Effect of temperature and substrate. Cardiovasc Res 14:435–445, 1980.

182. Gwathmey JK, Morgan JP. Altered calcium handling in experimental pressure-overload hypertrophy in the ferret. Circ Res 57:836–843, 1985.

183. Brutsaert DL, Rademakers FE, Sys SU, et al. Analysis of relaxation in the evaluation of ventricular function of the heart. Prog Cardiovasc Dis 28:143–163, 1985.

184. White WB, Schulman P, Dey HM, Katz AM. Effects of age and 24-hour ambulatory blood pressure on rapid left ventricular filling. Am J Cardiol 63:1343–1347, 1989.

185. Franchi F, Fabbri G, Monopoli A, et al. Left ventricular diastolic filling improvement obtained by intravenous verapamil in mild to moderate essential hypertension: A complex effect. Cardiology 76:32–41, 1989.

186. Betocchi S, Cuocolo A, Pace L, et al. Effect of intravenous verapamil administration of left ventricular diastolic function in systemic hypertension. Am J Cardiol 59:624–629, 1987.

187. De Simone G, Devereux RB, Koren MJ, et al. Midwall left ventricular mechanics: An independent predictor of cardiovascular risk in arterial hypertension. Circulation 93:259–265, 1996.

188. De Simone G, Devereux RB, Roman MJ, et al. Assessment of left ventricular function by the midwall fractional shortening/end-systolic stress relation in human hypertension. J Am Coll Cardiol 23:1444–1451, 1994 [Published erratum appears in J Am Coll Cardiol 24:844, 1994].

189. Schussheim AE, Diamond JA, Jhang JS, Phillips RA. Midwall fractional shortening is an independent predictor of left ventricular diastolic dysfunction in asymptomatic patients with systemic hypertension. Am J Cardiol 82:1056–1059, 1998.

190. Udelson JE, Bacharach SL, Cannon RO, Bonow RO. Minimum left ventricular pressure during β-adrenergic stimulation in human subjects: Evidence for elastic recoil and diastolic "suction" in the normal heart. Circulation 82:1174–1182, 1990.

191. Rademakers FE, Buchalter MB, Rogers WJ, et al. Dissociation between left ventricular untwisting and filling: Accentuation by catecholamines. Circulation 85:1672–1581, 1992.

192. MacGowan GA, Haber HL, Cowart TD, et al. Direct myocardial effects of OPC-18790 in human heart failure: Beneficial effects on contractile and diastolic function demonstrated by intracoronary infusion with pressure-volume analysis. J Am Coll Cardiol 31:1344–1351, 1998.

193. Harrison TR, Dixon K, Russell RO, et al. The relation of age to the

duration of contraction, ejection, and relaxation of the normal human heart. Am Heart J 67:189–199, 1964.

194. Miyatake K, Okamoto M, Kinoshita N, et al. Augmentation of atrial contribution to left ventricular inflow with aging as assessed by intracardiac Doppler flowmetry. Am J Cardiol 64:315–323, 1984.

195. Phillips RA, Krakoff LR, Coplin NL, et al. Normal aging produces left ventricular diastolic abnormalities detectable by Doppler echocardiography. Clin Res 34:336A, 1986.

196. Van Dam I, Fast T, DeBoo J, et al. Normal diastolic filling patterns of the left ventricle. Eur Heart J 9:165–171, 1988.

197. Spirito P, Maron BJ. Influence of aging on Doppler echocardiographic indices of left ventricular diastolic function. Br Heart J 59:672–679, 1988.

198. Arora RR, Machac J, Goldman ME, et al. Atrial kinetics and left ventricular diastolic filling in the healthy elderly. J Am Coll Cardiol 9:1255–1260, 1987.

199. Benjamin EJ, Plehn JF, D'Agostino RB, et al. Mitral annular calcification and the risk of stroke in an elderly cohort. N Engl J Med 327:374–379, 1992.

200. Psaty BM, Furberg CD, Kuller LH, et al. Isolated systolic hypertension and subclinical cardiovascular disease in the elderly: Initial findings from the Cardiovascular Health Study. JAMA 268:1287–1291, 1992.

201. Sagie A, Benjamin EJ, Galderisi M, et al. Echocardiographic assessment of left ventricular structure and diastolic filling in elderly subjects with borderline isolated systolic hypertension (the Framingham Heart Study). Am J Cardiol 72:662–665, 1993.

202. Nicolino A, Ferrara N, Longobardi G, et al. Left ventricular diastolic filling in elderly hypertensive patients. J Am Geriatr Soc 41:217–222, 1993.

203. Levy WC, Cerqueira MD, Abrass IB, et al. Endurance exercise training augments diastolic filling at rest and during exercise in healthy young and older men. Circulation 88:116–126, 1993.

204. Fleg JL, Shapiro EP, O'Connor F, et al. Left ventricular diastolic filling performance in older male athletes. JAMA 273:1371–1375, 1995.

205. Voutilainen S, Kupari M, Hippelainen M, et al. Factors influencing Doppler indexes of left ventricular filling in healthy persons. Am J Cardiol 68:653–659, 1991.

206. Weiss JL, Frederiksen JW, Weisfeldt ML. Hemodynamic determinants of the time-course of fall in canine left ventricular pressure. J Clin Invest 58:751–760, 1976.

207. Grossman W, McLaurin LP. Diastolic properties of the left ventricle. Ann Intern Med 84:316–326, 1976.

208. Hess OM, Ritter M, Schneider J, et al. Diastolic stiffness and myocardial structure in aortic valve disease before and after valve replacement. Circulation 69:855–865, 1984.

209. Spirito P, Maron BJ, Bonow RO. Noninvasive assessment of left ventricular diastolic function: Comparative analysis of Doppler echocardiographic and radionuclide angiographic techniques. J Am Coll Cardiol 7:518–526, 1986.

210. Shapiro LM, Mackinnon J, Beevers DG. Echocardiographic features of malignant hypertension. Br Heart J 46:374–379, 1981.

211. Kitabatake A, Inoue M, Asao M, et al. Transmitral blood flow reflecting diastolic behavior of the left ventricle in health and disease—A study by pulsed Doppler technique. Jpn Circ J 46:92–102, 1982.

212. Chenzbraun A, Pinto FJ, Popylisen S, et al. Filling patterns in left ventricular hypertrophy: A combined acoustic quantification and Doppler study. J Am Coll Cardiol 23:1179–1185, 1994.

213. Hanrath P, Mathey DG, Siegert R, Bleifeld W. Left ventricular relaxation and filling pattern in different forms of left ventricular hypertrophy: An echocardiographic study. Am J Cardiol 45:15–23, 1980.

214. Nakashima Y, Nii T, Ikeda M, Arakawa K. Role of left ventricular regional nonuniformity in hypertensive diastolic dysfunction. J Am Coll Cardiol 22:790–795, 1993.

215. Smith VE, Schulman P, Karimeddini M, et al. Rapid left ventricular filling in left ventricular hypertrophy II. Pathological hypertrophy. J Am Coll Cardiol 5:869–874, 1985.

216. Spirito P, Maron BJ. Doppler echocardiography for assessing left ventricular diastolic function. Ann Intern Med 109:122–126, 1988.

217. Choong CY, Abascal VM, Thomas JD, et al. Combined influence of ventricular loading and relaxation on the transmitral flow velocity profile in dogs measured by Doppler echocardiography. Circulation 78:672–683, 1988.

218. Himura Y, Kumada T, Kambayashi M, et al. Importance of left ventricular systolic function in the assessment of left ventricular diastolic function with Doppler transmitral flow velocity recording. J Am Coll Cardiol 18:753–760, 1991.

219. Appleton CP. Left ventricular diastolic function. In Murphy JG (ed): Mayo Clinic Cardiology Review. Armonk, NY, Futura, 1997; pp 43–56.

220. Benjamin EJ, Levy D, Anderson KM, et al. Determinants of Doppler indexes of left ventricular diastolic function in normal subjects (the Framingham Heart Study). Am J Cardiol 70:508–515, 1992.

221. Laufer E, Jennings GL, Dewar E: Prevalence of cardiac structural and functional abnormalities in untreated primary hypertension. Hypertension 13:151–162, 1989.

222. Ishida Y, Meisner JS, Tsujioka K, et al. Left ventricular filling dynamics: Influence of left ventricular relaxation and left atrial pressure. Circulation 74:187–196, 1986.

223. Appleton CP, Carucci MJ, Henry CP, Olajos M. Influence of incremental changes in heart rate on mitral flow velocity: Assessment in lightly sedated, conscious dogs. J Am Coll Cardiol 17:227–236, 1991.

224. Nishimura RA, Schwartz RS, Holmes DR Jr, Tajik AJ. Failure of calcium channel blockers to improve ventricular relaxation in humans. J Am Coll Cardiol 21:182–188, 1993.

225. Raine AEG, Erne P, Burgisser E, et al. Atrial natriuretic peptide and atrial pressure in patients with congestive heart failure. N Engl J Med 315:533–537, 1986.

226. Eison HB, Rosen MJ, Phillips RA, Krakoff LR. Determinants of atrial natriuretic factor in the adult respiratory distress syndrome. Chest 95:1040–1045, 1988.

227. Rodeheffer RJ, Tanaka I, Imada T, et al. Atrial pressure and secretion of atrial natriuretic factor into the human central circulation. J Am Coll Cardiol 8:18–26, 1986.

228. Matsuda Y, Toma Y, Matsuzaki M, et al. Change of left atrial systolic pressure waveform in relation to left ventricular end-diastolic pressure. Circulation 82:1659–1667, 1990.

229. Rossvoll O, Hatle LK. Pulmonary venous flow velocities recorded by transthoracic Doppler ultrasound: Relation to left ventricular diastolic pressures. J Am Coll Cardiol 21:1687–1696, 1993.

230. Appleton CP, Galloway JM, Gonzales MS, et al. Estimation of left ventricular filling pressures using two-dimensional and Doppler echocardiography in adult patients with cardiac disease. Additional value of analyzing left atrial size, left atrial ejection fraction and the differences in duration of pulmonary venous and mitral flow velocity at atrial contraction. J Am Coll Cardiol 22:1972–1982, 1993.

231. Pai RG, Suzuki M, Heywood JT, et al. Mitral A velocity wave transit time to the outflow tract as a measure of left ventricular diastolic stiffness: Hemodynamic correlations in patients with coronary artery disease. Circulation 89:553–557, 1994.

232. Pai RG, Shakudo M, Yoganathan AP, Shah PM. Clinical correlates of the rate of transmission of transmitral "A" wave to the left ventricular outflow tract in left ventricular hypertrophy secondary to system hypertension, hypertrophic cardiomyopathy or aortic valve stenosis. Am J Cardiol 73:831–834, 1994.

233. Stugaard M. Color M-mode Doppler improves the diagnosis of diastolic dysfunction in coronary artery disease. [Abstract] Circulation 88:1170, 1993.

234. Stugaard M, Smiseth OA, Risöe C, Ihlen H. Intraventricular early diastolic filling during acute myocardial ischemia: Assessment by multigated color M-mode Doppler echocardiography. Circulation 88:2705–2713, 1993.

235. Garcia MJ, Thomas JD, Klein AL. New Doppler echocardiographic applications for the study of diastolic function. J Am Coll Cardiol 32:865–875, 1988.

236. Derumeaux G, Ovize M, Loufoua J, et al. Doppler tissue imaging quantitates regional wall motion during myocardial ischemia and reperfusion. Circulation 97:1970–1977, 1998.

237. Galiuto L, Ignone G, DeMaria AN. Contraction and relaxation velocities of the normal left ventricle using pulsed-wave tissue Doppler echocardiography. Am J Cardiol 81:609–614, 1998.

238. Oki T, Tabata T, Yamada H, et al. Clinical application of pulsed Doppler tissue imaging for assessing abnormal left ventricular relaxation. Am J Cardiol 79:921–928, 1997.

239. Temporelli PL, Corra U, Imparato A, et al. Reversible restrictive left ventricular diastolic filling with optimized oral therapy predicts a more favorable prognosis in patients with chronic heart failure. J Am Coll Cardiol 31:1591–1597, 1998.

240. Aronow WS, Kronzon I. Effect of enalapril on congestive heart failure treated with diuretics in elderly patients with prior myocardial infarction and normal left ventricular ejection fraction. Am J Cardiol 71:602–604, 1993.

241. Setaro JF, Zaret BL, Schulman DS, et al. Usefulness of verapamil for congestive heart failure associated with abnormal left ventricular diastolic filling and normal left ventricular systolic performance. Am J Cardiol 66:981–986, 1990.

242. Given BD, Lee TH, Stone PH, Dzau VJ. Nifedipine in severely hypertensive patients with congestive heart failure and preserved ventricular systolic function. Arch Intern Med 145:281–285, 1985.

243. Andersson B, Caidahl K, di Lenarda A, et al. Changes in early and late diastolic filling patterns induced by long-term adrenergic beta-blockade in patients with idiopathic dilated cardiomyopathy. Circulation 94:673–682, 1996.

244. Gaasch WH. Diagnosis and treatment of heart failure based on left ventricular systolic or diastolic dysfunction. [Comments] JAMA 271:1276–1280, 1994.

245. Packer M. Abnormalities of diastolic function as a potential cause of exercise intolerance in chronic heart failure. Circulation 81:78–86, 1990.

246. The Fifth Report of the Joint National Committee on Detection, Evaluation, and Treatment of High Blood Pressure (JNC V). Arch Intern Med 153:154–183, 1993.

247. Lorell BH, Isoyama S, Grice WN, et al. Effects of ouabain and isoproterenol on left ventricular diastolic function during low-flow ischemia in isolated, blood-perfused rabbit hearts. Circ Res 63:457–467, 1988.

248. The Digitalis Investigation Group. The effect of digoxin on mortality and morbidity in patients with heart failure. N Engl J Med 336:525–533, 1997.

249. Brutsaert DL, Sys SU, Gillebert TC. Diastolic failure: Pathophysiology and therapeutic implications. J Am Coll Cardiol 22:318–325, 1993 [published erratum appears in J Am Coll Cardiol 22:1272].

250. Clements IP, Bailey KR, Zachariah PK. Effects of exercise and therapy on ventricular emptying and filling in mildly hypertensive patients. Am J Hypertens 7:695–702, 1994.

251. Zusman RM, Christensen DM, Higgins J, Boucher CA. Nifedipine improves left ventricular function in patients with hypertension. J Cardiovasc Pharmacol 18:843–848, 1991.

252. Szlachcic J, Tubau JF, Vollmer C, Massie BM. Effects of diltiazem on left ventricular mass and diastolic filling in mild to moderate hypertension. Am J Cardiol 63:198–201, 1989.

253. Topol EJ, Traill TA, Fortuin NJ. Hypertensive hypertrophic cardiomyopathy of the elderly. N Engl J Med 312:277–283, 1985.

254. Zusman RM, Christensen DM, Federman EB, et al. Nifedipine, but not propranolol, improves left ventricular systolic and diastolic function in patients with hypertension. Am J Cardiol 64:51F–61F, 1989.

255. Fouad FM, Slominski MJ, Tarazi RC, Gallagher JH. Alterations in left ventricular filling with beta-adrenergic blockade. Am J Cardiol 51:161–164, 1983.

256. Schunkert H, Dzau VJ, Tang SS, et al. Increased rat cardiac angiotensin-converting enzyme activity and mRNA expression in pressure overload left ventricular hypertrophy. J Clin Invest 86:1913–1920, 1990.

257. Esper RJ, Burrieza OH, Cacharrón JL, et al. Left ventricular mass regression and diastolic function improvement in mild and moderate hypertensive patients treated with lisinopril. Cardiology 83:76–81, 1993.

258. Strauer BE. The concept of coronary flow reserve. J Cardiovasc Pharmacol 19(suppl 5):S67–S80, 1992.

259. Bache RJ. Effects of hypertrophy on the coronary circulation. Prog Cardiovasc Dis 31:403–440, 1988.

260. Anversa P, Sonnenblick EH. Ischemic cardiomyopathy: Pathophysiologic mechanisms. Prog Cardiovasc Dis 32:1–22, 1990.

261. Greene AS, Tonellato PJ, Lui J, et al. Microvascular rarefaction and tissue vascular resistance in hypertension. Am J Physiol 256:H126–H131, 1989.

262. Rakusan K. Microcirculation in the stressed heart. In Legato MJ (ed). The Stressed Heart. Boston/Dordrect/Lancaster, Martinus Nijhoff, 1987; pp 107–123.

263. Marcus ML, Harrison DG, Chilian WM, et al. Alterations in the coronary circulation in hypertrophied ventricles. Circulation 75(suppl I):I19–I25, 1987.

264. Breisch EA, White FC, Nimmo LE, Bloor CM. Cardiac vasculature and flow during pressure-overload hypertrophy. Am J Physiol 251:H1031–H1037, 1986.

265. DePuey EG. Myocardial perfusion imaging with thallium-201 to evaluate patients before and after percutaneous transluminal coronary angioplasty. Circulation 94(suppl I):I59–I65, 1991.

266. Smolich JJ, Walker AM, Campbell GR, Adamson TM. Left and right ventricular myocardial morphometry in fetal, neonatal, and adult sheep. Am J Physiol 257:H1–H9, 1989.

267. Rakusan K, Flanagan MF, Geva T, et al. Morphometry of human coronary capillaries during normal growth and the effect of age in left ventricular pressure-overload hypertrophy. Circulation 86:38–46, 1992.

268. Tomanek RJ. Effects of age and exercise on the extent of the myocardial capillary bed. Anat Rec 167:55–62, 1970.

269. Noon JP, Walker BR, Webb DJ, et al. Impaired microvascular dilatation and capillary rarefaction in young adults with a predisposition to high blood pressure. J Clin Invest 99:1873–1879, 1997.

270. D'Amore PA, Thompson RW. Mechanisms of angiogenesis. Annu Rev Physiol 49:453–464, 1987.

271. Hudlicka O. What makes blood vessels grow? J Physiol 444:1–24, 1991.

272. Nakano N, Moriguchi A, Morishita R, et al. Role of angiotensin II in the regulation of a novel vascular modulator, hepatocyte growth factor (HGF), in experimental hypertensive rats. Hypertension 30:1448–1454, 1997.

273. Short D. Morphology of the intestinal arterials in chronic human hypertension. Br Heart J 28:184–192, 1966.

274. James TN. Morphologic characteristics and functional significance of focal fibromuscular dysplasia of small coronary arteries. Am J Cardiol 65:126–136, 1990.

275. Tomanek RJ, Plamer PY, Pfeiffer GL, et al. Morphologic characteristics and functional significance of focal fibromuscular dysplasia of small coronary arteries, arterioles and capillaries during hypertension and left ventricular hypertrophy. Circ Res 58:38–46, 1986.

276. Schwartzkopff B, Motz W, Knauer S, et al. Morphometric investigation of intramyocardial arterioles in right septal endomyocardial biopsy of patients with arterial hypertension and left ventricular hypertrophy. J Cardiovasc Pharmacol 20:2–7, 1992.

277. Strauer BE. The concept of coronary flow reserve. J Cardiovasc Pharmacol 19(suppl 5):S67–S80, 1992.

278. Korsgaard N, Aalkjaer C, Heagerty AM, et al. Histology of subcutaneous small arteries from patients with essential hypertension. Hypertension 22:523–526, 1993.

279. d'Uscio LV, Barton M, Shaw S, et al. Structure and function of small arteries in salt-induced hypertension: Effects of chronic endothelin-subtype-A-receptor blockade. Hypertension 30:905–911, 1997.

280. Barton M, d'Uscio LV, Shaw S, et al. ET(A) receptor blockade prevents increased tissue endothelin-1, vascular hypertrophy, and endothelial dysfunction in salt-sensitive hypertension. Hypertension 31:499–504, 1998.

281. Force T, Bonventre JV. Growth factors and mitogen-activated protein kinases. Hypertension 31:152–161, 1998.

282. Chien S, Li S, Shyy YJ. Effects of mechanical forces on signal transduction and gene expression in endothelial cells. Hypertension 31:162–169, 1998.

283. Rizzoni D, Porteri E, Castellano M, et al. Endothelial dysfunction in hypertension is independent from the etiology and from vascular structure. Hypertension 31:335–341, 1998.

284. Gilligan JP, Spector S. Synthesis of collagen in cardiac and vascular walls. Hypertension 6:44–49, 1984.

285. Iwatsuki K, Cardinale GJ, Spector S, Udenfriend S. Reduction of blood pressure and vascular collagen in hypertensive rats by β-aminoproprionitrile. Proc Natl Acad Sci U S A 74:360–362, 1977.

286. Isoyama S, Ito J, Sato K, Takishima T. Collagen deposition and the reversal of coronary reserve in cardiac hypertrophy. Hypertension 20:491–500, 1992.

287. Furchgott RF, Zaqadski JV. The obligatory role of endothelial cells in the relaxation of arterial smooth muscle by acetylcholine. Nature 288:373–376, 1980.

288. Raij L. Relationship with renal injury and left ventricular hypertrophy. Hypertension 31:189–193, 1998.

289. Brush JE, Faxon DP, Salmon S, et al. Abnormal endothelium-dependent coronary vasomotion in hypertensive patients. J Am Coll Card 19:809–815, 1992.

290. Motz W, Vogt M, Rabenau O, et al. Evidence of endothelial dysfunction in coronary resistance vessels in patients with angina pectoris and normal coronary angiograms. Am J Cardiol 68:996–1003, 1991.

291. Panza JA, Quyyumi AA, Brush JE, Epstein SE. Abnormal endothelium-dependent vascular relaxation in patients with essential hypertension. N Engl J Med 323:22–27, 1990.

292. Treasure CB, Klein JL, Vita JA, et al. Hypertension and left ventricular hypertrophy are associated with impaired endothelium-mediated relaxation in human coronary resistance vessels. Circulation 87:86–93, 1993.

293. Vrints CJ, Bult H, Hilter E, et al. Impaired endothelium-dependent cholinergic coronary vasodilation in patients with angina and normal coronary arteriograms. J Am Coll Cardiol 19:21–31, 1992.

294. Jameson M, Dai F-X, Lüscher T, et al. Endothelium-derived contracting factors in resistance arteries of young spontaneously hypertensive rats before development of overt hypertension. Hypertension 21:280–288, 1993.

295. Groves P, Kurz S, Just H, Drexler H. Role of endogenous bradykinin in human coronary vasomotor control. Circulation 92:3424–3430, 1995.

296. Gauthier-Rein KM, Rusch NJ. Distinct endothelial impairment in coronary microvessels from hypertensive Dahl rats. Hypertension 31:328–334, 1998.

297. Strauer BE. Coronary hemodynamics in hypertensive heart disease. Basic concepts, clinical consequences, and experimental analysis of regression of hypertensive microangiopathy. Am J Med 84(suppl 3A):45–54, 1988.

298. Strauer BE. Ventricular function and coronary hemodynamics in hypertensive heart disease. Am J Cardiol 44:999–1006, 1979.

299. Cannon RO III. Dynamic limitation of coronary vasodilator reserve in patients with dilated cardiomyopathy and chest pain. J Am Coll Cardiol 10:1190–1200, 1987.

300. Pichard AD, Smith H, Holt J, et al. Coronary vascular reserve in left ventricular hypertrophy secondary to chronic aortic regurgitation. Am J Cardiol 51:315–320, 1983.

301. Villari B, Hess OM, Moccetti D, et al. Effect of progression of left ventricular hypertrophy on coronary artery dimensions in aortic valve disease. J Am Coll Cardiol 20:1073–1079, 1992.

302. Rouleau J, Boerboom LE, Surjadhana A, Hoffman JIE. The role of autoregulation and tissue diastolic pressures in the transmural distribution of left ventricular blood flow in anesthetized dogs. Circ Res 45:804–815, 1979.

303. Guyton RA, McClenathan JH, Michaelis LL. Evolution of regional ischemia distal to a proximal coronary stenosis: Self-propagation of ischemia. Am J Cardiol 40:381–392, 1977.

304. Mosher P, Ross J, McFate PA, Shaw RF. Control of coronary blood flow by an autoregulatory mechanism. Circ Res 14:250–258, 1964.

305. Driscol TE, Moir TW, Eckstein RW. Autoregulation of coronary blood flow: Effect of intra-arterial pressure gradients. Circ Res 15:103–111, 1964.

306. Hoffman JI. A critical view of coronary reserve. Circulation 75 (suppl I):I6–I11, 1987.

307. DeFily DV, Chilian WM. Regulation of myocardial blood flow: Coordination of the responses of vascular microdomains in the coronary circulation. *In* Cardiology in Review. Baltimore, Williams & Wilkins, 1994; pp 67–76.

308. Berne RM, Rubio R. Cardiac nucleotides in hypoxia: Possible role in regulation of coronary blood flow. Am J Physiol 204:317–322, 1963.

309. Marcus ML. Metabolic regulation of coronary blood flow. *In* The Coronary Circulation in Health and Disease. New York, McGraw-Hill, 1983; pp 84–85.

310. Dole WP, Nuno DW. Myocardial oxygen tension determines the degree and pressure range of coronary autoregulation. Circ Res 59:202–215, 1986.

311. Samaha FF, Heineman C, Ince J, et al. ATP-sensitive potassium channel is essential to maintain basal coronary vascular tone in vivo. Am J Physiol 262:C1220–C1227, 1992.

312. Avontuur JA, Bruining HA, Ince C. Nitric oxide causes dysfunction of coronary autoregulation in endotoxemic rats. Cardiovasc Res 35:368–376, 1997.

313. Bayliss WM. On the local reaction of the arterial wall to changes in internal pressure. J Physiol 28:220–231, 1902.

314. Folkow B. Intravascular pressure as a factor regulating the tone of the small vessels. Acta Physiol Scand 17:289–310, 1949.

315. Marcus ML. Myogenic regulation of coronary blood flow. *In* The Coronary Circulation in Health and Disease. New York, McGraw-Hill, 1983; pp 147–154.

316. Johnson PC. The myogenic response. *In* Borh DF, Somlyo AP, Sparks HV (eds). The Cardiovascular System. Handbook of Physiology, vol 2. 1980; pp 409–442.

317. Chilian WM. Coronary microcirculation in health and disease: Summary of an NHLBI workshop. Circulation 95:522–528, 1997.

318. Wu CC, Feldman MD, Mills JD, et al. Myocardial contrast echocardiography can be used to quantify intramyocardial blood volume: New insights into structural mechanisms of coronary autoregulation. [Comments] Circulation 96:1004–1011, 1997.

319. Hoffman JIE. Maximal coronary flow and the concept of coronary vascular reserve. Circulation 70:153–159, 1984.

320. Cleary RM, Ayon D, Moore NB, et al. Tachycardia, contractility and volume loading alter conventional indexes of coronary flow reserve, but not the instantaneous hyperemic flow versus pressure slope index. J Am Coll Cardiol 20:1261–1269, 1992.

321. Rossen JD, Winniford MD. Effect of increases in heart rate and arterial pressure on coronary flow reserve in humans. J Am Coll Cardiol 21:343–348, 1993.

322. O'Keefe DD, Hoffman JI, Cheitlin R, et al. Coronary blood flow in experimental canine left ventricular hypertrophy. Circ Res 43:43–51, 1978.

323. Bretschneider HJ. Pharmakotherapie coronarer durchblutungsstorungen mit kreislaufwirksamen subtanzen. Deutsch Ges Med 69:583, 1963.

324. Opherk D, Mall G, Zebe H, et al. Reduction of coronary reserve: A mechanism for angina pectoris in patients with arterial hypertension and normal coronary arteries. Circulation 69:1–7, 1984.

325. Prichard AD, Gorlin R, Smith H, et al. Coronary flow studies in patients with left ventricular hypertrophy of the hypertensive type: Evidence for an impaired coronary vascular reserve. Am J Cardiol 47:547–554, 1981.

326. Goldstein RA, Haynie M. Limited myocardial perfusion reserve in patients with left ventricular hypertrophy. J Nucl Med 31:255–258, 1990.

327. Diamond JA, Machac J, Henzlova M, et al. Quantitative adenosine-thallium perfusion imaging for assessing coronary flow reserve in arterial hypertension [Abstract] J Am Coll Cardiol 21(suppl A):288A, 1993.

328. Houghton JL, Frank MJ, Carr AA, et al. Relations among impaired coronary flow reserve, left ventricular hypertrophy and thallium perfusion defects in hypertensive patients without obstructive coronary artery disease. J Am Coll Cardiol 15:43–51, 1990.

329. Marcus ML, White CW. Coronary flow reserve in patients with normal coronary angiograms. J Am Coll Cardiol 6:1254–1256, 1985.

330. Houghton JL, Prisant M, Carr AA, et al. Racial differences in myocardial ischemia and coronary flow reserve in hypertension. J Am Coll Cardiol 23:1123–1129, 1994.

331. Gould LK, Martucci JP, Goldberg DI, et al. Short-term cholesterol lowering decreases size and severity of perfusion abnormalities by positron emission tomography after dipyridamole in patients with coronary artery disease: A potential noninvasive marker of healing coronary endothelium. Circulation 89:1530–1538, 1994.

332. Quillen JE, Rossen JD, Oskarsson HJ, et al. Acute effects of cigarette smoking on the coronary circulation: Constriction of epicardial and resistance vessels. J Am Coll Cardiol 22:642–647, 1993.

333. Celermajer DS, Sorensen KE, Georgakopoulos D, et al. Cigarette smoking is associated with dose-related and potentially reversible impairment of endothelium-dependent dilation in healthy young adults. Circulation 88:2149–2155, 1993.

334. Nasher PJ, Brown RE, Oskarsson H, et al. Maximal coronary flow reserve and metabolic coronary vasodilation in patients with diabetes mellitus. Circulation 91:635–640, 1995.

335. Celermajer DS, Sorensen KE, Spiegelhalter DJ, et al. Aging is associated with endothelial dysfunction in healthy men years before the age-related decline in women. J Am Coll Cardiol 24:471–476, 1994.

336. Zeiher AM, Drexler H, Saurbier B, Just H. Endothelium-mediated coronary blood flow modulation in humans: Effects of age, atherosclerosis, hypercholesterolemia, and hypertension. J Clin Invest 92:652–662, 1993.

337. Vitullo JC, Penn MS, Rakusan K, Wicker P. Effects of hypertension and aging on coronary arteriolar density. Hypertension 21:406–414, 1993.

338. Antony I, Nitenberg A, Foult J-M, Aptecar E. Coronary vasodilator reserve in untreated and treated hypertensive patients with and without left ventricular hypertrophy. J Am Coll Cardiol 22:514–520, 1993.

339. Levy D, Garrison RJ, Savage DD, et al. Prognostic implications of echocardiographically determined left ventricular mass in the Framingham Heart Study. N Engl J Med 322:1561–1566, 1990.

340. Harrison DG, Florentine MS, Brooks LA, et al. The effect of hypertension and left ventricular hypertrophy on the lower range of coronary autoregulation. Circulation 77:1108–1115, 1988.

341. Koyanagi S, Eastham CL, Harrison DG, Marcus ML. Increased size of myocardial infarction in dogs with chronic hypertension and left ventricular hypertrophy. Circ Res 50:55, 1982.

342. Dellsperger KC, Clothier JL, Hartnett JA, et al. Acceleration of the wavefront of myocardial necrosis by chronic hypertension and left ventricular hypertrophy in dogs. Circ Res 63:87–96, 1988.

343. Taylor AL, Murphree S, Buja LM, et al. Segmental systolic responses to brief ischemia and reperfusion in the hypertrophied canine left ventricle. J Am Coll Cardiol 20:994–1002, 1992.

344. Polese A, DeCesare N, Montorsi P, et al. Upward shift of the lower range of coronary flow autoregulation in hypertensive patients with hypertrophy of the left ventricle. Circulation 83:845–853, 1991.

345. MacMahon S, Peto R, Cutler J, et al. Blood pressure, stroke, and coronary heart disease. Part 1: Prolonged differences in blood pressure: Prospective observational studies corrected for the regression dilution bias. Lancet 335:765–774, 1990.

346. Collins R, Peto R, MacMahon S, et al. Blood pressure, stroke, and coronary heart disease. Part 2: Short-term reductions in blood pressure: Overview of randomized drug trials in their epidemiological context. Lancet 335:827–838, 1990.

347. Cruickshank JM, Thorp JM, Zacharias FJ. Benefits and potential harm of lowering high blood pressure. Lancet 1:581–584, 1987.

348. Alderman MH, Ooi WL, Madhavan S, Cohen H. Treatment-induced blood pressure reduction and the risk of myocardial infarction. JAMA 262:920–924, 1989.

349. Farnett L, Mulrow CD, Linn WD, et al. The J-curve phenomenon and the treatment of hypertension. Is there a point beyond which pressure reduction is dangerous? JAMA 265:489–495, 1991.

350. Fletcher AE, Bulpitt CJ. How far should blood pressure be lowered? N Engl J Med 326:251–254, 1992.

351. McCloskey LW, Psaty BM, Koepsell TD, Aagaard GN. Level of blood pressure and risk of myocardial infarction among treated hypertensive patients. Arch Intern Med 152:513–520, 1992.

352. Weinberger MH. Do No Harm. Antihypertensive therapy and the "J" curve. Arch Intern Med 152:473–476, 1992.

353. Lindblad U, Rastam L, Ryden L, et al. Control of blood pressure and risk of first acute myocardial infarction: Skaraborg hypertension project. BMJ 308:681–686, 1994.

354. Hansson L. Future goals for the treatment of hypertension in the elderly with reference to STOP-hypertension, SHEP, and the MRC trial in older adults. Am J Hypertens 6(suppl):40S–43S, 1993.

355. Walker WG, Neaton JD, Cutler JA, et al. Renal function change in hypertensive members of the Multiple Risk Factor Intervention Trial: Racial and treatment effects. JAMA 268:3085–3091, 1992.

356. Klocke FJ, Ellis AK, Canty JM Jr. Interpretation of changes in coronary flow that accompany pharmacologic interventions. Circulation 75(suppl V):V34–V38, 1987.

357. Jeremy RW, Links JM, Becker LC. Progressive failure of coronary flow during reperfusion of myocardial infarction: Documentation of the no reflow phenomenon with positron emission tomography. J Am Coll Cardiol 16:695–704, 1990.

358. Uren NG, Marraccini P, Gistri R, et al. Altered coronary vasodilator reserve and metabolism in myocardium subtended by normal arteries in patients with coronary artery disease. J Am Coll Cardiol 22:650–658, 1993.

359. Uren NG, Crake T, Lefroy DC, et al. Reduced coronary vasodilator function in infarcted and normal myocardium after myocardial infarction. N Engl J Med 331:222–227, 1994.

360. Di Carli MF, Tobes MC, Mangner T, et al. Effects of cardiac sympathetic innervation on coronary blood flow. N Engl J Med 336:1208–1215, 1997.

361. Anderson PG, Bishop SP, Digerness SB. Vascular remodeling and improvement of coronary reserve after hydralazine treatment in spontaneously hypertensive rats. Circ Res 64:1127–1136, 1989.

362. Canby CA, Tomanek RJ. Role of lowering arterial pressure on

363. Ishihara K, Zile MR, Nagatsu M, et al. Coronary blood flow after the regression of pressure-overload left ventricular hypertrophy. Circ Res 71:1472–1481, 1992.

364. Sato F, Isoyama S, Takishima T. Normalization of impaired coronary circulation in hypertrophied rat hearts. Hypertension 16:26–34, 1990.

365. Heagerty AM, Bund SJ, Aalkjaer C. Effects of drug treatment on human resistance arteriole morphology in essential hypertension: Direct evidence for structural remodelling of resistance vessels. Lancet 2:1209–1212, 1988.

366. Vogt M, Motz WH, Schwartzkopf B, Strauer BE. Pathophysiology and clinical aspects of hypertensive hypertrophy. Eur Heart J 14:2–7, 1993.

367. Yamada H, Fabris B, Allen AM, et al. Localization of angiotensin-converting enzyme in the rat heart. Circ Res 68:141–149, 1991.

368. Rossen JD, Simonetti I, Marcus ML, et al. The effect of diltiazem on coronary flow reserve in humans. Circulation 80:1240–1246, 1989.

369. Vrolix MC, Sionis D, Piessens J, et al. Changes in human coronary flow reserve after administration of intracoronary diltiazem. J Cardiovasc Pharmacol 18(suppl 9):S64–S67, 1991.

370. Diamond JA, Machac J, Henzlova MJ, et al. Effect of long-term calcium channel blocker antihypertensive therapy on coronary physiology. J Am Coll Cardiol 256A, 1994.

371. Merrill G, Young M, Dorell S, Krieger L. Coronary interactions between nifedipine and adenosine in the intact dog heart. Eur J Pharmacol 81:543–550, 1982.

372. Pohlman AG. The course of the blood through the heart of the fetal mammal, with a note on the reptilian and amphibian circulations. Anat Rec 3:75–109, 1909.

373. Wagner HNJ, Rhodes BA, Sasaki Y, et al. Studies of the circulation with radioactive microspheres. Invest Radiol 4:374–386, 1969.

374. Wagner HNJ, Sabiston DCJ, Iio M, et al. Regional pulmonary blood flow in man by radioisotope scanning. JAMA 187:601–603, 1964.

375. Wagner HNJ, Jones E, Tow DE, et al. A method for the study of the peripheral circulation in man. J Nucl Med 6:150–154, 1965.

376. Rhodes BA, Zolle I, Buchanan JW. Preparation of metabolizable radioactive human serum albumin microspheres for studies of the pulmonary circulation. Radiology 92:1453–1460, 1969.

377. Zolle I, Rhodes BA, Wagner NHJ. Preparation of metabolizable radioactive human serum albumin microspheres for studies of the circulation. Int J Appl Radiat Isot 21:155–167, 1970.

378. Heymann MA, Payne BD, Hoffman JI, Rudolph AM. Blood flow measurements with radionuclide-labeled particles. Prog Cardiovasc Dis 20:55–79, 1977.

379. Hales JRS. Radioactive microsphere techniques for studies of the circulation. Clin Exp Pharmacol Physiol 1:31–46, 1974.

380. Skiegekoto K, Van Heerdan PD, Tohru M, Wagner HNJ. Measurement of distribution of cardiac output. J Appl Physiol 25:696–700, 1968.

381. Warren DJ, Ledingham JGG. Measurement of cardiac output distribution using microspheres: Some practical and theoretical considerations. Cardiovasc Res 8:570–581, 1974.

382. Gould KL, Schelbert HR, Phelps ME, Hoffman EJ. Noninvasive assessment of coronary stenoses with myocardial perfusion imaging during pharmacologic coronary vasodilation. Am J Cardiol 43:200–208, 1979.

383. Mullani NA, Goldstein RA, Gould KL, et al. Myocardial perfusion with rubidium-82. I: Measurement of extraction fraction and flow with external detectors. J Nucl Med 24:898–906, 1983.

384. Goldstein RA, Mullani NA, Marani SK, et al. Myocardial perfusion with rubidium-82. II: Effects of metabolic and pharmacologic interventions. J Nucl Med 24:907–915, 1983.

385. Schelbert HR, Phelps ME, Hoffman EJ, et al. Regional myocardial pergusion assessed with N-13 labeled ammonia and positron emission computerized axial tomography. Am J Cardiol 43:209–218, 1979.

386. Schelbert HR, Phelps ME, Huang S, et al. N-13 ammonia as an indicator of myocardial blood flow. Circulation 63:1259–1272, 1981.

387. Bellina RC, Parodi O, Camici PA, et al. Simultaneous in vitro and in vivo validation of nitrogen-13 ammonia for the assessment of regional myocardial blood flow. J Nucl Med 31:1335–1343, 1990.

388. Hutchins GD, Schwaiger M, Rosenspire KC, et al. Noninvasive quantification of regional blood flow in the human heart using N-13

maximal coronary flow with and without regression of cardiac hypertrophy. Am J Physiol 257:H1110–H1118, 1989.

ammonia and dynamic positron emmision tomographic imaging. J Am Coll Cardiol 15:1032–1042, 1990.

389. Gould LK, Martucci JP, Goldberg DI, et al. Short-term cholesterol lowering decreases size and severity of perfusion abnormalities by positron emission tomography after dipyridamole in patients with coronary artery disease: A potential noninvasive marker of healing coronary endothelium. Circulation 89:1530–1538, 1994.

390. Yokoyama I, Ohtake T, Momomura S, et al. Reduced coronary flow reserve in hypercholesterolemic patients without overt coronary stenosis. Circulation 94:3232–3238, 1996.

391. Laine H, Raitakari OT, Ninikoski H, et al. Early impairment of coronary flow reserve in young men with borderline hypertension. J Am Coll Cardiol 32:147–153, 1998.

392. Dayanikli F, Grambow D, Muzik O, et al. Early detection of abnormal coronary flow reserve in asymptomatic men at high risk for coronary artery disease using positron emission tomography. Circulation 90:808–817, 1994.

393. Parker JA, Beller GA, Hoop B, et al. Assessment of regional myocardial blood flow and regional fractional oxygen-extraction in dogs, using O-15 water and O-15 hemoglobin. Circ Res 42:511–518, 1978.

394. Merlett P, Mazoyer B, Hittinger L, et al. Assessment of coronary reserve in man: Comparison between positron emission tomography with oxygen-15 labeled water and intracoronary Doppler technique. J Nucl Med 34:1899–1904, 1993.

395. Porter TR, D'Sa A, Turner C, et al. Myocardial contrast echocardiography for the assessment of coronary blood flow reserve: Validation in humans. J Am Coll Cardiol 21:349–355, 1993.

396. Cheirif J, Zoghbi WA, Raizner AE, et al. Assessment of myocardial perfusion in humans by contrast echocardiography. I: Evaluation of regional coronary reserve by peak contrast intensity. J Am Coll Cardiol 11:735–743, 1988.

397. Jayaweera AR, Matthew TL, Sklenar J, et al. Method for the quantitation of myocardial perfusion during myocardial contrast two-dimensional echocardiography. J Am Soc Echocardiogr 3:91–98, 1990.

398. Wei K, Jayaweera AR, Firoozan S, et al. Quantification of myocardial blood flow with ultrasound-induced destruction of microbubbles administered as a constant venous infusion. Circulation 97:473–483, 1998.

399. Mulvagh SL, Foley DA, Aeschbacher BC, et al. Second harmonic imaging of an intravenously administered echocardiographic contrast agent: Visualization of coronary arteries and measurement of coronary blood flow. J Am Coll Cardiol 27:1519–1525, 1996.

400. Mundigler G, Zehetgruber M, Christ G, Siostrzonek P. Comparison of transesophageal coronary sinus and left anterior descending coronary artery Doppler measurements for the assessment of coronary flow reserve. Clin Cardiol 20:225–231, 1997.

401. Stoddard MF, Prince CR, Morris GT. Coronary flow reserve assessment by dobutamine transesophageal Doppler echocardiology. J Am Coll Cardiol 25:325–332, 1995.

402. Zehetgruber M, Mortl D, Porenta G, et al. Comparison of transesophageal Doppler coronary flow reserve measurements with thallium-201 single-photon emission computed tomography imaging in assessment of left anterior descending artery stenoses. Clin Cardiol 21:247–252, 1998.

403. Iliceto S, Marangelli V, Memmola C, Rizzon P. Transesophageal Doppler echocardiography evaluation of coronary blood flow velocity in baseline conditions and during dipyridamole-induced coronary vasodilation. Circulation 83:61–69, 1991.

404. Hozumi T, Yoshida K, Ogata Y, et al. Noninvasive assessment of significant left anterior descending coronary artery stenosis by coronary flow velocity reserve with transthoracic color Doppler echocardiography. Circulation 97:1557–1562, 1998.

405. Hozumi T, Yoshida K, Akasaka T, et al. Noninvasive assessment of coronary flow velocity and coronary flow velocity reserve in the left anterior descending coronary artery by Doppler echocardiography: Comparison with invasive technique. J Am Coll Cardiol 32:1251–1259, 1998.

406. Legrand V, Hodgson JM, Bates ER, et al. Abnormal coronary flow reserve and abnormal radionuclide exercise test results in patients with normal coronary angiograms. J Am Coll Card 6:1245–1253, 1985.

407. Rossen JD, Winniford MD. Effect of increases in heart rate and arterial pressure on coronary flow reserve in humans. J Am Coll Cardiol 21:343–348, 1993.

408. Nielson AT, Morris KG, Murdock R, et al. Linear relationship between the distribution of thallium-201 and blood flow in ischemic and non-ischemic myocardium during exercise. Circulation 61:797, 1980.

409. Beanlands R, Muzik O, Nguyen N, et al. The relationship between myocardial retention of technetium-99m teboroxime and myocardial blood flow. J Am Coll Cardiol 20:712–719, 1992.

410. Sinusas AJ, Shi QX, Saltzberg MT, et al. Technetium-99m-tetrofosmin to assess myocardial blood flow: Experimental validation in an intact canine model of ischemia. J Nucl Med 35:664–671, 1994.

411. Diamond JA, Gharavi AG, Roychoudhury D, et al. Effect of longterm eprosartan versus enalapril antihypertensive therapy on left ventricular mass and coronary flow reserve in stage I–II hypertension. Curr Med Res Opin 15:1–8, 1999.

412. Machac J, Diamond JA, Vallabhajosula S, et al. Validation of a noninvasive method of measuring coronary blood reserve: A split dose thallium-201 rest/stress imaging. J Am Coll Cardiol 1994, p 256A.

413. Lien DC, Araujo LI, Budinger T, Alavi A. Quantification of myocardial blood flow can be obtained with technetium-99m-teboroxime and fast dynamic SPECT scanning. J Am Coll Cardiol 21:376A, 1993.

414. Pepine CJ, Faich G, Makuch R. Verapamil use in patients with cardiovascular disease: An overview of randomized trials. Clin Cardiol 21:633–641, 1998.

415. Rumberger JA, Bell MR, Sheedy PF, Stanson AW. In vivo quantification of intramyocardial blood volume by ultrafast computed tomography. Circulation 78:II-398, 1988.

416. Weiss RM, Otoadese EA, Noel MP, et al. Quantitation of absolute regional myocardial perfusion using cine computed tomography. J Am Coll Cardiol 23:1186–1193, 1994.

417. Bogren HG, Buonocore MH. Measurement of coronary artery flow reserve by magnetic resonance velocity mapping in the aorta. Lancet 342:899–900, 1993.

418. Clarke GD, Eckels R, Chaney C, et al. Measurement of absolute epicardial coronary artery flow and flow reserve with breath-hold cine phase-contrast magnetic resonance imaging. Circulation 91:2627–2634, 1995.

419. Hundley WG, Lange RA, Clarke GD, et al. Assessment of coronary arterial flow and flow reserve in humans with magnetic resonance imaging. Circulation 93:1502–1508, 1996.

420. Davis CP, Liu PF, Hauser M, et al. Coronary flow and coronary flow reserve measurements in humans with breath-held magnetic resonance phase contrast velocity mapping. Magn Reson Med 37:537–544, 1997.

421. Grist TM, Polzin JA, Bianco JA, et al. Measurement of coronary blood flow and flow reserve using magnetic resonance imaging. Cardiology 88:80–89, 1997.

422. Poncelet BP, Weisskoff RM, Wedeen VJ, et al. Time of flight quantification of coronary flow with echo-planar MRI. Magn Reson Med 447–457, 1993.

423. Nagel E, Hug J, Bornstedt A, et al. Magnetic resonance techniques for the noninvasive determination of coronary blood flow velocity. [Abstract] J Am Coll Cardiol 31:165A, 1998.

424. Oyre S, Ringgaard S, Kozerke S, et al. Accurate noninvasive quantitation of blood flow, cross-sectional lumen vessel area and wall shear stress by three-dimensional paraboloid modeling of magnetic resonance imaging velocity data. J Am Coll Cardiol 32:128–134, 1998.

425. Frohlich ED, Apstein C, Chobanian AV, et al. Medical progress: The heart in hypertension. N Engl J Med 327:998–1008, 1992.

426. Benjamin EJ, Levy D, Anderson KM, et al. Determinants of Doppler indexes of left ventricular diastolic function in normal subjects (the Framingham Heart Study). Am J Cardiol 70:508–515, 1992.

427. Phillips RA, Goldman ME, Ardeljan M, et al. Determinants of abnormal left ventricular filling in early hypertension. J Am Coll Cardiol 14:979–985, 1989.

428. Kaul S. A glimpse of the coronary microcirculation with myocardial contrast echocardiography. [Abstract] J Invest Med 43:345–362, 1995.

429. Jones EC, Devereux RB, O'Grady MJ, et al. Relation of hemodynamic volume load to arterial and cardiac size. J Am Coll Cardiol 29:1303–1310, 1997.

430. Schmieder RE, Langenfeld MR, Friedrich A, et al. Angiotensin II related to sodium excretion modulates left ventricular structure in human essential hypertension. Circulation 94:1304–1309, 1996.

431. Devereux RB, Drayer JIM, Chien S, et al. Whole blood viscosity as

a determinant of cardiac hypertrophy in systemic hypertension. Am J Cardiol 54:592–595, 1986.

432. Rossi GP, Sacchetto A, Visentin P, et al. Changes in left ventricular anatomy and function in hypertension and primary aldosteronism. Hypertension 27:1039–1045, 1996.

433. De la Sierra A, Coca A, Paré JC, et al. Erythrocyte ion fluxes in essential hypertensive patients with left ventricular hypertrophy. Circulation 88:1628–1633, 1993.

434. Nosadini R, Semplicini A, Fioretto P, et al. Sodium-lithium countertransport and cardiorenal abnormalities in essential hypertension. Hypertension 18:191–198, 1991.

435. Akhter SA, Milano CA, Shotwell KF, et al. Transgenic mice with cardiac overexpression of alpha1B-adrenergic receptors. In vivo

alpha$_1$-adrenergic receptor–mediated regulation of beta-adrenergic signaling. J Biol Chem 272:21253–21259, 1997.

436. Choi DJ, Koch WJ, Hunter JJ, Rockman HA. Mechanism of beta-adrenergic receptor desensitization in cardiac hypertrophy is increased beta-adrenergic receptor kinase. J Biol Chem 272:17223–17229, 1997.

437. Casale PN, Devereux RB, Milner M, et al. Value of echocardiographic measurement of left ventricular mass in predicting cardiovascular morbid events in hypertensive men. Ann Intern Med 105:173–178, 1986.

438. Levy D, Savage DD, Garrison RJ, et al. Echocardiographic criteria for left ventricular hypertrophy: The Framingham Heart Study. Am J Cardiol 59:956–960, 1987.

CHAPTER 28

Stroke and Hypertension

J. David Spence and Kelly B. Zarnke

Severe stroke is a personal devastation for the patient and family; it is also a significant economic problem for most developed nations. The annual cost of stroke in the United States exceeds a billion dollars.[1] The incidence of stroke rises steeply with age,[1] so with the aging of the population this problem will take a steeply rising toll unless we learn to do a better job of prevention.

Most disabling strokes are preventable. Strokes due to high blood pressure can be prevented by effective detection and treatment of hypertension.[2] Strokes due to atherosclerosis are not prevented by lowering of blood pressure, so to prevent the residual strokes we must pay more attention to measures that can be taken to prevent atherosclerotic strokes.[3, 4] The prevention of stroke has two phases: primary prevention of hypertensive stroke by effective detection and control of hypertension in all patients, and secondary prevention to prevent atherosclerotic strokes by aggressive medical and surgical intervention in patients who have experienced a transient ischemic attack (TIA).

The abbreviation for *cerebrovascular accident*, CVA, all too often stands for "cursory vascular analysis." Too often, muddy thinking about stroke leads to missed opportunities for preventing a catastrophe. Although hypertensive intracerebral hemorrhages are now clearly distinguishable by computed tomography, there is much confusion about ischemic stroke. Cerebral ischemia due to hypertensive arteriolar disease (lacunar infarctions caused by hyaline degeneration and fibrinoid necrosis) is often lumped together with emboli from the heart; paradoxical emboli; atheromatous emboli (either platelet clumps, i.e., white thrombus, or chunks of plaque debris) from the aortic arch or vertebral arteries, common or internal carotid; or occlusion of the carotid or vertebral arteries by atherosclerotic plaque events, such as plaque rupture or intraplaque hemorrhage, or dissection; and so-called cerebral thrombosis. This is an oversimplification and reflects lack of knowledge of pathophysiology (Table 28–1).

Primary thrombosis (formation of red thrombus, meaning a fibrin polymer with entrapped red cells and platelets) occurs not in the setting of fast-flowing arterial blood but rather in conditions of stasis, after arterial occlusion (e.g., by plaque rupture), or in the setting of stasis, in deep veins or in the auricle of a fibrillating atrium or a ventricular aneurysm. Emboli from the heart and paradoxical emboli can be prevented with anticoagulants; platelet clumps (white thrombus) can be prevented with antiplatelet agents, but embolization of atheromatous debris from a carotid ulcer can be prevented only by endarterectomy or stenting. Atherosclerotic strokes will probably also be reduced by effective antiatherosclerotic therapies that stabilize plaque in the aortic arch and extracranial arteries. Thus, in a given case, choosing the right treatment to prevent a recurrent

Table 28–1 Types of Stroke

NONHYPERTENSIVE HEMORRHAGIC STROKE
Berry aneurysm
Vascular malformations
   Arteriovenous malformation
   Cavernous angioma
Amyloid angiopathy

HYPERTENSIVE STROKE (Located in the Vascular Centrencephalon)
Hypertensive intracerebral hemorrhage due to rupture of arterioles from hyaline degeneration or microaneurysms
Lacunar infarction due to occlusion of arterioles from fibrinoid necrosis or hyaline degeneration

CARDIOEMBOLIC STROKE (Embolization of Red Thrombus)
Atrial fibrillation
Ventricular aneurysm
Paradoxical embolism
   Atrial septal defect or propatent foramen ovale
   Pulmonary arteriovenous fistula

ATHEROSCLEROTIC STROKE
Occlusion of an extracranial or intracranial artery
   Intraplaque hemorrhage with occlusion
   Plaque rupture with occlusion
Embolization of platelet clumps ("white thrombus") or atheromatous debris from ulcerated plaques in
   Extracranial arteries
   Aortic arch

stroke critically depends on recognizing the cause of the TIA or nondisabling stroke with which the patient presented.

To make a success of dealing with the impending wave of stroke that looms over us with the aging of the population, physicians need to get better at sorting out the cause of stroke. This chapter deals, first, with understanding the difference between hypertensive and atherosclerotic strokes, and second, with the issue of when and how to reduce blood pressure in the setting of hypertensive encephalopathy and acute stroke. It then goes on to interventions that will reduce the burden of atherosclerotic stroke.

CEREBRAL CONSEQUENCES OF HYPERTENSION

As described by Pickering,[5] high blood pressure causes small vessel disease. Hyaline degeneration (Fig. 28–1) and fibrinoid necrosis (Fig. 28–2) in the short straight arteries with few branches at the base of the brain cause lacunar infarctions and hypertensive intracerebral hemorrhages (Fig. 28–3). Hachinski[6] explains the distribution of hypertensive strokes by the concept of the "vascular centrencephalon" (Fig. 28–4). In essence, the ancient part of the brain is exposed to the full brunt of arterial pressure, with a major drop in pressure over a very short distance, damaging the small resistance arteries and arterioles. In the neocortex, the long arteries with many branches act as a step-down transformer, protecting the cortex from the effects of hypertensive small vessel disease. For this reason, hypertensive strokes affect the internal capsule, basal ganglia, brain stem, and cerebellum, not the cortex. Other cerebral consequences of hypertension include hypertensive encephalopathy and, rarely, arterial ectasia.[4] The cerebrovascular consequences of high blood pressure are reviewed elsewhere.[3, 4]

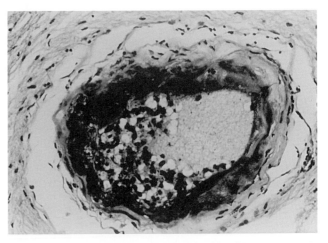

Figure 28–2. Fibrinoid necrosis, also the result of high pressure in small resistance vessels, contributes to lacunar infarction. (Reprinted from Spence JD, Arnold JMO, Gilbert JJ. Vascular consequences of hypertension and effects of antihypertensive therapy. *In* Robertson JIS [ed]. Clinical Hypertension. Vol 15 of Birkenhäger WH, Reid JL [eds]. Handbook of Hypertension. Copyright 1992, pp 621–654, with permission from Elsevier Science.)

WHAT KINDS OF STROKE ARE PREVENTED BY TREATMENT OF HYPERTENSION?

Between 1977 and 1984, we observed in London, Ontario, Canada, the effect of improved blood pressure detection and control of stroke prevention.[2] The Department of Family Medicine at the University of Western Ontario conducted a clinical trial from 1978 to 1983 to determine whether a practice assistant focusing on hypertension could improve detection and treatment of hypertension.[7] What

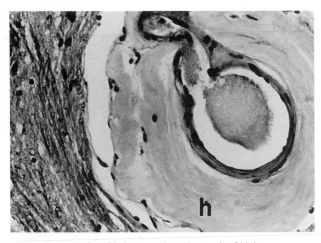

Figure 28–1. Hyaline (h) degeneration, the result of high pressures on small resistance vessels, contributes to lacunar infarction and hypertensive intracerebral hemorrhage. (Reprinted from Spence JD, Arnold JMO, Gilbert JJ. Vascular consequences of hypertension and effects of antihypertensive therapy. *In* Robertson JIS [ed]. Clinical Hypertension. Vol 15 of Birkenhäger WH, Reid JL [eds]. Handbook of Hypertension. Copyright 1992, pp 621–654, with permission from Elsevier Science.)

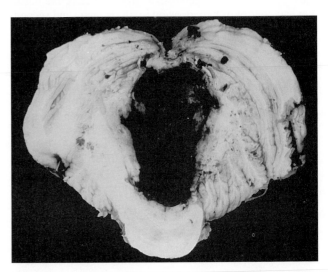

Figure 28–3. Hypertensive hemorrhage into the cerebellum. Hypertensive intracerebral hemorrhages have a characteristic location in the internal capsule, basal ganglia, thalamus, brain stem, and cerebellum. The hemorrhage shown here is a particularly important example because cerebellar hemorrhages, by causing brain stem compression, are often fatal (as in this case), and they respond well to timely surgical treatment. (Courtesy of Dr. Rob Hammond, London Health Sciences Centre.)

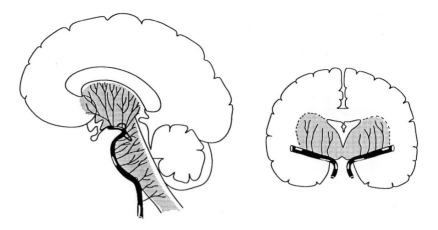

Figure 28–4. Vascular centrencephalon. Hypertensive strokes appear to occur in their characteristic distribution because short arteries with few branches transmit the full brunt of arterial pressure to the small resistance vessels. In contrast, the cortex is supplied by long arteries with many branches, which act as a step-down transformer. (From The Acute Stroke by VC Hachinski, JW Norris. Copyright © 1985 by Oxford University Press, Inc. Used by permission of Oxford University Press, Inc.)

happened was remarkable and may have been a manifestation of the Hawthorne effect. Detection and treatment of hypertension improved not only in the 34 family practices involved in the study but also in the entire community. By 1984, in Middlesex County, which surrounds London, 94% of hypertensives were detected; 92% were on treatment, and 72% were controlled.[8] Strokes were reduced by half. Remarkably, strokes due to hypertension were reduced from 50% of cases to less than 10%; strokes due to atherosclerosis were unchanged, increasing from 35% of 500 cases per year to 70% of 250 cases per year.[2] Thus, as predicted by Russell,[8a] treating high blood pressure prevented only hypertensive small vessel strokes.

This observation has been confirmed in the North American Symptomatic Carotid Endarterectomy Trial (NASCET).[9] In that study, 691 patients with severe carotid stenosis (>70%) and 2226 patients with moderate stenosis (<70%) were randomized to carotid endarterectomy with best medical care or to best medical care alone. Best medical care included blood pressure control to a systolic less than 160 mm Hg and diastolic less than 95 mm Hg. Despite the fact that the patients, who were arteriopaths, had a higher than usual prevalence of renovascular hypertension, blood pressure control among patients with moderate carotid stenosis was achieved better than in most communities: Only 5.4% of patients had diastolic pressures above 95 mm Hg, and only 28.9% had systolic pressures above 160 mm Hg. The result of this degree of blood pressure control was that only 1.7% of the strokes in the moderate stenosis group were due to intracerebral hemorrhage and 14.9% were thought to be lacunar.[10] As lacunar strokes were defined by the clinical presentation regardless of blood pressure, the number of true lacunes was probably less. (Usually hemorrhages represent about one quarter of hypertensive strokes, so the number of true lacunes was probably not more than 10% of all strokes, and the proportion of strokes due to hypertensive small vessel disease was probably 12% or less.) These observations lead to the conclusion that to prevent strokes due to small vessel disease, it is only necessary to control hypertension. Then it is necessary to focus on atherosclerosis to prevent a large proportion of the residual strokes.

HYPERTENSIVE ENCEPHALOPATHY

Hypertensive encephalopathy, now increasingly rare with better rates of blood pressure control, is a syndrome in which the patient develops headache, drowsiness, confusion, and if untreated, cortical blindness and seizures owing to forced vasodilatation of the cerebral vasculature in the setting of very high blood pressure. This condition has been, and continues to be, incorrectly attributed to cerebral arteriolar spasm. The pathogenesis of the syndrome was clearly elucidated in 1973, when Skinhoj, Strandgaard, Lassen, and associates[11, 12] showed that hypertensive encephalopathy is due to forced vasodilatation with breakthrough of cerebral autoregulation. Giese[13] had shown that the segment of the arteriole that appears to be in spasm in hypertensive encephalopathy is the normal segment of the artery; it constricts in response to high pressure to maintain constant cerebral blood flow despite high pressure. The segments that are blown open are damaged and leaky, contributing to cerebral edema.

Contrary to common belief, patients with hypertensive encephalopathy do not all have papilledema, which takes some time to develop. Furthermore, hypertensive encephalopathy can occur at blood pressures as low as 160/100 if there is an abrupt rise in pressure in a patient whose pressure was previously low (e.g., young women with eclampsia).

Treatment of hypertensive encephalopathy, as with any hypertensive emergency, must be done with the knowledge that if blood pressure is lowered abruptly below the threshold for cerebral autoregulation, the brain will suffer. It is imperative, therefore, that blood pressure be lowered in a controlled fashion with parenteral drugs by infusion. Intravenous diazoxide has the advantage that it does not increase intracranial pressure or interfere with diagnosis. A large proportion of patients presenting with severe hypertension have secondary hypertension, and an effective way to guide diagnosis is with a stimulated plasma renin level.[14–16] The main disadvantage of intravenous β-blockers such as propranolol or labetolol is that they suppress plasma renin and thereby delay diagnosis. Intravenous nitroprusside does not interfere with diagnosis but is much more difficult to use. My own practice in hypertensive emergencies is, when possible, to administer a dose of furosemide (0.5 mg/kg) and then start an infusion of diazoxide, aiming for a mean arterial pressure of ~120 mm Hg (~160 to 180/90 to 100 mm Hg). After 30 minutes, a plasma renin level can be drawn to guide diagnosis. A variety of options, including labetolol by infusion, or a combination of intravenous β-blocker with a vasodilator, such as hydralazine, nitroglycerine, or nitroprusside, is then appropriate for blood pressure control. This approach should not be used in patients with myocardial ischemia or aortic dissection, in whom β-blockers are preferred. In all cases, care must be taken to avoid dropping the pressure too low in order to avoid cerebral ischemia.

The popular practice of using "sublingual" nifedipine for hypertensive encephalopathy and other hypertensive crises should be avoided, since blood pressure cannot be controlled; once the dose is given, it cannot be retrieved. (The notion that the drug is being given sublingually is a myth; it is rapid absorption of swallowed liquid nifedipine that accounts for the abrupt reduction in pressure.[17]) I am aware of three strokes that occurred because of this practice, and there is a growing literature indicating that the use of capsular nifedipine is dangerous.[18] Many practitioners argue that the practice is safe, as they have not yet seen a problem; this argument is simply an admission of limited experience.

SHOULD BLOOD PRESSURE BE TREATED IN PATIENTS WITH ACUTE STROKE?

The issue of whether high blood pressure should be treated in patients with acute stroke remains controversial.[19] The statement that high blood pressure should *never* be treated in the setting of acute stroke is overly simplistic. There are some patients with acute stroke in whom the blood pressure *must* be treated. For example, patients with stroke due to aortic dissection that involves the origin of a carotid artery must have their blood pressure controlled in order to prevent progression of the dissection and even aortic rupture. Approximately 8% of ischemic strokes are due to embolism from the heart in the setting of a recent myocardial infarction. These patients, and many others, are also in critical need of blood pressure control. The question, then, is not *whether* blood pressure should be treated in patients with acute stroke, but *when* and *how* the blood pressure should be treated. This is a matter that requires clinical judgment and individualization of therapy. In general, the level at which blood pressure should be treated, the target blood pressure, and the choice of therapy are guided by the principles discussed previously with regard to hypertensive encephalopathy. Patients with previous severe long-standing hypertension have hypertrophy of their cerebral arterioles, with a rightward shift of their cerebral autoregulation curves (Fig. 28–5). They can withstand higher pressures, and cannot tolerate as low a pressure, as patients with no previous history of hypertension. Patients with severe intracranial hypertension with massive edema and a midline shift require a higher perfusion pressure than those who do not have those conditions.

Little evidence from randomized controlled trials is available to guide the management of elevated blood pressure after acute stroke.[20] On the one hand, lowering blood pressure may (1) prevent further vascular damage and stroke expansion, particularly in hemorrhagic stroke; (2) decrease the risk of conversion of ischemic stroke to hemorrhagic stroke; and (3) decrease the formation of periinfarct edema and thus avoid a worsening of the neurological deficit.[19] On the other hand, there may be a loss of autoreg-

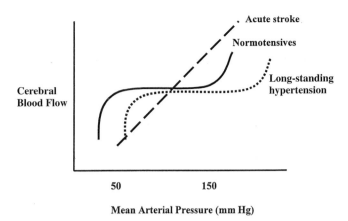

Figure 28–5. Cerebral autoregulation. Normally, cerebral blood flow is autoregulated through a wide range of perfusion pressures, from approximately 50 to 150 mm Hg (mean arterial pressure). In patients with severe long-standing hypertension, the autoregulation curve is shifted to the right because of arteriolar thickening; patients with that condition therefore can tolerate higher pressures than normotensives and do not tolerate as low a pressure as normotensives. In the region of cerebral ischemia, cerebral autoregulation is lost. The principles illustrated here are the reason that acute hypertension should not be treated with drugs that cannot be controlled, such as "sublingual" nifedipine.

ulation in ischemic regions of the brain, and lowering blood pressure may decrease perfusion pressure to the ischemic penumbra surrounding the stroke, thereby exacerbating ischemic damage in this vulnerable area.[21] Lowering systemic blood pressure might further decrease blood flow in the territory of a partially occluded cerebral vessel. Stroke patients with chronic hypertension may be more vulnerable to falls in blood pressure because of the rightward shift of their cerebral blood flow autoregulation curves toward higher blood pressures.[22]

EFFECTS OF LOWERING BLOOD PRESSURE IN HYPERTENSIVE STROKE PATIENTS

Data on which to base treatment decisions are limited, in spite of the high incidence of elevated blood pressure in patients with acute stroke. List and colleagues[23] randomized 16 hypertensive stroke patients to oral nicardipine, clonidine, captopril, or placebo. They observed no relationship between change in mean arterial pressure and change in National Institutes of Health stroke score and a negative correlation between fall in mean arterial pressure and change in the ratio of middle cerebral artery (MCA) blood flows measured by single-photon emission computed tomography over 3 days. Treated subjects did not achieve lower blood pressures than controls, and MCA ratios "improved" in the treated groups, especially the non–calcium channel blocker groups, but not in controls. The clinical rationale for the use of MCA ratio as an outcome is unclear, as it does not quantify regional cerebral blood flow. Patients were enrolled as late as 3 days after stroke, and thus, the opportunity to intervene may have been lost.

Fagan and coworkers[24] randomized 29 acute ischemic stroke patients to nimodipine or placebo. They included normotensive patients and reported only systemic blood pressure changes, not clinical status or cerebral blood flow estimates. In another small double-blinded randomized controlled trial, 28 hypertensive patients with acute cerebral ischemia were randomly assigned to perindopril or placebo 2 to 7 days after their event.[25] Blood pressure was effectively lowered without reductions in estimates of MCA and internal carotid artery blood flow, whereas improvements in National Institutes of Health stroke scores were similar in both groups. This study has a variety of limitations, including small size, inclusion of patients who entered the study later than the usual time of decision about antihypertensive treatment, and assessment of only global, not region-specific, blood flow.

In a study of 112 patients with acute stroke and increased blood pressure who were randomized to withdrawal of antihypertensive treatment after 72 hours, Popa and associates[26] found no differences between groups in modified Rankin score and mortality. However, these investigators failed to achieve better blood pressure control with treatment and all subjects were treated during first 72 hours, which may be the period of greatest importance after stroke.

EFFECTS OF INCIDENTAL LOWERING OF BLOOD PRESSURE IN STROKE PATIENTS

The results of randomized trials in acute ischemic stroke employing drugs that lower blood pressure as a side effect (as opposed to the primary intent, such as a cytoprotective effect) have been reported. Lifarizine, an ion channel modulator with putative neuroprotective effects, was studied in a randomized controlled trial involving 147 patients with acute ischemic stroke.[27] Blood pressure was lowered in the lifarizine group. Overall, mortality was lower in the treatment group, but a greater fall in blood pressure was associated with a lower likelihood of functional independence. Similarly, the Intravenous Nimodipine West European Stroke Trial (INWEST), which employed nimodipine in acute ischemic stroke for its proposed cytoprotective effects, was terminated early because of safety concerns after 295 patients were enrolled.[28] Adverse effects in that trial were attributed to hemodynamic consequences of the drug but are unlikely to be the sole reason for poorer outcomes, since neurological outcomes continued to diverge weeks after the time at which blood pressure differences were observed. Further, the relationship between blood pressure fall and neurological outcome was much weaker than between treatment assignment and outcome. As with the lifarizine trial, normotensive patients were included. In the INWEST trial, enrollment mean arterial pressure was only 113 mm Hg, and it was as low as 93 mm Hg in the higher-dose nimodipine group. These trials cannot address the hypothesis that high blood pressure may be treated safely and with benefit in patients with acute ischemic stroke because of the (1) confounding treatment effects of these drugs and (2) relatively normal blood pressure of subjects at enrollment.

CHOICE OF DRUGS FOR PHARMACOLOGICAL INTERVENTION

Short-acting intravenous blood pressure–lowering drugs should be used to reach blood pressure targets and to allow for safety should blood pressure drop precipitously (i.e., the drug can be stopped and hypotensive effects are rapidly reversed). Sodium nitroprusside and esmolol (a short-acting β-adrenergic blocker) meet this efficacy and safety criterion.[29, 30] Reports of the effects of these drugs on cerebrovascular autoregulation are mixed. Stånge and colleagues[31] reported that sodium nitroprusside causes a dose-dependent impairment of autoregulation. However, this study was conducted in pigs and used high doses to achieve mean arterial pressures as low as 61 mm Hg. In contrast, Sivarajan and coworkers[32] reported no change in cerebral blood flow at nitroprusside-mediated mean arterial pressures of 55 mm Hg in rhesus monkeys. Similarly, no change in regional cerebral blood flow was found in patients during cerebral aneurysm surgery when mean arterial pressure as low as 40 mm Hg was induced with nitroprusside.[33] Whereas fewer reports have been published describing the effects of esmolol on cerebrovascular autoregulation, most studies of the effects of β-adrenergic blockers on cerebral autoregulation have described a neutral effect on cerebral blood flow when the drugs were administered systemically.[34] Dyker and associates[25] and List and colleagues[23] reported no change in cerebral blood flow during oral administration of an angiotensin-converting enzyme inhibitor. Thus, the literature supports the hypothesis that nitroprusside, esmolol, and angiotensin-converting enzyme inhibitors can lower blood pressure while preserving cerebral blood flow. Data from randomized controlled trials are insufficient to make recommendations on the basis of evidence.

Pending the results of clinical trials, a prudent approach is as follows: In patients with acute ischemic stroke who do not appear to be at increased risk from high blood pressure, mild and moderate elevations of blood pressure can be left untreated in most cases. In such patients, if the blood pressure is very high (e.g., >230 mm Hg systolic or 125 mm Hg diastolic), blood pressure should be lowered cautiously toward a mean arterial pressure of 130 mm Hg while observing the patient for deterioration. In patients with special reasons for treatment of high blood pressure (aortic dissection, pulmonary edema, recent myocardial infarction, cerebral berry aneurysm), hypertension should be treated cautiously, as described previously under Hypertensive Encephalopathy.

STROKE PREVENTION: BEYOND BLOOD PRESSURE CONTROL

Atherosclerotic strokes occur in patients whose hypertension is effectively treated; this form of stroke is not reduced by antihypertensive therapy. It therefore becomes increasingly important, in patients under treatment for hypertension, to pay attention to other therapies that can reduce atherosclerotic and embolic strokes. These include carotid endarterectomy, antiplatelet agents, anticoagulants, treat-

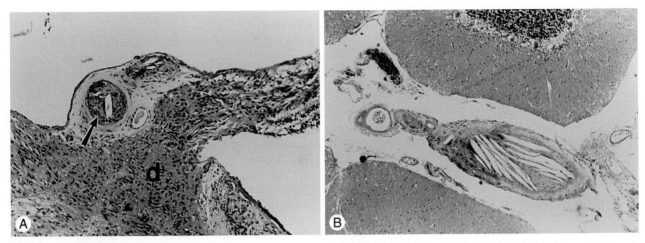

Figure 28–6. Atheromatous emboli. **A**. Optic disc. The retinal artery is occluded by atheromatous debris, including cholesterol crystals *(arrow)*. d, retina. The retina is artefactually torn away. 100×. **B**. Cholesterol crystals in an artery in the subarachnoid space of the cerebellum. (**A** and **B**, Reprinted from Spence JD, Arnold JMO, Gilbert JJ. Vascular consequences of hypertension and effects of antihypertensive therapy. *In* Robertson JIS [ed]. Clinical Hypertension. Vol 15 of Birkenhäger WH, Reid JL [eds]. Handbook of Hypertension. Copyright 1992, pp 621–654, with permission from Elsevier Science.)

ments for hyperlipidemia and hyper-homocyst(e)inemia, and postmenopausal hormone replacement therapy.

Carotid Endarterectomy

Major advances in stroke prevention have been provided by the findings of the North American Symptomatic Carotid Endarterectomy Trial (NASCET)[9] and the Asymptomatic Carotid Atherosclerosis Study (ACAS) trial.[35] The main benefit of endarterectomy is likely the prevention of atheromatous emboli (Fig. 28–6). Patients with symptomatic severe carotid stenosis (>70% by NASCET method) benefit so greatly from endarterectomy that they should be operated on if possible: The risk of subsequent stroke without surgery is approximately three times that with surgery. The perioperative risk of disabling stroke or death is 1% for each; i.e., the risk of bad outcomes is 2%, in the hands of experienced surgeons. This operation should not be done in centers with a history of bad outcomes, nor by surgeons who perform it only occasionally.[35a] Patients with symptomatic carotid stenosis between 50 and 70%[10] or severe asymptomatic stenosis[35] have only a marginal benefit from surgery, and are probably better off with aggressive medical therapy, reserving surgery for those with recurrent symptoms. Contralateral occlusion and male sex appear to increase the benefit of surgery (i.e., the risk is higher without surgery in those patients). Symptomatic patients with less than 50% stenosis appear to be better off without surgery, unless they have recurrent symptoms despite aggressive medical management.

Table 28–2 gives the number of patients who need to be treated (NNT) with endarterectomy to prevent one ipsilateral stroke in 5 years. For prevention of disabling stroke, the numbers are higher; for asymptomatic patients, or for symptomatic patients with less than 50% stenosis, the NNT is approximately 1000. For this reason, and because the likelihood is approximately 80% that the next stroke with expectant (medical) management will be non-disabling,[10] expectant management with aggressive medical

treatment is indicated except in patients with symptomatic severe stenosis, who clearly benefit from surgery.

Medical Management

Antiplatelet Agents and Anticoagulants

In high-risk patients of both sexes, antiplatelet agents reduce risk of stroke.[36, 37] For patients with no history of TIA, it is appropriate to prescribe daily aspirin (ASA). In patients who have failed ASA therapy (i.e., have experienced a TIA despite daily ASA therapy), it is probably best to *add*, rather than substitute, ticlopidine[38, 39] or clopidogrel[40] on the basis of studies in patients with coronary stents, which showed that the combination was substantially more effective than either ASA or ticlopidine alone.[41] Ticlopidine is expensive and toxic (1% of patients experience severe neutropenia; 12% have diarrhea, and the average increase in plasma cholesterol is ~10%) and, therefore, should be reserved for patients who cannot take ASA or who have failed on ASA. Because of widespread treatment of *Helicobacter pylori* infection,[42] the proportion of patients who cannot take ASA is remarkably less than in the past. A large Belgian study[43] showed a substantial benefit with the combination of ASA with dipyridamole compared with either agent alone in patients with TIA. For patients who

Table 28–2 Carotid Endarterectomy: Number of Patients That Need to Be Treated to Prevent One Ipsilateral Stroke in 5 Years

	Degree of Stenosis (%)	NNT
Symptomatic	70–99	8
	50–69	15
	<50	26
Asymptomatic	>60	18

Abbreviation: NNT, number of patients that need to be treated.

cannot take ticlopidine, dipyridamole may be an alternative.

Other studies have shown that patients with lone atrial fibrillation should be anticoagulated long-term if they are over age 65 years or have other stroke risk factors, such as hypertension or congestive heart failure.[44–46] Reluctance to use anticoagulation long-term based on historical bad experiences before the international normalized ratio (INR) was used to control therapy has led to significant underutilization of this therapy. This is inappropriate: INR makes anticoagulation much safer than in the past, and the risk for patients with atrial fibrillation and other stroke risk factors is much higher without anticoagulants.

Treatment of Hyperlipidemia in Cerebral Vascular Disease

It is commonly believed that the risk factors for stroke and myocardial infarction are very different. This belief is based on failure to distinguish different kinds of stroke. When strokes due to hypertensive small vessel disease are lumped with atherosclerotic strokes, the importance of hypertension is highlighted, and the importance of hyperlipidemia is deemphasized. Hyperlipidemia is a significant risk factor for stroke, as demonstrated by the experience in London, Ontario, Canada, where hypertensive strokes have largely been eliminated by the effective detection and treatment of hypertension.[47]

There is little evidence of secondary prevention of stroke with treatment of hyperlipidemia, but there is evidence of reduced stroke in patients treated with lipid-lowering drugs for other indications. In the Cholesterol and Recurrent Events (CARE) study, stroke was reduced by treatment with pravastatin in patients with coronary artery disease.[48] It is prudent to aggressively treat patients with carotid stenosis with diet and pharmacological therapy to lower their low-density lipoprotein to the same consensus targets as for patients with coronary artery disease (CAD) because patients with carotid stenosis have a coronary risk that is as high as or higher than in those with established CAD. For example, even patients with asymptomatic carotid stenosis have a higher coronary risk than that in patients with previous myocardial infarction or angina who benefited from simvastatin in the Scandanavian Simvastatin Survival Study (4S) Trial.[49] Chimowitz and associates[50] showed in the Veterans Administration Asymptomatic Carotid Endarterectomy trial that patients with both carotid stenosis and a history of CAD had a 40% 4-year risk of coronary events; patients with carotid stenosis alone had a 33% 4-year risk of CAD, which is substantially higher than the 24% 6-year risk of the patients in the 4S trial randomized to placebo. The 6-year NNT[51] is therefore lower for patients with carotid stenosis than it was for coronary patients in 4S: approximately 6.5 for carotid stenosis patients with coronary disease, and approximately 8.5 for patients with asymptomatic carotid stenosis alone, compared with 10.5 for coronary patients in the 4S trial. Few patients with carotid stenosis will have levels of low-density lipoprotein at the consensus target for coronary patients (<2.5 mmol/L or 100 mg/dl), so most will require lipid-lowering therapy.

In addition to medication for hyperlipidemia, dietary treatment is much more important than is generally recognized. Diet reduces *fasting* lipids by only about 5% on average, but *postprandial* lipids, largely determined by diet, may be more important determinants of atherosclerosis than are fasting lipids.[52–55] Patients with vascular disease should adhere to a step II National Cholesterol Education Program (NCEP) diet, which includes no egg yolks (egg whites or egg substitutes can be used in most recipes that call for eggs) and only 4 oz of red meat every other day, with avoidance of fried foods. (A large serving of fries at McDonald's contains about 200 cal of potato and 300 cal of fat; a single potato chip contains about 1 cal of potato and 9 cal of fat.)

Hyper-Homocyst(e)inemia

Homocystinuria was first recognized in 1962.[56] This rare condition (heterozygotes represent <1% of the population) is due to a deficiency of cystathionine β-synthase, which responds to treatment with its cofactor, pyridoxine (vitamin B_6). Hyper-homocyst(e)inemia, a recently defined risk factor for atherosclerotic disease, is more common and has a different cause. In 1985, a report from Holland indicated that about 30% of patients with premature atherosclerosis had hyper-homocyst(e)inemia;[57] this was confirmed by an Irish study in 1991.[58] Approximately 50% of the population are heterozygous, and 11% homozygous, for a mutation in methylenetetrahydrofolate reductase that causes hyper-homocyst(e)inemia, which responds to folate supplementation.[59] There are also mutations of methionine synthase, for which the cofactor is vitamin B_{12}. In addition, deficiency of folate, B_6, or B_{12} will cause hyper-homocyst(e)inemia. Such a vitamin deficiency can be nutritional or, in the case of vitamin B_{12}, can be due to malabsorption. An increasingly common cause of vitamin B_{12} deficiency is achlorhydria due to proton pump inhibitors such as omeprazole;[60] fortunately, crystalline vitamin B_{12} supplements do not require gastric acid for absorption.[61]

There are thus six main ways to develop hyper-homocyst(e)inemia, and the condition has a much higher prevalence than was previously suspected: 20% of the population have plasma homocyst(e)ine levels greater than 14 μmol/L, and 33% have levels above 10.5 μmol/L. Among patients with unexplained atherosclerosis (those whose carotid plaque area is not explained by age, sex, systolic pressure, cholesterol:high-density lipoprotein ratio, smoking, hypertension, or hyperlipidemia), 47% have plasma homocyst(e)ine levels above 14 μmol/L, and 60% have levels above 12 μmol/L.[62] In 1997, two key studies showed that plasma homocyst(e)ine levels above 10.2 μmol/L were associated with a doubling of coronary risk,[63] and that plasma homocyst(e)ine levels in the range from 5 to 20 μmol/L showed a steep dose-response, with coronary risk increasing eight-fold over that range.[64] The mechanisms by which hyper-homocyst(e)inemia causes hypercoagulability and accelerates atherosclerosis include increased production of hydrogen peroxide and consumption of nitric oxide, with impairment of endothelial function.[65]

Hyper-homocyst(e)inemia is an important risk factor not only because it is so common but also because it is so easily treated. Either folate or vitamin B_6 alone normalizes plasma homocyst(e)ine in 50% of cases; a combination of the two vitamins normalizes plasma homocyst(e)ine in 95% of cases and restores endothelial function.[66, 67] A combination of folic acid and vitamins B_6 and B_{12} is used for treatment. Vitamin B_{12} is added because it not only increases the activity of methionine synthase but also guards against the problem of masked vitamin B_{12} deficiency. A simple approach to that issue is to measure serum vitamin B_{12} levels a month after initiation of therapy to verify absorption.

We recently reported that a combination of folic acid 2.5 mg, vitamin B_6 25 mg, and vitamin B_{12} 250 μg daily halted the progression of carotid atherosclerosis in patients with plasma homocyst(e)ine levels over 14 μmol/L.[68] A clinical trial (the Vitamin Intervention for Stroke Prevention [VISP] trial) is now under way to test the hypothesis that vitamin therapy with similar doses of the three cofactors will prevent stroke, myocardial infarction, and death in patients with a previous nondisabling stroke.

Postmenopausal Hormone Replacement Therapy

One of the most intriguing, and possibly most important, features of vascular biology is the protection from vascular disease enjoyed by premenopausal women. Because women begin only at menopause to be subject to the same risk as men, their vascular problems are delayed by an average of 15 years. One hundred women survive to age 90 years for every 33 men who attain that age. Strong epidemiological evidence indicates that postmenopausal hormone replacement therapy (HRT) reduces vascular risk by 44%.[69] The degree of protection cannot be explained by the beneficial effect of estrogen on lipid profiles.[70] It appears that estrogen increases nitric oxide production[71] and reduces endothelin production.[72] Sublingual estrogen improves treadmill exercise tolerance in postmenopausal women with angina,[73] and estrogen improves coronary responses to stress[71, 74, 75] and endothelial function[71] in surgically menopausal monkeys.

Figure 28–7 shows the 6-year vascular risk with and without postmenopausal HRT (assuming the benefits reported in the Nurses Health Study[69]) for women with asymptomatic carotid stenosis and coronary disease,[50] CAD alone,[49] carotid stenosis with TIAs,[9] and for comparison, the 6-year incremental risk of breast cancer attributable to HRT for women ages 50 to 70 years.[76] A major meta-analysis showed that the incremental risk of breast cancer with HRT is only 1.2% over 15 years.[76] Pending the results of a major randomized trial of HRT, it appears likely that postmenopausal women with vascular disease should be taking HRT in the absence of strong contraindications.

CONCLUSION

Hypertension causes, and treatment of high blood pressure prevents, strokes characterized by small vessel disease: lacunar infarctions due to hyaline degeneration and fibrinoid necrosis and intracerebral hemorrhages due to hyaline degeneration. In the setting of hypertensive encephalopathy and in patients with acute stroke who require lowering of blood pressure because of either very high pressures or concomitant conditions necessitating blood pressure control, it is important to avoid treatments, such as "sublingual" nifedipine, that may abruptly drop pressure below the limits of autoregulation. Intravenous infusion of short-acting drugs is a fundamental principle of management in these situations.

Approximately 50% of strokes can be eliminated by effective detection and control of hypertension. To reduce the burden of the residual strokes, most of which are due to atherosclerosis, it is necessary to aggressively treat atherosclerosis in patients at high risk. Treatment includes carotid endarterectomy for patients with symptomatic severe stenosis, as well as antiplatelet agents, anticoagulants for atrial fibrillation, treatment of hyperlipidemia, and treatment of hyper-homocyst(e)inemia.

Acknowledgment

We are indebted to Dr. Joe Gilbert for the fine illustrations of hypertensive small vessel disease and atherosclerotic emboli.

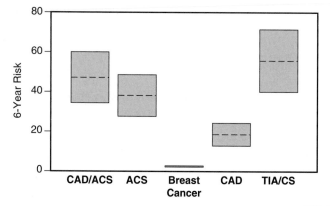

Figure 28–7. Six-year risk with and without postmenopausal hormone replacement therapy (HRT). The *bars* show the risk reduction with HRT for women with vascular disease and the increase in risk of breast cancer with HRT. The incremental risk of breast cancer is very small compared with the reduction in risk for women with coronary artery disease (CAD), carotid stenosis (CS), or transient ischemic attacks (TIA). ACS, asymptomatic carotid stenosis.

References

1. Kurtzke JF, McDowell FH, Caplan LR (eds). Cerebrovascular Survey Report: Epidemiology of Cerebrovascular Disease. Bethesda, MD, National Institute of Neurological and Communicative Disorders and Stroke, 1985; pp 1–34.
2. Spence JD. Antihypertensive drugs and prevention of stroke. Stroke 17:808–810, 1986.
3. Spence JD. Cerebral consequences of hypertension. *In* Laragh JH, Brenner BM (eds). Hypertension: Pathophysiology, Diagnosis, and Management, 2nd ed. New York, Raven, 1995; pp 741–753.
4. Spence JD, Hachinski VC. Neurological complications of hypertension. *In* Goetz CG, Tanner CM, Aminoff MJ (eds). Systemic Diseases: Part I. Amsterdam, Elsevier Science, 1993; pp 71–91.
5. Pickering G. Hypertension: Causes, Consequences and Management. London, Churchill Livingstone, 1974; pp 40–62.
6. Hachinski VC, Norris JW. The vascular infrastructure. *In* The Acute Stroke. Philadelphia, FA Davis, 1985; pp 27–40.
7. Bass MJ, McWhinney IR, Donner A. Do family physicians need medical assistants to detect and manage hypertension? Can Med Assoc J 134:1247–1255, 1986.
8. Birkett NJ, Donner A. Prevalence and control of hypertension in an Ontario county. Can Med Assoc J 132:1019–1024, 1985.

8a. Russell RWR. How does high blood pressure cause stroke? Lancet 2:1283–1285, 1975.

9. North American Symptomatic Carotid Endarterectomy Trial Collaborators. Beneficial effect of carotid endarterectomy in symptomatic patients with high-grade carotid stenosis. N Engl J Med 325:445–507, 1991.

10. Barnett HJM, Taylor DW, Eliasziw M, et al. Benefit of carotid endarterectomy in patients with symptomatic moderate or severe stenosis. N Engl J Med 339:1415–1425, 1998.

11. Skinhoj E, Strandgaard S. Pathogenesis of hypertensive encephalopathy. Lancet 1:461–462, 1973.

12. Strandgaard S, Olesen J, Skinhoj E, Lassen NA. Autoregulation of brain circulation in severe arterial hypertension. BMJ 1:507–510, 1973.

13. Giese J. Acute hypertensive vascular disease. 2: Studies on vascular reaction patterns and permeability changes by means of vital microscopy and colloidal tracer technique. Acta Pathol Microbiol 62:497–517, 1964.

14. Spence JD. Government guidelines for treatment of hypertension. Am J Hypertens 8:541, 1995.

15. Spence JD. Management of hypertensive emergencies. Can J Diagn 9:72–93, 1992.

16. Spence JD. Stepped care for hypertension is dead, but what will replace it? Can Med Assoc J 140:1133–1136, 1989.

17. van Harten J, Burggraaf K, Danhof M, et al. Negligible sublingual absorption of nifedipine. Lancet 2:1363–1365, 1987.

18. Grossman E, Messerli FH, Grodzicki T, Kowey P. Should a moratorium be placed on nifedipine capsules for hypertensive emergencies and pseudoemergencies? JAMA 276:1331, 1996.

19. Spence JD, Del Maestro RF. Hypertension in acute strokes: treat. Arch Neurol 42:1000–1002, 1985.

20. Blood Pressure in Acute Stroke Collaboration (BASC). Blood pressure management in acute stroke. Part 1: Assessment of trials designated to alter blood pressure. In Warlow C, van Gijn J, Sandercock P, et al (eds). Stroke Module of The Cochrane Database of Systematic Reviews. [Updated quarterly; updated June 3, 1997] Available from The Cochrane Library [database on disk and CD-ROM]. The Cochrane Collaboration, Issue 3. Oxford, Update Software, 1997. Accessed August 1997.

21. Meyer JS, Shimazu K, Fukuuchi Y, et al. Impaired neurogenic cerebrovascular control and dysautoregulation after stroke. Stroke 4:169–186, 1973.

22. Strandgaard S, Paulson OB. Cerebral blood flow and its pathophysiology. Am J Hypertens 2:486–492, 1989.

23. Lisk DR, Gortta JC, Lamki LM, et al. Should hypertension be treated after acute stroke? A randomized controlled trial using single photon emission computed tomography. Arch Neurol 50:855–862, 1993.

24. Fagan SC, Gengi FM, Bates V, et al. Effect of nimodipine on blood pressure in acute ischemic stroke in humans. Stroke 19:401–402, 1988.

25. Dyker AG, Grosset DG, Lees K. Perindopril reduces blood pressure but not cerebral blood flow in patients with recent cerebral ischemic stroke. Stroke 28:580–583, 1997.

26. Popa G, Voiculescu V, Popa C, et al. Stroke and hypertension: Antihypertensive therapy withdrawal. Rom J Neurol Psychiatr 33:29–36, 1995.

27. Squire IB, Lees KR, Pryse-Phillips W, et al. The effects of lifarizine in acute cerebral infarction: A pilot safety study. Cerebrovasc Dis 6:156–160, 1996.

28. Wahlgren NG, MacMahon DG, De Keyser J, et al. Intravenous Nimodipine West European Stroke Trial (INWEST) in the treatment of acute ischemic stroke. Cerebrovasc Dis 4:204–210, 1996.

29. Gray RJ, Bateman TM, Czer LSC, et al. Comparison of esmolol and nitroprusside for acute post-cardiac surgical hypertension. Am J Cardiol 59:887–891, 1987.

30. Ornstein E, Young WL, Ostaplovich N, et al. Deliberate hypotension in patients with intracranial arteriovenous malformations: Esmolol compared with isoflurane and sodium nitroprusside. Anesth Analg 72:639–644, 1991.

31. Stånge K, Lagerkranser M, Sollevi A. Nitroprusside-induced hypotension and cerebrovascular autoregulation in the anesthetized pig. Anesth Analg 73:745–752, 1991.

32. Sivarajan M, Amory DW, McKenzie SM. Regional blood flows during induced hypotension produced by nitroprusside or trimethaphan in the rhesus monkey. Anesth Analg 64:759–766, 1985.

33. Pinaud M, Souron R, Lelausque JN, et al. Cerebral blood flow and cerebral oxygen consumption during nitroprusside-induced hypotension to less than 50 mmHg. Anesthesiology 70:255–260, 1989.

34. Edvinsson L, MacKenzie ET, McCulloch J. Cerebral Blood Flow and Metabolism. New York: Raven, 1993.

35. Executive Committee for the Asymptomatic Carotid Atherosclerosis Study. Endarterectomy for asymptomatic carotid artery stenosis. JAMA 272:1421–1428, 1995.

35a. Chassin R. Appropriate use of carotid endarterectomy. N Engl J Med 339:1468–1471, 1998.

36. Barnett HJM, Eliasziw M, Meldrum H. Drugs and surgery in the prevention of ischemic stroke. N Engl J Med 332:238–248, 1995.

37. Antiplatelet Trialists' Collaboration. Collaborative overview of randomised trials of antiplatelet therapy. I: Prevention of death, myocardial infarction, and stroke by prolonged antiplatelet therapy in various categories of patients. BMJ 308:81–106, 1994.

38. Hass WK, Easton JD, Adams HP Jr, et al. A randomized trial comparing ticlopidine hydrochloride with aspirin for the prevention of stroke in high-risk patients. N Engl J Med 321:501–507, 1989.

39. Gent M, Blakely JA, Easton JD, et al. The Canadian American Ticlopidine Study (CATS) in thromboembolic stroke. Lancet 1:1215–1220, 1989.

40. Caprie Steering Committee. A randomised, blinded, trial of clopidogrel vs aspirin in patients at risk of ischaemic events. Lancet 348:1329–1339, 1996.

41. Schömig A, Neumann F-J, Kastrati A, et al. A randomized comparison of antiplatelet and anticoagulant therapy after the placement of coronary-artery stents. N Engl J Med 334:1084–1089, 1996.

42. Goodwin CS, Mendall MM, Northfield TC. Helicobacter pylori infection. Lancet 349:265–269, 1997.

43. Diener HC, Cunha L, Forbes J, et al. European Stroke Prevention Study 2. Dipyridamole and acetylsalicylic acid in the secondary prevention of stroke. J Neurol Sci 143:1–13, 1996.

44. Atrial Fibrillation Investigators. Risk factors for stroke and efficacy of antithrombotic therapy in atrial fibrillation. Arch Intern Med 154:1449–1457, 1994.

45. Rosendaal FR. The Scylla and Charybdis of oral anticoagulant treatment. N Engl J Med 335:587–589, 1996.

46. Hylek EM, Skates SJ, Sheehan MA, Singer DE. An analysis of the lowest effective intensity of prophylactic anticoagulation for patients with nonrheumatic atrial fibrillation. N Engl J Med 335:540–546, 1996.

47. Hachinski VC, Graffagnino C, Beaudry M, et al. Lipids and stroke: A paradox resolved. Arch Neurol 53:303–308, 1996.

48. Plehn JF, Rouleau J, Pfeffer M, et al. Reduction of stroke incidence following myocardial infarction with pravastatin: The CARE study. [Abstract] Stroke 29:287, 1998.

49. Scandinavian Simvastatin Survival Study Group. Randomized trial of cholesterol lowering in 4444 patients with coronary heart disease: The Scandinavian Simvastatin Survival Study (4S). Lancet 344:1383–1389, 1994.

50. Chimowitz MJ, Weiss DG, Cohen SL, et al. Cardiac prognosis of patients with carotid stenosis and no history of coronary artery disease. Stroke 25:759–765, 1994.

51. Laupacis A, Sackett DL, Roberts RS. An assessment of clinically useful measures of the consequences of treatment. N Engl J Med 318:1728–1734, 1988.

52. Hanefeld M, Temelkova-Kurktschiev T. The postprandial state and the risk of atherosclerosis. Diabet Med 14(Suppl 3):S6–S11, 1997.

53. Ebenbichler CF, Kirchmair R, Egger C, Patsch JR. Postprandial state and atherosclerosis. Curr Opin Lipidol 6:286–290, 1995.

54. Gronholdt ML, Nordestgaard BG, Nielsen TG, Sillesen H. Echolucent carotid artery plaques are associated with elevated levels of fasting and postprandial triglyceride-rich lipoproteins. Stroke 27:2166–2172, 1996.

55. Steiner G. Triglyceride-rich lipoproteins and atherosclerosis, from fast to feast. Ann Med 25:431–435, 1993.

56. McKusick VA. Homocystinuria. In Online Mendelian Inheritance in Man. 1997. [Generic] Available at: http://www3.ncbi.nlm.gov/htbin-post/Omim/dispmim?236200. Accessed December 14, 1998.

57. Boers GHJ, Trijbels FJM, Fowler B, et al. Heterozygosity for homocystinuria in premature peripheral and cerebral occlusive arterial disease. N Engl J Med 313:709–714, 1985.

58. Clarke R, Daly L, Robinson K, et al. Hyperhomocysteinemia: An independent risk factor for vascular disease. N Engl J Med 324:1149–1155, 1991.

59. Rozen R. Molecular genetic aspects of hyperhyper-homocyst(e)-inemia and its relation to folic acid. Clin Invest Med 19:171–178, 1996.
60. Marcuard SP, Alabernaz L, Khazanie PG. Omeprazole treatment causes malabsorption of cyanocobalamin (vitamin B$_{12}$). Ann Intern Med 120:211–215, 1994.
61. Saltzman J, Kemp JA, Golner BB, et al. Effect of hypochlorhydria due to omeprazole treatment or atrophic gastritis on protein-bound vitamin B$_{12}$ absorption. J Am Coll Nutr 13:584–591, 1994.
62. Spence JD, Barnett PA, Hegele RA, et al. Plasma homocyst(e)ine predicts carotid plaque better than methylenetetrahydrofolate reductase genotype. [Abstract] Stroke 29:285, 1998.
63. Graham IM, Daly L, Refsum H, et al. Plasma homocysteine as a risk factor for vascular disease. JAMA 277:1775–1781, 1997.
64. Nygård O, Nordrehaug JE, Refsum H, et al. Plasma homocysteine levels and mortality in patients with coronary artery disease. N Engl J Med 337:230–236, 1997.
65. Stamler JS, Osborne JA, Jaraki O, et al. Adverse vascular effects of homocysteine are modulated by endothelium-derived relaxing factor and related oxides of nitrogen. J Clin Invest 91:308–318, 1993.
66. Van den Berg M, Franken DG, Boers GH, et al. Combined vitamin B$_6$ plus folic acid therapy in young patients with arteriosclerosis and hyperhomocysteinemia. J Vasc Surg 20:933–940, 1994.
67. Van den Berg M, Boers GH, Franken DG, et al. Hyperhomocysteinaemia and endothelial dysfunction in young patients with peripheral arterial occlusive disease. Eur J Clin Invest 25:176–181, 1995.
68. Peterson JC, Spence JD. Vitamins and progression of atherosclerosis in hyper-homocyst(e)inemia. Lancet 351:263, 1998.
69. Stampfer MJ, Golditz GA, Willett WC, et al. Postmenopausal estrogen therapy and cardiovascular disease. Ten-year followup from the Nurses Health Study. N Engl J Med 325:756–762, 1991.
70. Bush TL, Barrett-Connor E, Cowan LD, et al. Cardiovascular mortality and noncontraceptive use of estrogen in women: Results from the Lipid Clinics Program follow-up study. Circulation 75:1102–1109, 1987.
71. Williams JK, Adams MR, Herrington DM, Clarkson TB. Short-term administration of estrogen and vascular esponses of atherosclerotic coronary arteries. Circulation 81:1680–1687, 1990.
72. Polderman KH, Stehouwer CDA, van Kamp GJ, et al. Influence of sex hormone on plasma endothelin levels. Ann Intern Med 118:429–432, 1993.
73. Rosano GMC, Sarrel PM, Poole-Wilson PA, Collins P. Beneficial effect of oestrogen on exercise-induced myocardial ischemia in women with coronary artery disease. Lancet 342:133–136, 1993.
74. Williams JK, Adams MR, Klopfenstein HS. Estrogen modulates responses of atherosclerotic coronary arteries. Circulation 81:1680–1687, 1990.
75. Williams JK, Kaplan JR, Manuck SB. Effect of psychosocial stress on endothelium-mediated dilation of atherosclerotic arteries in cynomolgus monkeys. J Clin Invest 92:1819–1823, 1993.
76. Collaborative Group on Hormonal Risk Factors in Breast Cancer. Breast cancer and hormone replacement therapy: Collaborative re-analysis of data from 51 epidemiological studies of 52,705 women with breast cancer and 108,411 women without breast cancer. Lancet 350:1047–1057, 1997.

CHAPTER 29

Chronic Renal Insufficiency in Hypertension: Slowing Its Progression

Samuel Spitalewitz, Pierre F. Faubert, and Jerome G. Porush

The prevalence of hypertension in patients with chronic renal insufficiency (CRI) varies with the underlying cause and increases linearly as renal function deteriorates.[1, 2] Hypertension is present in approximately 60 to 80% of patients with moderate to severe tubulointerstitial disease but occurs in more than 90% of patients with chronic glomerulonephritis who have similar levels of renal function. Regardless of the etiology of the renal insufficiency, as patients approach end-stage renal disease (ESRD), virtually all are hypertensive.[3] In addition, although the exact incidence is unknown, the incidence of renal failure caused by essential hypertension is substantial, with African Americans, males, and the elderly at highest risk. It is imperative to lower blood pressure (BP) in hypertensives with CRI, regardless of whether the hypertension is the cause of the renal dysfunction or the result of a primary, underlying renal disease.

Many studies have demonstrated that treatment of essential hypertension diminishes morbidity and mortality from cardiovascular disease, even in the elderly.[4–6] There is now substantial evidence that lowering BP will slow the inexorable decline in renal function in patients with CRI.[7] Nevertheless, at a time when morbidity and mortality from cardiovascular disease are declining, the incidence of ESRD is increasing dramatically, particularly among African Americans, the elderly, and diabetic hypertensive patients.[8, 9] There is no single explanation for this, but several pertinent issues are examined here.[6]

1. Should the general therapeutic approach to hypertension (nonpharmacological and pharmacological) differ between patients with CRI and those with essential hypertension without renal insufficiency?
2. Will lowering dietary salt intake impact favorably on hypertension and renal function?
3. Will lowering BP to levels below the current goal of 140/90 mm Hg, or a mean arterial pressure (MAP) of 107 mm Hg, better preserve renal function without increasing undesirable consequences?
4. Are there specific classes of antihypertensive drugs that are renoprotective over and above their effect on BP?
5. Finally, in addition to hypertension, are there other modifiable factors that alter the progression of renal disease?

PATHOGENESIS OF HYPERTENSION IN CHRONIC RENAL INSUFFICIENCY

The hypertension of CRI is secondary to the salt and water retention caused by the decrease in renal excretory function, which leads to intravascular volume expansion as well as to increased vascular tone and peripheral resistance. Several factors are responsible for the increase in peripheral vascular resistance. Studies done in normotensive and hypertensive subjects with renal insufficiency have revealed increases in cytosolic calcium and sodium concentrations associated with a depressed sodium pump and an increase in calcium ATPase activity. These abnormalities of cellular metabolism are aggravated if salt intake is increased.[10] Circulating plasma epinephrine levels are similar in hypertensives with normal kidney function and those with CRI; however, plasma norepinephrine is higher in the latter group.[11] Debrisoquin, a postganglionic sympathetic blocker, reduces BP much more in hypertensive dialysis patients than in controls or normotensive dialysis patients.[12] Plasma renin activity and angiotensin are elevated in CRI and correlate with the blood pressure.[13] Angiotensin II is capable of increasing peripheral vascular resistance directly by inducing smooth muscle hypertrophy or indirectly by potentiating the vasoconstrictive effect of norepinephrine. Other vasoactive agents, such as arginine vasopressin, atrial natriuretic peptide, and endothelin, are elevated in patients with CRI.[14] Their roles in the pathogenesis of hypertension associated with CRI remain to be elucidated, however.[15]

Finally, it should be noted that secondary hyperparathyroidism, commonly associated with CRI, may also contribute to the increase in peripheral vascular resistance by increasing intracellular calcium.[16] Also, erythropoietin therapy of anemic patients with CRI may cause hypertension or aggravate preexisting hypertension. Erythropoietin administration in such patients induces a rise in resting and stimulated intracellular calcium levels, resulting in resistance to the vasodilator effect of nitric oxide.[17]

Nonpharmacological Therapy

The same general measures useful in the treatment of essential hypertension can be applied to patients with hypertension and CRI. Because salt and water retention is an important contributor to the hypertension in CRI, sodium restriction is particularly important and is the single most important nonpharmacological intervention used with these patients.[3] In fact, sodium restriction is more effective in controlling BP in patients with CRI than it is in controlling BP in those without CRI, as only half of the latter group are salt-sensitive.[18] In addition to directly lowering BP by diminishing extracellular volume and vascular reactivity, dietary sodium restriction also potentiates the effects of other antihypertensive agents, particularly angiotensin-converting enzyme (ACE) inhibitors and angiotensin II receptor blockers (ARBs).[6, 19]

Interestingly, sodium restriction is as effective as protein restriction or ACE inhibition in preventing glomerular injury in uninephrectomized, spontaneously hypertensive rats and in remnant rat kidneys and may provide more renal protection than do diuretics.[6, 20, 21] In the remnant rat kidney model, sodium restriction appears to provide this protective effect not by reducing glomerular capillary pressure but rather by diminishing mesangial compensatory growth.[21] In addition, animal data suggest that high dietary sodium intake increases proteinuria not only by raising systemic BP but also by directly increasing glomerular hypertrophy.[6, 22]

As sodium intake is increased in humans, the antiproteinuric effects of an ACE inhibitor and a nondihydropyridine calcium antagonist are markedly blunted.[23, 24] Patients on a stable dose of lisinopril experienced a 52% reduction in protein excretion in the presence of only a 3% reduction in BP when placed on a low sodium diet.[6, 23] Thus, available data in both animals and humans[25] suggest that there is a benefit from sodium restriction in addition to its antihypertensive effect. Further clinical trials are necessary to more definitively assess whether sodium restriction alone can favorably affect the rate of progression of renal disease or modify the outcome of other therapeutic interventions.[6]

Sodium restriction and achieving the optimal hydration status ("dry weight") must be accomplished gradually. Rapid and marked reduction of sodium intake may result in severe volume contraction and worsening renal function, as the failing kidney is unable to rapidly accommodate to a decrease in sodium intake. Irreversibly worsening renal function may ensue unless sodium restriction to 1500 to 2000 mg/day is introduced gradually.[3]

Pharmacological Therapy

Diuretics

Given the central role of volume expansion in renal parenchymal hypertension, diuretic therapy is usually necessary if the patient is unwilling or unable to adhere to a sodium-restricted diet.[3] Either a loop-active or thiazide diuretic may be used, with the choice generally determined by the level of renal function. As glomerular filtration rate (GFR) falls below 35 ml/min (serum creatinine approximately 2.5 mg/dl), thiazides become ineffective and if used, should be combined with a loop-active diuretic. Even if adequately secreted (see later section), thiazides are not sufficiently potent to increase sodium excretion in a patient with a GFR of less than 35 ml/min. Even repeated doses of thiazides throughout the day would be inadequate unless combined with a loop-active diuretic, which has the potential to cause excretion of 25% of the filtered sodium. Combinations of the two types of diuretics have been successful in lowering BP in patients with renal failure who have been resistant to both when used alone.[26, 27]

It is important to note that almost all diuretics are protein-bound (primarily to albumin). Because they exert their action within the tubular lumen, they must be secreted, at least in part.[26] With a decline in renal function, organic acids accumulate and block the secretion of diuretics into the tubular lumen, which reduces their effectiveness and necessitates higher doses of drug.[26] In patients with a GFR of less than 20 ml/min, the plateau of the dose-response curve is approximately 160 mg of furosemide (or its equivalent as bumetanide or torsemide), given intravenously, or 320 to 400 mg given orally.[3] Of the three available loop-active diuretics, torsemide is the one that is best absorbed when given by mouth, so that in patients in whom intestinal absorption is impaired (e.g., patients with edematous bowel associated with nephrotic syndrome), it is the drug of choice.[28]

The response to diuretics is highly individual, and the

dose must be altered as the clinical response dictates. The initial response to the diuretic is loss of plasma volume, which is replaced by mobilization of peripheral edema. If edema is substantial, removal of 2 to 3 L/day is usually not hazardous. However, because there is a substantial risk of intravascular volume contraction with potentially irreversible worsening of renal function, close supervision of diuretic therapy is mandatory and must include monitoring of BP (including orthostatics) and timely evaluation of renal function and electrolytes.[3]

The antihypertensive agents used in essential hypertension are also effective in patients with CRI. As in patients with essential hypertension, certain circumstances dictate the use of specific drugs in patients with CRI.[29] For instance, patients with CRI and hypertension with associated benign prostatic hypertrophy or dyslipidemia may benefit most from an α-blocker. For those with associated hyperthyroidism, migraine headache, essential tremor, atrial arrhythmias, or angina, a β-blocker may be most desirable. After a myocardial infarction, patients would benefit most from a β-blocker, an ACE inhibitor, or both. Guidelines are provided elsewhere for appropriate reductions in doses of renally metabolized drugs such as atenolol, nadolol, hydralazine, clonidine, and captopril in patients with CRI.[29]

Caution must be exercised with α_1-adrenergic blockers, which have been reported to produce significant orthostatic hypotension, particularly in patients with autonomic neuropathy associated with CRI. Frequent monitoring of renal function is necessary when guanethidine is used, as it decreases renal blood flow and GFR and can reversibly worsen renal function. Centrally acting α_2-adrenergic agonists may cause marked lethargy in patients with GFRs less than 20 ml/min and should be administered at reduced doses.[6] Although they may be particularly effective in patients with CRI, ACE inhibitors (and probably ARBs) should be used cautiously in patients with proven or suspected bilateral renal artery stenosis or arterial stenosis in an isolated kidney, as they may precipitate acute renal insufficiency. Such an occurrence is an indication to look for what has been called "ischemic nephropathy."[30]

In the most recent Joint National Committee report (VI), two specific recommendations were made regarding the treatment of patients with hypertension and CRI. First, BP should be lowered to at least 130/85 mm Hg (and perhaps even to 125/75 mm Hg) in patients with proteinuria with protein excretion levels in excess of 1 g per 24 hours. Second, patients with hypertension who have renal insufficiency should receive, unless contraindicated, an ACE inhibitor both to control hypertension and to slow the progression of renal failure.[29, 31–35]

What Should the Goal Blood Pressure Be for Patients With Chronic Renal Insufficiency?

Although numerous studies have demonstrated the importance of hypertension as a risk factor for the progression of renal failure in diabetic and nondiabetic CRI,[9, 36–41] will lowering BP to the levels suggested (unrelated to the drugs used) slow the progression of renal disease without undesirable side effects? In essential hypertension, no large-scale, prospective, randomized studies have been designed to determine whether lowering BP prevents or slows the pro-

gression of renal failure. Furthermore, the appropriate goal BP has not been established.[9] However, data from a variety of studies suggest that aggressive treatment of essential hypertension, even with traditional therapy such as diuretics and β-blockers, can stabilize renal function as assessed by the serum creatinine.[6, 9]

In the Hypertension Detection and Follow-up Program,[42] the stepped-care group, which achieved a mean BP of 129/86, significantly lower than the usual-care group (139/90), showed stabilization of renal function after 1 year of aggressive treatment. Specifically, the stepped-care group showed a slower rate of development of an elevated serum creatinine compared with the less aggressively treated usual-care group.

Similarly, in the Multiple Risk Factor Intervention Trial (MRFIT),[43] a more rapid decline in renal function (assessed by the slope of the reciprocal of the serum creatinine) was observed over a 7-year follow-up period in 5061 non-African Americans with mild to moderate hypertension whose diastolic BP (DBP) was maintained above 95 mm Hg. A positive slope, reflecting stabilization or improvement in renal function, was observed in those patients whose DBP was maintained at less than 95 mm Hg. However, in African American men ($n = 463$), no such relationship between declining renal function and DBP was demonstrated. In fact, a negative reciprocal creatinine slope was noted down to a follow-up DBP of 75 mm Hg. Although the risk for renal dysfunction was highest in men with more severe hypertension (stage 3 or 4), there was also an increased risk in men with a DBP of 85 to 90 mm Hg compared with men with systolic BP (SBP) less than 120 mm Hg and a DBP less than 80 mm Hg, suggesting that the lower the BP the greater the renal protection and that the traditional target BP of 140/90 mm Hg may be too high.[6] In addition, in non-African Americans, declining renal function most closely correlated with the level of SBP. Those subjects with a follow-up SBP above 140 mm Hg had the most rapid decline in renal function, again suggesting that an SBP below the traditional 140 mm Hg may be desirable.

Tierney et al,[44] in a retrospective analysis of 6880 hypertensive patients, 72% of whom were African American and ≥60% of whom had essential hypertension (i.e., were nondiabetic), also demonstrated over an average follow-up period of 5.2 years that the strongest predictor of loss of renal function in treated hypertensive patients was the SBP. The threshold value for declining renal function in this study was an SBP of 130 to 140 mm Hg.

In another large study, Perry et al[45] monitored renal function in over 11,500 hypertensive men, with approximately 10,000 treated with antihypertensive medications and followed for a minimum of 13.9 years. An increased risk of progressive renal failure was associated with a high pretreatment SBP, with the risk of ESRD increasing progressively as the SBP increased from 165 to more than 180 mm Hg. However, reducing SBP by more than 20 mm Hg resulted in an almost two-thirds reduction in the rate of development of ESRD. There was a smaller but significant reduction in the risk for ESRD with lesser decrements in SBP.

Several smaller-scale studies, such as those of Brazy and Fitzwilliam,[46] Locatelli et al,[47] Rostand et al,[48] and Rosansky et al,[49] have demonstrated progressive renal functional deterioration in treated hypertensives in whom DBP was not reduced to less than 90 mm Hg or in whom an MAP of less than 107 mm Hg was not achieved. These data are highly suggestive that a lower MAP, a lower DBP, or both may be necessary for renal protection.[6]

Toto et al[50] prospectively studied 87 patients (68 of whom were African American) with hypertensive nephrosclerosis and randomized them into two groups to determine whether strict DBP control (65 to 80 mm Hg) compared with usual DBP control (80 to 90 mm Hg) is associated with a slower rate of decline in renal function. Over a 40-month follow-up period, the rate of loss of GFR was negligible and was similar in both groups. The level of BP control achieved was an MAP of approximately 104 mm Hg (mean DBP 87 mm Hg) in the usual control group and an MAP of 98 mm Hg (mean DBP 81 mm Hg) in the strict control group, suggesting that usual control, that is, a reduction of DBP to levels just below 90 mm Hg, is sufficient to prevent deterioration in renal function. Perhaps because of the small difference between groups (6 mm Hg) and because the lower BP group was not low enough, a difference between groups was not noted. Moreover, the strict control group started with a lower mean GFR (35 ml/min) than in the usual control group (42 ml/min), and the slope of loss of GFR was slightly better (but not significantly so) in the strict control group than in the usual control group, suggesting that strict control is more desirable.[9] The study was conducted with an ACE inhibitor as primary therapy and, as discussed later, this class of drugs may possess greater renoprotective effects than those of other classes of drugs and obviate the need to reduce BP to lower than usual levels.[6] In this as well as in the other studies cited, lower BP was not associated with an increase in cardiovascular or other adverse events.

The on-going African American Study of Kidney Disease (AASK) trial is designed to determine the optimum BP to prevent worsening renal function in African Americans with hypertensive nephrosclerosis and to determine the effects of an ACE inhibitor, calcium antagonist, or β-blocker on the progression of CRI in these subjects, independent of the level of BP.[51] Until the results of this trial are known, it appears reasonable to lower SBP to less than 135 mm Hg and DBP to less than 85 mm Hg in patients with essential hypertension and nephrosclerosis.[9]

Hypertension is a risk factor for the progression of renal disease of various etiologies.[36–41] The rate of progression of renal disease appears to correlate directly with the MAP down to the low end of the normal range.[9, 41, 49, 52] The Modification of Diet in Renal Disease (MDRD) study evaluated the benefits of aggressive reduction of BP (in addition to dietary protein restriction) in patients with a variety of primary renal diseases.[52] This large, prospective, randomized trial compared the effects of usual BP control (defined as an MAP less than 107 mm Hg in patients younger than 60 years of age and less than 113 mm Hg for those older than 60 years), with strict control (an MAP of 92 and 97 mm Hg for the two age groups, respectively).

A group of 840 patients with various levels of renal insufficiency (GFR range of 13 to 55 ml/min) were studied. Patients were preferentially treated with ACE inhibitors or calcium channel blockers (CCB), with diuretic therapy added as necessary. When the study groups were taken as a whole, aggressive control of BP added no benefit in

protecting renal function. However, only a 4.7 mm Hg MAP difference was observed between the two groups (97 vs. 92 mm Hg MAP). This difference may have been too small to detect a difference in the rate of renal functional deterioration. In addition, the less aggressively treated group's MAP was lower than the customary goal (MAP $\cong$ 107) in usual clinical practice, and these patients as a group did better than had been predicted when the study was initiated.

The patients with better renal function (GFR 25 to 55 ml/min) in the strict control group had a more rapid initial decline in renal function during the first 4 months of therapy than did the usual-care group. This decline in renal function is believed to be functional. Overall, patients in this group with a lower BP had a slower loss (29%) in renal function, as assessed by the terminal GFR slope (measured from the fourth month of follow-up visits and projected to 3 years of follow-up).[53] In fact, a study by Apperloo and coworkers[54] suggests that the initial "functional" drop in indexes of renal function with antihypertension treatment may be a marker for a long-term beneficial effect on renal function. There was no beneficial effect of the lower BP in patients with a GFR between 13 and 24 ml/min in the MDRD study.

The beneficial effect on the GFR slope in the low BP group in patients with an initial GFR of 25 to 55 ml/min was significantly correlated with the urinary protein excretion at baseline.[53] Patients with protein excretion levels of more than 3 g/day and the lower BP demonstrated a slower rate of renal functional decline than did the higher BP group after only about 1 year of follow-up. In contrast, those with lesser amounts of proteinuria (1 to 3 g/day) showed a slowing in the decline of GFR after an average follow-up of about 2 years. A longer follow-up period would have been necessary to determine whether lower BP is beneficial in patients with urinary protein excretion levels of only 0.25 to 1.00 g/day. It is important to note that, in general, this large cohort of patients had a slower rate of decline in renal function than expected, perhaps in part because of the overall excellent BP control observed in both the usual-care and the low BP groups at both levels of renal function,[9] similar to that observed by Toto and colleagues[50] in patients with hypertensive nephrosclerosis. Two types of patients with CRI did not benefit from more aggressive BP reduction in the MDRD study: those with adult polycystic kidney disease and those with chronic interstitial nephritis.

Support for the MDRD findings relative to BP control and proteinuria is provided by the Northern Italian Cooperative Study Group, which evaluated more than 400 nondiabetic patients with CRI and included a 30-month follow-up period.[47] They noted that an MAP greater than 107 mm Hg and associated with increasing levels of proteinuria predicted a worse outcome. Lowering the MAP to <107 mm Hg correlated with a diminution in proteinuria and prolonged renal survival compared with those with a higher MAP.

Several other smaller studies suggest that treatment of hypertension in nondiabetic patients with CRI slows progression of renal failure.[55–57] In 28 patients with CRI of diverse etiology and creatinine clearances ranging from 12 to 66 ml/min, Alvestrand et al[56] demonstrated a significant correlation between the decrement in MAP and a slowing of progression of CRI as well as a decrement in urinary protein excretion. In the group of patients who achieved a decrease in MAP from 109 mm Hg to 102 mm Hg, proteinuria was significantly lower, and the rate of progression of CRI was reduced by approximately 50%. In a larger study of 142 hypertensive patients with CRI and an average protein excretion of 1.8 g in 24 hours, Zucchelli and associates[58] randomized the patients into two groups; one group received captopril and the other nifedipine as the primary antihypertensive drug. BP was reduced in both groups from a mean pressure of 165/100 to a mean of 140/90. This reduction in BP reduced the rate of progression of renal failure by 47% over a 3-year period as assessed by the slope of the reciprocal of the serum creatinine. The groups were further subdivided into patients with an MAP persistently equal to or greater than 110 mm Hg and those in whom the MAP was consistently less than or equal to 100 mm Hg. In the group with the lower MAP, the rate of decline in renal function was decreased by 49%, and proteinuria decreased by 40% compared with those with an MAP greater than or equal to 110 mm Hg.

For the most part, the above studies excluded patients with diabetic nephropathy. In general, the results of studies in patients with diabetic nephropathy also suggest that renal function deteriorates more slowly with more aggressive lowering of BP and concomitant reduction of protein excretion. The beneficial effect of lower BP is continuous down to a SBP of approximately 130 mm Hg and a DBP of 70 mm Hg.[33, 59–65]

Mogensen[59] was the first to demonstrate that therapy with conventional antihypertensives, that is, a thiazide and a β-blocker with or without hydralazine, reduced the rate of deterioration in renal function from a GFR loss of 1.23 to 0.49 ml/min/mo in five insulin-dependent diabetic patients with persistent proteinuria. There was a positive correlation between the rates of fall of the GFR and the DBP as well as of urinary albumin excretion. The level of BP achieved was approximately 140/90. Walker[61] demonstrated that more aggressive BP control was important in diabetics. The longitudinal study of 131 patients with diabetes in the MRFIT demonstrated that the patients whose SBP was consistently controlled to less than 140 mm Hg had no deterioration in renal function, whereas those with a higher BP did.

Parving and coworkers[62] demonstrated that reducing BP in 11 patients with type 1 diabetic nephropathy from 143/96 to 129/84 decreased the rate of decline of renal function by almost 90% (from 0.94 to 0.10 ml/min/mo), which was also associated with a decline in albuminuria of more than 50%. β-Blockers, diuretics, and hydralazine were the only antihypertensives used during the 6-year follow-up.

In the collaborative study group of 409 patients with type 1 diabetic nephropathy, the mean systolic BP was lower in the patients who experienced remission in nephrotic-range proteinuria compared with those who did not remit.[65] When the MAP was reduced to 95 mm Hg or lower, the benefit of the lower BP was observed regardless of whether or not an ACE inhibitor was used. Specifically, the rate of doubling of serum creatinine was the same in the placebo and captopril groups when the MAP was 95 mm Hg or lower (unpublished observations). In the patients with higher MAP, the renoprotective effect of captopril was clearly demonstrated.

In a retrospective analysis, Dillon[60] demonstrated a close relationship between BP and progression of diabetic renal disease in 59 patients with both type 1 and type 2 diabetes mellitus with nephropathy and hypertension. More rapid decline in GFR, as estimated by the Cockcroft and Gault formula, was strongly correlated with higher DBP. This benefit was continuous down to a DBP of 70 mm Hg and also correlated (but less so) with SBP down to 130 mm Hg.[52] In a meta-analysis of 100 studies involving patients with diabetic nephropathy, Kasiske et al[64] noted that reduction in BP, regardless of type of antihypertensive agent used, was associated with relatively higher GFR; that is, the GFR was 3.7 ml/min higher for each 10 mm Hg decrease in MAP. In none of the studies reported were there more cardiovascular or other adverse events in patients with the lower BP.

Are There Renoprotective Antihypertensive Drugs?

ACE Inhibitors

Although patients with CRI and hypertension generally respond to the same classes of antihypertensives as do patients without renal disease, ACE inhibitors are particularly suited for use in patients with CRI and hypertension in whom the renin angiotensin system is activated.[3] It has also been suggested that this class has a specific renoprotective effect distinct from its effect on BP in its lowering of intraglomerular hydrostatic pressure (P_{GC}), which is elevated in experimental CRI and appears to contribute to the progression of renal failure.[66, 67] ACE inhibitors favorably alter intrarenal hemodynamics by preventing the formation of angiotensin II (Ang II) (and perhaps also by increasing kinin activity), thereby reversing the Ang II–induced increase in resistance at the efferent arteriole and lowering P_{GC}.

The decrease in Ang II formation accomplished by ACE inhibition may also prevent other deleterious effects of Ang II on renal function. Ang II promotes mesangial growth via enhanced release of transforming growth factor-β, matrix protein, and platelet-derived growth factor. Diminishing Ang II production by ACE inhibition may, therefore, minimize glomerular hypertrophy, which results in a smaller capillary radius (and lower P_{GC}) and may also reduce extracellular matrix and collagen production by mesangial and tubular cells, thereby reducing glomerular and tubular interstitial fibrosis.[68, 69] In addition, ACE inhibitors may directly improve the size-selective properties of the glomerulus, thereby preventing the accumulation in the mesangium of macromolecules or protein that could increase mesangial matrix production.[70]

Studies of proximal tubular and glomerular mesangial cells in culture have disclosed striking similarities between the effects of exposure to a high glucose medium and to Ang II on the growth properties of these cells. Both glucose and Ang II appear to increase growth and promote cytokine production. There may also be an additive effect of Ang II and high glucose on activation of protein kinase C and transforming growth factor-β that can promote hypertrophic and profibrotic effects in the mesangium and interstitium.[71] Thus, by favorably altering hemodynamics and diminishing cellular hypertrophy and fibrosis, ACE inhibition may be particularly protective in patients with diabetic nephropathy or with nondiabetic CRI.

Zucchelli et al[58] evaluated the effects of an ACE inhibitor (captopril) and of a slow-release dihydropyridine CCB, nifedipine, in 121 patients with nondiabetic CRI. The numbers of patients reaching ESRD at the end of a 2-year follow-up were similar in both groups. During the third year of treatment, however, the group treated with an ACE inhibitor had significantly fewer patients reaching ESRD compared with the CCB group, even though BP values were similar in both groups. At the end of 3 years, 11 of the 46 patients remaining in the CCB group and only 2 of the 44 patients remaining in the ACE inhibitor group reached ESRD ($p < .005$), indicating an advantage of long-term ACE inhibitor therapy in preserving renal function.

At the end of a 15-month follow-up, Hannedouche et al[72] demonstrated a renoprotective effect of ACE inhibition versus β-blockade in a group of 100 patients with varying levels of renal dysfunction and a variety of renal diseases. Of the group that took the ACE inhibitor (enalapril), 19% reached ESRD, compared with 35% of the group that took a β-blocker, despite similar BP controls in both groups (approximately 150/90).

A benefit of ACE inhibition was demonstrated by Maschio et al[34] in the Angiotensin-Converting Enzyme Inhibition in Progressive Renal Insufficiency (AIPRI) study in 583 patients with CRI. Three hundred patients were treated with benazepril, an ACE inhibitor, and the remainder with placebo plus other antihypertensive medications (including CCBs but excluding ARBs). The authors found the following: the ACE inhibitor–treated group had a greater reduction in DBP than did the placebo group—a reduction of 3.5 to 5.0 mm Hg vs. an increase of 0.2 to 1.5 mm Hg. Progression to a primary endpoint (a doubling of the serum creatinine or progression to ESRD) occurred in only 31 (10%) of 300 patients treated with ACE inhibitors vs. 57 (20%) of 283 in the placebo group. The overall risk reduction for these endpoints was 53%, with a 71% reduction in those who began with a creatinine clearance above 45 ml/min, and a lesser benefit (46%) in those with a baseline creatinine clearance of less than 45 ml/min. The greatest protection was observed in those with chronic glomerular diseases, including diabetic nephropathy. The greatest risk reduction occurred in patients with baseline 24-hour urinary protein excretion rates greater than 1 g. The decrease in urinary protein excretion was greater in the benazepril-treated group than in the placebo group. No conclusions regarding hypertensive nephrosclerosis patients could be drawn because too few such patients were studied. The protective effect of the ACE inhibitor remained after an adjustment was made for a slightly lower BP in the ACE inhibitor–treated group.

The Gruppo Italiano di Studi Epidemiologici in Nefrologia (GISEN)[73] similarly studied the effect of an ACE inhibitor (ramipril) vs. placebo in patients with nondiabetic chronic renal disease. The degree of BP control was the same in both groups (144.6/88.2 mm Hg in the ramipril group, compared with 144.6/88.9 in the placebo group). Again, only ARBs were excluded as additional antihypertensive drugs. The patients were divided into two strata according to baseline proteinuria: stratum 1: 1 to 3 g/24 hr; stratum 2: ≥ 3 g/24 hr. The trial was terminated early in the group with heavier proteinuria because of the significant benefit provided by ACE inhibition, which dramatically reduced the rate of decline of renal function compared with placebo (0.53 vs. 0.88 ml/min/mo, respectively). Ramipril halved the incidence of the predetermined endpoint of the study, the combined risk of doubling the serum creatinine and ESRD.

The Ramipril Efficacy in Nephropathy (REIN) trial also demonstrated that patients with baseline urinary protein excretion of less than 3.0 g/24 hr had slow rates of renal deterioration, whereas those with baseline urinary protein excretion of more than 3.0 g/24 hr had more rapid declines in renal function.[73, 74] Ramipril-induced early reduction in 24-hour urinary protein excretion correlated with the long-term effect on GFR decline and was the only covariate that predicted the drug's renoprotective effect. This reduction in decline of renal function was greatest in patients with the highest degree of baseline proteinuria and was not dependent on the initial degree of renal impairment or baseline or follow-up BP control, which was similar in both groups. Because the renoprotective actions of ramipril were not explained by its effect on systemic BP, an additional renoprotective mechanism was clearly implied.[73]

In the AIPRI study there was no decrease in the number of patients who progressed to ESRD on ACE-inhibitor treatment, whereas the percent of patients receiving the ACE inhibitor who progressed to ESRD was decreased in the REIN trial. However, in the AIPRI study, few patients, particularly those without clinical proteinuria, showed progression to ESRD.[34, 73] In the REIN trial, the overall mortality rates and the numbers of serious nonfatal cardiovascular events were similar in the two study groups. Moreover, there were fewer cardiac deaths in both treatment groups than previously reported in a similar patient population.[72] Patients in the AIPRI trial also had a lower mortality rate than in patients in previous studies, but there was a significantly higher short-term absolute death rate in the ACE inhibitor–treated group. This apparent imbalance in mortality between the two groups was not seen in the long-term AIPRI extension study.[75] In addition, at 6 years, many patients from the original treatment groups (64% for benazepril and 61% for placebo) had begun receiving the ACE inhibitor, suggesting that long-term use of an ACE inhibitor did not increase mortality.

At the end of the initial REIN trial, the core study patients who were originally on ramipril were continued on the drug, and those initially on placebo were switched to ramipril.[76] The follow-up study was designed to determine if late therapy with ramipril would slow deterioration in renal function and if longer-term therapy in those on the drug in the initial trial would continue to be beneficial. Of the initial 166 randomized patients, 97 participated in the extension trial; 51 continued on ramipril, and 46 were switched to ramipril. Continued ramipril treatment slowed the rate of GFR decline and limited progression to ESRD even more than had been observed during the original study. This suggests that the earlier ACE inhibitor treatment is started, the more renoprotection may be seen. At the end of the follow-up study (4.5 years), the patients initially randomized to ramipril had a renal survival rate three times better than the rate for those who were originally randomized to placebo and then were switched to ramipril. The original study had shown that ramipril was significantly better than placebo only for the combined endpoints (doubling of baseline serum creatinine and ESRD), but in the follow-up study the incidence of ESRD alone was significantly reduced. It is important to note that the patients who were switched to ramipril also had a significant reduction in the rate of decline in GFR (from 0.81 in the initial study to 0.14 ml/min/mo in the follow-up study), even though ACE-inhibitor treatment was started late—that is, when their GFRs were approximately 30 ml/min.

In a meta-analysis that excluded the REIN trials, Giatras et al[35] reported that ACE inhibitors are more effective than other antihypertensive agents in reducing the development of ESRD in nondiabetic renal disease, but they do not decrease mortality. It could not be determined from the analysis whether this renoprotective effect is due to the greater decline in BP associated with ACE inhibition or is caused by other effects. The REIN trials appear to establish that renoprotective mechanisms other than BP lowering may contribute to the beneficial effects of ACE inhibition. These beneficial effects might not extend to patients with the DD genotype for the ACE gene.[77, 78] Patients with DD polymorphism of the ACE gene appear to be more likely to have progressive renal disease whether or not they have an antiproteinuric response to ACE inhibitors.

In the meta-analysis of 100 studies of both type 1 and type 2 patients with diabetic nephropathy referred to earlier,[64] a reduction in BP per se was associated with relative protection of renal function. However, compared with other agents, ACE inhibitors had an additional favorable effect on GFR that was independent of BP.

Subsequent studies have also suggested that ACE inhibitors have a specific renoprotective effect in diabetic nephropathy.[33, 79–81] Of these, the prospective, randomized, double-blind collaborative study of 409 patients with type 1 diabetic nephropathy with mild to moderate renal insufficiency is the most impressive and has firmly established that ACE inhibition significantly reduces the rate of doubling of serum creatinine at usual levels of BP control.[33] Other studies suggest that the early use of ACE inhibition in incipient diabetic nephropathy (microalbuminuria) without hypertension reduces the rate of appearance of overt nephropathy (macroalbuminuria).[55, 82–85]

On the basis of the available data, an ACE inhibitor should be administered in both incipient and overt diabetic nephropathy (with or without hypertension). An ACE inhibitor is also the drug of choice for patients with other forms of chronic renal disease and hypertension. In nondiabetic patients without hypertension but with significant proteinuria, it may be prudent to administer an ACE inhibitor to decrease the degree of proteinuria. However, further studies delineating the possible nephrotoxic effects of proteinuria are necessary before a firm recommendation can be made.

Angiotensin II Receptor Blockers

ARBs are a new class of drugs that block the renin-angiotensin system at a site different from the site blocked by ACE inhibitors, and they may offer substantial promise as renoprotective drugs.[6, 86–88] These drugs selectively block the binding of Ang II to the type 1 angiotensin (AT_1)

receptor on the cell membrane.[89] The AT_1 subtype mediates the vasoconstrictor effect of Ang II, as well as Ang II–induced growth in the left ventricle and arterial wall. ARBs may, therefore, provide a renoprotective effect similar to that observed with ACE inhibitors. However, the two classes of drugs differ in several respects. Inhibition of Ang II formation by an ACE inhibitor diminishes activation of all subtypes of Ang II receptors. In contrast, ARBs block only the AT_1 receptor. ACE inhibitors, but not ARBs, also inhibit kinin inactivation, and potentiation of bradykinin may contribute to some of the beneficial effects of ACE inhibition. It is therefore unclear at present if ARBs will have the same benefits as conferred by ACE inhibitors in CRI.

There are, however, promising observations regarding a possible role for ARBs as renoprotective drugs. One study found that an ARB was as effective as an ACE inhibitor in reducing protein excretion in patients with chronic renal disease.[90] In this short-term trial, 11 patients with nondiabetic proteinuria and hypertension were studied for 7 months while receiving placebo or a high or low dose of losartan or enalapril. On both doses of losartan and enalapril, proteinuria and BP decreased and renal function remained unchanged. The values for percent decrease in urinary protein excretion were similar, 50%, with the high dose of either losartan (100 mg) or enalapril (20 mg). The antiproteinuric effect of ARBs has also been demonstrated in animal models, although some studies show that the antiproteinuric effect seen with ARBs is not as great as that seen with ACE inhibitors.[87, 91–94]

Because ACE inhibitors and ARBs act through different mechanisms, it is intriguing to consider whether the combination of the two classes of drugs will have an additive effect on urinary protein excretion and renal function in patients with CRI.[94, 95] A preliminary report by Russo et al[96] suggests that the combination of the two classes diminishes protein excretion more than either alone.

Calcium Channel Blockers

There is experimental evidence that CCBs have class-specific actions that may help slow the progression of CRI. However, the data have not been consistent,[97–103] in part because all CCBs do not dilate the efferent arteriole, because there was lack of equivalence of BP control in the studies, and because more than one mechanism may be operative in the renoprotection provided by CCBs.[99, 102, 103] Nifedipine, for example, may protect the glomerulus by reducing hypertrophy, thus diminishing stress on the glomerular capillary wall without lowering intraglomerular hydrostatic pressure.[103] Other mechanisms suggested include modulation of mesangial traffic of macromolecules, reduction in metabolic activity of remnant kidneys and in free radical formation, and amelioration of uremic nephrocalcinosis.[102]

Verapamil and diltiazem consistently lower urinary protein excretion, at least in diabetic nephropathy.[104] Bakris and colleagues[105] studied 34 African Americans with type 2 diabetes, renal insufficiency, and proteinuria who were randomized to therapy with either verapamil or atenolol. Goal BP was 140/90, with additional antihypertensive agents (excluding ACE inhibitors and ARBs) added as necessary to control BP. After a mean follow-up of

54 ± 6 months, the CCB group had a slower rate of decline in creatinine clearance and a greater reduction in proteinuria than in the atenolol group. In addition, a greater proportion of the atenolol group had a 50% or more increase in serum creatinine compared with the CCB group. The results were not explained by differences in BP control between the two groups.

Vellusi and coworkers[106] compared the effects of an ACE inhibitor (cilazapril) with those of a dihydropyridine CCB (amlodipine) on GFR and albumin excretion in 44 hypertensive type 2 diabetics, 26 of whom were normoalbuminuric and 18 microalbuminuric. After 3 years of follow-up, the GFR decline and albumin excretion in both groups were the same, regardless of whether the patients received CCBs or ACE inhibitors. These results are similar to those of Zucchelli and associates[58] in nondiabetic patients with CRI during the first 2 years of follow-up.

In a recent interim report, Rossing and colleagues[107] demonstrated a striking dissociation between antiproteinuric effects and effects on GFR in 49 patients with hypertension and type 1 diabetes receiving either a dihydropyridine CCB (nisoldipine) or an ACE inhibitor (lisinopril) after a 1-year follow-up. Albuminuria decreased by 47% in the lisinopril group as opposed to no decrement in the nisoldipine group. However, the CCB-treated group had a slower decline in GFR, suggesting that the protective mechanism of the dihydropyridine was independent of microcirculatory effects. In a similar trial, Janssen and coworkers[108] recently found that, in 21 patients with nondiabetic CRI studied for only 16 weeks, amlodipine did not affect protein excretion or GFR, whereas lisinopril lowered GFR despite its antiproteinuric effect.

Theoretical considerations suggest that ACE inhibitors and CCBs should work in concert and should protect renal function more effectively when given together than when either class is given alone.[102] Several animal studies have supported this concept.[101, 109–111] To date only two trials have examined the efficacy of this combination in protecting renal function in humans.[112, 113] Both were conducted in diabetic patients, and both demonstrated an additive effect for an ACE inhibitor combined with a CCB (verapamil) in reducing proteinuria and slowing the decline in renal function.

In summary, treatment of hypertension in patients with renal insufficiency is indicated at any stage of the disease. It would appear that the goal BP should be an MAP of 90 to 95 mm Hg and that an ACE inhibitor is the drug of choice. Treatment should be started early. Diuretics are probably the second-line choice of drugs. A CCB (preferably diltiazem or verapamil) should be added to achieve goal blood pressure, but a dihydropyridine CCB may be necessary. Additional antihypertensive agents should be added as necessary. The role of ARBs has not been well defined, but these agents may be as useful as ACE inhibitors or, possibly, may even be useful additions to regimens with ACE inhibitors.

OTHER FACTORS THAT MAY ALTER THE PROGRESSION OF CHRONIC RENAL INSUFFICIENCY

Dietary Protein Excretion

Protein restriction has been shown in animals to decrease intraglomerular pressure mainly through afferent arteriolar vasoconstriction.[114] In a recent meta-analysis of several published studies, Pedrini and associates[115] have determined that protein restriction slows the progression of renal failure in both diabetic and nondiabetic patients with CRI. The recommended approach is to reduce protein intake to approximately 0.8 mg/kg/day for patients with GFRs greater than 25 ml/min/1.73 m². Compliance with therapy can be determined by a 24-hour urine collection using the following formula:[116]

Estimated protein intake (g/day) =
urea nitrogen intake (g/day) × 6.25

Nonsteroidal Anti-Inflammatory Drugs

Nonsteroidal anti-inflammatory drugs (NSAIDs) lower urinary protein levels via afferent vasoconstriction and a subsequent decrease in GFR as well as by having a direct effect on the permeability of the glomerular barrier.[117] Insofar as decreasing the degree of proteinuria is beneficial per se, as is suggested by some studies,[73–76] NSAIDs may be used as an addition to ACE inhibitors or ARBs. Their potential benefit for patients with CRI may be limited, however, by their adverse side effects (e.g., gastrointestinal bleeding, acute renal failure, and hyperkalemia).

Treatment of Dyslipidemia

Experimental and clinical evidence in both diabetic and nondiabetic patients suggests that abnormal lipid metabolism, a relatively common finding in patients with CRI, may be an independent risk factor in the pathogenesis and progression of renal disease.[119, 120] Changes in glomerular permeability increase the filtration of lipoproteins. The accumulation of lipoproteins in the mesangial cells may stimulate them to proliferate and produce excess basement membrane material.[121] Hyperlipidemia may also increase platelet aggregation, with subsequent release of a platelet growth factor capable of binding to receptors on the mesangial cells and inducing cellular proliferation.[122] The use of 3-hydroxy-3-methylglutaryl coenzyme A (HMG CoA) reductase inhibitors in a small number of diabetic and nondiabetic subjects has been associated with a reduction in the rate of decline in renal function.[123–125] The possible beneficial effect of lipid-lowering therapy on renal function remains to be confirmed in larger randomized trials.[126] However, given the currently available data concerning the cardiovascular benefits of treating lipid disorders in the general population, as well as the possible beneficial effect of the HMG CoA reductase inhibitors on mesangial cellularity and proximal tubular cell proliferation, independent of their cholesterol-lowering properties,[119] patients with CRI should be screened and treated aggressively with these agents.

Heparin

Heparin has been shown both in vitro and in vivo to mitigate proteinuria, renal insufficiency, and hypertension in experimental glomerulonephritis and the renal ablation model.[127–129] The mechanisms of these effects are not known but do not depend on either the anticoagulant properties of heparin or its action on intraglomerular hemodynamics.[128, 129] Preliminary evidence suggests that heparin binds to transforming growth factor-β, which is known to stimulate mesangial cell growth and fibronectin production.[130] Such binding could modulate the activity of transforming growth factor-β, resulting in both decreased mesangial matrix synthesis and increased degradation.[131] Increased mesangial matrix production is known to contribute to the progression of renal disease.[132] A role for the currently available oral heparinoid in the progression of chronic renal disease is yet to be determined.

References

1. Vertes V, Cangiano JL, Berman LB, Gould A. Hypertension in end-stage renal disease. N Engl J Med 280:978–981, 1969.
2. Buckalew VM Jr, Berg RL, Want SR, et al. Prevalence of hypertension in 1,795 subjects with chronic renal disease: The Modification of Diet in Renal Disease Study baseline cohort. Am J Kidney Dis 28:811–821, 1996.
3. Spitalewitz S, Porush JG. Hypertension primer. *In* Izzo Jr, Black HR (eds). Treatment of Hypertensive Patients with Chronic Renal Insufficiency. Dallas, American Heart Association, 1994; pp 354–357.
4. MacMahon S, Peto R, Cutler J, et al. Blood pressure, stroke and coronary heart disease. Part 1: Prolonged differences in blood pressure: Prospective observational studies corrected for the regression dilution bias. Lancet 335:765–774, 1990.
5. SHEP Cooperative Research Group: Prevention of stroke by antihypertensive drug treatment in older patients with isolated systolic hypertension. JAMA 265:3255–3264, 1991.
6. Weir MR, Dworkin LD. Antihypertensive drugs, dietary salt, and renal protection: How low should you go and with which therapy? Am J Kidney Dis 32:1–22, 1998.
7. National High Blood Pressure Education Program Group: 1995 update of the Working Group reports on chronic renal failure and renovascular hypertension. Arch Intern Med 156:1938–1947, 1996.
8. U.S. Renal Data System. USRDS 1994 Annual Data Report. Bethesda, MD, National Institutes of Health, National Institute of Diabetes and Digestive and Kidney Diseases, 1994.
9. Porush JG. Hypertension and chronic renal failure: The use of ACE inhibitors. Am J Kidney Dis 31:177–184, 1998.
10. Schiffl H, Kuchle C, Lang S. Dietary salt, intracellular ion homeostasis and hypertension secondary to early-stage kidney disease. Miner Electrolyte Metab 22:178–181, 1996.
11. Cotone S, Panepinto N, Vadala A, et al. Sympathetic overactivity and 24-hour blood pressure pattern in hypertensives with chronic renal failure. Ren Fail 17:751–758, 1995.
12. Schohn D, Weidmann P, Jahn H, Baretta-Piccoli C. Norepinephrine-related mechanism in hypertension accompanying renal failure. Kidney Int 28:814–822, 1985.
13. Sinclair AM, Isles CG, Brown I, et al. Secondary hypertension in a blood pressure clinic. Arch Intern Med 147:1289–1293, 1987.
14. Jensen LW, Pedersen EB. Nocturnal blood pressure and relation to vasoactive hormones and renal function in hypertension and chronic renal failure. Blood Press 6:332–342, 1997.
15. Preston RA, Singer I, Epstein M. Renal parenchymal hypertension: Current concepts of pathogenesis and management. Arch Intern Med 156:602–611, 1996.
16. Goldsmith DJA, Covic AA, Venning MC, Ackrill P. Blood pressure reduction after parathyroidectomy for secondary hyperparathyroidism: Further evidence implicating calcium homeostasis in blood pressure regulation. Am J Kidney Dis 27:819–825, 1996.
17. Ni Z, Wang XQ, Vaziri ND. Nitric oxide metabolism in erythropoietin-induced hypertension: Effect of calcium channel blockade. Hypertension 32:724–729, 1998.
18. Flack JM, Ensrud KE, Mascioli S, et al. Racial and ethnic modifiers of the salt–blood pressure response. Hypertension 17(suppl I):115–121, 1991.
19. Bakris GL, Weir MR. Salt intake and reductions in the arterial pressure and proteinuria. Am J Hypertens 9:200S–206S, 1996.
20. Benstein JA, Parker M, Feiner HD, Dworkin LD. Superiority of salt restriction over diuretics in reducing renal hypertrophy and injury in uninephrectomized SHR. Am J Physiol 258:F1675–1681, 1990.
21. Lax DS, Benstein JA, Tolbert E, Dworkin LD. Effects of salt restriction on renal growth and glomerular injury in rats with remnant kidneys. Kidney Int 41:1527–1534, 1992.
22. Dworkin LD, Benstein JA, Tolbert E, Feiner HD. Salt restriction inhibits renal growth and stabilizes injury in rats with established renal disease. J Am Soc Nephrol 7:437–442, 1996.
23. Heeg JE, de Jong PE, van der Hem GK, de Zeeuw D. Efficacy and variability of the antiproteinuric effect of ACE inhibition by lisinopril. Kidney Int 36:272–280, 1989.
24. Bakris GL, Smith AC. Effects of sodium intake on albumin excretion in patients with diabetic nephropathy treated with long-acting calcium antagonists. Ann Intern Med 125:201–204, 1996.
25. Cianciaruso B, Bellizzi V, Minutolo R, et al. Salt intake and renal outcome in patients with progressive renal disease. Miner Electrolyte Metab 24:296–301, 1998.
26. Suki WN. Use of diuretics in chronic renal failure. Kidney Int 51(suppl 59):S33–S35, 1997.
27. Fliser D, Schroter M, Neubeck M, Ritz E. Coadministration of thiazides increases the efficacy of loop diuretics even in patients with advanced renal failure. Kidney Int 46:482–488, 1994.
28. Oates J. Antihypertensive agents and the drug therapy of hypertension. *In* Handman JG, Gilman AG, Limbird LE (eds). Goodman & Gilman's The Pharmacological Basis of Therapeutics, 9th ed. New York, McGraw-Hill, 1995; 780–808.
29. Joint National Committee. The Sixth Report of the Joint National Committee on Detection, Evaluation and Treatment of High Blood Pressure. Arch Intern Med 157:2413–2446, 1997.
30. Reiser IW, Pallan TM, Spitalewitz S. How to treat renovascular hypertension: Medical therapy versus revascularization. J Crit Illness 13:409–424, 1998.
31. Lazarus JM, Bourgoinge JJ, Buckalew VM, et al for the Modification of Diet in Renal Disease Study Group. Achievement and safety of a low blood pressure goal in chronic renal disease: The Modification of Diet in Renal Disease Study Group. Hypertension 29:641–650, 1997.
32. Klag MJ, Whelton PK, Randall BL, et al. End-stage renal disease in African-American and white men: 16-year MRFIT findings. JAMA 277:1293–1298, 1997.
33. Lewis EJ, Hunsicker LG, Bain RP, Rohde RD for the Collaborative Study Group. The effect of angiotensin-converting-enzyme inhibition on diabetic nephropathy. N Engl J Med 329:1456–1462, 1993.
34. Maschio G, Alberti D, Janin G, et al for the Angiotensin-Converting Enzyme Inhibition in Progressive Renal Insufficiency Study Group. Effect of the angiotensin-converting enzyme inhibitor benazepril on the progression of chronic renal insufficiency. N Engl J Med 334:939–945, 1996.
35. Giatras I, Lau J, Levey AS for the Angiotensin-Converting Enzyme Inhibition and Progressive Renal Disease Study Group. Effect of angiotensin-converting enzyme inhibitors on the progression of non-diabetic renal disease: A meta-analysis of randomized trials. Ann Intern Med 127:337–345, 1997.
36. Epstein M, Sowers JR. Diabetes mellitus and hypertension. Hypertension 19:403–418, 1992.
37. Chavers BM, Bilons RW, Ellis EN, et al. Glomerular lesions and urinary albumin excretion in type I diabetes without overt proteinuria. N Engl J Med 320:966–970, 1989.
38. Christensen CK. Abnormal albumin and blood pressure rise in incipient diabetic nephropathy induced by exercise. Kidney Int 25:819–823, 1984.
39. Baldwin DS, Neugarten J. Blood pressure control and progression of renal insufficiency. *In* Brenner BM, Stein JH (eds). Contemporary Issues in Nephrology. New York, Churchill Livingstone, 1986; pp 81–110.
40. Bergstrom J, Alverstrand A, Bucht H, Guitierrez A. Stockholm clinical study on progression of chronic renal failure: An interim report. Kidney Int 27:110–114, 1989.
41. Brazy PC, Stead WW, Fitzwilliam JF. Progression of renal insufficiency: Role of blood pressure. Kidney Int 35:670–674, 1989.
42. Schulman NB, Ford CE, Hall WD, et al. Prognostic value of serum creatinine and effect of treatment of hypertension on renal function:

Results from the Hypertension Detection and Follow-up Program. The Hypertension Detection and Follow-up Program Cooperative Group. Hypertension 13(suppl 1):80–93, 1989.

43. Walker GW, Neaton JD, Cutler JA et al. for the MRFIT Research Group. Renal function change in hypertensive members of the Multiple Risk Factor Intervention Trial: Racial and treatment effects. JAMA 268:3085–3091, 1992.

44. Tierney WM, McDonald CJ, Luft FC. Renal disease in hypertensive adults: Effect of race and type II diabetes mellitus. Am J Kidney Dis 13:485–493, 1989.

45. Perry HM, Miller JP, Formoff JR, et al. Early predictors of 15-year end-stage renal disease in hypertensive patients. Hypertension 25:587–594, 1995.

46. Brazy PC, Fitzwilliam JF. Progressive renal disease. Role of race and antihypertensive medications. Kidney Int 37:1113–1119, 1990.

47. Locatelli F, Marcelli D, Comelli M, et al for the Northern Italian Cooperative Study Group. Proteinuria and blood pressure as causal components of progression to end-stage renal failure. Nephrol Dial Transplant 11:461–467, 1996.

48. Rostand SG, Brown G, Kirk KA, et al. Renal insufficiency in treated essential hypertension. N Engl J Med 320:684–688, 1989.

49. Rosansky SJ, Hoover DR, King L, Gibson J. The association of blood pressure levels and change in renal function in hypertensive and non-hypertensive subjects. Arch Intern Med 150:2073–2076, 1990.

50. Toto RD, Mitchell HC, Smith RD, et al. "Strict" blood pressure control and progression of renal disease in hypertensive nephrosclerosis. Kidney Int 48:851–859, 1995.

51. Wright JT, Kusek JW, Toto RD, et al. Design and baseline characteristics of participants in the African-American Study of Kidney Disease and Hypertension (AASK) pilot study. Control Clin Trials 17(suppl 4):3S–16S, 1996.

52. Klahr S, Levey AS, Beck GJ, et al. The effects of dietary protein restriction and blood-pressure control on the progression of chronic renal disease. Modification of Diet in Renal Disease Study Group. N Engl J Med 330:877–884, 1994.

53. Klahr S. Role of dietary protein and blood pressure in the progression of renal disease. Kidney Int 49:1783–1786, 1996.

54. Apperloo AJ, de Zeeuw D, de Jong PE. A short-term antihypertensive treatment-induced fall in glomerular filtration rate predicts long-term stability of renal function. Kidney Int 51:793–797, 1997.

55. Wight JP, Brown CB, el Nahas AM. Effect of control of hypertension on progressive renal failure. Clin Nephrol 39:305–311, 1993.

56. Alvestrand A, Gutierrez A, Bucht H, Bergstrom J. Reduction in blood pressure retards the progression of chronic renal failure in man. Nephrol Dial Transplant 3:624–631, 1988.

57. Bergstrom J, Alvestrand A, Bucht H, Gutierrez A. Progression of chronic renal failure in man is retarded with more frequent clinical follow-ups and better blood pressure control. Clin Nephrol 25:1–6, 1986.

58. Zucchelli P, Zuccalà A, Borghi M, et al. Long-term comparison between captopril and nifedipine in the progression of renal insufficiency. Kidney Int 42:452–458, 1992.

59. Mogensen CE. Progression of nephropathy in long-term diabetics with proteinuria and effect of initial antihypertensive treatment. Scand J Clin Lab Invest 36:383–388, 1976.

60. Dillon JJ. The quantitative relationship between treated blood pressure and progression of diabetic renal disease. Am J Kidney Dis 22:798–802, 1993.

61. Walker WG. Hypertension-related renal injury: A major contributor to end-stage renal disease. Am J Kidney Dis 22:164–173, 1993.

62. Parving H-H, Smidt UM, Hommel E, et al. Effective antihypertensive treatment postpones renal insufficiency in diabetic nephropathy. Am J Kidney Dis 22:188–195, 1993.

63. Mathiesen ER, Hommel E, Giese J, Parving H-H. Efficacy of captopril in postponing nephropathy in nomotensive insulin-dependent diabetic patients with microalbuminuria. BMJ 303:81–87, 1991.

64. Kasiske BL, Kalil RSN, Ma JZ, et al. Effects of antihypertensive therapy on the kidney in patients with diabetes: A meta-regression analysis. Ann Intern Med 118:129–138, 1993.

65. Hebert LA, Bain RP, Verne D, et al. for the Collaborative Study Group. Remission of nephrotic range proteinuria in type I diabetes. Kidney Int 46:1688–1693, 1994.

66. Anderson S, Rennke HG, Brenner BM. Therapeutic advantage of converting enzyme inhibitors in arresting progressive renal disease associated with systemic hypertension in the rat. J Clin Invest 77:1993–2000, 1986.

67. Keane WF, Anderson S, Aurell M, et al. Angiotensin converting enzyme inhibitors and progressive renal insufficiency: Current experience and future directions. Ann Intern Med 111:503–516, 1989.

68. Wolf G, Neilson EG. Angiotensin II is a renal growth factor. J Am Soc Nephrol 3:1531–1540, 1993.

69. Border WA, Noble NA. Interactions of transforming growth factor-β and angiotensin II in renal fibrosis. Hypertension 31:181–188, 1998.

70. Remuzzi A, Puntorieri S, Battaglia C, et al. Angiotensin-converting enzyme inhibition ameliorates glomerular filtration of macromolecules and water and lessens glomerular injury in the rat. J Clin Invest 85:541–549, 1990.

71. Wolf G, Ziyadeh FN. The role of antiogensin II in diabetic nephropathy: Emphasis on nonhemodynamic mechanisms. Am J Kidney Dis 29:153–163, 1997.

72. Hannedouche T, Landais P, Goldfarb B, et al. Randomized controlled trial of enalapril and β-blockers in non-diabetic chronic renal failure. BMJ 309:833–837, 1994.

73. Gruppo Italiano di Studi Epidemiologici in Nefrologia. Randomized placebo-controlled trial of effect of ramipril on decline in glomerular filtration rate and risk of terminal renal failure in proteinuric, non-diabetic nephropathy. Lancet 349:1857–1863, 1997.

74. Ruggenenti P, Perna A, Mosconi L, et al on behalf of Gruppo Italiano di Studi Epidemiologici in Nefrologia (GISEN). Proteinuria predicts end-stage renal failure in non-diabetic chronic nephropathies. Kidney Int 52(suppl 63):S54–S57, 1997.

75. Locattelli, F, Carbarns IRI, Maschio G, et al and the Angiotensin-Converting-Enzyme Inhibition in Progressive Renal Insufficiency Study Group. Long-term progression of chronic renal insufficiency in the AIPRI Extension Study. Kidney Int 52(suppl 63):S63–S66, 1997.

76. Ruggenenti P, Perna A, Gherardi G, et al on behalf of Gruppo Italiano di Studi Epidemiologici in Nefrologia (GISEN). Renal function and requirement for dialysis in chronic nephropathy patients on long-term ramipril: REIN follow-up trial. Lancet 352:1252–1256, 1998.

77. van Essen GG, Rensma PL, de Zeeuw D, et al. Association between angiotensin-converting-enzyme gene polymorphism and failure of renoprotective therapy. Lancet 347:94–95, 1996.

78. Parving H-H, Jacobsen P, Tarnow L, et al. Effect of deletion polymorphism of the angiotensin-converting enzyme gene on progression of diabetic nephropathy during inhibition of angiotensin-converting enzyme: Observational follow-up study. BMJ 313:591–594, 1996.

79. Nielsen FS, Rossing P, Gall MA, et al. Impact of lisinopril and atenolol on kidney function in hypertensive NIDDM subjects with diabetic nephropathy. Diabetes 43:1108–1113, 1994.

80. Lacourcière Y, Nadeau A, Poirier L, Tancréde G. Captopril or conventional therapy in hypertensive type II diabetics: Three-year analysis. Hypertension 21:786–794, 1993.

81. Liou H-H, Huang T-P, Campese VM. Effect of long-term therapy with captopril on proteinuria and renal function in patients with non-insulin dependent diabetes and with non-diabetic renal disease. Nephron 69:41–48, 1995.

82. Dongall ML, Moore WV. Effect of angiotensin-converting enzyme inhibition on renal function and albuminuria in normotensive type I diabetic patients. Diabetes 41:62–67, 1992.

83. Ravid M, Savin H, Jutrin I, et al. Long-term stabilization effect of angiotensin-converting enzyme inhibitor on plasma creatinine and on proteinuria in normotensive type II diabetic patients. Ann Intern Med 118:577–581.

84. Romero R, Salinas I, Lucas A, et al. Renal function changes in microalbuminuric normotensive type II diabetic patients treated with angiotensin-converting enzyme inhibitors. Diabetes Care 16:597–600, 1993.

85. Viberti G, Mogensen CE, Groop LC, et al. Effect of captopril on progression to clinical proteinuria in patients with insulin-dependent diabetes mellitus and microalbuminuria. JAMA 271:275–279, 1994.

86. Weir MR. Angiotensin-II receptor antagonists: A new class of antihypertensive agents. Am Fam Physician 53:589–594, 1996.

87. Gansevoort RT, de Zeeuw D, Shahinfar S, et al. Effects of the angiotensin II antagonist losartan in hypertensive patients with renal disease. J Hypertens 12(suppl 2):S37–S42, 1994.

88. Ichikawa I. Will angiotensin II receptor antagonists be renoprotective in humans? Kidney Int 50:684–692, 1996.

89. Goodfriend TL, Elliot ME, Catt KJ. Angiotensin receptors and their antagonists. N Engl J Med 334:1649–1654, 1996.

90. Gansevoort RT, de Zeeuw D, de Jong PE. Is the antiproteinuric effect of ACE inhibition mediated by interference in the renin-angiotensin system? Kidney Int 45:861–867, 1994.

91. Lafayette RA, Mayer G, Park SK, Meyer TW. Angiotensin II receptor blockade limits glomerular injury in rate with reduced renal mass. J Clin Invest 90:766–771, 1992.

92. Kakinuma Y, Kawamura T, Bills T, et al. Blood pressure–independent effect of angiotensin inhibition on vascular lesions of chronic renal failure. Kidney Int 42:46–55, 1992.

93. Zoja C, Donadelli R, Corna D, et al. The renoprotective properties of angiotensin-converting enzyme inhibitors in a chronic model of membranous nephropathy are solely due to the inhibition of angiotensin II: Evidence based on comparative studies with a receptor antagonist. Am J Kidney Dis 29:254–264, 1997.

94. Hutchison FN, Cui X, Webster SK. The antiproteinuric action of angiotensin-converting enzyme is dependent on kinin. J Am Soc Nephrol 6:1216–1222, 1995.

95. Schmitt F, Natov S, Martinez F, et al. Renal effects of angiotensin II-receptor blockade and angiotensin convertase inhibition in man. Clin Sci 90:205–213, 1996.

96. Russo D, Pisani A, De Nicola L, et al. Additive antiproteinuric effect of converting enzyme inhibitor and losartan in normotensive patients with IgA nephropathy. [Abstract A0503] J Am Soc Nephrol 9:15P, 1998.

97. Dworkin LD, Feiner HD, Parker M, Tolbert E. Effects of nifedipine and enalapril on glomerular structure and function in uninephrectomized spontaneously hypertensive rats. Kidney Int 39:1112–1117, 1991.

98. Harris DCH, Hammond WS, Burke TJ, Schrier RW. Verapamil protects against progression of experimental chronic renal failure. Kidney Int 31:41–46, 1987.

99. Saruta T, Kanno Y, Hayashi K, Konishi K. Antihypertensive agents and renal protection: Calcium channel blockers. Kidney Int 49(suppl 55):S52–S56, 1996.

100. Bakris GL. The effects of calcium antagonists on renal hemodynamics, urinary protein excretion, and glomerular morphology in diabetic states. J Am Soc Nephrol 2(suppl 1):S21–S29, 1991.

101. Griffin KA, Picken MM, Bidani AK. Deleterious effects of calcium channel blockade on pressure transmission and glomerular injury in rat remnant kidney. J Clin Invest 96:793–800, 1995.

102. Epstein M. Calcium antagonists and the progression of chronic renal failure. Curr Opin Nephrol Hypertens 7:171–177, 1998.

103. Dworkin LD, Benstein JA, Parker M, et al. Calcium antagonists and converting enzyme inhibitors reduce renal injury by different mechanisms. Kidney Int 43:808–814, 1993.

104. Gansevoort RT, Sluiter WJ, Hemmelder MH, et al. Antiproteinuric effect of blood-pressure-lowering agents: A meta-analysis of comparative trials. Nephrol Dial Transplant 10:1963–1974, 1995.

105. Bakris GL, Mangrum A, Copley JB, Sadler R. Effect of calcium channel or β-blockade on the progression of diabetic nephropathy in African Americans. Hypertension 29:744–750, 1997.

106. Vellusi M, Brocco E, Frigato F, et al. Effects of cilazapril and amlodipine on kidney function in hypertensive NIDDM patients. Diabetes 45:216–222, 1996.

107. Rossing P, Tarnow L, Boelskifter S, et al. Differences between nisoldipine and lisinopril on glomerular filtration rates and albuminuria in hypertensive IDDM patients with diabetic nephropathy during the first year of treatment. Diabetes 46:481–487, 1997.

108. Janssen JJ, Gans RB, van der Meulen J, et al. Comparison between the effects of amlodopine and lisinopril on proteinuria in nondiabetic renal failure: A double-blind, randomized prospective study. Am J Hypertens 11:1074–1079, 1998.

109. Amann K, Tornig J, Nichols C, et al. Effect of ACE inhibitors, calcium channel blockers and their combinations on renal and extra-renal structures in renal failure. Nephrol Dial Transplant 10(suppl 9):33–38, 1995.

110. Brown S, Walton C, Crawford P, Bakris GL. Long-term effects of different antihypertensive regimens on renal hemodynamics and proteinuria. Kidney Int 43:1210–1218, 1993.

111. Münter K, Hergenröder S, Jochims K, Kirchengast M. Individual and combined effects of verapamil or trandolapril on glomeruloprotection in the stroke-prone rat. J Am Soc Nephrol 7:681–686, 1996.

112. Bakris GL, Barnhill BW, Sadler R. Treatment of arterial hypertension in diabetic humans: Importance of therapeutic selection. Kidney Int 41:912–919, 1992.

113. Bakris GL, Weir MR, De Quattro V, et al. Renal hemodynamic and antiproteinuric response to an ACE inhibitor, trandolapril, or calcium antagonist, verapamil, alone or in fixed dose combination in patients with diabetic nephropathy: A randomized multicentered study. [Abstract] J Am Soc Nephrol 7:1546, 1996.

114. de Jong P, Anderson S, de Zeeuw D. Glomerular preload and afterload reduction as a tool to lower urinary protein leakage: Will such treatments also help to improve renal function outcome? J Am Soc Nephrol 3:1333–1341, 1993.

115. Pedrini MT, Levey AS, Lau J, et al. The effect of dietary protein restriction on the progression of diabetic and non-diabetic renal diseases: a meta-analysis. Ann Intern Med 124:627–632, 1996.

116. Goodship THJ, Mitch WE. Nutritional approaches to preserving renal function. Adv Intern Med 33:337–357, 1988.

117. Golbetz H, Black V, Shemesh O, Myers BD. Mechanism of the antiproteinuric effect of indomethacin in nephrotic humans. Am J Physiol 256:F44–F51, 1989.

118. Remuzzi G, Bertani T. Pathophysiology of progressive nephropathies. N Engl J Med 339:1448–1456, 1998.

119. Massy ZA, Guijarro C, O'Donnell MP, et al. Lipids, 3-hydroxy-3-methylglutaryl coenzyme A reductase inhibitors and progression of renal failure. Adv Nephrol 27:39–56, 1998.

120. Capelli P, DiLiberato L, Albertazzi A. Role of dyslipidemia in the progression of chronic renal disease. Ren Fail 20:391–397, 1998.

121. Moorhead JF, El-Nahas M, Chan MK, Varghese Z. Lipid nephrotoxicity in chronic progressive glomerular and tubulointerstitial disease. Lancet 2:1309–1311, 1982.

122. GuiJarro C, Keane WF. Effects of lipids on the pathogenesis of progressive renal failure. Miner Electrolyte Metab 22:147–152, 1996.

123. Lam KSL, Cheng IKP, Janus ED, Pang RWC. Cholesterol-lowering therapy may retard the progression of diabetic nephropathy. Diabetologia 38:604–609, 1995.

124. Fuiano G, Esposito C, Sepe V. Effects of hypercholesterolemia on renal hemodynamics: Study in patients with nephrotic syndrome. Nephron 73:430–435, 1996.

125. Scanferla F, Landini S, Fracasso A. Risk factors for the progression of diabetic nephropathy: Role of hyperlipidemia and its correction. Acta Diabetol 29:268–272, 1992.

126. Attman P-O, Samuelsson O, Alanpovic P. Progression of renal failure: Role of apolipoprotein B–containing lipoproteins. Kidney Int 52:S98–S101, 1997.

127. Wang ZQ, Liang KH, Pahl MV, Vaziri ND. Effect of heparin on mesangial cell growth and gene expression on matrix proteins. Nephrol Dial Transplant 13:3052–3057, 1998.

128. Cade JR, DeQuesada AM, Shires DL, et al. The effect of long-term high-dose heparin treatment on the course of chronic proliferative glomerulonephritis. Nephron 8:67–71, 1971.

129. Diamond JR, Karnovsky MJ. Non-anticoagulant protective effect of heparin in chronic aminonucleoside nephrosis. Renal Physiol 9:366–374, 1986.

130. Peten EP, He CJ, Patel A, et al. Non-anticoagulant heparin suppresses ∝ 1 collagen mRNA and reduces laminin β₁ mRNA expression in sclerotic glomeruli from mice transgenic for growth hormone (GH). [Abstract] J Am Soc Nephrol 4:780, 1993.

131. Striker GE, Lupia E, Elliot S, et al. Glomerulosclerosis, arteriosclerosis, and vascular graft stenosis: Treatment with oral heparinoids. Kidney Int 52(suppl 63):S120–S123, 1997.

132. Johnson RJ. Cytokines, growth factors and renal injury: Where do we go now? Kidney Int 52(suppl 63):S2–S6, 1997.

Diagnosis

CHAPTER 30

Initial Evaluation and Follow-Up

Lawrence R. Krakoff

For acute disease processes, the initial evaluation, or workup, is often considered the definitive assessment that reveals the likely cause of disease, needed diagnostic tests, and appropriate treatment. Typically, it consists of a medical history, physical examination, and various tests that generally can be grouped as biochemical, or laboratory, tests, and imaging. The latter now includes some combination of radiologic, ultrasonographic, and radionuclear approaches. For hospitalized patients, the workup is often complete within 48 hours, and for uncomplicated illnesses, the admission ends within a few days and with successful treatment. In offices or clinics, many problems are similarly evaluated comprehensively and treated effectively at the first or second visit.

High arterial pressure, or hypertension, is a highly prevalent disorder of the adult population in the United States and other nations with Western cultures for which the initial evaluation is better seen from a perspective different from that of acute illness. First, a specific cause for hypertension, although possible, is rarely found. Second, the management of nearly all hypertensive patients takes place over an extended period of time, usually many years or decades. During this long interval, many changes can be anticipated as the patient's status becomes the result of evolution of disease states, changes due to treatment, alterations in treatment strategies, and aging. Hence, periodic reevaluation of hypertensive patients is a much more important part of management than for those with self-limited illnesses.

In the past few years, there has been increasing recognition that in adults, and to some extent, in younger patients as well, high blood pressure occurs in many individuals who have other predictors and risk factors for future cardiovascular disease. Smoking, overweight, hyperlipidemia, and either noninsulin dependent diabetes mellitus or impaired fasting glucose, in varying combinations, accompany hypertension in a substantial fraction of patients seen in a typical practice. In addition, middle-aged and older hypertensive individuals often have evidence of target organ damage that has already led to symptoms or impairment and also predicts likelihood of additional disease in the future. The absolute risk of future cardiovascular disease is a composite of reversible risk factors, mainly hypertension, elevated low-density lipoprotein (LDL)-cholesterol, diabetes, target organ damage, and unavoidably, the age of the patient. This concept is depicted in Figure 30–1.

Comprehensive evaluation of hypertensive patients takes into consideration all relevant factors that may contribute to the patient's current status and future risk, yet needs to be efficient and practical because of the limited time and resources available to busy clinicians. This is the guiding approach summarized in this chapter.

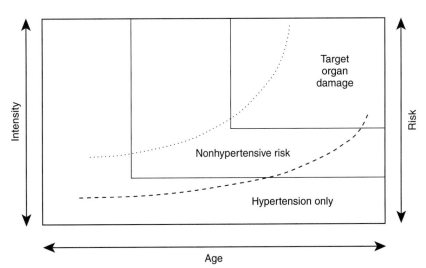

Figure 30–1. Schematic representation for assessing the absolute risk of future cardiovascular disease in hypertensive patients. The likelihood of a fatal or nonfatal stroke or myocardial infarction is related to the patient's age, the "intensity" of each risk factor (e.g., level of blood pressure or of low-density lipoprotein cholesterol), and the absence or presence of target organ damage (e.g., left ventricular hypertrophy). The *dashed lines* indicate that for any combination of risk factors and target organ damage, age will increase the risk.

WHEN IS HYPERTENSION PRESENT?

Arterial Pressure and Risk

Epidemiologists, statisticians, and clinicians have grappled with the problem of defining *hypertension* for many years. Some studies provide simplifying and practical concepts. For the broad range of blood pressure found in large populations, the risk of future cardiovascular disease (stroke or coronary heart disease) begins to increase when average diastolic pressures exceed 80 mm Hg,[1, 2] and for the middle-aged and older patient, systolic pressures exceed 130 to 135 mm Hg.[3, 4] Similarly, the risk of end-stage renal disease begins to increase when blood pressure is only minimally above the normal range, but it increases steeply when the pressure is very high.[5] Systemic arterial hypertension is high arterial pressure.[6] Most recently, ranges of blood pressure have been grouped into "high-normal pressure" and stages I to III, in the sixth report of the Joint National Committee on Prevention, Detection, Evaluation, and Treatment of Hypertension (JNC VI).[7] A modified version of these ranges is given in Table 30–1 as a basis for considering levels of blood pressure in relation to diagnosis and treatment.

Some have suggested that the average level of arterial pressure is not the only determinant of cardiovascular pathology and future risk, but that the *variability* of the pressure also contributes to disease. A cross-sectional study of intraarterial pressures suggests that excessive variation in pressure is correlated with target organ damage.[8] However, as a predictor of future disease in prospective studies and a basis for treatment, variability per se has yet to be shown to be an independent risk factor when adjusted for other factors.[9]

Accurate Measurement, Errors, and Bias

When arterial pressure is either well within the normal range (systolic pressure < 130 mm Hg and diastolic pressure < 80 mm Hg) or markedly elevated (systolic pressure > 180 mm Hg and diastolic pressure > 110 mm Hg), even an inaccurate method of blood pressure measurement will approximate the true range of the patient's blood pressure, so the likelihood of a false-positive or false-negative diagnosis of hypertension is very small.[10] However, most people with high-normal pressure or hypertension have average or usual pressures that fall in the ranges of 130 to 160 mm for systolic pressure or 80 to 105 mm Hg for diastolic pressure. Blood pressures measured by the ordinary clinical method (stethoscope and cuff with either a mercury or an anaeroid manometer) may be inaccurate or misrepresentative to the extent that an incorrect diagnosis or classification is made.[10, 11] When the average pressures are close to one of the dividing points for diagnosis, i.e., high-normal pressure versus JNC VI stage 1, there is greater potential for misclassification. Attention needs to be paid to: (1) correct cuff size, (2) accuracy of the manometer, (3) training and reliability of the observer,[12] and (4) sufficient number of measurements for a reasonable approximation of the average pressure.[10]

Supplemental Pressures

Obtaining additional blood pressure measurements outside of the clinic may be helpful in arriving at an average pressure. Supplemental pressures can help to determine the diagnosis, i.e., whether the patient has high-normal pressure or is indeed hypertensive, and can also assist in defining a response to treatment when clinic pressures are inconsistent. The use of either ambulatory blood pressure monitoring or self-measured or home blood pressures has gained recognition.[13, 14] Such measurements may reveal white-coat hypertension, in which blood pressure elevation is limited to the clinic or office, or its opposite state, when clinic pressures are lower than average daily pressures. These topics are discussed in Chapters 31, Blood Pressure Measurement Issues, and 32, White-Coat Hypertension.

NONHYPERTENSIVE RISK FACTORS

Definition of a Risk Factor

A small fraction of the hypertensive population has *only* high blood pressure as the basis for their increased risk of future cardiovascular or renal disease. Many patients have some combination of raised pressure and other, independent predictors of either stroke, coronary heart disease, or renal insufficiency. For the purposes of this discussion, the term *risk factor* incorporates the concepts of a quantifiable predictor and reversible cause that, if decreased or eliminated, will reduce the likelihood of future cardiovascular or renal disease. Thus, candidate risk factors are supported by evidence from epidemiology, pathophysiology, and therapeutic intervention, i.e., clinical trials. Table 30–2 lists those risk factors that should be taken into consideration during the

Table 30–1 Recommended Evaluation and Initial Management for Various Blood Pressure Levels*	
Blood Pressure Level	**Recommendations**
Systolic ≥ 220 mm Hg or Diastolic ≥ 115 mm Hg	Rapid evaluation by comprehensive history, physical examination, and laboratory tests; start treatment within 24 hr
Systolic ≥ 180 mm Hg or Diastolic ≥ 105 mm Hg	Comprehensive evaluation within 1 wk; begin treatment if pressure remains at this level
Systolic ≥ 160 mm Hg or Diastolic ≥ 100 mm Hg	Comprehensive evaluation within 2–4 wk; treatment decision depends on overall status
Systolic 140–159 mm Hg or Diastolic 90–99 mm Hg	Comprehensive evaluation within 1 mo; initiate lifestyle changes; ordinarily withold drug treatment for 1–6 mos; supplemental pressure, ambulatory monitoring, or self-measurement may be helpful

*Found at initial clinic measurement of *asymptomatic* adult subjects. For *symptoms* or *abnormal findings on physical examination,* individual decisions are more appropriate. The blood pressure levels approximately correspond to stages I–III of the sixth report of the Joint National Committee on the Prevention, Detection, Evaluation, and Treatment of High Blood Pressure.[7]

Table 30–2 Best-Established Nonhypertensive Risk Factors, by Evidence-Based Criteria for Causal Relationship and Results of Clinical Trials

Major Risk Factors	Comment
Smoking status	Cessation of smoking reduces risk of CHD within 2 yr by 50%; stroke and peripheral vascular disease can be prevented
Serum LDL-cholesterol concentration	Benefit of reducing LDL-concentrations is firmly established HDL-cholesterol and triglyceride levels add useful information, but changes induced by treatment remain to be shown fully effective in trials Other lipid or lipoprotein fractions, e.g., apoproteins and Lp(a), remain interesting probes for research
Diabetes mellitus	Presence of diabetes increases risk for future disease in virtually all studies; available trial evidence supports the importance of correcting glucose intolerance, but additional trials are needed for type II diabetes

Abbreviations: CHD, coronary heart disease; LDL, low-density lipoprotein; HDL, high-density lipoprotein; Lp(a), lipoprotein(a).

initial and continuing evaluation of *every* hypertensive patient, based on the best and most comprehensive evidence, usually including clinical trials. Table 30–3 includes some examples of predictors and causative factors that are associated with cardiovascular disease for which the totality of the evidence is limited to epidemiological correlations and/

Table 30–3 Useful and Some Recently Characterized Candidate Risk Factors, Not Yet Proved by Evidence-Based Criteria (Interventional Trials)

Risk Factor	Comment
Overweight and increased waist:hip ratio	Overweight and obesity are clearly related to cardiovascular disease; causal relationships are not entirely certain and trials of weight reduction with change in disease endpoints have yet to be conducted; evidence is limited to epidemiological association
Excess alcohol use	Clearly associated with increased blood pressure and likelihood of disease; evidence is limited to epidemiological association
Reduced aerobic exercise	Evidence limited to epidemiological association
Plasma renin activity	Evidence for association with risk *within hypertensive groups;* effectiveness for blockade is indirect, primarily in congestive heart failure, left ventricular dysfunction, and diabetic nephropathy

or pathophysiological studies, as randomized clinical trials are not available. Each of the items in Tables 30–2 and 30–3 is discussed later.

Smoking

A history of current or recent cigarette smoking nearly doubles the risk of stroke and coronary heart disease and is correlated with the likelihood of peripheral arterial disease. Smoking is also related to the occurrence of malignant hypertension.[15, 16] Cessation of smoking can rapidly reduce risk of coronary heart disease within a few years.[17] Ongoing counseling alone may reduce smoking behavior as demonstrated in the Multiple Risk Factor Intervention Trial (MRFIT).[18] More recently, pharmacological options have become available, including nicotine chewing gum, nicotine transcutaneous patches, and bupropion. Whether these strategies can achieve sustained elimination of smoking behavior and thus reduce long-term risk of stroke, coronary heart disease, and peripheral vascular disease remains to be proved.

Lipids and Lipoproteins

Many serum lipoprotein patterns have been associated with increased cardiovascular risk, and the list of possible candidates is increasing. Increased LDL and reduced high-density lipoprotein (HDL)-cholesterol are well-accepted predictors. The pattern of metabolic syndrome X, associated with insulin resistance, low HDL-cholesterol, and elevated serum triglyceride concentration, appears to be a predictor of coronary heart disease.[19] Increased lipoprotein-(a) (Lp[a]) levels are also correlated with increased cardiovascular risk. However, clinical trials that have included hypertensive patients have thus far been limited to showing that reduction of LDL-cholesterol by one of the statin drugs is effective for the prevention of coronary heart disease[20, 21] and perhaps for stroke as well. For practical purposes, measurement of the cholesterol or lipid profile, i.e., serum total, HDL, and LDL (calculated)-cholesterol fractions and triglyceride concentration, is sufficient to evaluate and manage hypertensive patients.

Diabetes, Glucose and Insulin Resistance

Every hypertensive patient not already known to be diabetic needs to be assessed for the presence of hidden type II diabetes or the borderline elevation of fasting glucose levels. The importance of diabetes and even high-normal fasting glucose levels in adding to potentially reversible risk in the hypertensive population and in those with high normal blood pressure cannot be overemphasized.[22]

Within the hypertensive population, a sizable fraction of patients have normal fasting glucose and glucose tolerance but the syndrome of insulin resistance.[23, 24] It is not yet certain that this state, apart from its frequent correlates of obesity and altered serum lipoprotein pattern, syndrome X mentioned earlier, confers independent risk. Furthermore, insulin resistance is not easily defined outside of research settings.

For ordinary clinical purposes, the fasting serum glucose is all that is needed to define the metabolic state of most patients. However, new definitions of both type II diabetes and the borderline state of impaired fasting glucose have been reached through an evidence-based process and the consensus of experts, and these should be used to classify hypertensive patients.[25] The diagnosis of type II diabetes is now based on an *average fasting glucose* (two or more separate measurements) of 125 mg/dl or greater (or ≥ 7 mM). When the average falls between 100 and 126 mg/dl, *impaired fasting glucose* is the correct label; such patients should be reevaluated at 1- to 2-year intervals for possible conversion to type II diabetes. If a patient is known to have had diabetes for several years, additional evaluation for complications of the diabetic state need to be undertaken to detect retinopathy, neuropathy, nephropathy, and evidence of peripheral macrovascular and microvascular disease, e.g., foot ulcers.

Weight, Build, and Overweight

Measurement of weight and height should be part of the initial assessment of all patients. At a glance, one can tell whether the body build is slim, muscular, mildly overweight, obese, or morbidly obese. It is useful, however, to have a single and simple calculation that gives a numerical counterpart to the clinical impression. The calculated body mass index (BMI) is widely used in clinical studies to convey body build that relates weight to height. The calculation for BMI is weight (in kilograms) divided by height in meters square (kg/m^2). For those measuring height in inches and weight in pounds, the formula for BMI, equivalent to using metric units with a correction factor, is 705 $\times$ lb/inches[2]. Generally, desirable BMI is 25 or less, mild overweight is 25 to 29, and definite overweight is 30 or higher or 20% or more above desirable weight.

Weight distribution may also predict future cardiovascular disease and the likelihood of hypertension or the tendency to diabetes. The "apple" shape is relatively incriminated, whereas the "pear" shape is less so. These adjectives are reflected in a simple measurement, the waist:hip ratio, which is usually well below 0.9. As the ratio increases in overweight patients, the body build becomes the apple or high-risk type.[26]

Overweight hypertensives may be considered to have a reversible disorder, whose correction, i.e., weight loss, not only may lower their blood pressure but also may improve their nonhypertensive risk status (elevated serum LDL-cholesterol, impaired glucose metabolism, or type II diabetes) as well. Unfortunately, national trends suggest that overweight is relentlessly increasing in the United States.[27]

Exercise Pattern—Fitness

Those who engage in regular aerobic exercise, as a part of their normal lifestyle, seem to have less cardiovascular disease in prospective studies.[28–30] As part of the initial evaluation, some analysis of exercise pattern is advisable, along with the suggestion that exercise, if feasible, may reduce blood pressure.[31, 32]

Alcohol Use or Overuse

Appraisal of day-to-day ingestion of alcohol is part of the initial and recurring assessment of hypertensive patients for several reasons. Low-level alcohol intake may be a preventive measure for future cardiovascular disease.[33, 34] However, higher consumption may contribute to both hypertension and cardiovascular disease.[34–37] Furthermore, evidence of very high sustained alcohol intake suggests that compliance with antihypertensive therapy will be difficult to achieve.

Renin as a Risk Factor and Renin Profiling

The renin-angiotensin-aldosterone system participates in control of arterial pressure and fluid-volume balance. Furthermore, several components of the system, most notably plasma renin activity and aldosterone production, can be assessed with widely available clinical measurements. Classification of hypertensive patients into low-, normal-, and high-renin subgroups has prognostic significance in that the low-renin subgroup tends to have less coronary heart disease, in both an observational study[38] and a prospective cohort analysis,[39] in contrast to higher rates of coronary heart disease in normal- and high-renin groups.

Despite controversy, some have recommended that hypertensive patients, in general, might benefit from determining their renin profile, in relation to sodium excretion, before initiating treatment. This is based on the prognostic significance of the renin profile and its predictive value for choosing therapy and the occasional clue to secondary hypertension that might not be found in other ways. A high plasma renin might suggest renovascular hypertension in a patient whose bruit was not heard. Alternatively, a very low plasma renin activity might prompt reevaluation for mineralocorticoid excess, as not all such patients have consistent hypokalemia.

Even if the decision is made not to perform a renin profile initially, knowledge of the pathophysiological role of this system is important for understanding response to treatment. An unusually good response to treatment with either an angiotensin-converting enzyme inhibitor or angiotensin I receptor blocker implies an overactive renin system. By contrast, a good response to diuretic treatment, but with appearance of hypokalemia, suggests the possibility of primary aldosteronism or a related state of mineralocorticoid excess.

If a clinician chooses to assess the renin system, patients should be withdrawn from medication for at least 1 week. Collection of a complete 24-hour urine for sodium and potassium excretion is absolutely necessary for interpreting the level of plasma renin activity in relation to published nomograms.[39] Blood samples for plasma renin activity (and serum aldosterone, if desired) are drawn at midday with the patient having been upright (not lying down) for 3 hours. Assessment of aldosterone production (serum aldosterone or 24-hour excretion of aldosterone conjugate) is warranted for any patient with unexplained hypokalemia.

Since the blood pressure response to rapid blockade of the renin system should also reflect whether this system is overactive or suppressed in hypertensive patients, tests were devised using either an injectable angiotensin II receptor antagonist[40, 41] or an angiotensin-converting enzyme inhibitor such as captopril.[42–46] The blood pressure response, alone, to such interventions may not be definitive. Greater accuracy for assessing the renin system is achievable if blood samples for plasma renin activity are obtained before and 1 to 2 hours after drug administration.[46] If samples are obtained for aldosterone as well, the captopril test can be useful for detection of mineralocorticoid excess states.[43]

Other Potential Risk Factors

Each year brings new candidates as predictors or possible participating causes of cardiovascular disease. The level of serum homocysteine has been been correlated with stroke[47] and coronary heart disease.[48] Homocysteine levels are partly related to the availability and normal metabolism of folic acid and vitamin B_{12} via methylation pathways.[49] An adequate dietary supply of folic acid is needed to minimize homocysteine concentration. Whether supplementation of dietary folic acid will prove to be beneficial for preventing cardiovascular disease through reduction of serum homocysteine is not yet established.

The plasma level of serum C-reactive protein (CRP),

a nonspecific manifestation of inflammation, is another proposed candidate risk factor for coronary and peripheral arterial disease.[50, 51] It has been suggested that the atherosclerotic process includes a low-grade inflammation, which can significantly elevate CRP and other markers of inflammation.[52, 53] Thus, an elevated CRP might be viewed as a reflection of target organ damage, rather than a candidate risk factor. The overall effect of aspirin in reducing risk of coronary heart disease[54] might then include an antiinflammatory effect (on atherogenesis) in addition to its antithrombotic action. At present, CRP measurement remains a research issue, as there is need for additional prospective epidemiological study before considering it to be a clinically useful marker.

TARGET ORGAN DAMAGE

Experimental and clinical studies amply demonstrate that a sustained period of high arterial blood pressure leads to pathology of the heart, kidneys, and vasculature—target organ damage. Detection of target organ damage in hypertensive patients is a crucial, yet highly feasible diagnostic enterprise for both initial evaluation and subsequent interval reassessments. Both the medical history and the pertinent physical examination are clearly useful to detect some forms of target organ damage. Relevant and cost-effective imaging and biochemical testing is, nonetheless, needed for improving precision in many instances. Table 30–4 lists the major sites of target organ damage to be surveyed, how these are to be assessed in the initial medical history and

Table 30–4 Assessment of Target Organ Damage to Be Suspected in Hypertensive Patients With or Without Other Risk Factors

Site/Pathology	Detection by History and Examination	Pertinent Additional Tests
Retina: arteriolar thickening, hemorrhage, exudates, papilledema	Opthalmoscopy	Flourescein angiography rarely needed
Carotid artery stenosis	Auscultation for bruits	Carotid ultrasound assessment
Left ventricular hypertrophy; diastolic, systolic dysfunction	History of dyspnea, fatigue; examination for S_4 sound, increased S_2; cardiac enlargement: left ventricular heave	ECG, echocardiogram for selected cases
Coronary artery disease	History of angina or previous myocardial infarction	ECG, stress tests*
Cerebrovascular disease	History of stroke or transient ischemic attack, screening neurologic examination	Carotid ultrasound assessment;* additional imaging with CT scan or MRI sometimes appropriate
Renal pathology	History of renal disease or diabetes >5 yr; unexplained edema	Urinalysis for protein, abnormal sediment; 24-hr urine for microalbumin or total protein;* serum creatinine, calculated creatinine clearance as estimate of glomerular filtration rate
Abdominal aortic aneurysm	History of abdominal mass or discomfort, detection of pulsatile mass on physical examination	Ultrasound of abdomen;* CT scan, MRI, MRA
Peripheral arterial stenosis	History of claudication, reduced pulses	Measurement of arm and calf pressures for ankle-arm index*

Abbreviations: ECG, electrocardiogram; CT, computed tomography; MRI, magnetic resonance imaging; MRA, magnetic resonance angiography.
*Indicated as an initial test, when history or physical examination reveals positive findings.

physical examination, and the tests or imaging procedures most commonly used for confirmation.

INITIAL ASSESSMENT OF HYPERTENSIVE PATIENTS

Ordinarily hypertension first presents during periodic checkup visits or as part of ordinary screening when patients are seen for unrelated minor illnesses. However, whenever elevated blood pressure is encountered, there should be a clinical reflex question: Is this a hypertensive emergency? In nearly all cases, the answer will be "no," and diagnostic assessment will proceed down the left-hand side of Figure 30–2. If the pressure is very high, stage 3 or more, and there are other signs of a hypertensive emergency, patients will usually be hospitalized, often in an intensive care unit, for immediate blood pressure reduction with appropriate rapidly acting medications (see Chap. 82, Hypertensive Crisis).

For the vast majority of hypertensives who will be managed at clinic or office visits, the initial evaluation should consist of (1) a careful medical history, (2) an appropriately comprehensive physical examination, and (3) the necessary laboratory assessments. Once the initial evaluation is completed, the issues given in Table 30–5 can be addressed. In most cases, management will be focused on the first two rows of Table 30–5, determining overall risk and then addressing the patient's potential for successful long-term commitment to antihypertensive treatment. Nonetheless, the possibility of secondary hypertension should not be overlooked, just because the reversible forms of secondary hypertension (as defined in Section IX) are so rare. Many forms of secondary hypertension can be detected through a careful history and physical examination. Table 30–6 provides a guideline for initial evaluation of patients for secondary causes of hypertension. Characteristics of most of the diagnostic tests frequently used to detect secondary hypertension have been calculated with

Table 30–5 Information to Be Derived From Initial Assessment of Hypertensive Patients	
Clinical Issue	Relevant Information
Overall risk status	Composite of: Average blood pressure level Nonhypertensive risk factors Target organ damage
Likelihood of secondary hypertension	Clues provided by history, physical examination, necessary tests
Assessment for management strategy	Potential for education, change in lifestyle, compliance with medication
Plan for treatment and follow-up	Decisions for nondrug (lifestyle) changes and/or medications, follow-up interval, rescreening.

regard to sensitivity, specificity, and predictive value.[55] When secondary hypertension is considered likely on clinical grounds, combinations of tests used judiciously may provide the greatest accuracy.[55, 56]

If secondary hypertension is not suggested, what imaging and chemical tests should be performed on recently discovered hypertensives? Practicality and considerations of cost-effectiveness have their impact on this process. No easy generalization is tenable, given the heterogeneity within the hypertensive population. My own choices and strategy for testing a *middle-aged, asymptomatic hypertensive patient, who has no evident target organ damage on examination are*:

1. Electrocardiogram: Is there evidence for left ventricular enlargement or ischemic disease?
2. Fasting glucose, serum creatinine, and electrolytes (Na^+, K^+, Cl^-, HCO_3^-): To assess for diabetes, hypokalemia, and renal function.
3. Serum lipid profile: HDL-, LDL-cholesterol fractions—a total cholesterol alone is not precise enough for risk stratification.
4. Urinalysis: Is proteinuria or an abnormal renal sediment present?
5. Consideration of a renin profile: It may guide treatment or unmask secondary hypertension.

Nothing else is absolutely necessary *unless*—and there are so many "unlesses." Here are only a few examples: (1) With a history of smoking, dyspnea, or cough, a chest x-ray becomes important. (2) A suggestion of angina in the review of systems introduces the prospect of coronary heart disease and need for a stress test. (3) The finding of a carotid bruit, even without neurological symptoms, may lead to ultrasound assessment of the carotid arteries. (4) A borderline low serum potassium implies increased aldosterone secretion that might be due to a primary adrenal cortical abnormality or to a secondary elevated renin, as in renovascular hypertension. Many more examples might be given. However, the main point is that the heterogeneity of the hypertensive population implies that guidelines for initial evaluation need to be broadly structured with ample flexibility for an appropriate diagnostic strategy for any one patient.

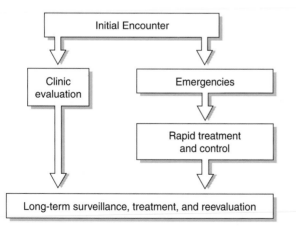

Figure 30–2. Simplified flow diagram for management of hypertensive patients after their initial detection. The few hypertensive emergencies will be rapidly evaluated and treated. Most patients will be evaluated entirely in clinic or office settings. All patients should be kept under observation with reevaluation, adjustment in treatment, and appropriate diagnostic assessment for as long as possible.

Table 30–6 Initial Assessment for Secondary Hypertension, Some Examples of More Well Known Forms

Specific Disease	Findings by History and Physical Examination	Usual Screening or Initial Tests
Coarctation of the aorta	Decreased pulsation and pressure in legs, radial femoral-pulse delay, interscapular bruit	Chest x-ray for abnormal aortic contour (three-sign) and rib notching
Cushing's syndrome	Obesity, "moon" face, "buffalo hump" of cervical fat pad, acne, bruises, purple abdominal striae	24-hr free cortisol and overnight dexamethasone suppression test
Primary aldosteronism, other forms of mineralocorticoid excess	Normal appearance, vague symptoms, fatigue, weakness, rarely tetany	Hypokalemia and low or suppressed renin profile; lack of blood pressure response with low nonresponsive renins in captopril test
Renal artery stenosis	Subcostal bruit, signs of widespread atherosclerotic arterial disease	High renin profile, positive captopril test; captopril renal scan; duplex Doppler study of renal arteries
Polycystic kidney disease	History of familial hypertension and renal disease, palpable flank masses	Ultrasound of kidneys
Chronic renal disease	History of abnormal urinalysis, known connective tissue disease, e.g., lupus erythematosis, edema, hematuria, recurrent urinary tract infections or stones	Complete urinalysis; increased serum creatinine, low creatinine clearance, 24-hr albumin/protein excretion; ultrasound of kidneys
Pheochromocytoma	Highly variable pressure, symptoms of paroxysmal palpitations, anxiety, sweating, headache, constipation or diarrhea, weight loss, family history of endocrine disease or "birthmark" diseases	24-hr urine metanephrine excretion most sensitive, specific, and available; other biochemical tests may be needed in special circumstances; imaging for localization of tumor
Drug reactions: diet pill overdose, cocaine use, drug (including some antihypertensives) or alcohol withdrawal	Often abrupt increase in blood pressure with headaches, *accurate history is crucial,* including recent use of any drugs	Chemical screens for amphetamines, cocaine, alcohol levels

Line 1 of Table 30–5 indicates that the initial assessment should reveal the overall absolute cardiovascular risk of each patient, as portrayed in Figure 30–1. Line 2 of Table 30–5 indicates that some estimate of the likelihood of secondary hypertension should be made after the initial assessment (including laboratory tests). Most often there will be no symptoms, physical findings, or abnormal tests, so that secondary hypertension (apart from obesity) is a remote possibility. Line 3 of Table 30–5 emphasizes those features derived from the medical history that are often overlooked in overviews and guidelines for patient management and yet are crucial in establishing a strategy for long-term management of hypertensive patients. The individual patient's ordinary activities, socioeconomic status, ability to understand his or her status, comprehension of what may be a complex medical regimen, and support systems are pertinent to management. Will this patient be compliant with medication and reliable about follow-up visits and reporting symptoms? What financial burdens can he or she deal with for tests and medications? Accurate assessment of these issues may determine whether or not a patient benefits from medical management designed to reduce cardiovascular risk using the usual interventions—change in lifestyle and medication. Line 4 of Table 30–5 states that the initial workup will lead to a plan that will include recommendations for treatment and for appropriate follow-up evaluations, to be dealt with in the next sections.

PLAN FOR INITIAL MANAGEMENT

After evaluating hypertensive patients, decisions will be made regarding goals for treatment and the strategy for achieving these goals. In general, some combination of lifestyle change and drug therapy will be recommended. For those with blood pressures in the range of 140 to 150 mm Hg/90 to 100 mm Hg, without target organ damage, nonpharmacological choices, particularly weight reduction, with or without reduced salt intake, are appropriate. When the blood pressure is higher, drug treatment will be started immediately. At the outset, if nonhypertensive risk factors (such as smoking, increased LDL-cholesterol, or diabetes) are most prominent, attention to these may be as important or more so than blood pressure reduction.

Apart from the detailed protocols used in clinical trials and the general advice given in guidelines or consensus documents, there is surprisingly little information in the medical literature about specific strategies for getting each patient to the goal of a reduced overall risk of cardiovascular disease. The patient's ability to understand and comply with treatment needs attention, as well as his or her various personal, social, and economic characteristics. In setting a plan for management, the time frame for achieving specific goals needs to be discussed with the patient. It is my impression that trying to do too much in too short a time often leads to frustration and less optimal compliance, compared with a gradual introduction of one intervention at a time over several visits, spaced out over many months.

REEVALUATION AND FOLLOW-UP

After the initial workup and period of observation, management of hypertension and cardiovascular risk ought to become a long-term partnership between doctor and patient in which periodic surveillance and reassessment are coupled with continuing motivation and education. The success of randomized clinical trials in demonstrating the efficacy of antihypertensive drug therapy and cholesterol reduction has depended on maintaining a high percentage of patients on treatment and willing to remain enrolled under observation. Most patients with well-controlled blood pressure after 6 to 9 months of treatment remain stable for long periods and, in my view, can be seen every 6 months thereafter. Even this frequency may be a demanding program for many patients who work or have family responsibilities and are free of symptoms, unless a highly convenient medical care system is available. Perhaps more patients can be effectively treated in situations in which there are adjunct resources such as work-site clinics.[57] Self-measurement of blood pressure, at home and elsewhere, has the potential for reducing need for office or clinic visits,[58] but there is a need for definitive studies showing that such a method improves outcomes.

Broad guidelines can be drawn for the frequency of follow-up and which follow-up tests should be performed at various intervals for uncomplicated or "usual" patients. My own suggestions are given in Table 30–7. There are, however, many exceptions or intercurrent changes that warrant highly individual choices. Even when hypertension and other risk factors are well controlled, over long periods of observation, hypertensive patients remain likely to develop cerebrovascular and cardiovascular disease.[59] Thus, clinicians should be aware that the syndromes of cerebrovascular disease or coronary heart disease are ever in the background despite effective therapy. This implies that screening tests for arterial vascular disease, particularly cardiac stress tests and ultrasound examinations of the carotid artery and the abdominal aorta, may be useful for hypertensives treated for many years, especially if they are older (>55 years) or have wide pulse pressures and any prior cardiovascular disease. More studies are needed to assess the efficacy and cost-effectiveness of such strategies.

Secondary hypertension occasionally develops in patients with essential hypertension during prolonged management. The most frequent form of secondary hypertension in this setting is atherosclerotic renal artery stenosis that tends to evolve when there are multiple risk factors for atherosclerosis, e.g., smoking, hypercholesterolemia, and diabetes. Patients with atherosclerotic renal artery stenosis often have evidence of atherosclerosis elsewhere, namely the carotid, coronary, and peripheral arteries. Development of renal insufficiency in elderly patients who used to be hypertensive, but now have congestive heart failure with lower arterial pressure, should raise the suspicion of renal arterial disease and ischemic nephropathy.[60, 61]

The high prevalence of essential hypertension in older populations implies that the rare diseases, pheochromocy-

Table 30–7 Suggested Follow-Up Assessment for Hypertensive Patients, Based on Level of Absolute Risk and Response to Treatment*	
Measurement or Procedure	**Comment**
Sitting pressure	Every visit
Weight	Every visit
Standing pressure	Initial visit, if patient dizzy, if tendency to orthostatic hypotension known or suspected
Listen for carotid bruit, cardiac examination, peripheral vascular assessment	Annual, unless new symptoms or abnormalities present in past
For nondiabetic patients: fasting glucose, lipid profile	For stable patients without abnormalities at baseline, every 2 yr For overweight patients, or unusual change in weight, recheck glucose and lipids more often
Patients with drug-treated hyperlipidemia	Monitor serum lipids every 6–12 mo
Diabetic patients	Glucose, HgbA$_1$C, serum lipids initially as often as necessary for optimal management; once stable, every 6–12 mo; check for microalbuminuria annually after 5 yr
Electrocardiogram	Every 2 yr unless new symptoms or known abnormalities at baseline
Renal function: creatinine, urine for microalbumin, electrolytes	Every 1–2 yr, unless abnormal at baseline or high-dose diuretics prescribed
Echocardiography, cardiac stress test, creatinine clearance	Only for change in status from baseline suspected by new symptoms
Workup for secondary hypertension	Only if pressure difficult to control, new symptoms, hypokalemia, impaired renal function

Abbreviation: HgbA$_1$C, hemoglobin A$_1$C.
*Suggestions are based on several current guidelines and clinical experience, but individual patients may require different kinds of ongoing assessment.

toma, Cushing's syndrome, and perhaps primary aldosteronism, will occur with the same frequency in those with prior essential hypertension as in those without it. Hypothyroidism is another cause of increased blood pressure more common in the elderly, in whom there is a tendency to higher pulse pressures with slower heart rates, as is often seen in isolated systolic hypertension of the elderly. Use of the highly sensitive assay for serum thyroid stimulating hormone has greatly enhanced detection of this disorder.

Each follow-up visit of a hypertensive patient not only is a reevaluation of medical status but also can be viewed as an opportunity to maintain or enhance the goals of optimal preventive care. Brief and focused emphasis on reinforcing positive changes in lifestyle, education about risk, and value of compliance with treatment may enhance the patient's commitment to staying on treatment. The message to be conveyed is that such periodic evaluations are part of the long-range plan for reducing the odds of cardiovascular disease through an effective partnership between doctor and patient.

SUMMARY

The initial and follow-up evaluations of hypertensive patients are, taken together, a complex scheme for preventing or reversing cardiovascular and renal disease over intervals from years to decades. The tools available to clinicians for workup include a wide spectrum of the most basic skills (the medical history and physical examination) to sophisticated imaging techniques and biochemical assay. It is now possible with reasonable cost and efficiency to predict absolute risk of future cardiovascular disease with far greater precision when many factors are taken together, and not rely on blood pressure alone. Such a strategy can lead to more rational therapy focused on risk factors and reversible pathology, as revealed from clinical trials. Secondary hypertension, although rare, can now be detected with more precise, but less invasive, methods owing to progress in diagnostic technology. Nonetheless, for most hypertensive patients, it is the sustained surveillance and reassessment, coupled with strategies for education and motivation to achieve their active participation in optimal treatment, that will be the crucial determinants in reducing the likelihood of stroke, coronary heart disease, congestive heart failure, and progression to end-stage renal disease.

References

1. Hypertension Detection and Follow-Up Program Cooperative Group. The Hypertension Detection and Follow-Up Program: A progress report. Circ Res 40(suppl 1):106–110, 1977.
2. MacMahon S, Peto R, Cutler J, et al. Blood pressure, stroke, and coronary heart disease. Part 1: Prolonged differences in blood pressure: Prospective observational studies corrected for the regression dilution bias. Lancet 335:765–774, 1990.
3. Lichtenstein MJ, Shipley MJ, Rose G. Systolic and diastolic blood pressure as predictors of coronary heart mortality in the Whitehall study. BMJ 291:243–245, 1985.
4. Glynn RJ, Field TS, Rosner B, et al. Evidence for a positive linear relation between blood pressure and mortality in elderly people. Lancet 345:825–829, 1995.
5. Klag MJ, Whelton PK, Randall BL, et al. Blood pressure and end-stage renal disease in men. N Engl J Med 334:13–18, 1996.
6. Pickering G. The Nature of Essential Hypertension. New York, Grune & Stratton, 1961.
7. Joint National Committee on Prevention, Detection, Evaluation, and Treatment of High Blood Pressure. The Sixth Report. Arch Intern Med 157:2413–2445, 1997.
8. Parati G, Pomidossi G, Albini F, et al. Relationship of 24-hour blood pressure mean and variability to severity of target-organ damage in hypertension. J Hypertens 5:93–98, 1987.
9. Verdecchia P, Borgioni C, Ciucci A, et al. Prognostic significance of blood pressure variability in essential hypertension. Blood Press Monit 1:3–11, 1996.
10. Perry HMJ, Miller JP. Difficulties in diagnosing hypertension: Implications and alternatives. J Hypertens 10:887–896, 1992.
11. Schechter CB, Adler RS. Bayesian analysis of diastolic blood pressure measurement. Med Decis Making 8:182–190, 1991.
12. Bruce NG, Shaper AG, Walker M, Wannamethee G. Observer bias in blood pressure studies. J Hypertens 6:375–380, 1988.
13. Appel LJ, Stason WB. Ambulatory blood pressure monitoring and blood pressure self-measurement in the diagnosis and management of hypertension. Ann Intern Med 118:867–882, 1993.
14. Sheps SG, Pickering TG, White WB, et al. Ambulatory blood pressure monitoring. J Am Coll Cardiol 23:1511–1513, 1994.
15. Isles C, Brown JJ, Cumming AMM, et al. Excess smoking in malignant-phase hypertension. BMJ 1:579–581, 1979.
16. Bloxham CA, Beevers DG, Walker JM. Malignant hypertension and cigarette smoking. BMJ 1:581–583, 1979.
17. Rosenberg L, Kaufman DW, Helmrich SP, Shapiro S. The risk of myocardial infarction after quitting smoking in men under 55 years of age. N Engl J Med 313:1511–1514, 1985.
18. Multiple Risk Factor Intervention Trial Research Group. Multiple Risk Factor Intervention Trial: Risk factor changes and mortality results. JAMA 248:1465–1477, 1982.
19. Zavaroni I, Bonora E, Pagliara M, et al. Risk factors for coronary artery disease in healthy persons with hyperinsulinemia and normal glucose tolerance. N Engl J Med 320:702–706, 1989.
20. Scandinavian Simvastatin Survival Study Group. Randomised trial of cholesterol lowering in 4444 patients with coronary heart disease: The Scandinavian Simvastatin Survival Study (4S). Lancet 344:1383–1389, 1994.
21. Shepard J, Cobbe SM, Ford I, et al. Prevention of coronary heart disease with pravastatin in men with hypercholesterolemia. N Engl J Med 333:1301–1307, 1995.
22. Gerstein HC, Yusuf S. Dysglycemia and risk of cardiovascular disease. Lancet 347:949–950, 1996.
23. Saad MF, Knowler WC, Pettitt DJ, et al. Insulin and hypertension—Relationship to obesity and glucose intolerance in Pima Indians. Diabetes 39:1430–1435, 1990.
24. Shen DC, Sheih SM, Chen YD, Reaven GM. Resistance to insulin-stimulated glucose uptake in patients with hypertension. J Clin Endocrinol Metab 66:580–583, 1988.
25. The Expert Committee on the Diagnosis and Classification of Diabetes Mellitus. Report of the Expert Committee on the Diagnosis and Classification of Diabetes Mellitus. Diabetes Care 20:1183–1197, 1997.
26. Haffner SM, Miettinen H, Gaskill SP, Stern MP. Metabolic precursors of hypertension. The San Antonio Heart Study. Arch Intern Med 156:1994–2000, 1996.
27. Kuszmarski RJ, Flegel KM, Campbell SM, Johnson CL. Increasing prevalence of overweight among U.S. adults: The National Health and Nutrition Surveys, 1960–1991. JAMA 272:205–211, 1994.
28. Paffenbarger RSJ, Hyde RT, Wing AL, Hsieh C. Physical activity, all-cause mortality, and longevity of college alumni. N Engl J Med 314:605–613, 1986.
29. Ekelund L, Haskell WL, Johnson JL, et al. Physical fitness as a predictor of cardiovascular mortality in asymptomatic North American men. N Engl J Med 319:1379–1384, 1988.
30. Fries JF, Singh G, Morfield D. Running and the development of disability with age. Ann Intern Med 121:502–509, 1994.
31. Nelson L, Jennings GL, Esler MD, Korner PI. Effect of changing levels of physical activity on blood-pressure and haemodynamics in essential hypertension. Lancet 2:473–476, 1986.
32. Kokkinos PF, Narayan P, Colleran JA, et al. Effects of regular exercise on blood pressure and left ventricular hypertrophy in African-American men with severe hypertension. N Engl J Med 333:1462–1467, 1995.
33. Gill JS, Zezulka AV, Shipley MJ, et al. Stroke and alcohol consumption. N Engl J Med 315:1041–1046, 1986.
34. Stampfer MJ, Colditz GA, Willett WC, et al. A prospective study of moderate alcohol consumption and the risk of coronary disease and stroke in women. N Engl J Med 319:267–273, 1988.
35. Beilin LJ. The fifth Sir George Pickering memorial lecture: Epitaph to essential hypertension—A preventable disorder of known aetiology? J Hypertens 6:85–94, 1988.
36. Puddey IB, Parker M, Beilin LJ, et al. Effects of alcohol and caloric restrictions on blood pressure and serum lipids in overweight men. Hypertension 20:533–541, 1992.
37. Marmot MG, Elliott P, Shipley MJ, et al. Alcohol and blood pressure: The INTERSALT Study. BMJ 308:1263–1267, 1994.
38. Brunner HR, Laragh JH, Baer L, et al. Essential hypertension: Renin, and aldosterone, heart attack and stroke. N Engl J Med 286:441–449, 1972.
39. Alderman MH, Madhavan S, Ooi WL, et al. Association of the renin-sodium profile with the risk of myocardial infarction in patients with hypertension. N Engl J Med 324:1098–1104, 1991.

40. Dalakos TG, Elias AN, Anderson GH, et al. Evidence for an angiotensinogenic mechanism of the hypertension in Cushing's syndrome. J Clin Endocrinol Metab 46:114–118, 1978.

41. Krakoff LR, Ribeiro AB, Gorkin JU, Felton KR. Saralasin infusion in screening patients for renovascular hypertension. Am J Cardiol 45:609–613, 1980.

42. Muller FB, Sealey JE, Case DB, et al. The captopril test for identifying renovascular disease in hypertensive patients. Am J Med 80:633–644, 1986.

43. Lyons DF, Kem DC, Brown RD, et al. Single dose captopril as a diagnostic test for primary aldosteronism. J Clin Endocrinol Metab 57:892–896, 1983.

44. Postma CT, van der Steen PHM, Hoefnagels WHL, et al. The captopril test in the detection of renovascular disease in hypertensive patients. Arch Intern Med 150:625–628, 1990.

45. Frederickson ED, Wilcox CS, Bucci CM, et al. A prospective evaluation of a simplified captopril test for the detection of renovascular hypertension. Arch Intern Med 150:569–572, 1990.

46. Gerber LM, Mann SJ, Muller FB, et al. Response to the captopril test is dependent on baseline renin profile. J Hypertens 12:173–178, 1994.

47. Perry IJ, Refsum H, Morris RW, et al. Prospective study of serum total homocysteine concentration and risk of stroke in middle-aged British men. Lancet 346:1395–1398, 1995.

48. Nygard O, Nordrehaug JE, Refsum H, et al. Plasma homocysteine levels and mortality in patients with coronary artery disease. N Engl J Med 337:230–236, 1998.

49. Mayer EL, Jacobsen DW, Robinson K. Homocysteine and coronary atherosclerosis. J Am Coll Cardiol 27:517–527, 1996.

50. Ridker PM, Cushman M, Stampfer M, et al. Inflammation, aspirin, and the risk of cardiovascular disease in apparently healthy men. N Engl J Med 336:973–979, 1997.

51. Ridker PM, Cushman M, Stampfer MJ, et al. Plasma concentration of C-reactive protein and risk of developing peripheral vascular disease. Circulation 97:425–428, 1998.

52. Grau AJ, Buggle F, Becher H, et al. The association of leukocyte count, fibrinogen, and C-reactive protein with vascular risk factors and ischemic vascular disease. Thromb Res 82:245–255, 1996.

53. Danesh J, Collins R, Appleby P, Peto R. Association of fibrinogen, C-reactive protein, albumin, or leukocyte count with coronary heart disease: Meta-analyses of prospective studies. JAMA 279:1477–1482, 1998.

54. Steering Committee of the Physician's Health Study Research Group. Final report on the aspirin component of the ongoing Physician's Health Study. N Engl J Med 321:129–135, 1989.

55. Krakoff LR. Secondary or curable hypertension. In Management of the Hypertensive Patient. New York, Churchill Livingstone, 1995; pp 75–86.

56. Pauker SG, Kopelman RI. Interpreting hoofbeats: Can Bayes help clear the haze? N Engl J Med 327:1009–1013, 1992.

57. Foote A, Efurt JC. Hypertension control at the work site: Comparison of screening alone, referral and follow-up, and on-site treatment. N Engl J Med 308:809–813, 1983.

58. Soghikian K, Casper SM, Fireman BH, et al. Home blood pressure monitoring: Effect on use of medical services and medical care costs. Med Care 30:855–865, 1992.

59. Alderman MH, Cohen H, Madhavan S. Distribution and determinants of cardiovascular events during 20 years of successful antihypertensive treatment. J Hypertens 16:761–769, 1998.

60. Rimmer JM, Gennari FJ. Atherosclerotic renovascular disease and progressive renal failure. Ann Intern Med 118:712–719, 1993.

61. MacDowell P, Kalra PA, O'Donoghue DJ, et al. Risk of morbidity from renovascular disease in elderly patients with congestive cardiac failure. Lancet 352:13–16, 1998.

CHAPTER

31 Blood Pressure Measurement Issues

Thomas G. Pickering

Hypertension can be identified only by measuring the blood pressure, but the conventionally used methods for its detection are notoriously unreliable. There are three main reasons for this: inaccuracies in the methods, some of which are avoidable; the inherent variability of blood pressure; and the tendency for blood pressure to increase in the presence of a physician (the so-called white-coat effect). For clinical practice, the gold standard is measurements made by a physician using the Korotkoff sound technique and a mercury sphygmomanometer, but there is increasing evidence that this may lead to the misclassification of large numbers of individuals as hypertensive who in actuality do not deserve such categorization. Neither the distribution of blood pressure in the population nor the relationship between blood pressure and cardiovascular morbidity provides any justification for a rigid separation between normotension and hypertension,[1] but for clinical purposes, a threshold level of blood pressure above which antihypertensive treatment is recommended has to be established. Thus, the accurate measurement of blood pressure is of extreme importance.

It is generally assumed that the adverse effects of high blood pressure on the circulation are caused by the average, or "true," level of blood pressure, for which the clinic or casual blood pressure is taken as a surrogate measure.

Recent advances in the techniques of measuring blood pressure, particularly ambulatory monitoring, have begun to provide the opportunity to examine the pathological role of other measures of blood pressure, such as abnormalities of the diurnal rhythm and short-term variability. At the present time, however, the clinical significance of these variables remains conjectural.

BASIC TECHNIQUES OF BLOOD PRESSURE MANAGEMENT

The Auscultatory Method

It is surprising that 90 years after it was first discovered, and after the subsequent recognition of its limited accuracy, the Korotkoff technique for measuring blood pressure has continued to be used and that there has been no substantial improvement in technique. The Korotkoff sound method tends to give values for systolic pressure that are lower than the intra-arterial pressure and diastolic values that are higher, but there is no obvious superiority for phase 5 over phase 4.[2–5] The range of discrepancies is quite striking; one author commented that the two methods might indicate a

Table 31–1 Patient- and Physician-Related Factors That Lead to a Discrepancy Between Clinic and True Blood Pressure		
	Clinic BP Overestimates True BP	Bidirectional Error	Clinic BP Underestimates True BP
Physician	Inadequate cuff size	Digit preference	
Patient	White coat effect/ anxiety	Spontaneous BP variability	Smoker
	Talking		Recent exercise
	Recent ingestion of pressor substances		

Abbreviation: BP, blood pressure.

Table 31–2 Cuff Sizes Recommended by the American Heart Association			
Cuff	Arm Circumference (cm)	Bladder Width (cm)	Bladder Length (cm)
Newborn	<6	3	6
Infant	6–15	5	15
Child	16–21	8	21
Small adult	22–26	10	24
Adult	27–34	13	30
Large adult	35–44	16	38
Adult thigh	45–52	20	42

difference of as much as 25 mm Hg in some individuals.[6] There is still no universal agreement about which phase of the Korotkoff sounds should be used for recording diastolic pressure. The official recommendation of organizations such as the American Heart Association (AHA)[7] and the British Hypertension Society (BHS)[8] is to use the fifth phase except in children and other patients in whom the disappearance of sounds cannot reliably be determined.[7] Most of the large-scale clinical trials that have evaluated the benefits of treating hypertension have used the fifth phase.

Sources of Error With the Auscultatory Method

Some of the major causes of discrepancy between the conventional clinical measurement of blood pressure and the true blood pressure are listed in Table 3–1. The measurement of blood pressure typically involves an interaction between the patient and the physician (or whoever is taking the reading), and factors related to both may lead to a tendency to either overestimate or underestimate the true blood pressure or to act as a source of bidirectional error, as shown in Table 31–1.

A number of factors may lead to inaccuracies with the Korotkoff sound technique.

CUFF SIZE. The size of the cuff relative to the diameter of the arm is critical. The most common mistake is to use a cuff that is too small, which will result in an overestimation of the blood pressure.[9–11] In general, the error can be reduced by using a large, adult-sized cuff for all but the thinnest arms. The BHS[8] recommends that if the arm circumference exceeds 33 cm, a large, adult cuff should be used (width 12.5 to 13 cm, length 35 cm). In the United States, the most widely advocated protocol for the selection of the appropriate cuff size is the one recommended by the AHA, as shown in Table 31–2.

ARM POSITION. Blood pressure measurements are also influenced by the position of the arm.[12, 13] As shown in Figure 31–1, there is a progressive increase in the pressure of about 5 to 6 mm Hg as the arm is moved down from the horizontal to the vertical position. These changes are exactly what would be expected based on the changes in hydrostatic pressure.

OBSERVER ERROR AND OBSERVER BIAS. Differences in auditory acuity among those using sphygmomanometers may lead to consistent errors, and digit preference is very common; most observers record a disproportionate number of readings ending in 5 or 0 (Fig. 31–2).[14] The average

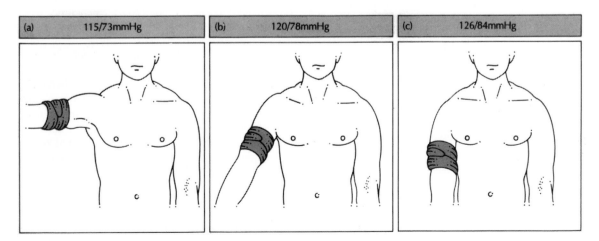

Figure 31–1. A–C. The effects of change in the position of the arm on the blood pressure recorded by a sphygmomanometer. (Data from Mitchell PL, Parlin RW, Blackburn H. Effect of vertical displacement of the arm on indirect blood pressure measurement. N Engl J Med 271:72–74, 1964.)

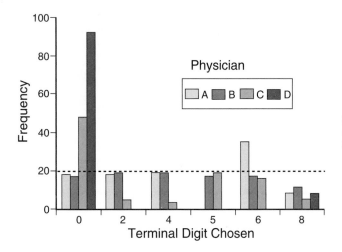

Figure 31–2. The percentage of terminal digits chosen by four physicians in a hypertension clinic during routine blood pressure measurement. Note the marked preference for zeros in physicians C and D.

values of blood pressure, as recorded by trained individual observers, have been found to vary by as much as 5 to 10 mm Hg.[15] The level of pressure that is recorded may also be profoundly influenced by behavioral factors related to the effects of the observer on the subject, the best known of which is the presence of a physician. It has been known for more than 40 years that blood pressures recorded by a physician can be as much as 30 mm Hg higher than pressures taken by the patient at home using the same technique and maintaining the same posture.[16] Also, physicians record higher pressures than do nurses or technicians.[17, 18] In our own population of patients with mild hypertension (diastolic pressures between 90 and 104 mm Hg), we have estimated that approximately 20% have "white-coat hypertension," that is, pressures that are consistently high when in the presence of a physician but normal at other times.[18] Other factors that influence the pressure that is recorded may include both the race and the sex of the observer.[19, 20] The extent to which interobserver differences in blood pressure are due to differences in technique as opposed to the white-coat effect can be assessed by having two observers take simultaneous readings with a double-headed stethoscope.

RATE OF CUFF INFLATION AND DEFLATION. The rate of inflation has no significant effect on the blood pressure,[21] but with very slow rates of deflation (2 mm Hg per second or less) the intensity of the Korotkoff sounds is diminished, resulting in slightly higher diastolic pressures. This effect has been attributed to venous congestion that reduces the rate of blood flow during very slow deflation.[22] The generally recommended deflation rate is 2 to 3 mm Hg per second. The rates of inflation and deflation are of crucial importance during self-monitoring of blood pressure because the isometric exercise involved in inflating the cuff produces a transient elevation of pressure of about 10 mm Hg.[23] This lasts for only about 20 seconds, but if the cuff is deflated too soon, the pressure may not have returned to baseline, so that a spuriously high systolic pressure is recorded.

AUSCULTATORY GAP. This can be defined as the loss and reappearance of Korotkoff sounds that occur during cuff deflation between systolic and diastolic pressures, in the absence of cardiac arrhythmias. Thus, if its presence is not recognized, spuriously high diastolic or low systolic pressures may be registered. This may occur because of phasic changes in arterial pressure or in patients who have faint Korotkoff sounds.[24] The auscultatory gap may pose a problem for automatic recorders that operate by the Korotkoff sound technique and may result in gross errors in the measurement of diastolic pressure.[25] Oscillometric devices are less susceptible to this problem.[25] The gap's presence is of clinical significance because it is associated with an increased prevalence of target organ damage.[26]

CUFF-INFLATION HYPERTENSION. Although in most patients the act of inflating a sphygmomanometer cuff does not itself change the blood pressure, as shown by intra-arterial[27] and Finapres[23] recordings, in occasional patients there may be a transient but substantial increase of up to 40 mm Hg coinciding with cuff inflation.[28] This condition appears to be distinct from white-coat hypertension in which the increase in pressure both precedes the act of inflation and outlasts it. This should also be distinguished from the transient increase in blood pressure that occurs during self-measurement due to the muscular act of inflating the cuff.

TECHNICAL SOURCES OF ERROR. There are also technical sources of error with the auscultatory method, although these usually occur less commonly when a mercury column is used than when many of the semiautomatic methods are used (see later section). These include the position of the column, which should be at approximately the level of the heart, and the mercury, which should read zero when no pressure is applied and should fall freely when the pressure is reduced (this may not occur if the mercury is not clean or if the pin-hole connecting the mercury column to the atmosphere is blocked). It is essential that aneroid meters be checked against a mercury column both at zero pressure and when pressure is applied to the cuff. Surveys of such devices used in clinical practice have often shown them to be inaccurate.[29]

The Oscillometric Technique

The oscillometric technique was first demonstrated by Marey in 1876,[30] and it was subsequently shown that when the oscillations of pressure in a sphygmomanometer cuff are recorded during gradual deflation, the point of maximal oscillation corresponds to the mean intra-arterial pressure.[31–33] The oscillations begin at approximately systolic pressure and continue below diastolic, so that systolic and diastolic pressure can be estimated only indirectly, according to some empirically derived algorithm. One advantage of the method is that no transducer need be placed over the brachial artery, so that placement of the cuff is not critical. Other potential advantages of the oscillometric method for ambulatory monitoring are that it is less susceptible to external noise (but not to low-frequency mechanical vibration) and that the cuff can be removed and replaced by the patient, for example, to take a shower. The main disadvantage is that such recorders do not work well during physical activity, when there may be considerable movement artifact.

The oscillometric technique has been used successfully in ambulatory blood pressure monitors (such as the Spacelab recorders) and home monitors. It should be pointed out that different brands of oscillometric recorders use different algorithms, and there is no generic oscillometric technique. However, comparisons of several different commercial models with intra-arterial and Korotkoff sound measurements have shown generally good agreement.[34–37]

Ultrasound Techniques

Devices incorporating ultrasound use a transmitter and receiver placed over the brachial artery under a sphygmomanometer cuff. As the cuff is deflated, the movement of the arterial wall at systolic pressure causes a Doppler phase shift in the reflected ultrasound, and diastolic pressure is recorded as the point at which diminution of arterial motion occurs.[38] A variation of this method detects the onset of blood flow at systolic pressure, which has been found to be of particular value for measuring pressure in infants and children.[39, 40]

The Finger Cuff Method of Penaz

This interesting method, first developed by Penaz,[41] works on the principle of the unloaded arterial wall. Arterial pulsation in a finger is detected by a photoplethysmograph under a pressure cuff. The output of the plethysmograph is used to drive a servoloop that rapidly changes the cuff pressure to keep the output constant so that the artery is held in a partially opened state. The oscillations of pressure in the cuff are measured and have been found to resemble the intra-arterial pressure wave in most subjects. This method gives an accurate estimate of the changes in systolic and diastolic pressure, although both may be underestimated (or overestimated in some subjects) when compared to brachial artery pressures.[41] The cuff can be kept inflated for up to 2 hours. It is now commercially available as the Finometer (formerly Finapres) and Portapres recorders, and has been validated in several studies that compared its readings with intra-arterial pressures.[42–44]

MEASUREMENT IN A VARIETY OF SITUATIONS

Clinic Measurement

The recent interest in alternative methods of measuring blood pressure has served to emphasize some of the potentially correctable deficiencies of the routine clinic measurement of blood pressure. By increasing the number of readings taken per visit and the number of visits, as well as by attempting to eliminate sources of error such as digit preference, the reliability of clinic pressure for estimating the true blood pressure and its consequences can be greatly increased. Despite this, it must be remembered that there are a substantial number of subjects with white-coat hypertension in whom clinic readings will continue to give unrepresentative values, no matter how many measurements are taken.

EFFECTS OF POSTURE. There is no consensus as to whether blood pressure should routinely be measured when the patient is sitting or supine, although most guidelines recommend sitting.[7, 8] In a survey of 245 subjects of different ages, Netea and associates[45] found that systolic pressures were the same in both positions, but that there was a systematic age-related discrepancy in diastolic pressure that was more marked in younger than in older subjects, as shown in Figure 31–3.

Self-Monitoring of Blood Pressure

The potential advantages of having patients take their own blood pressure are twofold: The distortion produced by the white-coat effect is eliminated, and multiple readings can be taken over prolonged periods of time. The potential

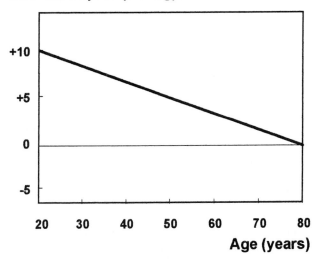

DBP Sit-Supine (mmHg)

Figure 31–3. The average difference between sitting and supine diastolic blood pressure (DBP) as a function of age. (Adapted from Netea RT, Smits P, Lenders JWM, Thien T. Does it matter whether blood pressure measurements are taken with subjects sitting or supine? J Hypertens 16[3]:263–268, 1998.)

disadvantages are that relatively little information is available concerning the diagnostic and prognostic significance of home readings, and there is an even greater potential for observer error than with physician readings. Exclusive reliance on self-monitored readings is not recommended, but they can provide a useful adjunct to clinic readings, both for the initial evaluation of newly diagnosed patients and for monitoring response to treatment.

When home monitoring was first used, the majority of studies used aneroid sphygmomanometers.[46] Although inexpensive, such devices do require a certain degree of training and dexterity on the part of the patient, and the dials are not always accurate; in one survey, 30% of aneroid dials had errors greater than 4 mm Hg.[47] The mercury sphygmomanometer has been the gold standard for clinical blood pressure measurement since the technique was introduced, but it has never been considered very suitable for home use, partly because of its expense but also because of concerns about the toxicity of mercury.[48] In the past few years, automatic electronic devices have become increasingly popular. The early versions were for the most part inaccurate,[49, 50] but the currently available ones are quite satisfactory.[51–53] Unfortunately, only a few have been subjected to proper validation tests such as the Association for the Advancement of Medical Instrumentation (AAMI) and the BHS protocols.[54] The advantages of electronic monitors have begun to be appreciated by epidemiologists,[55] who have always been greatly concerned about the accuracy of clinical blood pressure measurement and have paid much attention to the problems of observer error, digit preference, and the other causes of inaccuracy described above. Cooper and colleagues have made the case that the ease of use of the electronic devices and their relative insensitivity to the person actually taking the reading can outweigh any inherent inaccuracy when they are compared to the traditional sphygmomanometer.[55] Electronic devices now available take blood pressure from the upper arm, wrist, or finger. The use of the more distal sites may be more convenient, but measurement of blood pressure from the arm (the brachial artery) has always been the standard method and is likely to remain so for the foreseeable future.

The standard type of monitor for home use is now an oscillometric device that records pressure from the brachial artery. Oscillometric monitors have the advantage of being easy to use, as cuff placement is not as critical as it is with devices that use a Korotkoff sound microphone, and the oscillometric method has, in practice, been found to be as reliable as the Korotkoff sound method.

Wrist monitors have the advantage of being smaller than the arm devices, and they can be used by obese people, as the wrist diameter is little affected by obesity. A potential problem with wrist monitors is the systematic error introduced by the hydrostatic effect of differences in the position of the wrist relative to the heart,[12, 13] as shown in Figure 31–1. This can be avoided if the wrist is always at heart level when the readings are taken, but there is no way of knowing retrospectively whether this was complied with when a series of readings are reviewed. Wonka and coworkers[56] compared the Omron digital wrist monitor (Omron Healthcare, Vernon Hills, IL) with conventional sphygmomanometry and found that the wrist systolic pressure was 2 to 3 mm Hg lower than the arm readings;

diastolic pressures were close. The device scored grade C on the BHS protocol. Wrist monitors have potential, but should be evaluated further.[57]

Finger monitors are convenient but so far have been found to be inaccurate. The pressure waveform in the finger is different from the brachial artery trace because of the effects of wave reflection. Thus the systolic peak is shorter and higher; hence, finger monitors would be expected to overestimate the brachial artery systolic pressure by about 4 mm Hg.[58] In practice, there may be little systematic disagreement between finger blood pressure measurement and conventional sphygmomanometry, but the scatter of individual readings is excessively high.[59]

Ambulatory Monitoring

First developed more than 30 years ago, ambulatory blood pressure monitoring is only now beginning to find acceptance as a clinically useful technique. Technological advances over the past few years have led to the introduction of monitors that are small and relatively quiet and can take up to 100 blood pressure readings over 24 hours while patients go about their normal activities. These monitors are reasonably accurate when the patient is at rest but are less so during physical activity. When last systematically surveyed (in 1995), there were 43 different devices on the market; only 18 had been validated according to the AAMI or BHS criteria, and of those, only 9 satisfied the criteria for accuracy (Table 31–3).[60] Ambulatory monitors can, in theory, provide information about the three main measures of blood pressure—the average level, the diurnal variation, and the short-term variability. Because the currently available monitors take readings intermittently rather than continually and are unreliable during exercise, they can provide only a very crude estimate of the short-term variability of blood pressure.

In the majority of hypertensive patients, the average ambulatory pressure is lower than the clinic pressure and in some cases may be within the normal range, leading to a diagnosis of white-coat hypertension. Given the discrepancy between the clinic and ambulatory pressures, it is reasonable to suppose that the prediction of risk would be

Table 31–3 ABPM Devices That Have Fulfilled BHS and AAMI Criteria for Accuracy

Device	AAMI Grade	BHS Grade
CH-Druck	Pass	A/A
Profilomat	Pass	B/A
Nissei DS-240	Pass	B/A
Quiet Ttak	Pass	B/B
SpaceLabs 90202	Pass	B/B
SpaceLabs 90207	Pass	B/B
AND TM-2420 model 6	Pass	B/B
AND TM-2410 model 7	Pass	B/B
AND TM-2421	Pass	B/A

Data from O'Brien E, Atkins N, Staessen J. State of the market: A review of ambulatory blood pressure monitoring devices. Hypertension 26:835–842, 1995. *Abbreviations:* ABPM, ambulatory blood pressure monitoring; AAMI, Association for the Advancement of Medical Instrumentation; BHS, British Hypertension Society.

different. There are now more than 30 cross-sectional studies relating the extent of cardiovascular damage to both clinic and ambulatory pressures.[61] Almost all have shown that the correlation coefficients are higher for ambulatory pressure, although in many instances the differences have been small. The superiority of ambulatory pressure in this respect may be attributed at least in part to the larger number of readings and also to their more representative nature.

There are now four prospective studies showing that ambulatory pressure is a better predictor of risk than is clinic pressure, and more studies are on the way. The first, published by Perloff and associates,[62, 63] used noninvasive monitoring performed during the day only and reported that those whose ambulatory pressure was low in relation to their clinic pressure were at lower risk of morbidity. The second, by Verdecchia and colleagues,[64] followed a group of 1187 normotensive and hypertensive individuals for 3 years; hypertensives were classified as having white-coat or sustained hypertension. The morbid event rate was 0.49 per 100 patient-years in white-coat hypertensives (similar to the rate of 0.47 in the normotensives), whereas it was 1.79 in hypertensive dippers, who constituted the majority of the study's subjects, and 4.99 in nondippers. The third study, the pilot for a population study in Ohasama, Japan,[65] reported that ambulatory pressure was a better predictor of morbidity than was screening pressure; no attempt was made to classify individuals as having white-coat hypertension. The fourth[66] is a study of patients with refractory hypertension, defined as a diastolic pressure above 100 mm Hg while on three or more antihypertensive medications. Patients were classified into three groups according to their daytime ambulatory pressures; those in the lowest tertile (below 88 mm Hg) had a significantly lower rate of morbidity over the next 4 years despite similar clinic pressures. Thus, although these four prognostic studies differ widely in their designs, ranging from a population study to a study of refractory hypertensives, the results all point in the same direction, namely that ambulatory pressure provides a better assessment of prognosis after controlling for clinic pressure. The corollary of this is that patients with white-coat hypertension have a more benign prognosis than do those with sustained hypertension.

HOW SHOULD THE VARIOUS TECHNIQUES OF MEASUREMENT BE USED?

Which Measures of Blood Pressure Are Clinically Important?

In clinical practice, a patient's blood pressure is typically characterized by a single value for systolic and diastolic pressures that denotes the average level. Such readings are normally taken in a clinical setting, but there is extensive evidence that in hypertensive patients, clinic pressures are consistently higher than the average 24-hour pressures recorded with ambulatory monitors.[67] This overestimation by clinic readings of the true pressure at high levels of pressure and the underestimation at low levels has been referred

to as the *regression dilution bias*. This means that the slope of the line relating blood pressure and cardiovascular morbidity should be steeper for the true blood pressure than for the clinic pressure.[68]

There is a pronounced diurnal rhythm of blood pressure, with a decrease of 10 to 20 mm Hg during sleep and a prompt increase on waking and getting up in the morning. The highest blood pressures are usually seen between 6 AM and noon, which is also the period during which cardiovascular morbid events tend to occur most commonly.[69] The pattern of blood pressure during the day is to a large extent dependent on the pattern of activity, with pressures tending to be higher during the hours of work and lower when at home.[70]

In hypertensive patients, the diurnal blood pressure profile is reset at a higher level, with preservation of the normal diurnal rhythm in the majority. The short-term blood pressure variability is increased in hypertensives as compared to normotensives when expressed in absolute terms (mm Hg), but the percentage of change is not different. Thus, hypertension can be regarded as a disturbance of the set point, or tonic level, of blood pressure but a maintaining of normal short-term regulation. Antihypertensive treatment reverses these changes by moving the set point toward normal but having little effect on short-term variability.

The normal diurnal rhythm of blood pressure is disturbed in some hypertensive individuals, who do not experience the normal nocturnal fall of pressure. This has been observed in a variety of conditions, including malignant hypertension, chronic renal failure, several types of secondary hypertension, preeclampsia, and conditions associated with autonomic neuropathy.[67] There are potentially three measures of blood pressure that contribute to the adverse effects of hypertension. The first is the average, or "true," level; the second is the diurnal variation; and the third is the short-term variability. At the present time, epidemiological and clinical data are available only for the average level of blood pressure. It has been suggested that hypertensive patients whose pressures remains high at night (nondippers) have more target organ damage than do patients who show the normal pattern (dippers) and that in women, nondippers are at greater risk of cardiovascular morbidity than are dippers[64]; however, these findings are not sufficiently well established to be applied in routine clinical practice. Even less information is available for studies of the clinical significance of blood pressure variability, although it may be a risk factor for cardiovascular morbidity.

The Combined Use of Clinic, Home, and Ambulatory Monitoring

For the foreseeable future, measurement of blood pressure in clinics by conventional sphygmomanometry will continue to be the principal method of evaluation. A cardinal rule is that as the blood pressure approaches the threshold level at which treatment will be started, more readings should be taken over more visits before a decision about treatment is made. In patients who have persistently elevated clinic pressure and evidence of blood pressure–related target organ damage, it is usually unnecessary to

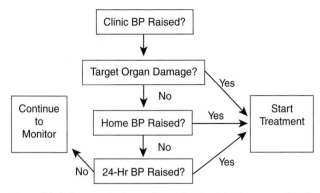

Figure 31–4. Proposed schema for evaluating blood pressure (BP) in patients with suspected hypertension using clinic, home, and ambulatory monitoring.

supplement the clinic readings with other types of measurement before reaching a therapeutic decision. When an elevated blood pressure is the only detectable abnormality, however, the possibility that the clinic pressure may overestimate the true pressure should be considered. Whether this is so may be determined by self-monitoring or by ambulatory monitoring. A schema for the use of the various means of measuring blood pressure when evaluating a newly diagnosed hypertensive patient is shown in Figure 31–4. If self-monitoring is chosen and reveals pressures comparable to the clinic values, treatment may be appropriate, but home readings that are much lower than clinic readings do not rule out the possibility that the blood pressure may be elevated at work. This is the advantage of ambulatory monitoring, which gives the best estimate of the full range of blood pressure experienced during everyday life.

MEASUREMENT OF BLOOD PRESSURE IN SPECIAL POPULATIONS AND CIRCUMSTANCES

Infants and Children

The Korotkoff sound technique is recommended as the standard for children above the age of 1 year; it may make systematic errors when measuring the pressures of infants, in whom the sounds are very difficult to hear and in whom the true systolic pressure may be underestimated.[71] In infants, the best indirect measurement technique is an ultrasonic flow detector.[72]

A particular problem associated with blood pressure measurement in children of various ages is knowing which size cuff to choose. The BHS recommends three cuff sizes—4 × 13 cm, 8 × 18 cm, and 12 × 35 cm (adult cuff)—and suggests using the widest cuff that will fit the arm.[73] The AHA[7] has recommended that the cuff size be standardized to the circumference of the arm.

Pregnant Women

In normal pregnancy there is a fall in blood pressure together with an increase in cardiac output and a large decrease in peripheral resistance. As a result of this hyperkinetic state, Korotkoff-like sounds may be heard over the brachial artery even if no pressure is applied to the cuff. These sounds are probably due to turbulent flow in the artery. Consequently, the use of phase 4 is commonly recommended for registering diastolic pressure in pregnant women,[74] as it may be 12 mm Hg higher than phase 5.[75] The National High Blood Pressure Education Program Working Group report recommends recording both phase 4 and phase 5 throughout pregnancy.[76]

Elderly Subjects

Some older people show an increase in systolic pressure without a corresponding increase in diastolic pressure (isolated systolic hypertension). These readings have been attributed to the diminished distensibility of the arteries that occurs with increasing age. In extreme cases, it may result in diminished compressibility of the artery by the sphygmomanometer cuff, so that falsely high readings may be recorded; this is often referred to as *pseudohypertension of the elderly*.[77] These patients represent the exception rather than the rule, however, because studies of healthy elderly subjects have shown no greater discrepancy between direct and indirect measurements of pressure than have studies of younger subjects.[78, 79]

Obese Subjects

Because the accurate estimation of blood pressure using the auscultatory method requires an appropriate match between cuff size and arm diameter, in obese subjects, the regular adult cuff (12 × 23 cm) may seriously overestimate blood pressure.[80] The effects of arm circumference on the measurement of blood pressure when using a cuff were studied systematically by King.[10]

Exercise

During dynamic exercise, the auscultatory method may underestimate systolic pressure by up to 15 mm Hg, whereas during recovery it may overestimate systolic pressure by as much as 30 mm Hg.[81, 82] Errors in diastolic pressure are unlikely to be as large except during the recovery period, when falsely low readings may be recorded.[82] This is the reason the AHA recommends taking the fourth phase of the Korotkoff sounds after exercise.[7]

References

1. Pickering GW. High Blood Pressure. London, Churchill, 1968.
2. Regan C, Bordley J. The accuracy of clinical measurements of arterial blood pressure, with a note on the auscultatory gap. Bull Johns Hopkins Hosp 69:504–528, 1941.
3. Kotte JH, Iglauer A, McGuire J. Measurements of arterial blood pressure in the arm and the leg: Comparison of sphygmomanometric and direct intra-arterial pressures, with special attention to their relationship in aortic regurgitation. Am Heart J 28:476–490, 1944.
4. Roberts LN, Smiley JR, Manning GW. A comparison of direct and indirect blood pressure determinations. Circulation 8:232–242, 1953.

5. Holland WW, Humerfelt S. Measurement of blood pressure: Comparison of intra-arterial and cuff values. BMJ 2:1241–1243, 1964.

6. Breit SN, O'Rourke MF. Comparison of direct and indirect arterial pressure measurements in hospitalized patients. Aust N Z J Med 4:485–491, 1974.

7. Perloff D, Grim C, Flack J, et al. AHA Medical/Scientific Statement Special Report. Human blood pressure determination by sphygmomanometry. Circulation 88:2459–2470, 1993.

8. Petrie JC, O'Brien ET, Littler WA, De Swiet M. British Hypertension Society recommendations on blood pressure measurement. BMJ 293:611–615, 1986.

9. Maxwell MH, Waks AV, Schroth PC, et al. Error in blood pressure measurement due to incorrect cuff size in obese patients. Lancet 2:33–35, 1982.

10. King GE. Errors in clinical measurement of blood pressure in obesity. Clin Sci 32:223–237, 1967.

11. Van Montfrans GA, Van Der Hoeven GMA, Karemaker JM, et al. Accuracy of auscultatory blood pressure measurement with a long cuff. BMJ 295:354–355, 1987.

12. Mitchell PL, Parlin RW, Blackburn H. Effect of vertical displacement of the arm on indirect blood pressure measurement. N Engl J Med 271:72–74, 1964.

13. Webster J, Newnham D, Petrie JC, Lovell HG. Influence of arm position on measurement of blood pressure. BMJ 228:1574–1575, 1984.

14. Padfield PL, Jyothinagaram SG, Watson DM, et al. Problems in the measurement of blood pressure. J Hum Hypertens 4 (suppl 2):3–7, 1990.

15. Eilersten E, Humerfelt S. The observer variation in the measurement of arterial blood pressure. Acta Med Scand 184:145–157, 1968.

16. Ayman P, Goldshine AD. Blood pressure determinations by patients with essential hypertension. I. The difference between clinic and home readings before treatment. Am J Med Sci 200:465–474, 1940.

17. Mancia G, Bertini G, Grassi G, et al. Effects of blood pressure measurement by the doctor on patients' blood pressure and heart rate. Lancet 2:695–697, 1983.

18. Pickering TG, James GD, Boddie C, et al. How common is white-coat hypertension? JAMA 259:225–228, 1988.

19. Comstock GW. An epidemiologic study of blood pressure levels in a biracial community in the southern United States. Am J Hyg 65:271–315, 1957.

20. McCubbin JA, Wilson JF, Bruehl S, et al. Gender effects on blood pressures obtained during an on-campus screening. Psychosom Med 53:90–100, 1991.

21. King GE. Influence of rate of cuff inflation and deflation on observed blood pressure by sphygmomanometry. Am Heart J 65:303–306, 1963.

22. Wilkins R, Bradly SE. Changes in arterial and venous blood pressure and flow distal to a cuff inflated on a human arm. Am J Physiol 147:260–269, 1946.

23. Veerman DP, Van Montfrans GA, Wieling W. Effects of cuff inflation on self-recorded blood pressure. Lancet 335:451–453, 1990.

24. Blank SG, West JE, Muller FB, et al. The characterization of auscultatory gaps using wideband external pulse recording. Hypertension 17:225–233, 1991.

25. Imai Y, Abe K, Sasaki S, et al. Clinical evaluation of semiautomatic and automatic devices for home blood pressure measurement: Comparison between cuff-oscillometric and microphone methods. J Hypertens 7:983–990, 1989.

26. Cavallini MC, Roman MJ, Blank SG, et al. Association of the auscultatory gap with vascular disease in hypertensive patients. Ann Int Med 124:877–883, 1996.

27. Parati G, Pomidossi G, Casadei R, Mancia G. Lack of alerting reactions to intermittent cuff inflations during noninvasive blood pressure monitoring. Hypertension 7:597–601, 1985.

28. Mejia AD, Egan BM, Schork NJ, Zweifler AJ. Artefacts in measurement of blood pressure and lack of target organ involvement in the assessment of patients with treatment-resistant hypertension. Ann Int Med 112:270–277, 1990.

29. Burke MJ, Towers HM, O'Malley K, et al. Sphygmomanometers in hospital and family practice: Problems and recommendations. BMJ 285:469–471, 1982.

30. Marey E-J. Pression et vitesse du sang. Physiologie Expérimentale. Paris, Pratique des hautes études laboratoire de M. Marey, 1876.

31. Mauck GB, Smith CR, Geddes LR, Bourland JD. The meaning of the point of maximum oscillations in cuff pressure in the indirect measurement of blood pressure: II. J Biomech Eng 102:28–33, 1980.

32. Ramsey M. Noninvasive automatic determination of mean arterial pressure. Med Biol Eng Comput 17:11–18, 1979.

33. Yelderman M, Ream AK. Indirect measurement of mean arterial pressure in the anesthetized patient. Anesthesiology 50:253–256, 1979.

34. Borow KM, Newburger JW. Noninvasive measurement of central aortic pressure using the oscillometric method for analyzing systemic artery pulsatile blood flow: Comparative study of indirect systolic, diastolic, and mean brachial artery pressure with simultaneous direct ascending aortic pressure measurements. Am Heart J 103:879–886, 1982.

35. Colan SD, Fuji A, Borow KM, et al. Noninvasive determination of systolic, diastolic, and end-systolic blood pressure in neonates, infants, and young children: Comparison with central aortic measurements. Am J Cardiol 52:867–870, 1983.

36. Wiinberg N, Walther-Larsen S, Eriksen C, Nielsen PE. An evaluation of semi-automatic blood-pressure monitors against intra-arterial blood pressure. J Ambul Mon 1:303–309, 1988.

37. Cates EM, Schlussel YR, James GD, Pickering TG. A validation study of the Spacelabs 90207 ambulatory blood pressure monitor. J Ambul Mon 3:149–154, 1990.

38. Ware RW, Laenger CJ. Indirect blood pressure measurement by Doppler ultrasonic kinetoarteriography. Proc 20th Ann Conf Eng Med Biol 9:27–30, 1967.

39. Elseed AM, Shinebourne EA, Joseph MC. Assessment of techniques for measurement of blood pressure in infants and children. Arch Dis Child 48:932–936, 1973.

40. Steinfeld L, Dimich I, Reder R, et al. Sphygmomanometry in the pediatric patients. J Pediat 92:934–938, 1978.

41. Penaz J. Photo-electric measurement of blood pressure, volume and flow in the finger. Digest 10th Int Conf Med Biol Eng Dresden, 1973, p 104.

42. Wesseling KH, deWit B, Settels JJ, Klawer WH. On the direct registration of finger blood pressure after Penaz. Funkt Biol Med J 245:245–250, 1982.

43. Van Egmond J, Hasenbos M, Crul JF. Invasive v. non-invasive measurement of arterial pressure: Comparison of two automatic methods and simultaneously measured direct intra-arterial pressure. Br J Anesthes 57:434–444, 1985.

44. Parati G, Casadei R, Groppelli A, et al. Continuous non-invasive finger blood pressure monitoring at rest and during laboratory testing: Evaluation by intra-arterial recording. J Hypertens 13:647–655, 1989.

45. Netea RT, Smits P, Lenders JWM, Thien T. Does it matter whether blood pressure measurements are taken with subjects sitting or supine? J Hypertens 16:263–268, 1998.

46. Kleinert HD, Harshfield GA, Pickering TG, et al. What is the value of home blood pressure measurement in patients with mild hypertension? Hypertension 6:574–578, 1984.

47. Burke MJ, Towers HM, O'Mally K, et al. Sphygmomanometers in hospital and family practice: Problems and recommendations. BMJ 285:469–471, 1982.

48. O'Brien E. Where are we now? Sphygmomanometry in the 20th century. Blood Press Mon 1 (suppl 2):S9–S13, 1996.

49. Pickering TG, Cvetkovski B, James GD. An evaluation of electronic recorders for self-monitoring of blood pressure. J Hypertens 4 (suppl 5):S328–S330, 1986.

50. Van Egmond J, Lenders JWM, Weernik E, Thien T. Accuracy and reproducibility of 30 devices for self-measurement of arterial blood pressure. Am J Hypertens 6:873–879, 1993.

51. Foster C, McKinlay S, Cruickshank JM, Coats AJS. Accuracy of the Omron HEM 706 portable monitor for home measurement of blood pressure. J Hum Hypertens 8:661–664, 1994.

52. Jamieson MJ, Webster J, Witte K, et al. An evaluation of the A&D UA-751 semi-automated cuff-oscillometric sphygmomanometer. J Hypertens 8:377–381, 1990.

53. Pannarale G, Monti F, Collauto F, et al. A statistical contribution to the clinical evaluation of blood pressure monitors. J Ambul Mon 8:231–237, 1995.

54. O'Brien E, Atkins N. A comparison of the British Hypertension Society and Association for the Advancement of Medical Instrumentation protocols for validating blood pressure measuring devices: Can the two be reconciled? J Hypertens 12:1089–1094, 1994.

55. Cooper R, Puras A, Tracy J, et al. Evaluation of an electronic blood pressure device for epidemiologic studies. Blood Press Mon 2:35–40, 1997.

56. Wonka F, Thummler M, Schoppe A. Clinical test of a blood pressure measurement device with a wrist cuff. Blood Press Mon 1:361–366, 1996.

57. Eckert S, Gleichmann S, Gleichmann U. Blood pressure self-measurement in upper arm and in wrist for treatment control of arterial hypertension compared to ABPM. Z Kardiol 85 (suppl 3):109–111, 1996.

58. Wesseling KH, Gizdulich P, Bos WJW. Whither continuous blood pressure measurement? *In* Abbott D, Campbell N, Carruthers-Czyzewski P, et al (eds). Guidelines for Measurement of Blood Pressure, Follow-Up, Lifestyle Counselling. Can J Pub Health 85 (suppl 2):S29–S35, 1994.

59. Sesler JM, Munroe WP, McKenney JM. Clinical evaluation of a finger oscillometric blood pressure device. DICP Ann Pharmacother 25:1310–1314, 1991.

60. O'Brien E, Atkins N, Staessen J. State of the market: A review of ambulatory blood pressure monitoring devices. Hypertension 26:835–842, 1995.

61. Devereux RB, Pickering TG. Ambulatory blood pressure in assessing the cardiac impact and prognosis of hypertension. *In* E O'Brien, K. O'Malley (eds). Handbook of Hypertension, vol. 14. Amsterdam, Elsevier Science 1991; pp 261–286.

62. Perloff D, Sokolow M, Cowan R. The prognostic value of ambulatory blood pressure. JAMA 249:2793–2798, 1983.

63. Perloff D, Sokolow M, Cowan RM, Juster RP. Prognostic value of ambulatory blood pressure measurements: Further analyses. J Hypertens 7 (suppl 3):S3–S10, 1989.

64. Verdecchia P, Porcellati C, Schillaci G, et al. Ambulatory blood pressure: An independent predictor of prognosis in essential hypertension. Hypertension 24:793–801, 1994.

65. Ohkubo T, Imai Y, Tsuji I, et al. Prediction of mortality by ambulatory blood pressure monitoring versus screening blood pressure measurements: A pilot study in Ohasama. J Hypertens 15:357–364, 1997.

66. Redon J, Campos C, Narciso ML, et al. Prognostic value of ambulatory blood pressure monitoring in refractory hypertension: A prospective study. Hypertension 31:712–718, 1998.

67. Pickering TG. Ambulatory Monitoring and Blood Pressure Variability. London, Science, 1991.

68. Pickering TG. The ninth Sir George Pickering memorial lecture. Ambulatory monitoring and the definition of hypertension. J Hypertens 10:401–409, 1992.

69. Pickering TG. Diurnal rhythms and other sources of blood pressure variability in normal and hypertensive subjects. *In* Laragh J, Brenner B (eds). Hypertension: Pathophysiology, Diagnosis and Management, vol I. New York, Raven, 1990; pp 1397–1405.

70. Clark LA, Denby L, Pregibon D, et al. A quantitative analysis of the effects of activity and time of day on the diurnal variations of blood pressure. J Chron Dis 40:671–681, 1987.

71. Elseed AM, Shinebourne EA, Joseph MC. Assessment of techniques for measurement of blood pressure in infants and children. Arch Dis Child 48:932–936, 1973.

72. Reder RF, Dimich I, Cohen ML, Steinfeld L. Evaluating indirect blood pressure measurement techniques: A comparison of three systems in infants and children. Pediatrics 62:326–330, 1978.

73. DeSwiet M, Dillon MJ, Littler W, et al. Measurement of blood pressure in children. Recommendations of a working party of the British Hypertension Society. BMJ 229:497, 1989.

74. De Swiet M. The physiology of normal pregnancy. *In* Rubin PC (ed). Handbook of Hypertension, vol 10. Hypertension in Pregnancy. Elsevier. Amsterdam. pp 1–15.

75. Villar J, Repke J, Markush L, et al. The measuring of blood pressure during pregnancy. Am J Obstet Gynecol 161:1019–1024, 1989.

76. Working Group Report on High Blood Pressure in Pregnancy. National High Blood Pressure Education Program. NIH Publication No. 90-3029, 1990.

77. Spence JD, Sibbald WJ, Cape RD. Direct, indirect and mean blood pressures in hypertensive patients: The problem of cuff artifact due to arterial wall stiffness, and a partial solution. Clin Invest Med 2:165–173, 1980.

78. Finnegan TP, Spence JD, Wong DG, Wells GA. Blood pressure measurements in the elderly: Correlation of arterial stiffness with differences between intra-arterial and cuff pressures. J Hypertens 3:231–235, 1985.

79. O'Callaghan W, Fitzgerald DJ, O'Malley K, O'Brien E. Accuracy of indirect blood pressure measurement in the elderly. BMJ 286:1545–1546, 1983.

80. Nielsen PE, Janniche H. The accuracy of auscultatory measurement of arm blood pressure in very obese subjects. Acta Med Scand 195:403–409, 1974.

81. Henschel A, DeLaVega F, Taylor HL. Simultaneous direct and indirect blood pressure measurements in man at rest and work. J Appl Physiol 5:506–508, 1954.

82. Gould BA, Hornung RS, Altman DG, et al. Indirect measurement of blood pressure during exercise testing can be misleading. Br Heart J 53:611–615, 1985.

CHAPTER 32

White-Coat Hypertension

George A. Mansoor and William B. White

The introduction of a methodology to monitor blood pressure in ambulant patients has generated considerable interest in blood pressure behavior, including variability and reactivity.[1] One type of reactivity commonly observed in many patients is the pressor response in the medical care environment. Indeed, in a proportion of newly diagnosed hypertensive subjects (based on office-measured blood pressure), out-of-office blood pressure will be entirely normal. This has been called *isolated office* or *white-coat* hypertension.[1] Another manifestation of the same reactivity is a persistently higher office than ambulatory blood pressure in *treated* hypertensive subjects; this is called *white-coat effect* or *white-coat phenomenon*. The latter subjects are hypertensive, but office blood pressure readings overestimate their true blood pressure. These findings question the most basic principle in the treatment of hypertension,

that office blood pressure is the best indicator of overall blood pressure and, hence, predictor of risk for that individual.[2] The clinical importance of white-coat hypertension has been recognized, and most consensus statements on ambulatory blood pressure monitoring have indicated that white-coat hypertension is the prime indication for such monitoring.[3]

The implications of detecting white-coat hypertension include (1) if these patients do not require drug therapy, substantial cost savings may accrue over time; (2) better diagnostic and prognostic risk assessment may be made for individual patients; and (3) clinical drug studies using ambulatory blood pressure monitoring can exclude white-coat hypertensives, who may not respond to drug therapy in the same fashion as sustained hypertensive patients do.[4]

Table 32–1 Prevalence of White-Coat Hypertension in Large Studies

First Author (ref)	Patients (n)	Mean Age (Yr)	ABPM Criterion	Prevalence (%)
Verdecchia (8)	1333	51	<131/86 (men) <136/87 (women)	19
Palatini (9)	942	33	<130/80 <135/85 <140/90	16 35 60
Pickering (10)	292	47	<134/90	21
Pierdomenico (11)	255	49	<135/85	21
Waeber (12)	245	40	<90	56

Abbreviation: ABPM, ambulatory blood pressure monitoring.

BACKGROUND AND DEFINITION

A higher blood pressure in the physician's presence compared with home blood pressure was reported in 1940.[5] This difference was reported to persist over time. Today, physicians are familiar with the fact that office blood pressure may be higher than out-of-office blood pressure. It is, therefore, important to study whether office or ambulatory blood pressure is more indicative of an individual patient's overall hypertensive burden and which parameter is more useful in deciding when to initiate treatment and monitor responses to drug therapy.

A substantial number of patients have white-coat hypertension. Because of variations in definitions among studies, the prevalence of white-coat hypertension has been reported to range from 10 to 60% of all newly diagnosed hypertensive patients.[6–13] Most larger studies that have found a higher prevalence have used higher cutoff levels of ambulatory blood pressure (Table 32–1). Verdecchia and coworkers[7] demonstrated that the prevalence of white-coat hypertension and left ventricular hypertrophy varied severalfold when different ambulatory blood pressure cutoff criteria were used (Fig. 32–1). When conservative criteria were used (e.g., <130/80 mm Hg), the prevalence of white-coat hypertension was approximately 12% and the incidence of left ventricular hypertrophy was similar to that in normotensive subjects (3%). Staessen and colleagues[14] compared two strategies of hypertension treatment guided by office blood pressure or ambulatory blood pressure (Ambulatory Blood Pressure Monitoring and Treatment of Hypertension Trial [APTH]). In the APTH study, 419 patients whose untreated clinic diastolic blood pressure averaged at least 95 mm Hg were randomized to identical antihypertensive drug titration based on either clinic or ambulatory blood pressure. All subjects underwent serial echocardiography and ambulatory blood pressure monitoring, but the latter data were used only in the titration of the ambulatory guided treatment arm. Drug titration by a blinded physician used either clinic or daytime diastolic blood pressure of 90 mm Hg or more to increase dose, 80 to 89 mm Hg to make no changes, and less than 80 mm Hg to reduce or stop drug therapy. After a median follow-up of about 6 months, 26% of the patients were able to discontinue drug therapy based on ambulatory blood pressure. No increase in left ventricular mass was detected in this group, which was found to have white-coat hypertension.

To standardize research in this field, analyses should be consistent and clinically based. The cutoff ambulatory blood pressure chosen to define white-coat hypertension should include both systolic and diastolic blood pressures and should reflect population normative values. This requirement is necessary because both systolic and diastolic blood pressure are important in the genesis of hypertensive complications. Home blood pressure measurements[1] alone should not be used to diagnose white-coat hypertension, especially in employed subjects, who often have higher blood pressure averages at work than at home.[15] Furthermore, single-visit office blood pressure readings are not adequate to diagnose hypertension, and therefore, several (at least three) office visits with blood pressure readings should be used to confirm the diagnosis of white-coat

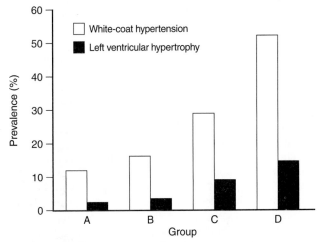

Group A: Daytime BP < 136/87 mm Hg (men) and 131/86 mm Hg (women)
Group B: Daytime BP < 134/90 mm Hg
Group C: Daytime BP < 146/91 mm Hg
Group D: Daytime BP by age and sex

Figure 32–1. Relationship between various criteria used in the diagnosis of white-coat hypertension and the prevalence of white-coat hypertension and left ventricular hypertrophy. BP, blood pressure. (Adapted from Verdecchia P, Schillaci F, Zampi I, Porcellati C. Variability between current definitions of normal ambulatory blood pressure. Hypertension 20:555–562, 1992.)

hypertension. These multiple office readings eliminate subjects who become normotensive over several visits. For example, in one random sample of 50 men who underwent 10 clinic blood pressure measurements over five visits and ambulatory blood pressure measurements, white-coat hypertension was reported to be rare.[16] In addition, patients with white-coat hypertension should have normal average ambulatory blood pressure, blood pressure loads, and awake-sleep variation.

The most comprehensive clinical studies of hypertensive target organ damage are those that included a group with defined white-coat hypertension, a group with ambulatory hypertension, and a normotensive control group. Ideally, such cross-sectional comparative studies should be performed on treatment-naive patients, since effects of previous therapy on hypertensive target organ damage complicate data analyses. The difference between clinic and daytime ambulatory blood pressure has been used by most researchers as an indicator of the white-coat effect, but this has recently been challenged.[17] Unfortunately, no easily measurable substitute for the office-ambulatory blood pressure difference is available, and it will likely continue to be used.

PATHOPHYSIOLOGY OF THE WHITE-COAT OR ALERTING REACTION

The cause of the pressor response in white-coat hypertension is difficult to study and poorly understood. Suggestions about its cause have included increased blood pressure reactivity to the stress of clinical visits, as well as a conditioned response to the medical care environment.[1] Several groups[13, 18–20] could not find any substantial increase in blood pressure variability in white-coat hypertensives compared with essential hypertensives. Furthermore, no consistent psychological or behavioral factors have been identified among white-coat hypertensives.[13, 18, 19] No differences have been found among white-coat hypertensives in a battery of psychometric tests of anger and hostility and anxiety and depression.[18] One recent small study of Japanese women that used home blood pressure to define white-coat hypertension demonstrated greater increases in blood pressure to mental arithmetic in white-coat hypertensives than in essential hypertensives.[21] A similar study that used the clinic-home blood pressure difference as an index of white-coat hypertension could also not find any relation with psychological distress.[22] It is plausible that anxiety may cause at least an initial rise in blood pressure at the first office visit compared with subsequent visits.[23] However, changes in blood pressure over one or two visits do not satisfy the definition of white-coat hypertension, which refers to persistent elevation of office blood pressure over normal out-of-office blood pressure.

It was initially reported that patients with white-coat hypertension were more likely to be younger and female.[10] However, subsequent studies have shown that a marked exaggeration of blood pressure in the clinic setting may also occur in older patients irrespective of gender[24, 25] and is common in older patients with isolated systolic hypertension.[26] In a small subset of generally older patients, reproducible dramatic elevations of systolic blood pressure have been demonstrated in the office.[27]

Office blood pressure is typically higher when measured by a physician than by a nurse or technician.[28, 29] This difference may be substantially reduced if at least 10 minutes pass from the entry of the patient into the office setting to the time of blood pressure measurement.[25] Furthermore, nurse-measured blood pressure is not a reliable indicator of white-coat hypertension.[29] The effects of patient and physician gender, race, and attitude are not well studied.

CROSS-SECTIONAL HYPERTENSIVE TARGET ORGAN STUDIES

Most studies of the risks of white-coat hypertension have used a cross-sectional design; have included white-coat hypertensives, normotensives, and ambulatory or sustained hypertensives; and have measured a hypertensive disease endpoint. Because left ventricular mass is easily and reliably determined echocardiographically, this measurement has been used most often in evaluating white-coat hypertension. Other indicators of hypertensive disease damage that have been studied include microalbuminuria, arterial compliance (as an index of vascular damage), and magnetic resonance imaging (MRI)–detected cerebral white matter lesions as indicators of silent cerebrovascular damage.[30]

Cardiac Studies

Left Ventricular Mass

Many of the studies attempting to measure the effects of the transient increases in office blood pressure have appropriately used measures of left ventricular mass or indirect measures of systolic and diastolic function. Despite the relative ease of measurement of left ventricular mass, there has been marked variability in the results. Some studies have found that left ventricular mass index in white-coat hypertensives is similar to that in age- and gender-matched normotensive subjects but lower than that in matched ambulatory hypertensives.[31–35] One of the first studies in this area[31] compared three groups of matched and never-treated hypertensive patients—office hypertensives ($n = 18$; office blood pressure > 140/90 mm Hg, and awake blood pressure < 130/80 mm Hg); normotensives ($n = 18$; office blood pressure < 135/85 mm Hg, and awake blood pressure < 130/80 mm Hg); and sustained hypertensives ($n = 18$; office blood pressure > 140/90 mm Hg, and awake blood pressure > 140/90 mm Hg)—using left ventricular mass index and wall thicknesses as indices of target organ damage. Office blood pressure was similar for white-coat hypertensives and sustained hypertensives, and ambulatory blood pressure was similar in normotensives and white-coat hypertensives. Left ventricular mass index was similar in the normotensive and white-coat groups but significantly less than in the sustained hypertensive group (Fig. 32–2). However, other researchers have found that white-coat hypertensives tend to have higher left ventricular mass than do normotensives but

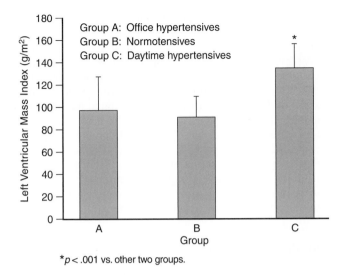

*p < .001 vs. other two groups.

Figure 32–2. Left ventricular mass index (g/m²) in three groups of matched patients, normotensive subjects (group A), white-coat hypertensives (group B), and ambulatory hypertensives (group C). (Adapted from White WB, Schulman P, McCabe EJ, Dey HM. Average daily blood pressure, not office blood pressure determines cardiac function in patients with hypertension. JAMA 26:873–877, 1989. Copyright 1989, American Medical Association.)

lower left ventricular mass than do sustained hypertensives, perhaps placing them at intermediate risk.[36–42] Some of the latter studies used an ambulatory diastolic blood pressure of 90 mm Hg, a value likely to include many subjects with mild hypertension, as the cutoff for white-coat hypertension.

Recently, Palatini and associates[9] reported data from the Hypertension and Ambulatory Recording Venetia Study (HARVEST), in which 942 never-treated subjects with office blood pressure 140 to 159/90 to 99 mm Hg were studied with echocardiography and ambulatory blood pres-

sure monitoring. The authors were very careful to use three different criteria for isolated office hypertension: (1) daytime blood pressure less than 130/90 mm Hg; (2) less than 135/85 mm Hg; and (3) less than 130/80 mm Hg. They found that irrespective of the criterion used, left ventricular mass index and wall thickness were higher in both the white-coat and the sustained hypertensive groups compared with the normotensive group. There was a gradual increase in left ventricular mass from the normotensive group to the white-coat hypertensive group and then the sustained hypertensive group, suggesting that the white-coat group is at intermediate risk.

The main debate has been about whether the white-coat effect or the office awake ambulatory blood pressure difference imparts additional risk above ambulatory blood pressure. Two initial studies[6, 43] could not find any relationship between the white-coat effect and left ventricular mass, whereas a more recent study[39] found that the white-coat effect was related to left ventricular mass, and it was more pronounced in subjects with higher levels of blood pressure.

The conflicting findings discussed previously are difficult to explain entirely on the basis of different cutoffs for diagnosing white-coat hypertension. The effects of previous antihypertensive treatment are likely to be a major confounder, since even short-term drug therapy may reduce left ventricular mass. If only studies of never-treated patients that included both sustained hypertensive and normotensive control groups are examined (Table 32–2), white-coat hypertensives either have left ventricular mass similar to that of normotensives or are intermediate between normotensives and sustained hypertensives.

Left Ventricular Function

All studies have uniformly found normal systolic function in white-coat hypertensives compared with normotensives.

Table 32–2 Echocardiographic Studies of Never-Treated Patients With White-Coat Hypertension (B) that Included a Normotensive (A) and Sustained Hypertensive Control Group (C)

First Author (ref)	Subjects (n)		Age (yr)	Office BP (mm Hg)	Ambulatory BP Criterion (mm Hg)	Left Ventricular Mass (g/m²)
Soma (38)	A	32	48	DBP < 90		102
	B	26	46	DBP > 90	<140/90	106
	C	22	48	DBP > 90	≥90	126*†
Palatini (9)	A	95	32	<140/90	<130/80	82.1
	B	119	32.6	>140/90	≥130/80	88.0*
	C	603	33.6	>140/90		92.9*†
Cardillo (19)	A	18	41.7	<140/90		81.9
	B	20	42.9	DBP > 90	<134/90	102.9*
	C	36	48.3	DBP > 90	≥134/90	121.6*†
White (31)	A	18	43.6	<135/85	≤130/80	91
	B	18	49.6	>140/90	≤130/80	97
	C	18	46.7	>140/90	≥140/90	135*
Pose-Reino (42)	A	51	42.7	<140/90		106
	B	27	46.3	>140/90	<135/85	132*
	C	24	46.7	>140/90	≥135/85	142*†

Abbreviations: BP, blood pressure; DBP, diastolic blood pressure.
*Significantly different from A.
†Significantly different from B.

Diastolic left ventricular function has also been evaluated in these patients by the early diastolic velocity wave:late diastolic wave (E:A) ratio on echocardiography or with radionuclide ventriculography. Similar to the studies with left ventricular mass, these studies have found normal[31, 36] or impaired[32, 37–39] left ventricular diastolic function in white-coat hypertensives. Most studies reported that white-coat hypertensives had either normal diastolic function or evidence for dysfunction, placing them at a slightly higher risk than normotensives but less than sustained hypertensives. However, the effects of aging on diastolic left ventricular function are sufficient to blur the superimposed effects of mild hypertension,[44] limiting the interpretation of small comparative studies. In summary, the available studies do not allow definite conclusions regarding cardiac damage in white-coat hypertension. Whether the minor changes in diastolic function observed in some studies have prognostic relevance is yet to be determined.

Renal Studies

A possible indicator of hypertensive renal damage is microalbuminuria. This marker is indicative of nephropathy in diabetic subjects and may also have some predictive value in hypertensive patients. Hoegholm and colleagues[45] compared albumin excretion in 111 patients with white-coat hypertension (daytime diastolic blood pressure < 90 mm Hg and office blood pressure > 90 mm Hg); 173 patients with established hypertension (office and daytime ambulatory diastolic blood pressure > 90 mm Hg); and 127 normotensive controls (both office and ambulatory diastolic blood pressure < 90 mm Hg). There was a graded increase in albumin excretion from normotensives to white-coat hypertensives to sustained hypertensives. These findings were not confirmed by Palatini and coworkers[39] or Pierdomenico and associates,[46] who reported that white-coat hypertensives had microalbumin levels identical to those of normotensives and lower than those of ambulatory hypertensives.

Burnier and coworkers,[47] and Marchesi and associates[48] sounded a cautionary note when they found that renal sodium handling was similar in white-coat hypertensives and sustained hypertensives and different from that in normotensive controls. A limitation of this study is that only 13 white-coat hypertensives were studied, and a high daytime ambulatory blood pressure (<140/90 mmg) was used in the definition. Nevertheless, other studies of sodium handling in white-coat hypertensives are warranted.

Vascular Studies

A third target of inquiry has been the vasculature; the rationale being that if white-coat hypertension is innocent, vascular involvement should be less than that in sustained hypertensive patients and similar to that in normotensives. The carotid artery is amenable to examination by ultrasound, and commonly derived parameters of injury are intima-media thickness, estimated extent of atherosclerosis, and compliance. Cavallini and colleagues[33] reported the first study of carotid artery structure in white-coat hyperten-

sives, normotensives, and sustained hypertensives. They found that sustained hypertensives had significantly increased intima-media thickness compared with the white-coat hypertensives and the normotensives. The results of Cuspidi and associates[40] were similar, although this study did not include a normotensive control group. A third study by Ferrara and coworkers[41] also found no differences among the three groups in intima-media thickness. In contrast, Glen and colleagues[32] concluded that both white-coat and sustained hypertensive subjects had abnormalities of elasticity, compliance, and stiffness that were different from the normotensive group. It is doubtful whether assessment of carotid artery structure and compliance is a sensitive indicator of early hypertensive damage.

Studies of the Brain

Early effects of hypertension on cerebrovascular structures are difficult to measure, but MRI studies can detect minor changes due to small vessel occlusive disease. The two most common cerebrovascular lesions detected by MRI in hypertensives are lacunae and periventricular white matter lesions. Lacunae are small infarcts, and hypertensive small vessel disease is believed to play a role in the genesis of periventricular white matter lesions.

One group has used these two MRI patterns as indicators of silent cerebrovascular disease and compared their prevalence in elderly patients with sustained and white-coat hypertension and normotensives.[30] None of the study subjects had a history of overt stroke. They underwent ambulatory blood pressure monitoring and MRI of the brain, as well as office blood pressure measurements. From the overall group of 73 patients, three age-matched groups were defined as follows: (1) sustained hypertensives ($n = 26$; office blood pressure $\geq$ 140/90 mm Hg; 24-hour blood pressure $\geq$ 135/80 mm Hg); (2) white-coat hypertensives ($n = 14$; office blood pressure $\geq$ 140/90 mm Hg; 24-hour blood pressure < 135/80 mm Hg); and (3) normotensives ($n = 28$; office blood pressure < 140/90 mm Hg; 24-hour blood pressure < 135/80 mm Hg). MRI studies were graded by a neuroradiologist unaware of the blood pressure data. The number of lacunae and the grade of periventricular white matter hyperintensities were similar in the white-coat hypertensive and normotensive groups and significantly less than in the sustained hypertensive group. This was true even though the white-coat hypertensive group had higher diastolic ambulatory blood pressure than the normotensive group.

CONCOMITANT CARDIOVASCULAR RISK FACTORS

Additional cardiovascular risk factors are common in patients with sustained hypertension. Therefore, several authors have measured cardiovascular risk factors in white-coat hypertensives. Pierdominico and associates[46] and Marchesi and coworkers[48] found no metabolic derangements among white-coat hypertensives, but Weber and associates[36] found that white-coat hypertensives had slightly higher insulin, renin, aldosterone, and norepinephrine levels than did normotensives. Similar metabolic perturbations were described in the white-coat hypertensive group of the Tecumseh study.[49] However, in this study, the difference in home blood pressure and office blood pressure was the criterion used to define the white-coat group, and ambulatory blood pressures were not performed.

PROGNOSTIC STUDIES USING AMBULATORY BLOOD PRESSURE MONITORING

No truly prospective morbidity and mortality endpoint studies have been completed using ambulatory blood pressure as a guide to antihypertensive therapy. There are, however, two studies using ambulatory and office blood pressures at one point in time and then retrospectively ascertaining cardiovascular outcomes several years later.[50, 51] Despite these limitations and the conflicting data presented previously, these studies provide some reassurance that the long-term risk of white-coat hypertension may not greatly exceed that of normotensives.

Perloff and coworkers[50] used a patient-activated ambulatory blood pressure monitor to study daytime blood pressure in 1076 hypertensive patients. Ambulatory blood pressure was referenced according to the regression equation of clinic versus ambulatory blood pressure for all subjects. The residual around this line of regression was calculated from the observed and the predicted blood pressure. Using a Cox proportional hazards model and controlling for a number of other clinical variables, the authors found that the patients in whom ambulatory blood pressure was significantly lower than clinic blood pressure had a lower risk of a cardiovascular event. This finding was true for patients both with and without a previous cardiovascular event. However, there was no normotensive control group in this study, making its results somewhat inconclusive.

Verdecchia and colleagues[51] studied 1187 patients with newly diagnosed essential hypertension and 205 healthy normotensive subjects and, then, after a mean of 3.2 years, retrospectively obtained cardiovascular endpoints. They defined the white-coat hypertension cutoff as daytime ambulatory blood pressure less than 136/87 mm Hg for men and less than 131/86 mm Hg for women. Subjects were followed by their own physicians with the goal of reducing their office blood pressure to less than 140/90 mm Hg. The ambulatory blood pressure data were available to the physicians but likely played only a small role in their management. At the time of the study, telephone interviewers unaware of the ambulatory blood pressure results assessed the cardiovascular complications of hypertension. Complete follow-up data were obtained on 99.1% of subjects who had initially been studied with both office and ambulatory blood pressure monitoring. Combined cardiovascular morbidity and mortality per 100 patient-years were 0.47 in the normotensive group (4 events in 205 subjects), 0.49 in the white-coat hypertension group (3 events in 228 subjects), 1.79 in dippers with ambulatory hypertension (37 events in 693 subjects), and 4.99 in nondippers with ambulatory hypertension (45 events in 266 subjects) (Fig. 32–3).

To conduct a trial to evaluate the risk of white-coat

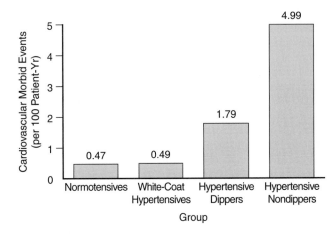

Figure 32–3. Incidence of major cardiovascular morbid events in four categories of patients: normotensives, white-coat hypertensives, hypertensive dippers, and hypertensive nondippers. (Adapted from Verdecchia P, Porcellati C, Schillaci G, et al. Ambulatory blood pressure: An independent predictor of prognosis in essential hypertension. Hypertension 24:793–801, 1994.)

hypertension is a complex matter. Because event rates are low in this group of patients,[51] the study would have to be large and have extended follow-up to show significant differences compared with normotensives. Furthermore, pharmacological therapy of white-coat hypertension may lead to reductions of office but not ambulatory blood pressure,[52, 53] further complicating the ability to conduct the trial and interpret the results.

BLOOD PRESSURE EVOLUTION IN UNTREATED PATIENTS WITH WHITE-COAT HYPERTENSION

The natural history of white-coat hypertensives is not well known. One approach has been to follow untreated patients over several years to see whether ambulatory blood pressure increases over time or whether a surrogate marker of hypertension (e.g., left ventricular mass) changes. If white-coat hypertension is a prehypertensive state, subjects should evolve into sustained hypertensives over time in excess of an age-matched normotensive group and may show increases in left ventricular mass. Polonia and associates[54] prospectively evaluated 36 untreated patients with white-coat hypertension (office blood pressure > 140/90 mm Hg; awake blood pressure < 132/84 mm Hg) and a control group of 52 normotensives (clinic blood pressure < 140/90 mm Hg; awake blood pressure < 132/84 mm Hg). Subjects underwent repeat ambulatory and office blood pressure studies after a mean interval of 3.5 years. The two groups showed similar rates of evolution to sustained hypertension (22% and 15%, respectively). Seventeen of the original 58 patients studied at baseline had been started on drug therapy, making it difficult to determine whether they remained in the white-coat hypertensive group or evolved into sustained hypertensives.

White and coworkers[55] reported similar results, showing that when a restrictive definition of white-coat hypertension is used (awake ambulatory blood pressure < 135/85 mm

Hg), the rate of evolution to sustained hypertension is similar to that in age-matched normotensives (12% versus 15%). Verdecchia and colleagues[56] repeated clinic and ambulatory blood pressure and echocardiographic cardiac evaluation on 83 untreated subjects defined with white-coat hypertension after a mean period of 2.5 years. They found that 37% of the patients became ambulatory hypertensives. In the group that evolved into sustained hypertension, there was a rise in left ventricular mass of 6.2%, whereas in the patients that remained in the white-coat hypertensive group, there was a small decrease in left ventricular mass. This study had no control group, so the proportion of age-matched normotensives who evolved into sustained hypertension could not be ascertained. Other authors have found a high rate of progression from white-coat to sustained hypertension, but this study suffers from liberal definition of white-coat hypertension and lack of a control group.[57]

COST-EFFECTIVENESS OF SCREENING FOR WHITE-COAT HYPERTENSION

If white-coat hypertensives can avoid drug therapy, their identification may result in reductions in the cost and adverse effects of antihypertensive medications. Some work shows that this is possible if only borderline hypertensives are studied and the cost of the ambulatory monitoring is minimized.[11, 58–60]

CONCLUSIONS

The final commentary on the prognosis of white-coat hypertension cannot be written today. Nevertheless, most investigators in the field agree to a few general principles concerning the care of patients with white-coat hypertension. A strict definition is necessary to avoid misclassification of patients as white-coat hypertensives when they are actually sustained hypertensives. The best defense against this starts with multiple office blood pressure measurements obtained in a standardized fashion. Ambulatory blood pressure criteria should use conservative cutoffs and include both systolic and diastolic parameters (e.g., daytime blood pressure < 130/80 mm Hg). Lastly, although there are conflicting data in the cross-sectional studies performed to date, the two completed studies with cardiovascular events as endpoints suggest a relatively benign prognosis for white-coat hypertensives; no studies have shown a worse outcome. It is, therefore, prudent to monitor such patients closely and reinforce lifestyle modifications while we await the results of a prospective trial of subjects with white-coat hypertension.

References

1. Pickering TG. Ambulatory monitoring and blood pressure variability. London, Science Press, 1991.
2. Mansoor GA, White WB. Ambulatory blood pressure and cardiovascular risk stratification. J Vasc Med Biol 5:61–68, 1994.
3. Pickering TG. A review of national guidelines on the clinical use of ambulatory blood pressure monitoring. Blood Press Monit 1:151–156, 1996.
4. Mansoor GA, White WB. Contribution of ambulatory blood pressure monitoring to the design and analysis of antihypertensive therapy trials. J Cardiovasc Risk 1:136–142, 1994.
5. Ayman D, Goldshine AD. Blood pressure determination by patients with essential hypertension: The difference between clinical and home readings before treatment. Am J Med Sci 200:465–470, 1940.
6. Gosse P, Bougaleb M, Egloff P, et al. Clinical significance of white-coat hypertension. J Hypertens 12(suppl 8):S43–S47, 1994.
7. Verdecchia P, Schillaci F, Zampi I, Porcellati C. Variability between current definitions of normal ambulatory blood pressure. Hypertension 20:555–562, 1992.
8. Verdecchia P, Schillaci G, Borgioni C, et al. White coat hypertension and white coat effect. Am J Hypertens 8:790–798, 1995.
9. Palatini P, Mormino P, Santonastaso M, et al, on behalf of the HARVEST Investigators. Target-organ damage in stage I hypertensive subjects with white-coat hypertension and sustained hypertension. Hypertension 31:57–63, 1998.
10. Pickering TG, James GD, Boddie C, et al. How common is white coat hypertension? JAMA 259:225–228, 1988.
11. Pierdomenico SD, Mezzetti A, Lapenna D, et al. White-coat hypertension in patients with newly diagnosed hypertension: Evaluation of prevalence by ambulatory monitoring and impact on cost of health care. Eur Heart J 16:692–697, 1995.
12. Waeber B, Jacot des Combes B, Porchet M, et al. Ambulatory blood pressure recording to identify truly hypertensive patients who truly need therapy. J Chron Dis 37:5–57, 1984.
13. Siegel WC, Blumenthal JA, Divine GW. Physiological, psychological, and behavioral factors and white coat hypertension. Hypertension 16:140–146, 1990.
14. Staessen JA, Byttebier G, Buntinx F, et al. Antihypertensive treatment based on conventional or ambulatory blood pressure measurement: A randomized controlled trial. JAMA 278:1065–1072, 1997.
15. Pieper C, Warren K, Pickering TG. A comparison of ambulatory blood pressure and heart rate at home and work on work and non-work days. J Hypertens 11:177–183, 1993.
16. Pearce KA, Grimm RH, Rao S, et al. Population-derived comparisons of ambulatory and office blood pressures. Arch Intern Med 152:750–756, 1992.
17. Parati G, Omboni S, Staessen J, et al, on behalf of the SYST-EUR Investigators. Limitations of the difference between clinic and daytime blood pressure as a surrogate measure of the white-coat effect. J Hypertens 16:23–29, 1998.
18. Lerman CE, Brody DS, Hui T, et al. The white-coat hypertension response: Prevalence and predictors. J Gen Intern Med 4:226–231, 1989.
19. Cardillo C, De Felice F, Campia U, Folli G. Psychophysiological reactivity and cardiac end-organ changes in white coat hypertension. Hypertension 21:836–844, 1993.
20. Ruddy MC, Bialy GB, Malka ES, et al. The relationship of plasma renin activity to clinic and ambulatory blood pressure in elderly people with isolated systolic hypertension. J Hypertens 6(suppl 6):S412–S415, 1988.
21. Nakao M, Shimosawa T, Nomura S, et al. Mental arithmetic is a useful diagnostic evaluation in white-coat hypertension. Am J Hypertens 11:41–45, 1998.
22. Donner-Branzhoff N, Chan Y, Szalai JP, Hilditch J. Is the clinic-home blood pressure difference associated with psychological distress? A primary care–based study. J Hypertens 15:585–590, 1997.
23. Carels RA, Sherwood A, Blumenthal JA. High anxiety and white-coat hypertension. JAMA 279:197–198, 1998.
24. Myers MG, Reeves RA. White coat phenomenon in patients receiving antihypertensive therapy. Am J Hypertens 4:844–849, 1991.
25. Mansoor GA, McCabe EJ, White WB. Determinants of the white-coat effect in hypertensive subjects. J Hum Hypertens 10:87–92, 1996.
26. Thijs L, Amery A, Clement D, et al. Ambulatory blood pressure monitoring in elderly patients with isolated systolic hypertension. J Hypertens 10:693–699, 1992.
27. Mansoor GA, White WB. The patient with an exaggerated white-coat effect. Blood Press Monit 1:75–79, 1996.
28. Mancia G, Parati G, Pomidossi G, et al. Alerting reaction and rise in blood pressure during measurement by physician and nurse. Hypertension 9:209–215, 1987.
29. Veerman DP, van Montfrans GA. Nurse-measured or ambulatory blood pressure in routine hypertension care. J Hypertens 11:287–292, 1993.
30. Shimada K, Kawamoto A, Matsubayashi K, Ozawa T. Silent cerebro-

vascular disease in the elderly: Correlation with ambulatory blood pressure. Hypertension 16:692–699, 1990.

31. White WB, Schulman P, McCabe EJ, Dey HM. Average daily blood pressure, not office blood pressure, determines cardiac function in patients with hypertension. JAMA 26:873–877, 1989.

32. Glen SK, Elliott HL, Curzio JL, et al. White-coat hypertension as a cause of cardiovascular dysfunction. Lancet 348:654–657, 1996.

33. Cavallini MC, Roman MJ, Pickering TG, et al. Is white coat hypertension associated with arterial disease or left ventricular hypertrophy? Hypertension 26:413–419, 1995.

34. Hoegholm A, Kristensen KS, Bang LE, et al. Left ventricular mass and geometry in patients with established hypertension and white-coat hypertension. Am J Hypertens 6:282–286, 1993.

35. Rizzo V, Cicconetti P, Bianchi A, et al. White-coat hypertension and cardiac organ damage in elderly subjects. J Hum Hypertens 10:293–298, 1996.

36. Weber MA, Neutel JM, Smith DHG, Graettinger WF. Diagnosis of mild hypertension by ambulatory blood pressure monitoring. Circulation 90:2291–2298, 1994.

37. Kuwajima I, Suzuki Y, Fujisawa A, Koramoto K. Is white-coat hypertension innocent? Hypertension 22:826–831, 1993.

38. Soma J, Wideroe TE, Dahl K, et al. Left ventricular systolic and diastolic function assessed with two-dimensional and Doppler echocardiography in white-coat hypertension. J Am Coll Cardiol 28:190–196, 1996.

39. Palatini P, Penzo M, Canali C, et al. Interactive action of the white-coat effect and the blood pressure levels on the cardiovascular complications in hypertension. Am J Med 103:208–216, 1997.

40. Cuspidi C, Marabini M, Lonati L, et al. Cardiac and carotid structure in patients with established hypertension and white-coat hypertension. J Hypertens 13:1707–1711, 1995.

41. Ferrara LA, Guida L, Pasanisi F, et al. Isolated office hypertension and end-organ damage. J Hypertens 15:979–985, 1997.

42. Pose-Reino A, Gonzalez-Juanatey JR, Pastor C, et al. Clinical implications of the white-coat hypertension. Blood Press 5:264–273, 1996.

43. Gosse P, Promax H, Durandet P, Clementy J. White coat hypertension: No harm for the heart. Hypertension 22:766–770, 1993.

44. White WB, Schulman P, Dey HM, Katz AM. Effects of age and 24-hour ambulatory blood pressure on rapid left ventricular filling. Am J Cardiol 63:1343–1347, 1989.

45. Hoegholm A, Bang LE, Kristensen KS, et al. Microalbuminuria in 411 untreated individuals with established hypertension, white-coat hypertension, and normotension. Hypertension 24:101–105, 1994.

46. Pierdomenico SD, Lapenna D, Guglielmi MD, et al. Target organ status and serum lipids in patients with white-coat hypertension. Hypertension 26:801–807, 1995.

47. Burnier M, Biollaz J, Magnin JL, et al. Renal sodium handling in patients with untreated hypertension and white-coat hypertension. Hypertension 23:496–502, 1993.

48. Marchesi E, Perani G, Falaschi F, et al. Metabolic risk factors in white-coat hypertensives. J Hum Hypertens 8:475–479, 1994.

49. Julius S, Mejia A, Jones K, et al. White-coat verus sustained borderline hypertension in Tecumseh, Michigan. J Hypertens 16:617–623, 1990.

50. Perloff D, Sokolow M, Cowan RM, Juster RP. Prognostic value of ambulatory blood pressure measurements: Further analyses. J Hypertens 7(suppl 3):S3–S10, 1989.

51. Verdecchia P, Porcellati C, Schillaci G, et al. Ambulatory blood pressure: An independent predictor of prognosis in essential hypertension. Hypertension 24:793–801, 1994.

52. Waeber B, Heynen G, Brunner HR. Analysis of ambulatory blood pressure monitoring: The problem of white-coat hypertension, responders and non-responders. Blood Press Monit 1:289–291, 1996.

53. Hoegholm A, Wiinberg N, Kristensen KS. The effect of antihypertensive treatment with dihydropyridine calcium antagonists on white-coat hypertension. Blood Press Monit 1:375–382, 1996.

54. Polonia JJ, Santos AR, Gama GM, et al. Follow-up clinic and ambulatory blood pressure in untreated white-coat hypertensive patients. Blood Press Monit 2:289–295, 1997.

55. White WB, Daragjati C, Mansoor GA, McCabe EJ. The management and follow up of patients with white-coat hypertension. Blood Press Monit 1(suppl 2):S33–S36, 1996.

56. Verdecchia P, Schillaci G, Borgioni C, et al. Identification of subjects with white-coat hypertension and persistently normal ambulatory blood pressure. Blood Press Monit 1:217–222, 1996.

57. Bidlingemeyer I, Burnier M, Bidlingemeyer M, et al. Isolated office hypertension: A prehypertensive state? J Hypertens 14:327–332, 1996.

58. Krakoff LR, Schechter C, Fahs M, Andre M. Ambulatory blood pressure monitoring: Is it cost-effective? J Hypertens 9(suppl 8):S28–S30, 1991.

59. Krakoff LR, Eison H, Phillips RH, et al. Effect of ambulatory blood pressure monitoring on the diagnosis and cost of treatment for mild hypertension. Am Heart J 116:1152–1154, 1988.

60. Sheps SG. Cost considerations of ambulatory blood pressure monitoring. J Hypertens 8(suppl 6):S29–S31, 1990.

SECTION 5

Treatment—General Considerations

33 Outcomes in Treating Hypertension

CHAPTER

Michael A. Weber and Paul Radensky

Hypertension is the most common chronic condition that physicians deal with. Indeed, the very frequency with which this diagnosis is made has led some physicians to discount its importance, and in some primary care practices, responsibility for managing this condition is often handed off to nonphysician personnel. The concept of hypertension appears straightforward. The measurement of blood pressure and the diagnosis of hypertension are relatively simple tasks, and there are a broad range of pharmacological agents and lifestyle modifications known to be helpful in controlling blood pressure. Moreover, it is now widely recognized, by both professionals and the lay public, that effective treatment of hypertension should result in a reduction in clinical cardiovascular events.

Frustratingly, this apparently simple goal is rarely attained. Even though a majority of the people with high blood pressure have been diagnosed, a large number of them are poorly treated or not treated at all. And despite the large number of efficacious agents in a variety of drug classes, it is still often quite difficult to reduce blood pressure to desirable levels. Even when this is achieved, symptomatic side effects or other complaints often jeopardize the long-term control of blood pressure.

Achieving meaningful patient compliance with antihypertensive therapy, especially beyond the initial treatment period, remains a daunting challenge. Despite clinical trials in hypertension that have shown encouraging reductions in such clinical endpoints as strokes and heart failure, coronary events—which remain the most common adverse outcome of hypertension—have been reduced only modestly.

It is clear that we are still confronting problems and unmet needs in the overall management of hypertension. In planning and assessing our attempts in this area, we are motivated by the need to provide long-term protection against major cardiovascular events. In devising strategies for individual patients, we must be guided by intermediate measures that can inform us whether our therapy is having the desired effects on the heart, kidneys, and other vital areas of the circulation.

But before we can even begin to assess these intermediate goals, we must first develop short-term strategies that will allow patients to start both treatment and the lifelong process of cardiovascular protection. This chapter reviews some of the principal short-term, intermediate, and long-term outcomes in hypertension treatment and discusses some of the strategies and issues involved in achieving these outcomes.

WHY TREAT HYPERTENSION?

Historically, hypertension was first recognized as a serious consequence of acute renal disease, often leading rapidly to fatal cardiovascular events. Malignant hypertension, of renal or nonrenal origins, dramatically reduced survival. More recently, data from life insurance and epidemiological sources have indicated that even mild forms of hypertension are predictive of cardiovascular events. The data in Figure 33–1 show that there are meaningful increases in risk at blood pressures as low as 140/90 mm Hg.[1]

Clinical trials have confirmed that treating hypertension reduces events. Although early studies with moderate or severe forms of hypertension showed the most dramatic benefits,[2] more recent studies in mild hypertension have also shown positive effects on clinical outcomes.[3, 4] The benefits of treatment are very evident in the elderly.[5, 6] Recently, much attention has been given to the economics of hypertension therapy. Although definitive economic models are still being established, long-term antihypertensive treatment appears to be a cost-effective undertaking.

A Broader Challenge

Hypertension is more than just a problem of high blood pressure alone. As shown in Table 33–1, it is a syndrome of metabolic and cardiovascular abnormalities.[7, 8] Further,

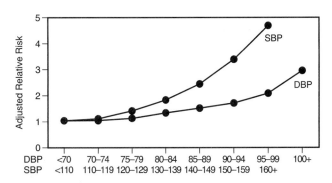

Figure 33–1. Adjusted relative risk of cardiovascular mortality in men screened for the Multiple Risk Factor Intervention Trial (MRFIT). SBP, systolic blood pressure; DBP, diastolic blood pressure. (Adapted from National High Blood Pressure Education Program Working Group. Report on primary prevention of hypertension. Arch Intern Med 153:186–208, 1993. Copyright 1993, American Medical Association.)

Table 33–1 Hypertension: A Syndrome of Abnormalities

High blood pressure
Increased susceptibility to the consequences of lipid
    abnormalities
Glucose intolerance and insulin resistance
Decreased renal function reserve
Altered left ventricular structure and function
Altered compliance of proximal and distal arteries

abnormalities in lipid, glucose, and insulin metabolism, as well as in left ventricular structure and function and renal function, appear to be inherited.[9] Careful management of these concomitant risk factors inevitably becomes part of overall hypertension treatment and must be included in clinical and economic outcome measures.

A second issue is the so-called coronary hypothesis,[10] which explains the high incidence of cardiac events in hypertensive patients on the basis of early intrinsic vascular abnormalities—probably genetically determined—that are exaggerated by concomitant risk factors and by the high blood pressure itself (Fig. 33–2). This model of hypertension indicates that optimal long-term prognosis for hypertensive patients requires treatment with multiple attributes. Ideally, antihypertensive drugs should have antiproliferative or other properties that can inhibit the vascular changes of atherosclerosis. In addition, they should not adversely affect metabolic parameters while lowering blood pressure effects. Although blood pressure reduction obviously is a critical first step or short-term outcome in hypertensive management, awareness of desirable intermediate and long-term outcomes inevitably must influence the selection of agents used for the control of blood pressure.

MEASURING OUTCOMES

Strategies to improve the prognosis of the hypertensive patient incorporate a number of scientific and practical short- and long-term issues. Consideration of the third National Health and Nutrition Examination Survey (NHANES III) data by the sixth report of the Joint National Committee on the Prevention, Detection, Evaluation, and Treatment of High Blood Pressure (JNC VI)[11] revealed that

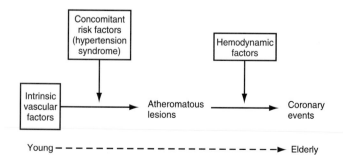

Figure 33–2. Coronary hypothesis. The high incidence of cardiac events in hypertensive patients is explained on the basis of early intrinsic abnormalities that are exaggerated by concomitant risk factors and by high blood pressure itself.

less than one quarter of hypertensive patients in the United States have blood pressures below 140/90 mm Hg and indicated that substantial attention must be focused on near-term outcomes. This also implies that important gains may be made by improving care of currently treated hypertensives as well as by screening for unidentified hypertensive patients.

It is axiomatic that outcomes must be measurable. It is also clear that blood pressure itself is only one of the short-term outcome measures. A variety of clinical and economic issues affect not only patients and doctors but also health plans, insurers, and the employers or government agencies that often pay for the care.

Short-Term Outcome Measures

The first few weeks or months of antihypertensive treatment are critical in overall management. During this preliminary period, physicians select or change drugs, titrate doses, and provide support and guidance in any of the lifestyle modifications that might have been selected. Keeping patients in therapy is pivotal. Beyond the blood pressure effects of treatment, physicians must also monitor symptomatic adverse effects, laboratory tests, and any other factors that might affect the success of the treatment program. In essence, the goal of spending short-term resources is to reduce long-term expenditures, although the effectiveness of this undertaking is difficult to assess.

The principal outcomes that are relevant and quantifiable during this first stage of treatment are listed in Table 33–2. They are described briefly in the following sections.

Blood Pressure

Control of blood pressure appears to be the most simple and obvious of all the outcome measures in treating hypertension. Recent publications have added even more emphasis to achieving blood pressure target values during treatment. The Hypertension Optimal Treatment (HOT) trial[12] has shown that patients whose diastolic blood pressures were reduced to the low 80s appeared to have a somewhat reduced frequency of clinical events when compared with those patients whose pressures were in the higher 80s. This was particularly true for hypertensives who also had diabetes. Another example is preservation of renal function, which appears to be best achieved when blood pressure is reduced below 125/75 mm Hg.[13] Not surprisingly, JNC VI[11] advocates that whereas blood pressure should be reduced to less than 140/90 mm Hg in uncomplicated hypertension, goals below 130/85 mm Hg are more appropriate for patients with major concomitant conditions or evidence for target organ damage. So, the easily measured short-term outcome of blood pressure lowering itself has reemerged as one of the most pivotal assessments of overall hypertension management.

Most physicians depend on blood pressure obtained during routine visits to the office or clinic, but readings obtained during such visits—often only a few hours after drug dosing—may not give an accurate portrayal of whether drugs are providing true 24-hour efficacy. Measuring blood pressure at the end of the dosing interval (most

Table 33–2 Short-Term Outcome Measures	
Outcome	How Measured
Blood pressure Office Indices of 24-hr efficacy	Numerical values (direct measure)
Symptomatic side effects	Present or absent Mild/moderate/severe or analogue scale
Quality of life: patient Perception of spouses or others	Numerical values: patients
Compliance with treatment	Yes/no Percentage achievement of optimal performance Drug utilization, self-reported Timely prescription refills Adherence to clinical appointments
Lifestyle modifications	Numerical values (direct measure or self-reported) Yes/no Weight control Weekly aerobic exercise Alcohol reduction Smoking cessation
Routine clinical chemistries Electrolytes Renal function Glucose	Numerical values (measured variables)
Number of drugs taken	Numerical value (measured variables)
Frequency of physician visits Complexity of treatment	Numerical value (measured variables)
Frequency of clinical tests	
Total direct medial costs of treatment*	Numerical value (calculated)
Indirect costs of treatment Travel expenses Loss of productivity Increased insurance costs	Numerical value (calculated cost and direct measure)
Global evaluation: patient Subjective perception of satisfaction	Analogue scale
Global evaluation: physician Subjective perception of satisfaction	Analogue scale

*Costs: Drug cost + monitoring cost + side effects cost − savings in management of underlying disease.

conveniently by having patients arrive for an early morning appointment after omitting that morning's dose) can be helpful in making this determination. Ambulatory blood pressure monitoring studies have emphasized the importance of blood pressure control during the early morning hours when patients are most vulnerable to cardiovascular events. Another area of interest is in whether or not night-time blood pressure values fall substantially below daytime values. This is a normal physiological event, and patients who fail to exhibit this pattern—sometimes termed *nondippers*—are believed to be more vulnerable to adverse clinical events. There are not yet sufficiently strong data,

however, for clear treatment guidelines to be established in this area.

Symptomatic Side Effects

The presence or absence of physical or emotional complaints during drug therapy can readily be documented. It is difficult to numerically quantify the severity of individual complaints, but adverse drug effects may be accurately divided into those that are truly minor (not likely to jeopardize long-term adherence to therapy) and those that are more severe (of sufficient concern that a change in therapy is necessary).

Quality of Life

Quality of life during antihypertensive treatment is influenced by symptomatic adverse effects and other obvious consequences of treatment. It has recently emerged as a comprehensive and quantifiable concept. Quality of life not only includes measures of the sense of general well-being but additionally may take into account a relatively detailed assessment of function in the social, domestic, and work settings. Some of these measurements are sufficiently sensitive to discriminate quality of life differences among classes of antihypertensive drugs.[14] It is likely that the perception of spouses or close relatives and friends concerning quality of life and function during treatment may differ from that of the patients themselves. This may represent an equally important outcome measure.

Compliance With Treatment

This may be the single most important factor in determining the result of antihypertensive treatment. Half of all patients started on antihypertensive therapy are no longer regularly taking their medications by 12 months[15] and, in many instances, are no longer keeping their clinic appointments. This may reflect difficulty in motivating patients who have an asymptomatic disorder or who lack understanding of long-term cardiovascular risk. Adverse effects and the costs and inconvenience of treatment can also weaken patient compliance.

Precise measurement of adherence to drug regimens is difficult. Self-reporting by patients is the most simple and obvious approach, although monitoring the regularity of prescription refills provides a more objective criterion. An index termed *medication possession ratio* has been used by pharmacoeconomists to describe treatment compliance estimated by analysis of pharmacy dispensing records.[16]

Prescription drug claims records indicate that compliance is greatest for relatively short treatment lengths of about 2 months, but it tends to decline with greater lengths of treatment. Adherence to scheduled clinic visits represents another readily quantifiable measure of compliance with treatment.

Lifestyle Modifications

Physicians sometimes advise their patients on nonpharmacological strategies that can contribute to blood pressure control. Weight loss is an effective method for reducing blood pressure and is directly measured by the physician. More subtle dietary modifications, e.g., to decrease sodium or increase potassium intake, are more difficult to measure unless patients undertake meticulous urine sample collections or are carefully interviewed by professional dietitians. Reducing alcohol intake to no more than 2 drinks daily is a further strategy for decreasing blood pressure, but this probably can be measured only by patient self-reporting. Aerobic exercise is a helpful technique for improving blood pressure control and probably can be accurately quantified—typically in terms of the frequency and duration of exercise sessions—by conscientious patients. Smoking cessation clearly is a critical part of overall management of hypertensive patients, and success or failure in achieving this goal can be directly documented.

Routine Clinical Chemistries

A wide variety of laboratory tests are relevant for the evaluation of hypertensive patients, and these can identify potential cardiovascular risk factors with long-term prognostic importance. But in assessing short-term outcomes, chiefly the effects of drugs or other forms of treatment, the most relevant measures are plasma electrolytes, glucose, and the indices of renal function. Abnormalities in these values can be directly measured and should lead to appropriate adjustments in treatment or the addition of appropriate therapies (e.g., potassium supplements for patients with hypokalemia) to compensate for unwanted changes.

Number of Drugs Taken

This includes the drugs prescribed for the control of blood pressure as well as any additional agents required to address metabolic abnormalities (e.g., electrolytes, glucose, or lipids) that are part of the baseline picture or have been induced by the antihypertensive therapy. This measure of outcome is important in at least two ways: It reflects on the complexity of the treatment regimen that patients are dealing with, and it affects the overall cost of treatment.

Frequency of Physician Visits

As with recording the number of drugs used, the frequency of physician visits is a measure of the difficulty and complexity of managing a patient with hypertension. It is influenced by the need to adjust treatment—such as the use of multiple titration steps to achieve goal blood pressures, the need to respond to changes in laboratory measurements, and the need to change treatment in response to symptomatic complaints by the patient. Again, this outcome measure has clear cost implications.

Frequency of Laboratory Tests

This measure is influenced by abnormalities that might exist at baseline in individual patients or that might result from antihypertensive therapy. Obviously, patients known to have conditions such as diabetes mellitus or renal insufficiency, which commonly accompany hypertension, will be monitored more closely than patients with apparently uncomplicated hypertension. The use of agents such as diuretics that produce changes in electrolytes and other metabolic measurements will increase the need for laboratory monitoring, especially in older patients or those with cardiac conditions that are vulnerable to such changes. Laboratory tests can be time-consuming and inconvenient as well as being an additional cost factor, and these are a major issue if sophisticated blood tests, echocardiograms, or other procedures become indicated.

Total Direct Medical Costs of Treatment

In evaluating the treatment of hypertension, it is possible to measure the direct costs of treatment. These include physician visits, laboratory tests, and antihypertensive drugs or other agents that are required for overall management. In addition, unscheduled office or emergency room visits and the need for more intensive diagnostic evaluations are included in calculating the overall direct medical cost.

Other Costs of Treatment

This is a more difficult measure that depends on difficult to quantify factors, e.g., the cost to the patient of making office visits (travel expenses or the need to find babysitters) and of being absent from work (either loss of pay or the need to use vacation entitlements). Furthermore, apart from the personal consequences to the patient, time away from work (including time taken in traveling to and from the doctor's office as well as the time for the appointment itself) can have a disrupting effect in the workplace, causing adverse financial consequences to employers and a loss of productivity that affects society as a whole.

Global Evaluation

Patient. This is an important concept, but again one that is difficult to quantify. Many factors play into a patient's perception of the success of treatment. Patients will be pleased that efficacious treatment is confronting an important risk factor, thereby reducing the likelihood of serious clinical events and potentially extending life. On the other hand, patients must take into account the costs, inconveniences, and discomforts of physician visits, laboratory tests, the need to take drugs on a long-term basis, and all the other commitments inherent in successful therapy. All of these issues can influence the patient's assessment of quality of life, which likely is the overall determining factor in patient satisfaction with treatment.

Patients are aware that a diagnosis of hypertension, despite the reassurances and optimism provided by the physician, is somehow indicative of a condition that takes away their right to describe themselves as being in "good health." Patients can be apprehensive that taking antihypertensive treatment, or being labeled as *hypertensive,* might affect their ability to buy life or health insurance and might even jeopardize their promotions to higher responsibilities at work. Although it is possible to have patients grade their perceptions on a continuous scale (e.g., a numerical analogue scale ranging from "highly dissatisfied" to "highly satisfied"), this area requires more research before we can have full confidence in the validity of numerical values.

Physician. The physician will be influenced by the success of therapy, in terms of both blood pressure–lowering efficacy and adverse effect profile. The physician may also be influenced by issues of cost. Physicians are sensitive to the degree of satisfaction with treatment expressed by their patients. Moreover, as we increase our understanding of the scientific issues that underlie hypertension and its cardiovascular consequences, physicians are intensifying their search for drugs or other forms of therapy that have the greatest potential for preventing vascular pathology as well as controlling hypertension and other clinical abnormalities. As with patients, the overall sense of satisfaction by physicians is complex and, until better understood, is probably best measured by simple scales such as those proposed for quantifying patient satisfaction.

Intermediate Outcome Measures

After the first few months of antihypertensive care, during which relatively frequent adjustments of treatment typically occur, patients move into a chronic phase. Because the ultimate effect of treatment on the incidence of major events or death cannot be gauged for several years, it is useful to have intermediate indices that provide guidance in determining whether treatment appears likely to achieve its protective goals. These intermediate outcome measures can be obtained typically after 6 months or more of antihypertensive treatment and are listed in Table 33–3. It must be emphasized that a firm causal link between intermediate outcomes and long-term clinical events has not been fully established in hypertension, although most experts in the field of hypertension regard these surrogates as useful predictors.

All Short-Term Clinical and Economic Outcomes

The measurements entailed in determining short-term outcomes remain relevant during the chronic phase of treatment and, thus, should be included in assessments of intermediate outcomes.

Concomitant Metabolic Risk Factors

Hypertension usually is a syndrome of metabolic and cardiovascular abnormalities, commonly including disorders of the lipid profile and glucose tolerance. Dealing with these abnormalities should be part of the overall management strategy. In addition, there can be treatment-induced abnormalities in these parameters, such as those produced by diuretics. The longer-term goals of treatment, however, must include reversal of metabolic abnormalities or, at the very least, an absence of deterioration. Thus, measurements of the lipid profile and of indices of glucose metabolism, such as fasting glucose or glycosylated hemoglobin, are important in assessing the status of concomitant coronary risk factors.

Table 33–3 Intermediate Outcome Measures

Outcome	How Measured
All short-term clinical and economic outcomes	See Table 33–1
Concomitant metabolic risk factors Lipid profile Glucose tolerance, HbA_{1C}	Numerical values (direct measure)
Renal outcome measures Renal function Proteinuria/microalbuminuria	Numerical values (direct measure)
Cardiac outcomes: ischemia	Present/absent: yes/no New findings: yes/no ECG changes
Cardiac outcomes: left ventricular structure and function	Numerical values (direct measure) Yes/no ECHO left ventricular mass Doppler diastolic function ECG left ventricular hypertrophy
Cardiac outcomes: arrhythmias	Present/absent Numerical values Symptoms ECG/ambulatory monitoring
Arterial compliance Noninvasive estimates of arterial stiffness	Numerical values (direct measure)
Clinical evidence of atherosclerosis	Present/absent: yes/no (or measure of severity of vascular changes) New-onset angina pectoris Findings of carotid stenosis Renovascular findings Changes in optic fundi
Patient days lost from work	Numerical value (measured variable)
Health resources utilization Related hospitalizations Clinic visits Advanced imaging or other tests	Numerical value

Abbreviations: HbA_{1C}, hemoglobin A_{1C}; ECG, electrocardiogram; ECHO, echocardiogram.

Renal Outcome Measures

Renal function can be assessed through measurements of plasma creatinine concentrations or creatinine clearance. Because of variability in these values, sequential measurements over a period of several months or years are helpful in establishing trends in renal function. Measurements of proteinuria or microalbuminuria are useful intermediate-term indices of renal function, especially as they appear to be predictive of long-term prognosis.

Cardiac Outcomes

Ischemia. The electrocardiogram (ECG) is a cost-effective method for determining the presence of myocardial ischemia during treatment of hypertension. Findings with this technique are not always specific, but at least the appearance of new abnormalities can be helpful in justifying the use of more sophisticated methods for evaluating coronary status. The ECG outcome measure is probably best expressed simply as the presence or absence of ischemic changes.

Left Ventricular Structure and Function. Left ventricular hypertrophy (LVH) occurs early in hypertension and is an independent predictor of cardiovascular events. LVH can be detected by the conventional ECG, but this method is less sensitive than echocardiography in diagnosing LVH.[17] Moreover, whereas the ECG simply provides a yes/no decision on LVH, echocardiography gives a numerical value of left ventricular muscle mass that can be used to measure trends during treatment. Doppler measurements allow quantification of mitral valve flow characteristics that can be used as an index of left ventricular diastolic function. As with LVH, abnormalities of diastolic function appear early in hypertension and changes can be monitored during treatment.

Arrhythmias. Arrhythmias, especially ectopic activity, are often associated with LVH or ischemia and are relatively common in hypertension. Sometimes, the arrhythmias produce symptoms, but more often, they are noted during physical examination or by ECG. As a simple outcome measure, it is possible to report on the presence or absence of arrhythmias. Ambulatory electrocardiography (Holter monitoring) would more precisely quantify the extent of rhythm abnormality but is not practical in routine hypertension care. Nor is it generally cost-effective, since in most cases, it is unlikely to lead to a beneficial intervention.

Arterial Compliance

Although studies of arteries in human hypertension do not as yet predict long-term events, the potential value of such measurements seems great. The molecular biology that anchors the coronary hypothesis of hypertension indicates that early proliferative and structural changes in the vasculature are a critical characteristic of hypertension that predict pathological changes and clinical episodes.[18] The development of reproducible and noninvasive measurements of arterial compliance appears to represent a logical and valuable outcome measure that, as with other relevant intermediate cardiovascular indices, can be used to monitor the effects of therapy.

Evidence for Clinical Atherosclerosis

Although the presence of atheromatous lesions, even in the coronary circulation, does not reliably predict when or whether major events will occur, clinical estimates of atherosclerosis are useful indicators of the success of antihypertensive therapy. In the absence of invasive imaging, simple clinical findings can be employed, such as the onset of clinical angina pectoris or other symptoms of ischemic heart disease. Likewise, clinical findings or symptoms suggestive of carotid disease are key findings.

Indirect clinical observations, such as a worsening of

blood pressure control, can be indicative of renal artery stenosis, a common and prognostically important form of atheromatous disease in hypertension. Examination of the optic fundi, albeit assessing a different type of circulation than the medium-sized arteries, is a further index. It could be argued, of course, that such clear clinical findings as new-onset angina pectoris or carotid symptoms could be regarded as long-term events rather than intermediate outcomes. Such findings should be anticipated throughout hypertension treatment.

Patient Days Lost From Work

This is a quantifiable economic outcome measure that may have a different basis during intermediate or long-term therapy than during the initial phase. During short-term treatment, it is likely that patient days lost from work largely reflect the time consumed in clinic visits or other activities associated with the initiation of therapy and achieving satisfactory blood pressure control. During longer-term treatment, it is more likely that days lost from work reflect complications of hypertension or adverse effects of the antihypertensive treatment itself. It could also reflect patient self-perceptions because hypertensive patients tend to have excessive sensitivity regarding their vulnerability to illness and, thereby, a tendency to be more self-protective during times of relatively minor ailments.

Health Resources Utilization

This depends chiefly on the office management of the hypertension. However, a certain percentage of patients will require additional hospital or other medical resources. This may be due to hypertension, or because these patients have increased exposure to health care professionals, it may reflect enhanced identification of unrelated problems. Thus, it is not always possible to quantify accurately the extent to which procedures or utilizations should be attributed to the hypertension. However, this type of outcome can be measured in a relatively straightforward fashion in monetary units.

Long-Term Outcome Measures

The goal of antihypertensive therapy is to prevent major cardiovascular events attributable to the hypertension syndrome. There is no clear definition of "success." In theory, antihypertensive therapy should be undertaken on a lifelong basis and can be proved to have achieved its goal only if a patient ultimately dies from a noncardiovascular cause and has not suffered a major cardiovascular event(s) during the course of treatment. Unlike short-term or intermediate outcomes, which can be measured in individual patients, long-term outcomes are best assessed from a population perspective. The principal measures, listed in Table 33–4, are as follows.

All Short-Term and Intermediate Clinical and Economic Outcomes

All the issues discussed previously as short-term and intermediate outcomes remain relevant during the full span

Table 33-4 Long-Term Outcome Measures	
Outcome	How Measured
All short-term and intermediate clinical and economic outcomes	Tables 33–1 and 33–2
Mortality Cardiovascular Noncardiovascular	Yes/no
Cardiac events Sudden death Myocardial infarction Angina pectoris Coronary artery bypass surgery Percutaneous transluminal coronary angioplasty Congestive heart failure Clinically significant arrhythmias	Yes/no

Cerebrovascular events	Yes/no
	Numerical value
	  Renal insufficiency
	  Renovascular disease

Aortic and peripheral vascular disease	Yes/no
Cost-effectiveness	Numerical value (calculated) Cost per year of life saved Cost of health resources Patient and indirect costs Costs of lost productivity

of therapy and, thus, also constitute long-term outcome measures.

Mortality

Death may be from either a cardiovascular cause, in which case it can be attributed—at least in part—to hypertension, or a noncardiovascular cause, in which case it could be assumed that antihypertensive therapy was effective during the patient's lifetime.

Cardiac Events

These outcomes generally are well defined and readily attributed to hypertension. The most common cardiac consequences of hypertension are sudden cardiac death, myocardial infarction, angina pectoris, a need for coronary bypass surgery or percutaneous transluminal coronary angioplasty, congestive heart failure, and clinically significant arrhythmias.

Cerebrovascular Events

Strokes, either hemorrhagic or thrombotic, are closely associated with hypertension. Clinical transient ischemic episodes are also associated with hypertension. There may be more subtle but equally important cerebrovascular outcomes of hypertension. For example, such conditions as multi-infarct dementia might be linked to inadequately managed hypertension.

Renal Events

Hypertension is one of the main causes of end-stage renal disease and is among the leading causes of disease in patients admitted to dialysis programs. This is especially true within the African American community. Renovascular disease, which leads not only to poorly controlled hypertension but also to renal insufficiency, is another result of hypertension.

Aortic and Peripheral Vascular Disease

These are further manifestations of the vascular abnormalities that characterize hypertension and, again, are readily diagnosed. Severe vascular outcomes rarely exist in just one part of the circulation, and patients with peripheral vascular or aortic disease are likely to have coronary or cerebrovascular insufficiency as well.

Cost-Effectiveness

This calculation is most readily performed in the long-term treatment context, for this allows adequate time to elapse to determine the costs of care and the effectiveness of that care in preventing or delaying major cardiovascular events or death. For cohorts of hypertensive patients sufficiently large to justify such statistics, it is possible to estimate the cost per year of life saved. Moreover, with the quality of life data and other information described earlier, it is possible to estimate the cost of quality-adjusted years of life saved. It is possible to make similar estimates of the cost of preventing major clinical events. Measuring long-term costs is highly complex and creates difficulties for health plan administrators responsible for figuring the true benefits of chronic therapy. Because hypertension is such a chronic condition and requires continuing interactions between patients and health care providers, the true costs are greater than can be attributed to health resources utilization. As discussed earlier, substantial costs are borne by the patient, the patient's family, and the patient's employer. These different financial risk holders inevitably will have their own perceptions of the cost-effectiveness of hypertension treatment.

PROS AND CONS OF OUTCOME MEASURES

The differing attributes of short-term, intermediate, and long-term outcomes of antihypertensive therapy are summarized in Table 33–5. As this chapter has stressed, only those outcomes that can be measured in an objective fashion have been included. Thus, all of the outcomes discussed can be measured and documented.

This approach to assessing hypertension does, however, have shortcomings. Even apparently successful achievement of short-term goals does not necessarily translate into success with intermediate or long-term measures. Moreover, accomplishment of such obvious early measures as blood pressure control itself may be regarded as an adequate endpoint, especially in a cost-sensitive environment, and the necessary resource investment to ensure long-term

Table 33–5 Attributes of Outcome Measures

	Pros	Cons
Long-term outcomes	Primary reason for treatment Clearly defined endpoints	Results not apparent for years or decades
Intermediate outcomes	Beneficial or adverse changes with treatment scientifically logical and readily measurable	Not proved that they are reliable surrogates for long-term outcomes Difficult to assess return on financial investment
Short-term outcomes	Well-defined measurements Readily assessed by primary care physicians Readily assessed by patients Inexpensive	Do not necessarily accomplish intermediate or long-term goals Concern that short-term success removes incentive to invest in longer-term management

protection may not be forthcoming. The situation is made more complex by the fact that even the intermediate outcome measures, interesting though they appear, do not necessarily predict long-term results.

Scientists and clinicians hypothesize that careful cardiovascular, renal, and metabolic measurements throughout the course of treatment provide helpful guidance and useful prognostic information; whereas health plan managers, motivated by a desire to limit spending, can point out that the treatment of hypertension is still a speculative and empirical undertaking and that the only proven strategy is the reduction of blood pressure.

SUMMARY

For the first time, JNC VI has classified treatment outcomes in hypertension under the headings of short-term, intermediate, and long-term. This allows a rational approach to evaluating hypertension at all stages of its management. The ultimate goal of treating hypertension is to prevent coronary disease, heart failure, strokes, and renal failure. But this long-term process inevitably must start with short-term goals. These include making an accurate diagnosis and selecting and modifying treatment to achieve desirable blood pressure control while avoiding unwanted symptomatic or metabolic effects. Preserving quality of life, satisfying both the patient and the physician, and achieving these goals in a cost-effective manner are all key components of the early phase of treatment. Because long-term protection typically takes several years to document, physicians and scientists must be guided by intermediate or surrogate endpoints. Measures of the structure and function of the heart, kidneys, and arteries are useful in this respect, as are measures of the lipid or glucose disorders that are commonly associated with the hypertension syndrome. The short-term, intermediate, and long-term outcomes of hypertension treatment all include objective and subjective evaluations by patients and physicians of clinical, personal, and economic factors. Outcome measures are of value only if they can be quantified in a specific fashion. National surveys in the United States have indicated that hypertension management frequently is suboptimal, and rigorous criteria for assessing the effectiveness of therapy in all its aspects are a necessary part of better understanding and caring for this condition. This chapter lists the principal outcome measures that can be employed to guide this task.

References

1. National High Blood Pressure Education Program Working Group. Report on primary prevention of hypertension. Arch Intern Med 153:186–208, 1993.
2. Veterans Administration Cooperative Study on Antihypertensive Agents. Effects of treatment on morbidity in hypertension. Results in patients with diastolic blood pressures averaging 115 through 129 mmHg. JAMA 202:1028–1034, 1967.
3. Australian Therapeutic Trial in Mild Hypertension. Report by the Management Committee. Lancet 1:1261–1267, 1980.
4. Medical Research Council Working Party. MRC trial of treatment in mild hypertension. Principal results. BMJ 291:97–104, 1985.
5. SHEP Cooperative Research Group. Prevention of stroke by antihypertensive drug treatment in older persons with isolated systolic hypertension: Final results of the Systolic Hypertension in the Elderly Program (SHEP). JAMA 265:3255–3264, 1991.
6. Dahlof B, Lundholm L, Hansson L, et al. Morbidity and mortality in the Swedish Trial in Old Patients with Hypertension (STOP-Hypertension). Lancet 338:1281–1285, 1991.
7. Naftilan AJ, Williams R, Burt D, et al. A lack of genetic linkage of renin gene restriction fragment length polymorphisms with human hypertension. Hypertension 14:614–618, 1989.
8. Weber MA, Smith DHG, Neutel JM, Graettinger WF. Cardiovascular and metabolic characteristics of hypertension. Am J Med 91:(suppl 1):1A–4S, 1991.
9. Neutel JM, Smith DHG, Graettinger WF, Weber MA. Heredity and hypertension. Impact on metabolic characteristics. Am Heart J 124:435–440, 1992.
10. Weber MA. Coronary heart disease and hypertension. Am J Hypertens 7(suppl):146S–153S, 1993.
11. Joint National Committee on Prevention, Detection, Evaluation and Treatment of High Blood Pressure. The sixth report. Arch Intern Med 157:2413–2446, 1997.
12. Hansson L, Zanchetti A, Carruthers SG, et al. Effects of intensive blood-pressure lowering and low-dose aspirin in patients with hypertension: Principal results of the Hypertension Optimal Treatment (HOT) randomised trial. HOT Study Group. Lancet 351:1755–1762, 1998.
13. Lazarus JM, Bourgoignie J, Buckalew VM, et al. Achievement and safety of a low blood pressure goal in chronic renal disease. The Modification of Diet in Renal Disease Study Group. Hypertension 29:641–650, 1997.
14. Croog SH, Levine S, Testa MA, et al. The effects of antihypertensive therapy on the quality of life. N Engl J Med 314:1657–1664, 1986.
15. Caldwell JR, Cobb S, Dowling MD, Dejongh D. The dropout problem in antihypertensive treatment. J Chron Dis 22:579–592, 1970.
16. Sclar DA, Skaer TL, Chin A, et al. Utility of a transdermal delivery system for antihypertensive therapy. Part 1. Am J Med 91(suppl):50S–56S, 1991.
17. Savage DD, Drayer JM, Henry WL, et al. Echocardiographic assessment of cardiac anatomy and function in hypertensive subjects. Circulation 59:623–632, 1979.
18. Weber MA. The changing focus of hypertension. Curr Opin Nephrol Hypertens 4:218–222, 1995.

34 Benefits of Treating Hypertension—Lessons From Clinical Trials

William J. Elliott and Henry R. Black

It is difficult for physicians practicing medicine near the year 2000 to understand the point of view expressed by experts less than 50 years ago, doubting whether lowering blood pressure (BP) would be not only possible but also beneficial in the long run. The main reasons why physicians and patients today are now convinced of the merits of lowering elevated BPs come directly from the results of randomized, blinded, prospective, multicenter, large clinical trials that have conclusively proved that active treatment with medications reduces cardiovascular risk.[1, 2]

In the 1950s and 1960s, there was emerging evidence from the Framingham Heart Study, other epidemiological surveys,[3] and several large insurance company databases that high BP is a powerful predictor of future cardiovascular events, especially stroke, acute myocardial infarction (MI), and death.[4, 5] Many, however, were less than favorably impressed with the few treatments available at that time to lower these "dangerous" BPs, since the armamentarium consisted mainly of a variety of low-salt diets, sedatives, *Rauwolfia* alkaloids, hydralazine, ganglionic-blocking agents, and/or mercurial diuretics. Great credit should be given to those in governmental organizations responsible for the public health (e.g., the National Institutes of Health and the Department of Veterans Affairs) who allocated resources and encouraged their constituents' participation in the now-classic clinical trials in hypertension that have proved that lowering BPs results in lower rates of serious cardiovascular events and even mortality from all causes.[6]

SHOULD DIASTOLIC HYPERTENSION BE TREATED?

There is abundant evidence from clinical trials that reducing elevated diastolic blood pressure (DBP) lowers cardiovascular risk. The impressive parade of data from placebo-controlled trials in diastolic hypertension are summarized in Table 34–1. These trials span the extremes of severity from the first Veterans' Administration study of patients with DBPs between 115 and 129 mm Hg after 6 days of inpatient hospitalization on a controlled-salt diet[7] to several nationwide studies of young patients with barely elevated DBPs (typically 90 to 99 mm Hg).[8, 9]

Perhaps because of the stronger and more direct relationship of stroke risk to easily understood hemodynamic factors (rupture of Charcot-Bouchard aneurysms due to chronic arterial wall stress from the barotrauma of higher perfusion pressure), as well as the multifactorial nature of atherosclerosis leading to coronary heart disease (which is also greatly affected by cigarette smoking, cholesterol, and diabetes, among other factors), it has been easier to demon-

strate reduced risk of cerebrovascular events than cardiac events with BP lowering. Recent meta-analyses of clinical trials have indicated that antihypertensive drug therapy lowers the risk of stroke by approximately 42% compared with placebo.[10] This approximates the benefit that would be expected from estimates derived from epidemiological studies for the difference in stroke rate achieved when the BP loads of those in the antihypertensive group are compared with the placebo or community controls.[11]

The beneficial effect of antihypertensive drug therapy on coronary heart disease has been more difficult to prove using results from the same clinical trials.[11] Although there are many reasons why a 5-year study may be unable to show major differences in coronary heart disease mortality (especially if the drugs used are associated with a temporary worsening of other risk factors for coronary atherosclerosis), including the decades needed to develop the lesions that lead to acute MI,[12] more recent trials, especially those in older persons,[1, 2] have demonstrated a significant reduction in coronary heart disease endpoints in the group randomized to active antihypertensive drug therapy. This has been seen in a recent meta-analysis of low-dose diuretic therapy,[10] as well as in both studies of isolated systolic hypertension, discussed later.[13, 14] The weight of the evidence indicates an improvement of approximately 16% in coronary heart disease endpoints with antihypertensive drug therapy. Whether this is equal to or less than the benefits estimated from epidemiological studies (20 to 25%) is still open to dispute.[15]

Often forgotten in the discussion of cardiovascular disease endpoints in clinical trials of hypertension are the more subtle progression of hypertension to higher stages and the prevention of heart failure. Both of these are clearly and substantially improved with antihypertensive drug therapy.[16] The prevention of heart failure has taken on more importance recently, as this condition has become the leading discharge diagnosis from American hospitals and is responsible for billions of dollars in health care expenditures. The recent meta-analysis of Psaty and colleagues indicates that the development of heart failure is reduced by 42% by either a low-dose diuretic or a β-blocker as first-line treatment.[10] Estimates from Moser and Hebert[16] indicate that in some placebo-controlled clinical trials,[17] the group randomized to active antihypertensive therapy had a 94% decreased risk of progressing to the higher stages of hypertension, which not only increases cardiovascular risk but also is more difficult and more expensive to treat.

Some of the most persuasive recent data supporting the value of antihypertensive drug therapy come from studies of diabetic patients and those with reduced renal function, who have a higher risk of progressing to renal failure, dialysis, or transplantation if their BPs are not controlled.

Table 34-1 Long-Term Outcome-Based Clinical Trials of Antihypertensive Agents

Trial Name	n	Year of Publication	Key Patient Characteristics	Primary Endpoint	Regimens	Primary Results	Key Findings
TRIALS USING PLACEBO CONTROLS							
VA Trial in Severe Hypertension	143	1967	Men with 115 ≤ DBP ≤ 129 mm Hg after 6 days in hospital at bedrest	Prespecified adverse complications of hypertension	HCTZ (± reserpine, hydralazine) vs. placebo	Deaths: 4 vs. 0 Complications: 23 vs. 2	Benefits of therapy became clear after <1.5 yr of follow-up
VA Cooperative Study	380	1970	Men with 90 ≤ DBP ≤ 114 mm Hg in outpatient department without target organ damage	Prespecified adverse complications of hypertension	HCTZ (± reserpine, hydralazine) vs. placebo	Deaths: 19 vs. 8 Complications: 37 vs. 14	Benefits of therapy demonstrated for age > 50 yr, or preexisting CV abnormality
U.S. Public Health Service Trial	389	1977	People aged 21–55 yr with DBP between 90–114 mm Hg without target organ damage	Hypertensive (ECG, CXR evidence of LVH) and atherosclerotic complications of hypertension	CTZ (± *Rauwolfia* alkaloids) vs. placebo	50% reduction in hypertensive complications (mostly LVH)	No difference in mortality (two in each group); no difference in atherosclerotic complications (e.g., MI)
VA-NHLBI Feasibility Study	1012	1978	Men aged 35–55 yr with DBP between 85–105 mm Hg without target organ damage	Hypertensive and atherosclerotic complications	Chlorthalidone (± reserpine) vs. placebo	Study stopped prematurely due to lack of resources to follow patients for 7.5 yr	Two deaths in active treatment group; none in placebo group
Australian National Blood Pressure Study	3427	1980	People aged 30–69 yr with DBP between 95–109 mm Hg without target organ damage	Prespecified complications of hypertension (death, stroke, MI, angina, CHF, dissecting aneurysm, grade 3 or 4 retinopathy, serum creatinine >2 mg/dl, encephalopathy)	CTZ (± methyldopa, propranolol, pindolol, hydralazine, clonidine) vs. placebo	Study stopped after 3 yr, with 30% fewer trial endpoints in treatment group	Excess morbidity in the placebo-treated group was limited to those with DBP > 100 mm Hg; for those with DBP <100 mm Hg, there was less morbidity on placebo than on active therapy
Medical Research Council Trial	17,354	1985	People aged 35–64 yr with DBP between 90–109 without severe target organ damage	Stroke, MI, CV death	Bendrofluazide or propranolol (each ± methyldopa, guanethidine) vs. placebo	Strokes were reduced by treatment, but not MI or total mortality	Smokers receiving propranolol had no significant benefit
European Working Party on Hypertension in the Elderly	840	1985	People aged > 60 yr with DBP between 90–119 without severe target organ damage	Stroke, MI, CV death	CTZ + triamterene vs. placebo	Significant reduction in CHD death, but no protection from stroke or nonfatal MI	No benefit seen in patients > 80 yr of age

Study	N	Year	Population	Endpoints	Comparison	Results	Comments
Medical Research Council Trial in The Elderly	4396	1992	People aged 65–74 yr with SBP between 180–209 and DBP < 115 mm Hg	Stroke, MI, CV death	Atenolol (25%) vs. HCTZ + amiloride (25%) vs. placebo (50%)	Only the diuretic group showed better reduction in overall and stroke morbidity than placebo	Few patients stayed on monotherapy during the entire 5.8 yr; many in the atenolol group were lost to follow-up
Swedish Trial of Old Patients (STOP) with Hypertension	1627	1991	People aged 70–84 yr with SBP between 180–230 or DBP between 105–120 mm Hg	Stroke, MI, CV death	Atenolol, metoprolol, or pindolol or diuretic (HCTZ + amiloride) vs. placebo	Total CV events reduced by about 33%, and stroke about 35%	Reduction in MI was not significant, but benefits were shown in all age groups, even 80–84 yr
Systolic Hypertension in the Elderly Program (SHEP)	4736	1991	People aged ≥ 60 yr with SBP between 160–219 and DBP < 90 mm Hg without major hypertensive complications	Fatal and nonfatal stroke	Low-dose chlorthalidone (± atenolol, methyldopa, hydralazine) vs. placebo	33% reduction in all stroke with active treatment after 4.5 yr (average)	50% reduction in CHF; 27% reduction in CV events; 41% of participants randomized to placebo were taking active medications after 4 yr
SYST-EUR	4695	1997	People aged ≥ 60 yr with SBP between 160–219 and DBP < 95 mm Hg without major hypertensive complications	Fatal and nonfatal stroke	Nisoldipine vs. placebo (± enalapril, HCTZ)	Stopped early due to 42–44% reduction with active treatment	All CV events, angina reduced; no increase in risk for developing cancer, bleeding, or death among patients treated with a CCB
TRIALS USING NO PLACEBO, BUT CONCOMITANT "NO TREATMENT"							
"The Oslo Trial"	785	1980	Men aged 40–49 yr with DBP between 95–109 or SBP ≥ 150 mm Hg, without target organ damage	Prespecified complications of hypertension	HCTZ (± methyldopa, propranolol) vs. no treatment	Overall no significant differences after 5 yr of follow-up	Significant 54% reduction in CV events if DBP > 100 mm Hg at entry; no differences for less severe hypertensives
Elderly Patients in Primary Care (Coope and Warrender)	884	1986	People aged 50–79 yr with DBP between 109–120 mm Hg	Fatal and nonfatal stroke	Atenolol (± bendroflazide) vs. no treatment	58% reduction in fatal and nonfatal stroke; no decrease in MI or total mortality	No benefit from therapy with isolated systolic hypertension

Abbreviations: VA, Veterans Administration; DBP, diastolic blood pressure; HCTZ, hydrochlorothiazide; CV, cardiovascular; CTZ, chlorothiazide; MI, myocardial infarction; NHLBI, National Heart, Lung, and Blood Institute; CHF, congestive heart failure; CHD, coronary heart disease; SBP, systolic blood pressure; SYST-EUR, Systolic Hypertension in Europe; CCB, calcium channel blocker. CXR, chest x-ray; LVH, left ventricular hypertrophy; ECG, electrocardiogram;

It has been known for many years that hypertension increases the risk of renal failure and renal replacement therapy, and recent data from the Multiple Risk Factor Intervention Trial (MRFIT) screenees and several other large databases indicate a generally improved prognosis in patients with lower BPs at baseline.[18, 19] Only recently have data from clinical trials shown that antihypertensive drug therapy improves prognosis in such patients.[20–23] Since end-stage renal disease, indexed by institution of dialysis, is the one area in cardiovascular medicine in which rates of morbidity and mortality have increased in recent years, this evidence from clinical trials has convinced those responsible for the sixth report of the Joint National Committee on Prevention, Detection, Evaluation, and Treatment of High Blood Pressure (JNC VI) that a lower treatment goal should be recommended for diabetics and patients with renal impairment.[24] The importance of choosing an appropriate agent to improve *both* BP and prognosis for diabetics with proteinuria has recently been demonstrated in two studies: the Appropriate Blood Pressure Control in Diabetes (ABCD) trial, and the Fosinopril Versus Amlodipine Cardiovascular Events Trial (FACET).[25, 26]

SHOULD ISOLATED SYSTOLIC HYPERTENSION BE TREATED?

Two trials completed in the 1990s have provided persuasive evidence of benefit of antihypertensive drug treatment in patients with elevated systolic blood pressures (SBPs) but DBPs below 90 mm Hg. Before 1993, the reports of the Joint National Committees had always defined hypertension only as a usual DBP greater than or equal to 90 mm Hg, but epidemiological data and especially clinical trial evidence from the Systolic Hypertension in the Elderly Program (SHEP) caused JNC V to reconsider the importance of elevations in SBP and to give equal weight to SBP and DBP.[27] In SHEP, 4736 patients over 60 years of age with SBPs of 160 mm Hg or greater and DBPs less than 90 mm Hg were randomized to either chlorthalidone 12.5 mg or placebo, with additional treatment (atenolol or reserpine) given until the SBPs were reduced to 160 mm Hg or less (if baseline SBP was ≥180 mm Hg) or by 20 mm Hg (if baseline SBP was 160 to 179 mm Hg).[13] After an average of 4.6 years of treatment, there were 33% fewer fatal or nonfatal strokes, 25% fewer coronary heart disease endpoints, 25% fewer cardiac events, and 32% fewer cardiovascular events in the group randomized to active treatment. All of these differences were statistically significant. These results are even more impressive, considering that at the end of the study, 44% of the patients randomized to placebo had been placed on active antihypertensive treatment because their BPs exceeded predetermined levels or because of other clinical indications. The results of SHEP show that antihypertensive drug therapy reduces cardiovascular risk in essentially all patient subgroups (men, women, older, younger, diabetic, nondiabetic,[28] initial SBP ≥ 180 mm Hg vs. 160 to 180 mm Hg, previously treated, and never-treated), even when only the SBP is elevated.[13]

Recent confirmation of the benefits of antihypertensive drug therapy for isolated systolic hypertension in older patients has been obtained in the Systolic Hypertension in Europe (SYST-EUR) study.[14] Patients ($n = 4695$) aged 60 years and older with SBPs 160 to 219 mm Hg and DBPs less than 95 mm Hg were randomized to placebo or active treatment beginning with nitrendipine, a moderately long-acting dihydropyridine calcium antagonist, followed by enalapril and hydrochlorothiazide (HCTZ) if needed to reach BP goal. This study was stopped early because, after an average of 2 years of follow-up, the Data Safety and Monitoring Board noted a significant (42 to 44%) reduction in stroke incidence among patients randomized initially to nitrendipine. Active treatment was also associated with a 26% reduction in sudden death, a 33% reduction in nonfatal cardiac endpoints, and a 31% reduction in all fatal and nonfatal cardiovascular events; all of these benefits were statistically significant.

The results of the SYST-EUR study were all the more important because these benefits accrued to those who received the active treatment regimen, which began with a dihydropyridine calcium antagonist. Concerns had been raised about this class of drugs after reports from retrospective reviews of databases gathered for other purposes had suggested that representatives of this antihypertensive drug class *increased* the risk for acute MI, death, bleeding, and cancer. The SYST-EUR data provide strong evidence (from a randomized, prospective clinical trial) that these potential problems tend to be *reduced* (although not significantly) in the group receiving a dihydropyridine calcium antagonist. The magnitude of the benefits and the similarity in reductions of secondary endpoints in SHEP and SYST-EUR are consistent with the concept that benefits accrue to patients whose BPs are reduced, independently of the type of agents used.

A study protocol identical to SYST-EUR was followed in the Chinese Trial on Isolated Systolic Hypertension in the Elderly (SYST-CHINA), except that allocation of treatment in the 2394 patients was by sequential alternate assignment rather than randomization. After 4 years, there was a significant 39% reduction in all-cause mortality, a 58% reduction in stroke mortality, a 37% reduction in all cardiovascular endpoints, and a 38% reduction in fatal and nonfatal stroke in the group allocated to active antihypertensive therapy.[29]

The true benefits of lowering BP are probably underestimated from clinical trial data.[30] Clinical trials are traditionally analyzed by intention-to-treat methodology, which provides estimates of the benefit of treatment by original assignment (the point in time when there is the least likelihood of bias) rather than by the treatment that was actually taken by the patient (which could be biased). During long-term placebo-controlled clinical trials like SHEP, some patients originally assigned to placebo begin taking open-label antihypertensive drug therapy (typically because their BPs exceed prespecified "escape" levels), and other patients originally assigned to active medication discontinue it owing to side effects or other intolerance. Each of these transitions leads to underestimation of the true benefit of prevention of stroke and other cardiovascular events due to active therapy versus placebo. In SHEP, 44% of patients in the placebo group began taking antihypertensive drug therapy by the end of the trial, and about 10% discontinued the active treatment. Thus, the true reduction in stroke due to therapy is undoubtedly greater than the 33% reported and probably is closer to the result of SYST-EUR (42 to 44%). In SYST-EUR, only 5.5% of patients had abandoned their placebo medications and switched to active treatment during the 2 years of follow-up. Both studies provide persuasive evidence that lowering elevated SBPs in older persons without elevated DBPs using drug therapy is beneficial.

IS BLOOD PRESSURE REDUCTION WITH MEDICATIONS MORE EFFECTIVE THAN LIFESTYLE MODIFICATIONS ALONE?

The benefits of BP reduction with medications discussed previously appear to be universal, applying to nearly all endpoints and nearly all subgroups of patients. However, several studies have shown that medications are not the only method of reducing BP, at least in the short term. Several diets, including the Dietary Approaches to Stop Hypertension (DASH) diet[31] and low-sodium–containing regimens,[32–35] have been shown in randomized clinical trials to result in lowered BP and other benefits (improved weights and lipid profiles). Several strategies directed toward weight loss and increased physical activity have also been shown in randomized, multicenter, prospective clinical trials to be associated with reduced BPs.[34–37]

The Treatment of Mild Hypertension Study (TOMHS) was undertaken largely because of concerns about the efficacy of some of the newer antihypertensive agents (angiotensin-converting enzyme [ACE] inhibitors, calcium antagonists, and peripheral α_1-adrenoceptor blocking agents) and what benefits they might offer over and above an aggressive strategy of lifestyle modifications.[38] This multicenter study compared five different antihypertensive agents combined with an aggressive program of weight, sodium, and alcohol restriction with placebo plus that lifestyle modification program for a 4-year treatment period. The rationale of the study was that if TOMHS showed equivalent benefit of lifestyle modifications compared with pharmacological therapy, a large number of hypertensive patients could be spared the risks and costs of drug therapy.

The results showed an impressively greater reduction in BPs, despite baseline BPs that were only barely elevated (140/91 mm Hg, on average), among the patients randomized to active drug therapy, over and above the reductions seen in patients treated with only lifestyle modifications (16/12 vs. 9/9 mm Hg).[38] The study was intended primarily as a pilot to see how well tolerated and effective the medications and lifestyle modification regimens were over the long term and did not have the statistical power to compare the ability of individual regimens to protect patients against cardiovascular events. Nevertheless, there was a statistically significant ($p < .05$) difference favoring the drug therapy group when all endpoints were pooled. TOMHS showed that the more recently introduced classes of antihypertensive medications (representatives of the classes were amlodipine, doxazosin, and enalapril) are well tolerated over a 4-year treatment period and, more importantly, that lifestyle modifications alone may not maximally reduce cardiovascular risk in otherwise low-risk patients with just barely elevated BPs. The results of this trial have led to the implementation of the largest antihyperten-

sive study ever done (with more than 42,000 participants), the Antihypertensive and Lipid Lowering to Prevent Heart Attack Trial (ALLHAT),[39] which uses four of the five drug therapies from TOMHS but does not include a lifestyle modification strategy alone.[40]

WHICH PATIENT GROUP IS MORE LIKELY TO BENEFIT FROM ANTIHYPERTENSIVE DRUG THERAPY?

Clinical trials have demonstrated that antihypertensive drug therapy lowers the risk of cardiovascular events better than placebo or lifestyle modifications alone. The challenge is how to implement programs that reduce cardiovascular risk in a cost-effective manner. Of the many suggestions that have been put forward, the one that has achieved acceptance in many countries (New Zealand, Canada, Belgium, and South Africa) is that high-risk patients ought to be treated more aggressively and more extensively than low-risk patients.[41] This approach has recently been recommended by JNC VI in its consideration of both low-risk patients (who are recommended to receive up to a year of lifestyle modifications alone before institution of antihypertensive drug therapy) and diabetic patients (who are recommended to be treated to a BP goal of <130/85 mm Hg compared with <140/90 mm Hg for lower-risk patients).[24] JNC VI recommends that hypertensives with renal disease and at least 1 g of proteinuria per day should have their BP reduced to less than 125/75 mm Hg.[24]

Much evidence from clinical trials indicates that given the same treatment, higher-risk patients benefit more than lower-risk patients.[42] The best recent review of this fundamental principle of preventive medicine is in the paper by Lever and Ramsay.[43] Figure 34–1 is a modified graph from

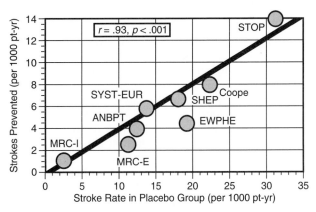

Figure 34–1. Relationship between baseline level of stroke risk (according to the stroke rate per 1000 patient-years in the group randomized to placebo) and the number of strokes prevented (per 1000 patient-years) by antihypertensive drug therapy. Each point represents the result of a single randomized clinical trial. MRC-I, Medical Research Council Trial in Mild Hypertension;[8] MRC-E, Medical Research Council Trial in Older Adults;[70] ANBPT, Australian National Blood Pressure Trial;[9] SYST-EUR, Systolic Hypertension Trial in Europe;[14] SHEP, Systolic Hypertension in the Elderly Program;[13] EWPHE, European Working Party on High Blood Pressure in the Elderly;[73] Coope, Coope and Warrender;[72] STOP, Swedish Trial in Old Patients with Hypertension.[44] (Adapted from Lever AF, Ramsay LE. Treatment of hypertension in the elderly. J Hypertens 13[6]:571–579, 1995.)

that article that includes SYST-EUR results and shows that the number of strokes avoided in a given trial depends on the baseline risk of stroke in the cohort studied. The correlation coefficient for this relationship is highly statistically significant ($p < .001$). Therefore, the high-risk, older patients with a higher level of baseline BP (e.g., those seen in the first Swedish Trial in Old Patients with Hypertension [STOP-Hypertension][44]) benefit far more (in terms of absolute reductions in stroke prevalence) than the young patients with lower baseline BPs studied in the first Medical Research Council (MRC) Trial in Mild Hypertension.[8]

The issue of how to implement this important principle in everyday medical practice is now being debated.[45, 46] Some health care systems (e.g., France) require low-risk patients to pay for the same therapies that higher-risk patients are provided without cost. Some systems have a sliding copayment system for pharmaceuticals that is based on a baseline risk assessment. Most American health care systems limit the lifetime payout for health care of any individual to US $1 million, which has the same impact over the lifetimes of enrollees but may have different consequences during shorter time spans.

HOW LOW SHOULD THE BLOOD PRESSURE GOAL BE FOR MOST PATIENTS?

Data from clinical trials suggest that a lower than usual BP goal, as recommended by JNC VI, is appropriate for higher-risk patients.[24] The Modification of Diet in Renal Disease (MDRD) study was a success more for the results of its BP intervention than for those obtained with dietary protein restriction.[47] A recent analysis of the prognosis of MDRD enrollees indicated that the group randomized to the lower BP goal had less diminution in renal function over the 2 years of follow-up.[22] Similar results were obtained in several other studies of patients with renal dysfunction and/or diabetes when antihypertensive treatment included an ACE inhibitor, as summarized in a recent meta-analysis.[23] Several ongoing clinical trials are attempting to assess which "high-risk" patients should be treated to a lower BP goal, in order to improve prognosis. The African American Study of Kidney Diseases (AASK) trial is the largest of the National Institutes of Health–sponsored trials that will randomize patients to different BP goals.

The issue of whether the traditional BP goal (<140/90 mm Hg) is low enough for *all* patients is an important and debatable point. Early data from the Hypertension Detection and Follow-up Program (HDFP) showed a 15 to 28% reduction in 5-year death rates in subgroups randomized to "stepped care" (in which the average DBP was 83 mm Hg) compared with those randomized to "referred care" (which achieved a DBP of 88 mm Hg).[48] Some have considered the possibility that there is a J-shaped curve with respect to coronary artery disease morbidity and mortality, especially in those with known preexisting ischemic heart disease. These authors have cautioned against excessive lowering of BP, based primarily on several post-hoc analyses of clinical trial data that showed an increase in morbidity and mortality in these patients whose BPs were in the lowest range.[49] Since this relationship has been seen

with multiple biological phenomena (e.g., blood cholesterol levels, weight) as well as in observational (i.e., nonintervention) studies and in placebo groups in clinical trials, there is a reasonable doubt that excessive risk results from increasing the intensity of treatment.[50]

Several clinical trials have attempted to determine whether a lower BP goal translates into reduced or increased cardiovascular risk. The first to be completed was the Behandla Blodtryck Battre (BBB) trial, which showed that although it was possible to treat BPs to a lower than typical goal, there appeared to be no real advantage to do so in terms of reduced cardiovascular events.[51] The results of the Hypertension Optimal Treatment (HOT) Study were recently reported.[52] This randomized trial of nearly 19,000 patients from 26 countries showed that DBP could be lowered from an average of 105 mm Hg to an optimal level of 83 mm Hg and that further lowering was safe, but not associated with further reductions in cardiovascular events. The original design of the trial was to randomize patients to three different DBP goals: 90 mm Hg or less, 85 mm Hg or less, or 80 mm Hg or less. Although there were fewer cardiovascular events than expected during the average 3.8 years of follow-up (only 3.8 cardiovascular deaths/1000 patient-years compared with 6.5/1000 in previous meta-analyses[15]), there was a progressive reduction in risk seen with each 5-mm decrement in achieved DBP from 100 mm Hg to 80 mm Hg, with the "optimum" at 83 mm Hg. The intention-to-treat analysis for 1501 diabetics in the HOT study also showed a statistically significant benefit of intensified treatment, with the greatest reductions in major cardiovascular events occurring in the group randomized to the lowest BP goal. These observations support the principle mentioned previously, that those at the highest risk benefit the most from effective therapy. There was no evidence for a J-shaped curve in the rates of cardiovascular morbidity and mortality for patients with known cardiovascular disease, and all patients appeared to tolerate the lower level of BP. The greatest improvement in quality of life scores occurred in those randomized to the lowest BP goal. The HOT study also showed that BP could be reduced to the goals recommended by JNC VI without significant risk or added complexity. Nearly two thirds of the participants in the HOT study required more than one drug to reach BP goal.

WHAT IS THE BEST WAY TO TREAT HYPERTENSION?

Because of the multitude of antihypertensive agents available, there is currently a great deal of uncertainty over which agent or class of agents should be used initially to lower elevated BP. Traditionally, diuretics or β-blockers have been used in most clinical trials as first-line therapy. Because of their proven benefit in reducing cardiovascular morbidity and mortality, they have been "preferred" in reports of the Joint National Committee.[24, 27] The recommendation to initiate therapy with a low-dose diuretic in older persons has recently been supported by a meta-analysis of clinical trials that began with a low-dose diuretic or β-blocker,[10] a meta-analysis of trials of β-blocker therapy in elderly hypertensives,[53] and the National High

Blood Pressure Education Program Working Group Report on Hypertension in the Elderly.[54]

Much effort is currently being directed to long-term comparative trials of representatives of the newer classes of antihypertensive agents, using morbidity/mortality endpoints. Many of these are comparisons of regimens involving initial therapy with either a diuretic or a β-blocker (as an example of an "agent with proven efficacy") in one treatment arm and a newer drug in the other treatment arm. ALLHAT compares chlorthalidone (the "gold standard diuretic") with amlodipine, doxazosin, and/or lisinopril over 5 years in more than 42,000 hypertensive patients, some of whom will concurrently receive lipid-lowering therapy as part of a substudy. Controlled ONset Verapamil INvestigation of Cardiovascular Endpoints (CONVINCE) will study the effectiveness of either a new formulation of verapamil designed to align its release with the circadian pattern of BP and pulse rate or a physician-directed choice of either atenolol or hydrochlorothiazide in 16,605 hypertensive patients with at least one additional cardiovascular risk factor.[55] Many other, smaller, long-term clinical trials comparing regimens of the newer antihypertensive agents on morbidity or mortality endpoints are summarized in Table 34–2.[56] It is estimated that, by 2003, there should be 8000 strokes and 12,000 coronary heart disease events recorded in current trials. This prospectively planned pooling of data should be sufficient to assess whether the newer antihypertensive drug classes are as effective as the older agents in improving cardiovascular prognosis in hypertensive patients and whether benefit is ubiquitous or specific to certain subgroups of patients.

These current, large clinical trials have another important purpose, which differs from the classical placebo-controlled clinical trials begun between 1960 and 1990. Because it is no longer ethical to give placebo in the long term to hypertensive patients, very large numbers of patients are needed to ensure sufficient statistical power in comparisons of treatment regimens. The newer clinical trials have, therefore, been designed to be performed in the offices of practitioners who are, in general, not as intensively trained or experienced in research practices. These newer trials are considered "effectiveness" trials, as opposed to "efficacy" trials (those done during the last several decades in specialized centers by highly trained, research-oriented investigators). It is expected that the results of the larger, more recent trials will be more easily generalizable to the population as a whole than results of efficacy trials.[57] For example, SHEP has been criticized because it enrolled only about 1% of the screened patients, whereas SYST-EUR enrolled nearly 60% of its screenees, presumably because there were many more clinical sites, each of which had a sizable roster of established patients who met the entry criteria.

ANTIHYPERTENSIVE MEDICATIONS MAY HAVE BENEFITS FAR BEYOND LOWERING OF BLOOD PRESSURE

The benefits of lowering BP are well documented in data from clinical trials. Some antihypertensive drugs have been shown in clinical trials to provide benefits to certain patient groups above and beyond their BP-lowering effects. The best recent example is the clinical trial demonstrating slowing of progression of diabetic retinopathy in young, normotensive type 1 diabetics given lisinopril.[58]

The recent clinical trials of various ACE inhibitors in patients with diabetes and renal insufficiency have generally shown that these agents are helpful in the prevention and/or delay of renal failure. In most of the trials, attempts were made in *both* treatment groups (ACE inhibitor vs. placebo as first-line treatment) to lower BPs. If the initial treatment (ACE inhibitor or placebo) was ineffective in lowering BP to goal, other antihypertensive medications were added (typically in stepwise fashion), so that the BPs of the two groups at the conclusion of the study were very similar. In many of these trials, calcium antagonists and ACE inhibitors other than the study medications could not be used. The recent ABCD trial, a prospective, randomized trial carried out in diabetic hypertensive patients, provided evidence that first-line treatment of BP with an ACE inhibitor appears to be more effective in preventing cardiovascular endpoints than the dihydropyridine calcium antagonist nisoldipine.[25] During the 5 years of this study, there was a 9.5-fold increase in the incidence of fatal and nonfatal MI in the group randomized to nisoldipine (25 of 235 patients) compared with the group initially treated with enalapril (5 of 235 patients). Whether this difference was due to the greater use of diuretics or β-blockers in the enalapril group, a worsened prognosis with the calcium antagonist, or chance is unclear.

FACET was designed to compare lipid levels and diabetes control in non-insulin–dependent diabetics treated over a 3.5-year period with a regimen starting with either the dihydropyridine calcium antagonist amlodipine or the ACE inhibitor fosinopril. If BP control was inadequate with either first-line drug, the second was added. No significant differences were found in biochemical measurements during treatment (the primary endpoint), but more patients (27 of 191) had adverse cardiovascular outcomes in the group randomized to amlodipine than in the fosinopril group (14 of 189, $p < .05$).[26] A post-hoc analysis showed that patients treated with a combination of *both* drugs had the best prognosis, perhaps owing to better BP control.[26] The probability of a chance finding is higher when a difference between groups is seen in a secondary endpoint but not in the primary endpoint. It is surprising and counterintuitive that the participants who needed two drugs did better than those whose BP was controlled with a single agent. The increased risk of coronary heart disease events in diabetics randomized to calcium antagonists has *not* been verified in subgroup analyses specifically undertaken for this purpose by the Data Safety and Monitoring Boards of larger trials involving 20 to 30 times more patients (ALLHAT and CONVINCE).[59]

In the landmark study of Lewis and coworkers, well over 90% of the patients were eventually treated with antihypertensive medications.[20] In two randomized controlled trials of the ACE inhibitors benazepril[21] and ramipril[60] in nondiabetic patients with renal impairment and proteinuria, benefits were seen in the group randomized to the ACE inhibitor, even though all patients were treated with other antihypertensive medications and, in the case of the ramipril study, to the same BP goal. Further clinical

Table 34–2 Long-Term Outcome-Based Clinical Trials of Antihypertensive Agents in Progress

Acronym (Name)	First-Line Agent	Comparator	Patients	Comments
ALLHAT (Antihypertensive and Lipid-Lowering to Prevent Heart Attack Trial)	Amlodipine, doxazosin, lisinopril	Chlorthalidone	42,565 in > 500 centers in United States and Canada	6-yr follow-up planned
ANBP-2 (Australian National Blood Pressure Trial #2)	ACE inhibitor	Diuretic	6000 65–84-yr-old Australians	5-yr follow-up planned
ASCOT (Anglo-Scandinavian Cardiac Outcomes Trial)	Calcium antagonist or ACE inhibitor	Diuretic or β-blocker	18,000 residents of Scandinavia or the United Kingdom	5-yr follow-up planned
CAPPP (Captopril Prevention Project)	Captopril	Diuretic or β-blocker	10,800 at 275 centers in Sweden and Finland	5-yr follow-up planned
CONVINCE (Controlled-Onset Verapamil Investigation of Cardiovascular Endpoints)	COER-verapamil	HCTZ or atenolol	15,000 in > 600 centers worldwide	5-yr follow-up planned
ELSA (European Lacidipine Study of Atherosclerosis)	Lacidipine	β-blocker	2251 European patients with known atherosclerosis	4-yr follow-up planned
HOT (Hypertension Optimal Treatment)	Felodipine	None	19,196 patients in 18 countries	Randomized to 1 of 3 BP goals
HYVET (Hypertension in the Very Elderly Trial)	ACE inhibitor (± diuretic)	Placebo	2100 patients > 80 yr old	5-yr follow-up planned
INSIGHT (International Nifedipine GITS Study Intervention as a Goal in Hypertension Treatment)	Nifedipine GITS	HCTZ + amiloride	6592 patients in 9 European countries	3-yr minimum follow-up planned
LIFE (Losartan Intervention for Endpoint Reduction)	Losartan	Atenolol	9194 patients in > 300 centers worldwide	ECG-LVH only; 4-yr follow-up planned
NICS-EH (National Intervention Cooperative Study in Elderly Hypertensives)	Calcium antagonist	Diuretic	1000 Japanese > 60 yr old	5-yr follow-up planned
NORDIL (Nordic Diltiazem Study)	Diltiazem	Diuretic or β-blocker	11,000 patients in 480 centers in Sweden and Norway	5-yr follow-up planned
SHELL (Systolic Hypertension in the Elderly Long-Term Lacidipine Trial)	Lacidipine	Diuretic	4800 Europeans with isolated systolic hypertension	Compares 3.5-yr incidence of cardiovascular morbidity/mortality
STOP-Hypertension 2 (Swedish Trial in Old Patients with Hypertension #2)	ACE inhibitor or calcium antagonist	Diuretic or β-blocker	6600 patients aged 70–84 yr in 300 centers in Sweden	4-yr minimum follow-up planned
SYST-CHINA (Systolic Hypertension in China Study)	Nitrendipine (± captopril, HCTZ)	Placebo	3379 Chinese with isolated systolic hypertension	Outcome: all strokes; follow-up ended in 1997
VALUE (Valsartan Amlodipine Long-Term Utilization Evaluation)	Valsartan (± HCTZ)	Amlodipine (± HCTZ)	14,400 patients in 1000 centers in 31 countries	6-yr follow-up, 1450 primary endpoints expected

Abbreviations: ACE, angiotensin-converting enzyme; COER, controlled onset-extended release; HCTZ, hydrochlorothiazide; BP, blood pressure; GITS, gastrointestinal therapeutic system; ECG, electrocardiogram; LVH, left ventricular hypertrophy.

trials will help to resolve the debate about which therapies offer specific advantages in certain patient populations.[59]

Analogous to the issue of how best to treat hypertension in patients with renal insufficiency and/or diabetes is the issue of which medications to recommend for patients who have survived a recent MI. Data from clinical trials indicate that β-blockers reduce the risk of death and of a second MI.[61] This was the conclusion of individual clinical trials (which varied with regard to how soon after MI the medications were begun and the degree of left ventricular dysfunction that was allowed for admission to the trial) and of a meta-analysis of 29 clinical trials that had a variety of designs and treatment regimens.[62] More recently, this conclusion has been corroborated and replicated in the New Jersey Medicare database, where the 21% of survivors of MI who were given β-blockers had a 43% improved 2-year survival compared with those who were given no β-blocker.[63]

ACE inhibitors have also been studied in heart failure[64] and in the post-MI state[65] and have been shown to reduce cardiovascular morbidity and mortality in high-risk patients (i.e., those with low ejection fractions or with manifest heart failure on presentation). It is likely that the benefit of ACE inhibitors in these settings is not due to treatment of hypertension—since it is not probable that elevated BPs would have gone untreated in people making frequent physician visits for heart failure or after an MI—but rather to specific effects of this drug class in patients with impaired ventricular function. Recent data from the Evaluation of Losartan In The Elderly (ELITE-1) trial suggest that these benefits may extend to the newest class of oral antihypertensive drugs, the angiotensin II receptor blockers (ARBs).[66] This finding needs to be replicated in similar studies with this and other ARBs. Such trials are in progress.

BENEFITS OF HYPERTENSION TREATMENT MAY DEPEND ON BEHAVIOR

Many recent data suggest that hypertension treatment and control in the population are suboptimal, due not to the unavailability of effective antihypertensive medications but rather to limitations in utilization of available treatment. One important predictor of good outcomes in several clinical trials has been the willingness and ability of the study participants to take the medications as prescribed. An analysis (done many years post hoc) of the Beta-Blocker Heart Attack Trial (BHAT) in post-MI patients indicated that patients who took more than 75% of their medications correctly had a 20 to 40% increase in event-free survival (to death or recurrent MI) than those who were less compliant, even if they were randomized to placebo.[67, 68] This has been seen in both men and women and may be generalizable to the entire population, even to hypertensive individuals treated with medications intended primarily to lower BP.[69] There are few analyses of the importance of medication compliance in antihypertensive clinical trials,[70] but it is likely that patients who are compliant with medications may also be more likely to keep appointments with physi-

cians, follow a proper diet, exercise regularly, and generally follow a healthier lifestyle.[71]

SUMMARY

Clinical trials have unequivocally demonstrated the benefits of antihypertensive drug therapy in reducing the risk of adverse cardiovascular and renal events. The challenge is to use these lessons to implement effective treatment strategies and reduce morbidity and mortality in the most cost-effective manner.[46]

References

1. Mulrow CD, Cornell JA, Herrera CR, et al. Hypertension in the elderly: Implications and generalizability of randomized trials. JAMA 272:1932–1938, 1994.
2. Insua AT, Sacks HS, Lau TS, et al. Drug treatment of hypertension in the elderly: A meta-analysis. Ann Intern Med 121:355–362, 1994.
3. Pooling Project Research Group. Relationship of blood pressure, serum cholesterol, smoking habit, relative weight, and ECG abnormalities to incidence of major coronary events: Final results of the pooling project. J Chronic Dis 31:201–306, 1978.
4. Gubner RS. Systolic hypertension: A pathogenetic entity. Significance and therapeutic considerations. Am J Cardiol 9:773–776, 1962.
5. Kannel WB, Schwartz MJ, McNamara PM. Blood pressure and risk of coronary heart disease: The Framingham Study. Dis Chest 56:43–52, 1969.
6. Roccella EJ, Lenfant C. Considerations regarding the cost and effectiveness of public and patient education programmes. J Hum Hypertens 6:463–467, 1992.
7. VA Cooperative Study Group on Antihypertensive Agents. Effects of treatment on morbidity in hypertension. Results in patients with diastolic blood pressures averaging 115 through 129 mm Hg. JAMA 202:1028–1034, 1967.
8. Medical Research Council Working Party. MRC trial of treatment of mild hypertension: Principal results. BMJ 291:97–104, 1985.
9. Management Committee. The Australian therapeutic trial in mild hypertension. Lancet 1:1261–1267, 1980.
10. Psaty BM, Smith NL, Siscovick DS, et al. Health outcomes associated with antihypertensive therapies used as first-line agents: A systematic review and meta-analysis. JAMA 277:739–745, 1997.
11. MacMahon S, Peto R, Cutler J, et al. Blood pressure, stroke, and coronary heart disease. Part 2: Short-term reductions in blood pressure: Overview of randomised drug trials in their epidemiological context. Lancet 335:827–838, 1990.
12. Black HR. The coronary artery disease paradox: The role of hyperinsulinemia and insulin resistance and implications for therapy. J Cardiovasc Pharmacol 15:S26–S38, 1990.
13. SHEP Cooperative Research Group. Prevention of stroke by antihypertensive drug treatment in older persons with isolated systolic hypertension. Final results of the Systolic Hypertension in the Elderly Program (SHEP). JAMA 266:3255–3264, 1991.
14. Staessen JA, Fagard R, Thijs L, et al, for the Systolic Hypertension—Europe (SYST-EUR) Trial Investigators. Morbidity and mortality in the placebo-controlled European Trial on Isolated Systolic Hypertension in the Elderly. Lancet 360:757–764, 1997.
15. Gueyffier F, Froment A, Gouton M. New meta-analysis of treatment trials in hypertension: Improving the estimate of therapeutic benefit. J Hum Hypertens 10:1–8, 1996.
16. Moser M, Hebert PR. Prevention of disease progression, left ventricular hypertrophy and congestive heart failure in hypertension treatment trials. J Am Coll Cardiol 27:1214–1218, 1996.
17. Kostis J, Davis BR, Cutler J, et al. Prevention of heart failure by antihypertensive drug treatment in older persons with isolated systolic hypertension. SHEP Cooperative Study Group. JAMA 278:212–216, 1997.
18. Perry HM Jr, Miller JP, Fornoff JR, et al. Early predictors of 15-year end-stage renal disease in hypertensive patients. Hypertension 25:587–594, 1995.
19. Klag MJ, Whelton PK, Randall BL, et al. End-stage renal disease in

African-American and white men: 16-year MRFIT findings. JAMA 277:1297–1298, 1997.

20. Lewis EJ, Hunsicker LG, Bain RP, Rohde RD. The effect of angiotensin converting enzyme inhibition in diabetic nephropathy. N Engl J Med 323:1456–1462, 1993.

21. Maschio G, Alberti D, Janin G, et al, for the Angiotensin-Converting Enzyme Inhibition in Progressive Renal Insufficiency Study Group. Effect of the angiotensin-converting enzyme inhibitor benazepril on the progression of chronic renal insufficiency. N Engl J Med 323:939–945, 1996.

22. Lazarus JM, Bourgoignie JJ, Buckalew VM, et al, for the Modification of Diet in Renal Disease Study Group. Achievement and safety of a low blood pressure goal in chronic renal disease: The Modification of Diet in Renal Disease Study Group. Hypertension 29:641–650, 1997.

23. Giatras I, Lau J, Levey AS. Effect of angiotensin-converting enzyme inhibitors on the progression of nondiabetic renal disease: A meta-analysis of randomized trials. Angiotensin-Converting Enzyme Inhibition and Progressive Renal Disease Study Group. Ann Intern Med 127:337–345, 1997.

24. Joint National Committee on Prevention, Detection, Evaluation, and Treatment of High Blood Pressure. The sixth report. Arch Intern Med 157:2413–2446, 1997.

25. Estacio RO, Jeffers BW, Hiatt WR, et al. The effect of nisoldipine as compared with enalapril on cardiovascular outcomes in patients with non-insulin dependent diabetes and hypertension. N Engl J Med 335:645–652, 1998.

26. Tatti P, Pahor M, Byington RB, et al. Outcome results of the Fosinopril versus Amlodipine Cardiovascular Events randomized Trial (FACET) in patients with hypertension and NIDDM. Diabetes Care 21:597–603, 1998.

27. Joint National Committee on Detection, Evaluation, and Treatment of High Blood Pressure. The fifth report. Arch Intern Med 153:154–186, 1993.

28. Curb JD, Pressel SL, Cutler JA, et al, for the Systolic Hypertension in the Elderly Program Cooperative Research Group. Effect of diuretic-based antihypertensive treatment on cardiovascular disease risk in older diabetic patients with isolated systolic hypertension. JAMA 276:1886–1892, 1996.

29. Liu L, Gong L, Wang J. Stroke incidence in the placebo-controlled Chinese Trial on Isolated Systolic Hypertension in the Elderly (SYST-CHINA). [Abstract] Am J Hypertens 11:245A, 1998.

30. Linjer E, Hansson L. Underestimation of the true benefits of antihypertensive treatment: An assessment of some important sources of error. J Hypertens 15:221–225, 1997.

31. Appel LJ, Moore TJ, Obarzanek E, et al, for the DASH Collaborative Research Group. A clinical trial of the effects of dietary patterns on blood pressure. N Engl J Med 336:1117–1124, 1997.

32. Stamler R, Stamler J, Gosch FC, et al. Primary prevention of hypertension by nutritional-hygienic means: Final report of a randomized, controlled trial. JAMA 262:1801–1807, 1989.

33. Trials of Hypertension Prevention Collaborative Research Group. The effects of nonpharmacologic interventions on blood pressure of persons with high normal levels: Results of the Trials of Hypertension Prevention, Phase I. JAMA 267:1213–1220, 1992.

34. Trials of Hypertension Prevention Collaborative Research Group. Effects of weight loss and sodium reduction intervention on blood pressure and hypertension incidence in overweight people with high-normal blood pressure: The Trials of Hypertension Prevention, Phase II. Arch Intern Med 157:657–667, 1997.

35. Cutler JA, Follman D, Allender PS. Randomized trials of sodium reduction: An overview. Am J Clin Nutr 65(suppl):643S–651S, 1997.

36. Kokkinos PF, Narayan P, Colleran JA, et al. Effects of regular exercise on blood pressure and left ventricular hypertrophy in African-American men with severe hypertension. N Engl J Med 333:1462–1467, 1995.

37. Whelton PK, Applegate WB, Ettinger WH, et al. Efficacy of weight loss and reduced sodium intake in the Trial of Nonpharmacologic Interventions in the Elderly (TONE). [Abstract] Circulation 94(suppl I):I-178, 1996.

38. Neaton JD, Grimm RH Jr, Prineas RJ, et al. Treatment of Mild Hypertension Study: Final results. JAMA 270:713–724, 1993.

39. Davis BR, Cutler JA, Gordon DJ, et al. Rationale and design for the Antihypertensive and Lipid Lowering Treatment to Prevent Heart Attack Trial (ALLHAT). Am J Hypertens 9:342–360, 1996.

40. Elliott WJ. ALLHAT: The largest and most important clinical trial in hypertension ever done in the U.S.A. [Editorial] Am J Hypertens 9:409–411, 1996.

41. Chatellier G, Ménard J. The absolute risk as a guide to influence the treatment decision-making process in mild hypertension. J Hypertens 15:217–219, 1997.

42. Alderman M. Blood pressure management: Individualized treatment based on absolute risk and the potential for benefit. Ann Intern Med 119:329–335, 1993.

43. Lever AF, Ramsay LE. Treatment of hypertension in the elderly. J Hypertens 13:571–579, 1995.

44. Dahlöf B, Lindholm LH, Hansson L, et al. Morbidity and mortality in the Swedish Trial in Old Patients with Hypertension (STOP-Hypertension). Lancet 338:1281–1285, 1991.

45. Swales JD. Economics and the treatment of hypertension. J Hypertens 13:1357–1361, 1995.

46. Elliott WJ. The costs of treating hypertension. In Epstein M (ed). Calcium Antagonists in Clinical Medicine, 2nd ed. Philadelphia, Hanley & Belfus, 1998; pp 513–526.

47. Klahr S, Levey AS, Beck GJ, et al. The effects of dietary protein restriction and blood-pressure control on the progression of chronic renal disease: Modification of Diet in Renal Disease Study Group. N Engl J Med 330:877–884, 1994.

48. Hypertension Detection and Follow-up Program Cooperative Group. Five-year findings of the Hypertension Detection and Follow-up Program. II. Mortality by race, sex and age. JAMA 242:2572–2577, 1979.

49. Farnett L, Mulrow CD, Linn WD, et al. The J-curve phenomenon and the treatment of hypertension: Is there a point beyond which pressure reduction is dangerous? JAMA 265:489–495, 1991.

50. Fletcher AE, Bulpitt CJ. How far should blood pressure be lowered? N Engl J Med 326:261–264, 1992.

51. Hansson L. The BBB study: The effect of intensified antihypertensive treatment on the level of blood pressure, side-effects, morbidity and mortality in "well-treated" hypertensive patients. Behandla Blodtryck Battre. Blood Press 3:248–254, 1994.

52. Hansson L, Zanchetti A, Carruthers SG, et al, on behalf of the HOT Study Group. Effects of intensive blood pressure lowering and low-dose aspirin in patients with hypertension: Principal results of the Hypertension Optimal Treatment (HOT) randomised trial. Lancet 351:1755–1762, 1998.

53. Messerli FH, Grossman E, Goldboourt U. Are beta-blockers efficacious as first-line therapy for hypertension in the elderly: A systematic review. JAMA 279:1903–1907, 1998.

54. National High Blood Pressure Education Program Working Group. Report on hypertension in the elderly. Hypertension 23:275–285, 1994.

55. Black HR, Elliott WJ, Neaton JD, et al, for the CONVINCE Research Group. Rationale and Design for the Controlled ONset Verapamil INvestigation of Cardiovascular Endpoints (CONVINCE) Trial. Control Clin Trials 19:370–390, 1998.

56. World Health Organization—International Society of Hypertension Blood Pressure Lowering Treatment Trialists' Collaboration. Protocol for prospective collaborative overviews of major randomized trials of blood-pressure–lowering treatments. J Hypertens 16:127–137, 1998.

57. Black HR, Crocitto MT. Number needed to treat: Solid science or a path to pernicious rationing? Am J Hypertens 11:128S–134S, 1998.

58. Chaturvedi N. Effect of lisinopril on progression of retinopathy in normotensive people with type 1 diabetes. Lancet 351:28–31, 1998.

59. Nuvachuku CE, Cutler JA. The explosion of morbidity and mortality trials in hypertension. Curr Opin Nephrol Hypertens 6:230–236, 1997.

60. GISEN Group (Gruppo Italiano di Studi Epidemiologici in Nefrologia). Randomised placebo-controlled trial of effect of ramipril on decline in glomerular filtration rate and risk of terminal renal failure in proteinuric, non-diabetic nephropathy. Lancet 349:1857–1863, 1997.

61. Hennekens CH, Albert CM, Godfried SL, et al. Adjunctive drug therapy of acute myocardial infarction—Evidence from clinical trials. N Engl J Med 335:1660–1667, 1996.

62. Yusuf S, Wittes J, Friedman L. Overview of randomized clinical trials in heart disease. I: Treatments following myocardial infarction. JAMA 260:2088–2093, 1988.

63. Soumerai SB, McLaughlin TJ, Spiegelman D, et al. Adverse outcomes of underuse of beta-blockers in elderly survivors of acute myocardial infarction. JAMA 277:115–121, 1997.

64. Garg R, Yusuf S, for the Collaborative Group on ACE-Inhibitor

Trials. Overview of randomized trials of angiotensin-converting enzyme inhibitors on mortality and morbidity in patients with heart failure. JAMA 273:1450–1456, 1995.

65. Young JB. Angiotensin-converting enzyme inhibitors post-myocardial infarction. Clin Cardiol 13:379–390, 1995.

66. Pitt B, Segal R, Martinez FA, et al, for the ELITE Study Investigators. Randomised trial of losartan versus captopril in patients over 65 with heart failure (Evaluation of Losartan in the Elderly Study). Lancet 349:747–752, 1997.

67. Horowitz RI, Viscoli CM, Berkman L. Treatment adherence and risk of death after a myocardial infarction. Lancet 336:542–545, 1990.

68. Gallagher EJ, Viscoli CM, Horowitz RI. The relationship of treatment adherence to the risk of death after myocardial infarction in women. JAMA 270:742–744, 1993.

69. Acute Infarction Ramipril Efficacy (AIRE) Study Investigators. Effect of ramipril on mortality and morbidity of survivors of acute myocardial infarction with clinical evidence of heart failure. Lancet 342:821–828, 1993.

70. MRC Working Party. Medical Research Council trial of treatment of hypertension in older adults. Principal results. BMJ 304:405–412, 1992.

71. McDermott MM, Schmitt B, Wallner E. Impact of medication nonadherence on coronary heart disease outcomes: A critical review. Arch Intern Med 157:1921–1929, 1997.

72. Coope J, Warrender TS. Randomised trial of treatment of hypertension in the elderly in primary care. BMJ 293:1145–1151, 1986.

73. Amery A, Birkenhager W, Brixko P, et al. Mortality and morbidity results from the European Working Party on High Blood Pressure in the Elderly trial. Lancet 1:1349–1354, 1985.

35 Characteristics of Published, Ongoing, and Planned Outcome Trials in Hypertension

Jan A. Staessen and Ji G. Wang

At present, several outcome trials in younger and older hypertensive patients have irrefutably proven that antihypertensive drug treatment reduces the risk of stroke, coronary heart disease, and other fatal and nonfatal cardiovascular complications.[1–29] Other published trials assessed the efficacy of diuretics (DIUs) and β-blockers (BBs) as first-line antihypertensive agents.[7, 8, 30–34] In spite of the abundant evidence already available, several questions remain unanswered and are being addressed by ongoing or planned trials. First, several trials investigate whether the newer classes of drugs, such as the calcium channel blockers (CCBs), the angiotensin I–converting enzyme inhibitors (ACEIs), the angiotensin II–type 1 receptor blockers (AR1Bs), and the α-blockers (ABs), are superior to DIUs and BBs in improving the prognosis of hypertensive patients.[35–49] Other trials study whether specific classes of antihypertensive drugs, over and above their blood pressure–lowering effect, might exert a beneficial effect in specific subgroups of hypertensive patients. Furthermore, a number of studies aim to clarify whether antihypertensive treatment or specific antihypertensive drugs are indicated in special groups of patients, such as the very elderly (≥80 years),[50, 51] those who have normal blood pressure but are at high cardiovascular risk,[52–58] patients with type II diabetes,[56, 59–67] patients with mild hypertension,[68] or hypertensive patients of African American extraction.[69] Finally, to what level the blood pressure should be lowered once antihypertensive treatment is prescribed is also subject to further investigation.[59, 61, 62, 69, 70]

This chapter does not attempt to repeat the work of the many meta-analysts who estimated the pooled results of the published outcome trials[71–76] or who will attempt to do this for the ongoing trials.[60, 75] The purpose of this chapter is to compare the characteristics of the published and ongoing trials in hypertension and hypertension-related disorders and to assess the assumptions made in establishing the sample size. Only long-term studies with primary or secondary fatal and nonfatal endpoints will be reviewed, excluding some trials that concentrate almost exclusively on softer intermediate endpoints.[77–86]

PUBLISHED TRIALS

Published Trials That Proved the Efficacy of Antihypertensive Drug Treatment

Most published trials (Table 35–1) tested the hypothesis that antihypertensive drug treatment, compared with no treatment or with placebo, would reduce morbidity and mortality in hypertensive patients.[1–4, 7–12, 14–28, 87–89] Some trials addressed the same question by comparing a well-organized antihypertensive drug treatment schedule with a treatment scheme left to the discretion of the treating physician[5, 6, 13] or by lowering the elevated diastolic blood pressure to graded target levels within the normotensive range.[29, 90–93]

Among the 25 outcome trials falling into this category, 6 recruited younger adults (<60 years)[8, 18, 19, 22, 25, 26]; 11 enrolled only older (≥60 years) patients[2–4, 7, 9–13, 17, 20]; and 8 entered both younger and older subjects.[5, 14, 16, 21, 23, 24, 27] In most of the intervention studies, the entry criteria stipulated that the diastolic blood pressure had to be 90 mm Hg or higher.[2, 4, 5, 8, 14, 17, 18, 21–26, 29] Three trials recruited exclusively patients with isolated systolic hypertension;[9, 10, 12] five studies enrolled patients with systolic or diastolic hypertension;[3, 11, 13, 19, 27] and in two studies the randomized patients had either isolated systolic hypertension or systolic combined with diastolic hypertension.[7, 20]

In most trials that proved the efficacy of antihypertensive treatment, a stepped-care approach was applied to titrate the study medication. Active treatment was usually initiated with a thiazide DIU or a BB. Only in the Shanghai

Table 35–1 Published Outcome Trials in Hypertension

Trial	Full Name of Trial or Study Group	Reference
ATTMH	Australian Trial in Mild Hypertension	14
Barraclough		22
Carter		27
CASTEL	Cardiovascular Study in the Elderly	13
EWPHE	European Working Party on High Blood Pressure in the Elderly	1, 2
HAPPHY	Heart Attack Primary Prevention in Hypertension Trial	31
HEP	Hypertension in the Elderly Prevention Trial	3
HDFP	Hypertension Detection and Follow-up Program	5, 6
HSCSG	Hypertension-Stroke Cooperative Study Group	21
HOT	Hypertension Optimal Treatment	29, 90–93
IPPPSH	International Prospective Primary Prevention Study in Hypertension	30
Kuramoto		20
MAPHY	Metoprolol Atherosclerosis Prevention in Hypertensives	32, 33
MRC-MH	Medical Research Council Trial in Mild Hypertension	8, 96
MRC-OA	Medical Research Council Trial in Old Adults	7
Oslo Trial		19
PATS	Post-Stroke Antihypertensive Treatment Study	16
SHEP	Systolic Hypertension in the Elderly Program	9, 87
Sprackling		17
STONE	Shanghai Trial of Nifedipine Treatment in the Elderly	11
STOP	Swedish Trial in Old Patients with Hypertension	4
SYST-China	Systolic Hypertension in the Elderly in China Trial	10, 28, 88
SYST-EUR	Systolic Hypertension in the Elderly in Europe Trial	12, 15, 89
USPHS	United States Public Health Service Hospitals Cooperative Study Group	26
VA-I	Veterans Administration Cooperative Study on Antihypertensive Agents (diastolic blood pressure: 115–129 mm Hg)	23
VA-II	Veterans Administration Cooperative Study on Antihypertensive Agents (diastolic blood pressure: 90–114 mm Hg)	24
VA-NHLBI	Veterans Administration–National Heart, Lung and Blood Institute Study Group for Evaluating Treatment in Mild Hypertension (feasibility study)	18
Wolff		25

Trial of Nifedipine Treatment in the Elderly (STONE),[11] Systolic Hypertension in the Elderly in Europe (SYST-Eur),[12, 15, 89] and Systolic Hypertension in the Elderly in China (SYST-China)[10, 28] trials, was antihypertensive treatment started with a dihydropyridine CCB, one of the newer drug classes. In many trials, DIUs and BBs were combined in treatment-resistant patients. The second-line or third-line active study medications included centrally or peripherally acting antiadrenergic agents, vasodilators, ACEIs, or CCBs.

The design characteristics of the trials that, over time, established the efficacy of antihypertensive drug treatment are summarized in Table 35–2. Of the 25 studies, 13 had a properly randomized double-blind design,[2, 4, 9, 12, 16, 18, 20–26] and 10 studies had a randomized open design.[3, 5, 7, 8, 13, 14, 17, 19, 27, 29] In 2 Chinese studies, the patients were alternatingly assigned to placebo or active treatment, but both the patients and the doctors remained blinded with respect to the treatment allocation.[11, 28] A prospective randomized open design with blinded endpoint evaluation (PROBE) was recently put forward as a novel concept,[94] although it is likely that this approach must have been common practice in many of the earlier published open trials.

Sample-size calculations require the definition of desired levels of statistical significance (α) and power (β), an estimate of the risk in the control group, and a projection of the change of the rate of the primary endpoint in the active-treatment or experimental group or groups. The required number of patient-years may be accumulated by following a larger number of patients over a shorter period of time or vice versa. Ten trials formally reported the levels of significance and power used in the sample size calculations.[3–5, 7–10, 12, 14, 16] Significance was set at 5% in five trials,[3–5, 9, 14] at 2% in one trial,[7] and at a conservative 1% level in four studies.[8, 10, 12, 16] The sample size of nine trials provided 90% power[3–5, 7, 9, 10, 12, 14, 16] and that of the Medical Research Council Trial in Mild Hypertension (MRC-MH), 95%.[8] The primary endpoint was fatal and nonfatal stroke in eight trials[3, 7–10, 12, 16, 21] and total mortality in four trials.[5, 13, 17, 27] Other trials considered composite endpoints.[2, 4, 14, 19, 20, 22–26] The sample size actually recruited varied widely, ranging from under 100 to over 18,000 randomized patients. In general, the trials for which detailed sample size calculations have been published (see Table 35–2) were larger than the others and were also more likely to demonstrate a significant positive outcome for the primary endpoint.

A quantitative overview[71] of 14 unconfounded randomized trials, which mainly tested DIUs or BBs as first-line treatment, showed that a decrease in diastolic blood pressure of 5 to 6 mm Hg reduced stroke by 42%, coronary heart disease by 14%, and vascular death by 21%. In older patients with systolic combined with diastolic hypertension, antihypertensive treatment starting with a DIU or a BB decreased total mortality by 10 to 15%, cardiovascular mortality by 20 to 25%, stroke by nearly 40%, coronary heart disease by 15 to 20%, and cardiovascular morbidity and mortality by 30%.[72] More recently, a systematic review[73] classified active treatment into BB therapy and high-dose or low-dose DIU therapy. This meta-analysis demonstrated that BB therapy as well as high-dose DIU therapy

Table 35–2 Published Trials That Proved the Efficacy of Antihypertensive Drug Treatment

Trial*	Year†	Active Drugs‡	Endpoints§	Design‖	α¶	β¶	FU**	Risk††	Δ%††	Sample Size‡‡
ACTIVE TREATMENT VS. PLACEBO										
Wolff	1965	Reserpine	TM + CV	R, DB	—	—	1.4	323.0	70	87
VA-I	1967	HCTZ + reserpine + hydralazine	TM + CV§§	R, DB	—	—	1.5	200.0	95	143
VA-II	1970	HCTZ + reserpine + hydralazine	TM + CV§§	R, DB	—	—	3.3	54.5	73	380
Barraclough	1973	Bendrofluazide	CV	R, DB	—	—	2.0	121.0	79	116
HSCSG	1974	Deserpidine + methyclothiazide	Stroke recurrence	R, DB	—	—	3.0 (5.0)	64.0 (100)	17 (50)	452 (350)
USPHS	1977	HCTZ + rauwolfia	TM + stroke + MI	R, DB	0.05	0.95	7.0 (7.0)	7.0 (350)	10 (57)	389 (400–450)
VA-NHLBI	1977	Chlorthalidone	Feasibility study	R, DB	—	—	1.5	—	—	1012
ATTMH	1980	Chlorothiazide	TM + CV	R, SB	0.05	0.90	4.0 (5.0)	24.5	20 (30)	3427 (3640)
Kuramoto	1981	Trichlormethiazide	Stroke + cardiac events	R, DB	—	—	4.0	55.0	52	91
EWPHE	1985	HCTZ + triamterene	TM + CV	R, DB	—	—	4.7 (5.0)	—	—	840
MRC-MH	1985	Bendrofluazide, propranolol	Stroke + MHT	R, SB	0.01	0.95	4.9 (5.0)	2.6	45 (40)	17,354 (18,000)
SHEP	1991	Chlorthalidone	Stroke	R, DB	0.05	0.90	4.5 (5.0)	—	36 (32)	4736 (4800)
STOP	1991	Atenolol, metoprolol, pindolol, HCTZ + amiloride	CVM + stroke + MI	R, DB	0.05	0.90	2.0 (3.0)	55.5	40 (35)	1627 (2000)
MRC-OA	1992	HCTZ + amiloride, atenolol	Stroke	R, SB	0.02	0.90	5.8 (5.0)	10.8	25 (30)	4396 (5000)
PATS	1995	Indapamide	Stroke recurrence	R, DB	0.01	0.90	2.0 (2.0)	41.0 (50.0)	29 (25)	5665 (5000)
STONE	1996	Nifedipine	CV	A, DB	—	—	2.5	29.6	60	1632
Syst-Eur	1997	Nitrendipine	Stroke	R, DB	0.01	0.90	2.0 (5.0)	13.7 (17.0)	42 (40)	4695 (3000)
Syst-China	1998	Nitrendipine	Stroke	A, DB	0.01	0.90	3.0 (5.0)	20.8 (17.0)	38 (40)	2394 (3000)
ACTIVE TREATMENT VS. NO TREATMENT										
Carter	1970	Thiazides	TM	R, O	—	—	4.0	115.0	42.0	97
Oslo Study	1980	HCTZ	CV	R, O	—	—	5.5	16.3	31.0	785
Sprackling	1981	Methyldopa	TM	R, O	—	—	4.0	—	—	123
HEP	1986	Atenolol	Stroke, CHD	R, O	0.05	0.90	4.4 (5.0)	21.4 (30.0)	42.0 (33)	884 (800)
STANDARDIZED TREATMENT VS. USUAL CARE										
HDFP	1979	Chlorthalidone	TM	R, O	5.00	0.90	5.0 (5.0)	7.7	16.9 (40)	10,940 (10,500)
CASTEL	1994	Clonidine, nifedipine, Atenolol + Chlorthalidone	TM	R, O	—	—	7.0	49.9	36.0	655
MODERATE VS. VIGOROUS BLOOD PRESSURE LOWERING										
HOT	1998	Felodipine	CVM + stroke + MI	R, OBE	—	—	3.8 (2.5)	9.9 (30.0)	— (15)	18,790 (18,000)

*See Table 35–1 for acronyms.

†Year of (main) publication.

‡Only first-line antihypertensive drugs are listed. Alternative drugs are separated by a comma. A plus sign (+) indicates a fixed combination of drugs. HCTZ, hydrochlorothiazide.

§The primary endpoint used in the analysis or in the sample-size calculations. A plus sign (+) denotes a composite endpoint. CHD, coronary heart disease; CV, fatal and nonfatal cardiovascular endpoints; CVM, cardiovascular mortality; MHT, malignant hypertension leading to death; MI, myocardial infarction; TM, total mortality.

‖A, alternate treatment allocation; R, randomized; DB, double-blind; SB, single-blind; O, open treatment; OBE, open treatment with blinded endpoint evaluation.

¶Levels of significance (α) and power (β) used in the sample-size calculations.

**FU indicates the average or median follow-up in years.

††Risk indicates the rate per 1000 patient-years in the reference group (placebo, no treatment, usual care, or highest on-treatment blood pressure); Δ% refers to the percentage reduction of the reference rate by experimental treatment (active drugs, standardized treatment, or more vigorous blood pressure reduction).

‡‡Numbers in parentheses refer to projections made in the sample-size calculations.

§§Excludes myocardial infarction and minor cerebrovascular thrombosis, but includes severe hypertension and hypotension.

343

significantly reduced stroke and congestive heart failure. Low-dose DIU therapy not only reduced stroke by 34% and congestive heart failure by 42%, but also decreased coronary heart disease by 28% and total mortality by 10%.[73]

Published Trials That Assessed the Protection Conferred by Diuretics or β-Blockers

Many trials have demonstrated the efficacy of DIUs or BBs (Table 35–3). The International Prospective Primary Prevention Study in Hypertension (IPPPSH)[30] was a randomized, double-blind trial conducted in 6357 men and women aged 40 to 64 years, with uncomplicated hypertension (diastolic blood pressure 100 to 125 mm Hg). At the start of the study, 3185 patients received antihypertensive treatment based on oxprenolol, a nonselective BB with intrinsic sympathomimetic activity,[95] and in the remaining 3172 patients, oxprenolol was replaced by placebo. The study medication could be increased, and other, open-label non–β-blocking antihypertensive drugs could be added to the double-blind study medication with the aim of reducing the diastolic blood pressure to the target level of 95 mm Hg or lower. Total DIU use was 67% in the oxprenolol patients and 82% in the control group.

The Heart Attack Primary Prevention in Hypertension (HAPPHY) Trial[31] had an open, randomized design with blinded endpoint evaluation.[94] Initially, the patients were randomized to metoprolol or to a DIU (hydrochlorothiazide or bendroflumethiazide). The first patients were randomized in March 1976. Two years later, the protocol of the ongoing trial was changed, so that centers wishing to randomize patients to either the BB atenolol or to one of the two DIUs could also take part. Of the 184 centers, 70 used metoprolol. The first-line drugs, either a BB or a DIU, were not to be crossed over or to be given together. Of the randomized patients, approximately 85% remained on the scheduled treatment, nearly 20% were prescribed hydralazine as second-line drug, and 5% had spironolactone as third-line treatment. About 4% in both the DIU and the BB group were on the opposite drug, and 3% were on drugs other than those foreseen by the protocol.

The Metoprolol Atherosclerosis Prevention in Hypertensives (MAPHY) trial[32] was published after the HAPPHY study,[31] but both trials shared 3234 patients. Indeed, when the HAPPHY trial closed on 31 December 1985, 66 of the 70 centers using metoprolol decided to continue following their patients, with the goal of collecting more data on the possible cardiovascular protective effects of metoprolol. No information about endpoints was available at the time of the decision to continue the trial.

In the single-blind Medical Research Council (MRC) trial in mild hypertension,[8, 96] adult patients (35 to 64 years) were randomized to active treatment with either propranolol (up to 240 mg/day) or bendrofluazide (10 mg/day), or to placebo. The MRC trial in older adults (65 to 74 years)[7] used a similar design but tested low-dose DIU treatment and a cardioselective BB (atenolol) against placebo. An early substudy had assessed blood pressure control and biochemical effects of two different dose regimens of DIUs, either hydrochlorothiazide 50 mg/day combined with 5 mg amiloride, or hydrochlorothiazide 25 mg/day combined with 2.5 mg amiloride. As a result, all patients randomized to DIU treatment were eventually transferred to the lower dose. The daily dose of atenolol was 50 mg, but was doubled to 100 mg in 20% of the patients. When further blood pressure control was necessary, the alternative trial drug was used to supplement the active drug allocated by randomization. After this, the CCB nifedipine in doses of up to 20 mg/day or other supplementary drugs could be prescribed.

ONGOING OR PLANNED TRIALS

Trials That Compare Active Treatment With Placebo in Special Groups of Patients

Among the ongoing or planned trials,[35–70, 97–102] 12 have a double-blind design (Tables 35–4 and 35–5) and aim to test the efficacy of the newer antihypertensive drugs versus placebo in special target groups of patients, such as patients with coronary heart disease but with preserved left-ventricular function (three trials),[52, 54, 55] patients with type 2 diabetes with or without diabetic nephropathy (four trials),[56, 63–65] Chinese patients with high cardiovascular risk profiles (personal communication from Lisheng Liu, Beijing, 1998), patients with a history of a cerebrovascular accident,[57] or old (70 to 89 years)[68] to very old (≥80 years)[50] patients with mild[68] to more severe[50] hypertension.

Trials in Patients with Type 2 Diabetes

The Appropriate Blood Pressure Control in Diabetes-Normotensive Cohort (ABCD) trial[65–67, 70, 99] is a prospective randomized clinical trial of 950 patients with type II diabetes. It was designed to evaluate the effects of blood pressure control on the prevention and progression of diabetic nephropathy, retinopathy, cardiovascular disease, and neuropathy and to compare the CCB nisoldipine (10 to 60 mg/day) with the ACEI enalapril (5 to 40 mg/day) as first-line antihypertensive agents. After the placebo run-in period, the 950 patients were stratified according to their mean baseline diastolic blood pressure, determined at two separate visits, into 480 normotensive (80 to 89 mm Hg) and 470 hypertensive (≥90 mm Hg) patients. In the normotensive cohort, the patients were randomly assigned to intensive treatment with the goal of decreasing the diastolic blood pressure by 10 mm Hg from the mean baseline value (with further random assignment to receive either nisoldipine or enalapril), or to moderate treatment with no intended change in the baseline diastolic blood pressure (these patients were randomly assigned to receive placebo). Thus, in the normotensive group, 50% of the patients received placebo, 25% nisoldipine, and 25% enalapril. A similar approach was used for the patients with hypertension. Patients were randomly assigned either to intensive treatment, with a target diastolic blood pressure of 75 mm Hg, or to moderate treatment, with a target diastolic blood pressure of 80 to 89 mm Hg. Unlike the normotensive group, however, all the patients with hypertension received active treatment (50% nisoldipine and 50% enalapril). The

Table 35–3 Published Trials That Assessed the Protection Conferred by Diuretics or β-Blockers

Trial*	Year	Drugs Tested	Endpoints	Design	α	β	FU	Risk†	Δt	Sample Size
IPPPSH	1985	Oxprenolol vs. placebo	Sudden death + MI	R, DB	0.05	0.90	4.0 (3–5)	8.4 (15)	9 (35–50)	6357 (5000)
MRC-MH	1985	Bendrofluazide vs. propranolol	Stroke + MHT	R, SB	—	—	4.9 (5.0)	1.9	58	8700 (9000)
HAPPHY	1987	Atenolol, metoprolol, propranolol vs. HCTZ, bendroflumethiazide	CHD death + MI	R, OBE	0.05	0.90	3.8 (5.0)	9.48 (20)	−12 (30)	6569 (4000)
MAPHY	1988	Metoprolol vs. HCTZ, bendroflumethiazide	TM	R, OBE	—	—	5.0	6.2	30	3234
MRC-OA	1992	HCTZ + amiloride vs. atenolol	Stroke	R, SB	—	—	5.8 (5.0)	9.0	19	2183 (2500)

*See Table 35–1 for acronyms.
†Risk indicates the rate in the reference group on placebo or thiazide diuretics; Δ refers to the percentage risk reduction in the group randomized to β-blockade.
See Table 35–2 for further explanation.

Table 35–4 Ongoing Trials in Hypertension or Hypertension-Related Disorders

Trial	Full Name of Trial or Study Group	References
AASK	African-American Study of Kidney Disease and Hypertension	69, 98
ABCD	Appropriate Blood Pressure Control in Diabetes—Normotensive Cohort	65–67, 70, 99
ALLHAT	Antihypertensive and Lipid Lowering to Prevent Heart Attack Trial	45, 114, 122
ANBP2	Australian National Blood Pressure Study—2	40
ASCOT	Anglo-Scandinavian Cardiac Outcome Trial	47
BENEDICT	Bergamo Nephrologic Diabetes Complication Trial	63
CAPPP	Captopril Prevention Project	41, 43, 97, 102
CLEVER	Chinese Lacidipine Event Reduction Trial	
CONVINCE	Controlled Onset Verapamil Investigation for Cardiovascular Endpoints	46, 116
CSGTEI	Collaborative Study Group Trial on Effect of Irbesartan	64
DIAB-HYCAR	Diabetes Hypertension Cardiovascular Morbidity-Mortality and Ramipril	56
HDS	Hypertension in Diabetes Study	59, 61, 62
HOPE	Heart Outcomes Prevention Evaluation Study	52
HYVET	Hypertension in the Very Elderly Trial	50, 51
INSIGHT	International Nifedipine GITS Study as a Goal for Hypertension Therapy	44
INVEST	International Verapamil-Trandolapril Study	49
LIFE	Losartan Intervention for Endpoint Reduction in Hypertension	36, 115
NICS-EH	National Intervention Cooperative Study in Elderly Hypertensives	39
NORDIL	Nordic Diltiazem Study	38
PEACE	Prevention of Events With Angiotensin-Converting Enzyme Inhibition	55, 101*
PROGRESS	Perindopril Protection Against Recurrent Stroke Study	57, 58
QUIET	Quinapril Ischemic Event Trial	53, 54, 100
RENAAL	Randomized Evaluation of NIDDM with the Angiotensin II Antagonist Losartan	60*
SCOPE	Study of Cognition and Prognosis in Elderly Patients with Hypertension	68
SHELL	Systolic Hypertension in the Elderly Lacidipine Long-Term Study	42, 113
STOP-2	Swedish Trial in Old Patients with Hypertension-2	35, 37
VALUE	Diovan Antihypertensive Long-Term Use Evaluation	48

*Specific reference not found at the time of writing.

study duration was 5 years and the study was scheduled to end in May 1998.[65]

The primary outcome measure in the ABCD trial was glomerular filtration rate as assessed by 24-hour creatinine clearance.[65] Secondary outcome measures were urinary albumin excretion, left-ventricular hypertrophy, retinopathy, neuropathy, and the incidence of cardiovascular morbidity and mortality. Recently, the Data and Safety Monitoring Committee of the ABCD trial recommended that nisoldipine treatment be terminated in the hypertensive group because the rate of fatal and nonfatal myocardial infarction was significantly higher among the hypertensive patients randomized to nisoldipine than among those assigned to enalapril.[99] The risk ratio was 9.5 (95% CI, 2.3 to 21.4). Among the 470 hypertensive patients, control of blood pressure, blood glucose and lipid concentrations, and smoking behavior were similar in the nisoldipine (235 patients) and enalapril (235 patients) groups throughout 5 years of follow-up. However, more patients in the enalapril group received DIUs ($p = .02$) or BBs ($p = .04$) as second-line treatment, and the first-line drug tended to be stopped more frequently in the nisoldipine group (142 vs. 129 patients). These findings suggest that cardiovascular protection by antihypertensive drug treatment may have been greater in the enalapril group. Moreover, the ABCD trial investigators did not report whether the hypertensive patients were still on nisoldipine or enalapril when they experienced a myocardial infarction. Similarly, the doses of nisoldipine and enalapril were not reported and the authors did not present a first-ever event survival analysis or a per-protocol analysis. Because the preliminary ABCD trial findings[99] involved a secondary endpoint, the investigators cautioned that their results should be balanced against the evidence of other reported or ongoing trials.[99] The trial continued in the normotensive group, and the overall final results will be reported later.

The Diabetes Hypertension Cardiovascular Morbidity-Mortality and Ramipril (DIAB-HYCAR) study[56] started from the supposition that microalbuminuria and proteinuria are strong independent predictors of increased cardiovascular mortality in patients with type 2 diabetes. In such patients, ACEIs retard the development of diabetic nephropathy,[103–107] but no data are currently available on the effects of ACEIs on cardiovascular endpoints. The aim of the DIAB-HYCAR study is to test the hypothesis that an ACEI at a low daily dose (1.25 mg ramipril), which has no significant effect on blood pressure, may reduce cardiovascular morbidity, mortality, or both, in normotensive or hypertensive patients with type 2 diabetes and persistent albuminuria. Selected and followed by general practitioners, 4000 patients will receive their usual oral antidiabetic treatment and, if necessary, antihypertensive treatment with the exclusion of ACEIs. In addition, in a randomized, double-blind trial they will be given either a placebo or 1.25 mg ramipril/day. The follow-up is currently scheduled to last 3 years. The efficacy of ACEIs will be assessed by the following major endpoints: cardiovascular death, sudden death, myocardial infarction, stroke, and renal replacement therapy.[56]

The Collaborative Study Group Trial on Effect of Irbesartan (CSGTEI)[64] is a double-blind clinical trial designed to compare the effects of the AR1B irbesartan, the CCB amlodipine, and placebo on morbidity, mortality, and renal function in hypertensive patients with diabetic nephropathy

Table 35–5 Ongoing Trials That Compare Antihypertensive Drugs with Placebo in Special Patient Groups

Trial*	Year†	Group‡	First-Line Active Drugs§	Endpoints||	Design¶	α**	β**	FU††	Risk‡‡	Δ%‡‡	Sample Size
PEACE	—	CHD	Trandolapril	CVM + MI	R, DB	—	—	5.0	—	—	14,000
QUIET	1995	CHD	Quinapril	Angiographic CHD, cardiac endpoints	R, DB	0.05	0.95	3.0	120.0	25	1700
ABCD	1998	NIDDM	Enalapril, nisoldipine	GFR, CVM, CVD	R, DB	—	—	—	—	—	950
DIAB-HYCAR	1999	NIDDM-N	Ramipril	CVM + SD + MI + stroke + kidney transplantation	R, DB	0.05	0.90	3.0	22.2	20	4000
CSGTEI	2000	NIDDM-N	Irbesartan, amlodipine	TM + RF	R, DB	—	—	3.0	—	—	1650
HOPE	2000	CHD	Ramipril	CVM + MI + stroke	R, DB	0.01	0.90	4.0	50.0	15	9000
BENEDICT	2001	NIDDM	Verapamil, trandolapril, verapamil + trandolapril	Diabetic nephropathy	R, DB	0.05	0.80	3.0	50.0	40	2400
CLEVER	2001	High risk	Lacidipine	Stroke	R, DB	0.05	0.80	3.0	14.0	30	10,000
PROGRESS	2001	CBV	Perindopril, perindopril + indapamide	Stroke	R, DB	0.05	0.90	4.0	20.0	30	6000
SCOPE	2001	Mild HT	Candesartan	CVM + MI + stroke, TM, dementia	R, DB	—	—	2.5	32.0	—	4000
RENAAL	2002	NIDDM-N	Losartan	Diabetic nephropathy	R, DB	—	—	4.0	—	—	1500
HYVET	2003	≥80 years	Indapamide	Stroke	R, DB	0.01	0.90	5.0	40.0	40	2100

*See Table 35–4 for acronyms.
†Year of intended publication.
‡Special groups eligible for recruitment: CBV, cerebrovascular disease, including transient ischemic attack and stroke; CHD, coronary heart disease; HT, hypertension; NIDDM, non-insulin–dependent diabetes mellitus (type 2 diabetes); NIDDM-N, non-insulin–dependent diabetic patients with nephropathy.
§Only first-line antihypertensive drugs are listed. Alternative drugs are separated by a comma. A plus sign (+) indicates a fixed combination of drugs.
||The primary endpoint used in the sample size calculations or the endpoint stated to be of major interest in the final analysis. A plus sign (+) denotes a composite endpoint and a comma separates alternative endpoints. CHD, coronary heart disease; CVM, cardiovascular mortality; CVD, cardiovascular morbidity; GFR, rate of decline of the glomerular filtration rate; MI, myocardial infarction; RF, renal failure defined as the doubling of serum creatinine; SD, sudden death; TM, total mortality.
¶R, randomized to treatment; DB, double-blind; SB, single-blind; O, open treatment; OBE, open treatment with blinded endpoint evaluation.
**Levels of significance (α) and power (β) used in the sample-size calculations.
††Projected duration of follow-up in years.
‡‡Risk indicates the rate in the placebo group; Δ% refers to the percentage reduction of the placebo rate on active treatment.

(type 2 diabetes mellitus). The primary outcome is the composite endpoint of time to doubling of entry serum creatinine concentration or death. Secondary outcomes include fatal and nonfatal cardiovascular endpoints. The goal is to recruit at 200 sites worldwide 1650 patients to be followed for at least 2 years. The eligibility criteria include: age 30 to 70 years; adult onset diabetes; urine protein excretion exceeding 0.9 g/day; and serum creatinine 1.0 to 3.0 mg/dl in women and 1.2 to 3.0 mg/dl in men. The target blood pressure in the three groups is defined as a sitting blood pressure below 135 mm Hg systolic and 95 mm Hg diastolic. These levels must be achieved using the three study medications as first-line treatment and additional antihypertensive drugs, excluding CCBs, ACEIs, and AR1Bs. The initial 765 patients were on average ($\pm$SD) 59 $\pm$ 8 years old. Their screening blood pressure was 159 $\pm$ 18 mm Hg systolic and 87 $\pm$ 10 mm Hg diastolic. Their urinary protein excretion was 4.3 $\pm$ 4.0 g/day and their serum creatinine 1.7 $\pm$ 0.6 mg/dl. Of the 765 patients, 67% were male; 72% were white and 15% African American; and 66% had diabetic retinopathy and 47% had neuropathy.

The Bergamo Nephrologic Diabetes Complication Trial (BENEDICT) is a prospective, randomized, double-blind, parallel-group study[63] that aims to investigate whether antihypertensive drug treatment would prevent diabetic nephropathy in 2400 hypertensive patients with type II diabetes. During the first phase of the trial, the patients will be randomized and treated for 3 years with the phenylalkylamine CCB verapamil in slow-release formulation (240 mg/day), the ACEI trandolapril (2 mg/day), the combination of these two drugs (verapamil 180 mg/day plus trandolapril 2 mg/day) or placebo. Other antihypertensive agents will be used to achieve and maintain in all patients systolic and diastolic blood pressure consistently below 140 and 90 mm Hg, respectively. The primary outcome variable of the first phase of the trial will be the progression to microalbuminuria. In the second phase, progression to macroalbuminuria will be assessed in the patients who became microalbuminuric during the first part of the trial. The latter patients will be rerandomized to 2 years of treatment with trandolapril (2 mg/day) alone or combined with verapamil (180 mg/day). The secondary outcome variables include the rate of increase in albuminuria; the rate of decline of glomerular filtration; the rate of progression of diabetic retinopathy; and the cumulative incidence of major cardiovascular endpoints and all-cause and cardiovascular mortality.

Randomized Evaluation of NIDDM [type II diabetes] with the Angiotensin II Antagonist Losartan (RENAAL) is a double-blind, placebo-controlled trial of the AR1B losartan in patients with type II diabetes and diabetic nephropathy. RENAAL was listed in the review article written by the World Health Organization–International Society of Hypertension Blood Pressure Lowering Treatment Trialists' Collaboration.[60] However, according to a Medline search in July 1998, published information on the RENAAL protocol did not seem to be available.

Trials in Patients with Previous Cardiovascular Disease

The primary objective of the Prevention of Events With Angiotensin-Converting Enzyme Inhibition (PEACE) trial[55, 101] is to determine whether addition of an ACEI (trandolapril, titrated to 4 mg/day) to standard therapy in patients with coronary artery disease and preserved left-ventricular function prevents cardiovascular mortality and reduces the risk of myocardial infarction. A secondary objective is to determine whether long-term ACEIs reduce cardiovascular death and hospital admissions for primary cardiovascular complications, including myocardial infarction, unstable angina, revascularization, cerebrovascular events, congestive heart failure, or arrhythmias.

The Quinapril Ischemic Event Trial (QUIET)[53, 54, 100] is a double-blind, placebo-controlled trial set up to investigate the long-term antiatherosclerotic effects of ACEIs in normotensive patients with angiographically documented coronary artery disease and normal left-ventricular systolic function. The hypothesis is that ACEIs will reduce the cardiac event rate by retarding or preventing coronary lesion progression, and that this can be documented by follow-up angiography in a subgroup of patients. Eligible patients are between 18 and 75 years old. They have all undergone successful percutaneous coronary transluminal angioplasty or atherectomy within 12 to 72 hours before enrollment, and have at least one major coronary artery that has not been subjected to intervention. Patients are required to have a low-density-lipoprotein cholesterol of 165 mg/dl or less without lipid-lowering drugs and to have an ejection fraction of at least 40%. After stratification for clinical center and for single versus multiple coronary heart disease, 1750 normotensive, normolipidemic subjects with normal left-ventricular systolic function were randomly assigned to receive 20 mg quinapril or matching placebo once daily for 3 years. The primary endpoint is the incidence of cardiac complications in the entire QUIET patient population on an intention-to-treat basis. The randomized patients have the following baseline characteristics (mean $\pm$ SD): age 58 $\pm$ 9 years; blood pressure 123 $\pm$ 15 mm Hg systolic and 74 $\pm$ 10 mm Hg diastolic; low-density-lipoprotein cholesterol 124 $\pm$ 27 mg/dl; high-density-lipoprotein cholesterol 37 $\pm$ 10 mg/dl; and triglycerides 167 $\pm$ 91 mg/dl. In addition, 81% are men, 22% are current smokers, and 49% gave a history of myocardial infarction.

The Heart Outcomes Prevention Evaluation (HOPE) trial[52] is a randomized, double-blind trial with a 2 $\times$ 2 factorial design. The study aims to investigate the efficacy of the ACEI ramipril and the antioxidant vitamin E in the prevention of myocardial infarction, stroke, or cardiovascular death. Eligible patients are men and women, aged 55 years or older, who have previous coronary heart disease, stroke, or peripheral vascular disease. Patients with diabetes mellitus also qualify if they have at least one other cardiovascular risk factor, such as hypertension (blood pressure equal to or higher than 160 mm Hg systolic or 90 mm Hg diastolic), total cholesterol higher than 200 mg/dl, high-density-lipoprotein cholesterol lower than 35 mg/dl, current cigarette smoking, known albuminuria, or any evidence of previous cardiovascular disease.

Patients eligible for randomization in the HOPE trial are identified via medical records, admissions to coronary care units, logs of invasive or noninvasive laboratory and relevant surgical procedures, screening in diabetic clinics, and referrals from physicians. About 3 weeks before randomization, a run-in visit is arranged. Eligible patients receive for 7 to 10 days 2.5 mg active ramipril per day followed by 10 to 14 days of placebo ramipril. Serum creatinine and potassium are determined between days 7 and 10 of the run-in phase (on active ramipril) to determine initial safety and tolerance of ACEIs. In total, 10,711 patients attended the eligibility visit. Of these, 135 were found ineligible and 10,576 entered the run-in phase; 1035 patients were withdrawn at the end of the run-in phase, and 9541 (90%) patients were randomized to ramipril (2.5 mg for 1 week, then 5 mg/day for 3 weeks), or matching placebo and vitamin E (400 IU/day), or matching placebo. At the first follow-up visit 1 month later, the dose of ramipril is increased to 10 mg/day. Further follow-up visits occur at 6 months and every 6 months thereafter up to the end of the study. The mean duration of follow-up is expected to be approximately 4 years. As of 1 January 1996, the study has completed randomizing 9541 patients. These include 2543 women, 7553 patients with previous cardiovascular disease, 3654 with diabetes mellitus, and 4406 with hypertension. Approximately half the patients are over 65 years of age. The primary endpoint in the HOPE trial is the incidence of myocardial infarction, stroke, and cardiovascular death combined. Major secondary endpoints include the following: total and cardiovascular mortality; the development of overt nephropathy or the need for dialysis among the patients with diabetes; hospitalization for congestive heart failure; unstable angina requiring hospitalization; all cardiovascular revascularization procedures; and fatal and nonfatal cancers.

For stroke mortality, most but not all reports have shown that the lowest rates are associated with the lowest treated systolic and diastolic blood pressures.[108, 109] The published observational studies suggest that the best target blood pressure for antihypertensive treatment would be at or below 130 mm Hg systolic and 85 mm Hg diastolic.[109] Along these lines, the Perindopril Protection Against Recurrent Stroke (PROGRESS) study,[57, 58] a randomized, double-blind placebo-controlled trial, aims to determine the effects of blood pressure reduction with an ACEI-based treatment regimen on the stroke risk of patients with a history of cerebrovascular disease. Eligible patients must have a history of transient ischemic attack (including amaurosis fugax), cerebral infarction, cerebral hemorrhage, or a stroke of unknown type. The qualifying event must have occurred within the past 5 years. Additionally, patients must have no clear indication for or against treatment with an ACEI and no disability likely to prevent regular attendance at the study's clinics. Both hypertensive and nonhypertensive patients are potentially eligible for inclusion. Before randomization, the patients receive open-label treatment with 2 mg perindopril/day for 2 weeks and then 4 mg perindopril/day for 2 additional weeks. At randomization, the patients are assigned to double-blind treatment with active perindopril (4 mg/day) with or without active indapamide (2.5 mg/day, except in Japan, where the dose will be 2 mg/day) or matching placebo or placebos. For patients without any indication for or against a DIU, the study treatment will comprise both perindopril and indapamide or matching placebos; for all other patients, the study treatment will comprise perindopril alone or matching placebo.

Allocation to active treatment or placebo will be performed by fax to the PROGRESS study randomization service.[57, 58] A minimization algorithm[101] stratifies treatment allocation by study center, sex, age (in decades), entry systolic blood pressure (in 20–mm Hg strata), inclusion diagnosis (transient ischemic attack, cerebral infarction, cerebral hemorrhage, stroke of an unknown type), and the intention to use combination therapy (perindopril plus indapamide or matching placebos) or monotherapy (perindopril alone or placebo). The primary study outcome is a stroke, defined as an acute disturbance of focal neurological function with symptoms lasting more than 24 hours and thought to be caused by cerebral ischemia or hemorrhage. Secondary study outcomes include a fatal or disabling stroke (with disability assessed 6 to 12 months after the stroke, using the Lindley classification system[110]); total major cardiovascular events (stroke, myocardial infarction, or cardiovascular death); death from cardiovascular disease; cognitive function (assessed at annual visits using the Mini-Mental State Examination[111] and dementia; and disability and dependency (assessed at annual visits using the Barthel and Lindley classification systems[110, 112]). After randomization, the patients will be assessed at 2 weeks, 1, 3, 6, 9, and 12 months, and thereafter at 6-month intervals until the scheduled end of the study in October 2000.

The Chinese Lacidipine Event Reduction (CLEVER) trial (personal communication by Lisheng Liu, Beijing, 1998) will include Chinese patients with documented cardiovascular disease or additional risk factors. The primary endpoint will be the incidence of fatal and nonfatal stroke, but further details on the protocol of this recently planned trial are not yet available.

Other Placebo-Controlled Trials

The Study of Cognition and Prognosis in Elderly Patients with Hypertension (SCOPE)[68] is a multinational, double-blind, prospective study that will evaluate the ability of antihypertensive treatment to improve cardiovascular prognosis and prevent cognitive impairment in elderly hypertensive patients. Approximately 4000 patients will be randomly assigned to treatment with the long-acting AR1B candesartan or to placebo. Patients are 70 to 89 years old and have systolic blood pressure rates of 160 to 179 mm Hg or diastolic blood pressure rates of 90 to 99 mm Hg, or both. Mean duration of follow-up will be 2.5 years. Any previous antihypertensive treatment will be standardized to hydrochlorothiazide 12.5 mg once daily, and the study drugs will be given in addition. The starting dose of candesartan is 8 mg/day; it is increased to 16 mg/day if necessary to control blood pressure. In patients with blood pressure rates continuously above 160 mm Hg systolic or 90 mm Hg diastolic, in either treatment group, additional antihypertensive treatment is recommended. The primary endpoint consists of the combined incidence of cardiovascular mortality, nonfatal myocardial infarction, and nonfatal stroke. Secondary endpoints include cognitive function measured by the Mini-Mental State Examination,[111] total mortality, renal function, hospitalization, quality of life, and health economics.

The Hypertension in the Very Elderly Trial (HYVET)[50] started as an open-label feasibility study. However, the main trial will have a randomized, double-blind, placebo-controlled design to detect a 35% difference in stroke incidence between placebo and active treatment in hypertensive patients aged 80 years or over. Patients will be eligible for the trial if they have sustained systolic blood pressures while on single-blind placebo of 160 to 199 mm Hg and at the same time diastolic (phase V) blood pressures of 90 to 109 mm Hg. The study requires that 2100 patients be followed for 5 years for a significance of 1% and 90% power. The patients will be randomized to active treatment starting with indapamide 1.5 mg/day in slow-release formulation or placebo. The goal blood pressure is a sitting systolic pressure of less than 150 mm Hg and a sitting diastolic pressure of less than 80 mm Hg. To achieve the goal pressure, indapamide may be combined with perindopril 2 to 4 mg/day.

Trials Assessing the Protection Conferred by Different Drug Classes

Several ongoing or recently planned trials[35–49, 113–116] will test the efficacy of various drug classes in the prevention of the cardiovascular complications of hypertension (Table 35–6). Most of these trials will compare the older drug classes (DIUs or BBs) with the newer classes (CCBs, ACEIs, or AR1Bs).

Trials Comparing Older with Newer Drug Classes

The National Intervention Cooperative Study in Elderly Hypertensives (NICS-EH)[39] is a double-blind, randomized clinical trial in older hypertensive patients in Japan. Its objectives are to compare the efficacy of nicardipine with that of trichlormethiazide in the prevention of cerebral or cardiovascular complications and to assess the effects of treatment on atherosclerotic risk factors and quality of life. Ambulatory patients of either sex with mild to moderate hypertension (systolic pressure 160 to 220 mm Hg or diastolic pressure < 115 mm Hg), aged 60 years or above and without cardiovascular complications are recruited. The qualifying blood pressure measurements must be taken in the sitting position after a minimum 2-week washout period and must satisfy the criteria at each of two separate visits separated by 2 to 4 weeks. Eligible patients are randomized to treatment with one 20-mg nicardipine sustained-release capsule plus one trichlormethiazide placebo in the morning and one 20-mg nicardipine capsule in the evening, or to treatment with one 2-mg trichlormethiazide tablet plus one nicardipine placebo capsule in the morning and one nicardipine placebo capsule in the evening (double-dummy technique). In treatment-resistant patients, the dose of the study medications may be doubled. Potassium supplements may also be administered as necessary, but no antihypertensive drugs other than the study medication should be prescribed. Enrollment is followed by an active treatment period of at least 5 years or until the occurrence of any specified major adverse event.

Between September 1989 and September 1991, 323 older hypertensive patients were recruited into the NICS-EH trial.[39] The original sample-size calculations called for 500 patients in each group, so enrollment was extended to March 1992, by which date a total of 423 patients had been randomized. Two thirds of the patients were female. Their ages were 60 to 69 years in 51%, 70 to 79 years in 40%, and 80 years or higher in 9%.[39] Interim results obtained in October 1992 showed that systolic and diastolic blood pressures were reduced to a similar degree in the two treatment groups after 1 year, and there was no change in the pulse rate. Because both recruitment and the event rate were lower than expected, it is unlikely that the NICS-EH trial will provide definitive results in the two drug comparison. However, the NICS-EH trial is the first nationwide, double-blind, long-term intervention study of elderly hypertensives in Japan, and it is therefore likely to provide very valuable information on cardiovascular complications, atherosclerotic risk factors, and quality of life.

The Captopril Prevention Project (CAPPP)[41, 43, 97, 102] is an open randomized trial with blinded endpoint evaluation[94] designed to investigate whether antihypertensive treatment with the ACEI captopril may reduce cardiovascular mortality and morbidity more than a therapeutic regimen that does not include an ACEI. Secondary objectives are to compare total mortality, the development or deterioration of ischemic heart disease, left-ventricular failure, atrial fibrillation, diabetes mellitus, and possible differences in renal function between the two groups. The initial sample-size calculations suggested that 7000 patients followed for an average of 5 years would be sufficient to demonstrate a 20% difference in cardiovascular mortality with a two-sided significance of 5% and 80% power. However, in total, 11,019 male and female patients with essential hypertension, aged 25 to 66 years, were randomized. Previously treated and untreated patients were eligible, provided that their diastolic blood pressures before treatment were at least 100 mm Hg on two separate occasions separated by at least 1 week. The target for antihypertensive treatment was a supine diastolic blood pressure of 90 mm Hg or lower. In the captopril group treatment was initiated with 50 mg captopril administered in one or more daily doses. The dosage could be increased to 100 mg/day. The ACEI could also be combined with other antihypertensive drugs, preferably including DIUs. In the non-ACEI group, treatment was started with a DIU or a BB. To achieve the target blood pressure, these two drug classes could be combined, or other antihypertensive drugs could be prescribed, with the exception of ACEIs. The CAPPP trial reported its final results in June 1998.[102]

The International Nifedipine GITS Study Intervention as a Goal for Hypertension Therapy (INSIGHT)[44] is a randomized, double-blind trial being conducted in nine countries (Denmark, France, Israel, Italy, the Netherlands, Norway, Spain, Sweden, and the United Kingdom). Its goal is to compare the rate of fatal and nonfatal cardiovascular endpoints in high-risk hypertensive patients randomized to the CCB nifedipine gastrointestinal therapeutic system (GITS) at (30 to 60 mg/day) and DIU treatment consisting of hydrochlorothiazide (25 to 50 mg/day) plus amiloride (2.5 to 5.0 mg/day). The primary endpoint includes the incidence during a 3-year follow-up period of stroke, intracerebral or subarachnoid hemorrhage, myocardial infarction, heart failure, or sudden death. The secondary endpoints are total mortality, cerebrovascular and cardiovascular mortality, and other events over the 3-year study period. In addition to the aforementioned cardiovascular

Table 35–6 Ongoing Trials Assessing the Protection Conferred by Different Drug Classes

Trial*	Year	Drugs Tested†	Endpoints‡	Design	α	β	FU	Risk§	Δ§	Sample Size
NICS-EH	1997	Nicardipine vs. trichlormethiazide	CVD + CBV	R, DB	—	—	5.0	—	—	1000
CAPPP	1998	Captopril vs. DIUs, BBs	CVM + CVD	R, OBE	0.05	0.90	4.0	18	20	11,000
INSIGHT	1999	Nifedipine vs. HCTZ + amiloride	SD + MI + stroke + CHF	R, DB	0.05	0.80	4.5	27	25	6600
SHELL	1999	Lacidipine vs. chlorthalidone	CVM + CVD + CBV	R, OBE	0.05	0.90	3.0–6.0	18	25	4800
STOP-2	1999	Enalapril, lisinopril vs. felodipine, isradipine vs. metoprolol, atenolol, pindolol, HCTZ + amiloride	CVM	R, OBE	0.05	0.90	4.0	18	25	6600
INVEST	2000	Verapamil vs. HCTZ, atenolol	TM + nonfatal MI + nonfatal stroke	R, DB	—	—	≥2.0	—	—	27,000
LIFE	2001	Losartan vs. atenolol	CVM + CVD	R, DB	0.05	0.80	4.0	30	15	8300
ALLHAT	2002	Chlorthalidone vs. amlodipine vs. lisinopril vs. doxazosin	CHD death + MI	R, DB	0.05	0.82	6.0	13	16	40,000
ANBP2	2002	Enalapril vs. DIUs	CVM + CVD	R, OBE	0.05	0.90	5.0	—	25	6000
CONVINCE	2002	Verapamil vs. HCTZ, atenolol	CVM + MI + stroke	R, DB	0.05	0.80	4.0	25–35	14–16	15,000
NORDIL	2002	Diltiazem vs. DIUs, BBs	CVM + MI + stroke	R, OBE	0.05	0.80	5.0	—	20	12,000
ASCOT	2003	Amlodipine vs. BBs	MI, TM	R, OBE	0.05	0.90	5.0	13	15	18,000
VALUE	2003	Valsartan vs. amlodipine	Cardiac death + MI + CHF	R, DB	0.05	0.90	4.0–6.0	25	15	14,000

*See Table 35–4 for acronyms.
†DIU, diuretic; BB, β-blocker; HCTZ, hydrochlorothiazide.
‡The primary endpoint used in the sample-size calculations or the endpoint stated to be of major interest in the final analysis. CBV, fatal and nonfatal cerebrovascular disease.
§Risk indicates the rate in the group randomized to the older class(es) of medication; Δ refers to the percentage reduction of the risk in the group randomized to the newer class(es).
See Table 35–5 for further explanation.

and cerebrovascular endpoints, the other events also include transient ischemic attack, worsening of existing angina pectoris or newly occurring angina, heart failure requiring fewer than 2 weeks of therapy, and renal failure.

Patients eligible for enrollment in the INSIGHT trial are between 55 and 80 years old and must have untreated or previously treated hypertension. The qualifying blood pressure after a 4-week treatment-free period must be 150 mm Hg systolic and 95 mm Hg diastolic, or the systolic blood pressure must be 160 mm Hg or higher, regardless of the diastolic blood pressure (mean of three readings). In addition, patients must have one or more of the following cardiovascular risk factors: be a current smoker ($\geq$10 cigarettes per day) or an ex-smoker who has stopped within the past year but previously smoked 10 or more cigarettes per day; have a total cholesterol level of 250 mg/dl or higher; have type 1 or type 2 diabetes mellitus; have stable angina or asymptomatic coronary heart disease confirmed by angiographic or electrocardiographic evidence (repolarization changes on exercise); have peripheral vascular disease; have ST-T segment alterations indicative of hypertension with left ventricular strain; have left ventricular hypertrophy confirmed by echocardiography; have a family history of cardiovascular disease (myocardial infarction in parent or sibling before the age of 50 years); have had a previous myocardial infarction; or have proteinuria (a positive dipstick result obtained at the first visit and proteinuria of at least 0.5 g/day confirmed by a 24-hour urine collection prior to the next visit).

The target blood pressure is defined as a level below 160 mm Hg systolic and 95 mm Hg diastolic, with decreases in blood pressure from the entry value of at least 20 mm Hg systolic and 10 mm Hg diastolic. To achieve the target blood pressure, the study medication may be combined first with atenolol (25 to 50 mg/day) or with enalapril (5 to 10 mg/day) if a BB is contraindicated and then with additional antihypertensive drugs chosen by the investigator. Sample-size calculations suggested that to demonstrate a 25% difference in the primary endpoint between the two treatment groups with 5% significance and 80% power, 2637 patients per treatment group would be required. To account for withdrawals and center effects in an international study, the number of patients was increased by 25%, resulting in a total of 6592 patients. Recruitment into the INSIGHT study started in September 1994 and was on target to end by 31 March 1996 with all patients completing a 3-year follow-up by 31 March 1999.[44]

The Systolic Hypertension in the Elderly Long-term Lacidipine Study (SHELL)[42, 113] has a randomized, open design with blinded evaluation of endpoints[94] and aims to assess the efficacy and tolerability of lacidipine compared with the DIU chlorthalidone in the treatment of isolated systolic hypertension in the elderly. The primary endpoint is the incidence of cardiovascular and cerebrovascular events. In particular, the SHELL trial is intended to determine whether lacidipine treatment will significantly reduce fatal myocardial infarction and total cardiovascular mortality.[113] The 115 Italian centers will enroll 4800 patients. The sample-size calculations were performed using the same assumptions as in the Swedish Trial in Old Patients with Hypertension-2 (STOP-2).[35, 37] Eligible male or female patients are at least 60 years old and have isolated systolic hypertension, defined as a systolic blood pressure of at least 160 mm Hg with a diastolic blood pressure below 95 mm Hg after a wash-out period from any previous treatment of at least 2 weeks. The patients are randomly allocated to either lacidipine-based or chlorthalidone-based treatment. Lacidipine is started at a dose of 4 mg and chlorthalidone at a dose of 12.5 mg once daily. After 1 month, patients whose systolic blood pressure has not fallen below 160 mm Hg with a reduction of at least 20 mm Hg (nonresponders) will be given an increased daily dose of either lacidipine (6 mg) or chlorthalidone (25 mg). After an additional month, nonresponders will be administered either a combination of lacidipine (4 mg) with the ACEI fosinopril (10 mg) or a combination of chlorthalidone (12.5 mg) with fosinopril (10 mg). In all patients, blood pressure will be measured monthly during the first 3 months (the titration period) and then at 3-month intervals. The follow-up will continue for 36 to 60 months, according to the actual incidence of events.

The STOP-2 trial[35, 37] is an open randomized trial with blinded endpoint evaluation.[94] It aims to compare the newer hypertension drug classes (ACEIs and CCBs) with the older classes (DIUs and BBs) in the prevention of cardiovascular morbidity and mortality in older hypertensive patients. The primary endpoint is the combined incidence of cardiovascular mortality, including fatal stroke, fatal myocardial infarction, sudden death, and other cardiovascular deaths. Secondary aims of the study are to analyze differences between the two treatment strategies with respect to the total incidence of cardiovascular disease, total mortality, new-onset diabetes mellitus, new cases of atrial fibrillation, the need for institutional care, tolerability and side effects, and cost-effectiveness. Eligible patients are untreated or previously treated hypertensive patients, men and women, aged 70 to 84 years, who on three separate occasions at intervals of at least 1 week maintain a supine blood pressure equal to or higher than 180 mm Hg systolic or 105 mm Hg diastolic.

In the control group of the STOP-2 trial, antihypertensive treatment was initiated with metoprolol controlled-release (100 mg), atenolol (50 mg), pindolol (5 mg), or hydrochlorothiazide (25 mg) plus amiloride (2.5 mg). In the other arm of the trial, half of the patients were started on a CCB (felodipine or isradipine 2.5 to 5.0 mg/day) and the other half on an ACEI (enalapril or lisinopril 10 to 20 mg/day). If the target blood pressure, defined as a level below 160 mm Hg systolic and 95 mm Hg diastolic, was not reached, DIUs and BBs were combined in the control group; in the patients on felodipine or isradipine at 5 mg/day, a BB was added, and in those on enalapril or lisinopril at 20 mg/day, the next treatment step involved the addition of hydrochlorothiazide at 12.5 mg/day. In patients who, after maximal dosing with any of the aforementioned treatment alternatives, maintained a supine blood pressure of 180 mm Hg systolic or 105 mm Hg diastolic or higher, an AB was the recommended third-line treatment. After randomization, the patients were examined at 1 and 2 months and thereafter every 6 months. Sample-size calculations indicated that 6600 patients followed for 4 years would be required to demonstrate a 25% difference in the primary endpoint between the new and the established therapies, with a two-sided significance of 5% and 90% power.

By the end of 1994, enrollment in the STOP-2 trial was completed, and 6628 hypertensive men (34%) and women (66%) had been recruited at 312 Swedish health centers. In the whole cohort, 11% had diabetes and 9% were smokers. Blood pressures were lowered from 194 mm Hg systolic and 98 mm Hg diastolic at entry to 167 mm Hg and 85 mm Hg, respectively, after 1 year of follow-up. At the end of 1995, 319 fatal events (all-cause mortality) had been reported, corresponding to a mortality rate of 21.3 per 1000 patient-years.

The International Verapamil-Trandolapril Study (IN-VEST)[49] is a trial to assess whether a CCB treatment strategy is equivalent to a non-CCB strategy in preventing adverse outcomes in 27,000 patients with hypertension and coronary heart disease. Patients are being enrolled at 1500 primary care sites using a novel electronic system for direct on-screen data entry, randomization, and drug distribution from a central mail-order pharmacy, all linked via the Internet. The entire system is backed up by facsimile and telephone. All study-related communications take place in cyberspace. The software has a high-level artificial intelligence to ensure adherence to the protocol and correct data entry and to permit physicians to customize drug combinations and dosing schedules within the randomly assigned treatment strategies. Pilot phase data on 150 patients from 15 sites have currently been collected.

The Losartan Intervention For Endpoint (LIFE) Reduction in Hypertension study[36, 115] is based on the hypothesis that the renin-angiotensin system plays a pivotal role in the pathogenesis of many cardiovascular complications and that AR1Bs may specifically counteract these disorders in high-risk hypertensive patients. The LIFE trial aims to compare the long-term effects ($\geq$ 4 years) of losartan and atenolol in hypertensive patients with documented left ventricular hypertrophy. The primary endpoint is the combined incidence of cardiovascular mortality and morbidity. Mortality is defined as death due to fatal myocardial infarction, fatal stroke, sudden death, progressive heart failure, or other cardiovascular causes; morbidity encompasses nonfatal acute myocardial infarction and nonfatal stroke. Among the secondary objectives, the LIFE investigators will assess the regression of electrocardiographic left ventricular hypertrophy in the two treatment groups as well as the relationship between the regression of left ventricular hypertrophy and cardiovascular mortality and morbidity. Eligible patients are male or female, aged 55 to 80 years, with untreated or previously treated hypertension and with electrocardiographically documented left-ventricular hypertrophy. After a 1 to 2 week run-in period on single-blind placebo, eligible patients must have a sitting blood pressure averaging 160 to 200 mm Hg systolic or 95 to 115 mm Hg diastolic. Left ventricular hypertrophy in the LIFE trial is diagnosed electrocardiographically by a standard 12-lead electrocardiogram analyzed at the core laboratory before randomization. Left ventricular hypertrophy is defined according to the Cornell voltage-duration index (RaVL + SV_3) $\times$ QRS[117–119] with the sex adjustment for the Cornell voltage in women reduced from 8 to 6 mm.[120] Furthermore, the Sokolow-Lyon voltage index (SV_1 + RV_5 or RV_6)[121]

is accepted as an alternative criterion for left ventricular hypertrophy in both men and women.

Approximately 830 centers in the United States, the United Kingdom, and Scandinavia are actively participating in the study. The first patient was enrolled in June 1995 and by 30 April 1997, when inclusion was stopped, 9218 patients had been randomized. The double-blind antihypertensive medication is either losartan or atenolol. The patients initially receive 50 mg losartan plus atenolol placebo, or 50 mg atenolol plus losartan placebo (double-dummy technique). The target blood pressure is a level measured at trough below 140 mm Hg systolic and 90 mm Hg diastolic. After 2 months on double-blind therapy, 12.5 mg hydrochlorothiazide will be added to the treatment regimen if a patient's blood pressure is not at or below the goal blood pressure. If at month 4 the blood pressure is still not adequately controlled, the dose of the double-blind therapy will be doubled to 100 mg losartan or 100 mg atenolol plus 12.5 mg hydrochlorothiazide. In patients whose blood pressure is not controlled at month 6, additional open-label antihypertensive medication (including upward titration of hydrochlorothiazide) should be added to the double-blind treatment. Further titration with other open-label therapy is mandatory only if the blood pressure exceeds 160 mm Hg systolic or 95 mm Hg diastolic. The follow-up of the patients will continue for 4 years after the last patient is enrolled or until 1040 patients have experienced a primary cardiovascular event.

The Antihypertensive and Lipid Lowering to Prevent Heart Attack Trial (ALLHAT) is the largest and most important clinical trial ever undertaken in the United States.[114] It is sponsored by the National Heart, Lung and Blood Institute in conjunction with the Department of Veterans Affairs. ALLHAT[45, 114, 122] is a practice-based, randomized, double-blind outcome trial in 40,000 high-risk hypertensive patients. The trial is designed to determine whether the combined incidence of fatal coronary heart disease and nonfatal myocardial infarction differs among groups of persons randomized to DIU (chlorthalidone) treatment and each of three alternative treatments, namely a CCB (amlodipine), an ACEI (lisinopril), or an AB (doxazosin). Thus, the statistical design must account for three primary comparisons. To maximize statistical power for the antihypertensive drug trial, 1.7 times as many patients are assigned to the DIU arm as to each of its other three arms. The blood pressure eligibility criteria for the antihypertensive trial are based on the patient's current treatment status and on the average of two seated blood pressure measurements at each of two visits. For untreated patients, the criteria used are the Joint National Committee V definitions of diastolic and systolic hypertension (stages I to II).[123] For previously treated patients, the criteria are a reasonable degree of blood pressure control. The blood pressure levels must not exceed 160 mm Hg systolic and 100 mm Hg diastolic at the first run-in visits or 180 mm Hg systolic and 110 mm Hg diastolic at the qualifying visit, when medication may have been partially withdrawn. The other eligibility criteria are being 55 or older and having one or more additional risk factors for heart attack, such as having an old (>6 months) or age-indeterminate myocardial infarction or stroke, a history of a revascularization procedure, a documented atherosclerotic cardiovascular disease, type 2 diabetes mellitus (fasting plasma glucose > 140 mg/dl or nonfasting plasma glucose > 200 mg/dl or being on insulin or oral hypoglycemics), high-density-lipoprotein cholesterol less than 35 mg/dl at two or more determinations within the past 5 years, left ventricular hypertrophy on electrocardiogram or echocardiogram, or ST-T wave electrocardiogram changes indicative of ischemia, or being a current cigarette smoker.

After randomization, the blood pressure goal in the ALLHAT is to achieve levels below 140 mm Hg systolic and 90 mm Hg diastolic. The therapeutic goal is to achieve blood pressure control on the lowest possible dosage of the first-line study medication to which the patients were randomized. The daily dosage ranges of the first-line medications are 12.5 to 25.0 mg for chlorthalidone; 2.5 to 10.0 mg for amlodipine; 10 to 40 mg for lisinopril; and 1 to 8 mg for doxazosin. For patients in any of the four treatment arms who are unable to attain satisfactory blood pressure control on the maximal tolerable dosage of their first-line drug, a choice of second-line and third-line drugs is provided in open-label form for use in addition to (not substitution for) the first-line drug, unless the first-line drug is not tolerated. The choice of second-line drug or drugs is at the discretion of the treating study investigator: reserpine 0.05 to 0.2 mg; clonidine 0.1 to 0.3 mg; and atenolol 25 to 100 mg. Hydralazine is used as a third-line agent (at a dose of from 25 to 100 mg twice daily). Because the investigators are blinded to the identity of the first-line drug to which each patient is assigned, it is likely that the frequency of use of each of the second-line drugs will be similar among the four treatment arms. Although in special cases, investigators may choose to prescribe second-line antihypertensive drugs other than those provided by the study, thiazide DIUs, CCBs, ACEIs, and ABs are to be avoided, unless maximal tolerated doses of a three-drug regimen have been tried and are unsuccessful in controlling blood pressure.

ALLHAT also contains a randomized, open-label, lipid-lowering trial designed to determine whether lowering low-density-lipoprotein cholesterol in 20,000 moderately hypercholesterolemic patients (a subset of the 40,000) with a 3-hydroxy-methylglutaryl coenzyme A reductase inhibitor, pravastatin, will reduce all-cause mortality compared with a control group receiving usual care. For the lipid-lowering trial, participants must have a low-density-lipoprotein cholesterol of 120 to 189 mg/dl (100 to 129 mg/dl for patients with known coronary heart disease) and a triglyceride level below 350 mg/dl.

In ALLHAT, the mean duration of treatment and follow-up is planned to be 6 years. Recently, the ALLHAT investigators described 20,798 patients, who met the entry criteria.[122] Of 10,628 patients on monotherapy with blinded study medication, 1219 (63%) in the East of the United States, 1481 (61%) in the Midwest, 2906 (56%) in the South, and 721 (65%) in the West were at goal blood pressure; of the 15,557 on blinded therapy plus other medications, 1515 (58%), 2008 (56%), 3905 (51%), and 994 (60%) had attained the goal blood pressure in the East, Midwest, South, and West, respectively. Thus, there were regional differences in the proportion of ALLHAT patients who had reached the goal blood pressure.

The Australian National Blood Pressure Study—2 (ANBP2)[40] is an outcome trial comparing ACEIs and DIUs as first-line drugs in older hypertensive patients, using a prospective randomized open-label design with blinded assessment of endpoints.[94] The primary endpoint of interest is total cardiovascular events, including cardiovascular deaths. Secondary endpoints include death and coronary heart disease events. All comparisons between treatment phases will be on an intention-to-treat basis. The ANBP2 trial is being conducted in general practices throughout Australia and will recruit 6000 subjects over 2 to 3 years (3000 in each arm of the study) to provide 30,000 years of patient observation (5 years of follow-up). This will allow detection of a 25% difference in the primary outcome variable with 5% significance and 90% power. Eligible patients, untreated or previously treated, should be from 65 to 84 years old. During the screening phase of the study, their sitting untreated blood pressure should average at least 160 mm Hg systolic and/or 90 mm Hg diastolic.

After randomization in the ANBP2 trial, the general practitioners may administer antihypertensive drug treatment according to their usual practice, but they have to conform with the arm of the trial to which the patient has been randomized. Antihypertensive treatment must be initiated either with an ACEI, preferably enalapril to increase consistency of treatment in the ACEI arm, or with a DIU. BBs, CCBs, or ABs may be added as additional drugs in both treatment groups. In the ACEI group, DIUs may also be prescribed as third-line or fourth-line antihypertensive agents. For patients with an entry systolic blood pressure of 160 mm Hg or higher, the goal of treatment is to reduce systolic blood pressure by at least 20 mm Hg to less than 160 mm Hg, with a further reduction to less than 140 mm Hg, if tolerated; for patients with an entry diastolic blood pressure of 90 mm Hg or higher, a reduction of diastolic blood pressure by at least 10 mm Hg to less than 90 mm Hg is the goal, with a further reduction to less than 80 mm Hg, if tolerated. All drugs are being prescribed through the Australian Commonwealth Pharmaceutical Benefits Scheme, the national system of government subsidy for essential drugs. Once the target blood pressure is achieved, the general practitioners continue maintenance of antihypertensive drug treatment with the proviso that the patients must be seen at least twice a year.

The Controlled Onset Verapamil Investigation for Cardiovascular Endpoints (CONVINCE)[46, 116] is a randomized, double-blind, parallel-group, 5-year clinical trial involving 15,000 patients. CONVINCE will compare the incidence of fatal or nonfatal myocardial infarction, fatal or nonfatal stroke, or cardiovascular-disease–related death between two antihypertensive treatment regimens. One treatment arm begins with controlled onset-extended release verapamil, which has its major antihypertensive effect 6 to 12 hours after administration; the other arm (standard-of-care) begins with either hydrochlorothiazide or atenolol, one of which is preselected by the investigator for an individual patient prior to randomization. Secondary objectives include comparisons of the regimens for: each of the components of the primary endpoint (separately); all-cause mortality; death or hospitalization related to cardiovascular disease; efficacy in lowering blood pressure to goal; primary events occurring between 6 AM and noon; withdrawals from blinded therapy; cancer; and hospitalizations due to bleeding. Patients may be enrolled if they are hypertensive, are at least 55 years old, and have an established second risk factor for cardiovascular disease. Initial medications include verapamil (180 mg/day) and hydrochlorothiazide (12.5 mg/day) or atenolol (50 mg/day). Initial doses are doubled if the blood pressure does not decrease below 140 mm Hg systolic and 90 mm Hg diastolic. If blood pressure is not controlled by the higher dose of the initial medication, hydrochlorothiazide is added to verapamil, or the standard-of-care drug not initially selected is added in the control group. An ACEI is recommended (although nearly any open-label medication is allowed) as the third step for patients whose blood pressure is not adequately controlled or who have a contraindication to one of the two standard-of-care medications. Although most patients switch from an established antihypertensive medication to randomized treatment, untreated patients with stages I to III hypertension (systolic blood pressure between 140 and 190 mm Hg or diastolic blood pressure between 90 and 110 mm Hg) are also eligible. Enrollment began during the third quarter of 1996 and follow-up is to be completed in the third quarter of 2002.

During the first year of enrollment in the CONVINCE trial,[46] 6482 patients were randomized. Most (45%) were between 60 and 69 years of age; 55% were female; and 87% were taking antihypertensive drugs on enrollment. The most common second cardiovascular risk factor was obesity (25% or more over ideal body weight, 48%) followed by dyslipidemia (34%); known cardiovascular disease (21%); cigarette use (21%); type II diabetes mellitus (20%); left ventricular hypertrophy by echocardiogram or electrocardiogram (12%); prior acute myocardial infarction (9%); vascular bruit (6%); prior stroke (5%); and prior transient ischemic attack with hospitalization (2%). Of the 6482 patients, 51% had more than one risk factor.

The Nordic Diltiazem Study (NORDIL)[38] was started in September 1992. This is a randomized, open, parallel-group trial with blinded endpoint evaluation,[94] conducted in Norway and Sweden. The study is designed to evaluate the potential preventive effects of diltiazem compared with conventional antihypertensive drug treatment. The primary endpoints are cardiovascular mortality (fatal myocardial infarction, fatal stroke, sudden death, and other fatal cardiovascular disorders) as well as cardiovascular morbidity (nonfatal myocardial infarction and nonfatal stroke). Secondary endpoints are: total mortality; the development or deterioration of ischemic heart disease; congestive heart failure; atrial fibrillation; transient ischemic attack; new-onset diabetes mellitus; and renal insufficiency. Male and female patients, aged 50 to 69 years, with primary hypertension are randomly allocated to therapy starting with either diltiazem (180 to 360 mg/day) or conventional treatment (DIUs or BBs). Add-on therapy in the conventional treatment group excludes all types of CCBs. The supine diastolic blood pressure at randomization should be 100 mm Hg or more at two separate visits at least 1 week apart (in previously treated patients in the absence of antihypertensive drug treatment); to be eligible these patients should have at least one additional risk factor, such as diabetes mellitus, hypercholesterolemia, smoking, or left ventricular hypertrophy. In previously untreated patients without additional risk factors, the supine diastolic blood pressure at

entry should be 110 mm Hg or higher only if confirmed at two visits 1 week apart or 100 mm Hg or higher at three visits over 3 months. The goal of treatment will be a target diastolic blood pressure of 90 mm Hg or lower with at least a 10% reduction in the diastolic blood pressure. The NORDIL study will allow the detection of a 20% difference in cardiovascular mortality between the two treatment groups with a 5% significance and 90% power. A total of 12,000 patients will be recruited from about 480 primary health care centers or hospital-based hypertension units. Patients will be treated for an average of 5 years.

The Anglo-Scandinavian Cardiac Outcome Trial (ASCOT)[47] has 2 × 2 factorial design and combines an open randomized trial with blinded endpoint evaluation[94] in hypertension with a double-blind placebo-controlled trial of lipid-lowering. The primary objective of the ASCOT is to compare the long-term effects on total (fatal and nonfatal) myocardial infarction of two antihypertensive drug regimens. One regimen starts with a BB with the possible addition of a DIU; the other includes amlodipine with an ACEI as a second-line antihypertensive drug. In the lipid-lowering part of the ASCOT trial, patients with a lower total cholesterol than usually recommended for medical intervention in Europe (≤6.5 mmol/L; no lower limit) will be randomized to atorvastatin 10 mg/day or placebo (personal communication by Francesco Capuccio, London, 1998).

The fundamental entry criterion of the ASCOT is that the patient's own doctors consider there to be no clear indication for or no clear contraindication to any of the trial treatments. Eligible men and women are from 40 to 70 years old. Untreated hypertensives should have a systolic blood pressure of 160 mm Hg or more or a diastolic blood pressure of at least 100 mm Hg, or both; in hypertensive patients on treatment with one or more drugs, these thresholds should be 140 mm Hg and 90 mm Hg, respectively. In addition, eligible patients should have three or more of the following cardiovascular risk factors: male; 50 years old or more; abnormal electrocardiogram; left-ventricular hypertrophy; peripheral vascular disease; history of one or more cerebrovascular event, including transient ischemic attacks within 3 months before enrollment; microalbuminuria or proteinuria; smoking; a ratio of total to high-density-lipoprotein cholesterol exceeding 6. The target blood pressure in the nondiabetic patients is below 140 mm Hg systolic and below 90 mm Hg diastolic and in the diabetic patients below 130 mm Hg and 80 mm Hg, respectively. A total of 18,000 patients will be recruited in the United Kingdom, Ireland, and Scandinavia and followed for an average of at least 5 years or until 1150 primary endpoints have occurred. The study will have over 80% power to detect with 5% significance and 90% power, a 15% difference in the primary endpoint between the two antihypertensive treatment regimens, as well as a 20% difference in all-cause mortality in the lipid-lowering limb. The pilot study began in the winter of 1997 and the main study started in 1998.[47]

Trials Comparing Second and Third-Generation Antihypertensive Drugs

The double-blind Diovan Antihypertensive Long-Term Use Evaluation (VALUE) trial[48] will test the hypothesis that in high-risk hypertensive patients, for the same level of blood pressure control, the use of an AR1B compared with a dihydropyridine CCB would reduce the incidence of cardiac morbidity and mortality by 15%. The trial starts from the premise that DIUs, BBs, and CCBs have proved, but hitherto suboptimal, effects on cardiovascular mortality and morbidity in hypertension, because a stimulated renin-angiotensin system may cause cardiovascular damage. The latter may be specifically and selectively blocked by AR1B. Eligible patients are untreated or previously treated, have a blood pressure ranging from 160 to 210 mm Hg systolic or from 95 to 115 mm Hg diastolic, are at least 50 years old, and have a high risk of cardiovascular complications due to the presence of one or more a priori defined risk factors or diseases. A total of 14,400 patients will be recruited over 2 years and followed for 4 to 6 years. They will be randomized to valsartan 80 to 160 mg plus hydrochlorothiazide or amlodipine 5 to 10 mg once daily. The primary endpoint, the combined incidence of myocardial infarction, congestive heart failure, and cardiac mortality, is expected to occur in at least 1450 patients. Patient enrollment started in October 1997.[48]

Other Trials in Special Subgroups

The African American Study of Kidney Disease and Hypertension (AASK)[69] was the first multicenter, randomized clinical trial of renal disease and hypertension in African Americans. The pilot study sought to establish the feasibility of carrying out a long-term, multicenter clinical trial utilizing a 3 × 2 factorial design consisting of antihypertensive regimens containing the ACEI enalapril, the CCB amlodipine, and the BB atenolol and two different levels of blood pressure control based on mean arterial pressure (102 to 107 mm Hg vs. ≥ 92 mm Hg). Furosemide, doxazosin, clonidine, hydralazine, and minoxidil were added sequentially until the goal mean arterial blood pressure was achieved. The goals of the AASK pilot study were to evaluate recruitment techniques, adherence to prescribed antihypertensive drug regimens, ability of the antihypertensive regimens to achieve blood pressure goals, rates of participation in scheduled clinic visits and procedures, and variability of the measurements of the glomerular filtration rate. A further goal was to obtain renal biopsy data in at least 75% of the randomized study participants. Compared to the patient population with end-stage renal disease due to hypertension, women were underrepresented in the AASK. The AASK investigators recognized that most participants in the main trial would require treatment with multiple antihypertensive drugs, including DIUs, in order to achieve blood pressure control, especially to reach the lower target level of mean arterial pressure. Therefore, the goal of the full-scale trial is to evaluate the effect of antihypertensive drug regimens containing the randomized agents rather than to evaluate specifically the effect of each of the individual agents.

The Hypertension in Diabetes Study (HDS)[59, 61, 62] was a prospective, randomized controlled study of therapy of mild hypertension in 758 patients with type 2 diabetes who were followed for over 5 years. Patients were eligible if they had systolic blood pressure over 150 mm Hg or

diastolic blood pressure over 85 mm Hg while on antihypertensive treatment or, if not on therapy, they had systolic blood pressure over 160 mm Hg or diastolic blood pressure over 90 mm Hg. Their mean blood pressure at entry into the study was 160 mm Hg systolic and 94 mm Hg diastolic. Mean age was 57 years. The patients were allocated to tight blood pressure control (levels below 150 mm Hg systolic and 85 mm Hg diastolic) or to less tight control (less than 180 mm Hg and 105 mm Hg, respectively). Members of the tight-control group were allocated to first-line therapy either with a BB (atenolol) or with an ACEI (captopril), with addition of other agents as required. Over 5 years, the blood pressures in the tightly controlled group were significantly lower (systolic 143 vs. 154 mm Hg; diastolic 82 vs. 88 mm Hg; $p < .001$), but no difference in blood pressure control was noticed between those allocated to atenolol and those allocated to captopril. The proportion of patients requiring three or more antihypertensive drugs to maintain tight control in those allocated to atenolol or captopril was similar and increased from 15 to 16% at 2 years to 25 to 26% at 5 years; in the less tightly controlled group, these proportions were only 5 and 7%, respectively. The study is continuing to determine whether the improved blood pressure control will be beneficial in maintaining the health of patients by decreasing the incidence of major clinical complications, principally myocardial infarction and stroke, and microvascular disorders, such as severe retinopathy requiring photocoagulation and the deterioration of renal function.[59, 61, 62]

CONCLUSIONS

The combined results of previous placebo-controlled trials in hypertension[71–76] provide strong evidence that antihypertensive treatment reduces stroke by 42% and coronary heart disease by approximately 14%. In general, the adequately powered trials achieved statistical significance, at least on their primary endpoints. However, the underpowered trials often produced confusing or contradictory results. Previous trials comparing BBs with DIUs failed to demonstrate either superiority or equivalence.[7, 8, 30–34] As outlined in a commentary,[124] the J-curve controversy was not resolved by the Hypertension Optimal Treatment (HOT) study[29] because overall, there were no differences in the rates of cardiovascular complications among the three treatment groups (with progressively tighter control of diastolic blood pressure) to which the patients were randomized.

In the modern trials, to keep sample size within reasonable limits, the investigators often recruited high-risk hypertensive patients, proposed composite primary endpoints, or adopted both approaches. However, high-risk hypertensive patients are not necessarily a homogeneous group. Various risk factors may act through divergent pathophysiological mechanisms with which antihypertensive drugs may interact differently. Open designs, multiple drug treatments, and crossing-over the experimental treatment are other potential problems that weaken the chances that some of the ongoing trials will provide conclusive answers. It is interesting to compare the assumed benefit and the power and significance in the earlier placebo-controlled trials with those parameters in the ongoing trials, of which many follow only actively treated patients. In spite of the increasing sample size, it appears that some trials will never answer their primary research question in a definite way. It may be necessary to utilize post hoc subgroup analyses, for instance in diabetic patients, to come up with significant results.

References

1. Amery A, Birkenhäger W, Brixko P, et al. Efficacy of antihypertensive drug treatment according to age, sex, blood pressure, and previous cardiovascular disease in patients over the age of 60. Lancet 2:589–592, 1986.
2. Amery A, Birkenhäger W, Brixko P, et al. Mortality and morbidity results from the European Working Party on High Blood Pressure in the Elderly trial. Lancet 1:1349–1354. 1985.
3. Coope J, Warrender TS. Randomised trial of treatment of hypertension in elderly patients in primary care. BMJ 293:1145–1151, 1986.
4. Dahlöf B, Lindholm LH, Hansson L, et al. Morbidity and mortality in the Swedish Trial in Old Patients with Hypertension (STOP-Hypertension). Lancet 338:1281–1285, 1991.
5. Hypertension Detection and Follow-up Program Cooperative Group. Five-year findings of the Hypertension Detection and Followup Program. II: Mortality by race, sex, and age. JAMA 242:2572–2577, 1979.
6. Hypertension Detection and Follow-up Program Cooperative Group. Five-year findings of the Hypertension Detection and Follow-up Program. I: Reduction in mortality of persons with high blood pressure, including mild hypertension. JAMA 242:2562–2571, 1979.
7. Medical Research Council Working Party. Medical Research Council trial of treatment of hypertension in older adults: Principal results. BMJ 304:405–412, 1992.
8. Medical Research Council Working Party. Medical Research Council trial of treatment of mild hypertension: Principal results. BMJ 291:97–104, 1985.
9. SHEP Cooperative Research Group. Prevention of stroke by antihypertensive drug treatment in older persons with isolated systolic hypertension. Final results of the Systolic Hypertension in the Elderly Program (SHEP). *JAMA* 265:3255–3264, 1991.
10. Wang J, Liu G, Wang X, et al. Long-term blood pressure control in older Chinese patients with isolated systolic hypertension: A progress report on the Syst-China trial. J Hum Hypertens 10:735–742, 1996.
11. Gong L, Zhang W, Zhu Y, et al. Shanghai Trial of Nifedipine in the Elderly (STONE). J Hypertens 14:1237–1245, 1996.
12. Staessen JA, Fagard R, Thijs L, et al. Randomised double-blind comparison of placebo and active treatment for older patients with isolated systolic hypertension. Lancet 350:757–764, 1997 [Correction. Lancet 350:1636, 1997].
13. Casiglia E, Spolaore P, Mazza A, et al. Effect of 2 different therapeutic approaches on total and cardiovascular mortality in a Cardiovascular Study in the Elderly. Jpn Heart J 35:589–600, 1994.
14. Management Committee. The Australian Therapeutic Trial in Mild Hypertension. Lancet 1:1261–1267, 1980.
15. Staessen JA, Fagard R, Thijs L, et al. Subgroup and per-protocol analysis of the randomized European trial on isolated systolic hypertension in the elderly. Arch Intern Med 158:1681–1691, 1998.
16. PATS Collaborative Group. Epidemiology survey. Post-stroke antihypertensive treatment study: A preliminary result. Chin Med J 108:710–717, 1995.
17. Sprackling ME, Mitchell JRA, Short AH, Watt G. Blood pressure reduction in the elderly: A randomised controlled trial of methyldopa. BMJ 283:1151–1153, 1981.
18. Perry JHM, Goldman AI, Lavin MA, et al. Evaluation of drug treatment in mild hypertension: VA-NHLBI feasibility trial. Ann N Y Acad Sci 304:267–288, 1978.
19. Helgeland A. Treatment of mild hypertension: A five-year controlled drug trial. Am J Med 69:725–732, 1980.
20. Kuramoto K, Matsushita S, Kuwajima I, Murakami M. Prospective study on the treatment of mild hypertension in the aged. Jpn Heart J 22:75–85, 1981.
21. Hypertension-Stroke Cooperative Study Group. Effect of antihypertensive treatment on stroke recurrence. JAMA 229:409–418, 1974.
22. Barraclough M, Joys MD, MacGregor GA, et al. Control of moderately raised blood pressure: Report of a co-operative randomized controlled trial. BMJ 434:436, 1973.
23. Veterans Administration Cooperative Study Group on Antihypertensive Agents. Effect of treatment on morbidity in hypertension: Results in patients with diastolic blood pressure averaging 115–129 mm Hg. JAMA 202:116–122, 1967.
24. Veterans Administration Cooperative Study Group on Antihypertensive Agents. Effects of treatment on morbidity in hypertension. II: Results in patients with diastolic blood pressure averaging 90 through 114 mm Hg. JAMA 213:1143–1152, 1970.
25. Wolff FW, Lindeman RD. Effects of treatment in hypertension: Results of a controlled study. J Chron Dis 19:227–240, 1966.
26. U.S. Public Health Service Hospitals Cooperative Study Group (Smith WM). Morbidity and mortality in mild essential hypertension. Circ Res 31(suppl 2):110–124, 1972.
27. Carter AB. Hypotensive therapy in stroke survivors. Lancet 1:485–489, 1970.
28. Liu L, Wang JG, Gong L, et al for the Systolic Hypertension in China (Syst-China) Collaborative Group. Comparison of active treatment and placebo for older patients with isolated systolic hypertension. J Hypertens 16:1823–1829, 1998.
29. Hansson L, Zanchetti A, Carruthers SG, et al. Effects of intensive blood pressure lowering and low-dose aspirin in patients with hypertension: Principal results of the Hypertension Optimal Treatment (HOT) randomised trial. Lancet 351:1755–1762, 1998.
30. The IPPPSH Collaborative Group. Cardiovascular risk and risk factors in a randomised trial of treatment based on the beta-blocker oxprenolol: The International Primary Prevention Study in Hypertension (IPPPSH). J Hypertens 3:379–392, 1985.
31. Wilhelmsen L, Berglund G, Elmfeldt D, et al. Beta-blockers versus diuretics in hypertensive men: Main results from the HAPPHY trial. J Hypertens 5:561–572, 1987.
32. Wikstrand J, Warnold I, Olsson G, et al. Primary prevention with metoprolol in patients with hypertension: Mortality results from the MAPHY study. JAMA 259:1976–1982, 1988.
33. Wilhelmsen L, Staessen J, Fagard R, et al. Primary prevention with metoprolol in patients with hypertension. JAMA 260:1713–1716, 1988.
34. Staessen JA, Wang JG, Birkenhäger WH, Fagard R. Treatment with beta-blockers for the primary prevention of the cardiovascular complications of hypertension. Eur Heart J 20:11–24, 1999.
35. Dahlöf B, Hansson L, Lindholm LH, et al. STOP-Hypertension 2: A prospective intervention trial of "newer" versus "older" treatment alternatives in old patients with hypertension. Blood Press 2:136–141, 1993.
36. Dahlöf B, Devereux R, de Faire U, et al. The Losartan Intervention for Endpoint Reduction (LIFE) in hypertension study: Rationale, design and methods. Am J Hypertens 10:705–713, 1997.
37. Lindholm LH, Hansson L, Dahlöf B, et al. The Swedish Trial in Old Patients with Hypertension-2 (STOP-Hypertension-2): A progress report. Blood Press 5:300–304, 1996.
38. The NORDIL Group. The Nordic Diltiazem Study (NORDIL): A prospective intervention trial of calcium antagonist therapy in hypertension. Blood Press 2:312–321, 1993.
39. Kuramoto K, the National Intervention Cooperative Study Group. Treatment of elderly hypertensives in Japan: National Intervention Cooperative Study in Elderly Hypertensives. J Hypertens 12:S35–S40, 1994.
40. Management Committee on behalf of the High Blood Pressure Research Council of Australia. Australian comparative outcome trial of angiotensin-converting enzyme inhibitor and diuretic-based treatment of hypertension in the elderly (ANBP2): Objectives and protocol. Clin Exp Pharmacol Physiol 24:188–192, 1997.
41. The CAPPP group. The Captopril Prevention Project: A prospective intervention trial of angiotensin-converting enzyme inhibition in the treatment of hypertension. J Hypertens 8:985–990, 1990.
42. Zanchetti A. Evaluating the benefits of an antihypertensive agent using trials based on event and organ damage: The Systolic Hypertension in the Elderly Long-term Lacidipine (SHELL) trial and the European Lacidipine Study on Atherosclerosis. J Hypertens 13(suppl 4):S35–S39, 1995.
43. Hansson L, Hedner T, Lindholm L, et al. The Captopril Prevention Project (CAPPP) in hypertension-baseline data and current status. Blood Press 6:365–367, 1997.

44. Brown MJ, Castaigne A, Ruilope LM, et al. INSIGHT: International Nifedipine GITS Study Intervention as a Goal in Hypertension Treatment. J Hum Hypertens 10:S157–S160, 1996.

45. Davis BR, Cutler JA, Gordon DJ, et al. Rationale and design for the Antihypertensive and Lipid Lowering Treatment to Prevent Heart Attack Trial (ALLHAT). Am J Hypertens 9:342–360, 1996.

46. Black HR, Elliott WJ, Grandits G, Fakouhi TD for the CONVINCE study group. Baseline characteristics of the first 6482 patients enrolled in the CONVINCE study. [Abstract] Am J Hypertens 11:74, 1998.

47. Dahlöf B, Sever PS, Poulter NR, Wedel H on behalf of the ASCOT Steering Committee. The Anglo-Scandinavian Cardiac Outcome Trial (ASCOT). [Abstract] J Hypertens 16:S212, 1998.

48. Julius S, Brunner HR, Hansson L, et al. DioVan Antihypertensive Long-term Use Evaluation (The VALUE study). [Abstract] J Hypertens 16:S201, 1998.

49. Pepine CJ, Conlon M, Handberg-Thurmond E, et al. A "paper-less" study on optimal treatment strategies for hypertension and CAD: Pilot phase data from the INternational VErapamil-trandolapril STudy. [Abstract] J Am Coll Cardiol 31:211, 1998.

50. Bulpitt CJ, Fletcher AE, Amery A, et al. The Hypertension in the Very Elderly Trial (HYVET). Rationale, methodology and comparison with previous trials. Drugs Aging 5:171–183, 1994.

51. Bulpitt CJ, Fletcher AE, Amery A, et al. The hypertension in the very elderly trial (HYVET). J Hum Hypertens 8:631–632, 1994.

52. The Hope Study Investigators. The HOPE (Heart Outcomes Prevention Evaluation) study: The design of a large, simple randomized trial of an angiotensin-converting enzyme inhibitor (ramipril) and vitamin E in patients at high risk of cardiovascular events. Can J Cardiol 12:127–137, 1996.

53. Lees RS, Pitt B, Chan RC, et al. Baseline clinical and angiographic data in the Quinapril Ischemic Event (QUIET) Trial. Am J Cardiol 78:1011–1016, 1996.

54. Texter M, Lees RS, Pitt B, et al. The QUinapril Ischemic Event Trial (QUIET) design and methods: Evaluation of chronic ACE inhibitor therapy after coronary artery intervention. Cardiovasc Drugs Ther 7:273–282, 1993.

55. Pepine CJ. Ongoing clinical trials of angiotensin-converting enzyme inhibitors for treatment of coronary artery disease in patients with preserved left ventricular function. J Am Coll Cardiol 27:1048–1052, 1996.

56. Passa P, Chatellier G on behalf of the Diab-Hycar Study Group. The DIAB-HYCAR study. Diabetologia 39:1662–1667, 1996.

57. Neal B, MacMahon S on behalf of the PROGRESS Management Committee. The PROGRESS study: Nationale and design. J Hypertens 13:1869–1873, 1995.

58. Neal B, Anderson C, Chalmers J, et al for the PROGRESS Management Committee. Blood pressure lowering in patients with cerebrovascular disease: Results of the PROGRESS (Perindopril Protection Against Recurrent Stroke Study) pilot phase. Clin Exp Pharmacol Physiol 23:444–446, 1996.

59. UK Prospective Diabetes Study Group. UK Prospective Diabetes Study (UKPDS). VIII: Study design, progress and performance. Diabetologia 34:877–890, 1991.

60. World Health Organization–International Society of Hypertension Blood Pressure Lowering Treatment Trialists' Collaboration. Protocol for prospective collaborative overviews of major randomized trials of blood pressure lowering treatments. J Hypertens 16:127–137, 1998.

61. Hypertension in Diabetes Study Group. Hypertension in Diabetes Study III: Prospective study of therapy of hypertension in type 2 diabetic patients: Efficacy of ACE inhibition and beta-blockade. Diabetic Med 11:773–782, 1994.

62. Hypertension in Diabetes Study Group. Hypertension in Diabetes Study IV: Therapeutic requirements to maintain tight blood pressure control. Diabetologia 39:1554–1561, 1996.

63. Ruggenenti P, Remuzzi G on behalf of the Bergamo Diabetic Nephrologic Study Group. Primary prevention of renal failure in diabetic patients: The Bergamo Nephrologic Diabetes Complications Trial. J Hypertens 16:S95–S97, 1998.

64. Porush JG, Berl T, Anzalone DA, Rohde R. Multicenter collaborative trial of angiotensin II receptor antagonism on morbidity, mortality and renal function in hypertensive type II diabetic patients with nephropathy. [Abstract] Am J Hypertens 11:73A, 1998.

65. Savage S, Johnson Nagel N, Estacio RO, et al. The ABCD (Appropriate Blood Pressure Control in Diabetes) trial. Rationale and design of a trial of hypertension control (moderate or intensive) in type II diabetes. In Online J Curr Clin Trials Doc No 104, Nov 24, 1993.

66. Schrier RW, Estacio RO, Jeffers BW. Appropriate blood pressure control in NIDDM (ABCD) trial. Diabetologia 39:1646–1654, 1996.

67. Estacio RO, Savage S, Nagel NJ, Schrier RW. Baseline characteristics of participants in the Appropriate Blood Pressure Control in Diabetes trial. Control Clin Trials 17:242–257, 1996.

68. Hansson L for the SCOPE Group. Study on cognition and prognosis in the elderly (SCOPE). Design and objectives. [Abstract] J Hypertens 16:S246, 1998.

69. Wright JT, Kusek JW, Toto RD, et al. Design and baseline characteristics of participants in the African American Study of Kidney Disease and Hypertension (AASK) pilot study. Control Clin Trials 16:3S–16S, 1996.

70. Schrier RW, Savage S. Appropriate Blood Pressure Control in Type II Diabetes (ABCD trial): Implications for complications. Am J Kidney Dis 20:653–657, 1992.

71. Collins R, Peto R, MacMahon S, et al. Blood pressure, stroke, and coronary heart disease. Part 2: Short-term reductions in blood pressure: Overview of randomised drug trials in their epidemiological context. Lancet 335:827–838, 1990.

72. Thijs L, Fagard R, Lijnen P, et al. A meta-analysis of outcome trials in elderly hypertensives. J Hypertens 10:1103–1109, 1992.

73. Psaty BM, Smith NL, Siscovick DS, et al. Health outcomes associated with antihypertensive therapies used as first-line agents. A systematic review and meta-analysis. JAMA 277:739–745, 1997.

74. Gueyffier F, Boutitie F, Boissel JP, et al. Effect of antihypertensive drug treatment on cardiovascular outcomes in women and men. A meta-analysis of individual patient data from randomized, controlled trials. Ann Intern Med 126:761–767, 1997.

75. Gueyffier F, Boutitie F, Boissel JP, et al. INDANA: A meta-analysis on individual patient data in hypertension. Protocol and preliminary results. Thérapie 50:353–362, 1995.

76. Thijs L, Fagard R, Lijnen P, et al. Why is antihypertensive drug therapy needed in elderly patients with systolodiastolic hypertension? J Hypertens 12(suppl 6):S25–S34, 1994.

77. Devereux RB, Dahlöf B, Levy D, Pfeffer MA. Comparison of enalapril versus nifedipine to decrease left ventricular hypertrophy in systemic hypertension (the PRESERVE Trial). Am J Cardiol 78:61–65, 1996.

78. Phyllis Project Group. Plaque hypertension lipid-lowering Italian study (PHYLLIS): A protocol for non-invasive evaluation of carotid atherosclerosis in hypercholesterolaemic hypertensive subjects. J Hypertens 11:S314–S315, 1993.

79. Ludwig M, Stumpe KO, Heagerty AM, et al. Vascular wall thickness in hypertension: The Perindopril Regression of Vascular Thickening European Community Trial (PROTECT). J Hypertens 11:S316–S317, 1993.

80. Bond G, Dal Palú C, Hansson L, et al. The E.L.S.A. Trial: Protocol of a randomized trial to explore the differential effect of antihypertensive drugs on atherosclerosis in hypertension. J Cardiovasc Pharmacol 23(suppl 5):S85–S87, 1994.

81. Zanchetti A, Magnani B, Dal Palú C on behalf of the Verapamil-Hypertension Atherosclerosis Study (VHAS) Investigators. Atherosclerosis and calcium antagonists: The VHAS. J Hum Hypertens 6:S45–S48, 1992.

82. Zanchetti A on behalf of the VHAS Study Group. Vascular complications in hypertension: The VHAS Study. Cardiovasc Drugs Ther 9:529–531, 1995.

83. Stumpe KO, Ludwig M, Heagerty AM, et al. Vascular wall thickness in hypertension: The Perindopril Regression of Vascular Thickening European Community Trial: PROTECT. Am J Cardiol 76:50E–54E, 1995.

84. Teo KK, Burton JR, Buller C, et al. Rationale and design features of clinical trial examining the effects of cholesterol lowering and angiotensin-converting enzyme inhibition on coronary atherosclerosis: Simvastatin/Enalapril Coronary Atherosclerosis Trial (SCAT). Can J Cardiol 13:591–599, 1997.

85. Byington RB, Miller ME, Herrington D, et al. Rationale, design, and baseline characteristics of the Prospective Randomized Evaluation of the Vascular Effects of Norvasc Trial (PREVENT). Am J Cardiol 80:1087–1090, 1997.

86. Lonn EM, Yusuf S, Doris CI, et al. Study design and baseline characteristics of the Study to Evaluate Carotid Ultrasound Changes

in patients treated with Ramipril and Vitamin E: SECURE. Am J Cardiol 78:914–919, 1996.

87. The Systolic Hypertension in the Elderly Program Cooperative Research Group. Implications of the Systolic Hypertension in the Elderly Program. Hypertension 21:335–343, 1993.

88. Collaborative Group Coordinating Center. Systolic hypertension in the elderly: Chinese trial (Syst-China): Interim report. Chin J Cardiol 20:270–275, 1992.

89. Staessen JA, Thijs L, Fagard RH, et al. Calcium channel blockade and cardiovascular prognosis in the European trial on isolated systolic hypertension. Hypertension 32:410–416, 1998.

90. Hansson L, Zanchetti A. The Hypertension Optimal Treatment (HOT) study: 24-month data on blood pressure and tolerability, with special reference to age and gender. Blood Press 6:313–317, 1997.

91. The HOT Study Group. The Hypertension Optimal Treatment Study (The HOT Study). Blood Press 2:62–68, 1993.

92. Hansson L, Zanchetti A for the HOT Study Group. The Hypertension Optimal Treatment (HOT) Study—Patients' characteristics: Randomization, risk profiles, and early blood pressure results. Blood Press 3:322–327, 1994.

93. Wiklund I, Halling K, Rydèn-Bergsten T, Fletcher A on behalf of the HOT Study Group. Does lowering the blood pressure improve the mood? Quality-of-life results from the Hypertension Optimal Treatment (HOT) Study. Blood Press 6:357–364, 1997.

94. Hansson L, Hedner T, Dahlöf B. Prospective Randomized Open Blinded End-point (PROBE) study. A novel design for intervention trials. Blood Press 1:113–119, 1992.

95. Ahlquist RP. Propranolol in clinical medicine. Am Heart J 97:137–140, 1979.

96. Miall WE, Greenberg G on behalf of The Medical Research Council's Working Party on Mild to Moderate Hypertension. Mild Hypertension: Is There Pressure to Treat? Cambridge, Cambridge University Press, 1987.

97. Hansson L. The Captopril Prevention Project (CAPPP): Description and status. Am J Hypertens 7:82S–83S, 1994.

98. Jamerson K. The effect of blood pressure reduction on end-stage renal disease. Am J Hypertens 9:60S–64S, 1996.

99. Estacio RO, Jeffers BW, Hiatt WR, et al. The effect of nisoldipine as compared with enalapril on cardiovascular outcomes in patients with non-insulin–dependent diabetes and hypertension. N Engl J Med 338:645–652, 1998.

100. Lees RS, Dinsmore RE. Can ACE inhibition alter the course of coronary heart disease? J Cardiovasc Pharmacol 20(suppl B):S33–S35, 1993.

101. ACE inhibitor therapy for coronary heart disease. Heart Lung Blood Newsletter 10:47–50, 1994.

102. Hansson L, Hedner T, Lindholm LH, et al. The Captopril Prevention Project: Final results. [Abstract] J Hypertens 16(suppl 2):S22, 1998.

103. Marre M, Chatellier G, Leblanc H, et al. Prevention of diabetic nephropathy with enalapril in normotensive diabetics with microalbuminuria. BMJ 297:1092–1095, 1988.

104. Ravid M, Lang R, Rachmani R, Lishner M. Long-term renoprotective effect of inhibition of angiotensin-converting enzyme inhibition in non-insulin–dependent diabetes mellitus. A 7-year follow-up study. Arch Intern Med 156:286–289, 1996.

105. Mogensen CE, Keane WF, Bennett PH, et al. Prevention of diabetic renal disease with special reference to microalbuminuria. Lancet 346:1080–1084, 1995.

106. Ravid M, Savin H, Jutrin I, et al. Long-term stabilizing effect of angiotensin-converting enzyme inhibition on plasma creatinine and on proteinuria in normotensive type II diabetic patients. Ann Intern Med 118:577–581, 1993.

107. Lewis EJ, Hunsicker LG, Bain RP, Rohde RP for the Collaborative Study Group. The effect of angiotensin-converting enzyme inhibition on diabetic nephropathy. N Engl J Med 329:1456–1462, 1993.

108. Staessen JA. Potential adverse effects of blood pressure lowering—J-curve revisited. Lancet 348:696–697, 1996.

109. Fletcher AE, Bulpitt CJ. How far should blood pressure be lowered? N Engl J Med 326:251–254, 1992.

110. Lindley RI, Waddell F, Livingston M, et al. A simple and easy estimate of dependency and recovery after acute stroke: A blinded, randomized validation study. Cerebrovasc Dis 4:314–324, 1994.

111. Folstein MF, Folstein SE, McHugh PR. "Mini-Mental State": A practical method for grading the cognitive state of patients for the clinician. J Psychiat Res 12:189–198, 1975.

112. Mahoney FI, Barthel DW. Functional evaluation: The Barthel Index. Md State Med J 14:61–65, 1965.

113. Malacco E, Gnemmi AE, Romagnoli A, Coppini A on behalf of the SHELL Study Group. Systolic hypertension in the elderly: Long-term lacidipine treatment. Objective, protocol and organization. J Cardiovasc Pharmacol 23(suppl 5):S62–S66, 1994.

114. Elliott WJ. ALLHAT: The largest and most important clinical trial in hypertension ever done in the USA. Am J Hypertens 9:409–411, 1996.

115. Dahlöf B. Effect of angiotensin II blockade on cardiac hypertrophy and remodeling: A review. J Hum Hypertens 9:S37–S44, 1995.

116. Black HR, Elliott WJ, Neaton JD, et al. Rationale and design for the controlled onset verapamil investigation of cardiovascular endpoints (CONVINCE) trial. Control Clin Trials 19:370–390, 1998.

117. Molloy TJ, Okin PM, Devereux RB, Kligfield P. Electrocardiographic detection of left ventricular hypertrophy by the simple QRS voltage-duration product. J Am Coll Cardiol 20:1180–1186, 1992.

118. Okin PM, Roman MJ, Devereux RB, Kligfield P. Gender differences and the electrocardiogram in left ventricular hypertrophy. Hypertension 25:242–249, 1995.

119. Okin PM, Roman MJ, Devereux RB, Kligfield P. Electrocardiographic identification of increased left ventricular mass by simple voltage duration products. J Am Coll Cardiol 24:417–423, 1995.

120. Norman JE Jr, Levy D. Improved electrocardiographic detection of echocardiographic left ventricular hypertrophy: Results of a correlated data base approach. J Am Coll Cardiol 26:1022–1029, 1995.

121. Sokolow M, Lyon TP. The ventricular complex in left ventricular hypertrophy as obtained by unipolar precordial and limb leads. Am Heart J 37:161–186, 1949.

122. Nwachuku CE, Cutler JA, Payne GH, et al. Regional differences in attainment of goal blood pressure (BP) among treated hypertensive patients in the United States. [Abstract] J Hypertens 16(suppl 2):S22, 1998.

123. The Joint National Committee on Detection, Evaluation, and Treatment of High Blood Pressure. The fifth report of the Joint National Committee on Detection, Evaluation and Treatment of High Blood Pressure (JNC V). Arch Intern Med 153:154–183, 1993.

124. Kaplan N. Commentary. J-curve not burned off by HOT study. Lancet 351:1748–1749, 1998.

36 The Antihypertensive and Lipid-Lowering to Prevent Heart Attack Trial

Vasilios Papademetriou

WHAT IS ALLHAT?

The Antihypertensive and Lipid-Lowering to Prevent Heart Attack Trial (ALLHAT) is the largest randomized, double-blind trial ever carried out in patients with hypertension in North America. ALLHAT is sponsored by the National Heart, Lung, and Blood Institute in conjunction with the Department of Veterans Affairs. It is a practice-based, clinical trial that initially planned to randomize over 40,000 high-risk patients, 55 years or older, with hypertension, of whom 45% would be women and 55% would be African Americans. It has two parts: the antihypertensive and the lipid-lowering components. The primary hypothesis of the antihypertensive component is that the combined incidence of fatal coronary heart disease (CHD) and nonfatal myocardial infarction (MI) will be lower in patients randomized to receive as first-line therapy either amlodipine, lisinopril, or doxazosin, compared with the combined incidence in patients randomized to take the diuretic chlorthalidone as first-line therapy. To maximize the statistical power for the antihypertensive component, 1.7 times as many patients were to be randomized to the diuretic as to each of the other three agents.

The primary hypothesis of the cholesterol-lowering component is that treatment with pravastatin will result in lower all-cause mortality in a subset of hypertensive patients with low-density lipoprotein (LDL)–cholesterol between 120 and 189 mg/dl and no demonstrable CHD, or between 100 and 129 mg/dl for those with known CHD, compared with patients randomized to receive usual care.

WHY DO WE NEED ALLHAT?

Antihypertensive Component

Although some surveys indicated that the prevalence of hypertension is declining in the United States, still over 43 million Americans carry the diagnosis.[1] Hypertension is the most frequent cause for visits to the physician's office, accounting for over 28 million visits per year.[2] Understanding the role of hypertension as a major contributor to cardiovascular disease has been strengthened and expanded by recent publications from the Multiple Risk Factor Intervention Trial (MRFIT)[3] and the Framingham cohorts.[4] Hypertension is an established risk factor not only for strokes and myocardial infarction[5, 6] but also for congestive heart failure,[4] renal insufficiency,[3] and peripheral vascular disease.[7] An analysis of observational data[2] in over 360,000 persons with long-term follow-up indicated a strong association of systolic blood pressure (more so than diastolic)

with cardiovascular events, CHD mortality, total mortality, and renal insufficiency.

Although the beneficial effects of antihypertensive treatment have been demonstrated in numerous trials, the question remains whether β-blockers and diuretics provide maximal benefit.[6, 8] Reduction in cardiovascular complications was first demonstrated by the landmark Veterans Administration cooperative studies published by Freis and colleagues in the late 1960s and early 1970s.[9] Since then, another 17 trials were carried out asking the question whether lowering blood pressure results in reduction of strokes, MIs, congestive heart failure, and total mortality.[10] These trials utilized the then-available agents, β-blockers and diuretics, for the treatment arm. These studies were mostly placebo-controlled and targeted normalization of diastolic blood pressure. These 17 trials included 47,653 patients with an average age of 57 years and a mean entry blood pressure of 168/96 mm Hg. Analysis of outcome data indicated that compared with placebo, treated patients had an impressive 38% reduction in strokes, but only a 16% reduction in CHD events. The reduction in strokes was precisely what had been predicted, based on epidemiological data, but the reduction in coronary events was less than expected. Five of these trials included 12,483 older patients with a mean age of 72 years and a baseline pressure of 181/88 mm Hg. Overall, compared with placebo, treatment with diuretics resulted in significant reductions in total mortality, stroke, MI, and congestive heart failure. Treatment with β-blockers reduced only the occurence of strokes and episodes of congestive heart failure, but it had no effect on total mortality or CHD events.

Although these trials provide convincing evidence that lowering blood pressure with diuretics and β-blockers will reduce cardiovascular complications, the question remains whether these agents provide maximal benefit. These deficiencies in outcomes—the shortfall in reduction of CHD events and the inability of β-blockers to reduce total mortality and cardiac events in the elderly—have been used as a justification for alternative therapies as first-line agents in the management of hypertension. Angiotensin-converting enzyme inhibitor (ACEI) and calcium channel blocker (CCB) prescriptions have exceeded by far those of β-blockers and diuretics, despite the fact that trials demonstrating outcome benefits with these agents are lacking.[11]

Another reason for the underutilization of β-blockers and diuretics is their potential for causing "metabolic abnormalities."[12] However, the clinical significance of such abnormalities has been exaggerated. For example, diuretic-induced hypokalemia was of great concern in the 1980s and was thought to be associated with arrhythmias and increased sudden death. Although some initial studies demonstrated mild increases in arrhythmias after diuretic therapy, subsequent studies with adequate numbers of patients and appropriate design could not confirm those observations.[13]

Similarly, the changes in lipids associated with diuretic therapy have been shown in large studies to be mild and short-lived.[12, 13] The reduction in coronary end-points with diuretic treatment diminishes the relevance of such observations. The effects of β-blockers on LDL and high-density lipoprotein (HDL) cholesterol have also been exaggerated.[13] These lipid abnormalities are usually mild, occur more with noncardioselective β-blockers at higher doses, and are generally short-lived. The most significant and persistent changes are seen with triglycerides, but their clinical importance in uncertain.

The preference for the ''newer'' agents, ACEIs and CCBs is based on their presumed cleaner profile and lack of adverse effects. However, treating hypertension is to prevent cardiovascular disease and death, and studies testing the effects of ACEIs, CCBs, and α-adrenergic blockers on morbid and mortal cardiovascular end-points are limited or unavailable. Further, the superiority of the newer agents in efficacy and adverse effect profile has not been proved. Two large, long-term, randomized trials—the Veterans Administration Cooperative Study Group on Antihypertensive Agents[14] and the Treatment of Mild Hypertension Study (TOMHS)[15]—compared the efficacy and adverse effects of five commonly used antihypertensive drugs (one from each class) and placebo. Although these trials found some differences in blood pressure control, adverse effects, quality of life, and biochemical parameters, these differences did not present a pattern that favored one drug over another. In fact, the Veterans Administration study showed that a diuretic provided the best efficacy when combined with any other drug. Reduction of left ventricular hypertrophy—an independent predictor of morbidity and mortality—favored diuretic therapy in both studies.

Further concerns surround the use of CCBs in the management of hypertension.[16] Drugs of this class are very effective in reducing blood pressure, particularly in African Americans, are well tolerated, and are associated with no demonstrable metabolic effects when used in cardiovascular diseases, including hypertension. Retrospective case reports, publicized in early 1995, and subsequent publications raised concerns about potential increases in cardiac events in patients treated with CCBs. More recently, reports comparing ACEI to CCB therapy in hypertensive patients with diabetes mellitus showed markedly fewer cardiovascular events in patients treated with ACEIs.[17] Although these studies cannot claim that CCB treatment increased the risk of cardiac events, as opposed to the beneficial effects resulting from ACEI use, these reports increase concerns about the appropriateness of using CCBs in hypertension, particularly in the setting of diabetes mellitus.

ACEIs, on the other hand, are a very promising class of agents. Although specific outcome trials in hypertension using ACEIs have not yet been completed, available data are encouraging. ACEIs reduce morbidity and mortality in mild, moderate, and severe heart failure[18, 19] and in patients after MI.[20] These observations—along with other data showing improvement in surrogate end-points such as endothelial dysfunction, reduction of left ventricular hypertrophy,[21] and improvement in insulin resistance—raise the hope that this class of agents will improve outcomes in patients with hypertension. Similarly, α-adrenergeric blockers have favorable effects on lipid profiles,[15, 22] insulin resistance,[23] and platelet aggregation,[24] but outcome data are lacking.

There is an urgent need to compare these newer agents with older, time-honored treatments such as diuretics in large well-designed trials. This need will be fulfilled with ALLHAT. Although other studies have announced similar intentions, ALLHAT is likely to remain the largest, the most independent of potential conflict of interest, and the trial most likely to give valid results in a head-to-head comparison of representatives of three newer classes of agents (ACEIs, CCBs, and α-blockers) against the time-tested diuretics. Furthermore, by design, ALLHAT will provide badly needed information in African American patients and in women with hypertension.

African-Americans have a much higher prevalence of hypertension,[25] which presents at a younger age[26] and, for the same level of blood pressure, is associated with more target organ damage[27, 28] compared with white patients. The incidence of end-stage renal disease secondary to hypertension is nearly eightfold higher in African American than in white hypertensives.[28] The risks of left ventricular hypertrophy, stroke, and stroke mortality are higher in African Americans.[27] The questions asked in ALLHAT are relevant to this population, and this is the group most likely to benefit from this information. This is why ALLHAT was designed to include at least 55% African American participants.

Cholesterol-Lowering Component

Numerous studies have shown substantial reductions in cardiovascular events with cholesterol lowering, but most of those were carried out in middle-aged white persons, predominantly men. Similar information is lacking in minorities and the elderly. With the advent of 3-hydroxy-3-methylglutaryl coenzyme A (HMG CoA) reductase inhibitors, drugs that can reduce LDL cholesterol between 25 and 40% with few adverse effects, several studies showed benefits in patients with or without demonstrable coronary disease. The Scandinavian Simvastatin Survival Study (4S), a major trial that included women and older patients (up to the age of 70 years), randomized 4444 men and women with documented CHD and cholesterol levels of 212 to 309 mg/dl to treatment with simvastatin or placebo.[29] After 5.4 years of follow-up, compared with placebo simvastatin-treated patients had 30% fewer deaths, a 42% decrease in CHD mortality, and significant reductions in nonfatal MIs and all-cause mortality. This trial also demonstrated benefits in older patients (aged 60 to 70 years).

These results were not available when ALLHAT was designed.[30] When the results of 4S were released, the ALLHAT steering committee considered whether the cholesterol component should be stopped. The decision to continue was based on the fact that the two studies include entirely different populations. Only 3% of the ALLHAT patients satisfied the entry criteria for the 4S trial. A second reason not to stop the cholesterol component of ALLHAT was that ALLHAT allows usual cholesterol-lowering therapy in the control arm while the experimental group receives 40 mg of pravastatin. The only change that the steering committee made was to exclude patients with CHD and LDL cholesterol above 129 mg/dl. In the original protocol, the upper limit was 159 mg/dl.

OBJECTIVES AND DESIGN

The primary and secondary hypotheses of ALLHAT are shown in Table 36–1. The trial assumes that blood pressure control will be similar in all treatment groups and that any observed differences will be attributed to specific drug effects other than blood pressure reduction. Unlike the antihypertensive component, the cholesterol component focuses on the generic effects of cholesterol lowering rather than the effects of a specific drug or drug class, and its power does not diminish as a result of crossovers from pravastatin to other treatments producing equivalent lipid changes.

ELIGIBILITY FOR THE ANTIHYPERTENSIVE COMPONENT

Eligible patients are men and women aged 55 years or older with history of documented hypertension using these

Table 36–1 Primary and Secondary Hypotheses of ALLHAT

ANTIHYPERTENSIVE COMPONENT

Primary Hypothesis

Combined incidence of fatal CHD and nonfatal MI will be lower in hypertensive patients receiving amlodipine, lisinopril, or doxazosin as first-line therapy than in similar patients treated with chlorothalidone.

Secondary Hypotheses

Compared with patients treated with chlorothalidone, patients treated with amlodipine, lisinopril, or doxazosin will have a lower incidence of
  All-cause mortality
  Combined CHD + revascularization procedures + hospitalized
    angina
  Stroke
  Combined CHD + stroke + revascularization procedures + angina
    + CHF + peripheral arterial disease
  Left ventricular hypertrophy by ECG
  Renal disease
  Health-related quality of life

Cholesterol-Lowering Component

Primary Hypothesis

All-cause mortality will be lower in patients randomized to receive
  pravastatin than in those patients randomized to usual care.

Secondary Hypotheses

Compared with patients randomized to receive usual care, patients
treated with pravastatin will have a lower incidence of
  Combined incidence of CHD death and nonfatal MI
    MI determined by ECG
    Cause-specific mortality
    Total and site-specific cancer incidence
    Health-related quality of life

Abbreviations: ALLHAT, Antihypertensive and Lipid-Lowering to Prevent Heart Attack Trial; CHD, coronary heart disease; MI, myocardial infarction; CHF, congestive heart failure; ECG, electrocardiogram.

Table 36–2 Major ALLHAT Inclusion and Exclusion Criteria—Antihypertensive Component

INCLUSION CRITERIA

One or more manifestations of atherosclerotic cardiovascular disease
  Old myocardial infarction or stroke
  History of revascularization procedures
  Documented atherosclerotic cardiovascular disease
Type II diabetes mellitus by glucose or on insulin or oral hypoglycemics
HDL cholesterol <35 mg/dl
Left ventricular hypertrophy on ECG or echocardiogram
ST-T-wave ECG changes indicative of ischemia
Current cigarette smoking

EXCLUSION CRITERIA

Symptomatic myocardial infarction or stroke within the past 6 months
Symptomatic congestive heart failure or ejection fraction <35%, if
  known
Angina pectoris within the past 6 months
Serum creatinine ≥2 mg/dl
Requirement for thiazide-like diuretics, calcium antagonists, angiotensin-
  converting enzyme inhibitors, or α-blockers for reasons other than
  hypertension
Requirement for more than two antihypertensive drugs to achieve
  satisfactory blood pressure control
Sensitivity or contraindications to any of the first-line study medications
Factors suggesting a low likelihood of compliance with the protocol
Diseases likely to lead to noncardiovascular death over the course of the
  study
Blood pressure >180 mm Hg systolic or >110 mm Hg diastolic on two
  separate readings during screening of step-down

Adapted by permission of Elsevier Science from Davis BR, Cutler JA, Gordon DJ, et al. Rationale and design for the Antihypertensive and Lipid-Lowering to Prevent Heart Attack Trial (ALLHAT). Am J Hypertens, volume 9, pp 342–360, copyright 1996, by American Journal of Hypertension Ltd.
Abbreviations: ALLHAT, Antihypertensive and Lipid-Lowering to Prevent Heart Attack Trial; HDL, high-density lipoprotein; ECG, electrocardiogram.

criteria: patients receiving one or two antihypertensive medications for at least 3 years qualify if repeated blood pressure measurements are less than 160/100 mm Hg or patients who are untreated or who have received therapy for less than 2 months and who have blood pressures between 140/90 and 180/110 mm Hg. All potential participants must also meet the inclusion and exclusion criteria in Table 36–2.

ELIGIBILITY FOR THE CHOLESTEROL-LOWERING COMPONENT

To be eligible for the cholesterol-lowering component, participants must first be enrolled in the antihypertensive component and meet the inclusion and exclusion criteria listed in Table 36–3.

TREATMENT PROGRAM

Antihypertensive Component

Before initiating any study drug, all antihypertensive medications are tapered and discontinued. The duration of tapering is left to the judgment of the responsible investigator. Participants who are not receiving any antihypertensive medication or who are well controlled on one medication can be randomized immediately after the screening visit.

Table 36–3 Major ALLHAT Inclusion and Exclusion Criteria—Cholesterol-Lowering Component

INCLUSION CRITERIA
Enrollment in the antihypertensive trial
LDL cholesterol of 120–189 mg/dl (100–129 mg/dl for patients with
    known congestive heart disease) with a triglyceride level ≤350 mg/dl

EXCLUSION CRITERIA
Current use of prescribed lipid-lowering agents or large doses (≥500
    mg/day) of nonprescription niacin
Contraindications to HMG CoA reductase inhibitors (e.g., significant
    liver disease, ongoing immunosuppressive therapy, known allergy or
    intolerance to the study drug)
Known untreated secondary cause of hyperlipidemia
ALT >2.0 times the upper limit of normal

Adapted by permission of Elsevier Science from Davis BR, Cutler JA, Gordon DJ,
et al. Rationale and design for the Antihypertensive and Lipid-Lowering to Prevent
Heart Attack Trial (ALLHAT). Am J Hypertens, volume 9, pp 342–360, copyright
1996, by American Journal of Hypertension Ltd.
Abbreviations: ALLHAT, Antihypertensive and Lipid-Lowering to Prevent Heart
Attack Trial; LDL, low-density lipoprotein; HMG CoA, 3-hydroxy-3-methyl-
glutaryl coenzyme A; ALT, alanine aminotransferase

Participants are randomized to one of the four antihypertensive treatment arms. The assigned medication is initially given at a low dose and increased to higher doses as follows: chlorothalidone is started at 12.5 mg daily and increased to 25 mg; amlodipine is started at 2.5 mg and increased to 5 or 10 mg d; lisinopril is started at 10 mg and increased to 20 or 40 mg d; and doxazosin is started at 1 mg and increased to 2, 4, or 8 mg d.

The objective of treatment is to achieve goal blood pressure (<90 mm Hg diastolic and <140 mm Hg systolic) using the lowest possible dosage of the first-line drug. Patients not controlled on the highest dose of the initial drug can receive reserpine 0.05 to 0.2 mg daily, clonidine 0.1 mg to 0.3 mg twice daily, atenolol 25 to 100 mg daily, hydralazine 25 mg to 100 mg twice daily, or any combination of these drugs in order to achieve goal blood pressure. The number of study drugs prescribed is influenced by patient tolerability and clinical judgment. The identity of the first-line drug is blinded to the investigator and the patient at all doses.

Doses of first-line medication are increased at monthly intervals until goal blood pressure is achieved. The choice of second-line medications is left to the discretion of the investigator.

Cholesterol-Lowering Component

Patients who indicate interest in participating in the cholesterol-lowering component undergo a battery of tests, including liver function and lipid profile. Patients with LDL cholesterol of 120 to 189 mg/dl (100 to 129 mg/dl for patients with known CHD) and fasting triglycerides less than or equal to 350 mg/dl are eligible for this part of the study. Consenting patients are randomized to receive pravastatin 40 mg every evening or usual care. All patients are advised to follow the National Cholesterol Education Program (NCEP) step 1 diet. Cholesterol levels are measured at visit 4 and all annual visits for the pravastatin-treated patients and at the second, fourth, and sixth annual

visits for the usual-care patients. Complete lipid profiles will be done in a random sample of 10% in the pravastatin group and 5% in the usual-care group.

DETERMINATION OF END-POINTS

The end-points of the study are listed in Table 36–4. At each visit, the coordinator at each participating center will document events by completing a checklist and, when necessary, by supplying interim reports. Specific diagnoses will be supported by documentation in discharge summaries or death certificates. The cause of death will be determined by the physician-investigator at each site. For a random 10% subset of hospitalized MIs and strokes, the clinical trials center will request more detailed information, such as electrocardiograms from hospitalized patients and enzyme levels for MIs and neurologists' notes and computed tomography and magnetic resonance imaging reports for strokes.

The primary end-point for the antihypertensive component is combined fatal CHD and nonfatal MI. For the primary end-point and the secondary end-points all-cause mortality, stroke, combined coronary and cardiovascular outcomes, and end-stage renal disease, comparison will be made between each of the nondiuretic-treated groups and the diuretic-treated group. For the outcomes of left ventric-

Table 36–4 ALLHAT End-Points

DEATH
Definite myocardial infarction
Definite coronary heart disease
Possible coronary heart disease
Stroke
Congestive heart failure
Other cardiovascular disease
Cancer
Accident, suicide, or homicide
Other noncardiovascular cause
Unknown cause

MYOCARDIAL INFARCTION

STROKE

HOSPITALIZED OR TREATED
Angina
Congestive heart failure
Peripheral arterial disease
New cancer diagnosis
Accident or attempted suicide

*LEFT VENTRICULAR HYPERTROPHY (BIENNIAL STUDY,
    ELECTROCARDIOGRAM)*

RENAL FUNCTION
Slope of the reciprocal of serum creatinine level versus time
End-stage renal disease (initiation of chronic renal dialysis or kidney
    transplant)

QUALITY OF LIFE

MEDICAL CARE USE

Adapted by permission of Elsevier Science from Davis BR, Cutler JA, Gordon DJ,
et al. Rationale and design for the Antihypertensive and Lipid-Lowering to Prevent
Heart Attack Trial (ALLHAT). Am J Hypertens, volume 9, pp 342–360, copyright
1996, by American Journal of Hypertension Ltd.
Abbreviation: ALLHAT, Antihypertensive and Lipid-Lowering to Prevent Heart
Attack Trial.

Table 36–5 Patient Recruitment

MARCH 15, 1996
14,646 patients to antihypertensive component
3304 to cholesterol-lowering component
356 clinics randomizing

JANUARY 31, 1998
41,836 patients to antihypertensive component
8962 to cholesterol-lowering component
547 sites have randomized

Table 36–7 Risk Characteristics—Antihypertensive Component

21% are cigarette smokers
46% have ASCVD
35% are diabetic patients
10% have ST-T-wave abnormalities
13% have low HDL
16% have LVH by ECG
4% have LVH by echocardiogram*

Abbreviations: ASCVD, atherosclerotic cardiovascular disease; HDL, high-density lipoprotein; LVH, left ventricular hypertrophy; ECG, electrocardiogram.
*Only a small number of patients had echocardiograms available.

ular hypertrophy and health-related quality of life, differences between groups will be determined.

Primary and secondary end-points for the lipid-lowering component will be compared between the pravastatin and the usual-care groups. For the outcomes of combined fatal CHD and nonfatal MI, differences between men and women; between patients aged 65 years and older and those under 65 years old; between African Americans and non–African Americans; and between diabetics and nondiabetics will be examined.

BASELINE CHARACTERISTICS

As of January 31, 1998, the conclusion of the enrollment period, a total of 41,836 participants had been randomized into the antihypertensive component of the trial. Of these patients, 8962 were randomized into the cholesterol-lowering component. Patients were recruited from 547 sites in the United States, Puerto Rico, and Canada. Table 36–5 demonstrates recruitment at two time points.

Baseline characteristics are depicted in Table 36–6. The mean age of this patient population was 67 years with 6.4% of the patients over the age of 80 years. African Americans had a fair representation, making up 36.7% of randomized patients. This cohort also included 45.7% women. The average duration of education was 11.1 years. Many patients were on treatment when rolled over to the study regimen without obtaining baseline blood pressures, so mean blood pressure at randomization was 146/84 mm Hg. The study population is indeed high risk: 21% are cigarette smokers; 46% have a history of atherosclerotic cardiovascular disease; and 35% have diabetes. Over 10% of the patients have ST-T-wave abnormalities on electrocardiogram, and 13% have an HDL cholesterol less than 35 mg/dl. In addition, 16% have left ventricular hypertrophy on the 12-lead electrocardiogram, and in 4%, an existing

echocardiogram demonstrated left ventricular hypertrophy as well (Table 36–7).

Table 36–8 shows baseline characteristics of patients randomized into the lipid-lowering component. The average age of this subgroup is 67 years, and 5.5% are over 80 years. This group includes 39% African Americans and 47% women. The average duration of education is 11 years, and 22% are cigarette smokers.

Table 36–9 shows the baseline lipid profile of patients randomized into the lipid-lowering component. The average LDL cholesterol was 146 mg/dl; total cholesterol, 224 mg/dl; HDL cholesterol, 47 mg/dl; and fasting triglycerides, 152 mg/dl.

SUMMARY

In summary, ALLHAT is the largest antihypertensive trial ever done in North America. It was designed to address the crucial question of whether there is a specific drug effect on outcomes beyond lowering blood pressure. Representative agents of three "newer" classes of antihypertensives—CCBs (amlodipine), ACEIs (lisinopril) and α-adrenergic blockers (doxazosin)—will be compared with the time-honored diuretics (chlorothalidone). Besides the primary outcomes of combined fatal CHD and nonfatal MI, a number of other cardiovascular conditions, as well as the preservation of quality of life, will be assessed. The cholesterol-lowering component will also provide long-awaited answers to questions such as benefits from lowering moderately elevated LDL cholesterol in older patients and benefits in subpopulations such as African Americans and diabetics.

The baseline characteristics of participants indicate that the enrolled population is truly at high risk, guaranteeing that enough end-points will occur during the follow-up period to ensure valid statistical comparisons. The results of ALLHAT are expected to be available by the year 2002

Table 36–6 Baseline Characteristics—Antihypertensive Component

Mean age 67 years (6.4% age 80+)
36.7% African American
45.7% women
11.1 years of education
Mean blood pressure 146/84 mm Hg*

*Blood pressure was obtained without prior discontinuation of antihypertensive therapy and washout phase.

Table 36–8 Baseline Characteristics—Cholesterol-Lowering Component

Mean age 67 years (5.5% age 80+)
39% African American
47% women
11 years of education
22% current cigarette smokers

Table 36–9 Lipid Characteristics at Baseline— Cholesterol-Lowering Component

Mean LDL cholesterol 146 mg/dl
Mean total cholesterol 224 mg/dl
Mean HDL cholesterol 47 mg/dl
Mean fasting triglycerides 152 mg/dl

Abbreviations: LDL, low-density lipoprotein; HDL, high-density lipoprotein.

and will influence the way we treat patients for many years to come.

References

1. Burt VI, Cutler JA, Higgins M, et al. Trends in the prevalence, awareness, treatment, and control of hypertension in the adult US population: Data from the Health Examination Surveys, 1960 to 1991. Hypertension 26:60–69, 1995.
2. Joint National Committee on Prevention, Detection, Evaluation and Treatment of High Blood Pressure. The Sixth Report of the Joint National Committee on Prevention, Detection, Evaluation and Treatment of High Blood Pressure. Arch Intern Med 157:2413–2446, 1997.
3. U.S. Renal Data System. USRDS 1997 Annual Report. Bethesda, MD, U.S. Department of Health and Human Services, National Institute of Diabetes and Digestive and Kidney Disease, 1997; p X.
4. Levy D, Larson MG, Vasan RS, et al. The progression from hypertension to congestive heart failure. JAMA 275:1557–1562, 1996.
5. MacMahon SW, Cutler JA, Furberg CD, et al. The effects of drug treatment for hypertension on morbidity and mortality from cardiovascular disease: A review of randomized controlled trials. Prog Cardiovasc Dis 29(suppl 1):99–119, 1986.
6. Collins R, Peto R, MacMahon S, et al. Blood pressure, stroke, and coronary heart disease. Part 2: Short-term reductions in blood pressure: Overview of randomized drug trials in their epidemiological context. Lancet 335:827–838, 1990.
7. Papademetriou V, Narayan P, Rubins H, et al. Influence of risk factors on peripheral and cerebrovascular disease in men with coronary artery disease, low HDL-C and desireable LDL-C. Am Heart J 136:734–740, 1998.
8. MacMahon S, Peto R, Cutler J, et al. Blood pressure, stroke, and coronary heart disease. Part 1: Prolonged differences in blood pressure: Prospective, observational studies corrected for the regression dilution bias. Lancet 335:765–774, 1990.
9. Veterans Administration Cooperative Study Group on Antihypertensive Agents. Effects of treatment on morbidity in hypertension. II: Results of patients with diastolic blood pressure averaging 90 through 114 mm Hg. JAMA 213:1143–1151, 1970.
10. Cutler JA, Psaty BM, MacMahon S, Furberg CD. Public health issues in hypertension control: What has been learned from clinical trials. *In* Laragh JH, Brenner BM (eds). Hypertension: Pathophysiology, Diagnosis, and Management, 2nd ed. New York, Raven, 1995, pp 253–272.
11. Joint National Committee on Prevention, Detection, Evaluation and Treatment of High Blood Pressure. The Fifth Report of the Joint National Committee on Prevention, Detection, Evaluation, and Treatment of High Blood Pressure (JNC V). Arch Intern Med 153:154–183, 1993.
12. Freis E, Papademetriou V. Current drug treatment and treatment patterns with antihypertensive drugs. Drugs 52:1–16, 1996.
13. Freis E. Cardiotoxicity of diuretics: Review of the evidence. J Hypertens 8:S23–S32, 1990.
14. Materson BJ, Reda DJ, Cushman WC, et al, for the Department of Veterans Affairs Cooperative Study Group on Antihypertensive Agents. Single-drug therapy for hypertension in men: A comparison of six antihypertensive agents with placebo. N Engl J Med 328:914–921, 1993.
15. Neaton JD, Grimm RH Jr, Prineas RJ, et al, for the Treatment of Mild Hypertension Study Research Group. Treatment of Mild Hypertension Study: Final results. JAMA 1993;270:713–724.
16. Psaty BM, Heckbert SR, Koepseil TD, et al. The risk of myocardial infarction associated with antihypertensive drug therapies. JAMA 274:620–625, 1995.
17. Estacio RO, Jeffers BW, Hiatt WR, et al. The effect of nisoldipine as compared with enalapril on cardiovascular outcomes in patients with non–insulin-dependent diabetes and hypertension. N Engl J Med 338:645–652, 1998.
18. The SOLVD Investigators: Effect of enalapril on survival in patients with reduced left ventricular ejection fractions and congestive heart failure. N Engl J Med 325:293–302, 1991.
19. Pfeffer MA, Braunwald E, Moye LA, et al. The effect of captopril on morbidity and mortality in patients with left ventricular dysfunction following myocardial infarction. N Engl J Med 327:678–684, 1992.
20. The Acute Infarction Ramipril Efficacy (AIRE) Study Investigators. Effects of ramipril on mortality and mortality of survivors of acute myocardial infarction with clinical evidence of heart failure. Lancet 342:821–828, 1993.
21. Dahlof B, Pennert K, Hansson L. Reversal of left ventricular hypertrophy in hypertension patients: A meta-analysis of 109 treatment studies. Am J Hypertens 5:95–110, 1992.
22. Pool JL. Effects of doxazosin on serum lipids: A review of the clinical data and molecular basis for altered lipid metabolism. Am Heart J 121:251–259, 1991.
23. Lithell H. Effects of antihypertensive drugs on insulin, glucose and lipid metabolism. Diabetes Care 14:203–209, 1991.
24. Hernandez RH, Guerrero PJ, Carvajal AR, et al. Evidence of anti-platelet aggregation action of doxazosin patients with hypertension: An ex-vivo study. Am Heart J 121:395–401, 1991.
25. Hall WD, Ferrario CM, Moore MA, et al. Hypertension-related morbidity and mortality in the southeastern United States. Am J Med Sci 313:195–206, 1997.
26. Burt VL, Whelton P, Rocella EJ, et al. Prevalence of hypertension in the US adult population: Results from the third National Health and Nutrition Examination Survey, 1988–1991. Hypertension 25:305–313, 1995.
27. Singh GK, Kochanek KD, MacDorman MF. Advance report of final mortality statistics, 1994. Mon Vital Stat Rep 45(suppl):1–76, 1996.
28. Klag MJ, Whelton PK, Randal BL, et al. End-stage renal disease in African-American and white men: 16-year MRFIT findings. JAMA 277:1293–1298, 1997.
29. Scandanavian Simvastatin Survival Study Group: Randomized trial of cholesterol lowering in 4444 patients with coronary heart disease: The Scandanavian Simvastatin Survival Study (4S). Lancet 344:1383–1389, 1994.
30. Davis BR, Cutler JA, Gordon DJ, et al. Rationale and design for the Antihypertensive and Lipid-Lowering Treatment to Prevent Heart Attack Trial (ALLHAT). Am J Hypertens 9:342–360, 1996.

CHAPTER 37

The Losartan Intervention For Endpoint Reduction (LIFE) in Hypertension Study: Rationale, Design, and Characteristics of 9194 Patients With Left Ventricular Hypertrophy

Sverre E. Kjeldsen and Björn Dahlöf

Losartan was the first orally available selective antagonist of the angiotensin II type-1 (AT_1) receptor approved for the treatment of essential hypertension.[1-3] The existence of left ventricular hypertrophy (LVH) identifies patients at particularly high risk for cardiovascular complications of essential hypertension.[4-6] Studies in animals suggest that treatment with losartan may be beneficial for target organ protection and, more importantly, improve survival.[7-10] Promising results have now been seen with losartan on survival in heart failure.[11]

The Losartan Intervention For Endpoint Reduction (LIFE) in Hypertension Study is a multicenter, double-blind, double-dummy, randomized, prospective, active-controlled parallel group study designed to compare the effects of losartan with those of the β-blocker atenolol, both in doses of 50 to 100 mg q.d., on cardiovascular morbidity and mortality in patients with essential hypertension and LVH documented by electrocardiogram (ECG). Additional treatment may be given as open-label hydrochlorothiazide 12.5 to 25 mg and, if needed, any other antihypertensive medication except for other β-blockers, AT_1-receptor antagonists, or angiotensin-converting enzyme (ACE) inhibitors to reach a target blood pressure of less than 140/90 mm Hg. After the 2-week single-blind placebo run-in period, there will be at least a 4-year period of randomized active double-blind treatment until 1040 patients have experienced a *primary cardiovascular event,* defined as cardiovascular death, nonfatal clinically evident acute myocardial infarction, or nonfatal cerebral stroke. This study is endpoint-driven and has been calculated to have 80% power with 8300 patients enrolled to detect a 15% further reduction in the primary outcome rate from 15% in the atenolol group to 12.75% in the losartan group. The rationale, objectives, design, and methods of the LIFE study, including outcome measures and statistical methods, have been published.[12]

Altogether, 9223 eligible patients in Scandinavia, the United Kingdom, and the United States were randomized as of April 30, 1997. The LIFE study is the largest ever to be undertaken in patients with LVH and one of the largest intervention studies in essential hypertension. The LIFE study is also unique in that it utilized ECG criteria for LVH to recruit a large population of high-risk hypertensives. This report summarizes some of the baseline characteristics of the LIFE participants.[13]

METHODS

Subjects

Eligible patients were men and women between 55 and 80 years of age with previously untreated or treated essential

hypertension and LVH documented by ECG (see later). To be included, the patients had to have mean trough sitting diastolic blood pressure readings of 95 to 115 mm Hg and/or mean sitting systolic blood pressure readings of 160 to 200 mm Hg after 1 and 2 weeks on single-blind placebo treatment. Blood pressure and heart rate were taken with standardized technique after subjects had been seated for 5 minutes. Subjects were questioned about alcohol intake, smoking habits, exercise level, and employment status; weight and height were measured. Information on previous diseases and drug therapies was collected by the investigators before randomization, and a physical examination was performed to detect concomitant diseases. Laboratory tests performed in the central laboratory included determinations of hemoglobin, serum sodium, potassium, creatinine, uric acid, total cholesterol, high-density lipoprotein (HDL) cholesterol and glucose. Mean blood pressures for the randomized patients averaged 169.9/94.8, 172.6/96.6, and 174.4/97.8 mm Hg, respectively, at screening and after 1 and 2 weeks on placebo. Exclusion criteria included cardiovascular conditions and obvious noncardiac diseases that may limit long-term survival of the patient or increase the likelihood of nonadherence to study medication.[12]

Protocol

After a pilot phase at eight sites in Norway and Sweden in June through August 1995, 945 centers in Denmark, Finland, Iceland, Norway, Sweden, the United Kingdom, and the United States enrolled patients during the period from September 1995 through April 1997. The vast majority of the centers are active in primary care; however, in Denmark, most LIFE patients were referred from primary care physicians to hospital-based centers. An average of 9.7 (range 1 to 148) participants were enrolled in each center.

LVH was diagnosed electrocardiographically from standard 12-lead ECGs in all participants before randomization by the core laboratory at Sahlgrenska University Hospital/Östra in Göteborg, Sweden. LVH was identified by the core laboratory using criteria based on the Cornell voltage × QRS duration product:[14-16] (RaVL + SV_3) × QRS duration > 2440 mm × msec in men, and (RaVL + SV_3 + 8 mm) × QRS duration > 2440 mm x msec in women. Beginning on May 1, 1996, at which time 2375 patients had been enrolled, the gender correction of Cornell criteria in women was revised from 8 to 6 mm both based on data published after the LIFE design had been established[17] and due to an initial relative oversampling of women. From this date, an additional acceptance criterion was introduced

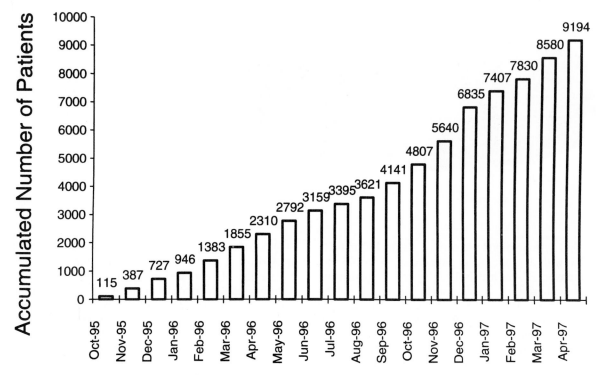

Figure 37–1. Accumulated number of patients from October 1995 through April 1997.

based on the Sokolow-Lyon voltage combination (SV_1 + RV_5 or V_6) > 38 mm.[18] The rationale for adding the Sokolow-Lyon criterion was based on the following assumption: Both Cornell and Sokolow-Lyon criteria (>35 mm) have specificities of about 95% in normal adults[19] but sensitivities of only approximately 30 to 40%. In reanalysis of published data sets,[14–16, 19] combining the two (and increasing Sokolow-Lyon voltage to >38 mm) increased the sensitivity by more than 10% without losing specificity.[14–18] The ECG criteria for LIFE participants will be further validated in a large echocardiographic substudy comprising about 12% of the LIFE study population.

Early in the process of preparing the final baseline database, irregularities were discovered at one center, and it was decided to remove the 29 patients randomized at this center.

Statistics

Results are presented as mean values ± SDs or as percentages of the total number of subjects. The statistical significance of the differences between men and women were assessed using the chi-squared test for categorical variables and the rank-sum test for continuous variables. An average 5-year risk of coronary heart disease was calculated according to the Framingham Risk Score.[20]

RESULTS

More than 33,000 screening ECGs were received, and approximately 19,000 ECGs were approved, meeting the study ECG-LVH criteria. Following these ECG approvals,

a total of 9223 patients met blood pressure and other inclusion and no-exclusion criteria and gave signed informed consent. Patients were enrolled from June 1995 through April 1997, when randomization was closed (Fig. 37–1). The number of patients in the seven participating countries are as follows (Fig. 37–2): Denmark (n = 1391 [15%]), Finland (n = 1485 [16%]), Iceland (n = 133 [1%]), Norway (n = 1415 [15%]), Sweden (n = 2245 [25%]), the United Kingdom (n = 817 [9%]), and the United States (n = 1708 [19%]). The great majority of the 945 study sites have relatively small numbers of patients (1 to 10 patients in 669 centers). The 25 larger centers with 40 or more patients enrolled 1621 patients, or 17.6% of the total population.

Many more women (61.3%) than men were enrolled through April 1996. After changing the gender correction from +8 to +6 mm on Cornell voltage, proportionately fewer women were randomized (51.5%), resulting in a total of 54.1% women in the study. Preliminary analysis showed that the proportion of subjects who qualified based on the Cornell voltage QRS duration product formula was approximately 66%; 21% qualified based on Sokolow-Lyon voltage; and 10% fulfilled both criteria.

The patients averaged 66.9 years of age at randomization. The women were older, had a higher body mass index, and were more likely to have isolated systolic hypertension. More men were working full time, and the men had higher Framingham Risk Scores for coronary heart disease than the women. However, the predicted 5-year event rate attributable to factors other than gender was only moderately higher ($p < .001$) in men (19.3%) than in women (17.1%).

More than 80% of patients were above the age of 60 years at randomization (Fig. 37–3). The majority of patients had moderate hypertension at the randomization visit

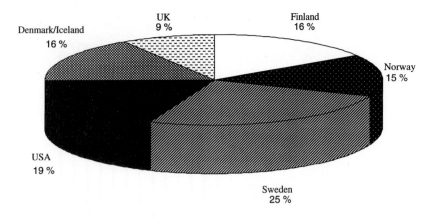

Figure 37–2. Patients from each participating country (%).

(55.9% with systolic blood pressure of 160 to 180 mm Hg and 53.7% with diastolic blood pressure of 95 to 105 mm Hg). Moreover, 27.4% had isolated systolic hypertension (systolic blood pressure ≥ 160 mm Hg and diastolic blood pressure < 95 mm Hg), and 9.5% were randomized based on diastolic hypertension only. Blood pressure levels were similar in all countries.

The overwhelming majority of subjects are white. Self-reported alcohol and tobacco use are moderate or low; 32.1% of men and 57.6% of women report that they never use alcohol, whereas 80.3% and 86.5%, respectively, do not smoke. Of men, 46.7% are previous tobacco smokers (Fig. 37–4). The average total cholesterol level was slightly above 6.0 mmol, somewhat compensated for by high HDL cholesterol and a total:HDL cholesterol ratio of 4.3. Both total cholesterol and HDL cholesterol were higher in women than in men. Although only 2.7% of participants were reported to have overt obesity, 21.3% had a body mass index of 30 to 35, 5.4% of 35 to 40, and 1.9% of 40 kg/m² or higher.

Approximately 15% of LIFE participants had one or more manifestations of coronary heart disease. Previous stroke and/or transient ischemic attack was reported by 7.7%, lipid disorders by 18.0%, and diabetes mellitus by 12.3% of patients. A variety of other disorders were less frequently reported.

Almost a third of the patients (28.9%) had been untreated for at least 6 months for their high blood pressure before the placebo period, whereas 39.6% were treated with one antihypertensive agent at the time of enrollment, 23.3% with two agents, and 8.1% with three or more antihypertensive agents. Diuretics were taken by 27.5%, more women (31.8%) than men (22.5%); β-blockers by 26.7%; calcium channel blockers by 24.3% (men 26.6%, women 22.3%); and ACE inhibitors by 25.2% (men 28.9%, women 22.1%). One of five patients (21.0%) was on aspirin; other drug therapies were less frequent. These included antiinflammatory drugs (7.1%), oral hypoglycemic agents (6.6%), cholesterol-lowering drugs (7.1%), antacids (5.2%), thyroxine (5.1%), nitrates (5.0%), digoxin (3.0%), and warfarin (1.4%). Eighteen percent of the women were on postmenopausal hormone replacement therapy.

The median number of days on placebo therapy was 14 in all participating countries. A limited number of patients, 724 men and 832 women, who entered the single-blind placebo phase of the study were not randomized. These subjects were fairly comparable with those who were randomized with respect to age and gender distribution. However, relatively more African Americans were not randomized. Blood pressure levels outside the windows that qualified for inclusion (29.9%) and nonapproved ECGs

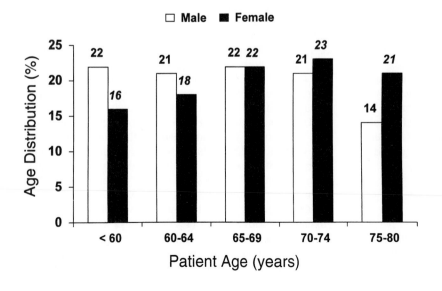

Figure 37–3. Age distribution for men and women (%).

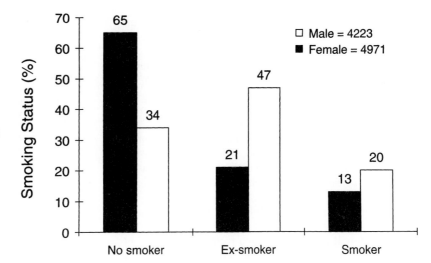

Figure 37–4. Nonsmokers, ex-smokers, and smokers for men and women (%).

(28.9%) were the most common reasons for not being randomized. Other common reasons for discontinuation during the placebo period were: exclusion criteria (14.7%), patient unwilling (10.8%), and clinical adverse experience (8.9%).

DISCUSSION

Nine hundred and forty-five centers in the Nordic countries, the United Kingdom, and the United States have, over a period of less than 2 years, applied some strict but simple 12-lead ECG criteria (Cornell voltage × QRS duration product > 2440 mm × msec and Sokolow-Lyon voltage combination >38 mm) to identify hypertensive patients between 55 and 80 years of age with LVH. Although aiming at a study population of 8300 patients, a total of 9223 patients were included and 9194 remain after exclusion of a site at which irregularities were discovered. This population of hypertensives with LVH comprises women and men, mostly retired, on average, overweight with relatively high prevalences of diabetes, lipid disorders, and coronary heart disease; and relatively low prevalence of active smoking. The population is predominantly white but includes 694 patients from other ethnic groups.

Investigators could submit 12-lead ECGs from any hypertensive patient between 55 and 80 years of age for approval by the ECG core laboratory. More than 33,000 ECGs were received, and more than 19,000 (57.6%) were approved. Preliminary results from a pilot study in Scandinavia showed that the prevalence of ECG-LVH in nearly 1500 hypertensive patients, most of whom were receiving antihypertensive treatment, who otherwise met eligibility criteria to be used in the LIFE study, was approximately 22%.[12] Although many investigators submitted unselected ECGs for scrutiny, an approval rate of 57.6% clearly suggests that most investigators accurately read ECGs according to the study's criteria before submitting them. The ability to enroll over 9000 hypertensive patients predominantly drawn from primary health care centers by this procedure supports the usefulness of ECG for identification of high-risk hypertensives and demonstrates the feasibility of this approach in general practice.

The patients who were randomized comprise about 28% of all patients screened for the study, and 48.5% of all those who were approved based on the ECG readings. The question of generalizability is important.[21] It is reasonable to consider the randomized patients in the LIFE study to be representative of hypertensive patients with ECG-LVH in the age group under study. Further, the demographic characteristics of those patients who entered the 2-week placebo run-in period were similar in nonrandomized patients and randomized patients except for specific exclusion criteria, i.e., either not approved ECG or blood pressure outside the range for inclusion.

Beginning on May 1, 1996, the gender correction of the Cornell voltage criteria in women was revised from 8 to 6 mm based on data published after initiation of LIFE recruitment,[17] owing to a relative oversampling of women. On this date, an additional acceptance criterion was introduced based on the Sokolow-Lyon voltage combination ($SV_1 + RV_5$ or V_6) above 38 mm.[19] After this change was implemented—i.e., subjects could fulfill the revised Cornell voltage criteria, the Sokolow-Lyon voltage, or a combination of both—51.5% of those randomized were women. Thus, ECG criteria used subsequent to May 1, 1996, are appropriate to achieve a balanced gender recruitment. Inclusion of participants with these ECG criteria has resulted in a high prevalence of left ventricular geometric abnormalities (82%) according to a preliminary analysis of baseline echocardiographic data in a substudy of 625 LIFE patients representative of the whole LIFE cohort.

The LIFE study population is at high risk for cardiovascular endpoints, with a 5-year probability of coronary morbid or mortal events of 22.3% according to the Framingham Risk Score. Although the Framingham composite risk score was not used to support the expected number of events in this study,[12] we have preliminarily assessed the usefulness of the score in relation to the first 301 reported primary endpoints. Men have a higher event rate than women (4.0% vs. 2.7%), and the event rate increases with age. The Framingham Risk Score appears to be useful in stratifying patients: patients in the lowest tertile have an event rate of 1.9%, the middle tertile 3.1%, and the highest tertile 4.9%.

Beyond high blood pressure and LVH, the subjects, on average, are elderly, are overweight, and have high prevalences of diabetes, lipid disorders, and previously known coronary heart disease. More than 27% have isolated systolic hypertension, a condition associated with particularly high cardiovascular risk.[21] Despite a surprisingly low total cholesterol:HDL cholesterol ratio of 4.3, total cardiovascular risk in the LIFE study is nearly as high as the risk in the recent successful Swedish Trial in Old Patients with Hypertension (STOP-Hypertension).[22] The lipid profiles of the LIFE participants and the low prevalence of statin use may have been due to selection bias, i.e., those with particular high cardiovascular risk and/or established cardiovascular disease were not eligible for enrollment.

The characteristics of the LIFE study population and the frequency of early endpoints suggest that the time-course of the study will not deviate much from projections,[12] i.e., a follow-up time of 4 years from enrollment of the last patient, at which time 1040 patients with primary endpoints will have been accumulated. However, the study included 894 more patients than initially planned. The study will thus have more than the planned 80% power after 4 years of follow-up on April 30, 2001, provided the discontinuation rate is kept at an acceptable level.

A surprising finding is that almost a third of the patients were untreated for their high blood pressure for at least 6 months when recruited into the LIFE study despite the recommendations in several recently published guidelines for detection, treatment, and follow-up of hypertension.[21–25] The low treatment rate is consistent with the findings of the Hypertension Optimal Treatment (HOT) Study,[26] in which 48% of participants were untreated at enrollment. Not so surprising are the gender differences in choice of antihypertensive drugs: More women were taking diuretics and fewer were taking calcium channel blockers and ACE inhibitors than was the case in men. Because of the high cardiovascular disease comorbidity, it is not surprising that 20% were taking aspirin, a treatment recently supported by the HOT study.[27] The blood pressure target in the LIFE study is less than 140/90 mm Hg, which seems appropriate in light of the high risk of the participants and the final results of the HOT study.[27]

Smoking and hypertension may be a deadly combination.[28] Cross-sectionally, there is less smoking with higher blood pressure.[29] The low prevalence of smoking in the LIFE study may be explained by selection/exclusion bias of smokers with concomitant diseases, such as myocardial infarction within 6 months, or need for open-label treatment with β-blockers, ACE inhibitors, or angiotensin-receptor antagonists. Another important reason for selection bias for smoking prevalence is that sicker patients are more likely to have stopped smoking owing to medical advice.

In conclusion, by applying simple 12-lead ECG criteria for LVH (Cornell voltage QRS duration product formula and/or Sokolow-Lyon voltage), it has been feasible to identify a large number of hypertensive patients with LVH. By using additional inclusion and exclusion criteria, it has been possible to select from the population and randomize into the LIFE study a total of 9194 high-risk patients with an average 5-year likelihood of coronary heart disease events of 22.3% by the Framingham Risk Score. This population will receive blood pressure–lowering treatment (aim < 140/90 mm Hg) according to the protocol for at least 4 years and until 1040 patients have experienced a primary endpoint.

References

1. Timmermans PB, Wong PC, Chiu AT, et al. Angiotensin II receptors and angiotensin II receptor antagonists. Pharmacol Rev 46:205–225, 1993.
2. Goldberg AL, Dunlay MC, Sweet CS. Safety and tolerability of losartan potassium, an angiotensin II receptor antagonist, compared with hydrochlorothiazide, atenolol, felodipine ER, and angiotensin-converting enzyme inhibitors for the treatment of systemic hypertension. Am J Cardiol 75:793–795, 1995.
3. Weber MA, Byyny RL, Pratt JH, et al. Blood pressure effects of the angiotensin II receptor blocker losartan. Arch Intern Med 155:405–411, 1995.
4. Levy D, Garrison RJ, Savage DD, et al. Prognostic implications of echocardiographically determined left ventricular mass in the Framingham Heart Study. N Engl J Med 322:1561–1566, 1990.
5. Koren MJ, Devereux RB, Casale PN, et al. Relation of left ventricular mass and geometry to morbidity and mortality in uncomplicated essential hypertension. Ann Intern Med 114:345–352, 1991.
6. Liao Y, Cooper RS, McGee DL, et al. The relative effects of left ventricular hypertrophy, coronary artery disease, and ventricular dysfunction on survival among black adults. JAMA 273:1592–1597, 1995.
7. Camargo MJF, von Lutterotti N, Pecker MS, et al. DuP 753 increases survival in spontaneously hypertensive stroke-prone rats fed a high sodium diet. Am J Hypertens 4(suppl):341S–345S, 1991.
8. von Lutterotti N, Camargo MJF, Mueller FB, et al. Angiotensin II receptor antagonist markedly reduces mortality in salt-loaded Dahl S rats. Am J Hypertens 4(suppl):346S–349S, 1991.
9. Schieffer B, Wirger A, Meybrunn M, et al. Comparative effects of chronic angiotensin-converting enzyme inhibition and angiotensin II type 1 receptor blockade on cardiac remodeling after myocardial infarction in the rat. Circulation 89:2273–2282, 1994.
10. de Simone G, Devereux RB, Camargo MJF, et al. Reduction of development of left ventricular hypertrophy in salt loaded Dahl salt-sensitive rats by angiotensin II receptor inhibition. Am J Hypertens 9:216–222, 1996.
11. Pitt B, Segal R, Martinez FA, et al. Randomized trial of losartan versus captopril in patients over 65 with heart failure (Evaluation of Losartan in the Elderly Study, ELITE). Lancet 349:747–752, 1997.
12. Dahlöf B, Devereux R, de Faire U, et al. The Losartan Intervention For Endpoint Reduction (LIFE) in Hypertension Study. Rationale, design, and methods. Am J Hypertens 10:705–713, 1997.
13. Dahlöf B, Devereux RB, Julius S, et al, for the LIFE Study Group. Characteristics of 9194 patients with left ventricular hypertrophy. The LIFE Study. Hypertension 32:989–997, 1998.
14. Molloy TJ, Okin PM, Devereux RB, Kligfield P. Electrocardiographic detection of left ventricular hypertrophy by the simple QRS voltage-duration product. J Am Coll Cardiol 20:1180–1186, 1992.
15. Okin PM, Roman MJ, Devereux RB, Kligfield P. Gender differences and the electrocardiogram in left ventricular hypertrophy. Hypertension 25:242–249, 1995.
16. Okin PM, Roman MJ, Devereux RB, Kligfield P. Electrocardiographic identification of increased left ventricular mass by simple voltage duration products. J Am Coll Cardiol 25:417–423, 1995.
17. Norman JE Jr, Levy D. Improved electrocardiographic detection of echocardiographic left ventricular hypertrophy: Results of a correlated data base approach. J Am Coll Cardiol 26:1022–1029, 1995.
18. Sokolow M, Lyon TO. The ventricular complex in left ventricular hypertrophy as obtained by unipolar precordial and link leads. Am Heart J 37:161–186, 1949.
19. Casale PN, Devereux RB, Alonso DR, et al. Improved sex-specific criteria of left ventricular hypertrophy for clinical and computer electrocardiogram interpretation. Circulation 75:565–572, 1987.
20. Anderson KM, Wilson PWF, Odell PM, Kannel WB. An updated coronary risk profile: A statement for health professionals. Circulation 83:356–362, 1991.
21. SHEP Cooperative Research Group. Prevention of stroke by antihypertensive drug treatment in older persons with isolated systolic hypertension. Final results of the Systolic Hypertension in the Elderly Program (SHEP). JAMA 265:3255–3264, 1991.

22. Dahlöf B, Lindholm LH, Hansson L, et al. Morbidity and mortality in the Swedish Trial in Old Patients with Hypertension (STOP-Hypertension). Lancet 338;1281–1285, 1991.
23. Sever P, Beevers G, Bulpitt C, et al. Management guidelines in essential hypertension: Report of the Second Working Party of the British Hypertension Society. BMJ 306:983–987, 1993.
24. Joint National Committee on Prevention, Detection, Evaluation, and Treatment of High Blood Pressure. The sixth report. Arch Intern Med 157:2413–2446, 1997.
25. Guidelines Sub-Committee of the WHO/ISH Mild Hypertension Liaison Committee: 1993 Guidelines for the management of mild hypertension: memorandum from a World Health Organization/International Society of Hypertension meeting. J Hypertens 11:905–918, 1993.
26. Hansson L, Zanchetti A, for the HOT Study Group. The Hypertension Optimal Treatment (HOT) Study—Patient characteristics: Randomization; risk profiles, and early blood pressure results. Blood Press 3:322–327, 1994.
27. Hansson L, Zanchetti A, Carruthers SG, et al, for the HOT Study Group. Effects of intensive blood-pressure lowering and low-dose aspirin in patients with hypertension: Principal results of the Hypertension Optimal Treatment (HOT) randomised trial. Lancet 351:1755–1762, 1998.
28. Omvik P. How smoking affects blood pressure. Blood Press 5:71–77, 1996.
29. Mundal R, Kjeldsen SE, Sandvik L, et al. Predictors of 7-year changes in exercise blood pressure: Effect of smoking, physical fitness and pulmonary function. J Hypertens 15:245–249, 1997.

CHAPTER 38

Changing Approaches to Diagnosis and Treatment of Hypertension

Norman M. Kaplan and C. Venkata S. Ram

The need for changing approaches to the diagnosis and treatment of hypertension is patently obvious when the most recent survey reveals that only 27% of U.S. hypertensives have adequate control of their condition, as indicated by blood pressures below 140/90 mm Hg.[1] As well reflected in the sixth report of the Joint National Committee on Prevention, Detection, Evaluation, and Treatment of High Blood Pressure (JNC VI),[1] multiple changes are being recommended in our attempt to treat hypertension in practice. Unfortunately, practitioners are often slow and hesitant in accepting these "expert" recommendations,[2] particularly if these entail more work on their part and less profit to managed care organizations and pharmaceutical companies. Nonetheless, changes in both diagnosis and treatment are needed and can be accomplished.

CHANGES IN DIAGNOSIS

Two are needed: more care in establishing the usual range of blood pressure by obtaining multiple out-of-the-office readings; and assessment of overall cardiovascular risk status to help determine the most appropriate therapy.

Multiple Out-of-the-Office Readings

Two characteristics inherent in the nature of hypertension—variability and reactivity—mandate multiple out-of-the-office readings. Too often, the diagnosis is made after only one or two office or clinic readings, resulting in the incorrect labeling of patients, with consequent financial and psychological costs and dangers from unneeded medications. JNC VI strongly supports the use of home blood pressure measurements with readily available, inexpensive, reliable, and easily used semiautomatic devices. If taken repeatedly during various life activities, these measure-

ments are similar to ambulatory monitoring while awake.[3] Since they overcome the alerting reaction that is responsible for the white-coat effect, they should avoid the mislabeling of 20 to 30% of patients with isolated office or white-coat hypertension. Conversely, the usually lower out-of-the-office readings mandate lower criteria for the diagnosis of hypertension, likely 130/85 mm Hg.[4]

Assessment of Cardiovascular Risk

Once the diagnosis is established, the multiple components of each patient's overall cardiovascular risk need to be ascertained (Table 38–1). These should be used along with the level of blood pressure to determine the urgency and appropriate course of therapy (Table 38–2). Some practitioners may believe that these JNC VI recommendations are too conservative; withholding drug therapy for 6 to 12 months in patients with blood pressure as high as 160/100

Table 38–1 Components of Cardiovascular Risk Stratification in Patients With Hypertension

Major Risk Factors	Target Organ Damage/Clinical Cardiovascular Disease
Smoking	Heart diseases
Dyslipidemia	Left ventricular hypertrophy
Diabetes mellitus	Angina/prior myocardial
Age older than 60 years	infarction
Gender (men and postmenopausal	Prior coronary revascularization
women)	Heart failure
Family history of cardiovascular	Stroke or transient ischemic
disease: women under age 65	attack
years or men under age 55	Nephropathy
years	Peripheral arterial disease
	Retinopathy

Table 38–2 Risk Stratification and Treatment*

Blood Pressure Stages (mm Hg)	Risk Group A (No Risk Factors; No TOD/CCD)	Risk Group B (At Least One Risk Factor, Not Including Diabetes; No TOD/CCD)	Risk Group C (TOD/CCD and/or Diabetes, With or Without Other Risk Factors)
High-normal (130–139/85–89)	Lifestyle modification	Lifestyle modification	Drug therapy†
Stage 1 (140–159/90–99)	Lifestyle modification (up to 12 mo)	Lifestyle modification‡ (up to 6 mo)	Drug therapy
Stages 2 and 3 (≥160/≥100)	Drug therapy	Drug therapy	Drug therapy

Abbreviation: TOD/CCD, target organ disease/clinical cardiovascular disease.
*Note: For example, a patient with diabetes and a blood pressure of 142/94 mm Hg plus left ventricular hypertrophy should be classified as having stage 1 hypertension with target organ disease (left ventricular hypertropy) and with another major risk factor (diabetes). This patient would be categorized as "Stage 1, Risk Group C," and recommended for immediate initiation of pharmacological treatment. Lifestyle modification should be adjunctive therapy for all patients recommended for pharmacological therapy.
†For those with heart failure, renal insufficiency, or diabetes.
‡For patients with multiple risk factors, clinicians should consider drugs as initial therapy plus lifestyle modifications.

mm Hg could be risky. Others may believe they are too liberal, indicating the need for drug therapy for some patients with blood pressure below 140/90 mm Hg. The evidence on which these recommendations are based supports such selectivity: On one hand, at least over the 3 to 6 years of most randomized controlled trials, little or no protection has been provided to low-risk patients with blood pressure below 150/100 mm Hg by drug therapy.[5] On the other hand, protection has been clearly documented in patients with blood pressure well below 140/90 mm Hg by using β-blockers after an acute myocardial infarction and for angiotensin-converting enzyme inhibitors (ACEIs) in diabetic nephropathy and congestive heart failure.[6]

CHANGES IN TREATMENT

Once therapy is indicated, based on adequate assessment of the usual range of blood pressure and the patient's overall risk status, lifestyle modifications alone or in combination with drug therapy should be instituted (Table 38–3). The value of these lifestyle modifications in lowering blood pressure in most patients who adopt them is widely recognized. However, many patients will not modify their lifestyle enough to achieve much of a lowering of blood pressure. Fortunately, when relatively small lifestyle changes are made in combination, significant falls in blood pressure can be seen. In the Treatment of Mild Hypertension Study (TOMHS),[7] an average fall of 8.6/8.6 mm Hg occurred over a 4-year follow-up, although the patients reduced daily sodium intakes by only 30 mmol, decreased body weight by only 7.8 pounds, increased physical activity by 30%, and reduced alcohol consumption by only 1 drink per week.

Reductions in blood pressure by lifestyle changes have not been shown to reduce morbidity or mortality, and in view of the difficulty in monitoring small changes in many thousands of subjects over many years, they likely will never be proved to do so. Nonetheless, lifestyle changes also reduce other cardiovascular risks while they lower blood pressure. If patients are highly motivated, reinforced by the persistent oversight of health care providers, and encouraged to use various services available in the community, such as Weight Watchers and SmokEnders, many may achieve meaningful reductions in blood pressure and overall cardiovascular risk.

Table 38–3 Lifestyle Modifications for Hypertension Prevention and Management

Lose weight if overweight
Limit alcohol intake to no more than 1 oz (30 ml) of ethanol (e.g., 24 oz [720 ml] of beer, 10 oz [300 ml] of wine, or 2 oz [60 ml] of 100-proof whiskey) per day for men and heavier people or 0.5 oz (15 ml) of ethanol per day for women and lighter people
Increase aerobic physical activity (30–45 min most days of the week)
Reduce sodium intake to no more than 100 mmol/day (2.4 g of sodium or 6 g of sodium chloride)
Maintain adequate intake of dietary potassium (approximately 90 mmol/day)
Maintain adequate intake of dietary calcium and magnesium for general health
Stop smoking and reduce intake of dietary saturated fat and cholesterol for overall cardiovascular health

Table 38–4 Considerations for Individualizing Antihypertensive Drug Therapy

Angina	β-Blockers, CAs
Atrial tachycardia and fibrillation	β-Blockers, CAs (non-DHP)
Cyclosporine-induced hypertension	CAs
Diabetes mellitus (types 1 and 2) with proteinuria	ACEIs (preferred), CAs
Diabetes mellitus (type 2)	Low-dose diuretics
Dyslipidemia	α-Blockers
Essential tremor	β-Blockers (non-CS)
Heart failure	Carvedilol, losartan
Hyperthyroidism	β-Blockers
Migraine	β-Blockers (non-CS), CAs (non-DHP)
Myocardial infarction	Diltiazem, verapamil
Osteoporosis	Thiazides
Preoperative hypertension	β-Blockers
Prostatism (BPH)	α-Blockers
Renal insufficiency (caution in renovascular hypertension and creatinine level ≥ 3 mg/dl)	ACEIs

Abbreviations: BPH, benign prostatic hyperplasia; CAs, calcium antagonists; non-DHP, nondihydropyridine; ACEIs, angiotensin-converting enzyme inhibitors; CS, cardioselective.

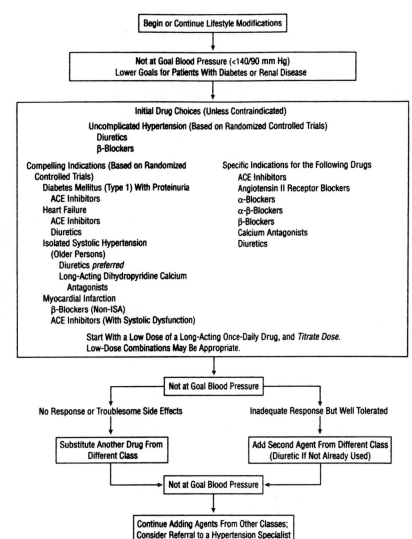

Figure 38–1. Algorithm for pathways for the initial choice of drug therapy if blood pressure remains above the goal of treatment despite attempts to modify lifestyle. ACE, angiotensin-converting enzyme; ISA, intrinsic sympathomimetic activity. (Adapted from Joint National Committee on Prevention, Detection, Evaluation, and Treatment of High Blood Pressure. The sixth report. Arch Intern Med 157:2413–2446, 1997. Copyright 1997, American Medical Association.)

Initial Choice of Drug Therapy

Unlike the single recommendations in prior reports, the JNC VI algorithm provides three pathways for the initial choice of drug therapy if the blood pressure remains above the goal of treatment despite attempts to modify lifestyles (Fig. 38–1). For those patients below age 65 years with uncomplicated hypertension, a diuretic or β-blocker is recommended, based on the evidence from all of the randomized controlled trials (RCTs) that utilized these drugs.[8]

For those patients with coexisting conditions in which specific drugs have been shown to reduce morbidity and mortality, the choice of these drugs is "compelling," that is, they should always be used unless strong contraindications are present. The compelling indications shown in Figure 38–1 are widely recognized, with the possible exception of long-acting dihydropyridine (DHP) calcium antagonists (CAs) for elderly patients with isolated systolic hypertension (ISH). Although diuretics are preferred for such patients based on five RCTs in the elderly, two of which involved patients with ISH,[9] the Systolic Hypertension—Europe (SYST-EUR) trial documented an

equal if not greater protection from strokes with therapy based on the long-acting DPH-CA nitrendipine compared with a placebo.[10] Since nitrendipine is not marketed in the United States, JNC VI advocates the use of the other long-acting DHP-CAs that are available, particularly in view of reductions in cardiovascular mortality shown with them in other trials.[11, 12]

The third path recommends the choice of various drugs that have been found to provide favorable effects on a variety of coexisting conditions but without the strength of data from RCTs to document that they will reduce mortality (Table 38–4). As examples, a β-blocker or CA is recommended for hypertensives with angina, an α-blocker for one with coexisting prostatism, and a diuretic in the presence of osteoporosis. In view of the compelling indication for a diuretic in an elderly hypertensive with ISH, a low-dose of a diuretic might logically be combined with a low-dose of an α-blocker if prostatism is present.

OTHER GUIDELINES

With whatever drug is chosen, two principles should be followed: Start with a low dose to avoid symptoms from too rapid and too great a fall in blood pressure; and use a long-acting formulation to give 24-hour coverage with a single daily dose. The second step will improve compliance while providing smoother control of the blood pressure and better protection from the cardiovascular consequences of the morning surge in blood pressure after arising from sleep. Despite the temptation to use less expensive, generic, short-acting formulations, the multiple benefits of once-daily therapy should always be kept in mind, even if the preparations are more expensive. Moreover, the better control of hypertension provided by once-daily formulations has been shown to translate into overall lower costs than the use of less expensive, multiple-dose formulations.[13]

Another general principle that should often be followed is the use of low-dose combinations, providing greater efficacy with fewer side effects than larger doses of single drugs. This principle applies particularly to combinations with only 6.25 mg of hydrochlorothiazide.[14] Even such low doses of diuretic clearly enhance the efficacy of other antihypertensive drugs. Therefore, JNC VI recommends that if another class of drug was chosen for initial therapy and if only a partial response has been achieved, the second drug should usually be a diuretic. The putative dangers of diuretics that caused many practitioners to avoid them are rarely seen at the currently recommended lower doses.[15] Without a definite contraindication, a low dose of a thiazide diuretic should be either the first or the second drug for most patients. Even in hypertensive patients with diabetes mellitus, who have been thought to be adversely affected by diuretics, diuretic use has been shown to protect against coronary disease to an even greater degree than in nondiabetic hypertensives.[16]

The remainder of the JNC VI treatment algorithm is little changed from prior reports. In order to give the patient the full benefit of antihypertensive treatment, blood pressure should be lowered to levels below 140/90 mm Hg in most patients and to levels below 130/85 in those at high risk because of concomitant nephropathy, heart failure, or coronary disease.

Hypertensive Urgencies

A last change in therapy is related to the use of short-acting CAs, in particular the liquid preparation of nifedipine, either sublingual or swallowed. In view of the rare but potential danger of tissue hypoperfusion after the abrupt and marked fall in blood pressure that may follow the use of liquid nifedipine,[17] this practice should be curtailed. Those few patients truly in need of an immediate reduction in blood pressure should be given a parenteral agent with constant monitoring. The larger number of patients with markedly elevated blood pressure but no impending target organ damage may be more safely given one or more oral agents in order to begin to reduce blood pressure within 30 to 60 minutes and to achieve a goal of less than 180/120 mm Hg in 2 to 4 hours. Multiple short-acting agents are available including a diuretic, furosemide; a β-blocker, propranolol; an ACEI, captopril; a CA, felodipine. Once the pressure is brought down to a safer level while the patient is under observation, long-acting once-daily formulations of the drugs chosen initially should be started for

long-term management. The patient should be closely followed and seen again within a few days to ensure that the therapy is working.

The potential hazards of short-acting CAs are not believed to apply to the appropriate use of long-acting preparations, which have been repeatedly blamed for multiple problems based on retrospective, uncontrolled observations.[18] The protection against coronary disease shown for long-acting CAs in the SYST-EUR prospective RCT was accompanied by a slight decrease in cancer and no increase in gastrointestinal bleeding.[10]

CONCLUSION

The changes in diagnosis and therapy recommended in JNC VI are not revolutionary or markedly different from practices that have been previously recommended. Nevertheless, these changes are important because current practices have not given the protection to millions of patients that can be provided by appropriate antihypertensive therapy.

References

1. Joint National Committee on Prevention, Detection, Evaluation, and Treatment of High Blood Pressure. The sixth report. Arch Intern Med 157:2413–2446, 1997.
2. Siegel D, Lopez J. Trends in antihypertensive drug use in the United States. JAMA 278:1745–1748, 1997.
3. Mancia G, Sega R, Milesi C, et al. Blood-pressure control in the hypertensive population. Lancet 349:454–457, 1997.
4. Pickering T, Kaplan NM, Krakoff L, et al. Recommendations for the use of home (self) and ambulatory blood pressure monitoring. Am J Hypertens 9:1–11, 1995.
5. Hoes AW, Grobbee DE, Lubsen J. Does drug treatment improve survival? Reconciling the trials in mild-to-moderate hypertension. J Hypertens 13:805–811, 1995.
6. Kaplan NM. Treatment of hypertension. *In* Clinical Hypertension, 7th ed. Baltimore, Williams & Wilkins, 1998.
7. Neaton JD, Grimm RH Jr, Prineas RJ, et al, for the Treatment of Mild Hypertension Study Research Group. Final results. JAMA 270:713–724, 1993.
8. Psaty BM, Smith NL, Siscovick DS, et al. Health outcomes associated with antihypertensive therapies used as first-line agents: A systematic review and meta-analysis. JAMA 277:739–745, 1997.
9. Collins R, MacMahon S. Blood pressure, antihypertensive drug treatment and the risks of stroke and of coronary heart disease. Br Med Bull 50:272–298, 1994.
10. Staessen JA, Fagard R, Thijs L, et al., for the Systolic Hypertension—Europe (SYST-EUR) Trial Investigators. Randomised double-blind comparison of placebo and active treatment for older patients with isolated systolic hypertension. Lancet 350:757–764, 1997.
11. Gong L, Zhang W, Zhu Y, et al. Shanghai Trial of Nifedipine in the Elderly (STONE). J Hypertens 14:1237–1245, 1996.
12. Packer M, O'Connor CM, Ghali JK, et al. Effect of amlodipine on morbidity and mortality in severe chronic heart failure. N Engl J Med 335:1107–1114, 1996.
13. Sclar DA, Tessler GC, Skaer TL, et al. Effect of pharmaceutical formulation of diltiazem on the utilization of Medicaid and health maintenance organization services. Curr Ther Res 55:1136–1149, 1994.
14. Frishman WH, Bryzinski BS, Coulson LR, et al. A multifactorial trial design to assess combination therapy in hypertension. Arch Intern Med 154:1461–1468, 1994.
15. Carlsen JE, Køber L, Torp-Pedersen C, Johansen P. Relation between dose of bendrofluazide, antihypertensive effect, and adverse biochemical effects. BMJ 300:974–978, 1990.

16. Curb JD, Pressel SL, Cutler JA, et al. Effect of diuretic-based antihypertensive treatment on cardiovascular disease risk in older diabetic patients with isolated systolic hypertension. JAMA 276:1886–1892, 1996.

17. Grossman E, Messerli FH, Grodzicki T, Kowey P. Should a moratorium be placed on sublingual nifedipine capsules given for hypertensive emergencies and pseudoemergencies? JAMA 276:1328–1331, 1996.

18. Ad Hoc Subcommittee of the Liaison Committee of the World Health Organization and the International Society of Hypertension. Effects of calcium antagonists on the risks of coronary heart disease, cancer and bleeding. J Hypertens 15:105–115, 1997.

39 Critical Assessment of Hypertension Guidelines

John D. Swales

CHAPTER

There have probably been more guidelines developed for treating hypertension than for any other clinical condition. There are probably three reasons for this. First, hypertension is a condition of very high prevalence in the developed world and of increasing prevalence in the developing world. It imposes a high economic and social burden on society, and for the same reason, the economic cost of prevention and treatment is high. The second reason conducive to guidelines is the fact that the evidence base for decision-making is very strong. The risks have been quantified by a large body of actuarial and epidemiological data, and the efficacy of treatment has been demonstrated by a substantial number of high-quality endpoint trials. Lastly, the diagnosis is comparatively straightforward; management is largely carried out by nonspecialists in primary care who welcome guidance and who are very susceptible to advice based on numerical analysis.

WHY GUIDELINES?

Guidelines for the treatment of most common conditions are now widely disseminated. Often, they have been produced by specialist professional societies. In other cases, governmental bodies commission them from professional experts; examples include the work of small local groups of professionals or health care purchasers produced for their own use. In the United Kingdom, it has been estimated that over 2000 sets of guidelines or protocols have been developed in recent years to inform professional audit.[1] The guidance that emerges is variable in quality and frequently conflicting in important respects. Nevertheless, the ubiquity of the phenomenon of guideline construction across the world suggests that there is a fundamental need that has to be met, however flawed some of the attempts to meet that need may be. The nature of this need is not too difficult to identify. Powerful evaluative tools in the form of clinical trials have identified efficacious treatments for many common diseases. By contrast, ample data show that this evidence is not consistently being translated into practice: Treatment of common diseases is suboptimal in all systems for health care delivery that have been examined. This conclusion applies particularly to treatment afforded by generalists, but even specialist clinics often fall short of the ideal.

Another potent influence has increased concerns about the quality of health care: The success of medical science has caused a massive increase in demand. Suboptimal or ineffective treatment is clearly unacceptable, since it is incompatible with the fundamental purpose of health care. All this is undeniable, but by no means the whole story. Identifying satisfactory standards cannot easily be separated from resources and rationing. Net benefit from a treatment is rarely an either/or phenomenon: Much more commonly, there is a gradient of benefit. At one end, there may be high clinical returns from a treatment, whereas at the other end of the spectrum, modest benefit for a few may be obtained only at inordinate cost in time, effort, and money. A decision has to be made about what is worthwhile.[2] This obviously has to recognize how much can be afforded, since no health care system has unlimited resources. Since expenditure on one treatment prevents the use of that money for another patient, the use of guidelines that define appropriate care implies that the doctor sacrifices possible benefit for the individual he or she is treating for the good of others whose treatment is being funded from the same source. This substitution of distributive ethics for the traditional individual ethic is, for many doctors, a violation of the Hippocratic oath.[3] Doctors' education and training teaches them to give an absolute priority to the patient who confronts them in their clinic and in their office. The suggestion that, in some circumstances, the interests of that individual should be of secondary importance to wider interests is highly distasteful.

There is an additional perceived conflict between guidelines that seek to define the most appropriate clinical action in particular circumstances and the professional ethos.[4, 5] The individual and social values that inform clinical practice are not reducible to an algorithmic protocol. Attempts to define practice in all-embracing guidance ignore other essential components of the interaction between a doctor and her or his patient. These components are judgmental in nature. Two different judgments are involved. First, most clinical situations are characterized by a degree of scientific uncertainty, i.e., available evidence is insufficient, and as a consequence, there is a legitimate disagreement among experts. A rigid protocol is inappropriate in such circumstances and likely to provoke justifiable professional rejection.

Even where relevant evidence is abundant, however,

there is still a subjective element in decision-making determined by professional and patient values that cannot be subsumed in a prescriptive protocol for treatment.[5] An identical risk profile in two patients may require management in quite different ways, and each management regimen may be perfectly defensible. For instance, even when a doctor subscribes to national guidelines, he or she may well defer drug treatment in a patient who meets the stated criteria in the light of the patient's particular circumstances, previous treatment experience, and preferences. The competent professional knows when to accede, and when not to accede, to a patient's wishes. This assessment reflects professional education and experience; at times, it has an intuitive element to it.[5] Kassirer summarized current concerns when he referred to the "growth industry" of clinical guidelines, writing: "From a system dominated by intelligent and thoughtful decision-making, we seem to be embarking on a path to codify medicine."[4]

These anxieties are amplified when guidelines are used for purposes other than guiding clinicians. Governments, service commissioners, health care insurers, and malpractice lawyers have all developed an active interest in guidelines.[6] This may have particularly worrying consequences for both content and implementation. It has been argued that some hypertension guidelines have been influenced by unstated economic constraints.[7] This becomes a matter of even greater significance when guidelines are enforced through contracts and financial penalties in managed care systems. The possible legal consequences of justifiable nonadherence to guidelines may also be serious.[8] Some authorities have suggested that guidelines provide a suitable basis for resolving malpractice litigation.[9]

There is no ready answer to these genuine concerns, which in many ways are the result of the social and economic pressures under which doctors act. The pressing requirement is for openness. On what basis are recommendations being made? How far is there a division of opinion among experts? Are guidelines simply defining the minimal levels of acceptable care in order to ensure appropriate quality? Are the expert committees that compile the guidelines clear as to how they are to be used, and are these constructed and presented in an appropriate way for that purpose? If cost is a factor in treatment recommendations (as it almost inevitably will be, even if not acknowledged), this should be made clear so that it can be debated. This is of crucial importance, not least for those who receive care and who are, ultimately, either directly or indirectly responsible for funding it. Where there is a legitimate difference of opinion or sheer uncertainty, it is misleading to present firm conclusions as though they were definitive. Where there is agreement on what is acceptable practice and what is not, guidelines offer an appropriate benchmark, and it would be churlish to reject them. The sensitive and complex nature of these issues has had the unfortunate consequence that most guidelines fall well short of the ideal.

THE PROCESS OF GUIDELINE DEVELOPMENT

Certain aspects of medical treatment are now beyond reasonable dispute, and it is likely that any group of motivated and knowledgeable experts will reach similar conclusions about the advice that can be offered. Unfortunately, much medical practice does not easily fit into this category. It is a "gray area" in which extrapolation from epidemiological associations, cohort studies, and even pathophysiological processes is required to draw a conclusion. Where persuasive conclusions based on such evidence end and where legitimate disagreements begin is debatable. Divergent advice for cholesterol screening in the United States by two learned bodies has been attributed to a fundamental difference of approach.[10] Evidence-based guidelines were based on a critical comprehensive review, whereas consensus-based guidelines relied on a panel of experts' views on "clinical and biological plausibilities." The former gave more selective advice about appropriate target populations than the latter. The distinction is to some extent an arbitrary one and misses the point. The concept of "evidence-based guidelines," if it is taken to imply exclusion of subjective "expert" judgment, does not bear scrutiny. Evidence of efficacy cannot be automatically translated into firm guidance: A judgment about social cost and value has to be made (of which economic cost is only one component). This requires informed input from a number of sources, including consumers of health care. But there will also almost invariably be a need for expert interpretation in extrapolating clinical trial evidence to the "real world" in which care will be given to patients who are likely to differ in important respects (e.g., compliance, the presence of comorbidity, race, gender, and age) from those recruited to the trial.

An exercise of debate and judgment is an essential part of any process that leads to the development of guidelines, whether the final process is consensus-based or not. Such debate clearly has to be evidence-based: A systematic objective literature review (perhaps accompanied by meta-analysis) is the preferred option for informing that debate, although this is often conspicuously lacking in national guidelines. However, even the technique of meta-analysis involves an exercise of scientific judgment in the selection of trials and the analysis of data. Striking inconsistencies in the outcomes of meta-analyses in the same field testify to the subjectivity of such judgments.[11] The Canadian Hypertension Society Guidelines explicitly recognize the varying quality and relevance of the evidence on which advice has to be given,[12] using a numerical grading system that ranges from large randomized controlled trials (RCTs) (level 1) at one end to small case series at the other (level 5). The latest U.S. guidelines annotate cited references according to the level of evidence they provide.[13] The strength of the recommendations in the Canadian guidelines are graded according to the level of evidence on which they are based. The apparently mechanistic nature of this process tends to disguise the fact that there is often a divergence between conviction that an intervention is of value and the level of evidence supporting it. The recommendation to stop smoking is an example of this, treatment of malignant hypertension is another. Occasionally, the dictates of commonsense are such that it would be unethical to carry out a controlled trial. The concept that there is a hierarchy of evidence that can determine the strength of recommendations for evidence-based guidelines is not persuasive.

The dilemma presented by combining an evidence-based approach with consensus expert judgment in constructing guidelines is evident when different recommendations are compared. The sixth report of the Joint National Committee on Prevention, Detection, Evaluation, and Treatment of High Blood Pressure (JNC VI), e.g., recommends diuretic or β-blocker first-line therapy "because numerous RCTs have shown a reduction in morbidity and mortality."[13] This follows recommendations on lifestyle modifications for which there is no such evidence, only evidence for efficacy in reducing a surrogate risk factor, hypertension. The same arguments could presumably be applied to justify the use of all licensed antihypertensive drugs. The position taken by JNC VI is an eminently reasonable one, but the slight inconsistency in argument emphasizes the inadmissibility of a mechanistic view of what the evidence does and does not show. Elsewhere, JNC VI states the problem admirably in a rather specific context. After listing the difficulties in basing advice simply on outcomes of RCTs, it states: "Because of these limitations, the executive committee extrapolated treatment effects beyond the duration of the clinical trials based on physiological and epidemiologic data."

Since all guidelines, whether admitting the fact or not, depend on a degree of consensus in areas in which there is legitimate debate, the process of reaching that consensus assumes central importance. In these debatable areas of hypertension (such as the choice of drug, the blood pressure threshold for treatment, or the importance attached to treatment in the elderly), final consensus can be reached in only one of three ways: by the use of general language that avoids the specifics in dispute; by compromise and group dynamics; or by selection of experts whose views concur. The alternative is to admit that there has been a fundamental difference of opinion. This option is rarely taken, although the 1993 British Hypertension Society Guidelines stated openly that the committee "was divided on the question of prescribing newer drugs instead of diuretics and β-blockers as first line treatment."[14]

The alternative of a "broad-brush" approach has been employed in many consensus publications and is not necessarily flawed if it conveys to the practitioner the advice that there is a broad framework of acceptable practice within which she or he has to make her or his own judgment. Occasionally, such language may rob guidelines of all value, however. In refusing to publish some National Institutes of Health consensus statements on management, the *New England Journal of Medicine* referred to "bland generalities and points so mild, so far from the cutting edge of progress and so well established that surely everyone must know them."[15] The use of compromise and group interpersonal dynamics may produce unforeseen results. The expert committee that produced the 1993 World Health Organization/International Society of Hypertension (WHO/ISH)[16] guidelines included members who had also signed off on national guidelines that differed from the WHO/ISH guidelines in important respects. Composition of the committee may also be all important. The most recent British Hypertension Society report that admitted to a division of opinion about first-line drug therapy had been preceded by 4 years by one that was unanimous in its opinion.[17]

There is another problem with guidelines, particularly when they are developed by specialist bodies working in isolation: This relates to equity. Where, either implicitly or explicitly, levels of risk are being targeted (as in the case of hypertension), these are selected without reference to levels of risk being targeted by guidelines for treating other conditions. JNC VI recommends rechecking blood pressure in normotensive individuals (blood pressure < 130/85 mm Hg) every 2 years.[13] The yield obtained by this policy in terms of complications prevented is not stated. Is it of the same order as the benefit from screening every 3 years of the over 45-year-olds for diabetes,[18] or adopting the recommended screening intervals for mammographic detection of breast cancer in healthy women. In all of these situations, there is a gradient of risk and benefit and a judgment about what is a reasonable level of risk at which to intervene. It is notable that other guidelines specifically reject population screening for blood pressure on the grounds of low yield.[19] Failure to ask questions about risk-benefit relationships can create worrying anomalies. The guidelines for treatment of hypertension by British physicians prepared by the British Hypertension Society[14] implicitly target a risk level for cardiovascular events of about 6% per annum. The recommendation given by the British Department of Health based on expert advice for the use of statin drugs to lower cholesterol in high-risk patients targets an annual risk of 3%.[20, 21] Such anomalies are an inevitable outcome of the way in which guidelines are currently produced and testimony to the hidden value judgments that have to be made in their production.

GUIDELINES AND THE COST OF RECOMMENDATIONS

The avoidance of this issue, except in the most general way, is a conspicuous feature of published guidelines. JNC VI, e.g., has a section headed "Economic Considerations."[13] This, however, refers only to the cost of specific classes of drugs, which we are told should be an "important consideration" in selection. If this is true of drug selection, it is also presumably true of the selection of a treatment threshold for drug therapy, which determines the size of the population recommended for treatment, or lifestyle modification, which may throw a considerable burden of cost on the individual. The 1996 WHO report recommends that cost-effectiveness analyses of hypertension control should seek "to assess the balance between benefits and burdens in terms of both health outcomes and of resources."[22] This compares with a considerably more equivocal statement in the joint WHO/ISH guidelines of 1993, where we read that "the choice of the initial therapy for an individual hypertensive patient is a challenge to the physician and should not be restricted on theoretical or economic grounds, to any one or two of the various classes of drug which have so far been tested, although it is the responsibility of the physician to give due consideration to the cost of drugs."[16]

Chalmers pointed out that economic considerations, masquerading as scientific judgments, play a role in some recommendations for management of hypertension.[7] I share this view, although unlike Chalmers, I think it is inevitable because, at some point, the magnitude of the social consequences of the recommendations has to be set against the magnitude of the benefit for the individual.[2, 23] No discussion of clinical care can ignore such considerations. There comes a point in, e.g., the diagnosis of secondary hypertension when it becomes absurd to advocate costly screening procedures to detect a very small number of patients who may benefit.

By failing to carry out a detailed analysis of the economic costs of treatment, guidelines miss the opportunity to describe the social costs of treatment failure, which enormously strengthens the case for vigorous programs of prevention and treatment with policy makers. Sometimes, the consequences of poorly treated ill-health fall on others—the patient's relatives and caregivers and social security systems. Apparent savings for health care providers through not treating may result in much greater expenditure by others. It is interesting to note that JNC VI, for the first time, alludes to the cost-effectiveness of treating hypertension in the context of managed care but does not relate this in any way to the recommendations made. Cost-effectiveness, like blood pressure, is not a dichotomous variable: It tends to increase in direct relation to the level of risk being targeted. In some low-risk, hypertensive patients cost-effectiveness is extremely low, and the case for treatment becomes correspondingly weaker.[2, 24]

IMPLEMENTATION

If guidelines are aimed at the practitioner, how effective are they in improving the level of practice? There is strong evidence that dissemination of nationally produced guidelines without further attempts at implementation is ineffective. Hill and coworkers surveyed a group of Maryland practitioners before and 1 year after the 1984 JNC III guidelines were issued.[25] Although 81% of practitioners were aware of the guidelines, only 17% admitted to any change in practice as a result. Even this may be an exaggeration. A clinician may provide an overoptimistic assessment of the impact of guidelines on clinical practice. Another group examined the impact of widely disseminated

guidelines for cesarean section on Canadian practitioners.[26] Although a third stated that their practice had been influenced, knowledge of the content of the guidelines was poor, and objective data on the incidence of cesarean section showed very little change. This is consistent with other evidence based on prescribing data. The recommendation of JNC V that diuretics and β-blockers should normally be first-line treatment for hypertension had no discernible impact on the prescription of calcium antagonists and angiotensin-converting enzyme inhibitors for hypertension, which continued to climb while prescriptions for the older agents declined.[27]

It is possible that such studies underestimate the impact of guidelines on practice, where guidelines remain the subject of continued discussion and education of practitioners. Entry into the culture of medicine can be a slow process. RCTs showed that low-dose diuretic regimens were equally effective in blood pressure control as high-dose preparations, and had a lower incidence of metabolic side effects. However, data (Fig. 39–1) showed a slowly progressive trend toward prescription of lower doses over the next 5 years, accompanied by only a slight decline in prescriptions of the higher doses, probably reflecting a reluctance to change dosage in patients on treatment.[28]

There is a growing body of research on methods for translating the findings of clinical research into routine practice. A systematic review of these methods confirms that passive dissemination without specific strategies to encourage implementation is likely to be ineffective.[29] More successful approaches include educational outreach visits and active participation in discussions and workshops, with reminders in the form of decision support systems and patient-mediated interventions.[29]

PRESENTATION

Appropriate presentation of guidelines is clearly essential to securing active participation and awareness of relevant evidence. The interpretation of this objective varies widely, as is shown by the length of the final published documents,

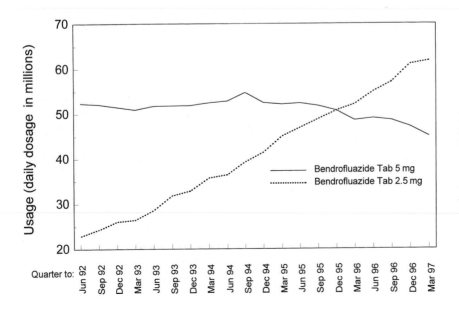

Figure 39–1. Trends in usage of bendrofluazide preparations in England and Wales (1992–1997). Data show a steady rise in lower-dose preparations after trial evidence demonstrated efficacy in blood pressure lowering of the agents. (From Prices and Prescription Authority. Annual Report 1998. London, Department of Health, 1998.)

Bendrofluazide Tab 5 mg
Bendrofluazide Tab 2.5 mg

which varies from 5 to 32 pages of published text.[13, 14] This reflects, to some extent, the degree to which expert groups have attempted to provide prescriptive advice for most eventualities with the level of detail one would expect of a textbook (and in some cases, well beyond that level). Indeed, all published guidelines to some extent reach conclusions in gray areas of hypertension treatment where there is still legitimate debate. None limits the task to defining a minimal level of acceptable care, although some stray farther from this ideal than others. The real danger of this, as I have argued previously, is when guidelines are used for different purposes from those originally intended. This may also impede adoption by the professional. When doctors feel moved to challenge the advice being presented to them, the likelihood of implementation recedes.

There are more specific problems with presentation of guidelines. JNC VI briefly refers to the importance of presentation if guidelines are to aid clinicians in their daily work. Focus groups recommended that guidelines must be succinct and user-friendly.[13] Clarity and user-friendliness are of crucial importance in the preparation of guidelines. It is difficult to reconcile this with the length and detail of the final product, in the case of JNC VI, or with the form in which these and other guidelines are presented. The extreme variation in length and detail suggest that, if considered at all, radically different conclusions have been reached about optimal presentation to meet the intended objective. Advice is often presented in a non–user-friendly form. Few guidelines present evidence of efficacy, e.g., as the numbers needed to treat to prevent one event, although this is more easily interpreted by the practicing physician than are more complex statistical data.[30] Expert committees producing guidelines seem to have taken the view that their task ends with defining the guidance. In some cases, this judgment may be unfair because summary documents explaining key points in an appropriately usable form may have been produced. Reference to such documents would have been desirable.

The process of guideline construction cannot be carried out in isolation. If adherence to good guidelines is fostered by the patient prompting the physician, parallel consistent information targeted at the patient is very helpful. More user-friendly documents for the physician are also helpful. Patient information booklets that make use of guidelines are often developed independently, but the guideline reports do not refer to such additional work. A clear statement of strategy to assist implementation would help to improve uptake of advice. As it is, frequent references to failure to implement best practice are not followed up by discussions on how the gap between evidence and care can be bridged or how guidelines are to be employed to improve the situation.

AGREEMENT IN GUIDELINES

It is not surprising, in view of the element of subjective judgment involved in their construction, that guidelines exhibit significant divergence in the advice they provide. The review of similarities and differences presented here is confined to national guidelines, written in English and freely accessible in the literature. Five of these are national,

Table 39–1 Areas of Agreement in Published Guidelines

Assessment of absolute risk, with early or urgent treatment of high-risk patients
Period of observation before treating lower-risk patients with medication
Nonpharmacological therapy (lifestyle modification) as first approach in lower-risk hypertensives
Importance of other cardiovascular risk factors in determining the blood pressure threshold for medication
Importance of systolic and diastolic criteria for treatment

presented either as guidelines or as consensus statements.[12–14, 19, 31] One is international, initially presented as joint WHO/ISH recommendations,[16] subsequently expanded and slightly modified as a WHO report.[22]

It is gratifying that there are several points of general agreement in all the guidelines (Table 39–1). All advise, e.g., that patients with the mildest hypertension and at lowest risk should be observed for a period of time while lifestyle modifications are employed before antihypertensive medication is used. Likewise, all recommend pharmacological treatment immediately after evaluation for the patients at highest risk. The period of observation recommended is inversely proportional to the estimated risk, so that there is an extended period of observation for those at lowest risk. The observation period recommended for lower-risk patients ranges up to 6 months in most guidelines and up to 12 months in the case of JNC VI.[13]

Where guidelines differ is in the relationship between the level of risk and the observation period. The two ends of the treatment profile are represented by the British and U.S. guidelines.[13, 14] Adopting the former would result in a period of observation for substantial numbers of hypertensive patients who would be treated immediately after the initial evaluation by adopting the latter. Thus, patients with uncomplicated hypertension and a diastolic blood pressure in the range of 100 to 109 mm Hg will be followed for 4 to 6 months according to the British guidelines,[14] whereas JNC VI recommends treatment after initial evaluation for patients with blood pressures equal to or above 160/100 mm Hg. The New Zealand guidelines closely resemble the British in this respect.[19] The WHO guidelines (together with the Australian Consensus Report[31]) in this, as other contexts, adopt an intermediate position, recommending treatment "without delay" of patients with a systolic blood pressure greater than 180 mm Hg and a diastolic blood pressure greater than 105 mm Hg.[21] It is notable that all guidelines (as distinct from their predecessors) now use both systolic and diastolic criteria for treatment.

All guidelines recommend that the level of risk should be assessed by the presence of other risk factors, such as target organ damage, smoking, dyslipidemia, and diabetes. The level of risk should then be a determinant of the nature and urgency of treatment. The most detailed profiling is used in the New Zealand guidelines, in which tabular cardiovascular risk data are presented separately for men and women, based on the Framingham Study.[19] The New Zealand recommendations are unique in another respect: They are the only ones to state explicitly an absolute level of cardiovascular risk for intervention with drug therapy.[19]

The recommendation is also qualified with the phrase "as a starting point for discussion with patients." Interestingly, risk profiling is used only for the "mild" range of blood pressures. Drug treatment is recommended for patients with blood pressure above 170/100 mm Hg irrespective of other cardiovascular risk factors:[19] This presumably represents a compromise in the face of strong professional perceptions about treatment of higher blood pressures, even though the absolute risk at this level in younger, uncomplicated hypertensives is well below the threshold adopted for other categories. JNC VI, although referring to databases for calculating absolute risk, develops a simplified system of risk factor profiling based on a matrix of three risk groups and four levels of blood pressure.[13] Other guidelines are much less detailed but recommend reducing the threshold in the presence of other cardiovascular risk factors. All guidelines recognize the importance of treating the elderly hypertensive, although only a minority spell out the consequences of age as a major cardiovascular risk factor in lowering the threshold for drug treatment.[14, 19]

DIFFERENCES IN GUIDELINES

Guidelines differ in content just as they do in style and presentation. There is a significant divergence in three major recommendations: the blood pressure threshold at which drug therapy should be initiated; the selection of first-line therapy in uncomplicated hypertension; and the target level of blood pressure at which treatment should be directed.

Recommended diastolic thresholds for pharmacological treatment range between 90 mm Hg[13] and 100 mm Hg[14] (Table 39–2); systolic thresholds vary between 140 mm Hg[13] and 160 mm Hg.[14] Taking into account the weighting attached to other risk factors in determining the final figure, and the different recommended periods of observation, strict adherence to the advice offered would result in substantially different populations receiving medication, with one exception. The Australian Consensus Statement on the Management of Hypertension[31] adheres closely to the WHO/ISH recommendations,[16] reproducing the WHO/ISH treatment algorithm.

Although the differences in terms of absolute blood pressure values are small, their consequences for unselected

populations are large, as values lie closer to the mode of the blood pressure distribution curve than to the tail. Fahey and Peters attempted to assess the magnitude of these differences by applying criteria for hypertension treatment to a population of 876 Oxfordshire hypertensive patients.[32] The proportions who met the criteria for controlled hypertension varied between 17.5% for JNC V criteria and 84.6% for the Canadian criteria. Figures for the New Zealand, British, and WHO/ISH criteria were 57.8%, 46.8%, and 28.9%, respectively. In many cases, therefore, although patients were under treatment, observed blood pressures still met the recommended criteria for requiring additional medication. Although there can be no questioning the impact of differing criteria, this study almost certainly exaggerates the differences, since blood pressures obtained from a primary care database cannot be equated with blood pressures at the end of recommended periods of observation. Nevertheless, the differences among recommendations have major impact on the proportion of patients who will be treated.

On what grounds do expert committees select systolic and diastolic criteria? All use some measure of absolute risk, which is clearly more relevant to the needs of the individual patient than is relative risk. The difficulty here is that a dichotomous classification (treat or do not treat with medication) is being introduced into a continuous spectrum of epidemiological risk. Does the existence of trial data provide the necessary evidence to do this? All guidelines cite trial evidence, but they also refer to the need to extrapolate. Although RCT evidence is available, it is clearly not sufficient to specify the precise blood pressure threshold for three reasons:

1. It would be arbitrary to select figures just because trial designers, on equally arbitrary grounds, selected those particular values. This is particularly relevant because other advice (e.g., for the use of lifestyle modification) is given when there are no supporting endpoint trials.

2. Blood pressures measured after prolonged observation periods cannot be equated with blood pressures at randomization into an RCT at the end of a shorter run-in period.

3. As Robertson pointed out, in the case of multiple risk factors and/or target organ damage, there are no trial data that help to specify a lower blood pressure threshold for treatment.[33] The systolic criterion for treatment in most guidelines (140 mm Hg) differs significantly from that used to recruit patients into the two relevant trials (see later). Epidemiological data are employed, and their use is implicit in much of the guidance given.

If trial evidence provides no justification for selection of a break point in the continuous distribution of risk and benefit, on what grounds is a threshold selected? One possibility is that treatment would have harmful effects that would more than counterbalance benefits in low-risk patients. Attempts to calculate such a point from trial data have, however, not been successful because numbers are small and confidence limits wide: None of the guidelines attempts this. Another relevant determinant might be the size of the population that would be exposed to drug treatment as a result of a particular recommendation. Such socioeconomic considerations are clearly important but are

Source	Diastolic Blood Pressure (mm Hg)	Systolic Blood Pressure (mm Hg)
Canadian[12]	100	160
United States[13]	90	140
British[14]	100	160
New Zealand[19]	2% annual risk or 100	2% annual risk or 170
World Health Organization[22]	95	160
Australian[31]	95	160

Table 39–2 Threshold Blood Pressures for Medication in Uncomplicated Hypertension Without Other Risk Factors

not mentioned in this context. Perhaps they can be deduced from the claim that particular guidelines are "cost-effective,"[13] if it is assumed that more liberal recommendations would not be cost-effective. However, the absence of discussion about the implications of the size of the population being recommended for treatment supports Chalmers' concerns about a hidden economic agenda.[7] In the absence of more direct evidence of the reasoning behind selection of thresholds, it seems likely that this represents an overall judgment by experts of what is worthwhile in the light of trial and epidemiological data on the one hand and social and economic cost on the other. The important differences in advice among experts indicates the essentially subjective nature of this judgment.

The difficulty with the use of absolute risk as a criterion is apparent in the impact it has on the treatment of hypertension in relation to age. All guidelines recognize that an elderly hypertensive patient is at greatly increased absolute risk. Some recommend lowering of the threshold for treatment on these grounds.[13, 14] Apart from the New Zealand guidelines, none adjusts the threshold for age before the patient enters the elderly category. Since the gradient of cardiovascular events with age is a steep one (as shown in the New Zealand tables), this process militates against treatment in the older age groups. This raises a further important issue. Can the same weight be attached to a cardiovascular event in a woman of 40 years compared with a man of 70 years? Strict adherence to the absolute-risk criterion assumes this. The results of such a policy are impressive. Even a blood pressure of 180/105 mm Hg in the woman is associated with an annual risk of a cardiovascular event of less than 2%, whereas a blood pressure of 140/90 mm Hg puts the older man into this absolute-risk category. Simpson argued that this is contrary to accepted values and that some adjustment should be made.[34] One suggestion is that treatment should be recommended on the basis of "marginal risk," i.e., the difference in absolute risk between a hypertensive and a normotensive individual of the same age sharing the same risk factors. Life expectancy and years of disease-free survival[35] have been suggested as alternative strategies to redress the balance in favor of treating the elderly.

This debate overlooks two key issues, one of economics and one of social values. The omission of any detailed discussion of cost-effectiveness removes a highly relevant argument.[36] Treatment of hypertension in the elderly, high-risk patient is highly cost-effective and, according to one analysis, can result in a net return to society through a reduction in the burden of strokes and heart attacks.[24] Thus, there would seem to be no rational argument for withholding treatment if the patient wishes it. More important than this, however, is the implicit value judgment in modifying recommendations for the elderly. Is generalization possible, and is it appropriate for an expert group to make recommendations based on their implicit assessment of individual and social values? If the value of preventing a stroke in a younger woman with children is rated highly, should this conclusion be modified in an alcoholic, homeless woman without dependents and perhaps with significant comorbidity? Most professionals would shrink at the attempt to make general judgments of this sort, but such arguments are not qualitatively different from

Table 39–3 Recommendations for First-Line Medical Therapy in Uncomplicated Hypertension

Source	Diuretics/β-Blockers Only	All Classes
Canadian[12]	+	−
United States[13]	+	−
British[14]	+	+
	("divided")	("divided")
New Zealand[19]	+	−
World Health Organization[22]	−	+
Australian[31]	−	+

discussions of the value of treating elderly hypertensives. They underline the need for guidelines to avoid too-great specificity, defining of acceptable care, and providing relevant evidence to inform the clinician in making a decision about the specific needs of the individual patient. The attempt to present prescriptive comprehensive advice (even with caveats about "flexibility") when the ultimate decision is an intensely individual one creates dilemmas of this sort.

The disagreement among guidelines on the choice of initial drug therapy has provoked intense debate (Table 39–3). The Canadian, U.S., and New Zealand guidelines[12, 13, 19] recommend diuretics or β-blockers in cases in which newer agents (angiotensin-converting enzyme inhibitors, angiotensin receptor blockers, calcium antagonists, or α-blockers) are not specifically indicated. The WHO and Australian reports recommend any class of drug.[22, 31] The most recent British expert committee was divided.[14] As discussed previously, both JNC guidelines and the British guidelines have changed their position on this despite the absence of significant new evidence. The key point at issue is the legitimacy of extrapolating from the known antihypertensive efficacy of the newer agents to efficacy in reducing endpoints: JNC VI states its reliance on RCT evidence quite clearly in this context.[13] For some of the other guidelines, this line of reasoning is less persuasive. The main argument in favor of newer agents would be greater efficacy or fewer adverse effects in reducing cardiovascular disease; if the agents were equal in these respects, the case for using them when older, cheaper agents could be used would seem weak. The absence of RCT evidence clearly cannot be an absolute barrier, since it is not a barrier elsewhere. The scientific judgment of the validity of non-RCT evidence will remain disputed until better data become available.

Bearing in mind that the primary objective of treating hypertension is to lower blood pressure, it is surprising that so little discussion has been devoted to the goal blood pressure (Table 39–4). This may reflect the paucity of directly relevant trial evidence, since the guidelines reviewed here were constructed before the Hypertension Optimal Treatment (HOT) trial reported.[37] Incorporation of the HOT data may result in some convergence in target diastolic pressures, since the outcomes suggested little advantage in targeting a diastolic blood pressure below 85 to 90 mm Hg. The recommendation to reduce systolic pressure to less than 140 mm Hg in some guidelines[13, 16, 31]

Table 39–4 Goal Blood Pressures Targeted in Treating Uncomplicated Hypertension

Source	Diastolic Blood Pressure (mm Hg)	Systolic Blood Pressure (mm Hg)
Canadian[12]	—	—
United States[13]	<90	<140
British[14]	80–90	<160
New Zealand[19]	70–80	120–140
World Health Organization[22]	<90 (80 in younger)	<140 (120–130 in younger)
Australian[31]	<90 (80 in younger)	<140 (120–130 in younger)

extrapolates beyond the RCT evidence provided by the two relevant trials that used a more modest goal.[38, 39] The HOT trial provides only the most indirect supportive evidence for a figure of 140 mm Hg from post hoc analyses of achieved systolic pressures:[37] This seems likely to remain a field of uncertainty until stronger trial evidence becomes available.

CONCLUSIONS

Guidelines for the treatment of hypertension can offer valuable advice for defining what is acceptable and what is unacceptable practice and for offering a relevant framework for professional decision-making. When guidelines attempt more than this, they encounter significant difficulty. The inconsistencies in the final products represent the outcome of two implicit misguided strategies. The first attempts to resolve the unresolvable by defining practice where scientific evidence is insufficient. The second seeks to make judgments of value on behalf of society and the individual that are the prerogative of others and that are not, in any case, susceptible to definitive resolution. The dangers of attempts to provide a systematic prescriptive code of practice extend beyond rejection by professionals to misuse of guidelines for purposes for which they are not intended.

References

1. Jackson R, Feder G. Guidelines for clinical guidelines. BMJ 317:427–428, 1998.
2. Swales JD. The growth of medical science: The lessons of Malthus. The Harveian Oration of 1995. London, Royal College of Physicians, 1995.
3. Kassirer JP. Managed care—Should we adopt a new ethic? N Engl J Med 339:397–398, 1998.
4. Kassirer JP. The quality of care and the quality of measuring it. N Engl J Med 329:1263–1265, 1993.
5. Tanenbaum SJ. What physicians know. N Engl J Med 329:1268–1271, 1993.
6. Feder G. Clinical guidelines in 1994. Let's be careful out there. BMJ 309:1457–1458, 1994.
7. Chalmers J. The National Consensus Conference—Not always what it seems. Blood Press 7:877–885, 1994.
8. Felsenthal B. Doctors' own guidelines hurt them in court. Wall St J 19:B1–16, 1994.
9. Garnick DW, Hendricks AM, Brennan TA. Can practice guidelines reduce the number and costs of malpractice claims? JAMA 266:2856–2860, 1991.
10. Garber AM, Browner WS. Cholesterol screening guidelines. Consensus, evidence and common sense. Circulation 95:1642–1645, 1997.
11. Swales JD. Meta-analysis as a guide to clinical practice. J Hypertens 11(Suppl 5):S59–S63, 1993.
12. Carruthers G, Larochelle P, Haynes B, et al. Report of the Canadian Hypertension Society Consensus Conference. Can Med Assoc J 149:289–292, 409–418, 575–584, 815–820, 1993.
13. Joint National Committee on Prevention, Detection, Evaluation, and Treatment of High Blood Pressure. The sixth report. Arch Intern Med 157:2413–2446, 1997.
14. Sever P, Beevers G, Bulpitt C, et al. Management guidelines in essential hypertension: Report of the Second Working Party of the British Hypertension Society. BMJ 306:983–987, 1993.
15. Rennie D. Consensus statements. N Engl J Med 304:665–666, 1981.
16. WHO/ISH Guidelines Committee. 1993 guidelines for the management of mild hypertension: Memorandum from a WHO/ISH meeting. J Hypertens 11:905–918, 1993
17. Swales JD, Ramsay LE, Coope JR, et al. Treating mild hypertension. BMJ 298:694–698, 1989.
18. Expert Committee on the Diagnosis and Classification of Diabetes Mellitus. Report. Diabetes Care 20:1183–1197, 1997.
19. The management of mildly raised blood pressure in New Zealand. Wellington, New Zealand, National Advisory Committee on Core Health and Disability Support Services, 1994.
20. Standing Medical Advisory Committee. The use of statins. London, Department of Health, 1997.
21. Haq IU, Ramsay LE, Pickin DM, et al. Lipid-lowering for prevention of coronary heart disease: What policy now? Clin Sci 91:399–413, 1996.
22. World Health Organization. Hypertension control. Report of a WHO Expert Committee. Geneva, World Health Organization, 1996.
23. Swales JD. Economics and the treatment of hypertension. J Hypertens 13:1357–1361, 1995.
24. Johannesson M. The cost-effectiveness of hypertension treatment in Sweden. Pharmacoeconomics 7:242–250, 1995.
25. Hill MN, Levine DM, Whelton PK. Awareness, use and impact of the 1984 Joint National Committee Consensus report on high blood pressure. Am J Public Health 78:1190–1194, 1988.
26. Lomas J, Anderson GM, Domnick-Pierre K, et al. Do practice guidelines guide practice? The effect of a consensus statement and practice of physicians. N Engl J Med 321:1306–1311, 1989.
27. Siegel D, Lopez J. Trends in antihypertensive drug use in the United States: Do the JNC V recommendations affect prescribing? JAMA 278:1745–1748, 1997.
28. National Prescribing Authority. Report 1997. London, Her Majesty's Stationery Office, 1997.
29. Bero LA, Grilli R, Grimshaw J, et al. Closing the gap between research and practice: An overview of systematic reviews of interventions to promote the implementation of research findings. BMJ 317:465–468, 1998.
30. Jackson R, Sackett D. Guidelines for managing raised blood pressure: Evidence-based or evidence burdened? BMJ 313:64–65, 1996.
31. Consensus Panel. The management of hypertension: A consensus statement. Med J Aust 16(suppl):S1–S16, 1994.
32. Fahey TP, Peters TJ. What constitutes controlled hypertension? Patient based comparison of hypertension guidelines. BMJ 313:93–96, 1996.
33. Robertson JIS. Guidelines for the treatment of hypertension: A critical review. Cardiovasc Drugs Ther 8:665–672, 1994.
34. Simpson FO. Guidelines for antihypertensive therapy: Problems with a strategy based on absolute risk. J Hypertens 14:683–689, 1996.
35. MacMahon S. Guidelines for antihypertensive therapy. J Hypertens 14:691–693, 1996.
36. Swales JD. Treating hypertension. J Hypertens 14:813–815, 1996.
37. Hansson L, Zanchetti A, Carruthers SG, et al. Effects of intensive blood pressure lowering and low dose aspirin in patients with hypertension: Principal results of the Hypertension Optimal Treatment (HOT) randomised trial. Lancet 351:1755–1762, 1998.
38. SHEP Cooperative Research Group. Prevention of stroke by antihypertensive drug treatment in older persons with isolated systolic hypertension. JAMA 265:3255–3264, 1991.
39. Staessen JA, Fagard R, Thijs L, et al. Randomised double-blind comparison of placebo and active treatment for older patients with isolated systolic hypertension. Lancet 350:757–764, 1997.

40 Current Prescribing Practices

J. Jaime Caro and Jeanne L. Speckman

That clinical decisions should be rational and based on the best evidence possible is the keystone of modern scientific medicine. Finding reality wanting, however, opinion leaders have increasingly called for a more determined effort to ensure that actual practice meets this standard. Chapter 35 is devoted to a discussion of *evidence-based medicine*. Criteria that have been proposed for the selection of studies that will provide this evidence emphasize the randomized clinical trial as a gold standard.[1, 2] A physician faced with a common—and very well studied—condition such as hypertension is expected to turn to randomized trials (or corresponding meta-analyses), and the guidelines based on these, for information on which to base treatment choices.

In Chapter 38, Changing Approaches to Diagnosis and Treatment of Hypertension, and Chapter 39, Critical Assessment of Hypertension Guidelines, the guidelines for hypertension treatment in the United States[3] were discussed. These guidelines suggest that once the decision to begin pharmacotherapy has been made, the physician should choose a diuretic or β-blocker in the absence of special patient characteristics that indicate use of a specific drug. Guidelines from the World Health Organization, although less directly recommending diuretics or β-blockers, do put these two classes at the top of the recommended list.[4] The sixth report of the Joint National Committee on Prevention, Detection, Evaluation, and Treatment of High Blood Pressure (JNC VI) guidelines further suggest that a series of steps be followed, including adding or switching medications, if the response to the initial treatment is insufficient.

In this chapter, we examine how current physician practices accord with these recommendations. We also review evidence that suggests possible reasons for choosing to start treatment with drugs other than diuretics or β-blockers (referred to as *group 1* in this chapter). Only data from articles published since 1988 are included.

INITIAL TREATMENT CHOICES

United States

In the United States, antihypertensive treatment practice appears quite varied (Fig. 40–1). For example, in a study of 377 newly diagnosed patients carried out in the Midwest over an 18-month period (1991 to 1992),[5] 55% received monotherapy but only about a third started on a group 1 drug. The most common initial therapy was a calcium channel blocker (CCB) given to 30%, followed by an angiotensin-converting enzyme inhibitor (ACEI) in 22%. Sequential monotherapy was used in 18% of the patients, and stepped therapy (with more than one class of drug given at some point) in 22%; 5% were started on more than one drug.

The picture was very different in patients beginning antihypertensive therapy who were part of a cohort of approximately 1700 patients examined annually between 1989 and 1993.[6] Consistently, about half started with regimens that incorporated a group 1 drug (55% of the 157 patients seen in 1989 to 1991; 49% of the 142 seen in 1990 to 1992; and 56% of the 120 seen in 1991 to 1993). CCBs slightly led ACEIs among the rest.

In contrast to these studies of actual practice, surveys of physicians find that they report much greater adherence to published treatment guidelines. For example, 69% of 128 family physicians and primary care internists in Iowa in 1988 reported choosing a group 1 drug as initial therapy for patients under 40 years of age.[7] Most of the rest (27%)

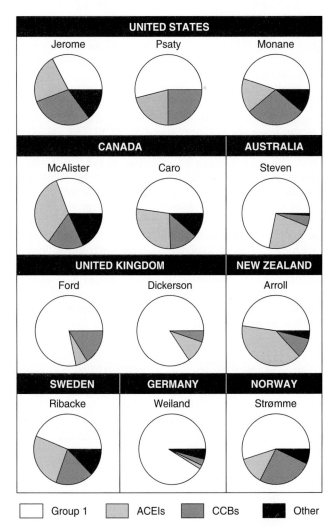

Figure 40–1. Distribution of the four major classes of medication prescribed to new hypertensive patients by country. ACEIs, angiotensin-converting enzyme inhibitors; CCBs, calcium channel blockers.

would choose an ACEI. Similar results were obtained for older patients in a survey of more than 1000 New Jersey physicians in 1985: 78% reported choosing a group 1 drug as the initial treatment for patients older than 60 years with isolated systolic hypertension.[8] Even greater adherence to official guidelines was reported in a survey of 274 physicians in Minnesota in 1987,[9] where 91% stated that a group 1 drug was their first choice of medication.

Factors such as age and gender of the patient can influence the choice of antihypertensive treatment in the United States. Among 183 Minnesota physicians surveyed about initial therapy in 1992,[10] no drug class predominated as first choice, but group 1 drugs were more frequently selected for a 48-year-old man (30%) than for a 65-year-old (25%). Choice of a CCB was much less common for the younger man (16% vs. 36%), whereas ACEIs were more common (44% vs. 37%). For older women, however, the preferences were evenly distributed.

Studies have revealed changes in the level of adherence to the guidelines over time. A review of 8428 people aged 65 years and older, whose records were in the New Jersey Medicaid and Medicare databases from 1982 to 1988, found that the proportion starting treatment with a group 1 drug dropped from about 70% to 45%—most of the decline occurring in diuretic prescriptions.[11] Use of a CCB increased from 7% to 28%, and of an ACEI from 0.3% to 16%, during the same 6-year period. Diuretic use was more common in patients older than eighty-five years, women, and African Americans.

Similar declines in preference for group 1 drugs were found among 241 primary care physicians in the Midwest surveyed in 1987 and again in 1989[12]—from 90 to 62%. In the latter survey, 30% chose an ACEI and the rest a CCB or other class. Physicians were also asked for their preferences for a group 2 medication. In 1987, 84% stayed within group 1, whereas only 60% did so by 1989, with ACEIs chosen by about one quarter of physicians.

In a structured care setting, changes in preferences appear to parallel the treatment guidelines. This is evident in a study of 550 union members during the first year of a union-sponsored hypertension screening and follow-up program carried out between 1986 and 1992.[13] In the period before JNC IV guidelines, physicians treated 87% of their patients with group 1 drugs. After JNC IV (which recommended all four classes), 90% of patients were started with a CCB or an ACEI, whereas publication of JNC V (which

recommended group 1 drugs for initial treatment) saw practice even out to about 25% for each major class.

Canada

Evidence from Canada also indicates some practice variations, but with a greater tendency to disregard the practice guidelines. In a review of the medical records of 711 newly diagnosed hypertensive patients seen in Edmonton, Alberta, between 1993 and 1995,[14] less than one third (31%) of those receiving medicines (531) were started on a group 1 drug. This remained under 50% even when patients with a documented contraindication to one of these drugs were excluded. ACEIs were the most common first choice (44%), whereas only 23% used a CCB. These prescribing patterns were reported to be very similar among physicians in many different types of practice. However, family physicians were found to choose the recommended classes of medication more often than did internists.

In a study of the records of more than 27,000 new patients in the neighboring province of Saskatchewan, carried out from 1990 through 1994,[15] nearly half (48%) were found to have started on a group 1 drug. Indeed, among the 24 different drugs prescribed initially to at least 100 patients each, the combination of triamterene and hydrochlorothiazide in a single tablet was more than three times more common than any given ACEI or CCB. ACEIs, however, were the second most frequent initial drug class, whereas only 13% of new patients began on a CCB.

The initial choice of drug among new patients varied according to the age and gender of the patient (Table 40–1). In females and older males, group 1 drugs remained the most frequent choice, with diuretics predominating. By contrast, in younger men, an ACEI was as common as a group 1 drug. Although choice of a β-blocker was infrequent in all groups, it was relatively more common in younger patients.

There was little variation over the 5 years of the study, however, with group 1 drugs consistently representing the initial choice in about 45% of new patients (Fig. 40–2). ACEIs also remained the second most common initial choice throughout the study period. Use of CCBs, other single drugs, combination drugs, and multiple drugs also remained stable during the study period.

These data on actual practice confirm the results of a

Table 40–1 Distribution of Class of Index Antihypertensive Prescriptions in New Patients by Age and Gender

| Drug Class | Male (%) | | Female (%) | | Overall (%) |
	Under 60 yr* (n = 5262)	60+ yr (n = 6653)	Under 60 yr (n = 6046)	60+ yr (n = 9403)	(n = 27364)
Diuretics	23	36	41	45	38
β-Blockers	15	8	13	8	10
ACEIs	38	28	25	25	29
CCBs	14	16	11	13	13
Other single agent	3	4	5	3	4
Combinations	3	3	3	2	3
Multiples	4	5	3	4	4

Abbreviations: ACEIs, angiotensin-converting enzyme inhibitors; CCBs, calcium channel blockers.
*Differences in distribution within gender and age group *p* < .001.

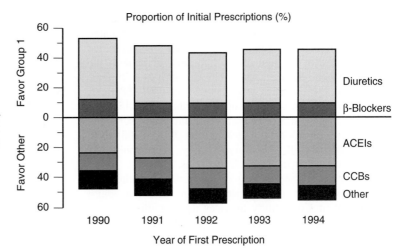

Figure 40–2. Distribution of index drug by calendar year for new patients (*n* = 27,364). Chi-square = 300.6; *p* < .001. ACEIs, angiotensin-converting enzyme inhibitors; CCBs, calcium channel blockers.

survey of physicians' preferences in the province of Alberta in 1995.[16] In that study, physicians were asked for their choice of initial therapy for several hypothetical cases. In the case of a lower-risk patient, group 1 drugs were prescribed by 44% of physicians, ACEIs by 46%, and CCBs by 5%. As risk factors increased, group 1 drugs dropped to 20%, ACEIs increased to 67%, and CCBs increased to 10%. Only in the case of a patient with target organ damage, left ventricular hypertrophy, and previous myocardial infarction did the preference shift to group 1 drugs (62%), primarily β-blockers (56%).

The choice of medication can vary, as expected, with the clinical condition.[17] When isolated systolic hypertension was the issue, the majority of 281 physicians surveyed in 1995 in Edmonton, Alberta, reported their choice of antihypertensive treatment to be a diuretic—74% among internists and 58% among family physicians; only 10% of internists and 26% of family physicians would choose an ACEI first in this situation.

New Zealand

Physicians in New Zealand also reported less preference for group 1 drugs. In a 1992 survey of 100 physicians, only 48% would choose a group 1 drug for a 60-year-old man with essential hypertension and no contraindications.[18] Most of the remainder (39%) would choose an ACEI (9% chose a CCB).

Actual practice data do not clearly address the issue of initial treatment choices, as they do not distinguish between new and established patients. For example, a 1988 survey of 37 general practitioners that included information on 2 months of prescriptions[19] found that nearly half of patients (44%) were receiving more than one drug. Thus, although diuretics were used in 47% and β-blockers in 48%, it is uncertain what their first prescription was. This problem applies as well to surveys in 1982 and 1987,[20] in which the use of diuretics was high initially but dropped between surveys (64% to 47%), whereas β-blocker use remained constant (52% to 55%), and use of CCBs (3% to 13%) and ACEIs increased (0% to 13%).

United Kingdom

In the United Kingdom, actual practice seems to be quite different in that it conforms much more to guidelines—at least, according to surveys of physicians' opinions. In one survey of 360 general practitioners in Leicestershire, England, in 1991,[21] 62% reported they would start treatment with a thiazide diuretic in a 70-year-old hypertensive patient without target organ damage. Among the remainder, 17% reported they would use nonpharmacological treatment. Another survey of 200 physicians in England (East Anglia) in 1993 found similar results: 85% of the respondents indicated that in the absence of contraindications, they would start therapy with a group 1 drug—nearly two thirds of these with a diuretic. Only 10% chose an ACEI and 5% a CCB.[22] The tendency to favor a diuretic was even more pronounced among 92 physicians surveyed in Northamptonshire in 1993:[23] 83% reported that a thiazide diuretic would be their initial choice for a 70-year-old patient with no end-organ damage; another 5% reported choosing a β-blocker first.

Although there are some differences according to the type of physician, the preference for group 1 drugs persists. For example, a 1992 survey of 214 general practitioners and 127 hospital physicians in the northern region of England found that the former would choose a group 1 drug for an otherwise well, 75-year-old male nonsmoker 79% of the time, whereas the latter would do so only 62% of the time.[24] For the remainder, the split was similar, with a CCB chosen almost three times as often as an ACEI.

These reported preferences for group 1 drugs are supported by actual practice data, although they are not specific to new patients. In a review of the database records of over 37,000 hypertensive patients seen in 1992 to 1993, new courses of treatment were considered.[25] Among the 10,222 patients starting a new type of treatment, 86% received a group 1 drug, 32% a CCB, and 27% an ACEI. The numbers add to more than 100%, as over a third of patients received multiple new drugs.

Australia

Survey data published in 1992 on 132 randomly selected general practitioners in South Australia indicate similarly high adherence to the guidelines: About three quarters would choose a group 1 drug for treating an uncomplicated moderately hypertensive patient.[26] Although this preference varied little with the age of the hypothetical patient, the balance between diuretics and β-blockers did: In a 75-year-old patient, the diuretics were heavily favored (68% vs. 9%) compared with a more even distribution for a 45-year-old patient (41% vs. 31%). Most of the physicians surveyed in Australia (80%) also indicated that if they failed to achieve control with the initial therapy, they would add another drug rather than switch therapies.

These reported preferences differ from the findings of an analysis over an 11-year period of the Commonwealth Department of Community Services and Health database, which covers 80% of community prescriptions (not including hospital dispensings or those paid by private insurance). According to these data, the use of diuretics decreased by nearly one third from 1982 to 1987, whereas the use of ACEIs increased dramatically.[27] Unfortunately, as in the United Kingdom, the analysis did not distinguish new from established patients, and thus it is impossible to say whether this change in prescription patterns reflects a shift in the choice of initial medication or in the drugs used subsequently.

Germany

Physicians in Germany also reported remarkable adherence to published guidelines in the choice of initial therapy. In a 1988 survey of 315 general practitioners, 93% reported choosing a group 1 drug for a 45-year-old man; in contrast to the United Kingdom and Australia, nearly all (92%) would select a β-blocker.[28] Only 3% chose a CCB and 1% an ACEI. For a 65-year-old man, a group 1 drug was chosen 71% of the time; the vast majority, however, chose a diuretic. A CCB was chosen by 21%; an ACEI by 2%. The overall pattern of prescribing was very similar for internists and was not affected by the physician's age.

Again, these reported preferences are somewhat at odds with actual data—this time gathered in the Monitoring of Trends and Determinants of Cardiovascular Disease (MONICA) Augsburg project, which surveyed 3324 hypertensive men and women in 1984 to 1985 and again in 1987 to 1988.[29] There were 167 patients treated for hypertension in the second survey who were untreated in the first. Although these patients were considered "newly treated" by the authors, it is unlikely that the prescription information obtained consistently represented the first medication used. Thus, by the time they were surveyed, only 25% of these patients were on a β-blocker and just as many were on triple-agent therapy. Among men, CCBs, singly or in combination with another agent, accounted for one third of prescriptions, whereas among women, diuretics and diuretic combinations accounted for one third of prescriptions reported.

Sweden

β-Blockers were reported to be the favorite in a survey of 126 general practitioners and specialists in the Uppsala-Örebro region in 1991.[30] The physicians were asked for their first choice of therapy for each of six hypothetical hypertensive patients. For a healthy, nonsmoking, 44-year-old man with a family history of diabetes and blood pressure of 180/100, 40% indicated that they would choose a β-blocker, whereas less than 1% chose a diuretic. ACEIs were the second most common choice (24%), but more so among specialists (34% vs. 18%). CCBs were the choice of 18%, and 17% would not choose pharmacotherapy. In only two of the six hypothetical cases did diuretics account for more than 10% of the choices, and neither of these was a new patient.

This preference for β-blockers was reported to be even stronger in a 1991 survey of 236 physicians.[10] For an otherwise healthy 48-year-old male patient, 72% chose a β-blocker. The preference for a β-blocker was less pronounced for older patients and women: 57% of physicians chose a β-blocker for a 65-year-old man, but only 52% did for a 65-year-old woman. Preference for diuretics increased from less than 5% for a 48-year-old male patient to 20% for a 65-year-old man and 27% for older women. Physicians were surveyed about the hypothetical 48-year-old male patient again in 1993, and treatment preferences were found to have changed little.[31]

Norway

Preferences for β-blockers did not hold in Norway. A 1989 survey of 235 Oslo physicians found that 51% would choose diuretics for an asymptomatic 75-year-old hypertensive man;[32] CCBs were a second choice at 25%. ACEIs accounted for only 13%, and β-blockers and others accounted for the remaining 11%. Physicians over 50 years of age were more apt to prescribe a diuretic, whereas a CCB was more commonly chosen by physicians under age 40 years and by specialists. Female physicians were significantly less apt to choose an ACEI than were males.

Other Countries

Marked differences between countries were reported in a 1992 survey of general practitioners in Indonesia, Italy, United Kingdom, Croatia, Panama, France, and Belgium (each represented by at least 18 physicians).[33] Asked for their first choice for treating mild hypertension in the absence of contraindications, 63% of Italian physicians and 93% of Croatian physicians chose diuretics, compared with Indonesia and Belgium, where 40% and 94%, respectively, chose β-blockers.

EFFECTS OF INITIAL TREATMENT CHOICES

The recommendations to choose group 1 drugs initially depend, at least in part, on two key assumptions. One is that at the start of therapy there is *no reason to expect that any one therapy will do better than others*. The second is that the initial treatment choice is not so important because, if it is not successful, changes can be made to optimize the regimen for a given patient and these *modifications will have no detrimental effects*. If these two assumptions hold, it makes sense to choose a drug from a class proved to reduce cardiovascular risk and with a lower acquisition cost. If they prove untenable, however, the appropriate first choice might turn out to be quite different. This might be the case if the likelihood of patients remaining compliant—and, thus, benefiting from treatment—differs according to the class of drug chosen initially. This could happen if the side effect profile of a class were less well tolerated by patients who, in the context of an otherwise asymptomatic condition, tend to stop treatment or if the therapeutic "turbulence" generated by changes in the regimen to deal with side effects or to achieve blood pressure control bothers the patient in excess of the perceived benefits. The patient may ask, Why put up with what appears to be troublesome trial and error to treat a condition with nebulous menace?

The assumptions underlying the choice of group 1 drugs may seem reasonable to the physician, but they have been implemented without testing in actual practice. The evidence for equivalent expectations is limited and almost entirely based on short-term, highly controlled clinical trials. The evidence that treatment modifications will have no detrimental effects is even more scant. Moreover, clinical trials designed to assess efficacy are unable to address these assumptions because the very procedures implemented to ensure valid efficacy data so alter compliance that the trials no longer reflect routine practice.

The essence of these two assumptions—that the drug classes are equivalent in the proportion of patients who can be expected to stay on therapy and thus achieve blood pressure control—was tested in a study using the health care databases of Saskatchewan.[34] Saskatchewan Health funds the health care system of the province, including a prescription drug plan.[35] The records were examined of 27,364 Saskatchewan residents with a diagnosis of essential hypertension who received at least one antihypertensive agent listed in the Saskatchewan formulary between November 1, 1989, and December 31, 1994, but had no record of treatment in the preceding year. Men and women over age 40 years without a diagnosis of malignant hypertension or hepatic, renal, or cardiovascular diseases other than hypertension were eligible.

The outpatient prescription drug plan database yielded all dispensings of an antihypertensive drug identified by its generic name, as well as the dispensing date, quantity, strength, and drug form. The database did not include information on the actual prescription nor on blood pressure. A patient was considered persistent with therapy if it was estimated, based on an a priori algorithm used to assess the dispensing records, that he or she still had antihypertensive medication to take on the last day of follow-up. Whether the patient actually took the medication, or if it had been discontinued following physician's advice, could not be determined.

Persistence was analyzed for the 22,918 patients who were observed in the database for at least 6 months and who began treatment with one of the four major classes of medication. Almost one quarter of patients had discontinued all antihypertensive therapy within a year of starting

it. The rate of persistence varied with class of drug: 74% of patients who started treatment with a diuretic were persistent at 1 year; the persistence rate among patients starting on a β-blocker was 78%; 81% for those starting on a CCB; and 84% for those starting on an ACEI. At 2 years, persistence rates were even lower: 64% for a diuretic; 69% for a β-blocker; 71% for a CCB; and 74% for an ACEI. Four years after starting antihypertensive therapy, only 46% of those starting on a diuretic were still on antihypertensive therapy; this figure was 54% for a β-blocker, 53% for a CCB, and 58% for an ACEI. The increased persistence over time associated with ACEIs compared with group 1 drugs remains significant, even when controlling for differences in age, gender, and use of health care resources in the prior year.

A higher frequency of changes in the therapeutic regimen was also significantly associated with decreasing persistence in each of the first 3 years of therapy ($p < .05$). For example, subjects who had two or more changes to their therapeutic regimen in any 6-month interval were 25% less likely to persist with medication in the next 6 months, and even a single change decreased persistence by 7%. These data indicate that the choice of first antihypertensive agent is an important determinant of the likelihood that the patient will continue with therapy. The premise of therapeutic guidelines that suggest that changes in medication can be made without detriment must, therefore, be questioned. Thus, data from actual practice suggest that two key assumptions required to support the initial choice of group 1 drugs may not be tenable.

SUMMARY

The choice of initial medication for treatment of hypertension varies by country and by practitioner. Whereas in some countries, such as Germany and the United Kingdom, a diuretic or β-blocker is frequently used, an ACEI or CCB is more common in others (United States, Canada, Sweden). For patients without comorbidities, known drug sensitivity, or other factors that drive the decision, current guidelines suggest that treatment be started with a group 1 drug and that changes be made thereafter as needed. Data from actual practice studies, such as the Saskatchewan analysis, indicate that there may be disadvantages to this process. An increased probability of achieving blood pressure control, by ensuring that patients remain on medication, could justify the initial choice of one of the newer agents, such as an ACEI or one of the more recently developed angiotensin II receptor antagonists.

References

1. Evidence-Based Medicine Working Group. Evidence-based medicine: A new approach to teaching the practice of medicine. JAMA 268:2420–2425, 1992.
2. Editorial Staff. Purpose and procedure. Evidence-Based Med 1:98–99, 1996.
3. Joint National Committee on Prevention, Detection, Evaluation, and Treatment of High Blood Pressure. The sixth report. Arch Intern Med 157:2401–2402, 1997.
4. WHO/ISH Guidelines Sub-Committee: 1993 Guidelines for the management of mild hypertension: Memorandum from a WHO/ISH meeting. Bull World Health Organ 71:503–517, 1993.

5. Jerome M, Xakellis GC, Angstman G, et al. Initial medication selection for treatment of hypertension in an open-panel HMO. J Am Board Fam Pract 8:1–6, 1995.

6. Psaty BM, Koepsell TD, Yanez ND, et al. Temporal patterns of antihypertensive medication use among older adults, 1989 through 1992. JAMA 273:1436–1438, 1995.

7. Carter BL, Kriesel HT, Steinkraus L, et al. Antihypertensive drug-prescribing patterns of internists and family physicians. J Fam Prac 29:257–262, 1989.

8. Breckenridge MB, Kostis JB. Isolated systolic hypertension in the elderly: Results of a statewide survey of clinical practice in New Jersey. Am J Med 86:370–375, 1989.

9. Kofron PM, Råstam L, Pirie PL, et al. Physician practice for cardiovascular disease risk-factor reduction in six upper midwestern communities. J Fam Pract 32:49–55, 1991.

10. Troein M, Arneson T, Råstam L, et al. Reported treatment of hypertension by family physicians in Sweden and Minnesota: A physician survey of practice habits. J Intern Med 238:215–221, 1995.

11. Monane M, Glynn RJ, Gurwitz JH, et al. Trends in medication choices for hypertension in the elderly. Hypertension 25:1045–1051, 1995.

12. Bostrick RM, Luepker RV, Kofron PM, et al. Changes in physician practice for the prevention of cardiovascular disease. Arch Intern Med 151:478–484, 1991.

13. Alderman MH, Madhavan S, Cohen H. Antihypertensive drug therapy. The effect of JNC criteria on prescribing patterns on patient status through the first year. Am J Hypertens 9:413–418, 1996.

14. McAlister FA, Teo KK, Lewanczuk RZ, et al. Contemporary practice patterns in the management of newly diagnosed hypertension. Can Med Assoc J 157:23–30, 1997.

15. Caro JJ, Salas M, Speckman JL, et al. Persistence with treatment for hypertension in actual practice. Can Med Assoc J 160:31–37, 1999.

16. McAlister FA, Laupacis A, Teo KK, et al. A survey of clinician attitudes and management practices in hypertension. J Hum Hypertens 11:413–419, 1997.

17. McAlister FA, Teo KK, Laupacis A. A survey of management practices for isolated systolic hypertension. J Am Geriatr Soc 45:1219–1222, 1997.

18. Arroll B, Jenkins S, North D, et al. Management of hypertension and the core services guidelines: Results from interviews with 100 Auckland general practitioners. N Z Med J 108:55–57, 1995.

19. Kawachi I, Malcolm LA, Purdie G. Variability in antihypertensive drug therapy in general practice: Results from a national survey. N Z Med J 102:307–309, 1989.

20. Sinclair B, Jackson R, Beaglehole R. Patterns in the drug treatment of hypertension in Auckland, 1982–7. N Z Med J 102:491–493, 1989.

21. Fotherby MD, Harper GD, Potter JF. General practice: General practitioners' management of hypertension in elderly patients. BMJ 305:750–752, 1992.

22. Dickerson JEC, Garratt CJ, Brown MJ. Management of hypertension in general practice: Agreements with and variations from the British Hypertension Society guidelines. J Hum Hypertens 9:835–839, 1995.

23. Fahey T, Silagy C. General practitioners' knowledge of and attitudes to the management of hypertension in elderly patients. Br J Gen Pract 44:446–449, 1994.

24. Ford GA, Asghar MN. Management of hypertension in the elderly: Attitudes of general practitioners and hospital physicians. Br J Clin Pharmacol 39:465–469, 1995.

25. Jones JK, Gorkin L, Lian JF, et al. Discontinuation of and changes in treatment after start of new courses of antihypertensive drugs: A study of a United Kingdom population. BMJ 311:293–295, 1995.

26. Steven ID, Wilson DH, Wakefield MA, et al. South Australian hypertension survey. General practitioner experiences with drug treatment. Med J Aust 156:641–644, 1992.

27. Hurley SF, Williams SL, McNeil JJ. Trends in prescribing of antihypertensive drugs in Australia, 1977–1987. Med J Aust 152:259–266, 1990.

28. Weiland SK, Keil U, Spelsberg A, et al. Diagnosis and management of hypertension by physicians in the Federal Republic of Germany. J Hypertens 9:131–134, 1991.

29. Hense HW, Tennis P. Changing patterns of antihypertensive drug use in a German population between 1984 and 1987. Eur J Clin Pharmacol 39:1–7, 1990.

30. Ribacke M. Treatment preferences, return visit planning and factors affecting hypertension practice amongst general practitioners and internal medicine specialists. J Intern Med 237:473–478, 1995.

31. Troein M, Gardell B, Selander S, et al. Guidelines and reported practice for the treatment of hypertension and hypercholesterolemia. J Intern Med 242:173–178, 1997.

32. Strømme HK, Botten G: Factors relating to the choice of antihypertensive and hypnotic drug treatment in old patients. Scand J Prim Health Care 10:301–305, 1992.

33. Avanzini F, Tognoni G, Alli C, et al., on behalf of the International Society of Drug Bulletins. How informed general practitioners manage mild hypertension: A survey of readers of drug bulleting in 7 countries. Eur J Clin Pharmacol 49:445–450, 1996.

34. Caro JJ, Speckman JL, Salas M, et al. The effect of initial drug choice on persistence with antihypertensive therapy: The importance of actual practice data. Can Med Assoc J 160:41–46, 1999.

35. Malcolm E, Downey W, Strand LM, et al. Saskatchewan Health's linkable data bases and pharmacoepidemiology. Post Marketing Surveillance 6:175–264, 1993.

41 Calcium Channel Blockers in the Treatment of Hypertension

Julie E. Buring, Robert J. Glynn, and Charles H. Hennekens

With respect to drug treatment and hypertension, since the early 1970s, a totality of evidence has emerged that includes large randomized trials and their overviews. Hypertensive patients prescribed drugs, most commonly diuretics and β-blockers, have decreased risks of myocardial infarction, stroke, and vascular mortality. During this period, antihypertensive drug therapy has increased dramatically in the United States;[1, 2] average blood pressure levels have declined; and control of hypertension has increased in both middle-aged and elderly hypertensive patients.[3–5] These trends have likely contributed substantially to the decline in cardiovascular mortality in the United States.

During the decade from 1985 to 1995, the use of diuretics and β-blockers has declined substantially, while the use of calcium channel blockers (CCBs) and angiotensin-converting enzyme (ACE) inhibitors has increased.[1, 5–9] These changes occurred through a preference of health care providers and patients for these newer agents for initial therapy as well as a trend toward switching treatments in previously diagnosed hypertensive patients. In 1995, CCBs accounted for 38% of antihypertensive drug prescriptions in the United States, compared with 33% for ACE inhibitors, 11% for β-blockers, and 8% for diuretics.[9] Although CCBs clearly reduce blood pressure, concerns have been raised about their possible adverse effects on myocardial infarction, bleeding, and cancer. In this chapter we review the available evidence that CCBs used to treat hypertension alter risk of developing cardiovascular disease, cancer, and bleeding as well as suggest future research directions to clarify their benefit:risk ratio.

CONTRIBUTIONS OF DIFFERENT TYPES OF EVIDENCE

As has been the case with CCBs in the treatment of hypertension, advances in knowledge proceed on several fronts, optimally simultaneously.[10, 11] Basic researchers provide biological mechanisms to answer the crucial question of why an agent has an effect. Clinicians provide enormous benefits to affected patients through advances in diagnosis and treatment and formulate hypotheses from their clinical experiences, namely in case reports and case series. Clinical investigators address the relevance of basic research findings to affected patients and healthy individuals. Epidemiologists and statisticians formulate hypotheses from descriptive studies and test them in analytical studies, both observational case-control and cohort and, where necessary, randomized trials. These answer the equally crucial and complementary question of whether an agent has an effect. Thus, each discipline and, indeed, every strategy within a discipline provide relevant and complementary information to the totality of evidence on which rational clinical decisions for individual patients and policy decisions for the health of the general public can be safely based. Each discipline has unique strengths and limitations, so it is crucial to consider the contributions of each to the totality of evidence. Given the existing controversies on the safety of CCBs in the treatment of hypertension, this seems particularly important.

Basic research has the unique strength of precision—achieving virtually complete control of exposures, environment, and even genetics—and provides mechanisms to explain findings from applied research in humans. However, basic research also has the disadvantage of questionable relevance to free-living humans owing to differences in species-specificity as well as doses and routes of administration of exposures.[12, 13] Nonetheless, the precision possible in such research provides unique information crucial to setting priorities to test their relevance in studies of free-living humans. Thus, basic research is crucial but so, too, is direct, straightforward observation of what actually happens in human populations.

Epidemiology is based directly on observations of free-living humans and has the unique advantage of relevance. Epidemiological studies also, however, have the unique disadvantage of imprecision. Epidemiology is crude and inexact, since observations in free-living humans can never take place under the controlled conditions possible to achieve in the laboratory. Nonetheless, epidemiology makes essential contributions to the totality of evidence, which can support a judgment of cause and effect. Making such a judgment involves several steps, the first being to establish whether there is, in fact, a valid statistical association. In order to conclude that an association is valid, alternative explanations for the finding, including the potential roles of chance, bias, and confounding, must be ruled out. If a valid statistical association is present, the question becomes a judgment of cause and effect. To render this judgment, the totality of evidence from all sources must be considered, with particular attention to the strength of the association, the consistency of the evidence from different studies, and the existence of plausible biological mechanisms to explain the findings.

A number of specific analytical epidemiological study design options can be employed. These can be divided into two broad design strategies: observational and intervention (i.e., randomized trials). In observational studies, the investigator observes the natural course of events, noting who self-selects to be exposed and nonexposed and who has and has not developed the outcome of interest. In randomized clinical trials, the investigators themselves allocate the exposure and then follow the subjects for the subsequent development of disease.

There are two basic types of observational analytic investigations: the case-control and the cohort study. In a case-control study, a case group or series of patients who have a disease of interest and a control, or comparison, group of individuals without the disease are selected for investigation, and the proportions with the exposure of interest in each group are compared. In contrast, in a cohort study, subjects are classified on the basis of the presence or absence of exposure to a particular factor and then followed for a specified period of time to determine the development of disease in each exposure group. Case-control and cohort studies are often criticized because of the potential for bias and confounding inherent in the fact that the design is observational. Since the use of a particular drug or treatment, for example, or the adoption of a certain lifestyle is self-selected, individuals who use that drug or adopt that lifestyle may be systematically different from those who do not in ways that will affect the outcome of interest. Moreover, since the outcome of interest has already occurred at the time exposure is assessed, case-control studies have unique potential for bias in the selection of individuals into the study and in their recall of prior events. In a cohort study, the often long latent period between exposure and disease can also lead to bias owing to losses to follow-up. However, despite these inherent limitations, observational epidemiological studies provide a crucial contribution to the totality of evidence.

There are two unique strengths of observational evidence. The first relates to the evaluation of exposures that require long duration; the second, to detect moderate- to large-sized effects (i.e., relative risks greater than 1.5).[14] When a very large effect is seen, such as the relative risk of 20 with smoking and lung cancer, the amount of uncontrolled confounding may affect the magnitude of the relative risk estimate, making it, for example, as high as 22 or as low as 18. However, it is unlikely that complete control of confounding would materially change the conclusion that there is a strong positive association between smoking and lung cancer. Even in the case of a relative risk of 1.8 for current smoking and coronary heart disease, although uncontrolled confounding may mean that the true relative risk is as small as 1.6 or as large as 2.0, that range of uncertainty does not materially affect the conclusion that current cigarette smoking increases the risk of coronary heart disease (CHD). On the other hand, when the most plausible effect size of benefit or harm is only 20 to 40%—as is the case with most drugs and interventions—a small amount of uncontrolled confounding in an observational study could mean the difference between a relative risk of 0.8 (indicating a 20% decreased risk), 1.0 (indicating no effect), or 1.2 (indicating a 20% increased risk).

Intervention studies, also referred to as experimental studies or randomized trials, may be viewed as a type of cohort study because participants are identified on the basis of their exposure status and followed to determine whether or not they develop the disease. The distinguishing feature of the intervention design is that the exposure status of each participant is assigned by the investigator. When exposure is assigned at random, intervention studies provide the most reliable evidence for small to moderate effects. This is due to the unique strength of randomization as a means of determining exposure status in a trial. When participants are allocated to a particular exposure group at random, such a strategy achieves, on average, control of all other factors that may affect disease risk. Whereas such variables, if they are known to the investigators, could be controlled in the design and/or analysis of observational studies, the unique feature of randomization is that it also, on average, controls the effects of risk factors that are unrecognized or unmeasurable. It is this ability to control both known and unknown confounders that makes the randomized trial such a powerful epidemiological strategy, especially for studying small to moderate effects. When well designed and conducted, intervention studies provide the most direct epidemiological evidence on which to judge whether an exposure causes or prevents a disease. If the treatments are allocated at random in a sample of sufficiently large size, intervention studies can provide a degree of assurance about the validity of a result that is not possible with any observational design option.

For many, perhaps most, hypotheses, randomized trials are neither necessary nor desirable. However, most often, the proposed benefit or harm of newer therapeutic or preventive measures is small to moderate, on the order of a 10 to 20% difference in disease outcomes. Such effects can be extremely important from a clinical or public health perspective, especially when the outcome of interest is mortality from common and serious diseases. Nonetheless, small to moderate differences are very difficult to establish reliably from observational studies, since the magnitude of the observed effect of treatment may be similar to the effect of uncontrolled and, indeed, uncontrollable confounding. This situation has been a particular problem for assessment of risks and benefits of drugs such as CCBs and for testing hypotheses where there is confounding by indication, namely, selective prescribing of an agent for patients with prior disease and/or cardiovascular risk factors that independently increase their risk of subsequent cardiovascular events. In these circumstances, the conduct of a randomized trial will yield the strongest and most reliable evidence on which to base a judgment of whether an observed association is one of cause and effect.

EFFECTS OF CALCIUM CHANNEL BLOCKERS ON CARDIOVASCULAR DISEASE RISK

Basic Research

Most CCBs act by blocking the L-type calcium channel.[15] There are three major classes of CCBs,[16] namely, phenylalkylamines (e.g., verapamil), benzothiazepines (e.g., diltiazem), and dihydropyridines (e.g., nifedipine, nicardipine, nimodipine, nitrendipine, nisoldipine, amlodipine, and felodipine). The original short-acting preparations have been replaced by long-acting ones.[17] Regardless of duration, the pharmacological effects of CCBs include coronary and peripheral vasodilatation and reduced myocardial contractility. The phenylalkylamines and benzothiazepines may slow heart rate and produce atrioventricular nodal blockade, whereas some dihydropyridines cause a reflex increase in heart rate.[17]

Clinical Research

CCBs reduce blood pressure and have become an attractive option for health care providers and their patients because of the perception that their side effects are far less common than those of the thiazides and β-blockers. Further, there is selective utilization in patients with hypertension who also have angina because these drugs prolong treadmill exercise time and reduce episodes of myocardial ischemia.[18] For these and other reasons, prescriptions of CCBs for hypertension have increased so markedly that they have become the most widely prescribed antihypertensive drug in the United States.[7] Despite their high frequency of use, however, data on the benefit:risk ratio of CCBs on clinically relevant outcomes in relation to other therapies for hypertension are not yet available from large-scale randomized trials.

Observational Epidemiological Studies

In some, but not all, observational epidemiological studies, both case-control and cohort, patients prescribed CCBs for hypertension appeared to have somewhat higher risks of cardiovascular disease, cancer, and bleeding than those prescribed other antihypertensive medications. Three case-control studies have reported data about the risks of myocardial infarction or death from CHD among hypertensive patients treated with a CCB. One observed an increased CHD risk in patients treated with a CCB[19] and two did not.[20, 21] Among those not reporting an increase in risk, one included about 200 cases and 800 controls[20] and the other included about 100 cases and 300 controls.[21] Both were too small to detect even a doubling in the risk of CHD with CCBs. The case-control study that reported an increase in risk involved about 600 cases and 2000 controls.[19] Among patients prescribed a CCB, the risk of a major CHD event was about 60% greater than that observed in patients treated with other drugs. The increased risk primarily reflected a higher risk of CHD events among those patients treated with a nondihydropyridine calcium antagonist. This study also showed that patients prescribed a CCB were more likely than others to have a previous history of CHD or other risk factors, such as diabetes. The higher risk of CHD events among patients treated with CCBs persisted after attempts to adjust for disease history and risk factor profile.

A further case-control study has recently reported data about the risks of a variety of cardiovascular events (but not CHD risks separately) among hypertensive patients treated with a CCB.[22] That study included about 200 cases and a similar number of controls and reported no overall increase in risk among patients prescribed a calcium antagonist (odds ratio 0.89, 95% Cl: 0.45 to 1.75). Although there was no evidence of increased risk among patients treated with a long-acting CCB, an increased risk was observed among patients taking a short-acting preparation (odds ratio 3.98, 95% Cl: 1.18 to 13.89). However, the prevalence of prior cardiovascular disease was much higher among patients receiving treatment with a short-acting CCB (63%) than among those receiving treatment with a long-acting CCB (38%) or another antihypertensive drug (21%). Although an increased risk of cardiovascular events among patients treated with a short-acting CCB was still evident among those patients without a cardiovascular disease history, the extremely high relative risk (12.4) and the small number of individuals in this subgroup treated with short-acting CCBs (nine cases and one control) severely limits the interpretability of this result.

In virtually all such observational studies, the decision to prescribe a CCB was frequently determined, at least in part, by factors associated with increased risk of CHD (e.g., disease history, age, risk factor levels). Thus, the use of hypertensive patients as controls will not necessarily avoid confounding by indication. Although the statistical analyses of these studies included adjustment for some potential confounding factors, this provides little reassurance that "indication bias" is not a plausible alternative explanation for the observed findings. Such statistical adjustment is likely to be incomplete owing to several factors. First, most studies were not designed to test the question. Second, there is a large error with which confounding factors (e.g., disease history or risk factor levels) were measured. Third, there was a limited number of potential confounding factors for which data were available (e.g., typically, few data were available about evidence of subclinical atherosclerotic or myocardial disease that may affect prescribing patterns). Comparisons of risk in patients treated with a CCB and patients treated with a β-blocker may not be free of indication bias. Although both treatments may be selectively given to high-risk patients (perhaps for the treatment of angina), there is no particular reason to expect that the average CHD risk (in the absence of treatment) in patients treated with a CCB should necessarily be the same as that in patients treated with a β-blocker. Moreover, the suggestion of a dose-response association, although consistent with the hypothesis of a true adverse effect of CCBs on CHD risk, could also be explained by the preferential use of higher doses of CCBs in very high-risk patients, perhaps for the control of higher blood pressures[23] or more refractory angina.

An increased risk of CHD events among hypertensive patients prescribed a calcium antagonist has also been reported in an analysis of a small subgroup of about 900 participants from a prospective study of more than 10,000 elderly individuals.[24] The subgroup for which data were reported included only patients treated with a single antihypertensive agent and excluded those treated with multiple agents as well as those not receiving antihypertensive therapy. In this subgroup, there was a total of about 50 CHD deaths observed during follow-up, and among those without a history of CHD, there were only about 60 fatal and nonfatal CHD events in total. The distribution of these events suggested a severalfold greater risk of CHD events among those treated with nifedipine or diltiazem (but not verapamil). As in some of the case-control studies described previously, patients prescribed a CCB were likely to have a higher-risk medical history and a worse risk factor profile than those treated with other drugs. The increased risk persisted after controlling for some potential confounding factors. Thus, it is once again likely that the observed higher risk of CHD events in patients treated with a CCB reflects, at least in part, the selection of higher-risk patients for such treatment. The magnitude of the risk observed among patients prescribed CCBs in this study population is implausibly large and inconsistent with the available results from randomized trials of CCBs in patients with CHD. This underlines the magnitude of the biases that can affect such nonrandomized studies.

Three other cohort studies have reported on the risk of all-cause mortality (but not specifically the risk of CHD events) among patients with a history of CHD receiving treatment with CCBs.[25–27] In one study of 1200 patients with myocardial infarction, overall mortality rates appeared to be higher among patients treated with either nifedipine or verapamil.[25] In another study of about 11,000 patients with established CHD, half of whom were treated with CCBs (half with nifedipine and a third with diltiazem), there was no clear increase in risk.[26] Once again, however, in both of these studies, there was evidence that patients prescribed CCBs tended to have a worse medical history and/or risk factor profile than did others, and the possibility that either of these results could have been importantly affected by confounding cannot be excluded. Further, a report on 7 years of follow-up in the Framingham Study provided no evidence of increased mortality among 400 hypertensive patients (half with a history of CHD) treated with a calcium antagonist.[27]

Most recently, the Nurses' Health Study assessed prospectively among 14,617 hypertensive female nurses or former nurses whether those prescribed CCBs had elevated rates of cardiovascular or total mortality.[28] This cohort study demonstrated the presence of confounding by indication. Compared with hypertensive women prescribed other agents, those prescribed CCBs had covariate-adjusted relative risks for cardiovascular mortality of 2.84 and 1.82 for total mortality before and 1.47 and 1.43, respectively, after exclusion of women with prior cardiovascular disease. The authors concluded that whether any remaining observed increase in relative risk is real, due to chance, or due to residual confounding by indication, cannot be resolved in observational data.

Randomized Trials

Data on the direct effects of CCBs on major CHD events are available from several small randomized trials in patients with hypertension, none of which was designed specifically to assess the effects of treatment on such outcomes. Some were placebo-controlled[29, 30] and some compared the effects of CCBs with other antihypertensive drugs.[29–32] Most of the trials investigated the effects of long-acting dihydropyridine drugs. Although these trials collectively involved a total of about 6000 patients, only about 50 cases of nonfatal myocardial infarction or death from CHD were observed during scheduled follow-up. Consequently, neither individually nor in combination did these trials document sufficient CHD events for the reliable determination of any plausible difference in risk between CCBs and placebo, let alone between CCBs and other drugs. So, although CHD events were similarly distributed among CCBs, other active treatment, and placebo groups in these trials, the results do not preclude real differences in outcome—in either direction—of moderate (or even large) magnitude. Thus, the available data from randomized trials of CCBs in patients with hypertension provide inadequate evidence from which to draw firm conclusions.

One nonrandomized trial of a long-acting formulation of nifedipine (which used alternate assignment to active treatment or placebo instead of proper random assignment) has been reported.[33] In that study, among 1632 Chinese patients, only 4 cases of myocardial infarction were reported during 30 months of follow-up; strokes appeared to be less frequent among patients treated with nifedipine (16 vs. 36, relative risk 0.43; 95% CI: 0.24 to 0.77). A similar effect on stroke was also observed in one of the randomized trials conducted in China (14 nifedipine vs. 28 controls; relative risk 0.49; 95% CI: 0.26 to 0.92) (T. Zhang, personal communication, 1996).

Among the subgroup of 415 patients with elevated glycosylated hemoglobin in the Multicenter Isradipine Diuretic Atherosclerosis Study (MIDAS), 15 patients assigned to isradipine had vascular events compared with 6 randomized to diuretic ($p = .04$).[34] This data-derived subgroup finding is limited by the small number of cases. The primary endpoint of the trial was progression of early atherosclerosis in carotid arteries, for which there were no treatment differences.[32]

Data from two additional trials indicated benefits of ACE inhibitors compared with CCBs in the treatment of diabetics with hypertension. In the Fosinopril versus Amlodipine Cardiovascular Events Randomized Trial (FACET), the 189 patients assigned fosinopril had 14 cardiovascular events compared with 27 among the 191 patients assigned amlodipine ($p = .03$).[35] The Appropriate Blood Pressure Control in Diabetes (ABCD) trial found a benefit of enalapril compared with nisoldipine.[36] In a subgroup of 470 diabetic hypertensive patients, 25 of 235 in the nisoldipine group had fatal or nonfatal myocardial infarctions, compared with 5 in the enalapril group ($p = .001$). Since there was no placebo group, it is unclear whether CCBs are deleterious or ACE inhibitors are simply more beneficial in reducing rates of myocardial infarction among diabetic patients with hypertension.

In the large Hypertension Optimal Treatment (HOT) trial of 18,790 patients, all received felodipine as initial therapy followed by additional drugs to achieve alternative target blood pressures.[37] This trial achieved substantially greater reductions in rates of cardiovascular events than expected from previous trials using alternative treatments. Further, treatment appeared particularly valuable among the 1501 diabetic patients.[38] The Systolic Hypertension in Europe (SYST-EUR) trial randomized 2398 elderly patients with isolated systolic hypertension to nitrendipine and 2297 to placebo. Those assigned active treatment had a 42% reduction in fatal or nonfatal stroke ($p = .003$) and a 26% reduction in fatal or nonfatal cardiac endpoints ($p = .03$).[39]

EFFECTS OF CALCIUM CHANNEL BLOCKERS ON CANCER RISK

In some but not all cohort studies, a modest direct association between blood pressure levels and the overall risk of death from cancer has been reported.[40] However, analyses based on the totality of evidence from a large number of cohort studies have not demonstrated such an association (Prospective Studies Collaboration, unpublished data, 1997). Although complete data on cancer incidence are not available from the earlier trials of antihypertensive treatment, those studies have demonstrated no change in the risk of death from nonvascular causes among patients assigned active treatment, mostly with diuretic- or β-blocker–based regimens.[41, 42] Similarly, no complete or reliable data on cancer incidence are available from the more recent randomized trials of CCBs in patients with hypertension or CHD. A review by the U.S. Food and Drug Administration (A. DeDelice, personal communication, 1997) of all the available evidence concerning rodent tumorigenicity concluded that there was no evidence of a direct carcinogenic effect of registered calcium antagonists in several strains of rats and mice and no indication of genotoxicity in a variety of bacterial and mammalian cells calibrated with known mutagens. Although there has been a report that verapamil increased the in vitro growth of human colon and breast cancer cell lines,[43] the main concerns about possible effects on cancer have arisen primarily from the results of some observational studies of patients treated with a CCB.

Two reports[44, 45] from part of the same parent cohort as the smaller study on CCBs and total mortality referred to previously[24] (and so involving some of the same people) describe a somewhat greater incidence of cancer among patients prescribed a CCB than among others in the population studied. This cohort study involved a total of 5052 elderly individuals followed for 4 years. The first report was based on a total of 61 cases of cancer, 27 of which occurred among patients treated with a CCB. Thus, neither report from this study involved sufficient cancer cases to reliably characterize any plausible modest association. Moreover, the two reports do not provide independent evidence about the association, since it appears that the cancer cases included in the first analysis were also included in the second, and in the report based on the larger number of cases, the observed increase in the crude rate of cancer among CCB-treated patients was of only borderline statistical significance ($p = .03$). Multivariate-adjusted analyses of the data suggested a greater increase in cancer risk with CCB use (adjusted odds ratio 1.72; 95% CI: 1.27 to 2.34). This increase in risk was observed in patients prescribed either nifedipine or verapamil but did not appear to reflect an increase in any one type of cancer (or subgroup of related cancers). As in some of the observational studies of CHD, there also appeared to be a direct association between the dose of CCB used and risk. It was suggested that these findings could be explained by a cancer-promoting effect of CCBs, mediated perhaps by inhibition of apoptosis. Although there is evidence that CCBs can inhibit experimentally induced apoptosis[46, 47] and increase the in vitro growth of certain human cancer cell lines,[43] other data on the effects of CCBs on apoptosis and growth in a tissue with increased proliferation indicate stimulation of apoptosis and inhibition of proliferation.[48]

A second prospective study, conducted among participants in the Cardiovascular Health Study, reported that women prescribed CCBs had an increased risk of cancer. This finding was based on 75 cases of incident invasive breast cancer,[49] of which 20 occurred among women prescribed CCBs. In analyses adjusted for measured confounders, women prescribed CCBs had a risk of breast cancer 2.57 times that of nonusers (95% CI: 1.47 to 4.49) and 2.91 times that of users of other antihypertensive medications (95% CI: 1.41 to 6.00). However, this study lacked information on duration of use of CCBs. Women prescribed CCBs tended to have greater comorbidity than women prescribed other antihypertensive agents, and some important measures of comorbidity and breast cancer risk factors, such as family history, were not assessed. By contrast, a far larger prospective cohort study, the Nurses' Health Study, showed no association between prescription of CCBs for hypertension and subsequent risk of breast cancer among 379 cases.[50]

Three case-control studies also showed no association between prescription of CCBs and cancer.[51–53] Jick and colleagues compared 446 incident cases of cancer with 1750 controls, all of whom were prescribed ACE inhibitors, CCBs, or β-blockers.[51] Overall, the risk of cancer among women prescribed CCBs was 1.27 times that of β-blocker users (95% CI: 0.98 to 1.63). However, the risk did not increase by duration. Rosenberg and coworkers compared 9513 incident cancer cases with 6492 hospitalized controls and found that women prescribed CCBs had 1.1 times the risk of cancer compared with nonusers (95% CI: 0.9 to 1.3).[52] Relative to women prescribed β-blockers, women prescribed CCBs had a relative risk of 0.9 (95% CI: 0.8 to 1.1). This study also showed no association between duration of CCB use and cancer risk. Neither of these case-control studies found an association between breast cancer and use of CCBs. One case-control study of colon cancer has reported an extreme increase in risk among patients treated with verapamil but not with other CCBs. However, only 11 patients in the entire study population reported prescription of verapamil.[53]

As in the observational studies of CHD, confounding by indication is a plausible alternative explanation of the findings from these observational studies of CCBs and cancer. At entry, there was evidence of a more frequent history of ill health among patients prescribed a CCB. Although the increased risk of cancer persisted after controlling for some aspects of medical history and a few other relevant factors that had been recorded (e.g., smoking, alcohol consumption, and body mass index), for reasons given earlier and elsewhere[54] such analyses cannot fully exclude confounding by indication as an alternative explanation. Residual confounding would be consistent with the observation that the association was not with just one or a few types of cancer but was with a generalized increase in most cancer types. Established exogenous causes of cancer typically affect particular sites selectively, and the apparently broad association of CCB use with cancer risk in this study population could be explained by more frequent use of these agents among sicker patients generally, including some whose symptoms were the consequence of undiagnosed cancer. Moreover, the apparent absence of the usual latent period between exposure and cancer development is also atypical of established exogenous causes of cancer, and this would once again suggest that residual confounding may be an explanation.

It has also been observed that sicker patients—as were the patients treated with a CCB in this study—are typically less likely to relocate than others who are in better health.[54] For this reason, it is possible that there may be a bias toward the less frequent detection not only of cancers but also of other conditions (e.g., myocardial infarction) among healthier individuals. Additionally, sicker patients could be more likely to receive diagnostic investigations that uncover malignancies, and this could also introduce detection bias, particularly over the short duration of these studies. Both of these sources of detection bias could result in a spurious apparent increase in risk among sicker patients, such as those prescribed a CCB.

EFFECTS OF CALCIUM CHANNEL BLOCKERS ON BLEEDING RISK

It has been suggested that CCBs might cause bleeding by inhibiting platelet aggregation while also preventing the normal vasoconstrictive response to bleeding.[55] A randomized, placebo-controlled trial of the dihydropyridine CCB nimodipine was stopped prematurely (after 149 of a scheduled 400 patients undergoing cardiac valve replacement had been recruited) owing to a few more deaths having been observed among those allocated nimodipine (8/75 [11%] vs. 1/74 [1%]).[56] As major bleeding during and after surgery appeared to occur often in that trial, analyses of bleeding were performed that indicated an excess of major bleeding with nimodipine (10 [13%] vs. 2 [3%]; $p = .03$). Subsequently, four observational studies explored the association between calcium antagonist use and bleeding.[55, 57–59] The first of these was a cohort study that included a total of 120 individuals with gastrointestinal bleeds, of which 47 were considered to be severe, among a total population of 1636 individuals aged 68 years or older prescribed β-blockers, CCBs, or ACE inhibitors for any indication.[55] Compared with β-blocker use, the use of any CCB was associated with an increased risk of any gastrointestinal bleeding (31 bleeds; relative risk 1.68; 95% CI: 1.03 to 2.74). Surprisingly, this was similar to the excess risk observed with aspirin use (relative risk 1.5) and with oral anticoagulants (relative risk 2.2). This apparent increase in any gastrointestinal bleeding was observed with the use of diltiazem (18 bleeds; relative risk 2.8; 95% CI: 1.24 to 3.82) and verapamil (13 bleeds; relative risk 2.39, 95% CI: 1.28 to 4.44) but not with nifedipine (9 bleeds; relative risk 1.04; 95% CI: 0.51 to 2.13).

A similar, although nonsignificant, increase in the risk of gastrointestinal bleeding was also observed among those prescribed CCBs (odds ratio 1.87; 95% CI: 0.79 to 4.41) in a study of 73 cases and 73 age- and gender-matched controls. However, in that study, 70 to 80% of patients treated with CCBs were using nifedipine.[57] By contrast, a large study comparing outcome between 2248 CCB-treated patients undergoing cardiac surgery and 2909 cardiac surgery patients not receiving these agents did not indicate any increases in transfusions (about 200 in total: 3% on CCB vs. 5% not) or reoperations for bleeding (about 100: 1% vs. 2%). There were significant trends toward fewer such bleeds with CCB use.[58] Similarly, in a small series of 120 patients undergoing coronary artery graft surgery, CCB use was not associated with any increases in postoperative bleeding or transfusions.[59]

CLINICAL IMPLICATIONS

In 1988, the fourth report of the Joint National Committee on the Detection, Evaluation, and Treatment of High Blood Pressure (JNC IV) recommended CCBs and ACE inhibitors as first-line choices for blood pressure treatment, in addition to diuretics and β-blockers.[60] Lack of comparative data on morbidity and mortality from randomized trials for CCBs and ACE inhibitors led national committees such as the JNC in 1993 (JNC V)[61] as well as the World Health Organization (WHO) and the International Society of Hypertension (ISH)[62] in 1997 to recommend diuretics and/or β-blockers as initial monotherapy for hypertension, and to reserve CCBs and ACE inhibitors as second-line choices when diuretics and β-blockers proved unacceptable or ineffective. The National Heart, Lung, and Blood Institute (NHLBI) stated that "short-acting nifedipine should be used with great caution (if at all), especially at higher doses, in the treatment of hypertension, angina, and MI [myocardial infarction]."[63] The JNC VI recommendations have reaffirmed diuretics and β-blockers as first-line choices and reserved CCBs for special indications.[64]

In general, data on drug efficacy and safety from observational studies should be interpreted with considerable caution because residual confounding by indication may remain even after careful consideration of other risk factors and comorbidity. In these circumstances, for small to moderate effects, randomized trials specifically designed to compare efficacies and adverse effects of the various antihypertensive medications are advantageous. The SYST-EUR trial indicated net cardiovascular benefit of the medium-acting CCB nitrendipine compared with placebo among patients with isolated systolic hypertension.[39] Because no comparison with other antihypertensives was made, inferences on the relative benefit or hazard of CCBs cannot be made from this trial.

Because short-acting CCBs have largely been supplanted by long-acting formulations in clinical practice, clinical trials that are currently under way are randomizing long-acting CCBs against other antihypertensive agents, including the first-line drugs—diuretics and β-blockers. Whether short-acting CCBs have harmful effects compared with other antihypertensive agents may never be completely resolved.

It should be reassuring to clinicians and their patients that most scientific organizations, including NHLBI[65] and WHO-ISH,[62] believe that the results of the several large ongoing trials will be necessary to complete the totality of evidence on the risk:benefit ratio of CCBs. The fact that these trials have not been terminated early suggests either that the results are null or that any beneficial or harmful effects must be far smaller than reported from the observational studies. In the meanwhile, the JNC VI guidelines provide a rational basis for clinical decisions for individual patients and policy recommendations for the health of the general public.

SUMMARY AND CONCLUSIONS

CCBs are used extensively throughout the world for the treatment of high blood pressure and angina. In Japan, they are prescribed for about three quarters of all treated hypertensive patients,[59] and in China, CCBs (mostly short-acting agents) are prescribed for about half of all such patients (L. Liu, personal communication, 1997). In these Far Eastern countries, the main objective of antihypertensive treatment is the prevention of stroke, since the risks of CHD are very much lower. For this reason, the concerns that have been raised about adverse effects of CCBs—particularly the short-acting agents—on CHD risk are less relevant to their use in the Far East than in the West. In Europe and the United States, CCBs are prescribed for a smaller but still substantial proportion of patients with high blood pressure.

The major objectives of antihypertensive treatment in these populations are the prevention of both stroke and CHD events. However, at the present time, data on stroke and CHD are available from only four small randomized trials of CCB use in patients with hypertension, and even in aggregate, the data do not provide sufficient, reliable information about effects of these drugs on these important outcomes of treatment with CCBs vs. other agents. There are more data on CHD events from trials of CCBs in patients with myocardial infarction or angina, but overviews of these trials do not show a clear overall effect of CCBs on risks of myocardial infarction or death from any cause. Subgroup analyses of trials with particular agents suggest the possibility of modestly beneficial effects of diltiazem and verapamil and modestly adverse effects of nifedipine. But these trends were not strong, and they could well be biased—both in favor of and against particular agents—as a consequence of the retrospective manner in which they were identified. The limited information available from trials of CCBs in patients with heart failure adds little to the assessment of the effects of these agents on the risk of CHD.

Although the data from randomized trials are limited, they do exclude the possibility of adverse effects of the extreme magnitude suggested in reports from some observational studies. For example, the upper 95% confidence limit of the estimated effect of nifedipine in randomized trials in patients with CHD includes a plausible adverse effect of 30 to 50%. This is substantially less than the 60 to 300% increases in risk suggested by some observational studies of hypertensive patients, underlining the very large potential for bias in such studies and suggesting that their results may be largely, perhaps wholly, due to residual confounding by indication rather than to drug effects. There is clear evidence from several studies that CCBs are preferentially prescribed to the sickest patients, including those with CHD and other high-risk conditions such as diabetes, and it is unlikely that statistical adjustment for confounding can entirely remove this source of bias.

The available evidence does not prove the existence of either beneficial or harmful effects of CCBs on the risks of major CHD events, including fatal or nonfatal myocardial infarctions and other deaths from CHD. This applies to the evidence for all CCBs considered collectively and to that for classes of these agents.

Evidence about the effects of CCBs on the risk of cancer is derived almost entirely from observational studies. The observed increases in cancer risk could reflect chance, systematic error, or a true adverse effect. The very small numbers of cancer cases on which the findings of increased risk were based and the modest level of statistical significance are consistent with chance being a plausible explanation. The results may well also have been affected by confounding by indication, since patients in poor health appear to be prescribed CCBs more frequently than other antihypertensive drugs. Detection bias may also have occurred, with adverse outcomes more likely to be detected among those prescribed CCBs, who as a consequence of their poorer state of health may be both less likely to relocate and more likely to receive diagnostic procedures. The possibility of residual confounding, even after statistical adjustment, is consistent with the observation that the increased risk appears to be distributed widely across cancer subtypes, as well as between other distinctly different disease entities (including gastrointestinal hemorrhage[55] and Parkinson's disease[66]). Although a biological mechanism has been proposed to account for the observed possible increased cancer risk in some observational studies, this is highly speculative and controversial.[67] The proposed mechanism is inconsistent with evidence from animal studies demonstrating no carcinogenicity of any CCB approved for use in the United States.

In considering the evidence about cancer risk, there is cause to reflect on earlier reports from observational studies raising concerns about possible adverse effects of reserpine,[68–70] another blood pressure–lowering drug, on breast cancer risk. The observation was subsequently shown to be the consequence of confounding.[71] Other reports of an increased cancer risk associated with atenolol[72] and enalapril[73] remain unconfirmed, but they too seem likely to have been the consequences of chance and selective post hoc emphasis. Thus, the available data from observational studies do not provide good evidence of an adverse effect of CCBs on cancer risk.

The available evidence on CCBs and bleeding does not indicate a consistent pattern of hazard. Excesses of bleeding among patients prescribed CCBs observed in some observational studies and randomized trials of small sample size have not been observed in other, larger studies. Moreover, in certain circumstances where the risks are high, no excesses of severe bleeding or adverse outcome due to bleeding were evident among patients prescribed CCBs. So, although it is not possible to rule out modest effects, the available evidence does not seem to be consistent with the large bleeding risk (i.e., similar to that associated with oral anticoagulants) that has been suggested by some investigators. Thus, the available data from observational studies and randomized trials do not provide clear evidence of an adverse effect of CCBs on bleeding risks.

It is unfortunate that pharmaceutical companies, regulatory authorities, and clinical researchers did not ensure the timely conduct of large-scale randomized trials to provide clinicians and patients with reliable evidence about both the safety and the efficacy of widely prescribed CCBs. Fortunately, a number of such trials are now under way. Some of these were ongoing at the time that concerns about safety of CCBs were raised, and others were initiated in direct response to the controversy. By early in the next decade, data should be available from trials involving about 100,000 patients with hypertension randomized to treatment with a CCB or a diuretic/β-blocker–based regimen. About half of these patients will be in trials of the newer slow-release or long-acting dihydropyridine agents, and the remainder will be in trials of nondihydropyridine drugs. These trials should be able to determine reliably whether CCB-based regimens have importantly different effects on CHD and major bleeding risks from those conferred by diuretic- or β-blocker–based regimens. Long-term follow-up of patients in these trials beyond the scheduled treatment period could also provide useful information about the effects of these agents, if any, on cancer risk. Such large-scale trials of efficacy and safety should *routinely* be initiated early in the development of new drug classes that are destined to be marketed for the treatment of common cardiovascular diseases.

It is also unfortunate that observational studies not even designed to test the questions have played a major role in generating public concerns about possible adverse effects of CCBs. Some investigators have even suggested that, in the absence of randomized trials, observational studies can provide a suitable basis for clinical and policy decisions.[74] Others, however, have acknowledged their limitations.[75] Specifically, the results of previous observational studies of medical interventions indicate that unless the observed effect of treatment is very large, the results of such studies cannot provide a reliable guide to the size, or even the direction, of the real treatment effects. This is probably, in large part, due to confounding by indication, but it may also reflect detection bias and publication bias. It is quite possible that there are a number of observational studies with data on both CCB use and cardiovascular and cancer outcomes that remain unpublished. Since null findings are less likely to be published than positive findings,[76] it is questionable whether the currently available data are representative of the totality of the observational data potentially available.

In conclusion, the available evidence about the effects of CCBs on the risks of CHD, cancer, and bleeding does not establish the existence of beneficial or harmful effects. This conclusion has few implications for current guidelines about the treatment of hypertension, since most already acknowledge the absence of reliable randomized evidence about the effects of CCBs on major morbidity and mortality. The results of this review similarly do not provide any strong reason to change recommendations for the treatment of angina. However, they do underline the large differences that exist in the strength of the evidence available about the effects of different classes of blood pressure–lowering drugs on major health outcomes. For patients with hypertension, there is now very strong evidence from randomized trials that treatment regimens involving diuretics and β-blockers (in combination with a wide variety of other older antihypertensive agents) are effective in reducing the risks of major CHD events and stroke; no effect on major nonvascular causes of death (of which there were, in aggregate, several hundred) was detected during the 5-year average duration of these trials.[41, 42] For patients with a history of myocardial infarction, there is strong evidence from randomized trials that treatment with a β-blocker reduces the risks of death and reinfarction.[77, 78] In the presence of left ventricular dysfunction or heart failure, there is clear evidence from randomized trials of beneficial effects of ACE inhibitors on overall mortality and heart failure–related morbidity[79] and emerging evidence of benefit for major CHD events.[80] However, for other patient groups (including those with hypertension), there is still no direct evidence from randomized trials of beneficial (or harmful) effects of calcium CCBs on major cardiovascular morbidity and mortality in any patient group. Although the trends for verapamil and diltiazem in patients with a history of myocardial infarction are suggestive of benefit and the trends for nifedipine are suggestive of harm, selective emphasis on these classes of agents was largely retrospective, and the trends could, therefore, be inflated (or produced entirely) by chance and selection bias. Hence, these findings require confirmation in further trials. For other newer agents, such as α-adrenergic receptor blockers and angiotensin II receptor blockers, there is no evidence whatsoever about their effects on major cardiovascular events in any patient group. Whether CCBs or the other newer agents have similar, lesser, or greater effects on major cardiovascular outcomes than the older established drugs will not be known for several more years, when the ongoing trials are completed.

References

1. Glynn RJ, Brock DB, Harris T, et al. Use of antihypertensive drugs and trends in blood pressure in the elderly. Arch Intern Med 155:1855–1860, 1995.
2. Burt VL, Whelton P, Roccella EJ, et al. Prevalence of hypertension in the U.S. adult population. Results from the Third National Health and Nutrition Examination Survey, 1988–1991. Hypertension 25:305–313, 1995.
3. National Center for Health Statistics. Blood pressure levels in persons 18–74 years of age in 1976–1980, and trends in blood pressure from 1960–1980 in the United States. Vital and Health Statistics, series 11, no. 234. DHHS Publication No. (PHS) 86-1684. Washington, DC, U.S. Government Printing Office, 1986.
4. Sprafka JM, Burke GL, Folsom AR, et al. Continued decline in cardiovascular disease risk factors: Results of the Minnesota Heart Survey, 1980–1982 and 1985–1987. Am J Epidemiol 132:489–500, 1990.
5. Glynn RJ, Field TS, Satterfield S, et al. Modification of increasing systolic blood pressure in the elderly during the 1980s. Am J Epidemiol 138:365–79, 1993.
6. Psaty BM, Savage PJ, Tell GS, et al. Temporal patterns of antihypertensive medication use among elderly patients. JAMA 270:1837–1841, 1993.
7. Manolio TA, Cutler JA, Furberg CD, et al. Trends in pharmacologic management of hypertension in the United States. Arch Intern Med 155:829–837, 1995.
8. Monane M, Glynn RJ, Gurwitz JH, et al. Trends in medication choices for hypertension in the elderly. The decline of the thiazides. Hypertension 25:1045–1051, 1995.
9. Siegel D, Lopez J. Trends in antihypertensive drug use in the United States. JAMA 278:1747–1748, 1997.
10. Hennekens CH, Buring JE. Epidemiology in Medicine. Boston, Little, Brown, 1987.
11. Hennekens CH. The increasing burden of cardiovascular disease: Current knowledge and future directions for research on risk factors. Circulation 97:1095–1102, 1998.
12. Cairns J. The treatment of diseases and the war against cancer. Sci Am 253:51–59, 1985.
13. Doll R, Peto R. The causes of cancer. New York, Oxford University Press, 1981.
14. Hennekens CH, Buring JE. Observational evidence. *In* Warren KS, Mosteller F (eds). Doing More Good Than Harm: The Evaluation of Health Care Interventions. Ann NY Acad Sci 703:18–24, 1993.

15. Katz AM. Calcium channel diversity in the cardiovascular system. J Am Coll Cardiol 28:522–529, 1996.

16. Godfraind T. Classification of calcium antagonists. Am J Cardiol 59:11B–23B, 1987.

17. Freedman DD, Walters DD. "Second generation" dihydropyridine calcium antagonists. Greater vascular selectivity and some unique applications. Drugs 34:578–598, 1987.

18. Waters D. Calcium channel blockers. In Hennekens CH, Buring JE, Manson JE, Ridker PM (eds). Randomized Trials in Cardiovascular Disease. Philadelphia, WB Saunders, 1999.

19. Psaty B, Heckbert S, Koepsell T, et al. The risk of myocardial infarction associated with antihypertensive drug therapies. JAMA 274:620–625, 1995.

20. Jick H, Derby L, Gurewich V, Vasilakis C. The risk of myocardial infarction in persons with uncomplicated essential hypertension. Pharmacotherapy 16:321–326, 1996.

21. Aursnes I, Litleskare I, Froyland H, Abdelnoor M. Association between various drugs used for hypertension and risk of acute myocardial infarction. Blood Press 4:157–163, 1995.

22. Alderman MH, Cohen H, Roque R, Madhavan S. Effect of long-acting and short-acting calcium antagonists on cardiovascular outcomes in hypertensive patients. Lancet 349:594–598, 1997.

23. Mancia G, Van Zwieten P. How safe are calcium antagonists in hypertension and coronary heart disease? J Hypertens 14:13–17, 1996.

24. Pahor M, Guralnik J, Corti M, et al. Long-term survival and use of antihypertensive medications in older persons. J Am Geriatr Soc 43:1–7, 1995.

25. Koenig W, Lowel H, Lewis M, Hormann A. Long-term survival after myocardial infarctions: Relationship with thrombolysis and discharge medication. Results of the Augsburg Myocardial Infarction Follow-up Study 1985 to 1993. Eur Heart J 17:1199–1206, 1996.

26. Braun S, Boyko V, Behar S, et al. Calcium antagonists and mortality in patients with coronary artery disease: A cohort study of 11,575 patients. J Am Coll Cardiol 28:7–11, 1996.

27. Abascal VM, Larson MG, Evans JC, et al. Calcium antagonists and mortality risk in men and women with hypertension in the Framingham Heart Study. Arch Intern Med 158:1882–1886, 1998.

28. Michels KB, Rosner BA, Manson JE, et al. Prospective study of calcium channel blocker use, cardiovascular disease, and total mortality among hypertensive women. The Nurses' Health Study. Circulation 97:1540–1548, 1998.

29. Neaton JD, Grimm RH, Prineas RJ, et al. Treatment of mild hypertension study. Final results. J Am Coll Cardiol 270:713–724, 1993.

30. Materson B. Department of Veterans Affairs single drug therapy of hypertension: Final results. Am J Hypertens 8:189–192, 1993.

31. The GLANT Study Group. A 12-month comparison of ACE-inhibitor and CA antagonist therapy in mild to moderate essential hypertension—The GLANT Study. Hypertens Res 18:235–244, 1995.

32. Borhani NO, Mercuri M, Borhani PA, et al. Final outcome results of the Multicenter Isradipine Diuretic Atherosclerosis Study (MIDAS): A randomized controlled trial. 276:785–791, 1996.

33. Gong L, Zhang W, Zhu Y, Zhu J, et al. Shanghai Trial of Nifedipine in the Elderly (STONE). J Hypertens 14:1237–1245, 1996.

34. Byington RP, Craven T, Furberg CD, Pahor M. Isradipine, raised glycosylated haemoglobin, and risk of cardiovascular events. Lancet 350:1075–1076, 1997.

35. Tatti P, Pahor M, Byington RP, et al. Outcome results of the Fosinopril Versus Amlodipine Cardiovascular Events Randomized Trial (FACET) in patients with hypertension and NIDDM. Diabetes Care 21:597–603, 1998.

36. Estacio RO, Jeffers BW, Hiatt WR et al. The effect of nisoldipine as compared with enalapril on cardiovascular outcomes in patients with non–insulin-dependent diabetes and hypertension. N Engl J Med 338:645–652, 1998.

37. Hansson L, Zanchetti A, Carruthers SG, et al, for the HOT Study Group. Effects of intensive blood pressure lowering and low-dose aspirin in patients with hypertension: Principal results of the Hypertension Optimal Treatment (HOT) randomised trial. Lancet 351:1755–1762, 1998.

38. Kaplan N. J-curve not burned off by HOT study. [Commentary] Lancet 351:1748–1749, 1998.

39. Staessen JA, Fagard R, Thijs L, et al., for the Systolic Hypertension in Europe (SYST-EUR) Trial Investigators. Randomised double-blind comparison of placebo and active treatment for older patients with isolated systolic hypertension. Lancet 350:757–764, 1997.

40. Hamet P. Cancer and hypertension—An unresolved issue. Hypertension 28:321–324, 1996.

41. Collins R, Peto R, MacMahon S, et al. Blood pressure, stroke, and coronary heart disease. Part 2: Short-term reductions in blood pressure: Overview of randomised drug trials in their epidemiological context. Lancet 335:827–838, 1990.

42. Collins R, MacMahon S. Blood pressure, antihypertensive drug treatment and the risks of stroke and of coronary heart disease. Br Med Bull 50:272–298, 1994.

43. Correale P, Tagliaferri P, Celio L, et al. Verapamil upregulates sensitivity of human colon and breast cancer cells to LA-cytotoxicity in vitro. Eur J Cancer 27:1393–1395, 1991.

44. Pahor M, Guralnik J, Salive M, et al. Do calcium channel blockers increase the risk of cancer? Am J Hypertens 9:695–699, 1996.

45. Pahor M, Guralnik J, Ferrucci L, et al: Calcium channel blockade and incidence of cancer in aged populations. Lancet 348:493–497, 1996.

46. Connor J, Sawczuk I, Benson M, et al: Calcium channel antagonists delay regression of androgen-dependent tissues and suppress gene activity associated with cell death. Prostate 13:119–130, 1988.

47. Ray S, Kamendulis L, Gurule M, et al. Ca²⁺ antagonists inhibit DNA fragmentation and toxic cell death induced by acetaminophen. FASEB J 7:453–463, 1993.

48. DeBlois D, Tea B, Dam T, Hamet P. Increased smooth muscle cell apoptosis during regression of vascular hypertrophy in the aorta of spontaneously hypertensive rats. Hypertension 29:340–349, 1997.

49. Fitzpatrick AL, Dalin JR, Furberg CD, et al. Use of calcium channel blockers and breast carcinoma risk in postmenopausal women. Cancer 80:1438–1447, 1997.

50. Michels KB, Rosner BA, Walker AM, et al. Calcium channel blockers, cancer incidence, and cancer mortality in a cohort of U.S. women. Cancer 83:2003–2007, 1998.

51. Jick H, Jick S, Derby LE, et al. Calcium-channel blockers and risk of cancer. Lancet 349:525–528, 1997.

52. Rosenberg L, Rao RS, Palmer JR, et al. Calcium channel blockers and the risk of cancer. JAMA 279:1000–1004, 1998.

53. Hardell L, Fredrikson M, Axelson O. Case control study on colon cancer regarding previous diseases and drug intake. Int J Oncol 8:439–444, 1996.

54. Ekbom A, Adama H. Kalciumantagonister och cancer—En oversikt. Inf Lakemedelsveket 7:3–5, 1996.

55. Pahor M, Guralnik J, Furberg C, et al. Risk of gastrointestinal haemorrhage with calcium antagonists in hypertensive persons over 67 years old. Lancet 347:1061–1065, 1996.

56. Wagenknecht L, Furberg C, Hammon J, et al. Surgical bleeding: Unexpected effect of a calcium antagonist. BMJ 210:776–777, 1995.

57. Pilotto A, Leandro G, Franceschi M, et al. Antagonism to calcium antagonists. Lancet 347:1761–1762, 1996.

58. Grodecki-DeFranco PV, Steinhubl SR, Taylor PC, et al. Calcium antagonist use and perioperative bleeding complications: An analysis of 5,157 patients. [Abstract] Circulation 94(suppl):I-476, 1996.

59. Hynynen M, Kurtunen A, Salmenpera M. Surgical bleeding and calcium antagonists. [Letter, comment] BMJ 312:313, 1996.

60. Joint National Committee on Detection, Evaluation, and Treatment of High Blood Pressure. The 1988 report. Arch Intern Med 148:1023–1038, 1988.

61. Joint National Committee on Detection, Evaluation, and Treatment of High Blood Pressure. The fifth report. Arch Intern Med 153:154–183, 1993.

62. Ad Hoc Subcommittee of the Liaison Committee of the World Health Organization and the International Society of Hypertension. Effects of calcium antagonists on the risks of coronary heart disease, cancer and bleeding. J Hypertens 15:105–115, 1997.

63. New Analyses Regarding the Safety of Calcium Channel Blockers: A Statement for Health Professionals From the National Heart, Lung, and Blood Institute. Rockville, MD, U.S. Department of Health and Human Services, 1995.

64. Joint National Committee on Prevention, Detection, Evaluation, and Treatment of High Blood Pressure. The sixth report. Arch Intern Med 157:2413–2446, 1997.

65. Cutler JA. Calcium-channel blockers for hypertension—Uncertainty continues. N Engl J Med 338:61–63, 1998.

66. Murros K, Furberg C. Calcium antagonists and extrapyramidal symptoms. Circulation 94(suppl):I-579, 1996.

67. Brown M. Calcium-channel blockers and cancer. Lancet 348:1166, 1996.

68. Boston Collaborative Drug Surveillance Program. Reserpine and breast cancer. Lancet 2:669–671, 1974.
69. Armstrong B, Stevens N, Doll R. Retrospective study of the association between use of *Rauwolfia* derivatives and breast cancer. Lancet 2:672–674, 1974.
70. Heinonen O, Shapiro S, Tuominen L, Turunen M. Reserpine use in relation to breast cancer. Lancet 2:675–677, 1974.
71. Horwitz R, Feinstein A. Exclusion bias and the false relationship of reserpine and breast cancer. Arch Intern Med 145:1873–1875, 1985.
72. MRC Working Party: Medical Research Council Trial of Treatment of Hypertension in Older Adults: Principal results. BMJ 304:405–412, 1992.
73. SOLVD investigators: Effect of enalapril on mortality and the development of heart failure in asymptomatic patients with reduced left ventricular ejection fractions. N Engl J Med 372:685–691, 1992.
74. Walker A, Stampfer M. Observational studies of drug safety. Lancet 348:489, 1996.

75. Buring J, Glynn R, Hennekens C. Calcium channel blockers and myocardial infarction. A hypothesis formulated but not yet tested. JAMA 274:654–655, 1995.
76. Easterbrook P, Berlin J, Gopalan R, Matthew D Publication bias in clinical research. Lancet 337:867–872, 1991.
77. Yusuf S, Peto R, Lewis J, et al. Beta-blockade during and after myocardial infarction. An overview of the randomized trials. Prog Cardiovasc Dis 27:335–371, 1985.
78. Hennekens CH, Albert CM, Godfried S, et al. Adjunctive drug therapy of acute myocardial infarction—Evidence from clinical trials. N Engl J Med 335:1660–1667, 1996.
79. Garg R, Yusuf S. Overview of randomized trials of angiotensin-converting enzyme inhibitors on mortality and morbidity in patients with heart failure. J Am Coll Cardiol 273:1450–1456, 1995.
80. Lonn EM, Yusuf S, Jha P, et al. Emerging role of angiotensin-converting enzyme inhibitors in cardiac and vascular protection. Circulation 90:2056–2069, 1994.

CHAPTER 42

Mild Hypertension: An Important Frontier in Therapy of Hypertension

Stevo Julius, Shawna D. Nesbitt, and Robert Brook

In spite of the clear demonstration that treatment of hypertension substantially reduces morbidity and mortality,[1, 2] essential hypertension remains a major public health problem. Recently, the Global Burden of Diseases Study,[3] which utilized World Health Organization (WHO) data, found that hypertension accounted for 5.8% of all deaths and globally ranked as the third most important risk factor for death after malnutrition (11.7%) and smoking (6%).

Much of the detrimental impact of hypertension reflects the failure to extend treatment to all patients and to decrease the blood pressure adequately in patients receiving treatment. In the most recent National Health and Nutrition Examination Survey (NHANES III) (phase 2 conducted from 1991 to 1994, cited in the sixth report of the Joint National Committee on Prevention, Detection, Evaluation, and Treatment of High Blood Pressure [JNC VI]), only 53% of hypertensive persons were receiving treatment, and the blood pressure was well controlled (<140/90) in only 27%. Similarly, 25% of patients treated by general practitioners in France had well-controlled hypertension.[4] The numbers are even less encouraging in Canada,[5] where only 39% were receiving treatment and only 16% had well-controlled blood pressure.

Most patients with elevated blood pressure have mild hypertension. Among 347,978 subjects aged 35 to 59 years whose blood pressure was measured during the screening process for the Multiple Risk Factor Intervention Trial (MRFIT),[6] 25.9% had mild stage 1 hypertension (140 to 159/90 to 99 mm Hg), 7.1% had stage 2, and only 1.9% had severe stages (3 or 4) of hypertension. Approximately 91,299,000 people in the United States are between the ages of 35 and 59 years.[7] If the MRFIT study percentage applies to the general population in this age group, then slightly less than 23,640,000 Americans have mild stage 1

hypertension. Therefore, most of the failure of blood pressure control found in NHANES III and other surveys occurs in patients with mild hypertension.

We could not find data on the percentage of adequate blood pressure control in patients with stage 1 hypertension. However, there are suggestions that undertreatment of mild hypertension is even a larger problem than undertreatment or inadequate control of the entire universe of hypertensives. The blood pressure response to antihypertensive treatment is directly proportional to the baseline blood pressure. An illustration of that phenomenon is given in Figure 42–1, which shows the blood pressure responses in the Hypertension Optimal Treatment (HOT) Study after 6 months of treatment: The higher the initial reading, the greater the blood pressure drop. It follows that in patients with a mild blood pressure elevation, the same dose of an antihypertensive agent will elicit less decrease in blood pressure than in patients with more severe forms of hypertension. It is therefore not surprising that in trials of mild hypertension, the effect of antihypertensive treatment was rather modest (Table 42–1). The average diastolic blood pressure response in these studies of mild hypertension was −4.9 mm Hg. This paradox is rarely conveyed to practitioners. In fact, the usual assumption is that because the blood pressure elevation is only mild, the blood pressure should be easy to control. On the contrary, bringing the blood pressure to the desirable level in stage 1 hypertension takes more work than one would presume. Given the dilemma of whether to further increase the treatment or to settle for a near goal blood pressure in a patient with "only mild hypertension," the physician frequently chooses to be conservative. The problem is further compounded by national and international guidelines. These guidelines outline a system of triage in which hypertensive

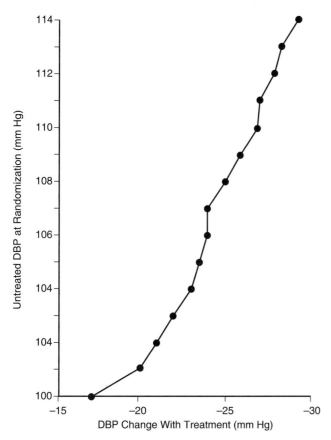

Figure 42–1. Baseline diastolic blood pressure (DBP) and DBP response to treatment in 16,000 patients in the Hypertension Optimal Treatment (HOT) study.[44] Blood pressure response at baseline is related to the blood pressure response after 6 months of treatment. At that point, approximately 40% of patients were receiving monotherapy with 5 mg felodipine. The curves for those on monotherapy showed the same strong relationship between the baseline and the blood pressure response. (Data from Hansson L, Zanchetti A, Carruthers SG, et al, for the HOT Study Group. Effects of intensive blood-pressure lowering and low-dose aspirin in patients with hypertension: Principal results of the Hypertension Optimal Treatment [HOT] randomised trial. Lancet 352:1755–1762, 1988.)

emergencies and severe hypertension are given priority. They suggest a very different (slower) time frame for management of stage 1 hypertension. Unfortunately, such algorithms unwittingly foster a lack of therapeutic vigor in mild hypertension.

PUBLIC HEALTH IMPACT OF MILD HYPERTENSION

The importance of a small blood pressure elevation as a precursor of hypertension and as a major cardiovascular risk factor has been well documented in the literature.[8–10] In one of the early reports from the Framingham Study,[11] Kannel pointed out that 30% of all men who died of cardiovascular disease had "borderline" hypertension (140 to 160/90 to 95) compared with 19% with lower blood pressure readings.

More recently, in the MRFIT study,[6] the cardiovascular mortality in mild hypertension was compared with the mortality of subjects with "optimal" blood pressure readings (<120/80). The data were adjusted for age, race, cholesterol, diabetes, and smoking. The adjusted relative risk for coronary death in stage 1 hypertension was 2.33, and for death from strokes, 3.58. However, the absolute rate of coronary deaths per 10,000 patient years was much higher (27.4) than for stroke (3.0). A similar picture of increased relative risk for coronary deaths (1.61) and deaths from strokes (2.14) was also obtained when subjects with "high-normal" blood pressure readings (130 to 139/85 to 89) were compared with those with "optimal" blood pressure values. Owing to the large number of subjects, the absolute impact of this modest excess of risk in the mild hypertension groups is huge. In the MRFIT study, over a period of 15 years, 35% of all deaths from strokes and coronary heart disease occurred among patients with stage 1 hypertension. Together, the high-normal and the stage 1 groups in the MRFIT study accounted for 54% of all coronary deaths and 51% of all fatal strokes. Nineteen percent of coronary deaths and 16% of deaths from strokes occurred in subjects with high-normal blood pressure, an impact similar to total deaths attributable to stage 2 hypertension (160 to 179/100 to 109), accounting for 14% and 17% of coronary and stroke deaths, respectively. Only 6.6% of coronary deaths and 10.6% of stroke deaths occurred in patients with severe stage 3 and stage 4 hypertension.

Combined, the impact of moderate and severe hypertension is less than that of stage 1 hypertension on coronary heart disease (10.6% vs. 35%). Even in regard to strokes, which are traditionally viewed as "pressure-dependent" and which can effectively be prevented with antihypertensive treatment,[12] more deaths are attributable to stage 1 (35% vs. 27%) than to all other forms of hypertension.

Admittedly, stating the statistical facts does not give a full picture. The issue is whether treating mild hypertension can effectively reduce cardiovascular mortality. We review results of some trials in mild hypertension and discuss their implications.

TRIALS OF ANTIHYPERTENSIVE TREATMENT IN MILD HYPERTENSION

Results of four major trials in mild hypertension, which were published between 1980 and 1993, a period we may as well call the "golden age of trials in mild hypertension," are presented in Table 42–1. Since the mid-1980s, outcome research focused entirely on high-risk hypertension (elderly and patients with target organ damage and/or various pro-atherosclerotic comorbidities). Demonstration research on the efficacy of nonpharmacological treatment in mild hypertension continues to be funded. These expensive and labor-intensive modalities generally achieve small, transient, blood pressure effects whose applicability to clinical practice remains obscure. In contrast, little research is being carried out and no new information is forthcoming on outcomes of pharmacological intervention in stage 1 hypertension despite the fact that it is a major contributor to cardiovascular mortality and that better tolerated and more effective medications are now available. Further, better techniques to select subjects and to monitor them during

Table 42–1 Effect of Antihypertension Treatment

	n	Age (yr)	Entry Criteria	Baseline BP	Placebo BP / DBP Difference From Placebo	Event Rates per 1000 pt/yr Actual	Event Rates per 1000 pt/yr Placebo	Reduction (%)	Significance	Patients Treated 1 yr to Prevent an Event
Australian Mild HTN	3427	50.4/4	DBP > 95 < 110 SBP < 200	DBP 100.5	DBP 93.9 / −5.6	1.1	2.6*	57	<.025	666
MRC	17,354	51/4.9	DBP 90–109 SBP < 200	158/98	148/92 / −5	1.4 6.7	2.6† 8.2‡	46 10.9	<.01 <.025	833 900
HDFP	7825	50.8/5	90–104	151/96	NA§ / −4.9	11.86	14.88‖	20	<.01	333
TOMHS	902	54.8/4	DBP 85–99	140.4/90.5	131/82 / 3.7	28	4.0¶	30	<.03	83

Abbreviations: BP, blood pressure; DBP, diastolic blood pressure; HTN, hypertension; SBP, systolic blood pressure; MRC, Medical Research Council; HDFP, Hypertension Detection and Follow-up Program; TOMHS, Treatment of Mild Hypertension Study.

*CV deaths.
†Strokes.
‡All CV events.
§Compared with "usual" care.
‖Calculated from cumulative mortality.
¶All CV events; calculated from 4 yr of cumulative rates.

study have become available: Measurement of target organ damage with new methods is feasible, and repetitive ambulatory blood pressure measurements have become common.

The four studies of mild hypertension presented in Table 42–1 have not been reported in a uniform fashion in regard to classification of endpoints or how the accumulated events have been calculated. We endeavored in Table 42–1 to highlight the most important features of these studies and to make them as comparable as possible. Some studies reported the event rates per 1000 patient-years of observations. We chose to recalculate all the data per 1000 patient-years. Clearly, since we did not have individual patient data, these calculations are only reasonable estimates. The data in Table 42–1 reflect experience from over 29,500 patients observed for 4 to 5 years. Three of the studies were placebo-controlled; one compared a more aggressive treatment with "usual care." The baseline characteristics of the four populations were similar: Patient's average age was between 50 and 54 years, and the untreated baseline blood pressure ranged from 140 to 158 systolic and 90 to 100 diastolic. A further reduction from the baseline blood pressure ranging from -10 to -9 systolic and -6 to -8 diastolic was observed in the three placebo groups. Thus, in the long term, patients in all four studies had very mild hypertension. At the extreme, in the Treatment of Mild Hypertension Study (TOMHS), the blood pressure of the placebo group, after nonpharmacological intervention, was 131/82. The effect of treatment was modest in all studies; the reduction of the diastolic blood pressure above that observed with placebo ranged from 3.7 to 5.6 mm Hg. Nevertheless, all studies reported statistically significant reductions in morbidity and/or mortality. Two studies disclosed mortality, but in the Hypertension Detection and Follow-up Program (HDFP),[12] total cumulative mortality was reported, whereas the Australian trial[13] gave data on cardiovascular deaths. In both instances, the reductions were significant. To provide a common frame of reference for these trials, we calculated the "number of patients that have to be treated in order to postpone one death per year." In the Australian study this amounted to 666, and in the HDFP, to 333 patients. This calculation exposes the weakness of the relative percent reduction, which is how some studies have chosen to report the data. Because of a smaller absolute incidence of events, the results of the Australian study suggested that many patients must be treated to avert an event. However, the relative mortality reduction was an impressive 57%. On the contrary, in the HDFP study, the relative reduction was only 20%, but because of a higher incidence of total deaths, a lesser number of patients had to be treated to postpone one death.

Both studies that reported on morbidity found a statistically significant reduction in events in the actively treated group, but the results are not comparable. In the British Medical Research Council (MRC) study,[14] the strongest effect was on strokes (46% reduction); a significant but lesser effect (11% reduction) was found for all cardiovascular events. The "number of patients treated for a year to save one event" was 833 for strokes and 900 for all cardiovascular events. In the TOMHS study,[15] the difference between active drug treatment and placebo (lifestyle modification only) groups was significant only when major and minor cardiovascular events were combined (32% re-

duction). Surprisingly, our calculation suggests that in these very mild hypertensive patients, one would have to treat only 86 patients to avoid one event per year. This unexpected high efficacy stems from the definition of endpoints, which in this study, in addition to "hard" endpoints, included transient ischemic attacks and questionnaires for angina and for intermittent claudication.

The overall impression from Table 42–1 is that treatment of mild hypertension is efficacious, but the results do not appear particularly cost-effective, as many patients must be treated to prevent a single event. We argue that these short-term trials cannot evaluate the true long-term potential of treating mild hypertension.

IMPLICATIONS FROM THE TRIALS

If left untreated, patients with borderline and mild hypertension eventually develop a more severe form of hypertension,[10] but the progression is neither linear nor uniform. That this progression is not linear has been shown by Lund-Johansen and associates,[16] who followed a group of patients with WHO stage 1 and 2 hypertension for 20 years. After 10 years, the average blood pressure of the group did not increase. However, after 20 years, almost all patients were receiving treatment, and when the drugs were withdrawn (in most cases for a period of 2 months), the patients were clearly hypertensive (160/100 mm Hg). That the progression is not uniform has been shown by the Australian Study of mild hypertension,[13] in which subjects qualified if their diastolic pressure was repeatedly between 95 and 110. After 3 years of follow-up, the blood pressure decreased below enrollment values in 59% of the 1119 subjects in the placebo group.

The nonlinear trend of blood pressure elevation and a substantial regression toward lower blood pressure values in the control group strongly suggest: (1) that the short time frame of trials in mild hypertension does not apply to the long-term potential of treatment and (2) that the yield in trials of mild hypertension could be improved, even over a short term, if patients whose blood pressure regressed toward normal were eliminated from the study. The first point is self-evident; with passage of time, most of subjects whose blood pressure initially fell will develop hypertension.[16] Treating them early may avert morbidity from the evolving hypertension. The second point, that the short-term efficacy of antihypertensive treatment could be enhanced if the treatment were reserved only for subjects who have "true" hypertension, is supported by epidemiological findings that target organ damage and mortality are directly correlated with average blood pressure. In the Tecumseh study,[17] we repeated blood pressure measurement and found that 51% of subjects with stage 1 hypertension were not hypertensive 3 years later. Blood pressure self-determination outside the physician's office (home blood pressure) proved useful in predicting future blood pressure trends in this study. An average home blood pressure of 128/83 mm Hg predicted sustained future hypertension with a 93% sensitivity but only a 48% specificity. A study using a similar algorithm to select "high-risk" patients with stage 1 hypertension is bound to yield more impressive results than previous trials in mild hypertension.

Clinicians are faced with a vexing paradox: A lifelong treatment is recommended for all forms of hypertension, but the indications are based on short therapeutic trials. The paradox can be best understood when one analyzes the long-term mortality in stage 1 hypertension. Figures 42–2 and 42–3 are derived from follow-up data on subjects screened before MRFIT.[6] Clearly, mortality from coronary heart disease and from strokes increases at a much steeper rate in stage 1 hypertension than in subjects with "ideal blood pressure" values. The first point in both graphs is at 5 years, which corresponds well to the average duration of outcome trials in Table 42–1. The difference in cumulative coronary deaths between the two groups was 0.04% at 5 years, 1.4% at 10 years, and 2.7% after 15 years. In the Australian study of mild hypertension,[13] fatal cardiovascular deaths were reduced by 57% after 4 years of treatment. This effect was statistically significant, but because of the low rate of events, the impact was considered to be of meager clinical relevance. However, if one assumes that the relative benefit shown in these studies would continue to accrue at the same rate, as Figures 42–2 and 42–3 suggest, with passage of time, the absolute impact of treatment would increase dramatically.

The assumption that long-term benefit is proportional to short-term mortality reduction is, in fact, conservative. Hypertension is a self-accelerating disease. Whereas over a short period of time the blood pressure may appear to improve in a substantial proportion of patients with stage 1 hypertension, the Bergen study[16] documented that after 20 years, everybody eventually develops greater hypertension. Importantly, in the Bergen study, the blood pressure reached hypertensive levels between the first and the sec-

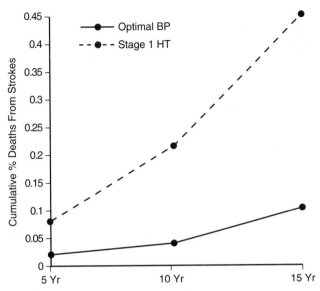

Figure 42–3. Time trends for stroke mortality in persons screened for the Multiple Risk Factor Intervention Trial (MRFIT). Optimal blood pressure (BP) was defined as systolic BP < 120 and diastolic BP < 80 mm Hg. Stage 1 hypertension (HT) was defined as 140–159 or 90–99. (Adapted from Neaton JD, Kuller L, Stamler J, et al. Impact of systolic and diastolic blood pressure on cardiovascular mortality. *In* Laragh JH, Brenner BM [eds]. Hypertension: Pathophysiology, Diagnosis, and Management. New York, Raven, 1995; pp 127–144.)

ond decade of observation, a period that coincides with acceleration of cardiovascular mortality, illustrated in Figures 42–2 and 42–3. Physiologically, this acceleration is best explained by vascular hypertrophy, which enhances vasoconstriction in resistance vessels while simultaneously decreasing the ability to vasodilate.[18] Hypertrophy of resistance vessels has been demonstrated in the mildest forms of hypertension.[19–22] It is impossible to predict on only statistical grounds the beneficial contribution of interrupting the acceleration of hypertension. Short-term early antihypertensive treatment can prevent hypertension in experimental animals.[23] Particularly impressive are studies in which antihypertensive treatment was given to pregnant spontaneously hypertensive rats in order to treat pups intra utero. The treatment prevented the usual development of hypertension after birth. This effect was present throughout the entire life span of the newborn generation, and lower blood pressure values were also seen in the offspring of the intra utero–treated animals.[24, 25]

Stage 1 hypertension is a complex pathophysiological condition, and preventing blood pressure acceleration is only one of the reasons to consider early treatment. In the Tecumseh study, we found significantly elevated cholesterol, triglyceride, glucose, and plasma insulin levels and decreased high-density lipoprotein levels in patients with borderline hypertension (average blood pressure in the clinic 131/94, at home 126/79).[26] Importantly, patients with clear-cut "white-coat" hypertension also had significant dyslipidemia and abnormal plasma insulin levels.[27] Dyslipidemia[28, 29] and high insulin levels[30, 31] are well-known independent coronary risk factors, and when they are combined with an elevated blood pressure, the increase in risk is additive. Furthermore, in the Tecumseh study,

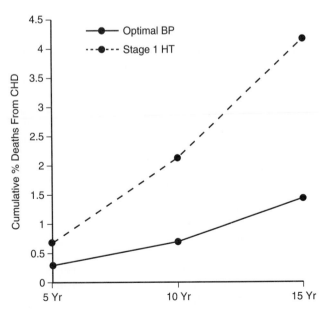

Figure 42–2. Time trends for coronary disease mortality in persons screened for the Multiple Risk Factor Intervention Trial (MRFIT). Optimal blood pressure (BP) was defined as systolic BP < 120 and diastolic BP < 80 mm Hg. Stage 1 hypertension (HT) was defined as 140–159 or 90–99. (Adapted from Neaton JD, Kuller L, Stamler J, et al. Impact of systolic and diastolic blood pressure on cardiovascular mortality. *In* Laragh JH, Brenner BM [eds]. Hypertension: Pathophysiology, Diagnosis, and Management. New York, Raven, 1995; pp 127–144.)

higher hematocrit levels were associated with higher blood pressures, and subjects with higher hematocrits also had significantly elevated plasma renin values.[32] High hematocrit[32] and elevated renin[33] are recognized predictors of coronary risk. Finally, about 30% of patients with stage 1 hypertension in the Tecumseh study had signs of enhanced sympathetic tone; their heart rates and plasma norepinephrine values were elevated. Rapid heart rate is a strong predictor of future increases in blood pressure, of coronary heart disease, and of coronary mortality.[34] Sympathetic stimulation favors vascular[35] and cardiac[36] hypertrophy that, in turn, enhances coronary risk. We have previously discussed the mechanism of this association[37] and its significance for coronary risk.[38] For the purposes of this presentation, it is important to recognize that abnormal metabolic, hormonal, and hemodynamic parameters are characteristic of stage 1 hypertension.

The Framingham study has repeatedly taught us that other risk cardiovascular factors greatly enhance the negative effects of mild hypertension.[28] It is inappropriate to determine just the blood pressure in a patient with stage 1 hypertension; metabolic risk factors must also be measured. Assessment of the combined cardiovascular risk can be used in practice to select candidates for early treatment.

Target organ abnormalities can be found in a proportion of patients with stage 1 hypertension even if blood pressure elevation is small. In the Tecumseh study,[26] patients whose clinic blood pressure was elevated but whose home blood pressure was normal had increased minimal forearm vascular resistance (a sign of arteriolar hypertrophy) and a stroke index and Doppler atrial outflow E:A ratio (early to late ventricular filling velocity) that suggested cardiac restructuring. These findings show that even very mild hypertension can cause structural cardiovascular alterations, but the complex methodology and a lack of normative data limit the usefulness of these measurements in clinical practice. However, standard echocardiography, which is widely used, may reveal cardiac hypertrophy in a small subgroup of patients with very mild hypertension. The prevalence rates of left ventricular hypertrophy (LVH) in such patients are in the range of 13% to 24%,[39–41] but figures as low as 4.4% have also been reported.[42] One study[40] suggested that the prevalence of LVH is somewhat higher in women, in whom, depending on the definition, it ranged from 20 to 45%. Since LVH is a strong predictor of poor cardiovascular outcomes,[11] its presence in a patient with mild hypertension mandates treatment. In a recent prospective study,[43] a decrease in cardiovascular risk was demonstrated by a reduction in left ventricular mass with antihypertensive therapy independent of blood pressure reduction. Early treatment of patients with mild hypertension and LVH with medications to reduce LVH may provide greater risk reduction than blood pressure lowering alone.

APPROACH TO THE PATIENT WITH STAGE 1 HYPERTENSION

Recent recommendations from JNC VI take into consideration blood pressure and the presence of both cardiovascular risk factors and target organ damage. Within that scheme, a patient with LVH and stage 1 hypertension

requires pharmacological treatment. If small studies quoted in this chapter are correct, anywhere between 4% and 25% of patients with mild hypertension who have LVH may require immediate drug treatment. However, echocardiographic measurements are not cost-effective in every patient with stage 1 hypertension. Therefore, indications for immediate treatment must be based on the presence of other easily determined signs of target organ damage (angina, prior myocardial infarction, prior coronary revascularization, congestive heart failure, stroke). If no target organ damage is present, risk factors for coronary heart disease (smoking, dyslipidemia, diabetes, and family history of heart disease) should be evaluated. JNC VI suggests that stage 1 hypertensive patients with at least one risk factor should be given pharmacological treatment if 6 months of nonpharmacological management had failed to correct the blood pressure. In a patient with stage 1 hypertension and no risk factors or target organ damage, treatment is initiated if 1 year of nonpharmacological treatment fails to lower the blood pressure. Based on the outcomes of a few short-term trials in mild hypertension, these recommendations are reasonable and well justified. However, we believe that these trials did not investigate the full potential of the treatment of mild hypertension. Future trials in this area are badly needed.

CONCLUSIONS

Because of its high prevalence (25.9% of the population), stage 1 hypertension is responsible for 35% of all deaths from strokes and 35% of all coronary deaths. Consequently, preventing cardiovascular events in mild hypertension should have a large impact on public health. Trials in stage 1 hypertension showed significant reductions of mortality and/or morbidity in the actively treated groups. However, absolute levels of reduction in these studies were rather meager: Between 333 and 666 patients must be treated per year to postpone 1 death. These studies were performed with first-generation antihypertensive agents (diuretics and β-blockers), and the diagnosis of stage 1 hypertension was based on a few repeat clinic readings. Future studies with better-tolerated, newer drugs and ambulatory or self-determined blood pressure, biochemical tests, and new methods of stratification by target organ status will likely yield better results. Such studies are needed to increase the cost-effectiveness of the treatment and to better define the target population. Present national guidelines provide a reasonable algorithm for management of stage 1 hypertension. However, in reality, stage 1 hypertension is not receiving sufficient attention and, along with other forms of hypertension, remains largely undertreated. This can be remedied only by renewed educational and organizational efforts to improve overall blood pressure control in the population and to reach more patients with stage 1 hypertension.

Acknowledgments

The Tecumseh Blood Pressure Study is supported by a grant from the National Heart, Lung, and Blood Institute (HL 37464). The biochemical analyses were performed at the Michigan Diabetes and Training Center, which is the recipient of a grant from the National Institutes of Health (DK 20572).

References

1. Collins R, Peto R, MacMahon S, et al. Blood pressure, stroke, and coronary heart disease. Part 2: Short-term reduction in blood pressure: Overview of randomised drug trials in their epidemiological context. Lancet 335:827–838, 1990.
2. MacMahon S, Peto R, Cutler J, et al. Blood pressure, stroke, and coronary heart disease. Part 1: Prolonged differences in blood pressure: Prospective observational studies corrected for the regression dilution bias. Lancet 335:765–774, 1990.
3. Murray CJL, Lopez AD. Global mortality, disability, and the contribution of risk factors: Global Burden of Disease Study. Lancet 349:1436–1442, 1997.
4. Poggi L, Chamontin B, Lang T, et al. An attempt to improve blood pressure control in the French population: Information and outcome awareness at the general practitioner level. Am J Hypertens 11:905–908, 1998.
5. Joffres MR, Ghadirian P, Fodor JG, et al. Awareness, treatment, and control of hypertension in Canada. Am J Hypertens 10:1097–1102, 1997.
6. Neaton JD, Kuller L, Stamler J, et al. Impact of systolic and diastolic blood pressure on cardiovascular mortality. *In* Laragh JH, Brenner BM (eds). Hypertension: Pathophysiology, Diagnosis, and Management. New York, Raven, 1995; pp 127–144.
7. U.S. Bureau of the Census, Population Division, release PPL-91. United States population estimates, by age, sex, race, and Hispanic origin, 1990–1997. Washington, DC, U.S. Bureau of the Census, 1998.
8. Kannel WB, Sorlie P, Gordon T. Labile hypertension: A faulty concept? The Framingham Study. Circulation 61:1183–1187, 1980.
9. Leitschuh M, Cupples LA, Kannel WB, et al. High-normal blood pressure progression to hypertension in the Framingham Heart Study. Hypertension 17:22–27, 1991.
10. Julius S, Schork MA. Borderline hypertension—A critical review. J Chronic Dis 23:723–754, 1971.
11. Kannel WB: Role of blood pressure in cardiovascular disease: The Framingham Study. Angiology 26:1–14, 1975.
12. Hypertension Detection and Follow-up Program Cooperative Group. Five-year findings of the Hypertension Detection and Follow-up Program. I: Reduction in mortality of persons with high blood pressure, including mild hypertension. JAMA 242:2562–2571, 1979.
13. Australian National Blood Pressure Study. The Australian Therapeutic Trial in Mild Hypertension. Lancet 1:1261–1267, 1980.
14. Esler M, Julius S, Zweifler A, et al. Mild high-renin essential hypertension: Neurogenic human hypertension? N Engl J Med 296:405–411, 1977.
15. Neaton JD, Grimm RH, Jr, Prineas RJ, et al. Treatment of Mild Hypertension Study. Final results. JAMA 270:713–724, 1993.
16. Lund-Johansen P, Omvik P. Hemodynamic patterns of untreated hypertensive disease. *In* Laragh JH, Brenner BM (eds). Hypertension: Pathophysiology, Diagnosis, and Management. New York, Raven, 1990; pp 305–327.
17. Nesbitt SD, Amerena JV, Grant E, et al. Home blood pressure as a predictor of future blood pressure stability in borderline hypertension. The Tecumseh Study. Am J Hypertens 10:1270–1280, 1997.
18. Folkow B. Physiological aspects of primary hypertension. Physiol Rev 62:347–503, 1982.
19. Conway J. A vascular abnormality in hypertension. A study of blood flow in the forearm. Circulation 27:520–529, 1963.
20. Sivertsson R, Sannerstedt R, Lundgren Y. Evidence for peripheral vascular involvement in mild elevation of blood pressure in man. Clin Sci Mol Med 51:65s–68s, 1976.
21. Egan B, Julius S. Vascular hypertrophy in borderline hypertension: Relationship to blood pressure and sympathetic drive. Clin Exp Hypertens [A] A7:243–255, 1985.
22. Egan B, Panis R, Hinderliter A, et al. Mechanism of increased alpha-

adrenergic vasoconstriction in human essential hypertension. J Clin Invest 80:812–817, 1987.
23. Harrap SB, Van der Merwe WM, Griffin SA, et al. Brief angiotensin-converting enzyme inhibitor treatment in young spontaneously hypertensive rats reduces blood pressure long-term. Hypertension 16:603–614, 1990.
24. Lee RM, Berecek KH, Tsoporis J, et al. Prevention of hypertension and vascular changes by captopril treatment. Hypertension 17:141–150, 1991.
25. Wu JN, Berecek KH. Prevention of genetic hypertension by early treatment of spontaneously hypertensive rats with the angiotensin-converting enzyme inhibitor captopril. Hypertension 22:139–146, 1993.
26. Julius S, Jamerson K, Mejia A, et al. The association of borderline hypertension with target organ changes and higher coronary risk. Tecumseh Blood Pressure Study. JAMA 264:354–358, 1990.
27. Julius S, Mejia A, Jones K, et al. "White coat" versus "sustained" borderline hypertension in Tecumseh, Michigan. Hypertension 16:617–623, 1990.
28. Kannel WB, Castelli WP, Gordon T. Cholesterol in the prediction of atherosclerotic disease. New perspectives based on the Framingham Study. Ann Intern Med 90:85–91, 1979.
29. Kannel WB. High-density lipoproteins: Epidemiologic profile and risks of coronary artery disease. Am J Cardiol 52:9–12, 1983.
30. Pyorala K, Savolainen E, Kaukola S, et al. Plasma insulin as a coronary heart disease risk factor: Relationship to other risk factors and predictive value during 9½ year follow-up of the Helsinki Policemen Study population. Acta Med Scand Suppl 701:38–52, 1985.
31. Ducimetiere P, Eschwege E, Papoz L, et al. Relationship of plasma insulin levels to the incidence of myocardial infarction and coronary heart disease mortality in a middle-aged population. Diabetologia 19:205–210, 1980.
32. Smith SD, Julius S, Jamerson K, et al. Hematocrit levels and physiologic factors in relationship to cardiovascular risk in Tecumseh, Michigan. Hypertension 12:455–462, 1994.
33. Kaplan NM. The deadly quartet. Upper body obesity, glucose intolerance, hypertriglyceridemia and hypertension. Arch Intern Med 149:1514–1520, 1989.
34. Palatini P, Julius S. Heart rate and the cardiovascular risk. J Hypertens 15:1–15, 1997.
35. Hart MN, Heistad DD, Brody MJ. Effect of chronic hypertension and sympathetic denervation on wall/lumen ratio of cerebral vessels. Hypertension 2:419–428, 1980.
36. Simpson P. Norepinephrine-stimulated hypertrophy of cultured rat myocardial cells is an alpha-1 adrenergic response. J Clin Invest 72:732–738, 1983.
37. Julius S. Coronary disease in hypertension: A new mosaic. J Hypertens 15:S3–S10, 1997.
38. Julius S. Sympathetic hyperactivity and coronary risk in hypertension (Corcoran Lecture). Hypertension 21:886–893, 1993.
39. Melina D, Colivicchi F, Guerrera G, et al. Prevalence of left ventricular hypertrophy and cardiac arrhythmias in borderline hypertension. Am J Hypertens 5:570–573, 1992.
40. Liebson PR, Grandits G, Prineas R, et al. Echocardiographic correlates of left ventricular structure among 844 mildly hypertensive men and women in the Treatment of Mild Hypertension Study (TOMHS). Circulation 87:476–486, 1993.
41. Lemne C, Lindvall K, Georgiades A, et al. Structural cardiac changes in relation to 24-h ambulatory blood pressure levels in borderline hypertension. J Intern Med 238:49–57, 1995.
42. Palatini P, Visentin P, Mormino P, et al, and the HARVEST Study Group. Structural abnormalities and not diastolic dysfunction are the earliest left ventricular changes in hypertension. Am J Hypertens 11:147–154, 1998.
43. Verdecchia P, Schillaci G, Borgioni C, et al. Prognostic significance of serial changes in left ventricular mass in essential hypertension. Circulation 97:48–54, 1998.
44. Hansson L, Zanchetti A, Carruthers SG, et al, for the Hot Study Group. Effects of intensive blood-pressure lowering and low-dose aspirin in patients with hypertension: Principal results of the Hypertension Optimal Treatment (HOT) randomised trial. Lancet 352:1755–1762, 1988.

Cost-Effectiveness in Treating Hypertension

Michael A. Weber and William J. Elliott

ESTIMATING COSTS

The economics of healthcare is drawing attention from governments, insurers, businesses, and the health professions. The practice of treating hypertension, although primarily an outpatient or office-based activity, is not immune to concerns over cost. Indeed, the sixth report of the Joint National Committee on Prevention, Detection, Evaluation, and Treatment of High Blood Pressure (JNC VI)[1] has dedicated a whole section to consideration of this issue. Managed care organizations, always sensitive to the cost of delivering services, have recognized that treatment of hypertension can be a meaningful part of their budgets. Older patients in the United States, whose health care is supported by Medicare, often have to pay out of pocket for their drugs and so are also sensitized to cost issues. And many physicians who provide care for their hypertensive patients express concern that cost could jeopardize effective treatment.

The national cost of treating hypertension is driven primarily by the large number of people who have this condition. Treatment of hypertension has become a major commitment for clinicians and organized health plans, especially as newer, more aggressive diagnostic and treatment guidelines, increased awareness, and an aging population have all served to increase the number of patients carrying this diagnosis.

It has been estimated that the annual cost of managing hypertension in the United States exceeds $20 billion,[2] not including the major contribution of hypertension to the more than $10 billion spent on end-stage renal disease. Because health care systems are changing so rapidly, these estimates depend as much on assumptions as on hard data. The cost of treating an individual hypertensive patient approximates $1000 during the first year: This includes a wide range of clinical and laboratory services and is not influenced to a major extent by the types of antihypertensive drugs initially selected.[3] The cost of drugs represents about 20% of the total expenditure on hypertension.[2]

Variable Costs

The principal factors contributing to the cost of managing hypertension are listed in Table 43–1. It is difficult to accurately quantify the cost of physician services: Some doctors charge traditional fees; others have negotiated with insurers to provide services at discounted fees; and still others provide services under capitated Health Maintenance Organizations (HMOs) in which the costs of treating an individual diagnosis, such as hypertension, cannot be separated from overall medical care.

Costs can vary widely even within small localities, and there may be variations in charges for managing hypertension within individual practices in which physicians care for patients with diverse insurance and health plans. A growing trend is for nonphysician professionals, particularly nurse practitioners and physician assistants, to play a key role in the management of conditions such as hypertension for which guidelines and algorithms can be constructed (see Chap. 44, Nursing Clinics in the Management of Hypertension.) As with professional services, the costs of providing laboratory and other forms of testing for hypertension, especially beyond routine initial studies, can depend on the policies of the payers.

Costs of Treatment

Although drugs account for only a relatively small part of the total cost of treating hypertension, the ease with which their prices can be ascertained has made them a frequent source of study by economists. Moreover, many of the traditional health insurance plans, including Medicare, have excluded the purchase of drugs from their coverage, thereby making patients selectively aware of this component of their hypertension management.

Influential advocates, including the Joint National Committee on Prevention, Detection, Evaluation, and Treatment of High Blood Pressure, have recommended lifestyle modifications such as weight loss, reduced sodium intake, and physical exercise as fundamental parts of hypertension management. Apart from a lack of outcome data to demonstrate clinical benefits of these strategies, they are also not inexpensive. Indeed, professional and patient-borne costs of lifestyle modifications may be greater than that of drug therapy.[4, 5]

Table 43–1 Cost of Treating Hypertension

DIRECT

Physician time
Other professional providers: nurses, physician assistants
Facilities overhead and nonprofessional staff
Laboratory and other tests
Antihypertensive drugs
Staff to oversee lifestyle modifications, e.g., dietitians
Adjunct treatments and drugs for anticipated concomitant risk factors, e.g., lipid agents
Unrelated comorbidities discovered through increased exposure to the medical setting
Major endpoints of hypertension: coronary events, heart failure, strokes, renal failure

INDIRECT

Loss of patient's work productivity
Travel and other costs of keeping appointments
Increased insurance premiums for patients, threats to job advancement or security
Special food requirements, exercise programs

Secondary Costs

The concept of total cardiovascular risk highlighted by JNC VI draws attention to the frequent coexistence of high blood pressure with other common and powerful cardiovascular risk factors such as lipid disorders. Comprehensive management of hypertension, therefore, will encompass the diagnosis and treatment—including drugs—of these abnormalities in a large proportion of patients. Long-term management of hypertension, which involves regular interactions between the patient and the health professionals, also leads to unanticipated costs. Common complaints such as joint pains, peptic ulcer symptoms, or sleep difficulties—which by themselves might not have prompted a visit to the doctor—will now be reported and add to the costs of tests and treatment.

Considering the global costs of managing hypertension, the greatest outlay is associated with the hospitalizations, intensive management, and long-term care necessitated by the heart disease, strokes, and renal insufficiency that result from unsuccessful antihypertensive treatment.[2] Providing thorough and comprehensive management of hypertension in its earlier stages is a wise investment that should reduce the high costs associated with managing major cardiovascular events.

Indirect Costs: The Patient

The indirect costs of treating routine hypertension are not high. For patients whose blood pressures and other risk factors are well controlled, and whose quality of life is maintained, there should be relatively little disruption of their work and other daily activities. There can be less obvious costs that could cause concern to patients. Although hypertension as a preexisting condition is now less likely to prevent individuals from obtaining health insurance, it is possible that life insurance premiums may be affected by this diagnosis.

Changes in lifestyle can be expensive, and such expenses are carried largely by the patient. Diets designed to promote weight loss and to reduce fat and sodium intake tend to be heavily dependent on fresh produce, which is often more expensive than other foods. Regular aerobic exercise, particularly for patients who live in extreme climates, can require joining health clubs or purchasing special equipment and clothing. Professionally supervised programs of lifestyle modification may be necessary for middle-aged or elderly patients and often requires the allocation and expense of trained personnel.

COST-EFFECTIVENESS

There are two major reasons why current estimates of cost-effectiveness ratios tend to be inaccurate. First, the paucity of clinical outcome studies in hypertension, particularly in the setting of multiple risk factors, makes it difficult to quantify the clinical benefits of therapeutic interventions. Second, as discussed earlier, the complexity of attributing costs for the management of hypertension, especially at a time of major changes in health care economics, also serves

---

Table 43–2   Cost-Effective Treatment of Hypertension

Verify the diagnosis: Confine treatment to true hypertensives
Use total-risk concept: Provide guidance on whether to treat milder forms of hypertension
Integrate the workup: Simultaneously identify target organ changes, concomitant risk factors, and possible causes of secondary hypertension
Utilize trained nonphysician professionals: Employ, e.g., nurse practitioners and physician assistants, who can ensure ready access to care and enhance compliance with therapeutic and lifestyle strategies
Optimize drug use: Choose antihypertensive agents that control blood pressure and have metabolic, cardiovascular, and renal effects appropriate to concomitant conditions
Utilize drugs efficiently: Explore different monotherapies before resorting to polypharmacy; consider fixed combinations that cost less than separate drugs

---

to make these measurements inaccurate. Inevitably, attempts to assess relationships between costs and benefits are highly dependent on assumptions and extrapolations. Even carefully constructed models such as the Coronary Heart Disease Policy Model that was used to compare the cost-effectiveness of differing antihypertensive drugs became the subject of controversy.[6–8]

Some principles, though, can define the most cost-effective care. Clearly, it is most efficient to treat high-risk patients. There is a greater return on the dollar from treating older rather than younger patients and from treating more severe rather than milder forms of hypertension.[9–11] This does not mean that younger patients with earlier stages of hypertension, particularly if other risk factors are present, should not be treated. Strategies that increase the efficiency of managing hypertension and can reduce costs without adversely affecting the goals of treatment are listed in Table 43–2.

Patient Selection

The effort involved in establishing that patients truly have hypertension is a critical first step. Studies of white-coat hypertension, using ambulatory blood pressure monitoring or other techniques, have shown that office hypertension cannot be confirmed at home or in other settings in a meaningful number of patients (see Chap. 31, Blood Pressure Measurement Issues, and Chap. 32, White-Coat Hypertension).[12, 13] It is possible that the cost of ambulatory blood pressure monitoring may yield a severalfold dividend by identifying individuals who might not require treatment.[14, 15] A related issue, discussed in depth in JNC VI, is basing the decision to treat on an estimate of overall risk (see Chap. 24, Total Risk). It may be appropriate to withhold treatment from a patient with modestly increased blood pressure but who, in the absence of other risk factors, appears to be at low absolute risk of major cardiovascular sequelae.

Practical Approaches

Effective long-term management of hypertension depends on frequent contacts between health professionals and patients. Trained nonphysician specialists such as nurse practitioners and physician assistants can play a pivotal part. Their salaries are usually lower than those of physicians. More importantly, they are able to focus more closely on achieving compliance with drugs and on encouraging lifestyle modifications. Moreover, the best control of hypertension is achieved with a high frequency of visits, shorter waits, more time dedicated to patient counseling, and a coordinated program of supervision that encompasses the entire clinical staff.[16] In pursuit of enhanced cost-effectiveness, it has been shown that more aggressive care of hypertensive patients, especially the elderly, decreases utilization of more expensive health care resources.[17]

JNC VI discusses in detail the optimal diagnostic workup of hypertensive patients. The principal goal of this process is the identification of target organ changes, concomitant risk factors, and possible causes of secondary hypertension. It is desirable to use laboratory panels and protocols that can integrate these objectives and thereby provide information in an economical fashion.

Optimizing the Use of Drugs

It is efficient and cost-saving to achieve treatment goals with the fewest numbers of drugs. Antihypertensive agents have differing effects on common concomitant risk factors such as lipoprotein levels, glucose tolerance, left ventricular hypertrophy, and renal dysfunction. Ideally, drugs should have beneficial effects or be neutral in their actions on these concomitant risk factors; certainly, drugs that exacerbate them should not be employed.

Cost-saving can be further enhanced by carefully selecting and, if necessary, exchanging initial therapies—sometimes termed *sequential monotherapy*—before resorting to combinations and polypharmacy. It is likely that many patients on multiple drug therapy are, in fact, receiving real benefit from only one or two of their drugs. When combination treatment is necessary, a host of newly available fixed-combination products incorporating a wide variety of different antihypertensive classes not only may simplify treatment but also may be less costly than multiple individual prescriptions.

Choosing drugs on the basis of cost alone may be inappropriate and, in the long run, may not reduce expenses. Although there are price differences among the drug classes, and among different brands within a class, these differences are not particularly conspicuous when considering the overall cost of managing hypertension. In general, the very cheapest or the most expensive drugs should not drive the overall cost of managing hypertension by more than 20% in either direction.[3] Although thoughtful selection of particular drugs can at times reduce costs, this should not be done by compromising optimal control of cardiovascular risk factors or quality of life.

Clinical pathways have been suggested as a solution to cost-effectiveness for a variety of medical conditions. In essence, JNC VI[1] is a clinical pathway for hypertension or, perhaps more accurately, a series of pathways for dealing with clinical management problems that can arise in the context of hypertension. Certainly JNC VI's recommendations on drug use, including the so-called compelling indi-

cations, emphasize that key comorbidities such as congestive heart failure, diabetes mellitus, and renal insufficiency should be managed in very specific ways. For example, the use of angiotensin-converting enzyme inhibitors or angiotensin receptor blockers in patients with congestive heart failure or diabetic nephropathy not only would promote better clinical outcomes but additionally, by reducing the need for hospitalizations or other expensive interventions, would markedly curtail costs.

MEASURING OUTCOMES IN HYPERTENSION

The development of managed care plans and the growing interest in cost-effectiveness and evidence-based medicine have all stimulated an interest in objectively measuring the outcomes of treating hypertension. JNC VI has accepted the proposal that outcomes be divided into three types: immediate, which encompass the findings during the initial few weeks or months of treatment; long-term, which deal with the effects of chronic treatment on survival and major clinical events; and intermediate or surrogate outcome measures, which provide guidance during the course of treatment.[18]

Chapter 33, Outcomes in Treating Hypertension, describes in detail the types of measurable variables and outcomes that can be classified as short-, intermediate-, or long-term. Interestingly, short-term outcomes have recently been reemphasized. In particular, JNC VI[1] points out that blood pressure remains critically important, and that for patients with meaningful comorbidities, it is desirable to bring blood pressure values below 130/85 mm Hg. JNC VI points out, moreover, that "optimal" blood pressure is below 120/80 mm Hg. Long-term outcomes are being addressed by a number of ongoing major clinical trials with a variety of drug interventions. Although the studies are of interest in providing guidance on therapeutic strategies, they do not necessarily help physicians in monitoring progress in individual patients. For this reason, intermediate endpoints that look at changes in the structure or function of the heart, kidneys, or blood vessels might ultimately be shown to be of considerable importance. Unfortunately, we do not yet have definitive data linking these intermediate measurements to long-term prognosis. If or when those data become available, we will be able to provide far more detailed guidance to clinicians on how to assess progress in their patients.

IMPACT OF MANAGED CARE

There is a continuing movement of medical services into various forms of managed care. It has not yet been possible to learn whether these changes are producing beneficial or adverse effects on the overall treatment of hypertension. Comparisons of short-term outcomes between HMOs and the traditional fee-for-service setting have been inconclusive.[19–21] Although there may be concern that aggressive managed care organizations may not provide the same level of service as conventional care, differences in the ages, economic and social status, and degree of illness among patients in the different types of systems make valid comparisons difficult.[22]

To help monitor the performance of the HMOs, the Health Plan Employer Data and Information Set (HEDIS) has been designed to provide a report card for these organizations.[23, 24] At this early stage, though, HEDIS is better able to study strategies and adherence to policies than to measure true outcomes.[25] It is likely, e.g., that HEDIS guidelines for hypertension will simply measure the percentage of hypertensive patients within a plan whose blood pressures have been controlled to an arbitrary level. It is not certain that a more thorough evaluation of hypertension services can be undertaken in the foreseeable future.

The Pros and Cons of Managed Care

There are some potential benefits that could result from well-run hypertension programs in the managed care setting (Table 43–3). HMOs have the ability to create their own clinical pathways for effective long-term management of hypertension and, through efficiencies of scale, can often provide nurse practitioners or other professionals to support their programs. Moreover, in a competitive environment, HMOs may be motivated to demonstrate their ability to meet or exceed national performance standards.

On the other hand, HMOs are business with a strong incentive to contain costs. Access to laboratory and other tests and to treatment with newer or more expensive drugs may be limited. Moreover, since many employers and individual patients frequently switch their allegiances among plans, it is not certain that HMOs are truly motivated to promote long-term outcomes.

In reality, it may not be easy to determine the true

Table 43–3 Hypertension in the Managed Care Setting

PROS

Plans profess awareness of long-term benefits of effective treatment (implicit in "health maintenance" concept)
Plans understand the role and value of nonphysician providers
Plans can design guidelines and clinical pathways that optimize care of their members
Plans are subject to external scrutiny of their performance (report card) in identifying and treating hypertensive patients

CONS

Cost-containment strategies can limit access to testing
Restricted drug formularies and rigid budgets can drive drug selection largely or entirely on cost basis
Attitudes toward treatment outcomes are short-term, especially when large numbers of enrollees frequently switch among plans

REALITIES

It is difficult to compare hypertension outcomes in traditional medicine and managed care owing to economic, employment, and demographic differences in the populations served
Because physicians now tend to join larger groups that work with multiple plans, standards of care in hypertension may be better judged locally than plan-wide
Ongoing transitions among staff model, capitation, and point-of-service plans limit generalizations about the performance of managed care organizations in hypertension

Table 43–4 Role of the Hypertension Specialist

1. Development of individualized clinical pathways
   Adaptation of guidelines to local demographics, cultures, economics, and logistics
   Guidance on new drugs and techniques
2. Consultation: WHEN TO REFER
   Workup of suspected secondary hypertension
   Difficulty in controlling blood pressure
      Owing to true treatment resistance
      Owing to unacceptable side effects
   The complex patient has
      Multiple risk factors that require therapy
      Concomitant conditions that make blood pressure control difficult or affect drug selection, e.g., diabetic nephropathy, congestive heart failure, angina pectoris
      Concomitant conditions that require conflicting drugs, e.g., arthritis, airway disease

impact of managed care on hypertension. As listed in Table 43–3, the rapidly changing nature of the HMOs and other forms of managed care makes it difficult to measure how hypertension is handled in these different settings.

THE HYPERTENSION SPECIALIST

Although the majority of hypertensive patients will be cared for in the primary care setting, the clinical hypertension specialist will continue to have key responsibility. The role of hypertension experts is summarized in Table 43–4. One major task for these specialists will be to adapt and customize treatment guidelines for local use. They will advise clinical pathway committees and help define optimal approaches for patients with differing economic and demographic characteristics. They will also assist in evaluating new drugs and interpreting new discoveries in the field of hypertension. On a more practical note, physicians will continue to refer their more difficult or complex hypertensive patients to the specialist. Patients with suspected secondary forms of hypertension, difficult to control blood pressure, and/or serious concomitant conditions or conflicting drug requirements are examples of appropriate referrals.

The American Society of Hypertension recently announced a program for identifying and certifying physicians in the United States who meet the criteria to be designated as *hypertension specialists*. JNC VI[1] clearly indicates that such individuals can have an important role in caring for patients with difficult hypertension problems. In addition, they should be capable of providing teaching services and, possibly, clinical pathway guidance to their institutions and communities.

References

1. Joint National Committee on Prevention, Detection, Evaluation and Treatment of High Blood Pressure. The sixth report. Arch Intern Med 2413–2446, 1997.
2. *Heart and Stroke Facts: 1996 Statistical Supplement.* Dallas, American Heart Association, 1996; p 23.
3. Hilleman DE, Mohiuddin SM, Lucas BD Jr, et al. Cost-minimization analysis of initial antihypertensive therapy in patients with mild-to-moderate essential diastolic hypertension. Clin Ther 16:88–102, 1994.

4. Johannesson M, Fagerberg B. A health-economic comparison of diet and drug treatments in obese men with mild hypertension. J Hypertens 10:1063–1070, 1992.

5. Edelson JT, Weinstein MC, Tosteson ANA, et al. Long-term cost-effectiveness of various initial monotherapies for mild-to-moderate hypertension. JAMA 263:408–413, 1990.

6. Kaplan NM: Cost-effectiveness of antihypertensive drugs: Fact or fancy? Am J Hypertens 4:478–480, 1991.

7. Goldman L, Weinstein MC. Reply to criticism. Am J Hypertens 5:666–668, 1992.

8. Kawachi I, Malcolm LA. The cost-effectiveness of treating mild-to-moderate hypertension: A reappraisal. J Hypertens 9:199–208, 1991.

9. Lindholm LH, Johannesson M. Cost-benefit aspects of treatment of hypertension in the elderly. Blood Press 3:11–14, 1995.

10. Bulpitt CJ, Fletcher AE. Cost-effectiveness of the treatment of hypertension. Clin Exp Hypertens 15:131–146, 1993.

11. Pickering TG, James GD, Boddie C, et al. How common is white-coat hypertension? JAMA 259:225–228, 1988.

12. Drayer JIM, Weber MA, Nakamura DK. Automated ambulatory blood pressure monitoring: A study in age-matched normotensive and hypertensive men. Am Heart J 109:1334–1338, 1985.

13. Krakoff LR. Ambulatory blood pressure monitoring can improve cost-effective management of hypertension. Am J Hypertens 6:2205–2245, 1993.

14. Yarows SA, Khoury S, Sowers JR. Cost effectiveness of 24-hour ambulatory blood pressure monitoring in evaluation and treatment of essential hypertension. Am J Hypertens 7:464–468, 1994.

15. Stason WB, Shepard DS, Perry HM Jr, et al. Effectiveness and costs of Veterans Affairs hypertension clinics. Am J Hypertens 32:1197–1215, 1994.

16. Reid DL, Johnson RE, Brody KK, Vogt TM. Medical care utilization among older HMO members with and without hypertension. J Am Geriatr Soc 43:222–229, 1995.

17. Weber MA, Radensky P. Measurement of short-term, intermediate, and long-term outcomes of treating hypertension. In Cullen JH (ed), Cardiology Clinics. Philadelphia, WB Saunders, 1995; pp 131–142.

18. Coffey E, Moscovice IP, Finch M, et al. Capitated Medicaid and the process of care of elderly hypertensives and diabetics: Results from a randomized trial. Am J Med 98:531–536, 1995.

19. Ware JR, Rogers WH, Davies AR, et al. Comparison of health outcomes at a health maintenance organization with those of fee for service care. Lancet 1:1017–1022, 1986.

20. Sloss EM, Keeler EB, Brook RH, et al. Effect of an HMO on physiologic health: Results from a randomized trial. Ann Intern Med 106:130–138, 1987.

21. Ware JE Jr, Bayliss MS, Rogers WH, et al. Differences in 4-year health outcomes for elderly and poor, chronically ill patients treated in HMO and fee-for-service systems. JAMA 276:1039–1047, 1996.

22. HEDIS 3.0 Draft for Public Comment: July 1996, Washington DC, National Committee for Quality Assurance, 1996.

23. Stephenson GM, Findlay, R: HEDIS: Almost ready for prime time. Bus Health 13:39, 42, 44, 46, 48, 50, 1995.

24. Schiff L, Service R (eds). Empowered patients buy more efficient care. Bus Health 14:35, 38–40, 42, 1996.

25. Weber MA. Impact on the pharmaceutical industry of changes in the American health care system: A physician's perspective. Seton Hall Law Review, vol 24. Newark, NJ, Seton Hall University, School of Law, 1994; pp 1290–1324.

CHAPTER 44

Nursing Clinics in the Management of Hypertension

Nancy Houston Miller and Martha N. Hill

Nearly one in four Americans has hypertension. Although the rates of awareness, treatment, and control of this condition have improved since the late 1970s, resulting in a reduction in both morbidity and mortality from stroke and coronary heart disease, significant numbers of hypertensive individuals lack appropriate treatment and follow-up. In addition, only half of all hypertensives under treatment achieve a goal blood pressure of less than 140/90 mm Hg as determined by the most recent National Health and Nutrition Examination Survey (NHANES III).[1] Finally, various subsets of patients, such as elderly white women, show rates of control of hypertension of only 19%, leaving them exposed to high risk for cardiovascular disease and congestive heart failure. Although the incidence of congestive heart failure has increased more than threefold from 1970 to 1994, research indicates that better control of hypertension could reduce this incidence by almost 50% and improve overall survival in those who ultimately suffer it.[2]

Management of an asymptomatic condition such as hypertension is challenging. Although a high proportion of individuals are aware of their high blood pressure, the first challenge is getting them to enter into and remain in treatment after initial screening. Many patients never make a first appointment or return for a follow-up appointment after the initial diagnosis is made. Others do not undertake lifestyle changes that could improve blood pressure control nor remain on medications that are costly and associated with side effects simply to reduce the uncertain risk of eventual chronic diseases. Lifestyle changes cannot be achieved without ongoing support during both the adoption and the maintenance of these behaviors. Research indicates that the most successful lifestyle change for the control of hypertension, that of weight reduction, is often one of the most difficult to achieve.[3] Effective pharmacological treatment of high blood pressure requires frequent rechecking with the patient to determine appropriate administration, side effects, compliance with the regimen, and whether or not the goal blood pressure—which could lower the patient's risk of future disease—has been achieved and maintained. Finally, for a patient to remain in care over years, there must be convenient office hours, personable staff, and appointment reminder systems. This chapter focuses on the success of nurses' managing hypertension clinics in which they care for patients in a variety of health care settings. Special emphasis is given to the components of a successful clinic.

Since the early 1970s, nurses and other nonphysician

health care providers have played an important role in managing patients with hypertension, primarily in inner city areas, academic health centers, and national multisite clinical trials. Whereas, in some instances, their work has been acknowledged, the improved outcomes that have been achieved in research and in clinical practice by nurses and health care teams working together have been largely unheralded. Perhaps because of the prevalence of hypertension and the perceived ease of treating it, this condition is the number one reason for an outpatient physician visit. However, in today's ever-changing health care environment, there is increased recognition of the need for effective services provided by nurses, such as screening, education, counseling, medication management, and follow-up of patients who must manage their hypertension and/or hypertension-related cardiovascular disease.

IMPLEMENTATION OF NURSE-RUN CLINICS

Since the early 1970s, nurses have played a very significant role in the management of patients with hypertension. In a landmark study by Runyan,[4] patients with hypertension, diabetes, or cardiac disease chose to be followed by specially trained nurses in decentralized clinics close to their homes or in a hospital outpatient clinic for chronic disease staffed by internists. These patients were similar with regard to sociodemographic and clinical characteristics. At the end of 2 years, patients treated by nurses had lower blood pressures in all age groups except among those aged 30 to 39 years and over 80 years. Moreover, by the end of the treatment period, patients treated in the nurse-run clinics had utilized approximately 50% fewer hospital admission days, whereas those treated in the outpatient clinics staffed by physicians showed an increase in hospital days for each of the disease categories. The author attributed the success of the nurse-run clinics to the greater follow-up and greater time devoted by nurses to helping patients manage their condition.

In a study conducted by Alderman and Schoenbaum,[5] nurses played the central role in the screening and follow-up of patients in a worksite setting in New York City. In this successful program, nurses performed screening and enrollment over an 11-day period in a New York department store. Hypertensive individuals who elected to participate in the program were followed by a nurse for 1 year. Nurses were responsible for taking the initial medical history and obtaining preliminary laboratory data and an electrocardiogram when a patient entered the program. Approximately 1 week later, the medical director took a history, performed a physical examination, and reviewed laboratory data. Working closely with the medical director and using treatment algorithms, nurses initiated drug therapy, then increased doses and numbers of drugs in a stepwise fashion until the blood pressure was less than 140/90 mm Hg. Diuretics were used as first-line therapy in treatment. Follow-up visits to the nurse were individualized based on the patient's needs and control of blood pressure. At these visits, which decreased in frequency to every 3 months once blood pressure was controlled, nurses monitored the blood pressure, reviewed therapy and potential complica-

tions, checked compliance, and helped to motivate patients by enhancing their participation in care. At the end of 1 year, the nurses' provision of care did not compromise program acceptability. In this worksite, 84% of the 1850 employees were screened, two thirds of those eligible for the treatment program sought treatment through the nurse program, and 97% of accepted patients remained in therapy, with 81% achieving acceptable blood pressure reduction. Moreover, the direct annual per patient cost of $100.00 offset the cost associated with hypertension, including time lost from work, and allowed the health payor to offer this program as a union membership benefit. Today, this model, which is still operational in New York City, has been replicated in numerous worksites.

In a study similar to that of Alderman and Schoenbaum, Logan and colleagues[6] found that hypertensive patients who were randomly allocated to receive care at work, compared with those receiving standard care, were significantly more likely to be put on antihypertensive medications (94.7% vs. 62.7%), to reach goal blood pressure in the first 6 months of therapy (48.5% vs. 27.5%), and to take prescribed medications (67.6% vs. 49.1%). The authors claimed that the improvement in blood pressure control was due to the fact that long-term care was more convenient, therapy was more vigorously applied, and compliance with therapy was more strongly encouraged by nurses.

Nurses have also made a major contribution to the management of hypertensive patients in national multisite clinical trials, many of which began in the late 1970s. The Hypertension Detection and Follow-up Program (HDFP)[7] and the Systolic Hypertension in the Elderly Program (SHEP)[8] are just two examples of large clinical trials conducted in the United States in which nurses provided screening, counseling, and medication management of hypertensive individuals. Whereas the excellent outcomes and treatment protocols in these trials have been widely disseminated, the fact that the care was delivered primarily by nurses has not been widely acknowledged. This has led to a lack of appreciation of the essential role of nurses in helping patients to enter care and remain in care as well as to achieve and maintain blood pressure control.

Evaluations of nurse-run clinics in which nurses saw patients alone or in collaboration with physicians show a level of blood pressure control comparable with that achieved by physicians.[9] Similar results are seen where case-mix adjustment indicates that nurses care for patients as complex as those seen by physicians.[10] Pheley and coworkers[11] reported on the screening, management, and outcomes of patients enrolled in a nurse-run hypertension management program in a large multispecialty practice in Minnesota. One year after entry into this program, the proportion of patients who had their blood pressure controlled to 140/90 mm Hg or less increased from 17 to 44%.

Nursing case management has recently been applied to hypertension. Nurses have taught patients to measure blood pressure at home and have managed them primarily by telephone, alleviating the logistical burden of visits to the clinic. In a study of 78 patients managed in this way, a single clinic encounter enabled nurses to provide education and counseling about lifestyle changes, begin medication management, and teach patients how to use the home blood pressure monitors. This session was followed by nurse-initiated telephone encounters of 10 minutes' duration that occurred on a biweekly and then monthly basis over the 6 months of the program. At the end of this period, systolic and diastolic blood pressures declined by 10% and 8%, respectively, or 15 mm Hg and 7 mm Hg in absolute terms. The proportion of patients reaching a goal blood pressure increased from 22 to 48%. Importantly, the mean weight loss of patients enrolled in the study was 3.5 kg.[12]

NURSE MANAGEMENT—CLINIC SETTINGS

Roles and Responsibilities

The goals of managing hypertensive individuals are the same, whether operationalized in specialty clinics, private practice offices, worksite settings, primary care clinics, or neighborhood clinics. A team approach, bringing together physicians and nurses as well as community health workers, often produces better outcomes than a traditional medical approach. If nurse practitioners are caring for the patients, they practice independently, using protocols developed jointly with the physician with whom they collaborate.[13] In settings in which the nurses do not have advanced practice credentials, physicians are responsible for making the diagnosis of hypertension and for determining secondary causes, which may influence decisions about appropriate treatment. Physicians help to formulate a treatment plan and provide consultation to nurses in managing complex cases. This arrangement allows physicians to use their time caring for sicker patients. In some of the oldest operating nurse clinics in the United States, patterned on the success of the Veterans Administration Cooperative Study,[14] physicians now see patients on only a limited basis: When a decision is made to treat patients with medication; when inadequate blood pressure control is achieved after optimizing drug therapy; if drug toxicity occurs; and when a significant complication of hypertension arises.

Nurses have shown that they can demonstrate critical clinical judgment in the management of patients within a hypertension clinic. In the worksite setting, they are often responsible for conducting screening programs to identify and refer hypertensive individuals. In programs to verify sustained elevated blood pressure, nurses are responsible for determining the appropriateness of patients' ongoing management. In the hypertension management program described by Pheley and coworkers,[11] e.g., more than three quarters of all patients referred for management of hypertension were deemed normotensive on the basis of a blood pressure reading of less than 140/90 mm Hg documented over three consecutive weekly screenings. Within this program, nurses were responsible for seeing patients weekly to determine their level of blood pressure and to provide the appropriate education for individuals with or at risk for hypertension. Screening and verification programs conducted by nurses enable them to identify individuals with sustained hypertension using standardized blood pressure techniques and to establish a database of individuals who can be followed for appropriate rescreening as is necessary. Such programs also help nurses identify patients who,

based on multiple blood pressure measurements, need lifestyle modification to lower high normal pressures. By having nurses measure blood pressure on multiple occasions, false-positive diagnoses of hypertension and unnecessary treatment can be avoided. This is important because previous studies have shown that physicians may base their treatment on a single measurement rather than making the diagnosis on at least two occasions with appropriate attention to technique.[15]

In managing a cohort of patients in a hypertension clinic, the nurse is responsible for taking a thorough medical history and for ordering appropriate blood chemistry tests, such as sodium, potassium, creatinine, blood urea nitrogen, cholesterol, and a complete blood cell count; a urinalysis; and an electrocardiogram. This allows physicians to devote their efforts during a subsequent visit to performing the physical examination and formulating an appropriate treatment plan based on extensive information and laboratory data provided by the nurse.

In the majority of hypertension clinics, nurses provide the education and counseling necessary to ensure that individuals are undertaking lifestyle changes that may favorably influence blood pressure. Weight loss, which may be the most successful nonpharmacological technique for lowering blood pressure, requires behavior change for both eating and physical activity patterns. Such nonpharmacological approaches include helping patients to initiate or maintain an aerobic exercise program and to limit sodium intake to 100 mmol/day and alcohol consumption to 1 to 2 drinks* per day.[16] In addition, many hypertensive individuals present to the clinic with multiple risk factors for cardiovascular disease. The nurse can also provide education and counseling for smoking cessation and lipid reduction to help patients lower their risk of cardiovascular disease. Why is the nurse's role so critical? Modifying lifestyle behaviors requires many clinical interventions: assessment of an individual's baseline behaviors; education about how to make the appropriate changes; counseling to develop strategies such as setting short-term goals and self-monitoring that will ensure the maintenance of the changes; constant rechecking with the individual to determine whether compliance is a problem and resolve barriers; and reinforcement of progress toward the goal of change in behavior.[17] Success with any of these changes requires frequent interaction with the patient. Additional exchange of information can be done by telephone, FAX, and/or a home visit, as well as a face-to-face clinic visit. This is often best accomplished by a health care provider such as the nurse who has the requisite time for the education and counseling necessary to change behavior. Moreover, it has been shown that individuals who receive education and counseling on hypertension management exhibit increased adherence.[18] The important aspects of education and counseling that should be incorporated into the management of individuals with hypertension are noted in Table 44–1.

In many settings, nurses are also responsible for the pharmacological aspects of hypertension management. Using well-defined protocols based on national guidelines such as the sixth report of the Joint National Committee on Prevention, Detection, Evaluation, and Treatment of

---

*A drink is defined as 1 oz of ethanol (e.g., 24 oz of beer, 10 oz of wine, or 2 oz of 100-proof whiskey).

Table 44–1 Strategies for Patient Education

IDENTIFY KNOWLEDGE, ATTITUDES, BELIEFS, AND EXPERIENCE
   Assess readiness to achieve blood pressure control
   Correct misinterpretations

EDUCATE ABOUT CONDITION AND TREATMENT
   Inform patient of the blood pressure level
   Identify alternative treatment plans
   Provide simple oral and written information
   Teach self-monitoring skills

TAILOR THE REGIMEN TO THE PATIENT
   Include patient in decision-making
   Agree on blood pressure goal
   Incorporate treatment into patient's daily lifestyle
   Simplify the regimen
   Prioritize critical aspects of the regimen
   Implement the treatment plan in stages
   Encourage self-monitoring of blood pressure in selected
      patients
   Encourage discussion of medication, side effects, and
      concerns
   Modify dosages or change medications to avoid side effects
   Minimize cost of therapy
   Schedule frequent visits for nonadherent patients

PROVIDE REINFORCEMENT
   Hold exit interviews
   Arrange home visits
   Use appointment reminders
   Contact patients who miss appointments
   Consider clinician-patient contracts

PROMOTE SOCIAL SUPPORT
   Include family and others in care
   Suggest group sessions

COLLABORATE WITH OTHER PROFESSIONALS
   Recognize shared practice goals
   Draw on the skills and knowledge of other providers

From Hill MH. Strategies for patient education. Clin Exp Hypertens Theory Pract A11:1187–1201, 1989.

High Blood Pressure (JNC VI),[16] advanced practice nurses and specially trained nurse case managers can prescribe and titrate medications and help patients to manage the numerous steps in medication-taking required for blood pressure control. In some settings, nurses have shown they can attain greater control of blood pressure than is achieved with standard care.[4, 6, 10] In many cases, the improved outcomes have resulted from nurses placing a greater number of patients on medications, altering drug regimens more frequently in response to inadequate blood pressure control, and prescribing more effectively. In some studies, nurses have also been noted to place a higher proportion of patients on multiple drug regimens in order to achieve greater control.[10, 14] Such changes may produce higher costs initially, as noted in a study conducted by Logan and associates.[19] However, if the goals of a clinic are to keep patients in treatment and achieve greater adherence and blood pressure control rates, obtaining the best regimen for the patient must be paramount.

Effective protocols for medication management allow achievement of blood pressure control, which can be a significant factor in helping to offset some of the costs of providing a clinic. For example, in the early work of the Veterans Clinics in over 6000 treated patients,[14] nurses successfully managed patients using the combination of a thiazide diuretic and other agents, such as methyldopa and reserpine. At the end of five treatment visits, half of all patients had diastolic pressures below 90 mm Hg, and two thirds of those who began treatment remained in treatment for at least 2.5 years. The total yearly cost for treating one patient was $221. Nurses have been shown to effectively manage other risk factors, such as dyslipidemia, using multiple drugs at lower cost.[20]

Another role of the nurse is to direct the efforts of other team members who may be providing direct consultation or are working within the clinic. Whereas collaborative teams of physicians and nurses provide care in a typical hypertension clinic, health care providers such as nutritionists, pharmacists, and community health care workers also practice in some clinics. A description of the role of community health care workers involved in underserved communities is noted in Chapter 45, Community Outreach. It may be the responsibility of the nurse to train other people, such as office assistants and receptionists, to take blood pressures, which can be helpful in screening and can also decrease costs. Receptionists can also play a helpful role in scheduling appointments, making reminder telephone calls, obtaining laboratory results, entering data to support evaluation of clinical outcomes, and assuring that referring physicians receive timely correspondence about their patient's management.

Clinic Needs and Setup

Most clinics undertaking hypertension management require no specialized equipment or space. An examination room and/or clinic office can be used to see patients and their families for education and counseling as well as for patient care. Using existing space within an operating facility avoids additional costs. Especially in underserved communities, neighborhood clinics minimize the burdens of transportation, enabling many individuals to remain in care who might not otherwise do so. This may require additional resources for rental space in a neighborhood.

Clinics must use accurately calibrated mercury sphygmomanometers to ensure adequate measurement of blood pressure. In addition, a clinic may benefit from providing patients with blood pressure monitors for home use, especially those patients whose blood pressure may need tighter control. Computers are necessary to track appointments and telephone contacts; collect medical, demographic, and billing information; and generate reports to physicians, payors, and patients. Moreover, documentation of clinical outcomes is becoming increasingly important and necessary. Tracking the frequency of visits, medications, compliance, hospitalizations, and blood pressures through a computer program enables rapid evaluation of clinical outcomes and the costs incurred in providing antihypertensive treatment. A simple checklist for use in developing a hypertension clinic is shown in Table 44–2.

Caseload Size

Several factors influence the capability of nurses and others to manage a caseload of patients within a clinic setting.

Table 44–2 Outpatient Hypertension Clinic Start-Up Checklist	
1. Establish need and cost benefits	7. Determine sequence and pathway of patient visit flow
2. Assess and establish staff support and qualifications	Schedule for new and return visit
3. Designate physician medical director and coordinator	Physician consultation schedule with new patients
4. Ensure efficient assessment and educational physical space	8. Develop patient data storage and tracking system
5. Develop written policies and procedures	Assess existing patient tracking software packages
Entry and referral criteria	Determine relevant patient data
Treatment algorithms	Develop protocol for monitoring clinical events and
Exit criteria	associated costs
Laboratory standards	9. Acquire and maintain patient education materials
Pricing	Pharmacological information
Fee-for-service schedule	Lifestyle information
Compute capitation rate or contribution to global rate for	Other resources
managed care contracts	10. Marketing and promotion plan
Billing and corrections policy	Internal marketing and promotion: Medical and ancillary staff
Operational budget and pro forma outcome measures (JNC	Patients
VI goals)	Referring physicians, PPOs, and HMOs
6. Develop standard forms	Business and industry
Patient information (medical history, lifestyle)	Alliances with hospitals, PPOs, and drug companies to
Initial assessment and treatment plan	form organized and efficient disease-management programs
Return visit and progress report	11. Develop continuing education schedule for clinic staff
Drug descriptions and patient administration instructions	New research funding
Individual lifestyle counseling prescription (dietary, exercise,	New reimbursement guidelines and legislation
stress management)	12. Develop link and network with national hypertension
Dietary and body fat assessment (BMI)	organizations

Adapted with permission from La Forge R, Thomas T. Outpatient management of lipid disorders. J Cardiovasc Nurs 11:39–53, © 1996, Aspen Publishers, Inc.
Abbreviations: JNC VI, the sixth report of the Joint National Committee on the Prevention, Detection, Evaluation, and Treatment of High Blood Pressure; BMI, body mass index; PPOs, Preferred Provider Organizations; HMOs, Health Maintenance Organizations.

Caseload size is strongly influenced by the characteristics of the patient population. Patients with more severe hypertension often require more frequent visits to regulate medications and manage target organ complications. Those with mild hypertension may require infrequent monitoring and reinforcement of education and counseling, which can be provided by both the nurse and a receptionist. Within the Veterans Hypertension Screening and Treatment Clinics, which have operated since the late 1970s, it is estimated that a staff of four (two nurses, a receptionist, and a quarter-time physician) can provide care including medication therapy to over 800 patients annually, initial screenings for 1800 patients, and rescreening for those 800 individuals with mild hypertension not requiring medication management. Data from this evaluation suggest that the average patient requires approximately five visits within a period of approximately 9 months in order to achieve goal blood pressure.[14] Experience of a large clinic in Glasgow suggests that a single nurse practitioner working with a physician can manage up to 700 to 900 patients per year.[21] Finally, within a worksite clinic, Alderman and colleagues note that a nurse can see an average of 16 patients per day.[5, 22] The capability of nurses and other personnel to shorten the length of clinic visits, order fewer unnecessary blood chemistry tests, lower the cost of medications, and creatively provide education within the clinic by offering some education and counseling through videotapes, written materials, and other vehicles in the waiting rooms enhances the efficiency of the clinic. Additional support can also be obtained by using volunteers to provide services that do not require the expertise of a nurse or physician.

REIMBURSEMENT FOR SERVICES

Issues about reimbursement are frequently discussed among nurses and physicians wanting to establish a hyper-
tension clinic. Much of what has been learned in the establishment of lipid clinics, anticoagulation monitoring services, and diabetic education programs applies to obtaining coverage for services provided within a hypertension clinic.[23] Although a hypertension clinic is not a covered service per se, many of the services provided within the clinic are covered under the guidelines set forth by the Health Care Finance Administration (HCFA) under Medicare. Hypertension clinic personnel should establish a fee structure using guidelines set forth by the HCFA Medicare Carriers Manual, Section 2050. Because the "incident to" guidelines under Medicare are nationally recognized, most of the insurance carriers follow the rules developed by HCFA. The guidelines indicate that nurses and other licensed personnel may provide services such as conducting physical examinations, taking medical histories, and providing medical decision-making as long as the service is provided under the direct supervision of the physician, in the same office setting, and he or she is immediately available to provide assistance. In these instances, the physician employs or contracts with the nurse and directly supervises the health care professional who provides the services. Some of the important issues that should be noted about following the "incident to" ruling under Medicare are noted in Table 44–3. Clinic personnel should recognize that each HCFA representative within a state may interpret the guidelines differently; therefore obtaining clarification through written guidelines is important to ensure that rules are followed and adequate coverage is obtained.

Several innovative mechanisms of payment may also provide a way to cover the costs incurred in running a hypertension clinic. Contracting to provide these services with a managed care organization may be a viable option. Working to develop relationships with pharmaceutical companies to conduct small research projects may offset some

Table 44–3 Medicare "Incident To" Billings
(What Is Important)

Service must be:

Integral part of physician's professional service

Commonly included in physician's bill

Furnished in physician's office or clinic under direct supervision

Furnished by individual qualifying as an "employee" acting under scope of state licensure laws

Services are billed:

Under supervising physician's provider number using same CPT codes

As one service per patient per day unless there is documentation of need

Documentation in the patient record to support level of service/coding is absolutely essential

Abbreviation: CPT, Current Procedural Terminology.

of the costs. Providing multiple services for cardiovascular disease management for patients with heart failure, lipid disorders, hypertension, and diabetes may also expand the scope and opportunities for success of specialized clinics.

In the mid-1970s, in two separate editorials,[24, 25] Finnerty suggested that asymptomatic patients would not remain under care and on medication without proper motivation. He noted that once the initial diagnosis of hypertension was made, the care of the patient was primarily related to education. He further suggested that we should recognize the value of specially trained nurses in managing hypertension, just as we have relied on such nurses in the coronary care unit. His suggestion was based on the reality that most physicians have been trained as diagnosticians responsible for managing complicated problems or treating the patient in an emergent situation. Recognizing that close to one third of patients drop out of care and that only a quarter of all treated hypertensive patients achieve a goal blood pressure of less than 140/90 mm Hg[1] should make us wake up and focus on the need for what Finnerty advocated and what we know improves patient care and outcomes. In a health care system that is highly focused on acute illness, on managing older, sicker patients, and on reducing costs, the use of nurses practicing collaboratively with physicians in the outpatient arena can be highly beneficial to large numbers of patients with hypertension and other chronic asymptomatic conditions, to the health care provider, and to the health care system.

References

1. Burt VL, Cutler JA, Higgins M, et al. Trends in the prevalence, awareness, treatment, and control of hypertension in the adult U.S. population: Data from the Health Examination Surveys, 1960–1991. Hypertension 26:60–69, 1995.
2. Levy D, Larson MG, Vasan RS, et al. The progression from hypertension to congestive heart failure. JAMA 275:1557–1562, 1996.
3. Kumanyika SK, Charleston JB. Lose weight and win: A church-based weight loss program for blood pressure control among black women. Patient Educ Couns 19:19–32, 1992.
4. Runyan KW Jr. The Memphis Chronic Disease Program. Comparisons in outcome and the nurse's extended role. JAMA 231:264–267, 1975.
5. Alderman MH, Schoenbaum EF. Detection and treatment of hypertension at the work site. N Engl J Med 293:65–68, 1973.
6. Logan AG, Milne BJ, Achber C, et al. Work-site treatment of hypertension by specially trained nurses. A controlled trial. Lancet 2:1175–1178, 1979.
7. Hypertension Detection and Follow-up Program Cooperative Group. Five-year findings of the Hypertension Detection and Follow-up Program. I: Reduction in mortality of persons with high blood pressure, including mild hypertension. JAMA 242:2562–2571, 1979.
8. SHEP Cooperative Research Group. Prevention of stroke by antihypertensive drug treatment in older persons with isolated systolic hypertension. JAMA 261:3255–3264, 1991.
9. Hill MN, Reichgott MJ. Achievement of standards for quality care of hypertension by physicians and nurses. Clin Exp Hypertens 1:665–684, 1979.
10. Reichgott MJ, Pearson S, Hill MN. The nurse practitioner's role in complex patient management: Hypertension. J Natl Med Assoc 75:1197–1204, 1983.
11. Pheley AM, Terry P, Pietz L, et al. Evaluation of a nurse-based hypertension management program: Screening, management, and outcomes. J Cardiovasc Nurs 9:54–61, 1995.
12. Miller NH. Nurse case management—The MULTIFIT Program. [Abstract] Am J Hypertens 9:194A, 1996.
13. Sox HC. Quality of patient care by nurse practitioners and physician's assistants: A ten-year perspective. Ann Intern Med 91:459–468, 1979.
14. Perry HM, Schnapner JW, Meyer G, Swatzell R. Clinical program for screening and treatment of hypertension in veterans. J Natl Med Assoc 74:433–444, 1982.
15. Stason WB. Opportunities to improve the cost-effectiveness of treatment for hypertension. Hypertension 18(suppl):I161–I166, 1991.
16. Joint National Committee on Prevention, Detection, Evaluation, and Treatment of High Blood Pressure. The sixth report. NIH Publication No. 98-4080. Bethesda, MD, U.S. Department of Health and Human Services, National Institutes of Health, 1998.
17. Miller NH, Taylor CB. Lifestyle Management for Patients With Coronary Heart Disease. Current Issues in Cardiac Rehabilitation, Monograph No. 2. Champaign, IL, Human Kinetics, 1995.
18. Levine DM, Green LW, Deeds SG, et al. Health education for hypertensive patients. JAMA 241:1700–1703, 1979.
19. Logan AC, Milne BJ, Flanagan PT, Haynes RB. Clinical effectiveness and cost-effectiveness of monitoring blood pressure of hypertensive employees at work. Hypertension 5:828–836, 1983.
20. DeBusk RF, Miller NH, Superko HR, et al. A case management system for coronary risk factor modification following acute myocardial infarction. Ann Intern Med 120:721–729, 1994.
21. Curzio JL, Beevers M. The role of nurses in hypertension care and research. J Hum Hypertens 11:541–550, 1997.
22. Wilson J. Nurse-run clinics for worksite treatment. [Abstract] Am J Hypertens 9:194A, 1996.
23. Cahill NE, Thomas T. Reimbursement Planning for Lipid Clinic Services. Princeton, NJ, Bristol-Myers Squibb, 1997.
24. Finnerty FA Jr. The nurse's role in treating hypertension. [Editorial] N Engl J Med 293:93–94, 1975.
25. Finnerty FA. The nurse and care of the hypertensive patient. Ann Intern Med 84:746, 1976.

45 Community Outreach

Martha N. Hill, Lee R. Bone, and David M. Levine

Community outreach is an essential component of comprehensive programs to promote health and prevent and/or control disease and related risk factors in populations. It complements other strategies to reach the entire population, including those who do not have access to care, who have discontinued care, or who need reinforcement in following treatment recommendations. From a public health perspective, community outreach offers the best opportunity to provide state-of-the-art treatment or prevention to the population at large as well as to individuals and families, with the goal of improving health. Outreach has been utilized successfully for a wide variety of health programs, including prenatal care, immunizations, and treatment for human immunodeficiency virus/acquired immunodeficiency disease syndrome (HIV/AIDS), tuberculosis, diabetes, and hypertension.

Effective hypertension management requires a comprehensive approach that integrates social, psychological, behavioral, and economic as well as biomedical considerations. Community outreach is a proven strategy that incorporates many of these approaches. Moreover, it links health professionals and health care organizations with current or potential patients and with resources in the patients' communities. From a clinical perspective, hypertension care and control programs that include community outreach provide three important lessons:

1. Clinicians can use resources in the community to directly enhance their care of patients, thus improving long-term control of hypertension and reducing associated target organ damage.
2. Community programs provide reinforcement of the clinician's recommendations and teaching efforts.
3. Physicians, nurse practitioners, and other clinicians can provide community service and leadership by accepting referrals, promoting outreach programs, and acting as consultants.

DEFINITION OF COMMUNITY OUTREACH

Community outreach is a health services, health education, and health promotion strategy. It is an activity in which medicine and public health interface, an area of practice that is the focus of community nursing. Outreach can be defined differently, depending on a program's purpose. Its goal, however, is to reach those who are not reached by usual methods for the purpose of increasing knowledge, information, and access to and utilization of health services. It inevitably has to address issues of health services availability, accessibility, acceptability, and affordability, focusing on removing geographic, cultural, administrative, and financial barriers to health care. Outreach has been an integral part of public health throughout the century. Traditionally, it has been a targeted approach to meeting the needs of the underserved. In the past few decades, hospitals and academic health centers have begun outreach as an extension of medical and nursing care, in part in response to needs broadly defined by the community. Outreach has thus become a way of providing community service to meet marketing and public relations as well as population needs and health promotion and disease prevention objectives. Comprehensive community health promotion programs are directed to entire populations as well as to specific high-risk and underserved groups.

Key principles of community outreach are active community participation and/or partnership, careful planning and diagnosis, program implementation, and evaluation. A needs assessment; definition of goals, aims, and strategies; and resources are essential for success. There is a wide variety of programs. Outreach is well recognized for its effectiveness, for example, in screening, case finding, referral, education, and monitoring. Effective interventions are a combination of persuasive communications, interpersonal relationships, skills training, and community organizing. Mass media can be used to deliver informative messages through dramas, documentaries, or public service announcements. Numerous types of outreach strategies include person-to-person contact by letter, telephone, home visit, mobile unit, and hot or warm lines. Outreach also can be provided at community events, such as health fairs, in the home by community health workers, in satellite clinics, or in nontraditional sites, such as churches and recreation centers.[1]

Community participation and partnership are essential ingredients for productive sustained outreach programs. A group of respected community leaders as an organizing or advisory committee can be constructive. Community organizers, politicians, physicians, clergy, and others with an interest can help design, implement, and evaluate a program that will be acceptable and responsive to the community and directed at meeting their needs. Community involvement is invaluable in deciding who should participate, what they should do, and how they should be recognized for their contributions. Whereas the good will and community service produced by many outreach activities are evident, it is important to evaluate the cost-effectiveness and efficiency of such activities to compare various approaches before replication. In spite of scarce resources, outreach programs need to demonstrate achievement of objectives and impact on clinical outcomes.

HISTORY OF OUTREACH PROGRAMS TO CONTROL HYPERTENSION

During the 1960s and the War on Poverty, outreach services became an integral part of many health and social service programs.[2] Grass roots organizing, community development, and more recently, economic development were seen as mechanisms to improve quality of life, including social, emotional, and physical well-being.[3] Many hypertension outreach programs targeted African Americans whose high blood pressure was detected, treated, and controlled at rates that continued to lag behind rates of whites.[4]

Case finding was recognized as an important outreach activity in the 1970s. The purpose was to motivate people to have their blood pressure measured at a familiar site for little or no cost. Organized blood pressure screenings in the community found that an accessible location, community participation, referrals to care, and follow-up reinforcement of people to complete referrals contributed to improved care and control of hypertension. Community-based screening programs grew in places, such as firehouses, churches, barbershops, and worksites, where people congregated and space was available for staff or volunteers to measure blood pressure and provide education and counseling.[5]

Early household and community surveys documented low rates of hypertension awareness, treatment, and control in Georgia, Virginia, Maryland, and Washington, DC.[6–10] In an effort to screen for undetected hypertension in inner-city Washington, DC, Finnerty and colleagues found house-to-house canvassing by trained interviewers to be ineffective, time-consuming, and dangerous. Encouraged by civic leaders, trained allied personnel screening in churches and supermarkets identified large numbers of hypertensive individuals and referred them for care. In several care settings, low rates of appointment attendance and blood pressure control and high rates of clinic dropouts were documented.[9, 10] Interviews with patients revealed three key findings affecting patients' attitudes about remaining in care: amount of time expended to receive care (transportation and waiting); understanding of all aspects of the disease; and "doctor/paramedical/patient" relationship. A new patient-centered hypertension care program was designed, including health aides trained to serve as patient advocates; deliver preappointment reminders by telephone, mail, or in person (which led to a doubling of attendance); and help resolve difficulties affecting compliance with visits and medication.

The Hypertension Detection and Follow-up Program (HDFP) was designed to test the effectiveness of a comprehensive treatment program to control high blood pressure and reduce complications compared with usual care in the community.[11, 12] Clinic and community outreach, free transportation and medication, a multidisciplinary team approach to care, and a very committed staff demonstrated that the pharmacological benefits of hypertension control could be generalized to the community. These methods have been incorporated into all major multisite hypertension treatment and prevention clinical trials, e.g., Multiple Risk Factor Intervention Trial (MRFIT), Treatment of Mild Hypertension Study (TOMHS), and Trials of Hypertension Prevention (TOHP).[13–16] Home visits were found to be an effective outreach strategy in a classic health education clinical trial to improve physician care of hypertension. Green, Levine, and coworkers used a factorial design to test three supplementary interventions: physician visit exit interview with the nurse; home visits to a person identified by the patient as a source of social support with health

matters; and group classes.[17, 18] The home visits were conducted by nurse-supervised high school students from the community. Worksite programs, an additional type of outreach, were found to be very successful in improving rates of hypertension care and control. Schoenbaum and Alderman, working with a labor union for department store employees, documented the high standard of care provided on site by nurse practitioners.[19] Foote and Erfut documented the value of worksite interventions at Ford Motor Company.[20]

A broad definition of community outreach encompasses the efforts of the National Heart, Lung, and Blood Institute's (NHLBI) National High Blood Pressure Education Program, founded in 1972. The recipients of these outreach activities are the public (through mass media campaigns), health care practitioners and organizations, industry, and individuals. Seven state programs supported by NHLBI demonstrated the value of mobilizing and coordinating community-wide resources to increase the rates of hypertension awareness, treatment, and control.[21–24] In Maryland, a coordinating council served as the hub for professional groups, academic health centers, voluntary nonprofit organizations, and others who wanted to improve high blood pressure care and control. Committees were formed to carry out aims of the project by providing outreach for many communities. Project efforts were numerous and varied: professional education; public information and communication; screening and monitoring at health departments, worksites, churches, and barbershops; and demonstration projects in inner-city and rural areas of the state.[25–27] Another type of national community outreach is professional education to disseminate consensus recommendations to improve practice and patient care. The Joint National Committee reports have focused increasingly on prevention, diagnosis, evaluation, and initial treatment with lessening amounts of content on community programs, multidisciplinary approaches, and adherence strategies.[28] Outreach information is available in separate documents disseminated primarily to the public health community.[29]

Three comprehensive community-based cardiovascular risk reduction studies were conducted: The Stanford Five-Cities Project,[30] The Minnesota Heart Health Program,[31] and The Pawtucket Heart Health Program.[32] These major community-based programs to reduce cardiovascular and stroke risk utilized state-of-the-art communication and education strategies in combination with community organization, outreach, and social support.[33] This application of knowledge drew from the social and behavioral sciences and complemented and supplemented knowledge from the biomedical sciences applied in medical settings.

Today, telecommunication technologies, including handheld and personal computers, telephone, FAX, FAX modems, and electronic mail, are being used to collect, transmit, and store data. These technologies provide opportunities for creative models of outreach. These models take advantage of patient self-monitoring and communication of information among patients in their homes, community laboratories, nurse case managers, primary care physicians, and specialist physicians. Extending home monitoring by the patient or a health provider on the telephone improves adherence by tailoring therapy promptly without office visits. Programs incorporating telecommunications, such as MULTIFIT, have earned high levels of patient and provider satisfaction and improved outcomes.[34, 35]

THE GAP BETWEEN RESEARCH AND PRACTICE

From the studies previously discussed and others, it is clear that a combination of lifestyle and, if necessary, pharmacological interventions contribute to hypertension control and reduce associated morbidity and mortality. These interventions are significantly more effective when based on appropriate patient, provider, and public education. The challenge in hypertension control is to extend the health benefits of these interventions to the population and, in particular, to more diverse, less select, high-risk groups to eliminate preventable disparities in health status. Despite our increased knowledge and subsequent improvements in the control of hypertension, national data as recent as 1995 indicate that the majority of Americans with hypertension do not have controlled blood pressures and that awareness, treatment, and control rates are dropping.[36] Community outreach, including grass roots advocacy and education by voluntary health organizations such as the American Heart Association, is necessary to eliminate gaps in the care and control of hypertension between the majority and the minority populations.[37] This will require renewed commitment and more clearly and strongly stated policy recommendations for effective community outreach. The evidence supports the value of community outreach activities designed with an understanding of the sociocultural context of patients' lives.

HOW COMMUNITY OUTREACH WILL NARROW THE GAP

Community–Health System Partnership

Community outreach has contributed importantly to the detection and control of prevalent chronic diseases by incorporating the priorities and strategies of both health professionals and the community.[38] This shared approach reflects a broader definition of health and its determinants, including the social, cultural, and economic context within which health is, or is not, promoted. Community–health system partnerships allow for individual and collective empowerment and participation of the community in identifying health problems and strategies for addressing those problems.

Advocacy is one such important partnership effort. Recognizing needs, identifying solutions, securing resources, and influencing policy makers have been shown to improve national and local hypertension control activities. Securing the availability of malls and high school tracks to promote walking and providing more low-fat and low-sodium foods in grocery stores are examples of advocacy outcomes. "Lose Weight and Win," a church-based weight-loss program for blood pressure control among African American women, is an example of a successful community-based outreach program that operated independently of health care settings but with the goal of modifying lifestyle to complement and supplement medical recommendations.[39]

Academic health centers and their neighboring communities are increasingly forming partnerships to address environmental and social needs. These efforts to build and maintain cohesive neighborhoods are an investment in health.[40] These partnerships are a particularly important solution to the national health care issues concerning underserved minority populations.[41] Opportunities abound for integrating education and research while providing patient care targeted to community health priorities. Such opportunities are readily available to improve hypertension care and control.

Ecological Multidisciplinary Approach

Hypertension care and control are complex and call for a comprehensive multidisciplinary approach. The numerous considerations are reflected in the five-level Ecological Model: intrapersonal; interpersonal; organizational; community; and societal.[42] To eliminate the disparities between what is beneficial in clinical trials and what occurs in practice, innovative outreach strategies are needed. Many people are without health insurance. The benefits of those who are insured cover fewer services, including preventive services such as screening and prescriptions to control cardiovascular risk factors. Outreach programs can inform uninsured and underinsured individuals about available services. However, policy makers must be influenced to provide coverage for all if the disproportionate burden of hypertension among the lower socioeconomic groups is to be addressed.

Physicians and other health professionals with responsibility for the care of hypertensive patients need to be aware and supportive of the social context of their patients' lives. If desired patient outcomes are to be achieved long-term, clinicians need to invest their expertise wisely. By joining with others in a multidisciplinary team, across geographic settings, physicians can maximize use of their medical expertise. We cannot afford to ignore the evidence supporting the contributions of nurses, nurse practitioners, physician assistants, pharmacists, nutritionists, health educators, and outreach workers.[43] The multilevel compliance challenge requires us to address behavior not only at the patient level but at the provider and health care organization levels as well.[44] Medicine and public health each have unique contributions to make and together can complement one another to eliminate the gap between what we know controls hypertension and reduces or minimizes its complications and what is happening daily in practice and in patients' lives.[37]

USE OF COMMUNITY HEALTH WORKERS

A particularly important aspect of community-based team approaches is the inclusion of community health workers. Also called *health aides* or *lay advisors,* they are receiving growing acceptance as valued members of the health care team.[45] Often viewed as nurse extenders, they provide basic primary care services in community settings, including the home, with which they are culturally familiar.[46–48] Their role focuses on improving access to and continuity of care, patient education, reinforcement of adherence to treatment, addressing needed human services, and promoting self-care skills and confidence. In research as well as service delivery programs, they strengthen the cultural understanding and acceptability, and thus the effectiveness, of many outreach activities, including hypertension care.[49, 50] They are trained to

1. Provide health information to improve knowledge and skills with appointments and recommended treatment;
2. Assist with referrals to community resources, including assistance with financial problems;
3. Monitor blood pressure and communicate with care providers in clinical settings; and
4. Facilitate the identification and involvement of a key support person to whom the patient turns to for help with health matters.

Functioning as health promoters, trained community health workers increase access to primary and preventive health services. Crucial qualifications include the desire to help others and to improve the community.[42] Often a member of the neighborhood, the worker understands the community's language, culture, and socioeconomic conditions and is able to help providers and patients better understand one another's expectations. This facilitates the development of an individualized plan for hypertension care that the patient can adhere to within the context of her or his daily life.

Currently, in inner-city Baltimore, a program of research has been developed to test the effectiveness of a nurse practitioner–community health worker–physician team approach to improving hypertension care and control in young African American men.[51] Lack of health insurance, a primary care physician, and compliance with antihypertensive treatment as well as dependence on emergency departments for episodic care contribute to low rates of hypertension care and control in this underserved high-risk population.[50–52] An additional program in another area of inner-city Baltimore focuses on testing the effectiveness of nurse practitioner–community health worker–physician delivered home-based interventions. The trained health workers are helpful members of the investigative team in improving hypertension care and control. Among their contributions is a community perspective and experience that has to be balanced with the inevitable tension between standardizing an intervention to meet protocol needs and providing individualized patient care and service.

CONCLUSION

We must seek to understand why U.S. rates of hypertension awareness, treatment, and control are declining. Community outreach offers proven strategies for complementing medical care and realizing the potential benefits of blood pressure control. Major efforts are needed to reverse declining trends by increasing entry into and remaining in continuous care as well as adherence to treatment recommendations. Community outreach offers new research

opportunities to investigate the most cost-effective and efficient strategies for diverse populations and those with the disproportionate burden of hypertension and its complications.

References

1. Lasater TM, Becker DM, Hill MN, Gans KM. Synthesis of findings and issues from religious-based cardiovascular disease prevention trials. Ann Epidemiol 7:S46–S53, 1997.
2. Colombo TJ, Freeborn DK, Mullooly JP, Burnham VR. The effect of outreach workers' educational efforts on disadvantaged preschool children's use of preventive services. Am J Public Health 69:465–468, 1979.
3. Rothman J, Erlick JL, Theresa JG. Promoting Innovation and Change in Organizations and Communities. New York, John Wiley & Sons, 1976.
4. Kong BW. Community-based hypertension control programs that work. J Poor Underserved 8:409–415, 1997.
5. Kong BW, Miller JM, Smoot RT. Churches as high blood pressure control centers. J Natl Med Assoc 74:920–923, 1982.
6. Wilber JA, Milward D, Baldwin A, et al. Atlanta community high blood pressure program methods of community hypertension screening. Circ Res 31:101–109, 1972.
7. Carey RM, Reid RA, Ayers CR, et al. The Charlottesville Blood-Pressure Survey. Value of repeated blood-pressure measurements. JAMA 236:847–851, 1976.
8. Entwistle G, Scott J, Apostoledes A, et al. A survey of blood pressure in the state of Maryland. Prev Med 12:695–708, 1983.
9. Finnerty FA Jr, Mattie EC, Finnerty FA III. Hypertension in the inner city. I: Analysis of clinic dropouts. Circulation 47:73–75, 1973.
10. Finnerty FA Jr, Shaw LW, Himmelsbach CK. Hypertension in the inner city. II: Detection and follow-up. Circulation 47:76–78, 1973.
11. Hypertension Detection and Follow-up Program Cooperative Group. The Hypertension Detection and Follow-up Program. Prev Med 5:207–215, 1976.
12. Hypertension Detection and Follow-up Program Cooperative Group. Five-year findings of the Hypertension Detection and Follow-up Program. I: Reduction in mortality of persons with high blood pressure, including mild hypertension. JAMA 242:2562–2571, 1979.
13. Multiple Risk Factor Intervention Trial Research Group. Multiple Risk Factor Intervention Trial (MRFIT). JAMA 248:1465–1477, 1982.
14. Multiple Risk Factor Intervention Trial Research Group. Multiple Risk Factor Intervention Trial: Risk factor changes and mortality results. JAMA 248:1465–1477, 1982.
15. Treatment of Mild Hypertension Study Research Group. Treatment of Mild Hypertension Study: Final results. JAMA 270:713–724, 1993.
16. Trials of Hypertension Prevention Collaborative Research Group. The effects of nonpharmacological interventions on blood pressure of persons with high normal levels: Results of the Trials of Hypertension Prevention, phase I. JAMA 267:1213–1220, 1992.
17. Levine DM, Morisky DE, Bone LR, et al. Data-based planning for educational interventions through hypertension control programs for urban and rural populations in Maryland. Public Health Rep 97:107–112, 1982.
18. Morisky DE, Levine DM, Green LW, et al. Five-year blood pressure control and mortality following health education for hypertensive patients. Am J Public Health 73:153–162, 1983.
19. Schoenbaum EE, Alderman MH. Organization for long-term management of hypertension: The recruitment, training, and responsibilities of the health team. Bull N Y Acad Med 52:699–708, 1976.
20. Foote A, Erfurt JC. Development and dissemination of model systems for hypertension control in organizational settings. Institute of Labor and Industrial Relations, The University of Michigan—Wayne State University, Ann Arbor, Michigan, 1974.
21. Ware D, Leonard A, Southard J, et al. A Coordination of statewide high blood pressure control activities: A study in four states. Prev Med 7:245, 1979.
22. Chiappini M, Henson M, Wilber J, McClellan W. Statewide community high blood pressure control programs. J Med Assoc Ga 70:357–360, 1981.
23. Medical Care Development, Inc. Statewide household survey of prevalence and control of hypertension in Maine. Monograph, May 1982.

24. Mills E (ed). Coordination of High Blood Pressure Control in Michigan: Final Report, vols I and II. Lansing, Michigan Department of Public Health, 1985.

25. Morisky D, Levine D, Green L, et al. The relative impact of health education for low- and high-risk patients with hypertension. Prev Med 9:550–558, 1980.

26. Shanker B, Russell R, Southard J, Schurman E. Patterns of care for hypertension among hospitalized patients. Public Health Rep 97:521–527, 1982.

27. Levine D, Bone L, Steinwachs D, et al. The physician's role in improving patient outcome in high blood pressure control. Md St Med J 32:291–293, 1983.

28. Joint National Committee on Prevention, Detection, Evaluation, and Treatment of High Blood Pressure. The sixth report. Arch Intern Med 157:2413–2446, 1997.

29. Community Guide to High Blood Pressure Control. U.S. Department of Health and Human Services. Public Health Service, National Institutes of Health, National Heart, Lung, and Blood Institute, National High Blood Pressure Education Program. NIH Publication No. 82-2333. May 1982.

30. Fortmann SP, Winleby MA, Flora JA, et al. Effect of long-term community health education on blood pressure and hypertension control: The Stanford Five-City Project. Am J Epidemiol 132:629–646, 1990.

31. Luepker RV, Murray DM, Jacobs DR, et al. Community education for cardiovascular disease prevention: Risk factor changes in the Minnesota Heart Health Program. Am J Public Health 84:1383–1393, 1994.

32. Carleton RA, Lasater TM, Assaf AR, et al. The Pawtucket Heart Health Program: An experiment in population-based disease prevention. R I Med J 70:533–538, 1987.

33. Weiss SM. Community health promotion demonstration programs: Introduction. In Matarrazo JD, Herd JA, Miller NE, Weiss SM (eds). Behavioral Health: A Handbook of Health Enhancement and Disease Prevention. New York, John Wiley & Sons, 1984; p 1137–1139.

34. DeBusk RF, Miller NH, Superko R, et al. A case-management system for coronary risk factor modification after acute myocardial infarction. Ann Intern Med 120:721–729, 1994.

35. Friedman RH, Kazis LE, Jette A, et al. A telecommunications system for monitoring and counseling patients with hypertension: Impact on medication adherence and blood pressure control. Am J Hypertens 9:285–292, 1996.

36. Burt VL, Cutler JA, Higgins M, et al. Trends in the prevalence, awareness, treatment, and control of hypertension in the adult US population: Data from the Health Examination Survey, 1960–1991. Hypertension 26:60–69, 1995.

37. Hill MN. Behavior and biology: The basic sciences for AHA action. Circulation 97:807–810, 1998.

38. Robertson A, Minkler M. New health promotion movement: A critical examination. Health Educ Q 2:295–312, 1994.

39. Kumanyika SK, Charleston JB. "Lose Weight and Win," a church-based weight loss program for blood pressure control among African American women. Patient Educ Couns 19:19–32, 1992.

40. Sampson RJ, Raudenbush SW, Earls F. Neighborhoods and violent crime: A multilevel study of collective efficacy. Science 277:918–924, 1977.

41. Levine DM, Becker DM, Bone LR, et al. Community-academic health center partnerships for underserved minority populations—One solution to a national crisis. JAMA 272:309–311, 1994.

42. McLeroy KR, Bibeau D, Steckler A, Glanz K. An ecological perspective on health promotion programs. Health Educ Q 15:351–377, 1988.

43. Hill MN, Miller NH. Compliance enhancement: A call for multidisciplinary team approaches. Circulation 93:4–6, 1996.

44. Miller NH, Hill MN, Kottke T, Ockene IS. The multilevel compliance challenge: Recommendations for a call to action. Circulation 95:1085–1090, 1997.

45. Pew Health Professions Commission. Community health workers: Integral yet often overlooked members of the health care workforce. San Francisco, UCSF Center for the Health Professions, 1994.

46. Scherer JL. Neighbor to neighbor: Community health workers educate their own. Hosp Health Netw 1994; pp 52–56.

47. Hill MN, Becker DM. Roles of nurses and health workers in cardiovascular health promotion. Am J Med Sci 310:S123–126, 1995.

48. Bray ML, Edwards LH. A primary care approach using Hispanic workers as nurse extenders. Public Health Nurs 11:7–11, 1994.

49. Hill MN, Bone LR, Butz AM. Maximizing the effectiveness of community health workers in research. Image J Nurs Sch 25:221–226, 1996.

50. Bone LR, Mamon J, Levine DM, et al. Emergency department detection and follow-up of high blood pressure: Use and effectiveness of community health workers. Am J Emerg Med 7:16–20, 1989.

51. Hill MN, Bone LR, Hilton SC, et al. A clinical trial to improve high blood pressure care in young urban black men. Am J Hypertens 12:548–554, 1999.

52. Shea S, Misra D, Ehrlich MH, et al. Predisposing factors for severe, uncontrolled hypertension in an inner-city minority population. N Engl J Med 327:776–781, 1992.

Medication Compliance for Antihypertensive Therapy

CHAPTER 46

Peter Rudd

Hypertension remains a powerful contributor to cardiovascular diseases, the most common cause of death in the United States. Calculated to be the fourth largest mortality risk factor, hypertension has been estimated to predict 6% of all deaths worldwide.[1] Since the late 1950s, the prevalence of hypertension has changed little despite improvements in its detection and treatment.[2] The importance of optimizing treatment adherence rises in proportion to the potential benefit from therapy. With successful treatment, the relative risks of fatal and nonfatal events fall by 38% for stroke and 16% for coronary heart disease.[3] Nationally, the data displayed in Figure 46–1 suggest the need for continued efforts, since less than 30% of American hypertensive patients are diagnosed, under treatment, and at goal blood pressure, leaving more than 10 million uncontrolled hypertensives in this country.[4]

The vast majority of clinical activity for managing hypertensive patients occurs in physicians' offices, clinics, and other ambulatory sites. Unlike hospitalized patients, whose every medication dose may be readily and objectively defined, charted, and administered, most hypertensive patients receive limited supervision and instruction from their prescribing clinicians. On most days in most settings for most doses of antihypertensive medication, the patients are on their own, as illustrated in Figure 46–2.

In essence, the sizable investment in diagnosing, evalu-

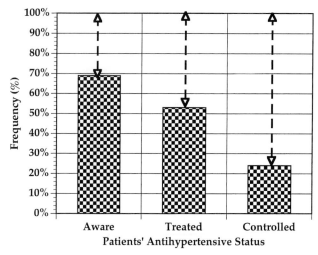

Figure 46–1. Status of antihypertensive management and opportunity for improvement, 1988 to 1991. Prevalence of hypertension by status of diagnosis, treatment, and blood pressure control from the Third National Health and Nutrition Examination Survey (NHANES III; 1988 to 1991),[4] based on a cross-sectional survey of the civilian, noninstitutionalized population of the United States after both an in-home interview and a clinical examination for 9901 participants above age 18 years.

ating, and prescribing treatment for individual hypertensive patients comes to depend on how well they follow the prescription: taking medications, modifying diet and activity, and making other lifestyle changes. These components make up the core of clinical adherence or compliance. The thoughtful clinician, concerned about optimizing outcomes for patients, brings focus, skills, and perseverance to the challenge of optimizing adherence to the prescription as well as to proper diagnosis and evaluation. The health plan administrator, in turn, seeks to optimize outcomes for both the individual patient and the group of patients with similar characteristics and conditions. In parallel, the pharmaceutical manufacturer wishes to differentiate her or his product from competitive medications for the optimal combination of therapeutic efficacy and quality of life, while minimizing symptomatic and biochemical toxicity.[5]

Each constituency (patient, clinician, administrator, manufacturer) has its special priorities. In this complex context, *patient compliance* refers to the willingness and ability of an individual patient to follow health-related advice, to take medication as prescribed, to attend sched-

uled clinic appointments, and to complete recommended investigations.[6] The subsequent discussion focuses on medication-taking behavior, with particular reference to hypertension.

THERAPEUTIC PARADIGM

Most clinicians titrate their patients' blood pressure to a therapeutic goal level, most commonly 140/90 mm Hg or lower. In the mid-1970s, Sackett and coworkers[7–9] formulated the clinician's dilemma as having to allocate the returning patient into one of four mutually exclusive categories, illustrated in Figure 46–3.

Some allocation is necessary to determine subsequent clinical prescription until the next visit. The clinician must decide whether to continue the current regimen, augment it, attenuate it, or withhold it altogether. For the busy clinician, the allocation may appear deceptively simple. If the clinician considers only two possibilities (the regimen is satisfactory *or* the regimen needs to be augmented), he or she is following a simplified strategy. At least two other conditions may escape detection: (1) the patient has achieved goal blood pressure despite not having fully complied with the prescription, and (2) the patient may have failed to achieve goal blood pressure, in part, because of imperfect adherence. All four possibilities make up a more comprehensive strategy.

Very limited data exist about the relative frequency distributions of the four groupings among ambulatory hypertensive patients. The McMaster group reported data from male steelworkers assessed by pill counts and home blood pressure assessments.[8–10] Silas and colleagues[11] used quantitative urinary assays after calibration as the adherence measure. Their data appear together in Table 46–1.

Despite different methodologies, the two studies offer remarkably similar patterns. Only a minority of studied patients achieved both goal blood pressure and optimal adherence at the same time. Indeed, only about half of each group achieved satisfactory blood pressure control. Perhaps most critically, more than half of those patients who failed to achieve goal blood pressure exhibited suboptimal medication compliance. Finally, a small but definable minority achieved goal blood pressure despite less than full adherence, perhaps because of overzealous diagnosis or prescription.

Table 46–2 enumerates some implications of these dis-

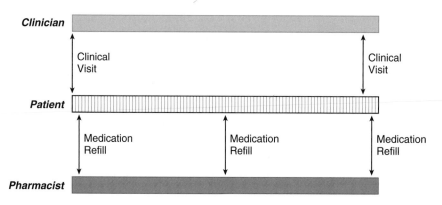

Figure 46–2. Relative contributions to adherent behaviors. The clinician, patient, and pharmacist all contribute to the frequency, consistency, and degree of adherence to the clinical prescription for ambulatory hypertensive patients. The relative contribution of the patient is the greatest, both overall and on a daily basis, despite the frequency of clinical visits and medication refills.

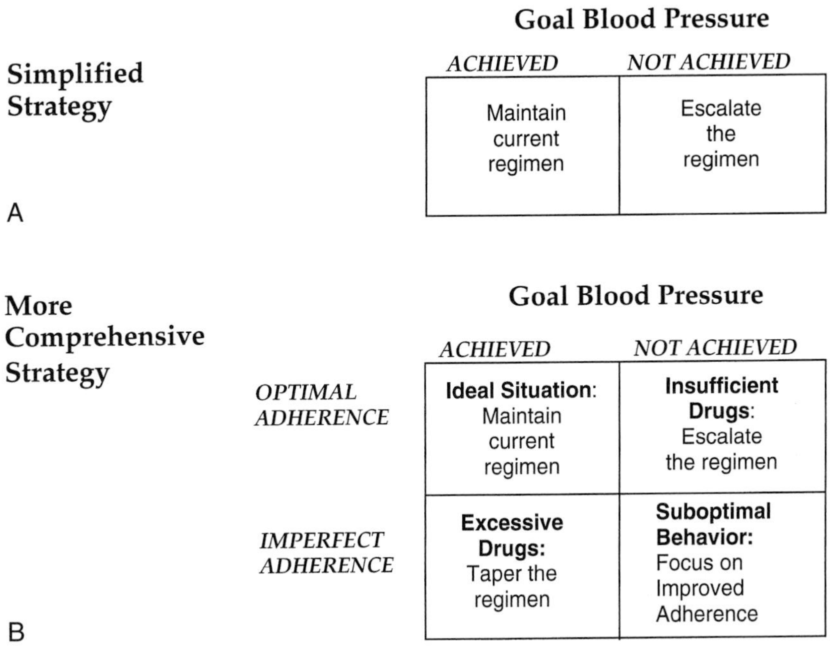

Goal Blood Pressure

ACHIEVED	NOT ACHIEVED
Maintain current regimen	Escalate the regimen

Simplified Strategy

A

Figure 46–3. Interpreting the therapeutic experiment. The clinician faces a dilemma of interpretation each time a patient returns for reassessment after receiving prescribed medication. *A,* Using a "simplified strategy," the clinician may interpret the achievement of goal blood pressure as ideal and escalate the regimen if goal blood pressure is not achieved. *B,* In reality, the variability in outcomes may reflect adherent behaviors as well as the biology of the disease and the pharmacology of the regimen. (*A* and *B,* Adapted from Sackett DL, Haynes RB, Tugwell P. Compliance. *In* Clinical Epidemiology; A Basic Science for Clinical Medicine. Boston, Little, Brown, 1985; p 203.)

More Comprehensive Strategy

Goal Blood Pressure

	ACHIEVED	NOT ACHIEVED
OPTIMAL ADHERENCE	**Ideal Situation:** Maintain current regimen	**Insufficient Drugs:** Escalate the regimen
IMPERFECT ADHERENCE	**Excessive Drugs:** Taper the regimen	**Suboptimal Behavior:** Focus on Improved Adherence

B

tributions. The first implication is that optimal compliance with prescribed antihypertensive medications should not be assumed, since it seems not to occur about half the time. Second, the clinician should resist automatic escalation of the drug regimen if the patient fails to achieve goal blood pressure. About half the time, the reason for failure reflects suboptimal medication-taking behavior rather than the biology of the disease or the pharmacology of the regimen. Third, an important minority on chronic antihypertensive medication succeed at full compliance without special interventions to attain goal blood pressure levels. Finally, a small group achieves goal blood pressure despite poor compliance but needs special assessments for detection.

In essence, there are consequences if the clinician misclassifies the patient, both in terms of risking toxic levels of drug exposure when full compliance occurs and in failing to achieve consistent blood pressure reduction with imperfect cardiovascular risk reduction. The data indirectly support the conclusion that the impact of treatment, both positive and negative, is proportional to the amount of treatment actually received rather than to the amount prescribed.[12]

On the positive side, full compliance brings maximal reduction of blood pressure reduction and cardiovascular risk. On the negative side, full compliance also brings maximal drug-related side effects and other toxicities. All but the most naive patients quickly learn to carry out their own miniexperiments, seeking to optimize among positive and negative, short- and long-term, benefit and risk.[13] Not surprisingly, partial or complete nonadherence is a major contributor to "refractory" hypertension.[14]

APPLICATION TO HYPERTENSION

Several features of treating ambulatory hypertension provide special challenges to the treating physician. Most daily responsibilities for following the regimen rest squarely on the patient's shoulders, regardless of the amount of

Table 46–1 Distributions of Adherence by Blood Pressure Achievement

Adherence	Goal Achieved	Goal Not Achieved	Totals
Sackett et al[9]			
Pill count ≥80%	43 (32%)	32 (24%)	75 (56%)
Pill count <80%	21 (16%)	38 (28%)	59 (44%)
Totals	64 (48%)	70 (52%)	134 (100%)
Silas et al[11]			
[Debrisoquine]$_u$ ≥11 mg/day	15 (41%)	6 (16%)	21 (57%)
[Debrisoquine]$_u$ <11 mg/day	6 (16%)	10 (27%)	16 (43%)
Totals	21 (57%)	16 (43%)	27 (100%)

Adapted from Rudd P. Compliance with antihypertensive therapy: Raising the bar of expectations. Am J Managed Care 4:600–609, 1998.

Table 46–2 Implications of the Adherence Distributions

1. Optimal adherence to the antihypertensive prescription should not be assumed
   Nonadherence occurs about half the time
   Overprescribing coupled with underadhering may still produce satisfactory blood pressure control
2. Failure to achieve goal blood pressure despite an adequate regimen and adequate time to respond may result from biological, pharmacological, or behavioral factors, or a combination of all three components
   About half the time when goal blood pressure is not achieved, suboptimal medication-taking may be present
   Escalating the regimen in such a context will be incorrect half the time
3. Only an important minority attains full compliance without special interventions to achieve goal blood pressure in a consistent manner

instruction, guidance, and support provided by physician, nurse, pharmacist, or family members.

On a more subtle level, treatment of hypertension almost never occurs in isolation but arises as part of a more comprehensive strategy to reduce cardiovascular risk factors, such as dyslipidemia, cigarette smoking, glucose intolerance, and obesity.[2] Unfortunately, the multiplicity of interventions may diminish rather than enhance some patients' motivation, as clinicians seek to have them reduce salt, saturated fat, and alcohol intake at the same time as they increase regular physical exercise and decrease stresses. The sheer number of things to be changed may overwhelm all but the most focused, trusting, and dedicated patient.

Interactions among the treatments may create extra dilemmas and opportunities. As data emerge indicating circadian variation in cardiovascular risk, selection of specific antihypertensive agents and their optimal administration time becomes more complex.[15] The clinician must learn to choose drugs on the basis of ability to reduce overall cardiovascular risk as well as to optimize antihypertensive efficacy, safety, quality of life, and adherence.[16, 17] Partially abandoned, the old concept of "stepped care" has been largely replaced by evolving notions of more personalized, nearly customized treatment plans.[18]

Part of the rationale for more aggressive and presumably more effective treatment strategies is the growing appreciation of lost benefits and increased risks for poor antihypertensive management. Suboptimal compliance carries increased probabilities of extra hospitalizations,[19] sudden death,[20] and other cardiovascular morbidity, even when the elevated pressures are linked to "white-coat" phenomena.[21]

HISTORICAL PERSPECTIVES

These perspectives on adherence and hypertension have evolved slowly but with increasing rapidity since the late 1980s with improved measures of medication-taking behavior. With better measures, clinicians have learned to broaden their focus and seize new opportunities.

Measures

For centuries, the study of medication-taking was constrained by the frailty of its measurements, as illustrated in Table 46–3.[22–27] Allusions by Hippocrates and Plato to nonadherence underscored the long traditions but provided few metrics except for global patient self-report or clinician opinion. Both of these hoary techniques are easy and inexpensive but prone to subjectivity and easily distorted. They are examples of indirect measures, remote in time and space from the actual consumption of prescribed medication. Other measures similar in stature and similarly subject to error are short-recall patient self-report, self-monitoring by diary, and therapeutic outcome. The latter has the hidden complexity that other factors beside adherence may determine clinical outcomes, with little foundation for teasing out the separate contribution of compliance on its own.

The arrival of pill counts has been a mixed blessing. On the one hand, they appear to bring a degree of precision and quantitation to measuring adherence. On the other hand, the parking lots of many clinical study facilities may give evidence of pill-dumping as patients try to retain study eligibility.[28] Some cynics have argued that pill counts have

Table 46–3 Comparison of Available Measures of Medication Adherence

Compliance Measure	Marginal Cost	Difficulty of Use		Approximate, Related to "Gold Standard"		Comments
		Patient	Investigator	Sensitivity Noncompliance (%)	Specificity Compliance (%)	
Indirect						
Self-report	+	+	+	20–55	80–95	Unspecified versus short (1–2 day) recall
Self-monitoring	+	+ +	+ +	40–70	80–95	Prospective logging of drug-taking
Clinician opinion	+		+	50–65	40–80	Point estimates
Pill/packet count	+ +	+ +	+ + +	60–90	75–90	Pill vial return issues: nontrivial
Prescription refill	+ +		+ + +	60–90	60–90	Central pharmacy is critical
Therapeutic outcome	+		+	20–40	40–80	Key: Implicit versus explicit criteria
Medication monitor	+ + +	+ +	+ + +	85–95	85–95	Often needs supplemental pill count as well
Direct						
Direct supervision	+ +	+	+ + +	85–95	85–95	Parenteral administration versus oral drugs
Bioassay of drug concentration	+ + +	+ +	+ + +	60–90	80–95	Bioassays not always feasible or available
Pharmacological marker	+ + +	+ +	+ + +	60–90	80–95	Combination of marker and primary drug may need FDA approval

Adapted from Hasford J. Compliance and the benefit/risk relationship of antihypertensive treatment. J Cardiovasc Pharmacol S30–S34, 1992.
Abbreviation: FDA, U.S. Food and Drug Administration.

provided job security for a whole generation of research assistants without adding substantially to our knowledge of true compliance patterns.[29]

In contrast, several groups have confirmed the relative accuracy of prescription refill rates, especially when carried out over several months, compared with a home inventory.[30, 31] Important cautions, however, include discrepancies between the prescription and the medical record and using refill rates for periods less than 60 days.[32] Even more limiting is the need for a closed system of pharmacies for all refills and complete, computerized records.

Over nearly 30 years, several investigators explored the use of medication monitors, capable of recording vial openings or discrete dispensings.[26, 29, 33–49] For the first time, one could track the day-to-day dynamics of medication-taking rather than relying on an imprecise "average" over days, weeks, or months and also minimize the likelihood of patients misrepresenting their own "report card."[50] Lingering problems and disappointments include relatively high cost, need for vial returns or transmissions for downloading of data, and limited discreteness of tracking individual doses with some devices. Most clinicians and investigators quickly agreed that it was improbable that anyone would systematically dispense pills over several months, as tracked by the monitor, and then discard the doses without actually administering them. These indirect methods dramatically advanced our sophistication about the process of medication-taking.[51]

In contrast, the available direct measures like biological assays[52, 53] or tracer systems[54, 55] require collection of body fluids (e.g., blood, urine, saliva), discrete and sometimes expensive quantitative assays, and assumptions about hepatic and/or renal function. Such measures still do not permit retrospective review beyond several pharmacokinetic half-lives. They further suffer from relatively high cost and difficulties of administration in exchange for superior sensitivity and specificity over the short periods reflected by point estimates of drug concentrations.

Focus

Regardless of specific measures used, compliance investigators have expanded the focus of discussion beyond patients themselves to include both the prescribing clinicians and the health care system in which they function.

As long as imperfect adherence could be "blamed" solely on patients' misbehavior, there were limited opportunities for intervention. Some investigators classified patients according to their readiness to accept the diagnosis and undertake active participation: deniers versus acceptors versus pragmatists.[56] Others focused on the perceived "net" barriers to full adherence, especially prevalent among younger patients and those most recently initiating treatment.[57] An unpublished telephone survey by the Angus Reid Group among 301 Canadian hypertensives reported that 62% of respondents admitted to not taking their prescribed antihypertensive medication as prescribed. Fully 47% of respondents acknowledged side effects from these drugs, and only 41% were aware that stroke was a major risk of hypertension. Perhaps most intriguing were the types of magical thinking among some respondents, who

believed they could skip doses and remain protected, who rewarded themselves with drug holidays for good behavior, and who tended not to refill medications promptly because they were too busy.

As worrisome as these patterns appear, enlarging the focus to include prescribing physicians has challenged several existing myths.[58] Many clinicians accept little if any responsibility for the complexity of the prescribed regimens or for assisting their patients in minimizing drug-related side effects by regimen adjustments. They may overestimate their own prowess in preventing or detecting suboptimal adherence among their own patients and underestimate the several barriers that patients face in trying to comply.[59] Surprising to some has been the correlation of patients' adherence to lifestyle change recommendations and the prescribing physician's own style. Predictors of adherence include the physician's job satisfaction, the number of patients seen per week, the scheduling of follow-up appointments, and the tendency to answer patients' questions.[60]

Finally, the growing predominance of managed care has brought pharmacy benefit management in an array of forms and formats, sometimes helpful and sometimes exacerbating the hurdles with restrictive formularies, generic substitution of more frequently dosed preparations, and requiring mail-away prescription-filling despite frequent drug or dosage changes.[61, 62]

In short, enhancing medication-taking for better outcomes will require a higher degree of sensitivity and collaboration among the principal parties than has existed in the past.[63]

EPIDEMIOLOGY OF MEDICATION COMPLIANCE

Patterns of Medication-Taking Behavior

Constrained by imperfect adherence measures, early studies concluded that chronic preventive treatments, such as those for hypertension, exhibit compliance rates approximating 50%.[64] More discrete measures, especially electronic medication monitors, permit more granularity, clarity, and complexity from the data. Most deviation from the prescription occurs as dose omissions rather than as dose insertions or mis-scheduling.[65] The dose omissions occur more frequently as the dosing frequency increases, as illustrated in Figure 46–4. Medication-taking patterns improve significantly in the 5 days preceding and following scheduled appointments, compared with 30 days after appointments, generating a kind of white-coat compliance.[42, 66]

Perhaps intuitive, the prescribing of very simple regimens (e.g., one pill once daily) did not ensure consistent adherence,[67] even among those patients with relatively frequent, reinforcing visits with the clinician.[43] There remained a core of 10 to 40% of subjects displaying imperfect dosing. Nevertheless, the difference in compliance between once- and twice-daily dosing tends to be small in most studies, whereas adherence declines more dramatically as prescribed dosing frequency exceeds twice-daily.[43, 67]

As adherence data from other medical conditions

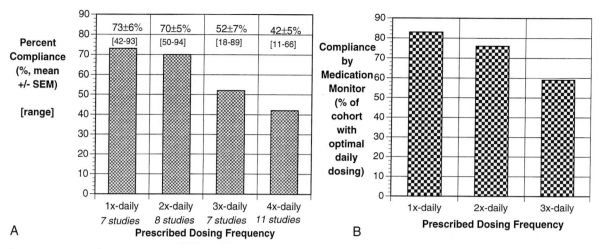

Figure 46–4. Compliance rate by dosing schedule. Compliance rates tend to fall as the frequency of daily doses increases. *A*, Greenberg[67] performed a literature review in 1984, reflecting adherence assessments primarily by self-report and pill count. *B*, Eisen and coworkers[43] employed an electronic medication monitor among hypertensive patients. Both studies support an inverse relationship between adherence and dosing frequency with more modest differences between once- and twice-daily dosing than with more frequent dosing schedules.

emerged, there appeared to be more similarities than differences for compliance distributions among patients with hypertension,[39, 43, 45, 68] seizure disorder,[29, 42] glaucoma,[40, 47, 69] and diverse conditions requiring hormone therapy and lipid-reducing agents.[70–72] Figure 46–5, although a hypothetical composite, reflects the similar J-shaped distributions reported by the respective investigator groups.

On the positive side, 50 to 60% of the patients are *full compliers* with trivial deviations from the prescription and

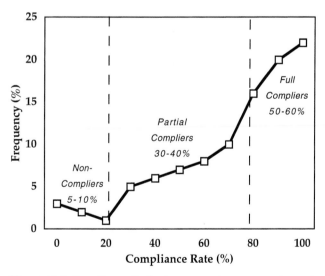

Figure 46–5. Compliance distribution composite: Hypertension, seizures, glaucoma, congestive heart failure. Several investigators have reported remarkably similar patterns of compliance among ambulatory patients monitored electronically for medication-taking behavior despite dissimilar diseases like hypertension, seizures, glaucoma, and congestive heart failure (see text for references). All the conditions exhibit three clusters, combined in a hypothetical composite: full compliers (50 to 60% of total); partial compliers (30 to 40%); and noncompliers (5 to 10%). (Adapted from Rudd P, Hagar RW. Hypertension: Mechanisms, diagnosis, therapy. *In* Topol E [ed]. Textbook of Cardiovascular Medicine. New York, Lippincott-Raven, 1997; pp 109–143.)

remarkably consistent medication-taking behaviors from day to day. At the other extreme, the *noncompliers* exhibit extremely imperfect adherence, although sometimes seeming to misrepresent their usual behavior with pill-dumping just before scheduled visits. In the middle lie the *partial compliers*. Rather than a simple intermediate point, the partial compliers show a complicated mixture of nearly perfect pill-taking interspersed with periods of marked deviation from the prescription. Such a pattern suggests that they understand what they are supposed to do but have difficulty in performing the tasks in a consistent manner.[73] Although not the predicted bell-shaped distribution, the average compliance for such groups approximates 60 to 75%, consistent with other reports.[74]

All but the full compliers display important gaps in medication-taking. The consequences of such nonadherence include subtherapeutic drug concentrations; imperfect blood pressure control; submaximal cardiovascular risk reduction; unnecessary and potentially dangerous treatment escalation; avoidable tests, procedures, and hospitalizations; and threats of withdrawal, rebound, and first-dose phenomena.[75] None of these bad outcomes should be surprising if one acknowledges that drugs act episodically in patients who dose episodically, inadequately or not at all in patients who underdose, and hazardously when dosed in intermittent patterns.[76] At a more extreme level, drugs cannot work (1) if they are never prescribed, (2) if the prescription is written but never filled, (3) if the drug is never taken by the patient, or (4) if the drug is taken but not absorbed. Overall, the pharmacological impact, whether beneficial or toxic, is proportional to the drug exposure and the dose received.

Classical Search for Predictors

Given the high stakes, many groups began intensive searches for predictors of noncompliance, so as to concentrate remedial interventions on the groups more needy of change. Early efforts quickly concluded that no simple nonadherent personality profile existed.[77] At the extremes of age, poverty, social isolation, and psychiatric dysfunction, increased noncompliance was observed. Symptom level, educational level, and objective seriousness of the medical condition provided little predictive value.

Despite limited success to date, the obvious broad areas for future focus include characteristics of the individual patient, the disease in question, the prescribed treatment, the patient-provider relationship, and the clinical setting.[78] Curtin and colleagues observed higher rates of nonadherence using electronic monitoring among younger than older hemodialysis patients with hypertension.[79] Similar patterns were observed by Morrell and coworkers except that the "old-old," ranging up to age 87 years in their series, also displayed inferior adherence.[80] Among an ambulatory hypertensive Medicaid population, Bailey and associates reported that prescription refill compliance varied by drug class (α-blockers > angiotensin-converting enzyme inhibitors > calcium channel blockers > diuretics).[81] Other independent predictors in their series included younger age, multiple daily doses, and fewer provider visits. In contrast, patient gender and regimen complexity held little predictive value.

Electronic monitoring confirmed that the dosing frequency varies inversely with adherence. Among 198 Canadian hypertensives randomized to diltiazem twice-daily versus amlodipine once-daily, those on a once-daily regimen display less dosing variability than those on twice-daily dosing.[82] Among diabetics on oral agents, the compliance rate monitored electronically fell from 79% on once-daily to 38% on three-times daily dosing.[65]

Knowledge about the disease and familiarity with the regimen are necessary but not sufficient to ensure high levels of adherence.[7, 83] Indeed, health professionals themselves are often cited as demonstration that knowledge and education are no guarantee of compliance. Each individual, whether or not sophisticated about the condition and its management, must make hard choices among risks and benefits, hardships and conveniences, costs and rewards. Commonly cited barriers include simple forgetfulness, drug side effects, financial costs, confusion about the regimen, and interference with daily schedules.[84, 85]

Some patients, especially the elderly, construct elaborate systems of locations and cues to facilitate remembering and adhering to the prescribed regimen.[84] Still others struggle with childproof vials, which functionally become person-proof.[58] Most of these coping mechanisms are highly personal and rarely emerge from routine clinical surveillance. Some advocates of patient self-management[86, 87] have argued that three issues are key to improving adherence: defining the key behaviors to be mastered and implemented, providing consistent guidance and reinforcement, and linking the behaviors to the desired clinical outcomes.

There appears to be something beneficial from compliant behaviors in general, even when they consist of administering placebo in clinical trials. Three of 12 studies comparing rates of hospitalization and mortality for chronic heart disease revealed better outcomes with adherence to placebo, suggesting that adherent behavior may be a marker for improved prognosis or confers a protective effect.[88]

Conversely, there are some definite negative consequences for nonadherence. Interruptions in antihypertensive prescription refills among California Medicaid patients greater than 40 years old were associated with higher costs, especially for hospitalization.[89] Among 602 women enrolled in the Beta Blocker Heart Attack Trial, nonadherence by appointment and medication adherence conferred a 2.4-fold (95% CI: 1.1 to 5.6) increase in post–myocardial infarction death rates. Those who complied had a 2.4-fold reduction in mortality, whether or not they were randomized to receive propranolol as the active drug.[90]

EVOLVING STRATEGIES FOR COMPLIANCE IMPROVEMENT

As we prepare to enter the next millennium, there are a cluster of discrete, effective, and feasible steps to detect, evaluate, and intervene among partial and noncompliant hypertensive patients, summarized in Table 46–4.[9] They represent challenges because few clinicians have received training in how to be educators, motivators, and coaches. For their part, many practices and medical institutions have not readily accepted responsibility for these critical efforts.[91]

Compliance-Enhancing Strategies for the Clinician

Watch for Nonattenders

Those patients who fail initial or follow-up appointments are most at risk for dropping permanently out of care. This is especially likely to occur in the first year of treatment but may occur at any time.[92] Once detected, such patients should receive special handling to maximize the likelihood of resuming regular visits and progress to goal.

Watch for Nonresponders

Most patients will respond to antihypertensive medications with a relatively prompt and sustained reduction in blood

Table 46–4. Compliance-Enhancing Strategies for Clinicians

1. Watch for nonattenders
2. Watch for nonresponders
3. Inquire nonconfrontationally about compliance barriers
4. Encourage the development and use of a medication-taking "system"
5. Provide simple, clear instruction
6. Simplify the regimen as much as possible
7. Provide substitutive and sequential steps
8. Monitor progress to goal, both in blood pressure and in compliance
9. Reinforce desirable behaviors and outcomes whenever possible
10. Apply useful, relevant information and help from all possible sources
11. Make explicit the potential value of the prescribed regimen and the impact of compliance
12. Emphasize the importance of dose-timing when appropriate
13. Seek to customize the regimen to the patient's needs and preferences

pressure, assuming a rational and suitably aggressive regimen is selected. Initial or secondary "resistance" to treatment carries its own differential diagnosis: secondary hypertension, interfering substances, biological factors, suboptimal regimen, and medication nonadherence.[14] Retaining a low threshold for these possibilities helps promptly detect, address, and hopefully resolve any noncompliance.

Inquire Nonconfrontationally About Compliance Barriers

The art may lie in establishing a collaboration rather than a confrontation. Few patients will openly admit to noncompliance if the clinician asks, "You're taking all your pills, aren't you?" Alternative phrasings might be, "Many people have difficulty taking their medications as prescribed. What kinds of problems have you had in taking the pills?" In one study of a community pharmacy, 549 prescriptions were not picked up over a 9-month interval. The stated reasons included transfer to another pharmacy, forgotten prescription, still had medication left over, or no longer needed the medication.[93] In another survey of general practice patients, prescribing physicians, and assisting nurses, imperfect knowledge of the medications occurred in up to 60% of patients.[94] After a suitable open-ended inquiry, some useful follow-up questions might include:

> "Some people experience awkward or embarrassing side effects, like leaking urine or having sexual problems. These problems may be hard to discuss.[95] Sometimes we can reduce or eliminate these problems if we know about them. Have you had any problems like these?"
>
> "Other people have trouble remembering the pills or find that pill-taking interferes with their normal schedule. What kind of system do you use at home or work to stay on track with your pills?"
>
> "I once had a patient who came to see me regularly but never mentioned that he could not afford the medications I prescribed. As soon as I gave him sample drugs, his blood pressure was promptly controlled. Have you had any problems filling the prescription, opening the vials, or swallowing the pills?"

Encourage the Development and Use of a Medication-Taking "System"

Cramer called for compliance enhancement by asking every patient at every visit about how the prescribed medications are taken.[96] The clinician may then encourage the selection of location, time, and/or activity cues, consistent with the patient's personal, daily routine. At each follow-up visit, the discussion may review how the selected method is working and lead to selective changes.

Provide Simple, Clear Instructions

Learning theory indicates that patients will often recall the first and last things they are told but retain little of what comes in between. Uncomplicated, unambiguous directions

are important, even when reinforced in writing or by review in the presence of the patient's significant other. Reliance on the pharmacist to provide more patient instruction, reinforcement, or reassurance may not always be realistic. On occasion, the addition of a pill dispenser aid facilitates following the instructions and highlights any missed doses.

Simplify the Regimen as Much as Possible

The number of dosings appears to be more of a stumbling block than the number of pills taken at any one time. In the elderly, such simplification may be particularly difficult but important when the reality is "polymedicine" for multiple, concurrent conditions rather than avoidable polypharmacy.[97, 98] One useful strategy involves selecting, whenever possible, one drug to serve more than one function, such as using an α_1-blocker for both prostatism and hypertension or an angiotensin-converting enzyme inhibitor for both congestive heart failure and hypertension.

Provide Substitutive and Sequential Steps

Too often, the well-intentioned patient may be overwhelmed by requests to change several medications, modify diet, and increase exercise all at the same time. In most cases, urgency is unnecessary. If possible, the clinician should identify one behavior to substitute for another rather than add to the large and daunting number of requests. Well-selected, the substitutive behavior takes no more work than the replaced behavior. The clinician can further assist by negotiating priorities for change in a manageable sequence rather than all at once.

Monitor Progress to Goal, Both in Blood Pressure and in Compliance

The clinician should specify the relation between prescribed medication and the attainment of goal blood pressure, laying the foundation for further inquiry about adherence if the goal is not achieved or not sustained.

Reinforce Desirable Behaviors and Outcomes Whenever Possible

The key behaviors to reinforce include keeping appointments, taking medications as prescribed, avoiding running out of medication, and remaining willing to work out medication-taking and other clinical problems in a collaborative way. Secret efforts to titrate one's medications down to minimize side effects is a double loss: loss of maximal cardiovascular protection and loss of the opportunity to reduce the symptoms by adjusting the regimen. Another strategy is to reinforce behaviors so that they produce discomfort or dysphoria when missed, such as feeling ill at ease when going to bed without brushing one's teeth or riding in an automobile when a seatbelt is not available. Patients may learn both the dysphoria and how to avoid it by adhering to the prescription.

Apply Useful, Relevant Information And Help From All Possible Sources

Family members and significant others may provide invaluable assistance and reinforcement for pill-taking, especially

Figure 46–6. Cholestyramine efficacy by compliance rate. The original report of the Lipid Research Clinics Coronary Primary Prevention Trial[119] included the now-famous relation of 10% reduction in cholesterol associated with 20% reduction in coronary risk. These data reflect the "average" level of adherence with cholestyramine packets. Maximal compliance (6 packets/day) led to nearly a 20% reduction in cholesterol and almost a 40% reduction in coronary risk. Thus, benefit may covary with compliance. (Adapted from Urquhart J. Patient compliance as an explanatory variable in four selected cardiovascular studies. *In* Cramer JA, Spilker B, [eds]. Patient Compliance in Medical Practice and Clinical Trials. New York, Lippincott-Raven, 1991; pp 305–306.)

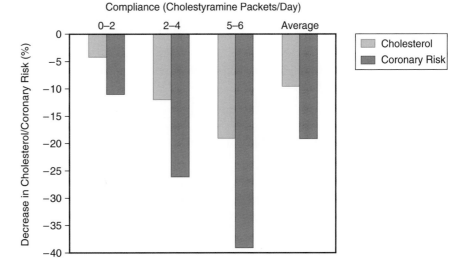

for patients with handicaps or cognitive impairment. For others, visiting nurse services and home health aides offer structure and support. Sometimes, important clues to nonadherence appear from failure to request prescription refills at indicated intervals. Other potential sources include symptoms, signs, or laboratory test changes linkable to the specific, prescribed medications.[99] Computer-based reminder systems have proved valuable in such settings.[100] On a more ambitious scale, several successful programs have used nurse-mediated services with decision support by algorithm and frequent telephone contacts to yield improved compliance and better cardiovascular control.[101, 102]

Make Explicit the Potential Value of the Prescribed Regimen and the Impact of Compliance

Several studies have quantified the difference between an "average effect," based on the mean level of adherence, and that achievable with maximal compliance.[103] Figure 46–6 illustrates the difference for lipid-lowering efficacy for cholestyramine at average and maximal levels of compliance.

Emphasize the Importance of Dose-Timing When Appropriate

Unless told and reminded, many patients will not pay much attention to the precise timing of doses. For some medications and some dosing times, electronic monitoring has confirmed the superiority of morning versus evening dosing.[104, 105]

Seek to Customize the Regimen to the Patient's Needs and Preferences

Most patients and most clinicians appear convinced that once-daily dosing will always be superior over more frequent dosing schedules. From a theoretical perspective, Levy argued that more frequent dosings reduce the likelihood of having drug concentrations fall to subtherapeutic levels when lapses in pill-taking occur.[106] Figure 46–7 illustrates the relationship for a hypothetical drug pre-

scribed once, twice, three, or four times daily. Empirically with electronic monitoring, Kruse and colleagues confirmed that once-daily dosing was more likely than twice-daily dosing to result in skipped days without any treatment, especially on weekends, and that evening doses were twice as likely as to be missed morning doses.[107]

Other Guiding Principles

Multifaceted Strategies

Despite these generalizing principles, the field of medication compliance has shown repetitively that one size does *not* fit all. Just as there is not a single cause for suboptimal

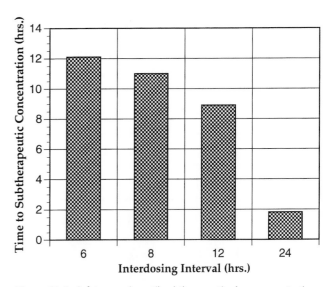

Figure 46–7. Safety margin until subtherapeutic drug concentrations for dosing intervals using a hypothetical drug. Levy[106] calculated the "safety margin" associated with different dosing intervals for a hypothetical drug with a half-life of 12 hours, volume of distribution of 1 L, dose of 10 mg/kg, 100% absorption, and minimal effective concentration of 3.0 mg/L. As dosing frequency decreases, the margin for error is reduced, even though drug concentrations remain therapeutic for once-daily dosing.

compliance, so there is no single fix. The reasons underlying noncompliance are multifaceted, and therefore, so must be the solutions.[108] As the field evolves, it has come to incorporate ethnocultural and psychosocial perspectives as well as traditional sociodemographic, clinical, pharmacological, and medical system issues. At the core of the broadened perspective is a realization that the patient with a chronic condition, even one with few symptoms such as hypertension, has special kinds of "work" to accomplish in living with the condition. The problem-solving by physicians, nurses, pharmacists, and other health professionals must go beyond the simplistic sender-message-receiver communication model used as a default. As the alternative, the patient should actively participate in the selection of therapeutic ingredients and the pace of treatment.[109]

New Skills and Collaboration

The effective prescriber-clinician should ask, simplify, tailor, and reinforce. Asking the patient for input early in the process immediately sets up a different and potentially far more useful dynamic than the traditional autocratic stance. Minimizing the total number of daily doses usually arises as a priority. Selecting the most useful cues and location for the particular patient's life and lifestyle provides an added "fit."[96]

Optimization will still require a melding of patients' personal preferences with clinical and pharmacological realities. Several recent reports emphasize the importance of effective 24-hour blood pressure control, smooth antihypertensive effect with decreased variability, reduced early morning surge in blood pressure, physiological diurnal variation in blood pressure, and minimal reflex activation of the sympathetic nervous system.[110] These characteristics assume even more prominence if medication-taking is imperfect and highly variable.

Pharmacokinetics as Guide for Adherence

A lively debate has arisen about the value and relevance of trough:peak variability in blood pressure in comparing one antihypertensive agent with another. Some have argued that the optimal drug is one with a smooth concentration-time profile and long elimination half-life to maintain stable drug concentrations and stable antihypertensive effect despite imperfect medication-taking.[111] In this context, the trough:peak ratio reflects the duration of drug's action relative to its dosage interval, avoiding the use of inappropriately large drug doses simply to extend the apparent duration of action. At least two different clusters of drugs have been identified. In the first group, the concentration-effect relationship is essentially linear, and the trough:peak ratio is almost invariably dose-independent and therefore more stable. In the second grouping, the concentration-effect relationship is sigmoid-shaped, and the trough:peak ratio becomes dose-dependent and highly affected by compliance.[112] The data from Meredith and Elliott illustrate some interdrug differences for several antihypertensive agents in Figure 46–8.[113]

Drugs with linear relationships are more "forgiving" of imperfect adherence. They achieve therapeutic sufficiency with desirable and sustained reductions in blood pressure in spite of variable pill-taking.[114] Using ambulatory blood pressure monitoring, Leenen and coworkers confirmed that once-daily amlodipine provided more effective and consistent antihypertensive effect than twice-daily diltiazem in the face of interrupted therapy.[115] Some authors have used the same arguments in support of newly introduced combination products, when one of the components is especially long-lasting.[116, 117]

The New Paradigm: Challenges for the Decade

Ultimately, the clinician is the expert on the disorder and its treatment in general, but the patient remains the expert on his or her own disorder and his or her own experience of the treatment.[118] The principal challenges for the next decade will be to (1) forge strong foundations for collaboration between patient and clinician, (2) reassess the traditional wisdoms about predictors of nonadherence and effective interventions, and (3) establish thresholds of therapeutic sufficiency for optimizing cardiovascular benefit to

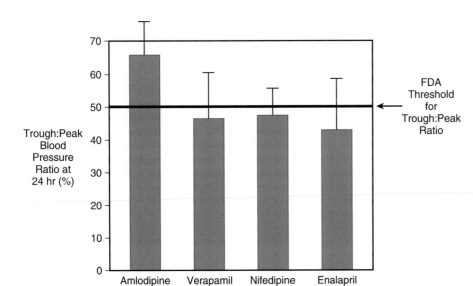

Figure 46–8. Trough:peak blood pressure ratios for selected antihypertensive agents. Trough:peak blood pressure ratios at 24 hours provide a useful index of sustained antihypertensive effect for once-daily medications. Meredith and Elliott[113] report the ratios for four antihypertensive agents compared with the U.S. Food and Drug Administration (FDA) benchmark of 50% at 24 hours.

hypertensive patients despite sometimes imperfect adherence.

References

1. Julius S. Current trends in the treatment of hypertension: A mixed picture. Am J Hypertens 10:300S–305S, 1997.
2. Kannel WB. Blood pressure as a cardiovascular risk factor: Prevention and treatment. JAMA 275:1571–1576, 1996.
3. Hebert PR, Moser M, Mayer J, et al. Recent evidence on drug therapy of mild to moderate hypertension and decreased risk of coronary heart disease. Arch Intern Med 153:578–581, 1993.
4. Burt VL, Whelton P, Roccella EJ, et al. Prevalence of hypertension in the US adult population. Results from the Third National Health and Nutrition Examination Survey, 1988–1991. Hypertension 25:305–313, 1995.
5. Urquhart J. Correlates of variable patient compliance in drug trials: Relevance in the new health care environment. Adv Drug Res 26:237–257, 1995.
6. Murphy J, Coster G. Issues in patient compliance. Drugs 54:797–800, 1997.
7. Sackett DL, Haynes RB, Gibson ES, et al. Randomized clinical trial of strategies for improving medication compliance in primary hypertension. Lancet 1:1205–1208, 1975.
8. Sackett D. Hypertension in the real world: Public reaction, physician response, and patient compliance. In Genest J, Koiw E, Kuchel O (eds). Hypertension: Physiopathology and Treatment. New York, McGraw-Hill, 1979; pp 1142–1149.
9. Sackett DL, Haynes RB, Tugwell P. Compliance. In Clinical Epidemiology: A Basic Science for Clinical Medicine. Boston, Little, Brown, 1985; pp 199–222.
10. Taylor D, Sackett D, Haynes R, et al. Compliance with antihypertensive drug therapy. Ann N Y Acad Sci 304:390–403, 1978.
11. Silas JH, Tucker GT, Smith AJ. Drug resistance, inappropriate dosing and non-compliance in hypertensive patients. Br J Clin Pharmacol 9:427–430, 1980.
12. Rudd P. Medication compliance: Correlation with clinical outcomes. Pharmacol Ther 19:10S–18S, 1994.
13. Wallenius SH, Vainio KK, Korhonen MJ, et al. Self-initiated modification of hypertension treatment in response to perceived problems. Ann Pharmacother 29:1213–1217, 1995.
14. Setaro JF, Black HR. Refractory hypertension. N Engl J Med 327:543–547, 1992.
15. Flack JM, Yunis C. Therapeutic implications of the epidemiology and timing of myocardial infarction and other cardiovascular diseases. J Hum Hypertens 11:23–28, 1997.
16. Schueler K. Cost-effectiveness issues in hypertension control. Can J Public Health 85:S54–S56, 1994.
17. Gandhi SK, Kong SX. Quality-of-life measures in the evaluation of antihypertensive drug therapy: Reliability, validity, and quality-of-life domains. Clin Ther 18:1276–1295, 1996.
18. Rudd P, Dzau VJ. Hypertension: Evaluation and management. In Loscalzo J, Creager MA, Dzau VJ (eds). Vascular Medicine. Boston, Little, Brown, 1996; pp 609–638.
19. Maronde RF, Chan LS, Larsen FJ, et al. Underutilization of antihypertensive drugs and associated hospitalization. Med Care 27:1159–1166, 1989.
20. Psaty BM, Koepsell TD, Wagner ED, et al. The relative risk of incident coronary heart disease associated with recently stopping the use of beta-blockers. JAMA 263:1653–1657, 1990.
21. Mezzetti A, Pierdomenico SD, Costantini F, et al. White-coat resistant hypertension. Am J Hypertens 10:1302–1307, 1997.
22. Dunbar J. Adherence measures and their utility. Controlled Clin Trials 5:515–521, 1984.
23. Mattson ME, Friedman LM. Issues in medication adherence assessment in clinical trials of the National Heart, Lung, and Blood Institute. Control Clin Trials 5:488–496, 1984.
24. Roth HP. Historical review: Comparison with other methods. Control Clin Trials 5:476–480, 1984.
25. Dunbar J, Dunning EJ, Dwyer K. Compliance measurement with arthritis regimen. Arthritis Care Res 2:16–24, 1989.
26. Spilker B. Methods of assessing and improving patient compliance in clinical trials. In Cramer JA, Spilker B (eds). Patient Compliance in Medical Practice and Clinical Trials. New York, Raven, 1991; pp 37–56.
27. Rudd P. The measurement of compliance: Medication-taking. In Krasnegor NA, Epstein L, Johnson SB, Yaffe SJ (eds). Developmental Aspects of Health Compliance Behavior. Hillsdale, NJ, Lawrence Erlbaum, 1993; pp 185–213.
28. Rudd P, Byyny RL, Zachary V, et al. Pill count measures of compliance in a drug trial: Variability and suitability. Am J Hypertens 1:309–312, 1988.
29. Cramer JA, Mattson RH, Prevey ML, et al. How often is medication taken as prescribed? A novel assessment technique. JAMA 261:3273–3277, 1989.
30. Lau HS, de Boer A, Beuning KS, et al. Validation of pharmacy records in drug exposure assessment. J Clin Epidemiol 50:619–625, 1997.
31. Steiner JF, Prochazka AV. The assessment of refill compliance using pharmacy records: Methods, validity, and applications. J Clin Epidemiol 50:105–116, 1997.
32. Christensen DB, Williams B, Goldberg HI, et al. Assessing compliance to antihypertensive medications using computer-based pharmacy records. Med Care 35:1164–1170, 1997.
33. Moulding TS. The potential uses of the medication monitor in the treatment of leprosy. Int J Lepr Other Mycobact Dis 47:601–606, 1979.
34. Norell SE. Accuracy of patient interviews and estimates by clinical staff in determining medication compliance. Soc Sci Med 15E:57–61, 1981.
35. Kass MA, Meltzer DW, Gordon M. A miniature compliance monitor for eyedrop medication. Arch Ophthalmol 102:1550–1554, 1984.
36. Norell SE. Methods in assessing drug compliance. Acta Med Scand Suppl 683:35–40, 1984.
37. Kass MA, Gordon M, Meltzer DW. Can ophthalmologists correctly identify patients defaulting from pilocarpine therapy? Am J Ophthalmol 101:524–530, 1986.
38. Spector SL, Kinsman R, Mawhinney H, et al. Compliance of patients with asthma with an experimental aerosolized medication: Implications for controlled clinical trials. J Allergy Clin Immunol 77:65–70, 1986.
39. Eisen SA, Hanpeter JA, Kreuger LW, et al. Monitoring medication compliance: Description of a new device. J Compliance Health Care 2:131–142, 1987.
40. Kass MA, Gordon M, Morley RJ, et al. Compliance with topical timolol treatment. Am J Ophthalmol 103:188–193, 1987.
41. Rudd P, Marshall G. Resolving problems of measuring compliance with medication monitors. J Compliance Health Care 2:23–35, 1987.
42. Cramer JA, Scheyer RD, Mattson RH. Compliance declines between clinic visits. Arch Intern Med 150:1509–1510, 1990.
43. Eisen SA, Miller DK, Woodward RS, et al. The effect of prescribed daily dose frequency on patient medication compliance. Arch Intern Med 150:1881–1884, 1990.
44. Kruse W, Schlierf G, Weber E. Monitoring compliance in clinical trials. [Letter; comment] Lancet 335:803–804, 1990.
45. Rudd P, Ahmed S, Zachary V, et al. Improved compliance measures: Applications in an ambulatory hypertensive drug trial. Clin Pharmacol Ther 48:676–685, 1990.
46. Cramer JA, Mattson RH. Monitoring compliance with antiepileptic drug therapy. In Cramer JA, Spilker B (eds). Patient Compliance in Medical Practice and Clinical Trials. New York, Raven, 1991; pp 123–137.
47. Gordon ME, Kass MA. Validity of standard compliance measures in glaucoma compared with an electronic eyedrop monitor. In Cramer JA, Spilker B (eds). Patient Compliance in Medical Practice and Clinical Trials. New York, Raven, 1991; pp 163–173.
48. Spector SL, Mawhinney H. Aerosol inhaler monitoring of asthmatic medication. In Cramer JA, Spilker B (eds). Patient Compliance in Medical Practice and Clinical Trials. New York, Raven, 1991; pp 149–162.
49. Rudd P, Ramesh J, Bryant-Kosling C, et al. Gaps in cardiovascular medication taking: The tip of the iceberg. J Gen Intern Med 8:659–666, 1993.
50. Straka RJ, Fish JT, Benson SR, et al. Patient self-reporting of compliance does not correspond with electronic monitoring: An evaluation using isosorbide dinitrate as a model drug. Pharmacotherapy 17:126–132, 1997.
51. Urquhart J. Role of patient compliance in clinical pharmacokinetics. A review of recent research. Clin Pharmacokinet 27:202–215, 1994.
52. Larkin JG, Herrick AL, McGuire GM, et al. Antiepileptic drug

monitoring at the epilepsy clinic: A prospective evaluation. Epilepsia 32:89–95, 1991.

53. Wiseman IC, Miller R. Quantifying non-compliance in patients receiving digoxin—A pharmacokinetic approach. S Afr Med J 79:155–157, 1991.

54. Hardy E, Kumar S, Peaker S, et al. A comparison of a short half-life marker (low-dose isoniazid), a long half-life pharmacological indicator (low-dose phenobarbitone) and measurements of a controlled release "therapeutic drug" (metoprolol, Metoros) in reflecting incomplete compliance by volunteers. Br J Clin Pharmacol 30:437–441, 1990.

55. Maenpaa H, Manninen V, Heinonen OP. Compliance with medication in the Helsinki Heart Study. Eur J Clin Pharmacol 42:15–19, 1992.

56. Adams S, Pill R, Jones A. Medication, chronic illness and identity: The perspective of people with asthma. Soc Sci Med 45:189–201, 1997.

57. Richardson MA, Simons-Morton B, Anneggers JF. Effect of perceived barriers on compliance with antihypertensive medication. Health Educ Q 20:489–503, 1993.

58. Rudd P. Maximizing compliance with antihypertensive therapy. Drug Ther 22:25–32, 1992.

59. Rudd P. Compliance with antihypertensive therapy: Raising the bar of expectations. Am J Managed Care 4:600–609, 1998.

60. DiMatteo MR, Sherbourne CD, Hays RD, et al. Physicians' characteristics influence patients' adherence to medical treatment: Results from the Medical Outcomes Study. Health Psychol 12:93–102, 1993.

61. Sanchez LA. Pharmacoeconomics and formulary decision making. Pharmacoeconomics 1:16–25, 1996.

62. Strandberg LR. Pharmacy benefits management and ambulatory pharmacy services. Pharm Pract Manag Q 15:19–26, 1996.

63. Cramer JA. Relationship between medication compliance and medical outcomes. Am J Health Syst Pharm 52:S27–S29, 1995.

64. Sackett DL, Snow JC. The magnitude of compliance and noncompliance. In Haynes RB, Taylor DW, Sackett DL (eds). Compliance in Health Care. Baltimore, Johns Hopkins University Press, 1979; pp 11–22.

65. Paes AH, Bakker A, Soe-Agnie CJ. Impact of dosage frequency on patient compliance. Diabetes Care 20:1512–1517, 1997.

66. Feinstein A. On white-coat effects and the electronic monitoring of compliance. Arch Intern Med 150:1377–1378, 1990.

67. Greenberg RN. Overview of patient compliance with medication dosing: A literature review. Clin Ther 6:592–599, 1984.

68. Guerrero D, Rudd P, Bryant-Kosling C, et al. Antihypertensive medication-taking. Investigation of a simple regimen. Am J Hypertens 6:586–592, 1993.

69. Kass MA, Meltzer DW, Gordon M, et al. Compliance with topical pilocarpine treatment. Am J Ophthalmol 101:515–523, 1986.

70. Kruse W, Weber E. Dynamics of drug regimen compliance—Its assessment by microprocessor-based monitoring. Eur J Clin Pharmacol 38:561–565, 1990.

71. Kruse W, Effert-Kruse W, Rampmaier J, et al. Compliance with short-term high-dose ethinyl oestradiol in young patients with primary infertility. New insights from the use of electronic devices. Agents Actions Suppl 29:105–115, 1990.

72. Kruse WHH. Compliance with treatment of hyperlipoproteinemia in medical practice and clinical trials. In Cramer JA, Spilker B (eds). Patient Compliance in Medical Practice and Clinical Trials. New York, Raven, 1991; pp 175–186.

73. Rudd P. Clinicians and patients with hypertension: Unsettled issues about compliance. Am Heart J 130:572–579, 1995.

74. Urquhart J. Patient compliance with crucial drug regimens: Implications for prostate cancer. Eur Urol 2:124–131, 1996.

75. Rand CS, Wise RA. Measuring adherence to asthma medication regimens. Am J Respir Crit Care Med 149:S69–S78, 1994.

76. Urquhart J. Patient non-compliance with drug regimens: Measurement, clinical correlates, economic impact. Eur Heart J 17:8–15, 1996.

77. Haynes RB. Determinants of compliance: The disease and the mechanisms of treatment. In Haynes RB, Taylor DW, Sackett DL (eds). Compliance in Health Care. Baltimore, Johns Hopkins University Press, 1979; pp 49–62.

78. Ickovics JR, Meisler AW. Adherence in AIDS clinical trials: A framework for clinical research and clinical care. J Clin Epidemiol 50:385–391, 1997.

79. Curtin RB, Svarstad BL, Andress D, et al. Differences in older versus younger hemodialysis patients' noncompliance with oral medications. Geriatr Nephrol Urol 7:35–44, 1997.

80. Morrell RW, Park DC, Kidder DP, et al. Adherence to antihypertensive medications across the life span. Gerontologist 37:609–619, 1997.

81. Bailey JE, Lee MD, Somes GW, et al. Risk factors for antihypertensive medication refill failure by patients under Medicaid managed care. Clin Ther 18:1252–1262, 1996.

82. Leenen FH, Wilson TW, Bolli P, et al. Patterns of compliance with once versus twice daily antihypertensive drug therapy in primary care: A randomized clinical trial using electronic monitoring. Can J Cardiol 13:914–920, 1997.

83. Haynes RB, Sackett DL, Gibson ES, et al. Improvement of medication compliance in uncontrolled hypertension. Lancet 1:1265–1268, 1976.

84. Rudd P, Marshall G. Antihypertensive medication-taking behavior: Outpatient patterns and implications. In Rosenfeld J (ed). Hypertension Control in the Community. London, John Libbey, 1985; pp 232–236.

85. Col N, Fanale JE, Kronholm P. The role of medication noncompliance and adverse drug reactions in hospitalizations of the elderly. Arch Intern Med 150:841–845, 1990.

86. Bandura A. Self-efficacy mechanism in human agency. Am Psychol 37:122–130, 1982.

87. Lorig KR, Mazonson PD, Holman HR. Evidence suggesting that health education for self-management in patients with chronic arthritis has sustained health benefits while reducing health care costs. Arthritis Rheum 36:439–446, 1993.

88. McDermott MM, Schmitt B, Wallner E. Impact of medication nonadherence on coronary heart disease outcomes. A critical review. Arch Intern Med 157:1921–1929, 1997.

89. McCombs JS, Nichol MB, Newman CM, et al. The costs of interrupting antihypertensive drug therapy in a Medicaid population. Med Care 32:214–226, 1994.

90. Gallagher EJ, Viscoli CM, Horwitz RI. The relationship of treatment adherence to the risk of death after myocardial infarction in women. JAMA 270:742–744, 1993.

91. Miller NH, Hill M, Kottke T, et al. The multilevel compliance challenge: Recommendations for a call to action. A statement for healthcare professionals. Circulation 95:1085–1090, 1997.

92. Rudd P, Tul V, Brown K, et al. Hypertension continuation adherence: Natural history and role as an indicator condition. Arch Intern Med 139:545–549, 1979.

93. Hamilton WR, Hopkins UK. Survey on unclaimed prescriptions in a community pharmacy. J Am Pharm Assoc 3:341–345, 1997.

94. McCormack PM, Lawlor R, Donegan C, et al. Knowledge and attitudes to prescribed drugs in young and elderly patients. Ir Med J 90:29–30, 1997.

95. Lip GY, Beevers DG. Doctors, nurses, pharmacists and patients—The Rational Evaluation and Choice in Hypertension (REACH) survey of hypertension care delivery. Blood Press Suppl 1:6–10, 1997.

96. Cramer JA. Optimizing long-term patient compliance. Neurology 45:S25–S28, 1995.

97. Colley CA, Lucas LM. Polypharmacy: The cure becomes the disease. J Gen Intern Med 8:278–283, 1993.

98. Monane M, Monane S, Semla T. Optimal medication use in elders. Key to successful aging. West J Med 167:233–237, 1997.

99. Haynes RB, Taylor DW, Sackett DL, et al. Can simple clinical measurements detect patient noncompliance? Hypertension 2:757–764, 1980.

100. Rossi RA, Every NR. A computerized intervention to decrease the use of calcium channel blockers in hypertension. J Gen Intern Med 12:672–678, 1997.

101. DeBusk RF. MULTIFIT: A new approach to risk factor modification. Cardiol Clin 14:143–157, 1996.

102. West JA, Miller NH, Parker KM, et al. A comprehensive management system for heart failure improves clinical outcomes and reduces medical resource utilization. Am J Cardiol 79:58–63, 1997.

103. Urquhart J. Patient compliance as an explanatory variable in four selected cardiovascular studies. In Cramer JA, Spilker B (eds). Patient Compliance in Medical Practice and Clinical Trials. New York, Raven, 1991; pp 301–322.

104. Mengden T, Binswanger B, Spuhler T, et al. The use of self-

measured blood pressure determinations in assessing dynamics of drug compliance in a study with amlodipine once a day, morning versus evening. J Hypertension 11:1403–1411, 1993.

105. Vrijens B, Goetghebeur E. Comparing compliance patterns between randomized treatments. Control Clin Trials 18:187–203, 1997.

106. Levy G. A pharmacokinetic perspective on medicament noncompliance. Clin Pharmacol Ther 54:242–244, 1993.

107. Kruse W, Rampmaier J, Ullrich G, et al. Patterns of drug compliance with medications to be taken once and twice daily assessed by continuous electronic monitoring in primary care. Int J Clin Pharmacol Ther 32:452–457, 1994.

108. Crespo-Fierro M. Compliance/adherence and care management in HIV disease. J Assoc Nurses AIDS Care 8:43–54, 1997.

109. Lewis RK, Lasack NL, Lambert BL, et al. Patient counseling—A focus on maintenance therapy. Am J Health Syst Pharm 54:2084–2098; quiz 2125–2126, 1997.

110. Meredith PA, Perloff D, Mancia G, et al. Blood pressure variability and its implications for antihypertensive therapy. Blood Press 4:5–11, 1995.

111. Meredith PA, Elliott HL. Therapeutic coverage: Reducing the risks of partial compliance. Br J Clin Pract Symp Suppl 73:13–17, 1994.

112. Meredith PA, Elliot HL. Concentration-effect relationships and implications for trough-to-peak ratio. Am J Hypertens 9:66S–70S; discussion 87S–90S, 1996.

113. Meredith PA, Elliott HL. Amlodipine: Clinical relevance of a unique pharmacokinetic profile. J Cardiovasc Pharmacol 22:S6–S8, 1993.

114. Rudd P, Ahmed S, Zachary V, et al. Issues in patient compliance: The search for therapeutic sufficiency. Cardiology 1:2–10, 1992.

115. Leenen FH, Fourney A, Notman G, et al. Persistence of antihypertensive effect after "missed doses" of calcium antagonist with long (amlodipine) vs. short (diltiazem) elimination half-life. Br J Clin Pharmacol 41:83–88, 1996.

116. Waeber B, Brunner HR. Combination antihypertensive therapy: Does it have a role in rational therapy? Am J Hypertens 10:131S–137S, 1997.

117. Prisant LM, Doll NC. Hypertension: The rediscovery of combination therapy. Geriatrics 52:28–30, 33–38, 1997.

118. Frank E, Kupfer DJ, Siegel LR. Alliance not compliance: A philosophy of outpatient care. J Clin Psychiatry 1:11–16; discussion 16–17, 1995.

119. Lipid Research Clinics Program. The Lipid Research Clinics Coronary Primary Prevention Trial results. II: The relationship of reduction in incidence of coronary heart disease to cholesterol lowering. JAMA 251:365–374, 1984.

Lifestyle Modification

47 Diet—Micronutrients—Special Foods
Suzanne Oparil

Nonpharmacological interventions (lifestyle modifications) are generally beneficial in reducing a variety of cardiovascular risk factors, including high blood pressure, and in promoting good health and should therefore be used in all hypertensive patients, either as definitive treatment or as an adjunct to drug therapy.[1] Although permanent modifications in diet and lifestyle are difficult to achieve and have never been shown in controlled trials to reduce cardiovascular disease morbidity or mortality, they may lower blood pressure and obviate the need for drug treatment or reduce the dosage requirements of antihypertensive drugs to control blood pressure.

Therapy should be tailored to the individual characteristics of each patient, such as weight reduction and exercise for the overweight patient (Chaps. 22, Obesity-Hypertension; 48, Diet—Calories; and 50, Exercise and Hypertension) and moderation in alcohol consumption for the heavy drinker (Chaps. 23, Alcohol and Hypertension; and 49, Alcohol Consumption and the Management of Hypertension). A reasonable generalized approach for all patients includes (1) reduced dietary sodium and fat and increased calcium, potassium, magnesium, vitamins, and fiber from food sources; (2) weight loss for the overweight patient; (3) regular physical activity; (4) moderation of alcohol consumption; and (5) smoking cessation. Such an approach has been shown to produce significant sustained reductions in blood pressure while reducing overall cardiovascular risk.

Two clinical trials, one involving a comprehensive food plan that supplied the recommended dietary allowances of all of the major nutrients,[2] and the other involving a diet rich in fruits, vegetables, and low-fat dairy products and low in saturated and total fat,[3] produced reductions in blood pressure comparable to or greater than those usually seen with monotherapy for stage 1 hypertension. The Dietary Approaches to Stop Hypertension (DASH) trial showed reductions in blood pressure of 11.4/5.5 mm Hg in hypertensive persons on the diet rich in fruits, vegetables, and low-fat dairy products, compared with control subjects on a so-called usual American diet, while dietary sodium intake and weight were held constant (Fig. 47–1.)[3, 4] Further, the DASH combination diet produced reductions in blood pressure of 3.5/2.1 mm Hg in subjects without hypertension. As pointed out by the authors in a letter to *Science*, the success of the DASH diet in lowering blood pressure cannot be attributed to its micronutrient content (high in calcium, potassium, and magnesium) alone, because the foods that were included in the DASH trial contain complex combinations of minerals, macronutrients, fiber, phytochemicals, vitamins, and other factors that, alone or in combination, could lower blood pressure.[5] They further point out that translation of the results of the DASH trial

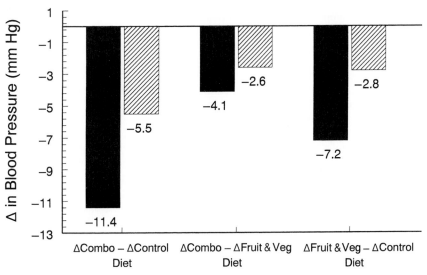

Figure 47–1. Effects on blood pressure of dietary modification in the 133 subjects with hypertension (systolic blood pressure ≥ 140 mm Hg, diastolic blood pressure ≥ 90 mm Hg, or both) in the Dietary Approaches to Stop Hypertension (DASH) trial. A control diet low in fruits, vegetables, and dairy products and containing 37% fat was fed for 3 weeks at the beginning of the study. Participants were then randomized to receive for 8 weeks (1) the control (usual American) diet, (2) a diet rich in fruits and vegetables, or (3) a combination diet rich in fruits, vegetables, and low-fat dairy products and with reduced saturated and total fat. Sodium intake and body weight were maintained constant. (Data from Appel LJ, Moore TJ, Obarzanek E, et al. The effect of dietary patterns on blood pressure: Results from the Dietary Approaches to Stop Hypertension [DASH] Clinical Trial. N Engl J Med 336:1117–1124, 1997.)

into advice for the general public (or for the universe of hypertensives) is more easily accomplished by recommending four servings of fruit, four servings of vegetables, and three servings of low-fat dairy products each day than by prescribing a specific daily intake of calcium, potassium, and magnesium. The paradigm shift toward recognition of the powerful role of total diet, rather than individual nutrients, in the prevention and treatment of hypertension in particular and cardiovascular disease in general deserves reemphasis.

Thus, in well-motivated patients with stage 1 or 2 hypertension, modifying lifestyle effectively lowers blood pressure and may be more important than the initial choice of antihypertensive drug. The same lifestyle-modification strategies that are effective in treating hypertensive patients may also be useful in the primary prevention of essential hypertension. The benefits of weight reduction (Chaps. 22 and 48), increased physical activity (Chap. 50), and moderation of alcohol intake (Chaps. 23 and 49) are discussed elsewhere in this volume. Accordingly, this chapter is confined to a discussion of the role of dietary micronutrients and of special foods that play a role in blood pressure control and in the modification of overall cardiovascular risk.

REDUCING DIETARY SODIUM

Historical Perspective

High dietary sodium chloride intake has been adduced as a cause of essential hypertension for over 4000 years.[6] Because neither blood pressure nor sodium intake and excretion could be measured directly, little progress was made in studying the relationship between dietary salt and blood pressure until the 20th century. In the early 1900s, two French physicians, Ambard and Beaujard, concluded, based on a study of several patients with hypertension and heart failure, that there was a positive relationship between chloride and blood pressure (they did not know how to measure sodium).[7] They restricted salt intake to almost nil in their patients and had them drink 2 L of milk every day. The result was a negative chloride balance and a decline in blood pressure, both of which were reversed when the patients were given salted bouillon in place of the milk.

Ambard and Beaujard also discovered the phenomenon of salt resistance. There was no change in blood pressure in one patient with an initial systolic blood pressure of 260 mm Hg who achieved a negative chloride balance on the salt-restricted and milk regimen. Even purgation with Seidlitz salts produced a negative chloride balance but only transiently decreased blood pressure. Ambard and Beaujard attributed the patient's persistent hypertension to "considerable saline impregnation of the tissues." Changes in blood pressure were observed when the regimens of extreme salt restriction were repeated in normotensive healthy subjects, leading the authors to conclude that there was a relationship between hypertension and salt intake, but only with extreme measures.[7]

The blood pressure lowering effects of extreme salt restriction were reconfirmed in the 1940s by Kempner, who observed normalization of blood pressure and reversal of

fundus changes in approximately 50% of patients with malignant hypertension who were placed on a diet of rice, fruit, and no salt.[8, 9] The remaining 50% of patients studied showed little change in blood pressure, indicating once again the lack of a universal response to restricted salt intake.

Dahl later popularized the notion that salt intake in a population is related to hypertension by showing a dramatic positive correlation between average salt intake and the percentage of hypertensive subjects in five populations (northern Japanese, southern Japanese, Americans, Marshall Islanders, and Eskimos from Alaska).[10] A review of 27 ecological studies published by Gleibermann and coworkers soon after the publication of the Dahl paper also concluded that there is a direct linear relationship between salt and blood pressure across populations.[11] These studies were flawed by numerous problems, including uncertainties about—and inconsistencies in—blood pressure measuring techniques and, in 16 of the 27 studies, a failure to measure salt intake directly. Further, other factors, including acculturation, industrialization, caloric intake, intake of fruits, vegetables, and dairy products, alcohol consumption, and exercise, also play important roles in determining mean blood pressure and the prevalence of hypertension in a population.

MODERN STUDIES OF SALT AND BLOOD PRESSURE

Observational Studies

The INTERSALT Study was a large observational trial that employed state-of-the-art techniques of measuring blood pressure and salt intake (24-hour urinary sodium excretion) in a very large sample (almost 11,000) of men and women aged 20 to 59 years from 52 centers in 39 countries around the world.[12] Within each center, 200 individuals, 100 men and 100 women, 50 from each decade of life between the ages of 20 and 60, were chosen at random from the population. The primary hypotheses of INTERSALT were that blood pressure would be directly and independently related to 24-hour urinary sodium excretion across the 11,000 participants in the study (the within-population hypothesis) and that for the 52 centers taken as individual population samples, median blood pressure would be directly related to median 24-hour urinary sodium excretion (the cross-population, or ecological, hypothesis).

There was no significant relationship between 24-hour urinary sodium excretion and blood pressure in an analysis of data from 48 acculturated populations (Figs. 47–2 and 47–3).[12] In contrast, body mass index and alcohol intake did correlate positively with blood pressure in this analysis. A weak but significant relationship between sodium excretion and blood pressure emerged only when four centers with nonacculturated populations (Yanomamo and Xingu tribes in Brazil and tribes in Kenya and Papua, New Guinea) that had extremely low intakes of salt and alcohol, as well as low body weight and low blood pressure, were included in the analysis (Figs. 47–2 and 47–3). A more robust association was found between salt intake and the increase in blood pressure with age, but the interpretation of the age/blood pressure relationship was clouded by its

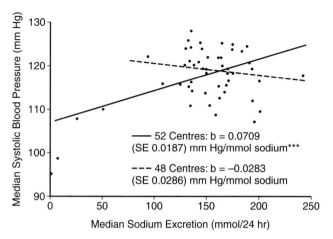

Figure 47–2. Cross-center plots of median systolic blood pressure and median sodium excretion (SE) and fitted regression lines for 52 and 48 centers standardized for age and sex. *** $p <$. 001. (From INTERSALT Cooperative Research Group. INTERSALT: An international study of electrolyte excretion and blood pressure: Results for 24-hour urinary sodium and potassium excretion. BMJ 297: 319–328, 1988.)

omission from the a priori hypotheses that appeared in prestudy publications.[13] A reanalysis of the data by the INTERSALT investigators with the stated purpose of correcting regression dilution bias yielded a stronger relationship between salt intake and blood pressure[14] but has been severely criticized on the grounds of assumptions unsupported by data and questionable statistical methods.[15, 16] Thus, the most contemporary, extensive, and rigorous observational study of the relationship between dietary salt and blood pressure has yielded results that have been the subject of controversy and variable interpretation.

A second large population study, the Scottish Heart Health Study, which also examined the relationship between 24-hour urinary sodium excretion and blood pressure in 11,629 Scottish men and women, found no correlation after correcting for confounding variables, including body mass and alcohol consumption.[17] An 8-year follow-up of the Scottish Heart Health Study showed no significant relationship between sodium excretion and coronary heart disease in men and a barely significant positive relationship for women (Fig. 47–4).[18] The relationship between sodium excretion and all-cause mortality was marginally significant in men and not significant in women. In contrast, potassium excretion was negatively correlated with all-cause mortality in both sexes and with coronary heart disease in men. Further, systolic blood pressure was positively correlated with both all-cause mortality and coronary heart disease in both sexes. Thus, in this large sample of representative men and women from the relatively high-risk Scottish population, sodium excretion (and presumably intake) had little predictive value for either coronary heart disease or all-cause mortality over an 8-year follow-up period.

Interventional Studies

Prospective, randomized, controlled trials of the effects of altering sodium intake on blood pressure would be ex-

pected to provide a firmer rationale than observational studies for therapeutic recommendations and public health policy. However, modifying salt intake, particularly restricting salt, in free-living persons is a complex intervention for a variety of reasons. (1) Sodium restriction generally results in altered intake of other nutrients, including calories, fat, protein, calcium, and potassium, which may have independent effects on blood pressure, other cardiovascular risk factors, and overall diet quality.[19] (2) Noncompliance with low-salt regimens is a major problem, particularly in long-term studies, and is frequently not taken into account in analyses. (3) Methods for quantitating salt intake are cumbersome and problematic, considering the substantial day-to-day variations in this parameter. Further, published studies in this area generally involve too few subjects and are of inadequate duration to provide the statistical power necessary to demonstrate a relationship between salt and blood pressure when analyzed on an individual basis. In addition, such studies are frequently not blinded or placebo-controlled and thus are subject to biases related to unintended interventions. Accordingly, a number of meta-analyses of published studies have been carried out in order to provide a larger database from which to assess the dietary salt/blood pressure relationship.

Three recent meta-analyses have shown small but consistent reductions in blood pressure in hypertensive individuals who participated in clinical trials of salt restriction. A meta-analysis of 32 trials (22 in hypertensives and 12 in normotensives) with outcome data for 2635 subjects showed mean blood pressure reductions of 4.8/2.5 mm Hg in hypertensive subjects and 1.9/1.1 mm Hg in normotensive subjects (Fig. 47–5) in association with median reductions in sodium excretion of 77 and 76 mmol/day, respectively.[20] Weighted linear regression analyses across trials showed dose responses, with calculated reductions in blood pressure/100 mmol sodium excretion/24 hr of 5.8/2.5 mm Hg in hypertensives and 2.3/1.4 mm Hg in normotensives. The authors commented that although the intervention ef-

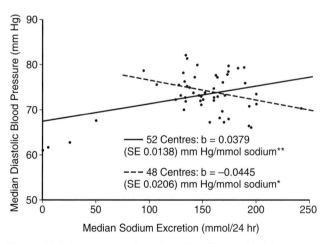

Figure 47–3. Cross-center plots of median diastolic blood pressure and median sodium excretion (SE) and fitted regression lines for 52 and 48 centers standardized for age and sex. ** $p <$.01, * $p <$ .05. (From INTERSALT Cooperative Research Group. INTERSALT: An international study of electrolyte excretion and blood pressure: Results for 24-hour urinary sodium and potassium excretion. BMJ 297: 319–328, 1988.)

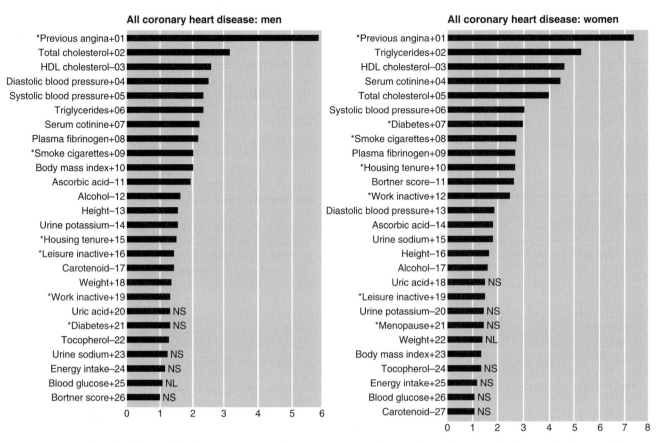

Figure 47–4. Ranking of risk factors for all coronary events in men and women by age-adjusted hazard ratios between highest and lowest category (fifths unless indicated). *Factors with fewer than five classes. NS, not significant; NL, not linear. (From Tunstall-Pedoe H, Woodward M, Tavendale R, et al. Comparison of the prediction by 27 different factors of coronary heart disease and death in men and women of the Scottish Heart Health Study: Cohort study. BMJ 315:722–729, 1997.)

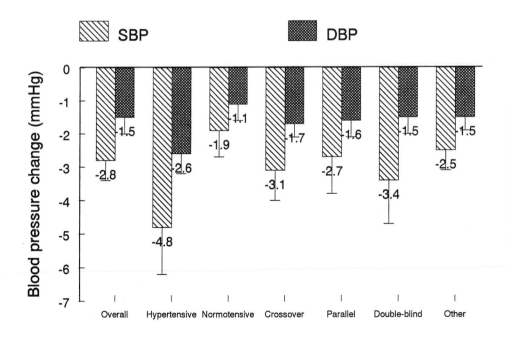

Figure 47–5. Mean net changes, with 95% CIs, pooled for all sodium-reduction trials and for various subsets. SBP, systolic blood pressure; DBP, diastolic blood pressure. (Redrawn from Cutler JA, Follman D, Allender PS. Randomized trials of sodium reduction: An overview. Am J Clin Nutr 65:643S–651S, 1997. © Am. J. Clin. Nutr. American Society for Clinical Nutrition.)

fect (reduction in sodium excretion) was reduced in the longer trials, the blood pressure effect was well maintained and, further, that the results were not confounded by concomitant changes in weight or potassium excretion. They concluded that the reduction in average blood pressure related to reduced sodium intake has great potential, especially when combined with other public health measures, for shifting the blood pressure distribution for the entire U.S. population. The importance to public health of this shift is illustrated by calculations based on associations of a 2 mm Hg reduction in diastolic blood pressure with improved cardiovascular disease outcomes: 15% fewer strokes and transient ischemic attacks and 6% fewer cases of coronary heart disease.[21]

A second meta-analysis included 56 randomized trials (28 in hypertensives and 28 in normotensives).[22] Most trials used a crossover design, and the median duration of intervention was 14 days. The median age of the study population in the normotensive trials was 26 years and in the hypertensive trials, 47 years. Only 15 studies provided information on race, and only 8 included blacks, who constituted only 2 to 39% of participants in these trials. Only 9% attrition was reported across studies, and 88% of studies achieved 80% or more of the sodium intervention target. Estimated mean reductions in sodium excretion across trials were 95 mmol/24 hr (range 71 to 119) for 1131 hypertensive subjects and 125 mmol/24 hr (range 95 to 156) for 2374 normotensive subjects. The unadjusted (for the marked variation in the dietary intervention effect, the change in urinary sodium excretion, among trials) effects on blood pressure were large in the hypertensive trials (mean 5.9 mm Hg, range 4.1 to 7.8 mm Hg) for systolic blood pressure ($p < .001$) and (mean 3.8 mm Hg, range 2.9 to 4.8 mm Hg) for diastolic blood pressure ($p < .001$). In the normotensive trials, there was a significant but smaller reduction ($p < .001$) in systolic blood pressure (mean 1.6 mm Hg, range 0.9 to 2.4 mm Hg) but no significant change in diastolic blood pressure (mean -0.5 mm Hg, range -0.1 to 1.2 mm Hg). After adjustment for measurement error, the mean decrease in blood pressure for a reduction in daily sodium excretion of 100 mmol was 3.7 mm Hg (range 2.4 to 5.1 mm Hg) for systolic ($p < .001$) and 0.9 mm Hg (range -0.1 to 1.9 mm Hg) for diastolic blood pressure ($p = .09$) in the hypertensive trials and 1.0 mm Hg (range 0.5 to 1.6 mm Hg) for systolic ($p < .001$) and 0.1 mm Hg (range -0.3 to 0.5 mm Hg) for diastolic blood pressure ($p = .64$) in the normotensive trials.

There was significant heterogeneity among trials in the effect of dietary sodium reduction on blood pressure, as illustrated by Figure 47–6, in which within-group blood pressure change was plotted against the within-group dietary sodium change for each group within a trial. This example from hypertensive trials shows that large between-group changes in urinary sodium excretion (horizontal axis) were associated in some trials with small changes in systolic blood pressure (vertical axis), whereas in others, small changes in urinary sodium excretion were accompanied by large changes in systolic blood pressure. Similar observations were made for diastolic blood pressure. The reasons for this heterogeneity are unknown. Furthermore, analysis of the data revealed evidence of confounding, resulting in

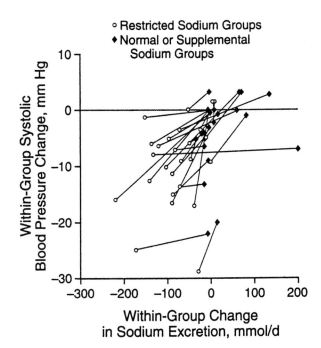

Figure 47–6. Plots of change in systolic blood pressure, outcome minus baseline, vs. change in urinary sodium excretion, outcome minus baseline, for each group. There is one plot for each study. (From Midgeley JP, Matthew AG, Greenwood CMT, Logan AG. Effect of reduced dietary sodium on blood pressure: A meta-analysis of randomized controlled trials. JAMA 275:1590–1597, 1996, Copyright 1996, American Medical Association.)

reductions in blood pressure unassociated with changes in sodium intake. Plausible confounding factors, such as changes in weight and changes in potassium intake or intake of other nutrients or alcohol, were not reported for most trials.

Subgroup analysis showed that the blood pressure response to dietary sodium reduction was larger in trials of older hypertensive subjects (mean age ≥ 45 years) than in all hypertensive trials together, confirming previous observations that older persons are more sensitive to dietary salt. The slope estimates were 6.3 mm Hg (range 4.1 to 8.4 mm Hg) per 100 mmol/day of sodium for systolic ($p < .001$) and 2.2 mm Hg (range 0.68 to 3.97 mm Hg) per 100 mmol/day of sodium for diastolic blood pressure ($p = .01$) in trials of older hypertensives. In trials of younger hypertensives, the decrease was much smaller for systolic and was negligible for diastolic blood pressure. Studies in which the methodology was classified as questionable because of imbalances in sex or in baseline urinary sodium excretion and studies that were smaller in size, were shorter in duration (2 weeks or less), or employed a crossover design tended to show a greater decrease in blood pressure with sodium reduction; larger studies employing optimal methodology tended to show smaller decreases in blood pressure.

Further, these authors pointed out that estimates of change in blood pressure normalized to 100-mmol/day reductions in sodium intake overstate what can be done in a free-living population. Mean baseline urinary sodium excretion in both normotensive and hypertensive subjects in most industrialized societies is approximately 160 mmol/day, and a 100-mmol/day decrease would require consumption of a diet containing 60 mmol/day, an unachievable goal for large populations. To attain the currently recommended goal of 2400 mg (104 mmol) sodium/day, an average reduction in sodium intake of only 60 mmol/day would be required. According to the Midgley meta-analysis, this would result in a blood pressure decrease of 2.2/0.5 mm Hg in hypertensive populations and 0.60/0.06 mm Hg in normotensive populations.[22]

The most recent meta-analysis of the effects of salt reduction on blood pressure included 58 trials of hypertensive and 56 trials of normotensive persons.[23] The effect of reduced sodium intake (mean 118 mmol/day) was a mean 3.9 mm Hg (95% CI 3.0 to 4.8 mm Hg) ($p < .001$) reduction in systolic blood pressure and a mean 1.9 mm Hg (95% CI 1.3 to 2.5 mm Hg) ($p < .001$) reduction in diastolic blood pressure in hypertensives (Fig. 47–7). In the trials of normotensives, the mean reduction in 24-hour urinary sodium excretion was 160 mmol, and the mean reductions in systolic and diastolic blood pressure were 1.2 mm Hg (95% CI 0.6 to 1.8 mm Hg) ($p < .001$) and 0.26 mm Hg (95% CI 0.3 to 0.9 mm Hg) ($p = 0.12$), respectively (Fig. 47–8).

The Graudal meta-analysis[23] took into account the neurohumoral consequences of sodium restriction (Table 47–1). All individual studies showed significant increases in plasma renin and aldosterone, and the magnitude of the increases in these parameters was related to the reduction in sodium excretion (Fig. 47–9). Renin and aldosterone responses to reduced sodium intake did not differ between normotensive and hypertensive populations, but plasma noradrenaline responses were more robust in hypertensive persons ($r = 0.76$; $p = .002$; $n = 13$ studies) than in normotensive persons ($r = 0.12$; $p = .64$; $n = 10$ studies). There were also significant increases in total and low-density lipoprotein cholesterol in the low sodium groups; other lipid parameters were not significantly changed. Plasma renin and aldosterone increased fivefold to sixfold in subjects in whom sodium excretion was less than 20 mmol/24 hr; in those who had reduced their sodium excretion only to 40 to 100 mmol/24 hr, these values increased twofold compared to baseline. This effect was sustained over time if the reduced sodium intake was maintained. The authors concluded that activation of the renin-angiotensin-aldosterone system and possibly of the sympathetic nervous

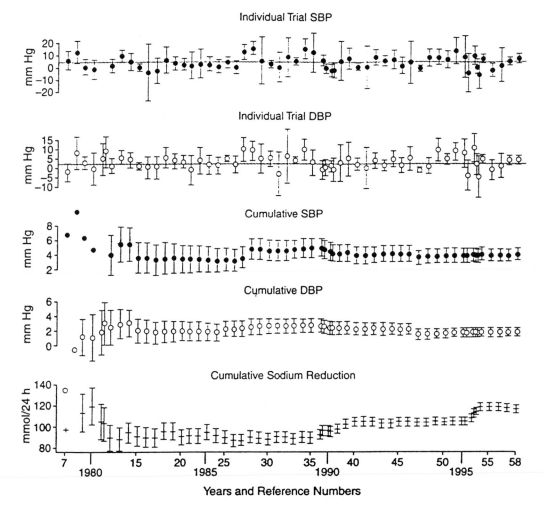

Figure 47–7. Meta-analysis of the effect of reduced sodium intake on systolic and diastolic blood pressure (SBP, DBP) in hypertensive populations ($n = 58$). The effect sizes (in millimeters of mercury [mm Hg]) and the 95% CIs for the individual trials, the cumulative meta-analyses, and the cumulative reduction of 24-hour urinary sodium excretion are shown. (From Graudal NA, Galloe AM, Garred P. Effects of sodium restriction on blood pressure, renin, aldosterone, catecholamines, cholesterols, and triglycerides. JAMA 279:1383–1390, 1998, Copyright 1998, American Medical Association.)

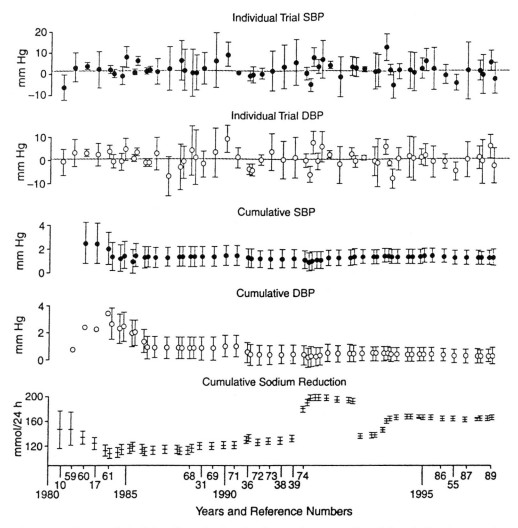

Figure 47–8. Meta-analysis of the effect of reduced sodium intake on systolic and diastolic blood pressure (SBP, DBP) in normotensive populations ($n = 56$). The effect sizes (in millimeters of mercury [mm Hg]) and the 95% CIs for the individual trials, the cumulative meta-analyses, and the cumulative reduction of 24-hour urinary sodium excretion are shown. (From Graudal NA, Galloe AM, Garred P. Effects of sodium restriction on blood pressure, renin, aldosterone, catecholamines, cholesterols, and triglycerides. JAMA 279:1383–1390, 1998, Copyright 1998, American Medical Association.)

Table 47–1 Meta-Analyses of the Effects of Sodium Reduction on Hormones and Lipids

	Number of Studies (Reference)	Number of Patients	Sodium Reduction, Mean (Range)	Duration Median (Range), day	Effect L/H* (SD)	p†	r‡	p
Renin	53 (37)	1110	182 (50–341)	7 (4–180)	3.63 (2.57)	<.001	0.66	<.001
Aldosterone	38 (26)	340	186 (61–341)	7 (4–180)	3.26 (1.59)	<.001	0.64	<.001
Noradrenaline	29 (18)	700	196 (72–328)	7 (4–180)	1.32 (0.27)	<.001	0.45	.02
Adrenaline	10 (8)	207	126 (72–178)	21 (7–180)	1.19 (0.18)	.02	−0.33	.35
Cholesterol	19 (13)	653	179 (56–280)	7 (7–90)	1.04 (0.04)	<.001	0.49	.03
High-density lipoprotein	15 (10)	573	186 (56–280)	7 (7–56)	1.01 (0.05)	.35	−0.17	.55
Low-density lipoprotein	13 (8)	517	203 (56–280)	7 (7–28)	1.05 (0.04)	.003	0.29	.34
Triglyceride	14 (9)	565	191 (56–280)	7 (7–56)	1.06 (0.11)	.05	0.33	.25

From Graudal NA, Galloe AM, Garred P. Effects of sodium restriction on blood pressure, renin, aldosterone, catecholamines, cholesterols, and triglycerides. JAMA 279:1383–1391, 1998, Copyright 1998, American Medical Association.
*L/H indicates value obtained during low-sodium diet/value obtained during high-sodium diet.
†$p < .005$.
‡Correlation coefficient, effect size vs. sodium reduction.

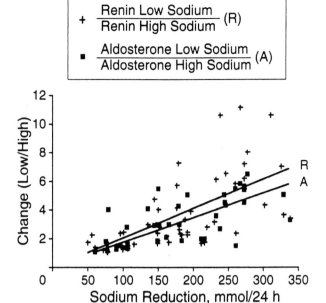

Figure 47–9. Regression analysis of the relation between sodium reduction and change in plasma renin (R) and change in plasma aldosterone (A) where R = 0.020 × [Sodium reduction] (95% CI, 0.018–0.022), r^2 = 0.43, and p <.001; A = 0.017 × [sodium reduction] (95% CI, 0.015–0.019), r^2 = 0.41, and p <.001. (From Graudal NA, Galloe AM, Garred P. Effects of sodium restriction on blood pressure, renin, aldosterone, catecholamines, cholesterols, and triglycerides. JAMA 279:1383–1390, 1998, Copyright 1998, American Medical Association.)

system in response to sodium restriction might account for the relatively small effect of reduced sodium intake on blood pressure. Further, elevations in plasma renin activity in the setting of hypertension have been related to increased target organ damage and coronary events[24, 25]; this finding suggests that sodium reduction may have adverse effects on cardiovascular outcomes. This concept will be discussed later in the chapter.

The hypothesis that lifestyle modification can prevent the progression from high normal blood pressure to frank hypertension has been tested in the Trials of Hypertension Prevention (TOHP).[26–29] Phase I of TOHP tested the short-term effect on blood pressure of selected nutritional and behavioral interventions and established the feasibility of a long-term clinical trial of methods designed to reduce the incidence of hypertension.[26, 27] TOHP-I consisted of three randomized, controlled, parallel-group trials with common source populations, eligibility criteria, and data collection and analytic methods (Fig. 47–10). Participants included 2132 men and women aged 30 to 54 years with diastolic blood pressures of 80 to 89 mm Hg. Seven interventions were tested: three lifestyle-change interventions (weight reduction, sodium reduction, and stress management) with an unmasked design but with blinded measurement of blood pressure as the endpoint, and four nutritional supplement interventions (calcium, magnesium, fish oil, and potassium supplements), with placebo-controlled, double-blind designs. The nutritional supplement component was divided into two stages, each of 6 months' duration, with an intervening washout period (Fig. 47–10). Participants in the nutritional supplement trial were allocated equally to

calcium carbonate, magnesium diglycine, or placebo (stage 1). After the washout period, participants were rerandomized to fish oil, potassium chloride, or placebo (stage 2).

Compliance with the various interventions was good. Weight reduction intervention produced a maximal mean weight loss of 5.7 kg (p < .01) at 6 months. Weight loss was reasonably well maintained at 18 months (3.9 kg, p < .01) compared to the control group. There were no significant differences in sodium excretion or in alcohol, calcium, or magnesium intake between the weight reduction and the control groups. The mean decrease in sodium excretion was 55 to 60 mmol/day at both 6 and 18 months in the sodium restriction group; the difference in sodium excretion between the sodium restriction and the control groups was only 44 mmol/day at 18 months because of a reduction in the control group compared to baseline levels. Compliance with the nutritional supplement and placebo protocols was monitored by pill count and appropriate biochemical testing and was found to be excellent except in the fish oil group due to gastrointestinal side effects of the intervention. Follow-up rates were high, and collection of blood pressure measurements was nearly complete (93% at final visits).

The primary outcome measure was change in diastolic blood pressure, and the major secondary outcome was change in systolic blood pressure from baseline to the last follow-up visit. The lifestyle change participants were followed for 18 months in order to provide a reasonable test of maintenance of behavioral changes over time. At 6 months of follow-up, significant reductions in systolic and diastolic blood pressure were seen in the weight reduction and sodium restriction groups only (Fig. 47–11). At 18 months of follow-up, very small but statistically significant reductions in systolic (1.7 mm Hg, p < .01) and diastolic (0.9 mm Hg, p < .05) blood pressure persisted in the sodium reduction group. Blood pressure effects were more robust (−2.9 mm Hg systolic, p < .01; −2.3 mm Hg diastolic, p < .01) in the weight reduction group. In contrast, the effects on blood pressure of stress management and of taking nutritional supplements were small, inconsistent in direction, and not statistically significant. The occurrence of hypertension during follow-up was significantly reduced only in the weight reduction group (relative risk [RR] 0.66; 95% CI 0.46 to 0.94). Despite the small number of participants who became hypertensive in the course of the study, the authors concluded that sodium reduction and weight loss could potentially have substantial benefit in preventing hypertension and cardiovascular morbidity and mortality, particularly if the effects on blood pressure are additive when the interventions are combined.

In contrast to the marginally positive results of sodium restriction on blood pressure in TOHP I, another large study published at the same time reported no effect of a low sodium/high potassium diet on blood pressure in patients with stage 1 hypertension recruited from the general population.[30, 31] The Trial of Antihypertensive Interventions and Management (TAIM) was designed to assess the relative value of the most commonly used approaches to antihypertensive drug therapy (thiazide diuretics and β-blockers) and diet therapy (weight loss, restricted sodium, and increased potassium intake) applied singly and in combination. An additional aim was to test the hypothesis that

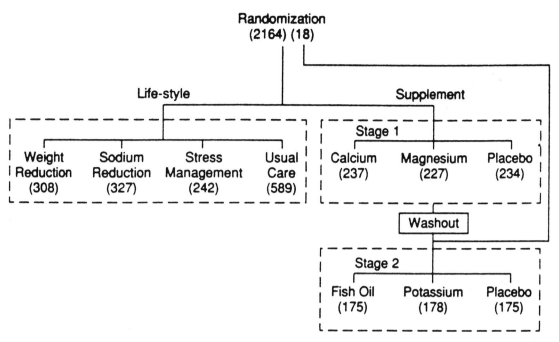

Figure 47–10. Schematic representation of randomization of participants into three component trials of the Trials of Hypertension Prevention, Phase I. Numbers in parentheses are sample sizes. Because of stratification by clinic and body mass index, the number of control subjects ("usual care") available for respective comparisons were, for sodium reduction, 417; for weight reduction, 256; and for stress management, 320. (From The Trials of Hypertension Prevention Collaborative Research Group. The effects of nonpharmacological interventions on blood pressure of persons with high normal levels: Results of the Trials of Hypertension Prevention [Phase I]. JAMA 267:1213–1220, 1992, Copyright 1992, American Medical Association.)

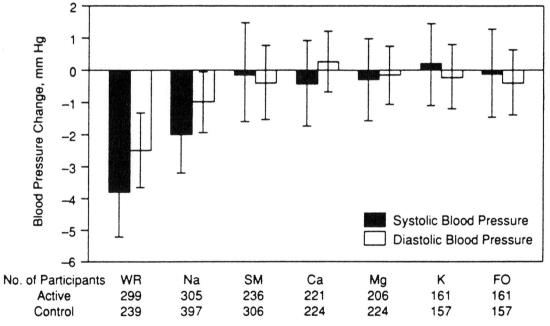

Figure 47–11. Net mean changes in systolic and diastolic blood pressure (baseline minus follow-up), with 95% CIs. WR, weight reduction; Na, sodium reduction; SM, stress management; Ca, calcium supplementation; Mg, magnesium supplementation; K, potassium supplementation; FO, fish oil supplementation. (From The Trials of Hypertension Prevention Collaborative Research Group. The effects of nonpharmacological interventions on blood pressure of persons with high normal levels: Results of the Trials of Hypertension Prevention [Phase I]. JAMA 267:1213–1220, 1992, Copyright 1992, American Medical Association.)

plasma renin activity predicts the blood pressure response to lifestyle modification therapy in patients with mild hypertension. Participants (878 patients at three centers) were assigned at random to a usual diet, a weight-loss diet, or a low sodium (90 mEq/day)/high potassium (80 mEq/day) diet and concurrently randomized to receive placebo, diuretic therapy (chlorthalidone, 25 mg/day) or β-blocker therapy (atenolol, 50 mg/day). Patients on the low sodium/high potassium diet plus placebo had a mean reduction in diastolic blood pressure of 7.9 mm Hg at 6 months, compared to reductions of 8.0 mm Hg for the usual diet plus placebo group and 8.8 mm Hg for the weight-loss group.[30] Patients with high renin hypertension at baseline had greater blood pressure responses to both the low sodium/high potassium and the weight-loss diets (Fig. 47–12). The low sodium/high potassium diet did not result in a greater reduction in blood pressure than did the usual diet, and it did not enhance the blood pressure effect of either drug. The mean urinary sodium excretion in the low sodium group at 6 months was 106 mEq/day, reflecting only a small reduction from baseline, and the authors suggested that this level might have been insufficient to affect extracellular fluid volume and blood pressure. In contrast, weight loss alone produced a beneficial effect on blood pressure, and adding weight loss to diuretic or β-blocker treatment enhanced the effect of drug treatment. The authors concluded that in the short-term management of mild hypertension, when diastolic blood pressure is the sole consideration, drugs outperform diet, and weight loss is beneficial, especially in combination with diuretics.

The second phase of TOHP (TOHP II) tested the hypotheses that sodium reduction and weight loss interventions, administered separately and in combination, could be sustained over time, could produce sustained reductions in systolic and diastolic blood pressure, and could prevent new-onset hypertension.[28, 29] This study enrolled 2382 moderately overweight (110 to 165% of desirable body weight) men and women age 30 to 54 years with high normal blood pressure (< 140/83 to 89 mm Hg) who were not taking antihypertensive medications. Participants were assigned at random to weight loss alone, sodium reduction alone, a combination of the two, or no active intervention (usual care). Follow-up was for 36 to 48 months. The study was carried out in nine academic centers. Importantly, counseling was intensive in the active intervention groups: weekly for the first 10 to 14 weeks, followed by a period of semiweekly or monthly sessions, depending on the intervention group. Intervention goals were a mean weight loss of at least 4.5 kg, a mean sodium intake of 80 mmol/day or less, or both in the first 6 months, to be maintained throughout the course of the study.

The sodium reduction and combined groups achieved estimated reductions in sodium excretion of 78 and 64 mmol/day, respectively, at 6 months, thus reaching estimated mean excretion levels of 104 and 124 mmol/day, substantially short of the target. More modest estimated reductions in sodium excretion occurred in the weight loss (18 mmol/day) and usual care (28 mmol/day) groups. At 6 months, the weight loss and combined groups lost a mean of 4.4 and 4.1 kg, respectively ($p < .001$ compared to the

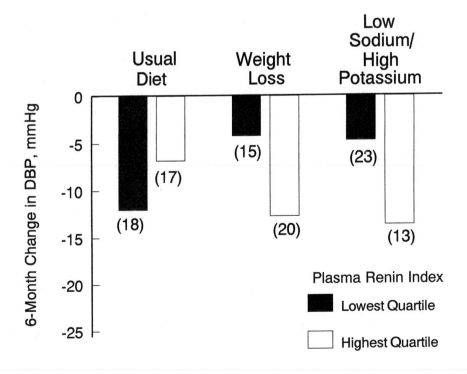

Plasma renin index = natural log plasma renin activity x natural log 24 hr urinary sodium excretion

Figure 47–12. Diastolic blood pressure (DBP) response for patients in the highest and lowest quartiles of plasma renin index values for each of the three diet groups. The number at the bottom of each bar is the number of subjects in that group. (From Blaufox MD, Lee HB, Davis B, et al. Renin predicts diastolic blood pressure response to nonpharmacologic and pharmacologic therapy. JAMA 267:1221–1225, 1992, Copyright 1992, American Medical Association.)

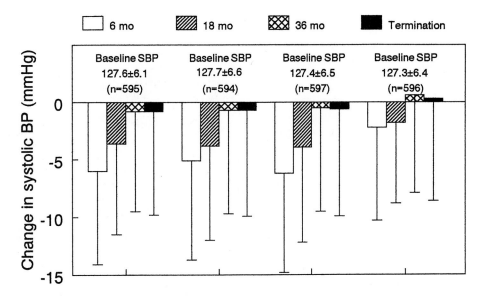

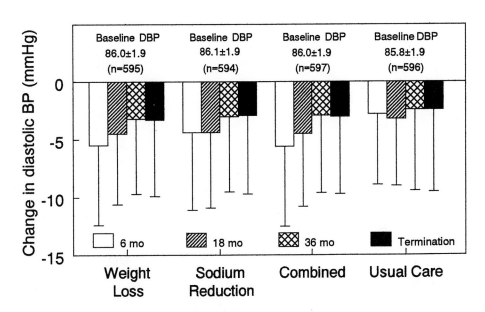

Figure 47–13. Baseline and change from baseline in systolic and diastolic blood pressure (BP) by intervention group. (From The Trials of Hypertension Prevention Collaborative Research Group. Effect of weight loss and sodium reduction intervention on blood pressure and hypertension incidence in overweight people with high-normal blood pressure: The Trials of Hypertension Prevention, Phase II. Arch Intern Med 157:657–667, 1997.)

usual care group), and the sodium reduction group also lost significant amounts of weight (1.1 kg, $p < .001$), compared to the usual care group. Both sodium excretion and weight increased significantly at 18 and 36 months of follow-up. Compared to the usual care group, estimated reductions in sodium excretion fell by 20% and 36%, respectively, at 36 months in the sodium reduction and combined groups. Differences from the usual care group were small (40 mmol/day for sodium reduction and 24 mmol/day for combined groups; $p < .001$) but significant for both groups.

Blood pressure reductions for the weight loss, sodium reduction, and combined groups were 3.7/2.7, 2.9/1.6, and 4.0/2.8 mm Hg, respectively, at 6 months ($p < .001$ for all) (Fig. 47–13). The main effects, which estimate the contributions of the single-modality intervention programs to the blood pressure change in the combined group, were 2.4/2.0 mm Hg for weight loss and 1.6/0.8 mm Hg for sodium reduction at 6 months. The effects of both interventions decreased over time until at 36 months, diastolic

blood pressure reductions were statistically significant for the weight loss group only (-0.9 mm Hg, $p < .04$), whereas systolic blood pressure reductions were small but statistically significant in both groups (1.3 and 1.2 mm Hg for the weight loss and sodium reduction groups, respectively, $p < .03$) (Fig. 47–13). Results were similar at termination of the study. None of the main effect estimates was significant for termination blood pressure.

Hypertension developed in 883 of 2250 participants, based on clinic blood pressures (381 based on systolic blood pressure, 140 based on diastolic blood pressure, 100 based on both) or on initiation of drug treatment for hypertension by a personal physician (262 participants) over the course of the 48-month study (Fig. 47–14). The incidence of hypertension increased steadily in all four experimental groups during the study: at 6 months, it was highest in the usual care group (7.3%), intermediate in the weight loss (4.2%) and sodium reduction (4.5%) groups, and lowest in the combined group (2.7%). The benefits of

Weight
Combined
Sodium
Usual Care
Incidence of Hypertension, %
0
10
20
30
40
50
0
6
12
18
24
30
36
42
48
Time, mo

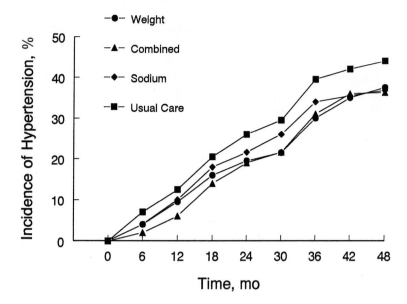

Figure 47–14. Plot of the incidence of hypertension for the respective randomized groups through 48 months of follow-up, from life-table analysis in the Trials of Hypertension Prevention, Phase II. (From The Trials of Hypertension Prevention Collaborative Research Group. Effect of weight loss and sodium reduction intervention on blood pressure and hypertension incidence in overweight people with high-normal blood pressure: The Trials of Hypertension Prevention, Phase II. Arch Intern Med 157:657–667, 1997.)

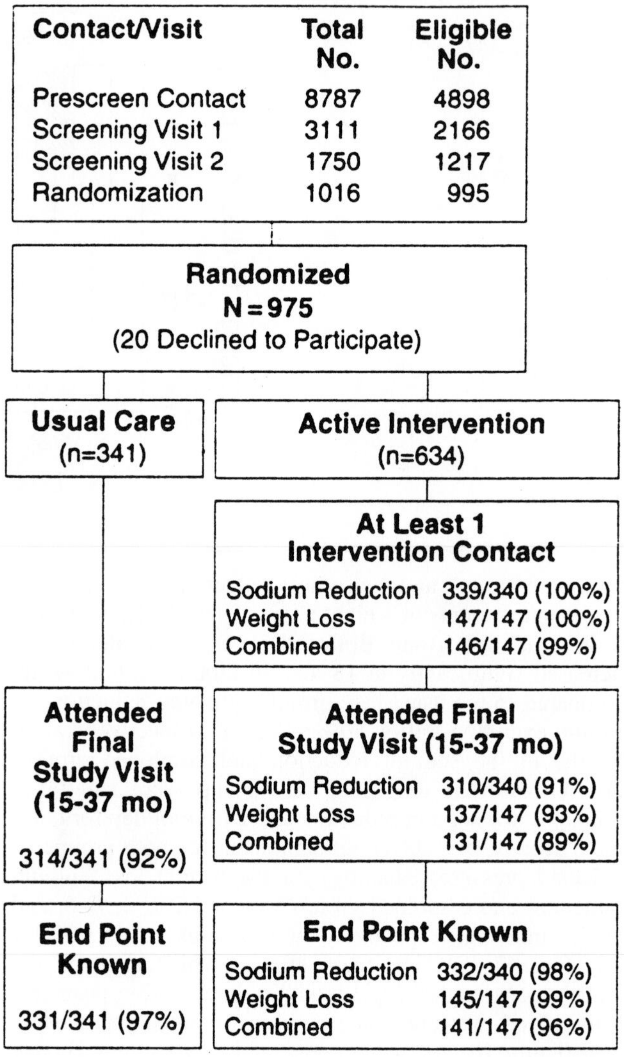

Contact/Visit
Total No.
Eligible No.
Prescreen Contact 8787 4898
Screening Visit 1 3111 2166
Screening Visit 2 1750 1217
Randomization 1016 995
Randomized
N=975
(20 Declined to Participate)
Usual Care
(n=341)
Active Intervention
(n=634)
At Least 1
Intervention Contact
Sodium Reduction 339/340 (100%)
Weight Loss 147/147 (100%)
Combined 146/147 (99%)
Attended Final Study Visit (15-37 mo)
314/341 (92%)
Attended Final Study Visit (15-37 mo)
Sodium Reduction 310/340 (91%)
Weight Loss 137/147 (93%)
Combined 131/147 (89%)
End Point Known
331/341 (97%)
End Point Known
Sodium Reduction 332/340 (98%)
Weight Loss 145/147 (99%)
Combined 141/147 (96%)

Figure 47–15. Participation in screening and follow-up in the Trial of Nonpharmacologic Interventions in the Elderly. (From Whelton PK, Appel LJ, Espeland MA, et al for the TONE Collaborative Research Group. Sodium reduction and weight loss in the treatment of hypertension in older persons. A randomized controlled trial of nonpharmacologic interventions in the elderly [TONE]. JAMA 279:839–846, 1998, Copyright 1998, American Medical Association.)

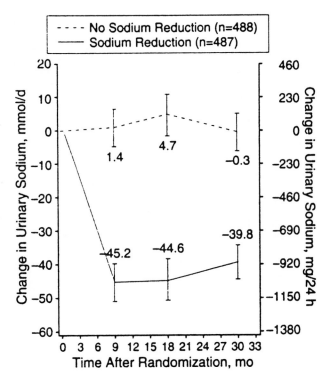

Figure 47–16. Mean change in 24-hour urinary sodium excretion among the 487 participants who were assigned and the 488 who were not assigned to the reduced sodium intake intervention of the Trial of Nonpharmacologic Interventions in the Elderly. *Error bars* indicate SEM. The numbers used in the figure are given in millimoles per day. (From Whelton PK, Appel LJ, Espeland MA, et al for the TONE Collaborative Research Group. Sodium reduction and weight loss in the treatment of hypertension in older persons. A randomized controlled trial of nonpharmacologic interventions in the elderly [TONE]. JAMA 279:839–846, 1998, Copyright 1998, American Medical Association.)

active intervention were attenuated over time, and by 48 months, the incidence of hypertension was similar in the three intervention groups (38%), slightly but significantly lower than in the usual care group (44%; $p = .02$ to .06).

Thus, the results of TOHP II tended to confirm those of TOHP I: both weight loss and sodium restriction reduce blood pressure in overweight adults with high normal blood pressure. Weight loss was more effective than sodium restriction as a solitary intervention, and the effects of both interventions dissipated with time. The combination of the two interventions had little additional effect on blood pressure, in part because participants found it difficult to adhere to both weight loss and sodium restriction regimens at the same time. Despite these difficulties, the incidence of hypertension was reduced slightly in all active intervention groups. The limitations in duration and size of these trials preclude any conclusions about the effects of these interventions on cardiovascular disease morbidity and mortality. Further, the high rates of recidivism in all intervention groups despite intensive and expert counseling raise questions about the general utility of lifestyle modification with sodium restriction, alone or combined with weight loss, in hypertension prevention for the general population.

The more recent Trial of Nonpharmacologic Interventions in the Elderly (TONE)[32] assessed the effects of nonpharmacological interventions (reduced sodium intake, weight loss, or both) on blood pressure in the population previously shown to be most responsive to sodium reduction, older persons with hypertension.[21] A total of 875 persons aged 60 to 80 years with hypertension controlled (<145/85 mm Hg) on a single antihypertensive medication were randomized (if obese) to reduced sodium intake, weight loss, both, or usual care or (if not obese) to reduced sodium intake or usual care (Fig. 47–15). Withdrawal of antihypertensive medication was attempted after 3 months

of intervention. The intervention program was intensive, as in TOHP II, and median follow-up was 29 months (range, 15 to 36 months). In contrast to results of trials in younger people, the effects of the sodium reduction and weight loss interventions were well maintained for the duration of the study (Figs. 47–16 and 47–17).

The primary endpoint of TONE was occurrence of high blood pressure at one or more follow-up visits after attempted withdrawal of antihypertensive medication, treatment with an antihypertensive medication, or occurrence of a cardiovascular event (myocardial infarction, angina, congestive heart failure, coronary artery bypass surgery, or angioplasty). A large majority of participants (87% of the usual care group and 93% of each intervention group) had antihypertensive therapy withdrawn an average of 3.2 months into the intervention. The percentage of participants remaining free of trial endpoints declined progressively during follow-up for all groups but was significantly greater for all three intervention groups than for usual care (Fig. 47–18). Based on Kaplan-Meier estimates, the proportions of randomized participants projected to be free of endpoints at 30 months were 34% (95% CI 25 to 43%) for sodium reduction, 37% (95% CI 28 to 46%) for weight loss, 44% (95% CI 32 to 55%) for sodium reduction and weight loss combined, and 16% (95% CI 5 to 27%) for usual care. The findings of TONE are remarkable in that they demonstrate the sustainability of moderate sodium reduction (mean decrease 40 to 45 mmol/day) and weight loss (mean decrease 4.5 to 5.0 kg) interventions in older persons with mild hypertension, along with blood pressure effects sufficient to reduce the need for antihypertensive medication by 30%. There were no differences in cardiovascular events among intervention groups. As suggested by the authors, the greater success of these interventions in older persons may have been due in part to a greater ability to achieve and

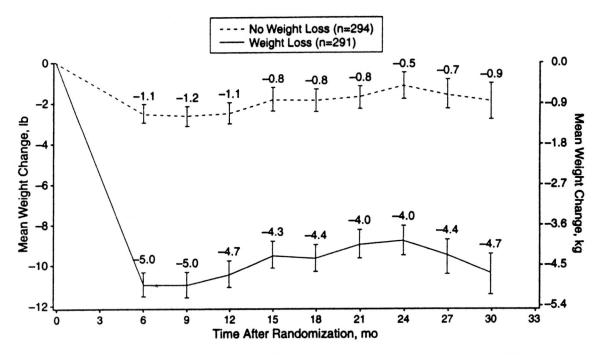

Figure 47–17. Mean change in body weight among the 294 obese participants who were assigned and the 291 who were not assigned to the weight loss intervention of the Trial of Nonpharmacologic Interventions in the Elderly. *Error bars* indicate SEM. The numbers used in the figure are given in kilograms. (From Whelton PK, Appel LJ, Espeland MA, et al for the TONE Collaborative Research Group. Sodium reduction and weight loss in the treatment of hypertension in older persons. A randomized controlled trial of nonpharmacologic interventions in the elderly [TONE]. JAMA 279:839–846, 1998, Copyright 1998, American Medical Association.)

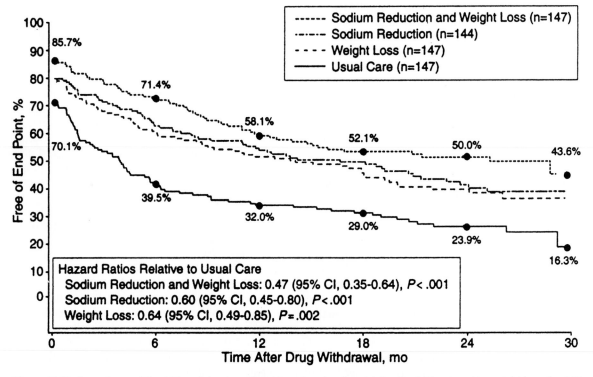

Figure 47–18. Percentages of the 144 participants assigned to reduced sodium intake, the 147 assigned to weight loss, the 147 assigned to reduced sodium intake and weight loss combined, and the 147 assigned to usual care (no lifestyle intervention) who remained free of cardiovascular events and high blood pressure and did not have an antihypertensive agent prescribed during follow-up. (From Whelton PK, Appel LJ, Espeland MA, et al for the TONE Collaborative Research Group. Sodium reduction and weight loss in the treatment of hypertension in older persons. A randomized controlled trial of nonpharmacologic interventions in the elderly [TONE]. JAMA 279:839–846, 1998, Copyright 1998, American Medical Association.)

maintain behavioral interventions in persons who are motivated to reduce their dependence on antihypertensive medication.

Potential Risks of Sodium Retention

Advocates of sodium restriction and other lifestyle modification strategies for hypertension treatment and prevention have repeatedly referred to its freedom from adverse effects. In fact, few studies have examined the effects of sodium restriction on other cardiovascular risk factors and on cardiovascular outcomes. The first study of the relationship between dietary sodium and cardiovascular disease outcomes was the cohort study of Alderman and colleagues which examined the relationship of urinary sodium excretion to subsequent morbidity and mortality in 2937 mildly and moderately hypertensive subjects who were participants in a worksite-based treatment program.[33] The 24-hour urinary excretion of sodium, potassium, and creatinine and plasma renin activity were measured following a 3- to 4- week period off antihypertensive medications at the time of entry into the study. Patients were treated with standard antihypertensive therapy without regard to their individual sodium excretion or plasma renin values. In addition, all participants were advised to avoid foods excessively high in salt throughout the course of treatment. During 3.5 years of median follow-up (range, 0.2 to 9.5 years), 282 events (221 morbid and 61 mortal) occurred. Of these, there were 117 cardiovascular disease events (55 myocardial infarctions, 23 strokes, 8 coronary [angioplasty/surgery] revascularizations, 9 unstable anginas, 6 congestive heart failures, and 16 other cardiovascular deaths) and 165 noncardiovascular disease events. Subjects were stratified according to sex-specific quartiles of urinary sodium excretion. Subjects in these strata were similar in race, prevalence of preexisting cardiovascular disease, family history of cardiovascular disease, smoking history, left ventricular hypertrophy by electrocardiogram, and initial and final antihypertensive drug use. Pretreatment and intreatment blood pressures were similar in all quartiles with the exception that systolic blood pressure in men in the lowest sodium quartile was 2 mm Hg lower than in the highest quartile ($p < .05$). Of the subjects, 80% had their blood pressure controlled on treatment.

Unadjusted overall incidence rates of myocardial infarction per 1000 person-years were inversely related to urinary sodium excretion for the total population, ranging from 8.1 (lowest quartile) to 2.9 (highest quartile), with an RR of 2.8 (95% CI 1.3 to 6.1). This was not true for stroke, noncardiovascular disease morbidity, or noncardiovascular disease deaths. A similar but stronger relationship between myocardial infarction and urinary sodium excretion was observed for men, with an RR of 5.2 (95% CI 2.0 to 13.5) for the lowest vs. the highest quartile. There was no relationship between urinary sodium excretion and myocardial infarction in women, who sustained only nine events in the course of the study. After adjustment for individual risk factors such as age, race, and left ventricular hypertrophy, the inverse relationship between sodium excretion and incidence of myocardial infarction in men persisted (Fig. 47–19). The magnitude of the relative risk of myocardial infarction in the lowest sodium quartile compared to the

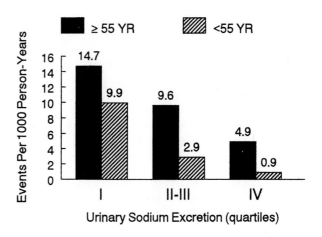

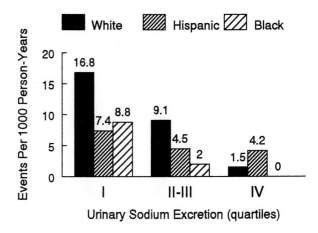

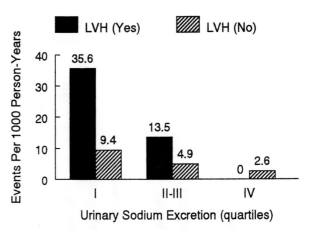

Figure 47–19. Bar graphs show incidence of myocardial infarction according to quartile of urinary sodium excretion and age, race, and left ventricular hypertrophy (LVH) in men. (From Alderman MH, Madhavan S, Cohen H, et al. Low urinary sodium is associated with greater risk of myocardial infarction among treated hypertensive men. Hypertension 25:1144–1152, 1995.)

higher quartiles varied according to the demographic or clinical characteristics of the participants.

As pointed out by the authors of both this article and the accompanying editorial commentary,[34] this study has a number of important limitations. First, the assessment of sodium intake was based on a single baseline measurement of 24-hour urinary sodium excretion and was linked to outcomes occurring many years later. Thus, it is not possible to know the stability of the measure over time, although the authors did provide some data to suggest that dietary intake tends to remain constant in middle-aged people over periods of years.[35, 36] Second, in this, as in any observational study, it is impossible to exclude the possibility that the observed associations are the result of undetected confounding. One possibility, not supported by the data reported, is that sicker subjects or those with a worse prognosis chose to eat less sodium. Inaccuracy in urine collection and random variation in eating habits were considered as other possible sources of error.

In a subsequent paper, the same investigators examined the relationship between dietary sodium intake as estimated by a single 24-hour dietary recall and subsequent all-cause and cardiovascular disease mortality rates in 11,346 participants in the first National Health and Nutrition Examination Survey (NHANES I).[37] There were 3923 deaths, of which 1970 were due to cardiovascular disease. All-cause mortality (per 1000 person-years, adjusted for age and sex) was inversely associated with sex-specific quartiles of sodium intake (lowest to highest quartile 23.18 to 19.01, $p <$ .0001) and total calorie intake (25.03 to 18.40, $p <$ .0001) and showed a weak positive association with quartiles of sodium:calorie ratio (20.27 to 21.71, $p = $ .14) (Fig. 47–20). The pattern for cardiovascular disease mortality was similar (sodium 11.80 to 9.60, $p <$ .0019; calories 12.80 to 8.94, $p <$ .0002; sodium:calorie ratio 9.73 to 11.35, $p = $ .017). In Cox multiple regression analysis, sodium intake was inversely associated with all-cause ($p = $ .0069) and cardiovascular disease mortality ($p = $ .086) and sodium:calorie ratio was directly associated with all-cause ($p = $ .0004) and cardiovascular disease mortality ($p = $ .0056).

The major limitation of this study is the unreliability of dietary recall as an index of sodium and calorie intake.

Dietary recall generally underestimates sodium and calorie intake.[38] As pointed out by critics of the paper, the dietary recall data used in this report obviously grossly underestimated true intake, as the lowest quartiles of sodium and calorie intake were in the range of 30 to 50 mmol sodium and 50% below the recommended daily allowance for calories.[39–41] Nevertheless, there is no a priori reason to believe that dietary recall was selectively inaccurate in the lowest quartile. These data by themselves are insufficient to justify the conclusion that dietary sodium reduction per se reduces life expectancy or increases cardiovascular events. Nevertheless, they are provocative and suggest a need for further examination of the relationship between dietary sodium and cardiovascular outcomes as well as study of likely pathogenic mechanisms linking sodium restriction and cardiovascular events.

Reducing sodium intake has a variety of effects, including activation of neurohormonal systems, that have the potential to adversely influence cardiovascular outcomes. For example, as previously discussed, plasma renin and aldosterone levels are increased in a dose-dependent fashion in response to sodium restriction in both hypertensive and normotensive subjects.[25, 42–45] Elevated plasma renin activity (PRA) has been put forward as an independent risk factor for cardiovascular disease events (both myocardial infarction and stroke), based on a longitudinal study of 219 untreated patients with moderate to severe hypertension.[24] Over a 5-year period of observation, patients with normal or high PRA had an 11% and a 14% incidence of myocardial infarction or stroke, respectively, whereas patients with low PRA had zero events. Subsequent studies showed that patients with low renin had better preservation of renal function than did those with normal or high PRA, despite comparable or greater severity and duration of hypertension.[46] Interestingly, the young black patients in this group, who tended to have more severe hypertension with vascular sequelae, generally fell into the high/medium renin group, whereas older blacks tended to have milder disease and low renin levels.[46]

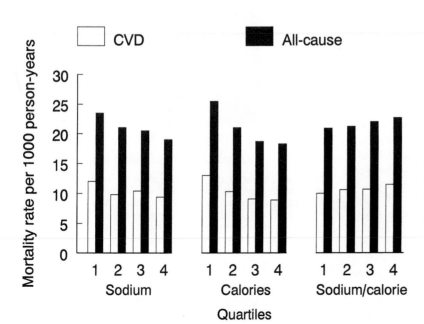

Figure 47–20. All-cause and cardiovascular disease (CVD) mortality rates per 1000 person-years according to quartile of daily sodium intake, total calorie intake, and sodium per calorie intake (adjusted for age and sex). (From Alderman MH, Cohen H, Madhavan S. Dietary sodium intake and mortality: The National Health and Nutrition Examination Survey [NHANES I]. Lancet 351[9105]:781–785, 1998.)

A more recent study from the same group, in which 1717 patients with mild hypertension were followed for 8 years, confirmed that baseline PRA is highly predictive of myocardial infarction.[25] PRA was an independent predictor of myocardial infarction in both sexes and races: in patients with concomitant diabetes, hypercholesterolemia, smoking, or all three, the myocardial infarction rate of high-renin patients was 3.2-fold higher than that of low-renin patients; in those without other risk factors, the risk was increased 7-fold (Fig. 47–21). This strong positive relationship between PRA and cardiovascular risk has not been reproduced by other groups, and no association between PRA and myocardial infarction or sudden cardiac death was seen in one careful study of normotensive men.[47] Nevertheless, the dramatic beneficial effects of the angiotensin-converting enzyme (ACE) inhibitors and perhaps angiotensin II receptor blockers in patients with myocardial infarction accompanied by systolic dysfunction, congestive heart failure, and diabetes with proteinuria provide powerful indirect evidence that angiotensin II has toxic effects on the heart and vasculature.[48–50] It has been hypothesized that the increases in PRA and angiotensin II levels that occur during dietary salt restriction and diuretic use may offset the blood pressure lowering effects of these interventions and increase cardiovascular risk, accounting for the less-than-predicted prevention of myocardial infarction by diuretics in clinical trials. Comparisons of diuretics with ACE inhibitors and angiotensin II receptor blockers in ongoing clinical trials (see Chap. 35, Characteristics of Published, Ongoing, and Planned Outcome Trials in Hypertension) will help to settle this question.

Additional mechanisms have been put forward to account for adverse effects of dietary sodium reduction, including activation of the sympathetic nervous system, as evidenced by elevations in plasma norepinephrine concentration.[23, 51] Elevated night-time plasma norepinephrine levels have been associated with sleep disturbances in human subjects on a sodium-restricted diet.[52] Increases in low-density lipoprotein cholesterol unaccompanied by increments in high-density lipoprotein cholesterol have been reported in a meta-analysis of studies of dietary sodium reduction and blood pressure[23] as well as in individual trials of salt restriction.[53–56] Salt-restricted diets may also be deficient in nutrients such as potassium, calcium, and vitamins that are necessary for good health and may be beneficial in lowering blood pressure and reducing other cardiovascular risk factors.[19, 33] Hemoconcentration associated with salt restriction has also been adduced as a risk factor for subsequent cardiovascular events because of consequent increases in blood viscosity, concentrations of clotting factors, and lipid levels. Finally, circulating insulin levels increase in the setting of dietary sodium restriction,[56, 57] and fasting plasma insulin levels have been correlated with subsequent cardiovascular events.[58] Although they have been dismissed by some as consequences of severe sodium restriction that are seldom achieved and almost never sustained in clinical practice, further study is needed to determine whether these counter-regulatory mechanisms are expressed at more modest levels of sodium reduction and attenuate the favorable effects of sodium reduction on blood pressure and cardiovascular outcomes.

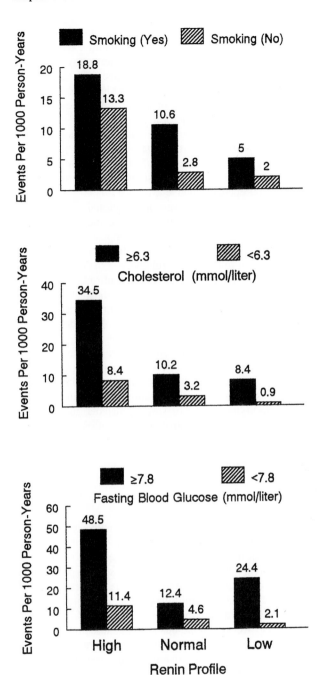

Figure 47–21. Bar graphs show incidence of cardiovascular events according to plasma renin status in hypertensive patients with concomitant risk factors. (From Alderman MH, Madhavan S, Ooi WL, et al. Association of the renin-sodium profile with the risk of myocardial infarction in patients with hypertension. N Engl J Med 324:1098–1104, 1991. Copyright © 1991 Massachusetts Medical Society.)

Recommendations

Based on the small but consistent effects on blood pressure that have been observed in clinical trials of dietary sodium reduction in hypertensive patients, particularly older patients, blacks, and women, avoidance of excessive sodium intake is recommended for all hypertensives. Additional benefits of sodium reduction include reduced diuretic-induced hypokalemia and greater ease of blood pressure control with diuretic therapy, protection from osteoporosis and fractures by reducing urinary calcium excretion, and favorable effects on left ventricular hypertrophy. A number of agencies have codified this recommendation as a reduction in daily consumption of sodium chloride to 6 g or less and of sodium to 2400 mg or less.[59–61] Whether this level of sodium reduction is helpful for the general population in preventing hypertension and related cardiovascular morbidity and mortality is a matter of debate, particularly considering the minimal effect of dietary sodium reduction on blood pressure in normotensives and the possibility of as yet unappreciated adverse effects.

The findings in two large observational studies of increased risk of heart attack and all-cause and cardiovascular disease mortality in persons who appeared to have restricted their sodium intake raises the possibility that sodium reduction may be harmful under some circumstances. These observations have not been confirmed in multiple cohorts or in prospective, controlled trials, and therefore do not justify modifying dietary recommendations for hypertensive patients or the public at large. They do, however, point to a need for further systematic study of possible adverse effects of sodium restriction on the cardiovascular system. Further, the impressive results of the DASH diet rich in fruits, vegetables, and low-fat dairy food in lowering blood pressure in hypertensive subjects may diminish the role of modifying intake of single nutrients, including sodium, in hypertension control and prevention.

POTASSIUM REPLETION

Observational Studies

Dietary potassium has been associated with blood pressure reductions since the time of Addison, who observed that adding potassium salt to the diet generally resulted in a reduction in blood pressure, whereas sodium salt usually produced an increase in pressure.[62] A subsequent study carried out in diabetic children showed that potassium salts lowered blood pressure even in the presence of high dietary salt intake.[63] Results of studies such as these and preclinical data in the rat demonstrated a clear inverse relationship between the effects of potassium and sodium on blood pressure: in essence, potassium protected against the adverse effects of a high-salt diet.[64] Subsequent population studies demonstrated an inverse relationship between potassium intake and blood pressure.[65–71] In some studies, potassium intake was more strongly correlated with blood pressure than any other dietary factor.[71] In the Evans County, Georgia, study, hypertension was more strongly associated with lower potassium intake in black adults than in white adults with similar sodium intakes.[72]

An inverse relationship between urinary potassium excretion and blood pressure has not been universally observed, however. For example, the Framingham study showed no such relationship.[73] In part, this may be related to concomitant consumption of sodium in the population under study, as there is strong evidence that the effect of potassium on blood pressure is influenced by sodium. The urinary sodium:potassium ratio is more strongly correlated with blood pressure than either sodium or potassium excre-

tion alone.[11, 74–76] The negative relationship between potassium intake and blood pressure is more sharply defined for hypertensives than normotensives and for persons with a family history of hypertension than for those without such a history.[77]

Importantly, an inverse relationship between potassium intake and cardiovascular events has also been observed. Several studies have shown that black men, women, and children in the United States consume considerably less potassium than do whites and have related this dietary pattern to an increased prevalence of hypertension and to hypertensive target organ damage, particularly stroke and renal failure, in blacks. Dietary potassium, estimated by 24-hour dietary recall at baseline, has been observed to be inversely related to death from stroke on 12-year follow-up in a cohort of 859 men and women aged 50 to 79 years living in southern California.[78] More recently, the Health Professionals Follow-up Study demonstrated a substantial reduction in the risk of stroke for men in the highest quintile of potassium intake (median, 4.3 g/day) compared to those in the lowest quintile (median 2.4 g/day) (RR 0.62; 95% CI 0.43 to 0.88).[79] In this large study, 43,738 U.S. men aged 40 to 75, without diagnosed cardiovascular disease or diabetes, were followed for 8 years, during which time 328 strokes (210 ischemic, 70 hemorrhagic, 48 unspecified) were documented. Intake of potassium and other nutrients was assessed using a food frequency questionnaire that also queried use of vitamin and mineral supplements. High potassium intakes were associated with reduced risk of ischemic but not of hemorrhagic stroke only in those participants who had a history of hypertension (Fig. 47–22). This was true whether potassium intake was derived from food sources or supplements. History of hypertension was a strong independent risk factor for stroke (RR 2.28; 95% CI 2.1 to 3.7) and was associated with the use of potassium supplements. For men taking diuretics, alone or in combination with other antihypertensive drugs, at baseline, RR of stroke for users of potassium supplements compared to nonusers was 0.36 (95% CI 0.18 to 0.72; $p = .004$). Intakes of magnesium and cereal fiber were also inversely related to stroke risk; calcium and sodium intakes were unrelated.

The authors postulated that biological mechanisms other than blood pressure lowering must have contributed to the large protective effect of potassium in this study, as results of controlled clinical trials have revealed significant but modest effects of increased potassium intake on blood pressure (vide infra). Men in the highest quintile of potassium intake had more health-promoting, disease-preventing behaviors (less smoking, lower alcohol and fat intake, more physical activity, and higher intakes of protein, magnesium, calcium, and fiber) than those in the lowest quintile, but adjustment for these covariants did not alter the association between potassium intake and risk of stroke. Interestingly, there was no difference in sodium intake between these groups. Preclinical studies have suggested that potassium may protect against vascular disease and events by inhibiting free-radical formation,[80] vascular smooth muscle cell proliferation,[81] and arterial thrombosis,[82] but the relevance of these observations to humans is uncertain. It is conceivable that high potassium intake increased serum potassium levels in some of these subjects, thereby reducing the risk

No History of Hypertension

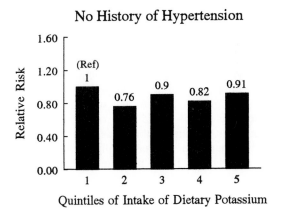

No History of Hypertension

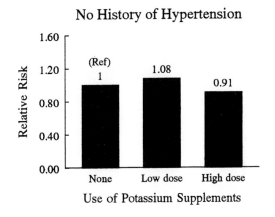

History of Hypertension

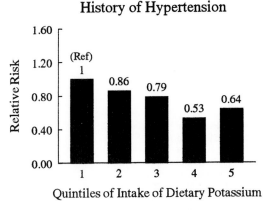

History of Hypertension

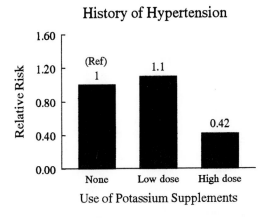

Figure 47–22. *Left panels:* Multivariate relative risk of total stroke according to intake of dietary potassium. *Top:* Men with no history of hypertension. *Bottom:* Men with history of hypertension. *Right panels:* Multivariate relative risk of total stroke according to intake of potassium supplements. *Top:* Men with no history of hypertension. *Bottom:* Men with history of hypertension. (From Ascherio A, Rimm EB, Hernan MA, et al. Intake of potassium, magnesium, calcium, and fiber and risk of stroke among U.S. men. Circulation 98:1198–1204, 1998.)

of hypokalemia, particularly in those on diuretic treatment. Hypokalemia induced by diuretics has been shown to increase the risk of ventricular dysrhythmia.[83, 84]

Interventional Studies

A recent meta-analysis of randomized, controlled clinical trials reviewed the effects of oral potassium supplementation on blood pressure in hypertensive and normotensive human subjects.[85] A total of 2609 participants in 33 randomized, controlled trials were included in the analysis; 21 of the trials were conducted in hypertensive subjects (1560 participants) and 12 in normotensive subjects (1005 participants). Trials were generally of short duration (median 5 weeks, range 4 days to 3 years) and involved potassium administration in doses of 60 or more mmol/day in the form of a pill, usually as a chloride salt. Of the trials, 24 were placebo-controlled; in the remainder, either the control groups were treated with potassium at lower doses than the intervention groups, or both intervention and control groups were maintained on similar diets, with the intervention group receiving potassium supplements concurrently. Average pretreatment urinary potassium excre-

tion ranged from 39 to 79 mmol/day (median 63 mmol/day); only three trials had average baseline potassium excretions less than 50 mmol/day. Average pretreatment sodium excretion ranged from 68 to 196 mmol/day (median 154 mmol/day) and was above 160 mmol/day in 11 trials.

Average net increases in urinary potassium excretion achieved in the intervention group compared to the control group ranged from 0 to 129 mmol/day (median 50 mmol/day). Net change in urinary sodium excretion for intervention vs. control groups ranged from −55 to +44 mmol/day (median 7 mmol/day), whereas mean change in body weight was negligible. The effects of the intervention on systolic and diastolic blood pressure are summarized in Figures 47–23 and 47–24. There was a trend toward a reduction in systolic blood pressure in the intervention group in 26 of 32 trials; this reduction was statistically significant in 11 trials. A similar trend was observed for diastolic blood pressure in 24 of 33 trials, and was statistically significant in 11 of these. Overall pooled estimates of the effect of potassium supplementation on systolic and diastolic blood pressure were significant ($p < .001$) for systolic (−3.1 mm Hg) and diastolic (−2.0 mm Hg) blood pressure even when the outlier trial[86] was excluded. Treatment effects were larger in trials in which the inter-

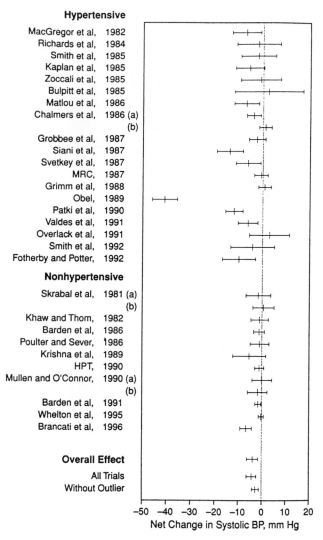

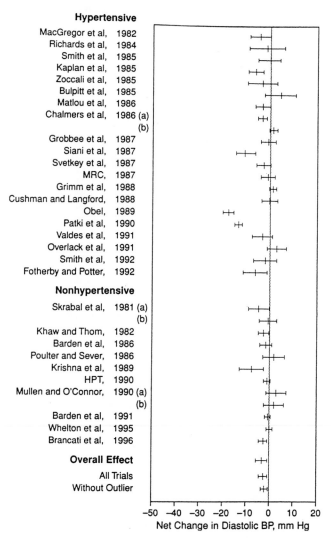

Figure 47–23. Average net change in systolic blood pressure (BP) and corresponding 95% CI after treatment with oral potassium supplementation in 32 randomized controlled trials. Net change was calculated as the difference of the baseline minus follow-up levels of BP for the intervention and control groups (parallel trials) or the difference in BP levels at the end of the intervention and control treatment periods (crossover trials). The overall effect represents a pooled estimate obtained by summing the average net change for each trial, weighted by the inverse of its variance. "All Trials" represents results from all 32 randomized trials; "Without Outlier" represents results after exclusion of an outlier trial.[86] MRC indicates Medical Research Council; HPT, Hypertension Prevention Trial. (From Whelton PK, Jiang H, Cutler JA, et al. Effects of oral potassium on blood pressure. JAMA 277:1624–1632, 1997, Copyright 1997, American Medical Association.)

positive relationship between average 24-hour urinary sodium excretion during follow-up in each trial and corresponding reductions in systolic ($p = .004$) and diastolic ($p = .003$) blood pressure. Treatment effects also appeared to be greater in blacks than in whites, as the effects of intervention on systolic blood pressure were significantly ($p = .03$) greater in the 6 trials with more than 80% black participants than in the 25 trials with more than 80% white participants. A similar trend was seen for diastolic blood pressure, but it was not statistically significant. Sample size and pretreatment blood pressure also contributed to the

Figure 47–24. Average net change in diastolic blood pressure (BP) and corresponding 95% CI after treatment with oral potassium supplementation in 33 randomized controlled trials. Net change was calculated as the difference of the baseline minus follow-up levels of BP for the intervention and control groups (parallel trials) or the difference in BP levels at the end of the intervention and control treatment periods (crossover trials). The overall effect represents a pooled estimate obtained by summing the average net change for each trial, weighted by the inverse of its variance. "All Trials" represents results from all 33 randomized trials; "Without Outlier" represents results after exclusion of an outlier trial.[86] MRC indicates Medical Research Council; HPT, Hypertension Prevention Trial. (From Whelton PK, Jiang H, Cutler JA, et al. Effects of oral potassium on blood pressure. JAMA 277:1624–1632, 1997, Copyright 1997, American Medical Association.)

vention succeeded in reducing urinary potassium excretion by 20 mmol/day or more and in which no antihypertensive medications were administered.

As indicated in Figures 47-23 and 47-24, there was significant variation across trials in the estimate of intervention-related average net change in blood pressure. A number of factors that contributed to this variation were identified. Most importantly, reductions in blood pressure tended to be greater in trials in which average urinary sodium excretion was higher during follow-up (Fig. 47–25). Linear regression analysis identified a significant, independent

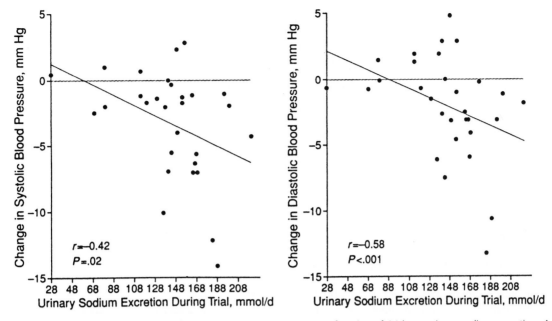

Figure 47–25. Net change in systolic and diastolic blood pressure as a function of 24-hour urinary sodium excretion. A significant inverse relationship was identified for both systolic ($p = .02$) and diastolic ($p < .001$) blood pressure. (From Whelton PK, Jiang H, Cutler JA, et al. Effects of oral potassium on blood pressure. JAMA 277:1624–1632, 1997, Copyright 1997, American Medical Association.)

variability in effect size of the intervention: there was a significant inverse relationship between sample size and treatment effect on systolic ($p < .001$) and diastolic ($p = .05$) blood pressure and a significant direct relationship between pretreatment diastolic blood pressure and treatment effect size for systolic blood pressure ($p = .02$). Interestingly, there was no relationship between study duration or treatment-related change in urinary potassium excretion and treatment effects on systolic or diastolic blood pressure. Further, the treatment effect was not significantly greater in hypertensive than in normotensive subjects.

Results of this meta-analysis confirmed previous findings from both observational and interventional studies that the ratio of urinary sodium:potassium excretion is more closely related to blood pressure than to either parameter individually.[69] There was no overall association between 24-hour urinary potassium excretion and blood pressure in this analysis, but a significant dose-response relationship between potassium and blood pressure emerged at higher levels of 24-hour urinary sodium excretion. Thus, potassium supplementation appears to be more effective in lowering blood pressure in persons with high sodium intake. This interpretation is consistent with the negative results of one large (287 participants) 2-year potassium supplementation trial that was cited by the authors but not included in the meta-analysis.[87] In this study, subjects were placed on a sodium-reduced diet concurrently with the potassium supplementation. The former intervention may have attenuated the effect of the latter.

An additional source of variability in blood pressure response to oral potassium supplementation is pretreatment potassium intake. As pointed out by Sacks and colleagues, a subset of the population that has a low intake of potassium and other minerals may be particularly responsive to supplementation.[88] Because most interventional trials have tested the effect of raising an average intake to a high

intake, such trials might tend to underestimate the true effect of potassium on blood pressure in the population. Accordingly, Sacks and colleagues tested the effects of potassium supplementation on blood pressure in 300 normotensive women in the Nurses Health Study II whose reported intake of potassium was between the 10th and 15th percentiles (62 ± 20 mmol/day).[88] Participants received potassium supplementation in the form of potassium chloride tablets (K-Dur 20 mmol b.i.d.) or placebo for 16 weeks. This dose was intended to raise potassium intake above the 90th percentile, as determined in the Nurses Health Study I.[89] Average sodium excretion was 135 mmol/day. Compared to the placebo group, both systolic and diastolic blood pressures (assessed as mean 24-hour ambulatory pressure) decreased significantly from baseline in the potassium group (-2.0 mm Hg, 95% CI -3.7 to -0.3 and -1.7 mm Hg, 95% CI -3.0 to -0.4, respectively). This decrease in blood pressure was fairly uniform throughout the 24 hours of monitoring, and the expected diurnal variation in blood pressure was preserved in the potassium-treated subjects. The authors contrasted their results with previous reports of minimal blood pressure effects of potassium supplementation, even at higher doses than used in their study, in normotensive persons who were not selected for low baseline potassium intake.[87, 90, 91] Taken together, these studies suggest that dietary potassium plays a role in blood pressure regulation in normotensive individuals with low levels of basal intake as well as in hypertensive individuals.

Recommendations

Maintenance of adequate potassium intake (> 100 mmol/day), preferably from dietary sources, is recommended for hypertensive persons and for those with high normal blood pressure. A diet rich in fruits and vegetables (the DASH diet) is superior to taking pills or other supplements as a potassium source, as these foods contain other nutrients, such as calcium, magnesium, and vitamins, which may also have beneficial effects on blood pressure. Further, it is clear that potassium supplements can be harmful.[92] Potassium supplements should be avoided or used only with extreme caution in patients with renal insufficiency, in diabetics, and in those receiving potassium-sparing diuretics, ACE inhibitors, or angiotensin II receptor blockers. Hypokalemia, whether caused by diuretic use or poor dietary intake, should be treated, particularly in patients receiving digoxin and those with known coronary artery disease, because it predisposes patients to arrhythmia.

CALCIUM REPLETION

Preclinical and Observational Studies

Studies in spontaneously hypertensive rats (SHRs) have generally shown that dietary calcium supplementation can prevent the development of hypertension, particularly salt-sensitive hypertension.[93, 94] Mechanisms that have been proposed to account for observed effects of dietary calcium on blood pressure include suppression of endogenous parathyroid hormone levels that are elevated due to a defect in calcium metabolism associated with calciuria; direct effects on vascular smooth muscle, calcium-regulating, and calcium-sensitive hormones; interactions between calcium and sodium-potassium transport; and increased appetite for sodium when calcium intake is low.[95, 96]

Reports that "hard" drinking water (containing calcium) was associated with reduced prevalence of cardiovascular disease provided indirect evidence for an association between dietary calcium and blood pressure.[97] This was supported by observations from the Puerto Rico Heart Health Program that individuals who drank no milk had twice the prevalence of hypertension as those who consumed a quart of milk or more per day.[98] An analysis of data from 5050 adults in southern California surveyed for heart disease risk factors as part of a Lipid Research Clinics population study indicated that hypertensive men, but not hypertensive women, had a significantly lower intake of calcium from milk than normotensive individuals.[99] In men, diastolic blood pressure decreased significantly with increasing milk consumption. Most of the subsequent observational studies that related dietary calcium to blood pressure found an inverse association between intake of calcium or calcium-rich foods and blood pressure or prevalence/incidence of hypertension.[100]

An analysis of the National Health and Nutrition Examination Survey I (NHANES I) data found an inverse association between dietary calcium and blood pressure: the higher blood pressures occurred at very low levels of calcium intake (300 to 600 mg/day) (Fig. 47–26).[101] Subsequent analyses of NHANES I and II data identified an inverse relationship between dietary calcium and blood pressure only among black males in NHANES I.[102] Other studies have failed to reveal such a relationship[103] and have identified methodological problems that complicate interpretation of these observational findings,[104] principally because of the strong correlations between dietary intakes

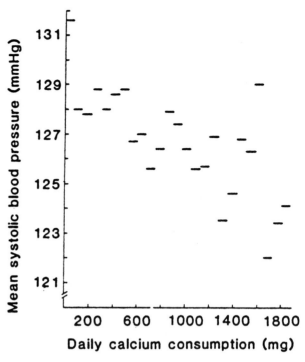

Figure 47–26. Daily intake of calcium versus systolic blood pressure for the entire cohort (National Health and Nutrition Examination Survey I). (Reprinted with permission from McCarron DA, Morris CD, Henry HJ, Stanton JL. Blood pressure and nutrient intake in the United States. Science 224:1392–1398, 1984. Copyright 1984, American Association for the Advancement of Science.)

of calcium and other nutrients that are thought to affect blood pressure, including potassium and magnesium. In contrast, the Nurses' Health Study, which employed a prospective design, suggested a significantly lower risk (RR 0.78) for self-reported hypertension associated with a dietary calcium intake of 800 mg/day compared to an intake of 400 mg/day.[105]

Similarly, the published literature describing the relationship between calcium intake and cardiovascular disease outcomes lacks consistency. The Health Professionals Follow-Up Study, which followed a cohort of 43,738 U.S. men 40 to 75 years old for 8 years found no relationship between calcium intake, assessed by a food frequency questionnaire, and stroke incidence.[79] The lack of association between calcium intake and stroke was present whether calcium was ingested as dairy foods or as supplements. These results contrast with previous findings of an inverse association between calcium intake from dairy sources and risk of stroke in middle-aged men in Honolulu[106] and subsequent findings of an inverse association between dietary calcium (RR for highest vs. lowest quartiles of total calcium intake was 0.67) and ischemic heart disease mortality in postmenopausal Iowa women.[107] In the latter study, vitamin D and dairy products were not associated with reduced risk.

Interventional Studies

Two recent meta-analyses of controlled clinical trials have shown that calcium supplementation (1000 to 2000 mg/

day) results in small but significant reductions in systolic but not diastolic blood pressure.[108, 109] A meta-analysis of 33 trials involving a total of 2412 participants showed an overall reduction in systolic blood pressure of 1.27 mm Hg (95% CI 2.25 to 0.29 mm Hg; $p = .01$) and diastolic blood pressure of 0.24 mm Hg (95% CI 0.92 to 0.44 mm Hg; $p = .49$).[108] Most trials were relatively brief (4 to 14 weeks in duration); only 5 had an intervention period of more than 6 months. Calcium was administered in pill form in most trials; only 7 used dietary interventions. In the 6 trials that classified participants as normotensive or hypertensive, there were differences in treatment effect between groups: in hypertensive patients, calcium supplementation was associated with a mean reduction in systolic blood pressure of 4.30 mm Hg (95% CI 6.47 to 2.13 mm Hg; $p < .001$) and in diastolic blood pressure of 1.50 mm Hg (95% CI 2.77 to 0.23 mm Hg; $p = .02$). For normotensive participants, mean reductions in systolic blood pressure were 0.27 mm Hg (not significant) and in diastolic blood pressure, 0.33 mm Hg (not significant). The authors did not interpret these results as evidence of a greater effect of calcium in hypertensive than in normotensive populations, however, because of problems with arbitrary and inconsistent definitions of hypertension and because there was no relationship across studies between initial blood pressure and blood pressure reduction due to calcium supplementation. They did not exclude the possibility that there may be subgroups of hypertensive patients (e.g., salt-sensitive hypertensives) that have exaggerated blood pressure responses to dietary calcium.[110, 111] Because of the absence of an effect on diastolic blood pressure and the uncertainty of the long-term impact of the intervention, the authors did not support the general use of calcium supplementation in the treatment of hypertensive patients but suggested that this therapy might be more useful in subjects (both normotensive and hypertensive) with inadequate baseline calcium intake and recommended that future interventional trials focus on this group.

A subsequent study tested the hypothesis that persons with low habitual intake might have particularly robust blood pressure responses to calcium supplementation.[88] In this study, 300 normotensive women in the Nurses Health Study whose reported intake of calcium was between the 10th and 15th percentiles for the population received supplementary calcium (30 mmol, 1200 mg) or placebo for 16 weeks. Mean dietary intake of calcium at baseline was 638 plus or minus 265 mg/day. Supplemental calcium in the form of calcium carbonate (Caltrate) 600 mg b.i.d. increased intake above the 90th percentile for the Nurses Health Study I.[105] Blood pressure effects were assessed by recording 24-hour ambulatory blood pressure and calculating the daily means. Changes in systolic and diastolic pressures from baseline in the calcium-supplemented vs. placebo groups were -0.6 (95% CI -2.2 to 1.0 mm Hg) and -0.7 (95% CI -2.0 to 0.6 mm Hg), respectively. Further, when calcium supplementation was added to potassium, the blood pressure lowering effect of potassium was not enhanced. Thus, increasing calcium intake via supplements did not lower blood pressure in normotensive women with low baseline intake, and adding calcium to supplemental potassium did not increase the blood pressure effect seen with potassium supplementation alone.

A second meta-analysis examined data from 26 randomized clinical trials, 13 of which included normotensive persons and 16 hypertensive persons.[109, 112] A total of 1231 participants were studied. Studies ranged from 1 week to 4 years in duration (median 8 weeks); calcium was administered in pill form as calcium carbonate in most trials. Average changes in blood pressure overall were -0.89 mm Hg systolic (95% CI -1.74 to -0.05 mm Hg) and -0.18 mm Hg diastolic (95% CI -0.75 to -0.40 mm Hg). Effect size for systolic blood pressure was slightly greater in hypertensives (mean -1.68 mm Hg; 95% CI -3.18 to -0.18 mm Hg) than in normotensives (mean -0.53 mm Hg; 95% CI -1.56 to $+0.49$ mm Hg). Diastolic blood pressure was not altered significantly in either group. Effect sizes were somewhat larger in older persons and in women. The authors concluded that calcium supplementation (median dose 1 g/day) has only a small and inconsistent effect on blood pressure and should not be recommended for the prevention of hypertension.

This meta-analysis has been criticized on grounds of inappropriate extraction and conversion of data from several studies and use of inappropriate statistical methods. Reanalysis of these studies revealed a stronger negative association between calcium intake and both systolic and diastolic blood pressure: differences in calcium intake of 1 g/day were associated with blood pressure changes of 0.5 to 4.0 mm Hg. The author put forth the caveat that potential confounding effects of age, body mass index, intake of alcohol and other nutrients, particularly sodium, should be considered before accepting any causal linkage between calcium intake and alterations in blood pressure.

Recommendations

Although there is insufficient evidence to recommend high intake of calcium for prevention or treatment of hypertension, calcium deficiency should be avoided.[60] It is important to note that 75 to 90% of adults in the United States fail to consume the recommended daily allowance of calcium (1200 to 1500 mg for adolescents and young adults and pregnant and nursing women; 1000 mg for mature adults younger than 65 years; 1500 mg for adults older than 65 years). Inadequate calcium intake is particularly common in populations that are at high risk for developing hypertension, including the elderly and African Americans.[113] Maintaining the recommended daily allowance for calcium, preferably from food sources, is beneficial for a variety of health reasons, such as preventing osteoporosis. Further, the DASH trial showed that a diet rich in low-fat dairy foods is associated with major reductions in blood pressure in both normotensive and hypertensive persons.[3, 4] The DASH trial was not designed to identify the specific components of the diet that are effective in reducing blood pressure. Nevertheless, it is likely that calcium and vitamin D derived from food sources contributed to the effects of the diet on blood pressure. Increased calcium intake has not been associated with major adverse effects. Although persons with a history of kidney stones may be at risk for recurrence with increased calcium intake, most persons can tolerate calcium intakes as high as 2000 mg/day without adverse effects.[109]

MAGNESIUM REPLETION

Preclinical and Observation Studies

Based in part on the early observation that magnesium salts lower blood pressure in patients,[114] the relationship between magnesium intake and blood pressure as well as cardiovascular morbidity and mortality has been examined. Magnesium is present along with calcium in hard water, and a number of ecological studies have demonstrated an inverse association between water hardness and cardiovascular death rates; between magnesium in tap water and hypertension and hypertensive heart disease mortality; and between water hardness and blood pressure.[100, 115–117] Further, magnesium-deficient rats have been shown to have both higher blood pressures and reduced diameters of microvessels.[118]

Most observational studies have found an inverse relationship between dietary magnesium intake and blood pressure or the development of hypertension.[100, 119–121] Hypertensive subjects have been shown to report lower dietary intake of magnesium than normotensives in cross-sectional studies, and in the prospective Nurses' Health Study, magnesium was the only dietary mineral that was a significant predictor of hypertension.[89] Further, low magnesium intake has been shown to be related to cardiovascular events. The

Health Professionals Follow-Up Study found a reduction in risk of stroke for men in the highest quintile of magnesium intake compared to those in the lowest quintile (RR 0.70; 95% CI 0.49 to 1.01).[79] The inverse relationship between magnesium intake and stroke risk was substantially weakened in regression models that included potassium and dietary fiber, however, because intakes of these nutrients were positively correlated. When participants were stratified by history of hypertension at baseline, an inverse association between magnesium intake and stroke risk was found only among hypertensive men (Fig. 47–27). This was true whether the magnesium was taken in the form of supplements or came from food sources.

As emphasized by Harlan, a major concern with observational studies relating blood pressure and magnesium intake from food sources is the lack of specificity for a nutrient effect.[122] Food is consumed, rather than nutrients, and it is seldom possible to separate the effects of the various nutrients contained in the food or to account for the effects of nutrients not consumed when a particular dietary pattern is followed. Furthermore, magnesium, calcium, and potassium are all abundant in commonly eaten foods such as vegetables, dairy products, cereals, fruits, and nuts. Accordingly, interventional studies using specific nutrient supplements and assessing food and nutrient intake

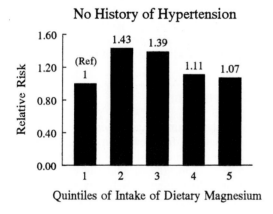

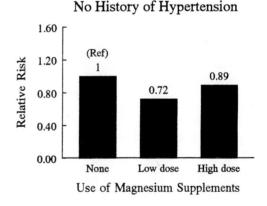

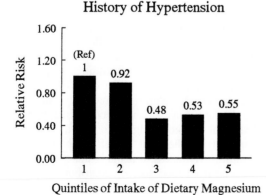

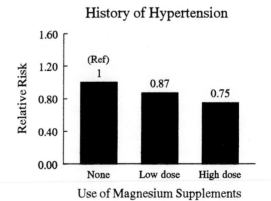

Figure 47–27. *Left panels:* Multivariate relative risk of total stroke according to intake of dietary magnesium. *Top:* Men with no history of hypertension. *Bottom:* Men with history of hypertension. *Right panels:* Multivariate relative risk of total stroke according to intake of magnesium supplements. *Top:* Men with no history of hypertension. *Bottom:* Men with history of hypertension. (From Ascherio A, Rumm EB, Hernan MA, et al. Intake of potassium, magnesium, calcium, and fiber and risk of stroke among U.S. men. Circulation 98:1198–1204, 1998.)

are necessary to assess the relationship between magnesium and blood pressure.

Interventional Studies

Results of controlled clinical trials investigating the effects of magnesium supplementation on blood pressure have been inconsistent, and the effects, when observed, have been modest.[122] Most trials showed downward trends in systolic and diastolic blood pressure with supplemental magnesium, but these reductions were not statistically significant and in many cases were confounded by concomitant use of antihypertensive medications and by a short duration of follow-up. Most of these studies lacked sufficient power to detect small differences in blood pressure. The largest study of the effects of magnesium supplementation on blood pressure was TOHP I, in which a 15 mmol magnesium supplement was given to 227 individuals with diastolic blood pressures between 80 and 89 mm Hg.[27] This treated group was compared with 234 individuals randomized to receive placebo. After 6 months of supplementation, no difference was found in the blood pressures of subjects on magnesium supplementation compared to those on placebo (see Fig. 47–11). Even when subjects deficient in basal magnesium intake have been selected for study, no significant effect of magnesium supplementation on blood pressure has been found in normotensive subjects.[88]

Recommendations

Based on the negative findings of controlled interventional trials and the difficulty in interpreting the association between magnesium intake and blood pressure, increasing magnesium intake from either food sources or supplements for the purpose of hypertension prevention or control cannot be recommended. However, consumption of the recommended daily allowance of approximately 300 mg/day (280 mg for women, 350 mg for men) from food sources is recommended for reasons of general health.

MACRONUTRIENT ALTERATION

A variety of macronutrients, including fiber, fish oils rich in omega-3 fatty acids, garlic, fat, carbohydrate, and protein have been related to blood pressure, based mainly on observations that populations that consume unusually large or small amounts of these nutrients have low blood pressures and a low prevalence of hypertension.[100] Careful observational studies in this area are few and have tended not to confirm the hypothesized relationships between macronutrient intake and blood pressure. Similarly, clinical trial data are sparse. Further study is needed before a judgment can be made regarding the utility of these interventions in the prevention or treatment of hypertension.

References

1. Oparil S. High blood pressure. *In* Goldman L, Bennett JC (eds). Cecil Textbook of Medicine, 21st ed. Philadelphia, WB Saunders, 2000.

2. McCarron DA, Oparil S, Chait A, et al. Nutritional management of cardiovascular risk factors: A randomized clinical trial. Arch Intern Med 175:169–177, 1997.
3. Appel LJ, Moore TJ, Obarzanek E, et al. The effect of dietary patterns on blood pressure: Results from the Dietary Approaches to Stop Hypertension (DASH) clinical trial. N Engl J Med 1336:1117–1124, 1997.
4. Svetkey LP, Simons-Morton D, Vollmer WM, et al. Effects of dietary patterns on blood pressure: Subgroup analysis of the Dietary Approaches to Stop Hypertension (DASH) randomized clinical trial. Arch Intern Med 159:285–293, 1999.
5. The DASH Steering Committee. "More Salt, Please." [Letter] Science 282:1049–1050, 1998.
6. Huang T, Nei C, Su W. The Yellow Emperor's Classic of Internal Medicine. Veith (trans). Baltimore, Williams & Wilkins, 1949.
7. Ambard L, Beaujard D. Causes de l'hypertension artérielle. Arch Gen Med 1:520–533, 1904.
8. Kempner W. Treatment of kidney disease and hypertensive vascular disease with rice diet. N Carolina Med J 5:125–133, 1944.
9. Kempner W. Treatment of hypertensive vascular disease with rice diet. Am J Med 4:545–577, 1948.
10. Dahl L. Salt and hypertension. Am J Clin Nutr 25:231–244, 1972.
11. Gleibermann L. Blood pressure and dietary salt in human populations. Ecol Food Nutr 2:143–156, 1973.
12. INTERSALT Cooperative Research Group. INTERSALT: An international study of electrolyte excretion and blood pressure: Results for 24-hour urinary sodium and potassium excretion. BMJ 297:319–328, 1988.
13. INTERSALT Cooperative Research Group. INTERSALT Study: An international cooperative study on the relation of blood pressure to electrolyte excretion in populations. I: Design and methods. J Hypertens 4:781–787, 1986.
14. Elliott P, Stamler J, Nichols R, et al for the INTERSALT Cooperative Research Group. INTERSALT revisited: Further analyses of 24-hour sodium excretion and blood pressure within and across populations. BMJ 312:1249–1253, 1996.
15. Hanneman RL. INTERSALT: Hypertension rise with age revisited. BMJ 312:1283–1284, 1996.
16. Davey Smith G, Phillips AN. Inflation in epidemiology: "The proof and measurement of association between two things" revisited. BMJ 312:1659–1664, 1996.
17. Smith WCS, Crombie IK, Tavendale RT, et al. Urinary electrolyte excretion, alcohol consumption, and blood pressure in the Scottish Heart Health Study. BMJ 297:329–330, 1988.
18. Tunstall-Pedoe H, Woodward M, Tavendale R, et al. Comparison of the prediction by 27 different factors of coronary heart disease and death in men and women of the Scottish Heart Health Study: Cohort study. BMJ 315:722–729, 1997.
19. Morris CD. Effect of dietary sodium restriction on overall nutrient intake. Am J Clin Nutr 65:687S–691S, 1997.
20. Cutler JA, Follman D, Allender PS. Randomized trials of sodium reduction: An overview. Am J Clin Nutr 65:643S–651S, 1997.
21. Cook NR, Cohen J, Hebert PR, et al. Implications of small reductions in diastolic blood pressure for primary prevention. Arch Intern Med 155:701–709, 1995.
22. Midgley JP, Matthew AG, Greenwood CMT, Logan AG. Effect of reduced dietary sodium on blood pressure: A meta-analysis of randomized controlled trials. JAMA 275:1590–1597, 1996.
23. Graudal NA, Galloe AM, Garred P. Effects of sodium restriction on blood pressure, renin, aldosterone, catecholamines, cholesterol, and triglycerides. JAMA 279:1383–1391.
24. Brunner HR, Laragh JH, Baer L, et al. Essential hypertension: Renin and aldosterone, heart attack and stroke. N Engl J Med 286:441–449, 1972.
25. Alderman MH, Madhavan S, Ooi WL, et al. Association of the renin-sodium profile with the risk of myocardial infarction in patients with hypertension. N Engl J Med 324:1098–1104, 1991.
26. Applegate WB, Borhani NO, Cohen J, et al for the Trials of Hypertension Prevention (TOHP) Collaborative Research Group. Trials of Hypertension Prevention, Phase I design. Ann Epidemiol 1:455–471, 1991.
27. The Trials of Hypertension Prevention Collaborative Research Group. The effects of non-pharmacological interventions on blood pressure of persons with high normal levels: Results of the Trials of Hypertension Prevention (Phase I). JAMA 267:1213–1220, 1992.

28. Hebert PR, Bolt RJ, Borhani NO, et al for the Trials of Hypertension Prevention (TOHP) Collaborative Research Group. Design of a multicenter trial to evaluate long-term lifestyle intervention in adults with high-normal blood pressure levels: Trials of Hypertension Prevention (Phase II). Ann Epidemiol 5:130–139, 1995.

29. The Trials of Hypertension Prevention Collaborative Research Group. Effect of weight loss and sodium reduction intervention on blood pressure and hypertension incidence in overweight people with high-normal blood pressure: The Trials of Hypertension Prevention, Phase II. Arch Intern Med 157:657–667, 1997.

30. Langford HG, Davis BR, Blaufox D, et al for the TAIM Research Group. Effect of drug and diet treatment of mild hypertension on diastolic blood pressure. Hypertension 17:210–217, 1991.

31. Blaufox MD, Lee HB, Davis B, et al. Renin predicts diastolic blood pressure response to nonpharmacologic and pharmacologic therapy. JAMA 267:1221–1225, 1992.

32. Whelton PK, Appel, LJ, Espeland MA, et al for the TONE Collaborative Research Group. Sodium reduction and weight loss in the treatment of hypertension in older persons. A randomized controlled trial of nonpharmacologic interventions in the elderly (TONE). JAMA 279:839–846, 1998.

33. Alderman MH, Madhavan S, Cohen H, et al. Low urinary sodium is associated with greater risk of myocardial infarction among treated hypertensive men. Hypertension 25:1144–1152, 1995.

34. Cook NR, Cutler JA, Hennekens CH. An unexpected result for sodium—causal or casual? [Editorial comment] Hypertension 25:1153–1154, 1995.

35. Jensen OM, Wahrendorf J, Rosenquist A, Geser A. The reliability of questionnaire-derived historical dietary information and temporal stability of food habits in individuals. Am J Epidemiol 120:281–290, 1984.

36. James GD, Sealey JE, Alderman MH, Laragh JH. Year-to-year stability of urine sodium, potassium, aldosterone and PRA in normotensive men and women. Am J Hypertens 6:86A–90A, 1993.

37. Alderman MH, Cohen H, Madhavan S. Dietary sodium intake and mortality: The National Health and Nutrition Examination Survey (NHANES I). Lancet 351:781–785, 1998.

38. Alaimo K, McDowell MA, Briefel RR, et al. Dietary intake of vitamins, minerals, and fiber of persons aged 2 months and over in the United States: Third National Health and Nutrition Examination Survey, Phase 1, 1988–91. Advance Data. Washington, DC, Department of Health and Human Services, 1994; vol 258, pp 1–28.

39. Engelman K. Sodium intake and mortality. [Letter] Lancet 351:1508–1509, 1998.

40. Karppanen H, Mervaala E. Sodium intake and mortality. [Letter] Lancet 351:1508–1509, 1998.

41. de Wardener HE. Salt reduction and cardiovascular risk: The anatomy of a myth. J Hum Hypertens 13:1–4, 1999.

42. Koolen MI, Brummelen P. Sodium sensitivity in essential hypertension: Role of the renin-angiotensin-aldosterone system and the predictive value of an intravenous frusemide test. J Hypertens 2:55–59, 1984.

43. Overlack A, Ruppert M, Kolloch R, et al. Divergent hemodynamic and hormonal responses to varying salt intake in normotensive subjects. Hypertension 22:331–338, 1993.

44. Jula AM, Karanko HM. Effects on left ventricular hypertrophy of long-term nonpharmacological treatment with sodium restriction in mild to moderate essential hypertension. Circulation 89:1023–1031, 1994.

45. Overlack A, Ruppert M, Kolloch R, et al. Age is a major determinant of the divergent blood pressure responses to varying salt intake in essential hypertension. Am J Hypertens 8:829–836, 1995.

46. Brunner HR, Sealey JE, Laragh JH. Renin as a risk factor in essential hypertension: More evidence. Am J Med 55:295–302, 1973.

47. Meade TW, Cooper JA, Peart WS. Plasma renin activity and ischemic heart disease. N Engl J Med 329:616–619, 1983.

48. Pfeffer MA, Braunwald E, Moye LA, et al on behalf of the SAVE Investigators. Effects of captopril on mortality and morbidity in patients with left ventricular dysfunction after myocardial infarction. N Engl J Med 327:669–677, 1992.

49. The SOLVD Investigators. Effect of enalapril on mortality and the development of heart failure in asymptomatic patients with reduced left ventricular ejection fractions. N Engl J Med 327:685–691, 1991.

50. Pitt B, Segal R, Martinez FA, et al on behalf of the ELITE Study Investigators. Randomized trial of losartan versus captopril in patients over 65 with heart failure (Evaluation of Losartan in the Elderly Study, ELITE). Lancet 349:747–752, 1997.

51. Egan BM, Weder AB, Petrin J, Hoffman RG. Neurohumoral and metabolic effects of short-term dietary NaCl restriction in men: Relationship to salt-sensitivity status. Am J Hypertens 4:416–421, 1991.

52. Vitiello MV, Prinz PM, Halter JB. Sodium-restricted diet increases nighttime plasma norepinephrine and impairs sleep patterns in man. J Clin Endocrinol Metab 56:553–556, 1984.

53. Ruppert M, Overlack A, Kolloch R, et al. Effects of severe and moderate salt restriction on serum lipids in nonobese normotensive adults. Am J Med Sci 307 (suppl 1):S87–S90, 1994.

54. Del Rio A, Rodriguez Villamil JL. Metabolic effects of strict salt restriction in essential hypertensive patients. J Intern Med 233:409–414, 1993.

55. Sharma AM, Arntz HR, Kribben A, et al. Dietary sodium restriction: Adverse effects on plasma lipids. Klin Wochenschr 68:664–668, 1990.

56. Ruppert M, Diehl J, Kolloch R, et al. Short-term dietary sodium restriction increases serum lipids and insulin in salt-sensitive and salt-resistant normotensive adults. Klin Wochenschr 69(suppl 25):51–57, 1991.

57. Lind L, Lithell H, Gustafsson IB, et al. Metabolic cardiovascular risk factors and sodium sensitivity in hypertensive subjects. Am J Hypertens 5:502–505, 1992.

58. Ruige JB, Assendelft WJJ, Dekker JM, et al. Insulin and risk of cardiovascular disease: A meta-analysis. Circulation 97:996–1001, 1998.

59. Joint National Committee on Prevention, Detection, Evaluation, and Treatment of High Blood Pressure. The sixth report. Arch Intern Med 157:2413–2446, 1997.

60. Kotchen TA, McCarron DA for the Nutrition Committee. Dietary electrolytes and blood pressure. Circulation 98:613–617, 1998.

61. Oparil S, Calhoun DA. High blood pressure. In Dale DC, Federman DD (eds). Scientific American Medicine, vol 1, sect 1, subsect 3. New York, Scientific American, 1997; pp 1–14.

62. Addison WLT. The use of sodium chloride, potassium chloride, sodium bromide and potassium bromide in cases of arterial hypertension which are amenable to potassium chloride. Can Med Assoc J 18:281–285, 1928.

63. McQuarrie I, Thompson WH, Anderson JA. Effects of excessive ingestion of sodium and potassium salts on carbohydrate metabolism and blood pressure in diabetic children. J Nutr 11:77–101, 1936.

64. Meneely GR, Battarbee HD. Sodium and potassium. Nutr Rev 34:225–235, 1976.

65. Walker WG, Whelton PK, Saito H, et al. Relation between blood pressure and renin, renin substrate, angiotensin II, aldosterone and urinary sodium and potassium in 574 ambulatory subjects. Hypertension 1:287–291, 1979.

66. Lever AF, Beretta-Piccoli C, Brown JJ, et al. Sodium and potassium in essential hypertension. BMJ 283:463–468, 1981.

67. Khaw KT, Rose G. Population study of blood pressure and associated factors in St. Lucia, West Indies. Int J Epidemiol 11:372–377, 1982.

68. Langford HG. Dietary potassium and hypertension: Epidemiologic data. Ann Intern Med 98:770–772, 1983.

69. Dai WS, Kuller LH, Miller G. Arterial blood pressure and urinary electrolytes. J Chron Dis 37:75–84, 1984.

70. Simpson FO. Monovalent and divalent cations in hypertension. Prev Med 14:436–450, 1985.

71. Reed D, McGee D, Yano K, Hankin J. Diet, blood pressure, and multicollinearity. Hypertension 7:405–410, 1985.

72. Grim CE, Luft FC, Miller JZ, et al. Racial differences in blood pressure in Evans County, Georgia: Relationship to sodium and potassium intake and plasma renin activity. J Chron Dis 33:87–94, 1980.

73. Dawber TR, Kannel WB, Kagan A, et al. Environmental factors in hypertension. In Stamler J, Stamler R, Pullman TN (eds). The Epidemiology of Hypertension. Proceedings of an International Symposium. New York, Stratton, 1967; 269–271.

74. McCarron DA, Morris CD, Henry HJ, Stanton JL. Blood pressure and nutrient intake in the United States. Science 224:1392–1398, 1984.

75. Khaw KT, Barrett-Connor E. The association between blood pressure, age, and dietary sodium and potassium: A population study. Circulation 77:53–61, 1988.

76. Morris RC, Sebastian A. Potassium responsive hypertension. *In* Laragh JH, Brenner BM (eds). Hypertension: Pathophysiology, Diagnosis, and Management, 2nd ed. New York, Raven, 1995;2715–2726, 1995.

77. Pietinen PI, Wong O, Altschul AM. Electrolyte output, blood pressure, and family history of hypertension. Am J Clin Nutr 33:87–94, 1979.

78. Khaw KT, Barrett-Connor E. Dietary potassium and stroke-associated mortality: A 12-year prospective study. N Engl J Med 316:235–240, 1987.

79. Ascherio A, Rimm EB, Hernan MA, et al. Intake of potassium, magnesium, calcium, and fiber and risk of stroke among US men. Circulation 98:1198–1204, 1998.

80. McCabe RD, Backarich MA, Srivastava K, Young DB. Potassium inhibits free radical formation. Hypertension 24:77–82, 1994.

81. McCabe RD, Young DB. Potassium inhibits cultured vascular smooth muscle proliferation. Am J Hypertens 7:346–350, 1994.

82. Lin H, Young DB. Interaction between plasma potassium and epinephrine in coronary thrombosis in dogs. Circulation 89:331–338, 1994.

83. Cohen JD, Neaton JD, Prineas RJ, Daniels KA for the Multiple Risk Factor Intervention Trial Research Group. Diuretics, serum potassium and ventricular arrhythmias in the Multiple Risk Factor Intervention Trial. Am J Cardiol 60:548–554, 1987.

84. Tsuji H, Venditti FJ Jr, Evans JC, et al. The associations of levels of serum potassium and magnesium with ventricular premature complexes (the Framingham Heart Study). Am J Cardiol 74:232–235, 1994.

85. Whelton PK, Jiang H, Cutler JA, et al. Effects of oral potassium on blood pressure. JAMA 277:1624–1632, 1997.

86. Obel AO. Placebo-controlled trial of potassium supplements in black patients with mild essential hypertension. J Cardiovasc Pharmacol 14:294–296, 1989.

87. Grimm RH, Neaton JD, Elmer PJ, et al. The influence of oral potassium chloride on blood pressure in hypertensive men on a low-sodium diet. N Engl J Med 322:569–574, 1990.

88. Sacks FM, Willett WC, Smith A, et al. Effect on blood pressure of potassium, calcium, and magnesium in women with low habitual intake. Hypertension 31:131–138, 1998.

89. Witteman JC, Willett WC, Stampfer MJ, et al. A prospective study of nutritional factors and hypertension among U.S. women. Circulation 80:1320–1327, 1989.

90. Miller JZ, Weinberger MH, Christian JC. Blood pressure response to potassium supplementation in normotensive adults and children. Hypertension 10:437–442, 1987.

91. Whelton PK, Buring J, Borhani NO, et al for the Trials of Hypertension Prevention (TOHP) Collaborative Research Group. The effect of potassium supplementation in persons with a high-normal blood pressure: Results from phase I of the Trials of Hypertension Prevention. Ann Epidemiol 5:85–95, 1995.

92. Kassirer JP, Harrington JT. Fending off the potassium pushers. N Engl J Med 312:785–787, 1985.

93. Ayachi S. Increased dietary calcium lowers blood pressure in the spontaneously hypertensive rat. Metabolism 12:1234–1238, 1979.

94. Oparil S, Chen YF, Jin H, et al. Dietary calcium prevents sodium-sensitive hypertension in spontaneously hypertensive rats via sympatholytic and renal effects. Am J Clin Nutr 54:227S–236S, 1991.

95. Hatton DC, McCarron DA. Dietary calcium and blood pressure in experimental models of hypertension: A review. Hypertension 23:513–530, 1994.

96. Hamet P. The evaluation of the scientific evidence for a relationship between calcium and hypertension. J Nutr 125:S311–S400, 1995.

97. Schroeder HA. Relation between mortality from cardiovascular disease and treated water supplies: Variations in states and 163 largest municipalities of the United States. JAMA 172:1902–1908, 1960.

98. Garcia-Palmieri MR, Costas R, Cruz-Vidal M, et al. Milk consumption, calcium intake and decreased hypertension in Puerto Rico: Puerto Rico Heart Health Program Study. Hypertension 6:322–328, 1984.

99. Ackley S, Barrett-Connor E, Juarez L. Dairy products, calcium and blood pressure. Am J Clin Nutr 38:457–461, 1983.

100. National High Blood Pressure Education Program Working Group. National High Blood Pressure Education Program Working Group report on primary prevention of hypertension. Arch Intern Med 153:186–206, 1993.

101. McCarron DA, Morris CD, Henry HJ, et al. Blood pressure and nutrient intake in the United States. Science 224:1392–1398, 1984.

102. Sempos C, Cooper R, Kovar MG. Dietary calcium and blood pressure in National Health and Nutrition Examination Surveys I and II. Hypertension 18:1067–1074, 1986.

103. Osborne CG, McTyre RB, Dudek J, et al. Evidence for the relationship of calcium to blood pressure. Nutr Rev 54:365–381, 1996.

104. Pryer J, Cappuccio FP, Elliott P. Dietary calcium and blood pressure: A review of the observational studies. J Hum Hypertens 9:597–604, 1995.

105. Witteman JCM, Willett WC, Stampfer MJ, et al. A prospective study of nutritional factors and hypertension among U.S. women. Circulation 80:1320–1327, 1989.

106. Abbott RD, Curb D, Rodriguez BL, et al. Effect of dietary calcium and milk consumption on risk of thromboembolic stroke in older middle-aged men: The Honolulu Heart Program. Stroke 27:813–818, 1996.

107. Bostick RM, Kushi LH, Wu Y, et al. Relation of calcium, vitamin D, and dairy food intake to ischemic heart disease mortality among postmenopausal women. Am J Epidemiol 149:151–161, 1999.

108. Bucher HC, Cook RJ, Guyatt GH, et al. Effects of dietary calcium supplementation on blood pressure: A meta-analysis of randomized controlled trials. JAMA 275:1016–1022, 1996.

109. Allender PS, Cutler JA, Follmann D. Dietary calcium and blood pressure: A meta-analysis of randomized clinical trials. Ann Intern Med 124:825–831, 1996.

110. Resnick LM, Muller FB, Laragh JH. Calcium-regulating hormones in essential hypertension: Relation to plasma renin activity and sodium metabolism. Ann Intern Med 105:649–654, 1986.

111. Weinberger MH, Wagner UL, Fineberg NS. The blood pressure effects of calcium supplementation in humans of known sodium responsiveness. Am J Hypertens 6:799–805, 1993.

112. Cappuccio FP, Elliott P, Allender PS, et al. Epidemiologic association between dietary calcium intake and blood pressure: A meta-analysis of published data. Am J Epidemiol 142:935–945, 1995.

113. Institute of Medicine, Food and Nutrition Board. Dietary Reference Intakes for Calcium, Phosphorus, Magnesium, Vitamin D, and Fluoride. Washington, DC, National Academy Press, 1997.

114. Blackfan KD, Hamilton B. Uremia in acute glomerular nephritis: The cause and treatment in children. Boston Med Surg J 193:617–628, 1925.

115. Schroeder HA. Municipal drinking water and cardiovascular disease death rates. JAMA 195:125–129, 1966.

116. Masironi R. Cardiovascular mortality in relation to radioactivity and hardness of local water supplies in the USA. Bull WHO 43:687–697, 1970.

117. Stitt FW, Clayton DG, Crawford MD, et al. Clinical and biochemical indicators of cardiovascular disease among men living in hard and soft water areas. Lancet 1:122–126, 1973.

118. Altura BM, Altura BT, Gebrewold A, et al. Magnesium deficiency and hypertension: Correlation between magnesium deficient diets and microcirculatory changes in situ. Science 223:1315–1317, 1984.

119. McCarron DA. Calcium and magnesium nutrition in human hypertension. Ann Intern Med 198:800–805, 1983.

120. Joffres MR, Reed DM, Yano K. Relationship of magnesium intake and other dietary factors to blood pressure: The Honolulu Heart Study. Am J Clin Nutr 45:469–475, 1987.

121. Whelton PK, Klag MJ. Magnesium and blood pressure: Review of the epidemiologic and clinical trial experience. Am J Cardiol 63:26G–30G, 1989.

122. Harlan WR, Harlan LC. Blood pressure and calcium and magnesium intake. *In* Laragh JH, Brenner BM (eds). Hypertension: Pathophysiology, Diagnosis, and Management, 2nd ed. New York, Raven, 1995;1143–1154.

Diet—Calories

Karen C. McCowen, Samuel Chan, and
George L. Blackburn

CHAPTER 48

Hypertension is a major public health problem, affecting 50 million Americans.[1] Although most hypertension is labeled *essential*, a myriad of epidemiological and cross-sectional data implicates obesity and simply being overweight in the development of elevated blood pressure. The high prevalence of obesity in Western societies, a 20th-century phenomenon, likely relates to both reduction in physical activity and ingestion of excess calories, since it has developed too abruptly to result from evolutionary changes. Although obesity, defined as a body mass index (BMI) greater than 30 kg/m², is present in 22.3% of U.S. adults, a full 55% are overweight (BMI > 25 kg/m²).[2] In addition to being high in calories, American and European diets are usually rich in sodium and typically low in fiber, phytochemicals, calcium and other minerals, and vitamins. It has been difficult to determine whether caloric excess, calories specifically from a particular form of fat or carbohydrate, and/or a deficiency in one or more micronutrients is/are the mechanism(s) responsible for blood pressure rising in parallel with weight gain.

This chapter presents evidence from studies that have examined the effects of changing caloric intake, weight loss, and substitution of calories from one food group for another on blood pressure. Specific micronutrient effects are considered in Chapter 47, Diet—Micronutrients—Special Foods. Studies of dietary manipulations in laboratory animals have usually shown effective blood pressure lowering with reductions in calories, fat, and sodium. Such work, although mechanistically interesting, may be of little relevance to the human problem of dietary change. As will be seen, long-term maintenance of weight loss is a difficult challenge for most people.

Weight-reducing diets as a therapy for hypertension in overweight persons, whatever the efficacy in blood pressure reduction, are likely to effect many significant health gains, such as reduction in incidence of impaired glucose tolerance; improved lipid profile; decreased degenerative joint disease, depression, and sleep apnea; and increased self-esteem, exercise tolerance, and quality of life. These additional benefits are unlikely to be seen in persons whose antihypertensive regimen consists entirely of medications, which may exacerbate lipid and glucose problems.

HYPERTENSION AND BODY WEIGHT: THE CONNECTION

The cause of the link between excess body weight and elevation in blood pressure has not been completely explained. Across the spectrum of epidemiological studies, this relationship is consistent. In the Framingham cohort, obese participants had twice the prevalence of hypertension of nonobese.[3, 4] The Intersalt cross-sectional study showed a direct correlation between BMI and blood pressure.[5] Some have questioned this simplistic relationship and put forward evidence that visceral fat, or its surrogate marker waist:hip ratio, has a closer correlation with blood pressure than BMI. In this way, hypertension is part of the metabolic syndrome (formerly known as *Syndrome X*) of insulin resistance, diabetes/impaired glucose tolerance, obesity, and dyslipidemia. The role of diet and obesity in the development of hypertension is more fully discussed in the earlier chapters on pathophysiology.

Increased understanding of the mechanism(s) by which blood pressure falls with weight reduction and is elevated in obesity might lead to the development of more specific targeting of dietary changes that would likely prove more acceptable to the population at risk. With our current "shotgun" approach of "low calorie/low salt" and reduction in various other constituents (total or saturated fat) or supplements of calcium, potassium, fiber, or fish oil, palatability of the diet is often low. Compliance with any dietary regime declines with time, and as lost weight is regained, valuable blood pressure–lowering effects are obliterated.

One pathophysiological explanation for the association between blood pressure and obesity may be hyperinsulinemia.[6] Skeletal muscle resistance to the action of insulin is present in obesity. In order to maintain normal glucose homeostasis, a compensatory elevation in circulating insulin concentrations occurs. Fasting and postprandial hyperinsulinemia are well described in the obese. Insulin may elevate blood pressure by effecting renal sodium retention and by activating the sympathetic nervous system, raising peripheral resistance and thus blood pressure. Cross-sectional studies demonstrate that circulating insulin concentrations correlate with blood pressure. If insulin levels can be lowered and insulin sensitivity enhanced by weight loss, this may represent a mechanism of blood pressure lowering.

THE EFFECT OF WEIGHT LOSS ON BLOOD PRESSURE CONTROL

Pharmacological therapy for mild hypertension is generally more efficacious than lifestyle intervention in lowering blood pressures, but these beneficial effects on blood pressure have not been translated into reductions in coronary heart disease morbidity and mortality. It has been proposed that some of the adverse effects of various antihypertensive medications, such as deleterious effects on serum lipids and insulin sensitivity, may negate some of the beneficial blood pressure effects on overall morbidity and mortality. Thus, blood pressure lowering through lifestyle changes without the use of such drugs is a vital research topic. Exercise, considered in Chapter 50, Exercise and Hypertension, has been compared with diet in a three-way randomized trial of diet, exercise, or the two combined over 12 weeks.[7] All three methods reduced blood pressure equally, without additive effects.

A number of intervention trials have focused on caloric restriction and consequent weight loss as a treatment for blood pressure. Information is available from as early as 1 to 2 weeks after the initiation of such diets to 4 years of follow-up. Many of these studies attempted to dissect the impact of sodium restriction from the effect of the weight loss on blood pressure. Some of the more recent and important of these are discussed later; the literature before the mid-1980s was reviewed by Haynes in an earlier publication.[8]

In the Trials of Hypertension Prevention (TOHP) multicenter study, 2250 overweight (BMI 24 to 37) men and women with high-normal diastolic blood pressure were randomized to sodium restriction, weight loss, the two interventions combined, or "usual care" and followed for 4 years (Table 48–1).[9] Although those randomized to weight loss lost an average of 5 kg in the early months, by 36 months they were only − 2 kg, although this was significantly different from controls. As the weight crept back on, early reductions in both systolic and diastolic blood pressure were not sustained. Weight loss to this degree lowered mean diastolic blood pressure by 0.9 mm Hg, systolic by 1.3 mm Hg. The incidence of hypertension was significantly reduced by all interventions at the 4-year mark. One very important result was that the addition of sodium restriction to the weight loss program did not effect any additional gain in blood pressure reduction, a recurrent theme among these trials.

A study of similar duration (Hypertension Control Program [HCP]) enrolled hypertensive patients ($n = 189$) already on drug therapy.[10] Entry criteria required being between 10 and 50% overweight and/or having high dietary sodium intake. Participants were randomized to three groups:

1. Stop antihypertensive drug, lifestyle modification (weight loss plus salt and alcohol reduction).
2. Stop antihypertensive drug, no lifestyle changes.
3. Continue antihypertensive drug.

Medications were reinitiated only as required for elevated diastolic blood pressures. Those given dietary advice had lost an average of 4 lb at 4 years, whereas controls gained 4 to 5 lb. Group 1 had a decreased need to restart antihypertensive drugs compared with group 2 (39% vs. 5% re-

mained medication-free) and had positive effects on lipids and blood sugar (see Table 48–1); group 3, remaining on pharmacotherapy, had the lowest blood pressures.

In a 3-year intervention study (Hypertension Prevention Trial [HPT]) involving 841 healthy people with high-normal blood pressure, those randomized to caloric reduction and weight loss had significant sustained positive effects on both systolic (− 2.4 mm Hg vs. controls) and diastolic (− 1.8 mm Hg) blood pressure (see Table 48–1).[11] This occurred despite only a modest weight loss (− 1.6 kg), although controls gained 1.8 kg. Some participants were randomized to reduce sodium or increase potassium intake, but neither of these had important effects on blood pressure. Interestingly, the group using weight loss plus salt restriction had less blood pressure reduction than the weight loss alone group, possibly signaling that a simple approach is more likely to have lasting effects because of problems with compliance. An alternative explanation is that weight loss is the more important effect and that coincident salt restriction lowers palatability of food to such an extent that noncompliance is increased.

In a multicenter study with follow-up for 1 year (TOMHS), 902 participants (aged 45 to 69 years) with mild diastolic hypertension were randomized to nutritional intervention plus either placebo or one of five antihypertensives (enalapril, doxazosin, chlorthalidone, amlodipine, or acebutolol).[12] A "usual diet" group was not included. The aim of the nutritional intervention was to lower weight (by 10% or to a desirable weight, whichever was lower) and reduce intake of fat, sodium, and alcohol. The weight loss at 1 year was substantial, averaging 4.7 kg, although only 21% achieved their weight loss goal. This was mirrored by blood pressure reductions in all groups, but those given an antihypertensive drug had greater success (systolic blood pressure − 18.6 vs. − 10.6 mm Hg in the "lifestyle modification plus placebo" group, diastolic blood pressure − 12.8 vs − 8.1 mm Hg). Of all of the medications, only chlorthalidone prevented the beneficial changes that were seen for low-density lipoprotein (LDL) and high-density lipoprotein (HDL) cholesterol in the dieters.[13] Diuretic therapy is often associated with a rise in LDL and a fall in HDL, but these were prevented in TOMHS by the concurrent dietary changes.

The Trial of Antihypertensive Interventions and Management (TAIM) study was very similar, enrolling 878 men and women with mild diastolic hypertension, all overweight, between 110 and 160% of ideal (see Table 48–1).[14] This study aimed to discriminate between the possible

Table 48–1 Effect of Weight Loss on Blood Pressure and Incidence of Hypertension Compared With "Usual Diet" Group in Recent Clinical Trials

Reference	Trial Name	Patients (n)	Duration (mo)	Weight Loss vs. Usual Care (kg)	BP Difference From Usual Diet (mm Hg)	Patients Remaining Normotensive vs. Placebo (%)
9	TOHP	2250	48	1.9	1.1 / 1	62% vs. 56%
10	HCP	189	48	1.8	0.6 / 1.5	39% vs. 5%
11	HPT	841	36	3.4	2.4 / 1.8	61.3% vs. 71.8%*
14	TAIM	878	6	4.76	2.8 / 2.5	

Abbreviations: BP, blood pressure; TOHP, Trials of Hypertension Prevention; HCP, Hypertension Control Program; HPT, Hypertension Prevention Trial; TAIM, Trial of Antihypertensive Interventions and Management.
*p = not significant.

beneficial effects of salt reduction/potassium supplementation and caloric restriction. Participants were randomized to receive one of three drugs—placebo, chlorthalidone, or atenolol—and randomized separately to one of three diets: "usual," weight loss, or low sodium/high potassium. With weight loss, blood pressure was lowered more than with either of the other two diets; as expected, either drug was better than placebo. The addition of weight loss to a drug resulted in yet lower blood pressure, −4 mm Hg for the diuretic and −2 mm Hg for the β-blocker. However, among those taking placebo pills, weight loss of more than 4.5 kg reduced blood pressure as effectively as either drug. The sodium/potassium intervention had little effect over usual diet on the outcome.

Another study with all 56 participants (BMI > 26) on a weight loss program compared the effects of either placebo antihypertensive pills or metoprolol.[15] Whereas both treatment groups had lower blood pressure at 6 months, only the weight loss group showed favorable effects on lipids and echocardiographic parameters of ventricular wall thickness. Endpoint of reduction in ventricular mass is of great potential significance, but unfortunately, such parameters have only rarely been the focus of clinical trials of nutrition interventions.

Remarkably, the positive effects of caloric restriction on blood pressure are often seen almost immediately, before weight has been lost. Some workers have seen this as an effect of lower salt intake. The early phase of fasting is associated with a rise in urinary sodium excretion, perhaps because insulin levels are lowered, whereas hyperinsulinemia stimulates renal tubular sodium retention. There has been some concern, therefore, that diets high in carbohydrate, which may promote higher insulin concentrations, might be associated with higher blood pressure. This was examined in a study published in 1986 in which short-term balance studies were performed in normotensive volunteers.[16] Low- and high-carbohydrate diets and their effects on urinary sodium, integrated insulin response, and blood pressure were compared. Energy levels, sodium, and protein were kept constant throughout the 4 weeks of the investigation, and diets were isocaloric by virtue of different amounts of fat. Switching from a low- (13% of calories) to a high- (52%) carbohydrate diet was associated with a transient reduction in urinary sodium that returned to baseline by the second week of the diet. As expected, integrated insulin response was elevated twofold by high-carbohydrate feeding. Despite this, the only significant change in blood pressure was a reduction in diastolic pressure on the high-carbohydrate diet. A limitation of the study is that the subjects were healthy normotensive men, possibly genetically free from traits that lead to elevations in blood pressure under circumstances of dietary differences.

Patients more likely to benefit from dietary intervention are those with features of the metabolic syndrome (essential hypertension, dyslipidemia, type II diabetes, or any combination of these metabolic disorders).[17] In a 10-week trial in such a population, participants were randomized either to self-selected diet or to prepared meals provided by the medical center. In the latter group, calories were reduced in those in whom weight loss was desired. The experimental meal plan provided 17% of calories as fat, 62% as carbohydrate, and 21% as protein, with recommended amounts of sodium, calcium, potassium, saturated fat, cholesterol, fiber, refined sugar, and complex carbohydrates. Most (85%) of the 560 patients were white, with an average age of 54 years. The experimental group had lower-fat and higher-carbohydrate intake than controls and had more pronounced blood pressure reduction, although when corrected for weight loss, the difference in blood pressure between the groups disappeared. Hence, for short-term dietary studies, weight loss via caloric reduction appears to have a more important effect than implementation of correct food choices.

Another study demonstrated the efficacy of a protein-sparing modified fast in obese (BMI > 28) persons.[18] In this rigorous diet, only 750 kcal/day were permitted (45% protein, 35% fat, and 20% carbohydrate), which led to a 47% dropout rate. Average weight loss for the remainder was 17.7 ± 7.9 kg (range 2 to 55.5 kg), mirrored by a significant change in mean arterial pressure (106.8 to 96.1). Surprisingly, there were no differences in urinary sodium between baseline and 6 months. Fasting and 2-hour postprandial blood glucose and insulin levels were substantially lower after weight loss. There have been many studies in persons with morbid obesity who were observed after gastric restrictive surgery. In one, preoperative hypertension resolved after 1 year or more in over 60% of persons, and the extent of blood pressure lowering could be predicted by the amount of weight lost.[19] In another study, there were significant improvements in cardiac function after weight loss with bariatric surgery.[20]

DIETARY FAT AND FISH OIL

Populations with the highest intakes of mono- or polyunsaturated fats have lower blood pressures than populations traditionally eating diets high in saturated fats. There is no easy way to determine whether the dietary fat per se, one of the myriad other dietary variables, or genetic differences are responsible for this phenomenon. A study in rats attempted to determine whether the hypertensive effect of a high-fat diet is caused by obesity.[21] Three isocaloric diets were compared over 10 weeks: two provided 66% of energy as fat, either polyunsaturated fatty acid (PUFA) or saturated (lard); the third provided 12% of energy as fat. The lard-fed but not the PUFA-fed rats became obese, but both fat-fed groups developed hypertension. This study has been difficult to repeat in humans.

Significant interest has been generated in the substitution of fish oils for the traditional long-chain fatty acids in diets. This was first considered because of the observation that the prevalence of hypertension and cardiovascular disease is low in populations in which large quantities of fish are consumed. In experimental animals such as the stroke-prone hypertensive rat, fish oil supplementation of a low-salt diet added further benefits to the antihypertensive effects of enalapril.[22] Some but not all human studies have shown similar benefits, and most of the early work was neither controlled nor blinded. In trials in which greater than 15 g/day of fish oil was given, a definite blood pressure effect was seen, although the incidence of side effects led subsequent authors to examine the use of smaller amounts. Thus far, the trials have used capsules to provide the oil. This may be a less-effective intervention than substituting fish for meat. Consumption of fish is associated with a higher percentage of linolenic acid in cell membranes. In one cross-sectional study published in the mid-1980s, higher linolenic acid content of adipose tissue in men presenting for routine physical examinations was correlated with lower blood pressure.[23] A 1% increase in linolenic acid was associated with a 5-mm Hg reduction in both systolic and diastolic blood pressure.

In one small, nonblinded study of men with mild diastolic hypertension, supplementation of diets with fish oil (15 g/day) was associated with a dramatic fall in blood pressure compared with other mixtures of PUFA common in the American diet or low doses of fish oil.[24] However, comparison of supplements of corn oil with fish oil (9 g/day of either) in a randomized, random-order, crossover blinded study in moderately hypertensive persons over age 60 years demonstrated a fall in blood pressure almost immediately, irrespective of the oil used.[25] This was most likely related to having received dietary advice, or even of regression to the mean. In an uncontrolled study that lasted 4 months and supplied a low dose (3 g/day) of fish oil to 24 hypertensives, ambulatory blood pressure monitoring demonstrated lack of effect on blood pressure.[25] Compliance was confirmed in this negative study by monitoring the effect of the supplement on changes in cell membrane constituents. Another study in slightly younger persons comparing fish oil (9 g/day) with olive oil (9 g/day) supplements in addition to the regular diet did show that fish oil reduced diastolic blood pressure, from 103 to 98 mm Hg, on average.[26] The only clue to the mechanism was that a fall in intracellular calcium was noted. Fish oil may need to be part of a salt-restricted program for its benefits to be fully realized: In a double-blind study of elderly normotensives, the combination of low-sodium diet and fish oil (4.2 g/day) was significantly better than either alone.[27] For diastolic blood pressure, the effect was more than merely additive, as it appeared to be for systolic pressure.

Thus, the evidence that fish oil supplementation lowers blood pressure is confusing and muddled. Similarly, it has been difficult to implicate fat, or a particular species of fat, in promoting hypertension. This is in marked contrast to the consistent benefits of weight loss through caloric restriction on blood pressure seen throughout the literature.

FRUITS AND VEGETABLES AND BLOOD PRESSURE TREATMENT

Observational studies indicate that vegetarians have lower blood pressures than omnivores.[28] There are reports that vegetarians fed meat for short periods developed elevations in blood pressure. A vegetarian diet contains more calcium, fiber, and magnesium and less saturated fat than an isocaloric diet more typical of Western societies. Attempts to discover which particular constituent of the vegetarian diet is most responsible for the lowering of blood pressure have been unsuccessful, and it has been considered that the positive effects of vegetarianism result from certain combinations of nutrients.

In 1995, a retrospective look was taken at over 500 patients in a live-in weight loss program.[29] Over a 12-day period, a vegetarian diet was provided that was composed of 5% fat, 12% protein, and 83% carbohydrate, with 60 g of fiber, no cholesterol, and less than 1000 mg of sodium/day. Although calories were not restricted in these overweight subjects, and no weight loss was seen within the first 12 days, there was a significant fall in blood pressure, on average 9/6 mm Hg, most prominent in those with baseline above 140/90. Since the low-salt intake might have been important in the blood pressure effect, the contribution of the added fruits and vegetables could not be ascertained. Another study attempted to compare a typical "heart-healthy" diet with its individual constituents added to a control diet.[30] A low-sodium, low-fat, high-fiber diet was instituted in one group of 193 hypertensives and compared with: (1) control diet, (2) low salt (40 to 50 mmol/day), (3) low fat (23 to 25% of calories), and (4) high fiber (40 to 45 g). After 8 weeks, the low-salt (nonsignificant) and low-fat (significant) diets reduced diastolic blood pressure; the combination diet produced highly significant reductions in both systolic and diastolic pressure. These changes were independent of weight loss, which did not correlate with blood pressure effects of the diets.

Thus, the recent publication of the Dietary Approaches to Stop Hypertension (DASH) study has been informative and of practical benefit.[31] The investigators' aim was to randomize all participants to a same-salt (3 g) eucaloric program, and on this background, compare the effect of a meal plan rich in fruits and vegetables or fruits, vegetables, and low-fat dairy products with a meal plan resembling a typical high-fat American diet. They succeeded in enrolling a diverse group of borderline or mild hypertensive subjects, 60% of whom were African American, the aim being to make the sample representative of hypertensives in the United States. For admission to the study, systolic blood pressure had to be below 160; diastolic, 80 to 95 mm Hg. During the 8 weeks of the specialized diets, all meals were provided to participants. Blood pressure fell within 2 weeks and reductions were maintained for the duration of the study. Whereas both experimental diets were successful in lowering blood pressure, the inclusion of extra low-fat dairy products was more effective (systolic −5.5 mm Hg and diastolic −3 mm Hg more than control diet). The greatest blood pressure lowering was seen in those with the highest values at entry. In the subgroup with stage 1 hypertension, blood pressure reductions as great as those produced by medications were found. Perhaps the most important facet of this excellent study is its emphasis on designing a meal plan that has a high level of acceptance, that allows for diverse cultural preferences, and that is likely to permit prolonged adherence and weight loss (Fig. 48–1).

CONCLUSIONS

In overweight persons with hypertension or high-normal blood pressure, weight loss through calorie restriction lowers blood pressure irrespective of changes in urinary sodium, indicating that weight loss is more important than reducing sodium intake in this population. Since over 50% of Americans are overweight, a diet that has taste and good nutrition and results in weight loss should be at the fore-

Food group	Daily servings	1 serving equals	Examples and notes
Grains and grain products 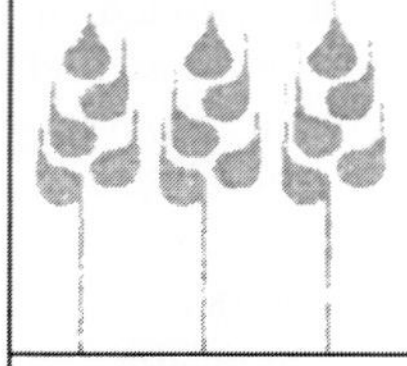	7–8	1 slice bread 1/2 cup dry cereal 1/2 cup cooked rice, pasta, or cereal	Whole-wheat breads, English muffin, pita bread, bagel, cereals and fiber, grits, oatmeal; provide energy and fiber.
Vegetables 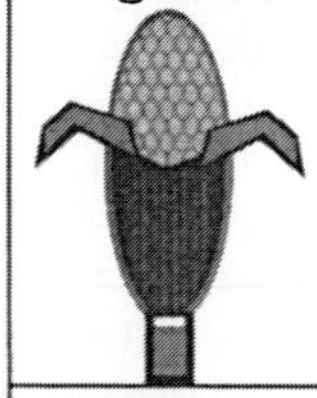	4–5	1 cup raw leafy vegetables 1/2 cup cooked vegetable 6 oz vegetable juice	Tomatoes, potatoes, carrots, peas, squash, broccoli, turnip greens, collards, kale, spinach, artichokes, beans, sweet potatoes; sources of potassium, magnesium, and fiber.
Fruit 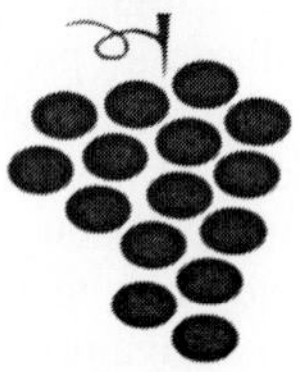	4–5	8 oz fruit juice 1 medium fruit 1/4 cup dried fruit 1/2 cup fresh, frozen, or canned fruit	Apricots, bananas, dates, grapes, oranges, orange juice, grapefruit, grapefruit juice, mangoes, melons, peaches, pineapples, prunes, raisins, strawberries, tangerines; provide potassium, magnesium, and fiber.
Low-fat and nonfat dairy foods 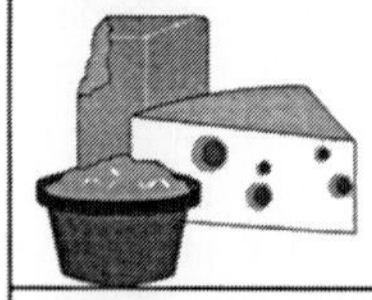	2–3	8 oz milk 1 cup yogurt 1 1/2 oz cheese	Skim or 1% milk, skim or low-fat buttermilk, nonfat or low-fat yogurt, part-skim mozzarella cheese, nonfat cheese; major sources of calcium and protein.
Meat, poultry, fish 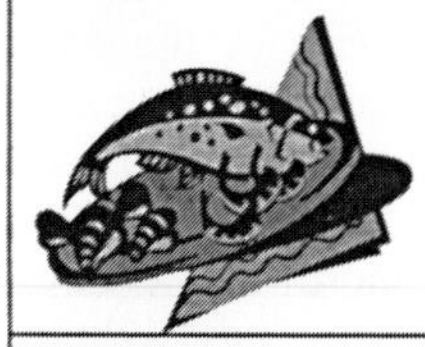	2 or fewer	3 oz cooked meats, poultry, or fish	Select only lean; trim away visible fats; broil, roast, or boil, instead of frying; remove skin from poultry. Rich sources of protein and magnesium.
Nuts 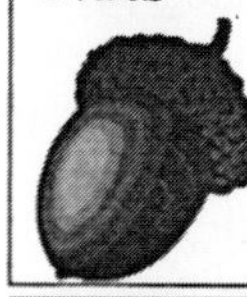	1/2	1 1/2 oz or 1/3 cup 2 tbs seed 1/2 cup cooked legumes	Almonds, filberts, mixed nuts, peanuts, walnuts, sunflower seeds, kidney beans, lentils; provide energy, protein, and fiber.

Tips on eating the DASH Way
* Start small. Make gradual changes in your eating habits.
* Center your meal around carbohydrates such as pasta, rice, beans, or vegetables.
* Treat meat as one part of the whole meal, instead of the focus.
* Use fruit or low-fat, low-energy foods such as sugar-free gelatin for desserts and snacks.

Figure 48–1. Food components of the Dietary Approaches to Stop Hypertension (DASH) diet, with daily servings, portion sizes, and examples and notes. In the DASH Study, researchers found that diet can reduce blood pressure as effectively as medication in many people. The recommended diet is rich in fruit, vegetables, low-fat dairy foods, and fiber but low in fat and cholesterol. The amounts shown are based on a daily recommended diet of 8368 kJ (2000 kcal). Depending on energy needs, the number of servings per day may vary. For restrained eating or weight loss and for relapse prevention, three-quarter-sized servings and portions can be used. (From Blackburn GL. Functional foods in the prevention and treatment of disease: Significance of the Dietary Approaches to Stop Hypertension Study. Am J Clin Nutr 66:1067–1071, 1997; data from Appel LJ, Moore TJ, Obarzanek E, et al. A clinical trial of the effects of dietary patterns on blood pressure. DASH Collaborative Research Group. N Engl J Med 336:1117–1124, 1997. © Am. J. Clin. Nutr. American Society for Clinical Nutrition.)

front of blood pressure–lowering strategies. Although small mean reductions in blood pressure in a dietary study may seem trivial, on a population basis these numbers can be translated into significant health care benefits and lead to reductions in stroke and other morbidities that are related to hypertension. It has been estimated, using data from the Framingham cohort studies, that a 2-mm Hg reduction in diastolic blood pressure can effect a 15% reduction in stroke and a 6% reduction in coronary disease.[32] Screening for high-normal blood pressure at routine physical examinations in overweight persons or those with adult weight gain will identify individuals who should be targeted for lifestyle change in diet and calorie intake.

Unfortunately, palatability of the typically recommended heart-healthy, meat-free diets is often unacceptable to many of those accustomed to a high-fat usual American diet. Studies that followed enrollees for several years generally showed that the lowest blood pressures were seen early when weight was at a nadir, before good compliance dissipated. New, creative approaches to dietary therapy that emphasize portion- and caloric-control, while maximizing taste and variety, are mandatory. What is most interesting about the diet used in the DASH study was the ease of acceptance by participants. This suggests that the way forward might be to focus on caloric manipulation by addition of fruits and vegetables, either fresh, frozen, or canned, and low-fat dairy products as an adjunct to a weight loss program.

A plethora of controlled trials has shown that weight loss in those with BMI greater than 25 kg/m^2 is the single most important lifestyle intervention that lowers blood pressure and prevents the onset of hypertension in those at risk. Those who succeed in sustained weight loss stand to accrue many other health benefits, in contrast to persons who have a similar blood pressure reduction with pharmacotherapy, which can be expensive and may lead to untoward effects. If the dietary regimen instituted is not enjoyable, simple, and culturally appropriate, the chances of success are slim. Sensible, balanced, and palatable foods, salted if necessary, can provide lasting health and blood pressure benefits.

References

1. Burt VL, Whelton P, Roccella EJ, et al. Prevalence of hypertension in the US adult population. Results from the Third National Health and Nutrition Examination Survey, 1988–1991. Hypertension 25:305–313, 1995.
2. Kuczmarski RJ, Carroll MD, Flegal KM, et al. Varying body mass index cutoff points to describe overweight prevalence among U.S. adults: NHANES III (1988 to 1994). Obes Res 5:542–548, 1997.
3. Garrison RJ, Kannel WB, Stokes J III, et al. Incidence and precursors of hypertension in young adults: The Framingham Offspring Study. Prev Med 16:235–251, 1987.
4. Kannel WB, Brand N, Skinner JJ Jr, et al. The relation of adiposity to blood pressure and development of hypertension. The Framingham Study. Ann Intern Med 67:48–59, 1967.
5. Elliott P, Marmot M, Dyer A, et al. The INTERSALT Study: Main results, conclusions and some implications. Clin Exp Hypertens A 11:1025–1034, 1989.
6. Ferrannini E, Natali A, Capaldo B, et al. Insulin resistance, hyperinsulinemia, and blood pressure: Role of age and obesity. European Group for the Study of Insulin Resistance (EGIR). Hypertension 30:1144–1149, 1997.
7. Gordon NF, Scott CB, Levine BD. Comparison of single versus multiple lifestyle interventions: Are the antihypertensive effects of exercise training and diet-induced weight loss additive? Am J Cardiol 79:763–767, 1997.
8. Haynes RB. Is weight loss an effective treatment for hypertension? The evidence against. Can J Physiol Pharmacol 64:825–830, 1986.
9. Trials of Hypertension Prevention Collaborative Research Group. Effects of weight loss and sodium reduction intervention on blood pressure and hypertension incidence in overweight people with high-normal blood pressure. The Trials of Hypertension Prevention, phase II. Arch Intern Med 157:657–667, 1997.
10. Stamler R, Stamler J, Grimm R, et al. Nutritional therapy for high blood pressure. Final report of a four-year randomized controlled trial—The Hypertension Control Program. JAMA 257:1484–1491, 1987.
11. Hypertension Prevention Trial Research Group. The Hypertension Prevention Trial: Three-year effects of dietary changes on blood pressure. Arch Intern Med 150:153–162, 1990.
12. Treatment of Mild Hypertension Research Group. The Treatment of Mild Hypertension Study. A randomized, placebo-controlled trial of a nutritional-hygienic regimen along with various drug monotherapies. Arch Intern Med 151:1413–1423, 1991.
13. Grimm RH Jr, Flack JM, Grandits GA, et al. Long-term effects on plasma lipids of diet and drugs to treat hypertension. Treatment of Mild Hypertension Study (TOMHS) Research Group. JAMA 275:1549–1556, 1996.
14. Wassertheil-Smoller S, Oberman A, Blaufox MD, et al. The Trial of Antihypertensive Interventions and Management (TAIM) Study. Final results with regard to blood pressure, cardiovascular risk, and quality of life. Am J Hypertens 5:37–44, 1992.
15. MacMahon S, Macdonald G. Treatment of high blood pressure in overweight patients. Nephron 47(suppl 1):8–12, 1987.
16. Affarah HB, Hall WD, Heymsfield SB, et al. High-carbohydrate diet: Antinatriuretic and blood pressure response in normal men. Am J Clin Nutr 44:341–348, 1986.
17. McCarron DA, Oparil S, Chait A, et al. Nutritional management of cardiovascular risk factors. A randomized clinical trial. Arch Intern Med 157:169–177, 1997.
18. Nobels F, van Gaal L, de Leeuw I. Weight reduction with a high protein, low carbohydrate, calorie-restricted diet: Effects on blood pressure, glucose and insulin levels. Neth J Med 35:295–302, 1989.
19. Foley EF, Benotti PN, Borlase BC, et al. Impact of gastric restrictive surgery on hypertension in the morbidly obese. Am J Surg 163:294–297, 1992.
20. Alaud-din A, Meterissian S, Lisbona R, et al. Assessment of cardiac function in patients who were morbidly obese. Surgery 108:809–818; discussion 818–822, 1990.
21. Kaufman LN, Peterson MM, Smith SM. Hypertensive effect of polyunsaturated dietary fat. Metabolism 43:1–3, 1994.
22. Marley AM, Rogers PF, Lungershausen YK, et al. Combined effects of dietary fish oil and sodium restriction on blood pressure in enalapril-treated hypertensive rats. Am J Hypertens 6:121–126, 1993.
23. Berry EM, Hirsch J. Does dietary linolenic acid influence blood pressure? Am J Clin Nutr 44:336–340, 1986.
24. Knapp HR, FitzGerald GA. The antihypertensive effects of fish oil. A controlled study of polyunsaturated fatty acid supplements in essential hypertension [see comments]. N Engl J Med 320:1037–1043, 1989.
25. Margolin G, Huster G, Glueck CJ, et al. Blood pressure lowering in elderly subjects: A double-blind crossover study of omega-3 and omega-6 fatty acids. Am J Clin Nutr 53:562–572, 1991.
26. Passfall J, Philipp T, Woermann F, et al. Different effects of eicosapentaenoic acid and olive oil on blood pressure, intracellular free platelet calcium, and plasma lipids in patients with essential hypertension. Clin Invest 71:628–633, 1993.
27. Cobiac L, Nestel PJ, Wing LM, et al. A low-sodium diet supplemented with fish oil lowers blood pressure in the elderly. J Hypertens 10:87–92, 1992.
28. Sacks FM, Rosner B, Kass EH. Blood pressure in vegetarians. Am J Epidemiol 100:390–398, 1974.
29. McDougall J, Litzau K, Haver E, et al. Rapid reduction of serum cholesterol and blood pressure by a twelve-day, very low fat, strictly vegetarian diet. J Am Coll Nutr 14:491–496, 1995.
30. Little P, Girling G, Hasler A, et al. A controlled trial of a low sodium, low fat, high fibre diet in treated hypertensive patients: The efficacy of multiple dietary intervention. Postgrad Med J 66:616–621, 1990.
31. Appel LJ, Moore TJ, Obarzanek E, et al. A clinical trial of the effects of dietary patterns on blood pressure. DASH Collaborative Research Group. N Engl J Med 336:1117–1124, 1997.
32. Cook NR, Cohen J, Hebert PR, et al. Implications of small reductions in diastolic blood pressure for primary prevention. Arch Intern Med 155:701–709, 1995.

49 Alcohol Consumption and the Management of Hypertension

William C. Cushman

There are many serious adverse health and psychosocial consequences of excessive alcohol intake, but there are also generally accepted positive psychosocial effects of drinking and beneficial effects on health, especially reduced atherothrombotic events and death, from regular alcohol consumption. One of the harmful effects attributed to alcohol is its association with hypertension.

In 1915, the French physician Lian called initial attention to a relationship between alcohol consumption and hypertension.[1] He reported that sailors who drank several liters of wine daily were more likely to have hypertension and that the prevalence of hypertension increased with increasing alcohol intake. Most of the epidemiological and clinical trial information concerning the relationship between alcohol intake and blood pressure (BP), however, has been reported since the late 1960s.

EPIDEMIOLOGY

Alcohol consumption has one of the strongest epidemiological associations with BP of the known potentially modifiable risk factors for hypertension.[2-6] Over 50 cross-sectional epidemiological studies from a variety of cultures have reported increasing average BP or a higher prevalence of hypertension with increasing levels of alcohol intake. Above an average intake of 2 drinks* per day, the higher the alcohol intake the higher the BP. This relationship usually persists as an independent effect even when controlling for age, body mass, sodium and potassium excretion or intake, cigarette smoking, and education, and has been demonstrated in Caucasians, Blacks, and Asians (see Chap. 23, Alcohol and Hypertension).[2-4]

In population studies, a J-shaped relationship is sometimes observed, with lower BP levels seen with low levels of alcohol intake compared with no drinking or consumption of 3 or more drinks per day on average.[2, 5] Sometimes low levels of alcohol intake have been associated with higher BP levels than no alcohol intake.[2, 7] Often, there is no difference in BP between nondrinkers and populations reporting 2 or fewer drinks per day.[2] However, the BP differences between these two groups, even when they are found, are usually small.

A reduction in BP is also associated with a reduction in alcohol consumption in prospective observational studies[8-10] and inpatient studies of cessation of alcohol intake in alcoholics.[11, 12] The hypertensive effect of alcohol appears to abate within several days of abstinence, and the

relationship between intake and BP is strongest for alcohol consumed within the previous 24 hours.[13] The pattern of drinking also affects BP. For example, weekend drinkers, but not daily drinkers, have significantly higher BPs on Monday than on Thursday.[14] In some studies, one type of alcoholic beverage, such as beer or liquor, is more strongly associated with BP than another, but no beverage type has been consistently incriminated or absolved. When all studies are taken together, it appears that the relationship between alcohol and BP is dependent on the amount of absolute alcohol ingested.

Excess alcohol intake has also been associated with resistance to antihypertensive therapy.[15] Although it is reasonable to assume that medication noncompliance in heavy drinkers contributes to this resistance, compelling data suggest true interference with the BP-lowering effects of medications taken appropriately.[16] Drinking 3 or more drinks of alcohol per day is associated with approximately a doubling of the prevalence of hypertension and has been estimated to account for 5 to 20% of hypertension in populations. However, this contribution will vary depending on the prevalence of heavy drinking in a population. The absolute impact also depends on the prevalence of hypertension in a population.

RANDOMIZED CONTROLLED TRIALS

From an evidence-based perspective, randomized controlled trials provide the highest level of evidence for the efficacy of an intervention. At least 12 randomized studies have been conducted to examine the effect of a reduction in alcohol intake on BP (Table 49–1).[14, 16–27] Although the majority of these studies included relatively few subjects, were of short duration, and were not designed as effectiveness trials, the results are generally consistent with the epidemiological evidence for the relationship of alcohol and BP.

The Prevention and Treatment of Hypertension Study (PATHS) is the largest and longest of the randomized controlled trials of the effects of alcohol reduction on BP.[26, 27] The National Heart, Lung, and Blood Institute (NHLBI), the National Institute on Alcohol Abuse and Alcoholism (NIAAA), and the Veterans Affairs (VA) Cooperative Studies Program collaborated in this multicenter trial. The primary objectives were to determine (1) whether alcohol intake could be reduced within 6 months and the reduction could be sustained for 2 years in order to determine (2) whether BP was lowered by sustained reductions in alcohol intake in 641 moderate to heavy drinkers with diastolic BP 80 to 99 mm Hg. Exclusions included evidence of alcoholism, medical complications of excess alco-

---

*A *standard drink* is defined as approximately 14 g of ethanol and is contained in a 12-oz glass of beer, a 5-oz glass of table wine, or 1.5 oz of distilled spirits.

Table 49–1 Randomized Controlled Trials of the Effect of Alcohol Reduction on Blood Pressure

First Author, Year	n	Age (yr) (mean ± SD or range)	Duration (wk)	Baseline BP (mm Hg)	Alcohol Intake Difference (drinks*/day)	BP Difference (mm Hg)	p Value
Puddey, 1985[17]	46	35 ± 8	6	133/76	3.7	3.8/1.4	<.001/<.05
Howes, 1985[18]	10	25–41	0.6	120/66	5.7	8/6	<.025/<.001
Puddey, 1987[16]	44	53 ± 16	6	142/84	4.0	5/3	<.001/<.001
Ueshima, 1987[19]	50	46 ± 7	2	148/93	2.6	5.2/2.2	<.005/ns
Wallace, 1988[20]	641	42 ± 20	52	136/82	1.0	2.1/?	<.05/ns
Parker, 1990[21]	59	52 ± 11	4	138/85	3.8	5.4/3.2	<.01/<.01
Cox, 1990[22]	72	20–45	4	132/73	3.4	4.1/1.6	<.05/<.05
Maheswaran, 1992[23]	41	40s	8	144/90	3.1	Not reported	ns
Puddey, 1992[24]	86	44	18	137/85	3.0	4.8/3.3	<.01/<.01
Ueshima, 1993[25]	54	44 ± 8	3	144/96	1.7	3.6/1.9	<.05/ns
Rakic, 1998[14] (pattern)							
Weekend	14	41	4	122/72	3.1	1/0	ns/ns†
Daily	41	48	4	124/77	2.6	2/2	<.05/<.01†
Cushman, 1998[26,27]	641	57 ± 11	104	140/86	1.3	0.9/0.6	.16/.10

Abbreviations: BP, blood pressure; ns, not significant.

*A standard drink is defined as 14 g of ethanol and is contained in a 12-oz glass of beer, a 5-oz glass of table wine, or a 1.5-oz serving of distilled spirits.

†Supine office BP; 24-hr ambulatory systolic BP (but not diastolic BP) was lowered by 3.1 mm Hg ($p < .001$) and 2.2 mm Hg ($p < .001$) in weekend and daily drinkers, respectively.

hol intake, significant cardiovascular or psychiatric diseases, secondary hypertension, and inability to stop any BP-lowering medication. Participants were randomized to a cognitive-behavioral alcohol-reduction intervention program or a control observation group and followed for 15 to 24 months. The goal of the intervention was a 50% reduction in intake or consumption of 2 or fewer drinks daily, whichever was lower. The differences in alcohol intake were highly significant from 3 to 24 months of follow-up (Fig. 49–1). However, the difference averaged only 1.3 drinks per day rather than the 2.0 drinks per day anticipated and estimated to provide the needed power to determine whether BP is lowered. This shortfall resulted in part because the control group lowered reported alcohol intake more than anticipated. The average difference in BP reduction of 0.9/0.6 mm Hg was not significantly different between the intervention and the control groups (Fig. 49–2). However, the effects of reducing alcohol intake on BP and the development or recurrence of hypertension were in the expected direction and quantitatively consistent with the BP changes seen in previous controlled studies in which larger differences in alcohol intake between treatment and control groups were achieved. Therefore, it is possible that greater differences in alcohol reduction between treatment groups in PATHS may have resulted in greater differences in BP reduction.

Larger BP differences between randomized groups were seen in most of the other controlled trials of alcohol reduction and BP compared with PATHS, perhaps related to higher baseline levels and larger reductions in alcohol intake (see Table 49–1). Average differences in alcohol intake in these randomized controlled studies ranged from 1.0 to 5.7 drinks per day and resulted in significant reductions in systolic BP or diastolic BP, or both, in all but two studies. Among these studies, five from Perth, Australia,[16, 17, 21, 22, 24] in normotensives and hypertensives are probably the best from which to derive a crude prediction of BP change. Their usual technique was to recruit middle-aged men who drank heavily and randomize them to continue

their usual intake of beer or to drink low-alcohol beer for the study periods, usually in a crossover design. In these studies, the difference in alcohol intake between randomized groups averaged 3.0 to 4.0 drinks per day and resulted in a 3.8- to 5.4-mm Hg average difference in systolic BP and a 1.4- to 3.3-mm Hg average difference in diastolic BP,

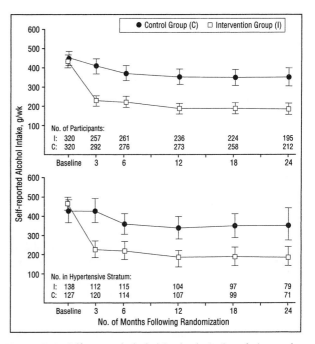

Figure 49–1. Self-reported alcohol intake (quintiles of change from baseline) and changes in biochemical markers of alcohol intake (mean ± 2 SEs) by treatment group from baseline to 6 months after randomization. Apo, apolipoprotein; GGT, γ-glutamyltransferase; HDL, high-density lipoprotein; inc, increase; dec, decrease. (From Cushman WC, Cutler JA, Hanna E, et al. Prevention and Treatment of Hypertension Study [PATHS]: Effects of an alcohol treatment program on blood pressure. Arch Intern Med 158:1197–1207, 1998. Copyright 1998, American Medical Association.)

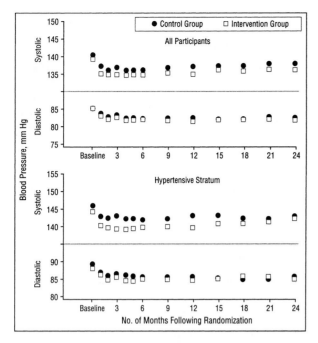

Figure 49–2. Average blood pressure at each period by randomized group for all participants *(top)* and for participants in the hypertensive stratum *(bottom)*. Blood pressure values have been imputed when measurement data were not available. (From Cushman WC, Cutler JA, Hanna E, et al. Prevention and Treatment of Hypertension Study [PATHS]: Effects of an alcohol treatment program on blood pressure. Arch Intern Med 158:1197–1207, 1998. Copyright 1998, American Medical Association.)

even though most of the participants were normotensives or treated hypertensives whose BP was controlled. In the initial two studies, a 3.0-drink per day net reduction in alcohol intake was associated with a 4.4-/2.2-mm Hg average reduction in BP.[27] Among all the studies, for every 1 drink per day reduction in alcohol intake in the intervention groups compared with the control groups, a 1-mm Hg decrease in systolic BP or diastolic BP, or both, was produced.

Overall, the randomized controlled trials give solid evidence that a reduction in alcohol intake in individuals who consume 3 or more drinks per day on average is effective in lowering BP. However, the results from PATHS, the primary effectiveness clinical trial in this area, do not support a recommendation that reduction of alcohol consumption should be the sole method for the prevention or treatment of hypertension in moderate to heavy drinkers.[27] Nevertheless, the recommendation from a variety of consensus committees to limit alcohol consumption to no more than 1 to 2 drinks per day is reasonable and prudent because of the potential efficacy of this intervention, the reduction in risk of a variety of other adverse consequences of drinking, and the apparent relative ease in achieving a reduction in alcohol intake in nondependent drinkers.[28, 29]

POTENTIAL MECHANISMS OF EFFECT ON BLOOD PRESSURE

A number of mechanisms have been proposed for the relationship between alcohol and elevated BP. Although

one of the immediate effects of alcohol consumption is vasodilatation in some vascular beds, sustained intake accompanied by high blood alcohol levels results in short-term elevation of BP.[30] In addition, as mentioned previously, BP correlates best with alcohol intake within the prior 24 hours and falls fairly rapidly after cessation or reduction in intake.[13, 14] Therefore, it is likely that the effect of alcohol on BP is not mediated by long-term structural alterations, but by neural, hormonal, or other reversible physiological changes.

It has been proposed that the hypertensive effect of alcohol results from a chronic state of alcohol withdrawal in frequent heavy drinkers, but there appears to be more evidence for a direct effect of alcohol. Suggested mediators of this direct effect include: (1) stimulation of the sympathetic nervous system, endothelin, renin-angiotensin-aldosterone system, insulin (or insulin resistance), or cortisol; (2) inhibition of vascular-relaxing substances; (3) calcium or magnesium depletion; (4) increased intracellular calcium or other electrolytes in vascular smooth muscle, possibly mediated by changes in membrane electrolyte transport; and (5) increased acetaldehyde.[31–33] There appears to be more evidence to support the role of the sympathetic nervous system or cellular transport of electrolytes, or both, than the other mechanisms suggested, but this remains an open question.

CARDIOVASCULAR PROTECTION

Compared with abstention, low to moderate levels of alcohol intake are associated with a reduced incidence of atherothrombotic events, such as myocardial infarction and atherothrombotic stroke.[34–36] These beneficial effects of alcohol appear to be, at least in part, attributable to increases in high-density lipoprotein cholesterol, apolipoproteins A_1 and A_2, and antioxidant effects and reduced platelet aggregability.[34–37] However, higher intake levels are associated with increased risk for hypertension, cardiomyopathy and other cardiac complications, hemorrhagic strokes, certain kinds of cancer, liver damage and other gastrointestinal pathology, suicides, accidents, violence, and alcohol abuse and dependence.[28, 31] Therefore, we should be cautious about encouraging initiation of alcohol consumption in hopes of reducing cardiovascular risk. However, for those who choose to drink and who have no contraindication, low levels of drinking can be recommended as prudent, as discussed later.

RECOMMENDATIONS

In light of the association between heavy drinking and hypertension, other detrimental health consequences, and adverse psychosocial effects, as well as the potential benefits of alcohol consumption, current public health recommendations in the United States are: For those who drink, average alcohol intake should not exceed 2 drinks per day in men and 1 drink per day in women, since women are generally smaller and have markedly reduced gastric alcohol-dehydrogenase compared with men.[28, 29] Many persons should not drink at all. These include pregnant women and individuals with a history of or who appear to be at risk of a drinking problem or serious medical complications from alcohol. For those who are not in one of these high-risk categories and who drink within the limits outlined previously, risk of developing hypertension is probably not increased and the beneficial effects of alcohol may predominate. However, anyone consuming an average of more than 1 to 2 drinks per day should be encouraged to reduce intake in order to reduce BP, the risk of developing hypertension, and the risk of other alcohol-related problems.

The majority of adults who drink more than 1 to 2 drinks per day do not have evidence for alcohol dependence and would have little difficulty in reducing drinking substantially. In the PATHS trial, for example, alcohol intake was reduced from an average of 6 drinks per day in the 6 months before screening by about 1.5 drinks per day during the week before randomization and before learning that the trial focused on alcohol intake.[26, 27] The intervention group reduced their intake a further 2.3 drinks per day for a net reported reduction of 4 drinks per day to approximately 2 drinks per day. In the studies performed in Perth, Australia, participants reduced their beer intake by 3 to 4 drinks per day for weeks at a time merely by substituting equal quantities of low-alcohol beer for their usual beer intake.

All hypertensive patients should be asked about quantities and frequency of drinking and drinking patterns. In addition, those who drink should be screened for alcohol dependence using an instrument such as the CAGE questions.* Effective cognitive-behavioral interventions, such as the one used in the PATHS trial, have been developed to reduce alcohol consumption in nondependent heavy drinkers.[26, 27, 38, 39] Although referral to treatment specialists may be necessary in some cases, especially if there is evidence of alcohol dependence or serious health consequences of drinking, primary care physicians, nurses, and other health care providers should discuss alcohol consumption with their patients and recommend limitation of excessive intake at each visit.

The BP lowering seen from reducing alcohol intake in randomized controlled trials is comparable with or greater than that found for most other effective lifestyle interventions.[40–42] For example, in the Trials of Hypertension Prevention, Phase I (TOHP-I), a long-term randomized controlled trial of lifestyle interventions and nutritional supplements in persons with high-normal BP, weight reduction was most effective in reducing BP (2.9/2.3 mm Hg), whereas sodium reduction also reduced BP (1.7/0.9 mm Hg) to an extent comparable with that seen with alcohol intervention in PATHS.[41] Stress management and various supplements in TOHP were associated with smaller nonsignificant differences. Exercise has also produced fairly consistent significant reductions in BP.[29, 43] Therefore, reduction in alcohol intake should be considered along with weight reduction, limitation of sodium intake, and exercise as the primary lifestyle changes to encourage in patients with or at risk for hypertension. If alcohol intake exceeds an average of 1 to 2 drinks per day, then reduction in alcohol consumption should be included in the initial management plan.

---

*CAGE, the official name of the screening questions for alcohol dependency, is an acronym that reminds one of the four questions: (1) Have you ever tried to Cut down your drinking level? (2) Does it Annoy you for others to talk about your drinking? (3) Have you ever felt Guilty about your drinking? (4) Do you ever need an Eye-opener drink in the mornings? Any positive answers should prompt further screening for alcohol dependence.

References

1. Lian C. L'alcoholisme, cause d'hypertension arterielle. Bull Acad Med 74:525–528, 1915.
2. MacMahon S. Alcohol consumption and hypertension. Hypertension 9:111–121, 1987.
3. Marmot MG, Elliott P, Shipley MJ, et al. Alcohol and blood pressure: The INTERSALT study. BMJ 308:1263–1267, 1994.
4. Glynn RJ, Bouchard GR, Hermos JA. Alcohol consumption, blood pressure and aging: Results from the Normative Aging Study. *In* Wood WG, Grant R (eds). Geriatric Clinical Pharmacology. New York, Raven, 1987.
5. Klatsky AL, Freidman GD, Siegelaub AB, Gerard MJ. Alcohol consumption and blood pressure. N Engl J Med 296:1194–1200, 1977.
6. Friedman GD, Klatsky AL, Siegelaub AB. Alcohol, tobacco, and hypertension. Hypertension 4:143–150, 1982.
7. Criqui MH, Mebane I, Wallace RB, et al. Multivariate correlates of adult blood pressures in nine North American populations: The Lipid Research Clinics Prevalence Study. Prev Med 11:391–402, 1982.
8. Gordon T, Kannel WB. Drinking and its relation to smoking, BP, blood lipids and uric acid. Arch Intern Med 143:1366–1374, 1983.
9. Kromhout D, Bosschieter EB, Coulander CL. Potassium, calcium, alcohol intake and blood pressure: The Zutphen Study. Am J Clin Nutr 41:1299–1304, 1985.
10. Gordon T, Doyle JT. Alcohol consumption and its relationship to smoking, weight, blood pressure, and blood lipids: The Albany Study. Arch Intern Med 146:262–265, 1986.
11. Saunders JB, Beevers DG, Paton A. Alcohol induced hypertension. Lancet 2:653–656, 1981.
12. Ashley MJ, Rankin JG. Alcohol consumption and hypertension: The evidence from hazardous drinking and alcohol populations. Aust N Z J Med 9:201–206, 1979.
13. Moreira LB, Fuchs FD, Moraes RS, et al. Alcohol intake and blood pressure: The importance of time elapsed since last drink. J Hypertens 16:175–180, 1998.
14. Rakic V, Puddey IB, Burke V, et al. Influence of pattern of alcohol intake on blood pressure in regular drinkers: A controlled trial. J Hypertens 16:165–174, 1998.
15. Henningsen NC, Ohlsson O, Mattiasson I, et al. Hypertension, levels of gamma-glutamyltranspeptidase and degree of blood pressure control in middle-aged males. Acta Med Scand 207:245–251, 1980.
16. Puddey IB, Beilin LJ, Vandongen R. Regular alcohol use raises blood pressure in treated hypertensive subjects: A randomized controlled trial. Lancet 1:647–651, 1987.
17. Puddey IB, Beilin LJ, Vandongen R, et al. Evidence for a direct pressor effect of alcohol consumption on blood pressure in normotensive men: A randomized controlled trial. Hypertension 7:707–713, 1985.
18. Howes LG. Pressor effect of alcohol. [Letter] Lancet 2:835, 1985.
19. Ueshima H, Ogihara T, Baba S, et al. The effect of reduced alcohol consumption on blood pressure: A randomized, controlled, single-blind study. J Hum Hypertens 1:113–119, 1987.
20. Wallace P, Cutler S, Haines A. Randomized controlled trial of general practitioner intervention in patients with excessive alcohol consumption. BMJ 297:663–668, 1988.
21. Parker M, Puddey IB, Beilin LJ, Vandongen R. Two-way factorial study of alcohol and salt restriction in treated hypertensive men. Hypertension 16:398–406, 1990.
22. Cox KL, Puddey IB, Morton AR, et al. Controlled comparison of effects of exercise and alcohol on blood pressure and serum high density lipoprotein cholesterol in sedentary males. Clin Exp Pharmacol Physiol 17:251–255, 1990.
23. Maheswaran R, Beevers M, Beevers DG. Effectiveness of advice to reduce alcohol consumption in hypertensive patients. Hypertension 19:79–84, 1992.
24. Puddey IB, Parker M, Beilin LJ, et al. Effects of alcohol and calorie

restrictions on blood pressure and serum lipids in overweight men. Hypertension 20:533–541, 1992.

25. Ueshima H, Mikawa K, Baba S, et al. Effect of reduced alcohol consumption on blood pressure in untreated hypertensive men. Hypertension 21:248–252, 1993.

26. Cushman WC, Cutler JA, Bingham SF, et al, for the PATHS Group. Prevention and Treatment of Hypertension Study (PATHS) rationale and design. Am J Hypertens 7:814–823, 1994.

27. Cushman WC, Cutler JA, Hanna E, et al, for the PATHS Group. The Prevention and Treatment of Hypertension Study (PATHS): Effects of an alcohol treatment program on blood pressure. Arch Intern Med 158:1197–1207, 1998.

28. U.S. Department of Health and Human Services. Nutrition and Your Health: Dietary Guidelines for Americans, 4th ed. Washington, DC, U.S. Department of Agriculture, 1995; pp 40–41.

29. Joint National Committee on Prevention, Detection, Evaluation, and Treatment of High Blood Pressure. The sixth report. Arch Intern Med 157:2413–2446, 1997.

30. Potter JF, Beevers DG. Two possible mechanisms for alcohol associated hypertension. Scand J Clin Lab Invest 176:92–99, 1985.

31. Beilin LJ. Alcohol, hypertension and cardiovascular disease. J Hypertens 13:939–942, 1995.

32. Cocoa A, Aguilera MT, Sierra AD, et al. Chronic alcohol intake induces reversible disturbances on cellular Na^+ metabolism in humans: Its relationship with changes in blood pressure. Alcohol Clin Exp Res 16:714–720, 1992.

33. Randin D, Vollenweider P, Tappy L, et al. Suppression of alcohol-induced hypertension by dexamethasone. N Engl J Med 332:1733–1737, 1995.

34. Klatsky AL, Armstrong MA, Friedman GD. Alcohol and mortality. Ann Intern Med 117:646–654, 1992.

35. Suh I, Shaten J, Cutler JA, Kuller LH. Alcohol use and mortality from coronary heart disease: The role of high-density lipoprotein. Ann Intern Med 116:881–887, 1992.

36. Thun MJ, Peto R, Lopez AD, et al. Alcohol consumption and mortality among middle-aged and elderly U.S. adults. N Engl J Med 337:1705–1714, 1997.

37. Renaud SC, Beswick AD, Fehily AM, et al. Alcohol and platelet aggregation: The Caerphilly Prospective Heart Disease Study. Am J Clin Nutr 55:1012–1017, 1992.

38. Hanna E. Approach to the patient with excessive alcohol consumption. *In* Goroll AH, May L, Mulley A (eds). Primary Care Medicine. Philadelphia, JB Lippincott, 1987; pp 916–927.

39. Sanchez-Craig M. Dealing with drinking. Steps to abstinence or moderate drinking. Toronto, Addiction Research Foundation, 1987.

40. Martin JE, Dubbert PM, Cushman WC. Controlled trial of aerobic exercise in hypertension. Circulation 81:1560–1567, 1990.

41. Trials of Hypertension Prevention Collaborative Research Group. The effects of nonpharmacologic interventions on blood pressure of persons with high normal levels: Results of the Trials of Hypertension Prevention, Phase I. JAMA 267:1213–1220, 1992.

42. Whelton PK, Appel LJ, Espeland MA, et al, for the TONE Collaborative Research Group. A randomized controlled trial of nonpharmacologic interventions in the elderly (TONE). JAMA 279:839–846, 1998.

43. Cushman WC. Extrinsic factors in essential hypertension: Physical activity/fitness. *In* Izzo JL, Black HR (eds). Hypertension Primer. Dallas, American Heart Association, 1993; pp 161–163.

CHAPTER 50 | Exercise and Hypertension

Angel H. Herrera and David T. Lowenthal

The current management of hypertension consists of lifestyle modifications and pharmacological treatment. Recommended lifestyle modifications are summarized in Table 50–1. Although physicians report making routine use of nonpharmacological therapies (lifestyle modifications) for hypertension,[1] many commonly use pharmacological management as initial treatment of hypertension. Lifestyle modification is the foundation for the management of hypertension and it is often overlooked. There are many links between fitness, physical exercise, blood pressure, and hypertension. Acute exercise increases blood pressure, heart rate, and cardiac output, whereas hemodynamic data on the chronic effects of aerobic exercise on blood pressure are somewhat conflicting. Whereas some studies of exercise in hypertensive patients have shown decreases in cardiac output,[2] others have shown that the hypotensive effects of training are due to a reduction in systemic vascular resistance[3] with a concomitant rise in stroke volume.

One of the major advances in health care since the late 1980s has been the proliferation of powerful scientific evidence that moderate amounts of physical activity and levels of physical fitness confer improvement in blood pressure control in hypertensive patients and protective benefit against all causes of mortality.[4–9] These investigations clearly and consistently demonstrate that the health benefits of exercise begin to accrue at a significant and measurable level when populations move from being sedentary to being only moderately active. As a result of these data, national guidelines have been proposed and disseminated by the Centers for Disease Control and Prevention (CDC), the American College of Sports Medicine (ACSM) and the National Institutes of Health (NIH) Consensus Development Conference on Physical Activity and Cardiovascular Health providing recommendations for

---

Table 50–1 Recommended Lifestyle Modifications for Hypertension Prevention and Management

Reduce weight; decrease dietary intake of cholesterol and saturated fat

Limit alcohol intake to no more than 1 oz (30 ml) of ethanol (e.g., 24 oz [720 ml] of beer, 10 oz [300 ml] of wine, 2 oz [60 ml] of 100-proof whiskey) per day or 0.5 oz (15 ml) of ethanol per day for women and lighter-weight people

Perform aerobic physical activity (30–45 min for at least 4 days/wk)

Reduce sodium intake to no more than 100 mmol/day (2.4 g of sodium or 6 g of sodium chloride)

Maintain adequate intake of dietary potassium (approximately 90 mmol/day); sources are dates, figs, bananas, avocados

Maintain adequate intake of dietary calcium and magnesium for normal bone and neuromuscular function

Stop smoking

Adapted from Joint National Committee on Prevention, Detection, Evaluation, and Treatment of High Blood Pressure. The sixth report. Arch Intern Med 157:2413–2446, 1997.

Americans about the desired frequency, quantity, and quality of physical activity.[7] The key concept in these recommendations is that individuals should accumulate between 30 and 40 minutes or more of moderately intense physical activity on most, but preferably all, days of the week.[7] The current guidelines differ from previous guidelines in that they pay more attention to the quantity and frequency of prescribed exercise and less attention to the intensity of exercise (VO_2; maximal aerobic capacity, heart rate).

Attention has been drawn recently to findings from three studies showing that cardiorespiratory fitness gains are similar when physical activity occurs in several short sessions (e.g., 10 minutes) to when the same total amount and intensity of activity occurs in one longer session (e.g., 30 minutes).[7, 10–13] Although, strictly speaking, the health benefits of such intermittent activity have not yet been demonstrated, it is reasonable to expect them to be similar to those of continuous activity. Moreover, for people who are unable to set aside 30 minutes for physical activity, shorter episodes are clearly better than none. Indeed, one study has shown greater adherence to a walking program among those walking several times per day than among those walking once per day, when the total amount of walking time was kept the same. For this reason, accumulating physical activity over the course of the day has been included in the recent recommendations from CDC and ACSM.

The most recent report by the Surgeon General[14] (in conjunction with CDC, the U.S. Department of Health and Human Services, and the National Center for Chronic Disease Prevention and Health Promotion) on the effects of physical activity on health and disease concluded that people of all ages, both male and female, undergo beneficial physiological adaptations to physical activity. These effects are summarized in Table 50–2.

The sixth report of the Joint National Committee on Prevention, Detection, Evaluation, and Treatment of High Blood Pressure (JNC VI) states that blood pressure can be lowered with moderately intense physical activity, such as 30 to 45 minutes of brisk walking on most days of the week. The report also states that regular aerobic physical

---

Table 50–2 Effects of Physical Activity on Health and Disease

Decreases mortality for both older and younger adults
Decreases the risk of cardiovascular disease in general (but particularly that of coronary artery disease)
Decreases blood pressure in people with hypertension
Prevents or delays the development of high blood pressure
Decreases risk of colon cancer
Decreases risk of developing diabetes mellitus type II
Benefits many people with arthritis
Helps to achieve and maintain peak bone mass in young adults through weight-bearing physical activity
Preserves the ability to maintain independent living status and reduces the risk of falling in older adults through strength training and other forms of exercise
Affects favorably body fat distribution
Relieves symptoms of depression and anxiety and improves mood
Improves health-related quality of life by enhancing psychological well-being and by improving physical functioning in persons compromised by poor health

---

activity (adequate to achieve at least a moderate level of physical fitness) can enhance weight loss and functional health status and reduce the risk for cardiovascular disease and all-cause mortality.[8, 15] When compared with their more active and fit peers, sedentary individuals with normal blood pressure have a 20 to 50% increased risk of developing hypertension.[16]

Most people can safely increase their level of physical activity without an extensive medical evaluation. Patients with cardiac or other serious health problems need a more thorough evaluation, sometimes including a cardiac stress test, and may need a referral to a specialist or medically supervised program.

HEMODYNAMIC RESPONSE DURING EXERCISE

Dynamic or aerobic (predominantly isotonic) and static (isometric) effort are two major forms of exercise. Insights on the hemodynamics of the acute response to exercise, as well as on the progression of hypertension, can be gained from the study of Lund-Johansen.[17] He followed the hemodynamics of 48 normotensive and 93 hypertensive subjects (World Health Organization, stage 1) of various ages over a 20-year period. The acute responses were obtained when the subjects performed periods of 50-, 100-, and 150-W steady-state exercise. When he compared the resting data from a cross-sectional perspective, the younger hypertensives (<40 years) had a profile of higher cardiac outputs with normal peripheral vascular resistance; the older hypertensives had higher cardiac outputs and higher peripheral vascular resistance. During exercise, the younger hypertensives exhibited lower cardiac outputs than their normotensive controls, which were attributed to a reduced stroke volume caused by decreased ventricular compliance. When these subjects were examined after 10 years, the resting and exercise blood pressure had increased slightly in the hypertensive group, whereas their indices for stroke volume and cardiac output had decreased by approximately 15% and their peripheral vascular resistance values increased by 20%. Because most of the hypertensive patients over 40 years of age were on medication, the investigators withdrew the drugs for 1 week before making the 20-year follow-up measurements. At that time, there was an increase in peripheral vascular resistance that was present both at rest and during steady-state exercise. Resting and exercise heart rate, cardiac index, and stroke index were markedly reduced, the latter two indices by approximately 20% compared with previous results. These data allowed for longitudinal and cross-sectional comparisons between younger and older hypertensive subjects, showing that aging significantly increased systolic blood pressure and peripheral vascular resistance and markedly reduced cardiac output.

There is a physiological increase in cardiac output and a decrease in systemic vascular resistance when hypertensive patients perform dynamic (isotonic) bicycle or treadmill exercise, as occurs in normal subjects. In patients with sustained essential hypertension, however, systemic vascular resistance remains higher than in normotensive control subjects at comparable levels of activity[18–20] and at maximal effort. The response of cardiac output is more variable. Whereas the exercise-induced increase in cardiac output was similar in hypertensives and normotensives in some studies or subgroups,[20, 21] the cardiac output response was less in some studies and in some subgroups of patients,[19, 21] probably related to differences in age, blood pressure, or other characteristics of the selected populations. Differences in cardiac output in response to exercise appear to be related to differences in stroke volume but not in heart rate.[19] Some studies have also demonstrated that repetitive isotonic exercise lowers blood pressure by decreasing sympathetic activity.[22] Table 50–3 summarizes the hemodynamic responses to dynamic exercise in normal male subjects and untreated, trained male borderline hypertensives. Studies in laboratory animals have shown a decrease in catecholamine production with chronic exercise that would, at least in part, account for a decrease in blood pressure.[23–25]

PHYSICAL ACTIVITY AND FITNESS

After regularly repeated aerobic (isotonic) exercise, the resting blood pressure is usually lowered. Although most studies on exercise and blood pressure have design faults, they almost uniformly show a reduction of 5 to 7 mm Hg for both systolic and diastolic blood pressure, independent of weight loss.[26] The validity of these overwhelmingly positive findings is supported by the significant association between the degree of fall in systolic pressure and the change in exercise capacity of both hypertensive and normotensive subjects.[27] An inverse relationship between blood pressure and regular physical activity has been demonstrated by both questionnaire and interview data[28, 29] and measured physical fitness.[30, 31] In addition, exercise[32] and fitness[33] are inversely related to the later development of hypertension. Elderly normotensives and hypertensives also experience a blood pressure–lowering effect from physical activity.[34, 35] In addition to the reduction of resting blood pressure, the degree of rise in blood pressure during exercise is blunted after regular physical training.[36, 37] Immediately after strenuous dynamic exercise, vasodilatation persists,[38] and the systolic blood pressure remains well below the preexercise level for a period that may be as long as 13 hours.[39] After enough repetitive exercise to reach a "conditioned state," resting and ambulatory blood pressure and heart rate usually are lower.[40] These lasting effects reflect a number of changes, including an increase in arterial compliance,[41] a decrease in sympathetic activity coupled with favorable changes in the baroreflex,[22] a decrease in activity of the endogenous Na^+-K^+ pump inhibitor,[42] and an improved glucose/insulin relationship.

One of the emerging concepts that links hypertension and type II diabetes mellitus is *Syndrome X*.[43, 44] This syndrome is defined as a common and underdiagnosed metabolic condition of insulin resistance that results in high blood pressure, glucose intolerance, hyperlipidemia, and central obesity. Exercise and physical activity improve the glucose/insulin relationship by increasing the glucose transporter level in muscle, thus increasing glucose utilization independent of insulin action,[45] increasing insulin sensitivity, and reducing insulin secretion.[46] Since hyperinsulinemia has a prohypertensive effect, regular physical activity may improve blood pressure as well as glycemic control in diabetic patients and in those with glucose intolerance. In a meta-analysis of controlled training studies, dynamic aerobic training resulted in weighted net changes in blood pressure of $-3/-3$ mm Hg in normotensives, $-6/-7$ mm Hg in borderline hypertensives, and $-10/-8$ mm Hg in hypertensives.[47]

ISOMETRIC EXERCISE/STRENGTH TRAINING

In normotensive subjects, strength training has been shown not to change blood pressure.[48] Despite reflex-mediated vasoconstriction during isometric exercise,[49] a fall in resting blood pressure has been observed after repetitive training using isometric contractions from 30 to 50% of maximal capacity.[50] For many years, physicians have advised hypertensive-prone or hypertensive populations not to perform static or weight-lifting activities. This has been a prudent recommendation because direct blood pressure measurements in humans have demonstrated that weight-lifting activities can elicit systolic blood pressure in excess of 200 mm Hg in normotensive subjects. More recent studies, however, have demonstrated that circuit weight training can be beneficial in hypertensive patients.[51–55] Better results follow circuit weight training involving aerobic effects by a continuing series of repetitive moderate weight lifts.[51]

Table 50–3 Hemodynamics in Unmedicated Males During Dynamic Exercise in Normal and Trained Borderline Hypertensives

	Normal*	Hypertensives*	Mechanism to Explain Difference
Heart rate	↑	↑↑	Greater adrenergic response and higher arteriovenous oxygen difference
Stroke volume	↑↑	↑	Progressively falls with age, leading to submaximal cardiac output
Cardiac index	↑↑	↑	As above
Total peripheral resistance	↓	↑↑	Higher at all ages and at all levels of work
Blood pressure	↑	↑↑	Resting blood pressure is lowered and the magnitude of the rise can be blunted with training
Arteriovenous oxygen	↑	↑↑	"Safety mechanism" for hypertensives to meet oxygen demand from skeletal muscle

*↑, slight increase; ↑↑, significant rise; ↓, slight decrease; ↓↓, marked reduction.

HYPERTENSION AND AMBULATORY BLOOD PRESSURE MONITORING

Noninvasive ambulatory blood pressure monitoring (ABPM) allows a 24-hour study of the effect of training on blood pressure. Most studies of ABPM have demonstrated that blood pressure measured during sleep does not change significantly in response to dynamic aerobic training. One study, however, demonstrated that when combined with caloric intake restriction, regular vigorous exercise exhibits a synergistic effect in reducing ambulatory blood pressure throughout a 24-hour period.[56] In borderline hypertensive subjects, studies have shown that daytime ambulatory blood pressure averaged 141/89 mm Hg in the unfit state and 136/81 mm Hg in the fit state.[57] Studies by Seals and Reiling[2] found that the lower systolic blood pressure observed after 12 months of training was entirely due to a decrease in daytime blood pressure from 142 to 135 mm Hg. In this study, ambulatory pressure was not altered after the first 6-month period, during which the patients exercised at a lower intensity. A more recent study demonstrated that the measurement of systolic and diastolic "load" (the percentage of pressures > 140/90 mm Hg during daytime hours and > 120/80 mm Hg during sleep) may be more sensitive than average systolic and diastolic blood pressure for the detection of 24-hour ambulatory blood pressure changes with exercise in borderline hypertension.[58]

HYPERTENSION AND EXERCISE PRESCRIPTION

Increased physical activity can benefit almost everyone. Since a large proportion of Americans have sedentary lifestyles (only 22% of adults in the United States engage regularly, five times a week for at least 30 minutes, in sustained physical activity of any intensity during leisure time),[14] exercise counseling should be a part of routine management of hypertension and health maintenance. Physicians need to provide patients with information about the specific benefits of exercise and motivate them to increase their physical activity. Physicians should encourage all adults to accumulate 30 to 45 minutes or more of moderately intense physical activity on most days of the week. Most high-risk adults (e.g., those with coronary artery disease [CAD], angina, acute congestive heart failure, or atrial or ventricular arrhythmias) require a complete history and physical examination, a cardiac stress test, and probably a subspecialist and a medically supervised program referral, but most hypertensive patients without other comorbid risk factors can safely start or increase their level of physical activity without an extensive medical evaluation.

Exercise testing (ET) has been employed for many years in the diagnosis, prognosis (i.e., predicting the likelihood that an individual with labile hypertension will go on to develop persistent, fixed hypertension), and treatment of hypertension.[59, 60] Controversy is substantial regarding the usefulness of ET in predicting future blood pressure.[61] However, abnormal systolic and/or diastolic responses during testing may be harbingers of underlying ischemic cardiomyopathy.[62, 63] Intraexercise and/or postexercise arrhythmia can be provoked with ET. Thus, ET should not be performed in persons with severe uncontrolled hypertension.

Use of ET in the screening before initiating exercise programs is a complex and important issue. The American College of Cardiology/American Heart Association[64] has considered the use of ET to be controversial, whereas ACSM has taken a more definitive stance.[12] The ACSM[12] recommends that high-risk persons submit to ET *before vigorous exercise* (not leisure walking). Such individuals include men over age 40 years and women over age 50, persons with more than one CAD risk factor, and especially those with known CAD. The Consensus Conference on Physical Activity and Cardiovascular Disease held at NIH[13] in December 1995 addressed the subject of ET before exercise training principally in relation to predicting CAD, not in relation to hypertension per se. The existing data indicate that a positive ET identifies persons who have hemodynamically significant coronary lesions but that routine ET is not effective in preventing acute coronary events even in high-risk populations, i.e., persons with a very high low-density lipoprotein cholesterol.[65] However, because hypertension and CAD often coexist, and since exercise-related alterations in blood pressure—i.e., a fall in systolic or a rise of greater than 10 mm Hg in diastolic pressure—can be associated with underlying occult coronary disease, there is justification for ET in patients with hypertension who want to undertake *vigorous* aerobic or resistance exercise.

A formal exercise prescription should include specific advice about the frequency, intensity, mode (type), duration (time), and progression of physical activity. It should also include a warm-up or stretching period and a cool-down or readjustment period. Once an exercise program has begun, injury prevention, compliance, and adherence to the program become important. Physical activity should include aerobic or cardiovascular endurance exercises (e.g., walking, bicycling, power or brisk walking, jogging, swimming, or treadmill). Frequency of exercise should begin at 3 to 4 times per week, but should progress to at least 5, if not all, days of the week. Duration of exercise should begin at 15 to 20 minutes daily, but should progress to at least 30 to 45 minutes daily. Intensity of exercise should begin at a comfortably paced walking program and progress to brisk or power walking or jogging. Another way to measure intensity is to calculate individual's target heart rate. All exercise programs should be adjusted or tailored for each individual patient and should include a warm-up and a cool-down period to prevent or reduce the risk of injuries. Individuals who are about to begin an exercise program should be advised to wear footgear with good traction to help prevent falls and cushioning to help prevent excessive wear on joints and injuries.

INTERACTIONS OF ANTIHYPERTENSIVE DRUGS WITH EXERCISE

Although dynamic physical activity may lower blood pressure in young or old[66, 67] and mild or borderline hypertensives,[66] even without weight loss,[66] the change is moderate

(5 to 10 mm Hg) and usually does not bring the blood pressure into the normal range. Thus, drug therapy must be considered as the standard form of antihypertensive treatment. Basically, no drug therapy is contraindicated in the mentally competent young or old hypertensive patient who wishes to exercise. Exercise is no contraindication to the administration of β-blockers to the patient with hypertension and CAD.[68] Training, using a scale of perceived exertion, can be accomplished under the influence of β-blockers, preferably β₁-selective antagonists.[69, 70] Similarly, the mental drive to succeed in the adolescent or young hypertensive adult can overcome any blunting of the exercise response observed with a β-antagonist.[71] Central α-agonists lower catecholamines[72, 73] but do not block their action at skeletal muscle receptor sites, the raison d'être, in part, for the muscle fatigue produced by β-blockade.

Diuretics

Diuretics are widely used antihypertensives. Their actions during exercise may vary.[74] Thiazides cause a drop in exercise blood pressure by decreasing peripheral resistance and plasma volume. The effects of loop diuretics on exercise blood pressure have not been well studied.

With any diuretic therapy, hypokalemia can become significant, resulting in moderate ST segment depression, cardiac irritability, and skeletal muscle fatigue. Skeletal muscle blood flow is in part dependent on normokalemia, indicating that total body potassium is not depleted. To ensure against potassium loss, patients on diuretics should receive potassium supplements and magnesium replacement, if deficient. Thus, diuretics result in a moderate decrease in the blood pressure response to exercise and, with adequate potassium supplementation, should not provoke any drug-related risks during physical activity.

Central α-Agonists

Guanfacine, guanabenz, clonidine, and α-methyldopa (methyldopa) decrease central and/or peripheral outflow of catecholamines. This results in reductions of plasma norepinephrine at rest and during exercise.[72, 75] All of these drugs can blunt the sympathetic response during exercise, but they have significantly different hemodynamic effects. In mild hypertensives, methyldopa, used less in the United States today than elsewhere, may decrease the blood pressure and heart rate responses to exercise.[76] Total peripheral resistance and cardiac output may[77] or may not[78] decrease. Clonidine differs from methyldopa in that it reduces blood pressure and heart rate at rest as well as during exercise.[73, 79] Central vagal stimulation results in decreased heart rate and cardiac output.[80] However, this is not considered a negative inotropic property, since cardiac output is normalized after chronic use. In contrast to clonidine, guanabenz does not decrease heart rate or cardiac output at rest or during dynamic exercise. Clonidine and methyldopa do not affect the changes in serum potassium, renin, and aldosterone that are normally observed in exercising healthy persons[72, 73, 81] or in those on β-blockers. No significant ST-T-wave changes occur during exercise in individuals using these drugs. The rise in diastolic blood pressure induced by isometric activity may be decreased with clonidine or methyldopa as long as resting blood pressure has been reduced.

β-Blockers

The most important effect of β-adrenergic blocking drugs is that cardiac output is reduced during exercise without any peripheral vascular effect because myocardial contractility and heart rate are reduced. Both of these effects prolong diastole, which allows for better coronary perfusion. This is an advantage for patients with CAD who are undergoing cardiac rehabilitation. With β-blockade, many such patients can exercise longer with less angina and fewer incidents of ST segment depression.[82] In patients with ischemic heart disease on propranolol, physical training can result in up to a 31% improvement in exercise capacity.[68, 83] Even the elderly and patients with atrial fibrillation can achieve a significant training effect while taking β-blocking drugs.[68] There is variability among β-blockers in their effects on heart rate and blood pressure during exercise.[84] Cardioselective β-blockers appear to be more effective than nonselective agents in blunting the exercise-induced increase in systolic blood pressure.

Propranolol and the cardioselective β-blockers atenolol and metoprolol have been studied in exercising normal volunteers. Heart rate and systolic blood pressure were reduced at maximal exercise,[72, 85] but there were no significant changes in diastolic blood pressure, Vo₂ or anaerobic threshold (that point at which oxygen consumption fails to increase in proportion to minute ventilation).[72, 85] This indicates that blood flow to the active muscles was unaltered.

Isometric exercise, such as trying to lift a heavy load that will not move, is known to increase both systolic and diastolic blood pressure. Antihypertensive therapy may decrease this response in persons with cardiovascular disease.[86] However, in patients with borderline hypertensive heart failure, metoprolol, with or without prazosin, did not abolish dangerous increases in blood pressure during isometric activity.[87–90]

The metabolic effects of β-blockade during exercise include an increase in serum potassium greater than that seen during dynamic exercise alone. Renin is decreased,[72] but plasma aldosterone does not appear to change. In contrast to the central α-agonists, which decrease plasma catecholamines, atenolol, propranolol, and metoprolol either increase resting plasma norepinephrine[91] or permit normal exercise-induced increases to occur. However, the response at the receptor level is blocked, thereby potentiating a greater rise in serum potassium than that seen with placebo, central α-agonists, calcium channel blockers, or angiotensin-converting enzyme inhibitors. Although β-blockade increases endurance in cardiac patients, it causes exercise fatigue in most individuals.[92] This appears to be due to substrate limitation-decreased blood levels of glucose, nonesterified fatty acids, and glycerol. Muscle glycogenolysis, a β₂-adrenoreceptor–mediated process, probably also decreases.

Neither propranolol nor metoprolol decreases the ventilatory response to CO_2 during physical activity.[93] This may be significant in the management of patients with chronic obstructive pulmonary disease in whom these drugs will not worsen CO_2 retention. In normal volunteers, a single dose of propranolol reduced Vo_2 at both submaximal and maximal effort.[94] Despite these metabolic and circulatory changes reported with β-blockade, Vo_{2max} increases with aerobic exercise, especially with β-selective drugs (atenolol, metoprolol, and betaxolol), and an overall training effect can be obtained.[68, 70, 95]

Plasma levels of both propranolol and acebutolol increase during exercise. This may be related to pH changes or to decreased hepatic blood flow during activity, which would affect those drugs with a high hepatic extraction ratio.

Vasodilators

The vasodilators, including hydralazine, minoxidil, prazosin, terazosin, doxazosin, and the calcium channel blockers, are used commonly in the treatment of hypertension. In normal volunteers, hydralazine decreases arterial blood pressure, with a resultant reflex tachycardia. This tends to increase cardiac output through an increase in sympathetic drive, which in a compromised heart, may lead to myocardial ischemia with angina and/or infarction.[96] However, hydralazine is useful as an afterload reducer in chronic heart failure patients.[97]

Prazosin is more of an atypical α-antagonist than a direct-acting vasodilator. It decreases mean arterial blood pressure and total peripheral resistance at rest and with dynamic work.[54, 98] In contrast to hydralazine, there is no reflex increase in heart rate or pressor response.[54, 99] During isometric activity, hydralazine neither improves skeletal muscle oxygen delivery in patients with heart failure[100] nor attenuates increases in sympathetic activity.[54, 87]

In heart failure patients, vasodilators are of interest during exercise. While increasing cardiac output by reducing afterload, hydralazine reduces both arterial and pulmonary wedge pressure and increases stroke volume. However, exercise tolerance appears not to improve unless nitrates are given concomitantly.[100] The vasodilator effect of hydralazine does not add to that of local metabolites.[100] There is a normal hemodynamic response to dynamic exercise with terazosin, prazosin, nifedipine, verapamil, and diltiazem. Pressor responses to controlled hand-grip are blunted by vasodilators, as long as a reduction in resting blood pressure is obtained.

Angiotensin-Converting Enzyme Inhibitors and Angiotensin II Receptor Antagonists

The effects of captopril on dynamic exercise have been studied extensively and the results differ among studies. Pickering and colleagues[101] found no changes in blood pressure or heart rate in subjects given captopril during graded treadmill exercise. Another study demonstrated significant reductions in systolic and diastolic pressures in response to captopril that were more pronounced during physical activity than at rest.[102, 103] Enalapril alone or with hydrochlorothiazide lowers blood pressure but permits an adequate cardiac response to dynamic exercise.[104] Saralasin, a partial antagonist of angiotensin II, has been shown to decrease blood pressure during dynamic exercise.[105] These findings suggest that angiotensin II is not a major determinant of blood pressure regulation during exercise in hypertensive patients. In fact, angiotensin-converting enzyme inhibition does not suppress the plasma angiotensin II increase during exercise in humans, nor does it influence the development of microalbuminuria with prolonged physical activity. This has significance in the management of the diabetic who has proteinuria, a manifestation of nephropathy.[106]

The effects of captopril on catecholamines, renin activity, angiotensin II levels, and plasma aldosterone during dynamic exercise have been studied, with somewhat conflicting results. After 4 or 5 days of high-dose captopril, both angiotensin II and plasma aldosterone levels were reduced significantly in patients at rest and during physical activity in one study.[102] In contrast, in another study, plasma renin activity increased over placebo both at baseline and at peak exercise during captopril administration, but the concentrations of norepinephrine and epinephrine remained unchanged.[106] Nonetheless, neither angiotensin-converting enzyme inhibitors nor angiotensin II receptor blockers, e.g., losartan, valsartan, limit dynamic exercise in hypertensive patients[107] and can blunt the pressor effects of mental stress.[108]

Calcium Antagonists

Calcium antagonists have been reported to reduce both systolic and diastolic blood pressure during exercise in hypertensive patients,[109, 110] probably by reducing systemic vascular resistance,[109–111] although cardiac and peripheral vascular mechanisms in tandem may explain the fall in blood pressure during exercise.[112] In normotensive, active volunteers, nifedipine and verapamil had little effect on systolic and diastolic blood pressure at rest and during treadmill exercise. Verapamil has been reported to have a slight blunting effect on diastolic blood pressure increases during isometric exercise.[113] Chronic treatment with long-acting calcium antagonists (i.e., isradipine and amlodipine) has been shown to lower blood pressure at rest and during exercise because of a reduction in systemic vascular resistance, a mechanism shared by all calcium antagonists.[114, 115]

Randomized clinical trials in progress with long-acting calcium antagonists in the treatment of hypertension will determine whether the problems of coronary ischemia and mortality seen with short-acting (immediate-release) formulations exist with the long-acting drugs.[116, 117] Nonetheless, based on the JNC VI report, long-acting calcium antagonists are recommended as antihypertensives for several specific indications.[116, 118]

SUMMARY

Epidemiological studies suggest an inverse relationship between physical activity or fitness and blood pressure. Regular aerobic exercise has been shown to reduce blood pressure by $-6/-7$ mm Hg in borderline hypertensives and by $-10/-8$ mm Hg in hypertensives. Reductions in blood pressure have also been observed during exercise and during daytime ABPM in physically active individuals. Regular aerobic exercise has also been shown to reduce the risk of cardiovascular disease and all-cause mortality. For this reason, JNC VI[118] recommended regular, moderately intense physical activity, including regular aerobic exercise, such as 30 to 45 minutes of brisk walking most days of the week, not only to improve blood pressure control but also to reduce the risk for cardiovascular disease and all-cause mortality. Antihypertensive treatment should include an exercise prescription for all hypertensive patients. Unfortunately, this is often overlooked.

References

1. Arroll B, Jenkins S, North D. Non-pharmacological management of hypertension: Results from interviews with 100 general practitioners. J Hypertens 14:773–777, 1996.
2. Seals D, Reiling M. Effect of regular exercise on 24-hour arterial pressure in older hypertensive humans. Hypertension 18:583–592, 1991.
3. Nelson L, Jennings G, Esler M, et al. Effect of changing levels of physical activity on blood-pressure and haemodynamics in essential hypertension. Lancet 2:473–476, 1986.
4. Lee I, Paffenbarger R, Hennekens C. Physical activity, physical fitness and longevity. Aging Clin Exp Res 9:2–11, 1997.
5. Tanaka H, Bassett D, Howley E, et al. Swimming training lowers the resting blood pressure in individuals with hypertension. J Hypertens 15:651–657, 1997.
6. Seals D, Silverman H, Reiling M, et al. Effects of regular aerobic exercise on elevated blood pressure in postmenopausal women. Am J Cardiol 80:49–55, 1997.
7. Pate R, Pratt M, Blair S, et al. Physical activity and public health—A recommendation from the Centers for Disease Control and Prevention and the American College of Sports Medicine. JAMA 273:402–407, 1995.
8. Paffenbarger R, Hyde R, Wing A, et al. The association of changes in physical-activity level and other lifestyle characteristics with mortality among men. N Engl J Med 328:538–545, 1993.
9. Blair S, Kohl H, Barlow C, et al. Physical fitness and all-cause mortality. JAMA 273:1093–1098, 1995.
10. Debusk RF, Stenestrand V, Sheehan M, et al. Training effects of long vs short bouts of exercise in healthy subjects. Am J Cardiol 65:1010–1013, 1990.
11. NIH Consensus Development Panel on Physical Activity and Cardiovascular Health. Physical Activity and Cardiovascular Health. JAMA 276:241–246, 1996.
12. American College of Sports Medicine. Position stand on the recommended quantity and quality of exercise for developing and maintaining cardiorespiratory and muscular fitness, and flexibility in healthy adults. Med Sci Sports Exerc 30:975–991, 1998.
13. Leon AS (ed). Physical Activity and Cardiovascular Health. A National Consensus. National Institutes of Health. Champaign, IL, Human Kinetics 1997.
14. U.S. Department of Health and Human Services. Physical activity and health. A report of the Surgeon General—Executive summary. Pittsburgh, Superintendent of Documents, 1996.
15. Kokkinos P, Narayan P, Colleran J, et al. Effects of regular exercise on blood pressure and left ventricular hypertrophy in African-American men with severe hypertension. N Engl J Med 333:1462–1467, 1995.
16. Blair S, Goodyear N, Gibbons L, et al. Physical fitness and incidence of hypertension in healthy normotensive men and women. JAMA 252:487–490, 1984.
17. Lund-Johansen P. Central haemodynamics in essential hypertension at rest and during exercise—A 20-year follow-up study. J Hypertens 7(suppl 6):S52–S55, 1989.
18. Miller D, Ruddy T, Zusman R, et al. Left ventricular ejection fraction response during exercise in asymptomatic systemic hypertension. Am J Cardiol 59:409, 1987.
19. Montain S, Jilka S, Ehsani A, et al. Altered hemodynamics during exercise in older essential hypertensive subjects. Hypertension 12:479, 1988.
20. Tochikubo O, Ishii M, Minamisawa K, et al. Fully automatic, noninvasive measurement of cardiac output by means of the CO_2 rebreathing method and its clinical application to hypertensive patients. Jpn Heart J 31:461, 1990.
21. Amery A, Julius S, Whitlock L, et al. Influence of hypertension on the hemodynamic response to exercise. Circulation 36:231, 1967.
22. Kingwell B, Dart A, Jennings G, et al. Exercise training reduces the sympathetic component of the blood pressure–heart rate baroreflex in man. Clin Sci 82:357–362, 1992.
23. Scarpace N, Lowenthal D. Sympathetic nervous system: Aging and exercise. South Med J 87(suppl):S42–S46, 1994.
24. Tumer N, Hale C, Lawler J, et al. Modulation of tyrosine hydroxylase gene expression in the rat adrenal gland by exercise: Effects of age. Mol Brain Res 14:51–56, 1992.
25. Tumer N, LaRochelle J, Yurekli M. Exercise training reverses the age-related decline in tyrosine hydroxylase expression in rat hypothalamus. J Gerontol 52A:B255–B259, 1997.
26. Arroll B, Beaglehole R. Does physical activity lower blood pressure? A critical review of the clinical trials. J Clin Epidemiol 45:439–447, 1992.
27. Fagard R, Bielen E, Hespel P, et al. Physical exercise in hypertension. In Brenner B, Laragh J (eds). Hypertension: Pathophysiology, Diagnosis and Management. New York, Raven, 1990; pp 1985–1998.
28. Folsom A, Caspersen C, Taylor H, et al. Leisure time physical activity and its relationship to coronary risk factors in a population-based sample. The Minnesota Heart Survey. Am J Epidemiol 121:570–579, 1985.
29. Reaven P, Barrett-Connor E, Edelstein S. Relation between leisure-time physical activity and blood pressure in older women. Circulation 83:559–565, 1991.
30. Cooper K, Pollock, Martin R, et al. Physical fitness levels vs selected coronary risk factors. A cross-sectional study. JAMA 236:166–169, 1976.
31. Hartung G, Kohl H, Blair S, et al. Exercise tolerance and alcohol intake. Blood pressure relation. Hypertension 16:501–507, 1990.
32. Paffenbarger R, Wing A, Hyde R, et al. Physical activity and incidence of hypertension in college alumni. Am J Epidemiol 117:245–257, 1983.
33. Blair S, Goodyear N, Gibbons L, et al. Physical fitness and incidence of hypertension in healthy normotensive men and women. JAMA 252:487–490, 1984.
34. Reaven P, Barrett-Connor E, Edelstein S. Relation between leisure-time physical activity and blood pressure in older women. Circulation 83:559–565, 1991.
35. Braith R, Pollock M, Lowenthal D, et al. Moderate- and high-intensity exercise lowers blood pressure in normotensive subjects 60 to 79 years of age. Am J Cardiol 73:1124–1128, 1994.
36. World Hypertension League. Physical exercise in the management of hypertension. J Hypertens 9:283–287, 1991.
37. Kaplan N. Treatment of hypertension: Nondrug therapy. In Retford D (ed). Clinical Hypertension, 6th ed. Baltimore, Williams & Wilkins, 1994; pp 171–189.
38. Cleroux J, Kouame N, Nadeau A, et al. Aftereffects of exercise on regional and systemic hemodynamics in hypertension. Hypertension 19:183–191, 1992.
39. Pescatello L, Fargo A, Leach C Jr, et al. Short-term effect of dynamic exercise on arterial blood pressure. Circulation 83:1557–1561, 1991.
40. Somers V, Conway J, Johnston J, et al. Effects of endurance training on baroreflex sensitivity and blood pressure in borderline hypertension. Lancet 337:1363–1368, 1991.
41. Cameron J, Dart A, Topham S. Effects of 4 weeks exercise training on arterial compliance in man. [Abstract] Circulation 86(suppl 1):276, 1992.
42. Koga M, Ideishi M, Matsusaki M, et al. Mild exercise decreases plasma endogenous digitalis-like substance in hypertensive individuals. Hypertension 19(suppl 2):231–236, 1992.
43. Reaven G. Insulin resistance, hyperinsulinemia and hypertriglyceridemia in the etiology and clinical course of hypertension. Am J Med 90(suppl 2A):75–125, 1991.

44. Kaplan N. The deadly quartet: Upper-body obesity, glucose intolerance, hypertriglyceridemia, and hypertension. Arch Intern Med 149:1514–1520, 1989.

45. Wasserman D, Geer R, Rice D, et al. Interaction of exercise and insulin action in humans. Am J Physiol 260:E37–E45, 1991.

46. DeFronzo R, Sherwin R, Kraemer N. Effect of physical training on insulin action in obesity. Diabetes 36:1379–1385, 1987.

47. Fagard R, Amery A. Physical exercise in hypertension. *In* Laragh J, Brenner B (eds). Hypertension: Pathophysiology, Diagnosis and Management, 2nd ed, vol 2. New York, Raven, 1995; pp 2669–2679.

48. Coconie C, Graves J, Pollock M, et al. Effect of exercise training on blood pressure in 70- to 79-yr-old men and women. Med Sci Sports Exerc 23:505–511, 1991.

49. Perez-Gonzalez J. Factors determining the blood pressure responses to isometric exercise. Circ Res 48(suppl 1):76–86, 1981.

50. Wiley R, Dunn C, Cox R, et al. Isometric exercise training lowers resting blood pressure. Med Sci Sports Exerc 24:749–754, 1992.

51. Stewart K. Weight training in coronary artery disease and hypertension. Prog Cardiovasc Dis 35:159–168, 1992.

52. Harris K, Holly R. Physiological responses to circuit weight training in borderline hypertensive subjects. Med Sci Sports Exerc 19:246–252, 1987.

53. Klemen M. Resistive training safety and assessment guidelines for cardiac and coronary prone patients. Med Sci Sports Exerc 21:675–677, 1989.

54. Goldbert A. Aerobic and resistive exercise modify risk factors for coronary heart disease. Med Sci Sports Exerc 21:669–674, 1989.

55. Lowenthal D, Dickerman D, Saris S, et al. The effect of pharmacologic interaction on central and peripheral alpha-receptors and pressor response to static exercise. Ann Sports Med 1:100–104, 1983.

56. Cox K, Puddey I, Morton A, et al. Exercise and weight control in sedentary overweight men: Effects on clinic and ambulatory blood pressure. J Hypertens 14:779–790, 1996.

57. Somers V, Conway J, Johnston J, et al. Effects of endurance training on baroreflex sensitivity and blood pressure in borderline hypertension. Lancet 337:1363–1368, 1991.

58. Wallace J, Bogle P, King B, et al. A comparison of 24-h average blood pressures and blood pressure load following exercise. Am J Hypertens 10:728–734, 1997.

59. Fagard R, Staessen J, Thijs L, et al. Prognostic significance of exercise versus resting blood pressure in hypertensive men. Hypertension 17:574–578, 1991.

60. Fixler DE, Laird WP, Dana K. Usefulness of exercise stress testing for prediction of blood pressure trends. Pediatrics 75:1071–1075, 1985.

61. Majahalme S, Turjanman V, Muomisto M, et al. Blood pressure responses to exercise as predictors of blood pressure level after 5 years. Am J Hypertens 10:106–116, 1997.

62. Sheps DS, Ernst JC, Briese FW, et al. Exercise-induced increase in diastolic pressure: Indicator of severe coronary artery disease. Am J Cardiol 43:708–712, 1979.

63. Hakki AH, Munley BM, Hadjimiltiades S, et al. Determinants of abnormal blood pressure response to exercise in coronary artery disease. Am J Cardiol 57:71–75, 1986.

64. Schlant RC, Blomqvist CG, Brandenberg RO, et al. Guidelines for exercise testing: A report of the Joint American College of Cardiology/American Heart Association Task Force on Assessment of Cardiovascular Procedures (Subcommittee on Exercise Testing). Circulation 74:653A–667A, 1986.

65. Siscovick DS, Ekelund LG, Johnson JL, et al. Sensitivity of exercise electrocardiography for acute cardiac events during moderate and strenuous physical activity: The Lip Research Clinics Coronary Primary Prevention Trial. Arch Intern Med 151:325–330, 1991.

66. Choquette G, Ferguson R. Blood pressures reduction in borderline hypertensives following physical training. Can Med Assoc J 108:699–703, 1973.

67. Hagberg J, Graves J, Limacher M, et al. Cardiovascular responses of 70–79 year old men and women to exercise training. J Appl Physiol 66:2589–2594, 1989.

68. Hare T, Lowenthal D, Hakki H, et al. Demonstration of training effect in elderly patients with coronary artery disease receiving beta adrenergic blocking drugs. Ann Sports Med 2:36–40, 1984.

69. Gordon N, Kruger P, van Rensburg J, et al. Effect of β-adrenoceptor blockade on thermoregulation during prolonged exercise. J Appl Physiol 58:899–906, 1985.

70. Gordon N, van Rensburg J, Russell H, et al. Effect of beta$_1$ selective adrenoceptor blockage on physiological response to exercise. Br Heart J 54:96–99, 1985.

71. Falkner B, Lowenthal D, Affrime M. The pharmacodynamic effectiveness of metoprolol in adolescent hypertension. J Pediatr Pharmacol 2:49–55, 1982.

72. Lowenthal D, Affrime M, Falkner B, et al. Potassium disposition and neuroendocrine effects of propranolol, methyldopa and clonidine during dynamic exercise. Clin Exp Hypertens [A] 4:1895–1911, 1982.

73. Lowenthal D, Affrime M, Rosenthal L, et al. Dynamic and biochemical responses to single and multiple dose clonidine during dynamic physical activity. Clin Pharmacol Ther 32:18–24, 1982.

74. Lund-Johansen P. Hemodynamic changes in long-term diuretic therapy of essential hypertension. A comparative study of chlorthalidone, polythiazide and hydrochlorothiazide. Acta Med Scand 1987:509–518, 1970.

75. Virtanen J, Janne J, Frick M. Response of blood pressure and plasma norepinephrine to propranolol, metoprolol and clonidine during isometric and dynamic exercise. Eur J Clin Pharmacol 21:275–279, 1982.

76. Sannerstedt R, Varnanses E, Werko L. Hemodynamic effects of methyldopa (Aldomet) at rest and during exercise in patients with arterial hypertension. Acta Med Scand 171:75–82, 1962.

77. Lund-Johansen P. Hemodynamic changes in long-term alpha methyldopa therapy of essential hypertension. Acta Med Scand 192:221–226, 1972.

78. Chamberlain D, Howard J. Guanethidine and methyldopa: A haemodynamic study. Br Heart J 26:528–536, 1964.

79. Lund-Johansen P. Hemodynamic changes at rest and during exercise in long-term clonidine therapy of essential hypertension. Acta Med Scand 195:111–117, 1974.

80. Onesti G, Schwartz A, Kim K, et al. Antihypertensive effect of clonidine. Circ Res 28(suppl 2):53–69, 1971.

81. Rosenthal L, Affrime M, Lowenthal D, et al. Biochemical and dynamic responses to single and repeated doses of methyldopa and propranolol during dynamic physical activity. Clin Pharmacol Ther 32:701–710, 1982.

82. Ellestad M. Stress Testing. Principles and Practice, 3rd ed. Philadelphia, FA Davis, 1986.

83. Pratt C, Welton D, Squires W, et al. Demonstration of training effect during chronic beta-adrenergic blockade in patients with coronary artery disease. Circulation 64:1125–1129, 1981.

84. Hartzell A, Freund B, Jilka S, et al. The effect of beta-adrenergic blockade on ratings of perceived exertion during submaximal exercise before and following endurance training. J Cardiopulm Rehabil 6:444–456, 1986.

85. Sklar J, Johnston D, Overlie P, et al. The effects of a cardioselective (metoprolol) and a nonselective (propranolol) beta-adrenergic blocker on the response to dynamic exercise in normal men. Circulation 65:894–899, 1982.

86. Lowenthal D, Saris S, Packer J, et al. The mechanisms of action and the clinical pharmacology of beta adrenergic blocking drugs. Am J Med 77(suppl 4A):119–127, 1984.

87. O'Hare J, Murnaghan D. Failure of antihypertensive drugs to control blood pressure rise with isometric exercise in hypertension. Postgrad Med J 57:552–555, 1981.

88. Nelson G, Donnelly G, Hunyor S. Haemodynamic effects of sustained treatment with prazosin and metoprolol, alone and in combination, in borderline hypertensive heart failure. J Cardiovasc Pharmacol 4:240–245, 1982.

89. Hansson B, Dymling J, Manhem P, et al. Long-term treatment of moderate hypertension with the beta$_1$-receptor blocking agent metoprolol. II: Effect of submaximal work and insulin-induced hypoglycemia on plasma catecholamines and renin activity, blood pressure, and pulse rate. Eur J Clin Pharmacol 11:247–254, 1977.

90. Lijnen P, Amery A, Fagard R, et al. The effect of beta-adrenoceptor blockade on renin, angiotensin, aldosterone and catecholamines at rest and during exercise. Br J Clin Pharmacol 7:175–181, 1979.

91. Christensen N, Brandsborg O. The relationship between plasma catecholamine concentration and pulse rate during exercise and standing. Eur J Clin Invest 3:299–306, 1973.

92. Lundborg P, Astrom H, Bengtsson C, et al. Effect of beta-adrenoceptor blockage on exercise performance and metabolism. Clin Sci 61:299–305, 1981.

93. Leitch A, Hopkin J, Ellis D, et al. Failure of propranolol and metoprolol to alter ventilatory responses to carbon dioxide and exercise. Br J Clin Pharmacol 9:493–498, 1980.

94. Twentyman O, Disley A, Gribbin H, et al. Effect of beta adrenergic blockade on respiratory and metabolic responses to exercise. J Appl Physiol 51:788–793, 1981.

95. Pollock M, Lowenthal D, Foster C, et al. Acute and chronic responses to exercise in patients treated with beta blockers. J Cardiopulm Rehabil 11:132–144, 1991.

96. Moyer J. Hydralazine (Apresoline) hydrochloride. Pharmacological observations and clinical results in the therapy of hypertension. Arch Intern Med 91:419–439, 1953.

97. Ginks W, Redwood D. Haemodynamic effects of hydralazine at rest and during exercise in patients with chronic heart failure. Br Heart J 44:259–264, 1980.

98. Lund-Johansen P. Hemodynamic changes at rest and during exercise in long-term prazosin therapy for essential hypertension. Postgraduate Medicine Symposium on Prazosin, November 1975; p 45.

99. Lowenthal D. Hypertension and exercise. In Bove A, Lowenthal D (eds). Exercise Medicine: Physiologic Principles and Clinical Applications. New York, Academic, 1984.

100. Wilson J, Untereker W, Hurshfeld J. Effects of isosorbide dinitrate and hydralazine on regional metabolic responses to arm exercise in patients with heart failure. Am J Cardiol 48:934–938, 1981.

101. Pickering TG, Base DB, Sullivan PA, et al. Comparison of antihypertensive and hormonal effects of captopril and propranolol at rest and during exercise. Am J Cardiol 49:1566–1568, 1982.

102. Manhem P, Bramnert M, Hulthen UL, et al. The effect of captopril on catecholamines, renin activity, angiotensin II and aldosterone in plasma during physical exercise in hypertensive patients. Eur J Clin Invest 11:389–395, 1981.

103. Fagard R, Lijnen P, Amery A. Hemodynamic response to captopril at rest and during exercise in hypertensive patients. Am J Cardiol 49:1569–1571, 1982.

104. Leon AS, McNally C, Casal D, et al. Enalapril alone and combined with hydrochlorothiazide in the treatment of hypertension: Effect on treadmill exercise performance. J Cardiopulm Rehabil 6:251–259, 1986.

105. Fagard R, Amery A, Reybrouck T, et al. Effects of angiotensin antagonism on hemodynamics, renin and catecholamines during exercise. J Appl Physiol 43:440–444, 1977.

106. Aldigier JC, Huang H, Calmay F, et al. Angiotensin converting enzyme inhibition does not suppress plasma angiotensin II increase during exercise in humans. J Cardiovasc Pharmacol 21:289–295, 1993.

107. Lang R, Elkayam U, Yellen L, et al. Comparative effects of losartan and enalapril on exercise capacity and clinical status in patients with heart failure. The Losartan Pilot Exercise Study Investigators. J Am Coll Cardiol 30:983–991, 1997.

108. Paran E, Neumann L, Cristal N, et al. Response to mental and physical stress before and during adrenoreceptor blocker and angiotensin-converting enzyme inhibitor treatment in essential hypertension. Am J Cardiol 68:1362–1366, 1991.

109. Andersen K, Vik-Mo H. Increased left ventricular emptying at maximal exercise after reduction in afterload. Circulation 69:492–496, 1984.

110. Yamakado T, Oonishi N, Kondo S, et al. Effects of diltiazem on cardiovascular responses during exercise in systemic hypertension and comparison with propranolol. Am J Cardiol 52:1023–1027, 1983.

111. Brod J, Fencl V, Hejl Z, et al. General and regional hypertension pattern underlying essential hypertension. Clin Sci 23:339–349, 1962.

112. Silke B, Goldhammer E, Sharma SK, et al. An exercise hemodynamic comparison of verapamil, diltiazem, and amlodipine in coronary artery disease. Cardiovasc Drug Ther 4:457–463, 1990.

113. Stein DT, Lowenthal DT, Porter RS, et al. Effects of nifedipine and verapamil on isometric and dynamic exercise in normal subjects. Am J Cardiol 54:386–389, 1984.

114. Cleroux J, Yardley C, Marshall A, et al. Antihypertensive and hemodynamic effects of calcium channel blockers with isradipine after acute exercise. Am J Hypertens 5:84–87, 1992.

115. Tarazi RC, Dustan HP. Beta-adrenergic blockade in hypertension: Practical and theoretical implications of long-term hemodynamic variations. Am J Cardiol 29:633–640, 1972.

116. Messerli F. Safety of calcium antagonists: Dissecting the evidence. Am J Cardiol 78(suppl 9A):19–23, 1996.

117. Psaty BM, Herkbert SR, Koepsell TD, et al. The risk of myocardial infarction associated with antihypertensive drug therapies. JAMA 274:620–625, 1995.

118. Joint National Committee on Prevention, Detection, Evaluation, and Treatment of High Blood Pressure. The sixth report. Arch Intern Med 157:2413–2446, 1997.

Pharmacological Treatment

CHAPTER 51

Initial Choices in the Treatment of Hypertension

Matthew R. Weir

Despite major advances in our understanding of the pathophysiology of hypertension and its treatment, a substantial conundrum exists in clinical practice: how to balance improved efficacy with enhanced tolerability and thereby improve long-term control rates.

Nonadherence to prescribed therapy is one of the most serious problems that physicians face. Since hypertension is usually an asymptomatic disorder, there is generally no symptomatic improvement in the condition that would merit continued use of a drug. This basic problem, coupled with inadequate education, a poor physician-patient relationship, and a lack of understanding of the pathophysiology of hypertension in a given patient, results in only a 40 to 50% long-term response rate to the major forms of pharmacotherapy currently being used.[1] The problems of nonadherence and poor response rates explain the National Health and Nutrition Examination Survey (NHANES) III (phase 2) findings that only one in four Americans with high blood pressure has satisfactory control, defined as blood pressure reduced to 140/90 mm Hg.[2] Even more concerning is the fact that there has been a subtle erosion in control rates since the NHANES III (phase 1) report was published.[1]

Efforts should be made not only to identify but also to educate hypertensive patients about the need for both hygienic measures and an optimal pharmacologic approach. The latter issue requires careful individualization, not generalization. No two patients are alike. Adverse events are not uncommon and may vary substantially among patients, not only for different drugs but also for different doses of medications. Discussions about initial choices of therapy must be tempered by the understanding that most patients would prefer not to change their lifestyle and would prefer the simplicity of a pill. Other patients rebel against the thought that they have a lifelong illness requiring medication and feel they can correct the problem with recommended hygienic measures. Thus, it is critical to individualize when making recommendations concerning both hygienic and pharmacological approaches to treating hypertension. Every patient is different and requires a unique set of recommendations, education, and support.

HYGIENIC MEASURES

Although we can all agree that reducing one's weight, exercising regularly, stopping smoking, and reducing di-

etary salt intake make sense, in real life, this is very hard to do for the vast majority of patients (Table 51–1). Not only is it impractical to rely on these approaches for controlling blood pressure, but also this may actually delay the use of appropriate therapy. Consequently, physicians must take the time to be honest with patients and find out how realistic lifestyle modifications will be in facilitating blood pressure control. Specifically, the physician should ask about salt and saturated fat intake, smoking, alcohol use, and physical activity.[1–3] He or she can then focus on the areas that might result in some success in an individual patient. Some reports have recommended that patients also focus on potassium, calcium, and magnesium.[4, 5] These recommendations, although theoretically appropriate, clearly hold little meaning for the vast majority of hypertensive patients, as well as most of their prescribing physicians. What makes more sense are general recommendations, such as in the Dietary Approaches to Stop Hypertension (DASH) diet, focusing on smaller portions and eating more slowly, centering meals around carbohydrates and vegetables eating more fruits and lower-calorie foods for desserts and snacks, and including low-fat dairy products.[6] These types of recommendations remove much of the constraining feeling of specific dietary regimens in which one must count all the salt, potassium, calcium, magnesium, and fat, as well as the calories.

Reduction of dietary salt intake can facilitate better blood pressure control in most hypertensive patients. Blood pressure sensitivity to salt is common in hypertensive individuals, particularly in the elderly, the obese, and diabetics. Salt sensitivity is also prevalent in the African American community. Epidemiological data demonstrate a positive association between dietary salt consumption and level of blood pressure.[3, 7–9] However, this is not an all-or-nothing phenomenon.[10] Graded reduction in dietary salt intake can

---

Table 51–1 Behavior Modification: Appropriate Hygienic Measures

Exercise regularly (30 min/day)
Achieve ideal body weight with exercise and improved eating habits
Avoid dietary salt modestly (<6 g NaCl/day)
Stop smoking
Limit alcohol to 1–2 drinks/day
Reduce dietary saturated fat

have a positive effect on reducing blood pressure in many patients, particularly of the salt-sensitive phenotype. Thus, a moderate dietary salt restriction should be the focus of lifestyle modification efforts in hypertensive patients. Experimental studies have demonstrated that some harm may result from drastic reductions in dietary salt restriction.[9] However, these studies used levels of dietary salt restriction that are almost impossible to obtain in free-living society. Modest salt reduction is the most accepted regimen, to allow time for adaptation in taste. Much of the benefit related to dietary salt reduction can be achieved simply by avoiding many of the processed foods that are currently available as fast foods and microwave cooking opportunities.

In summary, hygienic measures should always be recommended but not relied on for blood pressure control. Lifestyle modifications are safe and economical and complement pharmacological therapy in lowering blood pressure. They should always be considered as part of initial efforts to control blood pressure. However, recidivism is common and discouraging. Further, managed care systems generally afford few with opportunities to develop a systematic team approach with health care professionals to provide the necessary education and support for lifestyle modifications to be effective. Consequently, it makes little sense to delay appropriate pharmacological therapy based on the expectation that lifestyle modifications alone will be successful in controlling blood pressure.

PHARMACOLOGICAL THERAPY

Once the decision is made to pursue pharmacological therapy, one faces a key question. Is one therapy more effective or appropriate than another for controlling blood pressure in different types of patients? Since the pathophysiology of hypertension is so poorly understood, most initial choices of drug therapy are based on nonscientific grounds, anecdotal experience, or successful advertising and promotional efforts. For these reasons and perhaps others, a single agent chosen initially provides therapeutic success in only

40 to 50% of cases.[1] Consequently, improved strategies are needed to facilitate blood pressure control. This chapter deals with such issues, specifically focusing on whether we should be using lower doses of two or more drugs or higher doses of a single agent, special indications based on concomitant medical conditions, and demographic variables that can influence the response to antihypertensive therapy. This discussion focuses on the likelihood of achieving success with certain agents in different types of patients, realizing that every patient is different and will respond differently to a medication based on age, gender, race, body habitus, and of course, diet. These recommendations are generalizations and should be interpreted accordingly.

DEMOGRAPHIC ISSUES INFLUENCING INITIAL TREATMENT

Age

Important pathophysiological factors in age-related hypertension can influence our approach to treatment (Table 51–2). Functional and structural alterations of the cardiovascular system cause problems with some types of antihypertensive drugs and improve responsiveness to others. Aging is associated with reductions in left ventricular compliance and circulating blood volume, increased left ventricular wall thickness, and attenuated renin-angiotensin responses to various physiological stimuli.[11] Decreased elasticity and increased rigidity of large conduct arteries result in reduced vascular compliance and more rapid pulse wave transmission and earlier and greater pulse wave reflection in the aorta and its major tributaries (see Chap. 14, Arterial Stiffness).[11] This results in a widening of the pulse pressure (the difference between the systolic and the diastolic pressure). These structural changes also contribute to a reduction in baroreflex function, increased lability of blood pressure, and a propensity toward orthostatic hypotension.[11, 12] Thus, targeting elevated systolic blood pressure and the resultant widened pulse pressure in the

Table 51–2 Consideration for Initial Therapy in Older Patients With or Without Isolated Systolic Hypertension

Pathophysiology	Desirable Pharmacological Approach
Decreased vascular compliance and ↑ PVR	Vasodilator (e.g., HCTZ, ACEIs, ARBs, CCBs, α-blockers)
Isolated systolic hypertension and wider pulse pressure	Reduce systolic BP <160 mm Hg, or >20 mm Hg if systolic BP is 160–180 mm Hg before treatment (HCTZ [reduction in CVA, CHF, MI] CCBs [reduction in CVA])
Reduced LV compliance	Myocardial relaxation, ↓ HR (β-blockers, CCBs)
Impaired LV function	Preload, afterload reduction (ACEIs, HCTZ as necessary; ? β-blocker—carvedilol)
Impaired renal function and reduced renal blood flow	Vasodilator (e.g., HCTZ, ACEIs, ARBs, CCBs, α-blocker; avoid loop diuretics unless necessary)
Reduction of cardiovascular baroreflex function with BP lability	Avoid sympatholytics and volume depletion
Orthostatic hypotension	Consider using short-acting medications (<12-hr duration) at bedtime during recumbency
Reduced metabolic capability	Adjust all medications for renal/hepatic function—start at half dose
Prostatic hypertrophy (BPH)	Prostatic urethral dilatation (α-blockers)

Abbreviations: PVR, peripheral vascular resistance; HCTZ, hydrochlorothiazide; ACEIs, angiotensin-converting enzyme inhibitors; ARBs, angiotensin receptor blockers; CCBs, calcium channel blockers; BP, blood pressure; CVA, cerebrovascular accident; CHF, congestive heart failure; MI, myocardial infarction; LV, left ventricular; HR, heart rate; BPH, benign prostatic hypertrophy.

elderly is one of the most important facets of the treatment strategy. However, some older patients may have pseudohypertension (false elevations of blood pressure due to excessive vascular stiffness) and do not benefit from vigorous attempts to lower blood pressure.[13]

All therapeutic strategies, regardless of the age of the patient, should begin with behavior modification. Older patients, like younger patients, respond to modest dietary salt restriction, regular exercise, cessation of smoking and alcohol consumption, and weight loss. Frequently, goal blood pressure is not achieved with hygienic measures, and pharmacotherapy is required. In general, starting doses of drugs should be reduced by approximately 50% compared with usual doses for younger patients. This is required due to a diminution in hepatic and renal metabolism with age and a greater proclivity for antihypertensive drugs to induce postural hypotension.

Goal blood pressure should be similar in older and younger patients. Normal blood pressure is defined as less than or equal to 130/85 mm Hg, and optimal blood pressure as less than or equal to 120/80 mm Hg in older, as well as younger, patients.[1] However, in many elderly patients, systolic blood pressure elevation is the major problem and an interim goal of less than 160 mm Hg systolic may be necessary, particularly in those who start out with marked elevations in systolic blood pressure (>200 mm Hg). Growing evidence from large-scale clinical trials in patients with systolic hypertension indicates that reducing the systolic blood pressure closer to normal results in a greater survival benefit.[14–18] This is discussed in greater detail later in this chapter.

The major first-line medications are all effective in lowering blood pressure, but some may be more effective than others in certain patients. However, this can vary substantially depending on the doses used and the overall tolerability of the drugs. Some clinical trials demonstrate that drugs such as thiazide diuretics and calcium channel blockers are more universally effective than drugs that affect the renin-angiotensin system such as β-blockers or angiotensin-converting enzyme inhibitors (ACEIs).[15, 19] A limitation of these studies is that they have not uniformly assessed dietary salt consumption or evaluated full-dose titrations of the various drugs. Low doses of thiazide diuretics and calcium channel blockers do appear to be more effective than low doses of β-blockers and ACEIs in lowering blood pressure in older patients.

Adverse events are a critical problem with pharmacotherapy in the aged. This is particularly true for drugs that exaggerate postural changes in blood pressure, such as adrenergic blockers, α-blockers, or high-dose diuretics, and for therapies that can cause cognitive dysfunction, such as centrally acting agents and possibly β-blockers. Ankle edema may also be a problem in some patients and can be exaggerated by calcium channel blockers. This should not be treated with a diuretic, as it represents the end result of a capillary leak syndrome, not a manifestation of salt and water retention.[20] Constipation may also be worsened by some therapies.

Some therapies provide additional benefit in aged patients, particularly if there is concomitant medical illness. Low-dose diuretics are helpful for systolic blood pressure elevation; β-blockers or calcium channel blockers for angina or coronary disease; and ACEIs for systolic dysfunction and renal disease.[1] Older men who suffer from symptoms of prostatism may benefit substantially from the ability of α-blockers to dilate the prostatic urethra.[21]

Interactions with other commonly used medications can occur in the elderly. One of the most important of those is that nonsteroidal antiinflammatory drugs antagonize the antihypertensive properties of most drugs, with the exception of calcium channel blockers.[22] Salt substitutes containing potassium can cause undesirable increases in circulating potassium concentrations when coadministered with drugs that block the renin-angiotensin-aldosterone system. Aged individuals with high blood pressure are ideal candidates for use of lower doses of two or more medications in order to control blood pressure, thus avoiding the increased risk of drug accumulation and associated toxicity.

In summary, the physiology of aging requires us to modify our approach to the pharmacological treatment of hypertension. However, we should treat hypertension as aggressively in older as in younger patients because long-term clinical trials have demonstrated major cardiovascular benefits, with reductions in stroke, coronary heart disease, cardiovascular disease, heart failure, and all-cause mortality, from successful treatment of hypertension in the elderly.

Isolated Systolic Hypertension

Reduction of systolic blood pressure is one of the most difficult problems in the therapeutics of hypertension. Not only are the patients elderly and more susceptible to adverse events, particularly related to symptoms of orthostasis and fatigue, but there is also diminished renal and hepatic metabolism of drugs, which can accumulate and cause adverse events.[11, 12] Definitive evidence from large clinical trials has shown that reduction of systolic blood pressure is helpful in reducing both stroke- and cardiac-related morbidity and mortality in the elderly.[14–18] The Systolic Hypertension in the Elderly Program (SHEP)—employing low doses of diuretics and β-blockers, if necessary—demonstrated that lowering systolic blood pressure to less than 160 mm Hg, or by more than 20 mm Hg if pretreatment systolic blood pressure was between 160 and 180 mm Hg, resulted in substantial reductions in stroke, myocardial infarction, and congestive heart failure.[14] The more recent Systolic Hypertension in Europe (SYST-EUR) trial, employing a dihydropyridine calcium channel blocker–based therapy, demonstrated that lowering systolic blood pressure to less than 160 mm Hg substantially reduced the risk of stroke and produced statistically nonsignificant (presumably because the study was stopped early) reductions in myocardial infarction and congestive heart failure.[18]

Whether systolic blood pressure should be reduced to 150 or 140 mm Hg or less remains open to question. Studies are currently under way to address whether these more aggressive targets will result in morbidity and mortality benefits. Some have raised concerns about being overly aggressive in lowering diastolic blood pressure in patients with coronary disease.[23–25] It is likely that if these lower levels of systolic blood pressure can be achieved with safety, there will be some benefit. This additional benefit may be analogous to that observed in clinical trials involving patients with renal disease, in whom a consistent reduction of systolic blood pressure into the 120 to 130 mm Hg range was safely achieved without any increased risk of adverse events and resulted in delay of progression of renal disease.[26] However, the latter clinical trials involved younger patients. There is no evidence from the SHEP trial, even for the oldest patients (>80 years), that more aggressive blood pressure reduction resulted in increased risk of adverse events.[14] Similarly, a large trial in the United Kingdom demonstrated reduction in cerebrovascular disease with greater systolic blood pressure reduction in the elderly.[27]

The optimal treatment strategy for isolated systolic hypertension is to start with low doses of thiazide diuretics, as these have been employed in the majority of the large-scale clinical trials for this condition and have also shown the most definitive benefit with regard to morbidity and mortality.[1, 14–17, 28] However, two, possibly three or even four, drugs will likely be needed to control systolic hypertension in many patients, particularly the elderly. It makes excellent sense to employ lower doses of multiple agents that can be administered once daily in order to reduce the likelihood of adverse events and enhance compliance. Hygienic measures, particularly dietary salt reduction, should be encouraged, and one should always be mindful of orthostatic blood pressure changes and potential interference of drugs with cognitive function.

In summary, there are many reasons to intervene aggressively in elderly patients with systolic hypertension. Pharmacotherapy should include low doses of a thiazide diuretic in conjunction with low doses of other drugs as necessary to control blood pressure and, when needed, treat concomitant medical illnesses. Risks of orthostasis and drug accumulation need to be considered as medication doses are adjusted.

Gender

There are gender considerations in the pathophysiology and treatment of hypertension that may affect drug treatment selection (Table 51–3).[29] The incidence of coronary artery disease in women is one third that in men below the age of 55 years; the ratio declines rapidly after the menopause and approaches unity by age 75 years. Consequently hypertensive women, once they have reached menopause, are as much at risk for coronary disease as men.[29]

Hemodynamic differences between hypertensive men and women may be important in the selection of pharmacotherapy. In general, men have a lower resting heart rate, a longer left ventricular ejection time, and a lower pulse pressure, whereas women have lower total peripheral resistance and decreased blood volume.[30] When stressed, there is a 50% greater increase in pulse pressure and blood pressure in men compared with in women.[31] However, the stress response is greater in postmenopausal than in premenopausal women. The clinical expression of coronary artery disease differs substantially between genders. Women more commonly report chronic stable angina with discomfort during rest or sleep. Anginal equivalents are also more common in women than in men.[32] In addition, women are more prone to silent myocardial infarction.[33] Thus, the typical symptoms of ischemic chest pain are much more commonly seen in men than in women.

Large long-term clinical trials have not demonstrated substantial differences in response to blood pressure medications or in outcomes between genders.[34, 35] Thus, there should be no differences in goal blood pressures or types of medications based on gender. However, the incidence of certain adverse events differs between the genders and the requirement for estrogen replacement therapy also needs to be carefully considered.

Hypertension, itself, is not a contraindication to postmenopausal estrogen replacement therapy. Estrogen replacement has a beneficial effect on overall cardiovascular risk, and there is no evidence that blood pressure changes significantly with hormone replacement therapy in most women, either with or without hypertension.[29, 36, 37] However, some patients may experience increases in blood pressure with estrogen replacement, and consequently, once replacement therapy is started, blood pressure should be monitored more frequently.

In contrast, women who take oral contraceptives are likely to experience increases in blood pressure.[38] Hypertension is two to three times more frequent in women who

---

Table 51–3 Considerations for Initial Therapy Based on Gender

Pathophysiology	Desirable Pharmacological Approach
Men have ↓ resting HR, longer LVEF time, ↑ stressed pulse pressure than women	Vasodilator (e.g., HCTZ, ACEIs, ARBs, CCBs)
Women have ↓ TPR and ↑ blood volume than men	Vasodilator, HR reduction, less need for diuresis (HCTZ, ACEIs, ARBs, β-blockers, CCBs)
Postmenopausal women more frequently have CAD with atypical chest pain	Antianginal, HR reduction (β-blockers, CCBs)
Osteoporosis	Antagonize calciuria (HCTZ)
Pregnancy	Avoid teratogenic drugs (ACEIs, ARBs)
	Avoid drugs that may delay labor (CCBs)
	Avoid drugs that may cause ureteroplacental insufficiency (loop diuretics); optimal choices: α-methyldopa, hydralazine, β-blockers
Women report more pedal edema with CCBs and cough with ACEIs than men	Adjust medications if these symptoms are present

Abbreviations: HR, heart rate; LVEF, left ventricular ejection fraction; HCTZ, hydrochlorothiazide; ACEIs, angiotensin-converting enzyme inhibitors; ARBs, angiotensin receptor blockers; CCBs, calcium channel blockers; TPR, total peripheral resistance; CAD, coronary artery disease.

are using oral contraceptives, particularly if they are obese or older, compared with those who do not take these agents. This may also be a problem for women who smoke cigarettes. If hypertension does develop, or even if there is a substantial increase in blood pressure within the so-called normal range with oral contraceptives, it is advisable to discontinue them. In most cases, blood pressure will normalize over a period of months. However, if high blood pressure persists, pharmacological treatment may be required when hygienic measures are insufficient.

The recommendations concerning use of antihypertensive drugs in pregnancy have not changed substantially in recent years.[1] Centrally acting agents such as methyldopa or β-blockers appear to be safe, whereas ACEIs or angiotensin receptor blockers should never be used because of the risk of fetal abnormalities. Direct-acting vasodilators like hydralazine may also be used. Calcium antagonists may be effective but could synergize with magnesium sulfate to lead to a rapid fall in blood pressure and may delay labor. Low doses of diuretics may be helpful in some patients but should be used with caution to avoid volume depletion.

Adverse events are perhaps the most important issue in drug selection for women. Women more commonly have cough with ACEIs[39] and leg edema with calcium channel blockers.[40] These adverse events need to be considered carefully when these drugs are used. Lower doses of calcium channel blockers may be necessary to avoid the risk of pedal edema, which is dose related. All of the commonly used classes of drugs appear to have similar benefits in reducing blood pressure, although only traditional agents like thiazides and β-blockers have demonstrated morbidity and mortality benefits in women in long-term controlled clinical trials.[14–17, 41–45] Only one recent meta-analysis has addressed the relative morbidity and mortality benefits of long-term antihypertensive treatment in men and women.[46] This study demonstrated similar benefits in both genders. An improved understanding of mechanism of action, adverse effects, and potential interactions with estrogen replacement of the commonly used antihypertensive drugs is needed to guide therapy in women.

Because women tend to have a greater burden of osteoporosis than men, much emphasis has been placed on the use of thiazide diuretics to enhance bone mineral density by reducing the urinary excretion of calcium.[47–51] Clinical trials have yielded conflicting data about the metabolic effects of thiazides on bone.[50, 51] In general, the studies demonstrate an increase in bone mineral density with thiazide use, but the impact on the risk of fractures is unclear.[50, 51]

In summary, gender-specific considerations in the treatment of hypertension exist, particularly related to the increasing incidence of coronary disease after menopause, the use of estrogen replacement therapy or of birth control pills, and hypertension during pregnancy. There are also gender differences in adverse events that may dictate prescribing practices. Low-dose thiazides, alone or in combination with other drugs, may ultimately prove to have the most benefit for the treatment of hypertension in women, particularly if they reduce the occurrence of fractures in elderly women.

Race

Ethnicity has a substantial impact on the response to antihypertensive therapy. It has been observed for decades in clinical trials and in practice that there are differences in response rates to various antihypertensive drugs between white and African American populations. The biological basis for this difference remains obscure. The biological versus social concept of race and substantial interracial genetic pooling blur the issue. Thus, ethnic as opposed to biological racial differences are a more logical way of describing social, economic, and cultural factors that may influence the response to antihypertensive therapy. Ethnic minorities in the United States, particularly African Americans, have a greater frequency and intensity of hypertension associated with an increased risk of target organ damage.[52–56] In part, this is related to lower socioeconomic status and diminished access to health care. African Americans also have a greater propensity for renal disease, which may complicate the hypertension and make it more difficult to treat.[55] There are also ethnic differences in dietary patterns, propensity for obesity, and salt sensitivity.[56] These factors may explain why, for any given dietary salt consumption, blood pressure may be higher in an African American population compared with a white population. However, this does not fully explain racial differences in response to antihypertensive medication.[57]

African Americans receiving adequate antihypertensive treatment achieve similar overall reductions in cardiovascular morbidity and mortality.[58, 59] However, owing to lower socioeconomic status and delays in receiving proper treatment, target organ damage tends to be greater, in African Americans, resulting in a higher incidence of hypertension-associated morbidity and mortality, particularly end-stage renal disease.[52–56]

Lifestyle modification is particularly beneficial in African American populations, where obesity, type II diabetes, and increased salt sensitivity complicate the hypertensive process.[56, 60–62] But, as with all patients, lifestyle modifications, although often helpful, usually do not solve the hypertension problem in African Americans. Pharmacotherapy should focus on the basic pathophysiological problems observed in African Americans, including greater peripheral vascular resistance and salt sensitivity (Table 51–4).[63] Pharmacotherapies that induce vasodilatation are particularly helpful. Moreover, agents that have natriuretic properties may better facilitate blood pressure control. Diuretics and calcium channel blockers are among the most effective drugs for controlling blood pressure in African Americans. In contrast, African Americans may be less responsive to drugs that inhibit the renin-angiotensin system, perhaps owing to their lower-renin, more salt-sensitive pathophysiology.[19, 64] However, clinical trials to date have been flawed by the lack of full-scale titration of these drugs to vigorously assess whether there is a different dose response in patients with a low-renin physiology or greater salt sensitivity. Recent clinical trials have demonstrated that higher doses of ACEIs may overcome racial differences in responsiveness.[57, 65]

Because of the increased frequency of stage 3 hypertension in African American populations, as well as the greater proclivity for target organ injury, we should aim for normal

Table 51–4 Considerations for Initial Therapy in African American Patients

Pathophysiology	Desirable Pharmacological Approach
High PVR with associated reduction in cardiac output	Vasodilator (e.g., HCTZ, ACEIs, CCBs, ARBs)
Salt sensitivity	Natriuresis (HCTZ, ACEIs, ARBs, CCBs)
Variable blood volume (perhaps greater in some patients relative to ↑ PVR)	Natriuresis, diuresis (HCTZ; if creatinine >2.0, loop diuretic)
Cardiac disease	See Table 51–6
Renal disease	See Table 51–7

Abbreviations: PVR, peripheral vascular resistance; HCTZ, hydrochlorothiazide; ACEIs, angiotensin-converting enzyme inhibitors; CCBs, calcium channel blockers, ARBs, angiotensin receptor blockers.

blood pressure (≤130/85 mm Hg) when treating this group. In fact, 120/80 mm Hg may be a more appropriate blood pressure goal, particularly in patients with more advanced renal dysfunction. This has been demonstrated in patients with proteinuric renal disease[66] and is likely important in African Americans with hypertension and associated kidney disease.

Avoidance of adverse effects of cardiovascular drugs is a critical problem in minority populations. Overall, it makes sense to consider lower doses of more drugs to control blood pressure in patients who are younger and have more severe hypertensive disease, as this approach is more likely to both control blood pressure and reduce the possibility of adverse events. The use of low doses of thiazide diuretics or calcium channel blockers in concert with drugs that block the renin-angiotensin system and additional vasodilators may be an optimal strategy.

Other ethnic groups have not been as well studied as African Americans. Hispanic Americans have a lesser prevalence of hypertension than African Americans but do have a substantial risk of diabetes and dyslipidemia and a similar socioeconomic disadvantage, with delayed access to medical care.[56, 67] Based on limited data, there does not appear to be any substantial difference in response to the various antihypertensive drug classes between Hispanic Americans and whites.[57]

Native Americans have a much greater incidence of insulin resistance and type II diabetes.[67] Although their degree of blood pressure elevation and responsiveness to commonly used drugs do not differ from the general population, their concomitant diabetes and proclivity for renal disease deserve the attention of the clinician.

Asian Americans have not been well studied. The available literature indicates that their responses to calcium antagonists seem to be more favorable than to ACEIs and equivalent to their responses to diuretic and β-blocker therapy.[56] However, more clinical trials are needed. Thus, preference for the use of a specific drug class for the treatment of hypertension based on race or ethnicity should primarily be based on other key profiling factors, such as age, gender, obesity, diabetes, and concomitant cardiovascular risk factors.

Obesity

Essential hypertension is frequently associated with obesity and type II diabetes mellitus in westernized industrial societies, particularly with increasing patient age.[68–71] Coexis-

tent medical problems, such as dyslipidemia, degenerative joint disease, back pain, and immobility, are frequently found in obese patients. These patients almost always have an increased number of cardiovascular risk factors (Table 51–5).[72]

Consequently, therapeutic strategies for controlling blood pressure in obese patients should be targeted to both the pathophysiological processes underlying the hypertension and the coexistent cardiovascular risk factors. The primary clinical strategy should revolve around proper diet, exercise, and weight reduction, which can improve insulin sensitivity, help achieve consistent blood pressure reduction, and reduce salt sensitivity.

The pathophysiology of hypertension in obese patients includes increased salt sensitivity and a hyperdynamic circulation owing to increased activity of the sympathetic nervous system.[73–75] As in all forms of hypertension, increased peripheral vascular resistance also plays a substantial role in the elevation of blood pressure in obese individuals. These pathophysiological features suggest a number of different therapeutic targets. Low doses of diuretics are almost always helpful in reducing blood pressure in these patients and in correcting subtle abnormalities of blood volume. Diuretics may also help facilitate blood pressure control even in the face of slightly higher consumption of dietary salt. β-Blockers may also be useful in these patients because they can antagonize the sympathetic drive, which results in increased heart rate. Drugs that block the adrener-

Table 51–5 Considerations for Initial Therapy in Obese Hypertensives

Pathophysiology	Desirable Pharmacological Approach
Hyperdynamic circulation	Reduce HR and sympathoadrenal outflow (β-blocker)
Increased PVR	Vasodilator (e.g., HCTZ, ACEIs, ARBs, CCBs)
Salt sensitivity	Natriuresis (HCTZ, ACEIs, ARBs, CCBs)
NSAID (if DJD present)	Minimize use of NSAID (CCBs)
Expanded plasma volume	Diuresis (HCTZ, loop diuretic only if creatinine >2.0; note: edema in obese patients is usually due to structural problems as opposed to volume overload)

Abbreviations: HR, heart rate; PVR, peripheral vascular resistance; HCTZ, hydrochlorothiazide; ACEIs, angiotensin-converting enzyme inhibitors; ARBs, angiotensin receptor blockers; CCBs, calcium channel blockers; NSAID, nonsteroidal antiflammatory drug; DJD, degenerative joint disease.

gic nervous system, such as α-blockers, may also be useful, in that they antagonize the sympathetic nervous system and also function as vasodilators. Calcium antagonists may have beneficial effects, particularly because they facilitate blood pressure reduction even in the face of greater dietary salt consumption.[76] ACEIs are effective. Although primarily targeted toward the renin-angiotensin system, they also dampen the activity of the sympathetic nervous system[77] and facilitate natriuresis.[78] Thus, most of the major classes of drugs are useful in obese hypertensive patients.

The choice of specific drugs may depend on the patient's ability to tolerate the therapy and on coexistent medical problems. For example, for patients requiring concurrent nonsteroidal antiinflammatory drugs because of degenerative joint disease, a calcium channel blocker would be preferable because these agents are the least likely to have their antihypertensive efficacy offset by nonsteroidal antiinflammatory drugs. If the patient has concomitant diabetes, it may be appropriate to avoid β-blockade to not worsen glycemic control or, in the presence of proteinuria, to consider using ACEIs or nondihydropyridine calcium channel blockers because they have demonstrated antiproteinuric properties in hypertensive diabetic patients.[79–81] α_1-Adrenoreceptor blockers may have metabolic benefits in obese diabetic patients by improving insulin sensitivity and glucose utilization. They may also improve lipoprotein profiles. Male obese patients may also have prostatism, for which the α-blocker would be helpful.

Adverse events of antihypertensive drugs can limit efforts to control blood pressure in obese patients. Diuretics rarely cause problems with worsening of glycemic control unless hypokalemia occurs.[82] This is unusual if lower doses of diuretics are used. Calcium channel blockers may cause more edema in obese patients.

Thus, all classes of antihypertensive agents are appropriate for the obese hypertensive subject. These patients like all hypertensives, have specific issues that need to be addressed on a patient-by-patient basis in order to provide optimal therapy.

Heart Disease

Hypertensive patients with coronary artery disease need special attention to lifestyle modification, specifically with regard to proper diet, exercise, and maintenance of ideal body weight. They also have unique problems related to atherosclerosis of their coronary circulation. Hypertension, particularly systolic hypertension, increases the strain on the heart, leading to hypertrophic changes and subsequent left ventricular dysfunction.[83] Therefore, treatment of hypertension in a patient with coronary artery disease should focus not only on adequate blood pressure reduction but also on slowing of heart rate. Reducing heart rate increases coronary artery perfusion time during diastole, a factor that is particularly important if the coronary circulation is compromised. Regular exercise, owing to its vagal effects, will help reduce heart rate. Heart rate lowering drugs, such as β-blockers or nondihydropyridine calcium channel blockers, are also useful in this regard.

Conversely, drugs that increase heart rate should be avoided in patients with coronary artery disease. One cannot always predict which agents will cause this, and therefore it is appropriates to focus on individual heart rate responses when making therapeutic decisions. The recent discussion about myocardial infarction and antihypertensive therapy has revolved around heart rate responses to either oral or sublingual immediate-release nifedipine.[84, 85] Although a powerful antihypertensive agent, immediate-release nifedipine causes a rapid reduction in blood pressure that frequently results in a reflex increase in heart rate, and therefore should not be used in patients who are at risk for, or who have proven coronary artery disease. Heart rate increases may also occur in patients treated with nonspecific vasodilators, such as hydralazine or minoxidil, and even with long-acting dihydropyridine calcium channel blockers.

Another interesting issue in patients with coronary disease is how to effectively control heart rate and blood pressure in the early morning hours. Much of the interest in circadian patterns of heart rate and blood pressure has been fueled by observations that most strokes and heart attacks occur within the first 6 hours of waking in the morning.[86] Peak increases in heart rate and blood pressure also occur during this period. Thus, strategies to lower blood pressure and heart rate in synchrony with circadian patterns may be important for reducing ischemic events. Novel delivery systems for antihypertensive medications are enhancing our opportunity to realize this goal. Long-term outcome trials are under way to assess the importance of early morning heart rate and blood pressure reduction in reducing ischemic morbidity and mortality.

In summary, patients with coronary artery disease need close attention to all cardiovascular risk factors and aggressive control of both blood pressure and heart rate. Drugs that result in acute or sustained increases in heart rate should be avoided.

Left Ventricular Dysfunction

Patients who have symptoms of heart disease, such as shortness of breath or evidence of volume overload or ischemic chest pain, need a careful assessment of volume status and cardiac function for optimal selection of therapy. Heart rate–lowering drugs, particularly β-blockers, are beneficial in patients with active ischemic heart disease. Nondihydropyridine calcium channel blockers may be a suitable alternative. However, if there is evidence of systolic dysfunction (ejection fraction <30%), ACEIs alone or in conjunction with low doses of diuretics are the optimal therapeutic choice.[87–89] These agents not only unload the circulation and provide preload and afterload reduction but are also gentle diuretics.[78] Thus, thiazides should be used in concert with ACEIs in patients with early heart failure. Alternative therapeutic choices in patients with more advanced degrees of heart failure or who are intolerant of an ACEI include preload and afterload reduction with a nitrate and hydralazine, but all patients should be given the opportunity to receive ACEIs first. Additional trials are under way to study the use of β-blockers[90] and angiotensin receptor blockers[91] in these patients. There is evidence that inhibition of sympathetic nervous system or renin-angiotensin system activity with these drugs may be beneficial in

Table 51–6 Considerations for Initial Therapy in Patients With Heart Disease

Pathophysiology	Desirable Pharmacological Approach
Angina	HR reduction and antianginal therapy (reduce HR 10–20% or to 60–65 bpm) (β-blockers, CCBs)
LVH	Systolic blood pressure reduction (HCTZ, β-blockers, ACEIs, CCBs, ARBs—avoid nonspecific vasodilator or therapies that result in reflex ↑ HR)
Systolic dysfunction	Afterload reduction and natriuresis (ACEIs, HCTZ [avoid volume depletion; loop diuretic only if necessary or creatinine >2.0]) ?Sympathetic inhibitor → β-blockers (carvedilol, ?others)
Diastolic dysfunction	Improve myocardial compliance, reduce HR, avoid volume depletion (β-blockers, CCBs, avoid loop diuretics)
Myocardial infarction	HR reduction and reduction in myocardial oxygen demand (β-blockers, ACEIs if left ventricular dysfunction)

Abbreviations: HR, heart rate; CCBs, calcium channel blockers; LVH, left ventricular hypertrophy; HCTZ, hydrochlorothiazide; ACEIs, angiotensin-converting enzyme inhibitors; , ARBs, angiotensin receptor blockers.

improving symptoms and long-term outcome. Additional afterload and blood pressure reduction with the dihydropyridine calcium channel blockers amlodipine or felodipine has proved to be safe.[92, 93]

Patients with diastolic dysfunction require a different treatment strategy (Table 51–6). These patients have stiff noncompliant ventricles. Consequently, treatment strategies should be oriented toward enhancing myocardial relaxation during diastole and reducing heart rate.[94, 95] Optimal approaches include heart rate–lowering drugs like β-blockers or nondihydropyridine calcium channel blockers. Additional agents may be used as necessary to achieve optimal afterload reduction. One should avoid treatments that increase heart rate, as the reduction of time for diastolic filling in a noncompliant ventricle could impair cardiac output.

In summary, treatment strategies in patients with heart disease require careful evaluation of the underlying pathophysiology and function of the ventricle so that optimal treatments can be selected.

Renal Disease

Much has been learned in the last few years about how to optimally treat hypertension in patients with renal disease. One of the most helpful observations came from the Modification of Diet in Renal Disease (MDRD) Study,[66] which demonstrated that more aggressive reduction in blood pressure (to 125/75 mm Hg), particularly in patients who had more than 1 g of protein in their urine or in patients of African American descent, helped reduce the rate of progression of renal disease compared with traditional blood pressure control (to 140/90 mm Hg). Achieving a goal mean arterial pressure of 92 mm Hg (~125/75 mm Hg) in this study required intensive effort and usually three to four antihypertensive drugs. ACEIs, calcium channel blockers, and diuretics, as needed, were the preferred agents, but additional therapies such as α-blockers, β-blockers, and nonspecific vasodilators, such as minoxidil, were frequently needed. To control blood pressure in people with kidney disease, we need to mix and match several antihypertensive drugs and titrate them carefully so that they work optimally with one another without adverse events (Table 51–7).

Based on the MDRD trial, more aggressive antihypertensive approaches are needed, particularly targeted toward reducing systolic blood pressure. How to best achieve this goal is unclear because no two patients are alike and experimentation is frequently needed. Control of blood volume with a loop diuretic and the use of drugs to vasodilate the circulation and reduce cardiac output can be helpful.[96] There are also important indications for ACEIs, which reduce glomerular capillary pressure and proteinuria and delay the progression of renal disease more effectively than other commonly used antihypertensive drugs.[66, 79, 80, 96, 97] Even when employing these agents, it is still critical to achieve blood pressure reduction.[96–98] Calcium channel blockers may also offer benefits in delaying progression of renal disease that may be related to nonhemodynamic pathways.[90, 99, 100] Nondihydropyridine calcium channel blockers possess antiproteinuric properties that may work in concert with ACEIs to further reduce blood pressure and proteinuria.[81] Angiotensin II receptor blockers also reduce proteinuria to a greater extent than would be expected by blood pressure reduction alone.[101]

The ability of ACEIs to reduce both blood pressure and proteinuria may be particularly beneficial in delaying the progression of renal disease, as indicated by large collaborative studies in patients with diabetic and nondiabetic nephropathy.[66, 79, 80, 96–98] Increasing dietary salt offsets the

Table 51–7 Considerations for Initial Therapy in Patients With Renal Disease

Pathophysiology	Desirable Pharmacological Approach
Increased blood volume (common in glomerular diseases)	Reduce blood volume (loop diuretic [avoid HCTZ if creatinine >2.0])
Decreased blood volume (common in tubular diseases)	May require salt supplementation
Increased PVR	Vasodilator (ACEIs, CCBs, ARBs, α-blocker, minoxidil)
Proteinuria	Reduce proteinuria (ACEIs, ARBs, NDCCBs [BP systolic ≤125 mm Hg])
Diabetes	Control BP and glycemia (ACEIs, ?NDCCB, ?ARBs [BP systolic ≤125 mm Hg])

Abbreviations: HCTZ, hydrochlorothiazide; PVR, peripheral vascular resistance; ACEIs, angiotensin-converting enzyme inhibitors; CCBs, calcium channel blockers; ARBs, angiotensin receptor blockers; NDCCBs, nondihydropyridine calcium channel blockers; BP, blood pressure.

antihypertensive properties of most commonly used medications and the antiproteinuric properties of ACEIs and nondihydropyridine calcium channel blockers.[102] Consequently, it is critical to encourage dietary salt avoidance in hypertensive patients with renal disease.

One should not be concerned about using ACEIs in patients with renal disease because studies demonstrate benefit of these drugs in delaying progression of renal disease even in patients with significant renal insufficiency.[79] However, one needs to be cautious about monitoring the serum creatinine and potassium levels in such patients. A 15 to 20% increase in the serum creatinine is expected in response to an ACEI in patients with renal disease owing to the reduction in glomerular capillary pressure. If the serum creatinine increases by more than 25%, one should suspect diminished effective arterial blood volume due to excessive use of diuretics or anatomical renal artery stenosis.[103] Most ACEIs are largely eliminated by renal metabolism and need to be dosed accordingly in patients with advanced renal disease. Serum potassium frequently increases by approximately 0.5 mEq/L, not uncommonly into the 5 to 6 range with ACEI administration in these patients. One should not be concerned about potassium homeostasis unless there is a progressive rise to over 6 mEq/L.[104] This is unusual in the absence of significant type IV renal tubular acidosis.

In summary, in patients with renal disease, aggressive reduction of blood pressure is indicated, frequently with use of three to four or more antihypertensive drugs. Optimal control of volume is critical, and there are clear indications for using ACEIs, calcium channel blockers, and other drugs as necessary to optimally control blood pressure.

Diabetes Mellitus

In patients with hypertension and coexisting diabetes, the focus should be not only reducing blood pressure but also treating the attendant cardiovascular risk factors, as previously discussed. In addition, patients with diabetes frequently have autonomic dysfunction and associated orthostatic hypotension. Consequently, treatment strategies should be based on blood pressure determinations in the sitting and standing positions. Higher pressures in the supine position at night may require shorter-acting medications administered before bedtime that wear off by morning.

Both type I and type II diabetic patients may have insulin resistance related to a variety of factors, including obesity and peripheral vasoconstriction, that can limit the ability of insulin to find its receptors in skeletal muscle.[68] Thus, vasodilators make physiological sense in these patients. Volume contraction resulting from overzealous diuresis and hypokalemia may worsen insulin resistance. Clinical studies have demonstrated that prevention of diuretic-induced hypokalemia with potassium infusions preserves insulin sensitivity.[82] Thus, diuretics need to be used cautiously in diabetic hypertensives only as necessary to facilitate blood pressure control or volume reduction. β-blockers may interfere with peripheral blood flow and worsen insulin resistance.[105] These agents may also mask hypoglycemic symptoms and result in more prolonged hypoglycemia and associated morbidity. As previously discussed, ACEIs clearly have advantages in diabetic hypertensives, who have associated nephropathy or proteinuria, or both.

In summary, aggressive blood pressure reduction is indicated in diabetic hypertensives because there is so much coexistent cardiovascular risk. However, orthostasis may interfere with the intensity of antihypertensive efforts. Coexistent comorbidities may require use of a variety of antihypertensive drugs. Overall, however, vasodilators make the most physiological sense, and ACEIs in particular provide additional benefit with regard to the kidney. Individualization is critical in these high-risk patients in an effort to control the hypertension and associated comorbidities.

LOWER DOSES OF TWO VERSUS HIGHER DOSES OF ONE ANTIHYPERTENSIVE DRUG

The rationale behind employing two or more drugs in lower doses versus a single agent in higher doses stems from growing evidence that traditional strategies of using a single agent at higher dose has not been successful in controlling blood pressure in more than 50% of patients. Moreover, some hypertensives (diabetics and some patients with renal disease) may require greater reduction of systolic and diastolic blood pressure than what has been traditionally accepted (140/90 mm Hg).[66, 79] Traditional single-drug titration is associated with an increased incidence of dose-related adverse events that can interfere with tolerability. Essential hypertension is a complex and heterogeneous disorder whose underlying pathophysiology is unknown and likely varies substantially from patient to patient. Thus, it is impossible to predict which patient will respond to a given antihypertensive drug. Sequential therapeutic challenges take time and lead to substantial frustration and cost related to unused medication. Using lower doses of two or more drugs may provide greater efficacy through different therapeutic mechanisms of action, yet have a lower likelihood of inducing adverse events. Arguments against this strategy include that if the patient does not have a satisfactory response, one will not know which component to blame, and if there is an adverse event, one cannot be sure which drug is involved. However, more often than not, this has not been the case in clinical trials employing this therapeutic stratagem.

With six major classes of antihypertensive drugs available, one has a broad variety of combinations to use (Table 51–8). Most data available using drug combinations have been derived from studies in which one component is a thiazide diuretic. Clinical trials evaluating thiazides in combinations with other drugs have demonstrated a uniform benefit in lowering blood pressure that can be complimentary, additive, or even synergistic—the latter benefit usually occurring with drugs that inhibit the renin-angiotensin system, such as β-blockers, ACEIs, or angiotensin receptor blockers.[106]

The Veterans Affairs Cooperative Studies Group on Antihypertensive Agents has provided insightful data regarding the use of combination therapy in patients who did

Table 51–8 Common Forms of Combination Antihypertensive Therapy

THIAZIDE-BASED
Potassium-sparing diuretic/thiazide
β-Blocker/thiazide
ACEI/thiazide
Angiotensin II type 1 receptor blocker/thiazide

NON–THIAZIDE-BASED
ACEI/dihydropyridine CCB
ACEI/NDCCB

Abbreviations: ACEI, angiotensin-converting enzyme inhibitor; CCB, calcium channel blocker; NDCCB, nondihydropyridine calcium channel blocker.

not respond to a single agent.[107] The nonresponders in this study were randomly allocated to a second drug (initial therapy was either a thiazide, a β-blocker, an ACEI, a calcium channel blocker, or a centrally acting agent). The overall response rate to monotherapy in this study, defined as a diastolic blood pressure less than 90 mm Hg, was 57.7%. An additional 49.1% of the nonresponders achieved goal diastolic blood pressure with the addition of a second agent, resulting in an overall control rate of approximately 76%. If the combination regimen included a diuretic, 69% of nonresponders improved, compared with only 50% of the patients who received a nondiuretic combination. These data suggest a rationale for almost always including at least a low dose of a diuretic in most antihypertensive combinations, particularly with drugs that block the renin-angiotensin system.

There has been a major emphasis on the development of low-dose, fixed-combination antihypertensive therapies in the past few years. Traditional low-dose combinations of thiazides with β-blockers, ACEIs, and angiotensin receptor blockers as well as newer nondiuretic combinations including ACEIs and both dihydropyridine and nondihydropyridine calcium channel blockers are available.[106, 108–110] All of these low-dose, fixed-combinations demonstrate at least additive, if not synergistic, capabilities to lower blood pressure with an improved side effect profile compared with higher doses of the individual components.[111–114]

When more than one agent is used, there are no good clinical studies to show differences in blood pressure reduction based on the order of the two drugs employed. Additionally, some drugs may take longer to work with one another compared with other combinations. Consequently, decisions about adding another drug should be delayed for at least 6 to 8 weeks to give the initial agent time to have its maximal effect, unless clinical circumstances dictate otherwise. There are several options in combination therapy that physicians can consider, including starting with a single agent and adding another agent if the first drug does not achieve desired blood pressure control or starting with one agent and, if it fails to achieve desirable control, stopping the agent and starting treatment with an alternative drug. If this fails, it is appropriate to use the two in combination or to introduce one of the previously mentioned low-dose, fixed-combinations.

Other benefits may accrue from using lower doses of two or more drugs that reduce arterial pressure through different mechanisms. Besides the obvious ability to avoid dose-related adverse events, one drug may antagonize the adverse events induced by the other. For example, ACEIs or angiotensin receptor blockers may attenuate thiazide-induced hypokalemia, or an ACEI may reduce calcium channel blocker–induced pedal edema.[114] One drug may potentiate the antihypertensive properties of the other. For example, drugs that block the renin-angiotensin-aldosterone system are more effective during states of mild volume depletion and thus are potentiated by concomitant use of thiazides. Similarly, β-blockers may offset the reflex tachycardia induced by vasodilators and thus both agents facilitate blood pressure control and reduce the likelihood of adverse events that may stem from the increased heart rate.

Finally, lower doses of multiple drugs may have specific benefits with regard to target organ function above and beyond more effective blood pressure control and improved compliance. For example, drugs that more effectively attenuate left ventricular hypertrophy or improve diastolic function may provide benefit in patients with hypertrophic cardiomyopathy. Drugs such as an ACEI and a nondihydropyridine calcium channel blocker may potentiate the antiproteinuric properties of one another and thus be more effective in delaying the progression of renal disease.[79, 81] Consequently, there is substantial rationale for using lower doses of two or more agents as necessary to achieve satisfactory blood pressure control owing to both improved efficacy and improved tolerability. The Joint National Committee's Sixth Report endorses this approach as one form of initial antihypertensive therapy.[2]

Since all patients are different, the optimal combination of drugs is unknown. Substantial evidence and experience with diuretic-based combination therapy suggest that it makes the most sense. It certainly provides some of the best efficacy. However, data with some of the newer ACEI–calcium channel blocker combinations also demonstrate substantial potency. What we do not know is whether it is appropriate to use together two drugs of similar classes such as an ACEI with an angiotensin receptor blocker or a dihydropyridine calcium channel blocker with a nondihydropyridine channel blocker. More clinical trials are needed to answer these interesting questions. Additionally, more studies are needed to determine an optimal third drug to use in a low-dose regimen for patients with more complicated forms of hypertension.

CONCLUSIONS

Initial choices in the treatment of hypertension may vary substantially based on an individual patient's requirements. The Joint National Committee's Sixth Report encourages traditional therapies (low doses of thiazide diuretics or β-blockers) as initial treatment in patients with uncomplicated hypertension, based on longstanding experience with these drugs in reducing morbidity and mortality in large-scale clinical trials.[2] However, it is likely that sustained blood pressure reduction with other drugs will provide similar degrees of benefit. The key is not the drug so much as it is the ability to maintain long-term control based on satisfactory therapeutic efficacy and good tolerability. Nonadherence rates are extremely high, and there is no rationale for using one therapy versus another in patients who are free of comorbid conditions. Consequently, some degree of experimentation with the various classes of drugs will be necessary. This experimentation will involve which drug class, whether to titrate, whether to use lower doses of two versus higher doses of one, and how to mix and match therapies to achieve optimal control and deal with concomitant comorbidities.

Careful individualization, rather than generalization, is necessary. There are many good therapies that can be used. There are very few indications in which certain therapies should not be used. Nonpharmacological efforts should always be employed as best possible, with the realization that in many patients they will not be successful over the long term.

What is clear, however, is that more aggressive interventional strategies are needed because there is growing evidence that achieving lower levels of blood pressure may be optimal in preventing hypertensive morbidity and mortality.

Newer therapeutic strategies such as low-dose, fixed-combinations of drugs, the angiotensin receptor blockers, and renin inhibitors will soon be complementing our armamentarium. How to best use these therapies in conjunction with existing therapies that we have had more experience with will be an important test for practicing physicians over the next several years. However, our ability to better educate our patients and to work with them more closely about the need for medication will be a critical facet in achieving long-term control. In addition, we need to make clear to our patients that healthier lifestyle choices will reduce the dependence on medication for adequate blood pressure control. Optimally, every patient can be capably controlled if sufficient effort is made in choosing a therapeutic plan and providing the necessary background education.

References

1. Burt VL, Cutler JA, Higgins M, et al. Trends in the prevalence, awareness, treatment, and control of hypertension in the adult US population: Data from the Health Examination Surveys, 1960 to 1991. Hypertension 26:60–69, 1995.
2. Joint National Committee on Prevention, Detection, Evaluation, and Treatment of High Blood Pressure. The Sixth Report of the Joint National Committee on Prevention, Detection, Evaluation, and Treatment of High Blood Pressure. Arch Intern Med 157:2413–2446, 1997.
3. Messerli FH, Schmieder RE, Weir MR. Salt—A perpetrator of hypertensive target organ disease? Arch Intern Med 157:2449–2452, 1997.
4. Whelton PK, He J, Cutler JA, et al. Effects of oral potassium on blood pressure: Meta-analysis of randomized controlled clinical trials. JAMA 277:1624–1632, 1997.
5. Cappuccio FP, Elliott P, Allender PS, et al. Epidemiologic association between dietary calcium intake and blood pressure: A meta-analysis of published data. Am J Epidemiol 142:935–945, 1995.
6. Appel LJ, Moore TJ, Obarzanek E, et al. A clinical trial of the effects of dietary patterns on blood pressure. DASH Collaborative Research Group. N Engl J Med 336:1117–1124, 1997.
7. Elliott P, Stamler J, Nichols R, et al, for the Intersalt Cooperative Research Group. Intersalt revisited: Further analyses of 24 hour sodium excretion and blood pressure within and across populations. BMJ 312:1249–1253, 1996.
8. Cutler JA, Follmann D, Allender PS. Randomized trials of sodium reduction: An overview. Am J Clin Nutr 65(suppl):643S–651S, 1997.
9. Midgely JP, Matthew AG, Greenwood CMT, Logan AG. Effect of reduced dietary sodium on blood pressure: A meta-analysis of randomized controlled trials. JAMA 275:1590–1597, 1996.
10. Alderman MH, Madhavan S, Cohen H, et al. Low urinary sodium is associated with greater risk of myocardial infarction among treated hypertensive men. Hypertension 25:1144–1152, 1995.
11. Applegate WB, Sowers JR. Elevated systolic blood pressure: Increased cardiovascular risk and rationale for treatment. Am J Med 101(suppl 3A):3S–9S, 1996.
12. Ooi WL, Barrett S, Hossain M, et al. Patterns of orthostatic blood pressure change and their clinical correlates in a frail, elderly population. JAMA 277:1299–1304, 1997.
13. Messerli FH. Osler's maneuver, pseudohypertension, and true hypertension in the elderly. Am J Med 80:906–910, 1986.
14. SHEP Cooperative Research Group. Prevention of stroke by antihypertensive drug treatment in older persons with isolated systolic hypertension: Final results of the Systolic Hypertension in the Elderly Program (SHEP). JAMA 265:3255–3264, 1991.
15. MRC Working Party. Medical Research Council trial of treatment of hypertension in older adults: Principal results. BMJ 304:405–412, 1992.
16. Dahlöf B, Lindholm LH, Hansson L, et al. Morbidity and mortality in the Swedish Trial in Old Patients with Hypertension (STOP-Hypertension). Lancet 338:1281–1285, 1991.
17. Kostis JB, Davis BR, Cutler J, et al. Prevention of heart failure by antihypertensive drug treatment in older persons with isolated systolic hypertension. JAMA 278:212–216, 1997.
18. Staessen JA, Fagard R, Thijs L, et al, for the Systolic Hypertension in Europe (Syst-Eur) Trial Investigators. Randomised double-blind comparison of placebo and active treatment for older patients with isolated systolic hypertension. Lancet 350:757–764, 1997.
19. Materson BJ, Reda DJ, Cushman WC, et al, for the Department of Veterans Affairs Cooperative Study Group on Antihypertensive Agents. Single-drug therapy for hypertension in men: A comparison of six antihypertensive agents with placebo. N Engl J Med 328:914–921, 1993.
20. Iabichella ML, Dell'Omo G, Melillo E, Pedrinelli R. Calcium channel blockers blunt postural cutaneous vasoconstriction in hypertensive patients. Hypertension 29:751–756, 1997.
21. Hedlund H, Andersson KE, Ek AK. Effects of prazosin in patients with benign prostatic obstruction. J Urol 130:275–278, 1983.
22. Houston MC, Weir MR, Gray J, et al. The effects of nonsteroidal anti-inflammatory drugs on blood pressures of patients with hypertension controlled by verapamil. Arch Intern Med 155:1049–1054, 1995.
23. Farnett L, Mulrow CD, Linn WD, et al. The J-curve phenomenon and the treatment of hypertension: Is there a point beyond which pressure reduction is dangerous? JAMA 265:489–495, 1991.
24. Coope J, Warrender TS. Randomised trial of treatment of hypertension in elderly patients in primary care. BMJ 293:1145–1151, 1986.
25. Staessen J, Bulpitt C, Clement D, et al. Relation between mortality and treated blood pressure in elderly patients with hypertension: Report of the European Working Party on High Blood Pressure in the Elderly. BMJ 298:1552–1556, 1989.
26. Lazarus JM, Bourgoignie JJ, Buckalew VM, et al, for the Modification of Diet in Renal Disease Study Group. Achievement and safety of a low blood pressure goal in chronic renal disease: The Modification of Diet in Renal Disease Study Group. Hypertension 29:641–650, 1997.
27. Du X, Cruickshank K, McNamee R, et al. Case-control study of stroke and the quality of hypertension control in Northwest England. BMJ 314:272–276, 1997.
28. MacMahon S, Rodgers A. The effects of blood pressure reduction in older patients: An overview of five randomized controlled trials in elderly hypertensives. Clin Exp Hypertens 15:967–978, 1993.
29. Hanes DS, Weir MR, Sowers JR. Gender considerations in hypertension pathophysiology and treatment. Am J Med 101(suppl 3A):10S–21S, 1996.
30. Messerli FH, Garavaglia GE, Schmieder R. Disparate cardiovascular findings in men and women with essential hypertension. Ann Intern Med 107:158–163, 1987.
31. Stoney CM, Davis MC, Matthews KA. Sex differences in physiological responses to stress and coronary heart disease: A causal link? Psychophysiology 24:127–131, 1987.
32. Douglas PS, Ginsburg GS. The evaluation of chest pain in women. N Engl J Med 334:1311–1315, 1996.
33. Lerner DJ, Kannel WB. Patterns of coronary heart disease morbidity and mortality in the sexes. A 26-year follow-up of the Framingham population. Am Heart J 1:383–390, 1986.

34. National High Blood Pressure Education Program Working Group. National High Blood Pressure Education Program Working Group report on hypertension in the elderly. Hypertension 23:275–285, 1994.

35. Gueyffier F, Boutitie F, Boissel JP, et al, for the INDANA Investigators. Effect of antihypertensive drug treatment on cardiovascular outcomes in women and men: A meta-analysis of individual patient data from randomized, controlled trials. Ann Intern Med 126:761–767, 1997.

36. Schwartz J, Freeman R, Frishman W. Clinical pharmacology of estrogens: Cardiovascular actions and cardioprotective benefits of replacement therapy in postmenopausal women. J Clin Pharmacol 35:1–16, 1995.

37. The Writing Group for the PEPI Trial. Effects of estrogen or estrogen/progestin regimens on heart disease risk factors in postmenopausal women. The Postmenopausal Estrogen/Progestin Interventions trial. JAMA 273:199–208, 1995.

38. Woods JW. Oral contraceptives and hypertension. Hypertension 11(suppl II):II-11–II-15, 1988.

39. Os I, Bratland B, Daholf B, et al. Female preponderance for lisinopril-induced cough in hypertension. Am J Hypertens 7:1012–1015, 1994.

40. Weir MR. Antihypertensive combination therapy. Drugs Today 34:5–9, 1998.

41. Hypertension Detection and Follow-Up Program Cooperative Group. Five year findings of the Hypertension Detection and Follow-Up Program II. Mortality by race, sex, and age. J JAMA 242:2572–2577, 1979.

42. Schnall P, Alderman MH, Kern R. An analysis of the HDFP trial. Evidence of adverse effects of antihypertensive therapy on white women with moderate to severe hypertension. N Y State J Med 84:299–301, 1984.

43. Medical Research Council Working Party. MRC trial of treatment of mild hypertension: Principal results. BMJ 291:197–204, 1985.

44. The Australian Therapeutic Trial in Mild Hypertension. Report by the Management Committee. Lancet 1:1261–1267, 1980.

45. Treatment of Mild Hypertension in the Elderly. A study initiated and administered by the National Heart Foundation of Australia. Med J Aust 2:398–402, 1981.

46. Gueyffier F, Boutitie F, Boissel J, et al. Effect of antihypertensive drug treatment on cardiovascular outcomes in women and men: A meta-analysis of individual patient data from randomized, controlled trials. Ann Intern Med 126:761–767, 1997.

47. Hiedrich FE, Stergachis A, Gross KM. Diuretic drug use and the risk for hip fracture. Ann Intern Med 115:1–6, 1991.

48. Morton DJ, Barrett-Connor EL, Edelstein SL. Thiazides and bone mineral density in elderly men and women. Am J Epidemiol 139:1107–1115, 1994.

49. Wasnich R, Davis J, Ross P, Vogel J. Effect of thiazide on rates of bone mineral loss: A longitudinal study. BMJ 302:18, 1991.

50. Ray WA. Thiazide diuretics and osteoporosis: Time for a clinical trial. Ann Intern Med 115:64–65, 1991.

51. Jones G, Nguyen T, Sambrook PN, Eisman JA. Thiazide diuretics and fractures: Can meta-analysis help? J Bone Miner Res 10:106–111, 1995.

52. Hall WD, Ferrario CM, Moore MA, et al. Hypertension-related morbidity and mortality in the southeastern United States. Am J Med Sci 313:195–206, 1997.

53. Burt VL, Whelton P, Roccella EJ, et al. Prevalence of hypertension in the US adult population: Results from the third National Health and Nutrition Examination Survey, 1988–1991. Hypertension 25:305–313, 1995.

54. Singh GK, Kochanek KD, MacDorman MF. Advance report of final mortality statistics, 1994. Mon Vital Stat Rep 45(suppl 3):1–76, 1996.

55. Klag MJ, Whelton PK, Randall BL, et al. End-stage renal disease in African-American and white men: 16-year MRFIT findings. JAMA 277:1293–1298, 1997.

56. Jamerson K, DeQuattro V. The impact of ethnicity on response to antihypertensive therapy. Am J Med 101(suppl 3A): 22S–32S, 1996.

57. Weir MR, Chrysant SG, McCarron DA, et al. Influence of race and dietary salt on the antihypertensive efficacy of an angiotensin-converting enzyme inhibitor or a calcium channel antagonist in salt-sensitive hypertensives. Hypertension 31:1088–1096, 1998.

58. Hypertension Detection and Follow-Up Program Cooperative Group. Five-year findings of the Hypertension Detection and Follow-Up Program: Mortality by race-sex and blood pressure level. A further analysis. J Community Health 9:314–327, 1984.

59. Ooi WL, Budner NS, Cohen H, et al. Impact of race on treatment response and cardiovascular disease among hypertensives. Hypertension 14:227–234, 1989.

60. Weir MR, Tuck ML. Essential hypertension in blacks: Is it a metabolic disorder? Am J Kidney Dis 21(suppl 1):58–67, 1993.

61. Weir MR, Hanes DS. Hypertension in African Americans: A paradigm of metabolic disarray. Semin Nephrol 16:102–109, 1996.

62. Weir MR. Salt intake and hypertensive renal injury in African-Americans: A therapeutic perspective. Am J Hypertens 8:635–644, 1995.

63. Weir MR, Saunders E. Pharmacologic management of systemic hypertension in blacks. Am J Cardiol 61:46H–52H, 1988.

64. Saunders E, Weir MR, Kong BW, et al. A comparison of the efficacy and safety of a β-blocker, a calcium channel blocker, and a converting enzyme inhibitor in hypertensive blacks. Arch Intern Med 150:1707–1713, 1990.

65. Weir MR, Gray JM, Paster R, Saunders E. Differing mechanisms of action of angiotensin-converting enzyme inhibition in black and white hypertensive patients. The Trandolapril Multicenter Study Group. Hypertension 26:124–130, 1995.

66. Klahr S, Levey AS, Beck GJ, et al, for the Modification of Diet in Renal Disease Study Group. The effects of dietary protein restriction and blood-pressure control on the progression of chronic renal disease. N Engl J Med 330:877–884, 1994.

67. Havas S, Sherwin R. Putting it all together: Summary of the NHLBI Workshop on the Epidemiology of Hypertension in Hispanic American, Native American, and Asian/Pacific Islander American Populations. Public Health Rep 3(suppl 2):77–79, 1996.

68. Bakris GL, Weir MR, Sowers JR. Therapeutic challenges in the obese diabetic patient with hypertension. Am J Med 101(suppl 3A):33S–46S, 1996.

69. Bray GA. Obesity increases risk of diabetes. Int J Obesity 16(suppl 4):513–517, 1992.

70. Pi-Sunyer FX. Medical hazards of obesity. Ann Intern Med 119:655–660, 1993.

71. Sowers JR. Modest weight gain and the development of diabetes: Another perspective. Ann Intern Med 122:548–549, 1995.

72. Weir MR, Sowers JR. Physiologic and hemodynamic considerations in blood pressure control while maintaining organ perfusion. Am J Cardiol 61:60H–66H, 1988.

73. Messerli FH, Christie B, Decarvalho JGR, et al. Obesity and essential hypertension: Hemodynamics, intravascular volume, sodium excretion and plasma renin activity. Arch Intern Med 141:81–89, 1981.

74. Messerli FH, Sundgaard-Riise K, Reisin E, et al. Disparate cardiovascular effects of obesity and arterial hypertension. Am J Med 74:808–813, 1983.

75. Sowers JR, Whitfield LA, Catania RA, et al. Role of the sympathetic nervous system in blood pressure maintenance in obesity. J Clin Endocrinol Metab 54:1181–1185, 1982.

76. Romero JC, Raij L, Granger JP, et al. Multiple effects of calcium entry blockers on renal function in hypertension. Hypertension 10:140–151, 1987.

77. Zusman RM. Effects of converting enzyme inhibitors on the renin-angiotensin aldosterone, bradykinin, and arachidonic acid–prostaglandin systems: Correlation of chemical structure and biologic activity. Am J Kidney Dis 10(suppl 1):S13–S23, 1987.

78. Redgrave J, Rabinowe S, Hollenberg NK, et al. Correction of abnormal renal blood flow response to angiotensin II by converting enzyme inhibition in essential hypertensives. J Clin Invest 75:1285–1290, 1985.

79. Lewis EJ, Hunsicker LG, Bain RP, Rohde RD, for the Collaborative Study Group. The effect of angiotensin-converting-enzyme inhibition on diabetic nephropathy. N Engl J Med 329:1456–1462, 1993.

80. Giatras I, Lau J, Levey AS, for the Angiotensin-Converting Enzyme Inhibition and Progressive Renal Desease Study Group. Effect of angiotensin-converting enzyme inhibitors on the progression of nondiabetic renal disease: A meta-analysis of randomized trials. Ann Intern Med 127:337–345, 1997.

81. Bakris GL, Copley JB, Vicknair N, et al. Calcium channel blockers versus other antihypertensive therapies on progression of NIDDM–associated nephropathy. Kidney Int 50:1641–1650, 1996.

82. Helderman JH, Elahi D, Andersen DK, et al. Prevention of the

glucose intolerance of thiazide diuretics by maintenance of body potassium. Diabetes 32:106–111, 1983.

83. Franklin SS, Weber MA. Measuring hypertensive cardiovascular risk: The vascular overload concept. Am Heart J 128:793–802, 1994.

84. Furberg CD, Psaty BM, Meyer JV. Nifedipine: Dose-related increase in mortality in patients with coronary heart disease. Circulation 92:1326–1331, 1995.

85. Grossman E, Messerli FH, Grodzicki T, Kowey P. Should a moratorium be placed on sublingual nifedipine capsules given for hypertensive emergencies and pseudoemergencies? JAMA 92:1328–1331, 1996.

86. Smolensky MH. Chronobiology and chronotherapeutics. Am J Hypertens 9:11S–21S, 1996.

87. SOLVD Investigators. Effect of enalapril on survival in patients with reduced left ventricular ejection fractions and congestive heart faiure. N Engl J Med 325:293–302, 1991.

88. Pfeffer MA, Braunwald E, Moye LA, et al, for the SAVE Investigators. Effect of captopril on mortality and morbidity in patients with left ventricular dysfunction after myocardial infarction: Results of the survival and ventricular enlargement trials. N Engl J Med 327:669–677, 1992.

89. Garg R, Yusuf S, for the Collaborative Group on ACE Inhibitor trails. Overview of randomized trials of angiotensin-converting enzyme inhibitors on mortality and morbidity in patients with heart failure. JAMA 273:1450–1456, 1995.

90. Packer M, Bristow MR, Cohn JN, et al, for the U.S. Carvedilol Heart Failure Study Group. The effect of carvedilol on morbidity and mortality in patients with chronic heart failure. N Engl J Med 334:1349–1355, 1996.

91. Pitt B, Segal R, Martinez FA, et al, for the ELITE Study Investigators. Randomized trial of losartan versus captopril in patients over 65 with heart failure (Evaluation of Losartan in the Elderly Study, ELITE). Lancet 349:747–752, 1997.

92. Packer M, O'Connor CM, Ghali JK, et al, for the Prospective Randomized Amlodipine Survival Evaluation Study Group. Effect of amlodipine on morbidity and mortality in severe chronic heart failure. N Engl J Med 335:1107–1114, 1996.

93. Cohn JN, Ziesche S, Smith R, et al, for the Vasodilator-Heart Failure Trial. Effect of the calcium antagonist felodipine as supplementary vasodilator therapy in patients with chronic heart failure treated with enalapril: V-HeFT III. Circulation 96:856–863, 1997.

94. Cuocolo A, Sax FL, Brush JE, et al. Left ventricular hypertrophy and impaired diastolic filling in essential hypertension. Diastolic mechanisms for systolic dysfunction during exercise. Circulation 81:978–986, 1990.

95. Bonow RO, Dilsizian V, Rosing DR, et al. Verapamil-induced improvement in left ventricular diastolic filling and increased exercise tolerance in patients with hypertrophic cardiomyopathy: Short- and long-term effects. Circulation 72:853–864, 1985.

96. National High Blood Pressure Education Program Working Group. 1995 update of the Working Group reports on chronic renal failure and renovascular hypertension. Arch Intern Med 156:1938–1947, 1996.

97. Kasiske BL, Kalil RSN, Ma JZ, et al. Effect of antihypertensive therapy on the kidney in patients with diabetes. A meta-regression analysis. Ann Intern Med 118:129–138, 1993.

98. Weir MR, Dworkin LD. Antihypertensive drugs, dietary salt and renal protection: How low should you go, and with which therapy? Am J Kidney Dis 32:1–22, 1998.

99. Bakris GL, Mangrum A, Copley JB, et al. Effect of calcium channel or β-blockade on the progress of diabetic nephropathy in African Americans. Hypertension 29:744–750, 1997.

100. Velussi M, Brocco E, Frigato F, et al. Effects of cilazapril and amlodipine on kidney function in hypertensive NIDDM patients. Diabetes 45:216–222, 1996.

101. Gansevoort RT, de Zeeuw D, de Jong PE. Is the antiproteinuric effect of ACE inhibition mediated by interference in the renin-angiotensin system? Kidney Int 45:861–867, 1994.

102. Heeg JE, De Jong PE, van der Hem GK, de Zeeuw D. Efficacy and variability of the antiproteinuric effect of ACE inhibition by lisinopril. Kidney Int 36:272–279, 1989.

103. Textor SC. Renal failure related to angiotensin-converting enzyme inhibitors. Semin Nephrol 17:67–76, 1997.

104. Reardon LC, Macpherson DS. Hyperkalemia in outpatients using angiotensin-converting enzyme inhibitors. How much should we worry? Arch Intern Med 158:26–32, 1998.

105. Pollare T, Lithell H, Selinus J, Berne C. Sensitivity to insulin during treatment with atenolol and metoprolol: A randomized, double-blind study of effects on carbohydrate and lipoprotein metabolism in hypertensive patients. BMJ 298:1152–1157, 1989.

106. Neutel JM, Black HR, Weber MA. Combination therapy with diuretics: An evolution of understanding. Am J Med 101(suppl 3A):61S–70S, 1996.

107. Materson BJ, Reda DJ, Preston RA, et al, for the Department of Veterans Affairs Cooperative Study Group on Antihypertensive Agents. Response to a second single antihypertensive agent used as monotherapy for hypertension after failure of the initial drug. Arch Intern Med 155:1757–1762, 1995.

108. Prisant LM, Weir MR, Papademetriou V, et al. Low-dose drug combination therapy: An alternative first-line approach to hypertension treatment. Am Heart J 130:359–366, 1995.

109. Neutel JM, Rolf CN, Valentine SN, et al. Low-dose combination therapy as first line treatment of mild-to-moderate hypertension: The efficacy and safety of bisoprolol/HCTZ versus amlodipine, enalapril, and placebo. Cardiovasc Rev Rep 17:1–9, 1996.

110. Weir MR, Elkins M, Liss C, et al. Efficacy, tolerability, and quality of life of losartan, alone or with hydrochlorothiazide, versus nifedipine GITS in patients with essential hypertension. Clin Ther 18:411–428, 1996.

111. Gradman AH, Cutler NR, Davis PJ, et al: Combined enalapril and felodipine extended release (ER) for systemic hypertension. Am J Cardiol 79:431–435, 1997.

112. Messerli FH, Frishman WH, Elliott WJ, for the Trandolapril Study Group: Effects of verapamil and trandolapril in the treatment of hypertension. Am J Hypertens 11:322–327, 1998.

113. Cushman WC, Cohen JD, Jones RP, et al. Comparison of the fixed combination of enalapril/diltiazem ER and their monotherapies in stage 1–3 essential hypertension. Am J Hypertens 11:23–30, 1998.

114. Frishman WH, Ram CV, McMahon FG, et al. Comparison of amlodipine and benazepril monotherapy to amlodipine plus benazepril in patients with systemic hypertension: A randomized, double-blind, placebo-controlled, parallel-group study. J Clin Pharmacol 35:1060–1066, 1995.

52

CHAPTER

Dose-Response Relationships in Antihypertensive Treatment

Todd W. B. Gehr and Domenic A. Sica

Although there usually is a clearly defined pharmacokinetic relationship between the dose of a drug and the plasma drug concentration, the pharmacodynamic relationship between dose (or plasma concentration) and blood pressure response or efficacy is more problematic. The lack of understanding of this relationship has led to a variety of clinical problems, the most serious of which has been the introduction of antihypertensive medications to clinical practice at excessively high doses. Examples include thiazide diuretics,[1-4] β-blockers,[2,5,6] and captopril,[7] all of which are currently prescribed in dose ranges much lower than those originally recommended. As we approach a more individualized form of hypertension treatment, a thorough understanding of the determinants of this dose-response relationship will become essential.

DOSE-RESPONSE RELATIONSHIP

The assumption that the relationship between the plasma half-life of an antihypertensive medication and the duration and extent of its antihypertensive effect is very limited has only recently been questioned. The fundamental relationship in therapeutics exemplified by the typical dose-response curve applies to antihypertensive medications just as it does to other drugs. Although largely ignored in drug development, this concept is increasingly critical to a precise understanding of single and multidrug antihypertensive effects. Figure 52–1A depicts this fundamental relationship. Simply stated, a drug's effect or pharmacological response increases as the dose and, by extension, the concentration of the drug at its site of action rise. This dose-response relationship is commonly expressed as a log-linear dose-response relationship and assumes a characteristic S-shaped curve (Fig. 52–1B).

A particular antihypertensive's effect is dependent not

only on the size of the dose but also on the portion of the dose-response curve at which a particular drug dose falls. The importance of this relationship is exemplified by drugs that have been said to have "flat" dose-response curves (increasing doses produce little additional effect). For example, high doses of lisinopril[8] lead to high plasma concentrations, corresponding to antihypertensive effects at the plateau (maximal response) of the dose-response curve, whereas identifying lower-effect doses on the upward-going portion of the dose-response curve would likely expose a clear dose-response relationship.

Another important consideration in interpreting dose-response relationships is an understanding of the temporal relationship between dose or drug concentration and response.[9] For some drugs, there is little time-related correlation between plasma drug concentration and measured response, implying rapid penetration and equilibration from the plasma to the receptor site. For many drugs, however, this relationship is not simple, and the time course of drug effect is delayed and without a direct relationship to plasma concentrations. Interestingly, these temporal effects may be applicable to both intravenous and oral medications. A temporal delay in drug action may be related to the delay in entry of a drug or active metabolite into the compartment in which a particular effect is to be elicited. Figure 52–2 shows this delay in response as the drug moves into compartment 1. This lag in drug effect may be highly variable, since it is dependent on a number of factors, including the time taken for the drug-receptor interaction, delay in penetration to its receptor, or formation of an active metabolite.[10] This effect is expressed on the dose-response relationship as counterclockwise hysteresis (a particular plasma concentration elicits a variable, in this case, greater response with time) and is encountered frequently with intravenous drugs when there is a delay between the plasma concentration and the measured effect (Fig. 52–3). The

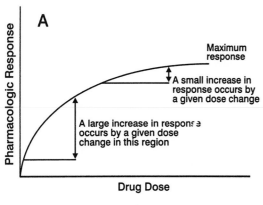

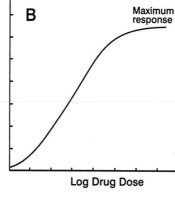

Figure 52–1. Schematics of examples of dose-response relationships. **A.** Linear drug dose concentration and the change in effect as drug dose is increased. **B.** Logarithmic dose-response relationship.

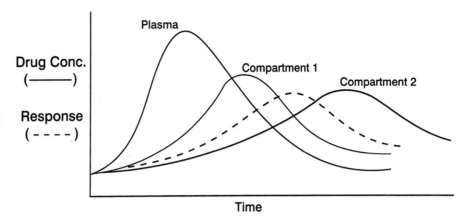

Figure 52–2. Schematic of the time dependency of drug response as the drug moves from its plasma compartment into its site of action (effect compartments).

opposite effect on the dose-response relationship is encountered with clockwise hysteresis in which a diminishing response is observed with the same drug concentration with time. This phenomenon occurs commonly with antihypertensive medications and diuretics, in which the particular blood pressure–lowering or diuretic response is blunted by the body's compensatory mechanisms such as tachycardia or salt retention.

Intraindividual variability in the pharmacokinetics and/or pharmacodynamics of antihypertensive drugs might thus confound interpretation of dose-response relationships derived from population-based studies. Indeed, many studies analyzing group data failed to define a dose-response relationship for particular antihypertensive drugs,[11] whereas a dose-response relationship is clearly identifiable from inspection of individual subject data.[12, 13] This discrepancy between group and individual dose-response data analysis is nicely illustrated by the α_1-adrenergic receptor antagonist doxazosin.[14] Figure 52–4A shows that there is no clear relationship between doxazosin concentration and its antihypertensive effect. In Figure 52–4B individual data sets plotted for three patients clearly show a concentration-effect relationship, with clockwise hysteresis apparent in each patient. In this particular case, the concentration-effect relationship is complex, and analysis of group data would

have yielded little information regarding the dose-response relationship of doxazosin.

The integration of pharmacokinetic and pharmacodynamic analysis (Fig. 52–5), often termed *concentration-effect analysis,* is best described by a number of mathematical models that discuss the complicated temporal effects of drugs on response.[15] In these models, building on established pharmacokinetic and pharmacodynamic principles, the measured effect (E) is related to the drug concentration in the effect compartment (C_e) at each time point by either a linear or a nonlinear model:

$$E = mC_e + i$$
$$E = E_{max} C_e/(C_e50 + C_e) \text{ (Langmuir)}$$
$$E = E_{max} C_e^\gamma/(C_e50 + C_e^\gamma) \text{ (Hill)}$$

where m is the slope of the relationship, i is the intercept, E_{max} is the maximal possible effect, C_e50 is the concentration required to produce 50% of E_{max}, and γ is the number influencing the slope of the curve. In practical terms, when antihypertensive effect is measured relative to drug concentrations on the steep portion of the dose-response curve, a linear model can be utilized that relates effect (millimeters of mercury fall in blood pressure) directly to plasma concentration. For a more thorough evaluation of a wider range of concentrations, the more rigorous E_{max} model should be utilized. Parameters such as m, E_{max}, and C_e50 provide simple numerical results that characterize an individual's pattern of antihypertensive response.[16] Most importantly, they can be standardized to account for variability in pharmacokinetics, the magnitude of the blood pressure response, placebo effects, and the circadian character of blood pressure variation. These standardized parameters can be used to compare a drug's effect in a variety of different circumstances, thus helping clarify the variability in blood pressure response.[16]

VARIABILITY IN ANTIHYPERTENSIVE DRUG RESPONSE

Before discussing those confounding factors that account for much of the variability in antihypertensive drug response, such as age, race, plasma renin activity, starting blood pressure, constancy of response, and counterregula-

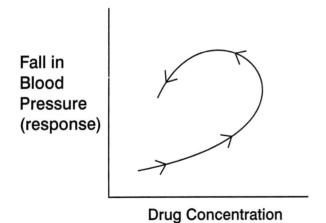

Fall in Blood Pressure (response)

Drug Concentration

Figure 52–3. Counter-clockwise hysteresis loop of concentration-response (fall in blood pressure) relationship represents the delay in equilibrium between the drug and its site of action.

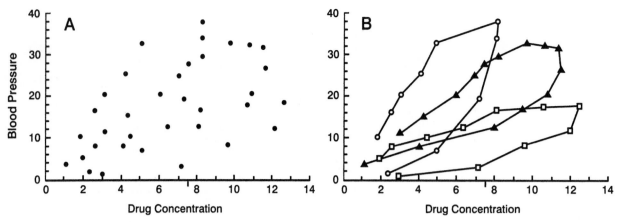

Figure 52–4. A. Plasma doxazosin concentrations relative to antihypertensive response for a group of three patients. **B.** Same data, but now individual patient data are connected sequentially, illustrating hysteresis. (**A** and **B**, From Meredith PA, Reid JL. The use of pharmacodynamic and pharmacokinetic profiles in drug development for planning individual therapy. *In* Laragh JH, Brenner BM [eds]. Hypertension: Pathophysiology, Diagnosis, and Management, 2nd ed, vol 2. Philadelphia, Lippincott-Raven, 1995; p 2774.)

tory mechanisms, a comment on blood pressure measurement is warranted. The timing of blood pressure measurement is critical in that it depicts both the magnitude and the duration of effect. In this regard, peak, trough, or peak:trough ratios for blood pressure response have been proposed as efficacy measures. Trough blood pressure readings whether obtained by home or 24-hour blood pressure monitoring, are particularly useful in defining whether blood pressure control has been effectively maintained throughout a dosing interval.[17, 18]

Although initially believed to be a major determinant of antihypertensive drug response,[19] age accounts for only a small part of the variation observed in this parameter.[20, 21] Much of the age variation in response is not pharmacodynamic but rather relates to pharmacokinetic changes characteristically seen in the elderly. Similarly, although plasma renin activity was once believed to be an important factor in determining blood pressure response,[22] it has since been shown not to be a reliable predictor of response in patients with uncomplicated mild or moderate essential hypertension on a normal salt intake.[23, 24] In studies that have

used concentration-effect analysis with either nifedipine or enalapril, age and plasma renin activity accounted for less than 10% of the variability in blood pressure response.[25]

The influence of race on blood pressure responsiveness is such that African American subjects appear to respond better to drugs such as diuretics and calcium channel blockers that produce a natriuretic response and poorly to β-blockers and angiotensin-converting enzyme inhibitors.[26] In a double-blind, randomized, placebo-controlled trial of the pharmacodynamics of trandolapril in white and black hypertensive subjects, black subjects required larger doses of trandolapril but did, in fact, attain blood pressure reductions similar to those of white subjects.[27] Racial differences in the underlying pathophysiology of hypertension probably account for this variability in the angiotensin-converting enzyme inhibitor dose-response relationship.

The importance of pretreatment blood pressure as a determinant of blood pressure response has been summarized for a variety of drugs in which concentration-effect parameters have been highly correlated with initial blood pressure.[28] A more relevant question relates to the relation-

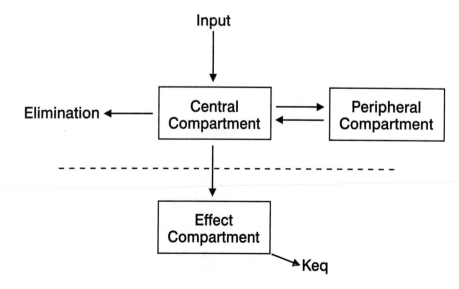

Figure 52–5. Extension of conventional compartmental pharmacokinetic models to include a pharmacodynamic or effect compartment with Keq representing the temporal relationship between concentration and effect.

ship between blood pressure responsiveness and duration of drug use. Although many factors may contribute to disparities between "acute" and "chronic" dose-response relationships, many studies have found a consistent relationship between drug responsiveness after 1 week and after 6 weeks of treatment;[9] suggesting that the acute hypotensive response to a drug can be used as a predictor of chronic antihypertensive efficacy. For example, the concentration-effect parameters derived after the first dose of enalapril have been used to predict individual blood pressure profiles during chronic dosing.[29] Similar correlation between acute and chronic responsiveness has been shown for nifedipine,[25] verapamil,[30] and amlodipine,[31] as well as other compounds.

Chronic blood pressure responsiveness is also influenced by counterregulatory mechanisms that tend to blunt the effect of an antihypertensive medication. Such factors include volume expansion secondary to renal sodium retention, tachycardia triggered by baroreceptor stimulation, and peripheral vasoconstriction resulting from activation of the renin-angiotensin and/or sympathetic system.

Clinically, it is sometimes difficult to gauge the extent to which counterregulatory systems are activated. Most typically, a loss of previously established blood pressure control should point to this possibility. A large number of such patients are unfortunately labeled as *resistant hypertensives*. Activation of the renin-angiotensin and/or sympathetic nervous system can be presumed by the known physiological effects of particular drug classes. Baseline pulse rates should be obtained when therapy is begun. A clinically relevant increase in pulse rate ($\sim$10%) should prompt consideration of either lowering the dose of the provoking agent or adding a pulse rate–lowering compound such as a β-blocker or clonidine.

Sodium retention, as a means by which blood pressure control is lost, is easy to recognize if peripheral edema develops; otherwise, the issue becomes more difficult. Weight gain is a rough and sometimes misleading clue to the degree of sodium retention. If sodium retention has developed secondary to a particular antihypertensive agent, volume depletion can generally be undertaken and the blood pressure response evaluated. Implementing these therapeutic stratagems will typically improve the dose-response relationship for a particular compound.

In summary, a multitude of factors are important in the complete evaluation of the dose/concentration-response/effect relationship for a particular antihypertensive drug. Only after a complete understanding of these factors is achieved will a more individualized approach to drug use be forthcoming. Table 52–1 summarizes these factors.

RELATIONSHIP BETWEEN DOSE AND ADVERSE EFFECTS

Early in the treatment of hypertension, it was not uncommon to use high doses of a single drug as the sole therapeutic modality. The price paid for this approach was frequent and severe, even fatal, side effects that were largely dose-related. Type A (augmented) reactions are common to all antihypertensive medication and are dose-dependent, whereas type B (idiosyncratic) reactions are usually bizarre,

---

Table 52–1 Factors Important to Understanding the Dose-Response Relationship

Study individual pharmacokinetic/pharmacodynamic relationship
Obtain enough data to characterize the full dose-response curve
Account for placebo effects
Account for the circadian variation in blood pressure
Study the time course of effect to determine the lag time for a particular effect
Correlate acute and chronic dosing
Take into account patient factors that might enhance or blunt the antihypertensive effect

---

unexpected effects that are not related to the drug's pharmacological action. Examples of type A reactions include the bronchospasm associated with β-blockers, the electrolyte abnormalities associated with thiazide diuretics, and the peripheral edema associated with dihydropyridine calcium channel blockers. Type A reactions are often predictable and follow a typical dose-response (side effect) relationship, although the side effect curve in this case falls to the right of the curve constructed for therapeutic effect.

A good example of how the maximally effective dose of a compound, without unacceptable side effects, can be identified can be seen in the history of how thiazide diuretics were utilized in the treatment of hypertension.[1–4] In past years, it was quite common to administer hydrochlorothiazide in doses ranging from 100 to 200 mg. It took several years to appreciate that the peak effect of this medication occurred at a dose of 25 mg. Unfortunately, when an excess of a thiazide diuretic is administered, it is not without risk. Although the dose-response relationship for blood pressure is plateaued at these higher doses ($>$25 mg), the dose–side effect relationship for hypokalemia continues to rise. Accordingly, the incidence rate of hypokalemia and hypomagnesemia is typically in excess of 50% with high-dose thiazide therapy; whereas, at lower doses, these electrolyte abnormalities occur with considerably less frequency. If the dose-response relationship had been adequately characterized before the introduction of thiazide diuretics into clinical practice, this pattern of serious electrolyte disturbance may have been avoided in many patients.

Another noteworthy example of the dissociation between the dose-response relationship and the dose–side effect relationship occurred with captopril. Most of the adverse effects of captopril observed during the initial investigations and after its introduction for the treatment of hypertension were related to dosage. Many of the early captopril-treated patients also had renal dysfunction, a factor that led to accumulation of captopril, since it is renally cleared from the circulation. With the high doses initially recommended, adverse reactions such as skin rashes, fever, arthralgias, bone marrow suppression, disturbances of taste, apthous ulcers, nephrotoxic reactions, and Raynaud's phenomenon occurred with regularity.[32] Adverse effects typically occurred in patients receiving doses over 150 mg/day. This among other factors prompted a reduction in the then-recommended dose.[7, 33]

These and other examples of excessive dosing led to the widely accepted stepped care approach to hypertension treatment. In the process, relatively low doses of rational drug combinations were employed to achieve a desired,

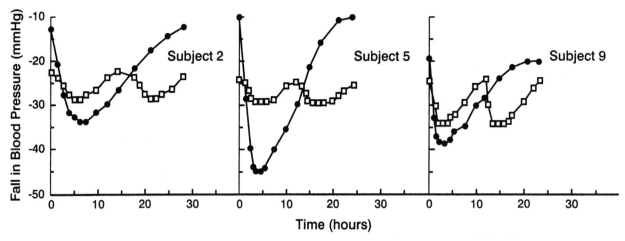

Figure 52–6. Simulated placebo-corrected blood pressure response profiles at steady state for enalapril 20 mg daily *(solid circles)* and 10 mg twice-daily *(open squares)*. (From Meredith PA, Donnelly R, Elliott HL, et.al. Prediction of the antihypertensive response to enalapril. J Hypertension 8[12]:1085–1090, 1990.)

additive antihypertensive effect. With the stepped care approach, a diuretic or β-blocker was initially opted for; in a second step, these drugs were combined; and lastly, a vasodilator was added. This approach was the foundation for a triple-drug regimen in common use in the 1980s that comprised hydralazine, propranolol, and hydrochlorothiazide. Since then, a number of equally effective and safe low-dose combinations, employing different drug classes, have come into common usage.

INDIVIDUALIZED ANTIHYPERTENSIVE THERAPY

Since all possible responses, both therapeutic and side effect, cannot possibly be gleaned from early clinical trials, utilization of concentration-effect analysis can supply vital information for individualizing antihypertensive therapy. This type of analysis can be used to predict drug effect utilizing various dosing regimens and during chronic dosing. Simulation of individual patient blood pressure response based on concentration-effect analysis has occurred with both once-a-day dosing with 20 mg of enalapril and twice-a-day dosing with 10 mg of enalapril. Figure 52–6 depicts these simulations in three patients and underscores the large interindividual variation in placebo-corrected fall in systolic blood pressure as well as the variations in peak: trough blood pressure responses.[29] This approach can also be applied early in drug development in order to optimize future study design and thereby minimize the time needed to bring the drug into clinical use.

References

1. Burris JF, Weir MR, Oparil S, et al. An assessment of diltiazem and hydrochlorothiazide in hypertension. JAMA 263:1507, 1990.
2. SHEP Cooperative Research Group. Prevention of stroke by antihypertensive drug treatment in older persons with isolated systolic hypertension: Final results of the Systolic Hypertensivion in the Elderly Program (SHEP). JAMA 265:3255, 1991.
3. Carlsen JE, Kober L, Torp-Pedersen C, et al. Relation between dose of bendrofluazide, antihypertensive effect, and adverse biochemical effects. BMJ 300:975, 1990.
4. McVeigh GE, Galloway D, Johnston D. The case for low dose diuretics in hypertension: Comparison of low and conventional doses of cyclopenthiazide. BMJ 297:95, 1988.
5. Serlin MJ, Orme ML, Baber NS, et al. Propranolol in the control of blood pressure: A dose-response study. Clin Pharmacol Ther 27:586, 1980.
6. Barritz DW, Marshall AJ: Beta blockade in essential hypertension: An analysis of response to oxprenolol. Br Heart J 39:825, 1977.
7. Aldigier JC, Plouin PF, Alexandre JM, et al. Dose dependency of captopril effects in severely hypertensive patients. J Cardiovasc Pharmacol 3:1229, 1981.
8. Gomez HJ, Sromovsky J, Kristianson K, et al. Lisinopril dose-response in mild to moderate hypertension. Clin Pharmacol Ther 37:198, 1985.
9. Donnelly R, Elliott HL, Merdith PA. Antihypertensive drugs: Individualized analysis and clinical relevance of kinetic-dynamic relationships. Pharmacol Ther 53:67, 1992.
10. Holford NHG, Sheiner LB. Understanding the dose-effect relationship: Clinical application of pharmacokinetic-pharmacodynamic models. Clin Pharmacokinet 6:429, 1981.
11. Kleinbloesem CH, van Brummelen P, Breimer DD. Nifedipine. Relationship between pharmacokinetics and pharmacodynamics. Clin Pharmacokinet 12:12, 1987.
12. Kelman AW, Reid JL, Milar JA. Concentration-effect modelling with converting enzyme inhibitors in man. Br J Clin Pharmacol 15:506, 1983.
13. Pasanisi F, Reid JL. Plasma nifedipine levels and fall in blood pressure in a 53 year old woman. Eur J Clin Pharmacol 25:143, 1983.
14. Donnelly R, Elliott HL, Meredith PA, et al. Concentration-effect relationships and individual responses to doxazosin in essential hypertension. Br J Clin Pharmacol 28:517, 1989.
15. Sheiner LB, Starski DR, Vozeh S, et al. Simultaneous modelling of pharmacokinetics and pharmacodynamics: Application to D-tubocurarine. Clin Pharmacol Ther 25:358, 1979.
16. Meredith PA, Reid JL. The use of pharmacodynamic and pharmacokinetic profiles in drug development for planning individual therapy. *In* Laragh JH, Brenner BM (eds). Hypertension: Pathophysiology, Diagnosis, and Management, 2nd ed, vol 2. Philadelphia, Lippincott-Raven, 1995; p 2771.
17. Zannad F. Duration of action of angiotensin converting enzyme inhibitors. Am J Hypertens 8:75S, 1995.
18. Conway J, Johnston J, Coats A, et al. The use of ambulatory blood pressure monitoring to improve the accuracy and reduce the numbers of subjects in clinical trials of antihypertensive agents. J Hypertens 6:111, 1988.
19. Buhler FR. Age and cardiovascular response: Determinants of an antihypertensive treatment concept previously based on beta blockers and calcium entry blockers. Hypertension 5(suppl 2):S94, 1983.
20. Wikstrand J, Berglund C. Antihypertensive treatment with beta blockers in patients over 65 years. BMJ 285:850, 1982.

21. Reid JL. Angiotensin converting enzyme inhibitors in the elderly. BMJ 295:943, 1987.
22. Cody RJ, Laragh JH, Case DB, et al. Renin system activity as a determinant of response to treatment in hypertension and heart failure. Hypertension 5(suppl 3):36, 1983.
23. Waeber B, Gavras I, Brunner HR, et al. Prediction of sustained antihypertensive efficacy of chronic captopril therapy: Relationships to immediate blood pressure response and control and plasma renin activity. Am Heart J 103:384, 1982.
24. Donnelly R, Meredith PA, Elliott HL, et al. Kinetic-dynamic relations and individual responses to enalapril. Hypertension 15:301, 1990.
25. Donnelly R, Elliott HL, Meredith PA, et al. Nifedipine: Individual responses and concentration-effect relationships. Hypertension 12:443, 1988.
26. Saunders E, Weir MR, Kong BW, et al. A comparison of the efficacy and safety of a beta-blocker, calcium channel blocker, and converting enzyme inhibitor in hypertensive blacks. Arch Intern Med 150:1707, 1990.
27. Weir MR, Gray JM, Paster R, Saunders E. Differing mechanisms of action of angiotensin-converting enzyme inhibition in black and white hypertensive patients. Hypertension 26:124, 1995.
28. Sumner DJ, Meredith PA, Howie CA, et al. Initial blood pressure as a predictor of response to antihypertensive therapy. Br J Clin Pharmacol 26:175, 1988.
29. Meredith PA, Donnelly R, Elliott HL, et al. Prediction of the antihypertensive response to enalapril. J Hypertens 8:1085, 1990.
30. Meredith PA, Elliott HL, Ahmed JA, et al. Age and the antihypertensive efficacy of verapamil: An integrated pharmacokinetic-pharmacodynamic approach. J Hypertens 5(suppl 5):S219, 1987.
31. Donnelly R, Meredith PA, Miller SHK, et al. Pharmacodynamic modelling of the antihypertensive response to amlodipine. Clin Pharmacol Ther 54:303, 1993.
32. Johnston GD. Dose-response relationships with antihypertensive drugs. Pharmacol Ther 35:53, 1992.
33. Henahan J. Captopril now for mild hypertension. JAMA 250:578, 1983.

CHAPTER 53

Low-Dose Fixed-Combination Antihypertensive Therapy

Domenic A. Sica and Elizabeth Ripley

Fixed-dose combination antihypertensive drugs have been available since the early 1960s. The first of these combined reserpine-hydralazine-hydrochlorothiazide (Ser-Ap-Es), α-methyldopa-hydrochlorothiazide (Aldoril), and soon thereafter, hydrochlorothiazide (HCTZ) with a potassium-sparing diuretic (Dyazide, Moduretic, Aldactazide). The 1970s and 1980s marked the arrival of innumerable fixed-dose combination products, in most instances diuretics combined with either β-blockers, centrally acting agents, or angiotensin-converting enzyme inhibitors (ACEIs) in high doses. Recently, fixed-dose combination products containing an ACEI/calcium channel blocker (CCB), or an angiotensin II receptor blocker (ARB)/diuretic have been approved for general use in the treatment of hypertension.

Academic opinion has vacillated regarding the advisability of fixed-dose combination antihypertensive therapy, even though this therapeutic approach offers a number of advantages (Table 53–1). The sixth report of the Joint National Committee on Prevention, Detection, Evaluation, and Treatment of High Blood Pressure (JNC VI) has for the first time included a listing of available fixed-dose combination products (29 compound mixtures) and the beginning thoughts concerning their use.[1, 2]

ADVANTAGES

Objectives

The objective of fixed-dose combination therapy is to procure better blood pressure (BP) control. Patients do not respond favorably to every antihypertensive drug class;[3] rather, individual patients respond in a somewhat random fashion, with certain drug classes clearly outperforming others.[4] Because of this therapeutic enigma, combination therapy, employing different classes of antihypertensives, often maximizes the likelihood of early and sustained therapeutic success.

An additional consideration in the management of hypertension is that long-term control of BP is coupled to the ease with which BP is normalized at the inception of therapy. Early therapeutic misadventures that contribute to poor long-term success in the control of BP include unnecessarily complex regimens, side effects either recognized or unrecognized, multiple class switches/dose titrations in seeking the one drug that works, and patient misperceptions arising from these prescribing exercises.[5] Even without consideration of the pathophysiological rationale behind combination therapy, a strong argument can be

Table 53–1 Fixed-Dose Combination Therapy: Advantages

↑ Compliance, simplified titration, and convenience of use
Potentiation of antihypertensive effects of a single compound
  Additive or synergistic effect
  Enhancing effect in specific populations
    Diuretic with an ACEI, ARB, or β-blocker in blacks
Reduction in side effects by giving lower doses of two drugs
Side effect attenuation
  ↓ In diuretic-induced metabolic derangements with ACEIs
  ↓ In CCB-related peripheral edema with ACEIs
Improved overall results, if the ratio of components is superior to what the physician has without the availability of a fixed-dose combination
Cost occasionally less than that of individual components

Adapted from Sica DA. Fixed-dose combination antihypertensive drugs. Do they have a role in rational therapy? Drugs 48:16–24, 1994.
Abbreviations: ACEI, angiotensin-converting enzyme inhibitor; ARB, angiotensin II receptor blocker; CCB, calcium channel blocker.

Table 53–2 Mechanistic Interruptions That Affect Blood Pressure Control During the Course of Combination Therapy

Class	Drug	Mechanism	Response	Blocking Class
Diuretic	HCTZ	Volume decrease	RAA, sympathetic activation	ACEI
Vasodilator	Minoxidil	Tachycardia, Na$^+$ retention	RAA, sympathetic activation	Diuretic, β-blocker
β-blocker	Propranolol	Na$^+$ retention	Decreased renal blood flow and/or cardiac output	Diuretic
Sympathetic inhibitor	Clonidine	Na$^+$ retention	Decreased renal blood flow and/or cardiac output	Diuretic

Abbreviations: HCTZ, hydrochlorothiazide; RAA, renin-angiotensin-aldosterone [axis]; ACEI, angiotensin-converting enzyme inhibitor.

advanced for the use of fixed-dose combination therapy when hypertension is first treated if BP control can be established quickly.

Rationale

The pathophysiological rationale for use of a fixed-dose combination drug is that its individual components neutralize counterregulatory mechanisms activated by one another. The result of this pharmacological partnering is typically a partially or fully additive, if not synergistic, effect on BP. Table 53–2 outlines the systemic responses to a second antihypertensive compound that might influence the degree to which BP is successfully reduced with a first drug.

BP can be readily controlled in most cases by a carefully selected prescription of two drugs.[1–2, 6] In general, drug classes interrupting the sympathetic nervous system (SNS) (e.g., clonidine or propranolol) result in salt and water retention and thereby a loss of BP control. Under these circumstances, BP control is typically restored by the addition of a diuretic. Control of BP by primary diuretic therapy (e.g., chlorthalidone) is occasionally lost because of the propensity for diuretics to activate the renin-angiotensin-aldosterone (RAA) axis and/or the SNS. Excess activity of these systems can be effectively curtailed by the complementary effects of an ACEI or an ARB, with a resultant drop in BP. Finally, nonspecific vasodilator therapy (e.g., hydralazine or minoxidil) causes salt and water retention, tachycardia, and activation of the RAA axis, responses that are prevented by combination therapy with diuretics and β-blockers.

Tolerability and Risk Factor Modification

Another aim of fixed-dose combination therapy is to lessen intolerance to individual components of the preparation by the use of low doses of each. Dose-dependent side effects can be neutralized by balancing actions of one or the other of the components. For example, when potassium-sparing diuretics or ACEIs are combined with a diuretic, the combination minimizes diuretic-induced hypokalemia and/or hypomagnesemia.[7] Similarly, when ACEIs are combined with CCBs, peripheral edema, a characteristic side effect of CCBs, diminishes dramatically.[8]

A final goal of fixed-dose therapy is to confer cardiovas-cular and/or cardiorenal protection by risk factor modification attributable to individual drug components.[9] Such is the case when the lipid-elevating effects of diuretics are tempered by the coadministration of an ACEI. In addition, it has been proposed that an ACEI and a CCB complement one another in regressing left ventricular hypertrophy (LVH), diminishing proteinuria, and/or slowing the progression of renal insufficiency.[2]

Pharmacology of Dose-Dependent Side Effects

A fundamental concept in therapeutics is that of the log-linear dose-response curve (Fig. 53–1). Simply stated, in the range of receptor occupancy from 0 to 100%, a drug's effect is related to the logarithm of the drug's concentration and, by extension, to the logarithm of the dose; thus, a tenfold dose increment is required to achieve a doubling of effect (Fig. 53–1) (e.g., point A → B). Doubling the dose of a medication will increase its effect by the logarithm of 2 (~30% change; point A → C).[10]

A corollary of this principle is that a drug exhibits a unique log dose-response curve for both its therapeutic and its toxic effects. The side effect curve is situated to the right of the therapeutic effect curve; thus, at any given

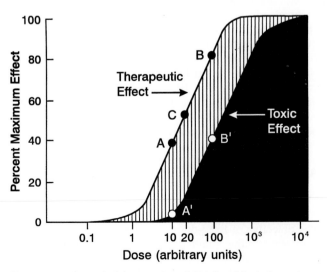

Figure 53–1. Theoretical therapeutic and toxic logarithmic-linear dose-response curves.

dose, the therapeutic effect will exceed the toxic effect (point B → B'). Decreasing the dose will diminish both the therapeutic and the toxic effects. It is possible to administer a small enough dose to remain at the early upward-going portion of the dose-response curve and yet not fall on the steep portion of the toxic effect curve (point A → A').[10]

Conventional teaching in the treatment of hypertension has suggested that a single drug be used and the dose increased until the desired effect is attained or side effect–limiting toxicity develops. Application of the pharmacological principles described previously suggests that an equally rational approach is combining two drugs at low doses. Each drug would exhibit an independent therapeutic effect on the low end of the dose-response curve (point A), and together they would generate an additive response (point C). Drug-specific side effects in each case would remain at a low point on the toxic dose-response curve (point A'), thus safely permitting treatment of hypertension.[10–12]

Prescription Strategy

There are several ways of approaching the use of antihypertensives in combination.[1–2, 12] First, two or three drugs can be prescribed as sequential monotherapy with dose titration of each;[6, 12] once BP is controlled, a suitable fixed-dose combination can be substituted. Alternatively, when two-drug treatment is considered from the onset of therapy, a fixed-dose combination product can be administered initially.[1, 2] Although the fixed-dose combinations of betaxolol/HCTZ, bisoprolol/HCTZ, and captopril/HCTZ are the only ones approved by the U.S. Food and Drug Administration for first-step treatment of hypertension, most fixed-dose combinations have been effectively employed in this fashion. With either approach, a rational theoretical basis exists for the use of a fixed-dose combination product (Table 53–3).[1, 12]

An inherent advantage of fixed-dose combination therapy is compliance enhancement because fewer pills are required.[13] Concentration-dependent side effects frequently diminish or disappear because lower amounts of the individual components are required for BP control.[14, 15] Fixed-dose combinations may also be cheaper than individually prescribed two-drug therapy. Market forces frequently dictate that the price of a fixed-dose combination remain well below that of the individual components purchased separately.

COMPLIANCE

Detailed management guidelines for the treatment of hypertension have been widely disseminated in the United States.[16] Despite such guidelines, a significant gap exists between ideal control rates and what is actually achieved in clinical practice. For example, the Third National Health and Nutrition Examination Survey (phase 2) found that only 27% of all hypertensives in the United States were at a target BP of less than 140/90,[16, 17] with control rates being equally poor in Europe.[18]

A number of factors can be implicated in the failure of current therapeutic regimens to successfully reduce BP in a more significant proportion of the population. Compliance/adherence is of utmost importance. Compliance studies typically show that patients have difficulty adhering to drug regimens that either are overly complex or produce side effects. Compliance can be improved by either simplifying the regimen or minimizing side effects as BP is reduced. Perhaps the most important compliance-enhancing maneuver available to physicians is to select a therapeutic regimen with the lowest frequency of dosing; therein lies the major advantage of fixed-dose combinations. Thus, the use of once-daily fixed-dose combinations improves compliance. Alternatively, this positive influence on compliance may disappear if twice-daily dosing of a fixed-dose combination is required or if the patient stops the medication because of an inability to exercise drug-specific compliance, as can occur with free-drug combination therapy.

DISADVANTAGES

A disadvantage of fixed-dose combinations is a lack of dosing flexibility, although physicians do not usually exploit the dosing flexibility inherent in the use of free combinations. With fixed-dose combination therapy, if additional amounts of either drug are required for BP control, the increased complexity of the regimen may negatively affect compliance. In addition, if the goal of fixed-dose combination therapy is for one component to provide adjunctive treatment of a concomitant nonhypertensive illness (e.g., a β-blocker/diuretic to lower BP while concomitantly treating angina), the amount of that component available from the fixed-dose combination may well prove inadequate for the treatment of the concomitant illness.

It has been suggested that fixed-dose combinations are pharmacokinetically irrational because of differing half-lives for individual components. This objection does not present an insurmountable hurdle to the use of fixed-dose combinations. Rather, this can be viewed as a therapeutic advantage if excessive peak reductions in BP are avoided. This is a serious consideration in the elderly, since an excessive early hypotensive effect from a fixed-dose combination can increase cardiovascular risk. Of primary im-

---

Table 53–3 Theoretical Requirements for a Rational Fixed-Dose Antihypertensive Combination

Each component should be safe and contribute to the overall effect
Results should be superior to those achieved with either individual agent at the same dose
Dosage form(s) should be optimized relative to
  Predictability of bioavailability
  Absence of unwanted pharmacokinetic interactions
Doses should be selected to maintain high trough:peak ratios
The dose-response relationship for the combination product should be clearly evident with a single dose and close to a maximal effect with two doses
Dose amounts should not create excessive hypotension when a fixed-dose product replaces monotherapy
A major proportion of the target population should respond
Physician education should be easily accomplished

Adapted from Sica DA. Fixed-dose combination antihypertensive drugs. Do they have a role in rational therapy? Drugs 48:16–24, 1994.

portance with a fixed-dose combination product is that its peak effect (achieved as the result of both components of the preparation) fairly closely approximates its trough effect (derived from the more long-acting of the two components) (trough:peak ratio > 50%).[8] On the surface, it would seem that this is a simple issue of pharmacokinetics when, in fact, other considerations exist. First, it has been commonly observed that the duration of action of an antihypertensive agent frequently bears a minimal relationship to its plasma half-life, whereas the peak response to an antihypertensive medication has a more direct drug concentration relationship. In this regard, a number of compounds routinely given twice or thrice daily as monotherapy (e.g., β-blockers, ACEIs) can safely be administered once daily in a fixed-dose combination because of the supporting effect of coadministered diuretics.[19] Second, the complementary nature of two drugs may reside in one modifying the counterregulatory response(s) induced by the other. Thus, pulse rate acceleration induced by either diuretics (volume contraction) or CCBs (SNS activation), if tempered by coadministration of either a β-blocker or an ACEI, can influence the degree to which BP declines in a pharmacokinetically independent fashion.[8]

FIXED-DOSE COMBINATIONS

In the past, many physicians were reluctant to prescribe fixed-dose combination antihypertensive therapy because most such combinations contained poorly tolerated rauwolfia compounds whose efficacy was limited. In addition, a number of the early fixed-dose combination products contained unnecessarily large doses of the individual components. However, since the late 1970s, a plethora of fixed-dose combinations have appeared, the majority of which contain a diuretic.[19] More recently, diuretic-free fixed-dose combinations composed of a CCB and an ACEI have become available.[8] In most instances, the drug doses found in these various combination products have been carefully selected on the basis of factorial design trials and response surface analyses. It is now apparent that low doses of many compounds are sufficient to effect significant BP reduction.[20, 21]

The most frequently employed fixed-dose combinations include a thiazide/potassium-sparing diuretic, a β-blocker/diuretic, an ACEI or ARB/diuretic, and a CCB/ACEI (Table 53–4). Other combinations such as β-blockers/dihydropyridine CCBs (e.g., felodipine/metoprolol [not available in the United States]), sympatholytics/diuretics, and nonspecific vasodilators/diuretics are available but have fallen out of favor with the advent of new low-dose combinations (Table 53–4). Three fixed-dose combinations are currently approved as first-line agents for the treatment of hypertension: betaxolol/HCTZ, bisoprolol (2.5/5.0/10.0 mg)/HCTZ 6.25 mg (Ziac), and captopril (25/50 mg)/HCTZ (15/25 mg) (Capozide).[16]

THIAZIDES AND POTASSIUM-SPARING DIURETICS

Fixed-dose combination products containing a thiazide/potassium-sparing diuretic typically reduce the potassium and magnesium wastage that accompanies thiazide use alone. The latter feature is important because diuretic-induced intracellular potassium deficiency is poorly corrected unless magnesium balance is first reestablished.[7, 22] A number of combination products exist in this category, including amiloride/HCTZ, spironolactone/HCTZ, and the most widely prescribed combination in this class, triamterene/HCTZ. Diuretic-diuretic fixed-dose combinations are of particular utility in the elderly.[23] The fixed-dose combination of amiloride and HCTZ is particularly efficient in the correction of diuretic-induced hypokalemia[24] and has been employed as adjunctive therapy in the treatment of calcium nephrolithiasis.[25]

β-BLOCKERS AND DIURETICS

The rationale for use of β-blocker/diuretic fixed-dose therapy is that β-blockers blunt both the tachycardia and the RAA axis activation induced by diuretics while the diuretic component reduces the dose-related sodium retention induced by β-blockers. β-blocker/diuretic combinations have additive but not synergistic effects and the combination restores the antihypertensive response to β-blockers in blacks.[26] The BP-lowering response to the combined α- and β-blocker labetalol is also favorably affected by combination with a diuretic. A number of potential advantages derive from the use of a fixed-dose β-blocker/diuretic combination when the β-blocker is given in low doses. These include a reduction in the risk of β-blocker–induced congestive heart failure and decreased concentration-dependent side effects. Other protective effects of β-blockers, such as attenuation of diuretic-induced hypokalemia and the associated arrhythmias and/or a possible cardioprotective effect, are less likely to occur at the low β-blocker doses employed in these fixed-dose combinations.

Although β-blocker/diuretic fixed-dose combinations lower BP in as many as 75% of treated subjects,[26, 27] their long-term usefulness is limited because they exhibit lipid-, glucose-, and uric acid–elevating effects and cause sexual dysfunction. Fortunately, the flat dose-response curve for thiazide diuretics in the presence of β-blockers suggests that high-dose diuretic therapy is not necessary.[28] Since the adverse metabolic consequences of diuretic/β-blocker therapy are dose-dependent, they can be minimized if the fixed-dose combination contains low doses of each component (Table 53–5).[28] Thus, side effects occur less frequently with new ultra–low-dose fixed-combinations such as bisoprolol, a cardioselective β1-blocker, and HCTZ (5.0/6.25 mg).[15] Clinical trials comparing bisoprolol/HCTZ (5.0/6.25 mg) with either amlodipine or enalapril have shown response rates that were comparable with those of amlodipine (70%) and superior to those of enalapril (45%).[29] Because this low-dose combination demonstrated superior efficacy in clinical trials with a side effect profile no worse than that of placebo, the Food and Drug Administration approved this combination as first-line therapy. A low dose of a β1-selective β-blocker, such as this, is also more likely to provide "true" cardioselectivity.

Table 53–4 Antihypertensives Available as a Fixed-Dose Combination Product

Class	Combination	Trade Name
β-Adrenergic blockers and diuretics	Atenolol 50–100 mg/chlorthalidone 25 mg	Tenoretic
	Bisoprolol 2.5–10 mg/HCTZ 6.25 mg	Ziac*
	Metoprolol 50–100 mg/HCTZ 25–50 mg	Lopressor HCT
	Nadolol 40–80 mg/bendroflumethiazide 5 mg	Corzide
	Propranolol 40–80 mg/HCTZ 25 mg	Inderide
	Propranolol ER 80–160 mg/HCTZ 50 mg	Inderide LA
	Timolol 10 mg/HCTZ 25 mg	Timolide
ACEIs and diuretics	Benazepril 5–20 mg/HCTZ 6.25–25 mg	Lotensin HCT
	Captopril 25–50 mg/HCTZ 15–25 mg	Capozide*
	Enalapril 5–10 mg/HCTZ 12.5–25 mg	Vaseretic
	Lisinopril 10–20 mg/HCTZ 12.5–25 mg	Zestoretic; Prinzide
Angiotensin II receptor blocker and diuretic	Losartan 50 mg/HCTZ 12.5 mg	Hyzaar
	Valsartan 80–160/HCTZ 12.5	Diovan HCT
Calcium antagonists and ACEIs	Amlodipine 2.5–5 mg/benazepril 10–20 mg	Lotrel
	Diltiazem 180 mg/enalapril 5 mg	Teczem
	Felodipine 5 mg/enalapril 5 mg	Lexxel
	Verapamil 180–240 mg/trandolapril 1–4 mg	Tarka
Other combinations	Clonidine HCl 0.1–0.3 mg/chlorthalidone 15 mg	Combipres
	Deserpidine 0.25–0.5 mg/methyclothiazide 5 mg	Enduronyl (Forte)
	Guanethidine 10 mg/HCTZ 25 mg	Esimil
	Hydralazine 25–100/HCTZ 25–50 mg	Apresazide
	Hydralazine 25 mg/reserpine 0.1 mg/HCTZ 15 mg	Ser-Ap-Es; Unipres; Tri-Hydroserpine
	Methyldopa 250 mg/chlorothiazide 150–250 mg	Aldoclor
	Methyldopa 250–500 mg/HCTZ 30–50 mg	Aldoril
	Prazosin 1–5 mg/polythiazide 0.5 mg	Minizide
	Rauwolfia 50 mg/bendroflumethiazide 4 mg	Rauzide
	Reserpine 0.125 mg/chlorthalidone 25 mg	Demi-Regroton
	Reserpine 0.125 mg/chlorothiazide 250–500 mg	Diupres
	Reserpine 0.125 mg/HCTZ 25–50 mg	Hydropres; Hydroserpin
	Reserpine 0.125 mg/hydroflumethiazide 50 mg	Salutensin (-Demi)
	Reserpine 0.25 mg/polythiazide 2 mg	Renese-R
	Reserpine 0.1 mg/trichlormethiazide 2–4 mg	Metatensin

Adapted from Joint National Committee on Prevention, Detection, Evaluation, and Treatment of High Blood Pressure. The sixth report. Arch Intern Med 157:2413–2446, 1997.
Abbreviations: HCTZ, hydrochlorothiazide; HCT, hydrochlorothiazide; ER, extended release; LA, long-acting; ACEIs, angiotensin-converting enzyme inhibitors.
*Approved for initial therapy of hypertension.

ANGIOTENSIN-CONVERTING ENZYME INHIBITORS OR ANGIOTENSIN II RECEPTOR BLOCKER ANTAGONISTS AND DIURETICS

Combining either an ACEI or an ARB with a diuretic in a fixed-dose combination results in a fairly potent combination product.[30–32] ACEIs or ARBs in combination with low-dose diuretics work synergistically to effectively lower BP in patients with low-, normal-, or high-renin hypertension.[30] The utility of these combinations is particularly evident in African Americans, in whom monotherapy with conventional doses of an ACEI or ARB is often unsuccessful.[33] Addition of a diuretic to either an ACEI or an ARB (e.g., losartan)[32] results in an extremely attractive treatment option. Response rates to a fixed-dose combination of an ACEI and a diuretic can exceed 80%[34] in mild-to-moderate hypertension and are typically better than those achieved with a β-blocker/diuretic combination given under similar conditions.[35, 36] With certain combinations (cilazapril 5.0 mg/HCTZ 12.5 mg), response rates as high as 96% have been reported in untreated mild hypertensives.[37] It should be noted that such high response rates may be specific to certain patient types and/or criteria employed to define response. Finally, although original thinking held that ACEI responses were optimized with a diuretic dose in the 12.5-

to 25.0-mg range,[31] more recent data suggest that even lower doses of HCTZ (6.25 mg), which produce minimal antihypertensive effects on their own, effectively lower BP if combined with an ACEI (Table 53–6).[30, 38]

Table 53–5 Mean Blood Pressure Reduction With Varying Doses of Hydrochlorothiazide Added to a β-Blocker

β-Blocker (mg)	HCTZ (mg)	Mean ↓ in SBP (mm Hg)	Mean ↓ in DBP (mm Hg)
Metoprolol			
200	50	24	12
200	25	21.5	12.5
200	12.5	16	11
Metoprolol			
100	12.5	16	12.4
Bisoprolol			
2.5	25	19.9	12.9
2.5	6.25	12.8	10.8
Bisoprolol			
10	25	23.5	15.4
10	6.75	16.4	13.4

Adapted from Am J Med, vol 101 (suppl 3A), Neutel JM, Black HR, Weber MA. Combination therapy with diuretics: An evolution of understanding, pp 61S–70S, Copyright 1996, with permission from Excerpta Medica Inc.
Abbreviations: HCTZ, hydrochlorothiazide; SBP, systolic blood pressure; DBP, diastolic blood pressure.

Table 53–6 Mean Blood Pressure Reduction With Varying Doses of Hydrochlorothiazide Added to Either an Angiotensin-Converting Enzyme Inhibitor or an Angiotensin Receptor Blocker

ACEI/ARB (mg)	HCTZ (mg)	Mean ↓ in SBP (mm Hg)	Mean ↓ in DBP (mm Hg)
Enalapril			
10	50	28	26
10	25	35.1	25.9
10	12.5	19.6	12.6
Enalapril			
20	50	35.7	25.4
20	25	19.8	15.0
20	12.5	24.7	15.7
20	6.25	11.5	7.3
Lisinopril			
10	25	22.8	14.3
10	12.5	21.9	17.1
Lisinopril			
20	25	—	15
20	12.5	22.7	15.4
20	6.25	—	12
Captopril			
100–150	50	23.2	13
Captopril			
50	50	32	18
50	25	19.9	16.5
Captopril			
25	50	33	14
25	25	20.5	16.9
25	15	15.7	15.2
25	12.5	24.3	19.7

Adapted from Neutel JM, Black HR, Weber MA. Combination therapy with diuretics: An evolution of understanding. Am J Med 101(suppl 3A):61S–70S, 1996.

Abbreviations: ACEI, angiotensin-converting enzyme inhibitor; ARB, angiotensin receptor blocker; HCTZ, hydrochlorothiazide; SBP, systolic blood pressure; DBP, diastolic blood pressure.

The synergy found with the combination of an ACEI or an ARB and a diuretic relates to the ability of the diuretic to stimulate the RAA axis by inducing volume contraction. This hypothesis is responsible for HCTZ doses of 25 mg or more; however, relevant volume contraction is much less likely when doses of HCTZ of 12.5 mg or less are administered. Thus, alternative mechanisms, such as activation of the tissue RAA axis, need to be considered to explain the utility of low diuretic doses (≤12.5 mg) in combination therapy. The addition of an ACEI or an ARB to a diuretic can effectively blunt metabolic derangements, such as hypokalemia, hypomagnesemia, and/or hypercholesterolemia, that are by-products of diuretic monotherapy.[19, 39] Recently, losartan, in a compound-specific fashion, has also been observed to blunt the hyperuricemia accompanying diuretic therapy.[40] This attenuation of the metabolic abnormalities induced by diuretic therapy derives from use of a lower diuretic dose because the ACEI or ARB therapy causes the RAA axis to become quiescent and, in the instance of losartan, because it has uricosuric properties.[41]

Fixed-dose combinations may also inhibit hypertension-related vascular remodeling, which may be facilitated by diuretic-induced increases in angiotensin II.[9] Thus, the fixed-dose combination of an ACEI/diuretic or an ARB/diuretic may be particularly useful in the hypertensive subject with LVH as well as the diabetic with nephropathy. Whether the dose of ACEI or ARB available in a fixed-dose combination is sufficient for target organ protection requires further clarification. In this regard, the pharmacodynamics of the ARB losartan suggest that 50 mg approaches a top-end dose for complete blockade of the AT$_1$ receptor.[42] Thus, if complete blockade of this receptor equates with target organ protection, the available fixed-dose combination of losartan/HCTZ (50/12.5 mg) could provide both BP control and target organ protection.

ANGIOTENSIN-CONVERTING ENZYME INHIBITORS AND CALCIUM-CHANNEL BLOCKERS

The rationale behind use of a fixed-dose combination of an ACEI and a CCB is that the ACEI buffers the SNS and RAA axis activation that may occur with a dihydropyridine CCB.[43] In addition, CCBs are natriuretic and thereby induce a state of negative sodium balance that further reinforces the antihypertensive effect of an ACEI.[21, 44] The use of factorial design and surface-response analysis will be necessary to determine optimal combinations of these drug classes[20, 45] and to identify the classes of CCBs that might most effectively combine with an ACEI.[8, 46, 47] It is likely that the typically more long-acting CCB component of these fixed-dose combinations will be the major determinant of effect.

The differing mechanisms of action of the available CCBs, both within the dihydropyridine class and among the nondihydropyridines, will require individual combinations to be evaluated independently,[48] particularly since combination regimens may not be any more effective than the CCB alone.[47] Finding effective fixed-dose combinations of these drug classes is of particular relevance, since in 1995, half of all antihypertensive prescriptions were from one of these drug classes.[21, 48] A fixed-dose combination of a CCB and an ACEI may prove particularly attractive because of the unique cardiac and renal effects of each class.[49] Whereas nondihydropyridine CCBs, such as verapamil or diltiazem, effectively lower pulse rate and cause regression of LVH, the persistent activation of the SNS seen with some of the dihydropyridines may limit the regression of LVH with CCBs.[50] This phenomenon may be effectively counterbalanced by addition of an ACEI, a maneuver that attenuates the increase in sympathetic outflow induced by dihydropyridine CCBs.[51] Combining an ACEI with a CCB also may lessen side effects such as CCB-related peripheral edema, either by a complementary venodilating action[8, 51] or because in combination a lower dose of the CCB is sufficient to effect BP control.[8, 14]

CONCLUSION

Use of fixed-dose combination antihypertensive therapy can reduce patient noncompliance, and this therapeutic stratagem will increase in popularity as additional combinations of drugs become available. The largest experience to date is with combination products containing a thiazide diuretic. Increasing experience with low-dose combination products suggests equivalent efficacy to high-dose combination therapy. More novel combinations, such as an ACEI and a CCB, promise to provide both greater treatment flexibility and more provider- and patient-friendly treatment regimens.

References

1. Sica DA. Fixed-dose combination antihypertensive drugs. Do they have a role in rational therapy? Drugs 48:16–24, 1994.
2. Epstein M, Bakris G. Newer approaches to antihypertensive therapy. Arch Intern Med 156:1969–1978, 1996.
3. Sever P. The heterogeneity of hypertension: Why doesn't every patient respond to every antihypertensive drug? J Hum Hypertens 9(suppl 2):S33–S36, 1995.
4. Materson BJ, Reda DJ, Cushman WC, et al. Single drug therapy for hypertension in men: A comparison of six antihypertensive agents with placebo. N Engl J Med 328:914–921, 1993.
5. Swales JD. Management guidelines for hypertension: Is anyone taking notice? J Hum Hypertens 9(suppl 2):S9–S13, 1995.
6. Dollery CT. Pharmacological basis for combination therapy of hypertension. Annu Rev Pharmacol Toxicol 17:311–323, 1977.
7. Davidov ME, Becker FE, Hollifield J. Serum magnesium and potassium levels in hypertensive patients after a therapeutic switch from hydrochlorothiazide plus a potassium supplement to Maxzide. Am J Med 82(suppl 3A):48–51, 1987.
8. Gradman AH, Cutler NR, Davis PJ, et al. Enalapril-felodipine ER in essential hypertension: A factorial design study of combination therapy. Am J Cardiol 79:431–435, 1997.
9. Dahlof B, Hansson L. The influence of antihypertensive therapy on the structural arteriolar changes in essential hypertension: Different effects of enalapril and hydrochlorothiazide. J Intern Med 234:271–279, 1993.
10. Fagan TC. Remembering the lessons of basic pharmacology. Arch Intern Med 154:1430–1431, 1994.
11. Brunner H, Menard J, Waeber B, et al. Treating the individual hypertensive patient: Considerations on dose, sequential monotherapy and drug combinations. J Hypertens 8:3–11, 1990.
12. Sica DA. Fixed-dose combination antihypertensive drugs: Principles and practice. Cardiovasc Rev Rep 9:28–46, 1997.
13. Eisen SA, Miller DK, Woodward RS, et al. The effect of prescribed daily dose frequency on patient medication compliance. Arch Intern Med 150:1881–1884, 1990.
14. Morgan TO, Anderson A, Jones E. Comparison and interaction of low dose felodipine and enalapril in the treatment of essential hypertension in elderly subjects. Am J Hypertens 5:238–243, 1992.
15. Lewen AJ, Lueg MC, Targum S, et al. A clinical trial evaluating the 24 hour effect of bisoprolol/hydrochlorothiazide 5 mg/6.25 mg combination in patients with mild to moderate hypertension. Clin Cardiol 16:732–736, 1993.
16. Joint National Committee on Prevention, Detection, Evaluation, and Treatment of High Blood Pressure. The sixth report. Arch Intern Med 157:2413–2446, 1997.
17. Burt VL, Whelton P, Roccella EJ, et al. Prevalence of hypertension in the US adult population. Result from the Third National Health and Nutrition Examination Survey, 1988–1991. Hypertension 25:305–313, 1995.
18. Hosie J, Wiklund I. Managing hypertension in general practice: Can we do better? J Hum Hypertens 9(suppl 2):S15–S18, 1995.
19. Ambrosini E, Borghi C, Costa FV. Captopril and hydrochlorothiazide: Rationale for their combination. Br J Clin Pharmacol 23:43S–50S, 1987.
20. Hung HMJ, Ng TH, Chi GY, et al. Response surface and factorial designs for combination antihypertensive drugs. Drug Inf J 24:371–378, 1990.
21. Menard J, Bellet M. Calcium antagonists–ACE inhibitors combination therapy: Objectives and methodology of clinical development. J Cardiovasc Pharmacol 21(suppl 2):S49–S54, 1993.
22. Dyckner T, Wester PO. Potassium/magnesium depletion in patients with cardiovascular disease. Am J Med 82(suppl 3A):11–17, 1987.
23. Ghosh AK, Mankikar G, Strouthidis T, et al. A single-blind, comparative study of hydrochlorothiazide/amiloride ("Moduretic" 25) and hydrochlorothiazide/triamterene ("Dyazide") in elderly patients with congestive heart failure. Curr Med Res Opin 10:573–579, 1987.
24. Naronde RF, Milgrom M, Vlachakis ND, et al. Response of thiazide-induced hypokalemia to amiloride. JAMA 249:237–241, 1983.
25. Maschio G, Tessitore N, D'Angelo A, et al. Prevention of calcium nephrolithiasis with low-dose thiazide, amiloride and allopurinol. Am J Med 71:623–626, 1981.
26. Veterans Administration Cooperative Study Group on Antihypertensive Agents. Efficacy of nadolol alone and combined with bendroflumethiazide and hydralazine for systemic hypertension. Am J Cardiol 52:1230–1237, 1983.
27. Veterans Administration Cooperative Study Group on Antihypertensive Agents. Propranolol in the treatment of essential hypertension. JAMA 237:2303–2310, 1977.
28. MacGregor GA, Banks RA, Markander ND, et al. Lack of effect of beta-blocker on flat dose response to thiazide combined with beta-blocker. BMJ 286:1535–1538, 1983.
29. Prisant LM, Weir MR, Papademetroiu V, et al. Low-dose drug combination therapy: An alternative first-line approach to hypertension treatment. Am Heart J 130:359–366, 1995.
30. Andren L, Weiner L, Svensson, et al. Enalapril with either a "very low" or "low" dose of hydrochlorothiazide is equally effective in essential hypertension. A double blind trial in 100 essential hypertensives. J Hypertens 1(suppl 2);384–386, 1983.
31. Chrysant SG. Antihypertensive effectiveness of low-dose lisinopril-hydrochlorothiazide combination: A large multi-center study. Arch Intern Med 154:737–743, 1994.
32. Schoenberger JA. Losartan with hydrochlorothiazide in the treatment of hypertension. J Hypertens 13(suppl 1):S43–S47, 1995.
33. Veteran Administration Cooperative Study Group on Antihypertensive Agents. Racial differences in response to low-dose captopril are abolished by the addition of hydrochlorothiazide. Br J Clin Pharmacol 14:97S–101S, 1982.
34. Johnston CI, Arnold L, Hiwatari M. Angiotensin converting enzyme inhibitors in the treatment of hypertension. Drugs 27:271–277, 1984.
35. Scholze J, Breitstadt A, Cairns V, et al. Ramipril and hydrochlorothiazide combination therapy in hypertension: A clinical trial of factorial design. J Hypertens 11;217–221, 1993.
36. Costa FV, Borghi C, Ambrosini E. Captopril and oxprenolol in a fixed combination with diuretics: Comparison of their antihypertensive efficacy and metabolic effects. Clin Ther 6:708–718, 1984.
37. Kellaway GSM, Inhibase General Study Group. A comparison of the efficacy of cilazapril versus cilazapril plus hydrochlorothiazide in patients with mild to moderate essential hypertension. Eur J Clin Pharmacol 44:377–379, 1993.
38. Neutel JM, Black HR, Weber MA. Combination therapy with diuretics: An evolution of understanding. Am J Med 101(suppl 3A):61S–70S, 1996.
39. Ratheiser K, Dusleag J, Seitl K, et al. A "lipo-protective" effect of a fixed combination of captopril and hydrochlorothiazide in antihypertensive therapy. Clin Cardiol 15:647–654, 1992.
40. Soffer BA, Wright JT, Pratt JH, et al. Effects of losartan on a background of hydrochlorothiazide in patients with hypertension. Hypertension 26:112–117, 1995.
41. Burnier M, Hagman M, Nussberger J, et al. Short-term and sustained renal effects of angiotensin II receptor blockade in healthy subjects. Hypertension 25:602–609, 1995.
42. Weber M, Byyny RL, Prat JH, et al. Blood pressure effects of the angiotensin-II receptor blocker, losartan. Arch Intern Med 155:405–411, 1995.
43. Bellet M, Sassano P, Guyene T, et al. Converting enzyme inhibition buffers the counter-regulatory response to acute administration of nicardipine. Br J Clin Pharmacol 24:465–472, 1987.
44. Leonetti G, Terzoli L, Rupoli L, et al. Renal effects of felodipine in hypertension. Drugs 34(suppl 3):59–66, 1987.
45. Hung HMJ, Chi GYH, Lipicky RJ. Testing for the existence of a desirable dose combination. Biometrics 49:85–94, 1993.
46. DeQuattro V, Lee D. Fixed-dose combination therapy with trandola-

pril and verapamil SR is effective in primary hypertension. Am J Hypertens 10(suppl 2):138S–145S, 1997.

47. Ferme I, Djiam J, Tcherdakoff P. Comparative study on monotherapy with sustained-release diltiazem 300 mg and enalapril 20 mg in mild to moderate arterial hypertension. J Cardiovasc Pharmacol 16(suppl 1):S46–S50, 1990.
48. Frishman WF, Landau A, Cretkovic A. Combination drug therapy with calcium-channel blockers in the treatment of systemic hypertension. J Clin Pharmacol 33:752–755, 1993.
49. Epstein M. The benefits of ACE inhibitors and calcium antagonists in slowing progressive renal failure: Focus on fixed-dose combination antihypertensive therapy. Ren Fail 18:813–832, 1996.
50. Leenen FHH, Holliwell DL. Antihypertensive effect of felodipine associated with persistent sympathetic nervous system activation and minimal regression of left ventricular hypertrophy. Am J Cardiol 69:639–645, 1992.
51. Guazzi MD, DeCesare N, Galli C, et al: Calcium channel blockade with nifedipine and angiotensin-converting enzyme inhibition with captopril in the therapy of patients with severe primary hypertension. Circulation 70:279–284, 1984.

CHAPTER 54

Chronotherapeutics in the Treatment of Hypertension

Joel M. Neutel and David H. G. Smith

Biological functions and processes are precisely organized in time, and physiological patterns such as growth, puberty, aging, menstruation, pregnancy, and jet lag confirm the presence of an internal pacemaker "clock" in the brain. Further, biological rhythms and their underlying mechanisms may have important influences on various disease processes. The study of these rhythms and their clinical applications is referred to as *chronobiology*. It has become obvious that biological patterns may be useful in the management of various disease processes. Using specifically formulated agents and drug delivery systems over 24 hours to provide drug concentrations that vary in synchrony with biological needs has the potential to improve the efficacy and safety of treatment. These agents have now been termed *chronotherapeutic agents*.

Ambulatory monitoring has clearly demonstrated that blood pressure has a very definite and reproducible circadian (diurnal) pattern over 24 hours.[1] This pattern of blood pressure coincides very closely with several patterns of cardiovascular disease, resulting in the belief that blood pressure may play an important role in precipitating some of the target organ damage associated with hypertension.[2–4] This has resulted in the development of new treatment modalities and innovative drugs to try to maximize blood pressure control at the time patients are most likely to have events.

CIRCADIAN RHYTHM OF BLOOD PRESSURE

Office-based blood pressure measurements with conventional sphygmomanometers have provided the basis of our understanding of the prognosis and natural history of hypertension. Office blood pressure measurements are clearly related to cardiovascular morbidity and mortality and underlie most decisions about clinical diagnosis and treatment, but ambulatory blood pressure monitoring (ABPM) has become a useful adjunct. ABPM permits detailed study of blood pressure variability and its potential effects on target organs, documentation of individual blood pressure variability (in both level and amplitude) and phasing (in nocturnal vs. diurnal hypertension), and clarification of diagnosis in patients with white-coat hypertension (Fig. 54–1) (see Chap. 31, Blood Pressure Measurement Issues, and Chap. 32, White-Coat Hypertension).

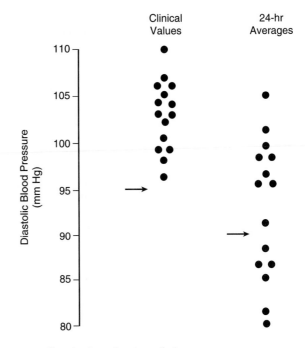

Figure 54–1. Clinical and 24-hour diastolic blood pressures in a group of 15 patients. In some, the average 24-hour blood pressures were normal despite consistently hypertensive readings during several clinical visits (white-coat hypertension). The criterion for diagnosing hypertension was decreased to 90 mm Hg to compensate for low nighttime levels included in the 24-hour average.

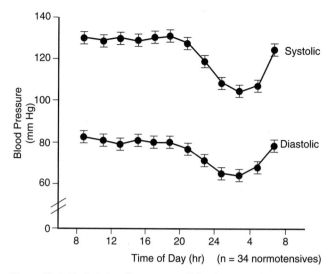

Figure 54–2. Typical circadian pattern of blood pressure in 34 normotensive individuals. The 24-hour period has been divided into 12 consecutive 2-hour periods, with each 2-hour value representing the average of all readings taken during that particular 2-hour period.

Data from both intraarterial and noninvasive ABPM have provided detailed evidence that, in most individuals, blood pressure has a characteristic and reproducible circadian pattern (Fig. 54–2).[1] Both systolic and diastolic blood pressure are highest during the day, fall steadily through the evening, and reach their lowest levels between midnight and 2 AM. Low nocturnal values then slowly rise again, frequently during sleep, until about 6 AM, when they abruptly and steeply increase to their higher daytime values with the assumption of upright posture and daily activity.

Frequently, blood pressure may overshoot, causing a shoulder of high blood pressure during the early morning hours.

Early studies, using intraarterial ABPM devices, established that 24-hour blood pressure curves are reproducible when studied on consecutive days and on separate days, weeks apart.[5] Similar findings were obtained when using noninvasive ABPM techniques both in hospitalized patients and in ambulatory patients participating in routine daily activities.[6, 7] Individual patients may experience variations from one day of monitoring to the next, particularly if engaging in different types of activities. In rotating-shift workers, the circadian pattern tends to reverse quickly, even by the first 24 hours of night work, with the highest blood pressure values occurring at night.[8]

Patients with secondary forms of hypertension generally do not have a circadian pattern to their blood pressure, which tends to remain constant (with no decrease during nighttime sleep) throughout the 24-hour period. The circadian pattern in patients with primary (essential) hypertension parallels that of normotensive individuals (Fig. 54–3), although at consistently higher blood pressure levels.[9] Antihypertensive treatment usually causes a downward shift of the curve, parallel to that of the pretreated levels.[10]

The main determinant of the circadian blood pressure pattern appears to be the sympathetic nervous system. Serial measurements of plasma catecholamines over 24 hours indicate that both norepinephrine and epinephrine have a circadian pattern very similar to that of blood pressure. The increase in sympathetic activity during arousal from sleep may be an important factor in producing the sharp, rapid, early morning blood pressure increase. Norepinephrine levels, in particular, appear to demonstrate a slight overshoot toward the end of the morning arousal process, similar to that seen with blood pressure.[7]

Figure 54–3. Systolic and diastolic blood pressure averages over 24 hours in 29 age-matched pairs of hypertensive and normotensive men. The 24-hour period has been divided into 12 2-hour intervals.

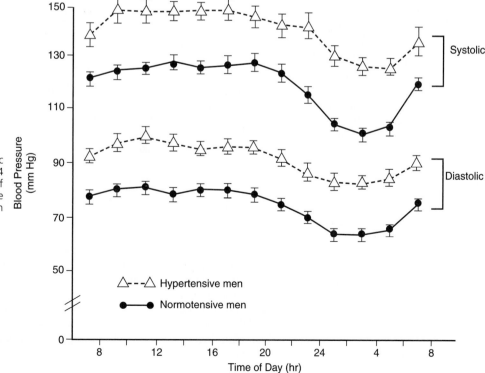

Studies using ABPM have shown that approximately 30 to 40% of African American hypertensive patients and approximately 30% of elderly hypertensive patients (over age 65 years), without evidence of secondary hypertension, do not experience a blood pressure decrease ("dip") during sleep.[11] Patients with this blood pressure pattern are referred to as *nondippers* and tend to exhibit more severe target organ damage than patients with similar mean blood pressures but with a more typical *dipper* pattern. These findings have generated a wide interest in the nighttime blood pressure, which may become more important in the diagnosis and treatment of hypertension in the future.

RELATIONSHIP OF BLOOD PRESSURE TO CARDIOVASCULAR EVENTS

The real importance of the circadian pattern of blood pressure is likely its relationship to cardiovascular events. The tendency for major cardiovascular events to occur during the early hours of the activity span is well recognized.[7–9] The incidence of myocardial infarction and sudden cardiac death rises steadily during the hours following awakening and tends to peak between 6 AM and 12 noon.[9, 12, 13] Studies of active patients using ambulatory electrocardiographic monitoring show that episodes of silent myocardial ischemia clearly have their highest incidence within the first few hours after awakening.[14] At least twice as many episodes of transient myocardial ischemia occur between 6 and 8 AM as during any other 2-hour period. Similarly, nonembolic strokes, to the extent that their timing can be determined, seem at least as likely as coronary events to occur in the early morning hours after arousal from sleep.

The relationship between the early morning blood pressure surge and the increased risk of cardiovascular disease has led investigators to question whether the rapid change in blood pressure may play a role in precipitating these early morning cardiovascular events. There is little doubt that other circadian rhythms in critical biological processes and functions contribute to the early morning increase in cardiovascular events after arousal from sleep.[14] Increased sympathetic nervous system activity, which causes a rapid rise in heart rate, increased cardiac output, and increased ventricular activity, may also have an impact on cardiovascular events. Increased whole-blood viscosity and platelet aggregability and reduced fibrinolytic activity make thrombogenesis more likely in the morning.[14, 15] All of these factors likely play a role in the increased cardiovascular events of the early morning hours.

There are now good data to show that sudden changes in blood pressure, as normally occur during arousal, may be directly involved in precipitating myocardial ischemia. Data from studies of patients with chronic stable angina undergoing simultaneous Holter monitoring and ABPM have suggested a causal relationship between blood pressure increases and silent myocardial ischemia, irrespective of what time of day they occur.[16] Patients in these studies typically experience a surge in blood pressure demonstrated on the ambulatory blood pressure monitor and then minutes later develop a clinically significant episode of ischemia, evidenced by ST segment depression on the Holter monitor. In a separate study, patients were divided into quintiles of

blood pressure and within each quintile were subdivided into patients with very labile blood pressure over the 24-hour period and those with a smooth blood pressure pattern over 24 hours.[17] Patients within each quintile with the labile pattern had significantly greater target organ damage than patients with consistent blood pressure, despite the fact that the mean 24-hour blood pressure in each of the subgroups was similar. These data also suggest that rapid changes in blood pressure are not well tolerated and that patients with smooth blood pressure patterns have less disease even though they have elevated blood pressures. A third study demonstrated that if adequate blood pressure control could be maintained during the early morning period, it may be possible to change the circadian pattern of heart disease.[4] Patients with well-controlled blood pressure during arousal from sleep did not show a peak incidence in myocardial infarction during the period 6 AM to 12 noon, but rather had an incidence of myocardial infarction that did not vary over the 24-hour period.[4]

A possible reason for the relationship between changing blood pressure and cardiovascular events may be plaque rupture.[18] Smooth plaques in the coronary arteries are generally well tolerated and frequently asymptomatic. Sudden blood pressure increases may rupture these plaques (as occurs with an angioplasty balloon), resulting in an irregular plaque surface that then becomes a nidus for platelet aggregation. This may result in a complex sequence of events promoting vessel occlusion and stenosis.

These data suggest that rapid surges of blood pressure play a role in precipitating cardiovascular events. Blood pressure physiologically increases rapidly in the early morning. This surge of blood pressure may play an important role in the pathogenesis of early morning cardiovascular events. Thus, this early morning period appears to be a time during which optimal blood pressure control is most desirable. Furthermore, it appears that utilizing drugs that have a smooth and continuous action, which may decrease blood pressure lability, may also be an important consideration in drug selection.

CHRONOTHERAPEUTICS IN THE TREATMENT OF HYPERTENSION

Achieving adequate blood pressure control in the morning is frequently difficult. Most antihypertensive drugs are taken in the morning and are at trough levels at the time when optimal blood pressure control is most desirable. These drugs then peak between 12 noon and 4 PM, several hours after the vulnerable period. Furthermore, many of the drugs that are marketed as once-a-day agents do not work for 24 hours and tend to lose efficacy during the last 4- to 6-hour period before the next dose.[10, 19] The time at which blood pressure increases due to reduced efficacy of the drug coincides with the time of the rapid circadian rise of blood pressure. The result may be a relatively greater risk of plaque rupture and thus cardiovascular disease.

Taking drugs at night may be one solution, but this also has some important problems. The gastrointestinal system also appears to have a circadian pattern, and absorption appears to be less effective at night than during the day.[20] Thus, to achieve similar drug levels at night, a larger dose of the drug may have to be given, which may be associated with an increase in side effect profile. Also, if a drug is taken at night, it frequently peaks at a time that blood pressure is physiologically at its lowest level. This is not a problem in patients with a relatively normal cardiovascular system, but in patients with underlying coronary artery disease and ventricular dysfunction, it may precipitate hypotension and ischemia.[15] In addition, the lower blood pressures at night are frequently associated with increased heart rate (compensatory mechanism to maintain a normal blood pressure). Increasing data suggest that heart rates that are elevated, especially chronically, may be associated with increased cardiovascular mortality.[21] Also, drugs that do not work for 24 hours and that are administered at night may lose efficacy at some stage during the daytime period (4 to 6 hours before the next dose). Although this may be less important than during the early morning period, it has been shown that target organ damage correlates with the length of time spent hypertensive and thus may be associated with target organ damage.[22]

Optimal treatment of hypertension would involve drugs that peak in the early morning and reach trough levels during the period between midnight and 4 AM. They should also have a consistent drug level in the plasma over the remaining 24-hour period to maintain smooth blood pressure control and true efficacy throughout the 24-hour dosing interval. The goal of chronotherapeutics is the development of drugs with pharmacokinetic/pharmacodynamic profiles that take into account chronobiological patterns of disease intensity over a 24-hour period. Current drug treatment strategies for once-a-day antihypertensive agents involve the application of drug delivery systems or drugs with long half-lives to achieve consistent blood levels of the drug throughout the 24-hour dosing interval in the hope that this will provide smooth blood pressure control throughout the 24-hour period. This approach assumes that the need for medication is consistent throughout the 24-hour period and that consistent blood levels of drug result in equal therapeutic responses. However, review of blood pressure patterns over a 24-hour period suggests that optimal treatment includes peak drug levels during the early morning period and trough levels during the time that blood pressure is physiologically at its lowest level (between 12 midnight and 4 AM). This is frequently difficult to achieve with once-a-day drugs, as those taken in the morning peak too late and those taken at night peak too early.

Attempts have been made to use once-a-day agents chronotherapeutically by varying the time of dosing to fit in with the circadian rhythm of blood pressure. It should be remembered that the development of once-a-day antihypertensive agents was directed at simplifying treatment regimens for hypertensive patients in the hope that these could result in increased patient compliance, and not at developing chronotherapeutic agents. Once-a-day agents have been successful in improving patient compliance and in many instances provide smooth blood pressure control over the entire 24-hour period. However, they do not provide peak and trough levels at the most desirable times during the dosing interval. Furthermore, in many cases, they fall short of providing efficacy throughout the dosing interval and are associated with blood pressure increases that coincide with the rapid early morning surge in blood

pressure.[10, 19] These patients may be relatively at greater risk of developing cardiovascular disease.

Recently, there has been an increased interest in developing antihypertensive agents that work in synchrony with circadian rhythms of blood pressure in the effort to maximize treatment at the time that it is most needed. The focus with these drugs has been an attempt to achieve peak drug levels during the early morning period, coinciding with arousal from sleep. Utilizing a delayed-release technology, these drugs are taken at night, and release of the drugs is then delayed by approximately 5 to 8 hours so that peak levels occur between 4 AM and 12 noon.[19, 23]

One such drug is a controlled-onset, extended-release formulation of verapamil that is taken at bedtime and peaks during the early morning period. The delivery system utilized with this drug is a variant of the gastrointestinal therapeutic system (GITS) but with an inner-tablet coating that delays drug release for 4 to 6 hours after administration. This allows lower drug concentrations during sleep and maximal drug delivery during the early morning hours. Studies with this agent have demonstrated maximal blood pressure reduction during the period 6 AM to 12 noon, the time at which cardiovascular events are most likely to occur (Fig. 54–4). Trough levels occur between midnight and 4 AM.[19]

Since rapid changes in blood pressure may play an important role in the pathogenesis of cardiovascular events, it is believed that changing the rate of rise of the early morning blood pressure may be important in decreasing events during this time period. Studies with ABPM have demonstrated that treatment of hypertension can eliminate the early morning surge of blood pressure. Blood pressure

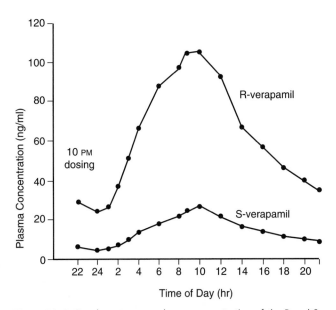

Figure 54–4. Steady-state mean plasma concentration of the R and S racemic isomers derived from verapamil HCl, controlled-onset, extended-release delivery system. Following 10 PM bedtime dosing with this formulation, a delay of 4 to 5 hours occurs in drug release. The most elevated levels of the R racemic isomer (affecting primarily the peripheral vasculature) and the S racemic isomer (affecting primarily cardiac impulse conduction) are achieved when typically most needed. Drug levels are intentionally minimized at night, when blood pressure naturally declines to its lowest level in uncomplicated hypertension.

has to increase from low early morning levels to higher daytime levels, as people could not function at the low nighttime blood pressure. However, it does appear that increasing the period of time over which the increase occurs (decreasing the rate of rise of blood pressure), which can be achieved with drugs that peak in the early morning, may affect cardiovascular events in these patients. A study comparing the delayed-release verapamil dosed at night to nifedipine GITS dosed in the morning demonstrated that both drugs were able to reduce the rate of rise of systolic and diastolic blood pressure compared with baseline.[24] Of note, the verapamil also resulted in a significant decrease in the rate of rise of early morning heart rate. This may be of clinical importance because recent epidemiological studies have shown that heart rate is an independent predictor of cardiovascular risk.[21]

Another meaningful measure of the impact of antihypertensive treatment is the heart rate–systolic blood pressure product, both over the 24-hour period and in the early morning. This measurement is an index of myocardial oxygen demand and one that parallels myocardial ischemia. In an assessment of the heart rate–systolic blood pressure product, it was shown that delayed-release mechanisms resulted in significant decreases in this measurement compared with placebo and nifedipine.[24]

Thus, the use of chronotherapeutic agents in hypertension has several important advantages:

1. It allows peak drug to be provided at a time when cardiovascular disease is most likely to occur, thus optimizing control and preventing events.
2. Trough drug levels can be achieved between 12 midnight and 4 AM, when blood pressure is physiologically at its lowest level.
3. Designing drugs to be most effective during the rapid early morning increase in blood pressure may allow smaller doses of drug to be used to achieve adequate control. This may result in a more favorable side effect profile.
4. It provides smooth blood pressure control over 24 hours and decreases blood pressure lability.
5. It provides adequate 24-hour blood pressure control throughout the dosing interval.
6. By adjusting dosing time, chronotherapeutic agents can be employed in usual disease presentations (such as patients with renal insufficiency who are nondippers) to try to normalize the blood pressure pattern.

Although chronotherapeutics appears to be an optimal means of treating hypertensive patients and preventing cardiovascular events, this still has to be demonstrated in long-term studies. Nonetheless, increasing numbers of chronotherapeutic agents are currently being developed, and they will provide a very exciting and likely very important addition to our armamentarium for the treatment of hypertension.

References

1. Drayer JI, Weber MA, Hoeger WJ. Whole-day BP monitoring in ambulatory normotensive men. Arch Intern Med 145:271–274, 1985.
2. Tofler GH, Brezinski D, Schafer AI. Concurrent morning increase in platelet aggregability and the risk of myocardial infarction and sudden cardiac death. N Engl J Med 316:1514–1518, 1987.
3. Marler JE, Price TR, Clark GL. Morning increase in onset of ischemic stroke. Stroke 20:473–476, 1989.
4. Muller JE, Stone PH, Turi ZG. Circadian variation in the frequency of onset of acute myocardial infarction. N Engl J Med 313:1315–1322, 1985.
5. Gould BA, Mann S, Davies AB. Can placebo therapy influence arterial blood pressure? Clin Sci 61(suppl 7):478S–490S, 1981.
6. Weber MA, Drayer JIM, Wyle FA. Reproducibility of the whole-day blood pressure pattern in essential hypertension. Clin Exp Hypertens A 4:1377–1390, 1982.
7. Graettinger WF, Lipson JL, Klein RC. Comparison of antihypertensive therapies by noninvasive techniques. Chest 96:74–79, 1989.
8. Sternberg H, Rosenthal T, Shamiss A, Green M. Altered circadian rhythm of blood pressure in shift worker. J Hum Hypertens 9:349–353, 1995.
9. Drayer JI, Weber MA, Nakamura DK. Automated ambulatory blood pressure monitoring: A study in age-matched normotensive and hypertensive men. Am Heart J 109:1334–1338, 1985.
10. Neutel JM, Smith DHG, Ram CVS, et al. Application of ambulatory blood pressure monitoring in differentiating between antihypertensive agents. Am J Med 94:181–187, 1993.
11. Harshfield GA, Hwang C, Grim CE. Circadian variation of blood pressure in blacks: Influence of age, gender and activity. J Hum Hypertens 4:43–47, 1990.
12. Willich SN, Linderer T, Wegscheider K. Increased morning incidence of myocardial infarction in the ISAM Study: Absence with prior β-adrenergic blockade. Circulation 80:853–858, 1989.
13. Willich SN, Levy D, Rocco MB. Circadian variation in the incidence of sudden cardiac death in the Framingham Heart Study population. Am J Cardiol 60:801–806, 1987.
14. Kario K, Matsuo T, Kobayashi H, et al: Nocturnal fall of blood pressure and silent cerebrovascular damage in elderly hypertensive patients. Hypertension 27:130–135, 1996.
15. Rocco MB, Barry J, Campbell S. Circadian variation of transient myocardial ischemia in patients with coronary artery disease. Circulation 75:395–400, 1987.
16. Deedwania PC, Nelson JR. Pathophysiology of silent myocardial ischemia during daily life: Hemodynamic evaluation by simultaneous electrocardiographic and blood pressure monitoring. Circulation 82:1296–1304, 1990.
17. Parati G, Pomidossi G, Albini F, et al. Relationship of 24-hour blood pressure mean and variability to severity of target-organ damage in hypertension. J Hypertens 5:93–98, 1987.
18. Muller JE, Tofler GH, Stone PH. Circadian variation and triggers of onset of acute cardiovascular disease. Circulation 79:733–743, 1989.
19. Neutel JM, Schnaper H, Cheung DG. Antihypertensive effects of β-blockers administered once-daily: 24-hour measurements. Am Heart J 120:166–171, 1990.
20. Reinberg A, Smolensky MH. Circadian changes of drug disposition in man. Clin Pharmacokinet 7:401–420, 1982.
21. Gillman MW, Kannel WB, Belanger A, D'Agostino RB. Influence of heart rate on mortality among persons with hypertension: The Framingham Study. Am Heart J 125:1148–1154, 1993.
22. White WB, Dey HM, Schulman P. Assessment of the daily blood pressure load as a determinant of cardiac function in patients with mild-to-moderate hypertension. Am Heart J 118:782–795, 1989.
23. White WB, Anders RJ, MacIntyre JM, and the Verapamil Study Group. Nocturnal dosing of a novel delivery system of verapamil for systemic hypertension. Am J Cardiol 76:375–380, 1995.
24. White WB, Black HR, Weber M, et al. Comparison of effects of controlled onset extended release verapamil at bedtime and nifedipine gastrointestinal therapeutics system on arising on early morning blood pressure, heart rate and heart rate–blood pressure product. Am J Cardiol 81:424–431, 1998.

Comorbid Conditions—Special Considerations

55 Comorbid Conditions

Gordon S. Stokes and Karen A. Duggan

PROFILING THE PATIENT

Taking account of comorbidity in management of the individual hypertensive patient is part of the broader exercise of patient profiling, in which antihypertensive drugs and other measures used in therapy are oriented to the particular needs of each patient. Global assessment of these needs includes consideration of gender, age, pregnancy risk, body mass, diet and exercise habits, and concurrent diseases.

Such diseases may be obvious, and their interaction with management of hypertension easily recognized. However, in the initial assessment of the patient, a careful history and physical examination will often reveal asymptomatic disorders that may be activated by the wrong choice of drug: e.g., asthma may be activated by β-blockers or gout by diuretics. Additionally, diagnostic tests undertaken to discover the basis of the hypertension or to determine the extent of hypertension-induced organ impairment may disclose factors that will condition the choice of therapy. This applies to nonpharmacological treatment as well as to drug therapy. For example, graded aerobic exercise is valuable as a primary measure in the control of mild to moderate hypertension in some subjects, but it might have to take a secondary and limited role in a hypertensive patient with hemodynamically significant cardiac valvular disease.

OBESITY

Generalized obesity is an important premorbid condition, associated with an increased incidence of hypertension and of hypertensive-ischemic cardiovascular disease. It may cause refractoriness to antihypertensive therapy. Weight loss through an appropriate dietary program is an essential part of the management of the obese hypertensive subject, and trials have shown significant falls in blood pressure with weight reduction.[1-3] However, failure to secure or maintain a decrease in weight is common. The physician should first exclude any primary metabolic cause of obesity, such as glucocorticoid excess or myxedema—a truncal disposition of adipose tissue may be an important clue here. Then questions should be directed at common problem areas in the diet that result from lack of awareness by the patient of the high calorie content of their food choices.

Intake of alcohol is a common "blind spot" in explaining weight reduction programs that fail. Nonalcoholic, sugar-containing drinks can also be a culprit, especially in climates and workplaces with high environmental temperatures that encourage excessive consumption. The physician should make a preliminary assessment of the patient's insight and motivation and set an appropriate body weight target. This target should be based on a table of ideal body weight in relation to height, and it should be reached in a time calculated by weight loss at a rate of 1 to 2 kg per month. Thorough assessment of the diet and implementation of a corrective program are the domain of the community-based nutritionist. Ideally, the nutritionist chosen should be located close to the patient's home or workplace to facilitate dietary follow-up, and she or he should consult the patient and spouse or partner jointly.

Exercise programs are of major benefit in the obese hypertensive patient. Not only does exercise assist weight loss, but it also contributes directly to lowering of blood pressure. A recent meta-analysis has indicated that dynamic aerobic training lowers both conventionally measured and ambulatory daytime blood pressure in hypertensive adults.[4]

METABOLIC DISORDERS

Diabetes Mellitus

Hypertension occurs twice as frequently in diabetic subjects as in the general population, affecting 25% of young patients with type 1 diabetes mellitus and 50% of patients with newly diagnosed type 2 diabetes.[5] By interacting with diabetes-induced microvascular disease in the kidney and retina, uncontrolled hypertension carries an extra penalty of morbidity in diabetics over and above that caused in nondiabetics. Moreover, in both type 1 and type 2 diabetes, hypertension is a well-recognized factor in the progression of diabetic nephropathy—now the most frequent single cause of all end-stage renal disease in the United States[6] and comparable countries.

Thus, along with glycemic control, prevention of dietary protein overload, cessation of smoking, and treatment of hyperlipidemia, the assiduous control of hypertension has a high priority in the management of diabetes.[5] Even when blood pressure is within the normal range, progression of diabetic retinopathy is faster in those patients with higher levels of blood pressure.[7] Since the late 1980s, target blood pressures in diabetics have been altered; from merely achieving a diastolic pressure less than 90 mm Hg, the target has now shifted to a lower level, less than 80 mm Hg in high-risk groups. The question of how far this process should be taken is unresolved. Preliminary studies suggest that the lower the blood pressure level, the greater the impact in decreasing proteinuria and delaying progression of nephropathy. For the present, the target blood pressure of 130/85 mm Hg given in the guidelines in the sixth report of the Joint National Committee on Prevention, Detection, Evaluation, and Treatment of High Blood Pressure (JNC VI)[8] should be used for patients with diabetes mellitus, except in patients with proteinuria in whom a slightly lower value would be appropriate.

Optimal antihypertensive drug therapy in diabetes should have three characteristics: (1) In addition to lowering systemic blood pressure, the agents chosen should have beneficial effects on the progression of diabetic nephropathy. (2) The agents chosen should not interfere with glycemic control. (3) The agents chosen should have a beneficial or neutral effect on the dyslipidemia of diabetes.

Both angiotensin-converting enzyme (ACE) inhibitors and calcium antagonists have been shown to reduce proteinuria and the rate of decline in renal function in type 1 and type 2 diabetic patients, with ACE inhibitors having the better documented efficacy on proteinuria. ACE inhibitors have been shown to slow the progression of nephropathy in type 1 and type 2 diabetic patients without hypertension, indicating that these agents have a nephroprotective activity beyond their capacity to lower blood pressure.[5] The reduction of the raised intraglomerular pressure characteristic of early diabetes by ACE inhibitors[9, 10] provides a rationale for their use even in the absence of hypertension and for their preferred use over other antihypertensive drug groups when systemic hypertension is present. ACE inhibitors may also benefit glomerular membrane permeability[11] and may slow proliferative changes by decreasing angiotensin II–induced mitogenic activity.[12] It is anticipated that angiotensin II receptor antagonists will confer similar benefit, although it is theoretically possible that they could confer more (through blockade of alternative pathways of angiotensin production, e.g., the chymase pathway[13]) or less (owing to lack of the kinin-mediated effects possessed by ACE inhibitors).

Whereas ACE inhibitors are generally of benefit in diabetic patients with relatively normal renal function, they may occasionally contribute to the decline in glomerular filtration rate in patients with more advanced disease. This is sometimes but not always attributable to concurrent renal ischemia. For this reason, renal function must be closely monitored with serial measurements of plasma creatinine and creatinine clearance.

Calcium antagonists do not reduce intraglomerular pressure, and their role in retarding the progression of diabetic renal failure is controversial.[14] The various classes of calcium antagonists appear to have different effects on renal function, and some have been associated with adverse cardiovascular outcomes. Verapamil and diltiazem may reduce diabetic proteinuria, whereas dihydropyridines generally do not.[15–17] The hypertensive arm of a large prospective trial designed to compare the nephroprotective efficacy of the calcium antagonist nisoldipine with the ACE inhibitor enalapril in hypertensive and normotensive patients with type 2 diabetes was terminated early because of an excess of fatal and nonfatal myocardial infarctions in those taking the calcium antagonist.[18] However, combined ACE inhibitor and calcium antagonist therapy appears to confer additive effects in reducing proteinuria and slowing renal failure in experimental and clinical diabetes.[5]

Of other commonly used antihypertensive agents, diuretics tend to produce renal vasoconstriction and do not reduce proteinuria; neither α- nor β-adrenoceptor blockers produce consistent changes in renal hemodynamics or proteinuria.[19]

In patients without insulin resistance or dyslipidemia, the commonly used antihypertensive agents do not interfere with glycemic control or blood lipid levels. ACE inhibitors, α-adrenoceptor blockers, and dihydropyridine calcium antagonists do not alter fasting glucose concentration or glycosylated hemoglobin in hypertensive type 2 diabetic patients after 12-week periods of treatment at therapeutically effective dosages[20] and tend to improve insulin sensitivity and dyslipidemia.[21] Therefore, they are the preferred drug groups in patients with such intercurrent disorders. However, thiazide diuretics, spironolactone, and β-blockers tend to impair insulin sensitivity and to worsen dyslipidemia, whereas diltiazem, verapamil, clonidine, methyldopa, and indapamide are neutral.[21, 22] β-blockers are also relatively contraindicated in treating hypertension in brittle diabetics because they may mask symptoms of hypoglycemia and inhibit reactive glycogenolysis. In type 2 diabetics, β₂-blockers have the added disadvantage of inhibiting residual insulin secretion.

It is important to allow for autonomic dysfunction in the assessment of blood pressure in diabetes. The nocturnal fall in blood pressure is blunted in patients with diabetic nephropathy, perhaps because of a lack of withdrawal of sympathetic tone during sleep.[23, 24] Thus, extra care is needed to ensure that such patients have adequate blood pressure control during the night. Medications given once daily in the morning, which may suffice to control hypertension in "dippers" (patients who demonstrate the nocturnal fall in blood pressure usual for uncomplicated hypertension), may be inadequate for 24-hour control in "nondippers." Conversely, one must safeguard against excessive blood pressure lowering in patients with orthostasis. To avoid attacks of postural hypotension in such patients, antihypertensive therapy may need to be titrated in relation to erect rather than supine or sitting blood pressure measurements. Additionally, postexercise blood pressure may need to be taken into account because autonomic dysfunction is associated with impaired work capacity.[25]

Hyperlipidemias

Dyslipidemias are more common in patients with essential hypertension than in the general population owing to a genetic linkage. They are also more common in diabetics and in persons with renal impairment. The combination of hypertension and hyperlipidemia in chronic renal failure kills more patients through cardiovascular disease than through the direct metabolic effects of uremia. Thus, dietary management of hypertensive patients should always include recognition and rigorous adjustment of excessive saturated fat intake, particularly in patients with known hyperlipidemia, renal impairment, or diabetes mellitus.

In the choice of antihypertensive drugs, diuretics and β-blockers (without intrinsic sympathomimetic activity [ISA]) are theoretically deleterious because they can raise blood concentrations of total cholesterol, low-density lipoproteins, and trigycerides. However, the Treatment of Mild Hypertension Study (TOMHS)[26] showed that chlorthalidone 15 mg/day given long term had no effect on plasma lipids. It is also clear that the effects of non-ISA β-blockers in preventing further cardiac events in patients with previous myocardial infarctions overrides whatever deleterious effect they may have on plasma lipids.[27] Alternatively, α-adrenoceptor blockers have the potentially beneficial actions of lowering atherogenic plasma lipids and raising high-density lipoproteins. However, some long-term trials with α-blockers have shown no sustained improvement in plasma lipid levels, and no long-term trials have shown significant outcome differences in morbid endpoints.

Hyperuricemia

Hyperuricemia, particularly if associated with clinical gout, is a relative contraindication to the use of thiazide and loop diuretics. If blood pressure cannot be controlled without diuretics in a patient with hyperuricemia, they should be used in combination with allopurinol.

AIRWAYS DISEASE

Airways disease associated with a tendency to bronchoconstriction is a risk factor for the use of β-blocker therapy, regardless of whether the drugs considered are β_1- or β_2-selective, have intrinsic sympathetic activity, or have combined β-blocking and vasodilator activity. Care must be taken even in subjects who have not had asthma since childhood; in such subjects, an adverse reaction to β-blockade may not occur until they develop an incidental respiratory tract infection. Thus, β-blockers are not the agents of choice in patients with airways disease. Nevertheless, in some circumstances, as when severe side effects or inefffectiveness precludes the use of other agents, it may be necessary to use them. In this event, a cardioselective β-blocker should be used—in low dose only, as at higher doses (e.g., greater than 200 mg/day for metoprolol), there is loss of cardioselectivity.

Other classes of antihypertensive drugs are usually safe in asthmatic patients or those with chronic airways disease. However, ACE inhibitors cause an irritating cough in 10 to 20% of all subjects, and asthmatic patients are more likely to be troubled by this symptom if it occurs. Obstructive sleep apnea may cause either a loss of the usual nocturnal decline in blood pressure or sustained diurnal hypertension.[28] Recognition and appropriate treatment of this disorder may be the key to the control of refractory hypertension. For patients with pulmonary hypertension requiring antihypertensive therapy, calcium antagonists are the agents of choice, as there is evidence that they provide pulmonary vasodilatation in addition to their systemic effects.[29]

CARDIAC DISEASE

Whether cardiac disease precedes or results from hypertension, uncontrolled systolic or diastolic hypertension has a deleterious effect on cardiac function. Because of increased afterload, the left ventricle hypertrophies and may then dilate. Left ventricular failure follows, and its progress is accelerated if coronary vascular perfusion is compromised secondary to hypertension and atherosclerosis. In subjects who have sustained a myocardial infarction, there is an increased risk of adverse outcomes associated with hypertension, whether antecedent[30] or after the infarction.[31]

With some exceptions, all classes of antihypertensive drugs achieve comparable decreases of afterload in relation to the reductions in blood pressure they produce. A minority of elderly patients with hypertension and concentric cardiac hypertrophy are prone to excessive hypotensive reactions with vasodilators, but respond well to β-blockers.[32] On the other hand, ACE inhibitors and β-blockers have specific cardioprotective effects after myocardial infarction.

The presence of coincidental cardiac valvular disease, or cardiac failure of any origin, should signal a lower decision-to-treat threshold with antihypertensive drugs. Not only will such treatment decrease the afterload on the already compromised left ventricle, but it may also confer beneficial effects through the ancillary actions of the drugs employed. These effects can be antiarrhythmic (e.g., β-blockers, diltiazem, verapamil) or can relate to ventricular perfusion and remodeling (e.g., ACE inhibitors). Long-acting nitrates may have a specific beneficial left ventricular unloading effect in elderly patients with systolic hypertension by reducing the augmentation of the systolic peak caused by pulse-wave reflectance.[33] In patients with pure aortic or mitral stenosis, assessment of the degree of stenosis needs to be made before instituting therapy. In patients with severe valvular stenosis, vasodilators should be used with caution, if at all; agents such as verapamil and β-blockers may be preferred.

Antihypertensive Treatment in Relation to Specific Cardiac Disorders

Cardiac Failure

Whether due to intercurrent cardiac disease or as a complication of uncontrolled hypertension, chronic left ventricular failure carries a poor prognosis in hypertensive patients unless it can be effectively controlled by therapy. The most successful therapies appear to be those that diminish the activity of the renin-angiotensin system and/or central sympathetic tone, both of which may be heightened in heart failure. In the Studies of Left Ventricular Dysfunction (SOLVD) project, ACE inhibitors proved effective in decreasing cardiovascular events and cardiac mortality in patients with congestive failure.[34] A retrospective subset analysis of hypertensive patients included in this trial showed treatment-induced risk reduction similar to that in the whole data set.[35] ACE inhibitors are now well established as the drug class of first choice in hypertensive heart failure, with diuretics having an ancillary role in symptom control. However, in a recent randomized trial, treatment of elderly heart failure patients with the angiotensin II receptor antagonist losartan was associated with lower mortality and fewer adverse effects than treatment with the ACE inhibitor captopril.[36] Further studies are required to ascertain whether this advantage holds with other patient groups and with other angiotensin II receptor antagonists. Clonidine, an antihypertensive agent that decreases sympathetic tone, has useful adjunctive effects when used with captopril in patients with congestive heart failure: Both preload and afterload parameters are improved more with the combined therapy than with captopril alone, and there is better neurohumoral suppression.[37]

Antihypertensive drugs with negative inotropic activity, such as β-blockers and the calcium antagonists verapamil and diltiazem, are generally considered to be contraindicated in uncontrolled heart failure. However, the possible role of β-blockade and some forms of calcium antagonist therapy as adjunctive treatment in hypertensive heart failure is under reappraisal. A dihydropyridine calcium antagonist[38] or β-blocker[39] can be useful when combined with ACE inhibitor, digitalis, and diuretic therapy, particularly when left ventricular diastolic dysfunction is suspected.[40]

Carvedilol, a β-blocker with vasodilating properties, has been shown in collaborative studies in the United States and Australasia to reduce mortality and hospitalization in heart failure.[41, 42] Although differences in hemodynamic and neuroendocrine effects between carvedilol and metoprolol have been reported[43, 44] that may reflect the vasodilator activity of carvedilol,[43] the prognostic significance of these differences remains to be determined.[44]

Left Ventricular Hypertrophy

Left ventricular hypertrophy is an independent risk factor for myocardial infarction and cardiac death.[45] Its presence in a newly diagnosed hypertensive patient indicates a need for particularly assiduous blood pressure control. In a patient with apparently well controlled hypertension, the presence of left ventricular hypertrophy is an indication for further diagnostic assessment. Ideally, assessment of left ventricular dimensions by echocardiography should be carried out in all severely hypertensive patients at their initial visit and at yearly intervals until their blood pressure is brought under good control. If left ventricular hypertrophy increases despite antihypertensive therapy, ambulatory blood pressure monitoring may be indicated to exclude the possibility of escape from blood pressure control during some part of the 24-hour cycle (commonly in the late afternoon). The possibility of hypertrophic obstructive cardiomyopathy should also be considered.

Coronary Vascular Disease

The presence of angina pectoris should not discourage the use of antihypertensive therapy, but should be taken into account in the choice of antihypertensive agent. β-Blockers and non–dihydropyridine calcium antagonists may relieve symptoms as well as lower blood pressure, whereas systemic vasodilators are best avoided because they can produce a coronary steal effect. Short-acting calcium antagonists have been associated with increased cardiac mortality and the possibility of coronary steal,[46] although this issue is still controversial.[47] In patients with a previous history of myocardial infaction, β-blockers, particularly those without intrinsic sympathomimetic activity, are preferred because they have been shown in numerous trials to decrease the risk of subsequent cardiac events and of sudden death.[48]

VASCULAR DISEASES

Cerebrovascular Disease

Acute Stroke

The desirability of reducing blood pressure in recent stroke is controversial (see Chap. 28, Stroke and Hypertension). Sudden reductions in blood pressure may be associated with critical falls in cerebral blood flow, which is already decreased in areas adjacent to the cerebral infarct because of either thrombosis with associated periinfarct edema or cerebral vasospasm secondary to a hemorrhagic lesion. Concern that lowering systemic blood pressure with antihypertensive agents may intensify brain damage in the absence of pharmacologically induced cerebral vasodilatation, led to trials with various candidate drugs. Initially, nimodipine was reported to increase perfusion after subarachnoid hemorrhage,[49] and subsequent work has tended to support the idea that this is a class effect of the calcium antagonist group. However, initial enthusiasm for calcium antagonists as the drugs of choice for lowering blood pressure in acute stroke has been tempered by concerns about adverse cardiovascular outcomes reported with these drugs in some studies.[18, 46, 47]

In the unconscious patient, clonidine intramuscularly can be used in modest doses, e.g., 75 μg every 4 hours, to lower blood pressure. Even at this modest dose and when used for short periods, care must be taken with clonidine, as rebound hypertension can occur. Other agents that have proved useful for parenteral administration include hydralazine intramuscularly or sodium nitroprusside given by intravenous infusion. The latter has the advantage of rapid offset of action should blood pressure fall too precipitously.

Chronic Cerebrovascular Disease

Prevention of stroke is a well-established benefit of long-term antihypertensive therapy, and preexisting stroke is not a contraindication to controlling blood pressure, using the same criteria as for uncomplicated hypertension.[50] However, care should be taken to reduce blood pressure gradually, particularly in patients with a history of transient ischemic attacks or known cerebrovascular insufficiency. The presence of a carotid artery bruit or of symptoms suggesting transient ischemic attacks is an indication for Doppler flow studies of the carotid arteries before lowering blood pressure.

Peripheral Vascular Disease

Vasodilators are preferred for antihypertensive treatment in patients with Raynaud's phenomenon, but do not appear to alleviate symptoms due to atherosclerosis or Buerger's disease. However, β-blockers can exacerbate claudication. If β-blockers are used in such patients, agents with β$_1$-selectivity or intrinsic sympathomimetic activity are preferred. Calcium antagonists inhibit atherogenesis in animal models. In patients with early ischemic heart disease treated with a calcium antagonist for 3 years, coronary artery plaque development was slowed.[51] The mechanism of this effect is not known, nor is it certain whether it is relevant to arresting progress of peripheral atherosclerotic vascular disease or the natural history of established coronary artery disease.

Migraine

In patients with hypertension and migraine, it is preferable to choose an antihypertensive agent that can also reduce the frequency of migrainous attacks. β-Blockers are preferred, whereas clonidine and verapamil may also be used.[52–59] All of these agents reduce the frequency of migraine.[55, 57–59] Peripheral vasodilators should be avoided, as they are likely to increase the severity of migrainous episodes by increasing extracerebral blood flow, with resultant increased cerebral ischemia.

RENAL DISEASE

Importance of Appropriate Management of Hypertension in Renal Disease

The management of hypertension in chronic renal disease is aimed not only at controlling the blood pressure but also at preserving renal function. In patients with impaired renal function, as in diabetes, good blood pressure control may delay the progression to end-stage disease. Historically, there was reluctance to treat hypertension because of fear of disturbing renal autoregulation. However, blood pressure reduction is clearly beneficial in chronic renal diseases such as polycystic kidneys and diabetic nephropathy.

As in diabetes mellitus, many forms of chronic renal disease are thought to progress because of altered intraglomerular hemodynamics as well as specific stimulatory effects of hormones such as angiotensin II on protein synthesis.[60, 61] On this basis, ACE inhibitors and possibly angiotensin II type 1 (AT-1) receptor blockers are the agents of choice for conserving renal function in renal parenchymal disease. These drugs have beneficial effects on glomerular hemodynamics, reducing single-nephron glomerular filtration rate in excess of what would be expected from their blood pressure–lowering effects; they also inhibit angiotensin-induced stimulation of protein synthesis.[62, 63] Present practice is that AT-1 blockers are reserved for patients in whom adverse effects, such as cough, prevent the use of ACE inhibitors; however, recent studies indicate that they are safe and effective in hypertensive patients with renal impairment.[64]

In patients with advanced renal impairment denoted by plasma creatinine concentrations greater than 0.20 mmol/L, care must be taken with both AT-1 blockers and ACE inhibitors because these agents can induce hyperkalemia and an accelerated decline in renal function. Plasma potassium and creatinine concentrations and creatinine clearance should be monitored. The possibility of undiagnosed ischemic renal disease, a potentially salvageable cause of renal failure,[65–67] must also be considered, particularly when the use of an ACE inhibitor precipitates acute renal failure, acute pulmonary edema, or progressive azotemia in an elderly atherosclerotic patient.[67] In patients with parenchymal renal disease and no recognizable renovascular disease, decreases in glomerular filtration rate of up to 30% are usually reversible on cessation of ACE inhibitor therapy; decreases of greater than 30% may not be reversible and dialysis may be required. The extent to which blood pressure should be lowered in chronic renal disease remains a matter of some controversy, although preliminary studies suggest that a diastolic pressure in the range of 70 to 75 mm Hg confers extra benefit when compared with the more commonly accepted goal of 80 to 90 mm Hg.[68, 69]

Hypertension and Renal Artery Stenosis

Unilateral or bilateral renal artery stenosis sufficiently severe to interfere with kidney perfusion may cause hypertension or exacerbate preexisting hypertension. Evidence of a functional perfusion deficit can be sought by isotope renography, renal venous renin determination, or other means. However, none of these is completely reliable. Thus, once a renal artery constriction of greater than 80% is discovered by angiography, a trial of transcutaneous perluminal balloon dilatation should be considered as a combined diagnostic and therapeutic technique. Placement of a stent to maintain patency after ballooning is advisable in some cases, particularly if the stenosis is due to atheroma, is within 1 cm of the renal artery origin, or is a restenotic lesion.

Pharmacotherapy for this disease differs from treatment for other forms of hypertension only in that special care must be taken in the use of ACE inhibitors and angiotensin II receptor antagonists. These drugs may be very effective in reducing blood pressure in renin-dependent states, such as renovascular hypertension, but can cause critical deterioration in renal function owing to their vasodilator effects on the postglomerular circulation; acute renal failure may occur in bilateral renal disease or unilateral renal artery stenosis in a solitary kidney.

Hypertension Due to Nonmineralocorticoid Sodium Retention

This group of disorders includes apparent mineralocorticoid excess (AME) syndrome,[70] Liddle's syndrome,[70] and Gordon's syndrome.[71] AME arises from 11β-hydroxylase deficiency, either congenital or induced, that allows endogenous cortisol to escape rapid conversion to cortisone and to act directly on renal mineralocorticoid receptors. AME induced by overingestion of licorice responds within days to the withdrawal of licorice or licorice-like compounds from the diet. The congenital form of AME responds to spironolactone therapy. Liddle's syndrome entails excessive sodium and water reabsorption through the renal epithelial sodium channel, which is due to mutations encoding the genes of the β- or γ-subunit of this channel. The hypertension of Liddle's syndrome responds well to amiloride, which acts selectively at this Na$^+$ transport site. The renal tubular reabsorption defect in Gordon's syndrome is not clearly established, but appears to respond well to thiazide diuretics.

End-Stage Renal Failure

Antihypertensive therapy improves survival in hemodialysis patients regardless of the level of blood pressure control.[72] In patients undergoing maintenance dialysis, an important cause of hypertension is fluid overload. The first step in managing such patients is an accurate assessment of their ideal body weight and attainment of that weight by fluid removal at subsequent dialyses. A small percentage of patients may require antihypertensive agents in addition. Many antihypertensive drugs are suitable, but the agent(s) of choice should be long-acting and not removable by dialysis. This will allow a minimal dose to be used, and fluctuations in blood levels to be avoided. ACE inhibitors may provide extra benefits because of their ability to reduce thirst and consequent interdialytic weight gain.[73]

Drugs Used in Renal Disease That Cause Hypertension

After renal transplantation, approximately 40% of patients develop hypertension. This may represent the effect of increased renin secretion by the native kidneys, rejection of the transplanted kidney, or rejection-induced stenosis in the artery of the transplant. Alternatively, and more commonly, hypertension develops after transplantation owing to immunosuppressive drugs, such as prednisone, cyclosporine, or tacrolimus. Hypertension may also develop during high-dose prednisone administration. Antihypertensive therapy may be reduced or even withdrawn when the dose of prednisone is reduced.

Cyclosporine is thought to cause hypertension by increasing the sensitivity of vascular smooth muscle cells to vasoconstrictors, such as angiotensin II, endothelin, and vasopressin.[74] Cyclosporine also increases the calcium response to vasoconstrictors.[75] Approximately 40% of patients treated with cyclosporine develop hypertension. Calcium channel blockers are the agents of choice in the treatment of cyclosporine-induced hypertension both because of the effects of cyclosporine on intracellular calcium and because cyclosporine dosage can be reduced by concomitant treatment with calcium channel blockers. Both cyclosporine and calcium channel blockers are metabolized by cytochrome P450. Studies in animals have suggested that cyclosporine-induced hypertension may be exacerbated by high dietary sodium intake,[76] and so appropriate dietary advice should be given as part of the treatment of affected patients.

Of the newer antirejection therapies, tacrolimus (FK-506) appears to cause a lower incidence of hypertension than cyclosporine.[77] In contrast, mycophenolate mofetil is believed not to be associated with hypertension.[78]

ADRENAL DISEASE

Primary Hyperaldosteronism

Approximately 30% of patients diagnosed as having primary aldosteronism have discrete adenomas of the adrenal zona glomerulosa (Conn's tumor). After tumor localization, most of these patients should undergo surgical removal of the lesion. Medical therapy is required during diagnosis and preoperatively to control hypertension and hypokalemia. Spironolactone, an agent useful for long-term management of primary aldosteronism, is contraindicated during the diagnostic process because it causes changes in the renin-aldosterone axis that are slow to reverse and can cause difficulty in interpretation of renin and aldosterone values. The same applies to β-blockers, which suppress plasma renin activity, and diuretics, ACE inhibitors, and angiotensin receptor antagonists, which increase it. The best drugs to use during the preoperative period are calcium antagonists, which may exert a specific effect on aldosterone release,[79] and amiloride, which prevents renal K$^+$ wasting.

For patients with Conn's syndrome in whom long-term pharmacotherapy rather than surgical ablation of the tumor is elected, the use of spironolactone is an important option. It is usually possible to control both hypertension and hypokalemia with a sufficient dose of this agent. Up to 400 mg/day or more may be required. However, in doses above 50 mg/day, spironolactone can cause menstrual disturbances in women and almost always causes troublesome breast tenderness and gynecomastia in men. Thus, therapy based on a well-tolerated dosage of a long-acting calcium antagonist to control hypertension together with either low-dose spironolactone or amiloride to control hypokalemia is recommended for these patients. Of the latter agents, spironolactone is preferred if an adjunctive antihypertensive effect is required.

For patients with primary aldosteronism without an identifiable discrete adenoma, familial glucocorticoid-suppressible hyperaldosteronism should be excluded. Medical treatment of the remaining cases, most of which are diagnosed by exclusion to have bilateral adrenocortical hyperplasia, is the same as that for Conn's syndrome.

Cushing's Syndrome

Medical treatment of the hypertension occurring in this condition is primarily that of the underlying endocrinopathy. Conventional antihypertensive agents can be used in addition. Care should be exercised in the case of diuretics not to precipitate hypokalemia or diabetes mellitus.

Pheochromocytoma

Pharmacotherapy for pheochromocytoma involves the use of combined α- and β-adrenoceptor blockade. Management initially requires α-adrenoceptor blocker therapy together with plasma volume replacement so that postural hypotension, which triggers catecholamine release, may be avoided. β-Blocker therapy is added if tachycardia develops. These measures help to prevent hypotension during subsequent surgery. However, intravenous vasodilator therapy combined with careful control of blood volume may still be required to prevent vasomotor collapse after removal of a catecholamine-secreting tumor.

PREGNANCY AND HORMONE REPLACEMENT THERAPY

Hypertension in Pregnancy

A number of double-blind placebo-controlled trials have demonstrated major benefit both to mother and to child by the early introduction of antihypertensive therapy.[80-84] Meta-analysis of these trials, in which the target diastolic blood pressure varied from less than 80 mm Hg to 90 mm Hg, showed a significant reduction in relative risk for severe hypertension requiring emergency delivery and for neonatal respiratory distress requiring ventilation.[85] Given these results, it is difficult to understand the reluctance in some centers to treat hypertension in pregnancy other than in the emergency situation. It is recommended that antihypertensive therapy be given at a diastolic blood pressure greater than 90 mmHg, even in the absence of proteinuria. The number of patients that are required to be treated in order to prevent one case of severe hypertension is 9, and the number requiring treatment to prevent one episode of neonatal respiratory distress is 13.[85]

First-line agents commonly used in the management of hypertension in pregnancy include β-blockers, combined α- and β-blockers, clonidine and, methyldopa. In keeping with the improved outcomes seen with carefully controlled blood pressure, a target diastolic blood pressure of less than 85 mm Hg is recommended, with therapy adjusted as necessary to maintain this level. Second-line agents include hydralazine and calcium antagonists, the latter restricted to the period after the 22nd week of gestation.[86] Patients require close monitoring of fetal growth as well as blood pressure. Because of the propensity of hypertension in pregnancy to become a multisystem disorder, other factors, such as urinary protein excretion, blood coagulation tests, and blood levels of creatinine, uric acid, hemoglobin, and platelets, also need to be monitored.

Recommendations for treatment regimens vary, but it is generally agreed that ACE inhibitors (and probably AT-1 receptor blockers) are probably best avoided throughout gestation. In the first and early second trimesters, some animal data suggest the possibility of teratogenicity.[87-90] In the late second and third trimesters, both experimental and human studies suggest that ACE inhibitors can cause acute renal failure in the fetus with consequent oligohydramnios, failure of pulmonary development, limb contractures, and eventual death.[91-93]

Hypertension and Hormone Replacement Therapy

Hypertension is not a contraindication to hormone replacement therapy (HRT). Prospective studies[94, 95] as well as double-blind placebo-controlled trials[96] have shown that HRT has no deleterious effect on blood pressure control. In contrast, data with combined oral contraceptive pills indicate a moderately increased risk of hypertension in current users.[97] Indeed, HRT appears to enhance the effects of antihypertensive drug therapy in some patients.[98] HRT may also improve the pulsatile afterload profile as determined by applanation tonometry of the carotid artery.[99] This potentially beneficial effect may not be detected by office sphygmomanometry[99] and may explain in part the improvement in cardiovascular morbidity ascribed to HRT.[100] The much lower dose of estrogen as well as the use of natural rather than synthetic estrogens may explain the difference in risk between HRT and the oral contraceptive pill. The route of administration of HRT appears to have no bearing on blood pressure, as both oral therapy and patches have been studied and found to have no effect on blood pressure.[95]

Thus, in patients with newly detected hypertension who are already receiving HRT, there is no need to discontinue this therapy. The benefits of antihypertensive therapy may summate with those of HRT to reduce the heightened incidence of myocardial infarction in postmenopausal women. The choice of antihypertensive agents in this group will be conditioned by the presence of comorbid conditions rather than by the concomitant HRT.

SPECIAL CONSIDERATIONS IN THE ELDERLY

The acceptance as normal of higher levels of blood pressure—particularly systolic blood pressure—in elderly than in younger subjects has been challenged by the results of treatment trials such as SHEP[101] and the Swedish Trial in Old Patients with Hypertension (STOP-Hypertension).[102] These trials have shown that, despite the risks associated with postural hypotension, appropriate blood pressure reduction in the elderly has beneficial effects overall. Stroke and other cardiovascular events are decreased.

The augmentation of systolic blood pressure seen in the elderly as a result of pulse-wave reflection is injurious to left ventricular function and to central blood vessels.[103] This augmentation is not a fixed abnormality caused by irreversible atherosclerotic changes in the major arteries, for it may be decreased with vasodilator therapy.[104] Further research is necessary to determine whether such therapy will prevent cardiovascular events.

Occasionally a rigid brachial artery may prevent occlusion by the sphygmomanometer cuff, giving rise to falsely high readings. This condition, called *pseudohypertension,* may be identified by palpation of the brachial or radial artery, which remains palpable during inflation of the sphygmomanometer cuff. Where necessary, a definitive diagnosis of pseudohypertension can be made by direct intraarterial measurement of blood pressure.

Atherosclerosis may also manifest in the elderly as a sudden rise in blood pressure due to renal artery stenosis. If the stenosis is bilateral, there may be a concurrent decrease in renal function, denoted by a rise in plasma creatinine concentration. These findings should sound a warning against the use of an ACE inhibitor or angiotensin

II receptor antagonist, which can accelerate the decline in renal function.

Decreased dietary salt intake, although often difficult to implement, may prove more effective in lowering blood pressure—especially systolic pressure—in the elderly than in younger patients, for salt sensitivity rises with age. This measure is preferable to diuretic use, which is prone to cause electrolyte disturbances in the elderly. However, if pharmacotherapy is required, it is recommended that a thiazide diuretic, with or without a β-blocker, should be used. This is based on the evidence that such treatment has been shown in numerous randomized controlled trials to reduce morbidity and mortality in elderly people with hypertension.[8]

References

1. Ramsay LE, Ramsay MH, Hettiarachchi J, et al. Weight reduction in a blood pressure clinic. BMJ 2:244–245, 1978.
2. Reisin E, Abel R, Modan M, et al. Effect of weight loss without salt restriction on the reduction of blood pressure in overweight hypertensive patients. N Engl J Med 298:1–6, 1978.
3. Weight reduction in hypertension. Lancet 1:1251–1252, 1985.
4. Fagard RH. The role of exercise in blood pressure control: Supportive evidence. J Hypertens 13:1223–1227, 1995.
5. Bretzel RG. Can we further slow down the progression to end-stage renal disease in diabetic hypertensive patients? J Hypertens 15(suppl 2):S83–S88, 1997.
6. U.S. Renal Data System. USRDS 1994 Annual Data Report. Incidence and causes of treated renal disease. Am J Kidney Dis 24(suppl 2):S48–S56, 1994.
7. Testa MA, Puklin JE, Sherwin RS, et al. Clinical predictors of retinopathy and its progression in patients with type I diabetes during CSII or conventional insulin treatment. Diabetes 34(suppl 3):61–68, 1985.
8. Joint National Committee on Prevention, Detection, Evaluation, and Treatment of High Blood Pressure. The Sixth Report. Arch Intern Med 157:2413–2446, 1997.
9. Hostetter TH, Troy JL, Brenner BM. Glomerular hemodynamics in experimental diabetes mellitus. Kidney Int 19:410–415, 1982.
10. Zatz R, Dunn BR, Meyer TW, et al. Prevention of diabetic glomerulopathy by pharmacological amelioration of glomerular capillary hypertension. J Clin Invest 77:1925–1930, 1986.
11. Morelli E, Loon N, Meyer TW, et al. Effects of converting-enzyme inhibition on barrier function in diabetic glomerulopathy. Diabetes 39:76–82, 1990.
12. Fugo A, Yoshida Y, Yared A, et al. Importance of angiogenic angiotensin II in the glomerular growth of maturing kidneys. Kidney Int 38:1068–1074, 1990.
13. Wolny A, Clozel JP, Rein J, et al. Functional and biochemical analysis of angiotensin II–forming pathways in the human heart. Circ Res 80:219–227, 1997.
14. Zanchi A, Brunner HR, Waeber B, et al. Renal haemodynamic and protective effects of calcium antagonists in hypertension. J Hypertens 13:1363–1375, 1995.
15. Bakris GL, Barnhill BW, Sadler R. Treatment of arterial hypertension in diabetic humans: Importance of therapeutic selection. Kidney Int 41:912–919, 1992.
16. Ferder L, Daccordi H, Martello M, et al. Angiotensin converting enzyme inhibitors versus calcium antagonists in the treatment of diabetic hypertensive patients. Hypertension 19:II237–II242, 1992.
17. Fogari R, Zoppi A, Pasotto C, et al. Comparative effects of ramipril and nitrendipine on albuminuria in hypertensive patients with non insulin dependent diabetes mellitus and impaired renal function. J Hum Hypertens 9:13–15, 1995.
18. Estacio RO, Jeffers B, Hiatt WR, et al. The effect of nisoldipine as compared with enalapril on cardiovascular outcomes in patients with non–insulin-dependent diabetes and hypertension. N Engl J Med 338:645–652, 1998.
19. Rodicio JL. Does antihypertensive therapy protect the kidney in essential hypertension? J Hypertens 14(suppl 2):S69–S76, 1996.
20. Giordano M, Sanders LR, Castellino P, et al. Effects of alpha-
adrenergic blockers, ACE inhibitors, and calcium channel antagonists on renal function in hypertensive non–insulin-dependent diabetic patients. Nephron 72:447–453, 1996.
21. Skyler JS, Marks JB, Schneiderman N: Hypertension in patients with diabetes mellitus. Am J Hypertens 8:100S–105S, 1995.
22. Teuscher AU, Weidmann PU. Requirements for antihypertensive therapy in diabetic patients: metabolic aspects. J Hypertens 15(suppl 2):S67–S75, 1997.
23. Baba T, Neugebauer S, Watanabe T. Diabetic nephropathy. Its relationship to hypertension and means of pharmacological intervention. Drugs 54:197–234, 1997.
24. Hansen HP, Rossing P, Tarnow L, et al. Circadian rhythm of arterial blood pressure and albuminuria in diabetic nephropathy. Kidney Int 50:579–585, 1996.
25. Barkai L, Peja M, Vamosi I. Physical work capacity in diabetic children and adolescents with and without cardiovascular autonomic function. Diabet Med 113:254–258, 1996.
26. Neaton JD, Grimm RH, Prineas RJ, et al. Treatment of Mild Hypertension Study. Final results. JAMA 270:713–724, 1993.
27. Yusuf S, Peto R, Lewis J, et al. Beta blockade during and after myocardial infarction: An overview of the randomized trials. Prog Cardiovasc Dis 27:335–371, 1985.
28. Weiss JW, Remsburg S, Garpestad E, et al. Hemodynamic consequences of obstructive sleep apnea. Sleep 19:388–397, 1996.
29. Woodmansey PA, O'Toole L, Channer KS, et al. Acute pulmonary vasodilatory properties of amlodipine in humans with pulmonary hypertension. Heart 75:171–173, 1996.
30. Haider AW, Chen L, Larson MG, et al. Antecedent hypertension confers increased risk for adverse outcomes after initial myocardial infarction. Hypertension 30:1020–1024, 1997.
31. Kannel WB, Sorlie P, Castelli WP, et al. Blood pressure and survival after myocardial infarction: The Framingham Study. Am J Cardiol 45:326–330, 1980.
32. Topol EJ, Traill TA, Fortuin NJ. Hypertensive hypertrophic cardiomyopathy of the elderly. N Engl J Med 312:277–283, 1985.
33. Westerhof N, O'Rourke MF. Haemodynamic basis for the development of left ventricular failure in systolic hypertension and for its logical therapy. J Hypertens 13:943–952, 1995.
34. SOLVD Investigators. Effect of enalapril on survival in patients with reduced left ventricular ejection fractions and congestive heart failure. N Engl J Med 325:293–302, 1991.
35. Kostis JB. The effect of enalapril on mortal and morbid events in patients with hypertension and left ventricular dysfunction. Am J Hypertens 8:909–914, 1995.
36. Pitt B, Segal R, Martinez FA, et al. Randomised trial of losartan versus captopril in patients over 65 with heart failure (Evaluation of Losartan in the Elderly Study, ELITE). Lancet 349:747–752, 1997.
37. Manolis AJ, Olympios C, Sifaki M, et al. Combined sympathetic suppression and angiotensin-converting enzyme inhibition in congestive heart failure. Hypertension 29:525–530, 1997.
38. Messerli FH, Michalewicz L. Effects of combination therapy on the heart. J Hum Hypertens 11:29–33, 1997.
39. Dilenarda A, Gregori D, Sinagra G, et al. Metoprolol in dilated cardiomyopathy: Is it possible to identify factors predictive of improvement? The Heart Muscle Disease Study Group. J Card Fail 2:87–102, 1996.
40. Spencer KT, Lang RM. What primary care physicians need to know. Postgrad Med 101:63–65, 1997.
41. Dunn CJ, Lea AP, Wagstaff AJ. Carvedilol. A reappraisal of its pharmacological properties and therapeutic use in cardiovascular disorders. Drugs 54:161–185, 1997.
42. Packer M, Bristow MR, Cohn JN, et al. The effect of carvedilol on morbidity and mortality in patients with chronic heart failure. U.S. Carvedilol Heart Failure Study Group. N Engl J Med 334:1349–1355, 1996.
43. Gilbert EM, Abraham WT, Olsen S, et al. Comparative hemodynamic, left ventricular functional, and antiadrenergic effects of chronic treatment with metoprolol versus carvedilol in the failing heart. Circulation 94:2817–2825, 1996.
44. Weber K, Bohmeke T, van der Does R, et al. Comparison of the hemodynamic effects of metoprolol and carvedilol in hypertensive patients. Cardiovasc Drugs Ther 10:113–117, 1996.
45. Levy D, Garrison RJ, Savage DD, et al. Prognostic implications of echocardiographically determined left ventricular mass in the Framingham Heart Study. N Engl J Med 322:1561–1566, 1990.

46. Furberg C, Psaty B, Meyer J. Nifedipine. Dose-related increase in mortality in patients with coronary heart disease. Circulation 92:1326–1331, 1995.

47. Report: Effects of calcium antagonists on the risks of coronary heart disease, cancer and bleeding. J Hypertension 15:105–115, 1997.

48. Yusuf S, Wittes J, Probstfield J. Evaluating effects of treatment in subgroups of patients within a clinical trial: The case of non–Q-wave infarction and beta blockers. Am J Cardiol 66:220–222, 1990.

49. Petruk KC, West M, Mohr G, et al. Nimodipine treatment in poor-grade aneurysm patients: Results of a multicenter double-blind placebo-controlled trial. J Neurosurg 68:505–507, 1988.

50. Veterans Administration Cooperative Study Group on Antihypertensive Agents. Effects of treatment on morbidity in hypertensive patients: Results in patients with diastolic blood pressure averaging 115 through 129 mm Hg. JAMA 202:1028–1034, 1967.

51. Lichtlen PR, Hugenholtz PG, Rafflenbeul W, et al. Retardation of angiographic progression of coronary artery disease by nifedipine. Lancet 335:1109–1113, 1990.

52. Weersuriya K, Patel L, Turner P. Beta-adrenoceptor blockade and migraine. Cephalgia 2:33–45, 1982.

53. Andersson KE, Ving E. Beta-adrenoceptor blockers and calcium channel antagonists in the prophylaxis and treatment of migraine. Drugs 39:355–373, 1990.

54. Wober C, Wober-Bingal C, Koch G, Wessely P. Long-term results of migraine prophylaxis with flunarizine and beta-blockers. Cephalgia 11:251–256, 1991.

55. Stensrud P, Sjaastad O: Clonidine (Cataprisan)—Double-blind study after long-term treatment with the drug in migraine. Acta Neurol Scand 53:233–236, 1976.

56. Solomon GD. Verapamil in migraine prophylaxis—A five-year review. Headache 29:425–427, 1989.

57. Marbley HG. Verapamil and migraine prophylaxis: Mechanisms and efficacy. Am J Med 90:485–535, 1991.

58. Taylor MD, McQueen KD. Verapamil as migraine prophylaxis. DICP 25:1076–1077, 1991.

59. Ablad B, Dahlof C. Migraine and beta-blockade: Modulation of sympathetic neurotransmission. Cephalgia 6:S7–S13, 1986.

60. Gomez-Garre D, Ruiz-Ortega M, Ortego M, et al. Effects and interactions of endothelin-I and angiotensin II on matrix protein expression and synthesis and mesangial cell growth. Hypertension 27:885–892, 1996.

61. Orth SR, Weinreich T, Bonisch S, et al. Angiotensin II induces hypertrophy and hyperplasia in adult human mesangial cells. Exp Nephrol 3:23–33, 1995.

62. Ruiz-Orteg M, Gonzalez S, Seron D, et al. ACE inhibition reduces proteinuria, glomerular lesions and extracellular matrix production in a normotensive rat model of immune complex nephritis. Kidney Int 48:1778–1791, 1995.

63. Madhun ZT, Ernsberger P, Ke FC, et al. Signal transduction mediated by angiotensin II receptor subtypes expressed in rat mesangial cells. Regul Pept 44:149–157, 1993.

64. Toto R, Schultz P, Raij L, et al. Efficacy and tolerability of losartan in hypertensive patients with renal impairment. Hypertension 31:684–691, 1998.

65. Sheil AGR, May J, Stokes GS, et al. Reversal of renal failure by revascularisation of kidneys with thrombosed renal arteries. Lancet 2:865–866, 1970.

66. Greco BA, Breyer JA. Atherosclerotic ischemic renal disease. Am J Kidney Dis 29:167–187, 1997.

67. Preston RA, Epstein M. Ischemic renal disease: An emerging cause of chronic renal failure and end-stage renal disease. J Hypertens 15:1365–1377, 1997.

68. Hunsieber LG, Adler S, Caggiula A, et al. Predictors of the progression of renal disease in the Modification of Diet in Renal Disease Study. Kidney Int 51:1908–1919, 1997.

69. Herbert LA, Kusek JW, Greene T, et al. Effects of blood pressure control on progressive renal disease in blacks and whites. Modification of Diet in Renal Disease Study Group. Hypertension 30:428–435, 1997.

70. Lifton RP. Molecular genetics of human blood pressure variation. Science 272:676–680, 1996.

71. Arnold JE, Healy JK. Hyperkalemia, hypertension and systemic acidosis without renal failure associated with a tubular defect in potassium excretion. Am J Med 47:461–472, 1969.

72. Salem MM, Bower J. Hypertension in the hemodialysis population:

73. Oldenburg B, Macdonald GJ, Shelley S. Controlled trial of enalapril in patients with chronic fluid overload undergoing dialysis. BMJ 296:1089–1091, 1988.

Any relation to one-year survival? Am J Kidney Dis 28:737–740, 1996.

74. Lo Russo A, Passaquin AC, Ruegg UT. Mechanisms of enhanced vasoconstrictor hormone action in vascular smooth muscle cells by cyclosporin A. Br J Pharmacol 121:240–252, 1997.

75. Lo Russo A, Passaquin AC, Ruegg U. Cyclosporin A potentiates receptor-activated [Ca²⁺] increase. J Recept Signal Transduct Res 17:149–161, 1997.

76. Mervaala EM, Pere AK, Lindgrin L, et al. Effects of dietary sodium and magnesium on cyclosporin A–induced hypertension and nephrotoxicity in spontaneous hypertensive rats. Hypertension 29:822–827, 1997.

77. Williams R, Neuhaus P, Bismuth H, et al. Two-year data from the European multicentre tacrolimus (FK506) liver study. Transplant Int 9(suppl 1):S144–S150, 1996.

78. Simmons WD, Rayhill SC, Sellinger HW. Preliminary risk-benefit assessment of mycophenolate mofetil in transplant rejection. Drug Saf 17:75–92, 1997.

79. Stimpel M, Ivens K, Wambach G, et al. Are calcium antagonists helpful in the management of primary aldosteronism? J Cardiovasc Pharmacol 12(suppl 6):S131–S134, 1988.

80. Hogstedt S, Lindeberg S, Axelson O, et al. A prospective controlled trial of metoprolol-hydralazine treatment in hypertension during pregnancy. Acta Obstet Gynecol Scand 64:505–510, 1985.

81. Pickles CJ, Symonds EM, Pipkin FB. The fetal outcome in a randomised double-blind controlled trial of labetalol versus placebo in pregnancy-induced hypertension. Br J Obstet Gynaecol 96:38–43, 1989.

82. Sibai BM, Gonzalez AR, Mabie WC, et al. A comparison of labetalol plus hospitalisation versus hospitalisation alone in the management of pre-eclampsia remote from term. Obstet Gynecol 70:323–327, 1987.

83. Plouin PF, Breast G, Llado J, et al. A randomised comparison of early with conservative use of antihypertensive drugs in the management of pregnancy-induced hypertension. Br J Obstet Gynecol 97:134–141, 1990.

84. Phippard AF, Fischer WE, Horvath JS, et al. Early blood pressure control improves pregnancy outcome in primigravid women with mild hypertension. Med J Aust 154:378–382, 1991.

85. Duggan KD. Personal communication, 1993.

86. Danielsson BR, Danielson M, Reiland S, et al. Histological and in vitro studies supporting decreased uteroplacental blood flow as explanation for digital defects after administration of vasodilators. Teratology 41:185–193, 1990.

87. Pryde PG, Sedman AB, Nugent CE, Barr M. Angiotensin-converting enzyme inhibitor fetopathy. J Am Soc Nephrol 3:1575–1582, 1993.

88. Kumar D, Moss G, Primhak R, Coombs D. Congenital renal tubular dysplasia and skull ossification defects similar to teratogenic effects of angiotensin converting enzyme (ACE) inhibitors. J Med Genet 34:541–545, 1997.

89. al-Shabanah OA, al-Harbi MM, al-Gharably NM, Islam MW: The effect of maternal administration of captopril on fetal development in the rat. Res Commun Chem Pathol Pharmacol 73:221–230, 1991.

90. Valdes G, Marinovic D, Falcon C, et al. Placental alterations, intrauterine growth retardation and teratogenicity associated with enalapril use in pregnant rats. Biol Neonate 61:124–130, 1992.

91. Mastrobattista JM. Angiotensin converting enzyme inhibitors in pregnancy. Semin Perinatol 21:124–134, 1997.

92. Lavoratti G, Serocini D, Fiorini P, et al. Neonatal anuria by ACE inhibitors during pregnancy. Nephron 76:235–236, 1997.

93. Alderma CP. Adverse effects of the angiotensin-converting enzyme inhibitors. Ann Pharmacother 30:55–61, 1996.

94. Lind T, Cameron EC, Hunter WM, et al. A prospective, controlled trial of six forms of hormone replacement therapy given to post-menopausal women. Br J Obstet Gynaecol 86(suppl 3):1–30, 1979.

95. Lip GY, Beevers M, Churchill D, et al. Hormone replacement therapy and blood pressure in hypertensive women. J Hum Hypertens 8:491–494, 1994.

96. Kornhauser C, Malacara JM, Garay ME, et al. The effect of hormone replacement therapy on blood pressure and cardiovascular risk factors in menopausal women with moderate hypertension. J Hum Hypertens 11:405–411, 1997.

97. Chasan-Taber L, Willett WC, Manson JE, et al. Prospective study of oral contraceptives and hypertension among women in the United States. Circulation 94:483–489, 1996.

98. Amoroso A, Garzia P, Ferri GM, et al. Hypertension and menopausal syndrome: Effects of hormone replacement therapy and antihypertensive drugs. Riv Eur Sci Med Farmacol 18:149–152, 1996.

99. Hayward SH, Knight DC, Wren BG, et al. Effect of hormone replacement therapy on noninvasive cardiovascular haemodynamics. J Hypertens 15:987–993, 1997.

100. Stampfer MJ, Colditz GA, Willett WA, et al. Postmenopausal estrogen therapy and cardiovascular disease. Ten year follow-up from the Nurses' Health Study. N Engl J Med 325:756–762, 1991.

101. SHEP Co-Operative Research Group: Prevention of stroke in older persons with isolated systolic hypertension: Final results of the Systolic Hypertension in the Elderly Program (SHEP). JAMA 256:3255–3264, 1991.

102. Dahlof B, Lindholm LH, Hansson L, et al. Morbidity and mortality in the Swedish Trial in Old Patients with Hypertension (STOP-Hypertension). Lancet 338:1281–1285, 1991.

103. Westerhof N, O'Rourke MF. Haemodynamic basis for the development of left ventricular failure in systolic hypertension and for its logical therapy. J Hypertens 13:943–952, 1995.

104. Stokes GS, Ryan M. Can extended-release isosorbide mononitrate be used as adjunctive therapy for systolic hypertension? An open study employing pulse-wave analysis to determine effects of antihypertensive therapy. Am J Geriatr Cardiol 6:11–19, 1997.

CHAPTER 56

Diabetes and Syndrome X: Focus on Reduction of Cardiovascular and Renal Events

Imelda P. Villarosa and George L. Bakris

The incidence and prevalence of diabetes have been steadily increasing in the United States since 1980. Approximately 16 million people have diabetes, but only 63% are diagnosed.[1] These numbers are expected to increase with the recent change in diagnostic criteria for diabetes, i.e., fasting glucose 126 mg/dl or higher.[1, 2] Certain racial and ethnic groups tend to have a higher incidence of type 2 diabetes, i.e., African Americans, Hispanic/Latin Americans, and Native Americans.[1, 3] These groups also have the highest incidence of renal failure secondary to diabetes.

One hundred percent of individuals with diabetes who progress to end-stage renal disease (ESRD) have hypertension.[3] A large proportion of such patients also have hyperlipidemia and hyperuricemia, components of syndrome X.[1, 3] However, not all subjects with insulin resistance have the associated components of syndrome X. Studies in normotensive offspring of hypertensive nondiabetic parents demonstrate the presence of insulin resistance.[4] This is also true for nondiabetic first-degree relatives of patients with type 2 diabetes.[5] Thus, a genetic predisposition is needed to develop this associated syndrome.

One reason for the high prevalence of diabetic renal disease may relate to control of blood pressure. Although the awareness of high blood pressure has increased slightly over the last few years, the percentage of patients whose blood pressure is controlled to 140/90 mm Hg or less has remained unchanged (Fig. 56–1).[6] Moreover, the recent sixth report of the Joint National Committee on Prevention, Detection, Evaluation, and Treatment of High Blood Pressure (JNC VI) has recommended that patients with diabetes and hypertension should have their blood pressure lowered to less than 130/85 mm Hg in order to slow renal disease progression.[7] Thus, the inability to adequately lower arterial pressure may have resulted in more people living longer but with a substantially greater morbidity.[6, 7]

This chapter focuses on various aspects of type 2 diabe-

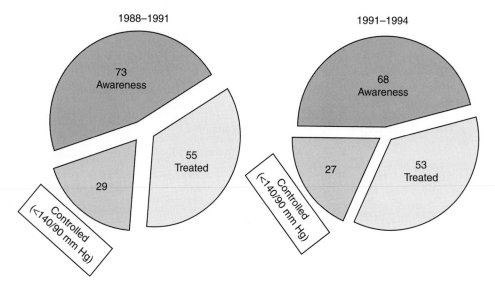

1988–1991

73 Awareness

55 Treated

29

Controlled (<140/90 mm Hg)

1991–1994

68 Awareness

53 Treated

27

Controlled (<140/90 mm Hg)

Figure 56–1. The percentage of the hypertensive population surveyed by the third National Health and Nutrition Examination Survey (NHANES III) over two distinct periods of time who were aware, treated, and controlled. *Note:* There was no improvement or deterioration in the number controlled or treated. (Data from Tarif N, Bakris GL. Pharmacologic treatment of essential hypertension. *In* Johnson R, Freehally J [eds]. Principles of Nephrology. London, CV Mosby, 1999.)

tes, which accounts for 90 to 95% of all diagnosed cases. Type 2 diabetes is most commonly seen among obese individuals and results from an inability to utilize glucose in the periphery, i.e., insulin resistance.[2] Death most commonly occurs in such patients from cardiovascular causes before the development of renal disease.[3] Although it is clear that reductions in blood pressure, lipids, and glucose are the keys to preserving the integrity of the vasculature and target organs, we concentrate on the consequences of inadequate blood pressure reduction.

FACTORS PREDISPOSING TO VASCULAR DISEASE IN DIABETICS

Hyperinsulinemia and hyperglycemia "set a fire," by creating a milieu in which activation of cytokines, matrix proteins, and other related factors accelerates cellular injury. Blood pressure elevation (>130/85 mm Hg) is like "adding gasoline to the fire." The increased shear stress on the vessels and target organs stimulates processes similar to the effects of hyperinsulinemia.[8-10] Thus, there is a synergy of adverse events that ultimately leads to vascular and target organ injury.

Some key factors that contribute to the pathogenesis of vascular disease in diabetes are summarized in Table 56–1. Most of these factors make up syndrome X. An in-depth discussion of these factors and their contributions to the pathogenesis of vascular disease is beyond the scope of this chapter. The reader is referred to reviews on the topic.[8-10] We focus on elevated blood pressure and hyperglycemia/hyperinsulinemia.

Elevated Arterial Pressure

A number of factors, including insulin resistance and hyperinsulinemia, contribute to the pathogenesis of hypertension in diabetes mellitus. Hyperinsulinemia causes sodium

retention and other vascular effects such as cellular proliferation and matrix expansion.[10] In the presence of hyperinsulinemia, neurohumoral factors such as angiotensin II, endothelin, and vasopressin potentiate proliferation of cells and matrix.[8-10] These factors can potentiate injury to the vasculature and target organs in a person genetically predisposed to develop nephropathy.[10-12]

Genes that have been implicated in predisposing diabetic patients to nephropathy include the angiotensinogen gene (hypertension); glycogen synthetase gene, associated with insulin resistance; DQB1 haplotype, which may increase the risk of hypertension in type 1 diabetes; and the DRV1 haplotype, which may protect against type 1 diabetes in hypertensive subjects.[10-13] Studies in African Americans with type 2 diabetes show an eightfold increase in the risk of developing ESRD if their first-degree relatives had ESRD.[11] These studies further demonstrate a familial aggregation of ESRD with an independence from glycemic control. This familial predisposition or "clustering" also applies to albuminuria development in white patients with type 2 diabetes.[14] Angiotensin-converting enzyme (ACE) genotypes may also contribute to development of diabetic nephropathy.[12] Studies comparing type 1 patients with and without nephropathy show a higher prevalence of D allele frequency in the subgroup with nephropathy. Moreover, the Génétique de la Néphropathie Diabétique (GENEDIAB) trial involving type 1 diabetic subjects concluded that the relative risk of developing diabetic nephropathy was 42% higher in the presence of an ACE D allele.[12] Interestingly, among type 2 diabetics, ACE genotypes are much stronger predictors of cardiovascular disease than of nephropathy progression.[15]

Regardless of genetic predisposition, aggressive reduction of arterial pressure with either an ACE inhibitor or an angiotensin II receptor antagonist clearly prevents development of the morphological and surrogate markers of diabetic nephropathy, i.e., mesangial matrix expansion and microalbuminuria.[16] A detailed discussion of the pathogenesis of hypertension in diabetes is beyond the scope of this chapter but is presented elsewhere.[10]

Hyperglycemia/Hyperinsulinemia

Table 56–2 summarizes the pharmacological effects of diabetes on the kidney. Mesangial matrix expansion is the earliest histopathological hallmark of diabetic nephropathy.[16] These alterations usually occur after 5 to 15 years of type 1 diabetes and within 3 to 5 years of type 2 diabetes.[17] Changes in intrarenal hemodynamics in diabetic patients include a loss of intrarenal autoregulation; increased efferent arteriolar tone secondary to angiotensin II and possibly vasopressin; and increases in afferent arteriolar tone secondary to hyperglycemia and hyperinsulinemia. Together, these increase intraglomerular capillary pressure.[18, 19] Additionally, vascular reactivity to catecholamines and angiotensin II is increased. Normally, the glomerular capillary wall is an efficient barrier to the passage of proteins, including albumin. However, the increases in capillary pressure and membrane permeability secondary to hyperglycemia impair this function and microalbuminuria ensues. Aggressive control of blood sugar reduces this

Table 56–1 Factors Involved in the Development of Vascular Disease in Diabetes

Factors	Cellular/Vascular Effects
Hyperglycemia	Increased permeability to molecules, apoptosis, AGE products; increased cytokine and matrix protein production by cells; intrarenal vasodilatation; loss of autoregulation
Hyperinsulinemia	Sodium retention; increased activity of AII, ET-1, and other vasoactive peptides; decreased activity of natriuretic hormones; increased sympathetic tone
Elevated pressure	Increased intraglomerular pressure; increased shear stress on vessels
Dyslipoproteinemia	Increased free radical production; increased collagen production and matrix; decreased factor Xa and thrombin,* increased PAI-1*

Abbreviations: AGE, advanced glycosylation end-products; AII, angiotensin II; ET-1, endothelin-1; PAI-1, plasminogen-activating factor inhibitor.
*Both insulin and glucose contribute to these processes.

Table 56–2 Pharmacological Effects of Different Classes of Antihypertensive Agents on Surrogate Markers of Cardiovascular Disease*

	Central Agonists	α-Blockers	α, β-Blockers	Vasodilators	β-Blockers	ACEIs	ARBs	CAs	Diuretics
METABOLIC									
Cholesterol									
LDL	→	→	→	→	→†↑	→	→	→	→↑
HDL	→	↑	→	→	→↓	→	→	→	→
Insulin resistance	→	↓	→↑	→↑	→↑	→↓	→↓	→	→↑
Glucose control	→	→	→	→	→↓	→↑	→	‡↓→	→↓
CARDIOVASCULAR									
Left ventricular hypertrophy	↓	↓	↓	→↑	↓	↓	↓	↓	→↓
RENAL									
Microalbuminuria	→	→	→↓	→↑	→↓	↓↓	↓↓	§↓→	→↓

Adapted from Tarif N, Bakris GL. Pharmacologic treatment of essential hypertension. *In* Johnson R, Freehally J (eds). Principles of Nephrology. London, CV Mosby, 1999.
Abbreviations: ACEIs, angiotensin-converting enzyme inhibitors; ARBs, angiotensin II receptor antagonists; CAs, calcium antagonists; LDL, low-density lipoprotein; HDL, high-density lipoprotein; →, no effect; ↑, increase; ↓, decrease.
*Note: This table summarizes the general trends in the literature.
†Only β-blockers with intrinsic sympathomimetic activity.
‡Only when used in high doses (e.g., 480 mg/day diltiazem, 480 mg/day verapamil, 90 mg/day nifedipine).
§Only nondihydropyridine CAs (verapamil, diltiazem).

increase in membrane permeability, in part, through reducing advanced glycosylation endproducts and, hence, preserving glomerular membrane charge selectivity.

Table 56–2 summarizes the effects of various antihypertensive drug classes on cardiovascular, renal, and metabolic factors associated with syndrome X.

Glycated Albumin

Albuminuria is an important contributor to the progression of diabetic renal disease because diabetic patients have high circulating levels of glycated albumin secondary to their high blood sugars. Albuminuria itself has been postulated to increase progression of renal disease independent of elevated arterial pressure.[20, 21] This is predominantly true in diabetics in whom albumin is glycated and shown to be directly toxic to cells.[20–22] If one subscribes to the hypothesis that the level of albuminuria contributes directly to the progression of diabetic nephropathy, then both microalbuminuria and albuminuria should have independent predictive value for progression to renal mortality.[22, 23]

Microalbuminuria is the amount of albumin in the urine above the normal value of 30 mg/day or lower and below the detectable limit by urine dipstick of 300 mg/day.[22] Based on epidemiological studies, microalbuminuria has a prevalence between 12 and 16% among patients with essential hypertension and 10 and 28% among patients with diabetes who are normotensive.[15, 22, 23] Microalbuminuria may be a marker of both insulin resistance and hypertension rather than a direct pathogen in nondiabetic subjects.[22] Hypertensive nondiabetic patients with microalbuminuria show a marked hyperinsulinemic response to an oral glucose load over their normoalbuminuric counterparts.[24] This decrease in insulin-induced glucose uptake is also seen in type 2 diabetics with hypertension or microalbuminuria, or both. Moreover, a 6-year follow-up study showed that diabetics with insulin resistance had a higher incidence of hypertension and microalbuminuria than diabetics with normal insulin sensitivity.[25] Thus, insulin resistance, at least

of the extrahepatic tissues, might precede the development of both microalbuminuria and hypertension.

Cross-sectional studies demonstrate that nondiabetic subjects with microalbuminuria have increased levels of insulin, triglycerides, and blood pressure with lower high-density lipoprotein cholesterols, compared with patients without microalbuminuria.[26] This and other studies confirm the observation that microalbuminuria may be a marker of the prediabetic state. Moreover, in type 2 diabetes, a recent meta-analysis demonstrated an overall odds ratio of 1.8 for cardiovascular morbidity and mortality and 2.5 for total mortality.[15] Thus, microalbuminuria in association with the insulin resistance syndrome clearly indicates an increased risk of cardiovascular morbidity and mortality.[15, 27]

Studies have also implicated microalbuminuria at baseline as an independent predictor of both cardiovascular and all-cause mortality in type 1 diabetics.[28] In this 10-year observational follow-up study involving 939 type 1 diabetic adults, other predictors of cardiovascular mortality that were observed included age, smoking, overt nephropathy, and hypertension.

TREATMENT OF HYPERTENSION IN DIABETES

Goals of Therapy

The goal of treatment for any disease process associated with diabetes mellitus is reduction in the incidence of long-term complications as well as mortality. It is fortunate that by reducing arterial pressure in diabetes, both cardiovascular and renal disease progression are reduced.[6, 13, 29] JNC VI recommends a goal blood pressure of below 130/85 mm Hg for hypertensive diabetics in order to slow progression of nephropathy maximally.[7] This is based on both prospective studies and post hoc analyses of clinical trials

Table 56–3 Groups That Require Blood Pressure Reduction to < 130/85 mm Hg to Optimally Protect Against Renal Disease Progression

Patient Group	Desired Blood Pressure	Data Supporting Specific Agents in "Antihypertensive Cocktail"*
African Americans	<130/85 mm Hg	?Verapamil/ACE inhibitors
Diabetics	<130/85 mm Hg	ACE inhibitors or ?AT₁ receptor antagonists†
Renal insufficiency (>1.4 mg/dl) + proteinuria (>1 g/day)	<130/85 mm Hg	ACE inhibitors

Adapted from Tarif N, Bakris GL. Pharmacologic treatment of essential hypertension. *In* Johnson R, Freehally J (eds). Principles of Nephrology. London, CV Mosby Summer, 1999.
Abbreviations: ACE, angiotensin-converting enzyme; AT₁, angiotensin 1.
Antihypertensive cocktail refers to the concept that more than one antihypertensive agent must be used to control blood pressure to the prescribed levels. Moreover, the agents selected should have complementary effects on mechanisms that reduce pressure.
†It is not yet proved whether AT₁ receptor antagonists are as efficacious as ACE inhibitors in slowing diabetic nephropathy progression.
?Very little data are available regarding the effects of specific agents on renal protection in diabetic African Americans. The data that do exist support verapamil and ACE inhibitors, but data from ongoing trials will definitively answer the question.

Table 56–4 Summary of Effects on Cardiovascular and Renal Events/Outcomes/Mortality by Different Classes of Antihypertensive Agents Among Those Patients With Diabetic Renal Disease*

Antihypertensive Agent	Cardiovascular	Renal
α-Blockers	→	→†
β-Blockers	⇓	⇓‡
Diuretics	⇓	⇓
ACE inhibitors	⇓	⇓
Angiotensin receptor blockers	↓ ?	?
Calcium channel blockers		
Non-DHP	⇓	⇓
DHP	→ ↑ ?[48, 49]	→
KCOs (hydralazine/minoxidil)	→	→

Abbreviations: ACE, angiotensin-converting enzymes; DHP, dihydropyridine; KCOs, potassium channel openers; GFR, glomerular filtration rate; ?, only short-acting calcium channel blockers increase cardiovascular mortality.
*Positive effects are indicated by double arrows.
†Based on only one randomized trial with 2-year follow-up looking at rate of decline in GFR.
‡Although β-blockers clearly slow progression of nephropathy, the degree of slowing is not as significant as either ACE inhibitors on non-DHP calcium channel blockers at blood pressure levels between 135 and 140/84 and 88 mm Hg.

that either randomized or stratified the group studied to different levels of blood pressure control (Table 56–3). These analyses also show that at this lower blood pressure value, safety was not compromised, i.e., there were no differences in stop points, hospitalizations, or deaths compared with the usual blood pressure group, those at a mean arterial pressure between 102 and 106 mm Hg.[30]

Pharmacological Therapy

All clinical trials to date have controlled blood pressure to levels of approximately 140/90 mm Hg. Using data from these trials, one could ask, are there agents with specific effects on reducing progression of renal disease independent of blood pressure level? A meta-analysis of all clinical trials in diabetic nephropathy to date suggests that ACE inhibitors clearly provide this benefit.[31] This is further echoed by the recommendations of JNC VI.[7] Table 56–4 lists the effects of different classes of agents on renal and cardiovascular outcomes.

Randomized, controlled trials in type 1 diabetics with nephropathy have shown that ACE inhibitors significantly reduce the rate of serum creatinine doubling compared with patients whose blood pressure was controlled without an ACE inhibitor.[30] ACE inhibitors also slow progression of nephropathy in microalbuminuric, normotensive type 2 diabetics. Ravid and colleagues[31] in a randomized, double-blind, placebo-controlled trial showed significant stabilization of both albuminuria and serum creatinine in the ACE inhibitor–treated group.[32] In fact, ACE inhibition offered an absolute risk reduction of 42% for the development of macroalbuminuria and nephropathy over a 7-year period. Reductions in baseline elevated glomerular filtration rates

and renal size with ACE inhibition have also been demonstrated in normotensive diuresis.[33] The mechanisms by which ACE inhibitors preserve the kidney are multiple, including a reduction in membrane permeability to glycated albumin, a marked reduction in mesangial matrix expansion, and lastly, a reduction in intraglomerular pressure.[16, 20, 22]

During initial therapy with an ACE inhibitor, monitoring kidney function is appropriate. Patients with bilateral renal artery stenosis may experience an acceleration of renal insufficiency. However, the most common cause of an elevated creatinine after initiation of an ACE inhibitor is intravascular volume depletion. Hyperkalemia may also ensue in patients with more advanced renal dysfunction (Cr ≥ 3.5 mg/dl) as well as in patients with type IV renal tubular acidosis (hyporeninemic hypoaldosteronism).

The effects of calcium antagonists (CAs) on renal function and structure are shown in Table 56–5. From the

Table 56–5 Effects of Calcium Antagonists on Outcomes in Renal Function and Morphology in Diabetes

	Short-Acting		Long-Acting	
	DHP	Non-DHP	DHP	Non-DHP
HEMODYNAMICS				
Autoregulation	↓	→	↓	→
Sympathetic tone	↑ ↑	→	→ ↑	↓
Albuminuria	→	↓	→	↓
MORPHOLOGY				
Glomerular scarring	→	↓	→	↓
Mesangial expansion	→	↓	→	↓

Abbreviation: DHP, dihydropyridine; ↓, decrease; →, no effect; ↑, increase; ↑ ↑, marked increase.

available data, it is apparent that dihydropyridine calcium antagonists (DHPCAs) neither slow progression of nephropathy nor reduce cardiovascular events in patients with hypertension and established nephropathy.[19, 31] Conversely, the nondihydropyridine calcium antagonists (NDHPCAs) verapamil and diltiazem significantly attenuate increases in proteinuria and confer better overall preservation of renal function, similar to ACE inhibitors, in these patients.[34–36] The reasons for differences between these two subgroups of CAs are reviewed elsewhere.[19]

The use of *low-dose* thiazide diuretics (≤25 mg hydrochlorothiazide) is appropriate in diabetics with hypertension, since these agents have been shown to reduce cardiovascular events and renal disease progression.[37, 38] At these doses, adverse effects on lipids and carbohydrate metabolism, as well as electrolyte disturbances such as hypokalemia and hypomagnesemia, are uncommon.[6] Diuretics are efficacious antihypertensive agents in diabetics, since these patients are generally volume-expanded and "salt-sensitive."[39] Additionally, diuretics are vasodilators and increase activity of the renin-angiotensin system. Thus, adding diuretics to ACE inhibitors can potentiate blood pressure reduction in this population. This type of combination therapy is key to potentiating the antihypertensive effect of a single drug and maintaining compliance.

β-Blockers also effectively reduce cardiovascular events in diabetics. However, they are associated with adverse effects on glucose and lipid levels, hypoglycemia unawareness, and vasospasm that may compromise peripheral blood flow. Thus, β-blockers should be used in diabetic patients only when angina is present or after myocardial infarction.[6] β-Blockers significantly slow the progression of diabetic nephropathy, albeit to a lesser degree than ACE inhibitors or NDHPCAs.[31] African Americans with diabetic nephropathy treated with NDHPCAs had a 62% slower decline in renal function compared with the atenolol-treated group at 5 years.[40]

According to JNC VI, α_1-blockers may also be used as antihypertensive therapy for diabetics.[7] These agents improve both lipid profiles and glucose utilization.[6, 39] Unfortunately, α_1-blockers do not consistently reduce proteinuria or preserve renal morphology in spite of blood pressure control in diabetic patients.[41, 42] These agents are relatively contraindicated in patients with autonomic neuropathy.

Angiotensin receptor blockers (ARBs) are the newest class of antihypertensive agents. Their blood pressure–lowering efficacy is similar to that of ACE inhibitors. These agents specifically block the angiotensin-1 (AT_1) receptor that is responsible for most of the effects of angiotensin II.[43] ARBs have a much better side effect profile than ACE inhibitors, with an incidence of cough similar to that of placebo. Initial studies with ARBs in small numbers of hypertensive type 2 diabetics demonstrated no adverse effects on glucose and lipid profiles.

In conclusion, we need to be much more aggressive in reducing arterial pressure in individuals with either type 1 or type 2 diabetes in order to preserve renal function. This cannot generally be done with one drug alone. Thus, to reduce arterial pressure to the newly prescribed goals, i.e., 130/85 mm Hg or lower, by the least obtrusive means possible, one should consider the use of fixed-dose combination therapy of an ACE inhibitor/diuretic or an ACE

inhibitor/CA. Recent evidence from small clinical studies supports the following observations about fixed-dose combination therapy in diabetes: First, an ACE inhibitor/NDHPCA combination reduced insulin resistance and had additive effects on reducing albuminuria.[44, 45] Moreover, the use of an ACE inhibitor/DHPCA combination yielded the same effects on proteinuria as an ACE inhibitor alone.[45] Hence, use of an ACE inhibitor with a DHPCA in patients with type 2 diabetes, hypertension, and nephropathy provides some protection against the lack of effect on proteinuria seen with a DHPCA alone.[46, 47] This relative lack of protection by a DHPCA has also been observed with regard to cardiovascular events in hypertensive type 2 diabetic patients with nephropathy.[48] This finding could not be explained by differences in blood pressure control between the two groups. Hence, use of combination therapy, i.e., ACE inhibitor/DHPCA, increases the likelihood of achieving blood pressure control with a lower side effect profile and better compliance.[44, 46] This approach should reduce cardiovascular and renal events when compared with dihydropyridine alone in diabetic patients with renal insufficiency.[47, 49] Moreover, both classes of agents either improve or have neutral effects on the components of syndrome X.

It is the job of every health care provider to make sure that adequate blood pressure control is achieved within the newly recommended guidelines of JNC VI. In this way, we can reduce both mortality and the tremendous human and economic cost of morbidity associated with cardiovascular and renal disease in diabetic patients.

References

1. American Diabetes Association. National Diabetes Fact Sheet, December 1997. www.diabetes.org/ada/c20f.html
2. Expert Committee on the Diagnosis and Classification of Diabetes Mellitus. Report of the Expert Committee on the Diagnosis and Classification of Diabetes Mellitus. Diabetes Care 20:S5–S19, 1997.
3. Sowers JR, Epstein M. Diabetes mellitus and associated hypertension, vascular disease and nephropathy: An update. Hypertension 26:869–879, 1995.
4. Andersen UB, Dige-Petersen H, Frandsen EK, et al. Basal insulin-level oscillations in normotensive individuals with genetic predisposition to essential hypertension exhibit an irregular pattern. J Hypertens 15:1167–1173, 1997.
5. Forsblom CM, Eriksson JG, Ekstrand AV, et al. Insulin resistance and abnormal albumin excretion in non-diabetic first-degree relatives of patients with NIDDM. Diabetologia 38:363–369, 1995.
6. Tarif N, Bakris GL. Pharmacologic treatment of essential hypertension. *In* Johnson R, Freehally J (eds). Principles of Nephrology London, CV Mosby, 1999.
7. Joint National Committee on Prevention, Diagnosis, Evaluation, and Treatment of High Blood Pressure. Sixth report. Arch Intern Med 157:2413–2446, 1997.
8. Stehouwer CDA, Lambert J, Donker AJM, Van Hinsbergh VWM. Endothelial dysfunction and pathogenesis of diabetic angiopathy. Cardiovasc Res 34:55–68, 1997.
9. Bakris GL, Walsh MF, Sowers JR. Endothelium/mesangium interactions: Role of insulin-like growth factors. Sowers JR (ed). Endocrinology of the Vasculature Totowa, NJ, Humana, 1996; pp 341–356.
10. Bakris GL. Pathogenesis of hypertension in diabetes. Diabetes Rev 3:460–476, 1995.
11. Freedman BI, Tuttle AB, Spray BJ. Familial predisposition to nephropathy in African-Americans with non-insulin–dependent diabetes mellitus. Am J Kidney Dis 25:710–713, 1996.
12. Marre M, Jeunemaitre X, Gallois Y, et al. Contributions of genetic polymorphism in the renin-angiotensin system to the development of renal complications in insulin-dependent diabetes. J Clin Invest 99:1585–1595, 1997.

13. Bakris GL, Mehler P, Schrier R. Hypertension and diabetes. *In* Schrier RW, Gottschalk CW (eds). Diseases of the Kidney, 6th ed. Boston, Little, Brown, 1996; pp 1455–1464.
14. Faronato PP, Maioili M, Tonolo G, et al, on behalf of the Italian NIDDM Nephropathy Study Group. Clustering of albumin excretion rates abnormalities in Caucasian patients with NIDDM. Diabetologia 40:816–823, 1997.
15. Dinneen SF, Gerstein HC. The association of microalbuminuria and mortality in non-insulin–dependent diabetes mellitus: A systematic overview of the literature. Arch Intern Med 157:1413–1418, 1997.
16. Gaber L, Walton C, Brown S, Bakris GL. Effects of different antihypertensive treatments on morphologic progression of diabetic nephropathy in uninephrectomized dogs. Kidney Int 46:161–169, 1994.
17. Nelson RG, Meyer TW, Myers BD, Bennett PH. Clinical and pathological course of renal disease in non-insulin–dependent diabetes mellitus: The Pima Indian experience. Semin Nephrol 17:124–131, 1997.
18. Perna A, Remuzzi G. Abnormal permeability to proteins and glomerular lesions: A meta-analysis of experimental and human studies. Am J Kidney Dis 27:34–41, 1996.
19. Tarif N, Bakris GL. Preservation of renal function: The spectrum of effects by calcium-channel blockers. Nephrol Dial Transplant 12:2244–2250, 1997.
20. Cohen MP, Sharma K, Jin Y, et al. Prevention of diabetic nephropathy in db/db mice with glycated albumin antagonists. A novel treatment strategy. J Clin Invest 95:2338–2345, 1995.
21. Vlassara H. Recent progress on the biologic and clinical significance of advanced glycosylation end products. J Lab Clin Med 124:19–30, 1994.
22. Bakris GL. Microalbuminuria: Prognostic implications. Curr Opin Nephrol Hypertens 5:219–223, 1996.
23. Parving HH. Microalbuminuria in essential hypertension and diabetes mellitus. J Hypertens 14(suppl 2):S89–S94, 1996.
24. Bianchi S, Bigazzi R, Galava AQ, et al. Insulin resistance in microalbuminuric hypertension: Sites and mechanisms. Hypertension 26:789–795, 1995.
25. Nosadini R, Solini A, Velussi M, et al. Impaired insulin-induced glucose uptake by extrahepatic tissue is the hallmark of NIDDM patients who have or will develop hypertension and microalbuminuria. Diabetes 43:491–499, 1994.
26. Mykkanen L, Haffner SM, Kuusisto J, et al. Microalbuminuria precedes the development of NIDDM. Diabetes 43:552–557, 1994.
27. Skov Jensen J, Borch-Johnsen K, Jensen G, Feldt-Rasmussen B. Atherosclerotic risk factors are increased in clinically healthy subjects with microalbuminuria. Atherosclerosis 112:245–252, 1995.
28. Rossing P, Hougaard P, Borch-Johnsen K, Parving H. Predictors of mortality in insulin dependent diabetes: 10 year observational follow up study. BMJ 313:779–784, 1996.
29. National High Blood Pressure Education Program Working Group. 1995 Update of the Working Group Reports on Chronic Renal Failure and Renovascular Hypertension. Arch Intern Med 156:1938–1947, 1996.
30. Lazarus JM, Bourgoignie JJ, Buckalew VM, et al, for the Modification of Diet in Renal Disease Study Group. Achievement and safety of a low blood pressure goal in chronic renal disease. Hypertension 29:641–650, 1997.
31. Remuzzi G, Ruggenenti P, Benigni A. Understanding the nature of renal disease progression. Kidney Int 51:2–15, 1997.
32. Ravid M, Lang B, Rachmani R, Lishner M. Long-term renoprotective effect of angiotensin-converting enzyme inhibition in non-insulin-dependent diabetes mellitus: A 7-year follow-up study. Arch Intern Med 156:286–289, 1996.
33. Bakris GL, Slataper R, Vicknair N, Sadler R. ACE inhibitor mediated reductions in renal size and microalbuminuria in normotensive, diabetic subjects. J Diabetes Complications 8:12–16, 1994.
34. Maki DD, Ma JZ, Louis TA, Kasiske BL. Long-term effects of antihypertensive agents on proteinuria and renal function. Arch Intern Med 155:1073–1080, 1995.
35. Kilaru PK, Bakris GL. ACE inhibition or calcium-channel blockade: Renal implications of combination therapy versus a single agent. J Cardiovasc Pharmacol 28(suppl 4):S34–S44, 1996.
36. Bakris GL, Copley JB, Vicknair N, et al. Calcium channel blockers versus other antihypertensive therapies on progression of NIDDM associated nephropathy. Kidney Int 50:1641–1650, 1996.
37. Walker WG, Hermann JA, Anderson JE. Randomized double-blinded trial of enalapril vs. hydrochlorothiazide on glomerular filtration rate in diabetic nephropathy. [Abstract] Hypertension 22:410, 1993.
38. Curb JD, Pressel SL, Cutler JA, et al, for the Systolic Hypertension in the Elderly Program (SHEP) Cooperative Research Group. Effect of diuretic-based antihypertensive treatment on cardiovascular disease risk in older diabetic patients with isolated systolic hypertension. JAMA 276:1886–1892, 1996.
39. Bakris GL, Weir MR, Sowers JR. Therapeutic challenges in the obese diabetic patients with hypertension. Am J Med 101:33S–46S, 1996.
40. Bakris GL, Mangrum A, Copley JB, et al. Effect of calcium channel or β-blockade on the progression of diabetic nephropathy in African Americans. Hypertension 29:744–750, 1997.
41. Kirk JK, Konen JC, Shihabi Z, et al. Effects of terazosin on glycemic control, cholesterol and microalbuminuria in patients with NIDDM and hypertension. Am J Therapeutics 3:32–35, 1994.
42. Rachmani R, Levi Z, Slavachevsky I, et al. The effect of an alpha adrenergic blocker, an ACE inhibitor and hydrochlorothiazide on blood pressure and on renal function in type 2 diabetic patients with hypertension and albuminuria. Nephron 80:175–182, 1998.
43. Tarif N, Bakris GL. Angiotensin II receptor blockade and progression of renal disease in nondiabetic patients. Kidney Int 52(suppl 63):S67–S70, 1997.
44. Bakris GL. Combination therapy for hypertension and renal disease in diabetes. *In* Mogensen CE (ed). The Kidney and Hypertension in Diabetes Mellitus, 4th ed. Boston, Kluwer Academic, 1998.
45. Bakris GL, Weir MR, DeQuattro V, McMahon FG. Effects of an ACE inhibitor/calcium antagonist combination on proteinuria in diabetic nephropathy. Kidney Int 54:1283–1289, 1998.
46. Epstein M, Bakris GL. Newer approaches to antihypertensive therapy: Use fixed dose combination therapy. Arch Intern Med 156:1969–1978, 1996.
47. Bakris GL, Griffin KA, Picken MM, Bidani AK. Combined effects of an angiotensin converting enzyme inhibitor and a calcium antagonist on renal injury. J Hypertens 15:1181–1185, 1997.
48. Estacio RO, Jeffers BW, Hiatt WR, et al. The effect of nisoldipine as compared with enalapril on cardiovascular outcomes in patients with non–insulin-dependent diabetes and hypertension. N Engl J Med 338:645–652, 1998.
49. Tatti P, Guarisco R, Pahor M. Outcome results of the fosinopril versus amlodipine cardiovascular events randomized trial (FACET) in patients with hypertension and NIDDM. Diabetes Care 21:597–602, 1998.

57 Renal Disease

Gerjan Navis, Paul E. de Jong, and Dick de Zeeuw

The first observation of an association between hypertension and renal disease dates back to more than 150 years ago, when Bright reported the postmortem finding of a correlation between small, shrunken kidneys and cardiac enlargement. Today, renal parenchymal disease is still a main cause of secondary hypertension, accounting for some 5% of the cases of hypertension in a secondary referral clinic or, stated otherwise, for half of the cases of secondary hypertension.[1] The treatment of hypertension is considered a cornerstone of therapy in renal patients, as hypertension contributes not only to the extremely high cardiovascular risk among renal patients[2] but also to the progression of renal function loss.[3] In this chapter, we give a brief overview of hypertension in nondiabetic renal disease with a focus on its role in the progression of renal function loss and implications for therapy. Hypertension in diabetes, renal vascular disease, and end-stage renal disease are discussed elsewhere.

PREVALENCE

Hypertension is common in chronic renal disease. Its prevalence appears to be related to the underlying disorder as well as to the severity of renal function loss. Prevalences vary considerably among reports, even within the same diagnostic category. Nevertheless, in primary glomerular disorders, hypertension is more common than in tubulointerstitial disease.[4] A prevalence of approximately 60% is reported for patients with glomerular disorders,[5] whereas in patients presenting with chronic tubulointerstitial nephropathy, some 33% are hypertensive.[6] When renal function loss has progressed toward end-stage renal failure, some 85 to 90% of patients are hypertensive.

PATHOGENESIS

Impairment of renal sodium excretion leading to an increase in extracellular fluid volume (ECV) appears to be a central, albeit not the exclusive, mechanism of hypertension in renal disease. Nevertheless, cross-sectional studies in patients with early renal function impairment found that an elevated total peripheral resistance rather than increased cardiac output accounted for the elevated blood pressure.[7] Longitudinal data in patients with early renal function impairment followed for 2 to 8 years, however, suggested that the rise in total peripheral resistance is preceded by an elevation in cardiac output.[8]

The interaction between sodium intake, body fluid status, and hypertension in chronic renal failure was elegantly demonstrated by Koomans and colleagues.[9] They found that the rise in blood pressure induced by a shift from a low to a high sodium intake (i.e., the salt sensitivity of

blood pressure) is inversely proportional to renal function. That is, the more renal function is impaired, the more blood pressure rises in response to a high sodium intake. The rise in blood pressure correlated with the extent of ECV expansion (Fig. 57–1). It is interesting that, in severe renal function impairment, the rise in blood pressure *for any given rise* in ECV was larger than in moderate renal function impairment. This indicates not only that the rise in blood pressure is due to ECV expansion, but also that other factors associated with renal function impairment must be involved in the sodium-induced rise in blood pressure.

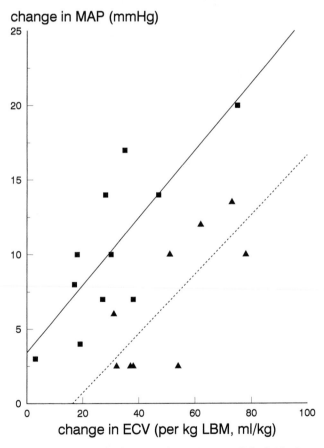

Figure 57–1. Relationship between the rise in extracellular fluid volume (ECV) per kilogram of lean body mass (LBM) and the rise in mean arterial pressure (MAP) induced by a high salt intake in 20 renal patients. *Solid triangles* and *broken line* show patients with moderate renal function impairment (creatinine clearance 32 to 75 ml/min); *solid squares* and *continuous line* show patients with severe renal function impairment (creatinine clearance 3 to 22 ml/min). Patients with salt-losing conditions were excluded from this study. (Adapted from Koomans HA, Roos JC, Boer P, et al. Salt sensitivity of blood pressure in chronic renal failure. Evidence for renal control of body fluid distribution in man. Hypertension 4:190–197, 1982.)

Enhanced activity of vasopressor systems as well as decreased function of vasodepressor systems have been implicated in the pathogenesis of hypertension in renal disease. Circulating levels of components of the renin-angiotensin-aldosterone system (RAAS) have been reported to be inappropriately high for the state of sodium balance in renal patients.[10, 11] Other studies, however, were unable to confirm these findings.[7, 12] Increased pressor sensitivity to angiotensin II, attributed to volume expansion, was reported in advanced renal failure,[13] illustrating that RAAS effects can be involved even without elevation of circulating hormone levels. Taken together, the evidence supports a role of increased RAAS effects in advanced renal disease and/or malignant hypertension,[14] whereas the role of the RAAS in hypertension in early renal disease is less well documented. Further, some (but not all) studies[9, 15] reported elevated plasma catecholamines in hypertensive patients with mild to moderate renal failure and/or a correlation with blood pressure, suggesting a role for enhanced sympathetic activity. Moreover, in early renal failure, pressor sensitivity to norepinephrine appears to be enhanced.[16] The correlation between catecholamines and plasma renin activity in hypertensive renal patients[13] suggests that sympathetic overactivity contributes to enhanced RAAS activity in these patients. Endothelin levels appear to be elevated in renal failure as well, possibly owing to decreased endothelin breakdown in the tubular brush border.[17, 18]

Decreased levels of kidney-derived vasodilator substances, such as renomedullary lipids, kinins, and vasodilator prostaglandins,[19] have been reported in patients with renal function impairment. Further, Vallance and coworkers[20] reported increased plasma levels of an endogenous nitric oxide synthase inhibitor in patients with renal failure, which could account for impaired endothelium-dependent vasodilatation.

Taken together, the available evidence suggests a multifactorial pathogenesis for hypertension in renal disease, with involvement of volume expansion as well as a disturbed balance between vasoconstrictor and vasodepressor systems. The relative contribution of each of the previously discussed mechanisms in an individual patient depends on the severity of renal function impairment, the nature of the underlying renal disease, and sodium intake.

TARGET ORGAN DAMAGE IN RENAL PATIENTS

Cardiovascular Target Organ Damage

Patients with renal function impairment have a considerably elevated cardiovascular risk. This is presumably due, first, to common cardiovascular risk factors that are also present in nonrenal populations, such as hypertension,[2] hyperlipidemia, and smoking. Moreover, in renal patients, the vascular susceptibility to hypertensive damage appears to be increased, as is apparent from the higher prevalence of hypertensive retinopathy for any given level of blood pressure compared with essential hypertensives.[21] Multiple metabolic abnormalities are presumed to be involved in the increased vascular susceptibility in renal patients. These include the accumulation of an array of uremic toxins or the metabolic abnormalities elicited by proteinuria, or a combination of these.

Proteinuria appears to be a potent cardiovascular risk factor: Proteinuric patients have a five- to sixfold increased risk for myocardial infarction compared with the general population.[22] Dyslipidemia presumably contributes to this high cardiovascular risk.[23] Hyperlipidemia is usually proportional to the severity of proteinuria[24] with, moreover, a particularly atherogenic lipid profile due to the elevation of lipoprotein(a).[25] Additional metabolic derangements in renal patients include the accumulation of advanced glycosylation end products[26] and hyperhomocysteinemia. Endothelial dysfunction may constitute a common pathway for cardiovascular morbidity in renal patients, as not only hypertension[27] but also renal function impairment[20] and proteinuria are associated with endothelial dysfunction.[28]

Renal Target Organ Damage

In renal patients, hypertension is associated with a poor renal outcome.[29, 30] Both systemic and glomerular hypertension may be involved in the pathogenesis of progressive renal damage.[31] Brenner and associates[31] hypothesized that reduction of nephron mass due to any cause elicits an adaptive response in the remaining nephrons. In these remnant nephrons, preglomerular vasodilatation leads to enhanced transmission of systemic blood pressure to the glomerular capillaries. The ensuing glomerular hypertension and hyperfiltration in these nephrons serve to maintain overall glomerular filtration rate and sodium balance in the short term but also lead to progressive hypertensive glomerular damage, glomerular protein leakage, and renal function loss in the long term. Thus, according to this hypothesis, loss of preglomerular autoregulatory vascular tone renders patients with impaired renal function particularly susceptible to hypertensive renal damage. Subsequent investigators suggested that once proteinuria occurs, it may be a main factor in the vicious circle of ongoing renal damage, as proteinuria is a powerful predictor of long-term renal function loss.[32, 33] Both intrarenal toxicity of leaked proteins and the systemic sequelae of proteinuria, such as hyperlipidemia, may be involved in proteinuria-associated renal damage.[34]

Remarkably, the risk factors for progressive renal function loss tend to parallel those for cardiovascular morbidity, as summarized in Table 57–1. In addition to the risk factors

Table 57–1 Common Risk Factors for Cardiovascular and Renal Target Organ Damage in Renal Patients

	Cardiovascular Damage	Renal Damage	Specific Intervention Available
Hypertension	+	+	+
Glomerular hypertension		+	+
Proteinuria	+	+	+
Hyperlipidemia	+	+	+
Genetic factors	+	+	To be investigated
Smoking	+	+	+

discussed previously, recent data suggest a common genetic predisposition to progressive cardiovascular and renal function loss conveyed by an insertion/deletion (I/D) polymorphism of the gene encoding for angiotensin-converting enzyme (ACE). Homozygosity for the deletion genotype, DD, is associated with a more rapid rate of renal function loss irrespective of the initial cause of renal damage.[35] In hypertensive patients without overt primary renal disease, the DD genotype appears to predispose to hypertensive nephrosclerosis.[36] Increasing evidence suggests that gene-gene interaction with other genetic polymorphisms of the RAAS, as well as gene-environment interaction, is involved in the impact of ACE genotype on renal and cardiovascular prognosis.

Finally, increasing evidence indicates that smoking is a risk factor not only for cardiovascular disease but also for progressive renal function loss.[37] The similarity of cardiovascular and renal risk factors presumably reflects the involvement of common pathophysiological pathways in target organ damage.

ANTIHYPERTENSIVE TREATMENT IN RENAL PATIENTS

The management of hypertension in renal patients should be part of a treatment regimen that aims at overall risk reduction. This includes not only reduction of the increased cardiovascular risk but also prevention of progressive renal function loss. Intervention in the risk factors mentioned previously provides a rational basis for therapy of hypertensive renal patients.

Blood Pressure Reduction

Blood pressure reduction slows the rate of long-term renal function loss. The Modification of Diet in Renal Disease (MDRD) trial demonstrated that the presence of proteinuria deserves specific consideration.[38] As expected, long-term renal function loss was most rapid in proteinuric patients. Interestingly, the long-term renal benefit of blood pressure reduction was more pronounced in proteinuric patients irrespective of the class of antihypertensive drug. Moreover, the MDRD data suggest that for effective long-term renoprotection, target blood pressure should be lower in proteinuric patients than in their nonproteinuric counterparts.[39] In patients with proteinuria, the lowest mean arterial pressure (MAP) attained (≤92 mm Hg, corresponding to 125/75 mm Hg) resulted in additional renoprotection, without signs of a J-shaped pattern,[40] whereas this low target level did not confer additional renoprotection in nonproteinuric patients (Fig. 57–2).

Intraglomerular Pressure Reduction

Reduction of intraglomerular pressure has been shown in animal experiments to confer specific renoprotection in addition to the lower blood pressure. In humans, interestingly, the early renal hemodynamic response to antihyper-

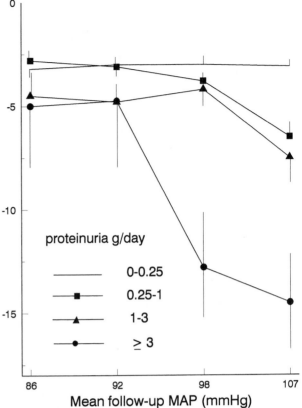

Figure 57–2. Mean glomerular filtration rate (GFR) decline and achieved blood pressure (mean arterial pressure [MAP]) during follow-up in the Modification of Diet in Renal Disease (MDRD) study for patients with different severity of proteinuria at baseline. (From Peterson JC, Adler S, Burkart JM, et al. Blood pressure control, proteinuria and the progression of renal disease. The Modification of Diet in Renal Disease Study. Ann Intern Med 123:754–762, 1995.)

tensive therapy predicts its long-term renoprotective efficacy irrespective of the class of drug used. A slight drop in glomerular filtration rate at onset of treatment—assumed to reflect a reduction in glomerular hydrostatic pressure—predicts a favorable long-term course of renal function, suggesting that reduction of glomerular pressure may be relevant to long-term renoprotection (Fig. 57–3).[41] In animal experiments, ACE inhibitors lower glomerular pressure more effectively than other agents of similar antihypertensive potency, suggesting that ACE inhibitors may provide specific renoprotection in addition to the lower blood pressure. In humans, several studies found that ACE inhibitors retarded renal function loss more effectively than other antihypertensives,[42] but other studies found no differences in renoprotection between ACE inhibitors and other antihypertensive agents.[43] These discrepancies may be related to different trial designs and to differences between study populations. A specific benefit of ACE inhibition was more readily apparent in populations with a rapid rate of renal function loss, such as those with overt proteinuria.[43]

Proteinuria Reduction

Reduction of proteinuria, whether elicited by antihypertensive treatment or other measures, such as dietary protein

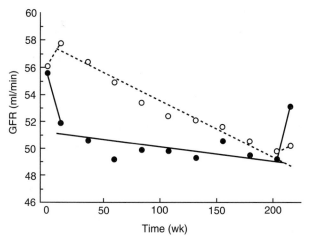

Figure 57–3. Time course of glomerular filtration rate (GFR) before, during, and after withdrawal of antihypertensive therapy in renal patients. *Closed circles* and *continuous lines* show patients who initially showed a distinct fall in GFR (*n* = 20); *open circles* and *broken lines* show patients in whom GFR did not fall after the start of treatment (*n* = 20). After withdrawal of therapy, a rise in GFR occurs in patients with an initial drop only, demonstrating the functional nature of the initial drop in GFR. Interestingly, withdrawal of treatment reveals that GFR is better preserved in the patients with the initial drop. (From Apperloo AJ, de Zeeuw D, de Jong PE. A short-term antihypertensive treatment–induced fall in glomerular filtration rate predicts long-term stability of renal function. Used with permission from Kidney International, volume 51, pages 793–797, 1997.)

restriction, may confer long-term renoprotection as well. A recent important study in patients with proteinuria greater than 3 g/day showed that an ACE inhibitor reduced proteinuria and the rate of renal function loss more effectively than other antihypertensives with a similar blood pressure–lowering action.[44] Interestingly, the reduction in proteinuria at onset of antihypertensive therapy predicts the subsequent rate of long-term renal function loss (Fig. 57–4). This predictive value is independent of the class of drug used,[41, 45–47] and also holds true for intervention by dietary protein restriction.[48] Animal data demonstrated that a reduction in proteinuria also predicts protection against renal structural damage.[49] These data suggest that the reduction in proteinuria is causally involved in long-term renoprotection and that, accordingly, proteinuria may be used as a parameter to monitor and titrate therapy in order to achieve effective long-term renoprotection.[50]

Lipid Profile

Lipid profile is improved by reduction of proteinuria. As reviewed recently, antiproteinuric treatment elicits an improvement in lipid profile irrespective of the class of antiproteinuric drug.[51] The reduction in cholesterol during antiproteinuric treatment is quantitatively related to the reduction in proteinuria (Fig. 57–5).[52–56] Notably, reduction of proteinuria also leads to a reduction in lipoprotein(a), an effect that is not obtained with current lipid-lowering drugs. Animal data demonstrated that reduction of hyperlipidemia may play a role in the prevention of progressive renal function loss. In humans, conclusive evidence that lipid lowering improves renal prognosis is not available.

Nevertheless, the poor cardiovascular risk profile of renal patients warrants aggressive treatment of dyslipidemia in this population.

Genetic Factors

Genetic factors may be involved in responsiveness to antihypertensive therapy. For instance, in essential hypertensives the response of blood pressure to diuretic therapy is greater in subjects with a Gly 460 Trp polymorphism of the gene encoding for α-adducin.[57] In renal patients, interest has focused on the ACE (I/D) genotype and the response to ACE inhibition. Data from various studies appear to be conflicting, as the responses of blood pressure and proteinuria in patients with the DD genotype were reported to be either better than, similar to, or worse than in heterozygotes (I/D) or in patients homozygous for the I-allele (II genotype). Interactions with environmental and genetic factors likely account for the discrepancies between studies. For instance, we demonstrated that a high sodium intake elicits differences in the responses of blood pressure and proteinuria to ACE inhibitors between patients with different ACE (I/D) genotypes. That is, a poor response in the

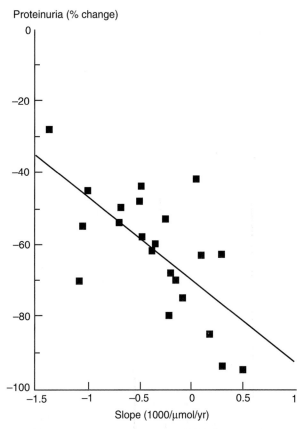

Figure 57–4. Correlation between the initial antiproteinuric response to antihypertensive treatment (reduction in proteinuria after 2 months of treatment; percent change from baseline) and the subsequent rate of renal function loss (slope of inverse serum creatinine levels) during follow-up in 21 patients. (Adapted from Gansevoort RT, de Zeeuw D, de Jong PE. Long-term benefits of the antiproteinuric effect of ACE-inhibition in non-diabetic renal disease. Am J Kidney Dis 2:202–206, 1993.)

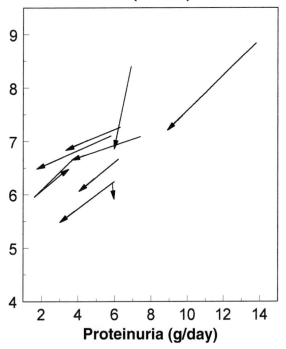

total cholesterol (mmol/l)

Proteinuria (g/day)

Figure 57–5. The relationship between reduction in proteinuria and reduction in cholesterol during antihypertensive treatment in various studies.[52-56] *Each arrow* represents the mean value from a specific intervention study.

DD genotype compared with II and I/D genotypes was apparent only in individuals on a high sodium intake, whereas no differences between genotypes were found among individuals on a low sodium intake.[58]

GUIDELINES FOR TREATMENT

In renal patients, blood pressure can effectively be reduced by any of the currently available classes of drugs, as reviewed in Section 9, Individual Drug Classes. For the choice of therapy as well as for subsequent dose titration, the presence of proteinuria is important. For patients without proteinuria, no specific advantage of any particular antihypertensive agent or class has been demonstrated thus far, i.e., renoprotection is provided by the reduction of blood pressure per se. For proteinuric patients, however, the antiproteinuric potential of the particular class of antihypertensive drug is relevant. Two recent meta-analyses addressed the antiproteinuric effect of ACE inhibition versus other antihypertensives.[59, 60] These studies found, first, that reduction in blood pressure per se leads to a significant, albeit small, fall in proteinuria. This held true for all antihypertensive agents except nifedipine. Second, for a given fall in blood pressure, the reduction in proteinuria is considerably larger with ACE inhibitors, indicating that specific renal effects of ACE inhibition are involved in the reduction in proteinuria. These effects may account for the greater renoprotective benefit of ACE inhibitors compared with other antihypertensives in patients with overt proteinuria.[44] This strongly suggests that in proteinuric patients,

ACE inhibitors are preferred as a first step of treatment. The short-term renal effects of angiotensin I receptor blockade—another mode of blocking the RAAS—are similar to those of ACE inhibition (Fig. 57–6),[61] but their long-term effects on renal and cardiovascular protection are still under investigation.

Furthermore, target blood pressure should be lower in proteinuric patients than in nonproteinuric patients. From the MDRD data, it can be inferred that for patients with proteinuria of 1 to 3 g/day, target MAP should be approximately 98 mm Hg (corresponding to 135/80 mm Hg), whereas for patients with proteinuria greater than 3 g/day, target MAP should be as low as 92 mm Hg (corresponding to 125/75 mm Hg).

Proteinuria reduction is important for long-term renoprotection, and the antiproteinuric response to ACE inhibition can be improved in several ways. First, the top of the dose-response for proteinuria reduction appears to be higher than for blood pressure reduction.[61, 62] Next, correction of volume overload by either dietary sodium restriction[63] or cotreatment with a diuretic[64] appears to be required to obtain the full therapeutic benefit of ACE inhibition (Fig. 57–7). Moreover, dietary protein restriction,[53] as well as cotreatment with indomethacin,[65] selectively enhances the antiproteinuric effect of ACE inhibitor treatment without a further reduction in blood pressure.

Treatment Schedule

ACE inhibition is a logical first step for antihypertensive drug therapy in renal patients, in particular for patients with overt proteinuria (>1 g/day). However, evidence for class-specific renal benefits of ACE inhibition in nonproteinuric patients is lacking, and cardiovascular comorbidity may provide reasons to select another class of drugs such as β-blockers or calcium entry blockers in these patients. Considering the important role of sodium status in renal patients, correction of volume is usually necessary to obtain a satisfactory therapeutic response. It should be noted that proteinuric patients tend to be volume-expanded even in the absence of renal function impairment. Restriction of dietary sodium intake (to 3 to 5 g daily) and diuretic treatment are therefore usually needed. If blood pressure is not reduced sufficiently by this regimen, it is worthwhile to check compliance with dietary sodium restriction, and if necessary, to attempt to improve it by dietary counseling. Further reduction of blood pressure may be obtained by combining diuretics with other classes of antihypertensives. Angiotensin I receptor blockers may be used in patients in whom ACE inhibitor therapy is not tolerated owing to side effects, such as cough or skin rash.

Special Considerations for Antihypertensive Drug Treatment in Renal Patients

A rise in serum creatinine often occurs in renal patients at the onset of antihypertensive treatment. As mentioned previously, this may reflect a drop in glomerular hydrostatic pressure that is favorable in the long run and therefore can be considered a favorable prognostic sign. It should be

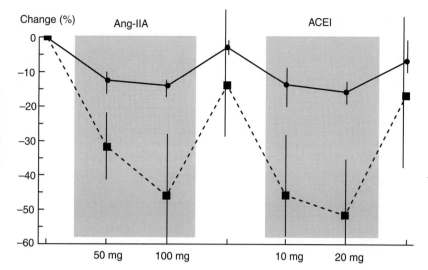

Figure 57–6. The effects of losartan, 50 and 100 mg daily, and enalapril, 10 and 20 mg daily, on blood pressure *(continuous lines)* and proteinuria *(broken lines)*. (From Gansevoort RT, de Zeeuw D, de Jong PE. Is the antiproteinuric effect of ACE inhibition mediated by interference in the renin-angiotensin system? Used with permission from Kidney International, volume 45, pages 861–867, 1994.)

noted, however, that in patients in whom the clinical signs are compatible with the presence of renal artery stenosis, a rise in serum creatinine at the onset of treatment (in particular with ACE inhibitors or angiotensin I receptor antagonists) should prompt the clinician to consider the possibility of renovascular hypertension. The diagnostic approach for renovascular hypertension is discussed in Chapter 77, Renovascular Hypertension: Diagnosis and Treatment.

Most antihypertensives used in essential hypertension can be safely used in renal patients, provided the dosage is adjusted to the renal function impairment whenever appropriate (see Sect. 9, Individual Drug Classes). For diuretics, in contrast to all other drugs excreted by the kidney, dosage should be increased in renal function impairment, in order to permit sufficient tubular delivery to exert an effect. When the creatinine clearance is below 30–40 ml/min, loop diuretics are preferred. Potassium-sparing diuretics should in general be avoided in renal patients. Particularly in patients treated with an ACE inhibitor or angiotensin I receptor blocker, potassium-sparing diuretics may induce severe hyperkalemia. In addition to the reduction of blood pressure, reduction of proteinuria is a treatment objective in proteinuric renal patients and may provide an important contribution to the reduction of renal (and cardiovascular) risk in these patients.

CONCLUSIONS

Hypertensive renal patients are at high risk for cardiovascular and renal target organ damage, particularly when proteinuria is present. Antihypertensive treatment is a corner-

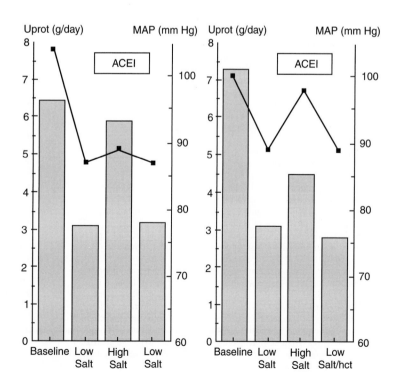

Figure 57–7. The effect of sodium status on the responses of proteinuria (Uprot; *bars*) and blood pressure (mean arterial pressure [MAP]; *lines*) to angiotensin-converting enzyme inhibition (ACEI). *Left,* The effect of ACEI compared with pretreatment values during low- and high-salt diets, with an almost complete blunting of the antiproteinuric effect during high salt intake. *Right,* The effect of a shift from a low to a high salt intake during chronic ACEI, with subsequent addition of hydrochlorothiazide (hct). Addition of the diuretic restored the responses of proteinuria and blood pressure to levels obtained during low salt intake. (*Left,* Adapted from Heeg JE, de Jong PE, van der Hem GK, de Zeeuw D. Efficacy and variability of the antiproteinuric effect of lisinopril. Used with permission from Kidney International, volume 36, pages 272–279, 1989. *Right,* Adapted from Buter H, Hemmelder MH, Navis GJ, et al. The blunting of the antiproteinuric efficacy of ACE inhibition can be restored by hydrochlorothiazide. Nephrol Dial Transplant 7:1682–1685, 1998. By permission of Oxford University Press.)

stone of risk reduction in renal patients. By virtue of their specific renoprotective effects, ACE inhibitors are drugs of choice in hypertensive renal patients, particularly in those with proteinuria. Correction of volume status by dietary sodium restriction and diuretic therapy is usually required to obtain an effective therapeutic response. In proteinuric patients, additional renoprotective benefit is obtained by a lower target blood pressure.

References

1. Sinclair AM, Isles CG, Brown I, et al. Secondary hypertension in a blood pressure clinic. Arch Int Med 147:1289–1293, 1987.
2. Ritz E, Koch M. Morbidity and mortality due to hypertension in patients with renal failure. Am J Kidney Dis 21(suppl 2):113–118, 1993.
3. Alvestrand A, Gutierrez A, Bucht H, Bergstrom J. Reduction of blood pressure retards the progression of chronic renal failure in man. Nephrol Dial Transplant 3:624–631, 1988.
4. Brown MA, Whitworth JA. Hypertension in human renal disease. J Hypertens 10:701–712, 1992.
5. Danielson H, Kornerup HJ, Olsen S, Posborg V. Arterial hypertension in chronic glomerulonephritis. An analysis of 310 cases. Clin Nephrol 19:284–287, 1987.
6. Arze RS, Ramos JM, Owen JP, et al. The natural history of chronic pyelonephritis in the adult. Q J Med 51:396–401, 1982.
7. Valvo E, Gammaro L, Bedogna V, et al. Hypertension in primary immunoglobulin A nephropathy (Berger's disease): Hemodynamic alterations and mechanisms. Nephron 45:219–223, 1987.
8. Brod J, Bahlmann J, Cachovan M, Pretschner P. Development of hypertension in renal disease. Clin Sci 64:141–152, 1983.
9. Koomans HA, Roos JC, Boer P, et al. Salt sensitivity of blood pressure in chronic renal failure. Evidence for renal control of body fluid distribution in man. Hypertension 4:190–197, 1982.
10. Beretta-Piccoli C, Weidmann P, de Chatel R, Reubi FC. Hypertension associated with early stage kidney disease: Complementary roles of circulating renin, the body sodium/volume state and duration of hypertension. Am J Med 61:739–747, 1976.
11. Levitan D, Massry SG, Romoff M, Campese V. Plasma catecholamines and autonomic nervous system function in patients with early renal insufficiency and hypertension: effect of clonidine. Nephron 36:24–29, 1984.
12. Mitas JA, Levy S, Holle R, et al. Urinary kallikrein in the hypertension of renal parenchymal disease. N Engl J Med 299:162–165, 1978.
13. Schalekamp MADH, Schalekamp-Kuyken MPA, de Moor Fruytier M, et al. Interrelationships between blood pressure, renin, renin substrate and blood volume in terminal renal failure. Clin Sci 45:417–428, 1973.
14. Davies DL, Beevers G, Briggs JD, et al. Abnormal relationship between exchangeable sodium and renin-angiotensin system in malignant hypertension and in hypertension with chronic renal failure. Lancet 1:683–686, 1973.
15. Ishii M, Ikeda T, Takagi M, et al. Elevated plasma catecholamines in hypertensives with primary glomerular disease. Hypertension 5:545–551, 1983.
16. Beretta-Piccoli C, Weidmann P, Schiffl H, et al. Enhanced cardiovascular pressor reactivity to norepinephrine in mild renal parenchymal disease. Kidney Int 22:297–303, 1982.
17. Koyama H, Nishzawa Y, Tabata T, et al. Plasma endothelin levels in patients with uraemia. Lancet 1:991–992, 1989.
18. Abassi ZA, Tate JE, Golomb E, Keiser HR. Role of neutral endopeptidase in the metabolism of endothelin. Hypertension 20:89–95, 1992.
19. Kishimoto T, Terada T, Okahara T, et al. Correlation of blood prostaglandins and blood pressure in chronic renal failure. Nephron 47:49–55, 1987.
20. Vallance P, Leone A, Calver A, et al. Accumulation of an endogenous inhibitor of nitric oxide synthesis in chronic renal failure. Lancet 339:572–575, 1992.
21. Heidbreder E, Huller U, Schafer B, Heidland A. Severe hypertensive retinopathy in hypertension. Increased incidence in renoparenchymal hypertension. Am J Nephrol 7:394–400, 1987.
22. Ordonez JD, Hiatt RA, Killebrew EJ, Fireman BH. The increased risk of coronary heart disease associated with the nephrotic syndrome. Kidney Int 44:638–642, 1993.
23. Radhakrishnan J, Appel AS, Valeri A, Appel GB. The nephrotic syndrome, lipids, and risk factors for cardiovascular disease. Am J Kidney Dis 22:135–142, 1993.
24. Moorhead JF. Lipids and pathogenesis of kidney disease. Am J Kidney Dis 17:65–70, 1991.
25. Karadi O, Romics L, Palos G, et al. Lp(a) lipoprotein concentration in serum of patients with heavy proteinuria of different origin. Clin Chem 35:2121–2123, 1989.
26. Vlassara H. Serum advanced glycosylation end products: A new class of uremic toxins? Blood Purif 12:54–59, 1994.
27. Higashi Y, Oshima T, Ozono R, et al. Aging and severity of hypertension attenuate endothelium-dependent renal vascular relaxation in humans. Hypertension 30:252–258, 1997.
28. Stroes ESG, Joles JA, Chang PC, et al. Impaired endothelial function in patients with nephrotic range proteinuria. Kidney Int 48:544–550, 1995.
29. Brazy PC, Fitzwilliam JF. Progressive renal disease: Role of race and antihypertensive medications. Kidney Int 37:1113–1119, 1990.
30. Orofino L, Quereda C, Lamas S, et al. Hypertension in primary chronic glomerulonephritis: Analysis of 288 biopsied patients. Nephron 45:22–26, 1987.
31. Brenner BM, Meyer TW, Hostetter TW. Dietary protein and the progressive nature of kidney disease: Role of hemodynamically mediated glomerular injury in the pathogenesis of progressive glomerular sclerosis of aging, renal ablation and intrinsic renal disease. N Engl J Med 307:652–659, 1982.
32. Remuzzi G, Bertani T. Is glomerulosclerosis a consequence of altered glomerular permeability to macromolecules? [Editorial] Kidney Int 38:384–394, 1990.
33. Williams PS, Fass G, Bone JM. Renal pathology and proteinuria determine progression in untreated mild/moderate chronic renal failure. Q J Med 67:343–354, 1988.
34. de Boer E, Navis GJ, Tiebosch ATM, et al. Systemic factors are involved in proteinuria-associated focal glomerulosclerosis. J Am Soc Nephrol 8:613A, 1997.
35. van Essen GG, Rensma PL, de Zeeuw D, et al. Association between angiotensin converting enzyme gene polymorphism and failure of renoprotective therapy. Lancet 347:94–95, 1996.
36. Kario K, Kanai N, Nishiuma S, et al. Hypertensive nephropathy and the gene for angiotensin converting enzyme. Hypertension 17:252–256, 1997.
37. Orth SR, Ritz E, Schrier RW. The renal risks of smoking. Kidney Int 51:1669–1677, 1997.
38. Klahr S, Levey AS, Beck GJ, et al. The effects of dietary protein restriction and blood pressure control on the progression of chronic renal disease. N Engl J Med 330:877–884, 1994.
39. Peterson JC, Adler S, Burkart JM, et al. Blood pressure control, proteinuria and the progression of renal disease. The Modification of Diet in Renal Disease Study. Ann Intern Med 123:754–762, 1995.
40. Lazarus JM, Bourgoignie JJ, Buckalew VM, et al, for the Modification of Diet in Renal Disease Study Group. Achievement and safety of a low blood pressure goal in chronic renal disease. Hypertension 29:641–650, 1997.
41. Apperloo AJ, de Zeeuw D, de Jong PE. A short-term antihypertensive treatment–induced fall in glomerular filtration rate predicts long-term stability of renal function. Kidney Int 51:793–797, 1997.
42. Giatras I, Lau J, Levey AS, on behalf of the Angiotensin Converting Enzyme Inhibition and Progressive Renal Disease Study Group. Effect of angiotensin-converting enzyme inhibitors on the progression of non-diabetic renal disease: A meta-analysis of randomized trials. Ann Intern Med 127:337–345, 1997.
43. Navis GJ, de Zeeuw D, de Jong PE. ACE-inhibitors, panacea for progressive renal disease? Lancet 349:1852–1853, 1997.
44. The GISEN Group. Randomised placebo-controlled trial of effect of ramipril on decline in glomerular filtration rate and risk of terminal renal failure in proteinuric, non-diabetic nephropathy. Lancet 349:1857–1863, 1997.
45. Apperloo AJ, de Zeeuw D, de Jong PE. Short-term antiproteinuric response to antihypertensive therapy predicts long-term GFR decline in patients with non-diabetic renal disease. Kidney Int 45(suppl 45):S174–S178, 1994.
46. Gansevoort RT, de Zeeuw D, de Jong PE. Long-term benefits of the antiproteinuric effect of ACE-inhibition in non-diabetic renal disease. Am J Kidney Dis 2:202–206, 1993.
47. Praga M, Hernández E, Montoyo C, et al. Long-term beneficial

effects of angiotensin-converting enzyme inhibition with nephrotic proteinuria. Am J Kidney Dis 20:240–248, 1992.

48. El Nahas AM, Masters-Thomas A, Brady SA, et al. Selective effect of low protein diet in chronic renal diseases. BMJ 289:1337–1341, 1984.

49. Wapstra FH, Goor H van, Navis GJ, et al. Short-term antiproteinuric effect of ACE-inhibition predicts renal protection in rats with established adriamycin nephrosis. Clin Sci 90:393–400, 1996.

50. Navis GJ, de Zeeuw D. Titrating for antiproteinuric efficacy: The clue to renoprotection? J Hum Hypertens 10:669–673, 1996.

51. Navis GJ, Buter H, Dullaart RPF, et al. Effects of symptomatic antiproteinuric treatment on lipid profile in proteinuric patients. In Keane WF, Horl WH, Kasiske BL (eds). Lipids and the Kidney. Contrib Nephrol 20:88–96, 1997.

52. Gansevoort RT, Heeg JE, Dikkeschei FD, et al. Symptomatic antiproteinuric treatment decreases serum lipoprotein(a) concentration in patients with glomerular proteinuria. Nephrol Dial Transplant 9:244–250, 1994.

53. Gansevoort RT, de Zeeuw D, de Jong PE. Additive antiproteinuric effect of ACE inhibition and a low-protein diet in human renal disease. Nephrol Dial Transplant 10:497–504, 1995.

54. Praga M, Hernandez E, Montoyo C, et al. Long term beneficial effects of angiotensin converting enzyme inhibition in patients with nephrotic syndrome. Am J Kidney Dis 20:240–248, 1992.

55. Keilani T, Schlueter WA, Levin ML, Battle DC. Improvement of lipid abnormalities associated with proteinuria with using fosinopril, an angiotensin converting enzyme inhibitor. Ann Intern Med 118:246–254, 1993.

56. de Zeeuw D, Gansevoort RT, Dullaart RPF, de Jong PE. Angiotensin II antagonism improves the lipoprotein profile in patients with the nephrotic syndrome. J Hypertens 13(suppl 1):S53–S58, 1995.

57. Cusi D, Barlassina A, Azzani T, et al. Polymorphisms of alpha-adducin and salt sensitivity in patients with essential hypertension. Lancet 349:1353–1357, 1997.

58. van der Kleij FGH, Schmidt A, Navis GJ, et al. ACE I/D polymorphism and short term response to ACE inhibition; role of sodium status. Kidney Int 52(suppl 63):S23–S26, 1997.

59. Gansevoort RT, Sluiter WJ, Hemmelder MH, et al. Antiproteinuric effect of blood-pressure lowering agents: A meta-analysis of comparative trials. Nephrol Dial Transplant 10:1963–1974, 1995.

60. Maki DD, Ma JZ, Louis TA, Kasiske BL. Long-term effects of antihypertensive agents on proteinuria and renal function. Arch Intern Med 155:1073–1080, 1995.

61. Gansevoort RT, de Zeeuw D, de Jong PE. Is the antiproteinuric effect of ACE inhibition mediated by interference in the renin-angiotensin system? Kidney Int 45:861–867, 1994.

62. Palla R, Panichi V, Finato V, et al. Effect of increasing doses of lisinopril on proteinuria of normotensive patients with IgA nephropathy and normal renal function. Int J Clin Pharmacol Res 14:35–43, 1994.

63. Heeg JE, de Jong PE, van der Hem GK, de Zeeuw D. Efficacy and variability of the antiproteinuric effect of lisinopril. Kidney Int 36:272–279, 1989.

64. Buter H, Hemmelder MH, Navis GJ, et al. The blunting of the antiproteinuric efficacy of ACE inhibition can be restored by hydrochlorothiazide. Nephrol Dial Transplant 7:1682–1685, 1998.

65. Heeg JE, de Jong PE, Vriesendorp R, de Zeeuw D. Additive antiproteinuric effect of the NSAID indomethacin and the ACE inhibitor lisinopril. Am J Nephrol 10:S94–S97, 1990.

58 Hypertension in Patients on Renal Replacement Therapy

CHAPTER

Madhukar Misra, Garry P. Reams, and John H. Bauer

Hypertension is considered to be an important factor governing morbidity and mortality in the dialysis population.[1–5] The concepts surrounding hypertension in dialysis patients are believed to be based on a few "well-established" facts. For example, hypertension is believed to be an important risk factor for cardiovascular disease in the dialysis population, similar to that in the general population. In addition, the major cause of hypertension in dialysis patients is considered to be excessive interdialytic weight gain. It is generally believed that high blood pressure in a majority of dialysis patients can be managed by controlling volume alone. Therefore, the best way to achieve a lower predialysis blood pressure in hypertensive dialysis patients is to lower the target weight. To determine whether these concepts are "facts" or "myths" requires a reassessment of the evidence that associates hypertension with cardiovascular mortality in this population.

The risks of hypertension in the general population have been well described in a variety of large-scale epidemiological studies. A meta-analysis, performed utilizing the major studies relating the level of diastolic blood pressure to the incidence of stroke and coronary heart disease, has demonstrated a direct and independent association between the level of diastolic blood pressure and the risk of stroke and coronary heart disease.[6] There was no apparent lower threshold level of diastolic blood pressure that was not associated with a lower risk of either stroke or coronary heart disease.[6] Nevertheless, it has been suggested that lowering diastolic blood pressure to levels below 85 mm Hg in hypertensive subjects with ischemic heart disease may be associated with lower survival, the J-curve phenomenon.[7] Since the J-curve hypothesis has not been supported by data from prospective clinical trials, it has fallen out of favor. Elevations in systolic blood pressure have also been shown to correlate with the risk of stroke and coronary heart disease.[8, 9] Indeed, over a 30-year interval in the Framingham Study, elevations in systolic blood pressure were more predictive of risk of stroke and coronary heart disease than were elevations in diastolic blood pressure.[10]

Other interesting trends have been observed. Women aged 35 to 64 years have demonstrated lower mortality rates at any level of blood pressure compared with men.[10] African Americans tend to have higher levels of blood pressure than non–African Americans and substantially higher mortality rates at all levels of blood pressure.[11]

However, several perplexing observations regarding racial differences in blood pressure and hypertension-related cardiovascular disease have been made. In African American men with diastolic blood pressures above 90 mm Hg, the mortality rate from coronary heart disease was lower compared with white men, whereas the mortality rate for stroke was higher.[12] In addition, mortality related to coronary heart disease in the United States is lower in Hispanic men compared with non-Hispanic white men despite higher cardiovascular risk profiles and poorer blood pressure control.[13, 14] The reasons for these apparent discrepancies are unclear.

Considerable epidemiological and clinical evidence supports the concept that reducing elevated blood pressure results in reductions in cardiovascular and cerebrovascular disease and overall mortality. However, it is important to remember that the mortality rate, particularly from coronary disease, is higher in hypertensive patients receiving therapy with antihypertensive agents than in untreated subjects with similar levels of blood pressure.[15–18] An important issue to be addressed is whether these concepts concerning hypertension in a general population are operational in patients undergoing renal replacement therapy (RRT).

HYPERTENSION IN PATIENTS ON DIALYSIS

The prevalence of *hypertension,* defined as a sitting blood pressure greater than 140/90 mm Hg in patients with chronic renal failure, is approximately 80%.[19] Approximately 80 to 90% of patients starting dialysis have hypertension, compared with 15 to 20% of the general population.[20] Even after 1 year of dialysis therapy, 50% of patients on hemodialysis (HD) and 30% of patients on peritoneal dialysis (PD) remain hypertensive on casual blood pressure recordings.[21, 22] Data from ambulatory blood pressure monitoring indicate a much higher prevalence of hypertension in this group. In a study of HD patients using ambulatory blood pressure monitoring, only 15% of patients were found to maintain a blood pressure of less than 150/90 mm Hg over a 48-hour period.[23]

The prevalence of hypertension in patients on RRT probably varies with gender and race, being higher in men and in African Americans.[19] Surprisingly, hypertension in African American patients on dialysis appears to be associated with reduced mortality.[24] The reasons for this are unknown.

International registry data show that cardiovascular disease is the major cause of morbidity and mortality in patients with end-stage renal disease (ESRD).[25–29] Unlike the general hypertensive population in which there has been a 53% reduction in age-adjusted death rate from coronary heart disease and a 60% reduction in age-adjusted death rate from stroke since the late 1960s,[30, 31] no such decline in cardiovascular mortality has been observed in the dialysis population, with nearly half of deaths now ascribed to cardiac causes.[32] In patients with ESRD, the probability of death from cardiac or cerebrovascular disease is approximately 10% per year.[33]

Evidence relating hypertension and cardiovascular mor-

tality in dialysis patients is conflicting. Whereas some studies either have shown no adverse effect of hypertension on survival or have demonstrated an independent association between lower blood pressures and higher mortality,[34–36] others support the concept that lower blood pressures correlate with improved survival in the dialysis population.[37–39] This controversy may be explained, in part, by differences unique to each study, such as comorbidities, design, outcome measures, and cohort size. However, these differences alone are probably not sufficient to totally explain the apparent inconsistencies in the data.

In the general population, the relationship between level of blood pressure and cardiovascular mortality is likely linear, with lower blood pressure levels associated with a lower cardiovascular risk.[40] Since the dialysis patient has a unique cardiovascular risk profile that includes hypertension, diabetes mellitus, volume overload, left ventricular hypertrophy, hypercirculatory state, hyperlipidemia, and a "uremic" myocardium more susceptible to hypertensive damage,[41] it could be argued that the target blood pressure should be lower in dialysis patients than in the general population. In a select cohort of patients with ESRD on dialysis, lower blood pressure has been associated with lower cardiovascular mortality.[42] In a separate cohort of long-term ESRD survivors, the prevalence of hypertension declined to approximately 29% compared with 80% in the incident patients enrolled in the U.S. ESRD registry.[43]

In another prospective study, the observed inverse relationship between mortality and blood pressure was believed to reflect the presence of cardiac failure.[4] Low blood pressure appears to be the single greatest predictor of death in patients with cardiac failure.[4] Since many patients with renal failure suffer from ischemic heart disease at the start of RRT, and a significant number develop de novo disease while on RRT, concerns relating to excessive lowering of blood pressure may be reasonably valid. However, the presence of hypertension may worsen the clinical outcome in ESRD patients who do not yet have heart failure.[4] Hypertension is still considered one of the most important and potentially reversible risk factors for ischemic heart disease and cardiac failure in dialysis patients.[44]

The relationship between blood pressure and cardiac mortality may be bimodal in that very high as well as very low levels may adversely affect survival in ESRD patients.[41] The level of blood pressure that reduces mortality risk in dialysis patients is largely undetermined owing to the paucity of long-term clinical outcome studies.[44] There is no standard definition of what constitutes good control in these patients. Lower blood pressure may be highly desirable, at least before the onset of systolic dysfunction. Blood pressure targets may need to be different in patients with and without cardiac dysfunction.

It is unclear which blood pressure values have the greatest impact on cardiovascular risk—systolic, diastolic, or mean. Predialysis blood pressure is often considered related to the extracellular volume accumulated during the interdialysis period. The postdialysis blood pressure is probably affected by a number of variables, including choice of dialysate buffer and osmolality, removal of antihypertensive drugs and vasoactive hormones during dialysis, and stimulation of the renin-angiotensin axis with ultrafiltration. Some workers have found no relationship between predialysis and postdialysis blood pressure and ambulatory blood pressure values,[45] whereas others have reported a strong correlation between the ambulatory systolic and diastolic blood pressure and both predialysis systolic and postdialysis diastolic blood pressure.[46, 47] Postdialysis blood pressure (office) readings have been reported to correlate with average interdialytic blood pressure in HD patients.[47] Blood pressure is elevated in almost half of HD patients during the interdialytic period,[10] highlighting the importance of interdialytic blood pressure measurement.

The prevalence of hypertension in dialysis patients may vary depending on the method of RRT. Theoretically, patients on PD have considerable hemodynamic advantage over HD patients, including absence of arteriovenous fistula causing a hypercirculatory state, absence of large volume shifts affecting cardiac preload, and more predictable pharmacokinetics of antihypertensive drug elimination. In the short term, blood pressure control on continuous ambulatory PD may be better than HD as long as patients maintain residual renal function and ultrafiltration capacity.[48] The initial beneficial effects seen in continuous ambulatory PD may be a consequence of slow, continuous fluid removal.[49] This early-phase reduction is seen chiefly in the systolic blood pressure.[50] In the long term, these initial benefits may be lost, and antihypertensive drug requirements may increase.[51]

PATHOGENESIS

The pathogenesis of hypertension in patients on RRT is believed to be multifactorial. Traditionally, two types of hypertension were described in patients on dialysis.[52–56] The first type was characterized by normal to low plasma renin activity with a reduction in blood pressure associated with a reduction in body weight resulting from salt depletion. The second type was characterized by high plasma renin activity and resistance to salt depletion and body weight reduction. In the latter situation, bilateral nephrectomy resulted in blood pressure control. The first type was termed *volume-dependent hypertension;* the second, *renin-dependent hypertension.* Much is known about the various hemodynamic and hormonal parameters associated with hypertension in patients on dialysis, but the heterogeneity of the patients receiving RRT makes meaningful interpretation of the available data difficult.

Mean arterial pressure is the product of cardiac output and peripheral vascular resistance. There are various control mechanisms for each parameter. Dialysis patients have some unique features that may influence the development of hypertension, including the presence of an arteriovenous fistula, anemia, and more recently, the use of erythropoietin. When terminal renal failure develops, an increase in cardiac output is likely to be found resulting from chronic anemia.[57–59] The changes in cardiac output can be attenuated by correcting the anemia.[60] With the correction of the anemic state, the increase in blood pressure is related to an increase in vascular resistance.[52–56] Also, with the onset of terminal renal failure, the level of exchangeable sodium rises associated with an increase in both extravascular and intravascular volume.[55, 57, 61–65] Most, but not all, studies demonstrate a positive correlation between blood volume

and peripheral vascular resistance;[66–68] a rise in blood pressure occurs when the vascular tree cannot accommodate volume excess through vasodilatation.

As described earlier, the pathogenesis of hypertension is likely multifactorial, ranging beyond the issue of volume excess alone. Among other mechanisms that can lead to alteration in vascular resistance in patients with ESRD are the activation of neurohumoral factors. The "dialysis-resistant" form of hypertension is believed to be renin-dependent, a concept supported by the normalization of blood pressure in dialysis-resistant patients with bilateral nephrectomy or by the use of specific agents that block the pressor effect of angiotensin II.[69–71] In addition to the renin-angiotensin system, an enhanced neurogenic system has been postulated. Overactivity of the sympathetic system, as measured by excessive catecholamine release and/or an increase in sympathetic nerve discharge, has been described in dialysis patients.[72–75]

Other factors that may contribute to the hypertensive state represent markers of hypertensive damage or that may accumulate due to diminished renal metabolism vs. excretion have been identified. Nitric oxide metabolism is altered in patients on dialysis.[76–78] Circulating levels of nitric oxide synthesis inhibitor have been shown to accumulate in terminal renal failure.[79] Changes in blood pressure during HD are inversely correlated with exhaled nitric oxide concentration, higher nitric oxide levels being associated with a decrease in blood pressure and lower nitric oxide levels with an increase in blood pressure during dialysis.[80] Other proposed mechanisms include the loss of vasodepressor activity with progressive loss of renal function,[52] the presence of a circulatory inhibitor of Na^+-K^+ pump leading to an increase in vascular resistance,[81, 82] and disordered calcium metabolism with an increase in cytosolic free calcium as result of an increase in parathyroid hormone.[83]

The pathogenesis of hypertension in patients receiving RRT is difficult to unravel. There are multiple mechanisms for hypertension, with probable significant overlap. Cross-sectional comparisons may be misleading, given the heterogeneity of the dialysis population. Prospective, long-term studies following a sufficient patient population from predialysis through initiation and maintenance dialysis are not available. If antihypertensive therapy is to be directed against the principal pathogenic factors for hypertension, these types of investigations are needed.

MANAGEMENT OF HYPERTENSION IN PATIENTS ON RRT

Principles of Management

The goal of controlling hypertension in dialysis patients is to reduce overall cardiovascular morbidity and mortality. For the general population, the guidelines of the sixth report of the Joint National Committee on Prevention, Detection, Evaluation, and Treatment of High Blood Pressure (JNC VI) define *hypertension* as blood pressure greater than 140/90 mm Hg, a blood pressure level below 120/80 mm Hg being considered as optimal control.[84] Unlike in the general population with hypertension, there are insuffi-

Table 58–1 Candidates for Initial Drug Therapy of Hypertension in Patients on Renal Replacement Therapy

	ACE Inhibitors	α$_1$-Adrenergic Antagonists	Angiotensin II Receptor Antagonists	β$_1$-Adrenergic Antagonists	Calcium Antagonists
Peripheral vascular resistance	Decrease	Decrease	Decrease	Decrease	Decrease
Target organ function					
Heart rate, cardiac output	No change	May increase	No change	Decrease	Class-specific
Cerebral function	Preserve	Preserve	Preserve	Preserve	Preserve
Renin-angiotensin-aldosterone					
Plasma renin activity	Increase	No change	Increase	Decrease	No change
Plasma angiotensin II	Decrease	No change	Increase	Decrease	No change
Plasma aldosterone	Decrease/no change	No change	Decrease/no change	Decrease/no change	No change
Sympathetic activity	No change/decrease	Decrease	No change/decrease	Decrease	No change
Concurrent disease efficacy					
Coronary disease	No effect	No effect	No effect	Benefit	Benefit
Peripheral vascular disease	No effect	No effect	No effect	May aggravate	May benefit
Obstructive airway disease	No effect	No effect	No effect	May aggravate	No effect
Diabetes mellitus	May benefit	No effect	May benefit	May aggravate	May benefit
Dyslipidemia	No effect	Benefit	No effect	May aggravate	No effect
Systolic dysfunction	Benefit	No effect	Benefit	May benefit	?Effect

Abbreviation: ACE, angiotensin-converting enzyme.

cient data to define the blood pressure level at which antihypertensive drug therapy should begin in patients on RRT. Likewise, the goal blood pressure that reduces cardiovascular mortality in dialysis patients has yet to be defined by evidence-based medicine. Lifestyle modifications, such as restriction of salt intake (4 g of sodium/day), weight reduction, increased physical activity, and moderation of alcohol intake, should be recommended in association with a sustained effort to achieve and maintain "dry weight."

Role of Extracellular Volume

To address the issue of blood pressure control, it may be helpful at the outset to divide dialysis patients, based on the effect of ultrafiltration on their blood pressure, into volume-responsive and volume-unresponsive groups. In almost half of dialysis patients, blood pressure responds to volume control by ultrafiltration. This may be especially true of African Americans and diabetic patients.

Chronic volume overload tends to occur for several reasons. Loss of lean body mass may go unrecognized and, if the target dry weight remains unadjusted, volume overload may occur. *Dry weight* has traditionally been defined as the weight at which edema and overt signs of pulmonary venous congestion are absent and/or the weight that optimizes postdialysis blood pressure without concomitant symptomatic postural hypotension or clinical fluid overload.[85] More stringent criteria define dry weight as the weight at which blood pressure is controlled throughout the interdialysis period without the use of antihypertensive medications.[86] Objective methods used to estimate or measure volume status in dialysis patients, such as body plethysmography, blood volume measurements, or measurements of plasma atrial natriuretic peptide concentrations, have shown promise but have not found widespread clinical application. Atrial natriuretic peptide measurements have, however, provided insight into the relationship of volume and hypertension in HD patients; elevations in predialysis atrial natriuretic peptide levels that decline after fluid removal are present in hypertensive dialysis patients.[87, 88]

In addition to changes in lean body mass, excessive fluid and salt ingestion can cause chronic volume overload. Slow and gradual ultrafiltration by prolonged (24 hours a week) HD has been shown to improve blood pressure control;[89] a more recent study has shown that short dialysis sessions with efficient HD treatment are highly effective in blood pressure control.[90] In patients with large interdialytic weight gain or associated cardiac complications making fluid removal difficult, programmed stepwise reduction of dialysate sodium concentration during HD may lead to improved postdialysis blood pressure and decrease antihypertensive drug requirements.[91]

Blood pressure control may be better in patients receiving PD owing to smooth and gradual ultrafiltration.[92] In addition to improved volume control, loss of vasopressor molecules in the PD effluent may also contribute to blood pressure control.[93] The observed improvement in blood pressure control in PD vs. HD may only be temporary. Loss of ultrafiltration due to peritoneal membrane failure may result in fluid overload, making hypertension difficult to control. However, limited data are available on the prevalence of hypertension in patients comparing low with high transporters.

Although control of plasma volume generally improves blood pressure in dialysis patients, there is no direct relationship between interdialytic weight gain and blood pressure.[94, 95] In nonnephrectomized dialysis patients, factors other than volume may be operative in the regulation of blood pressure. When blood pressure fails to improve or even rises after ultrafiltration, a volume-independent form of hypertension should be suspected. This occurs in almost 30% of patients and often requires initiation of drug therapy.

Antihypertensive Drug Therapy

When volume control through ultrafiltration is ineffective, other therapeutic measures will be necessary. The pharmacological treatment of hypertension should be based on at least three principles. First and foremost, agents should be selected that oppose the mechanism of hypertension believed to predominate in an individual patient. This may be difficult to determine in many cases, however. Second, specific agents can be selected that modify known comorbid factors observed in this patient population. Patients on RRT have multiple comorbidities, including ischemic heart disease, hyperlipidemia, diabetes mellitus, left ventricular dysfunction, and peripheral vascular disease. The choice of antihypertensive medication for patients on RRT should address these associated comorbid factors (Table 58–1). In patients with systolic dysfunction, angiotensin-converting enzyme inhibitors may be especially beneficial. However, major anaphylactoid reactions have been reported with the use of angiotensin-converting enzyme inhibitors in patients being dialyzed with acrylonitrile 69 dialyzers.[96] In patients with diastolic dysfunction, nondihydropyridine calcium antagonists may be beneficial. β-Adrenergic antagonists may be helpful in dialysis patients with associated ischemic heart disease. Calcium antagonists are also attractive in this group of patients and in dialysis patients with peripheral vascular disease. Finally, hyperlipidemic patients may benefit from use of α_1-adrenergic antagonists. Although all of these antihypertensive regimens have unique benefits for the patient receiving RRT, adverse effects are also common. Combination drug therapies may also be beneficial. A rational scheme for combination therapy is given in Table 58–2. Unfortunately, few well-controlled studies in dialysis patients address these concepts. If patients remain

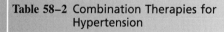

Table 58–2 Combination Therapies for Hypertension

Addition of the following agents after volume control via ultrafiltration
  ACE inhibitor
  β_1-Adrenergic antagonist
  α_1-Adrenergic antagonist
  Angiotensin II type I receptor antagonist
Classic triple-drug therapy
  Volume control via ultrafiltration
  β_1-Adrenergic antagonist
  Direct-acting vasodilator
ACE inhibitor plus calcium antagonist
β_1-Adrenergic antagonist plus α_1-adrenergic antagonist
β_1-Adrenergic antagonist plus dihydropyridine calcium antagonist

Abbreviation: ACE, angiotensin-converting enzyme.

hypertensive despite achieving dry weight on maximal anti-hypertensive treatment, careful investigation of the cause of this resistance is necessary. Patient adherence (dietary and drug) should be assured. Use of other drugs that blunt the efficacy of antihypertensive agents, such as nonsteroidal antiinflammatory drugs, cold remedies, amphetamines, and cocaine, should be determined. Secondary causes of hypertension may need to be ruled out.

Finally, since dialysis therapy may alter the pharmacological profile of a particular antihypertensive agent, selection should take into account drug metabolism and/or clearance on dialysis. For example, the properties of a particular drug as well as the dialyzer may affect final drug levels. Molecular weight, protein binding, volume of distribution,[97, 98] and water solubility of a particular drug also help determine final drug levels. In HD, material and surface area[99] of the dialysis membrane, along with the blood flow rate,[100] will affect dialyzability of a particular drug. In PD, dialysate flow rate, solute concentration, and pH may affect drug clearance.[101] Thus, both the pharmacokinetic and the pharmacodynamic profile of a drug may be affected by dialysis (Table 58–3).

Table 58–3 Pharmacokinetic Properties of Antihypertensive Agents in Patients With End-Stage Renal Disease

	Half-Life (hr)		Dose Change With ESRD	Removal With Dialysis	
	Normal	*ESRD*		*Hemodialysis*	*Peritoneal*
α-ADRENERGIC ANTAGONISTS					
Doxazosin	22		None	None	Unlikely
Prazosin	2–4		None	None	Unlikely
Terazosin	12		None	None	Unlikely
β-ADRENERGIC ANTAGONISTS					
Acebutolol	3–4	Prolonged	30–50%	Yes	?
Atenolol	6–7	Prolonged	25%	Yes	None
Bisoprolol	9–12	Prolonged	25%	Yes	None
Betaxolol	14–22	Prolonged	50%	Yes	?
Carteolol	5–6	Prolonged	25%	?	?
Labetalol	3–4		None	?	?
Carvedilol	7–10		None	None	?
Propranolol-LA	10		None	None	Unlikely
Propranolol	3–4		None	None	Unlikely
Metoprolol tartrate	3–7		None	Yes	?
Metoprolol succinate	3–7		None	Yes	?
Nadolol	20–24	Prolonged	25%	Yes	None
Pindolol	3–4		None	Unlikely	Unlikely
Timolol	3–4		None	None	None
Penbutolol	5		None	Unlikely	Unlikely
ANGIOTENSIN II TYPE 1 RECEPTOR ANTAGONISTS					
Irbesartan	11–15		No	?	?
Losartan	4–6		No	None	?
Valsartan	6		No	None	?
Candesartan	9–12		No	?	?
VASODILATORS					
Hydralazine	3–7	Prolonged	None	None	None
Minoxidil	4		None	Yes	Yes
ACE INHIBITORS					
Benazepril	10–11	Prolonged	25–50%	Unlikely	Unlikely
Captopril	2	Prolonged	50%	Yes	None
Enalapril	11	Prolonged	50%	Yes	None
Fosinopril	12		None	Yes	None
Moexipril	2–9	Prolonged	25–50%	?	?
Lisinopril	12	Prolonged	25–50%	Yes	?
Quinapril	25	Prolonged	25–50%	?	?
Ramipril	13–17	Prolonged	25–50%	Yes	None
Trandolapril	16–24	Prolonged	50%	?	?
CALCIUM ANTAGONISTS					
Amlodipine	30–50		None	None	Unlikely
Diltiazem	4–6		None	None	Unlikely
Felodipine	11–16		None	None	Unlikely
Isradipine	8		None	None	Unlikely
Nicardipine	8–9		None	None	Unlikely
Nifedipine	2		None	None	Unlikely
Nisoldipine	7–12		None	None	Unlikely
Verapamil	4–12		None	None	Unlikely

Abbreviations: ESRD, end-stage renal disease; LA, long-acting; ACE, angiotensin-converting enzyme.

CONCLUSION

Hypertension is a significant and widely prevalent problem in the dialysis population. It is multifactorial in cause, but volume overload is a major pathophysiological mechanism in many cases. The relationship between hypertension and risk of cardiovascular disease is controversial. High blood pressure is a significant risk factor in dialysis patients before the onset of cardiac failure, after which low blood pressure becomes the single greatest predictor of cardiac death. The target blood pressure in this population remains undefined. Although ambulatory blood pressure recordings correlate best with target organ damage, logistical and cost factors preclude their general use. Patients on PD may have somewhat better blood pressure control early, but with progressive loss of residual function, the initial blood pressure response may be lost. In addition to control of extracellular fluid volume, adjunctive antihypertensive therapy is often required in the management of these patients. Therapy should be tailored to each patient's associated comorbidities. Long-term prospective trials are needed to address the multiple remaining "myths" in our understanding of hypertension in patients receiving RRT.

References

1. Rostand SG, Kirk KA, Rutsky EA. Relationship of coronary risk factors in hemodialysis associated ischemic heart disease. Kidney Int 22:304–308, 1982.
2. Degoulet P, Legrain M, Reach I, et al. Mortality risk factors in patients treated by chronic hemodialysis: Report of the Diaphane collaborative study. Nephron 31:103–110, 1982.
3. Fernandez JM, Carbonell ME, Mazzuchi N, Petruccelli D. Simultaneous analysis of morbidity and mortality factors in chronic hemodialysis patients. Kidney Int 41:1029–1034, 1992.
4. Foley RN, Parfrey PS, Harnett JD, et al. Impact of hypertension on cardiomyopathy, morbidity and mortality in end-stage renal disease. Kidney Int 49:1379–1385, 1996.
5. Silzberg JS, Barre PE, Prichard SS, Sniderman AD. Impact of left ventricular hypertrophy on survival in end-stage renal disease. Kidney Int 36:286–290, 1989.
6. MacMahon S, Peto R, Cutler J, et al. Blood pressure, stroke, and coronary heart disease. Part I: Prolonged differences in blood pressure: Prospective observational studies corrected for the regression dilution bias. Lancet 335:765–774, 1990.
7. Cruickshank JM, Thorn JM, Zacharias FJ. Benefits and potential harm of lowering high blood pressure. Lancet 1:581–584, 1987.
8. Stassen J, Amery A, Fagard R. Isolated systolic hypertension in the elderly. J Hypertens 8:393–405, 1990.
9. Neaton JD, Wentworth D. Serum cholesterol, blood pressure, cigarette smoking, and death from coronary artery disease. Overall findings and differences by age for 316,099 white men. Arch Intern Med 152:56–64, 1992.
10. Vokonas PS, Kannel WB, Cupples LA. Epidemiology and risk of hypertension in the elderly: The Framingham Study. J Hypertens 6(suppl 1):S3–S9, 1988.
11. Neaton JD, Kuller LH, Wentworth D, Borhani NO. Total and cardiovascular mortality in relation to cigarette smoking, serum cholesterol concentration, and diastolic blood pressure among black and white males followed up for five years. Am Heart J 108:759–769, 1984.
12. Neaton JD, Wentworth D, Sherwin R, et al. Comparison of 10 year coronary and cerebrovascular disease mortality rates by hypertensive status for black and non-black men screened in The Multiple Risk Factor Interventions Trial (MRFIT). [Abstract] Circulation 80(suppl II):II-300, 1989.
13. Mitchell BD, Stern MP, Haffner SM, et al. Risk factors for cardiovascular mortality in Mexican Americans and non-Hispanic whites. San Antonio Heart Study. Am J Epidemiol 131:423–433, 1996.
14. Haffner SM, Morales PA, Hazunda HP, Stern MP. Level of control

15. Yano K, McGee D, Reed DM. The impact of elevated blood pressure upon 10-year mortality among Japanese men in Hawaii. The Honolulu Heart Program. J Chronic Dis 36:569–579, 1983.
16. Kannel WB, Cupples LA, D'Agostino RB, Stokes J III. Hypertension, antihypertensive treatment and sudden coronary death. The Framingham Study. Hypertension II(suppl II):II-45–II-50, 1988.
17. Strandberg TE, Solomaa VV, Naukkarinein VA, et al. Long-term mortality after 5-year multifactorial primary prevention of cardiovascular disease in middle-aged men. JAMA 266:1225–1229, 1991.
18. Clausen J, Jensen G. Blood pressure and mortality: An epidemiological survey with 10 years follow-up. J Hum Hypertens 6:53–59, 1992.
19. Buckalew VM Jr, Berg RL, Wang Shin-Ru, et al, and the MDRD Study Group. Prevalence of hypertension in 1,795 subjects with chronic renal disease. The Modification of Diet in Renal Disease Study baseline cohort. Am J Kidney Dis 28:811–821, 1996.
20. Faubert PF, Porush JG. Managing hypertension in chronic renal disease. Geriatrics 42:49–58, 1987.
21. HCFA—1995. 1995 Annual Report. ESRD Core Indicators project. Opportunities to Improve Care for Adult In-Center Hemodialysis Patients. Baltimore, Health Care Financing Administration, U.S. Department of Health and Human Services, January 1996.
22. Rocco MV, Flanigan MJ, Beaver S, et al. Report from the 1995 Core Indicators for Peritoneal Dialysis Study Group. Am J Kidney Dis 30:165, 1997.
23. Cheigh JS, Milite C, Sullivan JF, et al. Hypertension is not adequately controlled in hemodialysis patients. Am J Kidney Dis 5:453–459, 1992.
24. Salem MM, Bower JR. Hypertension in the hemodialysis population: Any relation to one year survival? Am J Kidney Dis 28:737–740, 1996.
25. U.S. Renal Data System: Causes of death. Am J Kidney Dis 30:S107–S117, 1997.
26. Disney APS (ed): ANZDATA Report 1996. Adelaide, South Australia, Australia and New Zealand Dialysis and Transplant Registry, 1996.
27. Annual Report 1996, vol 1: Dialysis and Renal Transplantation, Canadian Organ Replacement Register. Don Mills, Ontario, Canadian Institute for Health Information, 1996.
28. Raine AEG, Margreiter R, Brunner FP, et al. Report on management of renal failure in Europe XXII, 1991. Nephrol Dial Transplant Suppl 2:7–35, 1992.
29. An overview of regular dialysis treatment in Japan (as of December 31, 1994). Tokyo, Japanese Society for Dialysis Therapy, 1995.
30. National Heart, Lung, and Blood Institute. Fact Book Fiscal Year 1996. Bethesda, MD, U.S. Department of Health and Human Servicecs, National Institutes of Health, 1997.
31. Joint National Committee on Prevention, Detection, Evaluation, and Treatment of High Blood Pressure. The sixth report. Arch Intern Med 157:2413–2446, 1997.
32. U.S. Renal Data System. Causes of death. Am J Kidney Dis 32(suppl 1):S81–S88, 1998.
33. Greaves S, Sharpe D. Cardiovascular disease in patients with end-stage renal failure. Aust N Z J Med 22:153–158, 1992.
34. Duranti E, Imperiali P, Sasdelli M. Is hypertension a mortality risk factor in dialysis? Kidney Int 49(suppl 55):S173–174, 1996.
35. U.S. Renal Data System. 1992 Annual Report. IV: Comorbid conditions and correlations with mortality risk among 3,399 incident hemodialysis patients. Am J Kidney Dis 20(suppl 2):S32–S38, 1992.
36. Lowrie EG, Lew NL. Death risk in hemodialysis patients: The predictive value of commonly measured variables and an evaluation of death rate differences between facilities. Am J Kidney Dis 15:458–490, 1990.
37. Tomita J, Kimura G, Inoue T, et al. Role of systolic blood pressure in determining prognosis of hemodialyzed patients. Am J Kidney Dis 25:405–412, 1995.
38. Charra B, Calemard E, Ruffet M, et al. Survival as an index of adequacy of dialysis. Kidney Int 41:1286–1291, 1992.
39. Neff MS, Eiser AR, Slifkin RF, et al. Patients surviving 10 years of dialysis. Am J Med 74:996–1004, 1983.
40. Collins AJ, Hanson G, Umen A, et al. Changing risk factor demographics in end-stage renal disease patients entering hemodialysis and the impact on long-term mortality. Am J Kidney Dis 15:422–432, 1990.

of hypertension in Mexican Americans and non-Hispanic whites. Hypertension 21:83–88, 1993.

41. Ritz E, Koch M. Morbidity and mortality due to hypertension in patients with renal failure. Am J Kidney Dis 21(suppl 2):113–118, 1993.

42. Charra B, Calemard E, Laurent G. Importance of treatment time and blood pressure control in achieving long-term survival in dialysis. Am J Nephrol 16:35–44, 1996.

43. Owen WF, Madore F, Brenner BM. An observational study of cardiovascular characteristics of long-term end-stage renal disease survivors. Am J Kidney Dis 28:931–936, 1996.

44. Parfrey PS, Foley RN, Harnet JD, et al. Outcome and risk factors of ischemic heart disease in chronic uremia. Kidney Int 49:1428–1434, 1996.

45. Rodby RA, Vonesh EF, Korbet SM. Blood pressures in hemodialysis and peritoneal dialysis using ambulatory blood pressure monitoring. Am J Kidney Dis 23:401–411, 1994.

46. Conlon PJ, Walshe JJ, Heinle SK, et al. Predialysis systolic blood pressure correlates strongly with mean 24 hour systolic blood pressure and left ventricular mass in stable hemodialysis patients. J Am Soc Nephrol 7:2658–2663, 1996.

47. Kooman JP, Gladziwa U, Bocker G, et al. Blood pressure during the interdialytic period in hemodialysis patients: Estimation of representative blood pressure values. Nephrol Dial Transplant 7:197–923, 1992.

48. Saldanha LF, Weiler EW, Gonick HC. Effects of continuous ambulatory peritoneal dialysis on blood pressure control. Am J Kidney Dis 21:184–188, 1993.

49. Young M, Nolph K, Dutton S, Prowant BF. Antihypertensive drug requirements in continuous ambulatory peritoneal dialysis. Perit Dial Bull 4:85–88, 1984.

50. Stablien DM, Hamburger RJ, Lindblad AS, et al. The effect of CAPD on hypertension control: A report of the national CAPD registry. Perit Dial Int 8:141–144, 1988.

51. Faller B, Lameire N. Evolution of clinical parameters and peritoneal function in a cohort of CAPD patients followed over 7 years. Nephrol Dial Transplant 9:280–286, 1994.

52. de Leeuw PW. Pathophysiology of hypertension in patients in renal replacement therapy. Blood Purif 12:245–251, 1994.

53. Brown JJ, Durterdieck GO, Fraser R, et al. Hypertension and chronic renal failure. Br Med Bull 27:128–135, 1971.

54. Ledingham JM. Blood pressure regulation in renal failure. J R Coll Physicians 5:103–110, 1971.

55. Davies DL, Schalekamp MA, Beevers DG, et al. Abnormal relation between exchangeable sodium and the renin-angiotensin system in malignant hypertension and in hypertension with chronic renal failure. Lancet 1:683–686, 1973.

56. Thomson GE, Waterhouse K, McDonald HP, Friedman EA. Hemodialysis for chronic failure. Arch Intern Med 120:153–167, 1967.

57. Camgiano JL, Ramirez-Muzo O, Ramirez-Gonzales R, et al. Normal renin uremic hypertension. Study of cardiac hemodynamics, plasma volume, extracellular fluid volume, and the renin-angiotensin system. Arch Intern Med 136:17–23, 1976.

58. Kim KE, Onesti G, Schwartz AB, et al. Hemodynamics of hypertension in chronic end-stage renal disease. Circulation 46:456–464, 1972.

59. Tuckman J, Benninger JL, Reubi F. Haemodynamic and blood volume studies in long-term haemodialysis patients and in patients with successfully transplanted kidneys. Clin Sci Mod Med 45(suppl 1):155–157, 1973.

60. Neff MS, Kim KE, Persoff M, et al. Hemodynamics of uremic anemia. Circulation 43:876–883, 1971.

61. Safar ME, London GM, Weisis YA, Milliez PL. Overhydration and renin in hypertensive patients with terminal renal failure: A hemodynamic study. Clin Nephrol 5:183–188, 1975.

62. Leenen FHH, Galla SJ, Geyskes GG, et al. Effects of hemodialysis and saline loading on blood fluid compartments, plasma renin activity and blood pressure in patients on chronic hemodialysis. Nephron 18:93–100, 1977.

63. Beretta-Piccoli C, Weidmann P, DeChatel R, Reubi F. Hypertension associated with early stage kidney disease. Complementary roles of circulating renin, the body sodium/volume state and duration of hypertension. Am J Med 61:739–747, 1976.

64. Weidman P, Beretta-Piccoli C, Steffen F, et al. Hypertension in terminal renal failure. Kidney Int 9:294–301, 1976.

65. DePlunque BA, Mulder E, Dorhout Mess EJ: The behavior of blood and extracellular volume in hypertensive patients with renal insufficiency. Acta Med Scand 186:75–81, 1969.

66. Boer P, Koomans HA, Dorhourt Mess EJ. Renin and blood volume in chronic renal failure: A comparison with essential hypertension. Nephron 45:7–15, 1987.

67. Wilkinson R, Scott D, Uldall P, et al. Plasma renin and exchangeable sodium in the hypertension of chronic renal failure: The effect of bilateral nephrectomy. Q J Med 39:377–394, 1970.

68. Schultze G, Piefke S, Molzahn M. Blood pressure in terminal renal failure: Fluid spaces and the renin-angiotensin system. Nephron 25:15–24, 1980.

69. Lifschitz MD, Kirschenbaun MA, Rosenblatt SG, Gibner R. Effect of saralasin in hypertensive patients on chronic hemodialysis. Ann Intern Med 88:23–27, 1978.

70. Vaughn ED, Carey RM, Ayers CR, Peach MJ. Hemodialysis-resistant hypertension: Control with an orally active inhibitor of angiotensin-converting enzyme. J Clin Endocrinol Metab 48:869–871, 1979.

71. Mimran A, Shelden S, Barjon T, Mion C. The effect of angiotensin antagonist (saralasin) on arterial pressure and plasma aldosterone in hemodialysis-resistant hypertensive patients. Clin Nephrol 9:63–67, 1978.

72. McGrath BP, Ledingham JGG, Benedict CR. Catecholamines in peripheral venous plasma in patients on chronic hemodialysis. Clin Sci Mol Med 55:89–96, 1978.

73. Kobayashi K, Miura Y, Tomioka H, et al. Plasma catecholamine and dopamine-beta-hydroxylase activity in chronic renal failure. Clin Chim Acta 95:317–323, 1979.

74. Campese VM, Romoff MS, Levitan D, et al. Mechanisms of autonomic nervous system dysfunction in anemia. Kidney Int 20:246–253, 1981.

75. Schohn D, Weidmann P, John H, Beretta-Piccoli C. Noripinephrine-related mechanisms in hypertension accompanying renal failure. Kidney Int 28:814–822, 1985.

76. Yokokama K, Mankus R, Saklayen MG, et al. Increased nitric oxide production in patients with hypotension during hemodialysis. Ann Intern Med 123:35–37, 1995.

77. Beasley D, Brenner BM. Role of nitric oxide in hemodialysis hypotension. Kidney Int 42(suppl 38):96–106, 1992.

78. Amore A, Bonaudo R, Ghigo D, et al. Enhanced production of nitric oxide by blood-dialysis membrane interaction. J Am Soc Nephrol 6:1278–1283, 1995.

79. Vallare P, Leons A, Calver A, et al. Accumulation of an endogenous inhibitor of nitric oxide synthesis in chronic renal failure. Lancet 339:575–575, 1992.

80. Madore F, Prud'homme L, Austin JS, et al. Impact of nitric oxide in blood pressure in hemodialysis patients. Am J Kidney Dis 30:665–671, 1997.

81. Boero R, Guarena C, Berto IM, et al. Erythrocyte Na,K pump activity and arterial hypertension in uremic dialyzed patients. Kidney Int 34:691–696, 1988.

82. Izumo H, Izumo S, DeLuke M, Flier J. Erythrocyte Na,K pump in uremia. Acute correction of transport defect by hemodialysis. J Clin Invest 74:581–588, 1984.

83. Campese VM. Calcium, parathyroid hormone, and blood pressure. Am J Hypertens 2:345–445, 1981.

84. Joint National Committee on Prevention, Detection, Evaluation, and Treatment of High Blood Pressure. The sixth annual report. N.I.H. Publication No. 98-4080. Bethesda, MD, National Institutes of Health, 1997.

85. Abraham PA, Opsahl JA, Keshaviah PR, et al. Body fluid spaces and blood pressure in hemodialysis patients during amelioration of anemia with erythropoietin. Am J Kidney Dis 16:438, 1990.

86. Charra B, Laurent G, Chazot C, et al. Clinical assessment of dry weight. Nephrol Dial Transplant 11(suppl 2):S16–S19, 1996.

87. Fishbane S, Natke E, Maesaka JK. Role of volume overload in dialysis refractory hypertension. Am J Kidney Dis 28:257, 1996.

88. Lins RL, Elseviers M, Rogiers P, et al. Importance of volume factors in dialysis related hypertension. Clin Nephrol 48:29, 1997.

89. Chazot C, Charra B, Laurent G, et al. Interdialysis blood pressure control by long hemodialysis sessions. Nephrol Dial Transplant 10:831, 1995.

90. Velasquez MT, von Albertini B, Lew SQ, et al. Equal levels of blood pressure control in ESRD patients receiving high efficiency hemodialysis and conventional hemodialysis. Am J Kidney Dis 31:618–623, 1998.

91. Flanigan MJ, Khairullah QT, Lim VS. Dialysate sodium delivery can alter chronic blood pressure measurement. Am J Kidney Dis 29:383, 1997.

92. Hamburger RJ, Christ PG, Morris PA, Luft FC. Hypertension in dialysis patients: Does CAPD provide an advantage? Adv Perit Dial 5:91, 1989.
93. Weiler EW, Saldanha LF, Khalil-Manesh F, et al. Relationship of NA-K-ATPase inhibitors to blood pressure regulation in continuous ambulatory peritoneal dialysis and hemodialysis. J Am Soc Nephrol 7:454–463, 996.
94. Salem MM, Davis M. Effects of one year of hemodialysis on weight and blood pressure in 434 patients. Artif Organs 21:402–404, 1996.
95. Sherman RA, Daniel A, Cody RP. The effect of interdialytic weight gain on predialysis blood pressure. Artif Organs 17:770–774, 1993.
96. Brunet P, Jaber K, Berland Y, Baz M. Anaphylactoid reactions during hemodialysis and hemofiltration: Role of associating AN69

membrane and angiotensin I converting enzyme inhibition. Am J Kidney Dis 19:444, 1992.
97. Keller F, Wilms H, Schultze G, et al. Effect of plasma protein binding, volume of distribution and molecular weight on the fraction of drugs eliminated by hemodialysis. Clin Nephrol 19:201–205, 1983.
98. Lee CS, Marbury TC. Drug therapy in patients undergoing haemodialysis. Clinical pharmacokinetic considerations. Clin Pharmacokinet 9:42–66, 1984.
99. Surian M, Malberti F, Corradi B, et al. Adequacy of haemodiafiltration. Nephrol Dial Transplant 4:32–36, 1984.
100. Maher JF. Principles of dialysis and dialysis of drugs. Am J Med 62:475–481, 1977.
101. Golper TA. Drugs and peritoneal dialysis. Dial Transplant 8:41–43, 1979.

CHAPTER 59 Ischemic Heart Disease

Hal L. Chadow, Alan Feit, and Shahrokh Rafii

It is estimated that 13.5 million people in the United States have ischemic heart disease (IHD), with 1.5 million new cases diagnosed each year. IHD remains the leading cause of mortality in the United States today, resulting in approximately 500,000 deaths annually. Hypertension (HTN) and left ventricular hypertrophy (LVH) are major risk factors for cardiovascular disease.[1] HTN accelerates the onset and progression of atherosclerosis, and LVH aggravates the ischemic effects of obstructive coronary artery disease (CAD). The incidence of IHD increases with increasing blood pressure (BP). Other major risk factors for CAD include diabetes mellitus, hypercholesterolemia, cigarette smoking, and family history. The incidence of cardiovascular events is greater than would be predicted by the combined presence of HTN with diabetes mellitus or hypercholesterolemia, or both. Primary and secondary risk factor reduction, including effective treatment and control of BP, together with significant strides in the treatment of patients with IHD, have resulted in significant reductions in morbidity and mortality. In this chapter, we review the evaluation and management of the hypertensive patient with IHD.

NONINVASIVE CLINICAL EVALUATION

Clinical History

Physicians have long sought the ideal modality with which to diagnose patients with CAD and to predict prognosis. A thorough history is essential in identifying patients with, or at risk for, IHD and should include the list of modifiable risk factors for CAD. A history of IHD, including prior myocardial infarction(s) (MI), should be elicited. In a cohort of patients from the Multiple Risk Factor Intervention Trial (MRFIT) with a prior MI and elevated systolic BP, the cumulative risk of death from IHD, as well as all-cause mortality at 15 years of follow-up, was approximately 40% higher in men with a systolic BP of 140 mm Hg or higher.[2] The frequency, intensity, and duration of anginal

symptoms, including the patient's Canadian Cardiovascular Society (CCS) class of anginal symptoms,* should also be recorded. However, it should be recognized that silent ischemia is present in 2 to 4% of the general population, as well as 20% of patients after an MI, and these patients have an increased risk of recurrent cardiac events. Similarly, a history of congestive heart failure (CHF) is associated with an increased risk of cardiovascular death.

Electrocardiogram

The electrocardiogram (ECG) lacks the ability to diagnose LVH accurately in the majority of hypertensive patients. The ECG has a sensitivity of 25 to 50% with a specificity of 95% for the diagnosis of LVH.

The ECG is helpful in the diagnosis of acute MI. In addition, it can be used to predict in-hospital complications and the long-term prognosis of these patients. Sinus tachycardia on the initial ECG is the most powerful independent predictor of prognosis. Furthermore, the sum of the absolute ST segment deviation (both ST elevation and ST depression), ECG evidence of a prior MI, and QRS duration (especially with anterior infarctions) can also be used to identify patients with an increased mortality after an acute MI.[3] Similarly, the extent of ST segment resolution after thrombolytic therapy has been shown to correlate with mortality.[4] Transient or persistent ST segment depression on an ECG is also associated with an increased mortality in patients who had a prior MI.[5]

Echocardiography

Echocardiography remains the gold standard for the clinical diagnosis of LVH. In addition, echocardiography can be

---

*Class 1 patients have symptoms provoked only by strenuous or prolonged exertion. Class 2 patients develop symptoms during activities of daily living, such as climbing stairs, walking in cold weather, or emotional stress. Class 3 patients develop symptoms on minimal exertion. Class 4 patients experience angina at rest.

utilized to evaluate changes in left ventricular mass in response to antihypertensive medications.

Echocardiography is also capable of detecting myocardial ischemia by assessing regional wall motion. Ischemic myocardium may appear hypokinetic, whereas an infarcted zone appears akinetic and may exhibit loss of diastolic wall thickness. Echocardiography is also able to measure with accuracy ejection fraction and pulmonary artery systolic pressure, which is of greatest importance in the evaluation of patients with a recent MI or CHF, or both. In addition, the mechanical complications of an MI, including ventricular septal defect, severe mitral regurgitation secondary to papillary muscle ischemia, aneurysm or pseudoaneurysm formation, and apical thrombus can all be detected by echocardiography.

Exercise Stress Testing

Exercise stress testing has long been utilized to evaluate patients with known or suspected CAD and to predict the risk of future cardiac events. Exercise-induced ST segment depression, change in systolic BP with exercise, and exercise capacity have all been shown to predict future risk of cardiovascular death.[6] However, the sensitivity of an exercise ECG alone for the diagnosis of significant CAD as documented by coronary angiography has been reported to be 50 to 70%, with a specificity of 70 to 90%.[7] In addition, the presence of an abnormal resting ECG precludes a confident assessment of the ST segment response to exercise, as in the case of LVH, bundle branch block, and baseline ST-T abnormalities. Therefore, echocardiography or nuclear imaging techniques such as thallium scintigraphy are utilized in conjunction with an exercise ECG in the presence of an abnormal resting ECG, when a previous exercise ECG alone has been inconclusive or when the patient was unable to reach 85% of her or his maximal predicted heart rate.

Compared with an exercise ECG alone, the sensitivity of thallium scintigraphy is 68 to 96%, with a specificity of 65 to 100% for the diagnosis of significant CAD. Dobutamine echocardiography has a sensitivity and specificity similar to that of exercise thallium scintigraphy. Dobutamine echocardiography and thallium scintigraphy are also able to assess the viability of a previously infarcted area, which can aid the physician in making treatment decisions about revascularization. The risk of future cardiac events can be predicted from either modality. To illustrate this, a patient with multiple reperfusable defects on thallium scintigraphy, cavitary dilatation with exercise, or lung uptake of the isotope consistent with pulmonary congestion is more likely to have significant multivessel CAD and higher cardiac event rates. Similarly, patients with normal thallium scans have a low risk of recurrent cardiac events.

A fair number of patients are unable to exercise because of comorbid conditions such as severe pulmonary disease, peripheral vascular disease, previous stroke, or disabling arthritis. In such patients, dipyridamole (Persantine thallium) or dobutamine echocardiography may be employed.

CORONARY ANGIOGRAPHY

Coronary angiography remains the gold standard for the accurate diagnosis of CAD. It is utilized to decide on the optimal treatment strategy: medical therapy, percutaneous transluminal coronary angioplasty (PTCA), or coronary artery bypass graft (CABG) surgery. However, the risks associated with an invasive procedure in addition to cost constraints prevent the use of coronary angiography in all patients with suspected CAD. Furthermore, coronary angiography is inadequate to predict the site of a subsequent MI. It has been shown that the infarct-related artery is usually only mildly to moderately narrowed on the angiogram performed weeks to years before the index event. Therefore, the reader is referred to the detailed published guidelines for the performance of coronary angiography.[8]

Coronary angiography is generally performed in asymptomatic patients or patients presenting with atypical chest pain who have evidence of ischemia on noninvasive testing. Patients with atypical chest pain should be referred for coronary angiography if the results of noninvasive testing are equivocal or in the presence of persistent symptoms despite negative ECG or stress imaging studies, in which the presence or absence of CAD is necessary to guide appropriate therapy. Patients with severe left ventricular dysfunction should similarly be referred for coronary angiography to exclude an ischemic cause, as noninvasive imaging techniques, including stress thallium and dobutamine echocardiography, are unreliable in differentiating an ischemic cardiomyopathy from idiopathic cardiomyopathy. Revascularization can improve symptoms and prognosis of patients with ischemic cardiomyopathy.

Symptomatic patients at high risk for recurrent events should be referred for coronary angiography. This includes patients with an MI complicated by cardiogenic shock, CHF, severe mitral regurgitation, or ventricular septal defect causing heart failure, shock, postinfarction angina, or sustained ventricular arrhythmia, as well as patients presenting with unstable angina or non–Q-wave MI. Likewise, coronary angiography should be performed when anginal symptoms are not adequately controlled with medical therapy or recur after treatment with PTCA or CABG.

REVASCULARIZATION

After coronary angiography has been performed, a decision regarding the optimal treatment strategy, taking into account the risk:benefit ratio as well as comorbid conditions, can be made. The reader is referred to detailed guidelines published for PTCA and CABG.[9, 10] Increasing data support the use of coronary revascularization over medical therapy in selected patients with CAD (Fig. 59–1).

Percutaneous Transluminal Coronary Angioplasty

Since the first coronary angioplasty was performed by Andreas Grüntzig in September 1977, the technology and

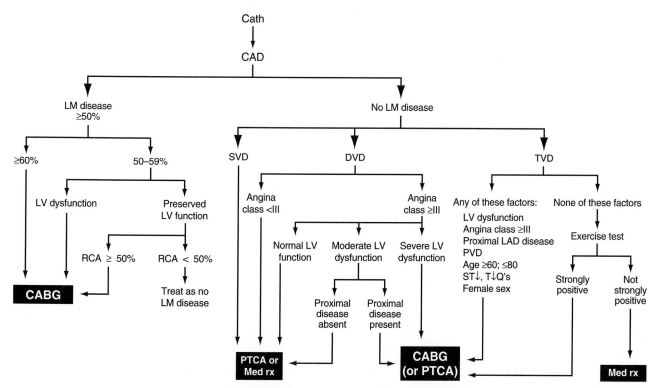

Figure 59–1. Algorithm for the selection of patients for revascularization. Coronary artery disease (CAD) is considered clinically important if the left main (LM) disease is of at least 50% severity or disease elsewhere is of at least 70% severity. Cath, cardiac catheterization; CABG, coronary artery bypass graft; LV, left ventricular; SVD, single-vessel disease; DVD, double (two)–vessel disease; TVD, triple (three)–vessel disease; PTCA, percutaneous transluminal coronary angioplasty; RCA, right coronary artery; Med rx, medical therapy; LAD, left anterior descending artery; PVD, peripheral vascular disease; ST, ST segment depression; T Q's, T-wave inversion and Q-waves in the baseline ECG. (From Nwasokwa ON, Koss JH, Friedman GH, et al. Bypass surgery for chronic stable angina: Predictors of survival benefit and strategy for patient selection. Ann Intern Med 114:1035, 1991.)

applications of PTCA have rapidly grown. It is the most common method of revascularization in patients with CAD today. It is estimated that approximately 1 million angioplasty procedures are performed annually. The ratio of PTCA:CABG is currently 3:2. As the technology has continued to improve and expand to include new devices, the ability to treat a greater number of patients with more complex lesions, resulting in better acute and long-term outcomes, has likewise grown. As a result, the indications for PTCA have expanded.

PTCA is currently the method of choice for the revascularization of appropriate patients with single-vessel disease as well as patients with double-vessel CAD and no significant left ventricular systolic dysfunction. Compared with medical therapy, PTCA results in less angina, improved exercise capacity, and the need for fewer antianginal medications with no difference in mortality or subsequent MI.[11] For selected nondiabetic patients with triple-vessel CAD and preserved left ventricular systolic function, several large clinical trials have shown that PTCA and CABG result in equivalent survival and freedom from MI. However, patients initially treated with CABG had less angina, required fewer repeat revascularization procedures, and were on less antianginal therapy.[12, 13]

Diabetic patients are known to have a higher incidence of recurrent cardiovascular events after revascularization procedures. Data from two large clinical trials have suggested that diabetic patients with triple-vessel CAD have a higher mortality with PTCA than with CABG.[14, 15] This risk appears to be greater in insulin-requiring diabetic patients. Therefore, extreme caution should be exercised in recommending interventional procedures in these patients. As a result, the majority of these patients are currently being treated with bypass surgery.

PTCA continues to have severe limitations and complications, including re-stenosis in 20 to 49% of patients, acute vessel closure in 4 to 8%, emergency CABG in 1 to 3%, nonfatal MI in 4%, and death in less than 1%. The decision to perform PTCA—which includes balloon angioplasty, directional and rotational atherectomy, coronary stents, laser devices, and extraction catheters—is based on several clinical and anatomical factors. Clinical factors associated with a worse outcome include advanced age, HTN, higher CCS class, unstable angina, diabetes mellitus, CHF, and previous PTCA. Anatomical factors include lesion severity and length, vessel size, proximal tortuosity, severity of distal disease, presence of thrombus, angulation of the vessel at the site of stenosis, and the presence of side branches at the site of dilatation, which increases the risk of side branch occlusion, bifurcation lesions, ostial lesions, and chronic total occlusions. All of these factors influence the degree of risk involved in the procedure. Patients deemed to be at high risk for recurrent cardiac events after PTCA should be considered for alternative forms of therapy, although this is not always feasible. Procedural maneuvers or adjunctive pharmacological therapy, or both, may be required to minimize the risk for these patients.

Coronary Artery Bypass Graft Surgery

Since the introduction of CABG in 1968, its use continues to grow with improved surgical techniques. CABG confers a survival advantage over medical therapy in patients with significant left main vessel disease, triple-vessel CAD with reduced left ventricular systolic function, double-vessel CAD with a proximal left anterior descending artery stenosis, or left ventricular aneurysm with heart failure symptoms.[16] In these patients, CABG is the method of choice for revascularization. In most other patient subsets, there is little or no survival advantage, and CABG is utilized for symptom relief in patients with unfavorable anatomy for PTCA.

CABG has been shown to be very effective in reducing myocardial ischemia and relieving anginal symptoms in most patients. However, its use is limited by perioperative complications, prolonged convalescence, and bypass graft failure, with 50% of saphenous vein grafts occluded at 10 years. Antiplatelet or anticoagulant therapy, or both, has not proved to be beneficial in maintaining saphenous vein graft patency. On the other hand, the internal mammary artery has a 90% patency rate at 10 years. Its use as a bypass conduit has resulted in a significant improvement in survival over saphenous vein grafts,[17] and therefore it is widely utilized in bypass operations.

MEDICAL THERAPY

Medical therapy for the hypertensive patient with IHD is aimed at lowering BP, reducing myocardial ischemia, alleviating anginal symptoms, and preventing recurrent cardiovascular events, regardless of whether the patient undergoes a revascularization procedure.

β-Blockers

β-Blockers without intrinsic sympathomimetic activity (ISA) are the single most important class of drugs in the treatment of patients with IHD. They exert their beneficial effects by decreasing heart rate, blood pressure, and contractility, with the net effect of decreasing myocardial oxygen demand. As primary preventive therapy, β-blockers have been shown to decrease total and cardiovascular mortality in hypertensive patients.[18] They can improve survival after an MI, limit infarct size, and reduce the risk for subsequent MI and the incidence of sudden cardiac death.[19] β-Blockers also improve symptoms and exercise capacity and decrease mortality in patients with CHF secondary to systolic dysfunction.[20] However, heart failure symptoms must first be controlled with angiotensin-converting enzyme (ACE) inhibitors and diuretics before initiation of β-blocker therapy, as β-blockers have a propensity for exacerbating symptoms of heart failure. Therefore, in the absence of contraindications, β-blockers should be a mainstay of therapy for patients with HTN and IHD.

Calcium Channel Blockers

If anginal symptoms or BP, or both, are not controlled on β-blockers, calcium channel blockers can be employed. Reports have suggested that short-acting calcium channel blockers can increase overall mortality in patients with CAD. However, studies with long-acting calcium channel blockers failed to support this claim, even in patients with a prior history of an MI.[21] Long-acting calcium channel blockers result in more stable plasma levels of drug levels and decrease the incidence of both silent and symptomatic ischemic episodes over a 24-hour period. BP control is more stable with the long-acting than with the short-acting calcium channel blockers. In patients with a non–Q-wave MI, diltiazem has been shown to decrease the incidence of postinfarction angina, early reinfarction, and death. However, the use of verapamil, diltiazem, and nifedipine should be avoided in patients with an acute MI, in the presence of CHF or severe left ventricular dysfunction.

Second-generation dihydropyridines (amlodipine, felodipine) are available for the treatment of HTN and angina. These agents reduce the incidence of ischemic events in patients with IHD and exert no significant negative inotropic or chronotropic effect on the heart. In the Prospective Randomized Amlodipine Survival Evaluation (PRAISE) study, amlodipine did not increase cardiovascular morbidity or mortality in patients with severely reduced systolic function.[22] Amlodipine can be used safely in these patients to control angina and HTN. Mibefradil, the first selective T-channel calcium channel blocker, was recently approved for the treatment of patients with HTN and angina. Its use is also being evaluated for symptomatic patients with moderate to severe heart failure in the Mibefradil in Patients with Congestive Heart Failure (MACH-1) trial, designed to evaluate whether the addition of mibefradil to standard therapy will reduce mortality.

β-Blockers and calcium channel blockers are frequently used in combination with other antianginal medications and are generally well tolerated. However, significant bradycardia, heart block, and hypotension have been reported in 10 to 15% of patients on verapamil and a β-blocker. Therefore, extreme caution should be exercised when using this combination. Similar concerns have been raised for mibefradil.

Antiplatelet Agents and Anticoagulants

Aspirin has long been shown to reduce the risk of major cardiovascular events in patients with IHD. In the Second International Study of Infarct Survival (ISIS-2), which evaluated the efficacy of aspirin given in the first 24 hours of an acute MI, aspirin had an impact on survival comparable to that of streptokinase, with a 23% reduction in mortality. The addition of aspirin to streptokinase resulted in a 45% reduction in mortality. In addition, aspirin reduced the incidence of nonfatal reinfarction by almost 50%.[23] In terms of absolute risk reduction, treating 1000 patients with an acute MI for 1 month prevents 38 fatal and nonfatal vascular events. The risk of MI and death has similarly been reduced in patients presenting with an acute coronary syndrome (unstable angina, non–Q-wave MI) by as much as 64% at 3 months and 48% at 1 year. Therefore, aspirin should be administered to every patient with IHD in the absence of contraindications.

Patients allergic to aspirin may be treated with ticlopidine or clopidogrel, antiplatelet agents that inhibit adenosine diphosphate–induced platelet aggregation. In the Studio della Ticlopidina nell' Angina Instabile (STAI) trial, ticlopidine reduced the incidence of MI and death by 53% at 6 months in patients presenting with unstable angina.[24] Clopidogrel has been shown to reduce the combined risk of MI, ischemic stroke, and vascular death compared with aspirin in patients with atherosclerotic vascular disease.[25]

A significant number of patients admitted with an acute coronary syndrome continue to have recurrent cardiac events for months after discharge, despite treatment with aspirin and heparin during the acute phase. This is due, in part, to activation of the coagulation system for months after the acute event, as well as reactivation of the coagulation system after unfractionated heparin has been discontinued. Therefore, prolonged treatment with anticoagulants such as low-molecular-weight heparin (LMWH) for several weeks after the acute event, in addition to aspirin, has the potential to decrease the risk of MI and death during this vulnerable time period. LMWH is an attractive option because it can be administered subcutaneously and does not require monitoring of the partial thromboplastin time. The significant reduction in risk of MI and death, as well as the feasibility of this strategy, has been confirmed in several clinical trials.[26]

Glycoprotein IIb/IIIa inhibitors, which inhibit the final common pathway of platelet activation and aggregation, have been evaluated in patients admitted with an acute coronary syndrome. They have also been shown to significantly lower the incidence of MI and death.[27] In an effort to sustain this benefit, oral glycoprotein IIb/IIIa inhibitors are currently being evaluated in clinical trials.

Nitrates

Topical and oral nitrates have long been a mainstay of therapy for patients with IHD, as they reduce the number of ischemic events. However, nitrates do not affect mortality or the incidence of MI in these patients. Care should be taken to ensure that patients have a daily nitrate-free interval to avoid the development of tolerance.

ACE Inhibitors

Large clinical trials have documented the benefit of ACE inhibitors in reducing cardiovascular morbidity and mortality in patients with severely reduced systolic function and large MIs.[28, 29] Whether ACE inhibitors have similar beneficial effects for patients with CAD and preserved systolic function is a matter under intense investigation. An ACE inhibitor should be a part of the medical regimen for the hypertensive patient with IHD who has CHF or an MI with severely reduced systolic function. In patients who are unable to tolerate, or have contraindications to an ACE inhibitor, an angiotensin II receptor antagonist can be substituted.[30]

ALTERNATIVE THERAPIES

Many patients with significant CAD are not candidates for revascularization because of unfavorable coronary anatomy and have significant anginal symptoms despite medical therapy. For these patients, there are currently two alternatives. The first is enhanced external counterpulsation. This consists of three sets of balloons wrapped around the calves and the lower and upper thighs, including the buttocks, that are inflated sequentially during diastole to improve coronary perfusion and increase cardiac output. After therapy, patients have noted significant improvement in their anginal symptoms, improved exercise capacity, and resolution or decrease in the area(s) of ischemia as judged by thallium scintigraphy.

The second alternative is transmyocardial revascularization. In this procedure, which is performed through a lateral thoracotomy, multiple small channels between the left ventricle and the ischemic myocardium are created using either a carbon dioxide or holmium:yttrium-aluminum-garnet laser system. The goal is to provide direct perfusion to the ischemic myocardium. The initial results appear promising, with a significant improvement in anginal symptoms accompanied by a reduction in ischemic wall motion abnormalities and hospital admissions. Clinical trials are now under way utilizing a percutaneous laser system.

SECONDARY PREVENTION

Modification of the known risk factors for CAD, including HTN, diabetes mellitus, hyperlipidemia, and smoking, has been shown to lower cardiovascular morbidity and mortality. In addition, family history, obesity, physical inactivity, homocysteinemia, alcohol consumption, and psychological conditions are important risk factors for cardiovascular disease. Identification of those risk factors present in each patient and implementation of an aggressive treatment strategy aimed at slowing the progression of CAD and preventing recurrent cardiovascular events are the goals of secondary prevention.

Hypertension

It is estimated that 50 million Americans have HTN, and the incidence increases with age. According to the third National Health and Nutrition Examination Survey (NHANES III), the strides made since the mid-1960s have been replaced with a trend toward slightly lower patient awareness, treatment, and control of high blood pressure.[31] This has happened despite the abundance of evidence linking HTN to the risk of CAD, MI, cerebrovascular disease, CHF, and sudden death. Even patients with borderline isolated systolic HTN have a greater risk of morbidity and mortality from cardiovascular disease than do normotensive patients.[32]

The treatment of HTN results in a 12% reduction in all-cause mortality, a 36% reduction in stroke mortality, a 25% reduction in fatal coronary events, a 35% reduction in nonfatal stroke, and a 15% reduction in nonfatal coronary events.[33] Therefore, control of high BP is essential in the secondary prevention of cardiovascular disease. Medical therapy for HTN is discussed in Section 5 of this text, Treatment—General Considerations, and is not reviewed here. However, the presence of other risk factors or comorbid conditions that can be adversely affected by certain antihypertensive medications needs to be considered when initiating medical therapy. For example, treatment with thiazide diuretics and β-blockers without ISA can have unfavorable effects on the lipid profile. In addition, β-blockers should be used cautiously in patients with asthma or emphysema. However, this should not discourage the use of these medications in appropriate patients. In the Systolic Hypertension in the Elderly Program (SHEP), diuretics reduced the incidence of cardiovascular and cerebrovascular events, even in patients with elevated lipid levels.[34] Likewise, β-blockers have a proven track record in the secondary prevention of cardiovascular events in patients with IHD.[19]

Hyperlipidemia

The importance of high cholesterol levels as a risk factor for cardiovascular disease and the benefit of cholesterol reduction in the secondary prevention of cardiovascular events have been well documented.[35] Reducing serum cholesterol levels by 10% has been shown to translate into a 20% reduction in mortality from coronary heart disease.[36] However, the mechanism(s) responsible for this benefit is not fully understood. Angiographic studies failed to show a significant change in the degree of stenosis in response to lipid-lowering therapy. However, lipid-lowering treatment does result in improved endothelium-dependent vasomotion in the coronary arteries of patients with atherosclerosis. The addition of an antioxidant such as probucol has been shown to further improve endothelial dysfunction. Moreover, lipid-lowering therapy may promote plaque stabilization by decreasing the accumulation of cholesterol in the atheromatous plaque or by reducing cholesterol content in an existing plaque, or both. This is accomplished by a process known as *reverse cholesterol transport,* whereby high-density lipoprotein (HDL) particles carry cholesterol away from the atherosclerotic plaque to the liver.[37] This may, in part, explain the beneficial effects of raising HDL cholesterol, independent of low-density lipoprotein (LDL)-cholesterol levels.

According to the National Cholesterol Education Program (NCEP) guidelines for the evaluation and treatment of patients with hyperlipidemia, lipid-lowering therapy should be initiated in patients with CAD when the LDL-cholesterol is greater than 130 mg/dl, and should always accompany a low-cholesterol diet (NCEP step 1 or 2).[38] The goal of therapy is to achieve an LDL-cholesterol of less than 100 mg/dl. More recently, the Cholesterol and Recurrent Events (CARE) trial demonstrated that reducing

average to low LDL-cholesterol levels with pravastatin in patients with CAD resulted in a 24% lower incidence of MI and death from coronary heart disease, and a 31% reduction in the incidence of stroke. The need for coronary angiography, PTCA, or CABG was also decreased.[39]

A low HDL-cholesterol level in patients with CAD is associated with an increased risk of cardiovascular events. Therefore, treatment to raise low HDL-cholesterol levels, including weight loss, exercise, smoking cessation, and medications such as niacin, should accompany therapy aimed at lowering LDL-cholesterol levels.

Diabetes Mellitus

Patients with diabetes mellitus have a higher incidence of CAD than nondiabetic patients, resulting in higher cardiovascular mortality. Several mechanisms work in concert to promote the aggressive atherosclerotic process commonly seen in diabetics. Hyperglycemia induces endothelial dysfunction by inactivating endothelium-derived relaxing factor (EDRF), reducing prostaglandin (PGI_2) synthesis, and increasing endothelin-1 production. Abnormalities in platelet function seen in diabetics include increased adhesiveness and hyperaggregability in response to agonists such as thrombin and epinephrine. Thromboxane A_2 production is also increased, facilitating platelet activation and aggregation. Abnormalities in the coagulation system that promote thrombus formation include increased levels of factor VII and fibrinogen, as well as decreased activity of antithrombin III and plasminogen activator inhibitor-1.[40] Good glycemic control may help correct the hypercoagulable state in diabetic patients.[41] In clinical trials, intensive treatment with insulin delays the onset and slows the progression of diabetic retinopathy, nephropathy, and neuropathy in insulin-requiring diabetic patients.[42] Future trials should address the vital issue of whether intensive therapy will have similar benefits for diabetic patients with CAD, especially those requiring revascularization with PTCA or CABG.

Medical Therapy

The benefit of long-term aspirin therapy in reducing the risk of MI, stroke, and vascular death in patients with documented cardiovascular disease has been shown in several clinical trials. This prompted the U.S. Food and Drug Administration to expand the indications for the use of aspirin therapy to include secondary prevention in all patients with a history of IHD and cerebrovascular disease.[43]

Hormone replacement therapy decreases the risk of cardiovascular disease in postmenopausal women. Treatment results in an improved lipid profile, reduced levels of fibrinogen and antithrombin III, and lower fasting glucose and insulin levels.[44] However, the widespread use of hormone replacement therapy has been limited by the lack of prospective, randomized clinical trials confirming its long-term benefit, coupled with the risk of endometrial and breast cancer. Furthermore, the appropriate duration of therapy is at present unknown. Over the next few years, the results of several large clinical trials designed to address these important issues will emerge.

Antioxidant therapy for secondary prevention in patients with cardiovascular disease has been evaluated in several clinical trials. Vitamin E decreased the incidence of nonfatal MI by 77% and the combined endpoint of nonfatal MI and cardiovascular death by 47% in the Cambridge Heart Antioxidant Study (CHAOS). However, there was a nonsignificant increase in the risk of cardiovascular death in the group treated with vitamin E.[45] Furthermore, an angiographic trial demonstrated the ability of vitamin E to reduce the progression of CAD.[46] Large, randomized clinical trials aimed at evaluating the use of vitamin E, vitamin C, and β-carotene in patients with cardiovascular disease have been initiated. Policy decisions concerning the use of antioxidants in patients with cardiovascular disease should await the results of these trials.

References

1. Kannel WB, Gordon T, Castelli WP, Margolis JR. Electrocardiographic left ventricular hypertrophy and risk of coronary heart disease: The Framingham Study. Ann Intern Med 72:813, 1970.
2. Flack JM, Neaton J, Grimm R, et al. Blood pressure and mortality among men with prior myocardial infarction. Circulation 92:2437, 1995.
3. Hathaway WR, Peterson ED, Wagner, GS, et al. Prognostic significance of the initial electrocardiogram in patients with acute myocardial infarction. JAMA 279:387, 1998.
4. Schroder R, Dissmann R, Bruggemann, et al. Extent of early ST segment resolution: A simple but strong predictor of outcome in patients with acute myocardial infarction. J Am Coll Cardiol 24:384, 1994.
5. Gheorghiade M, Shivkumar K, Schultz L, et al. Prognostic significance of electrocardiographic persistent ST depression in patients with their first myocardial infarction in the placebo arm of the Beta-Blocker Heart Attack Trial. Am Heart J 126:271, 1993.
6. Morrow K, Morris CK, Froelicher VF, et al. Prediction of cardiovascular death in men undergoing noninvasive evaluation for coronary artery disease. Ann Intern Med 118:689, 1993.
7. Gianrossi R, Detrano R, Mulvihill D, et al. Exercise-induced ST depression in the diagnosis of coronary artery disease: A meta-analysis. Circulation 80:87, 1989.
8. Ross J, Brandenburg RO, Dinsmore RE, et al. Guidelines for coronary angiography. A report of the American College of Cardiology/American Heart Association Task Force on Assessment of Diagnostic and Therapeutic Cardiovascular Procedures (Subcommittee on Coronary Angiography). J Am Coll Cardiol 10:935, 1987.
9. Ryan TJ, Bauman WB, Kennedy JW, et al. Guidelines for percutaneous transluminal coronary angioplasty. A report of the American College of Cardiology/American Heart Association Task Force on Assessment of Diagnostic and Therapeutic Cardiovascular Procedures (Subcommittee on Percutaneous Transluminal Coronary Angioplasty). J Am Coll Cardiol 22:2033, 1993.
10. Kirklin JW, Akins CW, Blackstone EH, et al. Guidelines and indications for coronary artery bypass graft surgery. A report of the American College of Cardiology/American Heart Association Task Force on Assessment of Diagnostic and Therapeutic Cardiovascular Procedures (Subcommittee on Coronary Artery Bypass Graft Surgery). J Am Coll Cardiol 17:543, 1991.
11. Parisi AF, Folland ED, Hartigan P, for the Veterans Affairs ACME Investigators. A comparison of angioplasty with medical therapy in the treatment of single vessel coronary artery disease. N Engl J Med 326:10, 1992.
12. King SB III, Lembo NJ, Weintraub WS, et al. A randomized trial comparing angioplasty with coronary bypass surgery: Emory Angioplasty versus Surgery Trial (EAST). N Engl J Med 331:1044, 1994.
13. Hamm CW, Reimers J, Ischinger T, et al. A randomized study of coronary angioplasty compared with bypass surgery in patients with symptomatic multivessel coronary disease. N Engl J Med 331:1037, 1994.
14. The BARI Investigators. Influence of diabetes on 5-year mortality and morbidity in a randomized trial comparing CABG and PTCA in patients with multivessel disease. The Bypass Angioplasty Revascularization Investigation (BARI). Circulation 96:1761, 1997.
15. CABRI Trial Participants. First-year results of CABRI (Coronary Angioplasty versus Bypass Revascularization Investigation). Lancet 346:1179, 1995.
16. Kaiser GC. CABG: Lessons from the randomized trials. Ann Thorac Surg 42:3, 1986.
17. Cameron A, Davis KB, Green G, et al. Coronary bypass surgery with internal thoracic grafts—Effects on survival over a 15-year period. N Engl J Med 334:216, 1996.
18. Wikstrand J, Warnold I, Olsson G, et al. Primary prevention with metroprolol in patients with hypertension: Mortality results from the MAPHY Study. JAMA 259:1976, 1988.
19. Antman E, Lau J, Kupelnick B, et al. A comparison of results of meta-analyses of randomized control trials and recommendations of clinical experts: Treatments for myocardial infarction. JAMA 268:240, 1992.
20. Packer M, Bristow MR, Cohn JN, et al. The effect of carvedilol on morbidity and mortality in patients with chronic heart failure. N Engl J Med 334:1349, 1996.
21. Braun S, Boyko V, Behar S, et al. Calcium antagonists and mortality in patients with coronary artery disease: A cohort study of 11,575 patients. J Am Coll Cardiol 28:7, 1996.
22. Packer M, O'Connor CM, Ghali JK, et al., for the Prospective Randomized Amlodipine Survival Evaluation Study Group. Effect of amlodipine on morbidity and mortality in severe chronic heart failure. N Engl J Med 335:1107, 1996.
23. ISIS-2 (Second International Study of Infarct Survival) Collaborative Group. Randomised trial of intravenous streptokinase, oral aspirin, both, or neither among 17,187 cases of suspected acute myocardial infarction: ISIS-2. Lancet 2:349, 1988.
24. Balsano F, Rizzon P, Violi F, et al. Antiplatelet treatment with ticlodine in unstable angina. A controlled multicenter clinical trial. The Studio della Ticlopidina nell' Angina Instabile Group. Circulation 82:17, 1990.
25. CAPRIE Steering Committee: A randomised, blinded, trial of clopidogrel versus aspirin in patients at risk of ischaemic events (CAPRIE). Lancet 348:1329, 1996.
26. Conti CR. Low molecular weight heparin for acute ischemic heart disease. Clin Cardiol 20:415, 1997.
27. Theroux P, Kouz S, Roy L, et al. Platelet membrane receptor glycoprotein IIb/IIIa antagonism in unstable angina: The Canadian Lamifiban Study. Circulation 94:899, 1996.
28. The SOLVD Investigators. Effects of enalapril on mortality in severe congestive heart failure. N Engl J Med 316:1429, 1987.
29. Pfeffer MA, Braunwald E, Moye LA, et al. Effect of captopril on mortality and morbidity in patients with left ventricular dysfunction after myocardial infarction. Results of the Survival and Ventricular Enlargement Trial. N Engl J Med 327:669, 1992.
30. Pitt B, Segal R, Martinez FA, et al., for the ELITE Study Investigators. Randomised trial of losartan versus captopril in patients over 65 with heart failure (Evaluation of Losartan in the Elderly Study, ELITE). Lancet 349:747, 1997.
31. Burt VL, Whelton P, Roccella EJ, et al. Prevalence of hypertension in the US adult population: Results from the third National Health and Nutrition Examination Survey, 1988–1991. Hypertension 25:305, 1995.
32. Sagie A, Larson MG, Levy D. The natural history of bordeline isolated systolic hypertension. N Engl J Med 329:1912, 1993.
33. Insua JT, Sacks HS, Lau TS, et al. Drug treatment of hypertension in the elderly: A meta-analysis. Ann Intern Med 121:355, 1994.
34. Frost PH, Davis BR, Burlando AJ, et al., for the Systolic Hypertension in the Elderly Research Group. Serum lipids and incidence of coronary heart disease: Findings from the Systolic Hypertension in the Elderly Program (SHEP). Circulation 94:2381, 1996.
35. Scandinavian Simvistatin Survival Study Group. Randomized trial of cholesterol lowering in 4444 patients with coronary heart disease: The Scandinavian Simvistatin Survival Study (4S). Lancet 344:1383, 1994.
36. Law MR, Wald NJ, Thompson SG. By how much and how quickly does reduction in serum cholesterol concentration lower risk of ischaemic heart disease? BMJ 308:367, 1994.
37. Levine GN, Keaney JF Jr, Vita JA. Cholesterol reduction in cardiovascular disease: Clinical benefits and possible mechanism. N Engl J Med 332:512, 1995.

38. Adult Treatment Panel II, National Cholesterol Education Program. Second report of the Expert Panel on Detection, Evaluation, and Treatment of High Blood Cholesterol in Adults. Circulation 89:1333, 1994.
39. Sacks FM, Pfeffer MA, Moye LA, et al. The effect of pravastatin on coronary events after myocardial infarction in patients with average cholesterol levels. N Engl J Med 335:1001, 1996.
40. Aronson D, Bloomgarden Z, Rayfield EJ. Potential mechanisms promoting restenosis in diabetic patients. J Am Coll Cardiol 27:528, 1996.
41. Aoki I, Shimoyama K, Aoki N, et al. Platelet-dependent thrombin generation in patients with diabetes mellitus: Effects of glycemic control on coagulability in diabetes. J Am Coll Cardiol 27:560, 1996.

42. Clark CM Jr, Lee DA. Prevention and treatment of the complications of diabetes mellitus. N Engl J Med 332:1210, 1995.
43. Hennekens CH, Dyken ML, Fuster V. Aspirin as a therapeutic agent in cardiovascular disease. Circulation 96:2751, 1997.
44. Nabulsi AA, Folsom AR, White A, et al. Association of hormone-replacement therapy with various cardiovascular risk factors in postmenopausal women. N Engl J Med 328:1069, 1993.
45. Stephens NG, Parsons A, Schofield PM, et al. Randomised controlled trial of vitamin E in patients with coronary artery disease: Cambridge Heart Antioxidant Study (CHAOS). Lancet 347:781, 1996.
46. Hodis HN, Mack WJ, LaBree L, et al. Serial coronary angiographic evidence that antioxidant vitamin intake reduces progression of coronary artery atherosclerosis. JAMA 273:18491, 1995.

CHAPTER

60 Hypertension in Women

Phyllis August and Suzanne Oparil

Hypertension is a major cause of cardiovascular disease in the United States and an important contributor to cardiovascular morbidity and mortality. Epidemiological, clinical, and experimental evidence indicates that men in the general population have higher diastolic blood pressures than women at all ages and also appear to have a higher prevalence of hypertension overall. Although men have a higher incidence of total cardiovascular endpoints at all ages, hypertensive men and women develop strokes, left ventricular hypertrophy, and renal dysfunction at similar rates.

GENDER DIFFERENCES IN BLOOD PRESSURE

Based on interviews and examinations of 9901 American adults 18 years of age or older, the Third National Health and Nutrition Examination Survey (NHANES III) found that overall mean arterial pressure is higher in both normotensive and hypertensive men than in women (Fig. 60–1).[1] Gender differences in blood pressure emerge during adolescence and persist through adulthood.[2, 3] In all ethnic groups, men tend to have higher mean systolic and diastolic blood pressure than women (by 6 to 7 mm Hg and 3 to 5 mm Hg, respectively), and through middle age, the prevalence of hypertension is higher among men than among women. NHANES III found that hypertension is more prevalent among women than among men after age 59 years. Furthermore, the Community Hypertension Evaluation Clinic (CHEC) Program, which screened 1 million Americans between 1973 and 1975, found that mean diastolic pressure was higher in men than in women at all ages, whereas mean systolic pressure was higher in men than in women

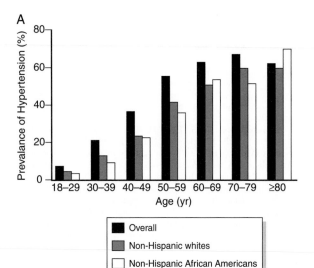

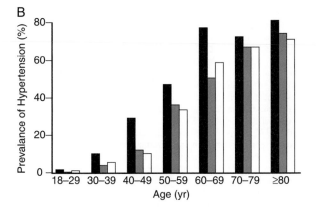

Figure 60–1. Prevalence of high blood pressure by age and race/ethnicity for men **(A)** and women **(B)** in the population of the United States aged 18 years or older. (**A** and **B**, Adapted from Burt VL, Whelton P, Rocella EJ, et al. Prevalence of hypertension in the US adult population: Results of the Third National Health and Nutrition Examination Survey, 1988–1991. Hypertension 25:305–313, 1995.)

until age 50 years for African Americans and age 65 years for whites and was higher in women thereafter.[4] The Hypertension Detection and Follow-up Program (HDFP) Cooperative Group screened 158,906 persons aged 30 to 69 years in 14 communities between 1973 and 1974 and found that hypertension was more prevalent in men than in women of both races.[5]

Whether there is a "crossover" in the relative prevalence of hypertension in men vs. women, with younger men and older women having more hypertension, is a point of controversy: The crossover has been reported in a number of cross-sectional studies[6] but was not apparent in the 30-year longitudinal data from the Framingham Study.[7] Mean systolic blood pressure in older women in Framingham approached that of older men but did not exceed it; mean diastolic blood pressure was lower in women at all ages and declined in both sexes after age 65 years.

The reasons for the gender differences in blood pressure are not known. It has been suggested, but not proved, that estrogen is responsible for the lower blood pressure in younger women. Data on blood pressure fluctuations during the life cycle lend some support to this hypothesis, but the evidence linking changes in blood pressure throughout the life cycle to levels of endogenous sex hormones remains circumstantial. A study of hemodynamic changes associated with the menstrual cycle reported lower blood pressure during the luteal phase compared with the follicular phase.[8] Not all investigators have found lower blood pressure in the luteal phase, and conflicting observations have been made.[9, 10] During normal pregnancy, when both estrogen and progesterone levels are 50 to 100 times higher than prepregnancy levels, blood pressure decreases dramatically. However, the time course of the maximal decrease in blood pressure does not coincide with the maximal rise in hormone levels, suggesting that the relationship between blood pressure and endogenous levels of hormones is complex and likely to be influenced by other factors.[11]

The influence of menopause on blood pressure is also controversial. Longitudinal studies have not documented a rise in blood pressure with menopause.[12–14] In contrast, cross-sectional studies have reported significantly higher systolic and diastolic blood pressures in postmenopausal women.[15, 16] Staessen and colleagues[15] reported a fourfold higher prevalence of hypertension in postmenopausal women than in premenopausal women. After adjusting for age and body mass index, postmenopausal women were still more than twice as likely to have hypertension than premenopausal women. The menopause-related increase in blood pressure described in some studies has been attributed to a variety of factors, including increases in weight, decreases in activity, and increases in alcohol intake. Whether reduced ovarian estrogen production plays a major role in the increase in blood pressure after menopause is controversial. It has now been well documented that exogenously administered estrogens, in the form of 17β-estradiol, promote endothelium-dependent vasodilatation.[17] Furthermore, studies of endothelial function utilizing acetylcholine-induced changes in forearm blood flow demonstrate diminished endothelium-dependent vasodilatation in association with menopause, suggesting a role for estrogen in blood pressure regulation.[18] Clinical studies have shown that estrogen may modulate blood pressure responses to stressful stimuli; postmenopausal women and men demonstrate larger stress-induced increases in blood pressure and higher ambulatory daytime blood pressure than do premenopausal women.[19] However, although postmenopausal women clearly have higher blood pressures than premenopausal women, the age-related increase in blood pressure in women is greatest after the age of 62 years, suggesting that loss of estrogen is not the primary cause.[1] Furthermore, a study from Finland that demonstrated that women who had undergone hysterectomy with ovarian preservation had higher blood pressures than age-matched women who had not undergone hysterectomy[20] highlights the importance of studying factors in addition to estrogen in relation to the pathogenesis of postmenopausal increases in blood pressure.

PATHOPHYSIOLOGY OF PRIMARY HYPERTENSION

Given the heterogeneity of essential hypertension, it is not surprising that few gender-specific pathogenic factors have been identified. Preliminary reports suggest that in premenopausal hypertensive women, resting heart rate, left ventricular ejection time, cardiac index, and pulse pressure are higher compared with age-matched men, and total peripheral resistance and blood volume are lower.[21] Both pre- and postmenopausal hypertensive women have been reported to have, on average, lower plasma renin levels than men.[22] Nordby and coworkers[23] reported lower serum estradiol levels in hypertensive premenopausal women compared with normotensives.

One aspect of hypertension in women that is worthy of emphasis from several different perspectives, including epidemiology, pathogenesis, and treatment, is obesity. Obesity is significantly more common in middle-aged women than in men, and there is evidence that body weight has a greater impact on blood pressure in females than in males.[24] Although the association between obesity and hypertension is firmly established, the mechanisms involved are not well understood. Nevertheless, a significant amount of hypertension in women is attributable to obesity, an observation that underscores the importance of dietary modification and exercise in treatment.

SECONDARY HYPERTENSION IN WOMEN

The causes of secondary hypertension in women are generally the same as in men, and similar considerations with respect to evaluation and treatment are applicable. Parenchymal renal disease should be considered and ruled out with urinalysis and serum creatinine levels. Collagen vascular diseases, such as systemic lupus erythematosis and systemic sclerosis, are more common in women, and the presence of hypertension in patients with these disorders suggests renal involvement. Renovascular hypertension due to fibromuscular dysplasia is primarily a disease of young women. Given the excellent results reported with renal angioplasty,[25] this condition should be ruled out in women under the age of 40 years with moderate to severe hypertension. It is particularly important to diagnose this disorder before pregnancy, since women with renovascular hypertension are more likely to have complicated pregnancies. Similarly, pheochromocytoma, although rare, is associated with considerable maternal morbidity and mortality during pregnancy and should be considered in young hypertensive women, particularly those with characteristic symptoms.

ORAL CONTRACEPTIVE HYPERTENSION

The most important and probably the most frequent form of secondary hypertension in women is that due to exogenous estrogen use, particularly in the form of oral contraceptive pills. A review of data accumulated since the mid-1970s suggests that most women taking oral contraceptives experience a small but detectable increase in both systolic and diastolic blood pressure.[26] The magnitude of the increase appears to vary depending on the population studied as well as on the dose of estrogen and progestin in the preparation. The large Walnut Creek Contraceptive Drug Study, based on data from 11,672 women, demonstrated a pressure elevation of 5 to 6 mm Hg systolic and 1 to 2 mm Hg diastolic in white women, and a lesser rise in African American women.[27] A study conducted in developing countries reported similar average changes after 1 year of oral contraceptive use.[28] However, in some centers, marked elevations (10 mm Hg systolic, 6.9 mm Hg diastolic) were reported.

Hypertension has been reported to be two to three times more common in women taking oral contraceptives than in age-matched women not taking these medications.[29] The risk of contraceptive-induced hypertension increases with age, duration of use, and perhaps with increased body mass. Oral contraceptives currently in use contain lower doses of ethinyl estradiol (30 to 35 μg) than those previously used. Available data suggest that there is a correlation between both estrogen and progestin dose and blood pressure.[26] Thus, the true incidence of oral contraceptive–induced hypertension may be less than that reported by earlier studies. Nevertheless, published data from the Nurses' Health Study[30] suggest that even oral contraceptives with lower doses of estrogen increase the risk of hypertension and that the risk increases with duration of use and with increased progestin potency.

The mechanism of the increase in blood pressure, or of the development of overt hypertension, due to oral contraceptives remains unclear. Increases in body weight, plasma volume, exchangeable sodium, plasma insulin, and insulin resistance, as well as increases in hepatic synthesis of angiotensinogen have been reported to be involved. Experimental evidence favors a role of the renin-angiotensin system in the hypertension induced by estrogen.[31] In a rat model of oral contraceptive hypertension, administration of estrogen alone (ethinyl estradiol) caused hypertension and an increase in angiotensinogen and angiotensin II levels.[32] The hypertension induced by estrogen responded to angiotensin-converting enzyme inhibitor treatment. Progestin administration alone also increased blood pressure, although the elevation in blood pressure was of lesser magnitude, of shorter duration, and associated with increased sodium retention.

In view of the preceding considerations, a prudent approach to oral contraceptive use is to monitor blood pressure at least every 6 months (dispense only 6 months of pills). If blood pressure rises, then a decision to discontinue the pill should be based on the degree of hypertension, the potential hazards of pregnancy, and overall cardiovascular risk profile. Although it is preferable to avoid oral contraceptives in individuals with elevated blood pressure, with careful monitoring of selected individuals, this modality of contraception can be considered when the risks of pregnancy appear greater than the risks of mild hypertension.

HORMONE REPLACEMENT THERAPY AND HYPERTENSION

The effects of hormone replacement therapy (HRT) on blood pressure are not as clearcut as the effects of oral contraceptive pills. Several reports of an association between estrogen therapy and hypertension in postmenopausal women were published in the 1970s and 1980s,[33–36] and until recently, many physicians considered hypertension to be a contraindication to HRT. Measurements of the components of the renin-angiotensin-aldosterone system implicated increased angiotensinogen generation, as well as increased sodium retention in the pathogenesis of HRT-induced hypertension.[37] In fact, estrogen preparations (e.g., Premarin, ethinyl estradiol) that have a greater ability to stimulate hepatic synthesis of angiotensinogen have been shown to raise blood pressure to a greater extent than those preparations that have a modest effect on angiotensinogen (natural estradiol, transdermal estrogen).[38, 39] The effects of synthetic progestins on blood pressure have not been extensively studied in postmenopausal women. However, preliminary evidence suggests that they may contribute to increases in blood pressure owing to increased sodium retention.[40]

Published data, obtained largely from prospective clinical trials, suggest that the risk of hypertension due to HRT is low, and some studies have even documented a decrease in blood pressure in patients treated with HRT.[41–43] The Postmenopausal Estrogen/Progestin Interventions (PEPI) trial evaluated cardiovascular risk factors in 875 normotensive postmenopausal women aged 45 to 64 years randomly assigned to treatment with a variety of different regimens of HRT. At 3 years of follow-up, there were no differences in systolic or diastolic blood pressure in any of the treatment groups compared with the placebo group. The patients in this clinical trial were normotensive to start, and it is not known whether hypertensive women would be more likely to develop increases in blood pressure while taking HRT. A prospective study of 75 hypertensive women treated with HRT failed to demonstrate an increase in blood pressure after 12 months of follow-up,[44] but data on larger numbers of patients are needed to determine whether HRT is a risk factor for blood pressure elevation in hypertensive postmenopausal women. A concern with respect to the existing data is that reporting mean changes in blood pressure in a population may mask individuals who have a blood pressure increase with HRT. In fact, a study of ambulatory blood pressure monitoring in normotensive women receiving either transdermal estrogen or oral estrogen showed that although the group as a whole did not have a rise in blood pressure, as many as one third of the individuals had a 4-mm Hg increase in diastolic blood pressure after 6 months of therapy.[39]

In summary, currently available data suggest that HRT is an uncommon cause of worsening hypertension in postmenopausal women. However, very few hypertensive subjects have been followed prospectively on HRT; thus, the incidence of HRT-induced increases in blood pressure in individuals with preexisting hypertension is not known. Subtle increases in blood pressure attributable to HRT might be difficult to detect in women already under treatment for hypertension, whose blood pressures may fluctuate with changes in body weight, level of activity, and diet. It is prudent to follow blood pressure closely in hypertensive women receiving HRT and to consider using preparations with minimal effects on hepatic production of angiotensinogen (transdermal estrogen) if blood pressure control becomes difficult.

GENDER ISSUES AND TREATMENT OF HYPERTENSION

Lifestyle Modifications

Analysis of results of the Treatment of Mild Hypertension Study (TOMHS) based on gender suggests that women may be less likely than men to have their blood pressure controlled with lifestyle interventions alone, perhaps because they are less successful in losing weight.[45] Weight reduction is of particular importance in women, given the high prevalence of obesity, particularly in African Americans. Although the effects of weight reduction on blood pressure have not been studied extensively in women, small clinical trials clearly demonstrate the expected benefit.[46] Decreased levels of physical activity have been associated with higher blood pressures in women, but prospective trials of the effects of exercise on blood pressure in women have not been performed. However, given the beneficial effects of exercise on weight control, prevention of osteoporosis, and insulin and glucose metabolism, it is justified to recommend increased activity for hypertensive women in the absence of unstable coronary artery disease.

Dietary recommendations for hypertensive women are similar to those for hypertensive men. Preliminary studies have suggested a greater depressor response to sodium restriction in women than in men.[47] Thus, sodium restriction should be encouraged in women who are likely to be salt sensitive (African Americans, individuals with low plasma renin).

Excessive (>2 to 3 drinks per day) alcohol intake is associated with increases in blood pressure. Thus, all hypertensive women should be advised to limit alcohol intake.

Drug Therapy

The effects of antihypertensive therapy on the cardiovascular complications of hypertension (heart attack, stroke, death) have not been studied separately in women. The large clinical trials of antihypertensive therapy (e.g., HDFP,

Medical Research Council [MRC], Australian Therapeutic Trial) have included variable proportions of women, and since certain subgroups (e.g., younger white women) have a low incidence of cardiovascular complications, there was insufficient power to detect a treatment effect in all groups (reviewed in ref. 48). The HDFP trial did demonstrate a reduction in stoke in all women receiving stepped care treatment; the effects on nonstroke outcomes were less clearcut. Benefits of treatment have been most clearly shown in African American women and elderly women. Analysis of the large clinical trials with respect to mortality in women has yielded conflicting results. The HDFP and MRC trials did not demonstrate a decrease in mortality in the active or stepped care treatment groups, whereas the Australian Therapeutic Trial did. Nevertheless, at present, the evidence is insufficient to warrant less aggressive treatment of hypertension in women, and it should be emphasized that African American women require particularly aggressive treatment. This view is supported by a meta-analysis of the effects of antihypertensive treatment on cardiovascular outcomes in women and men.[49] Antihypertensive treatment clearly reduced the incidence of stroke in women. A reduction in coronary events was not as apparent in women, although the investigators attributed this to lower absolute and relative risk in untreated women.

Side Effects

Adverse effects of antihypertensive medication are a major obstacle to treatment. A growing body of evidence suggests that there may be gender-specific side effect profiles (reviewed in refs. 22 and 45). In TOMHS, in which 902 men and women received nonpharmacological treatment plus treatment with a drug from each class of antihypertensive agent, women reported twice as many side effects as men, although the incidence of side effects in women was similar in placebo- and drug-treated individuals. Biochemical responses to drugs may be gender-dependent: Women are more likely to develop hyponatremia associated with diuretic therapy, whereas men are more likely to develop gout. Hypokalemia is more common in women taking diuretics. Angiotensin-converting enzyme inhibitor–induced cough has been reported to be twice as common in women as in men.[50] The effect of antihypertensive agents on lipid profiles has not been investigated extensively in women, although this is an important consideration with respect to cardiovascular risk. Preliminary evidence suggests that menopausal status may influence the effect of drugs on lipid profiles: High doses of diuretics have been shown to raise total cholesterol in men and postmenopausal women, but not in premenopausal women.[51]

Another area of relevance to drug treatment of hypertension is the effect of antihypertensive therapy on sexual function. This is a major obstacle to successful therapy of hypertension in men, and there is evidence that sexual dysfunction is a problem in hypertensive women as well. However, information regarding sexual dysfunction in women is seldom obtained in clinical trials or in clinical practice. Thus, this is an area clearly in need of further investigation.

SUMMARY

Hypertension is an important cardiovascular risk factor for women. Although younger, premenopausal women have lower blood pressures compared with age-matched men, population blood pressure rises with age, and the prevalence of hypertension is higher in older women. Oral contraceptive use increases the risk of hypertension in women, and women using this therapy should have blood pressure monitored twice yearly. The risk of hypertension is low in normotensive women receiving HRT. Few studies of HRT in hypertensive women have been performed, and more information is needed to assess risk of worsening hypertension in hypertensive postmenopausal women receiving this therapy. Investigations of gender differences in the pathophysiology of hypertension and response to antihypertensive treatment have not been extensively performed, and current evidence does not support gender-specific treatment of hypertension.

References

1. Burt VL, Whelton P, Rocella EJ, et al. Prevalence of hypertension in the US adult population: Results of the Third National Health and Nutrition Examination Survey, 1988–1991. Hypertension 25:305–313, 1995.
2. Himmelmann A, Svensson A, Hansson L. Influence of sex on blood pressure and left ventricular mass in adolescents: The Hypertension in Pregnancy Offspring Study. J. Hum Hypertens 8:485–490, 1994.
3. Yong LC, Kuller LH, Rutan G, Bunker C. Longitudinal study of blood pressure changes and determinants from adolescence to middle age. The Dormont High School Follow-Up Study, 1957–1963 to 1989–1990. Am J Epidemiol 138:973–983, 1993.
4. Stamler J, Stamler R, Riedlinger WF, et al. Hypertension screening of 1 million Americans. Community Hypertension Evaluation Clinic (CHEC) Program, 1973–1975. JAMA 235:2299–2306, 1976.
5. Hypertension Detection and Follow-up Program Cooperative Group. Blood pressure studies in 14 communities: A two-stage screen for hypertension. JAMA 237:2385–2391, 1977.
6. Kotchen JM, MacKean HE, Kotchen TA. Blood pressure trends with aging. Hypertension 4:III-128–III-134, 1982.
7. Vokonas PS, Kannel WB, Cupples LA. Epidemiology and risk of hypertension in the elderly. The Framingham Study. J Hypertens 6:3–9, 1988.
8. Chapman AB, Zamudio S, Woodmansee W, et al. Systemic and renal hemodynamic changes in the luteal phase of the menstrual cycle mimic early pregnancy. Am J Physiol 273:F777–F782, 1997.
9. Dunne FP, Barry DG, Ferriss JB, et al. Changes in blood pressure during the normal menstrual cycle. Clin Sci 81:515–518, 1991.
10. Karpanou EA, Vyssoulis GP, Georgoudi DG, et al. Ambulatory blood pressure changes in the menstrual cycle of hypertensive women. Significance of plasma renin activity values Am J Hypertens 6:654–659, 1993.
11. August P, Lenz T, Ales KL, et al. Longitudinal study of the renin angiotensin system in hypertensive women: Deviations related to the development of superimposed preeclampsia. Am J Obstet Gynecol 163:1612–1621, 1990.
12. Hjortland MC, McNamara PM, Kannel WB. Some atherogenic concomitants of menopause: The Framingham Study. Am J Epidemiol 103:304–311, 1976.
13. Matthews KA, Meilahn E, Kuller LH, et al. Menopause and risk factors for coronary heart disease. N Engl J Med 321:641–646, 1989.
14. Van Berensteyn ECH, Van'T Hof MA, De Waard H. Contributions of ovarian failure and aging to blood pressure in normotensive perimenopausal women: A mixed longitudinal study. Am J Epidemiol 129:947–955, 1989.
15. Staessen J, Bulpitt CJ, Fagard R, et al. The influence of menopause on blood pressure. J Hum Hypertens 3:427–433, 1989.
16. Weiss NS. Relationship of menopause to serum cholesterol and arterial pressure: The United States Health Examination Survey of Adults. Am J Epidemiol 96:237–241, 1972.

17. Lieberman EH, Gerhard MD, Uehata A, et al. Estrogen improves endothelium-dependent flow-mediated vasodilation in postmenopausal women. Ann Intern Med 121:936–941, 1994.
18. Taddei S, Virdis A, Ghiadoni L, et al. Menopause is associated with endothelial dysfunction in women. Hypertension 28:576–582, 1996.
19. Owens JF, Stoney CM, Matthews KA. Menopausal status influences ambulatory blood pressure levels and blood pressure changes during mental stress. Circulation 88:2794–2802, 1993.
20. Luoto R, Kaprio J, Reunanen A, Rutanenen EM. Cardiovascular morbidity in relation to ovarian function after hysterectomy. Obstet Gynecol 85:515–522, 1995.
21. Messerli FH, Baravaglia GE, Schmieder RE, et al. Disparate cardiovascular findings in men and women with essential hypertension. Ann Intern Med 107:158–161, 1987.
22. Lewis CE. Characteristics and treatment of hypertension in women: A review of the literature. Am J Med Sci 311:193–199, 1996.
23. Nordby G, Os I, Kjeldsen SE, Eide I. Mild essential hypertension in nonobese premenopausal women is characterized by low renin. Am J Hypertens 5:579–584, 1992.
24. Chaing BN, Perlman LV, Epstein FH. Overweight and hypertension. Circulation 39:403–421, 1969.
25. Sos TA, Pickering TG, Sniderman K, et al. Percutaneous transluminal renal angioplasty in renovascular hypertension due to atheroma or fibromuscular dysplasia. N Engl J Med 309:274, 1983.
26. Woods JW. Oral contraceptives and hypertension. Hypertension 11 (suppl II):II-11–II-15, 1988.
27. Ramcharan S, Pellegrin FA, Hoag EJ. The occurrence and course of hypertensive disease in users and nonusers of oral contraceptive drugs. In Ramcharan S (ed). The Walnut Creek Contraceptive Drug Study: A Prospective Study of the Side Effects of Oral Contraceptives, vol 2. U.S. Department of Health, Education, and Welfare Publication no. (NIH)76-563. Washington, DC, U.S. Government Printing Office 1976; pp 1–16.
28. WHO Task Force on Oral Contraceptives. The WHO Multicentre Trial of the Vasopressor Effects of Combined Oral Contraceptives. 1: Comparisons with IUD. Contraception 40:129–145, 1989.
29. Royal College of General Practitioners' Oral Contraception Study: Oral contraceptives and health. New York, Pitman, 1974.
30. Chasan-Taber L, Willett WC, Manson JE, et al. Prospective study of oral contraceptives and hypertension among women in the United States. Circulation 94:483–489, 1996.
31. Spellacy WN, Birk SA. The effect of intrauterine devices, oral contraceptives, estrogens, and progestogens on blood pressure. Am J Obstet Gynecol 112:912–919, 1972.
32. Byrne KB, Geraghty DP, Stewart BJ, Burcher E. Effect of contraceptive steroid and analapril treatment on systolic blood pressure and plasma renin-angiotensin in the rat. Clin Exp Hypertens 16:627–657, 1994.
33. Crane MG, Harris JJ, Winsor W III. Hypertension, oral contraceptive agents, and conjugated estrogens. Ann Intern Med 74:13, 1971.
34. Notelovitz M. Effect of natural oestrogens on blood pressure and weight in postmenopausal women. S Afr Med J 49:2251, 1975.
35. Utian WH. Effect of postmenopausal estrogen therapy on diastolic blood pressure and body weight. Maturitas 1:3, 1978.
36. Pfeffer RI. Estrogen use, hypertension and stroke in postmenopausal women. J Chron Dis 31:389–398, 1977.
37. Crane MG, Harris JJ. Estrogens and hypertension: Effect of discontinuing estrogens on blood pressure, exhangeable sodium, and the renin-aldosterone system. Am J Med Sci 276:33–55, 1978.
38. Wren BG, Routledge DA. Blood pressure changes Oestrogens in climacteric women. Med J Aust 2:528–531, 1981.
39. Akkad AA, Halligan AWF, Abrams K, Al-Azzawi F. Differing responses in blood pressure over 24 hours in normotensive women receiving oral or transdermal estrogen replacement therapy. Obstet Gynecol 89:97–103, 1997.
40. Oelkers W, Schoneshofer M, Blumel A. Effects of progesterone and four synthetic progetagens on sodium balance and the renin-aldosterone system in man. J Clin Endocrinol Metab 39:882–890, 1974.
41. Lind T, Cameron EC, Hunter WM, et al. A prospective, controlled trial of six forms of hormone replacement therapy given to postmenopausal women. Br J Obstet Gynaecol 86(suppl 3):1–29, 1979.
42. Elias AN, Meshkinpour H, Valenta LJ. Attenuation of hypertension by conjugated estrogens. Nephron 30:89–92, 1992.
43. PEPI Trial Writing Group. Effects of estrogen or estrogen/progestin

regimens on heart disease risk factors in postmenopausal women. The Postmenopausal Estrogen/Progestin Interventions (PEPI) trial. JAMA 3:199–208, 1995.

44. Lip GYH, Beevers M, Churchill D, Beevers DG: Hormone replacement therapy and blood pressure in hypertensive women. J Hum Hypertens 8:491–494, 1994.

45. Lewis CE, Grandits GA, Flack J, et al. Efficacy and tolerance of antihypertensive treatment in men and women with stage 1 diastolic hypertension. Arch Intern Med 156:377–385, 1996.

46. Kanai H, Tokunaga K, Fujioka S, et al. Decrease in intra-abdominal visceral fat may reduce blood pressure in obese hypertensive women. Hypertension 27:125–129, 1996.

47. Nestel PJ, Clifton PM, Noakes M, et al. Enhanced blood pressure response to dietary salt in elderly women, especially those with small waist:hip ratio. J Hypertens 11:1387–1394, 1993.

48. Anastos K, Charney P, Charon RA, et al. Hypertension in women: What is really known? Ann Intern Med 115:287–293, 1991.

49. Gueyffier F, Boutitie F, Boissel JP, et al. Effect of antihypertensive drug treatment on cardiovascular outcomes in women and men. A meta-analysis of individual patient data from randomized, controlled trials. The INDANA Investigators. Ann Intern Med 126:761–767, 1997.

50. Os I, Bratland B, Dahlof B, et al. Female sex as an important determinant of lisinopril-induced cough. Lancet 339:372, 1992.

51. Boehringer K, Wiedmann P, Mordasini R, et al. Menopause-dependent plasma lipoprotein alterations in diuretic-treated women. Ann Intern Med 97:206–209, 1982.

61 Hypertension in the Elderly

Koshy Abraham and David T. Lowenthal

In the United States, the elderly (aged 65 years and older) represent the most rapidly growing segment of the population. The elderly make up approximately 12% of the U.S. population, but they consume over one third of the health care dollars. These factors have helped to focus attention on hypertension in this population, since this condition is a major contributor to high morbidity and mortality with loss of functional capacity and decline in quality of life in this group.[1] Much attention is now being placed on the epidemiology, pathophysiology, and treatment of hypertension in the elderly.[2] In the elderly, hypertension is the single most potent remediable risk factor for cerebrovascular diseases, coronary artery disease, and congestive heart failure.[3] Heart disease and stroke remain the first and third leading causes of death, respectively, in the United States. The economic, social, and financial burdens placed on Americans (more than $259 billion in direct and indirect costs) for these disorders is a major public health concern,[4] so reducing the morbidity and mortality of cardiovascular disease, i.e., lowering blood pressure, can have an enormous impact on the social and economic climate in the United States.

DEFINITION

The risk of cardiovascular morbidity and mortality is independently related to both systolic blood pressure (SBP) and diastolic blood pressure (DBP). Risk increases in a continuous fashion as SBP or DBP rises, but the increase for each incremental rise in blood pressure becomes more pronounced with advancing age.[5] The sixth report of the Joint National Committee on Detection, Evaluation, and Treatment of High Blood Pressure (JNC VI) developed a useful classification of blood pressure in adults based on the average of two or more readings separated by 2 minutes. These criteria are for individuals who are neither on antihypertensive medications nor who have an acute illness. When the SBP and DBP fall into different categories, the higher category should be selected to classify the individual's blood pressure.[4]

EPIDEMIOLOGY

General Observations

Both SBP and DBP increase with age in the industrialized world. SBP continues to rise until age of 70 or 80 years, whereas DBP rises up to age 50 or 60 years and then levels off or may even decrease slightly. In the U.S. population, the average SBP will rise 5 to 10 mm Hg from age 40 to 70 years, whereas the DBP will increase 5 to 6 mm Hg. Peak blood pressure readings occur at a slightly younger age in men than in women. In African Americans, both SBP and DBP are higher than in whites after age 30 years. Persons with the highest blood pressures at younger ages will have the greatest increases in blood pressure as they get older. An increase in blood pressure is not an inevitable part of aging, however.[6–9] It is likely that environmental factors such as social and cultural habits play a major role. In many elderly individuals, blood pressure readings are normal and even low. Therefore, hypertension is a disease and not a right of passage through age.

Prevalence

The prevalence of hypertension and, in particular, isolated systolic hypertension (ISH) is considerable in the elderly population. As stated before, DBP rises up to age 50 to 60 years, and then levels off, but SBP continues to rise. Data from the Systolic Hypertension in the Elderly Program (SHEP) showed that 8% of those aged 60 to 69 years, 11% of those aged 70 to 79, and 22% of those over the age of 80 years had ISH.[10] There are differences in the prevalence of hypertension related to gender and ethnic group. The third National Health and Nutrition Examination Survey (NHANES III, 1988 to 1991) showed that at ages 65 to 74 years, the prevalence is highest in African Americans (71.8%) compared with non-Hispanic whites (52.9%) and Mexican Americans (54.9%). Men tended to have a higher prevalence than women (56.4% vs. 52.5%). The distribution of people aged 60 years and older with hypertension according to severity (Table 61–1) was 49.6% with stage 1, 18.2% with stage 2, and 6.5% with stage 3 or 4 hypertension. ISH was present in 64.8% of people aged 60 years or older.[11]

Risks

Elevation of both SBP and DBP is an important risk factor for cerebrovascular accidents (CVA), congestive heart failure (CHF), coronary artery disease (CAD), and end-stage renal failure.[12] At the age of 70 years, the risk of cardiovascular disease is three times higher if the SBP is 195 than if it is 105 mm Hg; the risk for CVA is three times higher as the SBP rises from less than 139 to greater than 160 mm Hg.[13] The risk of CHF is six times higher in hypertensives than in normotensives and SBP carries a higher risk for development of CHF than does DBP. This is true for both men and women.[14] In contrast, DBP is more closely related to the development of CAD in people younger than 45 years. After the age of 45, DBP becomes a less important risk factor; after age 60 years, SBP is a greater risk factor for CAD than is DBP.[15] The Chicago Stroke Study examined the risks of stroke in the elderly in relation to both SBP and DBP. SBP was a greater risk factor. Persons with an SBP greater than 179 mm Hg had a 3-year incidence of CVA that was three times greater than in persons with SBP less than 130 mm Hg.[16] The incidence of CVA has been shown to be twice as high in African Americans as in whites in all age groups, even when matched for socioeconomic status.[17]

Data from the Framingham Study showed SBP to be a better predictor of cardiovascular mortality than DBP. The risk associated with SBP increased rapidly with advancing age (Fig. 61–1).[12] The Framingham Study also showed ISH to be a risk factor for cardiovascular mortality. In a 20-year follow-up of men aged 55 to 74 years with ISH, mortality was twice that of normotensive individuals. The risk was 1.8 times greater for men and 4.7 times for women with ISH compared with normotensive individuals.[18] Data

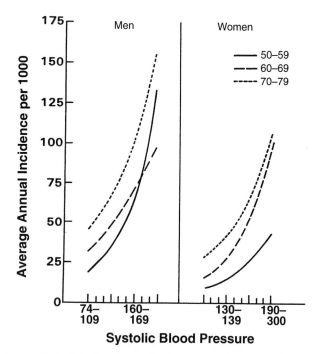

Figure 61–1. Risk of cardiovascular disease according to systolic blood pressure. Persons with diastolic blood pressure of 95 mm Hg or less: the Framingham study. (From Gavras H, Gavras I. Hypertension in the Elderly. Littleton, MA, PSG, 1983.)

from the Hypertension Detection and Follow-Up Program (HDFP) showed that for every 1 mm Hg increase in SBP, there was a 1% increase in mortality.[19]

PHYSIOLOGICAL AND PATHOLOGICAL CHANGES IN AGING

Anatomical/Hemodynamic

Although hypertension is not an inevitable fact of aging, there are cardiovascular changes that accompany aging. Many years ago, Starr and associates showed that there was a decrease in cardiac index of ~8.4 ml/min/m² per year.[20] Brandfonbrener and coworkers showed that there was a linear decrease in cardiac index with advancing age of about 1% per year.[21] If the arterial pressure remains unchanged, a reduction in cardiac output will result in an elevation of total peripheral resistance. This is seen in the normotensive elderly population. There is also a decline in responsiveness of the cardiovascular system to adrenergic stimuli, i.e., exercise, isoproterenol, so that aging confers an inability to appropriately increase heart rate and stroke volume.[22]

As the body ages, collagen becomes increasingly rigid, causing sclerosis and fibrosis of various tissues, including blood vessels, leaflets, and chordae of heart valves. The elastic fibers of the media gradually decrease in number as the collagen matrix increases, reducing the elasticity of the aorta and other arteries. Normally, the aortic wall absorbs the impact of systole and recoil during diastole and maintains pressure in the distal arterial tree, so that the difference between SBP and DBP is small, i.e., a narrow pulse

Table 61–1 Classification of Blood Pressure for Adults Aged 18 Years and Older

Category	Blood Pressure (mm Hg)		
	Systolic		*Diastolic*
Optimal	<120	and	<80
Normal	<130	and	<85
High-normal	130–139	or	85–89
Hypertension			
Stage 1	140–159	or	90–99
Stage 2	160–179	or	100–109
Stage 3	≥180	or	≥110

From Joint National Committee on Prevention, Detection, Evaluation, and Treatment of High Blood Pressure. The Sixth Report. Arch Intern Med 157:2413–2446, 1997.

pressure. With aging, the distensibility of the aortic wall is decreased during systole and the pressure cannot be absorbed by the aortic wall. Similarly, the recoiling ability during diastole is lessened. This causes a widening of the pulse pressure.[12] There is also an acceleration of pulse-wave velocity with aging. As aging stiffens the aorta, the left ventricle continues to eject the same amount of blood at the same rate. This results in the acceleration of blood down the arterial tree. Studies by Weisfeldt showed arterial vasodilating drugs such as nitroprusside can decrease aortic pulse-wave velocity, suggesting that the changes in the aorta are due to alterations in smooth muscle compliance, neurohormonal tone, or arterial wall thickness, or a combination, and not increased fibrosis or atherosclerosis.[23]

With aging, there is a reduction in body size, including a decrease in lean body mass (mostly muscle mass) and total body water, with an increase in fat per unit of body weight. By age 75 years, there is 18% less total body water than at age 30 years. There is a 40% reduction in extracellular fluid volume and a 8% reduction in plasma volume.[12] There is also a reduction in hepatic albumin synthesis and in the configuration of the albumin molecule, resulting in less protein binding. These aging changes have important implications for drug metabolism, particularly for acid organic compounds, resulting in increased levels of free drug available at the tissue/cellular level and increased pharmacodynamic action of the drug. There is also a gradual reduction in blood flow to the liver and kidney and decreased drug clearance. All of these factors may result in increased blood concentrations and increased pharmacological activity of highly water-soluble drugs. Conversely, highly lipid-soluble drugs will have longer pharmacological activity because of the increased volume of distribution and delay in clearance of the drug.[24] The reduction in total body water seen with aging puts the elderly at increased risk of dehydration when excess dosages of diuretics are used for the treatment of hypertension.

Humoral

The renin-angiotensin-aldosterone system becomes hyporesponsive with aging, in part as a result of reduced reactivity of the sympathetic nervous system. Plasma renin activity and levels of angiotensin II and aldosterone decrease with age, but it is not known what effect this has on the pathophysiology of hypertension in the elderly.[25] Plasma renin secretion or activity, or both, is also suppressed in the elderly population in response to sodium depletion,[26] diuretic administration,[27] upright posture,[28] and catecholamine stimulation.[29] Possible explanations for this include age-related thinning of the renal cortex, loss of renal mass, and hyposensitivity to circulating catecholamines. Although the number or density, or both, of β-receptors does not change, the sensitivity of these receptors decreases with aging. The elderly tend to be vulnerable to dehydration and orthostatic hypotension, in part because responses of neurohumoral mechanisms to reductions in effective blood volume are sluggish.[12]

The sympathetic nervous system is also altered with age. Plasma norepinephrine levels increase with age: The average level at age 70 years is twice that at age 20 (0.400

Table 61–2. Influences of Aging on Cardiac Structure and Function

MICROSCOPIC
Increased fat
Increased collagen
Increased lipofuscin
Increased amyloid
Decreased myocyte numbers
Increased myocyte size

ANATOMICAL
Increased aortic diameter
Increased left atrial dimension
Increased left ventricular cavity diameter
Annular calcification of mitral and aortic valve
Thickened aortic wall
Elongated aorta

PHYSIOLOGICAL
Myocyte
Decreased rate of relaxation
Decreased β-receptor sensitivity
Decreased inotropic response to cardiac glycosides
Increased duration of contraction

Left Ventricle
Normal systolic function (ejection fraction)
Decreased compliance
Abnormal diastolic filling (impaired early filling and enhanced filling with atrial contraction)

Aorta
Decreased elasticity
Increased systolic blood pressure
Increased pulse velocity

vs. 0.200 ng/ml, respectively). This does not result in a sustained hyperadrenergic state, since there is a decrease in β-receptor sensitivity as well as in α-receptor responsiveness in the elderly. There is also a decrease in concentration of catecholamines in the myocardium that, in conjunction with anatomical changes related to aging (Table 61–2), may explain the decreased myocardial contractility seen in the aged.[29] The mechanism of the elevation in norepinephrine levels in the elderly may relate to reduced hepatic clearance of these neurohormones as a person ages,[30] as well as to a compensatory response to the decreased sensitivity of adrenergic receptors.[12]

DIAGNOSIS AND CLINICAL ASSESSMENT

When evaluating the elderly hypertensive patient, there are three factors to consider: determining an accurate blood pressure, assessing for target organ damage, and evaluating for underlying conditions that may be responsible for the elevation in blood pressure. Blood pressure should be taken as the average of two or more readings with the patient seated comfortably. The first Korotkoff sound auscultated (phase I) represents the SBP, and the disappearance of sound (phase V) represents the DBP. One must avoid the auscultatory gap, which is seen more often in the elderly and may lead to the underestimation of SBP by as much as 50 mm Hg.[31] In order to avoid this, inflate the cuff to 250 mm Hg or more and deflate slowly. The measurement should be repeated with the patient supine and after 1 and

5 minutes standing. The diagnosis of hypertension can be made only after an average blood pressure of 140/90 mm Hg or greater is recorded on three successive visits. Initially, seated readings should be taken in both arms to rule out inaccurate measures due to local vascular/thrombotic disease.

Pseudohypertension is a falsely elevated blood pressure reading obtained with a blood pressure cuff while an intraarterial catheter reveals a normal blood pressure. This phenomenon is seen in thickened or calcified arteries that are not easily compressed by the blood pressure cuff. The Osler maneuver—in which the cuff is inflated above the SBP and the brachial or radial artery pulses, which should be obliterated, are still palpable—is helpful in diagnosing pseudohypertension.[32]

It is also important to check for orthostatic hypotension in the elderly. This condition is common in the elderly, and many of the prescribed antihypertensive treatments, i.e., sodium restriction and diuretics, may cause or exacerbate it. Medications such as tricyclic antidepressants, α-blockers, sedatives, and levodopa may contribute as well. This can be disabling and may have catastrophic consequences, such as a fall or a head injury.

The assessment of the hypertensive elderly patient should include several laboratory tests, including a hemogram, blood chemistry profile (serum creatinine, potassium, uric acid, and cholesterol), electrocardiogram, and urinalysis, looking for evidence of renal parenchymal diseases and vascular damage associated with diabetes mellitus. These tests are helpful in stratifying patients into risk groups and identifying important comorbid conditions (see under Pharmacological Therapy). The clinician should also rule out secondary causes of hypertension, even in the elderly.

EVIDENCE OF EFFICACY OF ANTIHYPERTENSIVE THERAPY

The benefits of treating hypertension in the elderly clearly outweigh the potential risks or adverse effects. The Veterans Administration Cooperative Study on Antihypertensive Agents was a multicenter double-blind placebo-controlled trial in men younger than age 75 years. The patients were treated with thiazides, reserpine, and hydralazine in sequence with a follow-up of 3.3 years. This study found a reduction in CVAs and CHF, but not CAD. Of the patients 60 years or older, morbid cardiovascular events occurred in 28.9% of the treatment group and 62.8% of the control group. ISH was not evaluated in this study.[33] The HDFP was another randomized clinical trial, with a duration of 5 years. A total of 2376 patients between ages 60 and 69 years were studied. This trial compared the efficacy of treatment in special care programs (stepped care) versus treatment in communities with existing patterns of care (referred care). Only 54% of referred care patients received antihypertensive therapy. In the stepped care patients with mild hypertension, there was a 17.2% reduction in overall mortality. Once again, ISH was not addressed specifically.[34]

The European Working Party on High Blood Pressure in the Elderly was a randomized trial in 840 patients older than 60 years. The treatment group received thiazide and triamterene, with methyldopa added if needed. There was

an 8-year follow-up with no reduction in overall mortality, but a 27% reduction in cardiovascular mortality. Again, ISH was not addressed.[35]

The Swedish Trial in Old Patients with Hypertension (STOP-Hypertension) evaluated 70- to 84-year-old patients. Three β-blockers and a thiazide diuretic were used in the treatment group, with a total of 1627 patients being randomized. At all ages studied, there was a reduction in CHF and CVAs in the treated group. Patients with ISH were excluded from this study.[36]

The Medical Research Council Trial of Treatment of Hypertension in Older Adults evaluated patients aged 65 to 74 years with a follow-up of 5 years. A total of 4396 patients entered the randomized, placebo-controlled single-blind study. The drug regimen consisted of either a β-blocker or a thiazide diuretic plus amiloride. When compared with placebo, the actively treated group had a 25% reduction in CVA, a 19% reduction in coronary events, and a 17% reduction in all cardiovascular events. Again, ISH was not specifically examined.[37]

MacMahon and Rodgers reviewed five of the randomized trials of treatment of hypertension in the elderly using meta-analysis (Fig. 61–2). Combining the results of these trials, the incidence of CVA was reduced by 34% and the incidence of CAD by 19%. None of these trials specifically addressed ISH.[38]

Before 1991, when the final results of the SHEP were published, studies had shown that treating diastolic hypertension had beneficial effects on cardiovascular morbidity and mortality.[39] Epidemiological studies had shown that ISH is a very important risk factor for cardiovascular disease, but no trials had been undertaken to test the benefits of treating this condition. SHEP was a double-blind randomized placebo-controlled trial of the treatment of ISH in patients older than 60 years. Active treatment consisted of chlorthalidone followed by atenolol or reserpine if necessary. A total of 4736 patients were randomized, with an average follow-up of 4.5 years. The incidence of CVA was reduced by 36% in the treated group, and the incidence of nonfatal myocardial infarction was 27% lower in the treated group. For all cardiovascular events, the incidence was reduced by 32%.[39] SHEP showed that a diuretic-based regimen reduced cardiovascular mortality in ISH.

In 1989, the Systolic Hypertension in Europe (SYST-EUR) Trial began. It was a randomized double-blind study comparing placebo with active treatment with medication that included nitrendipine (a long-acting dihydropyridine calcium channel blocker) with the possible addition of enalapril or hydrochlorothiazide, or both. This trial is particularly important in view of the current controversy over the use of short-acting calcium channel blockers in the treatment of hypertension. There was a median follow-up of 2 years with a reduction in all CVAs by 42%, sudden death by 26%, CHF by 29%, and myocardial infarction by 30%. All cardiovascular endpoints were reduced by 31%.[40]

Until this point, diuretics, specifically thiazides and β-blockers, were the primary medications studied in the prevention of cardiovascular mortality in hypertensive elderly. Clearly, these medications are of benefit, but the SYST-EUR trial showed that other medications such as angiotensin-converting enzyme inhibitors and calcium channel blockers could be considered in the treatment of this group.

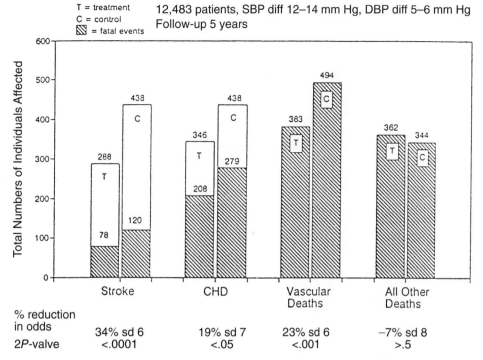

Figure 61–2. Effects of blood pressure reduction on stroke, coronary heart disease (CHD), vascular death, and nonvascular death in elderly patients. Combined results of five randomized trials of antihypertensive treatment in patients older than 60 years. SBP, systolic blood pressure; diff, differential; DBP, diastolic blood pressure; sd, standard deviation. (From MacMahon S, Rodgers A. The effects of blood pressure reduction in older patients: An overview of five randomized controlled trials in elderly hypertensives. Clin Exp Hypertens 15:967–978, 1993.)

Nonetheless, the adverse effects of angiotensin-converting enzyme inhibitors or calcium channel blockers, such as hyperkalemia, cough, gingival hyperplasia, edema, or constipation, may upset the fragile balance in a borderline functioning elderly person, particularly one with unsuspected reduced renal function.

In 1998, Messerli and associates called into question the use of β-blockers as a standard for the first-line therapy in the treatment of hypertension in the elderly. They reviewed selected randomized trials of at least 1 year's duration that were carried out between January 1966 and January 1998 using diuretics or β-blockers, or both, in the treatment of hypertension in the elderly. The results showed that β-blockers prevented cerebrovascular events, but were ineffective in preventing CAD, cardiovascular mortality, and all-cause mortality. In contrast, diuretic therapy was effective in preventing all of these.[41]

TREATMENT

The benefits of treating hypertension are clear. The choice of treatment should be based on risk stratification that takes into account risk factors for cardiovascular disease and the presence of target organ damage (Tables 61–3 and 61–4).[4]

Nonpharmacological Therapy

Lifestyle modifications are of proven benefit and may be the only therapy needed for stage 1 hypertension (Tables 61–5 and 61–6). Even when they are not adequate to control blood pressure by themselves, they can be used in conjunction with pharmacological therapy to help reduce the number and dosage of antihypertensive medications.[42]

Pharmacological Therapy

Many different classes of antihypertensive medications are available to the clinician. The recent JNC VI report recommends diuretics, specifically thiazide diuretics, and β-blockers as the initial choice for the treatment of hypertension in elderly patients without any comorbid conditions. Patients with comorbid conditions should have their therapy individualized. For example, in a patient with hypertension and diabetic nephropathy, an angiotensin-converting enzyme inhibitor would be the appropriate initial choice.

Table 61–3 Components of Cardiovascular Risk Stratification in Patients With Hypertension

MAJOR RISK FACTORS
Smoking
Dyslipidemia
Diabetes mellitus
Age >60 yr
Gender (men and postmenopausal women)
Family history of cardiovascular disease: women <65 yr or
  men <55 yr

TARGET ORGAN DAMAGE/CLINICAL CARDIOVASCULAR DISEASE
Heart diseases
  Left ventricular hypertrophy
  Angina or prior myocardial infarction
  Prior coronary revascularization
  Heart failure
Stroke or transient ischemic attack
Nephropathy
Peripheral arterial disease
Retinopathy

From Joint National Committee on Prevention, Detection, Evaluation, and Treatment of High Blood Pressure. The Sixth Report. Arch Intern Med 157:2413–2446, 1997.

Table 61-4 Risk Stratification and Treatment*

Blood Pressure Stage (mm Hg)	Risk Group A (No risk factors; no TOD/CCD†)	Risk Group B (At least 1 risk factor, not including diabetes; no TOD/CCD†)	Risk Group C (TOD/CCD† or diabetes, or both, with or without other risk factors)
High-normal (130–139/85–89)	Lifestyle modification	Lifestyle modification	Drug therapy‡
Stage 1 (140–159/90–99)	Lifestyle modification (up to 12 mo)	Lifestyle modification§ (up to 6 mo)	Drug therapy
Stages 2 and 3 (≥160/≥100)	Drug therapy	Drug therapy	Drug therapy

From Joint National Committee on Prevention, Detection, Evaluation, and Treatment of High Blood Pressure. The Sixth Report. Arch Intern Med 157:2413–2446, 1997.
* Note: For example, a patient with diabetes and a blood pressure of 142/94 mm Hg plus left ventricular hypertrophy should be classified as having stage 1 hypertension with target organ disease (left ventricular hypertrophy) and with another major risk factor (diabetes). This patient would be categorized as "Stage 1, Risk Group C," and recommended for immediate initiation of pharmacological treatment. Lifestyle modification should be adjunctive therapy for all patients recommended for pharmacological therapy.
† TOD/CCD, target organ disease/clinical cardiovascular disease.
‡ For those with heart failure, renal insufficiency, or diabetes.
§ For patients with multiple risk factors, clinicians should consider drugs as initial therapy plus lifestyle modifications.

Table 61-5 Lifestyle Modifications for Hypertension Prevention and Management

Lose weight if overweight
Limit alcohol intake to no more than 1 oz (30 ml) of ethanol (e.g., 24 oz [720 ml] of beer, 10 oz [300 ml] of wine, or 2 oz [60 ml] of 100-proof whiskey) per day or 0.5 oz (15 ml) of ethanol per day for women and lighter-weight people
Increase aerobic physical activity (30–45 min most days of the week)
Reduce sodium intake to no more than 100 mmol/day (2.4 g of sodium or 6 g of sodium chloride)
Maintain adequate intake of dietary potassium (approximately 90 mmol/day)
Maintain adequate intake of dietary calcium and magnesium for general health
Stop smoking and reduce intake of dietary saturated fat and cholesterol for overall cardiovascular health

From Joint National Committee on Prevention, Detection, Evaluation, and Treatment of High Blood Pressure. The Sixth Report. Arch Intern Med 157:2413–2446, 1997.

Table 61-6 The DASH Diet*

Food Group	Daily Servings (n)	Serving Sizes	Examples and Notes	Significance to the DASH Diet Pattern
Grains and grain products	7–8	1 slice bread ½ c (0.12 L) dry cereal ½ c (0.12 L) cooked rice, pasta, or cereal	Whole wheat bread, English muffin, pita bread, bagel, cereals, grits, oatmeal	Sources of energy and fiber
Vegetables	4–5	1 c (0.24 L) raw leafy vegetable ½ c (0.12 L) cooked vegetable 6 oz (180 ml) vegetable juice	Tomatoes, potatoes, carrots, peas, squash, broccoli, turnip greens, collards, kale, spinach, artichokes, beans, sweet potatoes	Sources of potassium, magnesium, and fiber
Fruits	4–5	6 oz (180 ml) fruit juice 1 medium fruit ½ c (0.06 L) dried fruit ¼ c (0.12 L) fresh, frozen, or canned fruit	Apricots, bananas, dates, grapes, oranges, orange juice, grapefruit, grapefruit juice, mangoes, melons, peaches, pineapples, prunes, raisins, strawberries, tangerines	Sources of potassium, magnesium, and fiber
Low-fat or nonfat dairy foods	2–3	8 oz (240 ml) milk 1 c (0.24 L) yogurt 1.5 oz (45 g) cheese	Skim or 1% milk, skim or low-fat buttermilk, nonfat or low-fat yogurt, part-skim mozzarella cheese, nonfat cheese	Sources of calcium and protein
Meats, poultry, and fish	≤2	3 oz (84 g) cooked meats, poultry, or fish	Select only lean meats; trim away visible fats; broil, roast, or boil, instead of fry; remove skin from poultry	Sources of protein and magnesium
Nuts, seeds, and legumes	4–5/wk	1.5 oz (42 g) or ⅓ c (0.08 L) nuts 0.5 oz (14 g) or 2 tbsp (3 ml) seeds ½ c (0.12 L) cooked legumes	Almonds, filberts, mixed nuts, peanuts, walnuts, sunflower seeds, kidney beans, lentils	Sources of energy, magnesium, potassium, protein, and fiber

From Joint National Committee on Prevention, Detection, Evaluation, and Treatment of High Blood Pressure. The Sixth Report. Arch Intern Med 157:2413–2446, 1997.
* From the Dietary Approaches to Stop Hypertension (DASH) clinical study. DASH's final results appear in the *New England Journal of Medicine* (336:1117–1124, 1997). The results show that the DASH "combination diet" lowered blood pressure and so may help prevent and control high blood pressure. The "combination diet" is rich in fruits, vegetables, and low-fat dairy foods and low in saturated and total fat. It also is low in cholesterol, high in dietary fiber, potassium, calcium, and magnesium, and moderately high in protein. The DASH eating plan shown is based on 2000 cal/day (8400 J/day). Depending on energy needs, the number of daily servings in a food group may vary from those listed.

An elderly man with hypertension and prostatism may benefit from a long-acting peripheral α-blocker, i.e., terazosin or doxazosin. A patient with a recent acute myocardial infarction should receive a β-blocker for the secondary prevention of cardiovascular mortality. Recently, the National Cooperative Cardiovascular Project showed that this drug class was grossly underutilized in this situation.[43] A postmenopausal woman with hypertension and osteoporosis may benefit from a thiazide diuretic, which lowers blood pressure and decreases urinary calcium excretion. Each class of antihypertensive drug has its own set of adverse effects, which are sometimes so severe that the clinician is forced to discontinue treatment and switch to a drug of a different class. β-Blockers can cause sleep disorders, nightmares, and depression. Central-acting α-agonists, such as clonidine, can cause dry mouth, drowsiness, and bradycardia. The elderly often have preexisting xerostomia and drowsiness, and the addition of clonidine may worsen these symptoms. Short-acting calcium channel blockers, such as sublingual nifedipine, can be dangerous in the elderly, as they drop the SBP to low levels without any control. In patients with CAD or cerebrovascular disease, this drop in SBP may reduce perfusion pressure to a critical level and cause a myocardial infarction or CVA. The clinician should decrease the SBP slowly and gradually. If an angiotensin-converting enzyme inhibitor or AT_1 receptor antagonist is prescribed, renal function must be monitored periodically, since patients with renal artery stenosis are at risk of acute renal failure when placed on these agents. In the coming years, newer classes of agents will become available and studies will need to be undertaken to ascertain their effectiveness and tolerability in the elderly population.[42]

CONCLUSION

Since hypertension in the elderly is a disorder with major target organ consequences, and not part of the normal aging process, therapy is needed to reduce target organ damage. It is particularly important to start with low doses of drugs and increase the doses slowly, since drug metabolism and excretion may be slowed in the elderly patient and target organ damage may sensitize the elderly patient to the adverse effects of drugs. In short, the addition of drug therapy can do as much harm as good if the physician is unaware of the complex interactions among age, hypertensive cardiovascular disease, and antihypertensive drugs.

References

1. Byyny RL. Hypertension in the elderly. *In* Laragh JH, Brenner BM (eds). Hypertension: Pathophysiology, Diagnosis, and Management. New York, Raven, pp 1869–1887, 1990.
2. Applegate WB. Hypertension in elderly patients. Ann Intern Med 110:901–905, 1989.
3. Kannel WB, Gordon T. Evaluation of cardiovascular risk in the elderly: The Framingham Study. Bull N Y Acad Med 54:573–591, 1978.
4. Joint National Committee on Prevention, Detection, Evaluation, and Treatment of High Blood Pressure. The Sixth Report. Arch Intern Med 157:2413–2446, 1997.
5. Kannel WB. Some lessons in cardiovascular epidemiology from Framingham. Am J Cardiol 37:269–274, 1976.
6. Maddocks I. Possible absence of hypertension in two complete Pacific Island populations. Lancet 2:396–399, 1961.
7. Prior IAM, Grimley EJ, Harvey HPB, et al. Sodium intake and blood pressure in two Polynesian populations. N Engl J Med 279:515, 1968.
8. Page LB, Damon A, Moellering RC. Antecedents of cardiovascular disease in six Solomon Islands societies. Circulation 49:1132–1146, 1974.
9. Lowenstein FW: Blood pressure in relation to age and sex in the tropics and subtropics. A review of the literature and an investigation in two tribes of Brazil Indians. Lancet 1:389, 1961.
10. Systolic Hypertension in the Elderly Program Cooperative Research Group. Implications of the Systolic Hypertension in the Elderly Program. Hypertension 21:335–343, 1993.
11. National High Blood Pressure Education Program Working Group. Report on hypertension in the elderly. Hypertension 23:275–285, 1994.
12. Gavras H, Gavras I. Hypertension in the Elderly. Littleton, MA, PSG, 1983.
13. Ostfeld AM. Elderly hypertensive patient. N Y State J Med 78:1125, 1978.
14. Kannel WB, Castelli WP, McNamara PM, et al. Role of blood pressure in the development of congestive failure: The Framingham Study. N Engl J Med 287:781–787, 1972.
15. Kannel WB, Gordon T. Systolic vs diastolic blood pressure and risk of coronary artery disease. Am J Cardiol 27:335, 1971.
16. Shekelle R, Ostfeld A. Hypertension and risk of stroke in an elderly population. Stroke 5:71–75, 1974.
17. Ostfeld AM, Shekelle RB, Klawans H, et al. Epidemiology of stroke in an elderly welfare population. Am J Public Health 64:450, 1973.
18. Kannel WB, Dawber T. Perspectives on systolic hypertension: The Framingham Study. Circulation 61:1179–1182, 1980.
19. Curb J, Curb JD, Borhani NO, et al. Isolated systolic hypertension in 14 communities. Am J Epidemiol 121:362–370, 1985.
20. Starr I, Donal JS, Margolies A, et al. Studies of the heart and circulation in disease: Estimations of basal cardiac output, metabolism, heart size and blood pressure in 235 subjects. J Clin Invest 13:561, 1934.
21. Brandfonbrener M, Landowne M, Shock NW. Changes in cardiac output with age. Circulation 12:557, 1955.
22. Port S, Cobb FR, Coleman RE, et al. Effect of age on the response of the left ventricular ejection fraction to exercise. N Engl J Med 303:1133, 1980.
23. Weisfeldt M. Aging changes in the cardiovascular system and responses to stress. Am J Hypertens 11:41S–45S, 1998.
24. Brest A (ed). Geriatric cardiology. *In* Cardiovascular Clinics. Philadelphia, FA Davis, 1997.
25. Crane MG, Harris JJ. Effect of aging on renin activity and aldosterone secretion. J Lab Clin Med 87:947, 1976.
26. Noth RH, Lassman MN, Tan SY, et al. Age and the renin-aldosterone system. Arch Intern Med 137:1414–1417, 1977.
27. Luft FC, Grim CE, Fineberg N, et al. Effects of volume expansion and contraction in normotensive whites, blacks, and subjects of different ages. Circulation 59:643, 1979.
28. Wiedman P, Beretta-Piccoli C. Age versus urinary sodium for judging renin, aldosterone and catecholamine levels. Kidney Int 14:619, 1978.
29. Vestal RE, Wood AJJ, Shand DG. Reduced beta adrenoceptor sensitivity in the elderly. Clin Pharmacol Ther 26:181, 1979.
30. Esler M, Skews H, Leonard P, et al. Age-dependence of noradrenaline kinetics in normal subjects. Clin Sci 60:217, 1981.
31. Niarchos AP, Laragh JH: Hypertension in the elderly. Mod Concepts Cardiovasc Dis 49:49, 1980.
32. Spence JD, Sibbald WJ, Cape RD. Pseudohypertension in the elderly. Clin Sci Mol Med 55:399s, 1978.
33. Veterans Administration Co-Operative Study on Antihypertensive Agents. Effects of treatment on morbidity in hypertension. III: Influence of age, diastolic pressure and prior cardiovascular disease. Circulation 45:991–1004, 1972.
34. Hypertension Detection and Follow-Up Program. Detection and treatment of hypertension in older individuals. Am J Epidemiol 121:371–376, 1985.
35. Amery A, Birkenhager W. Mortality and morbidity result from the European Working Party on High Blood Pressure in the Elderly Trial. Lancet 2:1349, 1985.

36. Dahlof B, Lindholm L, Hansson L, et al. Morbidity and mortality in the Swedish Trial in Old Patients with Hypertension (STOP-Hypertension). Lancet 338:1281–1285, 1991.
37. Medical Research Council Working Party. MRC Trial of Hypertension in Older Adults: Principal results. BMJ 304:405–412, 1992.
38. MacMahon S, Rodgers A. The effects of blood pressure reduction in older patients: An overview of five randomized controlled trials in elderly hypertensives. Clin Exp Hypertens 15:967–978, 1993.
39. SHEP Cooperative Research Group. Prevention of stroke by antihypertensive drug treatment in older persons with isolated systolic hypertension. JAMA 265:3255–3264, 1991.
40. SYST-EUR Trial Investigators. Randomized double-blind comparison of placebo and active treatment for older patients with isolated systolic hypertension. Lancet 350:757–764, 1997.
41. Messerli FH, Grossman E, Goldbourt U. Are β-blockers efficacious as first line therapy for hypertension in the elderly? JAMA 279:1903–1907, 1998.
42. Neaton JD, Grimm RH Jr, Prineas RJ, et al., for the Treatment of Mild Hypertension Study Research Group. Treatment of Mild Hypertension Study: Final results. JAMA 270:713–724, 1993.
43. Krumholz HM, Radford MJ, Wang Y, et al., for the National Cooperative Cardiovascular Project. National use and effectiveness of β-blockers for the treatment of elderly patients after acute myocardial infarction. JAMA 280:623–629, 1998.

CHAPTER 62

Hypertension in Blacks

John M. Flack and Beth A. Staffileno

EPIDEMIOLOGY

Clinical hypertension begins earlier in life and is more severe in African Americans than in whites. According to the sixth report of the Joint National Committee on Prevention, Detection, Evaluation, and Treatment of High Blood Pressure (JNC VI), the prevalence of stage 3 hypertension ($\geq$180/110 mm Hg) is approximately 8% in African Americans versus less than 1% in whites. The African Diaspora manifest a graded rise in hypertension prevalence with westward migration toward the United States. Hypertension prevalence is 33% and 50% greater in African American men and women, respectively, compared with gender-matched whites. Interestingly, and for unclear reasons, hypertension and its adverse clinical sequelae (e.g., stroke, renal disease) occur more commonly among African American residents of 13 southeastern states than among African Americans residing elsewhere in the United States. Similar to whites, African Americans experience an age-related rise in blood pressure (BP), particularly systolic BP. Isolated systolic hypertension (systolic BP $\geq$ 160 and diastolic BP < 90 mm Hg), the hypertension phenotype most closely linked to blood pressure–related morbidity and mortality, is preferentially manifested in older (>60 years) persons, particularly women, and is more prevalent in older African American women than in white women.

ANTECEDENTS OF HYPERTENSION

Why African Americans have higher rates of hypertension than whites and, as well, why there is a geographic predilection for hypertension and its adverse sequelae in African Americans residents of the southeastern United States are not trivial issues. A plethora of explanations have been put forth, including enhanced genetic susceptibility; excess obesity and low levels of physical activity (particularly in women); low dietary intake of potassium and calcium; and high levels of psychological stressors related to poverty, despair, and racism. Interestingly, the lifestyle attributes leading to hypertension and its adverse sequelae overlap substantially between African Americans and whites, despite the greater overall level of risk for these conditions in African Americans. Low birth weight is common in African Americans. Low birth weight has been linked to an increased risk of hypertension[1] and, therefore, might play a role in the excess hypertension rates in this high-risk population.

TARGET ORGAN DAMAGE

Virtually all forms of pressure-related target organ damage (TOD) and adverse clinical sequelae, including left ventricular hypertrophy, stroke, end-stage renal disease, and congestive heart failure, are more common in African Americans than in whites. African Americans in the southeastern United States have stroke rates that are 30 to 50% higher than African Americans residing in the rest of the country.[2, 3] Interestingly, stroke mortality rates for African American women are less than half those of Hungarian and Czechoslovakian women.[3] Coronary heart disease death rates for African Americans are, however, among the highest in the world.[4]

Pressure-related TOD has been increasingly recognized as more important than BP, per se, as a predictor of the absolute risk for future cardiovascular disease (CVD) complications (Table 62–1). In the Hypertension Detection Follow-up Program (HDFP), there was a threefold greater 5-year mortality among pressure-matched hypertensives with clinically manifest TOD in both the chlorthalidone (special care) and the usual care groups.[5] Moreover, a positive correlation exists in African Americans between BP level and TOD prevalence.[6] This relationship is stronger in men than in women. Thus, TOD and BP should not be considered as independent entities. In fact, TOD appears to correlate with an attenuation of the normal nocturnal decline in BP,[7, 8] leading to a greater 24-hour BP burden.

Table 62–1 Patterns and Clinical Manifestations Associated With Blood Pressure–Related Target Organ Damage*

PATTERNS OF BLOOD PRESSURE–RELATED TOD IN AFRICAN AMERICANS

Excess prevalence and incidence of
- LVH
- CHF
- CHD
- Renal insufficiency/failure
- Proteinuria
- Stroke

CLINICAL MANIFESTATIONS OF BLOOD PRESSURE–RELATED TOD

Cardiac remodeling/dysfunction
- LVH (ECG or ECHO)
- CHF
- ?Diastolic function

Cerebrovascular disease
- Abnormal imaging studies
- Stroke/TIA

Renal disease
- Microalbuminuria
- Proteinuria
- Hypercreatinemia
- ESRD

Severe retinopathy
- Hemorrhages
- Exudates
- Arteriolar narrowing, silver wiring, and segmental spasm
- Papilledema

Large vessel atherosclerosis
- Bruits
- MI
- Angina, claudication

Abbreviations: TOD, target organ damage; LVH, left ventricular hypertrophy; CHF, congestive heart failure; CHD, coronary heart disease; ECG, electrocardiogram; ECHO, echocardiogram; TIA, transient ischemic attack; ESRD, end-stage renal disease; MI, myocardial infarction.

*Although the absolute level of risk for some blood pressure–related sequelae (such as stroke and renal disease) is usually higher in African Americans compared with whites at a given blood pressure level, the fundamental association of blood pressure with pressure-related clinical sequelae is similar.

Observations we made in an early middle-aged cohort of 119 African Americans enrolled in the Sodium and Blood Pressure (SNAP) Study, with normal to high-normal BP (average BP 106/78 mm Hg) probably have relevance to the universe of hypertensive African Americans. Individuals with trace ($n = 32$) to 1+ ($n = 4$) dipstick proteinuria had substantially higher nocturnal systolic BP (121.6 vs. 116.9 mm Hg, $p = .07$) than those without proteinuria after dietary salt loading. The effect of dietary salt loading on daytime systolic BP was similar in the two groups, although it was less pronounced than the effect on nighttime systolic BP. Thus, even among normotensives, very low levels of proteinuria in African Americans correlate to a greater 24-hour BP burden, predominantly because of an attenuation of the normal nocturnal decline in BP. Interestingly, before randomization, cuff BP levels in the two groups with and without proteinuria were virtually identical. The salt-induced effect on nocturnal BP is likely to be even greater in African Americans with hypertension.

Some,[9–11] although not all,[12, 13] data suggest a greater susceptibility to TOD at a given BP level in African Americans compared with whites. It is reasonable to speculate that the total burden of vascular injury risk factors, not just BP per se, is greater in African Americans. The deleterious interaction of these risk factors with BP might explain, at least in part, the higher CVD risk at a given BP level in African Americans relative to whites.

MECHANISMS LEADING TO PRESSURE-RELATED TOD

"Low" renin status is the pathophysiological aberration that has been at the root of the ongoing speculations about the genetic basis of hypertension in African Americans. However, the genetics of the premature BP elevations and overexpression of pressure-related TOD in African Americans (or any other group) have not been elucidated. The recent emergence of powerful molecular genetic tools promises to shed light on this pathophysiological enigma.

The distribution of circulating renin levels is shifted downward in African Americans compared with whites. African Americans also manifest blunted hyperreninemia in response to provocative measures such as lasix-induced intravascular volume depletion or administration of angiotensin-converting enzyme (ACE) inhibition.[14] Thus, a *low-renin* label has been given to this population. It should, however, be noted that the majority of African Americans have normal to elevated circulating renin levels. An implicit assumption has been made that "low" renin status is a primary or genetic abnormality that reflects a diminished role of the renin-angiotensin-aldosterone system in the pathogenesis of hypertension and pressure-related TOD. However, the control of renin release from the juxtaglomerular cell, a specialized smooth muscle cell in the renal afferent arteriole, is a complex interplay of many factors (Fig. 62–1).

Renin synthesis and secretion can be suppressed by factors other than plasma volume expansion. Pressure-related stretch of the afferent arteriole, angiotensin II,[15] endothelin,[16] atrial natriuretic peptide,[17] and increased delivery of sodium to the specialized macula densa cells of the distal nephron all suppress renin synthesis and release.[18] Thus, "low" levels of circulating renin in African Americans could conceivably be a secondary phenomenon. The high burden of pressure-related TOD in African Americans (e.g., left ventricular hypertrophy), which has been closely linked to angiotensin II excess and/or kinin deficiency, lends circumstantial support to the thesis that "low" circulating renin may be a consequence of high renal tissue levels of angiotensin II.

Obesity is the major anthropometric correlate not only of hypertension but also of left ventricular hypertrophy[19] and albuminuria,[20, 21] two manifestations of pressure-related TOD. Obesity is disproportionately prevalent among African Americans, particularly in women,[22] as well as in African American residents of the 13 southeastern United States.[23] How does obesity raise BP? Obesity is associated with activation of the sympathetic nervous and renin-angiotensin-aldosterone-kinin systems, as well as with plasma volume expansion. In Jamaicans, obesity has been linked to increased circulating angiotensinogen levels and serum ACE activity.[24] Interestingly, circulating renin levels in

Site of synthesis: JG cells (modified smooth cells) in wall of afferent arteriole*

Factors affecting renin secretion:

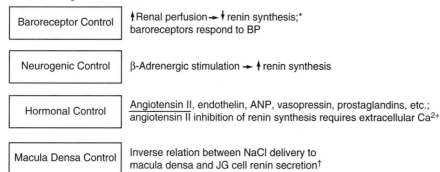

Baroreceptor Control	↑Renal perfusion → ↓renin synthesis;* baroreceptors respond to BP
Neurogenic Control	β-Adrenergic stimulation → ↑renin synthesis
Hormonal Control	<u>Angiotensin II, endothelin, ANP, vasopressin, prostaglandins, etc.;</u> angiotensin II inhibition of renin synthesis requires extracellular Ca^{2+}
Macula Densa Control	Inverse relation between NaCl delivery to macula densa and JG cell renin secretion†

*Main site for changes in vascular resistance mediating RBF autoregulation.

†Cl ion appears more important than Na ion.

Figure 62–1. Site of renin synthesis and factors affecting renin secretion. JG, juxtaglomerular; BP, blood pressure; ANP, atrial natriuretic peptide; RBF, renal blood flow. (Adapted from Lush DJ, King JA, Fray JC. Pathophysiology of low renin syndromes: Sites of renal renin secretory impairment and prorenin overexpression. Used with permission of Kidney International, volume 43, pages 983–999, 1993.)

obese hypertensives are not usually suppressed.[25] This probably reflects the increased renal sodium reabsorption in the distal (but proximal to the macula densa cells) nephron. The increased tubular reabsorption of sodium causes a rightward shift of the pressure-natriuresis curve (salt sensitivity). We have documented the linkage of obesity in African American women with normal to high-normal BP to both salt sensitivity and a reversible (with salt restriction) attenuation of the normal nocturnal decline in BP. This leads to higher nighttime BP and, therefore, a greater 24-hour BP burden. The greater 24-hour burden probably contributes to obesity-related TOD.

The kidney likely has a central role in the pathogenesis of hypertension in African Americans. In turn, the kidney in African Americans appears to have enhanced sensitivity to nephrotoxic exposures such as elevated BP, as indicated by the excess prevalence of renal injury and renal disease mortality across a broad BP range in African Americans compared with whites with similar BP levels.[9, 26] Depressed urinary excretion of renal vasodilators such as dopamine[27] and kallekrein[28] have also been documented in African Americans.

Hall and coworkers[29] have put forth a provocative hypothesis regarding how obesity might contribute to renal injury (Fig. 62–2). This hypothesis may have considerable relevance to African Americans, given their high rates of obesity (particularly among women), diabetes mellitus, renal insufficiency, end-stage renal disease, and renal mortality.[26] Hall and coworkers[29] postulate that renal compression by fat infiltration of the relatively noncompliant renal capsule leads to compression of the renal medulla, causing a reduction in renal blood and tubular urine flows. This sequence of events results in an increased fractional tubular reabsorption of sodium. Activation of the renin-angiotensin-aldosterone and sympathetic nervous systems also contributes to the increased tubular reabsorption of sodium. To overcome the increased tubular sodium reabsorption, there is intense renal vasodilatation, resulting in an increased renal plasma flow. Thus, glomerular hyperfiltration might contribute to renal glomerulosclerosis, particularly when elevated BP coexists with other nephrotoxic exposures, such as glucose intolerance, dyslipidemia, and cigarette smoking. This proposed mechanism of renal injury in obe-

sity merits consideration and, ultimately, careful investigation in African Americans.

Johnson and Schreiner[30] have proposed another intriguing hypothesis of salt-induced renal injury and elevated BP. They have suggested augmented renal tubuloglomerular feedback as a mechanism leading to renal ischemia, progressive tubulointerstitial disease, and salt-dependent hypertension. Increased sodium delivery to the distal nephron stimulates adenosine secretion from the specialized macula densa cells. Adenosine subsequently diffuses into the adjacent afferent arteriole, where it causes vasoconstriction; this reflexive afferent arteriolar vasoconstriction is further augmented by angiotensin II and low levels of nitric oxide. Moreover, sustained BP elevations can lead to structural remodeling of the afferent arteriole, thus contributing to further reductions in renal blood flow and poten-

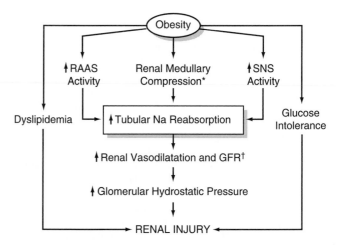

*Secondary to accumulation of adipose tissue around the kidney and increased intracellular matrix within the kidney.

†Occurs to compensate for ↑ tubular Na reabsorption.

Figure 62–2. Mechanisms by which obesity might contribute to the activation of neurohumoral systems and alterations in renal structure and function, thus leading to renal injury. RAAS, renin-angiotensin-aldosterone system; SNS, sympathetic nervous system; GFR, glomerular filtration rate. (Adapted from Hall JE, Brands MW, Henegar JR, et al. Abnormal kidney function as a cause and a consequence of obesity hypertension. Clin Exp Pharmacol Physiol 25:58–64, 1998.)

tially to renal ischemia and ultimately to reduced renal mass.

TREATMENT

The hypertensive African American presents to the clinician with difficult-to-treat hypertension more often than almost any other hypertensive subgroup, with the possible exceptions of diabetics, older persons, and those with renal insufficiency (Table 62–2). As previously stated, African American hypertensives are more likely than whites to have JNC VI stage 3 hypertension (≥180/100 mm Hg). Hypertensives of any race in the stage 3 BP range are considerably less likely to attain BP normalization with antihypertensive monotherapy of any drug class than are individuals with stage 1 or 2 disease. Thus, hypertensive African Americans will have more monotherapy "failures" (even after therapeutic trials of sufficient duration with adequate doses of drug) and will therefore more often need combination drug therapy to achieve BP normalization.

The presence of pressure-related TOD has profound implications for the timing of initiation of therapy as well as the BP goals. In individuals with heart failure, renal disease, and/or diabetes, according to the JNC VI report,[31] antihypertensive drug therapy should be initiated at a BP level of 130/85 mm Hg or higher rather than the traditional 140/90 mm Hg cutpoint. The rationale for this recommendation is the high level of absolute risk for CVD morbidity and mortality even at "high-normal" levels of BP in the presence of TOD and/or clinical CVD.

Based on our observations in the SNAP study, as well as those of others, the presence of obesity and/or TOD (e.g., proteinuria) correlates to a greater 24-hour BP burden, mostly attributable to higher nighttime BP, during dietary sodium loading. It should be noted that dietary sodium loading in studies such as SNAP results in dietary intake that is well within the range of usual sodium intake for free-living Americans. Thus, these observations likely have therapeutic relevance for African Americans in that attainment of BP normalization throughout the 24-hour dosing interval will be difficult to achieve during consumption of an ad libitum sodium diet, particularly during the latter period of the dosing interval near the trough BP drug effect.

A strong case can be made for a more thorough assessment of pressure-related TOD than is currently typical in African Americans because: (1) pressure-related TOD increases the absolute risk for CVD morbidity and mortality by a factor of three- to fourfold[6, 9] and (2) African-Americans have not only higher BP than whites but also an overall greater burden of pressure-related TOD at any given BP level. The most recent JNC VI report[31] keyed antihypertensive treatment recommendations more to the absolute risk of CVD complications than to absolute BP level, given the prominent consideration of TOD and clinical CVD status in determining the timing and intensity of therapy. Thus, amongst African Americans, timing of the initiation of antihypertensive therapy, as well as setting the most appropriate BP targets, depends on an accurate and comprehensive determination of pressure-related TOD.

Nondrug Therapy

A number of modifiable lifestyle characteristics contribute to the excess hypertension rates in African Americans. Clinical trial data have shown that in African Americans, lifestyle modification(s)—such as weight loss,[32] salt and alcohol restriction, and increase in physical activity, alone or in combination—lower BP. Interestingly, some beneficial interactions among various lifestyle modifications have been documented. For example, physical activity has been shown, over the short term, to augment urinary sodium excretion.[33] Moreover, weight loss attenuates the pressor response to dietary salt loading in white adolescents.[34] Although the impact of weight loss on salt sensitivity has not been studied, per se, in African Americans, we hypothesize a similar impact to that seen in whites, since body size and salt sensitivity have been linked in normotensive African Americans (Flack, unpublished data, 1998). In addition, concomitant weight reduction has been shown to amplify the benefits of physical activity not only by lowering BP but also by improving metabolic abnormalities and the CVD risk profile (improved insulin resistance, lower cholesterol and triglycerides, and higher high-density lipoprotein). With respect to pressure-related TOD, cigarette smoking is a major modifiable risk factor. The increased CVD risk attributable to cigarette smoking is, at least partially, mediated by short-term spikes in BP during smoking. Cigarette smokers also have a greater prevalence of microalbuminuria than nonsmokers (Flack, unpublished data, 1998).[35, 36]

Salt Restriction

Modest sodium restriction (<2 g of sodium intake/day) is recommended for most hypertensives. This is particularly

---

Table 62–2 Therapeutic Implications of Characteristics Associated With Hypertension in African Americans*	
Higher BP levels	More monotherapy failures
Longer duration of HTN	More short-term risk from rapid BP reduction; however, long-term benefits of BP normalization are greater
Greater burden of target organ damage	Need slow but aggressive BP control (<130/85 mm Hg); favor drugs with human data for TOP; greatly increased absolute risk for CVD
Obesity	More likely salt-sensitive leading to higher BP medication requirements; lower sodium intake, uptitrate ACE inhibitors, AT$_1$-receptor antagonists, β-blockers
Glomerular hyperfiltration	Aggressive BP control, favor ACEs, possibly AT$_1$-receptor antagonists
Reduced natriuretic capacity	More often need diuretics, especially in complex drug regimens; premium on reducing dietary sodium intake

Abbreviations: BP, blood pressure; HTN, hypertension; TOP, target organ protection; CVD, cardiovascular disease; ACE, angiotensin-converting enzyme; AT$_1$, angiotensin II type 1.
*More often, and more so than most other subgroups, the hypertensive African American presents to the clinician with difficult-to-treat hypertension.

relevant for the highly salt-sensitive hypertensive African American. Randomized clinical trials have shown BP-lowering effects of sodium-restricted diets in middle-aged and older African American hypertensives.[32, 37] Sodium consumption also exacerbates renal proteinuria.[38, 39] African Americans consume amounts of dietary sodium similar to whites,[37] although African Americans residing in the southeastern United States may consume more.[40]

Weight Loss

Weight loss is an important nonpharmacological intervention, particularly because of the higher prevalence of obesity among African Americans, especially women. A gradual 1- to 1.5-lb weight loss per week is recommended and can be achieved by following a low-fat and reduced-calorie diet combined with moderate amounts of regular physical activity. It is important to help individuals set realistic goals when modifying dietary habits. Smaller dietary changes may be accomplished more easily than large-scale changes. Cultural mores can often interfere with implementing healthy lifestyle changes. Therefore, it is important to encourage individuals to make favorable lifestyle changes within the context/framework of their cultural identity.

Physical Activity

Similar to obesity, the prevalence of physical inactivity is greatest among African Americans, particularly women.[41, 42] Physical activity is an important adjunctive treatment for hypertension. It has minimal side effects and (usually) costs and can also help control non-BP CVD risk factors (e.g., obesity, dyslipidemia, glucose intolerance) when performed on a regular basis. Numerous exercise training studies in hypertensive and normotensive individuals have shown a significant reduction in the average posttreatment resting BP that appears to be fully manifest within the first few weeks of training. Aerobic activity should be encouraged, whereas heavy weightlifting and isometric exercise should be avoided because of the striking exercise-induced BP elevations that occur during exercise and over the longer term.

Drug Therapy

Antihypertensive agents from all commonly used first-line drug classes as recommended by JNC VI will effectively lower BP in African Americans. There has been a long-held clinical belief that antihypertensive drugs (β-blockers, ACE inhibitors, angiotensin II type 1 antagonists) that have their predominant pharmacological effect on the renin-angiotensin-aldosterone system are ineffective hypotensive agents in African Americans. The data on BP-lowering efficacy of both β-blockers and ACE inhibitors suggest that when adequately dosed over a sufficient duration of time, monotherapy with these agents effectively lowers BP in African Americans.[14, 43, 44] Fewer published data are available for the angiotensin II type 1 antagonists. Thus, race should not be the sole or even primary criterion on which an antihypertensive drug class is avoided or selected.

Nevertheless, there are certain therapeutic caveats when using antihypertensive agents other than diuretics and calcium antagonists.

We have previously shown that high salt intake attenuates the antihypertensive efficacy of ACE inhibitors (enalapril) and calcium channel blockers (isradipine).[45] The salt-induced attenuation of the BP response was more pronounced with enalapril than with isradipine. The BP-lowering effects of diuretics and of all classes of calcium antagonists are less attenuated by high dietary sodium intake than those of other antihypertensive drug classes. Thus, there tends to be a greater reduction in BP with monotherapy using diuretics or calcium channel antagonists in African Americans. Increased body size also increases ACE inhibitor dosage requirements in African Americans. One study found no difference in BP response between African Americans and whites when drug dose was expressed as milligrams per kilogram of body weight. In addition, overweight, salt-sensitive, and/or hypertensive persons with TOD may pose a challenge in achieving 24-hour BP control, given their attenuated nocturnal fall in BP.

African American hypertensives often present with co-existing cardiovascular conditions such as dyslipidemia and diabetes mellitus. Thus, comprehensive CVD risk factor management (e.g., BP control, normalization of lipids and glucose) must be undertaken to achieve maximal CVD risk reduction.

References

1. Falkner B, Hulman S, Kushner H. Birth weight versus childhood growth as determinants of adult blood pressure. Hypertension 31:145–150, 1998.
2. Gillum RF. Stroke in blacks. Stroke 19:1–9, 1988.
3. Gillum RF, Ingram DD. Relation between residence in the southeast region of the United States and stroke incidence. The NHANES I epidemiologic followup study. Am J Epidemiol 144:665–673, 1996.
4. Gillum RF. Epidemiology of hypertension in African American women. Am Heart J 131:385–395, 1996.
5. Hypertension Detection and Follow-up Program Cooperative Group. The effect of treatment on mortality in "mild" hypertension. N Engl J Med 7:976–980, 1982.
6. Hypertension Detection and Follow-up Program Cooperative Group. Five year findings of Hypertension Detection and Follow-up Program. II: Mortality by race-sex and age. JAMA 242:2572–2576, 1979.
7. Bianchi S, Bigazzi R, Baldari G, et al. Diurnal variations of blood pressure and microalbuminuria in essential hypertension. Am J Hypertens 7:23–29, 1994.
8. Timio M, Venanzi S, Lolli S, et al. "Non-dipper" hypertensive patients and progressive renal insufficiency: A 3-year longitudinal study. Clin Nephrol 43:382–387, 1995.
9. Klagg ML, Whelton PK, Randall BL, et al. End-stage renal disease in African American and white men: 16-year MRFIT findings. JAMA 227:1293–1298, 1997.
10. Shulman NB, Ford CE, Hall WD, et al, for the Hypertension Detection and Follow-up Program Cooperative Group. Prognostic value of serum creatinine and effect of treatment of hypertension on renal function. Results from the Hypertension Detection and Follow-up Program. Hypertension 13:180–193, 1989.
11. Walker GW, Neaton JD, Cutler JA, et al. Renal function change in hypertensive members of the Multiple Risk Factor Intervention Trial. Racial and treatment effects. The MRFIT Research Group. JAMA 268:3085–3091, 1992.
12. Schmieder RE, Rockstroh JK, Luchters G, et al. Comparison of early target organ damage between blacks and whites with mild systemic arterial hypertension. Am J Cardiol 79:1695–1698, 1997.
13. Rockstroh JK, Schmieder RE, Schlaich MP, et al. Renal and systemic hemodynamics in black and white hypertensive patients. Am J Hypertens 10:971–978, 1997.

14. Weir MR, Gray JM, Paster R, et al. Differing mechanisms of action of angiotensin-converting enzyme inhibition in black and white hypertensive patients. The Trandolapril Multicenter Study Group. Hypertension 26:124–130, 1995.

15. Johns DW, Peach MJ, Gomez RA, et al. Angiotensin II regulates renin gene expression. Am J Physiol 259:F882–F887, 1990.

16. Letizia C, Cerci S, De Toma G, et al. High plasma endothelin-1 levels in hypertensive patients with low-renin essential hypertension. J Hum Hypertens 11:447–451, 1997.

17. Laragh JH. The endocrine control on blood volume, blood pressure and sodium balance: Atrial hormone and renin system interactions. J Hypertens Suppl 4:S143–S156, 1986.

18. Lush DJ, King JA, Fray JC. Pathophysiology of low renin syndromes: Sites of renal renin secretory impairment and prorenin overexpression. Kidney Int 43:983–999, 1993.

19. Gottdiener JS, Reda DJ, Materson BJ, et al. Importance of obesity, race and age to the cardiac structural and functional effects of hypertension. The Department of Veterans Affairs Cooperative Study Group on Antihypertensive Agents. J Am Coll Cardiol 24:1492–1498, 1994.

20. Anderson PJ, Chan JC, Chan YL, et al. Visceral fat and cardiovascular risk factors in Chinese NIDDM patients. Diabetes Care 20:1854–1858, 1997.

21. Metcalf PA, Scragg RK, Dryson E. Associations between body morphology and microalbuminuria in healthy middle-aged European, Maori and Pacific Island New Zealanders. Int J Obes Relat Metab Disord 21:203–210, 1997.

22. Kuczmarski R, Flegal K, Campbell S, et al. The increasing prevalence of overweight among US adults. The National Health and Nutrition Examination Surveys 1960 to 1991. JAMA 272:205–211, 1994.

23. Kumanyika S. Obesity in black women. Epidemiol Rev 9:31–50, 1987.

24. Cooper R, McFarlane-Anderson N, Bennett FI, et al. ACE, angiotensinogen and obesity: A potential pathway leading to hypertension. J Hum Hypertens 11:107–111, 1997.

25. Licata G, Scaglione R, Corrao S, et al. Heredity and obesity-associated hypertension: Impact of hormonal characteristics and left ventricular mass. J Hypertens 13:611–618, 1995.

26. Flack JM, Neaton JD, Daniels B, et al. Ethnicity and renal diseases: Lessons from the Multiple Risk Factor Intervention Trial and Treatment of Mild Hypertension Study. Am J Kidney Dis 21(suppl 1):31–40 ,1993.

27. Berenson GS, Webber LS, Srinivassan SR. Pathogenesis of hypertension in black and white children. Clin Cardiol 12(suppl 4):IV3–IV8, 1989.

28. Zinner SH, Margolius HS, Rosner B, et al. Familial aggregation of urinary kallikrein concentration in childhood: Relation to blood pressure, race and urinary electrolytes. Am J Epidemiol 104:124–132, 1976.

29. Hall JE, Brands MW, Henegar JR, et al. Abnormal kidney function as a cause and a consequence of obesity hypertension. Clin Exp Pharmacol Physiol 25:58–64, 1998.

30. Johnson RJ, Schreiner GF. Hypothesis: The role of acquired tubulointerstitial disease in the pathogenesis of salt-dependent hypertension. Kidney Int 52:1169–1179, 1997.

31. Joint National Committee on Prevention, Detection, Evaluation, and Treatment of High Blood Pressure. The sixth report. Arch Intern Med 157:2413–2446, 1997.

32. Whelton PK, Appel LJ, Espeland MA, et al, for the TONE Collaborative Research Group. Sodium reduction and weight loss in the treatment of hypertension in older persons: A randomized controlled Trial of Nonpharmacologic Interventions in the Elderly (TONE). JAMA 279:839–846, 1998.

33. Brown MD, Moore GE, Korythowski MT, et al. Improvement of insulin sensitivity by short-term exercise training in hypertensive African American women. Hypertension 30:1549–1553, 1997.

34. Rocchini AP, Key J, Bondie D, et al. The effect of weight loss on the sensitivity of blood pressure to sodium in obese adolescents. N Engl J Med 321:580–585, 1989.

35. Bruno G, Cavallo-Perin P, Bargero G, et al. Prevalence and risk factors for micro- and macroalbuminuria in an Italian population-based cohort of NIDDM subjects. Diabetes Care 19:43–47, 1996.

36. Chase HP, Garg SK, Marshall G, et al. Cigarette smoking increases the risk of albuminuria among subjects with type I diabetes. JAMA 265:614–617, 1991.

37. Neaton JD, Grimm RH, Prineas RJ, et al, for the Treatment of Mild Hypertension Study Research Group. Treatment of Mild Hypertension Study: Final results. JAMA 270:713–724, 1993.

38. Nesovic M, Stojanovic M, Nesovic MM, et al. Microalbuminuria is associated with salt sensitivity in hypertensive patients. J Hum Hypertens 10:573–576, 1996.

39. Hertzan-Levy S, Iaina A, Wollman Y, et al. Glomerular basement membrane polyanionic sites and nitric oxide in genetically salt-sensitive and -resistant hypertensive rats. Kidney Blood Press Res 20:218–224, 1997.

40. Hall WD, Ferrario CM, Moore MA, et al. Hypertension-related morbidity and mortality in the southeastern Unites States. Am J Med Sci 31:195–209, 1997.

41. Crespo C, Keteyian S, Heath G, et al. Leisure-time physical activity among US adults: Results from the Third National Health and Nutrition Examination Survey. Arch Intern Med 156:93–98, 1996.

42. Liu K, Ruth KJ, Flack JM, et al. Blood pressure in young blacks and whites: Relevance of obesity and lifestyle factors in determining differences. The CARDIA Study. Coronary Artery Risk Development in Young Adults. Circulation 93:60–66, 1996.

43. Saunders E, Weir MR, Kong BW, et al. A comparison of the efficacy and safety of a beta-blocker, a calcium channel blocker, and a converting enzyme inhibitor in hypertensive blacks. Arch Intern Med 150:1707–1713, 1990.

44. Drayer JI, Weber MA. Monotherapy of essential hypertension with a converting-enzyme inhibitor. Hypertension 5(suppl III):III-108–III-113, 1983.

45. Weir MR, Chrysant SG, McCarron DA, et al. Influence of race and dietary salt on the antihypertensive efficacy of an angiotensin-converting enzyme inhibitor or a calcium channel antagonist in salt-sensitive hypertension. Hypertension 31:1088–1096, 1998.

63

Resistant Hypertension

Donald G. Vidt

Hypertension is the most prevalent condition for which patients in North America seek medical care. Although hypertension is a potent cardiovascular risk factor, randomized, controlled, clinical trials have clearly shown that antihypertensive treatment reduces the risk of stroke; coronary artery disease events, including congestive heart failure; renal failure; and progression to higher levels of blood pressure.[1, 2]

Despite prolonged and extensive public and physician education programs, blood pressure in the majority of treated hypertensives remains above recommended treatment goals.[3] There are many recognized reasons why blood pressure, in the general population, is not controlled to the recommended level of 140/90 mm Hg or less. Most cases of resistant hypertension can be accounted for by reasons such as inadequate or inappropriate treatment regimens and patient noncompliance with treatment, including moderation of alcohol intake, salt restriction, weight reduction, and taking medications as prescribed. However, a number of compliant patients have hypertension unresponsive to appropriate medication and lifestyle modifications. A careful, structured evaluation will uncover a treatable cause for the resistance in most cases.

PREVALENCE

The true prevalence of resistant hypertension is difficult to determine. Studies have suggested a range from 3% in a carefully structured work control program to as high as 29% of patients seen in tertiary care hypertension clinics.[4–6] Added difficulties arise from differences in diagnostic criteria for both blood pressure and administered pharmacotherapy.

In view of the current availability of pharmacological agents for treatment of hypertension, blood pressure should be controllable to current recommended goals in the vast majority of patients. A definition offered by the recent guidelines in the sixth report of the Joint National Committee on Prevention, Detection, Evaluation, and Treatment of High Blood Pressure (JNC VI) appears appropriate.[1] Hypertension should be considered *resistant* if blood pressure cannot be reduced to below 140/90 mm Hg in patients who are adhering to an adequate and appropriate triple-drug regimen that includes a diuretic, with all three drugs prescribed in near-maximal recommended doses. For older patients with isolated systolic hypertension, *resistance* is defined as failure to reduce systolic blood pressure below 160 mm Hg with a similar regimen. Although definitions differ, there is general agreement regarding the numerous factors that can contribute to drug resistance (Table 63–1). One or several of these factors may play a role in individual patient responses. A systematic approach to each patient can provide a cost-effective assessment that identifies caus-

ative factors to guide therapy in the vast majority of resistant patients.

PSEUDORESISTANCE

A basic requirement of any hypertensive evaluation is the accurate measurement of blood pressure.[7, 8] A calibrated sphygmomanometer with an appropriate-size cuff should be utilized in a quiet environment. Measurements should be obtained after 5 to 15 minutes of relaxation, and at least

Table 63–1 Causes of Resistant Hypertension

PSEUDORESISTANCE
Office hypertension
Pseudohypertension

DRUG-RELATED
Inadequate dosages
Inappropriate combinations
Inappropriate diuretic therapy (e.g., loop diuretic with normal GFR or thiazide with renal insufficiency)
Volume overload
Inadequate diuretic dosage
Excess sodium
Progressive renal damage
Medication intolerance (objective with or without noncompliance)
Rapid inactivation (e.g., hydralazine)
Drug interaction
   Nonsteroidal antiinflammatory drugs
   Oral contraceptives
   Sympathomimetic drugs
   Corticosteroids
   Antidepressants
   Nasal decongestants
   Cocaine
   Cyclosporine
   Erythropoietin

ASSOCIATED CONDITIONS
Obesity/hyperinsulinemia
Alcohol abuse
Sleep apnea

NONADHERENCE TO THERAPY
Costs of medication
Levels of literacy or education
Complexity of regimen
Inconvenient dosing
Inadequate patient education
Memory deficits, dementia
Subjective drug intolerance

SECONDARY HYPERTENSION
Renal parenchymal disease
Renal artery stenosis
Primary aldosteronism
Thyroid disease
Pheochromocytoma

Abbreviation: GFR, glomerular filtration rate.

30 minutes after consuming coffee or smoking a cigarette, since both caffeine and nicotine can transiently elevate blood pressure.

In a condition called *pseudohypertension,* the cuff pressure is inappropriately high compared with intraarterial pressure because of extensive atheromatous and/or medial hyperplasia in the arterial tree.[9, 10] The prevalence is unknown, but it increases with age, and diagnosis requires a high index of suspicion. A positive Osler maneuver is of limited value as a bedside screening test for detecting pseudohypertension. The Osler maneuver is performed by inflating the blood pressure cuff above the systolic blood pressure; if a hard, cordlike radial artery can still be palpated, the maneuver is considered positive. Observations that should lead the clinician to suspect pseudohypertension are:

1. Marked hypertension in the absence of target organ damage
2. Antihypertensive therapy that produces symptoms consistent with hypotension (dizziness, fatigue) in the absence of excessive reduction in blood pressure
3. Radiological evidence of pipestem calcification in the brachial artery
4. Brachial artery pressure higher than lower extremity blood pressure
5. Severe and isolated systolic hypertension[9–11]

Another helpful maneuver in the patient with suspected pseudohypertension is the use of infrasonic or oscillometric measurements that appear to more closely approximate intraarterial blood pressure than is measured by indirect auscultatory sphygmomanometer.[12–14] Mejia and colleagues[15] have described another important artifact of measurement, that of "cuff inflation hypertension" resulting in marked rises in blood pressure with indirect sphygmomanometry. Unresolved issues in diagnosis will be clarified by intraarterial measurements of blood pressure.

Twenty to 50% of patients referred to specialty clinics for hypertension evaluation have normal blood pressure on ambulatory monitoring.[16, 17] This is a critical distinction to make, since patients may not require additional therapy if the blood pressure is elevated only in the clinic setting. Home blood pressure recordings with an inexpensive, calibrated digital device or ambulatory blood pressure monitoring can establish the diagnosis.[18] The clinician then must be comfortable in management and treatment recommendations based on out-of-office blood pressure readings.

DRUG-RELATED CAUSES

In a review of resistant hypertension in a tertiary care clinic, Yakovlevitch and Black[5] showed that the most frequent cause of resistance (43% of cases) was a suboptimal medical regimen. Blood pressure was subsequently controlled in most of those patients (74%) by optimizing the treatment regimen, particularly oral diuretics. Clinicians continue to demonstrate reluctance to use diuretics or prescribe them in appropriate doses, despite the demonstrated importance of controlling extracellular fluid and blood volume in the management of hypertension.[19] Some antihypertensive agents, particularly sympathetic antagonists and direct vasodilators, promote sodium and water retention if used in the absence of a diuretic, contributing to refractoriness or "pseudotolerance" to these agents.[20, 21]

Most newer antihypertensive agents have been developed for once-daily administration, yet some agents may fail to provide a duration of action of 24 hours or longer across the entire dosing range for that drug.[22, 23] Administration of a dose of an agent with a poor trough:peak ratio may lead to suboptimal control of blood pressure and apparent resistance. Use of an inappropriate combination of drugs, in most cases the use of two drugs from the same class of agents (e.g., two β-adrenergic blockers) or two agents with the same or similar mechanism of action (e.g., an angiotensin-converting enzyme inhibitor and an angiotensin II receptor antagonist) would seem inappropriate unless carefully controlled clinical trials have demonstrated specific benefits. In contrast, the use of appropriate agents in combination, including newer fixed combinations, can significantly improve response rates over those seen with either drug alone.[24–26]

In some patients, inability to control blood pressure can be due to typical adverse effects that often lead to drug intolerance. This form of objective drug intolerance can occur with multiple attempts to prescribe a variety of agents. For these patients, the search for combinations of agents that are well accepted and tolerated is often disappointing. Many patients have access to extensive information regarding adverse effects of drugs, and objectivity in evaluating symptoms can be difficult. A precise history characterizing past experience with agents in the same class, dosages, description of symptoms, and time of onset can be most helpful in assessment. On occasion, rechallenging the patient with a small dose of the same or a similar drug may be appropriate.

DRUG INTERACTIONS

Nonsteroidal Antiinflammatory Drugs

Nonsteroidal antiinflammatory drugs (NSAIDs) cause sodium retention, enhance the vasoconstrictor responses to pressor hormones, antagonize the effects of other antihypertensive drugs, and therefore may interfere with control of blood pressure.[27] Two NSAIDs that do not participate in this important drug interaction are aspirin and sulindac. NSAIDs have been said to antagonize the actions of all antihypertensive agents except the calcium channel blockers.[28] Since arthritis is such a common comorbid condition in older hypertensives, clinicians must be aware of the potential interaction of administered NSAIDs with the hypertension treatment regimen. Two meta-analyses have demonstrated that NSAIDs lead to increases in mean arterial pressure averaging 4 to 5 mm Hg.[29, 30]

Oral Contraceptives

Hypertension is two to three times more common in women taking oral contraceptives than in those not taking these agents.[31] It is especially common in obese and older oral contraceptive users who smoke, but blood pressure will normalize in most cases within several months of discontinuing the agent.

Cocaine, Amphetamines

The prevalence of recreational drug use mandates that cocaine abuse be considered in all patients presenting to an emergency department with hypertension-related problems.[32] Acute amphetamine toxicity is similar to that of cocaine, but longer in duration, lasting up to several hours. Paradoxical rises in blood pressure, as well as coronary vasoconstriction due to exaggerated catecholamine effects on unblocked α-receptors, can accompany the interaction of cocaine with β-adrenergic blockers.[33]

Sympathomimetic Amines

Over-the-counter nasal sprays, oral decongestants, and appetite suppressants contain vasoactive compounds such as phenylpropanolamine HCl, ephedrine, pseudoephedrine, and oxymetazoline HCl.[11, 34, 35] When used for prolonged periods, these agents can induce hypertension or interfere with otherwise optimal pharmacological treatment of hypertension. It is important that the clinician directly question patients regarding the use of these agents, since they are rarely reported when patients are asked to review their other prescription medications.

The effects of sympathomimetic amines are largely the result of α-adrenergic agonist activity resulting from both direct stimulation of α-adrenoreceptors and indirect facilitation of noradrenaline release from neuronal storage sites.[34] On the basis of their wide over-the-counter availability, sympathomimetic amines have considerable potential for interfering with the response to antihypertensive therapy.

Tricyclic Antidepressants

Tricyclic antidepressants antagonize the hypotensive effects of adrenergic blocking drugs such as guanethidine, and blood pressure overshoot to dangerous levels may occur. The tricyclics prevent the uptake of these antihypertensive drugs in adrenergic nerve endings, where they act to reduce sympathetic nerve output. Similar interactions have been described for drugs like clonidine and methyldopa.

Cyclosporine

Hypertension is a well-recognized adverse effect of cyclosporine therapy and has been reported in as many as 50 to 70% of patients undergoing renal, hepatic, or heart transplants. Enhanced renal vasoconstriction with decreased excretion of sodium and water and a volume-dependent type of hypertension are observed in patients with cyclosporine-induced hypotension.[36] Hypertension management can pose a problem in these patients as long as the cyclosporine administration is maintained. Diuretics are particularly effective, but they may exaggerate prerenal

azotemia, and calcium antagonists can also provide effective blood pressure control.

Corticosteroids

Similarly, the mineralocorticoid activity of corticosteroid hormones promote salt and water retention and a volume-dependent hypertension.

Recombinant Human Erythropoietin

Recombinant human erythropoietin increases blood pressure in one third of patients when used in the treatment of the anemia of end-stage renal disease. The hypertension is due to increased systemic vascular resistance, partly related to the direct vascular effects of erythropoietin.

VOLUME OVERLOAD

The most common physiological cause for resistant hypertension is volume overload. Several common associations are evident. Excessive dietary sodium intake raises blood pressure and can contribute to resistant hypertension in treated patients.[19, 37] With the possible exception of calcium channel blockers, all antihypertensive agents are more effective when patients follow a sodium-restricted diet.[38, 39] Treatment with direct vasodilators (minoxidil, hydralazine) or adrenergic-blocking drugs (β-blockers, α-blockers) can lead to volume expansion and acquired treatment resistance (pseudoresistance). Control of intravascular volume with an appropriate sodium-restricted diet and an oral diuretic in adequate dosage usually leads to improved blood pressure control.[19–21, 38]

It is distressing to note how many patients referred for resistant hypertension are not prescribed an appropriate diuretic, even when receiving a two- or three-drug regimen. In some cases, the choice of diuretic may be inappropriate. In patients with normal renal function, the administration of a single daily dose of a short-acting loop diuretic can represent inadequate therapy. Similarly, the administration of a long-acting thiazide-type diuretic can result in inadequate natriuresis and diuresis in patients with renal insufficiency (serum creatinine greater than 2.5 mg/dl).

When volume overload is suspected, the simple measurement of a 24-hour urine sodium will often uncover inadequate dietary restriction in patients who claim compliance with a sodium-restricted diet.[20] The measurement of plasma volume can provide an accurate assessment of the degree of volume overload and serve as a guide to enhance diuretic therapy. If this measurement is not readily available, a trial of increased diuretic therapy can be rewarding.[5, 40] In selected patients, particularly those with renal insufficiency, the careful administration of a combination of a long-acting diuretic such as metolazone together with a loop diuretic may be indicated in an effort to ensure optimal responsiveness to the antihypertensive regimen.[20]

ASSOCIATED CONDITIONS

Excessive Alcohol Intake

Excessive alcohol intake is the most common cause of reversible hypertension in our society and should be suspected in patients referred for resistant hypertension. Multiple North American studies have shown a significant positive association of blood pressure and alcohol consumption.[41] Limitation in the daily intake of alcohol to no more than 1 oz (30 ml) of ethanol is desirable.[42] Further limitation in intake may be desirable in women and in men of slight build.[1]

Cigarette Smoking

Cigarette smoking causes a transient rise in blood pressure. The duration of elevation may be influenced by the number of cigarettes smoked daily. Heavy smoking is associated with a persistent rise in blood pressure and increased blood pressure variability.[43] The antihypertensive efficacy of β-adrenergic blockers is blunted in hypertensive smokers, particularly African Americans.[44]

Obesity and Hyperinsulinemia

Obesity and hyperinsulinemia blunt the effectiveness of antihypertensive drug therapy and can contribute to resistant hypertension.[45] Obese, treatment-resistant hypertensives exhibit a greater degree of insulin resistance and have a higher degree of central obesity together with hypertrophied skeletal muscle fibers compared with well-controlled hypertensives matched for age, gender, and body mass index. It is hypothesized that insulin-induced hypertrophy of smooth muscle in resistance vessels could provide one explanation for the finding of increased vascular resistance in obese insulin-resistant patients with refractory hypertension.[46]

Obstructive Sleep Apnea

Obstructive sleep apnea should be considered in persistent hypertensives who present with obesity, excessive drowsiness, and observed apneic episodes during sleep.[47, 48] Ambulatory blood pressure monitoring will show that these patients do not experience the usual circadian dip in blood pressure at night, and studies at sleep centers confirm that they are experiencing multiple episodes of apnea and hypoxia per hour (i.e., a high apnea index). Appropriate therapy should improve both nocturnal and daytime blood pressures.[49] Hypertension, coronary ischemia, and cerebral infarction may contribute to the higher mortality rates seen in men with sleep apnea and a high apnea index.[50, 51]

NONADHERENCE TO ANTIHYPERTENSIVE THERAPY

Nonadherence to treatment regimens for hypertension is the single most important determinant of outcome, is directly associated with excess morbidity and mortality, and should be considered in all patients undergoing evaluation for refractory hypertension.[52, 53] Nonadherence with antihypertensive medications and/or lifestyle modifications is observed in upward of 50% of patients, including those involved in some clinical trials.[54, 55] Primary care physicians seem sensitized to compliance issues, since only 10% of patients referred to a specialized hypertension clinic were determined to be noncompliant.[5]

Multiple issues, including medication costs, inadequate patient education, complexity of the regimen, and convenience of dosing, together with cognitive deficits or dementia, must be considered in assessing issues of nonadherence.[1, 56] Direct inquiry of the patient remains the best means of identifying nonadherence. When nonadherence with the medication regimen and/or lifestyle modifications such as sodium restriction or alcohol intake are suspected, despite adamant patient denial, supervised drug administration should be considered.[57] A precipitous fall in blood pressure after administration of prescribed doses of medication under direct supervision can unmask noncompliance, yet this method is infrequently used. Adherence can be improved by establishing realistic, short-term objectives for specific components of treatment, such as weight control, salt intake, physical activity, alcohol consumption, and once-a-day medication administration linked to the patient's daily behavior pattern.[52]

SECONDARY CAUSES

Secondary hypertension may account for a significant proportion of resistant hypertensive patients, particularly those referred for evaluation to tertiary care centers.[5, 40, 58, 59] Resistance to treatment in a compliant patient may be a valuable clue to secondary hypertension that has been overlooked. Renal artery stenosis and primary hyperaldosteronism are among the more common secondary causes observed, particularly in older patients.[5, 60, 61] Hypertension secondary to pheochromocytoma often responds poorly, or even paradoxically, to antihypertensive therapy.[62] Occult hypothyroidism is increasingly common in older hypertensive patients and is easily ruled out by appropriate testing.[60] Thorough clinical evaluation and recommended screening studies should be sufficient to identify other secondary causes of hypertension, such as renal parenchymal disease, Cushing's syndrome, and the occasional patient with coarctation of the aorta.[63–65] Table 63–2 outlines clinical clues to the presence of the more common secondary causes of hypertension.

EVALUATION AND MANAGEMENT

In approaching a patient with resistant hypertension, a thorough, yet orderly and cost-effective evaluation should be undertaken. The attached algorithm should be helpful in this regard (Fig. 63–1). The algorithm addresses those initial, common causes of resistant hypertension in which a diagnosis should be suspected in the course of a careful history and clinical examination, then proceeds to review

	Table 63–2 Clinical Clues to Secondary Hypertension

RENAL PARENCHYMAL DISEASE
Increased creatinine (>1.3 mg/dl male, >1.1 mg/dl female)
Periorbital or pedal edema
Urinalysis with proteinuria, hematuria, cellular casts
Small kidneys (any radiological study)

RENAL VASCULAR DISEASE
Abrupt onset of hypertension at age < 30 or > 55 yr
Stage 3 hypertension
Azotemia induced by ACE inhibitors
Abdominal bruit, particularly in diastole
Continuous epigastric bruit
New-onset hypertension > 50 yr of age, with diffuse vascular disease
   (carotids, coronary, peripheral)
Unilateral small kidney (any radiological procedure)

PHEOCHROMOCYTOMA
Episodic symptoms or spells
Headache, palpitations, pallor, and perspiration
Unusual lability of blood pressure
Stage 3 hypertension
Pressor response to anesthesia or drugs
Suprarenal or midline abdominal mass

CUSHING'S SYNDROME
Truncal obesity, moon face, hirsutism
Typical purple skin, striae
Muscle weakness and fatigue
Emotional disturbances
Carbohydrate intolerance
Amenorrhea, loss of libido
Spontaneous fractures

PRIMARY ALDOSTERONISM
Hypokalemia, spontaneous or provoked
Muscle cramps, weakness
Polyuria, occasionally polydipsia

COARCTATION OF THE AORTA
Diminished femoral pulses
Systolic pressure gradient between arms (particularly right) and legs
Systolic murmur
Continuous bruits over intercostal arteries
Three sign on chest x-ray

THYROID DISEASE
Diffuse or nodular enlargement of gland
Hyperthyroidism
   Anxiety, tremor, sleep disorder
   Weight loss
   Proximal muscle weakness
   Amenorrhea (younger women)
   Dyspnea, palpitations, tachycardia
   Wide pulse pressure

HYPOTHYROIDISM
Lethargy, depression, constipation
Cold intolerance
Carpal tunnel syndrome
Weight increase
Hoarseness
Parkinson's disease, decreased mentation

Abbreviation: ACE, angiotensin-converting enzyme.

those additional causes that would require additional laboratory and/or diagnostic studies.[66]

A careful history should address prior medications and response to therapy and review current medications, dosages and frequency of administration, and blood pressure response.[1] This drug history should elucidate inadequate

dosages and/or inappropriate combinations of drugs. The absence of a diuretic or an inappropriate choice of dosage would suggest the possibility of volume expansion and pseudoresistance, the single most common drug-related cause of resistant hypertension. Alteration in the choice or dosage of diuretic will often resolve the problem of treatment resistance without the need for further studies.

It is important to look for symptoms and/or patient complaints that may indicate an adverse reaction to current medications. Even when patients report that they are taking their drugs, adverse reactions may contribute to irregular dosing with prescribed drugs. The clinician must determine whether the frequency of dosing of any and all antihypertensive agents is consistent with the duration of action of those medications.

In obtaining a medication history, it is critical to question the patient directly regarding over-the-counter drugs, such as NSAIDs and oral decongestants, as well as the use of recreational drugs. In younger women, the use of oral contraceptives should be questioned. Keep in mind that many patients will not volunteer information regarding nonprescription drugs unless questioned. Suboptimal therapy, together with objective medication intolerance, with or without noncompliance, and the occasional drug interaction account for 58% of patients seen and evaluated in a hypertension specialty referral clinic.[5]

If the regimen appears adequate and well tolerated and no drug interactions appear likely, the clinician should

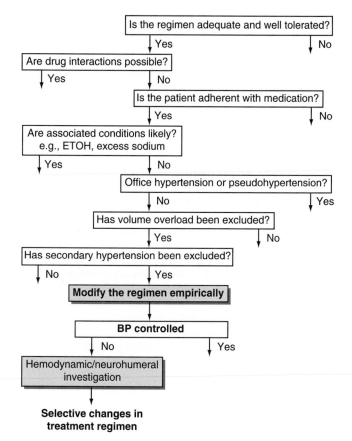

Figure 63–1. Algorithm for evaluating and treating a patient with resistant hypertension. ETOH, ethanol; BP, blood pressure.

proceed to address the issue of patient adherence to therapy. A direct and nonthreatening inquiry regarding patient adherence with prescribed drugs will usually bring a forthright response. Men and younger individuals are less likely to adhere to treatment, and inadequate adherence is more frequent in individuals who are less educated, unemployed, and more isolated.[52] Addressing the complexity of the regimen, the possible inconvenience of dosing, and the cost of medication in an open discussion will often uncover treatment inadequacies. Patients who complain of similar adverse effects with agents from different classes should alert the clinician to the possibility of a psychological aversion to medications. The same pattern of complaints is often noted with an initial dose or during the first several days of exposure to a given medication.

When a careful history does not clarify potential drug-related causes, one should look for clinical clues on physical examination. The absence of reflexive tachycardia in the occasional patient receiving minoxidil but no β-blocker or the absence of bradycardia in patients presumably compliant with moderate doses of a β-blocker should raise the question of poor adherence. The patient receiving a central α-agonist, such as clonidine, who voices no complaints of dry mouth or drowsiness and the patient on near-maximal doses of a dihydropyridine calcium antagonist without complaints of pedal edema would raise questions regarding optimal adherence with prescribed drugs. Appropriate adjustments in the antihypertensive regimen or changing to a better-tolerated agent may be all that is required in these common situations.

As the medication history and adherence to therapy are being questioned, the possibility of associated conditions should be considered. The chronicity of hypertension and the lack of associated symptoms lead many patients to fall short in the multiple lifestyle modifications required to optimize therapy. Whereas the presence of exogenous obesity, with or without carbohydrate intolerance, may be quite evident, daily alcohol and sodium usage will often be underestimated. Specific questions regarding type and frequency of alcoholic beverages as well as the makeup of the patient's diet are needed. The patient's spouse or significant other may provide insight regarding these conditions and may offer observations suggestive of the need for further evaluation of possible sleep apnea.

Evaluation of the resistant hypertensive patient to this point has been accomplished in the office, in the course of a careful history and clinical examination, and has required little to no additional laboratory evaluation. Careful attention to the issues previously discussed will have identified approximately 80% of patients presenting for evaluation of resistant hypertension. Drug treatment will have been appropriately altered and/or the clinician will have established realistic short-term therapeutic objectives to ensure adherence to both the drug regimen and appropriate lifestyle modifications. In the presence of several risk factors, it may be desirable to seek behavioral changes in a stepwise approach over time, so as not to overload the individual and exceed the clinician's expectations. Such an approach is particularly useful for anticipating and treating problems of adherence to antihypertensive therapy.[52]

Reported discrepancies between office blood pressure readings and those obtained at home or in other settings suggest the possibility of office or "white-coat" hypertension. Verification of home blood pressures using an inexpensive, well-calibrated digital recorder or 24-hour ambulatory blood pressure monitoring can establish the diagnosis.

For the occasional patient with pseudohypertension, the use of the Osler maneuver is unreliable, but intraarterial measurement of blood pressure will establish the diagnosis. As noted, infrasonic or oscillometric blood pressure monitors can also provide accurate readings.

If an explanation for the resistant hypertension is still in doubt, the clinician should reconsider the possibility of pseudoresistance due to volume overload. High-normal or modestly expanded plasma volume can induce pseudoresistance that may not have been apparent on earlier inquiries. A measurement of plasma volume at this point can provide guidance for more aggressive diuretic therapy, and 24-hour urine sodium content will reflect daily intake. If these tests are not easily available, a 1- to 2-week trial of increased diuretic treatment should be considered. If the patient is already on a long-acting thiazide-type diuretic, a small dose of a loop diuretic could be added two or three times daily. Changes in body weight as well as blood pressure may be used to monitor the response. Patients must also be observed closely for evidence of postural hypotension or volume depletion.

Having reached this point in the evaluation, it is appropriate to consider additional diagnostic studies in search of secondary causes of hypertension. Table 63–2 will be helpful in reassessing patients for a secondary cause that may be of recent onset or possibly missed during initial evaluation. Invasive diagnostic angiographic procedures should be avoided whenever possible in favor of noninvasive screening studies. The reported prevalence of secondary causes in patients with resistant hypertension ranges from 10 to 30% in series reviewed from tertiary care centers.

Renal Artery Stenosis

Renal artery stenosis is the most common cause of specifically treatable secondary hypertension and should be suspected particularly in those with recent-onset hypertension or hypertension that has become resistant to previously effective treatment. Captopril renography and renal arterial ultrasound are both sensitive procedures for demonstrating high-grade renal artery stenosis.[63] Magnetic resonance angiography, particularly when performed after an injection of gadolinium, provides excellent visualization of the aorta and main renal arteries.[67, 68]

Primary Aldosteronism

Upward of 30% of patients with primary aldosteronism present with resistant hypertension, many in the absence of hypokalemia. Renin:aldosterone ratios and urinary aldosterone excretion rates will help identify these patients.

Pheochromocytoma, Cushing's Syndrome

Plasma and/or urinary catecholamine determinations will identify patients with pheochromocytoma, and dexamethasone suppression will clarify a suspected diagnosis of Cushing's syndrome. Computed tomography scans can be helpful in localizing the lesion in patients with endocrine hypertension.

Progressive Renal Parenchymal Disease

Progressive renal parenchymal disease is heralded by abnormal renal function tests together with an abnormal urinalysis. Renal ultrasound provides an estimate of renal size and rules out calculus disease or obstruction.

If the evaluation to this point has not uncovered a likely cause for the resistance of blood pressure to treatment, it is appropriate to reevaluate the combination of drugs being used as well as the dosages. These patients should already be on a regimen of no less than three antihypertensive agents from different classes, including an oral diuretic in near-maximal dosages. Additional classes of agents may be considered, as well as further titration of dosages above the maximum usually recommended. Increasing dosages of selected agents is not so much an issue of safety as one of tolerability.

In selected patients, the direct-acting vasodilator minoxidil can provide a potent adjunct to the regimen. When this drug is used, associated fluid retention may mandate the addition of a loop diuretic, whereas reflexive tachycardia will require the presence of a β-adrenergic blocker as well. A central agonist, clonidine or guanfacine, can provide a potent addition to the regimen if the patient can tolerate the associated drowsiness and dry mouth. If small doses (0.1 to 0.3 mg b.i.d.) of oral clonidine prove effective, use of the transdermal preparation may lessen adverse effects.

All of the available classes of antihypertensive agents can be combined with one another, but not all combinations are equally effective, as well tolerated, or logical from a pharmacodynamic or hemodynamic viewpoint. Numerous studies have described the additional antihypertensive benefits of combining a β-blocker and a diuretic that can provide remarkably positive results in some patients.[69, 70] Similarly, the combination of a β-blocker and a dihydropyridine-derived calcium antagonist almost without exception offers improved efficacy.[71, 72] Conversely, combining a β-blocker and a nondihydropyridine calcium antagonist may be undesirable because of a possible increased risk of cardiac conduction abnormalities. Similarly the combination of an angiotensin-converting enzyme inhibitor and a thiazide-type diuretic is effective and potent.[73] Conversely, a β-blocker and an angiotensin-converting enzyme inhibitor used together appear to be a less optimal combination, with less pharmacological rationale. Available reports on two-drug combinations may not provide suitable direction to the clinician for patients on multiple-drug regimens, in which some trial and error are appropriate.

Modifications in the regimen can be made empirically, as discussed previously, or can be guided by the results of careful hemodynamic and neurohumoral evaluation. While the patient is receiving the ineffective regimen, a possible mechanism or mechanisms for the drug resistance may be identified to facilitate a more targeted addition or modification in the regimen (Table 63–3). These hemodynamic aberrations may represent the primary cause for the refrac-

Table 63–3 Hemodynamic Profile in Resistant Hypertension: Management Recommendations

Hemodynamic/Humeral Measurement	Management*
Cardiac output increase	β-Blocker
	NDHPCA
Peripheral resistance	ACE inhibitor, ARB
	DHPCA
	Minoxidil
	Hydralazine
Plasma volume increase	Loop diuretic
	Rigid NA restriction
Plasma catecholamine increase	Clonidine, guanfacine
	α-Blocker
Plasma renin activity increase	ACE inhibitor, ARB
	β-Blocker
Plasma/urinary aldosterone increase	Spironolactone
	Amiloride

Abbreviations: NDHPCA, nondihydropyridine calcium antagonist; ACE, angiotensin-converting enzyme; ARB, angiotensin receptor blocker; DHPCA, dihydropyridine calcium antagonist.
*If the patient is already taking drugs in this column, consider dosage increase.

toriness of hypertension or a compensatory reaction to other drugs in the regimen. Such observations may facilitate drug therapy through removal of potential protagonist effects (e.g., sodium and water retention from an α-blocker) and/or addition of agents capable of counteracting a given mechanism.

SUMMARY

Careful, systematic evaluation of patients with apparent resistant hypertension should, in the vast majority of cases, identify conditions and/or mechanisms of hypertension amenable to targeted therapy. The vast majority of cases of resistant hypertension will be unmasked by a cost-effective, office-based, and largely noninvasive evaluation. Few, if any, should elude a targeted hemodynamic evaluation designed to direct very focused treatment changes.

References

1. Joint National Committee on Prevention, Detection, Evaluation and Treatment of High Blood Pressure. The sixth report. Arch Intern Med 157:2413–2446, 1997.
2. Psaty BM, Smith NL, Siscovick DS, et al. Health outcomes associated with antihypertensive therapies used as first-line agents: A systematic review and meta-analysis. JAMA 277:739–745, 1997.
3. Burt VL, Whelton P, Roccella EJ, et al. Prevalence of hypertension in the US adult population: Results from the third National Health and Nutrition Examination Survey, 1988–1991. Hypertension 25:305–313, 1995.
4. Alderman MH, Budner N, Cohen H, et al. Prevalence of drug resistant hypertension. Hypertension 11:II-71–II-75, 1988.
5. Yakovlevitch M, Black HR. Resistant hypertension in a tertiary care clinic. Arch Intern Med 151:1786–1792, 1991.
6. Swales JD, Bing RF, Heagerty A, et al. Treatment of refractory hypertension. Lancet 1:894–896, 1982.
7. Prisant LM, Alpert BS, Robbins CB, et al. American National Standard for nonautomated sphygmomanometers. Summary report. Am J Hypertens 8:210–213, 1995.
8. Perloff D, Grim C, Flack J, et al. Human blood pressure determination by sphygmomanometer. Circulation 88:2460–2470, 1993.

9. Zuschke CA, Pettyjohn FS. Pseudohypertension. South Med J 88:1185–1190, 1995.

10. Messerli F. Osler's maneuver, pseudohypertension, and true hypertension in the elderly. Am J Med 30:906–910, 1986.

11. Messerli FH, Ventura HO, Amodeo C. Osler's maneuver and pseudohypertension. N Engl J Med 312:1548–1551, 1985.

12. Gandhi S, Santiesteban H. Resistant hypertension. Suggestions for dealing with the problem. Postgrad Med 100:97–102, 1996.

13. Hla KM, Vokaty KA, Feussner JR. Overestimation of diastolic blood pressure in the elderly. Magnitude of the problem and a potential solution. J Am Geriatr Soc 33:659–663, 1985.

14. Hla KM, Feussner JR. Screening for pseudohypertension. A quantitative, noninvasive approach. Arch Intern Med 148:673–676, 1988.

15. Mejia AD, Egan BM, Schork NJ, et al. Artefacts in measurement of blood pressure and lack of target organ involvement in the assessment of patients with treatment-resistant hypertension. Ann Intern Med 112:270–277, 1990.

16. Krakoff LR, Eison H, Phillips RH, et al. Effect of ambulatory blood pressure monitoring on the diagnosis and cost of treatment for mild hypertension. Am Heart J 116:1152–1154, 1988.

17. Waeber B, Scherrer U, Petrillo A, et al. Are some hypertensive patients overtreated? A prospective study of ambulatory blood pressure recording. Lancet 2:732–734, 1987.

18. Pickering T, for the American Society of Hypertension Ad Hoc Panel. Recommendations for the use of home (self) and ambulatory blood pressure monitoring. Am J Hypertens 9:1–11, 1996.

19. Dustan HP, Tarazi RC, Bravo EL. Dependence of arterial pressure on intravascular volume in treated hypertensive patients. N Engl J Med 286:861–866, 1972.

20. Gifford RW Jr, Tarazi RC. Resistant hypertension: Diagnosis and management. Ann Intern Med 88:661–665, 1978.

21. Finnerty FA Jr, Davidov M, Mroczek WJ, et al. Influence of extracellular fluid volume on response to antihypertensive drugs. Circ Res 27:71–82, 1970.

22. Meredith PA, Elliott HL. Concentration-effect relationships and implications for trough-to-peak ratio. Am J Hypertens 9:66S–70S, 1996.

23. Menard J, Belllet M, Brunner HR. Clinical development of antihypertensive drugs: Can we perform better? In Laragh JH, Brenner HR (eds). Hypertension: Pathophysiology, Diagnosis and Management. New York, Raven, 1990; pp 2331–2350.

24. Frishman WH, Bryzinski BS, Coulson LR, et al. A multifactorial trial design to assess combination therapy in hypertension. Treatment with bisoprolol and hydrochlorothiazide [see comments] [published erratum appears in Arch Intern Med 155:709, 1995]. Arch Intern Med 154:1461–1468, 1994.

25. Epstein M, Bakris G. Newer approaches to antihypertensive therapy. Use of fixed-dose combination therapy. Arch Intern Med 156:1969–1978, 1996.

26. Gradman AH, Cutler NR, Davis PJ, et al. Combined enalapril and felodipine extended release (ER) for systemic hypertension. Enalapril-Felodipine ER Factorial Study Group. Am J Cardiol 79:431–435, 1997.

27. Radack KL, Deck CC, Bloomfield SS. Ibuprofen interferes with the efficacy of antihypertensive drugs. A randomized, double-blind, placebo-controlled trial of ibuprofen compared with acetaminophen. Ann Intern Med 107:628–635, 1987.

28. MacFarlane LL, Orak DJ, Simpson WM. NSAIDs, antihypertensive agents and loss of blood pressure control. Am Fam Physician 51:849–856, 1995.

29. Pope JE, Anderson JJ, Felson DT. A meta-analysis of the effects of nonsteroidal anti-inflammatory drugs on blood pressure. Arch Intern Med 153:477–484, 1993.

30. Johnson AG, Nguyen TV, Day RO. Do nonsteroidal anti-inflammatory drugs affect blood pressure? A meta-analysis. Ann Intern Med 121:289–300, 1994.

31. Woods JW. Oral contraceptives and hypertension. Hypertension 11:II-11–II-15, 1988.

32. Brecklin C, Gopaniuk A, Kravetz T, et al. Chronic cocaine abuse causes acute but not chronic hypertension. [Abstract] J Am Soc Nephrol 7:1547, 1996.

33. Lange RA, Cigarroa RG, Flores ED, et al. Potentiation of cocaine-induced coronary vasoconstriction by beta-adrenergic blockade. Ann Intern Med 112:897–903, 1990.

34. Bravo EL. Phenylpropanolamine and other over-the-counter vasoactive compounds. Hypertension 11:II-7–II-10, 1988.

35. Joint National Committee on Detection, Evaluation, and Treatment of High Blood Pressure. The fifth report Arch Intern Med 153:154–183, 1993.

36. Textor SC, Taler SJ, Canzanello VJ, et al. Cyclosporine, blood pressure and atherosclerosis. Cardiol Rev 5:141–151, 1997.

37. Tarazi RC, Dustan HP, Frohlich ED, et al. Plasma volume and chronic hypertension. Relationship to arterial pressure levels in different hypertensive diseases. Arch Intern Med 125:835–842, 1970.

38. Frohlich ED. Classification of resistant hypertension. Hypertension 11:II-67–II-70, 1988.

39. Nicholson JP, Resnick LM, Laragh JH. The antihypertensive effect of verapamil at extremes of dietary sodium intake. Ann Intern Med 107:329–334, 1987.

40. Setaro JF, Black HR. Refractory hypertension. N Engl J Med 327:543–547, 1992.

41. MacMahon S. Alcohol consumption and hypertension. Hypertension 9:111–121, 1987.

42. Puddey IB, Beilin LJ, Vandongen R. Regular alcohol use raises blood pressure in treated hypertensive subjects. A randomised controlled trial. Lancet 1:647–651, 1987.

43. Groppelli A, Giorgi DM, Omboni S, et al. Persistent blood pressure increase induced by heavy smoking. J Hypertens 10:495–499, 1992.

44. Materson BJ, Reda D, Freis ED, et al. Cigarette smoking interferes with treatment of hypertension. Arch Intern Med 148:2116–2119, 1988.

45. Modan M, Almog S, Fuchs Z, et al. Obesity, glucose intolerance, hyperinsulinemia, and response to antihypertensive drugs. Hypertension 17:565–573, 1991.

46. Isaksson H, Cederholm T, Jansson E, et al. Therapy-resistant hypertension associated with central obesity, insulin resistance, and large muscle fibre area. Blood Press 2:46–52, 1993.

47. Hoffstein V, Chan CK, Slutsky AS. Sleep apnea and systemic hypertension: A causal association review. Am J Med 91:190–196, 1991.

48. Williams AJ, Houston D, Finberg S, et al. Sleep apnea syndrome and essential hypertension. Am J Cardiol 55:1019–1022, 1985.

49. Levinson PD, Millman RP: Sleep apnea: Management. In Izzo JL Jr, Black HR (eds). Hypertension Primer. Dallas, American Heart Association, 1993; pp 275–277.

50. He J, Kryger MH, Zorick FJ, et al. Mortality and apnea index in obstructive sleep apnea. Experience in 385 male patients. Chest 94:9–14, 1988.

51. Shepard JW Jr, Garrison MW, Grither DA, et al. Relationship of ventricular ectopy to oxyhemoglobin desaturation in patients with obstructive sleep apnea. Chest 88:335–340, 1985.

52. Levine DM. Adherence to antihypertensive therapy. In Izzo JL Jr, Black HR (eds). Hypertension Primer. Dallas, American Heart Association, 1993; pp 291–293.

53. Haynes RB. Determinants of compliance: The disease and mechanism of treatment. In Haynes RB, Sacket DL, Taylor DW (eds). Compliance in Health Care. Baltimore, Johns Hopkins University Press, 1979; pp 49–62.

54. Klein LE. Compliance and blood pressure control. Hypertension 11:II-61–II-64, 1988.

55. Sackett DL, Haynes RB, Gibson ES, et al. Randomised clinical trial of strategies for improving medication compliance in primary hypertension. Lancet 1:1205–1207, 1975.

56. Hill MN, Bone LR, Butz AM. Enhancing the role of community-health workers in research. Image J Nurs Sch 28:221–226, 1996.

57. Cronin CC, Higgins TM, Murphy MB, et al. Supervised drug administration in patients with refractory hypertension unmasking noncompliance. Postgrad Med J 73:239–40, 1997.

58. Isaksson H, Danielsson M, Rosenhamer G, et al. Characteristics of patients resistant to antihypertensive drug therapy. J Intern Med 229:421–426, 1991.

59. Davis BA, Crook JE, Vestal RE, et al. Prevalence of renovascular hypertension in patients with grade III or IV hypertensive retinopathy. N Engl J Med 301:1273–1276, 1979.

60. Anderson GH Jr, Blakeman N, Streeten DH. The effect of age on prevalence of secondary forms of hypertension in 4429 consecutively referred patients. J Hypertens 12:609–615, 1994.

61. Bravo EL, Tarazi RC, Dustan HP, et al. The changing clinical spectrum of primary aldosteronism. Am J Med 74:641–651, 1983.

62. Sheps SG. Pheochromocytoma: Evaluation. In Izzo JL Jr, Black HR (eds). Hypertension Primer. Dallas, American Heart Association, 1993; pp 268–270.

63. National High Blood Pressure Education Program (NHBPEP) Work-

ing Group: 1995 Update of the Working Group Reports on Chronic Renal Failure and Renovascular Hypertension. Arch Intern Med 156:1938–1947, 1996.

64. Rocchini AP. Coarctation of the aorta. *In* Izzo JL Jr, Black HR (eds). Hypertension Primer. Dallas, American Heart Association, 1993; pp 107–108.

65. Kaye TB, Crapo L. The Cushing syndrome: An update on diagnostic tests. Ann Intern Med 112:434–444, 1990.

66. Gifford RW Jr. An algorithm for the management of resistant hypertension. Hypertension 11:II-101–II-105, 1988.

67. Yucel EK, Kaufman J, Prince M, et al. Time of flight renal MR angiography. Utility in patients with renal insufficiency. Magn Reson Imaging 11:925–930, 1993.

68. Grist TM. Magnetic resonance angiography of renal artery stenosis. Am J Kidney Dis 24:700–712, 1994.

69. Hansson L. Drug treatment of hypertension. *In* Robertson JK (ed). Clinical Aspects of Essential Hypertension. Vol 1 of Handbook of Hypertension. Amsterdam, Elsevier Science, 1983; pp 397–436.

70. Dahlöf B, Lindholm LH, Hansson L, et al. Morbidity and mortality in the Swedish Trial in Old Patients with Hypertension (STOP Hypertension). Lancet 338:1281–1285, 1991.

71. Hansson L, Dahlöf B. Antihypertensive effect of a new dihydropyridine calcium antagonist (isradipine), combined with pindolol. Am J Cardiol 59(suppl B):127B–140B, 1987.

72. Hansson L, Dahlöf B, Gudbrandsson T, et al. Antihypertensive effect of felodipine or hydralazine when added to beta blocker therapy. J Cardiovasc Pharmacol 12:94–101, 1998.

73. Hansson L, Svensson A, Dahlöf B, et al. Drug treatment of hypertension. *In* Robertson JK (ed). Clinical Hypertension. Vol 15 of Handbook of Hypertension. Amsterdam, Elsevier, 1992; pp 658–708.

CHAPTER

64

Orthostatic Hypotension

Bojan Pohar and David Robertson

Patients with autonomic dysfunction present in quite diverse ways. These manifestations depend on which part of the autonomic nervous system is involved in the disease process. Some of these diseases have had a well-known pathophysiological substrate for many decades. Others are less understood, and their mechanisms are under intensive investigation. In this chapter, we focus on three major dysautonomic processes: *pure autonomic failure,* which has relatively clear clinical manifestations and was first described in 1925; *baroreflex failure,* which also produces a characteristic clinical syndrome and has a well-defined pathophysiological substrate; and *orthostatic intolerance,* which is much more common than the previous two, but is very poorly characterized in terms of pathophysiology. Clinical features of these autonomic disorders are shown in Table 64–1.

PURE AUTONOMIC FAILURE

This syndrome is also referred to as *idiopathic orthostatic hypotension* or the *Bradbury-Eggleston syndrome.*[1] These two authors in 1925 described the clinical presentation of severe autonomic failure. They described orthostatic hypotension with an unchanging heart rate, supine hypertension, reduced sweating, reduced basal metabolic rate, impotence, nocturia, constipation, and anemia. They demonstrated pharmacologically the failure of both sympathetic and parasympathetic nervous systems, together with denervation hypersensitivity to respective agonists. They also showed the therapeutic success of garments that prevented pooling of blood in the lower part of the body. Successful symptomatic pharmacotherapy with a sympathomimetic amine was soon reported.[2]

The orthostatic hypotension in pure autonomic failure is often extraordinarily severe (Fig. 64–1),[3] being greatest early in the day and after a large meal. In mildly affected individuals, orthostatic hypotension may be present only

after a meal. It may be present in the morning but not later in the day, after climbing stairs or walking up a hill, but not before. Even small body temperature elevation owing to infection greatly reduces blood pressure. Patients learn to avoid a hot environment because it also lowers blood pressure.[4]

The upright blood pressure may be 60/30 mm Hg or even lower in the most severely affected patients and cannot be accurately measured sphygmomanometrically. For this reason, it is useful to monitor disease severity with the *standing time.* It is defined as the length of time a patient can stand motionless before the onset of symptoms of orthostatic hypotension. As soon as the herald symptom of orthostatic hypotension appears, the patient is allowed to sit down and the time is recorded. If the patient is able to stand for 3 minutes without symptoms, a reliable blood

Table 64–1 Clinical Features of Autonomic Disorders

Feature	PAF	BF	OI
Orthostatic hypotension	+ + +	±	+
Postprandial hypotension	+ + +	−	−
Episodic hypotension	+	+ + +	+ +
Supine hypertension	+ +	+	±
Chronic hypertension	−	+ +	−
Labile hypertension	−	+ + +	±
Orthostatic tachycardia	−	+	+ + +
Episodic tachycardia	−	+ + +	+ +
Syncope	+ + +	+	+ +
Diaphoresis	−	+ + +	+
Flushing	−	+ + +	+
Emotional volatility	−	+ + +	+

Adapted from Robertson D. Disorders of autonomic cardiovascular regulation: Baroreflex failure, autonomic failure, and orthostatic intolerance syndromes. *In* Laragh JH, Brenner BM (eds). Hypertension: Pathology, Diagnosis and Management. Philadelphia, Lippincott-Raven, 1995; pp 941–959.
Abbreviations: PAF, pure autonomic failure; BF, baroreceptor failure; OI, orthostatic intolerance.

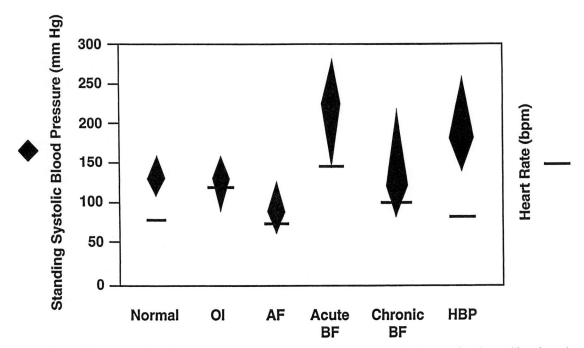

Figure 64–1. Representative standing systolic blood pressure and heart rate in normal subjects and patients with orthostatic intolerance (OI), autonomic failure (AF), acute baroreceptor failure (Acute BF), chronic baroreceptor failure (Chronic BF), and severe hypertension (HBP). The *widest part of each diamond* depicts the most common standing systolic blood pressure seen in typical patients, and the *height* depicts the range of pressures seen throughout the day. *Horizontal lines* depict the most common heart rate seen in typical patients. Patients with OI have orthostatic tachycardia. Patients with AF have the lowest standing blood pressure and heart rate. In acute BF, extremely high blood pressures are seen, in some cases even exceeding those seen in severe hypertension. Arterial hypertension and tachycardia occur together. After several months (Chronic BF), the standing systolic pressure is usually nearly normal, but great variability is still seen. (From Robertson D. Orthostatic intolerance and orthostatic hypotension. *In* Melmon KL, Morelli H [eds]. Clinical Pharmacology. New York, McGraw-Hill [in press].)

pressure determination can usually be obtained by sphygmomanometer.[5]

The standing time is primarily of value in monitoring patients who are not able to stand motionless for as long as 3 minutes. Many patients who have an increase in standing time from 30 to 120 seconds may have a substantial increase in functional capacity. It is important not to be overconcerned about a low standing blood pressure if the patient is without symptoms. Patients can sometimes tolerate a standing systolic blood pressure as low as 70 mm Hg without dizziness or syncope, probably because their cerebral blood flow is maintained at an adequate level because of the capacity of their cerebral circulation to undergo autoregulation.[6] A patient with a standing time under 30 seconds usually cannot live alone, whereas a patient with a standing time greater than 60 seconds generally can.

Many patients with pure autonomic failure also have supine hypertension, even when not taking pressor medications. Supine hypertension can be undetected if blood pressure is measured only in the seated position. In a recent study of 117 autonomic failure patients at our institution, we found that 56% had supine diastolic blood pressure of 90 mm Hg or greater and in 43% it was 95 mm Hg or greater.[7] Supine blood pressures as high as 228/140 mm Hg were observed. The results of this study show that supine hypertension is common in autonomic failure and frequently can be severe. The mechanisms responsible for supine hypertension in these patients are not known. It has

been reported that patients with autonomic failure have a normal plasma volume,[8] so an increase in intravascular volume cannot be responsible for supine hypertension. In a previous study, we found that autonomic failure patients with supine hypertension had a normal cardiac output.[9] Therefore, their hypertension was due to increased vascular resistance. As plasma norepinephrine and renin are low in these patients, it is unlikely that they play a substantial role in the increased vascular resistance. Other substances that increase vascular tone (vasopressin, endothelin, decreased nitric oxide production) need to be addressed in future studies.

Patients with asymptomatic orthostatic hypotension need no treatment, but should be closely observed for symptoms. Symptomatic patients can be treated nonpharmacologically by applying external support (by bandages firmly wrapped around the legs or by custom-fitted counterpressure support stockings) and by using physical countermaneuvers (leg-crossing, squatting, abdominal compression, bending forward, or placing one foot on a chair) to reduce venous pooling when in the upright position.[10] If orthostatic symptoms continue, pharmacological treatment, consisting of the mineralocorticoid fludrocortisone[11] and pressor drugs,[12] should be added. As patients with severe autonomic failure have a high incidence of anemia, which may contribute to their symptoms, erythropoietin treatment was tried and was found to reverse anemia and improve upright blood pressure.[13] An approach to treatment of orthostatic hypotension is shown schematically in Figure 64–2.[14] However,

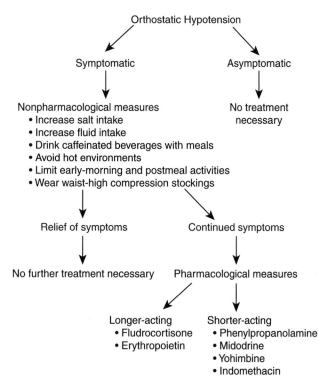

Figure 64–2. A useful strategy for the treatment of orthostatic hypotension. (Adapted from Jordan J, Shannon JR, Biaggioni I, et al. Contrasting actions of pressor agents in severe autonomic failure. Am J Med 105:116–124, 1998.)

the agents that are useful in treating orthostatic hypotension also aggravate supine hypertension. One approach for treating orthostatic hypotension in patients with supine hypertension is to use only short-acting pressor agents.[15] Transdermal nitroglycerin was found to be effective for the treatment of supine hypertension during the night. Patients are also encouraged to sleep with the head of the bed elevated 6 to 10 inches to avoid supine hypertension.[7]

BAROREFLEX FAILURE

Arterial baroreflexes maintain arterial pressure within a narrow range. The baroreflex arc can be damaged at any site: at the baroreceptors (stretch-receptors), in the vasculature (mainly in the carotid sinus), in the course of the glossopharyngeal or vagal nerves, or at the nuclei in the brain stem. In humans, baroreflex failure is a rare disorder, usually related to neck surgery, neck irradiation therapy for malignant tumors, brain stem infarction, or bilateral carotid body tumors.[5] Failure of the baroreflex at any point produces a characteristic clinical syndrome that is presumably caused by an inability to buffer supramedullary input to cardiovascular control centers in the brain stem.[16] Numerous animal and human studies have shown that complete denervation of the carotid and aortic baroreceptors is necessary to cause baroreflex failure, i.e., all baroreceptors, both glossopharyngeal and vagus nerves, and the brain stem nuclei have to be damaged.[16, 17]

At Vanderbilt University's Autonomic Dysfunction Center, we identified 11 patients with arterial baroreflex failure

(out of approximately 500 referred with severe disorders of autonomic function). Reasons for referral were evaluation of essential hypertension, suspicion of pheochromocytoma, uncontrolled severe hypertension, and assumption that glossopharyngeal or vagal nerves had been damaged. Among causes for baroreflex failure were surgery and irradiation of throat carcinoma in 3 patients; surgical section of the glossopharyngeal nerve for glossopharyngeal neuralgia in a patient with previously sustained injury to the contralateral glossopharyngeal and vagus nerves; the familial paraganglioma syndrome in 4 patients; and marked bilateral cell loss in the nuclei of the solitary tract (found at subsequent autopsy) in the setting of a degenerative neurological disease of medullary and higher structures in 1 patient. The familial paraganglioma syndrome is a genetic disorder in which affected individuals develop multiple benign non–catecholamine-producing tumors of the carotid body, glomus jugulare, and glomus vagale.[18] These tumors physically damage the glossopharyngeal and vagus nerves, leading to baroreflex failure. In 2 patients, no cause could be documented.

Patients with baroreflex failure usually present with arterial hypertension, either episodic or sustained. Patients who develop baroreflex failure more gradually (e.g., years after neck irradiation) usually have episodic hypertension but no initial phase of sustained hypertension. Sustained hypertension is especially severe in patients with acute interruption of the baroreflex arc (see Fig. 64–1). Hypertensive crises can be seen, with arterial pressures in the range of 170 to 280/110 to 135 mm Hg. The clinical picture is often similar to that of pheochromocytoma, in which arterial hypertension and tachycardia also occur together. Patients have the same subjective sensations of warmth or flushing, palpitations, headache, and diaphoresis. The diagnosis of pheochromocytoma[19] was seriously considered in the course of evaluation of almost all of our patients and was ruled out in some of them by computed tomography scanning, metaiodobenzylguanidine scanning, arteriography of the adrenal glands, and venous norepinephrine sampling. In addition, patients with baroreflex failure, in contrast to those with pheochromocytoma, show stability or improvement in hypertensive symptoms over time. There is sometimes emotional lability or nervousness in the history of patients with baroreflex failure, more prominent at the time of blood pressure elevation.[16]

The loss of the baroreflex buffering capacity causes much more pronounced effects of cortical influences on the vasomotor centers in patients with baroreflex failure. Pain, emotion, visual attention, and mental arithmetic may have a much greater effect in patients with baroreflex failure than in normal subjects. Hand pain (cold pressor test—placing the patient's hand in a combination of ice and water for 1 minute) in normal subjects caused an increase in systolic arterial pressure of 24 ± 7 mm Hg; in patients with baroreflex failure, increases of 56 ± 14 mm Hg were noted.[16] In normals, the increase in blood pressure abates over a few minutes once the hand is rewarmed. In patients with baroreflex failure, a significant increase in blood pressure may persist for more than 30 minutes (Fig. 64–3).

The diagnostic abnormality in patients with baroreflex failure is a large parallel increase in blood pressure and

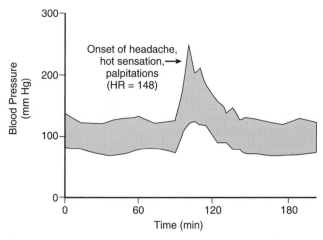

Figure 64–3. Blood pressure monitoring over a 200-minute period in a 43-year-old man approximately 2 weeks after surgical removal of a second carotid body tumor, 5 years after removal of the initial (contralateral) carotid body tumor. While blood pressure was being monitored at normal baseline levels, a cold pressor test with immersion of the hand in ice water for 60 seconds was performed. The blood pressure immediately rose and continued to rise for several minutes after the cold stimulus. The symptoms appeared during this time and resolved as blood pressure and heart rate (HR) returned to normal over the succeeding half hour. On some occasions, paroxysms of similar magnitude occurred without obvious exogenous causative stimuli. (From Robertson D, Hollister AS, Biaggioni I, et al. The diagnosis and treatment of baroreflex failure. N Engl J Med 329:1449–1455, 1993. Copyright © 1993 Massachusetts Medical Society. All rights reserved.)

heart rate with stress and a substantial decrease with sedation or rest. However, there is no reflex decrease in heart rate after pressor agents and no reflex increase in heart rate after vasodilators. In normal subjects, an increase in blood pressure of 20 mm Hg with phenylephrine will decrease the heart rate by 7 to 21 beats per minute, and a decrease in blood pressure of 20 mm Hg with sodium nitroprusside will increase the heart rate by 9 to 28 beats per minute. In contrast, patients with baroreceptor failure do not alter their heart rate by more than 4 beats per minute with either drug.[16]

Plasma norepinephrine levels parallel the blood pressure changes. During surges of sympathetic activity associated with hypertensive-tachycardic episodes, plasma norepinephrine levels as high as 2260 pg/ml have been seen. Many normal subjects cannot achieve such high levels even with potent sympathetic nervous stimulation, as in treadmill exercise.[5] During quiescent periods, norepinephrine levels may be normal (111 to 360 pg/ml). There can also be diagnostic confusion with orthostatic intolerance, because orthostatic intolerance is sometimes also associated with elevated catecholamines and volatile blood pressure.

Acute administration of clonidine decreases blood pressure, heart rate, and plasma catecholamine levels in such patients and is therefore useful as a diagnostic test to distinguish baroreflex failure from pheochromocytoma.[20] Clonidine is also the most effective drug in terms of decreasing the number and the severity of hypertensive crises. Diazepam is used to control stress.

In contrast to the majority of patients with nonselective (complete) baroreflex failure, parasympathetic control of the heart rate may be intact in occasional patients with this syndrome. These patients have a lesion involving only the afferent arc of the baroreflex (selective baroreceptor failure) and display not only undamped sympathetic but also undamped parasympathetic discharge and excessive vasotonic reactions. We have described a patient with episodes of severe hypertension and tachycardia alternating with prolonged episodes of severe bradycardia and asystole. Such patients require unique therapeutic strategies, including medications that attenuate sympathetic nerve traffic, medications that increase blood pressure, and in some cases, implantation of a cardiac pacemaker.[21]

ORTHOSTATIC INTOLERANCE

Orthostatic intolerance is the most common disorder of blood pressure regulation after essential hypertension, being found in approximately 500,000 Americans. It tends to occur in younger individuals, most under age 35 years, and most often in women. It has many causes. Homeostatic adjustments to the upright posture[22] in these patients for some reason fail, and disabling symptoms may occur.[23] These include dizziness, visual changes, discomfort in the head or neck, throbbing of the head, poor concentration, tiredness, or weakness. Palpitations, tremulousness, fatigue, and anxiety are also seen. Generally, there is little fall in blood pressure (see Fig. 64–1).[3] However, in the most severe cases, there are altered breathing patterns and orthostatic hypotension, associated with syncope. All these symptoms are attributed to inadequate perfusion of the central nervous system.

Orthostatic intolerance is very poorly characterized in terms of pathophysiology. In the 1920s, it was shown that orthostatic symptoms occur in patients now considered to have pure autonomic failure.[1] However, the diversity of presentations of orthostatic disorders was soon noted,[24] and in the intervening years, there has been much improvement in our understanding of the heterogeneity of orthostatic disorders and autonomic failure.[5] The contrasting features of pure autonomic failure and orthostatic intolerance are presented in Table 64–2. A classification of milder orthostatic disorders roughly calibrated by the severity of the impairment was proposed.[25] This patient population is heterogeneous, and their illness has been referred to by many names (Table 64–3). Each presentation has its own characteristic clinical pattern, but orthostatic tachycardia is the most constant feature. It is likely that a very large number of pathological processes have this presentation as their final common denominator.

Orthostatic tachycardia has caused investigators to con-

Table 64–2 Contrasting Features Between Pure Autonomic Failure and Orthostatic Intolerance

Pure Autonomic Failure	Orthostatic Intolerance
Hypotension	Tachycardia
Syncope early	Syncope late
Onset after age 50 years	Onset before age 35 years
Male = female	Female >> male
Low norepinephrine	High norepinephrine

Table 64–3 Syndromes Either Identical to or Overlapping the Syndrome of Orthostatic Intolerance

Hyperadrenergic orthostatic hypotension
Hyperadrenergic postural hypotension
Orthostatic tachycardia syndrome
Postural orthostatic tachycardia syndrome
Sympathotonic orthostatic hypotension
Mitral valve prolapse syndrome
Soldier's heart
Vasoregulatory asthenia
Neurocirculatory asthenia
Irritable heart orthostatic anemia
Chronic fatigue syndrome

sider several possibilities to explain the syncope. If there were a circulating vasodilator[26] or a reduced "effective" blood volume,[27–29] the orthostatic tachycardia might be an appropriate autonomic compensatory response mediated through the baroreflex to maintain adequate blood pressure and cardiac output.[30] However, this hemodynamic response may not be sufficient to adequately perfuse the central nervous system. A number of possible vasodilators have been investigated: bradykinin,[26] atrial natriuretic factor,[31] histamine, and prostaglandin D_2.[32] However, it does not appear that vasodilators are a common cause for this disorder.

These largely negative studies have caused investigators to look elsewhere to explain orthostatic intolerance. Some proposed that an abnormally sensitive cardiac β_1-adrenoreceptor could result in orthostatic tachycardia in situations in which the sympathetic nervous system is activated.[33] Orthostatic intolerance occurs in many patients with the mitral valve prolapse syndrome.[34] Some investigators reported an apparent "supercoupling" of β_2-adrenoreceptors: Although receptor number and affinity were not abnormal, activation of lymphocyte β_2-adrenoreceptors from patients resulted in greater cyclic adenosine monophosphate accumulation than in normal subjects,[35] suggesting an abnormal coupling of the receptors to the guanine nucleotide regulatory complex. These observations, together with those reported previously, strongly suggest that the major abnormality underlying orthostatic intolerance remains undiscovered.

The finding of high-normal and elevated plasma norepinephrine levels[36] and elevated urinary norepinephrine excretion[37] in some patients supports the view that increased sympathetic nervous system activation is responsible for the disorder. On the other hand, the observations of delayed recovery from the bradycardia of phase IV of the Valsalva maneuver and increased heart rate variability[34] suggest that there might be an imbalance in central autonomic regulation, a view that has been strengthened by evidence that there is increased muscle sympathetic nerve traffic even at rest in some patients with orthostatic intolerance.[38]

During recent years, suggestions began to emerge that orthostatic intolerance might also be explained, perhaps paradoxically, by an impairment in sympathetic function. Loss of the galvanic skin response (a sympathetic marker) on the soles of the feet has been noted.[39] The cause of orthostatic intolerance might thus be denervation of the lower extremities, allowing pooling of blood with upright posture. This hypothesis is based on an analogy to certain sensory and motor neurological disorders, in which selective impairment of neurons may occur distally, with or without more proximal progression. Viral and/or immunological causes could be operative.[40] In addition, patchy impairment of autonomic neuronal function could occur so that some areas remain intact. The heart might, e.g., remain normally innervated while the distal extremities could have impaired innervation.[41] Recent observations that there is reduced clearance of norepinephrine from the circulation in some patients with orthostatic intolerance supports this view.[42]

No contemporary pharmacotherapy of this disorder is broadly effective, although individual agents may be somewhat helpful in selected patients.[43] The most widely employed agents are the β-adrenoreceptor antagonists, which are given to attenuate the symptomatic tachycardia on standing. Another approach to minimize sympathetic activation is to use the α_2-adrenoreceptor class of drugs, e.g., clonidine.[44] Finally, in an attempt to increase blood volume and compensatorily reduce sympathetic activation, fludrocortisone, sometimes at doses above 0.4 mg daily, has been employed.[45] All of these drugs lower plasma renin activity in normal subjects. If low plasma renin activity contributes to the pathophysiology of orthostatic intolerance,[46] the currently used agents may be marginally effective because, along with the primary actions that constitute the rationale for their use, they also exert a counterproductive action at the level of the juxtaglomerular apparatus. This would mean that therapeutic alternatives that do not suppress renin should be sought. One alternative that is known to raise renin levels is exercise.[47] However, there has never been a prospective trial to assess the efficacy of exercise in orthostatic intolerance.

In summary, orthostatic intolerance is a final common clinical expression of multiple pathophysiological processes that alter the normal response to upright posture. Two pathophysiologies are expressed in a substantial proportion of patients: a partial dysautonomia due to impairment of the peripheral autonomic system and a hyperadrenergic orthostatic intolerance due to an abnormality in the central nervous system. With improved dissection of these and other pathophysiologies and improved matching of therapy with pathophysiology, improved therapeutic strategies for management of these patients may emerge.

References

1. Bradbury S, Eggleston C. Postural hypotension: A report of three cases. Am Heart J 1:75–86, 1925.
2. Ghrist DG, Brown GE. Postural hypotension with syncope: Its successful treatment with ephedrine. Am J Med Sci 175:336–349, 1928.
3. Robertson D. Orthostatic intolerance and orthostatic hypotension. *In* Melmon KL, Morelli H (eds). Clinical Pharmacology. New York, McGraw-Hill (in press).
4. Bannister R. Clinical features of autonomic failure. *In* Bannister R (ed). Autonomic Failure: A Textbook of Clinical Disorders of the Autonomic Nervous System, 2nd ed. Oxford, Oxford University Press, 1990; pp 267–281.
5. Robertson D. Disorders of autonomic cardiovascular regulation: Baroreflex failure, autonomic failure, and orthostatic intolerance syndromes. *In* Laragh JH, Brenner BM (eds). Hypertension: Pathology, Diagnosis and Management. Philadelphia, Lippincott-Raven, 1995; pp 941–959.

6. Bannister R, Mathias C. Management of postural hypotension. *In* Bannister R (ed). Autonomic Failure: A Textbook of Clinical Disorders of the Autonomic Nervous System, 2nd ed. Oxford, Oxford University Press, 1990; pp 569–595.

7. Shannon J, Jordan J, Costa F, et al. The hypertension of autonomic failure and its treatment. Hypertension 30:1062–1067, 1997.

8. Wilcox CS, Puritz R, Lightman SL, et al. Plasma volume regulation in patients with progressive autonomic failure during changes in salt intake and posture. J Lab Clin Med 104:331–339, 1984.

9. Kronenberg MW, Forman MB, Onrot J, et al. Enhanced left ventricular contractility in autonomic failure: Assessment using pressure-volume relations. J Am Coll Cardiol 15:1334–1342, 1990.

10. Weiling W. Nonpharmacological management of autonomic disorders. *In* Robertson D, Low PA, Polinsky RJ (eds). Primer on the Autonomic Nervous System. San Diego, Academic, 1996; pp 319–324.

11. Robertson D. Fludrocortisone. *In* Robertson D, Low PA, Polinsky RJ (eds). Primer on the Autonomic Nervous System. San Diego, Academic, 1996; pp 324–326.

12. Freeman R. Midodrine and other pressor drugs. *In* Robertson D, Low PA, Polinsky RJ (eds). Primer on the Autonomic Nervous System. San Diego, Academic, 1996; pp 326–332.

13. Biaggioni I, Robertson D, Krantz DS, et al. The anemia of primary autonomic failure and its reversal with recombinant erythropoietin. Ann Intern Med 121:181–186, 1994.

14. Jordan J, Shannon JR, Biaggioni I, et al. Contrasting actions of pressor agents in severe autonomic failure. Am J Med 105:116–124, 1998.

15. Biaggioni I, Onrot J, Stewart CK, et al. The potential pressor effect of phenylpropanolamine in patients with autonomic impairment. JAMA 258:263–239, 1987.

16. Robertson D, Hollister AS, Biaggioni I, et al. The diagnosis and treatment of baroreflex failure. N Engl J Med 329:1449–1455, 1993.

17. Cowley AW, Liard JF, Guyton AC. Role of the baroreceptor reflex in daily control of arterial blood pressure and other variables in dogs. Circ Res 32:564–576, 1973.

18. van Baars FM, Cremers CW, van den Broek P, et al. Familial non-chromaffinic paragangliomas (glomus tumors). Clinical and genetic aspects (abridged). Acta Otolaryngol (Stockh) 91:589–593, 1981.

19. Manger WM, Gifford RW Jr. Pheochromocytoma. New York, Springer-Verlag, 1977.

20. Shannon JR, Robertson D. The clinical utility of plasma catecholamines. J Lab Clin Med 128:450–451, 1996.

21. Jordan J, Shannon JR, Black BK, et al. Malignant vagotonia due to selective baroreflex failure. Hypertension 30:1072–1077, 1997.

22. Jacob G, Ertl AC, Shannon JR, et al. The effect of standing on neurohumoral responses and plasma volume in healthy subjects. J Appl Physiol 84:914–921, 1998.

23. Robertson D. Genetics and molecular biology of hypotension. Curr Opin Neurol 3:13–24, 1994.

24. Bjure A, Laurell H. Om abnorma statiska circulationsfenomen och därmed sammanhängande sjukliga symptom. Den arteriella orthostatiska anämin en försummad sjukdomsbild. Ups Läkarförenings Förh 33:1–23, 1927.

25. Streeten DHP. Orthostatic Disorders of the Circulation: Mechanisms, Manifestations, and Treatment. New York, Plenum, 1987.

26. Streeten DHP, Kerr LP, Kerr CB. Hyperbradykininism: A new orthostatic syndrome. Lancet 2:1048–1053, 1972.

27. Fouad FM, Tadena-Thome L, Bravo E, et al. Idiopathic hypovolemia. Ann Intern Med 104:298–303, 1986.

28. El-Sayed H, Hainsworth R. Relationship between plasma volume, carotid baroreceptor sensitivity and orthostatic tolerance. Clin Sci 88:463–470, 1995.

29. Jacob G, Biaggioni I, Mosqueda-Garcia R, et al. The relation of blood volume and blood pressure in orthostatic intolerance. Am J Med Sci 315:95–100, 1998.

30. Cryer PE, Silverberg AB, Santiago JV, et al. Plasma catecholamines in diabetes. The syndromes of hypoadrenergic and hyperadrenergic postural hypotension. Am J Med 64:407–416, 1978.

31. Hollister AS, Tanaka I, Imada T, et al. Sodium loading and posture modulate human atrial natriuretic factor plasma levels. Hypertension 8:II-106–II-111, 1986.

32. Roberts LJ, Oates JA. Mastocytosis. *In* Wilson JD, Foster DW (eds). Williams' Textbook of Endocrinology. Philadelphia, WB Saunders, 1985; pp 1363–1379.

33. Feldman RD, Limbird LE, Nadeau J, et al. Dynamic regulation of leukocyte beta adrenergic receptor agonist interactions by physiological changes in circulating catecholamines. J Clin Invest 72:164–170, 1983.

34. Coghlan HC, Phares P, Cowley M, et al. Dysautonomia in mitral valve prolapse. Am J Med 67:236–244, 1979.

35. Davies AO, Mares A, Pool JL, et al. Mitral valve prolapse with symptoms of beta-adrenergic hypersensitivity. Am J Med 82:193–201, 1987.

36. Low PA, Opfer-Gehrking TL, Textor SC, et al. Postural tachycardia syndrome. Neurology 45:519–525, 1995.

37. Boudoulas H, Reynolds JC, Mazzaferri E, et al. Metabolic studies in mitral valve prolapse syndrome. Circulation 61:1200–1205, 1980.

38. Furlan R, Jacob G, Snell M, et al. Chronic orthostatic intolerance: A primary central sympathetic disorder with discordant cardiac and vascular sympathetic control. Circulation 98:2154–2159, 1998.

39. Hoeldtke RD, Davis KM. The orthostatic tachycardia syndrome. J Clin Endocrinol Metab 73:132–139, 1991.

40. Fujii N, Tabira T, Shibasaki H, et al. Acute autonomic and sensory neuropathy associated with elevated Epstein-Barr virus antibody titre. J Neurol Neurosurg Psychiatry 45:656–657, 1982.

41. Streeten DHP. Pathogenesis of hyperadrenergic orthostatic hypotension. J Clin Invest 86:1582–1588, 1990.

42. Jacob G, Shannon JR, Costa F, et al. Abnormal epinephrine clearance and adrenergic receptor sensitivity in idiopathic orthostatic intolerance. Circulation 99:1706–1712, 1999.

43. Jacob G, Shannon JR, Black B, et al. Effects of volume loading and pressor agents in idiopathic orthostatic tachycardia. Circulation 96:575–580, 1997.

44. Gaffney FA, Lane LB, Pettinger W, et al. Effects of long-term clonidine administration on the hemodynamic and neuroendocrine postural responses of patients with dysautonomia. Chest 83:436–438, 1983.

45. Ertl AC, Schlegel TT, Mitsky VP, et al. The effect of fludrocortisone and salt loading on orthostatic tolerance following 7 days of 6 head-down bed rest. Clin Auton Res 5:326, 1995.

46. Jacob G, Robertson D, Mosqueda-Garcia R, et al. Hypovolemia in syncope and orthostatic intolerance. Role of the renin-angiotensin system. Am J Med 103:128–133, 1997.

47. Convertino VA. Blood volume: Its adaptation to endurance training. Med Sci Sports Exerc 12:1338–1348, 1991.

Individual Drug Classes

65

How Hypertensive Drugs Get Approved in the United States*†

Robert R. Fenichel

This chapter describes the means by which manufacturers gain permission to bring antihypertensive drugs to the U.S. market. Some of the chapter is applicable only to oral antihypertensive formulations intended for long-term use, but much of it applies equally well to intravenous antihypertensive formulations and, indeed, to drugs other than antihypertensives.

Before a drug may be promoted as an antihypertensive on the U.S. market, the claim of antihypertensive efficacy must be approved by the U.S. Food and Drug Administration (FDA). An antihypertensive product might theoretically avoid FDA jurisdiction by never appearing in interstate commerce, but the notion of "interstate commerce" has been so broadly construed that this option is more apparent than real.

Federal regulations do not prevent U.S. physicians from prescribing, or U.S. pharmacists from dispensing, medications (or other substances) for nonapproved uses. Medical insurers, however, frequently refuse to reimburse patients for the cost of such prescriptions. After medical misadventures, physicians may find it difficult to defend a therapeutic choice that was not FDA-approved. Perhaps for these reasons, and with the notable exception of immediate-release nifedipine preparations (approved in the United States only for the treatment of chronic stable angina, but widely prescribed as antihypertensives), unapproved products are not frequently prescribed as antihypertensives by U.S. physicians.

Would-be manufacturers have adequate incentives, then, to obtain FDA approval for an antihypertensive claim. To obtain that approval, the sponsor must demonstrate:

That the product is of known and stable composition, and can be reliably manufactured and distributed;

That there is an identifiable population in whom the product is reproducibly effective and reasonably safe; and

That it is possible to lay out evidence-based instructions for use of the product.

CHEMISTRY AND BIOPHARMACEUTICS

If a product is not of stable composition, then there is little point in discussing its clinical effects. In general, a drug's manufacturer is required to formalize the work of synthesis, compounding, packaging, and labeling, so that little is left to judgmental variation. The manufacturer is also required to establish a system of controls, to verify at various stages of manufacture that things are what they should be. The details of these requirements will not be of interest to most clinicians.

The proposed product must also be studied to determine the pharmacokinetics (absorption, distribution, metabolism, and excretion) of its active ingredient(s). Sometimes, development of the to-be-marketed formulation proceeds in parallel with clinical trials. In these cases, special bioavailability trials may need to be done to demonstrate that the to-be-marketed formulation is not substantially different from the formulation(s) tested in clinical trials. In addition, samples of the final product in final packaging must be shown to survive storage for the claimed shelf life.

TOXICOLOGY

FDA consent is required when a novel chemical substance is given experimentally to a human being in the United States. Before that time, the manufacturer of a new antihypertensive will generally have done studies to demonstrate that the new drug is antihypertensive in animals. Such studies are not required,* but in the case of antihypertensives, some such studies are almost always performed to reassure the manufacturer (and the FDA) that antihypertensive efficacy in humans can be plausibly anticipated, justifying the risks and costs of human trials. Once antihypertensive efficacy has been demonstrated in humans, the animal-efficacy data are no longer of great interest.

Toxicological studies in animals, unlike studies of antihypertensive efficacy, are strictly required. In general, human trials are permitted only after the FDA has reviewed animal studies in which maximal-tolerated doses were administered for as long as, or longer than, the proposed exposure in human trials. Unlike the efficacy studies in animals, some of these toxicology studies retain their im-

---

*The opinions expressed in this chapter are those of the author, and not necessarily those of the U.S. Food and Drug Administration.
†All material in this chapter is in the public domain, with the exception of any borrowed figures or tables.

*Because many human illnesses have no animal models, the FDA could not reasonably require demonstrations of efficacy in animals for all drug claims. Even in hypertension (where animal models are available), a drug effective in humans might conceivably not be effective in any nonhuman species.

portance throughout the development process and after approval. In particular, some toxicological studies (reproductive and carcinogenicity studies) are not analogous to any feasible human trials.

CLINICAL TRIALS

The earliest human trials are those that are traditionally called *phase I* trials. These studies may be unblinded and nonrandomized; their purpose is not to demonstrate antihypertensive efficacy, but rather to investigate human pharmacokinetics and metabolic pathways, to detect unanticipated adverse effects, and to begin the search for well-tolerated doses with some evidence of antihypertensive activity in humans. The subjects in phase I trials are conventionally healthy young adult volunteers; a typical trial might utilize only a dozen or so such volunteers, each exposed once or a few times to one or two doses. If the product is to be taken orally, there will be at least one study to determine the extent to which the rate and extent of absorption are affected by food. More complexly, if metabolism and elimination of the product's ingredients have been found to be dependent on renal function, or on the function of one or another of the cytochrome P-450 pathways in the liver or the gut, or if administration of the product results in induction or inhibition of those pathways, then other studies will need to investigate potential interactions between this product and at least a few of the important other products that interact with the same pathways.

Using the results of the phase I studies, the *phase II* studies are generally double-blind, randomized, placebo-controlled trials. In a typical trial, each of a few dozen patients is randomized to receive a few weeks of treatment with a regimen of placebo or the new drug. In other trials done around this time or a bit later, investigators recruit patients who are diabetic, who have hepatic or renal dysfunction, or who are receiving various unrelated drugs (e.g., antianginal drugs, cholesterol-lowering drugs, oral contraceptives) that are frequently received by reasonably large numbers of hypertensive patients. These various middle-stage trials greatly increase the total accumulated number of patient-days of exposure to the new drug, and sometimes they reveal adverse effects that were not apparent earlier. If all goes well, they suggest which regimens are most worth examining in the definitive trials.

As the phase II studies are completed, the trials that are intended to provide definitive proof of efficacy are designed and begun. These *phase III* trials are typically randomized, double-blind, placebo-controlled, parallel-group trials comparing two or three regimens of the new drug (different doses, different interdosing intervals) to placebo, with each trial following a few hundred hypertensive patients for 2 or 3 months. In the case of a combination product (e.g., a combination of an angiotensin-converting enzyme [ACE] inhibitor and a thiazide diuretic), the phase III trials are typically of parallel-group "factorial" design, in which patients are randomized to each of the possible combinations of (1) one dose from among several possible doses (including placebo) of the first drug and (2) one dose from among several possible doses (again, including placebo) of the second drug. The primary metric of each of these trials

is the placebo-corrected change in blood pressure, usually seated diastolic pressure, although systolic pressure is increasingly of equal importance. One of these trials is said to have succeeded when analysis shows that one or more regimens have effects that are significantly superior to those seen with placebo. Documentation of the phase III trials is usually the last-completed component of the package that an applicant submits to the FDA for marketing approval.

The phase I/phase II/phase III nomenclature is widely used, but the conventional distinctions are increasingly blurry. In recent years, for example, some investigators have done even their earliest trials using patients, healthy except for hypertension, instead of healthy volunteers.

SUBMISSION OF THE APPLICATION

A typical complete application comprises about 200,000 pages of text and tables, collected into volumes of about 500 pages each. A little more than half of the application is typically devoted to the clinical trials, which usually have involved a total of 1500 to 3000 patients.* Under the Prescription Drug User Fee Act of 1997, the application must be accompanied by a filing fee; for 1999, the fee is approximately $272,000.

Although FDA permission is required for human drug experiments within the United States, there is no requirement that a development program include any U.S. trials at all, so a program based entirely on non-U.S. trials might theoretically not come to the FDA's attention until the moment that the application was submitted. This theoretical possibility has never been realized; sponsors and investigators of new antihypertensives have always availed themselves of the opportunity to meet with the FDA on multiple earlier occasions during development. In an early meeting, the topic might be the order in which various potential claims might best be studied or what studies might be useful to estimate the importance of a worrisome toxicological finding. In later meetings, the sponsor and FDA might discuss which drug-drug interactions were most reasonable to explore or the design of the phase III trials. Still later, most sponsors visit the FDA to discuss the formatting of the application and the design of any computer-based aids for the FDA reviewers.

REVIEW OF THE APPLICATION

Some drug products are approved not on the basis of new toxicological and clinical data, but rather on the basis of chemical identity (and physical near-identity) to previously approved products. Applications describing such products

---

*No specific requirement for overall patient exposure is present in FDA regulations, but the FDA has accepted as "guidelines" the notions that there should be at least 1500 patients studied, at least 500 followed for at least 6 months, and at least 100 followed for a year or more. These numbers were the consensus recommendations of recent "harmonization" discussions among the FDA and its counterparts in Europe and Japan. This patient exposure greatly exceeds what is needed for a demonstration of antihypertensive efficacy, and it is determined by the desire to detect adverse effects that might not be apparent in smaller populations.

("generics") are handled by the FDA's Office of Generic Drugs (OGD). The pertinent chemical and biopharmaceutical criteria used by OGD are sufficient to guarantee that new drug/old drug differences are small compared with the expected interpatient and intrapatient variability. The details of those criteria will probably be of little interest to readers of this volume.

Applications for new antihypertensive drug products come to the FDA's Division of Cardio-Renal Drug Products (DCRDP). As of early 1999, the staff of DCRDP included 16 physicians, 15 toxicologists, and 11 administrative and technical personnel. In addition, there were at that time 11 chemists, 6 biopharmaceutical reviewers, and 4 statisticians who—although not formally members of DCRDP—were assigned full-time to the support of the DCRDP.

Filing

Within 60 days of the arrival of a new application, the DCRDP must decide whether the application is capable of being reviewed at all. Rarely, the DCRDP decides that an application is incomplete on its face,* so review would be impossible. In such cases, the DCRDP formally Refuses To File the application, and further processing is omitted. The Refusal to File action (like all others) is subject to appeal and reversal; in addition, a manufacturer may insist that an application be filed (and reviewed) despite the initial refusal by the Division.

Criteria of Approvability

Before a product is approved for marketing, the sponsor must have demonstrated to the FDA that the product is produced by a securely repeatable process and that its bioavailability has been described. The specific requirements in these areas are narrowly technical, and they are probably not of interest to most clinicians.

The clinical and toxicological requirements are of broader interest. The FDA does not look to the clinical trials for a useful estimate of the magnitude of antihypertensive effect. That magnitude varies, of course, from patient to patient. In the clinical treatment of hypertension, drugs are titrated to effect, and any given drug is used only in patients who appear to respond to it. If a treatment is effective in a given patient, then it is immaterial that its antihypertensive effect in other patients is small or even absent. But because natural variations in blood pressure are often similar in amplitude to the effects of therapy, the clinical trials may be the only setting in which active drugs can reliably be distinguished from placebos, and this distinction is at the center of the clinical review.

To demonstrate superiority to placebo, it is theoretically not necessary to do a placebo-controlled trial. If a new antihypertensive regimen were shown to be unequivocally *superior* to an approved regimen of an approved antihyper-

tensive agent, the new drug could be approved. If, on the other hand, trials seemed to show only that the new drug was *similar* to approved therapy, then interpretation would be much more difficult. Such results might reflect genuine shared superiority to placebo, but they might instead reflect only that the trials had been so poorly executed that even a totally ineffective new drug could not have been distinguished from the approved therapy. In any event, the FDA has never seen an application for approval of an antihypertensive drug in which the major phase III trials were not placebo-controlled.

The primary metric of each trial is usually the baseline-adjusted seated diastolic blood pressure, but other measurements of blood pressure (seated systolic, supine systolic and diastolic, standing systolic and diastolic) are also performed. Responder rates* are usually recorded, but (in part because of their necessarily arbitrary definitions, in part because of their statistical inefficiency) they have not been used as primary measures. Trials are usually powered to show that each of several doses of test drug is significantly superior to placebo, but sometimes the analysis uses a trend test to show only that taking all of the trial results together, the observed blood pressures cannot reasonably be believed to have been unrelated to the administered doses of test drug. In factorial trials, where individual cells of the randomization may each receive relatively few patients, a two-dimensional analogue of the trend test[1] is especially attractive.

From the widespread adoption of $p \leq .05$ as the threshold of meaningful statistical significance, and from the Federal regulations' requirement (21 CFR §314.126) that approvals be supported by "adequate and well-controlled studies" (note the plural), the FDA has come to expect that any approvable antihypertensive claim would be supported by at least two trials, each successful by the criterion of $p \leq .05$. A single trial with $p \leq .05 \times .05 \div 2 = .00125$† could in principle provide equally strong evidence,‡ but no antihypertensive application to date has ever rested its case on such an argument.§

FDA policy with respect to antihypertensives is derived from the landmark historical placebo-controlled trials that demonstrated the benefits of treatment with respect to the irreversible outcomes of stroke and similar hard endpoints. As described in Chapters 35, Characteristics of Published, Ongoing, and Planned Outcome Trials in Hypertension, and 39, Critical Assessment of Hypertension Guidelines, these trials employed antihypertensive medications of many

---

*For example, one application revealed that during a few months of storage, the to-be-marketed product came to contain large quantities of a degradation product whose carcinogenicity had not been studied in any species.

*For example, the fractions of patients whose last measured seated diastolic blood pressure was below 90 mm Hg *or* at least 10 mm Hg less than it had been at baseline.

†That is, two trials rejecting the null hypothesis with each $p \leq .05$ (.05 $\times$ .05), and both results in the *same* tail of the distribution ($\div 2$).

‡As could, e.g., four trials, each successful with $p \approx .3$.

§A treatment that is nontrivially antihypertensive in patients with mild to moderate hypertension can easily be distinguished from placebo in small, short trials (a few hundred patients for a few weeks), so these statistical thresholds (whatever their exact levels) are not much of a hurdle. They are much more of an issue in other clinical areas (e.g., congestive heart failure), and they may become important in hypertension if claims are sought on the basis of the large, hard-endpoint trials (see Chaps. 35, Characteristics of Published, Ongoing, and Planned Outcome Trials in Hypertension, and 39, Critical Assessment of Hypertension Guidelines) now under way.

different classes, always in stepped-therapy schemes, and usually starting with a diuretic or β-blocker. In every such trial with adequate statistical power to show a difference, antihypertensive therapy was seen to be superior to placebo. Whereas the fractional reduction in event rate was consistently large, the absolute benefit—at least in patients with mild or moderate disease—was generally small, typically only a few averted events per thousand years of patient treatment.

Because the benefits of antihypertensive treatment have been so consistent across such a wide range of regimens, the FDA believes that reduction of blood pressure—however achieved—can be expected to be associated with a reduction in the incidence of irreversible vascular events. Accordingly, the FDA considers antihypertensive efficacy to have been demonstrated when the regimen in question is shown to reduce blood pressure.

On the other hand, the small absolute benefit of antihypertensive treatment could easily be outweighed by a small incidence of unrelated toxic effects, possibly an incidence too small to be reasonably estimated from the total experience in a typical package of clinical trials. The clinical and toxicological reviewers must be satisfied that a new antihypertensive regimen is unlikely to be more toxic than those that, in the hard-endpoint trials, provided a net positive benefit.

Special additional criteria are imposed on fixed-dose combination products. Because any combination therapy exposes the patient to the potential adverse effects of each component, the FDA requires that each component of a combination product contribute to the antihypertensive effect and that there be well-defined situations in which the combination offers antihypertensive efficacy that is superior to that provided by monotherapy with one or another of the components. Some additional considerations related to fixed-dose combination products were described in a 1994 editorial.[2]

Why New Hard-Endpoint Trials Are Not Required

To avoid relying on uncertain predictions of long-term toxicity, the FDA could require that before any new antihypertensive regimens could be approved, net benefit would need to have been demonstrated in new hard-endpoint trials. The FDA's adoption of such a requirement has been proposed from time to time, and some of the difficulties of such a policy were discussed at the Cardio-Renal Advisory-Committee meeting of 20 October 1995.

Because most of the reported hard-endpoint trials were performed before the discovery of some currently available drugs, and especially because they predated our current knowledge of effective dosing of diuretics, limiting FDA approval to hard-endpoint trial–based therapy would not result in treatment recommendations that would be acceptable to most modern clinicians. The regimens tested in the hard-endpoint trials were shown to provide net benefit, but our knowledge of these regimens' toxicity* suggests that

current recommendations (although not strictly based on hard-endpoint data) are likely to provide greater net benefit.

Also, the very success of the hard-endpoint trials of the 1970s and 1980s makes it ethically impossible to perform similar placebo-controlled trials today. When interventions have been shown to prevent a substantial incidence of irreversible harm, it is no longer permissible to assign patients to inactive therapy.* Without placebo controls, and probably without control regimens identical to any of the creaky, now-disfavored regimens of the reported hard-endpoint trials, net benefit would be difficult to demonstrate.

Finally, many of the possible hazards of antihypertensive therapy can be reliably estimated from hard-endpoint trials in other clinical areas. Of course, it is always possible that an antihypertensive regimen will turn out to induce obscure organ toxicity (e.g., agranulocytosis, pancreatitis) whose net effect, integrated over the years of treatment, will negate the benefit of blood pressure reduction. To the extent, however, that the toxicity of antihypertensive therapy is likely to be directly related to cardiovascular effects (e.g., from excessive rate or extent of pressure reduction), that toxicity can often be assessed by looking at the results of relatively short hard-endpoint trials in which the same therapy was given to patients (e.g., those with myocardial infarctions or congestive heart failure) who might be expected to be unusually sensitive to such effects.

Primary Reviews

In the usual case, the application is formally accepted for filing, and the various sections of the application are reviewed more or less independently by specialists from the separate disciplines. In particular, separate primary reviews are contributed by a chemist, a toxicologist, and a biopharmaceutist. If the proposed product is to be administered parenterally, an additional review is provided by a microbiologist. In each of these disciplines, the primary reviewer's work is not considered complete until it has been cosigned by a supervisor. In many cases, the initial nonclinical reviews reveal various gaps in the manufacturer's documentation of its data and control procedures. The reviews lead to correspondence between the agency and the manufacturer, and thereafter to a (usually) convergent series of supplemental submissions and reviews.

Review of the clinical trials is handled differently. Sometimes, there are separate reviews by a statistician and a physician, but more often a statistician and a physician (or two or three physicians) jointly produce a single review, dividing the work among themselves under the direction

---

*They often used doses of hydrochlorothiazide and triamterene up to 100 and 300 mg/day, respectively, and often used hydralazine (up to 200 mg/day) and α-methyldopa (up to 2 g/day) as the first add-ons.

*Similar considerations are prominent in other clinical areas in which the goal of treatment is to reduce the incidence of irreversible harm. In congestive heart failure, e.g., patients in a typical placebo-controlled trial receive either an ACE inhibitor and placebo or an ACE inhibitor and the test drug. Omission of ACE inhibitors would be impermissible, since ACE inhibitors reduce mortality in this condition.

Despite the use of ACE inhibitors, patients with congestive heart failure have high mortality compared with age-matched controls, so the possibility of additional clinical benefit from an additional drug is not far-fetched. In hypertension, on the other hand, it may be unrealistic to expect that a new drug will provide additional hard-endpoint benefit when it is added to a regimen that is already providing blood pressure control that is believed to be adequate.

of a team leader who is then responsible for integrating the group's work into a coherent document. In addition to writing their review(s), the clinical reviewers will usually identify a few trial sites for routine audit by FDA field personnel. Like the nonclinical reviews, a clinical review often leads to correspondence intended to fill in gaps in documentation. In their conclusions, primary clinical reviews attempt to identify the clinical data whose interpretation should lead to approval or nonapproval, with suggestions for labeling in the event of approval.

Secondary Reviews

On average, each volume of an application submitted to DCRDP will cause the generation of about one page of primary review, so the several primary reviews add up to a few hundred pages of text. The primary reviews are then brought together by a team leader (always a physician), who prepares a secondary review of (typically) a few dozen pages, including overall recommendations for approval/nonapproval and labeling. The secondary reviewer's recommendations regarding approval and labeling may differ from those of the primary reviewers, but the primary reviews are not revised on this account. In this situation, the secondary reviewer will devote some of his or her review to discussion of the arguments that were raised by the primary reviewers.

Advisory Committee

At approximately this point in the review process, issues raised by the application may optionally be brought to a public meeting of the FDA's Cardio-Renal Advisory Committee. The Committee comprises 10 to 12 distinguished academic clinicians and statisticians, appointed for 4-year terms. In most years, the Committee will have three or four 2-day meetings, during which a total of 8 to 10 applications will be discussed. Sometimes the DCRDP turns to the Committee for help in reaching a difficult decision about a specific application, but Committee meetings are more often used to bring complex regulatory issues to public awareness, usually (not always) with initial reference to a pending application. At most meetings, the Committee ultimately discusses and votes on a series of formal questions posed to the Committee by the DCRDP. The decisions of the Committee are not binding on the FDA, but it is unusual for the FDA to contravene strong recommendations from the Committee.

Tertiary and Quaternary Reviews

After the Committee meeting (if any), a tertiary review (usually just a few pages long) is written by the Division Director. If the Division Director disagrees with the secondary reviewer or the Advisory Committee, then her or his review will generally explain the disagreement.

With two other divisions, DCRDP is a component of FDA's Office of Drug Evaluation I (ODE I). The FDA's decision authority about applications that come to DCRDP is held by ODE I, but this decision authority is often, on a case-by-case basis, delegated to DCRDP for applications (e.g., new formulations, new fixed-dose combinations) that do not involve new chemical substances. Applications for products containing new chemical substances are passed to ODE I for quaternary review.

Action Letters

The tertiary (or quaternary) review describes the FDA's decision as to whether or not the application is approvable, and an Action Letter is then sent to the sponsor of the application. An Action Letter describes the application as *Nonapprovable, Approvable*, or *Approval*.

A Nonapprovable letter must describe the deficiencies in the application that led to the FDA's negative conclusion. At the other extreme, an Approval letter is usually short and simple. The third type of Action Letter, the Approvable letter, is used for a product that appears to be safe and effective, but with respect to which there remain minor gaps in the chemistry description, unsettled portions of labeling, or other deficiencies that appear to be straightforwardly reparable. Marketing of the product is not permitted until the issuance of an Approval letter.

The total elapsed time from the DCRDP's receipt of the application to its issuance of the Action Letter has, in recent years, averaged about 14 months.

DEVELOPMENTS AFTER APPROVAL

Even after approval, a drug's sponsor is required to inform the FDA of the results of human trials and to report adverse drug reactions that come to its attention. Most approved applications are followed over months or years by various supplemental applications to amend the labeling with new claims, new dosing regimens, or new precautions or warnings.

References

1. Hung HMJ, Chi GYH, Lipicky RJ. On some statistical methods for analysis of combination drug studies. Commun Stat Theory Methods 23:361–376, 1994.
2. Fenichel RR, Lipicky RJ. Combination products as first-line pharmacotherapy. Arch Intern Med 154:1429–1430, 1994.

66 Diuretics

Jules B. Puschett

Over time, diuretics have proved to be safe and effective therapy for the treatment of essential hypertension. Although their predominant use as monotherapy has given way somewhat in recent years[1] to other classes of drugs, nevertheless, they remain a mainstay of therapy,[2, 3] especially in certain demographic groups[3]—African Americans, the obese, and the elderly. Patients in these groups behave as if their essential hypertension is largely mediated by volume expansion, hence, the utility of the diuretics. In this chapter, the following aspects of the use of diuretics in the therapy of hypertension are discussed: (1) How do diuretics reduce high blood pressure? (2) What is the evidence that therapy of hypertension with diuretics is beneficial with respect to the morbidity and mortality of this disease process? (3) What diuretics are currently available for use? (4) What are the complications of diuretic usage? (5) Finally, what are the therapeutic guidelines and suggestions for use of diuretics?

MECHANISM(S) OF ACTION OF DIURETICS IN HYPERTENSION

The pathogenetic mechanisms of essential hypertension may be divided into two broad general categories: volume expansion and vasoconstriction. This formulation is based on the physical expression relating blood pressure (P), blood flow (Q), and resistance to flow (R) as follows:

$$Q = P/R$$

Rearranging this equation to solve for blood pressure, one obtains the expression

$$P = Q \times R$$

Thus, one can perturb blood pressure by either altering blood flow through the vasculature or changing flow resistance, or both. If we concentrate for the moment on blood flow, we recognize that this parameter is represented in the human being by cardiac output. Furthermore, cardiac output is, in turn, dependent on venous return to the heart. The major determinant of venous return is the extracellular fluid volume. Thus, vascular flow is a function of body volume, and the relationship of extracellular fluid volume and blood pressure has been well documented (Fig. 66–1).[4] Theoretically, therefore, the ability of diuretics to lower blood pressure should depend on their capacity to cause volume depletion.[5] Acutely, this is certainly the case, as demonstrated by a number of workers.[6–11]

The longer-term effects of the diuretics are also mediated by a reduction in total peripheral resistance, which may assume a predominant role with extracellular fluid volume trending toward pretreatment levels (Table 66–1).[12–18] These changes are depicted diagrammatically in Figure 66–2. The possibility that diuretics may have a

direct vascular effect is supported by the data of Baumgart and coworkers.[19] These workers treated mild to moderate hypertensives with a nonnatriuretic dose of torsemide, a recently developed long-acting loop of Henle blocker (Table 66–2). They observed an average reduction in blood pressure of 15 mm Hg. Furthermore, the primary importance of volume depletion associated with sodium loss as the antihypertensive mechanism of diuretics is verified by studies performed by Wilson and Freis.[9] They treated a group of hypertensives with thiazide diuretics, achieving normalization of their blood pressure. They then continued the diuretic but acutely volume-expanded the patients, with the result that blood pressure returned to pretreatment levels and the antihypertensive effect of the diuretic was vitiated.

EFFECTS OF DIURETICS ON MORBIDITY AND MORTALITY

Beginning in the mid-1980s, and despite their long record (>30 years) of safe and effective use, questions began to be raised about potential risks of both the short-term and the long-term use of diuretics as monotherapy of essential hypertension.[20] The major concern raised by the Multiple Risk Factor Intervention Trial (MRFIT) was that hypertensive male subjects with abnormal baseline electrocardiograms had a higher death rate from coronary artery disease events when treated with diuretics. This was presumed to be related to the development of fatal arrhythmias believed

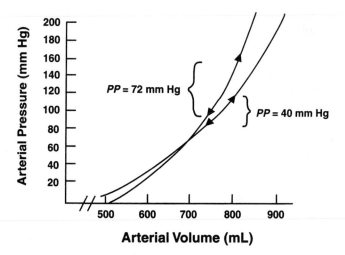

Figure 66–1. Relationship between vascular volume and blood pressure. PP, pulse pressure. (From Vari RC, Navar LG. Normal regulation of arterial pressure. *In* Jacobson HR, Striker GE, Klahr S [eds]. The Principles and Practice of Nephrology, 2nd ed. St. Louis, Mosby–Year Book, 1995; pp 354–361.)

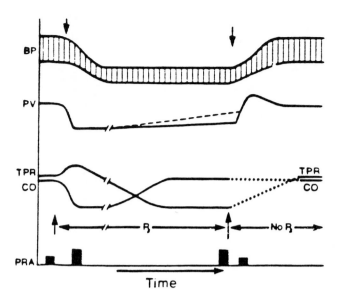

Figure 66–2. Diagrammatic representation of the effects of diuretic administration on blood pressure (BP), plasma volume (PV), total peripheral resistance (TPR), and cardiac output (CO). Therapy with a thiazide diuretic was begun at the *arrow* on the *left (top)* and discontinued at the *arrow* on the *right*. PRA, plasma renin activity. (From Puschett JB. Diuretics. *In* Izzo JL Jr, Black HR [eds]. Hypertension Primer. Dallas, American Heart Association, 1993; pp 294–296; adapted from Tarazi R, Dustan HP, Frohlich ED. Long-term thiazide therapy in essential hypertension. Circulation 41:709, 1970.)

to be caused by hypokalemia induced by the thiazides. A more recent case-control study from the Netherlands has also raised this issue.[21] Furthermore, it was subsequently proposed that diuretics, unlike other classes of antihypertensive drugs (most notably, the calcium channel blockers and angiotensin-converting enzyme inhibitors), do not cause the regression of left ventricular hypertrophy (specifically, a reduction in left ventricular muscle mass).[22–25] It was further proposed that this phenomenon renders diuretics less effective in preventing congestive heart failure, sudden death, and myocardial infarction. In addition, concerns were expressed that elevations in serum cholesterol associated with thiazide use[26, 27] could compromise the ability of these drugs to improve cardiovascular mortality.

Several events have combined to dispel the concerns previously raised about the use of diuretics as first-line therapy in the treatment of hypertension. Mortality from stroke and coronary artery events continues to decline, with the latest data indicating age-adjusted reductions of 60%

and 53%, respectively.[2] Second, the reduction in doses of thiazides that has taken place over the last several years has had a significant impact in reducing diuretic complications, particularly hypokalemia.[28–30] Results of several large trials have shown that lower doses of diuretics are effective in controlling hypertension as well as reducing the incidence of coronary artery disease and stroke.[31–35] In some of these clinical trials, either potassium supplementation or the addition of a potassium-sparing drug was used.

There is conclusive evidence that the thiazide diuretics cause reductions in both left ventricular hypertrophy and left ventricular muscle mass.[25, 34–37] Further, diuretics are effective in reducing the occurrence of congestive heart failure. In a recent analysis from the Systolic Hypertension in the Elderly Program (SHEP) Cooperative Research Group, the overall incidence of heart failure was reduced by 50%.[38] This dramatic benefit was observed whether or not patients had evidence of previous myocardial infarction.

Short-term elevations in serum cholesterol have been documented in association with thiazide use.[26, 27, 31 39] However, these increments have generally been small, and longer-term studies demonstrate that the values decline to pretreatment levels after 6 to 24 months of therapy.[40–44]

Based on these observations and others, consensus favors the concept that diuretics remain safe and effective first-line therapy for hypertension.[5, 45–50] In the era of managed care, the fact that these drugs are generally much less expensive than alternative therapies makes them attractive choices, especially in the economically disadvantaged patient. Finally, their use in those demographic groups that behave as if their hypertension is largely mediated by volume expansion (African Americans, the elderly, and the obese) recommends their use as first-line therapy in a substantial segment of the hypertensive population.

CURRENT DIURETIC THERAPY FOR HYPERTENSION

Table 66–2 is a list of diuretics that are currently available in the United States for the therapy of hypertension, along with brief descriptions of their key features and dosage guidelines. The mainstays of diuretic therapy of hypertension, as discussed extensively earlier, are hydrochlorothiazide, chlorthalidone, and their congeners. Although these agents are only moderately potent natriuretic agents, their utility resides in the fact that they are long-acting and can be given once-daily. Their long duration of action results in a persistent natriuretic effect and avoids the diuretic rebound[51] observed with the short-acting loop of Henle agents furosemide, bumetanide, and ethacrynic acid. For this reason, the short-acting loop of Henle agents are not good antihypertensive agents, unless one is prepared to prescribe them two or three times daily. An exception to this is the new loop of Henle agent torsemide, which has a long duration of action and is especially useful in patients with renal insufficiency in whom the thiazides are not effective. The potassium-sparing agents, alone or in combination with the thiazides or other diuretics, are chosen principally for their ability to reduce potassium excretion, thus minimizing the development of hypokalemia.

Table 66–1 Effects of Diuretics on Systemic Hemodynamics in Hypertensive Patients				
	BP	PV/BV	CO	TPR
Acute	↓	↓	↓	↑
Subacute	↓		↑, ↓	↑
Chronic	↓	N or ↓	↑, N, or ↓	↓

From O'Donovan RA, Muhammedi M, Puschett JB. Diuretics in the therapy of hypertension: Current status. Am J Med Sci 304:312–318, 1992.
Abbreviations: BP, blood pressure; PV, plasma volume; BV, blood volume; CO, cardiac output; TPR, total peripheral resistance; N, normal.

Table 66–2 Characteristics and Dosages of Diuretics Currently Available for Use in the Treatment of Hypertension

Drug Generic	Trade Name	Chemical Class	Potency*	Primary Nephron Site of Action†	Duration of Action	Dosage in Hypertension	Remarks
THIAZIDES AND THIAZIDE-LIKE AGENTS							
Hydrochlorothiazide	Hydrodiuril	Sulfonamide derivative	Moderately potent	Early distal convoluted tubule (site 3)	24 hr	12.5–50 mg, q.d.	Begin with 12.5 mg in the elderly; top dose is 25 mg; in other age groups, exceeding 50 mg/day considerably increases the likelihood of the development of hypokalemia and other metabolic side effects. Thiazides are not effective in patients with reduced glomerular filtration rate (<30–40 ml/min)
Chlorthalidone	Hygroton	Sulfonamide derivative	Moderately potent	Early distal convoluted tubule (site 3)	24–48 hr	12.5–50 mg, q.d.	Chlorthalidone is a member of the thiazide group of diuretics; it differs from hydrochlorothiazide in that it may act for up to 48 hr; otherwise, comments (above) for hydrochlorothiazide apply
Metolazone	Zaroxolyn, Diulo	Quinazoline-sulfonamide	Moderately potent	Early distal convoluted tubule (site 3)‡	24 hr	0.5–5.0 mg, q.d.	Metolazone differs from hydrochlorothiazide or chorthalidone in that it is effective in patients with marked reductions in glomerular filtration rate; however, in the latter group of patients, larger doses (10–20 mg) than those used in benign essential hypertension will often be required; because of its proximal activity,‡ metolazone has proved useful in combination therapy in advanced renal failure and in patients with hypertension who have resistant edema
LOOP OF HENLE DIURETICS							
Furosemide	Lasix	Sulfonamide derivative	Very potent	Loop of Henle (site 2)	4–6 hr	40–240 mg, b.i.d.	The loop of Henle drugs, typified by furosemide, have an advantage over the thiazides in that they cause substantially greater amounts of sodium to be excreted and are effective when given in incremental doses in patients with even advanced renal failure; however, with the exception of torsemide, they have the disadvantage that they are short-acting; thus, unless given more than once-daily, they are not effective antihypertensive drugs because they cause diuretic "rebound" to occur; in hypertensive patients with edema, the single effective dose should be determined, then repeated if necessary; in very edematous hypertensive patients, the intravenous route may initially be necessary, as is the case for patients with pulmonary edema; in patients with normal or only mildly impaired renal function, 40 mg b.i.d. is often sufficient; approximate dosage equivalents for the loop of Henle drugs: furosemide 40 mg ≅ bumetanide 1 mg ≅ ethacrynic acid 50 mg ≈ torsemide 20 mg

Generic name	Trade name	Chemical class	Potency	Nephron site†	Half-life	Dosage	Comments
Bumetanide	Bumex	Sulfonamide derivative	Very potent	Loop of Henle (site 2)	4–6 hr	0.5–5.0 mg, b.i.d.	Comments (above) for furosemide related to general properties of loop-active drugs apply to bumetanide as well; rather than continuing to escalate the dose in hypertensive patients with refractory edema, combination therapy ("sequential nephron blockade") is recommended (see text); in some cases, patients who do not respond to one of the other loop of Henle agents will respond to bumetanide, and vice versa
Ethacrynic acid	Edecrin	Substituted phenoxyacetic acid	Very potent	Loop of Henle (site 2)	4–6 hr	25.0–100.0 mg b.i.d.	See comments for furosemide and bumetanide (above)
Torsemide	Demadex	Sulfonamide derivative	Very potent	Loop of Henle (site 2)	12–24 hr	2.5–10.0 mg q.d.	Unlike the other loop of Henle drugs, torsemide need be given only once-daily; in hypertensive patients with pulmonary edema and in advanced renal failure, dosages of 100 mg and 200 mg, respectively, have been effectively utilized; in patients with normal renal function and no edema, 2.5–5.0 mg/day is often adequate
POTASSIUM-SPARING AGENTS							
Spironolactone	Aldactone	Steroid	Mildly potent	Late distal convolution and collecting duct (site 4a)	24–48 hr	25–100 mg, q.d.-b.i.d.	In hypertension, the potassium-sparing agents are used almost exclusively in combination with the thiazides to reduce the likelihood that hypokalemia will develop; fixed-dosage combination of the thiazides and triamterene (Maxzide, Dyazide) are available and are often employed, as are combinations of hydrochlorothiazide and spironolactone (e.g., Aldactazide) and hydrochlorothiazide with amiloride (Moduretic); spironolactone is a competitive inhibitor of aldosterone
Amiloride	Midamor	Pyrazine-carbonyl guanidine	Mildly potent	Late distal convolution and collecting duct (site 4b)	12–24 hr	5–10 mg, q.d.-b.i.d.	See general comments related to potassium-sparing agents; amiloride acts either by blocking sodium channels or by causing them to be open less frequently
Triamterene	Dyrenium	Pteridine derivative	Mildly potent	Late distal convolution and collecting duct (site 4b)	6–8 hr	50–150 mg q.d.-b.i.d.	Mechanism of action most likely same as for amiloride; potassium-sparing drugs should be used with caution or not at all in patients with renal insufficiency/failure

Modified from Puschett JB. Diuretics. *In* Izzo JL, Black HR (eds). Hypertension Primer. Dallas, American Heart Association, 1993; pp 294–296.

*Moderately potent, causes the excretion of 5–8% of filtered sodium load; mildly potent, causes the excretion of 2–3% of filtered sodium load; very potent, causes the excretion of 15–25% of filtered sodium load.

†For nephron site, see Figure 66–3.

‡Metolazone has proximal tubular activity as well. However, the proximally rejected ions are reabsorbed in the loop of Henle.

The primary site of action of each drug in the nephron is provided in Table 66–2. A detailed description of the actions of each drug on the transport system located at each of the nephron sites is beyond the scope of this discussion. The reader is directed to other reviews for a more complete analysis of this aspect of diuretic action.[52, 53] In hypertensive patients with resistant edema, the administration of more than one diuretic in order to block the proximal tubule, loop of Henle, and early distal convolutions sequentially and simultaneously will often result in a natriuresis when neither drug alone is effective.[54, 55]

DIURETIC COMPLICATIONS

Volume contraction results from the injudicious use of diuretics and represents an exaggeration of their therapeutic effect. This may manifest itself simply as an elevation in blood urea nitrogen or increments in both blood urea nitrogen and serum creatinine, with the former rising proportionately more than the latter ("prerenal azotemia"). More profound volume depletion will result in findings such as orthostatic hypotension, poor tissue turgor, tachycardia, and postural symptoms. In severe cases, supine hypotension and reduced urinary output can be present. Therapy of this complication ordinarily includes discontinuation of the diuretic and liberalization of sodium in the diet. In more severe cases, volume resuscitation with saline may be required.

Hypokalemia has been discussed extensively earlier. It results from the following phenomena:

1. Diuretics that act at nephron segments proximal to site 4 (Fig. 66–3) present additional amounts of sodium for exchange at this site. This occurs at an accelerated rate with a consequent secretion of potassium and hydrogen ions in exchange for sodium.
2. Diuretics that work in the proximal nephron and the loop of Henle interfere not only with the reabsorption of sodium but also with that of potassium.

3. When volume contraction is induced by the diuretic, activation of the sodium/potassium hydrogen transport locus (site 4) occurs because of stimulation of the renin-angiotensin-aldosterone system. Note, however, that only a portion of this transport mechanism (Fig. 68–3, site 4a) is under mineralocorticoid control. When potassium loss from the body exceeds intake, potassium depletion and hypokalemia supervene.

Hypokalemia is treated with either potassium supplementation (see also later) or the administration of a potassium-sparing diuretic.

Metabolic alkalosis is a consequence of the actions of the thiazides and the loop of Henle drugs. It results from the fact that these agents cause the excretion of proportionately more chloride than bicarbonate accompanying the excreted sodium. As volume contraction proceeds, serum bicarbonate concentration (reflected in the serum total CO_2) rises. These events are usually accompanied by the development of hypokalemia. For this reason, correction of hypokalemia and metabolic alkalosis should be accomplished with the provision of potassium as the *chloride* salt.

Hyperkalemia and *metabolic acidosis* are potential complications of the use of the potassium-sparing agents. These drugs, as is the case for all diuretics, may also cause *renal insufficiency*. This may be the result either of compromised renal plasma flow secondary to volume contraction or of actual anatomical damage (usually interstitial nephritis).

Hyperuricemia is a not uncommon complication of diuretic therapy. It is a consequence of two phenomena: (1) Volume contraction may impair renal plasma flow sufficiently to reduce the delivery of both uric acid and the diuretic to their tubular transport sites. (2) Uric acid competes with the diuretics for excretion along a secretory pathway in the proximal nephron. Furthermore, urate reabsorption is enhanced by volume depletion.

The sulfonamide-derivative diuretics have been reported to interfere with *glucose metabolism* when given in large doses (for review, see ref. 56). However, when these drugs are given in low doses, these adverse effects seem to be

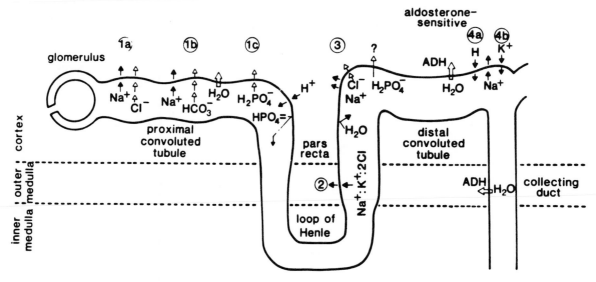

Figure 66–3. Major nephron sites of fluid and electrolyte reabsorption. ADH, antidiuretic hormone.

Table 66–3 Therapeutic Guidelines for Mild to Moderate Hypertension

SODIUM RESTRICTION

Except in special circumstances (see below) begin with low-dose diuretics (12.5 mg in elderly, 25 mg in others); top dose: 25 mg in elderly, 50 mg in other groups; diuretics especially helpful in African Americans, the obese, and the elderly

Special circumstances (examples); first choice may be
    Hypertension and congestive heart failure: ACE inhibitor, carvedilol
    Hypertension and diabetic nephropathy with proteinuria: ACE inhibitor
    Young white male: calcium channel blocker or β-blocker
    Hypertension and history of myocardial infarction: β-blocker
    Hypertension and angina: diltiazem (or verapamil) or β-blocker

If lowest BP not reached after patient is on top dose of diuretic for 3–4 wk, add a second agent

Diuretic often helpful when added to another agent that has been started as monotherapy

Monitoring
    Serum potassium: check at initial visit, after 3–4 wk of therapy, then at 2–3 mo, then 6-mo intervals; if stable, check annually; treat serum K <3.5 mEq/L with KCl or potassium-sparing agent; in patients taking digoxin or with MI history, treat levels <3.8 mEq/L
    Evaluate blood sugar, lipids, BUN, creatinine, and magnesium at first visit and every 6 mo; if lipids rise, institute low-fat diet

Abbreviations: ACE, angiotensin-converting enzyme; BP, blood pressure; MI, myocardial infarction; BUN, blood urea nitrogen

minimal or nonexistent.[56, 57] Thus, diuretics need not be avoided in the therapy of hypertension in patients with type 2 diabetes. Even in patients with type 1 diabetes, edema may be safely treated with sulfonamide-derivative diuretics. Careful blood sugar monitoring will be required and adjustments in insulin made. Generally speaking, this is a dose-related phenomenon.

Hyponatremia can result from diuretic therapy. There are both idiosyncratic and dose-related forms of this disorder. In the latter situation, interference by diuretics with the generation of solute-free water in the diluting segments of the nephron (Fig. 66–3, sites 2 and 3) is causative, as is the stimulus for the elaboration of antidiuretic hormone in the volume-contracted patient.

THERAPEUTIC GUIDELINES

Therapeutic recommendations are outlined in Table 66–3. Given the fact that diuretics owe at least their initial therapeutic effect to volume contraction, diuretic therapy must be accompanied by sodium restriction. In general, outpatients can achieve a 4-g *sodium* intake. This can be accomplished by asking the patient to avoid all obviously salty foods (e.g., pickles, pretzels, potato chips), fast foods, and the use of the salt shaker at the table. Salt should not be added in the cooking: instead, paprika and other spices should be substituted. Salt substitutes (which contain potassium) may be employed in patients who do not have compromised renal function. Diuretics are especially helpful in the demographic groups listed previously. In special circumstances (Table 66–3), other drugs may be better choices as first-line therapy. However, diuretics are excellent additions to nearly all other classes of antihypertensive agents. Monitoring suggestions are provided in Table 66–3.

References

1. Kaplan NM. Treatment of hypertension: Drug therapy. *In* Kaplan NB, Lieberman E (eds). Clinical Hypertension, 6th ed. Baltimore, Williams & Williams, 1994; pp 191–280.
2. Joint National Committee on Prevention, Detection, Evaluation, and Treatment of High Blood Pressure. The sixth report. Arch Intern Med 157:2413–2446, 1997.
3. Puschett JB. Diuretics. *In* Izzo JL, Black HR (eds). Hypertension Primer. Dallas, American Heart Association, 1993; pp 294–296.
4. Vari RC, Navar LG. Normal regulation of arterial pressure. *In* Jacobson HR, Striker GE, Klahr S (eds). The Principles and Practice of Nephrology, 2nd ed. St. Louis, Mosby–Year Book, 1995; pp 354–361.
5. O'Donovan RA, Muhammedi M, Puschett JB. Diuretics in the therapy of hypertension: Current status. Am J Med Sci 304:312–318, 1992.
6. Dustan HP, Cumming GR, Corcoran AC, et al. A mechanism of chlorothiazide-enhanced effectiveness of anti-hypertensive ganglioplegic drugs. Circulation 19:360–365, 1959.
7. Frohlich ED, Schnaper HW, Wilson IM, et al. Hemodynamic alterations in hypertensive patients due to chlorothiazide. N Engl J Med 262:1261–1263, 1960.
8. Gifford RW, Mattox VR, Orvis AL, et al. Effect of thiazide diuretics on plasma volume, body electrolytes, and excretion of aldosterone in hypertension. Circulation 24:1197–1205, 1961.
9. Wilson IM, Freis ED. Relationship between plasma and extracellular fluid volume depletion and the antihypertensive effect of chlorothiazide. Circulation 20:1028–1036, 1959.
10. Villarreal H, Exaire JE, Revollo A, et al. Effects of chlorothiazide on systemic hemodynamics in essential hypertension. Circulation 26:405–408, 1962.
11. Freis ED. How diuretics lower blood pressure. Am Heart J 106:185–187, 1983.
12. Conway, J, Lauwers P. Hemodynamic and hypotensive effects of long-term therapy with chlorothiazide. Circulation 21:21–27, 1960.
13. Lauwers P, Conway J. Effect of long-term treatment with chlorothiazide on body fluids, serum electrolytes, and exchangeable sodium in hypertensive patients. J Lab Clin Med 56:401–408, 1960.
14. Niarchos AP, Magrini F. Hemodynamic effects of diuretics in patients with marked peripheral edema and mild hypertension. Clin Pharmacol Ther 31:370–376, 1982.
15. O'Connor DT, Preston RA, Mitas JA, et al. Urinary kallikrein activity and renal vascular resistance in the antihypertensive response to thiazide diuretics. Hypertension 3:139–147, 1981.
16. Lund-Johansen H. Hemodynamic changes in long-term diuretic therapy of essential hypertension. Acta Med Scand 187:509–518, 1970.
17. Shah S, Khatri I, Freis ED. Mechanism of antihypertensive effect of thiazide diuretics. Am Heart J 95:611–618, 1978.
18. Vardan S, Mookherjee S, Warner R, et al. Systolic hypertension in the elderly. JAMA 250:2807–2813, 1983.
19. Baumgart P, Walger M v. Eiff, Achhammer I. Long-term efficacy and tolerance of torasemide in hypertension. *In* Krück F, Mutschler E, Knauf H (eds). Progress in Pharmacology and Clinical Pharmacology, vol 8, no. 1. Stuttgart, Gustav Fischer, 1990; pp 169–181.
20. Multiple Risk Factor Intervention Trial Group. Multiple Risk Factor Intervention Trial. JAMA 248:1465–1472, 1982.
21. Hoes AW, Grobbee DE, Lubsen J, et al. Diuretics, β-blockers, and the risk for sudden cardiac death in hypertensive patients. Ann Intern Med 123:481–487, 1995.
22. Messerli FH, Nunez BH, Nunez NM, et al. Hypertension and sudden death: Disparate effects of calcium entry blockers and diuretic therapy in cardiac dysrhythmias. Arch Intern Med 149:1263, 1989.
23. Drayer JIM, Gardia MJ, Weber MA, et al. Changes in ventricular septal thickness during diuretic therapy. Clin Pharmacol Ther 32:283–288, 1982.
24. Wollam GL, Hall WD, Pertra VD, et al. Time course of regression of left ventricular hypertrophy in treated hypertensive patients. Am J Med 75(suppl 3A):100–110, 1983.
25. Dahlöf B, Pennert K, Hansson L. Reversal of left ventricular hypertrophy in hypertensive patients. Am J Hypertens 5:95–110, 1992.
26. Schoenfeld MR, Goldberger E. Hypercholesterolemia induced by thiazides: A pilot study. Curr Ther Res Clin Exp 6:180–184, 1964.
27. Ames RP, Hill D. Elevations of serum lipids during diuretic therapy of hypertension. Am J Med 61:748–757, 1976.
28. McVeigh G, Galloway D, Johnson D. The case for low dose diuretics in hypertension: Comparison of low and conventional doses of cyclopenthiazide. BMJ 297:95–98, 1988.

29. Carlsen JE, Køber L, Torp-Pedersen C, Johansen P. Relation between dose of bendrofluazide, antihypertensive effect, and adverse biochemical effects. BMJ 300:975–978, 1990.

30. Johnston GD, Wilson R, McDermott BJ, et al. Low-dose cyclopenthiazide in the treatment of hypertension: A one-year commentary-based study. Q J Med 78:135–143, 1991.

31. SHEP Cooperative Research Group. Prevention of stroke by antihypertensive drug treatment in older persons with isolated systolic hypertension. Final results of the Systolic Hypertension in the Elderly Program (SHEP). JAMA 266:3255–3264, 1991.

32. Hypertension Detection and Follow-up Cooperative Research Group. The effect of anti-hypertensive drug treatment on mortality in the presence of resting electrocardiographic abnormalities at baseline. Circulation 70:996–1003, 1984.

33. Medical Research Council Working Party. Trial of treatment of hypertension in older adults: Principal research. BMJ 304:405–412, 1992.

34. Heaton JD, Grimm RHJ, Primas RJ, et al. Treatment of Mild Hypertension Study (TOMHS): Final research. JAMA 270:713–724, 1993.

35. Materson BJ, Reda DJ, Cushman WC, et al. Single drug therapy for hypertension in men: A comparison of six anti-hypertensive agents with placebo. N Engl J Med 328:914–921, 1993.

36. Carey PA, Sheridan DJ, de Cordoue A, et al. Effect of indapamide on left ventricular hypertrophy in hypertension: A meta-analysis. Am J Cardiol 77:17B–19B, 1996.

37. Curry CL, Robinson H, Brown R, et al. Regression of left ventricular hypertrophy in patients with essential hypertension. Results of 6 month treatment with indapamide. Am J Hypertens 9:828–832, 1996.

38. Kostis JB, David BR, Cutler J, et al. Prevention of heart failure in persons with systolic hypertension. JAMA 278:212–216, 1997.

39. Amery A, Birkenhager W, Brixko P, et al. Mortality and morbidity results from the European Working Party on High Blood Pressure in the Elderly trial. Lancet 1:1349–1354, 1985.

40. Veterans Administration Cooperative Study Group on Antihypertensive Agents. Comparison of propanolol and hydrochlorothiazide for the initial treatment of hypertension. I: Results of short-term titration with emphasis on racial differences in response. JAMA 248:1996–2003, 1982.

41. Veterans Administration Cooperative Study Group on Antihypertensive Agents. Comparison of propanolol and hydrochlorothiazide for the initial treatment of hypertension. II: Results of long-term therapy. JAMA 248:2004–2011, 1982.

42. Amery A, Birkenhager W, Bulpitt C, et al. Influence of anti-hypertensive therapy on serum cholesterol in elderly hypertensive patients. Results of trial by the European Working Party on High Blood Pressure in the Elderly (EWPE). Acta Cardiol 37:235–244, 1982.

43. Lasser NL, Grandits G, Caggiula AW, et al. Effects of antihypertensive therapy on plasma lipids and lipoproteins in the Multiple Risk Factor Intervention Trial. Am J Med 76:52–66, 1984.

44. Miettinen TA, Huttunen JK, Naukkarinen V, et al. Multifactorial primary prevention of cardiovascular diseases in middle-aged men. Risk factor changes, incidence, and mortality. JAMA 254:2097–2102, 1985.

45. Freis ED. The efficacy and safety of diuretics in treating hypertension. Ann Intern Med 122:223–226, 1995.

46. Kaplan NM. Diuretics: Cornerstone of antihypertensive therapy. Am J Cardiol 77:3B–5B, 1996.

47. Weir MR, Flack JM, Applegate WB. Tolerability, safety, and quality of life and hypertensive therapy: The case for low-dose diuretics. Am J Med 101(suppl 3A):83S–92S, 1996.

48. Flack JM, Cushman WC. Evidence for the efficacy of low-dose diuretic monotherapy. Am J Med 101(suppl 3A):53S–60S, 1996.

49. Valvo E, D'Angelo A, Maschio G. Diuretics in hypertension. Kidney Int 51(suppl 59):S36–S38, 1997.

50. Dorhout Mees EJ. Antihypertensive treatment with diuretics: Antediluvian or up to date? Nephrol Dial Transplant 11:587–592, 1996.

51. Loon NR, Wilcox CS, Unwin RJ. Mechanism of the impaired natriuretic response to furosemide during prolonged therapy. Kidney Int 36:682–689, 1989.

52. Puschett JB. Diuretics in hypertension. In Singh BN, Dzau VJ, Vanhoutte PM, et al (eds). Cardiovascular Pharmacology and Therapeutics. New York, Churchill Livingstone, 1994; pp 885–908.

53. Puschett JB, Winaver J. The effects of diuretics on renal function. In Windhager EE (ed). Handbook of Physiology. New York, Oxford University Press, 1992; pp 2335–2406.

54. Puschett JB, O'Donovan RM. Renal actions and uses of diuretics. In Massry SG, Glassock RJ (eds). Textbook of Nephrology, 3rd ed. Baltimore, Williams & Wilkins, 1995; pp 494–507.

55. Puschett JB. Clinical uses of diuretics. In Greger R, Knauf H, Mutschler E (eds). Handbook of Experimental Pharmacology, vol 117. Heidelberg, Springer-Verlag, 1995; pp 443–505.

56. Harper AB, Atkinson AB, Bell PM. Should we use thiazide diuretics in hypertensive patients with non–insulin-dependent diabetes mellitus? Q J Med 89:477–482, 1996.

57. Freis ED, Papademetriou V. Current drug treatment and treatment patterns with antihypertensive drugs. Drugs 52:1–16, 1996.

67 β-Adrenergic Blockers

CHAPTER

William H. Frishman and Ulrich Jorde

The sixth report of the Joint National Committee on Detection, Evaluation, and Treatment of High Blood Pressure (JNC VI) from the National High Blood Pressure Education Program of the National Heart, Lung, and Blood Institute has reiterated the recommendation of JNC III, IV, and V that β-adrenergic blockers are appropriate alternatives as first-line treatment for hypertension.[1] These recommendations are based on the reductions in morbidity and mortality when these drugs are used in large clinical trials. There is no consensus as to the mechanisms by which β-blocking drugs lower blood pressure, but some or all of the modes of action referred to in Table 67–1 are likely involved.[2]

Thirteen orally active β-adrenergic blockers are approved in the United States for treatment of hypertension (Table 67–2). In addition, intravenous labetalol is approved for the management of hypertensive emergencies. Oral bisoprolol in combination with a very low dose diuretic has received approval as a first-line antihypertensive treatment, the first such β-blocker combination so approved for the treatment of hypertension.[3]

The various agents differ in terms of the presence or absence of intrinsic sympathomimetic activity, membrane stabilizing activity, β_1-selectivity, α-adrenergic blocking activity, and relative potencies and duration of action. Nevertheless, all β-blockers studied to date appear to have favorable blood pressure–lowering effects when used in appropriate dosages .[4,5]

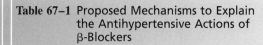

Table 67–1 Proposed Mechanisms to Explain the Antihypertensive Actions of β-Blockers

Reduction in cardiac output
Effect on central nervous system
Inhibition of renin
Reduction in venous return and plasma volume
Reduction in peripheral vascular resistance
Improvement in vascular compliance
Resetting of baroreceptor levels
Effects on prejunctional β-receptors: reduction in norepinephrine release
Attenuation of pressor response to catecholamines with exercise and stress

Adapted from Frishman WH. Clinical Pharmacology of the β-Adrenoceptor Blocking Drugs, 2nd ed. Norwalk, CT, Appleton-Century-Crofts, 1984.

PHARMACODYNAMIC PROPERTIES

Membrane Stabilizing Activity

At concentrations well above therapeutic levels, certain β-blockers have a quinidine-like or local anesthetic membrane stabilizing effect on the cardiac action potential. There is no evidence that membrane stabilizing activity is responsible for any direct negative inotropic effect of the β-blockers, since drugs with and without this property depress left ventricular function. However, membrane stabilizing activity can manifest itself clinically with massive β-blocker intoxications.[2, 4]

β₁-Selectivity

When used in low doses, β_1-selective blocking agents such as acebutolol, betaxolol, bisoprolol, atenolol, and metoprolol inhibit cardiac β_1-receptors but have less influence on bronchial and vascular β-adrenergic receptors (β_2). In higher doses, however, β_1-selective blocking agents also block β_2-receptors. Accordingly, β_1-selective agents may

be safer than nonselective β-blockers in patients with obstructive pulmonary disease, since β_2-receptors remain available to mediate adrenergic bronchodilatation. However, even selective β_1-blockers may aggravate bronchospasm in certain patients, so these drugs should generally not be used in patients with bronchospastic disease.[2, 4]

A second theoretical advantage is that unlike nonselective β-blockers, β_1-selective blockers in low doses may not block the β_2-receptors that mediate dilatation of arterioles. It is possible that leaving the β_2-receptors unblocked and responsive to epinephrine may be functionally important in some patients with asthma, hypoglycemia, hypertension, or peripheral vascular disease treated with β-adrenergic blocking drugs.[2, 4]

Intrinsic Sympathomimetic Activity or Partial Agonist Activity

Certain β-adrenergic receptor blockers possess partial agonist activity at β_1-adrenergic receptor sites or β_2-adrenergic receptor sites, or both. This causes slight cardiac stimulation that can be blocked by propranolol. β-blockers with this property slightly activate the β-receptor in addition to preventing the access of natural or synthetic catecholamines to the receptor. In the treatment of patients with arrhythmias, angina pectoris of effort, and hypertension, drugs with mild to moderate partial agonist activity appear to be as efficacious as β-blockers lacking this property. It is still debated whether the presence of partial agonist activity in a β-blocker constitutes an overall advantage or disadvantage in cardiac therapy. Drugs with partial agonist activity cause less slowing of the heart rate at rest than do propranolol and metoprolol, although the increments in heart rate with exercise are similarly blunted. β-Blocking agents with nonselective partial agonist activity reduce peripheral vascular resistance and may also cause less depression of atrioventricular conduction compared with drugs lacking this property.[2–6]

Table 67–2 Pharmacodynamic Properties of β-Adrenergic Blocking Drugs Used in Hypertension

Drug	β₁-Blockade Potency Ratio (Propranolol = 1.0)	Relative β₁-Selectivity	Intrinsic Sympathomimetic Activity	Membrane Stabilizing Activity
Acebutolol	0.3	+	+	+
Atenolol	1.0	+ +	0	0
Betaxolol	1.0	+ +	0	+
Bisoprolol*	10.0	+ +	0	0
Carteolol	10.0	0	+	0
Carvedilol†	10.0	0	0	+ +
Labetalol‡	0.3	0	+ ?	0
Metoprolol	1.0	+ +	0	0
Nadolol	1.0	0	0	0
Penbutolol	1.0	0	+	0
Pindolol	6.0	0	+ +	+
Propranolol	1.0	0	0	+ +
Timolol	6.0	0	0	0

Adapted from Frishman WH. Clinical Pharmacology of the β-Adrenoceptor Blocking Drugs, 2nd ed. Norwalk, CT, Appleton-Century-Crofts, 1984.
*Bisoprolol is also approved as a first-line antihypertensive therapy in combination with a very low-dose diuretic.
†Carvedilol has additional α_1-adrenergic blocking activity without peripheral β_2-agonism.
‡Labetalol has additional α_1-adrenergic blocking activity and direct vasodilatory activity (β_2-agonism); it is available for use in intravenous form for hypertensive emergencies.

Table 67-3 Pharmacokinetic Properties of β-Adrenoceptor Blocking Drugs Used in Hypertension

Drug	Extent of Absorption (% of Dose)	Extent of Bioavailability (% of Dose)	Dose-Dependent Bioavailability (Major First-Pass Hepatic Metabolism)	Interpatient Variations in Plasma Levels	β-Blocking Plasma Concentrations	Protein Binding (%)	Lipid Solubility*
Acebutolol	≈70	≈40	No	7-fold	0.3–2.0 μg/ml	25	Moderate
Atenolol	≈50	≈40	No	4-fold	0.2–5.0 μg/ml	<5	Weak
Betaxolol	>90	>80	No	2-fold	5–20 ng/ml	50	Moderate
Bisoprolol	>80	90	No		0.01–0.1 μg/ml	≈30	Moderate
Carteolol	≈90	≈90	No	2-fold	40–160 ng/ml	20–30	Weak
Carvedilol	>90	≈30	Yes	5–10-fold	10–100 ng/ml	98	Moderate
Labetalol	>90	≈33	Yes	10-fold	0.7–3.0 μg/ml	≈50	Weak
Metoprolol	>90	≈50	No	7-fold	50–100 ng/ml	12	Moderate
Long-acting metoprolol	>90	≈80	No	2-fold	70–400 ng/ml	12	Moderate
Nadolol	≈30	≈30	No	7-fold	50–100 ng/ml	≈30	Weak
Penbutolol	>90	≈90	No	4-fold	5–15 ng/ml	98	High
Pindolol	>90	≈90	No	4-fold	5–15 ng/ml	57	Moderate
Propranolol	>90	≈30	Yes	20-fold	50–100 ng/ml	93	High
Long-acting propranolol	>90	≈20	Yes	10–20-fold	20–100 ng/ml	93	High
Timolol	>90	≈75	No	7-fold	5–10 ng/ml	≈10	Weak

Adapted from Frishman WH. Clinical Pharmacology of the β-Adrenoceptor Blocking Drugs, 2nd ed. Norwalk, CT, Appleton-Century-Crofts, 1984.
*Determined by the distribution ratio between octanol and water.

α-Adrenergic Activity

Carvedilol and labetalol are β-blockers with antagonistic properties at both α- and β-adrenergic receptors and with direct vasodilator activity. Like other β-blockers, they are useful in the treatment of hypertension and angina pectoris. However, unlike most β-blocking drugs, the additional α-adrenergic blocking actions of carvedilol and labetalol lead to a reduction in peripheral vascular resistance that may maintain cardiac output. Whether concomitant α-adrenergic blocking activity is actually advantageous in a β-blocker remains to be determined.[2, 4]

PHARMACOKINETIC PROPERTIES

Although the β-adrenergic blocking drugs as a group have similar therapeutic effects, their pharmacokinetics are markedly different (Tables 67–3 and 67–4). Their varied aromatic ring structures lead to differences in completeness of gastrointestinal absorption, amount of first-pass hepatic metabolism, lipid solubility, protein binding, extent of distribution in the body, penetration into the brain, concentration in the heart, rate of hepatic biotransformation, pharmacological activity of metabolites, and renal clearance of a drug and its metabolites that may influence the clinical usefulness of these drugs in some patients.[2, 4]

The β-blockers can be divided by their pharmacokinetic properties into two broad categories: those eliminated by hepatic metabolism, which tend to have relatively short plasma half-lives, and those eliminated unchanged by the kidney, which tend to have longer half-lives. Both propranolol and metoprolol are lipid-soluble, are almost completely absorbed by the small intestine, and are largely metabolized by the liver. They tend to have highly variable bioavailability and relatively short plasma half-lives. A lack of correlation between the duration of clinical pharmacological effect and plasma half-life may allow these drugs to be administered once- or twice-daily.[2, 4]

In contrast, agents such as atenolol and nadolol are more water-soluble, are incompletely absorbed through the gut, and are eliminated unchanged by the kidney. They tend to have less variable bioavailability in patients with normal renal function, in addition to longer half-lives, allowing once-daily dosing. The longer half-lives may be useful in patients who find compliance with frequent β-blocker dosing a problem.[2, 4]

Extended-release formulations of metoprolol and propranolol are available that allow once-daily dosing of these drugs. Studies have shown that both long-acting propranolol and metoprolol provide much smoother curves of daily plasma levels than do comparable divided doses of conventional propranolol and metoprolol. Sublingual and nasal spray formulations that can provide immediate β-blockade are being tested in clinical trials.[2, 4]

Ultra-short-acting β-blockers are now available and may be useful where a short duration of action is desired (e.g., in patients with questionable congestive heart failure). One of these compounds, esmolol, a β$_1$-selective drug, has been shown to be useful in the treatment of perioperative hypertension and supraventricular tachycardias. The short half-life (approximately 15 minutes) relates to the rapid metabolism of the drug by blood and hepatic esterases. Metabolism does not seem to be altered by disease states.[7]

EFFECTS ON BLOOD PRESSURE

β-Adrenergic blockers, alone and in combination with other antihypertensives, reduce blood pressure in patients with combined systolic and diastolic hypertension and with isolated systolic hypertension.[8–10] The drugs are considered to be first-line treatment and are also indicated for patients having concomitant angina pectoris, hypertrophic cardiomyopathy, congestive cardiomyopathy, hyperdynamic circulations, essential tremor, and headaches.[2–6, 11] Some β-adrenergic blockers are also found to reduce the risk of mortality in survivors of acute myocardial infarction.[12] The drugs can be used with caution in pregnancy, and appear to be especially useful in treating perioperative hypertension.[13, 14]

Most antihypertensive drugs, including β-blockers, reduce left ventricular mass and wall thickness.[15] It is not known, however, whether reversal of hypertension-induced cardiac hypertrophy improves the independent risk of cardiovascular morbidity and mortality associated with left ventricular hypertrophy.

There is evidence that some β-adrenergic blockers (those not having partial agonist activity) may not be as effective as other antihypertensive treatments in black patients. However, when combined with a diuretic, β-blockers appear to be as effective as other combination treatment regimens in black patients.[2, 4]

The α-β-blocker labetalol is the only β-blocker indicated for parenteral management of hypertensive emergencies and for treatment of intraoperative and postoperative hypertension. It can also be used in oral form to treat patients with hypertensive emergencies.[2, 4]

ADVERSE EFFECTS AND CONTRAINDICATIONS

β-Adrenergic blockers should not be used in patients with asthma, chronic obstructive pulmonary disease, unstable congestive heart failure with systolic dysfunction, heart block (greater than first degree), and sick sinus syndrome.[2–6] The α-β-blocker carvedilol can be used to reduce morbidity and mortality in patients with hypertension and stable New York Heart Association class 2 and 3 heart failure who are receiving diuretics, angiotensin-converting enzyme inhibitors, and digoxin.[11] There are limited efficacy and safety experiences using other β-blockers in this population, and clinical studies are currently in progress.

β-Blockers should be used with caution in type 1 diabetes because they may worsen glucose intolerance and mask the symptoms of and prolong recovery from hypoglycemia. There is probably a shorter recovery period from hypoglycemia with β$_1$-selective adrenergic blockers.[2, 4] β-Blockers should not be discontinued abruptly in patients with known ischemic heart disease.[2–6]

β-Blockers may increase levels of plasma triglycerides and reduce those of high-density lipoprotein cholesterol.[16] Despite this effect, β-blockers without intrinsic sympatho-

Table 67–4 Elimination Characteristics of β-Adrenoceptor Blocking Drugs Used in Hypertension

Drug	Elimination Half-Life (hr)	Total Body Clearance (ml/min)	Urinary Recovery of Unchanged Drug (% of Dose)	Total Urinary Recovery (% of Dose)	Predominant Route of Elimination	Active Metabolites	Drug Accumulation in Renal Disease
Acebutolol	3–4*	480	≈40	>90	RE (≈40% unchanged & HM)	Yes	Yes
Atenolol	6–9	130	≈40	>95	RE	No	Yes
Betaxolol	15	350	15	>90	HM	No	Yes
Bisoprolol	9–12	260	50	>98	RE + HM	No	Yes
Carteolol	5–6	497	40–68	90	RE	Yes	Yes
Carvedilol	7–10	600†	<2	16	HM	Yes	No
Celiprolol	5	500	≈90	≈30	RE (≈50% unchanged & HM)	Yes	No
Labetalol	3–4	2700	<1	>90	HM	No	No
Metoprolol	3–4	1100	≈3	>95	HM	No	No
Long-acting metoprolol							
Penbutolol	27	350	50–70	>90	RE	No	No
Pindolol	3–4	400	≈40	>90	RE (≈40% unchanged & HM)	No	No
Propranolol	3–4	1000	<1	>90	HM	Yes	No
Long-acting propranolol	10	1000	<1	>90	HM	Yes	No
Timolol	4–5	660	≈20	65	RE (≈20% unchanged & HM)	No	No

Adapted from Frishman WH. Clinical Pharmacology of the β-Adrenoceptor Blocking Drugs, 2nd ed. Norwalk, CT, Appleton-Century-Crofts, 1984.
Abbreviations: RE, renal excretion; HM, hepatic metabolism.
*Acebutolol has an active metabolite with elimination half-life of 8–13 hr.
†Plasma clearance.

mimetic activity are the only agents conclusively shown to decrease the rate of sudden death, overall mortality, and recurrent myocardial infarction in survivors of acute myocardial infarction.[12] β-Blockers with intrinsic sympathomimetic activity or α-blocking activity have little or no adverse effects on plasma lipids,[16] but these agents have not been shown to have a protective effect after a myocardial infarction except in a limited study of high-risk patients.[12]

There are special considerations when β-blockers are combined with other drugs.[17] Combinations of diltiazem or verapamil with β-blockers may have additional sinoatrial and atrioventricular node depressant effects, and may also promote negative inotropy.[17] Combinations of β-blockers and reserpine may cause marked bradycardia and syncope. Combination with phenylpropanolamine, pseudoephedrine, ephedrine, and epinephrine can cause elevations in blood pressure due to unopposed α-receptor–induced vasoconstriction.

References

1. Joint National Committee on Prevention, Detection, Evaluation, and Treatment of High Blood Pressure. The sixth report. Arch Intern Med l57:2413–2446, l997.
2. Frishman WH, Sonnenblick EH. β-Adrenergic blocking drugs and calcium channel blockers. *In* Alexander RW, Schlant RC, Fuster V (eds). Hurst's The Heart, 9th ed. New York, McGraw-Hill, 1998; pp 1583–1618.
3. Frishman WH, Bryzinski BS, Coulson LR, et al. A multifactorial trial design to assess combination therapy in hypertension: Treatment with bisoprolol and hydrochlorothiazide. Arch Intern Med 154:1461–1468, 1994.
4. Frishman WH. Alpha- and beta-adrenergic blocking drugs. *In* Frishman WH, Sonnenblick EH (eds). Cardiovascular Pharmacotherapeutics. New York, McGraw-Hill, 1997; pp 59–94.
5. Frishman WH. Alpha- and beta-adrenergic blocking drugs. *In* Frishman WH, Sonnenblick EH (eds). Cardiovascular Pharmacotherapeutics Companion Handbook. New York, McGraw-Hill, 1998; pp 23–64.
6. Frishman WH. Clinical Pharmacology of the β-Adrenoceptor Blocking Drugs, 2nd ed. Norwalk, CT, Appleton-Century-Crofts, l984.
7. Frishman WH, Murthy VS, Strom JA, Hershman D. Ultrashort-acting β-adrenoreceptor blocking drug: Esmolol. *In* Messerli FH (ed). Cardiovascular Drug Therapy, 2nd ed. Philadelphia, WB Saunders, 1996; pp 507–516.
8. Systolic Hypertension in the Elderly Program Cooperative Research Group. Implications of the Systolic Hypertension in the Elderly Program (SHEP). Hypertension 21:335–343, 1993.
9. Materson BJ, Reda DJ, Cushman WC, et al, for the Department of Veterans Affairs Cooperative Study Group on Antihypertensive Agents. Single-drug therapy for hypertension in men: A comparison of six antihypertensive agents with placebo. N Engl J Med 328:914–921, 1993.
10. Psaty BM, Smith NL, Siscovick DS, et al. Health outcomes associated with antihypertensive therapies used as first-line agents: A systematic review and meta-analysis. JAMA 277:739–745, 1997.
11. Frishman WH. Carvedilol. N Engl J Med 339:1759–1765, 1998.
12. Frishman WH. Postinfarction survival: Role of β-adrenergic blockade. *In* Fuster V, Ross R, Topol EJ (eds). Atherosclerosis and Coronary Artery Disease. Philadelphia, Lippincott-Raven, 1996; pp 1205–1214.
13. Ngo A, Frishman WH, Elkayam U: Cardiovascular pharmacotherapeutic considerations during pregnancy and lactation. *In* Frishman WH, Sonnenblick EH (eds). Cardiovascular Pharmacotherapeutics. New York, McGraw-Hill, 1997, p 1309.
14. Hurst AK, Hoffman K, Frishman WH, Elkayam U: The use of β-adrenergic blocking agents in pregnancy and lactation. In Elkayam U, Gleicher N (eds). Cardiac Problems in Pregnancy, 3rd ed. New York, Wiley-Liss, 1998; pp 357–372.
15. Devereux RB. Do antihypertensive drugs differ in their ability to regress left ventricular hypertrophy? Circulation 95:1983–1985, 1997.
16. Frishman WH, Zimetbaum P. Lipid-lowering drugs. *In* Frishman WH, Sonnenblick EH (eds). Cardiovascular Pharmacotherapeutics. New York, McGraw-Hill, 1997; p 399.
17. Frishman WH. Calcium channel blockers. *In* Frishman WH, Sonnenblick EH (eds). Cardiovascular Pharmacotherapeutics. New York, McGraw-Hill, 1997; p 101.

68 α-Adrenoceptor Blockers

James L. Pool

α-ADRENOCEPTORS IN HYPERTENSION

Since the discovery of α- and β-adrenergic receptors by Ahlquist 50 years ago,[1] the dual impact of α-adrenoceptors on the circulatory system has become apparent. α-Adrenoceptors not only participate in the physiological regulation of vascular resistance, they also play a role in hypertension and other cardiovascular diseases. Hypertension has emerged as a complex syndrome of multiple hemodynamic, neuroendocrine, and metabolic abnormalities.[2] To understand the role of α-adrenoceptors and the modulation of receptor function in hypertension by α-adrenoceptor antagonists, it is necessary to be familiar with the contributions of the sympathetic nervous system (SNS) to the development of hypertension and cardiovascular diseases.

α-Adrenoceptors have been further classified into two types, α_1 and α_2.[3, 4] α_1-Adrenoceptor stimulation causes generalized vasoconstriction. These adrenoceptors are located postsynaptically, close to nerve terminals, and they mediate vasoconstriction through endogenously released norepinephrine (Fig. 68–1). In the borderline and early, mild phases of hypertension, there is evidence of increased SNS activity, including microneurographic recordings of increased sympathetic traffic in the peroneal nerve.[5] Patients with increased sympathetic tone and early hypertension have hyperdynamic circulation with elevated plasma norepinephrine, increased cardiac output, and faster heart rates. In a longitudinal study over 20 years, Lund-Johansen observed gradual transformation in such patients to established hypertension with normal cardiac output and increased vascular resistance.[6] The mechanisms that underlie this transition from high cardiac output to high vascular resistance involve modifications of SNS receptors and a dominant role for α-adrenoceptors. There is functional

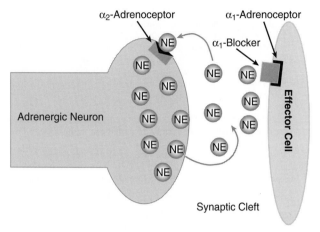

Figure 68–1. Postganglionic sympathetic neuron with synaptic cleft, presynaptic α_2-adrenoceptor, and postsynaptic α_1-adrenoceptor. NE, norepinephrine.

Table 68–1 Select α-Adrenoceptor Antagonists		
Antagonist Compound	α_1 Selective	α_1 and α_2 Nonselective
Alfuzosin	✔	
BMY-7378	✔	
Bunazosin	✔	
Chloroethylclonidine	✔	
Cyclazosin	✔	
Doxazosin	✔	
Phenoxybenzamine		✔
Phentolamine		✔
Prazosin	✔	
RS 17053	✔	
SK&F 105854	✔	
SNAP 5150	✔	
(+)Niguldipine	✔	
Tamsulosin	✔	
Terazosin	✔	
5-Methyl-urapidil	✔	
WB-4101	✔	

downregulation of β-adrenergic responsiveness in the heart[7] plus alteration of vascular anatomy and function,[8] followed by a steady increase in vascular resistance. An exaggerated response of blood vessels to adrenergic and nonadrenergic vasoconstrictors[9] develops in hypertensives that likely contributes to the steady increase in vascular resistance during the evolution of hypertension.

PHARMACOLOGY OF α-ADRENOCEPTOR ANTAGONISTS

Considering this early recognition of the contribution of the SNS to the control of vascular resistance and the evolution of hypertension, it follows that α-adrenoceptor antagonists were among the first drugs to be evaluated as antihypertensive agents. Phenoxybenzamine and phentolamine, the initial α-adrenoceptor antagonists, were disappointing because clinical investigations showed minimal reduction in supine blood pressure, rapid development of pharmacological tolerance, and unacceptable side effects such as orthostatic hypotension and tachycardia.[10] Prazosin, the first member of the quinazoline class of α-adrenoceptor antagonists, quickly became the accepted pharmacological agent for producing selective α₁-adrenoceptor blockade.[11] Clinical studies of prazosin showed sustained reductions in both supine and standing blood pressure without reflex tachycardia in hypertensive patients. Over the past 25 years, prazosin and two additional quinazolines, terazosin[12] and doxazosin,[13] which have longer duration of action with once-a-day dosing, have emerged as highly effective antihypertensive agents.

The receptor selectivity of the quinazolines, compared with the earlier nonselective phenoxybenzamine and phentolamine, appears to account for their enhanced efficacy as antihypertensive agents. The selectivity of the quinazolines for postsynaptic vascular α₁-adrenoceptors and the resultant lack of antagonist action at the presynaptic neuroinhibitory α₂-adrenoceptor allow normal feedback control of norepinephrine release from sympathetic nerve terminals (Table 68–1).[10] Nonselective α-adrenoceptor antagonists that also block the presynaptic neuroinhibitory α₂-adrenoceptor significantly elevate circulating catecholamines, thus counteracting the competitive blockade of postsynaptic vascular α₁-adrenoceptors and limiting their efficacy.

CLASSIFICATION OF α-ADRENOCEPTORS

As part of the classification of adrenergic receptors, the International Union of Pharmacology has published nomenclature for the α-adrenoceptors.[3, 4] In the past 3 decades, there has been a major expansion of α-adrenoceptor pharmacology, and subtypes of both α₁- and α₂-receptors have been discovered. α₁- and α₂-Adrenoceptors have been classified further, each having three subtypes (Table 68–2).[4] α₁-Adrenoceptors are selectively antagonized by prazosin, an accepted pharmacological criterion for distinguishing α₁- from α₂-adrenoceptors.[14] The α₁-adrenoceptor was identified as the type that mediates contraction of smooth muscle, including that of the prostate. The existence of subtypes of the α₁-adrenoceptor is therefore of potential clinical relevance to α-adrenoceptor blockade in vascular tissue and the prostate. Three α₁-adrenoceptors have been cloned and designated α₁ₐ, α₁ᵦ, and α₁𝒹, using the lower case letters to distinguish them from corresponding receptors found in native tissues, α₁ₐ, α₁ᵦ, and α₁𝒹. The relationship between the pharmacologically defined and the cloned subtypes has been the subject of much discussion,[15–17] but

Table 68–2 α_1-Adrenoceptor Subtypes			
Native Receptors	Cloned Receptors		Human Chromosome Location
1995 Classification		Cloned Receptors (Historical)	
α_{1A}	α_{1a}	α_{1a}	C8
α_{1B}	α_{1b}	α_{1b}	C5
α_{1D}	α_{1d}	$\alpha_{1a/d}$, α_{1a}	C20

the α_{1A}-adrenoceptor and the previously cloned α_{1c}-adrenoceptor are now known to be the same.[16]

After extensive characterization of cloned and native receptors in many tissues,[18, 19] it is still difficult to ascribe a definite clinical significance to each subtype of α_1-adrenoceptor. Early in vitro experiments have shown that the α_1-adrenoceptor that mediates smooth muscle contraction in human prostate tissue is the α_{1A} subtype.[16] There is currently no α-adrenoceptor antagonist selective for the α_{1A} subtype. There is some in vitro evidence that tamsulosin has a higher affinity for α_1-adrenoceptors in the prostate than in the aorta,[20] and there is some evidence from animal models of urethral and vascular hypertonia that alfuzosin has a higher affinity for genitourinary than for vascular α_1-adrenoceptors.[21] However, direct in vitro comparative studies suggest that all available agents have a similar affinity for the α_{1A}-adrenoceptor.[22]

TREATMENT OF HYPERTENSION

Numerous clinical studies have shown α_1-adrenoceptor antagonists to lower blood pressure through reduction of vascular resistance without significant effects on heart rate, cardiac output, or central hemodynamics.[23, 24] Long-term administration of long-acting α_1-adrenoceptor antagonists produces a reduction in blood pressure similar to that of other major classes of antihypertensive agents, such as diuretics, β-blockers, calcium channel antagonists, and angiotensin-converting enzyme inhibitors.[25] Effectiveness is irrespective of age, race, and renal function. Antihypertensive benefits have also been demonstrated in patients with concomitant illnesses, such as type 2 diabetes mellitus and chronic obstructive pulmonary disease, and in those taking additional medication. Blood pressure effects are not clinically significant in normotensive patients who have normal sympathetic tone and peripheral vascular resistance.[26] α_1-Adrenoceptor antagonists are recommended widely by a dozen national and international organizations for the initial treatment of hypertension.

α_1-Adrenoceptor antagonists have been well tolerated in the treatment of hypertension, with experience amounting to several billion patient-days of therapy. The majority of side effects reported have been mild to moderate, and their incidence has been similar to that of the side effects of other antihypertensive agents at doses producing similar reductions in blood pressure.

CONTROL OF HYPERTENSION AND MULTIPLE CORONARY ARTERY DISEASE RISK FACTORS

The goal of antihypertensive therapy is, ultimately, to reduce the death rate from cerebrovascular accident and coronary heart disease. Antihypertensive intervention has resulted in the expected fall in stroke incidence (around 40%), but the reduction in coronary heart disease has been only 60% of that expected from prospective data.[27] This disappointing result reflects the importance of other risk factors in the etiology of coronary heart disease and the

inability of most antihypertensive therapy to control these confounding factors.

Risk factors for coronary heart disease are highly prevalent in the general population. In fact, the clustering of metabolic disorders such as elevated lipids, insulin resistance, and glucose intolerance is common in patients with hypertension.[28] The majority of hypertensives have abnormal levels of serum lipids. Insulin resistance and glucose intolerance tend to be associated with hypertension.[29] For example, in the San Antonio Heart Study, which included 287 hypertensive patients, about 50% had type 2 diabetes or impaired glucose tolerance. Only 15% were free of glucose intolerance, lipid disorder, and obesity.[30]

Many antihypertensive drugs have an unfavorable effect on the serum lipid profile. β-Blockers and diuretics have adverse effects on both lipids and glucose. Angiotensin-converting enzyme inhibitors and calcium antagonists tend to be lipid-neutral, but only α_1-adrenoceptor antagonists have truly positive effects on lipids[31] and glucose.[32] Results from the Treatment of Mild Hypertension Study (TOMHS) demonstrate the long-term, beneficial effects of a long-acting α_1-adrenoceptor antagonist (doxazosin) on serum lipids.[25] β-Blockers and diuretics impair insulin sensitivity by 20 to 30% and 15 to 20%, respectively; calcium antagonists and angiotensin-converting enzyme inhibitors have no significant effects; but the selective α_1-adrenoceptor antagonist improves insulin sensitivity by 20 to 25%.[33]

MANAGEMENT OF HYPERTENSION AND LOWER URINARY TRACT SYMPTOMS IN BENIGN PROSTATIC HYPERPLASIA

Hypertension and benign prostatic hyperplasia (BPH) share a pathophysiology through the SNS that has important implications for clinical management. The coincidence of the two disorders, both of which cause substantial morbidity, may be more than a random association in aging men. Hypertension is common in most Western societies, although the exact incidence varies according to the precise definition employed. The prevalence of hypertension also increases with age. In older patients ($\geq$60 years), recent prevalence estimates for hypertension (blood pressure $\geq$ 140/90 mm Hg) from the National Health and Nutrition Examination Survey (NHANES) III in the United States are 60% of non-Hispanic whites, 71% of non-Hispanic blacks, and 61% of Mexican Americans.[34] Like hypertension, BPH is common and increases in prevalence with advancing age; 88% of prostates removed at autopsy from men 80 years of age or older showed signs of BPH, compared to 50% of prostates in men 60 years of age or older, and none in men under 30 years old.[35] Lower urinary tract symptom surveys show a lower prevalence but a similar pattern.[36]

In BPH, the urinary obstruction responsible for the distressing symptoms has two primary sources: the static pressure caused by the enlarged gland itself and the dynamic pressure exerted by the prostate smooth muscle.[37] This smooth muscle is constricted by the sympathetic adrenergic nerves innervating the lower urinary tract and is believed to account for about 50% of prostatic outflow obstruction.[38] Prostatic adrenoceptors have been characterized by using prostatic tissue from men undergoing prostate surgery, mainly for BPH. Prostatic smooth muscle has been shown to be contracted by adrenergic stimulation of α_1-adrenoceptor sites, but no significant effects are mediated by α_2-adrenoceptors. Radiographic localization showed that the α_1-adrenoceptor binding sites are located predominantly in the prostatic stroma and bladder neck, consistent with their presence mainly on smooth muscle fibers. Static pressure can be reduced only by surgical intervention, but the dynamic component can be antagonized by blocking the action of norepinephrine at α-adrenoceptors.

Guidelines from the Fourth International Consultation on BPH[39] and the U.S. Public Health Service Agency for Health Care Policy and Research[40] recommend α_1-adrenoceptor antagonists for treatment of BPH. Treatment with an α_1-adrenoceptor antagonist improves both symptom score and urinary flow in men with BPH. Long-term data derived from studies of up to 48 months of drug therapy indicate that these improvements are sustained. In a meta-analysis of the published literature, selective α_1-adrenoceptor inhibitors produced a 48% reduction in lower urinary tract symptom scores[41] as well as improvements in peak flow rate and postvoid residual volume, without any clinically significant risk of urinary incontinence.

The activity of the SNS increases with age.[42-45] Older subjects have higher plasma norepinephrine concentration[42-44] and urinary norepinephrine excretion[45] than younger people and these parameters increase with advancing age. These findings, using norepinephrine release as a proxy for sympathetic tone, have recently been confirmed by studies of muscular sympathetic nerve activity recorded directly from microelectrodes.[43] The SNS plays a role in both hypertension and BPH, each of which increases in prevalence with advancing age. The increase in sympathetic activity observed in older males may contribute to the simultaneous initiation and progression of both disorders. α_1-Adrenoceptor blockade thus offers the opportunity to improve two common conditions simultaneously.

References

1. Ahlquist RP. A study of the adrenotropic responses. Am J Physiol 153:586–600, 1948.
2. Weber MA, Laragh JH. Hypertension: Steps forward and steps backward. The Joint National Committee fifth report [Editorial, Commentary] Arch Int Med 153:149–152, 1993.
3. Bylund DB, Eikenberg DC, Hieble JP, et al. International Union of Pharmacology nomenclature of adrenoceptors. Pharmacol Rev 46:121–136, 1994.
4. Hieble JP, Ruffolo RR Jr. Subclassification and nomenclature of alpha 1- and alpha 2-adrenoceptors. Prog Drug Res 47:81–130, 1996.
5. Anderson EA, Sinkey CA, Lawton WJ, Mark AL. Elevated sympathetic nerve activity in borderline hypertensive humans: Evidence from direct intraneural recordings. Hypertension 14:177–183, 1989.
6. Lund-Johansen P. Central haemodynamics in essential hypertension at rest and during exercise: A 20-year follow-up study. Hypertens 7(suppl):S52–S55, 1989.
7. Trimarco B, Volpe M, Ricciardelli B, et al. Studies of the mechanisms underlying impairment of beta-adrenoceptor-mediated effects in human hypertension. Hypertension 5:584–590, 1983.
8. Sivertsson R. Structural adaptation in borderline hypertension. Hypertension 6:III103–III107, 1984.
9. Sivertsson R, Sannerstedt R, Lundgren Y. Evidence for peripheral vascular involvement in mild elevation of blood pressure in man. Clin Sci Molec Med 3(suppl):65S–68S, 1976.
10. Stokes GS, Marwood JF. Review of the use of alpha-adrenoceptor antagonists in hypertension. Methods Find Exp Clin Pharmacol 6:197–204, 1984.
11. Stanaszek WF, Kellerman D, Brogden RN, Romankiewicz JA. Prazosin update: A review of its pharmacological properties and therapeutic use in hypertension and congestive heart failure. Drugs 25:339–384, 1983.
12. Pool JL, Nunez E, Messerli FH. Terazosin. In Messerli FH (ed). Cardiovascular Drug Therapy, 2nd ed. Philadelphia, WB Saunders, 1996; pp 665–673.
13. Neutel JM, Taylor SH, Smith DGH, et al. Doxazosin. In Messerli FH (ed). Cardiovascular Drug Therapy, 2nd ed. Philadelphia, WB Saunders, 1996; pp 681–689.
14. Ruffolo RRJ, Nichols AJ, Stadel JM, Hieble JP. Structure and function of alpha-adrenoceptors. Pharmacol Rev 43:475–505, 1991.
15. Ford AP, Williams TJ, Blue DR, Clarke DE. Alpha 1-adrenoceptor classification: Sharpening Occam's razor. Trends Pharmacol Sci 15:167–170, 1994.
16. Forray C, Bard JA, Wetzel JM, et al. The alpha 1-adrenergic receptor that mediates smooth muscle contraction in human prostate has the pharmacological properties of the cloned human alpha 1c subtype. Molec Pharmacol 45:703–708, 1994.
17. Ruffolo RRJ, Hieble JP. Alpha-adrenoceptors. Pharmacol Ther 61:1–64, 1994.
18. Han C, Abel PW, Minneman KP. Alpha 1-adrenoceptor subtypes linked to different mechanisms for increasing intracellular Ca^{2+} in smooth muscle. Nature 329:333–335, 1987.
19. Hieble JP, Ruffolo RRJ. Recent advances in the identification of alpha$_1$- and alpha$_2$-adrenoceptor subtypes: Therapeutic implications. Exp Opin Invest Drugs 6:367–387, 1997.
20. Yamada S, Tanaka C, Kimura R, Kawabe K. Alpha 1-adrenoceptors in human prostate: characterization and binding characteristics of alpha 1-antagonists. Life Sciences 54:1845–1854, 1994.
21. Wilde MI, Fitton A, McTavish D. Alfuzosin: A review of its pharmacodynamic and pharmacokinetic properties, and therapeutic potential in benign prostatic hyperplasia. Drugs 45:410–429, 1993.
22. Kenny BA, Naylor, AM, Carter AJ, et al. Effect of alpha 1 adrenoceptor antagonists on prostatic pressure and blood pressure in the anesthetized dog. Urology 44:52–57, 1994.
23. Lund-Johansen P, Omvik P. Acute and chronic hemodynamic effects of drugs with different actions on adrenergic receptors: A comparison between alpha blockers and different types of beta blockers with and without vasodilating effect. Cardiovasc Drugs Ther 5:605–615, 1991.
24. Lund-Johansen P, Hjermann I, Iversen BM, Thaulow E. Selective alpha-1 inhibitors: First- or second-line antihypertensive agents? Cardiology 83:150–159, 1993.
25. Neaton JD, Grimm RHJ, Prineas RJ, et al. Treatment of Mild Hypertension Study: Final results. JAMA 270:713–724, 1993.
26. Lepor H, Kaplan SA, Klimberg I, et al. Doxazosin for benign prostatic hyperplasia: Long-term efficacy and safety in hypertensive and normotensive patients. The Multicenter Study Group. J Urol 157:525–530, 1997.
27. Collins R, Peto R, MacMahon S, et al. Blood pressure, stroke, and coronary heart disease. Part 2: Short-term reductions in blood pressure: Overview of randomised drug trials in their epidemiological context. Lancet 335:827–838, 1990.
28. Reaven GM, Lithell H, Landsberg L. Hypertension and associated metabolic abnormalities—the role of insulin resistance and the sympathoadrenal system. N Engl J Med 334:374–381, 1996.
29. Kannel WB, Wilson PW, Zhang TJ. The epidemiology of impaired glucose tolerance and hypertension. Am Heart J 121:1268–1273, 1991.
30. Mitchell BD, Stern MP, Haffner SM, et al. Risk factors for cardiovascular mortality in Mexican Americans and non-Hispanic whites. San Antonio Heart Study. Am J Epidemiol 131:423–433, 1990.
31. Pool JL, Lenz ML, Taylor AA. Alpha 1-adrenoreceptor blockade and the molecular basis of lipid metabolism alterations. J Hum Hypertens 4(suppl 3):23–33, 1990.
32. Lithell H. Metabolic aspects of the treatment of hypertension. J Hypertens 13(suppl):S77–S80, 1995.
33. Lithell HO. Effect of antihypertensive drugs on insulin, glucose, and lipid metabolism. Diabetes Care 14:203–209, 1991.
34. Burt VL, Whelton P, Roccella EJ, et al. Prevalence of hypertension in the U.S. adult population. Results from the Third National Health and Nutrition Examination Survey, 1988–1991. Hypertension 25:305–313, 1995.

35. Berry SJ, Coffey DS, Walsh PC, Ewing LL. The development of human benign prostatic hyperplasia with age. J Urol 132:474–479, 1984.

36. Chute CG, Panser LA, Girman CJ, et al. The prevalence of prostatism: A population-based survey of urinary symptoms. J Urol 150:85–89, 1993.

37. Kirby RS, Pool JL. Alpha adrenoceptor blockade in the treatment of benign prostatic hyperplasia: Past, present and future. Br J Urol 80:521–532, 1997.

38. Chapple CR, Aubry ML, James S, et al. Characterisation of human prostatic adrenoceptors using pharmacology receptor binding and localisation. Br J Urol 63:487–496, 1989.

39. Denis L, McConnell J, Yoshida O, et al. Recommendations of the International Scientific Committee: The Evaluation and Treatment of Lower Urinary Tract Symptoms (LUTS) Suggestive of Benign Prostatic Obstruction. In Denis L, Griffiths K, Khoury S, et al. (eds). Fourth International Consultation on Benign Prostatic Hyperplasia. Plymouth, UK, Plymbridge Distributors, 1998; 669–684.

40. Agency for Health Care Policy and Research. Benign Prostatic Hyperplasia: Diagnosis and Treatment. Rockville, MD, AHCPR Publication No. 94-0582, 1994.

41. Direct Treatment Outcomes—Symptom Improvement. In U.S. Department of Health and Human Services, Public Health Service Agency for Health Care Policy and Research. Benign Prostatic Hyperplasia: Diagnosis and Treatment. Rockville, MD: AHCPR Publication No. 94-0582, 1994; 83–89.

42. Blandini F, Martignoni E, Melzi dG, et al. Free plasma catecholamine levels in healthy subjects: A basal and dynamic study. The influence of age. Scand J Clin Laboratory Invest 52:9–17, 1992.

43. Ng AV, Agre JC, Hanson P, et al. Influence of muscle length and force on endurance and pressor responses to isometric exercise. J Appl Physiol 76:2561–2569, 1994.

44. Taylor JA, Hand GA, Johnson DG, Seals DR. Augmented forearm vasoconstriction during dynamic exercise in healthy older men. Circulation 86:1789–1799, 1992.

45. Jenner DA, Harrison GA, Prior IA, et al. 24-h Catecholamine excretion: Relationships with age and weight. Clin Chim Acta 164:17–25, 1987.

69 Angiotensin-Converting Enzyme Inhibitors

CHAPTER

Domenic A. Sica and Todd W. B. Gehr

Many therapeutic strategies have been employed in the treatment of hypertension over the past three decades. One such strategy has been to identify a presumed mediator of the hypertensive condition and then target this mediator with specific medications, providing so-called individualized therapy. This approach proved to be only variably successful, in part because hypertension was found to be much more heterogeneous in its origin than was first imagined. Another approach was to use so-called stepped-care therapy wherein treatment was initiated with either a diuretic or a β-blocker, irrespective of the cause of the hypertension. Stepped-care therapy was generally no more successful than individualized therapy, but for several reasons it was viewed more favorably. First and probably foremost, it was a less costly way to treat hypertension; in addition, diuretics and β-blockers had been shown in numerous randomized, controlled trials to reduce morbidity and mortality.[1]

Since the late 1970s, the renin-angiotensin-aldosterone (RAA) axis has been increasingly viewed as an important effector system for hypertension and thus has become an attractive target for pharmacological intervention. Treatment of hypertension with angiotensin-converting enzyme inhibitors (ACEIs) is perhaps the best example of an individualized therapeutic approach. The newfound enthusiasm for directing hypertension treatment at the RAA axis derived from the observation that ACEIs could be effective in both normal and low-renin forms of hypertension, particularly if appropriate doses were given. Of those drugs known to interrupt the RAA axis, by far the greatest treatment experience exists with ACEIs.

ACEIs have earned an important place in medical therapy since their discovery almost 20 years ago. This family of drugs has grown tremendously since the first compound in this class, captopril, was released in 1981. This compound proved to be an extremely effective blood pressure lowering agent in a number of renin-dependent models of hypertension.[2] The ACEI field quickly mushroomed; there are currently more than 14 ACEIs available in the world, 9 of them available in the United States.[3, 4] In addition to having vasodepressor properties, ACEIs were quickly recognized as being capable of slowing progressive renal, cardiac, and vascular disease processes. Thus, it was a logical step in their development to seek additional indications for ACEIs in the areas of congestive heart failure (CHF), post–myocardial infarction, and diabetic nephropathy (Table 69–1). A full description of the tissue-protective properties of ACEIs goes beyond the scope of this chapter. The reader is referred to a number of comprehensive reviews on these topics.[2, 5–10]

MECHANISM OF ACTION

An understanding of ACEIs requires an appreciation of how they interact with the RAA axis and how they differ from other compounds known to interrupt RAA axis activity. For example, ACEIs alter RAA axis activity by decreasing plasma angiotensin II production, as do β-blockers (β-blockers decrease plasma renin activity [PRA]), whereas angiotensin-receptor blockers inhibit angiotensin II effects by blocking the type I angiotensin receptor.[11]

The locus of activity of ACEIs within the RAA axis is at the angiotensin-converting enzyme (ACE). ACE is pluripotent in that it catalyzes the conversion of angiotensin I into angiotensin II and also effects the degradation of bradykinin as well as a range of other vasoactive peptides.[12] Although ACEIs effectively curtail the generation of angiotensin II from angiotensin I, they do not interfere with the production of angiotensin II by non–ACE-dependent

Table 69–1 U.S. Food and Drug Administration–Approved Indications for Angiotensin-Converting Enzyme Inhibitors

Drug	Hypertension	Congestive Heart Failure	Diabetic Nephropathy	Left Ventricular Dysfunction
Captopril	·	·		· (post-MI)
Benazepril	·			
Enalapril	·	·		· (asymptomatic)
Fosinopril	·	·		
Lisinopril	·	·		
Moexipril	·			
Quinapril	·	·		
Ramipril	·	·		
Trandolapril	·	· (post-MI)		· (post-MI)

Abbreviation: MI, myocardial infarction.

pathways.[13] Such pathways rely on chymase and other proteases to produce angiotensin II independently in myocardial and vascular tissue,[14] with the ensuing gradual rise in angiotensin II levels, despite continuation of ACEIs, being termed *angiotensin escape*.[15, 16]

When ACEIs are given, the temporary fall in angiotensin II levels disrupts the normal negative feedback that occurs in renin production and leads to increased renin secretion and subsequent angiotensin II formation.[17] This surplus of angiotensin I emerges as one source of substrate for the alternative pathways and provides a partial explanation for the phenomenon of angiotensin II escape. The rise in angiotensin I that accompanies ACE inhibition seems to derive from an enhanced release of active renin rather than from an accumulation of angiotensin I[18] and is blunted by β-adrenergic antagonism.[19]

ACEIs reduce angiotensin II levels only transiently (for days or weeks).[13, 15, 16] Therefore, other mechanisms of lowering blood pressure must come into play, particularly in light of the pattern of blood pressure response to an ACEI. When first administered, ACEIs transiently reduce blood pressure commensurate with the degree of RAA axis activation.[20] With long-term therapy, the relationship between the fall in blood pressure and the pretreatment level of angiotensin II fades.[21] This limits the practical value of renin profiling in predicting the degree to which an ACEI will reduce blood pressure in a particular patient.[22] Instead, the blood pressure response achieved shortly after the initiation of ACE inhibition appears to provide a better predictive index of long-term response. In many patients, sustained ACE inhibition lowers blood pressure to levels beyond those achieved at the beginning of therapy, despite the escape of angiotensin II mentioned earlier. Although the precise explanation for the persistent decline in blood pressure with ACEIs has not yet been identified, changes in bradykinin concentration appear to influence the process.[23]

How ACEIs interact with the kallikrein-kinin system is a matter of considerable interest. ACE processes peptides other than angiotensin I which, no doubt, has important functional implications. For example, bradykinin is broken down by kininases, one of which (kininase II) is identical to ACE. Thus, in theory, ACEI administration should elevate tissue and circulating bradykinin levels. In turn, bradykinin is known to stimulate the production of endothelium-derived relaxing factor (NO) and to induce the release of prostacyclin. Circulating bradykinin concentrations measured in ACEI-treated patients have been found to be inconsistently elevated.[24, 25] It is possible, though, that tissue bradykinin increases with ACEI therapy and thereby influences local vascular tone, which would provide a partial explanation for the chronically reduced blood pressure in ACEI-treated patients.[23]

The contribution of prostaglandins to the antihypertensive effect of ACEIs is still unknown. The evidence supporting a role for increased vasodilator prostaglandins in the blood pressure lowering effect of ACEIs is circumstantial at best.[26] Although circulating levels of prostaglandin E₂ and prostacyclin metabolites are not noticeably altered by ACEIs, it has been recognized for some time that nonsteroidal anti-inflammatory drugs blunt the blood pressure lowering effect of ACEIs.[27] Low-dose aspirin (100 mg/day or less) has no significant effect on ACEI-induced blood pressure reduction, but higher doses (>236 mg/day) can sometimes blunt the antihypertensive response to ACEIs.[28, 29]

The effect of ACEIs is thought to be due in part to reduced activity of the sympathetic nervous system. This is attributable to a change in both central and peripheral activity in the sympathetic nervous system as well as to an attenuation of sympathetically mediated vasoconstriction, although this has been variably observed.[30] ACEI administration does not produce a consistent change in circulating catecholamines. ACEIs also do not alter circulatory reflexes and therefore do not increase heart rate when blood pressure is lowered.[31] The latter property explains why ACEIs are rarely associated with postural hypotension. Finally, ACEIs improve endothelial function, facilitate vascular remodeling, and favorably alter the viscoelastic properties of blood vessels.[32] These additional attributes of ACEIs may help explain the observation that the long-term blood pressure reduction with ACEIs generally exceeds that observed in the short term.

PHARMACOLOGY

The first orally active ACEI was captopril, a sulfhydryl-containing compound with a rapid onset and brief duration of action. Subsequently, a longer-acting compound, enalapril became available. Enalapril, like all other ACEIs with the exception of lisinopril and captopril, undergoes metabolic conversion into an active diacid form, a process that occurs within the liver or the intestinal wall. An early theory held that the formation of the active metabolite of an ACEI could be inhibited in the presence of hepatic impairment, as in advanced CHF, but this has not proved to be the case.[33]

ACEIs are structurally heterogenous in the ways they bind to and diminish the activity of ACE, and they contain different side groups capable of binding to ACE. For example, the active chemical side group, or ligand, for captopril is a sulfhydryl group; for fosinopril, a phosphinyl group; each of the remaining ACEIs contains a carboxyl group. The side group of an ACEI is one factor likely to be responsible for differing pharmacological responses to these compounds. Thus, the sulfhydryl group on captopril is purported to act as a recyclable free radical scavenger, and for this reason, captopril may retard atherogenesis and protect patients from myocardial infarction and diabetes.[34] This possibility has not been clinically substantiated, however. In addition, captopril directly stimulates prostaglandin synthesis, whereas other ACEIs accomplish this indirectly by increasing bradykinin activity.[35] The sulfhydryl group is also believed to lead to a higher incidence of skin rashes and dysgeusia. The presence of a phosphinyl group on fosinopril has been proffered as the reason for the low incidence of cough[36] and its ability to improve diastolic dysfunction, perhaps because the phosphinyl group facilitates the myocardial penetration or retention of fosinopril.[37]

Although ACEIs can be distinguished from each other by differences in absorption, protein binding, half-life, and metabolic disposition, they behave quite similarly in terms of how they lower blood pressure. Rarely, beyond the issue of frequency of dosing, do pharmacological subtleties govern the selection of an ACEI (Table 69–2).[3] This said, two pharmacological considerations have generated considerable recent debate and warrant additional discussion.

The active diacid form of only two ACEIs, fosinopril and trandolapril, is eliminated to any significant degree by renal and hepatic routes.[38] For all other ACEIs, elimination is accomplished by renal clearance involving varying degrees of filtration and tubular secretion.[39] Combined renal and hepatic elimination typically minimizes accumulation of these compounds in renal failure, once patients have been dosed to steady state.[40] To date, although a direct adverse effect from ACEI accumulation has not been identified, the longer drug concentrations remain elevated, the more likely it is that blood pressure will remain low in responders to ACEIs. Thus, the major adverse consequence of drug accumulation may be that of prolonged hypotension and its organ-specific sequelae of hypotension.[41]

The second debated feature of the ACEIs concerns tissue binding. ACEIs such as quinapril and ramipril are highly lipophilic, so they bind to tissue sites for prolonged periods of time.[10] It was originally believed that lipophilicity could confer superiority relative to blood pressure control and end-organ protection. However, there have been few direct head-to-head comparisons between ACEIs that are highly tissue-bound and ACEIs with more limited tissue binding, and the results of those trials that have been carried out do not convincingly support the claim of overall superiority for lipophilic ACEIs.[10, 42]

In most details there is very little that truly separates one ACEI from another, so the cost of ACEIs has become a dominant issue.[43] The question of price neglects the fact that only a small number of ACEIs have been specifically studied for their ability to protect end organs. *Class effect* is a phrase often invoked to legitimize the use of a less costly ACEI when only a higher-priced agent has been specifically studied for a disease state such as CHF or diabetic nephropathy.[44, 45] The concept of class effect may be applicable in the treatment of diabetic nephropathy, in which the primary goals are reducing blood pressure and decreasing proteinuria. Substituting a less costly ACEI is reasonable if reductions in blood pressure and protein excretion are comparable to those achieved with a more costly ACEI. Thus, in renal disease, once dose equivalency is established, an ACEI is an ACEI. In contrast, in the case of CHF, blood pressure normalization is not a specific treatment goal; rather, maximal tissue effect is desired. Thus, recommendations for ACEIs such as enalapril and captopril may include titration to higher levels than those required for blood pressure control.[46] Thus, the success of an ACEI in CHF may derive from multiple properties other than ACE inhibition. Myocardial binding, reductions in plasma aldosterone, and increases in neuropeptides normally degraded by ACE may contribute to the overall cardioprotective effects of ACEIs.[47] All ACEIs have not been thoroughly studied in connection with CHF, particularly in terms of these secondary response parameters, so it is less likely that ACEIs are truly interchangeable in the treatment of CHF. Furthermore, true dose equivalence among the ACEIs has not been established for the treatment of CHF and myocardial infarction.

Table 69–2 Pharmacokinetic Parameters of Angiotensin-Converting Enzyme Inhibitors

Drug	Onset/Duration (hrs)	Peak Hypotensive Effect (hrs)	Protein Binding (%)	Effect of Food on Absorption	Serum Half-Life	Elimination
Benazepril	1/24	2–4	> 95	None	10–11	Renal, some biliary
Captopril	0.25/dose-related	1–1.5	25–30	Reduced	<2	Renal, as disulfides
Enalapril	1/24	4–6	50	None	11	Renal
Fosinopril	1/24	2–6	95	None	11	Renal = hepatic
Lisinopril	1/24	6	10	None	13	Renal
Moexipril	1/24	4–6	50	Reduced	2–9	Renal, some biliary
Quinapril	1/24	2	97	Reduced	2	Renal > hepatic
Ramipril	1–2/24	3–6	73	Reduced	13–17	Renal
Trandolapril	2–4/24	6–8	80–94	None	16–24	Renal > hepatic

HEMODYNAMIC EFFECTS

A number of well-described hemodynamic effects occur with the administration of an ACEI (Table 69–3).[3] The underlying disease commonly dictates the magnitude of change in many of these hemodynamic parameters. This is particularly evident in the treatment of CHF and renal failure. In addition, many of these hemodynamic changes are accentuated in the presence of an activated RAA axis, as may occur with diuretic therapy and a low-salt diet. The latter is a well-established risk factor for the occurrence of first-dose hypotension with an ACEI.[48]

The reduction in blood pressure resulting from an ACEI, occurs independently of either a decrease in cardiac output or an increase in heart rate.[31, 49] Occasionally, cardiac output increases with ACEI therapy, particularly if it was reduced before therapy began.[50] The fall in peripheral vascular resistance that occurs with ACEI therapy can be accompanied by a decrease in cardiac filling pressures.[31] Angiotensin II can actively participate in the regulation of coronary vascular tone and coronary blood flow if the RAA axis has been activated. Conversely, treatment with an ACEI can reverse this angiotensin II–mediated decline in coronary blood flow.[51] Several small trials, generally of short duration, that assessed the effects of ACEIs on the severity of angina or on objective measures of myocardial ischemia have reported conflicting results.[52]

ACEIs lower blood pressure without diminishing cerebral blood flow.[53] This phenomenon is considered a favorable effect of ACE inhibition on cerebral autoregulatory ability and is potentially relevant to the treatment of hypertension in the elderly.[54] Furthermore, ACEIs decrease capacitance vessel tone, which may explain why ACEIs can alleviate the peripheral edema associated with calcium channel blocker therapy.[55] ACEIs do not limit the peak heart-rate response to exercise, but they do effectively reduce the peak blood pressure response.[56] Addition of a diuretic to an ACEI does not alter the hemodynamic profile of ACE inhibition except in the instance of exercise, when the exercise-related increase in cardiac output may be blunted.[57]

ACEIs routinely increase effective renal plasma flow (ERPF) while maintaining the glomerular filtration rate (GFR). The rise in ERPF evoked by ACEIs is characterized by a preferential dilatation of the efferent arteriole.[58, 59] The arithmetic consequence of this is a drop in the filtration fraction (GFR/ERPF), a well-accepted marker of the effect of ACEIs on the kidney. When the GFR is heavily reliant on efferent arteriolar tone (as in CHF, dehydration, and renal artery stenosis), administration of an ACEI may result in a sudden decline in GFR.[60]

EFFECTS ON BLOOD PRESSURE

Diuretics and β-blockers are still commonly employed as first-step therapy for hypertension, although ACEIs are starting to be considered a suitable alternative.[61, 62] The enthusiasm for the use of ACEIs is not related to efficacy, for ACEIs have efficacy comparable to (and no better than) most other drug classes, with response rates ranging from 40 to 70% in stage 1 or 2 hypertension.[63] Clinical trial results do not reflect conditions in actual practice, where the favorable side effect profile of ACEIs and their proposed ability to protect target organs dominate the thinking of many practitioners. ACEIs are heavily prescribed because they are thought to be well tolerated drugs that patients will continue to take over a long period.[64] This enthusiasm may be somewhat misguided in cases of routine, uncomplicated hypertension. There is a paucity of

Table 69–3 Predominant Hemodynamic Effects of Angiotensin-Converting Enzyme Inhibitors

Hemodynamic Parameter	Effect	Clinical Significance
Cardiovascular		
Total peripheral resistance	Decreased	
Mean arterial pressure	Decreased	
Cardiac output	Increased or no change	
Stroke volume	Increased	These parameters contribute to a general decrease in systemic blood pressure
Preload and afterload	Decreased	
Pulmonary artery pressure	Decreased	
Right atrial pressure	Decreased	
Diastolic dysfunction	Improve	
Renal		
Renal blood flow	Usually increased	
Glomerular filtration rate	Variable, usually unchanged but may ↓ in renal failure	Contributes to the renoprotective effect of these agents
Efferent arteriolar resistance	Decreased	
Filtration fraction	Decreased	
Peripheral Nervous System		
Biosynthesis of noradrenaline	Decreased	
Reuptake of adrenaline	Inhibited	Enhances blood pressure lowering effect and resets baroreceptor function
Circulating catecholamines	Decreased	

Table 69–4 Dosage Strengths and Treatment Guidelines for Oral ACEIs

Drug	Strengths (mg)	Hypertension		Heart Failure	
		Mg	Frequency	Mg	Frequency
Benazepril	5, 10, 20, 40	20–40	q.d.–b.i.d.	Not FDA-approved	
Captopril	12.5, 25, 50, 100	50–450	b.i.d.–t.i.d.	18.75–150	t.i.d.
Enalapril	2.5, 5, 10, 20	10–40	q.d.–b.i.d.	5–20	q.d.–b.i.d.
Fosinopril	10, 20	20–40	q.d.–b.i.d.	20–40	q.d.
Lisinopril	2.5, 5, 10, 20, 40	20–40	q.d.	5–20	q.d.
Moexipril	7.5, 15	7.5–30	q.d.–b.i.d.	Not FDA-approved	
Quinapril	5, 10, 20, 40	20–80	q.d.–b.i.d.	20–40	q.d.–b.i.d.
Ramipril	1.25, 2.5, 5, 10	2.5–20	q.d.–b.i.d.	10	b.i.d.
Trandolapril	1, 2, 4	1–4	q.d.	1–4	q.d.

Abbreviation: FDA, U.S. Food and Drug Administration.

information concerning long-term cardiovascular morbidity and mortality in connection with ACEIs as opposed to conventional antihypertensive therapy. Where comparative data are available, ACEIs and conventional therapy have similar effects on cardiovascular and cardiorenal morbidity and mortality.[65, 66]

There are few predictors of response to ACEIs. When hypertension is accompanied by high PRA values, as in renal artery stenosis, the response to an ACEI can be profound.[67] In most other cases, there is little relationship between the PRA values before and after treatment and the depressor response to an ACEI. Certain categories of patients demonstrate lower response rates to ACEI monotherapy—low-renin, salt-sensitive individuals such as those with diabetes and African Americans and elderly individuals with hypertension.[4]

The low-renin state characteristic of the elderly hypertensive differs from other low-renin forms of hypertension in that it develops not as a response to volume expansion but because of senescence-related changes in PRA.[68] The elderly generally respond well to ACEIs in conventional doses,[54] although senescence-related renal failure, which slows the elimination of these drugs, complicates the interpretation of such treatment successes. African Americans with hypertension tend, as a group, to have lower PRA levels and are perceived to respond poorly to ACEI monotherapy when compared with whites.[69] Yet in many instances, if careful dose titration occurs, blood pressure will eventually be normalized.[70]

All nine ACEIs are approved by the U.S. Food and Drug Administration for the treatment of hypertension. ACEIs are now recognized by the Joint National Committee on the Prevention, Detection, Evaluation, and Treatment of High Blood Pressure as an option for first-line therapy in patients with essential hypertension, especially in those with diabetes accompanied by renal disease and in those with CHF.[1] Considerable dosing flexibility exists with the available ACEIs. Enalaprilat is the sole ACEI available in intravenous form (Table 69–4).[3]

Results from a number of head-to-head trials support the comparable antihypertensive efficacy and tolerability of the various ACEIs. However, there are differences among ACEIs in time to onset of effect and time to maximal blood pressure reduction. These differences do not translate into different response rates if comparable doses are given. Typical confounding variables that confuse the interpreta-

tion of study results have included differences in study design and methodology, dose frequency, and dose. ACEIs labeled "once daily" vary in their ability to reduce blood pressure for a full 24 hours, as defined by a trough:peak ratio greater than 50%.[71] The trough:peak ratio, as an index of duration of blood pressure control, often misrepresents the true blood pressure reduction achieved by a compound.[72] Because of this, dosing instructions for many of these compounds include the proviso to administer a second daily dose if the antihypertensive effect has dissipated by the end of the dosing interval. Additional prospective clinical trials will be required to clarify the issue of duration of effect for the various ACEIs.

The question is often raised as to what to do if an ACEI does not normalize blood pressure. One approach is simply to raise the dose; however, the dose-response curve for ACEIs, like most antihypertensive agents, is flat.[73] Responders to ACEIs typically do so at doses well below that necessary for prolonged 24-hour suppression of ACE. In addition, the maximal depressor response to an ACEI does not occur until several weeks after beginning therapy. Only with complete failure to respond to an ACEI or if an important adverse effect occurs should an alternative drug class be substituted. If a partial response has occurred, therapy with an ACEI can be continued in anticipation of an additional drop in blood pressure over several weeks. Alternatively, an additional compound such as a diuretic, calcium channel blocker or peripheral α-blocker can be combined with an ACEI to effect better blood pressure control.

ACEIs IN COMBINATION WITH OTHER AGENTS

The depressor effect of an ACEI is considerably enhanced by the simultaneous administration of a diuretic.[74, 75] This pattern of response has spurred the development of a number of fixed-dose combination products composed of an ACEI and a diuretic.[1, 76] The rationale for this combination of drugs derives from the observation that sodium depletion increases PRA and thereby shifts blood pressure into an angiotensin II–dependent mode. Very low-dose diuretic therapy such as 12.5 mg of hydrochlorothiazide can evoke this synergistic response, suggesting that even subtle alterations in sodium balance are sufficient to bolster the effect of an ACEI[75] (see Chap. 53, Low-Dose Fixed-Combination Antihypertensive Therapy). It is important to note that combining an ACEI and a diuretic eliminates the disparity in response to ACEIs between black and white patients.[77]

The rationale behind combining an ACEI and a β-blocker is that the β-blocker will presumably blunt the hyperreninemia induced by the ACEI.[76, 78] In practice, only a modest additional blood pressure response occurs when these two drug classes are combined.[79] In contrast, the addition of a peripheral α-antagonist such as doxazosin to an ACEI can be followed by a significant additional response.[80] The mechanism of this response remains to be elucidated. Finally, the blood pressure lowering effect of an ACEI is considerably enhanced by the coadministration of a calcium channel blocker.[55, 81] This seems to occur whether the calcium channel blocker is a dihydropyridine (e.g., felodipine or amlodipine)[55, 81] or a nondihydropyridine (e.g., verapamil),[82] and the response has spurred the development of a number of fixed-dose combination products composed of an ACEI and a calcium channel blocker.[83]

A number of studies have demonstrated the utility of ACEIs in the management of hypertensive patients otherwise unresponsive to drug combinations.[84, 85] Typically, such combinations have included a diuretic as well as minoxidil, a calcium channel blocker, and a peripheral α-blocker. The key, as with two-drug therapy, is to combine agents with different mechanisms of action. In addition, acute reduction in blood pressure can be achieved with oral or sublingual captopril, which begins to act 15 minutes after administration.[86] Another option for the management of hypertensive emergencies is parenteral therapy with enalaprilat.[87] Compounds that interrupt the RAA axis activity, as ACEIs do, should be administered cautiously to patients suspected of marked activation of the RAA axis (e.g, prior treatment with diuretics). In such subjects, sudden and extreme drops in blood pressure have occasionally been observed.[48]

ACEIs IN HYPERTENSION ASSOCIATED WITH OTHER DISORDERS

ACEIs effectively regress left ventricular hypertrophy during prolonged lowering of blood pressure.[88] This is an important feature in that left ventricular hypertrophy portends a significant risk of sudden death or myocardial infarction.[89] ACEIs can be safely utilized in patients with coronary artery disease. Although they do not specifically dilate coronary arteries, they do improve hemodynamic factors that dictate myocardial oxygen consumption and thereby reduce the risk of ischemia (see Table 69–3). For example, ACEIs, unlike other antihypertensive agents, do not increase myocardial sympathetic tone in hypertensive patients with angina.[90]

ACEIs are also useful in the treatment of isolated systolic hypertension and predominantly systolic forms of hypertension because they improve arteriolar compliance.[91] In addition, ACEIs are effective in the treatment of hypertensive patients with concomitant cerebrovascular disease because they maintain cerebral autoregulatory ability despite reducing blood pressure.[53, 92] This is particularly important in the treatment of the elderly hypertensive.[54]

ACEIs dilate both small and large arteries and can be used safely in patients with peripheral vascular disease; they may, on occasion, even lessen intermittent claudication.[93]

ACEIs are touted being the agents of choice for diabetic hypertensive patients, whether or not they have diabetic renal disease. Such enthusiasm should be tempered by the realization that these compounds, when admistered as monotherapy, do not effectively reduce blood pressure in many diabetics. This may relate to the fact that many diabetics have a low-renin, volume-expanded form of hypertension, which is generally less responsive to an ACEI. This hurdle can be overcome by adding a diuretic to the treatment regimen. Alternatively, a different class of antihypertensives may be used. The rationale for ACEI use is much stronger for the diabetic patient with renal involvement. The data are very impressive in support of using an ACEI as a major element of the treatment regimen, irrespective of its ability to reduce blood pressure.[94] A final consideration concerning use of ACEIs in hypertensive diabetics relates to their effect on hyperlipidemia and insulin resistance. ACEIs have not exhibited an unambiguous effect on serum lipids and insulin resistance in diabetic patients.[95–97]

TARGET ORGAN EFFECTS

Renal

The Sixth Report of the Joint National Committee on Prevention, Detection, Evaluation, and Treatment of High Blood Pressure recommends the use of ACEIs in patients with hypertension and chronic renal disease to control hypertension and to slow progressive renal failure.[1] Irrespective of the drug class being used to lower blood pressure, the most important component in the management of the patient with hypertension and renal disease remains tight blood pressure control. The report advises a goal blood pressure of 130/85 mm Hg, and an even lower value, 125/75, is advised for patients with proteinuria of more than 1 g/day.[1] Management of hypertension in the patient with renal failure is typically multifactorial, although in most instances, it is volume dependent. Because of the volume dependency of hypertension related to renal failure, ACEI therapy alone does not always provide the desired level of blood pressure control. Thus it is not uncommon for diuretics and other drugs to be added to the treatment regimen of such patients.

ACEIs have been found in clinical trials to be useful in established type 1 (insulin-dependent) diabetes mellitus nephropathy,[45] type 2 (noninsulin-dependent) diabetic mellitus nephropathy,[98] type 1 diabetes in patients with normal blood pressures and microalbuminuria,[99] type 2 diabetes normotensive patients with microalbuminuria and normal renal function,[100] and a variety of nondiabetic renal diseases,[101–103] especially in the setting of significant proteinuria.[100–104] ACEI regimens shown to slow the progression of renal failure include captopril 25 mg three times a day,[45, 99] enalapril 5 to 10 mg/day,[100] benazepril 10 mg/day[101] and ramipril 2.5 to 5.0 mg/day.[102] It is presumed that renal failure increases the pharmacological effects of these doses by reducing renal clearance of the ACEIs.[38, 40]

ACEIs have a number of effects that can be construed as being renoprotective, including but not limited to the following: (1) they decrease glomerular capillary pressure,[105] (2) they decrease protein excretion,[100–104] and (3) they transiently reduce GFR (see Table 69–3).[106] Early opinion attributed the renoprotective features of ACEIs to their ability to decrease glomerular capillary pressures.[105] Current opinion holds that the predominant renoprotective mechanism of ACEIs is their modification of tissue-based growth factors that are activated by prior or ongoing renal disease and stimulated by the presence of angiotensin II.[107] The renoprotective effect of ACEIs is most evident in patients with heavy proteinuria (>3 g/day) who, if left untreated, generally progress rapidly to end-stage renal failure.[100–104]

Three factors are potential modifiers of the renal response to ACEIs. First, low sodium intake enhances the antiproteinuric effect of ACEIs.[7, 108] Second, short-term studies suggest that dietary protein restriction complements the ACEIs' effect on protein excretion in nephrotic patients. This suggests that combining ACEIs and protein restriction might prove more effective than ACEIs alone in slowing the progression of renal failure.[109] A third factor is inherited variation in ACE activity. Two common forms of the ACE gene, I (insertion) and D (deletion), give rise to three potential genotypes—II, ID, and DD. The DD phenotype is associated with higher circulating ACE levels[110] and a greater pressor response to the infusion of angiotensin I compared with the II phenotype; the ID phenotype displays intermediate characteristics.[111] These phenotypic characteristics may be relevant to the response to ACE inhibition. The finding that DD patients are at increased risk for myocardial infarction and ischemic cardiomyopathy first established the clinical significance of the inherited variation in ACE activity.[112] Recent work suggests that GFR declines more rapidly in DD than in II patients and that such patients do not demonstrate significant reductions in proteinuria or slowing in the rate of progression of renal failure when administered ACEIs.[113, 114]

Cardiac

Data from both placebo-controlled and open trials suggest that ACEIs substantially reduce the risk of death and hospitalization because of CHF and improve its symptomatology.[8] These agents interfere with the neurohumoral deterioration that is characteristic of CHF.[115] Statistically significant reductions in mortality have been observed only with enalapril, but similar trends have been observed with other ACEIs, including captopril, ramipril, quinapril, and lisinopril.[8] Furthermore, these agents have demonstrated efficacy and tolerability in the treatment of CHF based on the endpoints of improved exercise tolerance and symptomatology. Although ACEIs are almost universally recommended as a cost-effective strategy for the treatment of CHF, physicians' prescribing practices are such that only about 50% of patients eligible for treatment with ACEIs actually receive them.[116, 117]

Enalapril, captopril, lisinopril, and trandolapril have been shown to reduce morbidity and mortality rates in patients with myocardial infarction and a wide range of ventricular function. Currently, insufficient data exist to determine whether clinically significant differences exist among the ACEIs in the post–myocardial infarction setting; there is a paucity of head-to-head trials among these agents, and studies have varied in length and duration.[118] At this time, only captopril and trandolapril have been approved for left ventricular dysfunction that occurs after myocardial infarction, although enalapril has been approved for asymptomatic left ventricular dysfunction. However, as in patients with CHF, numerous ACEIs have demonstrated benefits in patients after myocardial infarction, suggesting a class effect.[119]

Several dosing strategies have been shown to be effective in reducing morbidity and mortality in patients with systolic left ventricular dysfunction. Most importantly, a systematic effort must be made to reach the target doses shown to be effective in the randomized trials of ACEIs in CHF. Emerging data suggest that the doses of ACEIs used in clinical practice are less effective than the relatively high doses used in the randomized trials.[47, 120] Dose ranges used in community practice are typically in the range of 50 mg/day and 10 mg/day for captopril and enalapril, respectively. Randomized trials on the other hand, achieved their successes, with captopril and enalapril doses approaching 150 mg/day and 40 mg/day, respectively. The treatment of CHF should include sequential dose titration of the ACEI being used up to doses employed in randomized clinical trials. The ability to reach these doses in the CHF patient can sometimes be a vexing issue; a major deterrent is the development of systemic hypotension or a decline in GFR.[4] Thus, reaching goal ACEI doses necessitates a keen understanding of the critical relationship between volume status, blood pressure, and the final desired ACEI dose. The single most important variable in choosing effective dose titration is understanding the relationship between volume status and blood pressure.[41]

ADVERSE EFFECTS OF ACEIs

Soon after their release, a syndrome of functional renal insufficiency was observed as a class effect with ACEIs. This process was initially recognized in patients with both a solitary kidney and a renal artery stenosis or in the setting of bilateral renal artery stenosis. Since the original reports were issued, this phenomenon has been observed in a number of other conditions, too, including dehydration, CHF, and microvascular renal disease.[50, 60, 121] The theme common to all of these conditions is that GFR is dependent on angiotensin II–mediated constriction of the efferent arteriole. When the efferent arteriole is constricted, upstream hydrostatic pressures within the glomerular capillary bed remain normal or increased despite a decline in afferent arteriolar flow. The abrupt removal of angiotensin II causes this sustaining pressure increase to dissipate, and with this change, GFR rapidly diminishes. This phenomenon of functional renal insufficiency is best treated by discontinuation of the ACEI, careful volume repletion if intravascular volume contraction exists and, if it is suspected, investigation for the presence of renal artery stenosis. If these steps are taken, the process is self-limited in almost all cases.[122]

An additional adverse effect of ACEIs is hyperkalemia[123] which generally occurs only in predisposed patients such as diabetic or CHF patients with renal failure who are receiving potassium-sparing diuretics or potassium supplements.[121] ACEIs are known to lessen the degree of hypokalemia produced by diuretic therapy.[124]

A dry, nonproductive cough is common with ACEIs and is seen in as many as 20% of treated patients,[125] particularly among women and Chinese people.[126] It has been attributed to increased levels of bradykinin or other vasoactive peptides such as substance P, which may play a role as a second messenger in triggering the cough reflex. Although numerous therapies have been tried, few have successfully eliminated ACEI-induced cough. The cough usually disappears 1 to 2 weeks after the offending agent is stopped. Switching to a different agent in the class or reducing the dose generally does not alleviate the problem.[125] Nonspecific adverse effects are rare with ACEIs, except for taste disturbances, leukopenia, skin rash, and dysgeusia, which occur most often in captopril-treated patients[127] The sulfhydryl group found in captopril has been implicated in these effects.

Angioedema is a potentially life-threatening complication of ACEIs. Its incidence rate is less than 1% but it can occur quite unpredictably. Typically, it is not a first-dose phenomenon. It is easily recognized because of the characteristic involvement of the mouth, tongue, and upper airway.[128, 129] If angioedema occurs, it is a contraindication to the use of ACEIs. A final issue concerning ACEIs is their capacity to cause birth defects. ACEIs are not teratogenic; rather, when administered during the second and third trimesters of pregnancy, they can result in developmental defects, acute renal failure, or death in the fetus because the maturing fetus is heavily reliant on angiotensin II for development.[130, 131]

CLASS-SPECIFIC AND AGENT-SPECIFIC DRUG INTERACTIONS OF ACEIs

Several class-specific drug interactions occur with ACEIs.[132] Potassium supplements and potassium-sparing diuretics, when given with ACEIs, increase the probability of developing hyperkalemia.[133] Nonsteroidal anti-inflammatory drugs such as indomethacin reduce the antihypertensive effects of ACEIs, particularly in low-renin forms of hypertension.[27] The concurrent administration of lithium with ACEI is associated with a greater likelihood of lithium toxicity.[134] Combining an ACEI with allopurinol is associated with a higher risk of hypersensitivity reactions and there have been several cases of the Stevens-Johnson syndrome have been reported with the combination of captopril and allopurinol.[135] Quinapril reduces the absorption of tetracycline by about 35%, possibly because of the high magnesium content of quinapril tablets.

CONCLUSION

ACEIs treat hypertension by altering levels of both angiotensin II and bradykinin as well as by decreasing sympathetic outflow. Whereas early theories held that these drugs were only marginally effective in low-renin forms of hypertension, more recent information suggests otherwise. A plethora of ACEIs is available and distinctions among individual members of the class are sometimes quite subtle. Pharmacological properties proposed as distinguishing features among the ACEIs include their tissue-binding potential and mode of elimination (renal or renal and hepatic). ACEIs are of clearly proven benefit in slowing the progression of chronic renal failure and reducing the morbidity and mortality that attends progressive CHF. ACEIs have few adverse effects other than cough, which may occur in as many as 20% of patients. Other ACEI-associated adverse effects include hyperkalemia and a reversible form of renal failure attributable to diminished efferent arteriolar tone in an angiotensin II–dependent kidney, as occurs when ACEIs are given to patients with bilateral renal artery stenosis.

References

1. The Sixth Report of the Joint National Committee on Prevention, Detection, Evaluation, and Treatment of High Blood Pressure. Arch Intern Med 157:2413–2446, 1997.
2. Brunner HR, Waeber B, Nussberger J. Angiotensin-converting enzyme inhibitors. In Messerli F (ed). Cardiovascular Drug Therapy, 2nd ed. Philadelphia, WB Saunders, 1996; pp 690–711.
3. Sica DA, Ripley E. Angiotensin converting enzyme inhibitors. In Izzo JL, Black HR (eds). Hypertension Primer, 2nd ed. Baltimore, Williams & Wilkins, 1998; pp 372–376.
4. Cheng A, Frishman WH. Use of angiotensin-converting enzyme inhibitors as monotherapy and in combination with diuretics and calcium channel blockers. J Clin Pharmacol 38:477–491, 1998.
5. Giatras I, Lau J, Levey SS. Effect of angiotensin-converting enzyme inhibitors on the progression of nondiabetic renal disease: A meta-analysis of randomized trials. Ann Intern Med 127:337–345, 1997.
6. Navis G, Faber HJ, de Zeeuw D, de Jong PE. ACE inhibitors and the kidney. Drug Safety 15:200–211, 1996.
7. Navis G, de Jong PE, de Zeeuw D. Optimizing the renal response to ACE inhibition: A strategy toward more effective long-term renoprotection. Adv Nephrol 27:57–66, 1998.
8. Garg R, Yusuf S for the Collaborative Group on ACE Inhibitor Trials. Overview of randomized trials of angiotensin-converting enzyme inhibitors on mortality and morbidity in patients with heart failure. JAMA 273:1450–1456, 1995.
9. Lonn EM, Yusuf S, Jha P, et al. Emerging role of angiotensin-converting enzyme inhibitors in cardiac and vascular protection. Circulation 90:2056–2069.
10. Ruddy MC, Kostis JB, Frishman WH. Drugs that affect the renin-angiotensin system. In Frishman WH, Sonnenblick EH (eds). Cardiovascular Pharmacotherapeutics. New York, McGraw-Hill, 1996; pp 131–192.
11. Johnston C, Risvanis J. Preclinical pharmacology of angiotensin II receptor antagonists: Update and outstanding issues. Am J. Hypertens 10:306S–310S, 1997.
12. Carretero OA, Scicli AG. The kallikrein-kinin system as a regulator of cardiovascular and renal function. In Brenner BM, Laragh JH (eds). Hypertension: Pathophysiology, Diagnosis, and Management, 2nd ed. New York, Raven, 1995; pp 983–999.
13. Juillerat L, Nussberger J, Menard J, et al. Determinants of angiotensin II generation during converting enzyme inhibition. Hypertension 16:564–572, 1990.
14. Urata H, Nishimura H, Ganten D. Chymase-dependent angiotensin II forming system in humans. Am J Hypertens 9:277–284, 1996.
15. Swedberg K, Eneroth P, Kjekshus J, Wilhelmsen L. Hormones regulating cardiovascular function in patients with severe congestive heart failure and their relation to mortality. CONSENSUS Trial Study Group. Circulation 82:1730–1736, 1990.
16. Mooser V, Nussberger J, Juillert L, et al. Reactive hyperreninemia is a major determinant of plasma angiotensin II during ACE inhibition. J Cardiovasc Pharmacol 15:276–282, 1990.

17. Vander AJ, Geelhoed GW. Inhibition of renin secretion by angiotensin II. Proc Soc Exp Biol Med 120:399–403, 1965.
18. Nussberger J, Brunner DB, Waeber A, et al. Lack of angiotensin I accumulation after converting enzyme blockade with enalapril or lisinopril in man. Clin Sci 72:387–389, 1987.
19. Staessen J, Fagard R, Lijnen P, et al. The hypotensive effect of propranolol in captopril-treated patients does not involve the plasma renin-angiotensin-aldosterone system. Clin Sci 61:441S–444S, 1981.
20. Hodsman GP, Isles CG, Murray GD, et al. Factors related to the first dose hypotensive effect of captopril: Prediction and treatment. BMJ 286:832–834, 1983.
21. Case DB, Atlas SA, Laragh JH, et al. Use of first dose response or plasma renin activity to predict the long-term effect of captopril: Identification of triphasic pattern of blood pressure response. J Cardiovasc Pharmacol 2:339–346, 1980.
22. Brunner HR, Waeber B, Nussberger J. Does pharmacological profiling of a new drug in normotensive volunteers provide a useful guide to antihypertensive therapy? Hypertension 5(suppl III):101–107, 1983.
23. Gainer JV, Morrow JD, Loveland A, et al. Effect of bradykinin-receptor blockade on the response to angiotensin-converting enzyme inhibitor in normotensive and hypertensive subjects. N Engl J Med 339:1285–1292, 1998.
24. Ogihara T, Maruyama A, Hata T, et al. Hormonal responses to long-term converting enzyme inhibition I hypertensive patients. Clin Pharmacol Ther 30:328–335, 1981.
25. Gavras I. Bradykinin-mediated effects of ACE inhibition. Kidney Int 42:1020–1029, 1992.
26. Waeber B, Nussberger J, Brunner HR. Angiotensin-converting enzyme inhibitors in hypertension. In Laragh JH, Brenner BM (eds). Hypertension: Pathophysiology, Diagnosis, and Management, 2nd ed. New York, Raven, 1995; pp 2861–2875.
27. Salvetti A, Abdel-Hag B, Magagna A, et al. Indomethacin reduces the antihypertensive effect of enalapril. Clin Exp Hypertens 9:559–567, 1987.
28. Nawarskas JJ, Spinler SA. Does aspirin interfere with the therapeutic efficacy of angiotensin-converting enzyme inhibitors in hypertension or congestive heart failure? Pharmacotherapy 18:1041–1052, 1998.
29. Guazzi MD, Campodonico J, Celeste F, et al. Antihypertensive efficacy of angiotensin-converting enzyme inhibition and aspirin counteraction. Clin Pharmacol Ther 63:79–86, 1998.
30. Lang CC, Stein M, He HB, et al. Angiotensin-converting enzyme inhibition and sympathetic activity in healthy subjects. Clin Pharmacol Ther 59:668–674, 1996.
31. Fagard R, Amery A, Reybrouck T, et al. Acute and chronic systemic and hemodynamic effects of angiotensin-converting enzyme inhibition with captopril in hypertensive patients. Am J Cardiol 46:295–300, 1980.
32. Vanhoutte PM. Endothelial dysfunction and inhibition of converting enzyme. Eur Heart J 19(suppl J):J7–J15, 1998.
33. Cody R. Optimizing ACE inhibitor therapy of congestive heart failure: Insights from pharmacodynamic studies. Clin Pharmacokinet 24:59–70, 1993.
34. Salvetti A. Newer ACE inhibitors: A look at the future. Drugs 40:800–828, 1990.
35. Zusman RM. Effects of converting-enzyme inhibitors on the renin-angiotensin-aldosterone, bradykinin, and arachidonic acid-prostaglandin systems: Correlation of chemical structure and biological activity. Am J Kid Dis 10(suppl 1):13–23, 1987.
36. Punzi HD. Safety update: Focus on cough. Am J Cardiol 72:45H–48H, 1993.
37. Zusman RM. Angiotensin-converting enzyme inhibitors: More different than alike? Am J Cardiol 72:25H–36H, 1993.
38. Sica DA. Kinetics of angiotensin-converting enzyme inhibitors in renal failure. J Cardiovasc Pharmacol 20(suppl 10):S13–S20, 1992.
39. Hoyer J, Schulte K-L, Lenz T. Clinical pharmacokinetics of angiotensin-converting enzyme inhibitors in renal failure. Clin Pharmacokinet 24:230–254, 1993.
40. Sica DA, Cutler RE, Parmer RJ, et al. Comparison of the steady-state pharmacokinetics of fosinopril, lisinopril, and enalapril in patients with chronic renal insufficiency. Clin Pharmacokinet 20:420–427, 1991.
41. Sica DA, Deedwania PC. Renal considerations in the use of angiotensin-converting enzyme inhibitors in the treatment of congestive heart failure. Congest Heart Fail 3:54–59, 1997.
42. Leonetti G, Cuspidi C. Choosing the right ACE inhibitor: A guide to selection. Drugs 49:516–535, 1995.
43. Briscoe TA, Dearing CJ. Clinical and economic effects of replacing enalapril with benazepril in hypertensive patients. Am J Health Syst Pharm 53:2191–2193, 1996.
44. The SOLVD investigators. Effect of enalapril on survival in patients with reduced left ventricular ejection fractions and congestive heart failure. N Engl J Med 325:293–302, 1991.
45. Lewis EJ, Hunsicker LG, Bain RP, Rohde RD. The effect of angiotensin-converting enzyme inhibition on diabetic nephropathy: The Collaborative Study Group. N Engl J Med 329:1456–1462, 1993.
46. The American College of Cardiology/American Heart Association Task Force on Practical Guidelines (Committee on Evaluation and Management of Heart Failure). Guidelines for the evaluation and management of heart failure. Circulation 92:2764–2784, 1995.
47. Van Veldhuisen DJ, Genth-Zotz S, Brouwer J, et al. High- versus low-dose ACE inhibition in chronic heart failure: A double-blind, placebo-controlled study of imidapril. J Am Coll Cardiol 32:1811–1818, 1998.
48. Hodsman GP, Isles CG, Murray GD, et al. Factors related to first-dose hypotensive effect of captopril: Prediction and treatment. BMJ 286:832–834, 1983.
49. Muiesan G, Alicandri CL, Agabiti-Rosei E, et al. Angiotensin-converting enzyme inhibition, catecholamines, and hemodynamics in essential hypertension. Am J Cardiol 46:1420–1424, 1980.
50. Saragoca MA, Homsi E, Ribeiro AB, et al. Hemodynamic mechanism of blood pressure response to captopril in human malignant hypertension. Hypertension 5(suppl I):53–59, 1983.
51. Magrini F, Shimizu M, Roberts N, et al. Converting-enzyme inhibition and coronary blood flow. Circulation 75:1168–1174, 1987.
52. Yusuf S, Lonn E. Anti-ischemic effects of ACE inhibitors: Review of current clinical evidence and ongoing clinical trials. Eur Heart J 19(suppl J):J36–J44, 1998.
53. Waldemar G, Ibsen H, Strandgaard S, et al. The effect of fosinopril sodium on cerebral blood flow in moderate essential hypertension. Am J Hypertens 3:464–470, 1990.
54. Israili ZH, Hall WD, ACE Inhibitors: Differential use in elderly patients with hypertension. Drugs Aging 7:355–371, 1995.
55. Gradman AH, Cutler NR, Davis PJ, et al. Combined enalapril and felodipine extended release for systemic hypertension: Enalapril-Felodipine ER Factorial Study Group. Am J Cardiol 79:431–435, 1997.
56. Morioka S, Simon G, Cohn JN. Cardiac and hormonal effects of enalapril in hypertension. Clin Pharmacol Ther 34:583–589, 1988.
57. Omvik P, Lund-Johansen P. Combined captopril and hydrochlorothiazide therapy in severe hypertension: Long-term haemodynamic changes at rest and during exercise. J Hypertens 2:73–80, 1984.
58. Navis G, Faber HJ, de Zeeuw D, et al. ACE inhibitors and the kidney. Drug Saf 15:200–211, 1996.
59. Hollenberg N, Raij L. Angiotensin-converting enzyme inhibition and renal protection. Arch Int Med 153:2426–2435, 1993.
60. Toto RD, Mitchell HC, Lee HC, et al. Reversible renal insufficiency due to angiotensin-converting enzyme inhibitors in hypertensive nephrosclerosis. Ann Intern Med 115:513–519, 1991.
61. Siegel D, Lopez J, Meier J. Pharmacologic treatment of hypertension in the Department of Veterans Affairs during 1995 and 1996. Am J Hypertens 11:1271–1278, 1998.
62. Doyle JC, Mottram DR, Stubbs H. Prescribing of ACE inhibitors for cardiovascular disorders in general practice. J Clin Pharm Ther 23:133–136, 1998.
63. Materson BJ, Reda DJ, Cushman WC, et al. Single-drug therapy for hypertension in men: A comparison of six antihypertensives agents with placebo. N Engl J Med 328:914–921, 1993.
64. Caro JJ, Speckman JL, Salas M, et al. Effect of initial drug choice on persistence with antihypertensive therapy: The importance of actual practice data. Can Med Assoc J 160:41–46, 1999.
65. Hansson L, Lindholm L, Niskanen L, et al. Effect of angiotensin-converting-enzyme inhibition compared with conventional therapy on cardiovascular morbidity and mortality in hypertension: The Captopril Prevention Project (CAPPP) randomised trial. Lancet 353:611–616, 1999.
66. U.K. Prospective Diabetes Study Group. Efficacy of atenolol and captopril in reducing risk of macrovascular and microvascular complications in type II diabetes. BMJ 317:713–720, 1998.
67. Smith RD, Franklin SS. Comparison of effects of enalapril plus

hydrochlorothiazide versus standard triple therapy on renal function in renovascular hypertension. Am J Med 79(suppl 3C):14–23, 1985.

68. Weidmann P, De Myttenaere-Bursztein S, Maxwell MH. Effect of aging on plasma renin and aldosterone in normal man. Kidney Int 8:325–333, 1975.

69. Weinberger MH. Blood pressure and metabolic responses to hydrochlorothiazide, captopril, and the combination in black and white mild-to-moderate hypertensive patients. J Cardiovasc Pharmacol 7(suppl 1):52–55, 1985.

70. Weir MR, Gray JM, Paster R, et al. Differing mechanisms of action of angiotensin-converting enzyme inhibition in black and white hypertensive patients. Hypertension 25:124–130, 1995.

71. Zannad F. Trandolapril: How does it differ from other angiotensin-converting enzyme inhibitors? Drugs 46(suppl 2):172–182, 1993.

72. Omboni S, Fogari R, Palatini P, et al. Reproducibility and clinical value of the trough-to-peak ratio of the antihypertensive effect: Evidence from the Sample Study. Hypertension 32:424–429, 1998.

73. Sica DA, Gehr TWB. Dose-response relationship and dose adjustments. *In* Izzo JL, Black HR (eds). Hypertension Primer, 2nd ed. Baltimore, Williams & Wilkins, 1998; pp 342–344.

74. Veterans Administration Cooperative Study Group on Antihypertensive Agents: Low-dose captopril for the treatment of mild to moderate hypertension. Hypertension 5(suppl III):139–144, 1983.

75. Neutel JM, Black HR, Weber MA. Combination therapy with diuretics: An evolution of understanding. Am J Med 101:61S–70S, 1996.

76. Sica DA. Fixed combination antihypertensive drugs: Do they have a role in rational therapy? Drugs 48:16–24, 1994.

77. Veterans Administration Cooperative Study Group on Antihypertensive Agents. Racial differences in response to low-dose captopril are abolished by the addition of hydrochlorothiazide. Br J Clin Pharmacol 14:97S–101S, 1982.

78. Hansson L, Beta blockers with ACE inhibitors—a logical combination? J Hum Hypertens 3:97–100, 1989.

79. Belz GG, Essig J, Erb K, et al. Pharmacokinetic and pharmacodynamic interactions between the ACE inhibitor cilazapril and beta-adrenoreceptor antagonist propranolol in healthy subjects and in hypertensive patients. Br J Clin Pharmacol 27(suppl 2):317S–322S, 1989.

80. Brown MJ, Dickerson JE. Synergism between alpha-1 blockade and angiotensin-converting enzyme inhibition in essential hypertension. J Hypertens (suppl):S362–363, 1991.

81. Frishman WH, Ram CV, McMahon FG, et al for the Benazepril/Amlodipine Study Group: Comparison of amlodipine and benazepril monotherapy to amlodipine plus benazepril in patients with systemic hypertension: A randomized, double-blind, placebo-controlled, parallel-group study. J Clin Pharmacol 35:1060–1066, 1995.

82. DeQuattro V, Lee D. Fixed-dose combination therapy with trandolapril and verapamil SR is effective in primary hypertension. Am J Hypertens 10(suppl 2):138S–145S, 1997.

83. Sica DA. Fixed-dose combination therapy: Principles and practice. Cardiovasc Rev Rep 9:28–46, 1997.

84. Bevan EG, Pringle SD, Walker PC, et al. Comparison of captopril, hydralazine and nifedipine as third drug in hypertensive patients. J Hum Hypertens 7:83–88, 1993.

85. Dufloux JJ, Prasquier R. Chatellier G, et al. Effects of captopril and minoxidil on left ventricular hypertrophy in resistant hypertensive patients: A 6-month double-blind comparison. J Am Coll Cardiol 16:137–142, 1990.

86. Damasceno A, Ferreira B, Patel S, et al. Efficacy of captopril and nifedipine in black and white patients with hypertensive crisis. J Hum Hypertens 11:471–476, 1997.

87. Hirschl MM, Binder M, Bur A, et al. Impact of the renin-angiotensin-aldosterone system on blood pressure response to intravenous enalaprilat in patients with hypertensive crises. J Hum Hypertens 11:177–183, 1997.

88. Schlaich MP, Schmieder RE. Left ventricular hypertrophy and its regression: Pathophysiology and therapeutic approach. Am J Hypertens 11:1394–1404, 1998.

89. Koren MJ, Devereux RB, Casale PN, et al. Relation of left ventricular mass and geometry to morbidity and mortality in uncomplicated essential hypertension. Ann Intern Med 114:345–352, 1991.

90. Daly P, Mettauer B, Rouleau JL, et al. Lack of reflex increase in myocardial sympathetic tone after captopril: Potential antianginal mechanism. Circulation 71:317–325, 1985.

91. Chrysant SG. Vascular remodeling: The role of angiotensin-converting enzyme inhibitors. Am Heart J 135:S21–S30, 1998.

92. Frei A, Muller-Brand J. Cerebral blood flow and antihypertensive treatment with enalapril. J Hypertens 4:365–368, 1986.

93. Roberts DH, Tsao Y, McLoughlin GA, et al. Placebo-controlled comparison of captopril, atenolol, labetalol, and pindolol in hypertension complicated by intermittent claudication. Lancet 2:650–653, 1987.

94. Preston RA. Renoprotective effects of antihypertensive drugs. Am J Hypertens 12:19S–32S, 1999.

95. Malini P, Stochi E, Ambosini E, et al. Long-term antihypertensive, metabolic and cellular effects of enalapril. J Hypertens 2(suppl 2):101–105, 1984.

96. Lithell HO, Pollare T, Berne C. Insulin sensitivity in newly detected hypertensive patients: Influence of captopril and other antihypertensive agents on insulin sensitivity and related biological parameters. J Cardiovasc Pharmacol 15(suppl 5):S46–S52, 1990.

97. Tillmann HC, Walker RJ, Lewis-Barned NJ, et al. A long-term comparison between enalapril and captopril on insulin sensitivity in normotensive non-insulin dependent diabetic volunteers. J Clin Pharmacol Ther 22:273–278, 1997.

98. Lebovitz HE, Wiegmann TB, Cnaan A, et al. Renal protective effect of enalapril in hypertensive NIDDM: Role of baseline albuminuria. Kidney Int 45(suppl):S150–155, 1994.

99. Laffel LMB, McGill J, Gans D. The beneficial effects of angiotensin-converting enzyme inhibition with captopril on diabetic nephropathy in normotensive IDDM patients with microalbuminuria. Am J Med 99:497–503, 1995.

100. Ravid M, Lang R, Rachmani R, et al. Long-term renoprotective effect of angiotensin-converting enzyme inhibition in non-insulin dependent diabetes mellitus: A 7-year follow-up study. Arch Int Med 156:286–289, 1996.

101. Maschio G, Alberti D, Janin G, et al. Effect of the angiotensin-converting enzyme inhibitor benazepril on the progression of chronic renal insufficiency. N Engl J Med 334:939–945, 1996.

102. The Gisen Group: Randomized placebo-controlled trial of effect of ramipril on decline in glomerular filtration rate and risk of terminal renal failure in proteinuric, non-diabetic nephropathy. Lancet 349:1857–1863, 1997.

103. Uhle BU, Whitworth JA, Shahinfar S, et al. Angiotensin-converting enzyme inhibition in nondiabetic progressive renal insufficiency: A controlled double-blind trial. Am J Kidney Dis 27:489–495, 1996.

104. Giatras I, Lau J, Levey AS, et al for the Angiotensin-Converting-Enzyme Inhibition and Progressive Renal Disease Study Group: Effect of angiotensin-converting enzyme inhibitors on the progression of nondiabetic renal disease: A meta-analysis of randomized trials. Ann Intern Med 127:337–347, 1997.

105. Anderson S. Rennke HG, Brenner BM. Therapeutic advantage of converting enzyme inhibitors in arresting progressive renal disease associated with systemic hypertension in the rat. J Clin Invest 77:1993–2000, 1986.

106. Apperloo AJ, de Zeeuw D, de Jong PE. A short-term antihypertensive-treatment induced drop in glomerular filtration rate predicts long-term stability of renal function. Kidney Int 51:793–797, 1997.

107. Peters H, Border WA, Noble NA, Targeting TGF-β overexpression in renal disease: Maximizing the antifibrotic action of angiotensin II blockade. Kidney Int 54:1570–1580, 1998.

108. Heeg JE, de Jong PE, van der Hem GK, et al. Efficacy and variability of the antiproteinuric effect of ACE inhibition by lisinopril. Kidney Int 36:272–279, 1989.

109. Gansevoort RT, de Zeeuw D, de Jong PE. Additive antiproteinuric effect of ACE inhibition and a low protein diet in human renal disease. Nephrol Dial Transplant 10:497–504, 1995.

110. Rigat B, Hubert C, Alhenc-Gelas F, et al. An insertion/deletion polymorphism in the angiotensin I converting enzyme gene accounting for half the variance of serum enzyme levels. J Clin Invest 86:1343–1346, 1990.

111. Ueda S, Elliott HL, Morton JJ, et al. Enhanced pressor response to angiotensin I in normotensive men with the deletion genotype (DD) for angiotensin-converting enzyme. Hypertension 25:1266–1269, 1995.

112. Cambien F, Poirier O, Lecerf L, et al. Deletion polymorphism in the gene for angiotensin-converting enzyme is a potent risk factor for myocardial infarction. Nature 359:641–644, 1992.

113. van Essen GG, Rensma PL, de Zeeuw D, et al. Association between angiotensin converting enzyme gene polymorphism and failure of renoprotective therapy. Lancet 347:94–95, 1996.

114. Parving HH, Jacobsen P, Tarnow L, et al. Effect of deletion polymorphism of angiotensin-converting enzyme gene on progression of diabetic nephropathy during inhibition of angiotensin converting enzyme: Observational follow-up study. BMJ 313:591–594, 1996.

115. Remme WJ. Effect of ACE inhibition on neurohormones. Eur Heart J 19(suppl J):J16–J23, 1998.

116. Stafford RS, Saglam D, Blumenthal D. National patterns of angiotensin-converting enzyme inhibitor use in congestive heart failure. Arch Int Med 157:2460–2464, 1997.

117. Philbin EF, Andreou C, Rocco TA, et al. Patterns of angiotensin-converting enzyme inhibitor use in congestive heart failure in two community hospitals. Am J Cardiol 77:832–838, 1996.

118. Domanski MJ, Exner DV, Borkowf CB, et al. Effect of angiotensin converting enzyme inhibition on sudden cardiac death following acute myocardial infarction: A meta-analysis of randomized clinical trials. J Am Coll Cardiol 33:598–604, 1999.

119. Megarry M, Sapsford R, Hall AS, et al. Do ACE inhibitors provide protection for the heart in the clinical setting of acute myocardial infarction? Drugs 54(suppl 5):48–58, 1997.

120. The ATLAS Investigators. Comparative effects of low-dose versus high-dose lisinopril on survival and major cardiac events in chronic heart failure. [Abstract] Eur Heart J 19:142, 1998.

121. Textor SC. Renal failure related to angiotensin-converting enzyme inhibitors. Semin Nephrol 17:67–76, 1997.

122. Wynckel A, Ebikili B, Melin JP, et al. Long-term follow-up of acute renal failure caused by angiotensin converting enzyme inhibitors. Am J Hypertens 11:1080–1086, 1998.

123. Textor S, Bravo EL, Fouad FM, et al. Hyperkalemia in azotemic patients during angiotensin-converting enzyme inhibition and aldosterone reduction with captopril. Am J Med 73:719–725, 1982.

124. Weinberger MH. Influence of an angiotensin-converting enzyme inhibitor on diuretic-induced metabolic effects in hypertension. Hypertension 5(suppl III):132–138, 1983.

125. Israili ZH, Hall WD. Cough and angioneurotic edema associated with angiotensin-converting enzyme inhibitor therapy: A review of the literature and pathophysiology. Ann Intern Med 117:234–242, 1992.

126. Chan WK, Chan TYK, Luk WK. A high incidence of cough in Chinese subjects treated with angiotensin-converting enzyme inhibitors. Eur J Clin Pharmacol 44:299–300, 1993.

127. Chalmers D, Dombey SL, Lawson DH. Post-marketing surveillance of captopril (for hypertension): A preliminary report. Br J Clin Pharmacol 24:343–349, 1987.

128. Vleeming W, van Amsterdam JGC, Stricker BH, et al. ACE inhibitor–induced angioedema. Drug Saf 18:171–188, 1998.

129. Brown NJ, Snowden M, Griffin MR. Recurrent angiotensin-converting enzyme inhibitor-associated angioedema. JAMA 278:232–233, 1997.

130. Pryde PG, Sedman AB, Nugent CE, et al. Angiotensin-converting enzyme inhibitor fetopathy. J Am Soc Nephrol 3:1575–1582, 1993.

131. Burrows RF, Burrows EA. Assessing the teratogenic potential of angiotensin-converting enzyme inhibitors in pregnancy. Aust N Z J Obstet Gynaecol 38:306–311, 1998.

132. Mignat C, Unger T. ACE Inhibitors: Drug interactions of clinical significance. Drug Saf 12:334–347, 1995.

133. Ponce SP, Jennings AE, Madias NE, et al. Drug-induced hyperkalemia. Medicine 64:357–370, 1985.

134. Correa FJ, Eiser AR. Angiotensin-converting enzyme inhibitors and lithium toxicity. Am J Med 93:108–109, 1992.

135. Samanta A, Burden AC. Fever, myalgia, and arthralgia in a patient on captopril and allopurinol. Lancet 1:679, 1984.

70 Calcium Antagonists as Antihypertensives

P. A. van Zwieten

CHAPTER

HISTORICAL BACKGROUNDS

The now well-known calcium antagonist (CA) verapamil was originally but incorrectly believed to be a β-blocker because of its chemical structure (Fig. 70–1), which resembles that of the β-blocker class. In the 1960s, verapamil was recognized as an inhibitor of the transmembranous influx of calcium ions in myocardial and vascular smooth muscle cells.[1] Similar findings were described for drugs such as cinnarizine and lidoflazine.[2]

The concept of calcium antagonism was postulated independently and almost simultaneously by Godfraind[2, 3] and Fleckenstein[1] and their coworkers.

The term *calcium antagonists* for the drugs that cause vasodilatation by blockade of calcium entry in depolarized arteries was firmly established by Godfraind and Kaba in 1969[2] and has been used ever since. The term *calcium antagonist* has been defined as official nomenclature by the International Union of Pharmacology. Other terms sometimes encountered in the literature are calcium entry blockers, calcium slow channel blockers, and calcium blockers. The term *calcium antagonists* should be adhered to as the official nomenclature.

CAs, selective inhibitors of calcium influx in depolarized smooth muscle, have been recognized as useful agents in the treatment of hypertension and angina pectoris.

Verapamil may also be used as an antiarrhythmic agent or in the treatment of obstructive cardiomyopathy.

The present chapter emphasizes the use of CAs as antihypertensives.

CELLULAR ACTION

Transmembrane ion movements occur via selective ion channels. Ion channels that are selective for calcium, potassium, and sodium ions have been identified and characterized.[4–6]

Calcium channels may be identified by electrophysiological techniques. Over the years, different types of calcium channels have been identified and named *L-, T-,* and *N-channels.*[7] The differentiation of these channels is based on their sensitivity to membrane potential variation and to the time required to reach inactivation.

The L-type channels are the best-characterized and most important members of the class. L-type channels occur in myocardial cells, nodal tissues, and vascular smooth muscle. Their amino acid sequence has been clarified by means of cloning techniques;[8] their binding sites for calcium ions have been identified as well.[9] L-channels are activated by depolarization, thus facilitating the influx of extracellular

Figure 70–1. Chemical structures of the major subgroups of calcium antagonists (CAs): phenylalkylamines (verapamil and related drugs); benzothiazepines (diltiazem and related drugs); dihydropyridines (nifedipine and related drugs).

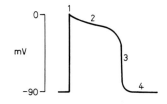

Figure 70–2. Effect of CAs on a cardiac cell, with a typical cardiac action potential *(top)*. The calcium (slow) inward current flows during the characteristic plateau phase (phase 2) of the action potential. This calcium influx is selectively inhibited by CA. Activation of the sarcoplasmic reticulum (SR) and other cellular calcium pools occur via Ca^{2+} and Na^+ that flow into the cell. The SR and other pools donate activator Ca^{2+} that stimulates the contractile proteins. The presence of tubular systems (invaginations), characteristic of cardiac tissues, causes considerable enlargement of the cellular surface, thus allowing an effective influx of Na^+ and Ca^{2+}. Inhibition of the calcium inward flux by a CA causes diminished activation of the contractile proteins.

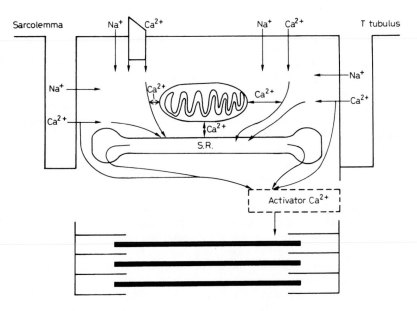

calcium ions into the cell. This influx causes, partly via the stimulated release of calcium ions from intracellular sources (e.g., sarcoplasmic reticulum, mitochondria), activation of contractile proteins, such as actin, myosin, and troponin.[8, 9] Conversely, blockade of the L-type channels by CAs causes vascular relaxation and a decrease in myocardial contractile activity (Fig. 70–2). Certain CAs, such as verapamil, mibefradil, and diltiazem, depress the activity of the nodal tissues, thus causing impaired atrioventricular (AV) conduction and reduced heart rate.

T-channels have been identified in nodal cardiac tissues.[10] Their electrophysiological characteristics are different from those of the L-channels: They require a different voltage to be opened, their time of opening is shorter than that of the L-channels, and their capacitance is lower, which means that they can transport fewer calcium ions per unit of time than the L-channels. T-channels have been proposed as the target of the newer CA mibefradil, which also has affinity for the L-channel.[11, 12] It seems likely, however, that most of the beneficial vasodilator effects of mibefradil can be explained by L-channel blockade.[13] The negative chronotropic activity of mibefradil is mediated in part by T-channel blockade.[12]

Mechanisms other than L-channel blockade may contribute to the vasodilator effect of the CAs. Stimulation of both α-adrenoceptors and angiotensin II receptors by their endogenous agonists (catecholamines and angiotensin II, respectively) causes the influx of calcium ions into vascular smooth muscle cells. Conversely, blockade of L-type calcium channels reduces this effect. This subtle interaction between CAs, α-adrenoceptors, and angiotensin II receptors is assumed to play a part in the vasodilator action of the CAs,[14–17] in particular when the sympathetic nervous system and/or the renin-angiotensin-aldosterone system is activated.

CLASSIFICATION OF CALCIUM ANTAGONISTS

Blockade of the voltage-operated, L-type calcium channel is the common mechanism shared by all subtypes of CAs. Classification of the various subtypes of CAs is based on their chemical structures (see Fig. 70–1). The three major subtypes of CAs are verapamil, gallopamil, and mibefradil (phenylalkylamines and derivatives); nifedipine and related drugs (dihydropyridine-CAs); and diltiazem and related drugs (benzothiazepines). The dihydropyridine-CA group has been expanded recently by the development of several new agents.

HEMODYNAMIC ACTIONS

Blood Pressure Lowering

Vasodilatation is a major property of the CAs, underlying most of their therapeutic actions. Vasodilatation occurs predominantly at the level of the resistance vessels (precapillary arterioles), thus causing a reduction in elevated peripheral resistance in hypertensive subjects.[18] In therapeutic doses, the CAs have no primary venodilator effect, thus

explaining the absence of orthostatic hypotension during treatment with these agents.[18–21] The fall in blood pressure and vascular resistance triggers a sinoaortic baroreflex-mediated rise in sympathetic activity, as reflected by the transient tachycardia associated with nifedipine and other dihydropyridine-CAs.[18, 21] The direct cardiac actions of verapamil and diltiazem, in addition to their interference with the baroreflex mechanism, prevent a rise in heart rate and cardiac output. As a result of a long-term adaptation process, heart rate and cardiac output return to values close to (dihydropyridines) or slightly below (verapamil, diltiazem) control levels (Fig. 70–3).[18, 21]

Vasodilatation is especially prominent in the skeletal muscle and coronary vascular beds.[18, 21] The gastrointestinal, cerebral, and renal vascular beds are also dilated, whereas the skin is only slightly affected, although facial flushes may occur as an adverse reaction to dihydropyridine-CAs. Vasodilatation in the coronary system, in particular the relaxation of coronary spasm, is a major component of the antiischemic activity of CAs in coronary heart disease. A mild natriuretic effect, probably at the renal tubular level, may explain why the CAs, although potent vasodilators, do not cause fluid retention.

Peripheral (ankle) edema, a well-known adverse effect of the dihydropyridine-CAs, does not reflect systemic fluid

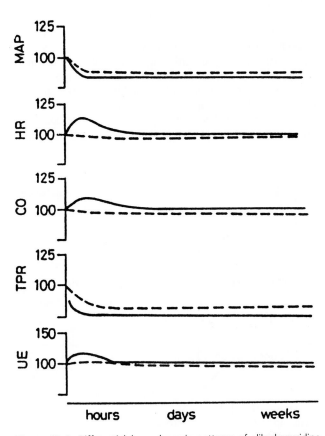

Figure 70–3. Differential hemodynamic patterns of dihydropyridine CA (nifedipine) and verapamil (or diltiazem). *Solid lines,* dihydropyridines; *dotted lines,* verapamil or diltiazem. Reflex tachycardia is evoked by the dihydropyridine CA and also a rise in sodium excretion. MAP, mean arterial pressure; HR, heart rate; CO, cardiac output; TPR, total peripheral resistance; UE, urinary excretion.

retention, but rather a direct effect on the microcirculation, and possibly also on the lymphatic circulation.[20]

From a hemodynamic point of view, established hypertension is characterized by a rise in peripheral vascular resistance and slowly decreasing cardiac output over the course of several years.[21] Since elevated peripheral resistance is the most consistent hemodynamic change in hypertensive disease, vasodilatation at the level of the arterioles (resistance vessels) appears to be a logical approach in treatment. All three classes of CAs are vasodilators that cause a reduction in peripheral resistance and a concomitant fall in blood pressure in hypertensives.[18, 19, 22] For instance, diltiazem treatment in hypertensives largely maintains the diurnal variations in pressure, although at a lower level than in normotensive subjects.[23] The antihypertensive activity of the various types of CAs is similar at appropriate doses, but different types have different effects on heart rate, as mentioned previously. With long-term use, CAs may induce a regression of myocardial and vascular hypertrophy.[24]

Antianginal Activity

The imbalance between myocardial oxygen supply and demand, which underlies myocardial ischemia and its sequelae in angina pectoris, may be improved by CAs via a reduction in peripheral vascular resistance and, in consequence, a reduction in cardiac afterload and left ventricular wall tension. These mechanisms will reduce myocardial oxygen consumption.[25–27] A further action of CAs is coronary vasodilatation, in particular the relaxation of coronary spasm, which improves the myocardial oxygen supply. These two mechanisms are brought about by all classes of CAs (dihydropyridines, verapamil, and diltiazem; Fig. 70–4).

A reduction in heart rate, as induced by verapamil or diltiazem, further contributes to the antianginal activity of

these two classes of compounds by reducing the oxygen consumption of the myocardium (see Figs. 70–3 and 70–4). The dihydropyridines, as mentioned, either cause reflex tachycardia (nifedipine in the nonretarded formulation) or leave the heart rate unchanged. At the cellular level, most CAs are believed to preserve adenosine triphosphate levels in the ischemic heart, as demonstrated in animal and biochemical experiments. However, there is no evidence that this cellular antiischemic mechanism is of clinical importance in the treatment of angina.[28]

Secondary Prevention After Acute Coronary Syndromes (Myocardial Infarction, Unstable Angina)

Verapamil is the only CA for which a clear protective effect has been shown in patients who have suffered an acute coronary syndrome. Increased survival and a lower reinfarction rate were found in the Second Danish Verapamil Infarction Trial (DAVIT II) in patients treated for 12 to 18 months after a myocardial infarction (verapamil vs. placebo).[29, 30] In a smaller study with diltiazem, the Diltiazem Multicenter Postinfarction Research Trial, a favorable trend was seen following a myocardial infarction in patients without pulmonary congestion after long-term treatment with diltiazem (compared with placebo).[31] Nifedipine has no protective effect in patients who have survived an acute coronary syndrome. In patients who had experienced unstable angina, the incidence of subsequent myocardial infarction has been shown to be higher in those treated with nifedipine compared with placebo. This negative effect of nifedipine was suppressed by simultaneous treatment with a β-blocker (Holland Interuniversity Nifedipine Trial [HINT]).[32] The mechanism of the cardioprotective effect of verapamil in the DAVIT II study has not been determined. It seems likely, however, that the reduction in heart rate may have been an important factor. Conversely, the reflex tachycardia provoked by nifedipine may explain the unfavorable effect of this CA in the HINT study.[32] The favorable effect of adding a β-blocker in this study was associated with the suppression of the nifedipine-induced reflex tachycardia.

Antiarrhytmic Activity

Verapamil and diltiazem may be used in the treatment of supraventricular tachyarrhythmias. This antiarrhythmic activity is related to impairment of electrical activity in the cardiac nodal tissues, causing delayed AV conduction and a reduction in heart rate. The dihydropyridine-CAs (nifedipine and related drugs) display no useful antiarrhythmic activity.

In clinical practice, verapamil may be used both intravenously and via the oral route. Atrial fibrillation is a major indication, including the atrial fibrillation frequently observed postoperatively after surgical valve reconstruction or coronary bypass surgery.

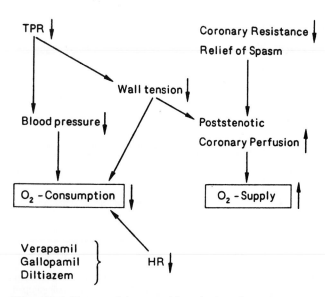

Figure 70–4. Diagram of the potential mechanism of CAs shows their beneficial effects in angina pectoris. The final result is an improvement in the imbalance between myocardial oxygen demand and supply. TPR, total peripheral resistance; HR, heart rate.

ADVERSE EFFECTS

The short-term adverse effects of the CAs differ with respect to the subtype (chemical class) of CA involved. The most important adverse effects are[33, 34]

Verapamil and related drugs: constipation; impaired AV conduction; vasodilatation, flushing, headache; reduced cardiac contractile force (not to be used in patients with heart failure).

Mibefradil does not cause constipation and displays no negative inotropic activity; the adverse reactions to *diltiazem* are very similar to those of verapamil, but constipation and impaired AV conduction occur less frequently than with verapamil.

Nifedipine and related dihydropyridines frequently cause ankle edema, probably reflecting a direct action on the local microcirculation, and possibly also the lymphatic circulation.

Headache and flushing are caused by vasodilatation.

Reflex tachycardia, induced by vasodilatation, may be felt by the patient as palpitations.

The adverse effect profile of the newer CAs is more favorable than that of nonretarded nifedipine, which is rapid and short-acting.

LONG-TERM SAFETY

The safety of long-term treatment with CAs has been challenged by three studies, 2 case-control studies in hypertensives,[35, 36] and a meta-analysis of 16 studies in which nifedipine was used as secondary prevention in patients with acute coronary syndromes.[37] From these studies, it was concluded that long-term treatment with CAs may be associated with a higher risk of cardiovascular morbidity and mortality. It has also been suggested that long-term use of CAs may elevate the risk of cancer in elderly populations[38] and that CAs enhance the risk of bleeding in the digestive tract[39] or during surgical interventions.[40]

Most of these studies have been subject to emotional and biased, premature publication in the media before they were published in appropriate scientific journals.

In the case-control studies in hypertension, CAs appeared to cause a modest increase in the risk of myocardial infarction, whereas the meta-analysis appeared to show that nifedipine was associated with increased mortality in patients with symptomatic coronary heart disease. However, all three studies have severe methodological flaws, and their interpretation has been strongly criticized[41–43] with respect to the following issues: erroneous calculations, conclusions drawn too "heavy" on the basis of too-meager statistics, confounding by indication. Further, the relevance of case-control studies is limited, especially if the difference between cases and controls is as modest (increase in risk of 60%) as in the aforementioned studies. As a rule, the relevance of case-control studies is considered valid if the difference between cases and controls is at least 300%, as in the large retrospective studies of the association between smoking cigarettes and lung cancer in the 1960s.

There is considerable uncertainty about the negative conclusions drawn from these studies, as reflected by the recent U.S. Food and Drug Administration (FDA) decision not to change the general policy toward the use of CAs as antihypertensive agents. Conversely, more and more data are beginning to emerge that challenge the validity and relevance of the aforementioned studies on CAs. In a case-control study by Aursnes and colleagues,[44] CAs did not increase the risk of cardiovascular morbidity or mortality and even proved protective. In a cohort study by Braun and associates[45] in 15,502 patients with coronary heart disease, the risk ratio of death was not influenced by CAs. In a case-control study by Alderman and coworkers,[46] hypertensive patients with a history of at least one major cardiovascular event were compared with correctly matched controls. Rapidly acting, nonretarded nifedipine increased the risk of death (RR = 3.88) when compared with a β-blocker. However, the more recently introduced slow-onset and long-acting CAs significantly reduced the risk of death (RR = 0.76) when compared with a β-blocker. In both the Shanghai Trial of Nifedipine in the Elderly (STONE) and the Systolic Hypertension in Europe (SYST-EUR) studies,[47, 48] total mortality was unchanged by CA treatment, whereas protection against cerebrovascular and cardiovascular events was evident, and there was no increased risk of cancer or gastrointestinal bleeding. A recent communication by Lever[49] reported that in the well-known West of Scotland Coronary Prevention (WOSCOP) trial,[50] survival, cardiovascular morbidity/mortality, and incidence of cancer were uninfluenced by the long-term use of CAs.

In conclusion, the challenge of the long-term safety of CAs that has been published in the literature is controversial and not convincing. The major, randomized ongoing studies (Swedish Trial in Old Patients with Hypertension [STOP-2], European Lacidipine Study on Atherosclerosis [ELSA], Verapamil Hypertension Atherosclerosis Study [VHAS], Nordic Diltiazem Study [NORDIL], Hypertension Optimal Treatment [HOT], and others) offer a decisive answer concerning the long-term safety of CAs. The data currently available do not condemn all CAs. However, considerable doubt has been cast on the safety of the rapidly and short-acting dihydropyridines, such as nonretarded nifedipine. This limitation seems particularly relevant in patients with ischemic heart disease, in whom reflex tachycardia is undesirable and possibly dangerous. It seems wise to replace this agent by the newer slow-onset and long-acting CAs. The efficacy and safety of these newer CAs are being tested in the aforementioned ongoing trials.

DRUG COMBINATIONS AND INTERACTIONS

CAs can be combined with several types of antihypertensives, with a synergistic antihypertensive effect in most cases, which for certain combinations will provoke hypotension.[51] The following combinations can be considered:

Verapamil or diltiazem + β-blocker: Effective antihypertensive combination, but an additive impairment of AV conduction and the risk of AV block.

Verapamil + angiotensin-converting enzyme inhibitor: Effective combination, registered as a combined preparation in several European countries.

Dihydropyridine-CAs (e.g., nifedipine) + β-blocker: Effective and logical combination. The reflex tachycardia caused by the dihydropyridine-CA is counteracted by the β-blocker. Conversely, the dihydropyridine-CA suppresses the cold hands and feet, a well-known side effect of β-blockers. Hypotension may occur.

Dihydropyridine-CAs + α₁-adrenoceptor blocker: This is a very effective antihypertensive combination, which may, however, cause hypotension. Other combinations between CAs and other antihypertensives may be useful as well.

Drug Interactions[51, 52]

Verapamil or diltiazem + β-blocker: Additive depression of AV conduction, bradycardia. This may be a particular problem if a patient treated with a β-blocker (long-term, orally) receives an intravenous injection of verapamil.

Verapamil + digoxin: Verapamil impairs the renal excretion of digoxin and hence raises the plasma level of the cardiac glycoside, thus increasing its toxicity.

Plasma levels and the risk of neurotoxicity of carbamazepine are enhanced by verapamil and diltiazem.

Plasma levels of cyclosporine are increased by verapamil, diltiazem, and nicardipine.

ANTIHYPERTENSIVE EFFICACY OF CALCIUM ANTAGONISTS

Nifedipine (Adalat) was introduced as an antihypertensive agent in the 1970s. Somewhat later, the antihypertensive efficacy of verapamil and diltiazem were recognized. Since then numerous newer CAs have been introduced as antihypertensives. The effective reduction of elevated blood pressure by CAs has been described in numerous communications and review papers (see, e.g., refs. 53 to 56). There is no specific category of hypertensive patients that should preferably be treated with CAs, or in which CAs should be avoided. An earlier hypothesis that CAs should preferably be used in elderly hypertensive patients[56] has been dismissed. Accordingly, CAs are effective antihypertensives in the following groups of patients:

Patients with essential hypertension[53–55]
Patients with renovascular hypertension[57]
Black patients with hypertension[58]
Patients with both hypertension and diabetes mellitus (since the CAs do not influence glucose tolerance or plasma lipids)[59]

CsA should be avoided in pregnant women with hypertension. Teratogenic effects of CAs in humans have not been clearly described, but animal experiments have demonstrated noxious effects of CAs on the fetus.[60]

CAs are clearly effective in lowering elevated blood pressure. Furthermore, large-scale outcome studies concerning protection by CAs against the complications of hypertension (stroke, myocardial infarction, heart failure, renal disease) are beginning to emerge.

Outcome Studies

The Treatment of Mild Hypertension Study (TOMHS) evaluated five classes of antihypertensive monotherapy and placebo, in comparison with lifestyle intervention in 902 mild hypertensives followed for 4 years.[61] Left ventricular mass was monitored in 844 of the 902 patients. The following drugs were used: chlorthalidone (diuretic); acebutolol (β-blocker); doxazosin (α₁-adrenoceptor antagonist); amlodipine (CA); and enalapril (angiotensin-converting enzyme [ACE] inhibitor). The five drugs were compared with nonpharmacological treatment, consisting of nutritional-hygienic intervention plus placebo. The drugs used (including the CA amlodipine) were virtually equieffective in lowering blood pressure and were more effective in lowering blood pressure than the nonpharmacological treatment.

STONE[47] was a single-blind study on the use of nonretarded nifedipine versus placebo in elderly Chinese hypertensives. In the active treatment arm of this study, nifedipine significantly reduced the overall risk of cardiovascular events (including stroke) by almost 60%. The rarity of myocardial infarction in the Chinese patient population may be considered as a weak point of the STONE study from a Western point of view. However, it is one of the very few studies in which the beneficial effect of a CA against placebo has been clearly demonstrated.

The SYST-EUR study was performed in 4695 patients age 60 years and older with isolated systolic hypertension.[48] The dihydropyridine-CA nitrendipine was compared with placebo. If necessary, enalapril or hydrochlorothiazide was added. The study was stopped prematurely after 2 years of follow-up because the active treatment with nitrendipine proved clearly beneficial when compared with placebo. In particular, the incidence of stroke was significantly and substantially reduced (−42%) by the treatment with nitrendipine.

Important ongoing studies of CAs in hypertensives include:

STOP-2[62]	Diuretics, β-blockers compared with ACE inhibitors and CAs in elderly hypertensives.
ELSA[63]	Lacidipine (a lipophilic CA) compared with atenolol on carotid wall thickness and atherosclerosis in elderly hypertensives.
VHAS[64]	Verapamil compared with (slow release) chlorthalidone on carotid wall thickness and atherosclerosis in hypertensives.
NORDIL[65]	Diltiazem compared with a β-blocker and/or a diuretic in hypertensives aged 50 to 60 years.
HOT[66]	Felodipine used in hypertensives aged 55 to 80 years; if necessary an ACE inhibitor or a β-blocker is added.

ALLHAT*[67]   Amlodipine used in hypertensives; blood pressure and lipid profile.

Most of these studies will be completed in by 2001, and their results are anxiously awaited.

CALCIUM ANTAGONISTS AND LEFT VENTRICULAR HYPERTROPHY

Left ventricular hypertrophy (LVH) is considered an important, virtually independent risk factor in hypertensives, as recognized in the Framingham Study.[68] It is, therefore, an important issue whether treatment with antihypertensive drugs will cause regression of LVH. Numerous animal experiments have indicated that CAs may cause regression of the LVH associated with hypertension. Most clinical investigations of this question have also shown that various types of CAs cause regression of LVH.[24, 61, 69–72] Attempts have been made to compare the efficacy of different types of antihypertensives in this respect.[73] ACE inhibitors and CAs appear to be the most efficacious antihypertensive drugs with respect to the regression of LVH in hypertensives, probably more effective than β-blockers or diuretics.[73] Existing studies do not allow a definite conclusion with respect to the differential efficacies of various types of drugs on LVH, mainly because of methodological difficulties in the quantitative determination of LVH in patients.[73] Trials designed to make quantitative comparisons between various drugs are in progress. Taken together, there are sound reasons to assume that long-term antihypertensive treatment with CAs will cause significant and relevant reduction of LVH. (For a review on this issue, see refs. 24 and 73.)

CALCIUM ANTAGONISTS AND ATHEROSCLEROSIS

In vitro and animal studies have strongly suggested that CAs impair lipid accumulation in the aorta. CAs inhibit a variety of processes that underlie atherosclerotic plaque formation, such as cholesterol deposition, cellular proliferation and migration, extracellular matrix formation, calcium overload, and platelet aggregation.[74] The antiatherogenic activity of CAs is not mediated by a reduction in plasma lipid levels, which are not influenced by CAs in therapeutic concentrations. Lipophilic CAs, such as lacidipine and lercanidipine, appear to be the more active antiatherogenic agents, at least in animal and biochemical experiments. It has been difficult to demonstrate an antiatherogenic effect of CAs in humans. Nifedipine was shown to impair the formation of new coronary artery lesions in patients with ischemic heart disease.[75] Large, established lesions, however, were not affected by nifedipine treatment, and nifedipine did not protect against acute coronary syndromes in these patients.[75] Comparable findings were obtained for nicardipine in the Montréal Heart Study.[76] In the Multicenter Isradipine Diuretic Atherosclerosis Study (MIDAS),

isradipine and hydrochlorothiazide were compared in mild to moderate hypertensives. Atherosclerotic plaque formation in the carotid artery was monitored by means of an ECHO-Doppler procedure. Data were inconclusive because of methodological difficulties.[77] In the ongoing ELSA study, 2300 hypertensive patients were randomized to lacidipine or atenolol, and the effects of the drugs on blood pressure and carotid artery plaque formation are being monitored.[63] In the similarly designed VHAS study, verapamil and captopril are being compared.[64]

In conclusion, the potential antiatherogenic activity of CAs is a most important issue. It remains to be demonstrated whether CAs protect against atherosclerosis in hypertensive patients who are being treated with these drugs.

CALCIUM ANTAGONISTS AND PERIOPERATIVE HYPERTENSION

Perioperative hypertension, predominantly caused by sympathetic stimulation, occurs frequently during and after thoracic surgery. This acute form of hypertension can usually be suppressed by using short-acting, intravenously administered antihypertensive drugs. Nitroglycerin, sodium nitroprusside, clonidine, urapidil, ketanserin, and short-acting β-blockers or CAs may be used for this purpose.[78] A theoretical argument in favor of using CAs in this condition is the antiischemic activity of this class of drugs, which may be helpful in patients with coronary artery disease undergoing surgery.[79] This antiischemic activity does not occur with other vasodilators, such as sodium nitroprusside, which may cause additional problems as a result of coronary "steal." However, the antiischemic activity of CAs, particularly when given intravenously, has been challenged by reports of a substantial risk of proischemic effects with the dihydropyridine class.[80]

Only the dihydropyridines, which are predominantly vasodilator agents with little or no cardiodepressant activity, have been studied in detail in surgical patients in an effort to counteract or prevent perioperative hypertension. Most of the studies have been limited to nifedipine and nicardipine; a few smaller studies have been performed with isradipine and diltiazem. Nifedipine and nicardipine are considered to be useful in the treatment of perioperative hypertension.[78, 81, 82]

NEW CALCIUM ANTAGONISTS

Several new CAs have been introduced as potential therapeutic agents in cardiovascular medicine. The majority of these compounds are dihydropyridines (Fig. 70–5), although an interesting verapamil derivative (mibefradil; Fig. 70–6) has been developed as well. Nifedipine, the prototype of the dihydropyridine-CAs, has been used on a very large scale for many years but is known to have a number of deficiencies, including negative inotropic activity and a short duration of action, thus requiring at least three daily doses in long-term treatment for hypertension or angina pectoris. In particular, the rapid development of its blood pressure–lowering effects, reflecting its kinetic characteris-

---

*ALLHAT, Antihypertensive and Lipid-Lowering to Prevent Heart Attack Trial.

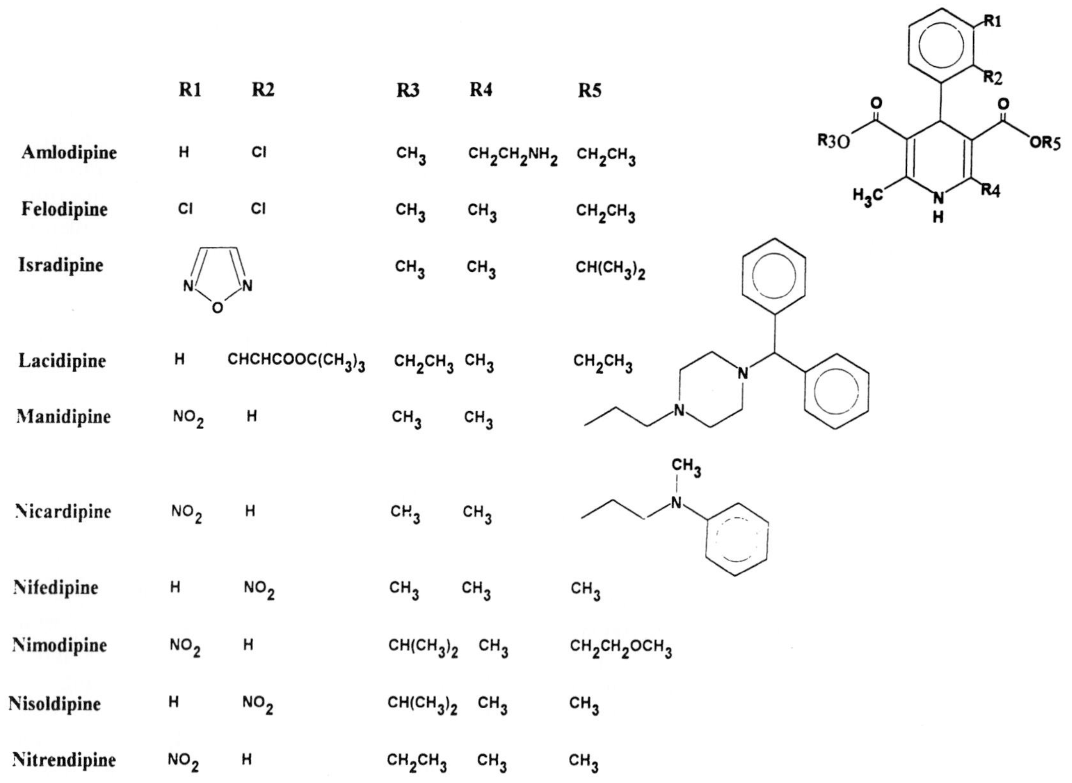

	R1	R2	R3	R4	R5
Amlodipine	H	Cl	CH_3	$CH_2CH_2NH_2$	CH_2CH_3
Felodipine	Cl	Cl	CH_3	CH_3	CH_2CH_3
Isradipine	(oxadiazole ring)		CH_3	CH_3	$CH(CH_3)_2$
Lacidipine	H	$CHCHCOOC(CH_3)_3$	CH_2CH_3	CH_3	CH_2CH_3
Manidipine	NO_2	H	CH_3	CH_3	
Nicardipine	NO_2	H	CH_3	CH_3	
Nifedipine	H	NO_2	CH_3	CH_3	CH_3
Nimodipine	NO_2	H	$CH(CH_3)_2$	CH_3	$CH_2CH_2OCH_3$
Nisoldipine	H	NO_2	$CH(CH_3)_2$	CH_3	CH_3
Nitrendipine	NO_2	H	CH_2CH_3	CH_3	CH_3

Figure 70–5. Chemical structures of dihydropyridine CAs, including several newer compounds.

tics, appears to trigger reflex tachycardia, which is potentially harmful as a proischemic process.

These disadvantages of nifedipine stimulated the development of dihydropyridine-CAs with less negative inotropic activity and a more favorable pharmacokinetic profile. These newer compounds are more vasoselective than nifedipine and have less depressant action on cardiac contractile force, combined with antihypertensive efficacy that is equal or superior to that of nifedipine. Attempts to develop CAs with selectivity for a particular vascular bed are currently under way. Further, newer CA preparations have been developed for several dihydropyridines and for verapamil, diltiazem, and mibefradil. These pharmacokinetic improvements are based on two principles: (1) the development of slow-release (retarded) preparations of rapid- and short-acting CAs, and (2) the development of CA molecules that are intrinsically slow-onset and long-acting.

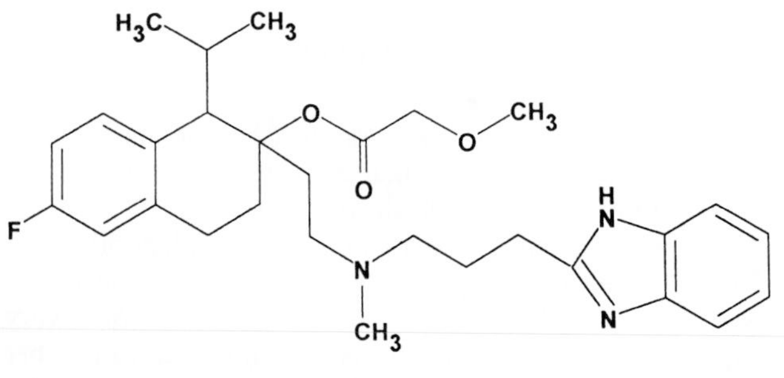

Pharmacokinetic Improvements

Slow-Release (Retarded) Preparations

Nifedipine was originally introduced as capsules, nonretarded, and characterized by a rapid onset and short action. Accordingly, this preparation had to be administered three to four times daily in order to obtain and maintain sufficient therapeutic activity over a period of 24 hours. Furthermore, substantial reflex tachycardia occurred, triggered by the rapid vasodilator effect of this preparation. This preparation, although still available, should not be used, not even in case of hypertensive emergency, since several alternative medications are available.

The nonretarded nifedipine capsules were replaced by a slow-release preparation that has to be administered twice-daily in order to obtain an acceptable control of blood pressure in hypertensives. Use of this preparation is associated with less intense reflex tachycardia compared with the nonretarded preparation. More recently, the nifedipine–gastrointestinal therapeutic system (GITS) was introduced.[83, 84] This preparation is based on the principle of an ALZET-minipump, which after oral ingestion, is compressed via an osmotic mechanism and hence slowly squeezes out the solution of nifedipine with zero-order kinetics into the intestinal lumen. Consequently, a constant, slow release of the active drug is achieved, thus leading to

Mibefradil (Ro 40-5967)

Figure 70–6. Chemical structure of mibefradil (Ro 40-5967), a benzimidazole derivative. This CA, a vasodilator, which also reduces heart rate, is virtually devoid of negative inotropic activity.

a slowly developing, long-lasting effect, high bioavailability, and stable blood levels, as well as a favorable trough:peak ratio.[83, 84] Felodipine, isradipine, nicardipine, verapamil, and diltiazem are also available as slow-release preparations, as well as the so-called coat core formulation of nisoldipine.[85] All of these preparations allow a once-daily administration with an acceptable or good trough:peak ratio, slow onset of action, and the virtual absence of reflex tachycardia or neuroendocrine activation.

Slow-Onset and Long-Acting Calcium Antagonists

A second way of improving the pharmacokinetic profile of CAs is to develop molecules that have an intrinsic slow onset and prolonged duration of action. Amlodipine, a dihydropyridine, was one of the first examples of such slow-onset and long-acting CAs. The kinetic characteristics of this molecule are explained by its strong affinity for the membranes of vascular smooth muscle.[86] Further, the molecule is stable, and hepatic degradation occurs but slowly.[86]

Lipophilic Calcium Antagonists

Several newer dihydropyridine-CAs are lipophilic. The lipid (fat) solubility of such compounds implies that they readily dissolve in lipid-rich depots, including those within the cell membrane (Fig. 70–7). From these depots, they are slowly released to reach their receptors, the L-type calcium channel. This phenomenon explains their slow onset of action and, therefore, the virtual absence of reflex tachycardia and sympathetic activation. The persistence of such

lipophilic CAs within cellular and other lipid depots also explains their long duration of action.[87, 88] The interaction between the lipophilic CAs and the cell membrane, as illustrated schematically in Figure 70–7, has been explored in detail for lacidipine and lercanidipine.[87–90] The slow onset of the effects of such drugs as well as their lack of reflex tachycardia in antihypertensive doses is illustrated in Figure 70–8. This figure demonstrates the antihypertensive action of lacidipine in patients over a period of 24 hours. The antihypertensive action after a single dose persists for 24 hours, and the circadian rhythm of blood pressure is maintained, although at a lower level. Interestingly, heart rate remains unchanged, in spite of the vasodilator/antihypertensive action of lacidipine, indicating that no reflex tachycardia is triggered. Similar findings have been obtained with lercanidipine, another lipophilic CA.[89, 90]

Vascular Selectivity

Amlodipine, barnidipine, felodipine, isradipine, lacidipine, manidipine, nicardipine, and nisoldipine are examples of dihydropyridine-CAs with vascular selectivity. The stronger effect of these agents on the vascular system than on the heart has been attributed to subtle differences between L-type calcium channels in the various tissues and organs. The vascular selectivity of nicardipine has been well demonstrated in a study in patients with coronary heart disease; when the drug was injected into a left main coronary artery, it did not depress cardiac contractile force, in spite of a clear dilator effect in the coronary system.[91] Based on in vitro experiments with isolated human and animal blood vessels, it has been suggested that nisoldipine

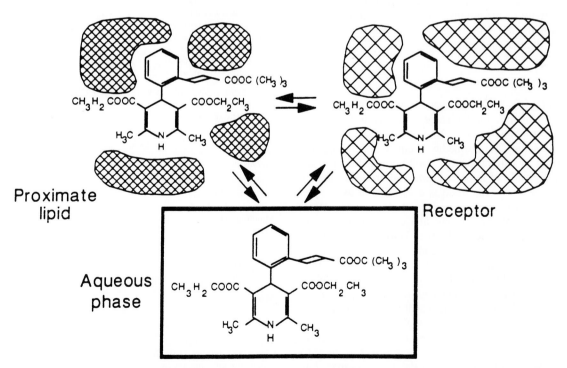

Figure 70–7. Diagrammatic representation of the three-compartment model of lacidipine, which may explain its slower onset and longer duration of action than that of most other calcium antagonists. (From Pfaffendorf M, Mathy MJ, van Zwieten PA. In vitro effects of nifedipine, nisoldipine, and lacidipine on rat isolated coronary small arteries. J Cardiovasc Pharmacol 21:496–502, 1993.)

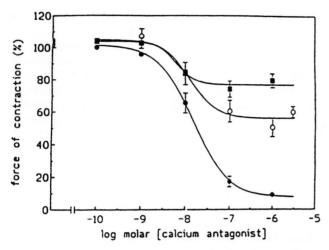

Figure 70–8. Concentration-response curves for the inhibitory effects of nifedipine *(open circles)*, nisoldipine *(solid squares)*, and manidipine *(solid circles)* on serotonin-induced contractions in isolated rat renal artery preparations. Note the strong antagonistic effect of manidipine. (From Pfaffendorf M, Mathy MJ, van Zwieten PA. In vitro effects of nifedipine, nisoldipine, and lacidipine on rat isolated coronary small arteries. J Cardiovasc Pharmacol 21:496–502, 1993.)

has the highest degree of vascular selectivity of all the dihydropyridine-CAs.[92] Claims that some CAs display moderate selectivity for a particular, specialized vascular bed have been made, generally based on rather meager evidence. The best evidence for such selectivity is available for manidipine, which shows the most potent dilator effects on renal vessels in intact animals and in vitro (see Fig. 70–8) and improves renal function in animal models of renal insufficiency.[93] Clinical data that support the claim of renal selectivity of manidipine are beginning to emerge.[94]

It goes without saying that a renal selective CA would be of great clinical and scientific interest.

Mibefradil

Mibefradil (Ro 40-5967) has been derived chemically from verapamil, although its molecule contains a few rather unusual substituents (see Fig. 70–6). Mibefradil appears to bind to the same [^{3}H]-desmethoxyverapamil-binding sites as verapamil in cardiac membrane homogenates. The hemodynamic profile of mibefradil may be briefly characterized as follows:[11, 12] Mibefradil is a vasodilator agent, predominantly at arteriolar sites (resistance vessels) with significant negative chronotropic and dromotropic activity. Importantly, cardiac contractile force is not reduced by this agent, as shown in isolated organs, animal models, and patients.[95] The vasodilator activity of mibefradil is fully explained by its blocking effect on L-type calcium channels.[13] Mibefradil has a stronger effect on T-type than on L-type calcium channels, and its negative chronotropic and dromotropic activities may be brought about, at least in part, by T-channel blockade in the sinus node and in the AV conduction system.[11, 12] Interestingly, it was recently demonstrated in isolated human atrial tissue preparations that mibefradil in therapeutically relevant preparations also blocks N-type calcium channels. Consequently, noradrenaline release from cardiac sympathetic nerves is suppressed

by mibefradil via N-channel blockade.[96] This property of mibefradil is unique among the CAs in clinical use, and it may contribute to the negative chronotropic activity of the drug in vivo.[96]

Mibefradil is an effective antihypertensive and antianginal agent, as confirmed in numerous clinical studies carried out in a large number of patients.[95, 97, 98] The antihypertensive action of mibefradil is largely explained by its vasodilator activity, based on L-type calcium channel blockade.[13] Its antianginal activity is largely explained by its negative chronotropic activity, together with its coronary and peripheral vasodilator actions. In patients with angina, mibefradil has a more beneficial influence on the double product (heart rate × pressure) than verapamil. Mibefradil has a kinetic profile that allows administration of a single daily dose for an adequate control of hypertension and angina. Its side effect profile appears to be favorable, although according to a recent FDA warning,[99] dangerous bradycardia may occur, in particular in patients who take another drug that could lower heart rate. In the same warning by the FDA,[99] it was stated that mibefradil may interfere with the biodegradation of certain statins, such as lovastatin and simvastatin, and possibly also atorvastatin and cerivastatin, thus resulting in an enhanced risk of rhabdomyolysis. For these reasons, mibefradil has been withdrawn.

Table 70–1 Survey of the Newer Calcium Antagonists*

SLOW-RELEASE PREPARATIONS OF CLASSIC AND NEWER CAs
Verapamil-SR (Isoptin)
Diltiazem-SR (Tildiem)
Nifedipine-SR (Adalat)
Nifedipine-GITS (Adalat-OROS)
Felodipine-SR (Plendil)
Isradipine-SR (Lomir)
Nicardipine-SR (Cardene)
Nisoldipine-CC (Sular)

NEWER DIHYDROPYRIDINES WITH A SLOW ONSET AND LONG DURATION OF ACTION
Amlodipine (Norvasc)
Lacidipine (Motens)
Lercanidipine (Lerdip)
Barnidipine
Manidipine

LIPOPHILIC CAs
Lacidipine (Motens)
Lercanidipine (Lerdip)
Mibefradil (Posicor)
Manidipine
Barnidipine

VASOSELECTIVE CAs
Lacidipine (Motens)
Lercanidipine (Lerdip)
Manidipine
Barnidipine
(Amlodipine [Norvasc] only partially)

MIBEFRADIL (POSICOR)
Vasodilator with negative chronotropic and dromotropic activity; no negative influence on cardiac contractile force

Abbreviations: CAs, calcium antagonists; SR, slow-release; GITS, gastrointestinal therapeutic system; OROS, oral osmotic; CC, Coat Core.
*Commercial names as in the Netherlands are used.

Overview

For an overview of the most relevant newer CAs, see Table 70–1.

References

1. Fleckenstein A, Fleckenstein-Grün G. Cardiovascular protection by Ca antagonists. Eur Heart J 1:15–21, 1980.
2. Godfraind T, Kaba A. Blockade or reversal of contraction induced by calcium and adrenaline in depolarized arterial smooth muscle. Br J Pharmacol 36:549–560, 1969.
3. Godfraind T, Miller RC, Wibo M. Calcium antagonism and calcium entry blockade. Pharmacol Rev 38:321–416, 1986.
4. Tsien RW, Tsien RY. Calcium channels, stores and oscillations. Annu Rev Cell Biol 6:715–760, 1990.
5. Hess P, Lansman JB, Tsien RW. Different modes of Ca-channel gating behaviour favoured by dihydropyridine Ca-agonists and -antagonists. Nature 311:538–544, 1984.
6. Hess P, Lansman JB, Tsien RW. Calcium channel selectivity for divalent and monovalent cations. J Gen Physiol 88:293–319, 1986.
7. Sher E, Biancardi E, Passafaro M, Clementi F. Physiopathology of neuronal voltage-operated calcium channels. FASEB J 5:2677–2683, 1991.
8. Catterall WA. Structure and function of voltage-gated ion channels. Trends Neurosci 16:500–506, 1993.
9. Godfraind T. Vasodilators and calcium antagonists. *In* van Zwieten PA, Greenlee WJ (eds). Antihypertensive Drugs. Amsterdam, Harwood Academic, 1997; pp 313–375.
10. Mishra SK, Hermsmeyer K. Selective inhibition of T-type Ca^{2+}-channels by Ro 40-5967. Circ Res 75:144–148, 1994.
11. Mehrke G, Zong XG, Flockerzi V, Hofmann F. The Ca^{++} channel blocker Ro 40-5967 blocks differently T-type and L-type Ca^{++} channels. J Pharmacol Exp Ther 271:1483–1488, 1994.
12. Lüscher TF, Clozel JP, Noll G. Pharmacology of the calcium antagonist mibefradil. J Hypertens 15(suppl 3):S11–S18, 1997.
13. Van der Lee R, Pfaffendorf M, van Zwieten PA. Effects of mibefradil and other calcium antagonists on microvessels of different end organs. 8th European Meeting on Hypertension, Milan, June 1997.
14. Van Meel JCA, de Jonge AJ, Kalkman HO, et al. Vascular smooth muscle contraction initiated by postsynaptic α_2-adrenoceptor activation is induced by an influx of extracellular calcium. Eur J Pharmacol 69:205–208, 1981.
15. Timmermans PBMWM, van Zwieten PA. α_2-Adrenoceptors. Classification, localisation, mechanisms and targets for drugs. J Med Chem 25:1389–1401, 1982.
16. Van Heiningen PNM, van Zwieten PA. Differential sensitivity to calcium entry blockade of angiotensin II–induced contractions of rat and guinea-pig aorta. Arch Int Pharmacodyn 296:118–130, 1988.
17. Van Zwieten PA, Timmermans PBMWM, van Heiningen PNM. Receptor subtypes involved in the action of calcium antagonists. J Hypertens 5(suppl 4):S21–S28, 1987.
18. Nayler WG. Calcium Antagonists. London, Academic, 1988, pp 1–347.
19. Opie LH. Clinical Use of Calcium Channel Antagonistic Drugs, 2nd ed. Boston, Kluwer Academic, 1990; pp 70–130.
20. Gray Ellrodt A, Singh BN. Clinical applications of slow channel blocking compounds. Clin Pharmacol Ther 23:1–43, 1983.
21. Struyker Boudier HAJ, de Mey JG, Smits JFM, Nievelstein HMNW. Hemodynamic actions of calcium entry blockers. *In* van Zwieten PA (ed). Clinical Aspects of Calcium Entry Blockers. Basel, S Karger, 1989; pp 21–66.
22. Muiesan G, Agabiti-Rosei E, Castellano M, et al. Antihypertensive and humoral effects of verapamil and nifedipine in essential hypertension. J Cardiovasc Pharmacol 4(suppl 3):S325–S329, 1982.
23. Kiowski W, Linder L, Bühler FR. Arterial vasodilator and antihypertensive effects of diltiazem. J Cardiovasc Pharmacol 16(suppl 6):S7–S10, 1990.
24. Agabiti-Rosei E, Muiesan ML, Rizzoni D, et al. Cardiovascular structural changes and calcium antagonist therapy in patients with hypertension. J Cardiovasc Pharmacol 24(suppl A):S37–S43, 1994.
25. Sever P. 1985, the year of the hypertension trials. Trends Pharmacol Sci 6:134–139, 1986.
26. Van Zwieten PA. Clinical aspects of calcium entry blockers. Progr Basic Clin Pharmacol 2:1–20, 1989.
27. Van Zwieten PA. Drug targets in unstable angina. *In* Hugenholtz PG (ed). Unstable Angina, Current Concepts and Management. Stuttgart, Schattauer, 1985; pp 151–157.
28. Nayler WG. Calcium antagonists and myocardial ischaemia. *In* Nayler WG (ed). Calcium Antagonists. New York, Academic, 1988; pp 157–176.
29. Danish Study Group on Verapamil in Myocardial Infarction. Effect of verapamil on mortality and major events after acute myocardial infarction (The Danish Verapamil Infarction Trial II—DAVIT II). Am J Cardiol 66:779–785, 1990.
30. Fischer Hansen J. Secondary prevention with calcium antagonists after acute myocardial infarction. Drugs 44:33–43, 1992.
31. Multicenter Diltiazem Postinfarction Trial Research Group. The effect of diltiazem on mortality and reinfarction after myocardial infarction. N Engl J Med 319:385–392, 1988.
32. Holland Interuniversity Nifedipine-Metoprolol Trial (HINT) Research Group. Early treatment of unstable angina in the coronary care unit: A randomised, double blind, placebo-controlled comparison of recurrent ischemia in patients treated with nifedipine or metoprolol or both. Br Heart J 56:400–413, 1986.
33. Van Zwieten PA, Lie KI. Long term efficacy and safety of calcium antagonists. Cardiologie 2:457–460, 1995.
34. Van Zwieten PA. Therapy update—What is new? Calcium antagonists. Neth J Cardiol 5:17–22, 1992.
35. Psaty BM, Heckbert SR, Koepsell TD, et al. The risk of myocardial infarction associated with antihypertensive drug therapies. JAMA 274:620–625, 1995.
36. Pahor M, Guralnik JM, Corti M, et al. Long-term survival and use of antihypertensive medications in older persons. J Am Geriatr Soc 43:1–7, 1995.
37. Furberg CD, Psaty BM, Meyer JV. Nifedipine. Dose-related increase in mortality in patients with coronary heart disease. Circulation 92:1326–1330, 1995.
38. Pahor M, Guralnik J, Salive M, et al. Do calcium channel blockers increase the risk of cancer? J Hypertens 9:695–699, 1996.
39. Pahor M, Guralnik J, Furberg C, et al. Risk of gastrointestinal haemorrhage with calcium antagonists in hypertensive persons over 67 years old. Lancet 347:1061–1065, 1996.
40. Wagenknecht L, Furberg C, Hammon J, et al. Surgical bleeding: Unexpected effect of a calcium antagonist. BMJ 310:776–777, 1995.
41. Tijssen JGP, Hugenholtz PG. Critical appraisal of recent studies on nifedipine and other calcium channel blockers in coronary heart disease and hypertension. Eur Heart J 17:1152–1157, 1996.
42. Mancia G, van Zwieten PA. How safe are calcium antagonists in hypertension and coronary heart disease? J Hypertens 14:13–17, 1996.
43. WHO-ISH Study. Ad hoc subcommittee of the Liaison Committee of the World Health Organization and the International Society of Hypertension. Effects of calcium antagonists on the risks of coronary heart disease, cancer and bleeding. J Hypertens 15:105–115, 1997.
44. Aursnes I, Litleskare I, Froyland H, Abdelnoor M. Association between various drugs used for hypertension and risk of acute myocardial infarction. Blood Press; 4:157–163, 1995.
45. Braun S, Boyko V, Behar S, et al. Calcium antagonists and mortality in patients with coronary artery disease: A cohort study of 11,575 patients. J Am Coll Cardiol 28:7–11, 1996.
46. Alderman MH, Cohen H, Roque R, Medhaven S. Effect of long-acting and short-acting calcium antagonists on cardiovascular outcomes in hypertensive patients. Lancet 349:594–598, 1997.
47. Gong L, Zhang W, Zhy Y, Zhu J. Shanghai Trial of Nifedipine in the Elderly (STONE). J Hypertens 14:1237–1245, 1996.
48. Staessen JA, Fagard R, Thijs L, et al. Randomised double-blind comparison of placebo and active treatment for older persons with isolated systolic hypertension. The Systolic Hypertension in Europe (SYST-EUR) Trial Investigators. Lancet 350:757–764, 1997.
49. Lever AF. Calcium antagonists and cancer. 8th European Meeting on Hypertension. Milan, June 1997.
50. Shepherd J, Cobbe SM, Ford I, et al. Prevention of coronary heart disease with pravastatin in men with hypercholesterolemia. West of Scotland Coronary Prevention Study Group. N Engl J Med 333:1301–1307, 1995.
51. Hansten PhD. Important drug interactions. *In* Katzung BG (ed). Basic and Clinical Pharmacology, 5th ed. Englewood Cliffs, NJ, Prentice-Hall, 1992; pp 931–942.
52. Stockley IH. Drug Interactions, 3rd ed. Oxford, Blackwell, 1994.

53. Müller FB, Ha HR, Hotz M, et al. Once a day verapamil in essential hypertension. Br J Clin Pharmacol 21(suppl 2):143S–147S, 1985.

54. Pedrinelli R, Fouad FM, Tarazi RC, et al. Nitrendipine, a calcium entry blocker: Renal and humoral effects in human arterial hypertension. Arch Intern Med 146:62–65, 1986.

55. Ribstein J, de Treglode D, Mimran A. Acute effects of nifedipine on arterial pressure in healthy subjects and hypertensives. Arch Mal Coeur 78:29–32, 1985.

56. Bühler FR. Antihypertensive care with calcium antagonists. *In* Laragh JH, Brenner BM (eds). Hypertension. Pathophysiology, Diagnosis and Management, 2nd ed. New York, Lippincott-Raven, 1995; pp 2801–2814.

57. Rodicio JL, Morales JM, Alcazar M, Ruilope LM. Calcium antagonists and renal protection. J Hypertens 11:S49–S53, 1993.

58. Dustan HP. Nitrendipine in black US patients. J Cardiovasc Pharmacol 9(suppl 4):267–271, 1987.

59. Henry PD. Calcium antagonists as anti-atherosclerotic agents. Arteriosclerosis 10:963–965, 1990.

60. Rubin P. Prescribing in Pregnancy, 2nd ed. London, BMJ Publishing Group, 1995; pp 99–102.

61. Liebson PR, Grandits GA, Dianzumba S, et al, for the Treatment of Hypertension Study Research Group. Comparison of five antihypertensive monotherapies and placebo for change in left ventricular mass in patients receiving nutritional-hygienic therapy in the Treatment of Mild Hypertension Study (TOMHS). Circulation 91:698–706, 1995.

62. Dahlöf B, Hansson L, Lindholm LH, et al. STOP-Hypertension-2: A prospective intervention trial of "newer" versus "older" treatment alternatives in old patients with hypertension. Blood Press 2:136–141, 1993.

63. Bond G, Dal Palu C, Hansson L, et al. European Lacidipine Study on Atherosclerosis (ELSA). J. Hypertens 11(suppl 5):S405, 1993.

64. Zanchetti A. Antiatherosclerotic effects of antihypertensive drugs: Recent evidence and ongoing trial. Clin Exp Hypertens 18:489–499, 1996.

65. NORDIL Study Group. The Nordic Diltiazem Study. A prospective intervention trial of calcium antagonist therapy in hypertension. Blood Press 2:312–321, 1993.

66. HOT Study Group. The Hypertension Optimal Treatment (HOT) Study. Blood Press 2:113–119, 1993.

67. Davis BR, Cutler JA, Gordon DJ, et al, for the ALLHAT-Research Group. Rationale and design for the Antihypertensive and Lipid Lowering Treatment to Prevent Heart Attack Trial (ALLHAT). Am J Hypertens 9:342–360, 1996.

68. Levy D, Garrison RJ, Savage DD, et al. Left ventricular mass and incidence of coronary heart disease in an elderly cohort: The Framingham Heart Study. Ann Intern Med 110:101–107, 1989.

69. Thürmann PA, Stephens N, Heagerty AM, et al. Influence of isradipine and spirapril on left ventricular hypertrophy and resistance arteries. Hypertension 28:450–456, 1996.

70. Schmieder RE, Messuli FH, Garavglio GE, Nunes BD. Cardiovascular effects of verapamil in essential hypertension. Circulation 76:1143–1155, 1987.

71. Malbantgil I, Önder R, Kill iccioglu B, et al. The efficacy of felodipine ER on regression of left ventricular hypertrophy in patients with primary hypertension. Blood Press 5:285–291, 1996.

72. Matsuzaki K, Mukai M, Sumimoto T, Murakami E. Effects of ACE-inhibitors versus calcium antagonists on left ventricular morphology and function in patients with essential hypertension. Hypertens Res 20:7–10, 1997.

73. Devereux RB. Do antihypertensive drugs differ in their ability to regress left ventricular hypertrophy? Circulation 95:1983–1985, 1997.

74. Catapano AL. Calcium antagonists and atherosclerosis. Experimental evidence. Eur Heart J 18(suppl A):A80–A86, 1997.

75. Lichtlen PR, Hugenholtz PG, Raffenbeul W, et al. Retardation of angiographic progression of coronary artery disease by nifedipine. Lancet 335:1109–1113, 1990.

76. Waters D, Lespérance J, Francetich M. A controlled clinical trial to assess the effect of a calcium channel blocker on the progression of coronary atherosclerosis. Circulation 82:1940–1953, 1990.

77. Borhani NO, Mercuri M, Borhani PA, et al. Final outcome results of the Multicenter Isradipine Diuretic Atherosclerosis Study (MIDAS). JAMA 276:785–791, 1996.

78. Van Zwieten PA, van Wezel HB. Antihypertensive drug treatment in the perioperative period. J Cardiothorac Vasc Anesth 7:213–226, 1993.

79. Underwood SM, Davies SW, Feneck RO, et al. Comparison of isradipine with nitroprusside for control of blood pressure following myocardial revascularization: Effects on hemodynamics, cardiac metabolism and coronary blood flow. J Cardiothorac Vasc Anesth 5:348–356, 1991.

80. Waters D. Proischemic complications of dihydropyridine calcium channel blockers. Circulation 84:2598–2600, 1991.

81. Kaplan JA. The role of nicardipine during anesthesia and surgery. Clin Ther 11:84–93, 1989.

82. Visser CA, Koolen JJ, van Wezel HB, et al. Effects of intracoronary nicardipine and nifedipine on left ventricular function and coronary sinus blood flow. Br J Clin Pharmacol 22(suppl 2):313S–318S, 1986.

83. Zanchetti A, on behalf of the Italian Nifedipine-GITS Study Group. The 24-hour efficacy of a new once-daily formulation of nifedipine. Drugs 49(suppl 1):23–31, 1994.

84. Brogden RN, McTavish D. Nifedipine gastrointestinal therapeutic system (GITS). Drugs 50:495–512, 1995.

85. Fodor JG. Nisoldipine CC: Efficacy and tolerability in hypertension and ischemic heart disease. Cardiovasc Drugs Ther 10:873–879, 1997.

86. Murdoch D, Heel RC. Amlodipine. Drugs 41:478–505, 1991.

87. Pfaffendorf M, Mathy MJ, van Zwieten PA. In vitro effects of nifedipine, nisoldipine, and lacidipine on rat isolated coronary small arteries. J Cardiovasc Pharmacol 21:496–502, 1993.

88. Leonetti G. Clinical position of lacidipine, a new dihydropyridine calcium antagonist, in the treatment of hypertension. J Cardiovasc Pharmacol 18(suppl 11):S18–S21, 1991.

89. Guarneri L, Sironi G, Angelico P, et al. In vitro and in vivo vascular selectivity of lercanidipine and its enantiomers. J Cardiovasc Pharmacol 29(suppl 1):S25–S32, 1997.

90. Cafiero M, Giasi M. Long-term (12-month) treatment with lercanidipine in patients with mild to moderate hypertension. J Cardiovasc Pharmacol 29(suppl 2):S45–S49, 1997.

91. Van Zwieten PA. The newer calcium antagonists. Cardiologie 5:4–13, 1998.

92. Plosker GL, Faulds D. Nisoldipine Coat-Core. A review of its pharmacology and therapeutic efficacy in hypertension. Drugs 52:232–253, 1996.

93. Van Zwieten PA, Pfaffendorf M. New aspects of the pharmacology of dihydropyridine calcium antagonists. JAMA SE Asia 15(suppl):9–19, 1994.

94. Rodicio JL. Renal effects of calcium antagonists with special reference to manidipine hydrochloride. Blood Press 5(suppl 5):10–15, 1996.

95. Portegies MCM, Schmitt R, Kraaij CJ, et al. Lack of negative inotropic effect of a new calcium antagonist Ro 40-5967 in patients with stable angina pectoris. J Cardiovasc Pharmacol 18:746–751, 1991.

96. Göthert M, Molderings GJ. Mibefradil and ω-conotoxin GVIA-induced inhibition of noradrenaline release from the sympathetic nerves of the human heart. Naunyn Schmiedebergs Arch Pharmacol 356:860–863, 1997.

97. Bernink PJLM, Prager G, Schelling A, Kobrin I, on behalf of the Mibefradil International Study Group. Antihypertensive properties of the novel calcium antagonist mibefradil (Ro 40-5967). Hypertension 27:426–432, 1996.

98. Muntinga HJ, van der Vring JAFM, Niemeijer MG, et al. Effect of mibefradil on left ventricular diastolic function in patients with congestive heart failure. J Cardiovasc Pharmacol 27:652–656, 1996.

99. FDA warns on calcium channel blockers. [Editorial] Lancet 351:44, 1998.

71 Angiotensin II Receptor Antagonists

Michael C. Ruddy and John B. Kostis

In the mid-1950s, Leonard Skeggs[1] and his group in Cleveland used hog renal renin and equine plasma renin substrate to show that there are two forms of the peptide product. The biologically inactive decapeptide angiotensin I was found to be quickly transformed in plasma by a chloride-dependent "converting enzyme" to the vasopressor octapeptide angiotensin II.[2] In rapid succession, the Cleveland group also determined the nature of the renin substrate molecule from which angiotensin is generated as well as the function of converting enzyme. They found three important biochemical properties of the converting enzyme: its anion dependence, its metalloprotein nature, and its ability to catalyze the hydrolytic cleavage of a dipeptide from the carboxyl terminus of its decapeptide substrate. By 1956, Skeggs and colleagues[3] had documented the precise amino acid sequences of angiotensin I and II.

Skeggs and his coworkers went on to suggest three possible avenues to therapeutically affect the renin-angiotensin system. The first possibility, that of direct inhibition of the action of renin on its substrate, remains to this day under study with several renin inhibitors currently undergoing investigation (see Chap. 74, Renin Inhibitors). A second proposal was to prevent the formation of the octapeptide hypertenin II (angiotensin II) from its decapeptide precursor by inhibition of the converting enzyme (see Chap. 9, Angiotensin-Converting Enzyme: Basic Properties, Distribution, and Functional Role). This strategy has since been extraordinarily successful through the development of orally active angiotensin-converting enzyme (ACE) inhibitors. (see Chap. 69, Angiotensin-Converting Enzyme Inhibitors).

A third technique suggested by Skeggs and associates in 1956[3] was to prevent the vasoconstrictive action of angiotensin II on smooth muscle, perhaps by analogues of angiotensin II. The present chapter outlines the products of this approach.

ANGIOTENSIN SYSTEM

Pathways for Angiotensin Generation

All of the known biological actions of the renin-angiotensin system are mediated by the angiotensin series of peptides. Of these, the octapeptide angiotensin II has the broadest range of activity and the greatest potency in circulatory regulation. Most angiotensin II is formed in two steps through the sequential catalytic action of renin and converting enzyme on the substrate angiotensinogen (Fig. 71–1). In addition, angiotensin II is formed in cardiac tissue through the action of other proteolytic enzymes such as chymase and cathepsin on the decapeptide angiotensin I.[4]

Actions of Angiotensin II

A primary function of the renin-angiotensin system is to maintain perfusion when the circulation is threatened by volume depletion or hypotensive stress.[5] In this respect, acute effects of angiotensin II production include vasoconstriction; increased aldosterone secretion with retention of salt, increased thirst, and release of antidiuretic hormone;[6] and amplification of sympathetic nervous system activity.[7]

Blood Vessels

Angiotensin II acts as a potent constrictor of precapillary arterioles and, to a lesser extent, postcapillary venules.[8] The direct action at the vascular smooth muscle site appears to account for most of the increase in peripheral resistance. The vasoconstrictor effect of angiotensin II is mediated primarily through direct binding to AT_1 receptors on vascular smooth muscle.[9] However, in certain vascular beds such as those perfusing skeletal muscle of the extremities of humans, α-adrenergic antagonists can appreciably attenuate the vasoconstrictor effect of infused angiotensin II.[10] This finding is consistent with an important role for sympathetic augmentation of the vascular action of angiotensin II. The vasoconstrictor effect of angiotensin II is greatest in the splanchnic, renal, and cutaneous vascular beds and is less in vessels of the brain, lung, heart (coronary), and skeletal muscle. In the latter regions, blood flow may actually

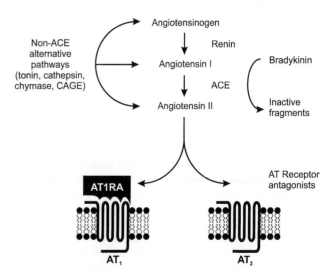

Figure 71–1. The renin-angiotensin system: areas of potential blockade. ACE, angiotensin-converting enzyme; CAGE, chymostatin-sensitive angiotensin II–generating enzyme; AT, angiotensin. (Reprinted by permission of Elsevier Science from Johnston CI, Risvanis J. Preclinical pharmacology of angiotensin II receptor antagonists: Update and outstanding issues. Am J Hypertens, vol 10, pp 306S–310S, copyright 1997 by American Journal of Hypertension Ltd.)

increase during low-dose infusions of angiotensin II owing to the stronger effect of elevated systemic blood pressure opposing the relatively weak vasoconstrictor response in these areas.[11]

Adrenal Cortex

Angiotensin II has an important role in the regulation of plasma volume through actions on the adrenal gland and kidney. Angiotensin II is the primary secretagogue for the synthesis and release of aldosterone by cells of the adrenal cortical zona glomerulosa. The cells of the zona glomerulosa have a high density of AT_1 receptors.[12] Aldosterone secretion can be elicited by concentrations of angiotensin II that are well below the threshold of a systemic pressor response.[12] Aldosterone acts on the distal tubule and collecting duct of the kidney to promote reabsorption of sodium in exchange for secretion of potassium and hydrogen ions. The effect of increasing aldosterone levels is preservation or expansion of total body sodium and plasma volume.

Kidney

The renal effects of angiotensin II have been observed in several distinct domains, including the microvasculature, the mesangium, and the tubular epithelium. Autoregulation of glomerular filtration rate (GFR) in response to variations in renal perfusion pressure is mediated predominantly, although not exclusively, through angiotensin II.[13] At the level of the pre- and postglomerular arterioles, angiotensin II acts as a vasoconstrictor. The glomerular efferent arterioles are highly sensitive to low concentrations of angiotensin II.[14] The afferent arterioles are less sensitive to the constrictor effects of angiotensin II, perhaps owing to differential production of vasodilator prostaglandins and nitric oxide.[15] Also, angiotensin II produces a direct contractile response in the glomerular mesangial cells, an effect that tends to decrease the effective surface area available for glomerular filtration.[16] Modest increases of tissue or circulating angiotensin II levels increase glomerular hydrostatic pressure and GFR by the dual effects of raised systemic perfusion pressure and heightened resistance of postglomerular outflow. At higher levels of angiotensin II, the less sensitive preglomerular afferent arterioles constrict, impeding glomerular perfusion. Reduced glomerular perfusion, combined with the direct contractile action of angiotensin II on the glomerular mesangium, may result in a significant impairment of renal blood flow and GFR.

The proximal tubular epithelial cells have a high density of AT_1 receptors on both the basolateral and the luminal membranes.[17] The density of receptors decreases from the most proximal to distal portions of the proximal tubule.[18] The effect of low to moderate concentrations of angiotensin II on the proximal tubule is to promote reabsorption of filtered sodium.[19] This is mediated through stimulation of the epithelial sodium-proton pump.[20] In contrast, high concentrations of angiotensin II inhibit tubular fluid reabsorption.[21] The mechanisms involved and the physiological implications of high-dose angiotensin II–induced inhibition of sodium reabsorption are not well understood. Angiotensin II in the usual physiological range may preserve or enhance net renal sodium retention by several mechanisms,

including direct actions on the proximal tubule, and indirect actions through stimulation of adrenal aldosterone release, promoting reabsorption in the distal tubule and collecting duct.

Nervous System

The effects of angiotensin II on the nervous system are complex. The earliest described action was the central pressor effect: Infusion of angiotensin II into the isolated cerebral circulation of dogs was associated with a rise in systemic blood pressure even though the angiotensin has no access to the systemic blood vessels.[22] Blockade of peripheral α-adrenergic receptors inhibited this central action of angiotensin II, indicating that sympathetic tone plays an important role.[23] Ablation of the area postrema inhibits the pressor effects of centrally administered angiotensin II, indicating that this structure mediates angiotensin II–induced stimulation of sympathetic outflow.[24] Angiotensin II also enhances the activity of peripheral noradrenergic nerve terminals by stimulating the release inhibiting the reuptake of norepinephrine at this site.[7]

Both intravenous and centrally administered angiotensin II provoke water intake and salt appetite and stimulate secretion of vasopressin and adrenocorticotropic hormone. These central actions of angiotensin II provide short- and intermediate-term defense of extracellular fluid volume in the hypovolemic or hypotensive animal. Although angiotensin II does not cross the blood-brain barrier, there is evidence that some of its central actions may be mediated through the subfornical organ.[26] Finally, neurons at various locations in the central nervous system are capable of synthesizing angiotensin II, presumably for local release as a neurotransmitter and/or neuromodulator.[23]

Structural Effects of Angiotensin II

Suppressor amounts of angiotensin II, when administered over days to weeks, can produce hypertrophy of the myocardium and vascular smooth muscle.[27] These effects can be attenuated or prevented altogether with angiotensin-converting enzyme (ACE) inhibitors and angiotensin II receptor antagonists. In vascular smooth muscle cell cultures, angiotensin II enhances production of extracellular matrix proteins, such as type V collagen and fibronectin.[28] Angiotensin II also can act as a mitogen by promoting a proliferative response in fibroblasts, adrenal cortical cells, and vascular smooth muscle cells.[29] The growth-promoting effects of low levels of angiotensin II occur despite "downregulation" of its receptors.

Distribution of Angiotensin II Receptors

Angiotensin II, like other peptide hormones, elicits its cellular actions by first binding to highly specific receptors located on the cell membrane (Table 71–1). At least three types of angiotensin II receptors have been identified, designated AT_1, AT_2, and AT_4 (see Chap. 10, The AT_1 and AT_2 Angiotensin Receptors).[30] In humans, only the first two of these receptor subtypes are known to exist. The AT_1 receptor appears to mediate most of the known actions of the angiotensins.

Table 71–1 Actions of Angiotensin II

Tissue	Action
Vasculature	Vasoconstriction
	Promotion of smooth muscle hypertrophy
Adrenal cortex	Stimulation of synthesis and secretion of aldosterone
Adrenal medulla	Increased release of epinephrine
Kidney	Vasoconstriction of the efferent and afferent arterioles
	Inhibition of renin release by the juxtaglomerular apparatus
	Stimulation of sodium reabsorption in the proximal tubule
Heart	Stimulation of myocardial hypertrophy and collagen synthesis
Brain	Stimulation of thirst and release of vasopressin
	Increased central sympathetic outflow
Peripheral sympathetic nerve terminals	Presynaptic augmentation of norepinephrine release

AT$_1$ receptors have been demonstrated in a large number of tissues, including vascular smooth muscle, adrenal zona glomerulosa, mesangial and tubular epithelial cells of the kidney, neuronal tissue, and choroid plexus.[30] The AT$_2$ receptor subtype has been found in abundance in fetal mesenchymal cells, brain tissue, adrenal medulla, and uterus.[30, 31] The physiological functions and intracellular signaling mechanisms of the AT$_2$ receptor protein remain poorly understood. There is evidence that the AT$_2$ receptor subtype can mediate an antiproliferative effect of angiotensin II.[32-34]

With the exception of the adrenal glomerulosa, prolonged exposure of target organs to angiotensin II reduces responsiveness, an effect that is associated with internalization and phosphorylation of the AT$_1$ receptor.[35]

DEVELOPMENT OF ANGIOTENSIN II ANTAGONISTS

Peptide Analogues of Angiotensin II

Detailed analyses of the structural requirements of angiotensin for binding to its receptor and studies of many analogues of angiotensin II eventually led to the development of saralasin, a potent angiotensin II receptor antagonist.[36] Saralasin is an octapeptide that differs in structure from angiotensin II at the first (sarcosine) and eighth (alanine) residues. Sarcosine is a nonmammallian amino acid that, when located at the N-terminal, was found to slow the degradation of the molecule. Saralasin was shown to lower blood pressure and aldosterone levels in humans in proportion to the circulating levels of angiotensin II.[37] Owing to its peptide nature, saralasin required intravenous administration, was expensive to manufacture, and had a short half-life. Initially, saralasin was approved only as a diagnostic probe for renin-dependent forms of hypertension.[38] Because of its weak agonist action, it occasionally produced a signficant pressor effect in patients with low-renin forms of hypertension.[39] The inconvenience and ex-

pense of administration, as well as the unpredictability of response, markedly limited the clinical usefulness of saralasin. Because of the limitations, along with the development of the orally active converting enzyme inhibitors in the early 1980s, saralasin was eventually withdrawn from the market.

Medicinal Chemistry of Nonpeptide Angiotensin II Receptor Antagonists

For several decades, investigators struggled to identify potent orally active angiotensin II receptor antagonists. An important breakthrough occurred in 1982, when Furakawa and coworkers,[40] in the laboratories of Takeda Limited in Japan, identified and patented several 1-benzylimidazole 5-acetic acid derivatives that had specific angiotensin II receptor binding activity.[40] However, these initial compounds had weak antihypertensive effects.[41] Investigators at the Dupont Merck Pharmaceutical Company postulated that the imidazole compounds and angiotensin II bound to the same receptor site, but the test molecules needed enlargement to better mimic angiotensin II at its points of attachment to the receptor.[30] The molecular model employed by these investigators suggested that there was overlap between the imidazole group and histidine at the six-position of angiotensin II. The lipophilic n-butyl group at the two-position was pointed at the ileucine at the five-position of angiotensin II. It was posited that the benzyl group of the Takeda compound extended in the direction of the N-terminal of angiotensin II. Elongation of the compound by building the molecule toward the tyrosine site at the four-position of angiotensin II might increase potency (Fig. 71–2).

Addition of a carboxylic moiety at the para-position of the benzene ring improved receptor binding 10-fold and lowered blood pressure when administered intravenously to renal hypertensive rat.[42] By enlarging the molecule with placement of a second acidic phenyl group linked by a single carbon atom to the first aromatic ring, binding affinity increased another 10-fold, and oral bioavailability was markedly enhanced.[43] A significant and final improvement in bioavailability and receptor binding was obtained when the carboxylic moiety located on the second phenyl group was replaced by a tetrazole at the ortho-position. Losartan, 2-butyl-4-chloro-1[p-(o-1H-tetrazole-5-ylphenyl)-benzyl]imidazole-5-methanol monopotassium salt, is the first of a new class of nonpeptide, orally active antihypertensive agents with specific binding to the AT$_1$ receptor subtype.[44] Maximal pharmacological action requires the oxidation of the 5-hydroxymethyl group on the imidazole ring to form EXP3174, the carboxylic acid metabolite of losartan.[45]

DISCOVERY OF NEWER ANGIOTENSIN II RECEPTOR ANTAGONISTS

A number of angiotensin II receptor antagonists have been approved for use in the treatment of hypertension, and more are undergoing preclinical and clinical investigation.

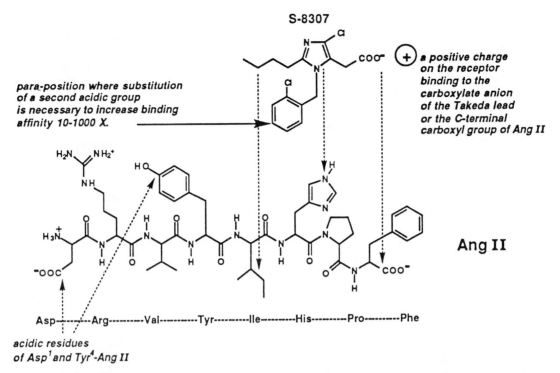

Figure 71–2. Hypothetical structural relations of angiotensin II and the Takeda nonpeptide antagonist S-8307. (From Timmermans PB, Duncia JV, Carini DJ, et al. Discovery of losartan, the first angiotensin II receptor antagonist. J Hum Hypertens 9 [suppl 5]:S3–S18, 1995.)

Development of these compounds has often but not always followed strategies based on the Takeda- and Dupont-Merck–lead benzylimidazole series of compounds.

The second AT_1 subtype angiotensin II receptor antagonist to gain approval for clinical use is valsartan. Investigators at Ciba (Novartis) in Switzerland employed a strategy to open up the imidazole ring and replace it with the acylated amino acid valine.[46] The acidic biphenyl tetrazole substituent is preserved. The carboxyl moiety of the valine serves to preserve oral bioavailability with high-affinity receptor binding. Thus, valsartan is, like EXP3174 (the active metabolite of losartan), a diacid. Unlike losartan, valsartan does not require metabolic oxidation to achieve maximal pharmacological effect.[47]

Irbesartan, 2-butyl-(1H-tetrazol-5-yl)[1,1′-biphenyl]-4-yl[methyl]-1,3-diazespiro[4,4] non-1-en, is the third nonpeptide, orally active angiotensin II antagonist that has received approval for clinical use in the United States. This compound was discovered by Sanofi Recherche of France and is being jointly developed with Bristol-Myers Squibb in the United States. These investigators incorporated an imidazolinone moiety in place of the imidazole heterocyclical ring. A carbonyl group functions as the hydrogen bond acceptor in place of the 5-hyroxymethyl group of losartan and the valine carboxylic acid group of valsartan.[48] Irbesartan possesses a high affinity and specificity for AT_1 receptors. Like valsartan, irbesartan does not require biotransformation to achieve its effects.[49]

Another successful approach has been to develop fused-ring imidazoles. Candesartan cilexetil is an ester carbonate benzimidazole prodrug that has been designed by Takeda Limited and is being jointly developed with Astra.[50] This agent is rapidly metabolized to CV-11974, a highly potent AT_1 receptor antagonist. The latter compound bears a C7 carboxyl group that is positioned in a fashion similar to the imidazole carboxyl moiety of EXP3174.[51]

The Boehringer Ingelheim/Thomae research team has followed a similar fused-ring approach but substituted a second phenylimidazole moiety at the six-position of the primary heterocycle.[52] This compound, telmisartan, incorporates a carboxylic acid as the biphenyl acidic group that achieves greater receptor antagonism than does the tetrazole analogue.[53]

Still another promising approach has been to replace the imidazole ring of losartan with a fused six-membered ring heterocycle to form quinazolinone derivatives of the biphenyl tetrazole. One such product, tasosartan, has been found to be a potent competitive antagonist and is under clinical development by Wyeth Ayerst.[54] This molecule has a carbonyl group on the quinazolinone ring that, like that of irbesartan, may serve as a mimic of the hydroxymethyl group of losartan (Fig. 71–3).[55]

Investigators at SmithKline Beecham devised an alternative model for the superimposition of the Takeda benzylimidazole antagonists with angiotensin II. As with the Dupont model, the 2-chlorobenzyl substituent of the Takeda lead was proposed to be spacially equivalent to the Tyr-4 position of angiotensin II, and the aliphatic butyl group pointed toward the Lle-5. However, the equivalence between the imidazole of the Takeda lead and the His-6 of angiotensin II was not assumed. Instead, the imidazole was believed to function as a scaffold for positioning of substituent groups toward the receptor.[56] This led to a different but also successful approach through refining the presentation of the carboxylic acid and greater filling of the binding pocket for the Phe-8 side chain of angiotensin II. Chain extension at the imidazole-5-position via a *trans*-acrylic acid group yielded the final product, eprosartan, which is 40,000 times more potent than the original Takeda lead[57] (Fig. 71–4).

EFFECTS OF ANGIOTENSIN II ANTAGONISTS

Hemodynamic Effects

Angiotensin II antagonists reduce peripheral resistance and systemic arterial pressure in hypertensive animals.[58] The depressor effect is more potent and more consistent in renin-angiotensin–dependent models such as 2-kidney 1-clip or angiotensin-infusion forms of hypertension.[59, 60] Volume expansion or bilateral nephrectomy appears to attenuate or abolish the antihypertensive effect of the angiotensin II antagonists.[61] In euvolemic normotensive animals and humans, angiotensin II antagonists have little effect.[30] In the majority of hypertensive humans, these agents produce a significant reduction of peripheral resistance and blood pressure.[62, 63]

Lowering of peripheral resistance is most likely due to several factors, especially direct binding to and antagonism of vascular angiotensin II receptor sites and reversal of angiotensin II–mediated vasoconstriction.[30, 61] Augmentation of this effect may occur through blockade of angiotensin II receptors on sympathetic nerve terminals, with consequent attenuation of sympathetically mediated vasoconstriction.[64]

Cardiac Effects

Despite the angiotensin antagonist–induced decline in peripheral resistance, heart rate is little affected or is reduced slightly in hypertensive euvolemic animals and humans.[30] This neutral effect on heart rate in the setting of lowered peripheral resistance may be due to antagonism of angiotensin II receptors at peripheral sympathetic sites as well as through centrally mediated actions of these agents.[65]

Based on several converging lines of evidence, it has been predicted that AT_1 antagonists would have an especially beneficial effect on cardiac and vascular hypertrophy. Plasma angiotensin II levels tend to increase during therapy with these agents, most likely as a result of AT_1 receptor–mediated disinhibition of renin release by cells of the renal juxtaglomerular apparatus.[66] Also, it has been found that the cardiac chymase-angiotensin system provides an alternate path for angiotensin II formation that is independent of converting enzyme.[67] Moreover, there is evidence that the AT_2 receptor subtype can mediate an antiproliferative effect on tissue growth.[68] Thus, administration of a selec-

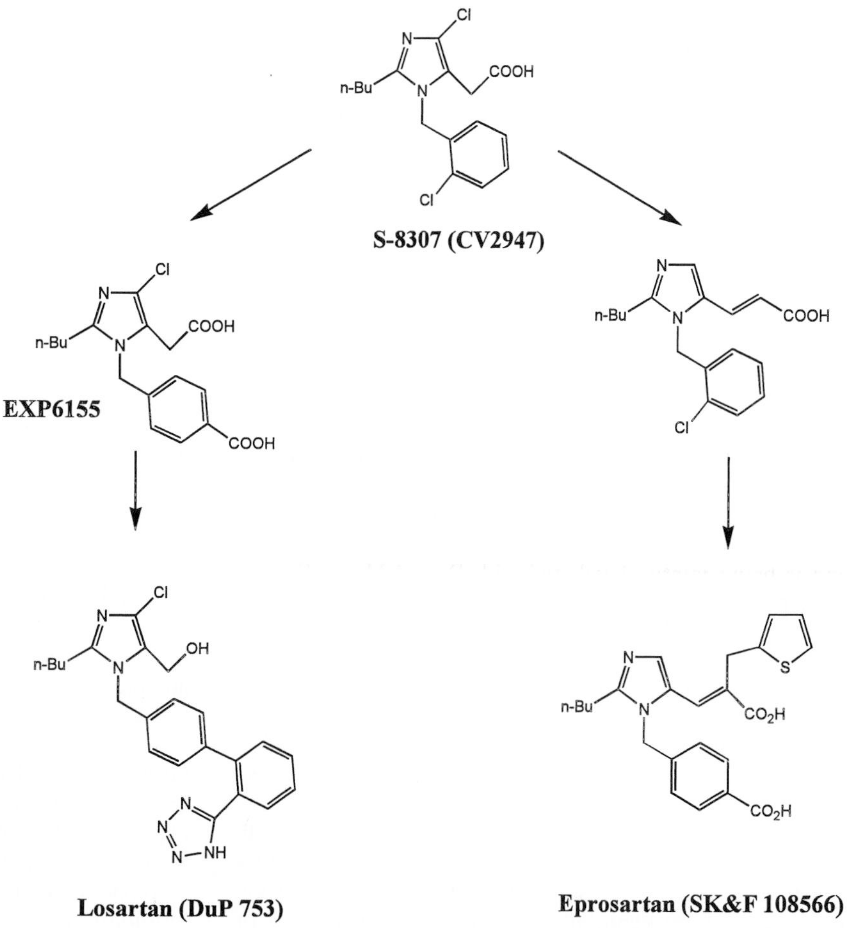

Figure 71–3. The development of losartan and eprosartan. (From Wexler RR, Greenlee WJ, Irvin JD, et al. Nonpeptide angiotensin II receptor antagonists: The next generation in antihypertensive therapy. J Med Chem 39:626–656, 1996.)

S-8307 (CV2947)

EXP6155

Losartan (DuP 753)

Eprosartan (SK&F 108566)

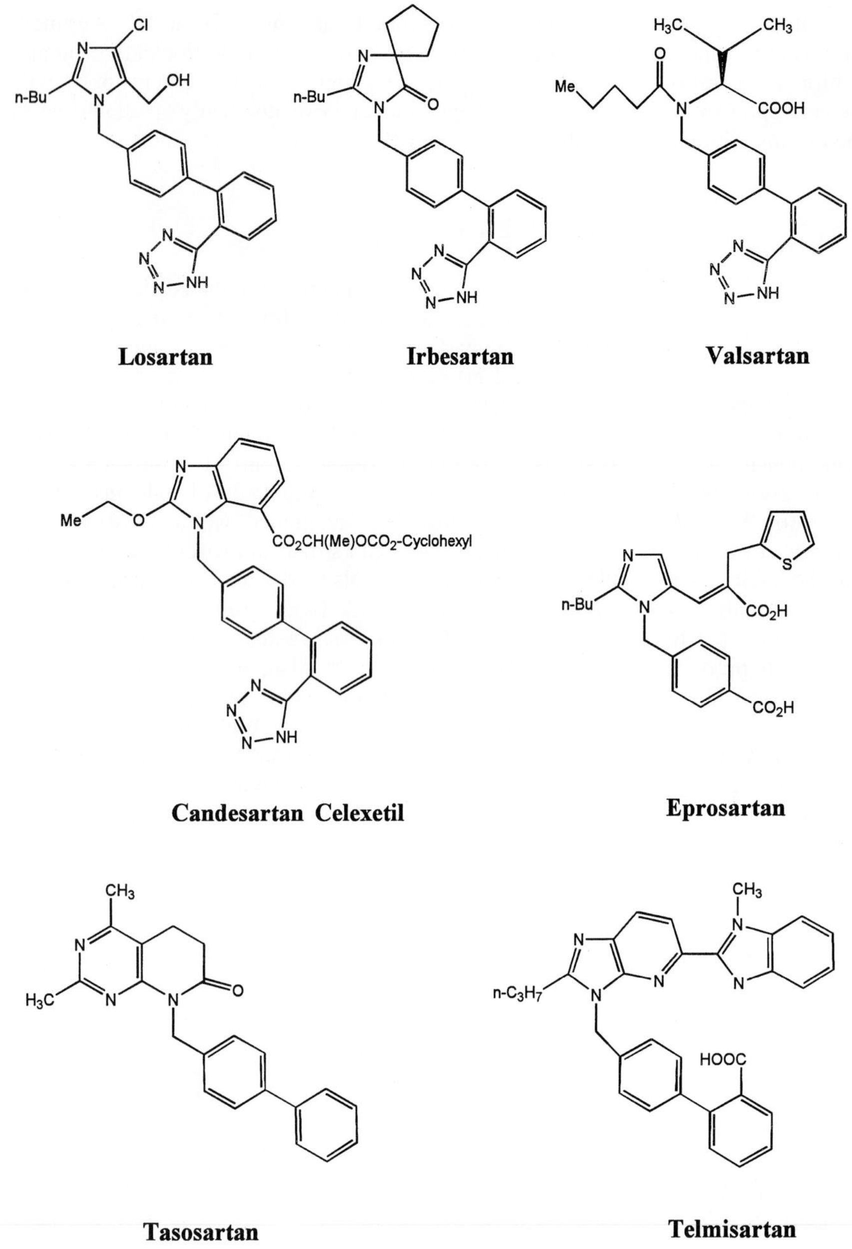

Losartan

Irbesartan

Valsartan

Candesartan Celexetil

Eprosartan

Figure 71–4. Chemical structures of nonpeptide angiotensin receptor antagonists currently available or in late clinical development.

Tasosartan

Telmisartan

tive AT_1 antagonist not only attenuates growth-promoting effects mediated by the AT_1 receptor but also, as angiotensin II levels rise, may enhance the antiproliferative effect mediated by the unblocked AT_2 receptor subtype.[68]

There is evidence that angiotensin II receptor antagonists prevent angiotensin II–mediated cardiac growth and remodeling.[69, 70] These effects may prove to be of special importance in the prevention or treatment of ischemic or hypertensive cardiomyopathies. In experimental models of coronary ischemia, losartan appears to have a beneficial effect on survival and myocardial growth and remodeling.[71, 72] Also, there is experimental evidence that angiotensin II receptor antagonists may improve coronary reserve in hypertensive animals concomitant with a reduction in cardiac mass.[73, 74] Alterations in coronary blood flow are a function of coronary vasomotor tone, diastolic perfusion pressure, and left ventricular end-diastolic pressure, all of

which may be affected by angiotensin II receptor antagonists.[75, 76] Thus, in the clinical setting, the effects of angiotensin II antagonists on coronary flow are expected to vary.

Renal Effects

In animal models such as the anesthetized dog or rat, angiotensin II antagonists produce renal vasodilatation and natriuresis with a small increase in GFR.[77, 78] In patients with essential hypertension, angiotensin II receptor antagonists generally have no discernible effect on GFR as assessed by creatinine clearance.[79] Renal blood flow is usually unaffected by angiotensin II receptor antagonists in the euvolemic animal or human.[80]

Because angiotensin II has the potential for growth-promoting effects at the mesangial tissue level, it has been speculated that angiotensin II receptor blockade may exert effects on glomerular filtration at the basement membrane filtration barrier site.[81] In hypertensive patients with proteinuric renal disorders, administration of losartan was associated with a decrease in urinary protein, an increase in effective renal blood flow, and stable GFR.[82]

In healthy men on a very low salt diet, it has been found that renal blood flow increases with eprosartan administration to an extent that equals or exceeds that following ACE inhibitor infusion.[83] In the clinical setting of salt or volume depletion, angiotensin II antagonists may produce a decline in GFR, perhaps by interference with glomerular blood flow autoregulation.[84]

In experimental models of unilateral renal artery stenosis, angiotensin receptor antagonists consistently produce a decline in GFR of the affected kidney.[85] Reported effects on glomerular filtration and renal blood flow in the contralateral kidney have been variable.[86] In patients with renal impairment and renovascular occlusive disease, reversible increases in serum creatinine have been reported following angiotensin II receptor antagonist administration.[84, 87]

Angiotensin II receptor antagonists produce a modest natriuretic action through blockade of proximal tubular angiotensin II receptor sites that mediate sodium reabsorption.[78, 79] This effect is most evident in the volume-depleted state in which the renin-angiotensin system is activated.[84, 88] An additional natriuretic action occurs through inhibition of aldosterone synthesis and release by the adrenal zona glomerulosa cells.[89, 90] Reduced aldosterone-mediated distal tubular sodium reabsorption may contribute to the diuretic effect of the angiotensin II receptor antagonists.

Among the angiotensin II receptor antagonists, losartan has the apparently unique property of exerting a modest uricosuric effect.[91] The effect is dose-dependent and has been documented in normotensive and hypertensive individuals with and without renal impairment. It does not appear to be dependent on the activity of the renin-angiotensin system and is not affected by changes in salt intake. Infusion of the active metabolite of losartan, EXP3174, has no effect on uric acid excretion, indicating that the uricosuric effect is specific to the parent drug losartan.[91] The mechanism is not known but may be related to renal tubular anion load competing with urate at the tubular transport sites.

Nervous System Effects

Angiotensin II antagonism appears to inhibit peripheral sympathetic activity via blockade of presynaptic angiotensin II receptors that normally amplify release of neurotransmitters.[92] When administered intracerebrally to experimental animals angiotensin II receptor antagonists appear to inhibit centrally mediated sympathetic nervous outflow at the level of the paraventricular nucleus.[93] Drinking behavior in animals and release of vasopressin are also suppressed following central administration of these agents.[94]

Behavior and Affect

In experimental animals, angiotensin II receptor antagonists have been shown to improve cognitive function and anxi-

ety-associated deficits (Table 71–2).[95] In humans, a randomized trial of amlodipine with losartan showed that the angiotensin antagonist–treated group had higher mean scores on the Psychological General Well-Being Index after 12 weeks of double-blind therapy despite equivalent blood pressure–lowering effects.[96]

CLINICAL PHARMACOLOGY

The angiotensin AT_1 receptor antagonists appear to occupy space among the seven-transmembrane helices of the receptor protein. Interaction with amino acid residues in these regions of the receptor molecule prevents the binding of angiotensin II to the receptor.[97] All currently available AT_1 receptor antagonists have been shown to attenuate the circulatory, renal, endocrine, and neurohumoral actions normally mediated by angiotensin II. Unlike the earlier nonselective peptide antagonist saralasin, these agents are devoid of partial agonist effect. The AT_1 receptor antagonists have been shown to cause a two- to threefold rise in plasma renin activity and a consequent rise in angiotensin II concentration.[98]

At this time, the angiotensin II receptor antagonists have U.S. Food and Drug Administration approval only for the treatment of hypertension. Clinical trials are under way for the treatment of patients with left ventricular hypertrophy, congestive heart failure, diabetic nephropathy, and other conditions.

It is important to note that angiotensin II receptor antagonists, as well as ACE inhibitors, are contraindicated during pregnancy. Several dozen cases of fetal and neonatal morbidity and death have been reported in conjunction with ACE inhibitor administration in the second or third trimester of pregnancy.[99] Abnormalities have included renal failure, oligohydramnios, fetal limb and craniofacial deformities, and hypoplastic lung development.

The angiotensin II receptor antagonists differ from one another somewhat in their oral bioavailability, rate of absorption, tissue distribution, metabolism, and rate of elimination. Several of these agents act as prodrugs with conversion to more biologically active metabolites.

Losartan Potassium

Losartan potassium, 2-butyl-4-chloro-1[p-(o-1*H*-tetrazol-5-ylphenyl)-benzyl]imidazol-5-methanol monopotassium

Table 71–2 Established Clinical Effects of AT_1 Receptor Antagonists
Arterial vasodilatation
Reduced serum aldosterone level
Increased plasma renin activity
Increased plasma angiotensin II
Peripheral sympathetic activity inhibition
Decreased peripheral resistance
Decreased blood pressure of hypertensives
Improved hemodynamic profile in heart failure
Improved exercise tolerance in heart failure

salt, is the first orally active angiotensin II receptor antagonist approved for clinical use.[100] The potassium salt of losartan is well absorbed orally with a systemic bioavailability of approximately 33%.[101–103] It is rapidly absorbed with peak plasma levels achieved in about 1 hour. Losartan has a relatively short terminal half-life of 1.5 to 2.5 hours.[104] It undergoes substantial first-pass metabolism by the cytochrome P-450 (CYP-450) enzymes 2C9 and 3A4.[105, 106] The methyl hydroxyl group of losartan located on the imidazole ring undergoes biooxidation to the carboxylated form of the compound, EXP3174.[105] Approximately 50% of orally administered losartan is converted to the active metabolite. EXP3174, with a potency 15 to 30 times greater than that of losartan, is responsible for most of the angiotensin II receptor antagonism.[104] EXP3174 reaches peak concentration in 3 to 4 hours and has a longer terminal half-life of 6 to 9 hours.[104] Food intake slows absorption of losartan and delays the time to peak concentration (C_{max}) but has little effect on the total area under the curve (AUC) of either losartan or EXP3174.[107]

Losartan is a competitive antagonist of angiotensin II in that it causes a rightward shift of the concentration-contraction curve without depression of the maximal pressor response to the octapeptide. In contrast, EXP3174 is a noncompetitive, so-called insurmountable antagonist in that it produces a nonparallel right shift in the concentration-contraction curve and reduces the maximal response to angiotensin II. The mechanism of the noncompetitive nature of drug-receptor interaction is not yet known. However, it seems likely that tight receptor binding by the active metabolite contributes to the prolonged biological activity of orally administered losartan.

In the plasma, losartan and its metabolites are highly protein bound (98.7 to 99.8%) in a nonsaturable mode. These compounds have been shown to penetrate the blood-brain barrier poorly, if at all. Biliary excretion plays a major role in the elimination of losartan and its metabolites.[107] A lower starting dose is recommended for patients with hepatic dysfunction. Somewhat less than one third of the absorbed drug and its metabolites is cleared by renal filtration.[107] Dose adjustment is not necessary in patients with renal impairment, including dialysis patients, unless they are volume depleted or have occlusive renovascular disease.[108] Neither losartan nor EXP3174 can be removed by hemodialysis.[106]

Losartan administration does not affect the pharmacokinetics of warfarin or digoxin.[109, 110] Coadministration of losartan with cimetidine led to about a 20% increase in the AUC of losartan but not its more potent metabolite.[106] Phenobarbital administration led to a reduction of about 20% in the AUC of both losartan and its carboxylated metabolite.[106] These interactions are not considered to be clinically significant.

The effects of potent inhibitors of CYP-450 3A4 and 2C9 have recently been assessed in healthy volunteers utilizing fluconazole, a CYP-450 2C9 inhibitor, and itraconazole, a CYP-450 3A4 inhibitor.[111] Administration of fluconazole but not itraconazole was found to inhibit the formation of EXP3174. This implies that CYP-450 2C9 is a major enzyme for the conversion of losartan to its more active metabolite. It is possible that concomitant use of other agents known to inhibit one of these oxidative enzymes may significantly attenuate the therapeutic effect of losartan.

Losartan is available in 25-mg and 50-mg tablets. The usual starting dose is 50 mg once daily, and the highest recommended dose is 100 mg per day. For patients with volume depletion or on diuretic therapy, the 25-mg dose may be safer.

Valsartan

Valsartan, 1-oxopentyl-*N*[[2'-(1*H*-tetrozol-5-yl)[1,1'-biphenyl]-4-yl]methyl]-L-valine, acts as a competitive antagonist of the AT_1 receptor.[47] Unlike losartan, valsartan is not a prodrug and its activity is independent of hepatic metabolism.[112] Oral bioavailability for the capsule formulation of valsartan is approximately 25% (range 10 to 35%).[113] The time to peak concentration in the plasma is 2 to 4 hours. Food intake decreases AUC by approximately 40% and peak plasma concentrations by about 50.%[114] Like losartan, valsartan is highly bound to serum proteins (95%), primarily albumin.[115] The volume of distribution of this compound is only 17 L, indicating that tissue distribution is not very extensive. For most patients, the onset of the antihypertensive effect occurs at about 2 hours, with the maximal reduction of blood pressure achieved in about 6 hours.[112, 114]

Elimination of valsartan is mainly (80%) in the unchanged form through the gastrointestinal tract.[113] Approximately 9% of the dose is metabolized to valeryl 4-hydroxy valsartan. This process does not appear to be CYP-450–dependent. Orally administered valsartan shows a biexponential decay curve with an elimination half-life of about 6 hours. The antihypertensive action of valsartan persists for 24 hours after oral administration. Valsartan does not appear to accumulate in plasma after repeated administration. However, patients with hepatic or biliary tract impairment have an increase in the AUC, indicating a slower plasma clearance rate.[116] The pharmacokinetics of valsartan do not appear to be appreciably affected by renal impairment. However, as with all agents that affect the renin-angiotensin system, the presence of renal insufficiency warrants careful monitoring of the patient's hemodynamic, renal, and electrolyte status.

Coadministration of valsartan with amlodipine, atenolol, cimetidine, digoxin, furosemide, glibenclamide, hydrochlorothiazide, indomethacin, or warfarin has failed to show any clinically significant pharmacokinetic interactions.[114] Valsartan, like other angiotensin II receptor antagonists and ACE inhibitors, is contraindicated in pregnancy. The extent to which this agent is excreted in human milk is not yet known. Dose adjustment does not appear to be necessary for the elderly, although careful clinical monitoring is prudent in this population group.[117]

Valsartan is available in capsule form as the 80-mg and 160-mg dose formulations. It is recommended to initiate valsartan therapy with 80 mg once daily. The dosage of valsartan may be increased as needed up to a total daily dose of 320 mg. It is prudent to reevaluate patients within one month after such a dose adjustment.

Irbesartan

Irbesartan, 2-butyl-3-[[2(1H-tetrazo 5yl)[1,1'-biphenyl]-4yl]methyl]-1,3 diazaspiro[4,4]-non-1en-4-olone, has an imidazolinone ring in which a carbonyl group functions as the hydrogen bond acceptor in place of the C-5 hydroxymethyl group of losartan.[48] Irbesartan has been shown to be an insurmountable noncompetitive antagonist of the AT_1 receptor (Fig. 71–5).[49,118] Irbesartan does not require biotransformation for its pharmacological action.[119]

Oral bioavailability of Irbesartan is relatively high at 60 to 80% and is not affected by food intake.[120] Peak plasma concentrations occur 1.5 to 2 hours after oral administration. Irbesartan is less protein bound than other angiotensin receptor antagonists and has a plasma half-life of approximately 11 to 15 hours.[120]

Irbesartan is metabolized by oxidation and glucuronide conjugation. Oxidation is mediated primarily through the 2C9 isoenzyme. Metabolism by 3A4 is negligible.[119] Irbesartan has no effect on the function of other CYP-450 oxidative isoenzymes such as 1A1, 1A2, 2A6, 2B6, and 2E1[99] and no demonstrated effects on the pharmacokinetics or pharmacodynamics of nifedipine, hydrochlorothiazide, warfarin, and digoxin.[119]

Irbesartan is eliminated from the body primarily through biliary excretion (75%) and to a lesser extent through the kidneys.[121] Drug accumulation does not appear to occur in the setting of hepatic or renal insufficiency, and dose adjustment is not required for these conditions.[119] Irbesartan is not dialyzable. In the elderly, C_{max} and AUC are increased by 20 to 50% and elimination half-life unchanged. Dose adjustment of irbesartan has not been found to be necessary in the elderly or for gender or race.[99, 119, 121]

Irbesartan is available in 75 mg, 150 mg, and 300 mg tablets. The usual starting dose is 150 mg once daily.[99] However, for patients receiving a diuretic or who are otherwise volume depleted, it may be prudent to begin with a lower initial dose such as 75 mg per day.

Candesartan Cilexetil

Candesartan, 2-ethoxy-1-[[2′-(1H-tetrazol-5-yl)biphenyl-4-yl]methyl]-1H-benzimidazole-7-carboxylic acid, is a potent angiotensin II receptor antagonist (Fig. 71–6).[122] Its structure is a biphenyl imidazole derivative that, like losartan, has a tetrazolyl moiety, a lipophilic side chain, and a carboxyl group. To overcome poor oral absorption, the

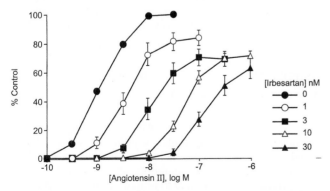

Figure 71–5. Dose-related inhibition of angiotensin II–induced contraction of rabbit aorta by irbesartan. (Reprinted by permission of Elsevier Science from Johnston CI, Risvanis J. Preclinical pharmacology of angiotensin II receptor antagonists: Update and outstanding issues. Am J Hypertens, vol 10, 306S–310S, copyright 1997 by American Journal of Hypertension Ltd.)

cilexetil ester prodrug form was synthesized. Candesartan cilexetil has been found to be rapidly and completely converted by hydrolytic cleavage to the active compound, candesartan, during gastrointestinal absorption.

Candesartan has a high affinity for the AT_1 receptor and dissociates slowly from its binding sites.[122] In the presence of angiotensin II, candesartan acts as an insurmountable antagonist for the AT_1 receptor. The effects of candesartan at the receptor level have been observed at low doses and are of long duration.[123]

The maximal serum concentration of candesartan is reached at approximately 4 hours after oral dosing, with a terminal half-life of about 9 hours.[124] The AUC of candesartan is linear throughout the dose range of 2 to 16 mg. In elderly healthy volunteers, steady-state concentrations of candesartan are approximately 30 to 50% higher than in younger subjects.[124] Oral bioavailability does not appear to be affected by food intake.[125] Most of the drug is excreted in the urine as candesartan, with a smaller fraction as an inactive metabolite.[126] Excretion through the biliary tract accounts for less than 40% of total drug elimination.

The pharmacokinetic profile of candesartan is not altered in patients with mild to moderate hepatic dysfunction.[127] In patients with renal impairment, the AUC, C_{max}, and terminal half-life were significantly greater than in healthy subjects. It may be prudent to employ lower starting doses in patients with severe renal dysfunction. The drug is not dialyzable.[127]

Coadministration of candesartan cilexetil with hydrochlorthiazide has caused a small but significant decrease in the AUC of the latter agent and a slightly higher bioavailability and C_{max} for candesartan itself.[128] Candesartan produces a small decrease in trough warfarin concentration but does not affect prothrombin time. There have been no significant interactions found when candesartan cilexetil has been coadministered with nifedipine, glibenclamide, digoxin, or estrogen-containing oral contraceptives.[128]

Candesartan cilexetil is available as 4-mg, 8-mg, 16-mg, and 32-mg tablets.

Eprosartan

Eprosartan, (E)-α-[[2-butyl-1-[(4-carboxyphenyl)methyl]-1H-imidazol-5-yl]methylene]-2-thiophenepropanoic acid, is a nonphenyl, nontetrazole angiotensin II receptor antagonist with a high degree of affinity of AT_1 receptor sites.[129] Eprosartan has incomplete oral absorption, with an oral bioavailability of 13 to 15%.[130] Maximal plasma concentrations of the drug are reached in 1 to 3 hours. Food intake appears to have unpredictable effects on C_{max} and time to C_{max}.[131] The bioavailability of eprosartan increases with age.[131]

Approximately 90% of orally administered eprosartan is found in the feces; the remainder, in the urine.[132] Only 20% of the excreted drug undergoes metabolism to its glucuronide form.[132] Both renal insufficiency and hepatic impairment delay the elimination of eprosartan. Eprosartan is not metabolized by the CYP-450 system and has not been shown to have significant drug interactions with glyburide and digoxin.[133] Eprosartan, like most of the currently available angiotensin II receptor antagonists, is highly pro-

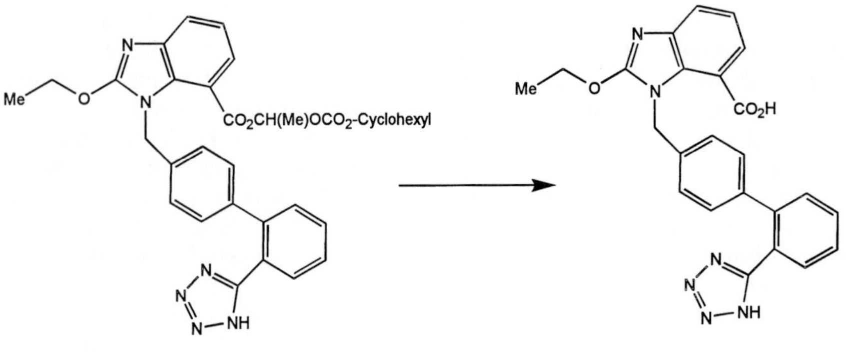

Candesartan Celexetil (TCV-116)   **Candesartan(CV-11974)**

Figure 71–6. Angiotensin II receptor antagonists with active metabolites.

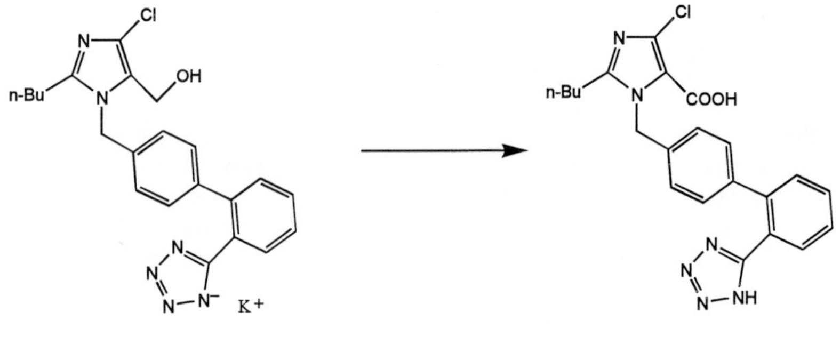

Losartan (DuP 753, MK-954)   **EXP3174**

tein bound in plasma (98%) but does not appear to affect the anticoagulant activity of warfarin.[132, 133]

Eprosartan has been approved for use in the United States and other countries. In several European countries, eprosartan is available in 200-mg, 300-mg, and 400-mg tablets for once-daily administration.

Telmisartan

Telmisartan, 4′-[(1,4′-dimethyl-2′-propyl[2,6′-bi-1H-benzimidazol]-1′-yl)methyl]-[1,1′-biphenyl]-2-carboxylic acid, is an orally active angiotensin II receptor antagonist with competitive affinity for the AT_1 receptor subtype.[175] Approximately one half of an orally administered dose is absorbed.[176] Oral bioavailability is somewhat dose dependent. Peak plasma concentrations of telmisartan are reached relatively rapidly, within 0.5 to 1.0 hours after oral ingestion.[175] Food intake reduces the AUC by 6 to 20%.[176] Unlike losartan and candesartan, telmisartan is not a prodrug.[175] Approximately 97% of an orally administered dose is eventually excreted unchanged through the biliary tract.[176] A very small proportion of telmisartan undergoes metabolism to the glucuronide form. The CYP-450 isoenzymes are not involved in the metabolism of telmisartan.[176]

Telmisartan is highly protein bound in plasma (>99.5%) and has a very large volume of distribution (~500 L), indicating additional tissue binding.[175] The terminal elimination half-life of telmisartan is approximately 24 hours.[176, 177] Owing to its biliary route of elimination, telmisartan should

be used with caution in patients with hepatic insufficiency.[176] Telmisartan and digoxin coadministration has been shown to be associated with significant increases in circulating digoxin levels.[176] It is recommended that digoxin levels be monitored when initiating, adjusting, and discontinuing telmisartan therapy to avoid possible over-digitalization. Telmisartan does not appear to alter the anticoagulant effect of warfarin.[176]

The antihypertensive effect of telmisartan is greater in patients with high plasma renin activity.[177] Telmisartan has been approved for use in the United States and other countries. It is available in the United States as 40-mg and 80-mg tablets for once-daily administration. The recommended starting dose for telmisartan is 40-mg once daily.[176]

Safety and Adverse Effects of the Angiotensin II Receptor Antagonists

Angiotensin II receptor antagonists are generally very well tolerated. With two important exceptions, these agents have a side effect profile that is similar to that of the ACE inhibitors. Like the ACE inhibitors, angiotensin II blockers may produce excessive and too-rapid fall of blood pressure in volume depleted or otherwise highly renin-dependent forms of hypertension. In patients with renal impairment, there is an increased risk of hyperkalemia owing to inhibition of aldosterone release. As with ACE inhibitors, patients with bilateral renovascular and renal parenchymal disease are at increased risk of deterioration of renal function that is usually but not always reversible.

Angiotensin II antagonists do not appear to have adverse effects on glucose or lipid metabolism. Losartan is unique among this class in its uricosuric effect. Of special note is that the incidence of cough with angiotensin II receptor antagonists is similar to that of placebo.[134–136] The incidence of angioedema appears to be very low, although cases have been reported.[137, 138] Indeed, among the currently available antihypertensive drug classes, angiotensin receptor antagonists appear to have the lowest incidence of adverse effects (Table 71–3).[139, 140]

CLINICAL APPLICATIONS OF THE ANGIOTENSIN II RECEPTOR ANTAGONISTS

Hypertension

All of the currently approved angiotensin II receptor antagonists have been demonstrated in randomized, placebo-controlled clinical trials to lower blood pressure in hypertensive individuals. Approximately 50 to 60% of hypertensive patients have a clinically significant response to these agents.[63, 141] This is comparable to monotherapy with diuretics, β-blockers, ACE inhibitors, and calcium antagonists.[142, 143]

The antihypertensive efficacy of the angiotensin II receptor antagonists seems to depend at least partially on the activity of the renin-angiotensin system. Approximately 80% of patients demonstrate a significant blood pressure–lowering response when losartan is combined with a thiazide diuretic. The antihypertensive response can be abolished in experimental animals following nephrectomy and is attenuated in humans following volume expansion.[30] The full therapeutic profile of the angiotensin II receptor antagonists has yet to be completely elucidated. These effects of age, race, and concomitant medical conditions on the antihypertensive efficacy of these agents await further clarification.

Several studies have compared the relative efficacy of the currently available angiotensin II antagonists. In general, the observed differences are rather small. In one double-blind parallel group study of 8 weeks' duration, candesartan cilexetil 8 mg per day was found to produce an antihypertensive effect equal to that of losartan 50 mg per day.[144] The 16-mg dose of candesartan cilexetil was found to be more effective than losartan 50 mg administered once daily. However, the use of microcrystalline cellulose back-filled gelatin capsules in the losartan group has been debated.[145, 146] In a double-masked, elective dose-titration study of 8 weeks' duration, irbesartan 150 to 300 mg once daily was found to produce a greater decline in trough seated diastolic blood pressure than did losartan 50 to 100 mg per day.[147] Also, a smaller proportion of patients on the starting dose of irbesartan (53%) as compared with the losartan group (61%) required uptitration at 4 weeks to reach the goal diastolic blood pressure of 90 mm Hg. Adding hydrochlorthiazide to both study drugs produced further reductions in blood pressure, with the greater effect seen in the irbesartan group compared with the losartan group.[147] The incidence of adverse effects in patients receiving either candesartan cilexetil or irbesartan were similar to that experienced by the patients receiving losartan.[144, 147]

Angiotensin II Receptor Antagonists in Cardiac Disease

Angiotensin II exerts many actions on the heart and the coronary circulation. In the vasculature, angiotensin II causes vasoconstriction as well as smooth muscle cell hyperplasia and enhances norepinephrine release, potentiating vasoconstriction. Angiotensin II also causes increased myocardial contractility and facilitates the development of left ventricular hypertrophy. The effects of angiotensin II on plasminogen activator inhibitor I, smooth muscle proliferation, and extracellular matrix formation may enhance the development of atherosclerosis.

The rationale for the use of angiotensin II receptor antagonists in heart failure is based on several hypotheses.[148] Because these agents reduce peripheral resistance, it has been posited that concomitant reduction in cardiac impedance would promote cardiac emptying with less left

Table 71–3 Pharmacological Characteristics of the Angiotensin II Receptor Antagonists

Characteristic	Losartan Potassium	Valsartan	Irbesartan	Candesartan Cilexetil	Telmisartan
Active metabolite	EXP3174	No	No	Candesartan	No
AT$_1$ receptor antagonism	Competitive/Insurmountable (EXP3174)	Competitive	Insurmountable	Insurmountable	Competitive
Bioavailability (%)	33	25	60–80	34–56	42–58
Absorption affected by food	Yes	Yes	No	No	Small
Protein binding (%)	98–99	95	90	99	99
Routes of elimination	70% biliary, 30% renal	80% biliary	75% biliary	60% renal	97% biliary
Half-life (hr)	1.5–2.5 (losartan) 6–9 (EXP3174)	6	11–15	9	24
Uricosuric	Yes	No	No	No	No
U.S. proprietary name	Cozaar	Diovan	Avapro	Atacand	Micardis
Available dosages	25, 50 mg	80, 160 mg	75, 150, 300 mg	4, 8, 16, 32 mg	40, 80 mg
Recommended starting dose	25–50 mg	80 mg	75–150 mg	16 mg	40 mg

ventricular wall stress. Also, blockade of the direct hypertrophic action of angiotensin II on the myocardium by the angiotensin II receptor antagonists might further augment the benefit. Intracardiac angiotensin II is also formed via a non–ACE-dependent mechanism. The latter effect might be expected to provide an advantage of angiotensin II receptor antagonist over ACE inhibitor therapy for treatment of heart failure.

In young healthy adults, plasma angiotensin II, lean body mass, and systemic blood pressure are related to left ventricular mass.[149] Moreover, in patients with heart failure, those who are on ACE inhibitor therapy have been shown to have higher plasma angiotensin II levels than controls, a finding consistent with non–ACE-mediated angiotensin II production in patients with failing hearts.[150]

In a study of the acute effects of angiotensin II receptor antagonists in patients with heart failure, these agents improved hemodynamic indices such as blood pressure, pulmonary wedge pressure, systemic vascular resistance, and cardiac output.[151] In patients with ischemic or idiopathic dilated cardiomyopathy, exercise V_{O_2} and exercise tolerance were found to increase during treatment with both the ACE inhibitor enalapril and the AT_1 receptor antagonist losartan.[152] In contrast to enalapril, the effect of losartan was not antagonized by aspirin.[152] In an earlier study, oral administration of losartan to patients with symptomatic heart failure resulted in beneficial hemodynamic effects with short-term administration and more enhanced benefits after 12 weeks of therapy.[153]

The Evaluation of Losartan in the Elderly (ELITE) Study was designed to determine whether the angiotensin receptor antagonist losartan offered advantages over the ACE inhibitor captopril in older patients with heart failure.[154] The primary endpoint of the study was persistent increase in serum creatinine equal to or greater than 0.3 mg/dL on therapy. The secondary endpoint was death or hospital admission for heart failure. In this randomized, double-blind study of 722 patients with heart failure and ejection fraction equal to or lower than 40%, losartan was titrated to 50 mg once a day and captopril was titrated to 50 mg three times a day for 48 weeks. The occurrence of the primary endpoint (persistent increase in serum creatinine) was the same in the two groups. However, fewer losartan patients than captopril patients discontinued therapy because of adverse experiences (12.2% vs. 20.8%). The losartan treatment group had a 46% lower risk of death, a 64% reduction in sudden death, and a 26% reduction in total hospitalization rate compared with the captopril-treated group. Improvement in symptoms was similar for the two groups, as was the rate of hospitalization for progressive heart failure. It remains unclear why the relative beneficial effect of losartan was so dramatic for sudden death and less so for symptoms of and hospitalization rates for heart failure. This unexpected lowering in mortality with losartan compared with captopril could be due to a better suppression of the effects of angiotensin II, the absence of bradykinin effects during losartan therapy, or the better compliance of patients on losartan. In order to confirm and clarify these results, a new trial evaluating losartan and captopril effects on morbidity and mortality (ELITE-2) has been initiated. In another study, where the effects of losartan and enalapril were compared in patients

with moderate or severe chronic heart failure, no significant differences between the groups in terms of exercise capacity or neurohormonal activation (plasma levels of N-terminal atrial natriuretic factor and norepinephrine) were observed.[154]

In patients with symptomatic heart failure receiving maximal doses of ACE inhibitors, the effects of add-on therapy with angiotensin II receptor antagonists has been studied.[155] The combination was found to be safe and to lead to a further decrease in cardiac afterload. It has been hypothesized that the combination will produce a greater suppression of angiotensin II effects by blocking both ACE- and non-ACE-dependent pathways while maintaining the effects of ACE inhibition in preventing bradykinin degradation. The potential clinical effects of adding an angiotensin II receptor antagonist to ACE inhibitor treatment continues to be investigated.[156]

The effects of angiotensin II receptor antagonists on left ventricular hypertrophy have been studied extensively. Findings from experimental and clinical studies suggest that the pharmacodynamic profile of the antihypertensive agent plays an additional role to that of blood pressure lowering in decreasing left ventricular mass. Losartan has been found to decrease cardiac mass and improve coronary flow reserve in spontaneously hypertensive rats and in left ventricular hypertrophy owing to volume overload induced by aortic insufficiency in Wistar rats.[157, 158] The effects of enalapril and losartan in rats after myocardial infarction appear to be divergent, with enalapril diminishing collagen content, while both agents prevent the myocyte hypertrophic response.[159] In fetal sheep, pressure overload induced (pulmonary artery banding) right ventricular hypertrophy was not affected by losartan, implying that angiotensin II may not play a role in this model.[160]

In a 10-month study of 89 hypertensive patients, losartan given as monotherapy or in association with hydrochlorthiazide produced not only a significant reduction in blood pressure but also a decrease in left ventricular mass by echocardiography.[161] General clinical application of these promising findings of the beneficial actions of angiotensin II receptor antagonists in cardiac disorders will need to await the completion of several clinical trials that are currently under way. For example, the Losartan Intervention For Endpoint Reduction in Hypertension (LIFE) Study, is designed to compare the effects of losartan with the β-blocker atenolol in a double-blind, parallel design in over 9000 patients with electrocardiographic evidence of left ventricular hypertrophy.[162] The primary endpoint of this ongoing study is cardiovascular morbidity and mortality.

Renal Disease

In animals with experimentally induced renal impairment from ablation[163, 164] or streptozotocin-induced diabetes,[165] angiotensin II receptor antagonists preserve renal function to a degree previously demonstrated for ACE inhibitor therapy. In stroke-prone spontaneously hypertensive rats, candesartan prevents the progression of glomerulosclerosis.[166] The results of the ELITE trial suggest that in humans with heart failure, long-term therapy with losartan has an effect comparable to that of captopril on renal function as assessed by serum creatinine levels.[154]

In nonhemodynamically mediated experimental renal disease, the experimental evidence is less consistent. For example, experimental puromycin nephrosis does not appear to be affected by the administration of AT_1 receptor antagonists.[167] In passive Heymann nephritis, a rat model of membranous nephropathy with proteinuria, angiotensin II receptor blockade had virtually no effect on urinary albumin excretion, as opposed to a markedly beneficial effect observed with enalapril.[168] However, in a model of antithymocyte serum-induced mesangioproliferative glomerulonephritis, angiotensin II receptor blockade attenuated histopathological changes and reduced renal transforming growth factor-β mRNA.[169]

In humans with nondiabetic renal disease and proteinuria, losartan has been found to be significantly reduce protein excretion in a dose-dependent manner comparable to that of enalapril.[170] Several long-term studies are under way to determine the effects of angiotensin II receptor antagonism on the progression of diabetic nephropathy.[171, 172]

Cerebrovascular and Neurological Disorders

In animal studies, activation of the renin-angiotensin system has been shown to increase the severity of neurological damage associated with experimental stroke. In animal models of hypertension, such as the stroke-prone spontaneously hypertensive rat, angiotensin II receptor blockers have been shown to decrease mortality from stroke.[173, 174] Furthermore, angiotensin II receptor antagonists have been shown to produce a favorable shift in cerebral autoregulation. Clinical trials are under way to determine the extent to which these agents prevent stroke in patients at higher than normal risk.

There has also been considerable interest in the potential for beneficial behavioral and congnitive effects of angiotensin II receptor antagonists. In experimental animals, losartan has been shown to have positive effects on a variety of mental functions, including learned helplessness and maze performance time.[30] In one double-blind clinical study, total Psychological General Well-Being Index scores were higher in hypertensive patients taking losartan or losartan plus hydrochlorthiazide compared with amlodipine.[96] However, the implication of this finding is difficult to assess in light of the overall lower incidence of adverse effects seen in the losartan-treatment groups.

SUMMARY

The angiotensin II receptor antagonists are playing an ever-more important role in the armamentarium available to the clinician treating patients with high blood pressure and related circulatory disorders. As a class, this group of agents has a high degree of specificity for the AT_1 receptor subtype. The angiotensin II receptor antagonists are effective antihypertensive agents in a broad range of patients and appear to have a lower incidence of adverse effects than other currently available agents. Furthermore, angiotensin blockers have become valuable pharmacological

probes for studying the renin-angiotensin system and angiotensin receptor functions. Additional clinical indications such as left ventricular hypertrophy, congestive heart failure, and renal insufficiency are under study.

Several angiotensin II receptor antagonists have been approved for the treatment of hypertension and more are likely to become available in the near future. It remains to be determined whether the demonstrated clinical effects of the angiotensin II receptor antagonists will translate into beneficial effects on cardiovascular and total morbidity and mortality in patients with hypertension and other disorders of the circulation.

References

1. Skeggs LT, Marsh WH, Kahn JR, Shumway NP. The existence of two forms of hypertensin. J Exp Med 99:275–282, 1954.
2. Skeggs LT, Kahn JR, Shumway NP. The preparation and function of hypertensin converting enzyme. J Exp Med 103:295–299, 1956.
3. Skeggs LT, Lentz KE, Kahn JR, et al. The amino acid sequence of hypertensin II. J Exp Med 104:193–197, 1956.
4. Urata H, Kinoshita A, Misono K, et al. Identification of a highly specific chymase as the major angiotensin II–forming enzyme in the human heart. J Biol Chm 265:22348–22357, 1990.
5. Sancho J, Re R, Burton J. The role of the renin-angiotensin-aldosterone system in cardiovascular homeostasis in normal human subjects. Circulation 53:400–412, 1976.
6. Ganong W. Neuropeptides in cardiovascular control. J Hypertens 2(suppl 3):15–22, 1984.
7. Zimmerman B, Sybertz E, Wong P. Interaction between sympathetic and renin-angiotensin system. J Hypertens 2:581–588, 1984.
8. Wood J. Peripheral venous and arteriolar responses to infusions of angiotensin in normal and hypertensive subjects. Circ Res 9:768–774, 1961.
9. Catt K. Angiotensin II receptors. In Robertson J, Nichols M (eds). The Renin-Angiotensin System. London, Gower Medical, 1993; pp 12.1–12.14.
10. Forsyth R, Hoffbrand B, Melmon K: Hemodynamic effects of angiotensin in normal and environmentally stressed monkeys. Circulation 44:119–125, 1971.
11. Fleming J, Joshua I. Mechanisms of the biphasic effect of angiotensin II on arteriolar response. Am J Physiol 247:H88–H98, 1984.
12. Quinn S, Williams G. Regulation of aldosterone secretion. In James VT (ed). The Adrenal Gland. New York, Raven, 1992; pp 159–189.
13. Dworkin L, Ichikawa I, Brenner B. Hormonal modulation of glomerular filtration function. Am J Physiol 244: F95–F106, 1983.
14. Edwards R. Segmental effects of norepinephrine and angiotensin II on isolated renal microvessels. Am J Physiol 244:F526–F535, 1983.
15. Hura C, Kunau R. Angiotensin II–stimulated prostaglandin production by canine renal afferent arterioles. Am J Physiol 254:F734–F745, 1983.
16. Andrews P. Investigations of cytoplasmic contractile and cytoskeletal elements in the kidney glomerulus. Kidney Int 20:549–559, 1981.
17. Mujais S, Kauffman S, Katz A. Angiotensin II binding sites in individual segments of the rat nephron. J Clin Invest 77:315–327, 1986.
18. Cogan MG. Angiotensin II: A powerful controller of sodium transport in the early proximal tubule. Hypertension 15:451–458, 1990.
19. Schuster V, Kokko J, Jacobson H. Angiotensin II directly stimulates sodium transport in rabbit proximal convoluted tubules. J Clin Invest 73:507–516, 1984.
20. Liu F, Cogan M. Angiotensin II stimulation of hydrogen ion secretion in rat early proximal tubule. J Clin Invest 82:601–610, 1988.
21. Chatsudthipong V, Chang YL. Inhibitory effect of angiotensin II on renal tubular transport. Am J Physiol 260:F340–F346, 1991.
22. Sweet C, Kadowitz P, Brody M. Arterial hypertension elicited by prolonged intervertebral infusion of angiotensin II in conscious dog. Am J Physiol 221:1640–1651, 1971.
23. Reid J, Rubin P. Peptides and central neural regulation of the circulation. Physiol Rev 67: 725–749, 1987.
24. Joy M, Lowe R. Evidence that the area postrema mediates the central cardiovascular response to angiotensin II. Nature 228:1303, 1970.

25. Simpson JB. The circumventricular organs and the central actions of angiotensin II. Neuroendocrinology 32:248–256, 1981.

26. Pardridge MW. Neuropeptides and the blood-brain barrier. Ann Rev Physiol 45:73–82, 1983.

27. Schelling P, Fischer H, Ganten D. Angiotensin and cell growth: A link to cardiovascular hypertrophy J Hypertens 9:3–15, 1991.

28. Kjato H, Suzuki H, Tajima S, et al. Angiotensin II stimulates collagen synthesis in cultured vascular smooth muscle cells. J Hypertens 9:17–22, 1991.

29. Zachary I, Woll P, Rozengurt E. A role for neuropeptides in the control of cell proliferation. Dev Biol 124:295–311, 1987.

30. Timmermans PB, Wong PC, Chiu AT, et al. Angiotensin II receptors and angiotensin II receptor antagonists. Pharmacol Rev 45:205–251, 1993.

31. Timmermans P, Smith R. Angiotensin II receptor subtypes: Selective antagonists and functional correlates. Eur Heart J 15:(suppl 1):79–87, 1994.

32. Kai H, Griendling KK, Lassegue B, et al. Agonist induced phosphorylation of the vascular type 1 angiotensin II receptor. Hypertension 24:523–527, 1994.

33. Metsarinne KP. Angiotensin II is antiproliferative for coronary endothelial cells in vitro. Pharm Pharmacol Lett 2:150–152, 1992.

34. Nakajima M, Horiuchi M, Morishita R, et al. Growth inhibitory function of type 2 angiotensin II receptor: Gain of function study by in vitro gene transfer. Hypertension 24:379, 1994.

35. Bottari SP, King IN, Reichlin S, et al. The angiotensin AT_2 receptor stimulates protein tyrosine phosphatase activity and mediates inhibition of particulate guanylate cyclase. Biochem Biophys Res Commun 183:206–211, 1992.

36. Pals D, Masucci F, Sipos F, Denning G. A specific competitive antagonist of the vascular action of angiotensin II. Circ Res 29:664–672, 1971.

37. Rosei E, Trust P. The effects of the angiotensin II antagonist on blood pressure and plasma aldosterone in man in relation to the prevailing plasma angiotensin II concentration. Prog Biochem Pharmacol 12:230–241, 1976.

38. Streeten D, Anderson G, Freiberg J, Dalakos T. Use of an angiotensin II antagonist (saralasin) in the recognition of angiotensinogenic hypertension. N Engl J Med 292:657–662, 1975.

39. Keeton TK, Campbell WB. The pharmacologic alteration of renin release. Pharmacol Rev 32:81–227, 1980.

40. Furakawa Y, Kishimoto S, Nishikawa K. Hypotensive imidazole derivatives and hypotensive imidazole 5-acetic acid derivatives. Patents issued to Takeda Chemical Industries Ltd., on July 20, 1982, and October 19, 1982, respectively, U.S. Patents 4,340,598 and 4,355,040, Osaka, Japan, 1982.

41. Wong PC, Chiu AT, Price WA, et al. Nonpeptide angiotensin II receptor antagonists. I: Pharmacological characterization of 2-N-butyl-4-chloro-1 (2-chlorobenzyl)imidazole-5-acetic acid, sodium salt (S-8307). J Pharmacol Exp Ther 247:1–7, 1988.

42. Chiu AT, Duncia JV, McCall DE, et al. Nonpeptide angiotensin II receptor antagonists. III: Structure-function studies. J Pharmacol Exp. Ther 250:867–874, 1989.

43. Carini DJ, Duncia JV, Aldrich PE, et al. Nonpeptide angiotensin II receptor antagonists: The discovery of a series of N-biphenylmethyl-imidazoles as potent orally active antihypertensives. J Med Chem 34:2525–2547, 1991.

44. Wexler RR, Greenlee WJ, Irvin JD, et al. Nonpeptide angiotensin II receptor antagonists: The next generation in antihypertensive therapy. J Med Chum 39:626–656, 1996.

45. Wong PC, Price WA, Chiu AT, et al. Nonpeptide angiotensin antagonists. IX: Pharmacology of EXP3174: An active metabolite of DuP 753, an orally active antihypertensive agent. J Pharmacol Exp Ther 255:211–217, 1990.

46. Buhlmeyer P, Furet P, Criscione L, et al. Valsartan, a potent, orally active angiotensin II antagonist developed from the structurally new amino acid series. Bioorg Med Chem Lett 4:29–34, 1994.

47. Criscione L, de Gasparo M, Buhlmeyer P, et al. Pharmacologic profile of CGP-48933, a novel, nonpeptide antagonist of AT_1 angiotensin II receptor subtype. Br J Pharmacol 110:761–771, 1993.

48. Bernhart CA, Perreaut PM, Ferrari BP, et al. A new series of imidazolones: Highly specific and potent nonpeptide AT_1 angiotensin II receptor antagonist. J Med Chem 36:3371–3380, 1993.

49. Cazaubon C, Gougat J, Bouscet F, et al. Pharmacologic characterization of SR 47436: A new nonpeptide AT_1 subtype angiotensin II receptor antagonist. J Pharmacol Exp Ther 265: 826–834, 1993.

50. Kobo K, Kohara Y, Imamya E, et al. Nonpeptide angiotensin II receptor antagonists. Synthesis and biologic activity of benzimidazolecarboxylic acids. J Med Chem 36:2182–2195, 1993.

51. Kubo K, Kohara Y, Yoshimura Y, et al. Nonpeptide angiotensin II receptor antagonists. Synthesis and biologic activity of potential prodrugs of benzimidazole-7-carboxylic acids. J Med Chem 36:2343–2349, 1993.

52. Ries UJ, Mihm G, Narr B, et al. 6-Substituted benzimidazoles as new nonpeptide angiotensin II receptor antagonists: Synthesis, biological activity, and structure activity relationships. J Med Chem 36:4040–4051, 1993.

53. Wienen W, Hauel N, Van Meel JC, et al. Pharmacologic characterization of the novel nonpeptide angiotensin II receptor antagonist. BIBR 277. Br J Pharmacol 110:245–252, 1993.

54. Hartupee D, White V, Rovnyak L, et al. In vivo characterization of WAY-ANA-756, an angiotensin II antagonist. FASEB J 8:A5, 1994.

55. Elingboe JW, Antane M, Nguyen TT, et al. Pyrido[2,3-d]pyrimidine angiotensin II antagonists. J Med Chem 37:542–550, 1994.

56. Samamen JM, Peishoff CE, Keenan RM, Weinstock J: Refinement of a molecular model of angiotensin II employed in the discovery of potent nonpeptide antagonists. Bioorg Med Chem Lett 3:909–914, 1993.

57. Keenan RM, Weinstock J, Finkelstein JA, et al. Potent nonpeptide angiotensin II receptor antagonists. 1-(carboxybenzyl)imidazole-5-acrylic acids. J Med Chem 36:1880–1892, 1993.

58. Cody RJ, Haas GJ, Binkley PF, Brown DM. Hemodynamic and vascular characteristics of Dup 753: A specific angiotensin II antagonist in the spontaneously hypertensive rat (SHR). J Am Coll Cardiol 17 (suppl A):202A, 1991.

59. Timmermans PB, Duncia JV, Carini DJ, et al. Discovery of losartan, the first angiotensin II receptor antagonist. J Hum Hypertens 9(suppl 5):S3–S18, 1995.

60. Lacour C, Canals F, Galindo G, et al. Efficacy of SR 47436 (BMS-186295), a nonpeptide angiotensin AT_1 receptor antagonist in hypertensive rat models. Eur J Pharmacol 264:307–316, 1994.

61. Messerli FH, Weber MA, Brunner HR. Angiotensin II receptor inhibition: A new therapeutic principle. Arch Intern Med 156:1957–1965, 1996.

62. Brunner HR, Delacretaz E, Nussberger J, et al. Angiotensin II antagonists DuP 753 and TCV 116. J Hypertens Suppl 12:S29–S34 1994.

63. Gradman AH, Arcuri KE, Goldberg Al, et al. A randomized, placebo controlled, double-blind, parallel study of various doses of losartan potassium compared with enalapril maleate in patients with essential hypertension. Hypertension 25:1345–1350, 1995.

64. Wong PC, Hart SD, Timmermans PB. Effect of angiotensin II antagonism on canine renal sympathetic nerve function. Hypertension 17: 1127–1134. 1991.

65. Reid IA. Interactions between ANG II, sympathetic nervous system, and baroreceptor reflexes in regulation of blood pressure. Am J Physiol 262:E763–E778, 1992.

66. Goldberg M, Tanaka W, Burchowsky A, et al. Effects of losartan on blood pressure, plasma renin activity and angiotensin II in volunteers. Hypertension 21:704–713, 1993.

67. Hussain A. The chymase-angiotensin system in humans. J Hypertens 11:1155–1159, 1993.

68. Dzau VJ, Sasamura H, Hein L. Heterogeneity of angiotensin synthetic pathways and receptor subtypes: Physiological and pharmacological implications. Curr Opin Hypertens 1:3–9, 1993.

69. Bunkenburg B, van Amelsvoort T, Roog H, Wood JM. Receptor-mediated effects of angiotensin II on growth of vascular smooth muscle cells from spontaneously hypertensive rats. Hypertension 20:746–754, 1992.

70. Raya TE, Morkin E, Goldman S. Angiotensin antagonists in models of heart failure. *In* Saavedra JM, Timmermans PB (eds). Angiotensin Receptors. New York, London, Plenum, 1994; pp 309–318.

71. Schieffer B, Wirger A, Meybrunn M, et al. Comparative effect of chronic angiotensin-converting enzyme inhibition and angiotensin II type 1 receptor blockade on cardiac remodeling after myocardial infarction in the rat. Circulation 89:2273–2282, 1994.

72. Smits JF, van Krimpen C, Schoemaker RG, et al. Angiotensin II receptor blockade after myocardial infarction in rats: Effects on hemodynamics, myocardial DNA synthesis, and interstitial collagen content. J Cardiovasc Pharmacol 20:772–778, 1992.

73. Dahlof B. Effect of angiotensin II blockade on cardiac hypertrophy

and remodeling: A review. J Hum Hyperten 9(suppl 5):S37–S44, 1995.

74. Kaneko K, Susic D, Nunez E, Frolich E. Losartan reduces cardiac mass and improves coronary flow reserve in the spontaneously hypertensive rat. J Hypertens 14:645–654, 1996.

75. Braunwald E, Sarnoff SJ, Case RB. Hemodynamic determinants of coronary flow: Effect of changes in aortic pressure and cardiac output on the relationship between myocardial oxygen consumption and coronary flow. Am J Physiol 192: 157–163, 1958.

76. Dietz R, Waas W, Haberbosch W, et al. Modulation of coronary circulation and the cardiac matrix by the renin-angiotensin system. Eur Heart J 12(suppl F):107–111, 1991.

77. Chan DP, Sandok EK, Aarhus LL, et al. Renal specific effects of angiotensin II receptor antagonism in the anesthetized dog. Am J Hypertens 5(suppl 2):354–360, 1992.

78. Xie MH, Liu FY, Wong PC, et al. Proximal nephron and renal effects of DuP 753, a nonpeptide angiotensin II antagonist. Kidney Int 38:473–479, 1990.

79. Burnier MJ, Brunner HR. Angiotensin receptor antagonists and the kidney. Opin Nephrol Hypertens 3:537–545, 1994.

80. Bauer JH, Reams GP. The angiotensin II type I receptor antagonists: A new class of antihypertensive drugs. Arch Intern Med 155:1361–1368, 1995.

81. Burnier M, Brunner H. Angiotensin II receptor antagonists and the kidney. Curr Opin Hypertens 1:92–100 1995.

82. Gansesvoort RT, de Zeeuw D, Shahinfar S, et al. Effects of the angiotensin II antagonist losartan in hypertensive patients with renal disease. J Hypertens Suppl 12:S37–S42, 1994.

83. Price DA, De'Oliveira JM, Fisher ND, Hollenberg NK. Renal hemodynamic response to an angiotensin antagonist, eprosartan, in healthy men. Hypertension 30:240–246, 1997.

84. Burnier M, Roch-Ramel F, Brunner HR. Renal effects of angiotensin II receptor blockade in normotensive subjects. Kidney Int 49:1787–1790, 1996.

85. El Amrani Al, Philippe M, Michel JB. Bilateral renal responses to the angiotensin II receptor antagonist losartan, in 2K-1C Goldblatt hypertensive rats. J Hypertens 10(suppl 4):206, 1992.

86. Lee JY, Blaufox MD. Renal effect of DuP 753 in renovascular hypertension. Am J Hypertens 4: 84A, 1991.

87. Same DR, Ahrens ER. Renal impairment associated with losartan. Ann Intern Med 124:775, 1996.

88. Fenoy FJ, Milicic I, Smith RD, et al. Effects of DuP 753 on renal function of normotensive and spontaneously hypertensive rats. Am J Hypertens 4:321S–326S, 1991.

89. Balla T, Bankal AJ, Eng S, Catt KJ. Angiotensin II receptor subtypes and biological responses in the adrenal cortex and medulla. Mol Pharmacol 40:401–406, 1991.

90. Goldberg MR, Bradstreet TE, McWilliams EJ, et al. Biochemical effects of losartan, a nonpeptide angiotensin II receptor antagonist, on the renin-angiotensin-aldosterone system in hypertensive patients. Hypertension 25:37–46, 1995.

91. Nakashima M, Uematsu T, Kosuge K, Kanamaru M. Pilot study of the uricosuric effect of DuP-753, a new angiotensin II receptor antagonist in healthy subjects. Eur J Clin Pharmacol 42:333–335, 1992.

92. Moan A, Hoieggen A Nordby G, et al. Effects of losartan on insulin sensitivity in severe hypertension: Connections through sympathetic nervous activity? J Hum Hypertens 9(suppl 5):S45–S50, 1995.

93. Stadler T, Veltmar A, Qadri F, Unger T. Angiotensin II evokes noradrenaline release from the paraventricular nucleus in conscious rats. Brain Res 569:117–122, 1992.

94. Blair-West JR, Denton DA, McKinley MJ, Weisinger RS. Thirst and brain angiotensin in cattle. Am J Physiol 262: R204–R210, 1992.

95. Martin P. Antidepressant-like effects of DuP753, a nonpeptide angiotensin II receptor antagonist in the learned helplessness paradigm in rats. Presented at the Third World Congress of Neuroscience, Montreal, 1991.

96. Dahlof B, Lindholm L, Carney S, et al. Main results of the losartan versus amlodipine (LOA) study on drug tolerability and psychological general well-being. J Hypertens 15:1327–1335, 1997.

97. Ji H, Leung M, Zhang Y, et al. Differential structural requirements for specific binding of nonpeptide and peptide antagonists to the AT$_1$ angiotensin receptor: Identification of amino acid residues that determine binding of the antihypertensive drug losartan. J Biol Chum 269: 16533–16536, 1994.

98. Azizi M, Chatellier G, Guyene T, et al. Additive effects of combined angiotensin converting enzyme inhibition and angiotensin II antagonism on blood pressure and renin release in sodium depleted normotensives. Circulation 92:825–834, 1995.

99. Avapro (irbesartan), U.S. product information. In Physician's Desk Reference, 52nd ed. Montvale, NJ, Medical Economics, 1998.

100. Beevers D. Losartan: The first angiotensin receptor antagonist in clinical use. J Hum Hypertens 9(suppl 5):S1–S3, 1995.

101. Munafo A, Christen Y, Nussberger J, et al. Drug concentration response relationships in normal volunteers after oral administration of losartan, an angiotensin antagonist. Clin Pharmacol Ther 51:513–521, 1992.

102. Weber MA. Clinical experience with the angiotensin receptor antagonist losartan: A preliminary report. Am J Hypertens 5:247S–251S, 1992.

103. Ohtawa M, Takayama F, Saitoh K, et al. Pharmacokinetics and biochemical efficacy after single and multiple oral administration of losartan, an orally active nonpeptide angiotensin receptor antagonist, in humans. Br J Pharmacol 35:290–297, 1993.

104. Burnier M, Waeber B, Brunner H. Clinical pharmacology of the angiotensin II receptor antagonist losartan in healthy subjects. J Hypertens 13(Suppl 1):S23–S28, 1995.

105. Stearns R. Chakravarty P, Chen R, Chiu S. Biotransformation of losartan to its active carboxylic acid metabolite in human liver microsomes. Role of cytochrome P450C and 3A subfamily members. Drug Metab Dispos 23:207–215, 1995.

106. Cozaar (losartan potassium), U.S. product information. In Physician's Desk Reference. 52nd ed. Montvale, NJ, Medical Economics. 1998.

107. Lo M, Goldberg M, McCrea J, et al. Pharmacokinetics of losartan, an angiotensin II receptor antagonist, and its active metabolite EXP3174 in humans. Clin Pharmacol Ther 58:641–649, 1995.

108. Sica D, Lo M, Shaw W, et al. The pharmacokinetics of losartan in renal insufficiency. J Hypertens 13(suppl 1):S49–S52, 1995.

109. Kong A, Tomasko L, Waldman S, et al. Losartan does not affect the pharmacokinetics and pharmacodynamics of warfarin. J Clin Pharmacol 35:1008–1015, 1995.

110. De Smet M, Schoors D, De Meyer G, et al. Effect of multiple doses of losartan on the pharmacokinetics of single doses of digoxin in healthy volunteers. Br J Clin Pharmacol 40:571–575, 1995.

111. Kaukonen K, Olkkola K, Neuvonen P. Fluconazole but not itraconazole decreases the metabolism of losartan to E-3174. Eur J Clin Pharmacol 53:445–449, 1998.

112. Muller P, Flesch G, de Gasparo M, et al. Pharmacokinetics and pharmacodynamic effects of the angiotensin I antagonist valsartan at steady state in healthy, normotensive subjects. Eur J Clin Pharmacol 52:441–449, 1997.

113. Flesch G, Muller P, Lloyd P. Absolute bioavailability and pharmacokinetics of valsartan, an angiotensin II antagonist, in man. Eur J Clin Pharmacol 52:115–120, 1997.

114. Markham A, Goa K. Valsartan. A review of its pharmacology and therapeutic use in essential hypertension. Drugs 54:299–311, 1997.

115. Colussi D, Parisot C, Rossolino M, et al. Protein binding in plasma of valsartan, a new angiotensin II receptor antagonist. J Clin Pharmacol 37:214–221, 1997.

116. Brookman L, Rolan P, Benjamin I, et al. Pharmacokinetics of valsartan in patients with liver disease. Clin Pharmacol Ther 62:272–278, 1997.

117. Sioufi A, Marfil F, Jaouen A, et al. The effect of age on the pharmacokinetics of valsartan. Biopharm Drug Dispos 19:237–244, 1998.

118. Johnston CL, Risvanis J. Preclinical pharmacology of angiotensin II receptor antagonists. Am J Hypertens 10:306S–310S, 1997.

119. Ruilope L. Human pharmacokinetic/pharmacodynamic profile of irbesartan: A new potent angiotensin II receptor antagonist. J Hypertens 15(suppl 7): S15–S20, 1997.

120. Marino M, Langenbacher K, Ford N, Uderman H. Safety, tolerability, pharmacokinetics (PK) and pharmacodynamics (PD) of irbesartan after single and multiple doses in healthy male subjects. Clin Pharmacol Ther 61:207, 1997.

121. Brunner H. The new angiotensin II receptor antagonist, irbesartan pharmacokinetic and pharmacodynamic considerations. Am J Hypertens 10:311S–317S, 1997.

122. Nishikawa K, Naka T, Chatani F, Yoshimura Y. Candesartan cilexetil: A review of its preclinical pharmacology. J Hum Hypertens 11(suppl 2):S9–S17, 1997.

123. Sever P. Candesartan cilexetil: A new, long-acting, effective angiotensin II type 1 receptor blocker. J Hum Hypertens 11(suppl 2):S91–S95, 1997.

124. Hubner R, Hogemann A, Sunzel M, Riddel J. Pharmacokinetics of candesartan after single and repeated doses of candesartan cilexetil in young and elderly healthy volunteers. J Hum Hypertens 11(Suppl 2):S19–S25, 1997.

125. Riddell JG. Bioavailability of candesartan is unaffected by food in healthy volunteers administered candesartan cilexetil. J Hum Hypertens 11(suppl 2):S29–S30, 1997.

126. van Lier JJ, van Heiningen PNM, Sunzel M. Absorption, metabolism and excretion of 14C-candesartan and 14C-candesartan cilexetil in healthy volunteers. J Hum Hypertens 11(suppl 2):S27–S28, 1997.

127. de Zeeuw D, Remuzzi G, Kirch W. Pharmacokinetics of candesartan cilexetil in patients with renal or hepatic impairment. J Hum Hypertens 11(Suppl 2):S37–S42, 1997.

128. Jonkman JHG, van Lier JJ, van Heiningen PNM, et al. Pharmacokinetic drug interaction studies with candesartan cilexetil. J Hum Hypertens 11(suppl 2):S31–S35, 1997.

129. Edwards RM, Aiyar N, Ohlstein EH, et al. Pharmacological characterization of the nonpeptide angiotensin II receptor antagonist, SK & F 108566. J Pharmacol Exp Ther 260:175–181, 1992.

130. Cox PJ, Bush BD, Gorycki PD, et al. The metabolic fate of eprosartan in healthy subjects. Exp Toxicol Pathol 48(suppl II):75–82, 1996.

131. Tenero D, Martin D, Chapelsky MC, et al. Pharmacokinetics and protein binding of eprosartan in healthy volunteers and in patients with varying degrees of renal impairment. Pharmacotherapy 17:1114, 1997.

132. Tenero D, Martin D, Miller A, et al. Effect of age and gender on the pharmacokinetics and plasma protein binding of eprosartan. [Abstract] Pharmacotherapy 17:114, 1997.

133. McClellan KJ, Balfour JA Eprosartan Drugs 55:713–718, 1998.

134. Benz J, Oshrain C, Henry D, et al. Valsartan, a new angiotensin II receptor antagonist: A double-blind study comparing the incidence of cough with lisinopril and hydrochlorthiazide. J Clin Pharmacol 37:101–07, 1997.

135. Ramsay L, Yeo W. ACE inhibitors, angiotensin II antagonists and cough. The Losartan Cough Study Group. J Hum Hypertens 9(suppl 5):S51–S54, 1995.

136. Pouleur HG. Clinical overview of irbesartan. Am J Hypertens 10:318S–324S, 1997.

137. Acker CG, Greenberg A. Angioedema induced by the angiotensin II blocker losartan. N Engl J Med 333:1572, 1995.

138. Frye C, Pettigrew T. Angioedema and photosensitive rash induced by valsartan. Pharmacotherapy 18:866–868, 1998.

139. Smith R, Aurup P, Goldberg A, Snavely D. Long term safety of losartan in open label trials with mild to moderate essential hypertension. Am J Hypertens 11:43A, 1998.

140. Moore M. Efficacy of AT₁ receptor blockade in hypertension. Am J Hypertens 11:251A, 1998.

141. Oparil S, Dyke S, Harris F, et al. The efficacy and safety of valsartan compared with placebo in the treatment of patients with essential hypertension. Clin Ther 18:797–810, 1996.

142. Oparil S, Barr E, Telkins M, et al. Efficacy, tolerability, and effects on quality of life of losartan, alone or with hydrochlorthiazide, versus amlodipine, alone or with hydrochlorthiazide, in patients with essential hypertension. Clin Ther 18:608–625, 1996.

143. Holwerda N, Fofari R, Angeli P, et al. Valsartan, a new angiotensin II antagonist for the treatment of essential hypertension: Efficacy and safety compared with placebo and enalapril. J Hypertens 14:1147–1151, 1996.

144. Andersson OK, Neldam S. The antihypertensive effect and tolerability of candesartan cilexetil, a new generation angiotensin II antagonist, in comparison with losartan. Blood Press 7:53–59, 1998.

145. Bunt T, Dumswala A. Candesartan vs. losartan. J Hum Hypertens 12:419, 1998.

146. Nyman L, Quintiles A, Cullberg K, et al. Encapsulation of commercially available losartan does not influence its bioavailability. Am J Hypertens 11:77A, 1998.

147. Oparil S, Guthrie R, Lewin A, et al. An elective-titration study of the comparative effectiveness of two angiotensin II-receptor blockers, irbesartan and losartan. Clin Ther 20:398–409, 1998.

148. Cody R. The clinical potential of renin inhibitors and angiotensin antagonists. Drugs 47:586–598, 1994.

149. Harrap SB, Dominiczak AF, Fraser R, et al. Plasma angiotensin II, predisposition to hypertension, and left ventricular size in healthy young adults. Circulation 93:1148–1154, 1994.

150. Pitt B. ACE inhibitors in heart failure: Prospects and limitations. Cardiovasc Drugs Ther 11(suppl 1):285–290, 1997.

151. Regitz-Zagrosek V, Neuss M, Fleck E. Effects of angiotensin receptor antagonists in heart failure: Clinical and experimental aspects. Eur Heart J 16(suppl N):86–91, 1995.

152. Guazzi M, Melzi G, Agostoni P. Comparison of changes in respiratory function and exercise oxygen uptake with losartan versus enalapril in congestive heart failure secondary to ischemic or idiopathic dilated cardiomyopathy. Am J Cardiol 80:1572–1576, 1997.

153. Crosier I, Ikram H, Awan N, et al. Losartan in heart failure. Hemodynamic effects and tolerability. Losartan Hemodynamic Study Group. Circulation 91:691–697, 1995.

154. Pitt B. Segal R, Martinez FA, et al. Randomized trial of losartan versus captopril in patients over 65 with heart failure (Evaluation of Losartan in the Elderly Study, ELITE). Lancet 349:747–752, 1997.

155. Hamroff G, Blaufarb I, Mancini D, et al. Angiotensin II-receptor blockade further reduces afterload safely in patients maximally treated with angiotensin-converting enzyme inhibitors for heart failure. J Cardiovasc Pharmacol 30:533–611, 1997.

156. Pitt B, Chang P, Grossman W, et al. Rationale. background, and design of the randomized angiotensin receptor antagonist–angiotensin-converting enzyme inhibitor study (RAAS). Am J Cardiol 78:1129–1131, 1996.

157. Kaneko K, Susic D, Nunez E, Frohlich ED. Losartan reduces cardiac mass and improves coronary flow reserve in the spontaneously hypertensive rat. J Hypertens 14:645–653, 1996.

158. Ishiye M, Umemura K, Uematsu T, Nakashima M. Effects of losartan, an angiotensin II antagonist, on the development of cardiac hypertrophy due to volume overload. Biol Pharm Bull 18:700–704, 1995.

159. Taylor K, Patten RD, Smith JJ, et al. Divergent effects of angiotensin-converting enzyme inhibition and angiotensin II-receptor antagonism on myocardial cellular proliferation and collagen deposition after myocardial infarction in rats. J Cardiovasc Pharmacol 31:654–660, 1998.

160. Segar JL, Scholz TD, Bedell KA, et al. Angiotensin AT₁ receptor blockade fails to attenuate pressure-overload cardiac hypertrophy in fetal sheep. Am J Physiol 273:R1501–R1508, 1997.

161. Tedesco MA, Ratti G, Aquino D, et al. The effectiveness and tolerability of losartan and effect on left ventricular mass in patients with essential hypertension. Cardiologia 43:53–59, 1998.

162. Dahlof B, Devereux R, de Faire U, et al. The Losartan Intervention For Endpoint reduction (LIFE) in Hypertension Study. Rationale, design, and methods. The LIFE Study Group. Am J Hypertens 10:705–713, 1997.

163. Pollack D, Divish B, Polakowski J, Opgenorth T. Angiotensin II receptor blockade improves renal function in rats with reduced renal mass. J Pharmacol Exp Ther 267:657–663, 1993.

164. Okada H, Suzuki H, Kanno H, Saruta T. Renal responses to angiotensin receptor antagonists and angiotensin-converting enzyme inhibitor in partially nephrectomized spontaneously hypertensive rats. J Cardiovasc Pharmacol 26:564–560, 1995.

165. Remuzzi A, Perico N, Amuchastegui C, et al. Short and long term effect of angiotensin II receptor blockade in rats with experimental diabetes. J Am Soc Nephrol 4:40–49, 1993.

166. Obata J, Nakamura T, Kuroyanagi R, et al. Candesartan prevents the progression of glomerulosclerosis in genetically hypertensive rats. Kidney Int Suppl 63:S229–S231, 1997.

167. Tarif N, Bakris GL. Angiotensin II receptor blockade and progression of nondiabetic-mediated renal disease. Kidney Int Suppl 63:S67–S70, 1997.

168. Hutchison FN, Webster SK. Effect of AII receptor antagonist on albuminuria and renal function in passive Heimann nephritis. Am J Physiol 263:F311–F318, 1992.

169. Zoja C, Abbate M, Corna D, et al. Pharmacology's control of angiotensin II ameliorates renal disease while reducing renal TGF-beta in experimental mesangioproliferative glomerulonephritis. Am J Kidney Dis 31:453–463, 1998.

170. Gansevoort R, de Zeeuw D, de Jong P. Is the antiproteinuric effect of ACE inhibition mediated by interference in the renin-angiotensin system? Kidney Int 45:861–867, 1994.

171. Hollenberg NK. Non–insulin-dependent diabetes mellitus, nephropathy, and the renin system. J Hypertens 15(suppl 7):S7–S13, 1997.
172. Porush JG, Berl T, Anzalone DA. Multicenter collaborative trial of angiotensin II receptor antagonism on morbidity, mortality and renal function in hypertensive type II diabetic patients with nephropathy. Am J Hypertens 11:73A, 1998.
173. Camargo M, von Lutterotti N, Pecker M, et al. DuP753 increases survival in spontaneously hypertensive stroke-prone rats fed a high sodium diet. Am J Hypertens 4:341S, 1991.
174. Nishikawa K. Angiotensin AT$_1$ receptor antagonism and protection against cardiovascular end-organ damage. J Hum Hypertens 12:301–309, 1998.
175. Wienen W, Hauel N, vanMeel JC, et al. Pharmacological characterization of the novel nonpeptide angiotensin II receptor antagonist BIBR 277. Br J Pharmacol 110:245–252, 1993.
176. Micardis Prescribing Information. Boehringer Ingelheim Pharmaceuticals, Inc., 1999.
177. Neutel JM, Smith DHG. Dose response and pharmacokinetics of telmisartan, a new angiotensin II receptor blocker. J Hypertens 16(suppl 2):S210, 1998.

72

CHAPTER

Other Adrenergic Inhibitors and the Direct-Acting Smooth Muscle Vasodilators

Edward D. Frohlich

Since the early 1970s, antihypertensive drug therapy has made a tremendous impact on morbidity and mortality from cardiovascular diseases. Nevertheless, despite the introduction of newer modalities of treatment and the claims of adverse effects related to the adrenergic inhibitors and the direct-acting smooth muscle vasodilators, improvement in cardiovascular outcomes seems to have stalled. End-stage renal disease and congestive heart failure, both related to hypertension, continue to increase unabated.

Whereas use of many of the agents discussed in this chapter has drastically decreased in the United States in favor of newer agents with different mechanisms of action, the older agents continue to be used broadly elsewhere around the world. No doubt this is related to availability of generic formulations of these agents and their lower cost.

Among the more potent antihypertensive drugs are those that inhibit sympathetic activity. This inhibition may be achieved at practically any anatomical level of adrenergic function. However, for these compounds to maintain their effectiveness over time, for the most part, they must be used in conjunction with diuretics. The following discussion reviews these adrenolytic agents, describing their mechanisms of action, hemodynamic effects, their clinical uses, and adverse effects.

Every direct-acting smooth muscle vasodilator and adrenergic inhibitor except the β-adrenergic receptor blockers and, perhaps, the α-adrenergic blockers will induce compensatory sodium and water retention and extracellular fluid volume expansion following reduction of arterial pressure.[1–3] The clinician must therefore recognize the need for concomitant diuretic therapy. The type of diuretic is relatively unimportant: Drastic dietary sodium restriction, a thiazide diuretic, or a loop diuretic can be employed. However, since it is most important to minimize potassium wastage and maintain persistent and steady contraction of the intravascular volume, a thiazide is generally the best choice for patients with relatively normal renal function because it has a longer duration of action than the loop diuretic. The diuretic enhances the antihypertensive action of the adrenergic inhibitor by maintaining the contraction of the extracellular and intravascular compartments.

ADRENERGIC INHIBITORS

Stress and anxiety can alter cardiovascular function, producing transient increases in heart rate and arterial blood pressure. However, these stimuli are generally not sufficient to cause hypertension, which requires persistent increased tension or tone of the arteriolar vascular smooth muscle for its maintenance. Confusion in terminology can confound any discussion of agents that inhibit neural function. The present discussion does not concern itself with agents that sedate, tranquilize, or minimize psychic stress through higher centers.

Central adrenergic efferent impulses pass through major cardiovascular centers in the hypothalamic, medullary, and other subcortical areas to the spinal cord to synapse with second neurons located in sympathetic ganglia at the thoracolumbar level of the spinal column. These more distal neurons are stimulated at the ganglion level by the release of acetylcholine from the terminals of the central neurons, thereby propagating the peripheral outflow of adrenergic impulses. Neural impulses, passing distally via the adrenergic neurons, reach the heart or blood vessels, where they release norepinephrine from nerve terminals. Norepinephrine stimulates the effector organ—heart, venule, or arteriole—by attachment to specific binding sites identified as either α- or β-adrenergic receptors.

Norepinephrine and other neurohumoral mediators, including epinephrine and dopamine, are synthesized in the adrenal gland and adrenergic neurons, but norepinephrine is the major neurotransmitter that is released from postganglionic nerve terminals. Norepinephrine synthesis begins with the essential amino acid, L-tyrosine, by hydroxylation with tyrosine hydroxylase to form L-hydroxyphenylalanine and then L-hydroxyphenylethylamine (dopamine). Dopamine β-hydroxylase and phenylethanolamine-N-methyltransferase continue the biosynthesis of the catecholamines to form L-norepinephrine and L-epinephrine, respectively. Norepinephrine is the major neurotransmitter and is most responsible for adrenergic receptor stimulation. Norepinephrine is found in the axon sheath and stored in the nerve terminals in vesicles that release it on nerve stimulation.

Norepinephrine is metabolized within the nerve terminal, by monoamine oxidase (MAO) in the mitochondria via a deamination process to form, initially, dihydroxymandelic acid and, later, vanillylmandelic acid. In contrast, the norepinephrine that finds its way extraneuronally is metabolized by the enzyme catechol O-methyltransferase to form 3-methoxy,4-hydroxymandelic acid or vanillylmandelic acid. These metabolic products can be measured in the laboratory as metanephrines and normetanephrines or vanillylmandelic acid, respectively. Consideration of these metabolic processes is important in the interpretation of laboratory tests utilized in the diagnosis of pheochromocytoma, particularly in the identification of therapeutic agents that may be responsible for false-positive or false-negative test results.

With the arrival of the adrenergic impulse at the nerve terminal, there is release of free norepinephrine. The neurotransmitter may bind to myocardial and/or vascular smooth muscle receptor sites, producing the adrenergic cardiovascular response. It may also be taken up by the nerve terminal for conservation and release at a later time or may be acted on by the extraneuronal enzymatic system to form the metabolites or to circulate freely within the vascular system. The normal circulating levels of epinephrine and norepinephrine are less than 100 pg/ml and less than 500 pg/ml, respectively; the daily urinary excretion rates of catecholamines and metabolites are shown in Table 72–1.

With the binding of norepinephrine at the effector site, several possible processes may occur. Stimulation of the α-adrenergic receptor will produce vasoconstriction of the arteriole and venule. Stimulation of the β-adrenergic receptor will promote peripheral vasodilatation and increased heart rate, myocardial contractility, and myocardial metabolism.

There are many loci at which antihypertensive agents may inhibit the adrenergic nerve stimulus, including afferent sensory pathways from the heart, vessels, and mechanoreceptors, centrally at the ganglion level, or at the nerve terminal. Antihypertensive agents can inhibit norepinephrine biosynthesis or block its action at the adrenergic receptor. The following discussion concerns the specifics of each class of adrenergic inhibitors.

Ganglion Blocking Drugs

MECHANISM OF ACTION. When the adrenergic preganglionic impulse arrives at the ganglion, acetylcholine is released from the nerve terminals, crosses the synaptic gap, and stimulates the postganglionic axons. The physiochemical action on the axon membrane is complex but, in simplest terms, involves the alteration of axon permeability. Thus, when acetylcholine attaches to receptor sites on the axon membrane, transmembrane ion flux is permitted, by which potassium ions move extracellularly and sodium ions intracellularly. When this depolarization process reaches an optimal rate, transmission of the neural impulse down the postganglionic neuron continues.[4]

One of the first major classes of antihypertensive drugs was the ganglion blockers.[5] These agents act by occupying receptor sites on the postganglionic axon to stabilize the membrane against acetylcholine stimulation; they have no effect on preganglionic neuronal acetylcholine release, cholinesterase activity, postganglionic neuronal catecholamine release, or vascular smooth muscle contractility.[4–6] Tetraethylammonium chloride was the first agent used; later, other compounds were synthesized, including hexamethonium chloride, pentolinium tartrate, mecamylamine hydrochloride, pempidine hydrochloride, and chlorisondamine chloride. In a controlled, prospective, double-blind study involving three of the more commonly used ganglion blocking drugs (at the time of their popular use), when equivalent doses of these agents were employed, all three agents were equally efficacious in reducing arterial blood pressure.[7]

Because interference with transmission of the autonomic impulse at the ganglion level impairs adrenergic and parasympathetic impulse transmission, clinical use of ganglion blockers was associated with severe side effects of unwanted parasympathetic inhibition. With the advent of more specific adrenergic blocking drugs, such as guanethidine sulfate and methyldopa, the ganglion blocking drugs were less frequently used, until at present they are mostly of academic interest.

The exception is trimethaphan camsylate, which is still useful as an antihypertensive agent because of its intravenous formulation and mode of action. Trimethaphan is infused by slow intravenous drip (1 mg in a 1-L solution with the addition of one or two additional 1000-mg ampules, if necessary).[8] Reduction of arterial blood pressure is immediate, and careful monitoring of pressure is essential. When the infusion is discontinued, return of arterial blood pressure to preinfusion levels is prompt. Therefore, when administering this agent to the severely hypertensive patient, the physician must initiate long-acting antihypertensive therapy before discontinuing the infusion. Further, as with any adrenergic inhibitor, volume contraction is associated with augmented hypotensive responses, and norepinephrine administration is associated with an enhanced pressor response. This phenomenon of denervation supersensitivity is extremely important in patients treated with sympatholytic agents.[9]

HEMODYNAMIC EFFECTS. Adrenergic transmission to the heart and vessels is impaired by ganglion blocking drugs, and reduced heart rate, myocardial contractility, and total peripheral resistance result. The fall in arterial pressure and resistance is not as great in the supine as in the upright position because the adrenergic venomotor effect is enhanced by the gravitational effect of pooling when the

Table 72–1 24-Hour Urinary Excretion Rate of Catecholamines and Metabolites	
CATECHOLAMINES	
Norepinephrine	0.100 μg
Epinephrine	0–25 μg
Dopamine	60–440 μg
METABOLITES	
HVA	0–15.0 mg
VMA	0–7.0 mg
Metanephrine	30–350 μg
Normetanephrine	50–650 μg

Abbreviations: HVA, homovanillic acid; VMA, vanillylmandelic acid.

patient is upright. As a result of a reduction in venomotor tone, the patient treated with ganglion blocking drugs or any other sympatholytic therapy will pool blood in the capacitance vessels of the dependent areas of the body. As a result, venous return to the heart is reduced in proportion to the degree of adrenergic inhibition and the degree of upright posture. This effect explains the phenomenon of orthostatic hypotension that, if carried to the extreme, can be associated with syncope.[10] Thus, the orthostatic fall in cardiac output is not predominantly the result of direct adrenergic inhibition of myocardial function but of reduced venous return. Since the orthostatic effect on arterial blood pressure is so important with sympatholytic therapy, the knowledgeable physician should measure blood pressure in the supine or sitting as well as in the standing position. The orthostatic hypotension should be considered an effect of treatment rather than a side effect. To enhance the antihypertensive effect of sympatholytic agents in the supine position, it is necessary to reduce intravascular (and extracellular fluid) volume.[2, 3, 11] Further, to artificially produce this orthostatic response, elevation of the head of the bed is a worthwhile maneuver. Since cardiac output is reduced with ganglion blocking therapy, there is at least a proportionate reduction of renal blood flow, which may be associated with a reduced creatinine clearance.[12, 13] Cerebral[14] and splanchnic[15] blood flows are also reduced.

SIDE EFFECTS. It is often stated that, with prolonged hypotensive therapy with trimethaphan (48 to 72 hours), the patient frequently becomes refractory to the treatment.[14] Although this may occur, expansion of intravascular volume is more likely, and better control of pressure may be achieved with introduction of a diuretic or more vigorous use of diuretics.[1, 2] Moreover, contraction of intravascular volume produces exaggerated hypotension and adrenergic stimulation (e.g., with norepinephrine). Since parasympathetic inhibition also results from ganglion blockade, tonic activity to the gastrointestinal tract will occur, and the physician is cautioned to consider development of a paralytic ileus or acute urinary retention as a possible side effect. Thus, abdominal pain with reduced bowel sounds, constipation, or reduced urinary output during ganglion blocking therapy in a patient with aortic dissection may not reflect extension of the dissecting aneurysm into the mesenteric or renal arteries, but instead may be a side effect of the medication.

CLINICAL USES. Although several other potent and rapidly acting parenteral antihypertensive agents are available, there is still a role for trimethaphan in the treatment of hypertensive emergencies. Thus, in producing controlled hypotension during surgery, in arteriography, or in acute aortic dissection, trimethaphan-induced hypotension may be more manageable than hypotension induced by an agent with a more prolonged action. Under these circumstances, ganglion blockade will not be associated with the secondary reflective stimulation of the heart that is found with other vasodilator therapy.

Postganglionic Adrenergic Inhibitors

When acetylcholine stimulates the postganglionic axon at the ganglion level, the impulse is propagated distally and culminates in the release of norepinephrine at the nerve terminal with stimulation of adrenergic receptors on the vascular smooth muscle membrane. This impulse can be interfered with pharmacologically by a variety of mechanisms, including depletion of neurohumoral stores at the nerve terminal, prevention of norepinephrine reuptake by the nerve terminal, inhibition of catecholamine biosynthesis, therapeutic introduction of false neurohumoral transmitters that bind to the adrenergic receptors on vascular smooth muscle, or blockade of the latter receptors. The following discussion concerns sympathetic blocking drugs that act through one or a combination of these mechanisms.

Rauwolfia Alkaloids

These agents, including reserpine and more than 20 related compounds, were initially introduced for the treatment of hypertension in the early 1950s. They deplete the myocardium, blood vessels, adrenergic nerve terminals, adrenal medulla, and brain of catecholamines and serotonin.[16, 17] By depleting the nerve terminal of norepinephrine stores and inhibiting norepinephrine reuptake, adrenergic transmission is altered so that vascular resistance falls. With prolonged treatment, the persistent arterial hypotension is associated with slight decreases in renal blood flow and glomerular filtration rate. This may be related to a reduction in cardiac output or a venodilator effect similar to that of ganglion blocking drugs.[17, 18] Although arterial dilatation with increased blood flow has been considered greatest in the skin, other vascular beds are also involved (e.g., nasal stuffiness, a frequent complaint, is ameliorated by nasally administered vasoconstrictors).[19, 20]

SIDE EFFECTS. Because the inhibitory effect of the rauwolfia alkaloids is selective for adrenergic function, parasympathetic activity remains unopposed. Thus, bradycardia, prolonged atrioventricular conduction, nasal dilatation and stuffiness, increased gastric acid secretion with possible secondary peptic ulceration, and frequency of bowel movements are adverse effects of these drugs.[20] These effects may be counteracted by parasympathetic inhibitors or by intranasally administered vasoconstrictors. As a result of depletion of brain catecholamines and serotonin, there may be behavioral alterations and subtle or overt depression, sometimes leading to suicide.[21]

CLINICAL USES. Reserpine and similar alkaloids are efficacious in reducing arterial pressure to normal levels when used with diuretics and/or hydralazine.[22, 23] When reserpine is used in doses of 0.10 to 0.50 mg/day (or with whole-root preparations, 50 to 100 mg), it synergizes the antihypertensive action of these two agents. Reserpine and other sympatholytic agents have been useful in treating hypertensive emergencies and the cardiovascular manifestations of thyrotoxicosis without altering thyroid function.[24, 25]

Guanethidine and Bretylium

These agents interfere with adrenergic neurotransmission at the postganglionic nerve terminals. Like reserpine, these compounds deplete nerve terminals, blood vessels, and myocardium of catecholamine stores. However, unlike reserpine, they have little effect on catecholamine stores in the adrenal and brain. Furthermore, even though they fail to deplete normal adrenal medullary catecholamines, they can release these substances from a pheochromocytoma, producing an alarming and dramatic hypertensive crisis. With catecholamine depletion and impairment of chemical neurotransmission, denervation supersensitivity of effector cells is achieved.[26, 27]

HEMODYNAMIC EFFECTS. After injection of guanethidine or bretylium, there is a transitory pressor phase associated with an increased heart rate and cardiac output related to catecholamine release. A prolonged period of cardiac, vascular, and nerve terminal catecholamine depletion follows, associated with progressive reductions in systemic and pulmonary arterial pressure. The pressure reduction, brought about through an interference in chemical neurotransmission, can be explained by a reduction in vascular resistance. This hypotension is not as great in the supine position as in the upright posture or with agents that simultaneously contract or prevent reexpansion of plasma volume.[1-3] Because of the coincidental inhibition of venous tone,[19] venous return to the heart is reduced by peripheral pooling of blood in dependent areas of the body with upright posture. As a result, cardiac output falls and enhances the hypotensive action of guanethidine by this effect (not a side effect) of orthostatic hypotension.[28, 29] As a result of diminished systemic blood flow, there is a proportionate reduction in organ blood flows.[29-32] The renal and splanchnic areas may receive a smaller proportion of the total cardiac output, but glomerular filtration rate and renal function appear to return toward normal with time.[30-33] With reduced skeletal muscle blood flow and adrenergic innervation to skeletal muscle, resting muscle weakness may result that can be exacerbated by diuretic treatment.[34, 35] This muscle weakness may be aggravated further during or immediately after exercise when, because of arteriolar dilatation, increased muscle flow, and passively increased peripheral pooling of blood, cardiac output becomes so reduced that the patient becomes symptomatic.[36]

SIDE EFFECTS. Many of the side effects of guanethidine (orthostatic hypotension, exercise hypotension, bradycardia, increased gastric secretion) result from unopposed parasympathetic activity and impaired adrenergic function. Similarly, diarrhea, retrograde ejaculation, and fluid retention may be explained by reduced adrenergic transmission. Many of these side effects may be counteracted by reduced guanethidine dosage, addition of parasympatholytic agents, or addition of a diuretic.[37] Because guanethidine acts by entering the nerve terminal and interfering with neurohumoral transmission, any agent that prevents this will block the action of guanethidine. This is the means by which the tricyclic antidepressants—imipramine, desipramine, and protriptyline compounds—act.[38, 39] Therefore, guanethidine, guanadrel, and bretylium should not be prescribed for any patient receiving these psychoactive agents.

CLINICAL USES. Because of the prolonged action of guanethidine, it need be prescribed only once daily (25 to 150 mg). Moreover, since sympathetic inhibition is usually maximal with bedrest, there is little to be gained by prescribing it in divided doses. Further, since fluid retention and expanded intravascular and extracellular fluid volumes

are most pronounced with potent adrenolytic agents, a diuretic is indicated for use with guanethidine with the caveat that patients should be observed carefully for hypokalemia and impaired renal excretory function. This phenomenon of fluid reexpansion explains most of the refractoriness to guanethidine and other sympatholytic therapy, since impairment in drug absorption over time seems unlikely.[37] Moreover, when a diuretic is added to guanethidine, care should be exercised to determine development of symptomatic orthostatic hypotension.

Methyldopa, Clonidine, Guanabenz, and Guanfacine

The mechanisms of the antihypertensive effects of these adrenergic inhibitors are different from those of the foregoing agents. Originally, the antihypertensive action of methyldopa was believed to be exerted through tissue depletion of biogenic amines via inhibition of dopa decarboxylase.[40] However, although methyldopa does inhibit dopa decarboxylase, that mechanism contributes minimally to its blood pressure–lowering effect. Instead, methyldopa lowers blood pressure by being converted to α-methyl-norepinephrine, a metabolite that displaces norepinephrine from the α-adrenergic receptor site, thereby preventing the neurotransmitter from producing vascular smooth muscle stimulation. Even more importantly, this metabolite of methyldopa as well as clonidine and the other agents in this group stimulate adrenergic receptors in central vasomotor centers (e.g., nucleus tractus solitarii), thereby inhibiting sympathetic outflow from the brain.[41-47]

HEMODYNAMIC EFFECTS. Shortly after their administration (by mouth or by injection), these agents cause a progressive decrease in arterial pressure and heart rate that is associated with a reduction in cardiac output or total peripheral resistance, or both.[37, 48] With time, the reduction in cardiac output becomes less apparent, and the renal blood flow is maintained.[49]

CLINICAL USES. Methyldopa has been useful in all types and degrees of severity of hypertension. It is effective in reducing supine pressure without associated orthostatic hypotension in doses from 250 mg to 2.0 g daily. This antihypertensive effect may diminish if methyldopa is used as monotherapy; its effectiveness can be restored and enhanced with a diuretic. Similar indications apply to clonidine and the other centrally active α-adrenergic receptor blockers. Another use for clonidine is in the diagnosis of pheochromocytoma: When 0.1 mg of clonidine is administered hourly for 3 doses, the plasma norepinephrine levels fall in patients with essential hypertension, but remain elevated in those with pheochromocytoma.[50] Further, clonidine can be administered via transdermal patches.

SIDE EFFECTS. As with any antihypertensive agent that inhibits sympathetic nervous system activity, most anticipated side effects (postural hypotension, weakness, fluid retention, gastrointestinal symptoms) may be related to its adrenolytic action or the resultant overriding of parasympathetic function, or both. Additional side effects characteristic of methyldopa, including somnolence and depressive reactions, may be related to its action on biogenic amine stores in the brain.[37] Methyldopa also may produce a flulike syndrome characterized primarily by a fever as high as 41°C (105°F);[51] when therapy is discontinued, the fever disappears. This problem may be related to hepatocellular damage without jaundice or development of a positive direct Coombs test that, rarely, may be associated with hemolytic anemia.[37, 52] In general, therapy may be maintained with methyldopa in the presence of a positive direct Coombs test; however, if anemia occurs, the therapy should be discontinued.[53] Other side effects attributable to agents of this class include dry mouth, somnolence, and depression.[54] Sudden withdrawal of clonidine therapy has been associated with severe rebound hypertension.[55]

Monoamine Oxidase Inhibitors

Although still prescribed by some physicians as antihypertensive agents, their inclusion is merited only because of their potentially dangerous side effects. The first therapeutic use of MAOs was administration of iproniazid for tuberculosis. It was soon learned that these compounds had mood-elevating effects[56] and ameliorated chest pain of coronary arterial insufficiency.[54] At present, their major role is in the treatment of mental depression,[54] but one compound, pargyline hydrochloride, was introduced primarily as an antihypertensive agent.[37] MAOs may actually aggravate hypertension by inhibiting norepinephrine metabolism.[54] Since MAO is inhibited in the postganglionic nerve terminal, several weakly pressor amines (e.g., dopamine, octopamine) accumulate at this site. These substances are believed to act as false neurohumoral transmitters, tending to elevate blood pressure.[57]

HEMODYNAMIC EFFECTS. Only a relatively few hypertensive patients have been studied, and the results have not been striking. One report claimed marked reduction in arterial pressure and vascular resistance and a moderate impairment in glomerular filtration.[58]

SIDE EFFECTS. In addition to mental/emotional reactions, including euphoria, insomnia, and acute psychoses, hepatocellular necrosis, blood dyscrasias, and symptoms of adrenergic inhibition occur.[37] Most important is the severe acute hypertensive crisis that has been observed repeatedly following the ingestion of certain foods containing tyramine (e.g., aged cheeses, beer, sherry, Chianti wine, and herring) while the patient is receiving MAOs (e.g., pargyline hydrochloride, tranylcypromine sulfate, phenelzine sulfate, nialamide, iproniazid).[59–61]

CLINICAL USES. Because of the potentially severe hypertensive crises that may be associated with these antihypertensive drugs, they should be considered primarily of academic interest in the treatment of hypertension.[37]

Veratrum Alkaloids

These compounds are of importance because of their availability, potent antihypertensive efficacy, and unusual mode of action. They alter the responsiveness of the vagal afferent nerve fibers in the coronary sinus, left ventricle, and carotid sinus so that any pressure stimulus will result in increased nerve traffic. This stimulus is interpreted in the medullary vasomotor centers as reflecting a higher pressure

than actually exists as a result of an induced delay in the vagal repolarization process.[62, 63]

HEMODYNAMIC EFFECTS. As a result of this altered afferent input to the central vasomotor centers, there is a reflexive fall in systolic and diastolic pressure and heart rate; the latter response may be abolished by atropine sulfate. Since adrenergic function is not blocked, only reset at a different pressure level, the usual postural and adrenergic reflective responses are not altered. The result is a significant fall in total peripheral resistance with little change in cardiac output despite the rather marked bradycardia. Cerebral and renal blood flow and glomerular filtration rate remain normal unless the hypotensive response is excessive.[63]

SIDE EFFECTS. Because of the narrow therapeutic index, the effective control of arterial pressure by the veratrum alkaloids is not infrequently associated with side effects, including nausea, vomiting, excessive salivation and diaphoresis, blurred vision, and mental confusion. These effects have been reduced slightly by combined use with other antihypertensives.

CLINICAL USES. Clinical use of the veratrum alkaloids has been restricted severely by their side effects. A parenteral agent (cryptenamine tannate [Unitensin], 1.0 mg) has been useful in the treatment of certain hypertensive emergencies, including eclampsia.

DIRECT-ACTING VASCULAR SMOOTH MUSCLE RELAXANTS

With the introduction of β-adrenergic blocking therapy, a resurgence in interest in direct-acting smooth muscle vasodilating drugs for hypertension occurred. These agents have also been used with varying success in patients with cardiac failure. Hydralazine and minoxidil act by decreasing arteriolar resistance. With the fall in total peripheral resistance and arterial pressure, a reflex stimulation of the heart occurs so that tachycardia and palpitations frequently result unless these cardiac reflexive responses are offset by an adrenergic inhibitor (e.g., a β-adrenergic receptor blocking drug). These agents should not be administered to patients with hypertension who have myocardial infarction, angina pectoris, or aortic dissection because the reflexive cardiac effects will aggravate these underlying cardiac conditions. Other side effects include headaches and nasal stuffiness—attributable to the local vasodilatation—and fluid retention and edema (i.e., pseudotolerance), which occurs more frequently with minoxidil.

A unique side effect of hydralazine is precipitation of a lupus erythematosus–like syndrome, which occurs more frequently in patients who are receiving more than 400 mg/day of hydralazine. A common side effect from minoxidil is hirsutism, which is particularly bothersome to women. When hydralazine is administered by injection (10 to 15 mg intravenously), a prompt reduction in pressure occurs.

Another parenteral vasodilator, diazoxide, is a nonnatriuretic thiazide congener that must be injected rapidly (in single-bolus doses of 300 mg or in successive pulsed-bolus divided doses) to prevent binding to circulating albumin.

Diazoxide should not be administered to the patient with hypertension who has cardiac failure, angina pectoris, myocardial infarction, or an active aortic dissection. However, it has been useful for the patient with hypertensive encephalopathy, intracranial hemorrhage, and severe malignant or accelerated hypertension (without cardiac failure) in whom rapid and immediate reduction in arterial pressure is mandatory.

References

1. Weil JV, Chidsey CA. Plasma volume expansion resulting from interference with adrenergic function in normal man. Circulation 37:54–61, 1968.
2. Dustan HP, Tarazi RC, Bravo EL. Dependence of arterial pressure on intravascular volume in treated hypertensive patients. N Engl J Med 286:861–866, 1972.
3. Dustan HP, Cumming GR, Corcoran AC, Page IH. A mechanism of chlorothiazide-enhanced effectiveness of antihypertensive ganglioplegic drugs. Circulation 19:360–365, 1959.
4. Patton WDM. Transmission and block in autonomic ganglia. Pharmacol Rev 6:59–67, 1954.
5. Smirk FH. Methonium compounds in hypertension. Lancet 2:477, 1950.
6. Patton WDM, Zaimis EJ. The methonium compounds. Pharmacol Rev 4:219–253, 1952.
7. Veterans Administration Cooperative Study on Antihypertensive Agents. Double-blind control study of antihypertensive agents. II: Further report on the comparative effectiveness of reserpine, reserpine and hydralazine, and three ganglion blocking agents, chlorisondamine, mecamylamine, and pentolinium tartrate. Arch Intern Med 110:222–229, 1962.
8. Bhatia S, Frohlich ED. A hemodynamic comparison of agents useful in hypertensive emergencies. Am Heart J 85:367–373, 1973.
9. Cannon WB, Rosenbleuth A. The Supersensitivity of Denervation Structures: A Law of Denervation. New York, Macmillan, 1949.
10. Freis ED, Rose JC, Partenope EA, et al. The hemodynamic effects of hypotensive drugs in man. II: Hexamethonium. J Clin Invest 32:1285–1298, 1953.
11. Takagi H, Dustan HP, Page IH. Relationship among intravascular volume, total body sodium, arterial pressure, and vasomotor tone. Circ Res 9:1233–1239, 1961.
12. Ford RV, Moyer JH, Spurr CL. Hexamethonium in the chronic treatment of hypertension: Its effects on renal hemodynamics and on the excretion of water and electrolytes. J Clin Invest 32:1133–1139, 1953.
13. Ullmann TD, Menczel J. The effect of a ganglion blocking agent (hexamethonium) on renal function and on excretion of water and electrolytes in hypertension and in congestive heart failure. Am Heart J 52:106–120, 1956.
14. Finnerty FA, Witkin L, Fazekas JF. Cerebral hemodynamics in acute hypotension. J Clin Invest 33:933, 1954.
15. Reynolds TB, Paton A, Freeman M, et al. The effect of hexamethonium bromide in splanchnic blood flow, oxygen consumption and glucose output in man. J Clin Invest 32:793–800, 1953.
16. Pletschet A, Shore PA, Brodie BB. Serotonin release as a possible mechanism of reserpine action. Science 122:374–375, 1955.
17. Brest AN, Onesti G, Swartz C, et al. Mechanisms of antihypertensive drug therapy. JAMA 211:480–484, 1970.
18. Moyer JH. Cardiovascular and renal hemodynamic response to reserpine (Serpasil) and clinical results of using this agent for treatment of hypertension. Ann N Y Acad Sci 59:82–94, 1954.
19. Gaffney TE, Bryant WM, Braunwald E. Effects of reserpine and guanethidine on venous reflexes. Circ Res 11:889–894, 1962.
20. Frohlich ED. Inhibition of adrenergic function in the treatment of hypertension. Arch Intern Med 133:1033–1048, 1974.
21. Freis ED. Metal depression in hypertensive patients treated for long periods with large doses of reserpine. N Engl J Med 251:1006–1008, 1954.
22. Veterans Administration Cooperative Study Group on Antihypertensive Agents. Effects of treatment in morbidity in hypertension: Results in patients with diastolic blood pressures averaging 115 through 129 mm Hg. JAMA 202:116–122, 1967.
23. Veterans Administration Cooperative Study Group on Antihypertensive Agents. Effects of treatment in morbidity in hypertension. II: Results in patients with diastolic blood pressure averaging 90 through 114 mm Hg. JAMA 213:1143–1152, 1970.
24. Canary JJ, Schaaf M, Duffy BJ Jr, Kyle LH. Effects of oral and intramuscular administration of reserpine in thyrotoxicosis. N Engl J Med 257:435–442, 1957.
25. Waldstein SS, West GH Jr, Lee WLY, Bronsky D. Guanethidine in hyperthyroidism. JAMA 189:609–612, 1964.
26. McCubbin JW, Kaneko Y, Page IH. The peripheral cardiovascular actions of guanethidine in dogs. J Pharmacol Exp Ther 181:346–354, 1961.
27. Emmelin N, Engstrom J. Supersensitivity of salivary glands following treatment with bretylium or guanethidine. Br J Pharmacol Chemother 16:315–319, 1961.
28. Frohlich ED, Freis ED. Clinical trial of guanethidine: A new type of antihypertensive agent. Med Ann D C 28:419–423, 1959.
29. Cohn JN, Liptak TE, Freis ED. Hemodynamic effect of guanethidine in man. Circ Res 12:298–307, 1963.
30. Villarreal H, Exaire JB, Rubio V, D'Avila H. Effects of guanethidine and bretylium tosylate on systemic and renal hemodynamics in essential hypertension. Am J Cardiol 14:633–640, 1964.
31. Gaffney TE, Braunwold E, Cooper T. Analysis of the acute circulatory effects of guanethidine and bretylium. Circ Res 10:83–88, 1962.
32. Novack P. The effect of guanethidine on renal, cerebral, and cardiac hemodynamics. In Brest AN, Moyer JH (eds). Hypertension, Recent Advances. Philadelphia, Lea & Febiger, 1961; pp 444–448.
33. Williams RL, Mains JE III, Pearson JE. Direct and systemic effects of guanethidine on renal function. J Pharmacol Exp Ther 177:69–77, 1971.
34. Bowman WC, Notts MW. Actions of sympathomimetic amines and their antagonists on skeletal muscle. Pharmacol Rev 21:27–72, 1969.
35. Chrysant S, Frohlich ED. Antihypertensive drugs: The pathophysiology of their side effects. Am Fam Physician 9:94–101, 1974.
36. Khatri IM, Cohn HN. Mechanism of exercise hypotension after sympathetic blockade. Am J Cardiol 25:329–338, 1970.
37. Page LB, Sidd JJ. Medical management of primary hypertension. N Engl J Med 287:967–967, 1018–1023, 1074–1081, 1972.
38. Mitchell JR, Arias L, Oates JA. Antagonism of the antihypertensive action of guanethidine sulfate by desipramine hydrochloride. JAMA 202:149–152, 1967.
39. Mitchell JR, Cavanaugh JH, Arias L, Oates JA. Guanethidine and related agents. III: Antagonism by drugs which inhibit the norepinephrine pump in man. J Clin Invest 49:1596–1604, 1970.
40. Oates JA, Gillespie L, Undenfriend S, Sjoerdsma A. Decarboxylase, inhibition and blood pressure reduction by α-methyl-3,4-dihydroxy-DL-phenylalanine. Science 131:1890–1891, 1960.
41. Kopin IJ. False adrenergic transmitters. Ann Rev Pharmacol 8:377–394, 1968.
42. Henning M, van Zwieten PA. Central hypotensive effect of α-methyldopa. J Pharm Pharmacol 20:409–417, 1968.
43. Ingenito AJ, Barrett JP, Procita L. A centrally mediated peripheral hypotensive effect of α-methyldopa. J Pharmacol Exp Ther 175:593–599, 1970.
44. Sattler RW, van Zwieten PA: Acute hypotensive action of 2-(2,6-dichlorophenylamino)-2-imidazoline hydrochloride (ST 155) after infusion into the cat's vertebral artery. Eur J Pharmacol 2:9–13, 1967.
45. Schmitt H, Boissier JR, Giudicelli JF. Centrally mediated decrease in sympathetic tone induced by 2-(2,6-dichlorophenylamine)-2-imidazoline (ST 155, Catapressan). Eur J Pharmacol 2:147–148, 1967.
46. Katie F, Lavery H, Lowe RD. The central action of clonidine and its antagonism. Br J Pharmacol 44:779–787, 1972.
47. Kobinger W, Walland A. Investigations into the mechanism of the hypotensive effect of 2-(2,6-dichlorophenylamine)-2-imidazoline HCl. Eur J Pharmacol 2:155–161, 1967.
48. Dollery CT, Harington M, Hodge JV. Haemodynamic studies with methyldopa: Effect on cardiac output and response to pressor amines. Br Heart J 25:670–676, 1963.
49. Mohammed S, Hanenson IB, Magenheim HG, Gaffney TE. The effects of α-methyldopa on renal function in hypertensive patients. Am Heart J 76:21–27, 1968.
50. Bravo EL, Tarazi RC, Fouad FM, et al. Clonidine suppression test: A useful aid in the diagnosis of pheodermocytoma. N Engl J Med 305:623–626, 1981.

51. Glontz GE, Saslaw S. Methyldopa fever. Arch Intern Med 122:445–447, 1968.
52. Norlledge SM, Carstairs KC, Dacie JV. Autoimmune haemolytic anemia associated with α-methyldopa therapy. Lancet 2:135–139, 1966.
53. Finnerty FA Jr. Drugs in the treatment of hypertension. Mod Concepts Cardiovasc Dis 42:33–36, 1973.
54. Jarvik MD. Drugs used in the treatment of psychiatric disorders. In Goodman LS, Gilman A (eds). The Pharmacological Basis of Therapeutics. New York, Macmillan, 1968; pp 159–214.
55. Hansson L, Hunyor SN, Julius S, Hoobier SW. Blood pressure crisis following withdrawal of clonidine (Catapres, Catapresan) with special reference to arterial and urinary catecholamine levels, and suggestions for acute management. Am Heart J 85:605–610, 1973.
56. Cohen RA, Kopin IJ, Creveling CR, et al. False neurochemical transmitters: Combined clinical staff conference at the National Institutes of Health. Ann Intern Med 65:347–362, 1966.
57. Onesti G, Novack P, Ramirez O, et al. Hemodynamic effects of pargyline in hypertensive patients. Circulation 30:830–835, 1964.
58. Richards DW. Paradoxical hypertension from tranylcypromine sulfate. Report of the Council on Drugs. JAMA 186:854, 1963.
59. Blackwell B. Hypertensive crisis due to monoamine oxidase inhibitors. Lancet 2:849–851, 1963.
60. Goldberg LI. Monoamine oxidase inhibitors: Adverse reactions and possible mechanisms. JAMA 190:456–462, 1964.
61. Dawes GS, Comroe JH Jr. Chemoreflexes from the heart and lungs. Physiol Rev 34:167–201, 1954.
62. Wang SC, Ngai SH, Grossman RG. Mechanism of vasomotor action of veratrum alkaloids: Extravagal sites of action of veriloid, protoveratrine, germitrine, neogermitrine, germerine, veratridine and veratramine. J Pharmacol Exp Ther 113:100–114, 1955.
63. Freis ED, Stanton JR, Partenope EA, et al. The hemodynamic effects of hypotensive drugs in man. I: Veratrum viride. J Clin Invest 28:353–368, 1949.

New Classes

CHAPTER 73

Endothelin Antagonists

Ernesto L. Schiffrin

ROLE OF ENDOTHELINS IN EXPERIMENTAL HYPERTENSION SUGGESTING THAT ENDOTHELIN ANTAGONISTS MAY BE USEFUL ANTIHYPERTENSIVE AGENTS

The endothelins (ETs), potent 21-amino acid vasoconstrictor peptides produced in many different tissues, particularly in the endothelium of blood vessels, have already been described in Chapter 15, Endothelin in Hypertension. ET-1 is the main isoform secreted by the endothelium, and it acts in a paracrine or autocrine fashion on adjacent cells (endothelial or smooth muscle). ET-1 acts on ET_A and ET_B receptors in smooth muscle cells to induce contraction, proliferation, and cell hypertrophy and on endothelial ET_B receptors, inducing release of nitric oxide and prostacyclin to elicit vasorelaxation. It is not known whether the vasoconstrictor or the vasorelaxant action of ETs is their most important physiological function, and this probably varies from one vascular bed to another. In the coronary circulation, the virtual absence of endothelial ET_B receptors[1] results in ETs behaving as vasoconstrictors. In other vascular beds, it is possible that ET-1 acts on smooth muscle cells as a paracrine constrictor and growth promoter only when it is overexpressed in endothelial cells under pathological conditions.

In the heart, ET-1 is produced by various cell types, including endothelial cells, smooth muscle cells, fibroblasts, and cardiomyocytes. Upregulation of the ET-1 gene may occur in these cells in response to angiotensin II, wall stretch, and ischemia. The ET_A receptor is the predominant subtype in cardiomyocytes, whereas a mixed population of ET_A and ET_B receptors is found in cardiac fibroblasts.[2] ETs stimulate expression of fetal genes, protein synthesis, and growth in cardiomyocytes. Expression of the ETs, the presence of ET_A and ET_B receptors, and the vasoconstrictor and salt-retaining effects of these peptides in kidney have been described in detail in Chapter 15, Endothelin in Hypertension.

Antagonists that are highly selective for the ET_A or the ET_B receptor, as well as agents that have a high affinity for both receptor subtypes, the so-called balanced or nonselective ET_A/ET_B receptor antagonists, have been developed (Table 73–1). It is unclear as yet whether the balanced or nonselective antagonists act through blockade of both

Table 73–1 Endothelin Antagonists

ET_A/ET_B	ET_A	ET_B
TAK-044	BQ-123	BQ-788
Bosentan	BQ-610	RES-701-1
PD145065	FR139317	RO-468443
L-744,453	IPI-725	
L-751,281	A-127722.5	
L-754,142	LU135252	
SB209670	PD155080	
SB217242	PD156707	
	BMS-182874	
	TBC11251	

Abbreviation: ET, endothelin.

receptor subtypes or predominantly via the ET_A receptor. Some of these agents can be administered only intravenously (e.g., TAK-044, BQ-123, BQ-610, FR139317, IPI-725, BQ-788, RES-701-1); others are orally active and are currently undergoing clinical development. The availability of subtype-selective and -nonselective antagonists of ET receptors has allowed the dissection of the physiological and pathophysiological roles of ETs mediated through these receptor subtypes in both experimental animals and humans.

Activation of the ET system has been demonstrated in salt-dependent models of hypertension, such as the deoxycorticosterone acetate (DOCA)–salt hypertensive rat and the DOCA-salt–treated spontaneously hypertensive rat (SHR). These models overexpress ET-1 in the endothelium,[3, 4] and respond with blood pressure lowering to ET antagonism with bosentan, an ET_A/ET_B receptor antagonist.[5] In contrast, the ET system appears not to be activated in SHRs.[3] When the activity of the vascular ET system is enhanced, growth of resistance arteries is accentuated, and administration of ET antagonists lowers blood pressure and induces regression of hypertrophic arterial remodeling.[5, 6] The actions of ET on the kidney of some of these hypertensive models may contribute to water and sodium retention, renal vasoconstriction and hypertension, and eventually renal failure.[7] In rats infused with angiotensin II, a known stimulant of ET-1 expression, ET antagonists lowered blood pressure and reduced cardiac and small artery hypertrophic remodeling.[8] Thus, the ET system seems to be activated more often in low-renin, salt-sensitive, and severe forms of hypertension, but may be also stimulated by exogenous angiotensin II, and presumably by endogenous angiotensin II, as well. Cyclosporine-induced hypertension has an ET-dependent component, and bosentan lowers blood pressure in rats and primates with this form of acquired hypertension.[9] ET may also play a role in hypertensive models with hyperinsulinemia and insulin resistance, in which chronic bosentan treatment reduced blood pressure.[10]

In all these salt-sensitive, severe, or exogenous angiotensin II–infused models of hypertension in which ET-1 expression has been shown to be enhanced, severe hypertrophy of small arteries is often a characteristic feature.[11] In those models in which overexpression of ET-1 occurs, bosentan or other ET antagonists reduced blood pressure and hypertrophic remodeling of small arteries and protected the kidney.[12] In some experimental models of hypertension, enhanced expression of ET-1 may be local rather than generalized; the endothelium of coronary arteries appears to be particularly vulnerable in this regard.[13] Enhanced production of ET-1, without compensatory vasodilatation because of absence of endothelial ET_B receptors,[1] could result in vasoconstriction of the coronary circulation and a significant role of ET in myocardial ischemia in hypertension. In the absence of overexpression of ET-1 in tissues, the ET system may still play a role, if not in blood pressure elevation, in perivascular fibrosis of the heart and in progression of renal dysfunction, as shown by the response to chronic bosentan treatment in SHRs.[14] Cardiac ET-1 expression increases in animal models of cardiac hypertrophy and chronic administration of either selective ET_A or mixed antagonists may reduce the development of left ventricular hypertrophy. Norepinephrine administered for 7 days increased expression of ET-1 in the heart of rats, mainly in cardiomyocytes and in endothelial cells, and bosentan administration has attenuated cardiac hypertrophy.[15] The ET system is activated in heart failure in rats, and infusion of the ET_A antagonist BQ-123 for a short period of time decreased the rate and force of contraction of the heart, indicating an inotropic action of the activated ET system in this model.[16] Prolonged infusion of BQ-123 significantly reduced mortality in the same rat model of heart failure.[17] Cardiac dysfunction secondary to activation of the cardiac ET system, ET-dependent vasoconstriction, and increased afterload in advanced heart failure may therefore respond favorably to ET receptor antagonism, as has been demonstrated in humans.[18]

PATHOPHYSIOLOGY OF THE CARDIOVASCULAR ENDOTHELIN SYSTEM AND USE OF ENDOTHELIN ANTAGONISTS IN HUMAN HYPERTENSION

Plasma ET levels are usually normal in human hypertension, although in some severely hypertensive patients, elevated ET immunoreactivity in plasma may be found (see references cited in ref. 11). Acute intravenous administration of the mixed ET_A/ET_B receptor antagonist TAK-044 induced an increase in forearm blood flow and slightly lowered blood pressure in healthy subjects.[19] This suggests that ET-dependent vascular tone may be present in normotensive humans. Enhanced plasma ET responses to mental stress have been reported in normotensive offspring of hypertensive parents,[20] suggesting the presence of genetically determined endothelial dysfunction in the early stages preceding the development of hypertension. Expression of preproET-1 mRNA in the endothelium of small arteries obtained from gluteal subcutaneous biopsies of patients with moderate to severe hypertension was significantly greater than in normotensive subjects or patients with mild hypertension.[21] This is in agreement with a report of increased ET-1 production by the endothelium of small arteries in experimental models with severe hypertension. Enhanced production of ET-1 could play a role in hypertrophic remodeling of small arteries in patients with moderate to severe hypertension in addition to contributing to elevation of blood pressure. In African Americans, in whom hypertension is often severe and salt-sensitive, activation of the ET system has been described.[22] Other forms of hypertension in which ETs may play a role are those associated with chronic renal failure, erythropoietin and cyclosporine administration, pheochromocytoma, and pregnancy (reviewed in ref. 11).

The role of ETs in the pathophysiology of hypertension is still unclear, and their place in the therapeutic armamentarium awaits clinical trials with the ET antagonists. These trials are ongoing, and a recent report in abstract form demonstrated that bosentan given to patients with mild hypertension over a period of 4 weeks at a dose of 0.5 g once or twice daily was as effective as 20 mg of enalapril daily and well tolerated.[23] In the same study, a blunting of reflex neurohormonal vasoconstrictor activation in patients with essential hypertension was reported following administration of bosentan.[24] If these results are reproduced with some of the newer ET antagonists, these agents may become an interesting addition to the arsenal of antihypertensive agents currently available.

We believe based on the data summarized in this chapter that it is likely that ET-1 is mainly involved in blood pressure elevation and vascular hypertrophy in moderate to severe hypertension, probably in salt-sensitive forms and perhaps in special populations. Worsening endothelial damage in hypertension may activate expression of ET in blood vessels and in the heart. ET activation may be initially beneficial by causing: (1) thickening of the blood vessel wall with resultant reductions in wall stress and (2) positive inotropic effects on the heart. However, progression of these actions generally has deleterious effects on the cardiovascular system. ET antagonists may prove useful at this point. ET antagonists may prove to be beneficial in human cardiovascular therapeutics, particularly in clinical situations such as moderate to severe hypertension, in subsets of patients such as salt-sensitive hypertensives or African Americans, in the prevention of progression of nephrosclerosis and development of renal failure in hypertension, in the protection from ischemic heart disease and stroke (reviewed in ref. 25), and in the treatment of heart failure.[18] ET antagonists may function in these conditions as disease-modifying agents more than as blood pressure–lowering agents. Whether balanced ET_A/ET_B antagonists, selective ET_A antagonists, or endothelin converting enzyme inhibitors will prove to be the preferred agents is as yet unclear. The clinical evaluation of these drugs will allow us to learn more about their therapeutic utility and about the pathophysiological implications of the ET system in human disease, as well as its role in the short- and long-term regulation of cardiovascular function.

References

1. Russell FD, Skepper JN, Davenport AP. Detection of endothelin receptors in human coronary artery vascular smooth muscle cells but not endothelial cells by using electron microscope autoradiography. J Cardiovasc Pharmacol 29:820–826, 1997.
2. Fareh J, Touyz RM, Schiffrin EL, et al. Endothelin-1 and angiotensin II receptors in cells from rat hypertrophied heart. Receptor regulation and intracellular Ca^{2+} modulation. Circ Res 78:302–311, 1996.
3. Larivière R, Thibault G, Schiffrin EL. Increased endothelin-1 content in blood vessels of deoxycorticosterone acetate-salt hypertensive but not in spontaneously hypertensive rats. Hypertension 21:294–300, 1993.
4. Day R, Larivière R, Schiffrin EL. In situ hybridization shows increased endothelin-1 mRNA levels in endothelial cells of blood vessels of deoxycorticosterone acetate-salt hypertensive rats. Am J Hypertens 8:294–300, 1995.
5. Li J-S, Larivière R, Schiffrin EL. Effect of a nonselective endothelin antagonist on vascular remodeling in DOCA-salt hypertensive rats. Evidence for a role of endothelin in vascular hypertrophy. Hypertension 24:183–188, 1994.
6. Schiffrin EL, Larivière R, Li J-S, et al. Enhanced expression of endothelin-1 gene in blood vessels of DOCA-salt hypertensive rats: Correlation with vascular structure. J Vasc Res 33:235–248, 1996.
7. Benigni A, Zoja C, Corna D, et al. Specific endothelin subtype A receptor antagonist protects against injury in renal disease progression. Kidney Int 44:440–444, 1993.
8. D'Uscio LV, Moreau P, Shaw S, et al. Effects of chronic ET_A-receptor blockade in angiotensin II-induced hypertension. Hypertension 29:435–441, 1997.
9. Bartholomeusz B, Hardy KJ, Nelson AS, et al. Bosentan ameliorates cyclosporin A-induced hypertension in rats and primates. Hypertension 27:1341–1345, 1996.
10. Verma S, Bhanot S, McNeill JH. Effect of chronic endothelin blockade in hyperinsulinemic hypertensive rats. Am J Physiol 269:H2017–H2021, 1995.
11. Schiffrin EL. Endothelin: Potential role in hypertension and vascular hypertrophy. [Brief invited review] Hypertension 25:1135–1143, 1995.
12. Li J-S, Schürch W, Schiffrin EL. Renal and vascular effects of chronic endothelin receptor antagonism in malignant hypertensive rats. Am J Hypertens 9:803–811, 1996.
13. Deng LY, Schiffrin EL. Endothelin-1 gene expression in blood vessels and kidney of spontaneously hypertensive rats (SHR), L-NAME-treated SHR, and renovascular hypertensive rats. J Cardiovasc Pharmacol 31(suppl 1):S380–S383, 1998.
14. Karam H, Heudes D, Bruneval P, et al. Endothelin antagonism in end-organ damage of spontaneously hypertensive rats—Comparison with angiotensin-converting enzyme inhibition and calcium antagonism. Hypertension 28:379–385, 1996.
15. Kaddoura S, Firth JD, Boheler KR, et al. Endothelin-1 is involved in norepinephrine-induced ventricular hypertrophy in vivo. Acute effects of bosentan, an orally active, mixed endothelin ET_A and ET_B receptor antagonist. Circulation 93:2068–2079, 1996.
16. Sakai S, Miyauchi T, Sakurai T, et al. Endogenous endothelin-1 participates in the maintenance of cardiac function in rats with congestive heart failure. Circulation 93:1214–1222, 1996.
17. Sakai S, Miyauchi T, Kobayashi M, et al. Inhibition of myocardial endothelin pathway improves long-term survival in heart failure. Nature 384:353–355, 1996.
18. Kiowski W, Sütsch G, Hunziker P, et al. Evidence for endothelin-1–mediated vasoconstriction in severe chronic heart failure. Lancet 346:732–736, 1995.
19. Haynes WG, Ferro CJ, O'Kane KPJ, et al. Systemic endothelin receptor blockade decreases peripheral vascular resistance and blood pressure in humans. Circulation 93:1860–1870, 1996.
20. Noll G, Wenzel RR, Schneider M, et al. Increased activation of sympathetic nervous system and endothelin by mental stress in normotensive offspring of hypertensive parents. Circulation 93:866–869, 1996.
21. Schiffrin EL, Deng LY, Sventek P, et al. Enhanced expression of endothelin-1 gene in endothelium of resistance arteries in severe human essential hypertension. J Hypertens 15:57–63, 1997.
22. Ergul S, Parish DC, Puett D, et al. Racial differences in plasma endothelin-1 concentrations in individuals with essential hypertension. Hypertension 28:652–655, 1996.
23. Krum H, Budde M, Charlon V. Endothelin contributes to blood pressure elevations in patients with mild-moderate essential hypertension: Evidence from treatment with a mixed endothelin receptor antagonist, bosentan. [Abstract] Circulation Suppl I:I-598, 1997.
24. Krum H, Budde M, Charlon V. Effect of endothelin receptor antagonism on reflex neurohormonal vasoconstrictor activation in patients with essential hypertension. [Abstract] Circulation Suppl I:I-406, 1997.
25. Schiffrin EL, Intengan HD, Thibault G, et al. Clinical significance of endothelin in cardiovascular disease. Curr Opin Cardiol 12:354–367, 1997.

74 Renin Inhibitors

Norman K. Hollenberg

Although it is a hundred years since Tigerstedt and Berg-man[1] first described renin and its remarkable ability to induce a sustained rise in blood pressure, it is only since the early 1970s, when pharmacological interruption of the renin-angiotensin system became a reality, that the importance of this system in biology and medicine has been fully appreciated. Haber[2] provided the mechanistic explanation: Pharmacological interruption of the renin system played the role of the crucial ablation experiment in proving that a hormone was responsible for a response. In the case of the renin system, where the kidney was both the source of the hormone and a major responding organ, the ablation experiment was limited.

Three locations in the renin-angiotensin cascade are available for blockade: The interaction of renin with its substrate, angiotensinogen; the enzyme responsible for conversion of angiotensin I (Ang I) to angiotensin II (Ang II); and the Ang II receptor site. Skeggs and associates in 1957[3] recognized these three possible sites and argued "since renin is the initial and rate-limiting substance in the renin-angiotensin system, it would seem that the [renin

inhibition] approach would be the most likely to succeed." No pharmacologist would have chosen the angiotensin-converting enzyme (ACE) step first as part of a planned approach to interrupting the renin system. The Ang II receptor provides an attractive site for a number of reasons, primarily because of the possibility of nonrenin and non-ACE-dependent Ang II generation.[4] Whatever the pathway of Ang II generation, blockade at the level of the Ang II receptor will be effective in preventing or reversing the response.

Two biochemical facts made the renin step a very attractive target. The first is that the interaction of renin with its substrate, angiotensinogen, is rate-limiting.[3] The second involves the remarkable specificity of renin for its substrate.[5] That remarkable specificity had implications for the renin inhibitors. In Figure 74–1, the species specificity of a renin inhibitor for human and marmoset plasma renin is contrasted with the inhibition of dog and rat renin. The marmoset is a primate. In the same figure, inhibition of human renin is contrasted with inhibition of other aspartic proteinases, pepsin and cathepsin-D, both of which are far less sensitive to the renin inhibitor.

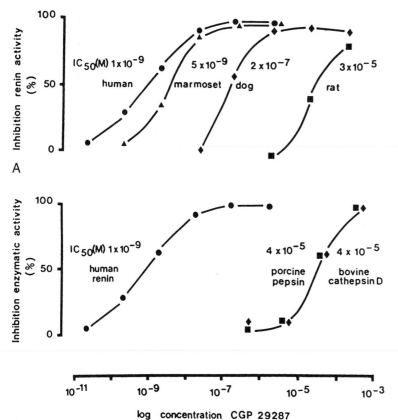

Figure 74–1. *A*, Species specificity of the renin inhibitor CGP 29287. Note that the two primate sources of renin, human and marmoset, were blocked with low concentrations of the inhibitor, whereas much higher concentrations were required to block canine and rat renin. *B*, Blockade of human renin with this agent is contrasted with the very poor efficacy on pepsin and cathepsin-D, other aspartic proteinases. (*A* and *B*, From Wood JM, Gulati N, Forgiarini P, et al. Effects of a specific and long-acting renin inhibitor in the marmoset. Hypertension 7:797–803, 1985.)

RELEVANT BIOCHEMISTRY OF THE RENIN SYSTEM AND RENIN INHIBITORS

Renin belongs to the aspartic proteinase family, which includes the enzymes pepsin, cathepsin-D, and chymosin.[5] This class of enzyme is named because of a crucial feature: Each enzyme has two aspartic acid residues in its active site that are necessary for catalytic activity. Three-dimensional models of human renin, based on x-ray crystal structure of other aspartic proteinases, reveal coplanar, symmetrically arranged β-carbonyl groups of the aspartic acid residues at 38 and 226, held in an intricate web of hydrogen bonds. The active site appears as a long, deep cleft that can accommodate seven amino acid units of substrate. The enzyme also contains a mobile flap that, when closed, lies across the cleft and probably holds substrate in the active site.[6] Renin has a bilobal structure consistent with the hypothesis that aspartic proteinases, including renin, arose from a common ancestral gene.[7] Their common catalytic mechanism involves hydrolysis, whereby water stereospecifically attacks the carbonyl of the scissile amide bond and the aspartate moieties act as anchors, mediating the appropriate proton transfer.[8]

Although the aspartyl proteinases have much in common, renins from different species vary in their specificity for angiotensinogens from other species. In all species, angiotensinogen is the only known physiological substrate for renin, conferring remarkable specificity.[5]

The development of renin inhibitors follows from the biochemical considerations described previously. Proof of principle, that blocking the renin step would produce a biologically important response, first came from an immunological approach. Antisera produced against crude renin extracts were used initially, followed by polyclonal and monoclonal antibodies against renin purified from multiple species.[9] The most potent inhibitor of human renin described so far had an IC_{50} of 10^{11M}.[5]

Pepstatin is a peptide derived from microbial metabolism that acts as a potent competitive inhibitor of most aspartic proteinases, with an IC_{50} of 0.05 nmol for pepsin, for example. Unfortunately, it proved to be a rather weak inhibitor of renin, with an IC_{50} of 10 nmol.[10] Statine, an unusual amino acid found in pepstatin, is believed to act as a "transition state" mimic, resembling the tetrahedral conformation of the natural substrate at the scissile bond after it has been bound to the enzyme and activated for cleavage.[11] This amino acid later proved to be an important part of the structure:function evolution.[12]

The approach that followed for synthesis of renin inhibitors involved two different pathways,[13] as summarized in Figure 74–2. One was based on the hypothesis that the prosegment of prorenin is capable of inhibiting enzyme activity by preventing access of the substrate. This pathway developed only weak inhibitors. The other approach was to synthesize peptide analogues of the N-terminal amino acid sequence of the substrate, angiotensinogen. Substitution of the amino acid at the scissile bond (positions 10 and 11) of octapeptide analogues resulted in active competitive inhibitors. The most effective, known as *renin inhibitory peptide*, had an inhibitory potency against human renin in the micromolar range and was sufficiently active to be useful for research.[14]

With further evolution, the amino acids at the scissile bond were replaced by noncleavable analogues, either a reduced peptide bond or a hydroxy-ethylene group.[5] By analogy with statine, described previously, the structural elements were believed to act as transition state mimics. The result was inhibitors with a potency in the nanomole range (see Fig. 74–2).

With increasing potency, emphasis shifted to the development of agents that would retain potency but that would also be bioavailable (see Fig. 74–2). The best of these agents, remikiren and enalkiren, were very potent and active on parenteral administration but showed oral bioavailability that was substantially less than 10%, more often in the 1% range.[13] Progress was being made in dealing with the bioavailability problem. The last three agents shown in Figure 74–2, FK-906, zankiren, and A-74273, all showed appreciable oral bioavailability and efficacy in animal studies and in humans.[13] At this crucial stage, all of the programs appear to have been canceled for commercial reasons. The rapid advance of the Ang II antagonists was believed by the decisionmakers to make ultimate commercial success unlikely.

INFLUENCE OF RENIN INHIBITION ON BLOOD PRESSURE

The ultimate goal of treating hypertension is reduction of morbidity and mortality and target organ damage, so that analysis restricted to blood pressure measurement is overly simplistic. Even in a simple model, however, there is substantial variation in response, reflecting the specifics of the pathogenesis of the disorder, the demographics of the patient, the state of sodium balance, and other issues such as genotype. A number of studies of blood pressure in various animal models have shown either equivalence of ACE and renin inhibition or a small advantage of one or the other.[5] The principle that blocking renin would reduce blood pressure was established early in humans. We restrict this review to those studies in which responses to an ACE inhibitor and to a renin inhibitor were assessed in the same patients.

Jeunemaitre and coworkers[15] compared CJP-38560A, a renin inhibitor, with captopril, both at apparently maximal doses—0.25 mg/kg of the renin inhibitor and 50 mg of captopril. Salt intake was unrestricted and presumably fairly high in a French population. The patients were selected because they had a marked fall in mean blood pressure after captopril (15.3 ± 1.5 mm Hg), but showed only a limited 6.4 ± 1.2-mm Hg mean blood pressure fall after the renin inhibitor. Thus, if this renin inhibitor had been administered at the maximal dose, captopril would have had an additional action unrelated to renin in these selected patients.

Neutel and colleagues[16] reported precisely opposite findings in a comparison of intravenous placebo, enalaprilat (1.25 mg IV) and enalkiren (in a dose range from 0.03 to 1 mg/kg) in hydrochlorothiazide-treated hypertensive patients with an activated renin system. The acute decrease in systolic blood pressure of 18.5 ± 0.4 mm Hg during enalkiren was substantially greater than the 12.6 ± 0.7 mm Hg during enalaprilat ($p < .01$). The fall in diastolic blood

Structure[a]	IC$_{50}$ (nM)[b]	Structure[a]	IC$_{50}$ (nM)[b]
Iva-Val-Val-Sta-Ala-Sta Pepstatin	20,000	A-64662, enalkiren	14
Pro-His-Pro-Phe-His-Phe-Phe-Val-Tyr-Lys RIP	2000	FK 906	0.58[d]
Pro-His-Pro-Phe-His-Leu^{R}Val-Ile-His-Lys H-142	10	A-72517, zankiren	1.1
Z-Arg-Arg-Pro-Phe-His-Sta-Ile-His-Lys(Boc) OMe CGP-29 287	1	A-74273	3.1
Boc-Pro-Phe-(Me)His-Leu^{OH}•Val-Ile-AMP U-71038, ditekiren	0.4		
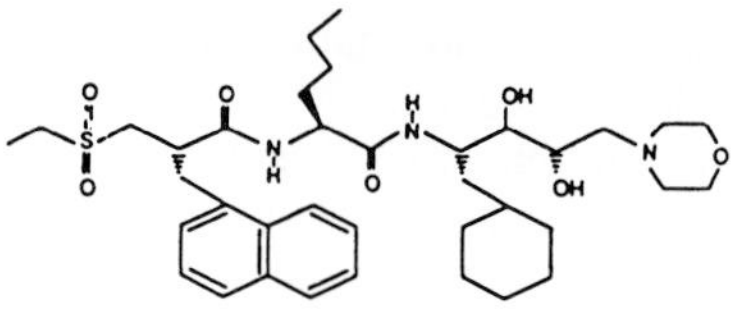 BW-175	3.3		
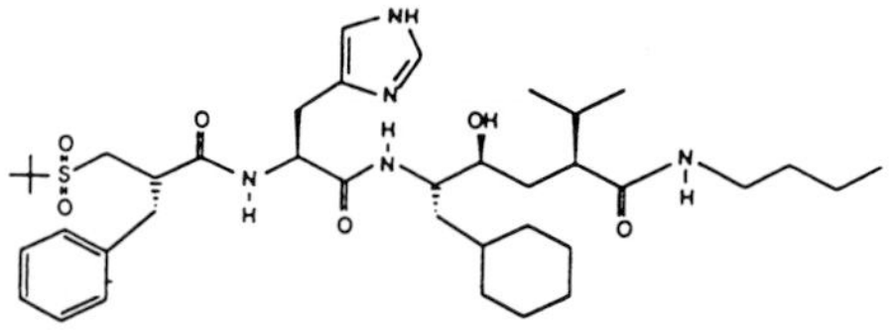 CGP 38 560	0.7		
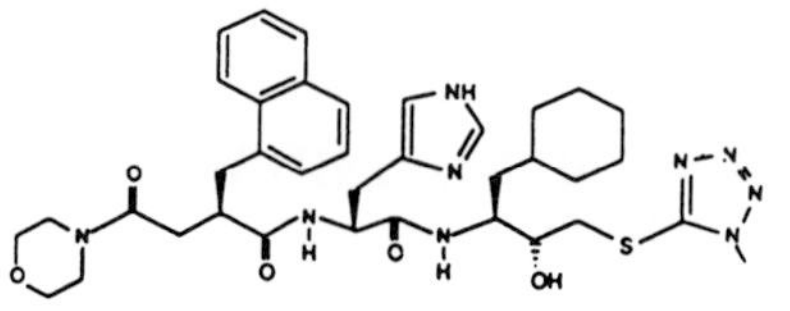 YM-21095	0.47[c]		
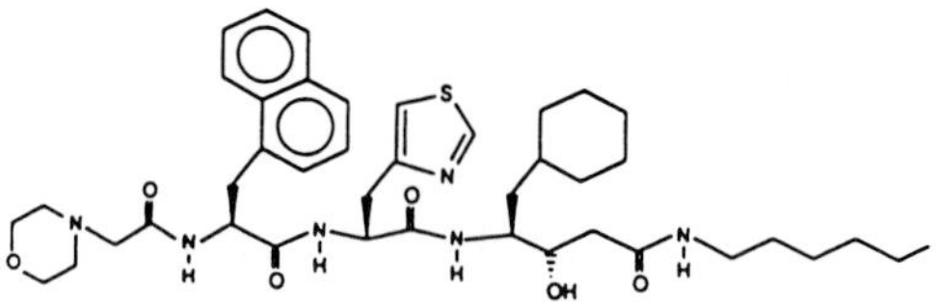 ES-8891	1.1		
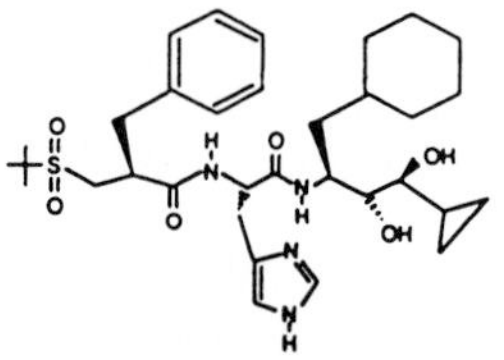 RO 42-5892, remikiren	0.7		

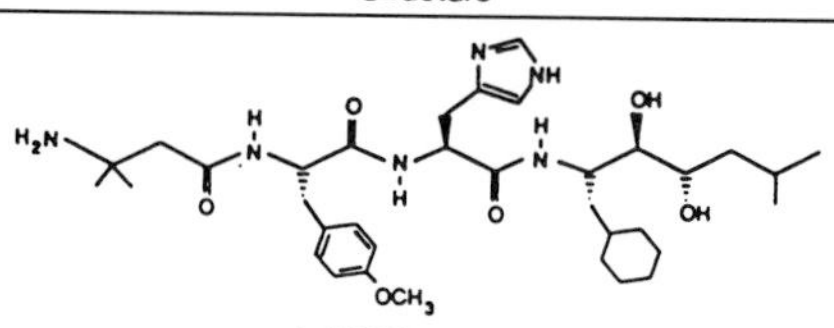

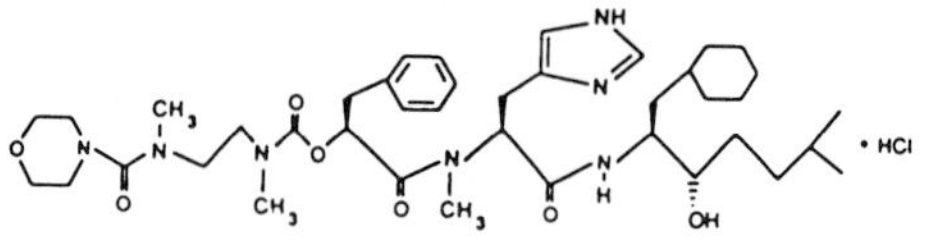

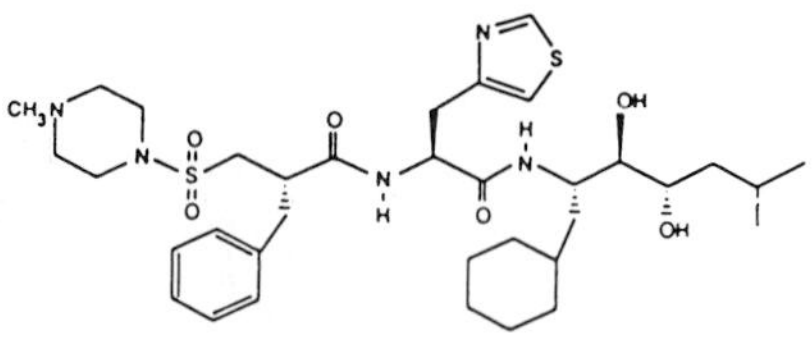

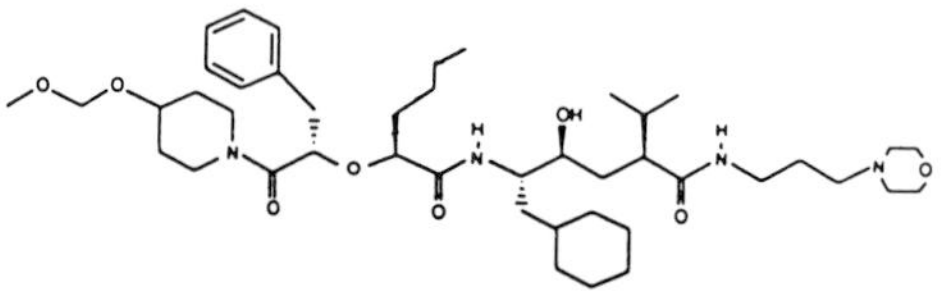

[a] Iva = isovaleryl; Sta = (3S,4S)-4-amino-3-hydroxy-6-methylheptanoic acid; R = (—CH$_2$—NH—); Z = carbobenzoxy; Boc = N-tert-butoxycarbonyl; OH = (—CHOHCH$_2$—); AMP = 2-aminomethylpyridine amide.
[b] Human renin, pH 7.0–7.4.
[c] pH 6.0.
[d] Ki.

Figure 74–2. Structure and potency of renin inhibitors developed, approximately, sequentially. (From Kleinert HD, Stein HH. Specific renin inhibitors: Concepts and prospects. *In* Laragh JH, Brenner BM [eds]. Hypertension, Pathophysiology, Diagnosis, and Management, 2nd ed, vol 2. New York, Raven, 1995; pp 3065–3077.)

pressure during enalkiren (11.9 ± 0.4 mm Hg) was also slightly greater than during enalaprilat (9.2 ± 0.4 mm Hg; p < .01). In the patients in whom plasma renin activity rose most, a similar pattern emerged, but the differences were not significant in the low or normal renin groups. This analysis might explain the findings described previously by Jeunemaitre and coworkers[15] in individuals on a liberal salt intake.

Kiowski and associates[17] compared another renin inhibitor, RO-42-5892, with captopril (50 mg). The renin inhibitor was given by mouth in a 600-mg dose. In normal individuals, captopril decreased diastolic blood pressure from 60 ± 5 to 51 ± 7 mm Hg but the renin inhibitor did not alter diastolic blood pressure. Salt intake was described as normal. RO-42-5892 was thought to be poorly bioavailable.

In none of the three studies was the ACE inhibitor added to the renin inhibitor or the renin inhibitor to the ACE inhibitor when a nadir in blood pressure had been reached. The conclusion of these studies is that the more renin-dependent the blood pressure, the larger the fall induced by renin inhibition. As there are no studies that go beyond very brief intervals of drug administration, the implications of these studies for therapeutics are limited.

RENAL RESPONSE TO RENIN INHIBITION

Ang II plays a crucial role in the control of the renal circulation and renal function. Moreover, the remarkable efficacy of ACE inhibition in limiting renal injury in patients with diabetes and other forms of nephropathy placed a high priority on examining the effects of renin inhibitors on the renal blood supply and kidney function. When our studies in humans began, there was already substantial experience in animal models to suggest that renin inhibitors would induce a robust renal vasodilator response.[18–21] The hypothesis of our first studies of the renal hemodynamic response to a renin inhibitor was straightforward.[22] To the extent that ACE inhibitors reduce kinin degradation and thereby induce vasodilator prostaglandin formation or activation of endothelial nitric oxide release, the renal vasodilator response to ACE inhibition should exceed the response to renin inhibition. We hypothesized that the difference in magnitude of the renal vascular responses would provide a measure of the magnitude of the contributions of other vasodilators compared with reduced Ang II formation. To our surprise, the renal vasodilator response to the renin inhibitor enalkiren exceeded expectations from our previous experience with ACE inhibitors.[22]

In a follow-up, three-arm study designed to compare placebo, enalkiren, and captopril, the placebo did nothing and captopril and enalkiren both led to striking renal vasodilatation.[23] The response to enalkiren was larger than the response to captopril in 6 of the 9 healthy subjects. The magnitude of the response to the renin inhibitor in this study confirmed our earlier observation, as did a more recent study with another renin inhibitor, zankiren, that induced a larger renal vasodilator response than could have been anticipated from the ACE inhibitor experience.[24]

The renal vascular response to renin inhibitor at the top of the dose-response curve in these three studies is summarized in Figure 74–3 in a meta-analysis format.[25] All studies were performed in healthy men who were less than 40 years of age and who were in balance on a 10-mEq sodium intake to activate the renin system. All were studied by the same group of physicians, nurses, dieticians, and technicians on the same metabolic ward utilizing the same techniques for measurement of p-aminohippurate clearance as the index of renal perfusion. Also shown in Figure 74–3 are responses to three ACE inhibitors, each study performed at the top of the dose-response curve for renal blood flow. All were performed over the same time interval and under the same conditions. In the special case of the captopril:enalkiren comparison, the same subjects were involved. By analysis of variance, no statistical difference was identified among the three ACE inhibitors or between the two renin inhibitors, but the striking difference between the ACE and the renin inhibitors was highly significant ($p < .001$). The renal vasodilator response to renin inhibition in healthy humans under these conditions, in the range of 140 to 150 ml/min/1.73 m^2, exceeded by more than 50% the response to ACE inhibitors, which

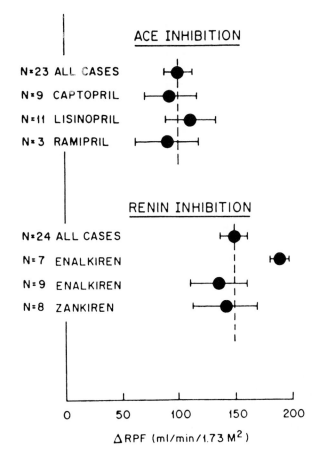

Figure 74–3. Change in renal plasma flow (RPF) in healthy young men studied when in balance on a 10-mEq sodium intake to activate the renin system. All of the subjects were studied on an identical ward with the same research team and on the same protocol. Each of the agents is compared at the top of the dose-response relationship for the kidney. Note that the three angiotensin-converting enzyme (ACE) inhibitors induced a maximal response in the 90 to 100 ml/min range, whereas the renin inhibitors induced a significantly larger response, in the 140- to 150-ml range. (From Hollenberg NK, Fisher NDL. Renal circulation and blockade of the renin-angiotensin system. Is angiotensin-converting enzyme inhibition the last word? Hypertension 26:602–609, 1995.)

averaged about 90 to 100 ml/min/1.73 m^2—when theory said it should be less.

In a subsequent study, el Amrani and coworkers[26] compared the renal vascular response to a renin inhibitor (R042-5892), an Ang II receptor antagonist (losartan), and an ACE inhibitor (lisinopril) in guinea pigs. Renin structure varies with species, and renin inhibitors display species specificity, so the guinea pig was selected as the experimental species in this study because this renin inhibitor developed for primates is effective in the guinea pig. Doses of the agents were adjusted to induce an identical small but unambiguous fall in blood pressure and were administered coded and in a random sequence. This careful, elegant study design revealed remarkable differences in the overall response to the three classes of agents. Despite an identical fall in blood pressure, the renin inhibitor induced a substantially larger increase in renal plasma flow, glomerular filtration rate, diuresis, and natriuresis—as in the humans.[26] The authors suggest that the potentiated response to renin

Table 74–1 The Biological Effects of Renin-Angiotensin System Blockers

Blockade	PRA and Plasma Ang II Concentration		Ang II Receptors Type 1	Ang II Receptors Type 2	Nonrenin/ Non–ACE-Dependent and Ang II Production	Bradykinin in Plasma and Tissue
	PRA	Ang II				
ACE inhibition	Up	Down	Not stimulated	Not stimulated	Not blocked	Increased
Renin inhibition	Down	Down	Not stimulated	Not stimulated	Not blocked	Unchanged
Ang II antagonists	Up	Up	Blocked	Not blocked	Blocked	Unchanged

Abbreviations: PRA, plasma renin activity; Ang II, angiotensin II; ACE, angiotensin-converting enzyme.

inhibition could reflect greater lipophilicity and tissue penetration, leading to a local intrarenal action at the site of Ang II production.[26] As an alternative, the guinea pig might share with humans substantial non–ACE-dependent conversion of Ang I to Ang II, perhaps via chymase.[4] The data suggest strongly that renin inhibition is far more effective than ACE inhibition in blocking Ang II formation in the kidney.

CONSEQUENCES OF PHARMACOLOGICAL INTERRUPTION OF THE RENIN SYSTEM: COMPARISON OF ACE INHIBITION, RENIN INHIBITION, AND BLOCKADE AT THE AT₁ RECEPTOR

A number of predictable consequences occur when the renin system is blocked at different levels. ACE inhibition will lead to an increase in plasma bradykinin concentration (Table 74–1); will not suppress non–ACE-dependent Ang II, and will lead to an increase in plasma Ang I concentration, proximal to the level of the block. As a consequence, other pathways, including generation of Ang_{1-7} and other metabolites, can come into play. Because plasma Ang II concentration is reduced, the AT_2 receptor will not be activated. Renin inhibitors, on the other hand, will reduce the production and plasma concentrations of both Ang I and Ang II, will leave bradykinin production unchanged, and as plasma Ang II concentration is reduced, will not stimulate either angiotensin receptor. The Ang II antagonists lead to an increase in renin release and, thus, increases in plasma Ang I and Ang II concentrations. Blockade of the AT_1 receptor is not matched by blockade of the AT_2 receptor, which is stimulated. Bradykinin is unchanged. All of these consequences are predictable and will have a major influence on the ultimate succes of blockade at the three levels.

CLINICAL IMPLICATIONS

At the moment, it appears that all renin inhibitor development programs have been closed, although hints periodically reappear to indicate that one company or another is pursuing a renin inhibitor. The decision to close programs seems to have reflected not the therapeutic potential of renin inhibitors but rather the cost of their synthesis, continuing problems with bioavailability, and the remarkable

success of the competitor class—the Ang II antagonists. The remarkable absence of adverse effects of the Ang II antagonist class makes that competition difficult. If the sustained increases in Ang I and Ang II generation and plasma concentrations induce an adverse effect, perhaps by way of the AT_2 receptor, renin inhibition would enjoy a new advantage likely to be exploited. At the moment, that jury is out.

References

1. Tigerstedt R, Bergman PG. 1897. The kidneys and the circulation. *In* Ruskin R, Nowinski WW (eds). Classics in Arterial Hypertension. Springfield, IL, Charles C Thomas, 1956; pp 274–287.
2. Haber E. The role of renin in normal and pathological cardiovascular homeostasis. Circulation 54:849–861, 1976.
3. Skeggs LT, Kahn JR, Lentz K, Shumway NP. Preparation, purification and amino acid sequence of a polypeptide renin substrate. J Exp Med 106:439–453, 1957.
4. Hollenberg NK, Fisher NDL, Price DA. Pathways for angiotensin II generation in the tissues of intact humans: Evidence from comparative pharmacological interruption of the renin system. Hypertension 32:387–392, 1998.
5. Wood JM, Stanton JL, Hofbauer KG. Inhibitors of renin as potential therapeutic agents. [Review article] J Enzyme Inhibition 1:169–185, 1987.
6. James MN, Sielecki A, Salituro F, et al. Conformational flexibility in the active sites of aspartyl proteinases revealed by a pepstatin fragment binding to penicillopepsin. Proc Natl Acad Sci U S A 79:6137–6141, 1982.
7. Tang J, James MNG, Hsu IN, et al. Structural evidence for gene duplication in the evolution of the acid proteases. Nature 271:618–621, 1978.
8. James MN, Sielecki AR. Stereochemical analysis of peptide bond hydrolysis catalyzed by the aspartic proteinase penicillopepsin. Biochemistry 24:3701–3713, 1985.
9. Dzau VJ, Devine D, Mudgett-Hunter M, et al. Antibodies as specific renin inhibitors: Studies with polyclonal and monoclonal antibodies and Fab fragments. Clin Exp Hypertens [A] 5:1207–1220, 1983.
10. Gross F, Lazar J, Orth H. Inhibition of the renin-angiotensinogen reaction by pepstatin. Science 175:656, 1972.
11. Ngo TT, Tunnicliff G. Inhibition of enzymic reactions by transition state analogs: An approach for drug design. Gen Pharmacol 12:129–138, 1981.
12. Blaine EH, Schorn TW, Boger J. Statine-containing renin inhibition. Dissociation of blood pressure lowering and renin inhibition in sodium-deficient dogs. Hypertension 6:111–118, 1984.
13. Kleinert HD, Stein HH. Specific renin inhibitors: Concepts and prospects. *In* Laragh JH, Brenner BM (eds). Hypertension, Pathophysiology, Diagnosis, and Management, 2nd ed, Vol 2. New York, Raven, 1995; pp 3065–3077.
14. Burton J, Cody RJ Jr, Herd JA, Haber E. Specific inhibition of renin by an angiotensinogen analog: Studies in sodium depletion and renin-dependent hypertension. Proc Natl Acad Sci U S A 77:5476–5479, 1980.
15. Jeunemaitre X, Menard J, Nussberger J, et al. Plasma angiotensin,

renin, and blood pressure during acute renin inhibition by CGP 38 560A in hypertensive patients. Am J Hypertens 2:819–827, 1989.

16. Neutel JM, Luther RR, Boger RS, Weber MA. Immediate blood pressure effects of the renin inhibitor enalkiren and the ACE inhibitor enalaprilat. Am Heart J 122:1094–1100, 1991.

17. Kiowski W, Linder L, Kleinbloesem C, et al. Blood pressure control of the renin-angiotensin system in normotensive subjects. Circulation 85:1–8, 1992.

18. Siragy HM, Lamb NE, Rose CE Jr, et al. Intrarenal renin inhibition increases renal function by an angiotensin II–dependent mechanism. Am J Physiol 363:F749–F754, 1988.

19. Verburg KM, Kleinert HD, Chekal MA, et al. Renal hemodynamic and excretory responses to renin inhibition induced by A-646622. J Pharmacol Exp Ther 252:449–455, 1989.

20. Hall JE, Mizelle HL. Control of arterial pressure and renal function during chronic renin inhibition. J Hypertens 8:351–359, 1990.

21. Verburg KM, Young GA, Rosenberg SH, Kleinert HD. Intrarenal renin inhibition: Renal hemodynamic and excretory actions of A-65317. J Hypertens 8(suppl 3):S25, 1990.

22. Cordero PL, Fisher NE, Moore TJ, et al. Renal and endocrine response to a renin inhibitor, enalkiren, in normal renin humans. Hypertension 17:510–516, 1991.

23. Fisher NDL, Allan D, Kifor I, et al. Responses to converting enzyme and renin inhibition: Role of angiotensin II in humans. Hypertension 23:44–51, 1994.

24. Fisher NDL, Hollenberg NK. Renal vascular responses to renin inhibition with zankiren in men. Clin Pharmacol Ther 57:342–348, 1995.

25. Hollenberg NK, Fisher NDL. Renal circulation and blockade of the renin-angiotensin system. Is angiotensin-converting enzyme inhibition the last word? Hypertension 26:602–609, 1995.

26. el Amrani A-I, Menard J, Gonzales MF, Michel JB. Effects of blocking the angiotensin II receptor, converting enzyme, and renin activity on the renal hemodynamics of normotensive guinea pigs. J Cardiovasc Pharmacol 22:231–239, 1993.

75

Vasopeptidase Inhibitors: A New Class of Cardiovascular Agents

Nick C. Trippodo and Ravi K. Saini

Vasopeptidase inhibitors simultaneously inhibit two key cardiovascular regulatory enzymes: the endopeptidase referred to as *endopeptidase 24.11* or neutral endopeptidase (NEP), and the dipeptidyl-carboxypeptidase, well known as *angiotensin-converting enzyme* (ACE). ACE inhibition blocks the formation of angiotensin II (Ang II) and hence attenuates this peptide's vasoconstricting, sodium-retaining, and growth-promoting activities. NEP inhibition blocks the inactivation of several regulatory peptides, including the natriuretic peptides, and thus augments vasodilatation, natriuresis, and cardioprotection through increased levels of atrial natriuretic peptide (ANP) and bradykinin. Bradykinin is also potentiated by ACE inhibition. The concept of minimizing the vasoconstricting, vascular and cardiac growth-promoting, and sodium-retaining actions of one regulatory system while simultaneously potentiating the vasodilator, antihypertrophic, and natriuretic effects of others, and the possibility that this would lead to greater beneficial effects than inhibition of NEP or ACE alone, has been the driving force behind the development of these single molecules that inhibit both ACE and NEP. This chapter gives an account of experimental studies and early clinical trials involved in the development of this new class of cardiovascular agents. Earlier reviews on vasopeptidase inhibitors are available.[1–4]

NEP INHIBITION

NEP, a cell-surface enzyme found in a number of tissues, degrades bioactive peptides and is a major pathway for the clearance of ANP and brain natriuretic peptide (BNP).[5] By protecting the natriuretic peptides and bradykinin from catabolism, it was reasoned that NEP inhibition, like ACE

inhibition, would shift the balance of endogenous hormonal factors from a vasoconstrictive, sodium-retaining, and hypertrophic range toward a more vasodilator, natriuretic, and cardioprotective level, and, hence, be effective as antihypertensive therapy. However, the findings in hypertensive patients have been mixed, with some reports on NEP inhibitors showing promising results[6, 7] and others displaying only marginal or negligible antihypertensive effects.[8, 9] The discordant findings may be partly due to the overriding effects of the renin-angiotensin system, neurohormonal activation, and attenuation of NEP-mediated catabolism of Ang II. Selective NEP inhibition produced increases in plasma Ang II, aldosterone, and catecholamines in hypertensive patients.[10, 11] As NEP has a broad substrate specificity, other endogenous vasoconstrictors may be protected by NEP inhibitors as well. For instance, candoxatril (a pure NEP inhibitor) increased circulating levels of endothelin in patients with heart failure[12] and in healthy men.[13] Moreover, in patients with heart failure, NEP inhibition leads to partial beneficial hemodynamic effects and inconsistent diuretic responses.[14] Thus, the efficacy of selective NEP inhibitors in the treatment of hypertension is in question, and their utility in heart failure requires further investigation.

RATIONALE

Several concepts provided the basis for the development of vasopeptidase inhibitors. Some early inhibitors of NEP or ACE displayed cross-reactivity toward both peptidases, suggesting that a single molecular structure could be optimized for activity against both enzymes. Both NEP and ACE contain zinc, thus providing a common pharmacophore. Their active sites are likely located at the cell surface, suggesting that inhibition of both enzymes in vivo could be readily achieved. Hence, from a standpoint of design, development of compounds that inhibit both ACE and NEP appeared feasible. The physiological interaction of the renin-angiotensin-aldosterone and natriuretic peptide systems provided biological grounds for simultaneously inhibiting NEP and ACE. NEP inhibition protects ANP and BNP from enzymatic inactivation and potentiates their biological actions,[4, 5, 14, 15] whereas ACE inhibition attenuates the formation of Ang II. Ang II acts as a physiological antagonist of ANP.[16] Moreover, ACE inhibition potentiates the acute cardiovascular[17, 18] and renal[19] responses to NEP inhibition in animal models of heart failure, presumably by mitigating the Ang II–mediated antagonsim of ANP. Combined NEP and ACE inhibition has greater antihypertensive effects than either selective inhibitor alone in spontaneously hypertensive rats (SHRs)[20, 21] and in patients with essential hypertension.[22] Therefore, potentiation of the vasodilator, natriuretic, and other effects of the natriuretic peptides by NEP inhibition acts synergistically with attenuation of the actions of Ang II by ACE inhibition.[23]

Protection of bradykinin by both ACE and NEP inhibition might also contribute to the interaction. Bradykinin contributed to the synergistic hemodynamic effects of combined NEP and ACE inhibition in cardiomyopathic hamsters.[23] Potential beneficial actions of bradykinin include natriuretic, vasodilator, and cardioprotective effects; antihypertrophic and antiarrhythmogenic effects; and improved glucose uptake by myocytes.[24] Substance P, another vasodilator cleaved by both ACE and NEP, acts as a partial counterregulatory mechanism against vasoconstriction in hypertension.[25] Plasma substance P was increased in heart failure patients by ACE inhibition.[26] Dual NEP and ACE inhibition might provide even greater protection of substance P. Two other vasodilators that are protected by NEP inhibition in vivo are C-type natriuretic peptide[27, 28] and calcitonin gene–related peptide.[12] Thus, NEP and ACE inhibition act synergistically by repressing vasoconstriction and sodium retention caused by Ang II while simultaneously unmasking and potentiating vasodilatation, cardioprotection, and natriuresis effectuated by several endogenous peptides.

INHIBITORS WITH AFFINITIES FOR BOTH ACE AND NEP

The promising results with the combination of NEP and ACE inhibition, together with the poor performance of selective NEP inhibition in patients, fostered the development of inhibitors with affinities for both ACE and NEP.[29–52] A key characteristic of vasopeptidase inhibitors is their capacity to lower blood pressure in animal models of hypertension irrespective of the sodium status or the activity of the renin-angiotensin system. Their ACE inhibitory activity lowers blood pressure in animals with high renin, whereas NEP inhibition decreases blood pressure in models with low renin; both activities may work in concert at intermediate levels of sodium and renin. They also activate biochemical markers of both NEP and ACE inhibition in vivo, such as plasma or urinary ANP (or cyclic guanosine monophosphate [cGMP], the second messenger

of ANP) and plasma renin activity (PRA), respectively. Moreover, these compounds reproduce the synergistic effects elicited by the coadministration of selective inhibitors of NEP and ACE.[53] A discussion of some vasopeptidase inhibitors follows (Fig. 75–1).

Aladotril (formerly alatriopril) is a diester prodrug that is equipotent against NEP and ACE in vitro (i.e., parent compound aladotrilat), but expresses weak ACE inhibitory activity orally.[29–31] Aladotril at 100 mg/kg PO inhibited the pressor response to Ang I in rats by 55 to 70%, whereas captopril at 10 mg/kg PO produced a maximal inhibition (>92%) for the 2-hour duration of the experiment.[29] In ganglion-blocked rats, aladotrilat produces the same inhibition of the Ang I pressor response as a 30-fold lower dose of captopril, yet the duration of action was less than that of the ACE inhibitor.[31] Intravenous administration of aladotrilat in transgenic rats with an extra renin gene resulted in increases in plasma ANP and cGMP and urinary cGMP and sodium.[31] Systolic blood pressure in the transgenic rats was decreased after oral administration of aladotril, but returned to baseline by 6 hours. In contrast, a nearly three-fold lower dose of the NEP inhibitor ecadotril decreased systolic blood pressure for the 6-hour duration of study.[31] Chronic treatment with aladotril in rats with myocardial infarction resulted in a greater reduction in cardiac hypertrophy than a 10-times lower dose of captopril;[29] however, this has not been firmly established.[30] At 100 mg b.i.d. for 6 weeks, aladotril lowered blood pressure in patients with essential hypertension.[32]

MDL 100,240 is a thioester prodrug of MDL 100,173.[33–35] After parenteral administration of either compound to rats, evidence of inhibition of both ACE and NEP was observed, including inhibition of the Ang I pressor response and enhancement of the effects of infused ANP on blood pressure, diuresis, and natriuresis.[34] Intravenous MDL 100,173 lowered blood pressure, increased urinary ANP, and increased PRA in spontaneously, deoxycorticosterone acetate (DOCA)–salt (low-renin) and renovascular (high-renin) hypertensive rats.[35] MDL 100,173, but not captopril, increased diuresis and natriuresis in the SHR and DOCA-salt rats. Oral MDL 100,240 lowered blood pressure in these two models with an inconsistent duration of action.[33] In healthy men, intravenous MDL 100,240 inhibited the blood pressure response to exogenous Ang I,[36] decreased systolic blood pressure, and increased urinary flow and ANP.[37] Whether MDL 100,240 would be effective as a once-a-day antihypertensive agent is not evident.

Mixanpril is a benzoylthioacetate prodrug of S21402 (RB105), which has been studied extensively in various rodent model.[38–40] S21402 given intravenously produced an array of cardiovascular, renal, and hormonal effects indicative of both NEP and ACE inhibition.[39] Moreover, S21402 decreased blood pressure similarly in DOCA-salt and renovascular rats and SHRs, indicating that the antihypertensive activity was independent of the status of the renin-angiotensin system. Despite the decreases in blood pressure, S21402 produced increases in urinary sodium excretion in the three hypertensive models. Mixanpril was antihypertensive in SHRs after repeat oral administration for 4 days.[38] The compound was administered twice a day and blood pressure was measured by tail-cuff 2 hours after dosing. Hence, the duration of the antihypertensive action

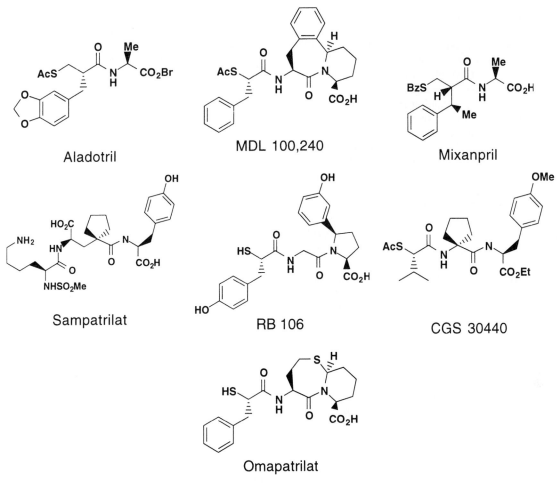

Figure 75–1. Inhibitors with affinities for both angiotensin-converting enzyme and neutral endopeptidase advanced to clinical or late-stage experimental evaluation.

of mixanpril was not reported. In rats with myocardial infarction, acute intravenous administration of S21402 decreased mean arterial pressure and increased PRA and urinary excretion of sodium, ANP, cGMP, and bradykinin.[40]

Sampatrilat (UK-81252), a dicarboxylic acid, reduced mean arterial pressure yet improved daily sodium excretion and increased renal blood flow in a dog model of heart failure when administered orally.[41] The increase in left ventricular mass seen in this model was abolished by sampatrilat.[41] In hypercholesterolemic rabbits, sampatrilat suppressed atherogenesis and improved endothelial function.[42] At a dose that inhibited the pressor response to Ang I by 80%, intravenous sampatrilat increased urinary sodium and cGMP excretion in rats with an aortovenocaval fistula.[43] The urinary responses were less than those induced by candoxatrilat, but blood pressure was decreased to a greater extent compared with the NEP inhibitor. The reduced renal response to sampatrilat was attributed to the acute hypotensive action of combined inhibition of NEP and ACE.[43] In patients with essential hypertension, single oral doses of 50 to 200 mg of sampatrilat lowered blood pressure for at least 24 hours and produced dose-dependent natriuresis.[44] Once-a-day treatment with sampatrilat at 50 to 200 mg for 10 days in hypertensive patients produced reductions in blood pressure similar to those of lisinopril 20

mg once daily, accompanied by increased urinary cGMP.[45] Sampatrilat exerted less inhibition of plasma ACE and less rise in renin activity than lisinopril. NEP inhibition may contribute to the antihypertensive effect of sampatrilat.[45]

RB 106 is a thiol-containing inhibitor that is very potent against NEP and ACE in vitro.[46] In a screening protocol, RB 106 at a low oral dose, produced a favorable time course of inhibition of renal NEP and lung ACE in mice. Intravenous RB 106 lowered blood pressure and increased sodium excretion in DOCA-salt rats. Repeat daily oral administration of RB 106 for 5 days in SHRs lowered blood pressure, and the antihypertensive effect lasted at least 24 hours.[46]

CGS 30440 is a thioacetate carboxylic acid ester prodrug with a long duration of antihypertensive action in SHRs.[47, 48] Oral CGS 30440 in rats potentiated the plasma ANP response to exogenous ANP. The pressor response to Ang I in rats was inhibited 4 hours after 3 mg/kg PO of CGS 30440 to about the same extent as after 10 mg/kg PO of captopril. Oral CGS 30440 lowered blood pressure in the renin-dependent aortic-ligated rat model and in SHRs.[47] After 8 weeks of once-daily oral administration in SHRs, CGS 30440 inhibited lung and kidney NEP and ACE activities.[48] CGS 30440 also increased urinary excretion of sodium and cGMP in the SHRs throughout treatment.

Mean arterial pressure measured with indwelling catheters at the conclusion of the 8 weeks of treatment with CGS 30440 was significantly lower than in vehicle-treated SHRs at both peak (1 hour after dosing) and trough (23 hours after dosing) periods.[48] CGS 30440 may have utility as a once-a-day antihypertensive agent.

Omapatrilat is a thiol-containing inhibitor that is long-acting and orally active as the free acid.[49, 50] Omapatrilat given orally inhibited the pressor response to Ang I in rats and monkeys with a duration of action similar to that of fosinopril, an ACE inhibitor currently prescribed as a once-a-day antihypertensive agent. Intravenous omapatrilat potentiated the natriuretic, cGMP, and ANP excretory responses to exogenous ANP in monkeys.[49] After single-dose administration, omapatrilat lowered mean arterial pressure (aortic catheter) at 24 hours in sodium-depleted SHRs (high renin), DOCA-salt rats, and SHRs.[50] During once-daily oral administration, omapatrilat consistently lowered systolic blood pressure (tail-cuff) in SHRs and DOCA-salt rats at 11 and 3 days of treatment, respectively; at 24 hours after dosing on days 12 and 4, respectively, mean arterial pressure (aortic catheter) was lower in the groups receiving omapatrilat than in those receiving vehicle.[49, 50] In healthy volunteers, single oral doses of omapatrilat (2.5 to 500 mg) increased urinary ANP and cGMP, indicating NEP inhibition, and increased PRA, indicating ACE inhibition. At 24 hours after administration, mean arterial pressure was decreased in a dose-related manner,[51, 52] an effect usually not seen with pure ACE inhibitors.

In hypertensive patients, dose-related decreases in 24-hour ambulatory and cuff blood pressures were observed with omapatrilat in short-term (up to 8 weeks) studies (unpublished data). The reduction in trough diastolic blood pressure observed with omapatrilat compared favorably with historical data with other commonly prescribed antihypertensive agents such as amlodipine, lisinopril, and losartan. Of note, omapatrilat appears to be particularly effective in lowering systolic blood pressure compared with ACE inhibitors and Ang II receptor antagonists, and appears to be equally efficacious in white and black subjects. Moreover, omapatrilat appears to be well tolerated in both hypertensive and heart failure subjects. Both the overall incidence of adverse events and the adverse event profile observed with omapatrilat were generally comparable with placebo or the active comparator(s). Clinical experience to date suggests that the incidence of cough is comparable with the active control groups that include ACE inhibitors. Overall, the adverse event profile compared favorably with those of the ACE inhibitors and amlodipine (unpublished data). Omapatrilat has potential as a once-a-day, broad-spectrum antihypertensive agent.

POTENTIAL DRAWBACKS

As with selective NEP inhibitors, enhanced activities of Ang II and endothelin may limit the efficacy of inhibitors with affinities for both ACE and NEP. However, the attenuation of Ang II formation by the ACE inhibitory component might minimize the impact of augmenting Ang II by NEP inhibition. Moreover, as endothelin is upregulated by Ang II, the contribution of endothelin may be lessened by

decreased Ang II formation. Indeed, early captopril treatment reduced plasma endothelin concentration in patients with myocardial infarction.[54] The overexpression of the endothelin gene observed in uninephrectomized SHRs was diminished by treatment with ACE inhibition.[55] ACE inhibition also attenuated endothelin secretion by effecting the accumulation of bradykinin in endothelial cells.[56] Further protection of bradykinin by vasopeptidase inhibitors may have a greater salutary influence on endothelin production. Nevertheless, although it is possible that ACE inhibition reduces the potentiation of Ang II and endothelin caused by NEP inhibition, the potential role of vasoconstrictor peptides during simultaneous inhibition of ACE and NEP requires investigation. Interestingly, mean arterial pressure was 20% lower in mice in which the NEP gene was deleted compared with wild-type mice,[57] suggesting that the net effect of NEP ablation shifts the balance of vasoactive agents to a hypotensive state.

POTENTIAL ADVANTAGES

Because of the synergistic effects of combining NEP and ACE inhibition, vasopeptidase inhibitors have several potential advantages over ACE inhibitors. Vasopeptidase inhibitors may have greater efficacy in lowering blood pressure, especially systolic blood pressure, by potentiating an ANP-induced decrease in arterial stiffness,[58] thus affording better end-organ protection. Because both NEP and ACE participate in the inactivation of bradykinin, their combined blockade may augment the cardioprotective and renal effects of bradykinin. Vasopeptidase inhibitors lower blood pressure in hypertensive models with varied levels of PRA and therefore should be effective in a broad range of patients irrespective of their sodium and renin status. The potential natriuretic effects of the protected natriuretic peptides and bradykinin may reduce the need for diuretics in some patients.

Acknowledgment

We thank Dr. Jeffrey A. Robl for his help in preparing this manuscript.

References

1. Flynn GA, French JF, Dage, RC. Dual inhibitors of angiotensin-converting enzyme and neutral endopeptidase: Design and therapeutic rationale. In Laragh JH, Brenner BM (eds). Hypertension. Pathophysiology, Diagnosis, and Management, 2nd ed., vol. 2. New York, Raven, 1995; p 3099.
2. De Lombaert S, Chatelain R, Fink C, Trapani A. Design and pharmacology of dual angiotensin-converting enzyme and neutral endopeptidase inhibitors. Curr Drug Design 2:443, 1996.
3. Fink CA. Recent advances in the development of dual angiotensin-converting enzyme and neutral endopeptidase inhibitors. Exp Opin Ther Patents 6:1147, 1996.
4. Robl JA, Trippodo NC, Petrillo EW. Neutral endopeptidase inhibitors and combined inhibitors of neutral endopeptidase and angiotensin-converting enzyme. In Van Zwieten PA, Greenlee WJ (eds). Antihypertensive Drugs, Amsterdam, Harwood Academic, 1997; p 113.
5. Roques BP, Noble F, Daugé V, et al. Neutral endopeptidase 24.11: Structure, inhibition, and experimental and clinical pharmacology, Pharmacol Rev 45:87, 1993.
6. Lefrançois P, Clerc G, Duchier J, et al. Antihypertensive activity of sinorphan. Lancet 336:307, 1990.

7. Ogihara T, Rakugi H, Masuo K, et al. Antihypertensive effects of the neutral endopeptidase inhibitor SCH 42495 in essential hypertension. Am J Hypertens 7:943, 1994.

8. Bevan EG, Connell JMC, Doyle J, et al. Candoxatril, a neutral endopeptidase inhibitor: Efficacy and tolerability in essential hypertension. J Hypertens 10:607, 1992.

9. Richards AM, Crozier IG, Espiner EA, et al. Acute inhibition of endopeptidase 24.11 in essential hypertension: SCH 34826 enhances atrial natriuretic peptide and natriuresis without lowering blood pressure. J Cardiovasc Pharmacol 20:735, 1992.

10. Richards AM, Wittert GA, Crozier IG, et al. Chronic inhibition of endopeptidase 24.11 in essential hypertension: Evidence for enhanced atrial natriuretic peptide and angiotensin II. J Hypertens 11:407, 1993.

11. Richards AM, Crozier IG, Kosoglou T, et al. Endopeptidase 24.11 inhibition by SCH 42495 in essential hypertension. Hypertension 22:119, 1993.

12. McDowell G, Coutie W, Shaw C, et al. The effect of the neutral endopeptidase inhibitor drug, candoxatril, on circulating levels of two of the most potent vasoactive peptides. Br J Clin Pharmacol 43:329, 1997.

13. Ando S, Rahman MA, Butler GC, et al. Comparison of candoxatril and atrial natriuretic factor in healthy men. Effects on hemodynamics, sympathetic activity, heart rate variability, and endothelin. Hypertension 26:1160, 1995.

14. Cleland JGF, Cowburn PJ, Struthers AD. Neutral endopeptidase inhibitors: Effects on peptide metabolism and potential therapeutic use in the treatment of heart failure. Heart Failure 12:73, 1996.

15. Wilkins MR, Unwin RJ, Kenny AJ. Endopeptidase-24.11 and its inhibitors: Potential therapeutic agents for edematous disorders and hypertension. Kidney Int 43:273, 1993.

16. Raya TE, Lee RW, Westhoff T, Goldman S. Captopril restores hemodynamic responsiveness to atrial natriuretic peptide in rats with heart failure. Circulation 80:1886, 1989.

17. Seymour AA, Asaad MM, Lanoce VM, et al. Systemic hemodynamics, renal function and hormonal levels during inhibition of neutral endopeptidase 3.4.24.11 and angiotensin-converting enzyme in conscious dogs with pacing-induced heart failure. J Pharmacol Exp Ther 266:872, 1993.

18. Trippodo NC, Fox M, Natarajan V. et al. Combined inhibition of neutral endopeptidase and angiotensin converting enzyme in cardiomyopathic hamsters with compensated heart failure. J Pharmacol Exp Ther 267:108, 1993.

19. Margulies KB, Perrella MA, McKinley LJ, Burnett JC Jr. Angiotensin inhibition potentiates the renal response to neutral endopeptidase inhibition in dogs with congestive heart failure. J Clin Invest 88:1636, 1991.

20. Seymour AA, Swerdel JN, Abboa-Offei B. Antihypertensive activity during inhibition of neutral endopeptidase and angiotensin converting enzyme. J Cardiovasc Pharmacol 17:456, 1991.

21. Pham I, Gonzalez W, Amrani AIKE, et al. Effects of converting enzyme inhibitor and neutral endopeptidase inhibitor on blood pressure and renal function in experimental hypertension. J Pharmacol Exp Ther 265:1339, 1993.

22. Favrat B, Burnier M, Nussberger J, et al. Neutral endopeptidase versus angiotensin converting enzyme inhibition in essential hypertension. J Hypertens 13:797, 1995.

23. Trippodo NC, Panchal BC, Fox M. Repression of angiotensin II and potentiation of bradykinin contribute to the synergistic effects of dual metalloprotease inhibition in heart failure. J Pharmacol Exp Ther 272:619, 1995.

24. Gavras I. Bradykinin-mediated effects of ACE inhibition. Kidney Int 42:1020, 1992.

25. Kohlmann O Jr, Cesaretti ML, Ginoza M, et al. Role of substance P in blood pressure regulation in salt-dependent experimental hypertension. Hypertension 29:506, 1997.

26. Valdemarsson S, Edvinsson L, Ekman R, et al. Increased plasma level of substance P in patients with severe congestive heart failure treated with ACE inhibitors. J Intern Med 230:325, 1991.

27. Seymour AA, Mathers PD, Abboa-Offei BE, et al. Renal and depressor activity of C-natriuretic peptide in conscious monkeys: Effects of enzyme inhibitors. J Cardiovasc Pharmacol 28:397, 1996.

28. Brandt RR, Mattingly MT, Clavell AL, et al. Neutral endopeptidase regulates C-type natriuretic peptide metabolism but does not potentiate its bioactivity in vivo. Hypertension 30:184, 1997.

29. Bralet J, Marie C, Mossiat C, et al. Effects of alatriopril, a mixed inhibitor of atriopeptidase and angiotensin I-converting enzyme, on cardiac hypertrophy and hormonal responses in rats with myocardial infarction. Comparison with captopril. J Pharmacol Exp Ther 270:8, 1994.

30. Marie C. Mossiat C, Lecomte JM, et al. Hemodynamic effects of acute and chronic treatment with aladotril, a mixed inhibitor of neutral endopeptidase and angiotensin I-converting enzyme, in conscious rats with myocardial infarction. J Pharmacol Exp Ther 275:1324, 1995.

31. Wegner M, Hirth-Dietrich C, Knorr A, et al. Cardiorenal consequences of dual angiotensin converting enzyme and neutral endopeptidase 24.11 inhibition in transgenic rats with an extra renin gene. Hypertens Res 19:151, 1996.

32. Laurent S, Boutouyrie P, Azizi M, et al. Random zero sphygmomanometer for evaluating the antihypertensive effect of alatriopril. A dual inhibitor of neutral endopeptidase and angiotensin converting enzyme. J Hypertens 15(suppl 4):S158, 1997.

33. Flynn GA, Beight DW, Mehdi S, et al. Application of a conformationally restricted Phe-Leu dipeptide mimetic to the design of a combined inhibitor of angiotensin I-converting enzyme and neutral endopeptidase 24.11. J Med Chem 36:2420, 1993.

34. French JF, Flynn GA, Giroux EL, et al. Characterization of a dual inhibitor of angiotensin I-converting enzyme and neutral endopeptidase. J Pharmacol Exp Ther 268:180, 1994.

35. French JF, Anderson BA, Downs TR, Dage RC. Dual inhibition of angiotensin-converting enzyme and neutral endopeptidase in rats with hypertension. J Cardiovasc Pharmacol 26:107, 1995.

36. Buclin T, Rousso P, Nussberger J, et al. Effects of MDL 100,240 on the response to angiotensin I and II challenges in healthy volunteers. Clin Pharmacol Ther 61:208, 1997.

37. Rousso P, Buclin T, Decosterd L, et al. Effects of MDL 100,240 on the glomerular filtration rate and renal tubular function in healthy volunteers under high and low sodium. Clin Pharmacol Ther 61:206, 1997.

38. Fournié-Zaluski MC, Gonzalez W, Turcaud S, et al. Dual inhibition of angiotensin-converting enzyme and neutral endopeptidase by the orally active inhibitor mixanpril: A potential therapeutic approach in hypertension. Proc Natl Acad Sci U S A 91:4072, 1994.

39. Vera WG, Fournié-Zaluski M-C, Pham I, et al. Hypotensive and natriuretic effects of RB 105, a new dual inhibitor of angiotensin converting enzyme and neutral endopeptidase in hypertensive rats. J Pharmacol Exp Ther 272:343, 1995.

40. Gonzalez W, Beslot F, Laboulandine I, et al. Inhibition of both angiotensin-converting enzyme and neutral endopeptidase by S21402 (RB105) in rats with experimental myocardial infarction. J Pharmacol Exp Ther 278:573, 1996.

41. Stevens TL, Borgeson DD, Redfield MM, et al. Dual inhibition of neutral endopeptidase and angiotensin converting enzyme delays the progression of experimental heart failure. J Am Coll Cardiol 272:257A, 1996.

42. Kullo IJ, Miller VM, Lawson GM, Burnett JC Jr. Dual inhibition of neutral endopeptidase (NEP) and angiotensin converting enzyme (ACE) suppresses atherogenesis and improves endothelial function in hypercholesterolemic rabbits. J Am Coll Cardiol 272:164A, 1996.

43. Kirk JE, Wilkins MR. Renal effects of concurrent E-24.11 and ACE inhibition in the aorto-venocaval fistula rat. Br J Pharmacol 119:943, 1996.

44. Ann Drug Data Report 18:235, 1996.

45. Ramsay LE, Hettiarachchi J. Efficacy and safety of sampatrilat, a novel combined inhibitor of angiotensin converting enzyme and neutral endopeptidase. J Hypertens 14:S223, 1996.

46. Fournie-Zaluski MC, Coric P, Thery V, et al. Design of orally active dual inhibitors of neutral endopeptidase and angiotensin-converting enzyme with long duration of action. J Med Chem 39:2594, 1996.

47. Fink CA, Carlson JE, McTaggart PA, et al. Mercaptoacyl dipeptides as orally active dual inhibitors of angiotensin-converting enzyme and neutral endopeptidase. J Med Chem 39:3158, 1996.

48. Webb RL, Abramson ML, Beil ME, et al. Effects of the novel dual inhibitor of neutral endopeptidase and angiotensin-converting enzyme, CGS 30440, on blood pressure and cardiac hypertrophy in spontaneously hypertensive rats. J Cardiovasc Pharmacol 30:632, 1997.

49. Robl JA, Sun CQ, Stevenson, J, et al. Dual metalloprotease inhibitors: Mercaptoacetyl-based fused heterocyclic dipeptide mimetics as inhibitors of angiotensin-converting enzyme and neutral endopeptidase. J Med Chem 40:1570, 1997.

50. Trippodo NC, Robl JA, Asaad MM, et al. Effects of omapatrilat in low, normal and high renin experimental hypertension. Am J Hypertens 11:363, 1998.

51. Liao W, Delaney C, Smith R, et al. Supine mean arterial blood pressure (MAP) lowering and oral tolerance of BMS-186716, a new dual metalloprotease inhibitor of angiotensin converting enzyme (ACE) and neutral endopeptidase (NEP), in healthy male subjects. Clin Pharmacol Ther 61:229, 1997.

52. Vesterqvist O, Liao W, Manning JA, et al. Effects of BMS-186716, a new dual metalloprotease inhibitor, on pharmacodynamic markers of neutral endopeptidase (NEP) and angiotensin converting enzyme (ACE) activity in healthy men. Clin Pharmacol Ther 61:230, 1997.

53. Trippodo NC, Robl JA, Asaad MM, et al. Cardiovascular effects of the novel dual inhibitor of neutral endopeptidase and angiotensin converting enzyme BMS-182657 in experimental hypertension and heart failure. J Pharmacol Exp Ther 275:745, 1995.

54. Pasquale PD, Valdes L, Albano V, et al. Early captopril treatment reduces plasma endothelin concentrations in the acute and subacute phases of myocardial infarction: A pilot study. J Cardiovasc Pharmacol 29:202, 1997.

55. Largo R, Gómez-Garre D, Liu XH, et al. Endothelin-1 upregulation in the kidney of uninephrectomized spontaneously hypertensive rats and its modification by the angiotensin-converting enzyme inhibitor quinapril. Hypertension 29:1178, 1997.

56. Momose N, Fukuo K, Morimoto S, Ogihara T. Captopril inhibits endothelin-1 secretion from endothelial cells through bradykinin. Hypertension 21:921, 1993.

57. Lu B, Figini M, Emanueli C, et al. The control of microvascular permeability and blood pressure by neutral endopeptidase. Nat Med 3:904, 1997.

58. Mourlon-Le-Grand MC, Poitevin P, Benessiano J, et al. Effect of a nonhypotensive long-term infusion of ANP on the mechanical and structural properties of the arterial wall in Wistar-Kyoto and spontaneously hypertensive rats. Arterioscler Thromb 13:640, 1993.

SECTION 10

Secondary Hypertension

CHAPTER

76 Obstructive Sleep Apnea

Douglas M. Kahn, Paul D. Levinson, and Richard P. Millman

Sleep-disordered breathing spans the spectrum from primary snoring without any evidence of sleep disruption or oxygen desaturation to obstructive sleep apnea.[1] In obstructive sleep apnea, there are repetitive episodes of partial or complete collapse of the posterior pharynx during sleep.[2] This may occur in the retropalatal (velopharynx), in the retroglossal portion of the oropharynx, or in the hypopharynx.[3, 4] The obstructive events lead to hypoxemia, hypercapnia, and acidosis. Respiratory events will continue without airflow until arousal from sleep eventually occurs. With the arousal from sleep, the oropharyngeal muscles contract, the airway opens, and respiration resumes. These recurrent arousals lead to sleep fragmentation and/or deprivation. Patients are believed to have obstructive sleep apnea syndrome (OSAS) when these obstructive events are accompanied by characteristic symptoms, specifically disruptive snoring, daytime hypersomnolence, and cognitive impairment resulting from this sleep fragmentation and hypoxemia.[2]

Risk factors clearly associated with the development of OSAS are upper body obesity and age. Other potential risk factors include male gender, a positive family history, nonwhite race, alcohol consumption, and tobacco use.[2] Although patients may rarely complain of choking arousals, apneas are witnessed frequently by the patient's bed partner and are strongly associated with the diagnosis of OSAS.[1] Findings on physical examination that heighten the possibility of sleep apnea are retrognathia, enlarged tonsils, a large soft palate and uvula, increased body mass index, upper body obesity, increased neck circumference, and the presence of hypertension (HTN).[5]

OSAS has been associated with many clinical consequences. Sleep fragmentation can cause excessive sleepiness, and there is an increased incidence of motor vehicle accidents in patients with severe OSAS.[1, 2, 6, 7] Patients may have problems with memory and concentration, and job performance and family functioning can be adversely affected.[1, 2, 6] There can be increased irritability and even depression.[1, 2, 6] Many cardiovascular complications are associated with OSAS, including a possible link between systemic HTN and OSAS. These are discussed later in the chapter.

PREVALENCE

The prevalence of OSAS in the middle-aged population is generally considered to be 2% in women and 4% in men.[8]

This prevalence increases in the elderly.[9, 10] This contrasts significantly to the prevalence of OSAS in populations of patients with HTN, in which the prevalence is reported to be between 22 and 48%.[11–15] The prevalence of HTN in the general population is approximately 15 to 20%,[16, 17] and in populations of patients with OSAS, it has been reported to exceed 40%.[18–20]

DIAGNOSIS

To establish a diagnosis of OSAS and determine severity, patients must undergo sleep testing. This can be performed with devices that vary in the number and type of recording channels. The most basic is a four-channel cardiorespiratory device that typically records airflow, respiratory effort, heart rate, and oxygen saturation. The most sophisticated devices are typically used in sleep disorder centers or laboratories in which complete polysomnography is performed. For the patient, this entails sleeping overnight while being monitored for electroencephalographic activity with two leads, eye movements (two leads), and chin electromyographic activity. These recordings allow the determination of sleep stage. Airflow can be assessed by using either a thermistor in the nose or mouth or a nasal pressure transducer. The latter is much more sensitive and can detect mild changes in upper airway resistance. Typically, one uses a snoring microphone as well. Respiratory effort is usually determined using chest and abdominal monitors and intercostal electromyographs. In some sleep disorder centers, respiratory effort is assessed using an invasive esophageal balloon. Electrocardiograms and oxygen saturation level measurements are typically performed as well. To exclude an alternative diagnosis of periodic limb movement disorder, anterior tibialis electromyographic activity is also recorded.[21]

The best test for a given patient is determined by pretest clinical suspicion. If there is a high clinical suspicion for sleep apnea with loud snoring in any position, observed apneas or choking arousals, daytime sleepiness, obesity, and HTN, the patients can be diagnosed by either basic or sophisticated sleep studies.[21] Sleep studies are not currently recommended for all hypertensive patients. Such evaluation appears to be appropriate if hypertensive patients have symptoms or conditions commonly associated with OSAS (Table 76–1), especially excessive daytime sleepiness, loud

657

Table 76–1 Clinical Features and Predisposing Factors Associated With Obstructive Sleep Apnea Syndrome

Clinical Features	Predisposing Factors
Snoring	Obesity
Observed apneas	Male sex
Choking arousals	Increasing age
Fragmented sleep	Enlarged tonsils and adenoids
Insomnia	Macroglossia
Daytime sleepiness	Retrognathia
Memory problems	Nasal obstruction
Poor attention and concentration	Evening alcohol or sedative ingestion
Personality changes	Acromegaly
Impotence	Hypothyroidism

snoring, or witnessed apneas.[20] Because patients who have resistant HTN or who are nondippers (lack the normal blood pressure decline with sleep) appear to have a somewhat higher risk of OSAS, the threshold for sleep testing in them should probably be set somewhat lower.[20] The combination of HTN, obesity (body mass index > 30), witnessed apneic episodes, and daytime somnolence predicts the diagnosis of OSAS with greater than 95% accuracy.[22]

In the presence of a high pretest clinical suspicion, a negative basic study does not exclude obstructive sleep apnea, and full polysomnography should be performed.[21] For patients with a lower probability for sleep apnea (e.g., patients who snore but have minimal sleepiness and no observed apneic episodes), full polysomnography using a nasal pressure transducer is probably the best way to assess mild sleep apnea.[21] Patients who present primarily with daytime sleepiness in whom snoring is only a mild component clearly need in-laboratory polysomnography and may need a special test during the daytime, a multiple sleep latency test, to assess the severity of the sleepiness as well as to exclude narcolepsy.[21]

A diagnosis of OSAS is made when a patient with the appropriate symptom complex undergoes overnight sleep testing and is found to have greater than five apneas or hypopneas per hour of sleep (this is known as an *apnea-hypopnea index* [AHI] > 5). An *apnea* is defined as a cessation of airflow for at least 10 seconds, whereas a *hypopnea* is usually described as a reduction in airflow associated with oxyhemoglobin desaturation or an arousal.[23] There has been considerable controversy regarding the appropriateness of this AHI threshold. In patients over the age of 65 years, it may be more appropriate to use a higher level.[24]

TREATMENT

The mainstay of treatment for OSAS is weight loss, as this has been clearly shown to improve OSAS.[25, 26] There is evidence that with even modest weight loss of approximately 10 kg, OSAS can be improved.[27] With extensive weight loss, patients with OSAS can even be cured.[25–27] The response to weight loss is directly determined by

anatomical abnormalities.[28] Treatment that can be used while weight loss is in progress can be divided into three categories: behavioral, medical, and surgical. Besides weight loss, behavioral therapy includes the cessation of alcohol consumption and sedative use, the avoidance of sleep deprivation, and sleep positioning to avoid the supine position. Obstruction occurs more frequently in the supine position in some patients.[29] Patients who sleep on a firm mattress can be trained to get off their backs. They can insert a regulation hard softball into a sock and can clip the top of the sock to the collar of their pajamas and the bottom of the sock to the mid back. Whenever the patient lies on his or her back, the ball will create discomfort and he or she will automatically go on to the side.

Medical therapies include the treatment of any associated medical condition, such as hypothyroidism or acromegaly. In addition, there are conservative therapies for sleep apnea, such as nocturnal continuous positive airway pressure (nCPAP).[30] nCPAP is usually delivered via a tightly fitted nasal mask, but other types of masks and adapters are available to fit the individual needs of patients. The headgear is connected by tubing to an air compressor that forces air down the nose and throat to keep the pharynx open, thus creating a pneumatic splint. Typically, pressures of 10 to 15 cm H_2O are required. The correct pressure is determined during a sleep study; pressure is titrated to obliterate snoring, apneas and hypopneas, oxygen desaturation, and arousals. Patients who have trouble tolerating high continual pressures may be tried on bilevel pressure, in which the pressure drop is typically 5 cm H_2O during exhalation. Compliance is the major problem with therapies that utilize positive airway pressure. Typically, there is irritation of the nasal mucosa, leading to excessive dryness or rhinitis. Steroid nasal sprays may help somewhat, but the best treatment appears to be heated humidification.

An alternative conservative therapy involves oral appliances.[31, 32] Typically, these devices advance the mandible and thrust the tongue forward. There is evidence that these devices enlarge both the posterior oropharynx and the velopharynx.[33] They are extremely successful in patients with mild to moderate disease and are preferred by some patients over nasal continuous positive airway pressure.[32]

In some patients, it is worthwhile to attempt a surgical cure.[34, 35] In children with sleep apnea, removal of tonsils and adenoids is the preferred treatment.[36] A uvulopalatopharyngoplasty procedure removes the uvula and part of the soft palate.[34] If it is combined with a genioglossal/mandibular advancement procedure, patients with mild to moderate sleep apnea may obtain a successful response approximately 70 to 78% of the time.[37]

BLOOD PRESSURE DURING SLEEP

Arterial blood pressure declines by 10 to 20% during sleep in normotensive persons without OSAS as well as in most persons with essential HTN. Blood pressure may decrease slightly with deeper stages of sleep; it tends to be higher and more variable during rapid eye movement sleep than during non–rapid eye movement sleep.[20, 38, 39]

Since 1972, many investigators have documented the unique pattern of hemodynamic changes that accompanies obstructive apneic episodes during sleep (Fig. 76–1).[40–42] At the start of a typical apnea, systemic pressure declines transiently, then increases gradually as the apnea continues. After arousal and the resumption of ventilation, blood pressure increases acutely, and often markedly, for 10 to 15 seconds before returning to baseline during the following 30 to 45 seconds. Pulmonary artery pressure follows a pattern similar to that of arterial pressure. Heart rate tends to decrease during the apnea, but accelerates as breathing resumes. The magnitude of the apnea-related blood pressure rise appears to depend in part on the duration and severity of the apnea, and probably other factors as well (see later in this chapter). In one study of six patients, maximal blood pressure increases averaged 48 ± 21/32 ± 14 mm Hg above presleep, awake blood pressures.[42] Effective treatment of OSAS, e.g., by nCPAP, reduces or eliminates both the recurrent apneas and the related circulatory changes.[43]

The apnea-related blood pressure changes described previously are the most frequent arterial pressure abnormality observed in OSAS. Investigators have also observed hypotensive readings (mean arterial pressure < 60 mm Hg) during sleep,[44] but these appear to be infrequent. In patients with severe OSAS, mean nocturnal blood pressure may equal or exceed waking blood pressure levels.[45, 46] Although some studies indicated that the absence of a nocturnal blood pressure "dip" during 24-hour ambulatory blood pressure monitoring was a sensitive diagnostic indicator of OSAS, other studies have not.[47, 48] Whereas some patients with OSAS (especially severe OSAS) may lose the normal nocturnal decline in blood pressure, many OSAS patients do not.

Blood pressure changes during apneas appear to result largely from the hemodynamic alterations associated with the markedly negative intrathoracic pressures generated by respiratory effort against a closed glottis. Peripheral vasoconstriction mediated by the sympathetic nervous system appears to cause the acute arterial pressure rise that occurs with apnea termination and resumption of breathing. Despite a great deal of research, the mechanism of sympathetic activation remains unclear. Several studies suggest that the brief arousals that end apneic episodes are the primary stimuli of sympathetic activation.[49–51] Stimulation of carotid and aortic chemoreceptors by hypoxemia also appears to activate brain stem cardiovascular centers and increase sympathetic outflow.[52] This reflex presumably overrides the direct vasodilator effect of hypoxemia in regional vascular beds. Increases in heart rate and intrapleural pressure that accompany the resumption of ventilation have also been postulated to cause the postapnea blood pressure increase, but few studies have assessed the importance of these mechanisms in human subjects. Humoral factors, e.g., prostaglandins or nitric oxide, have not been shown to play a role in the acute blood pressure changes associated with apneas. Increased atrial natriuretic peptide secretion during sleep may contribute to the nocturnal natriuresis and diuresis that has been observed in patients with OSAS.[53]

BLOOD PRESSURE IN THE AWAKE STATE

The relationship between OSAS and HTN has generated considerable controversy since the mid-1980s. Although theories support the contention that either condition may cause the other (or a third condition, e.g., obesity, may cause both), most attention has been given to the hypothesis that OSAS promotes the development of daytime, as well as nocturnal, HTN (see later). A recent population study of Wisconsin state workers showed that the severity of sleep-disordered breathing was independently correlated with both daytime and 24-hour ambulatory blood pressure.[54] Other population surveys tend to show minimal or no effect of sleep apneas on blood pressure, however.[55, 56]

A significant reduction in blood pressure during effective treatment of OSAS would provide strong support for OSAS as an independent risk factor for HTN. Whereas available data suggest that blood pressure decreases with nCPAP, the observed blood pressure reductions tend to be modest and inconsistent.[56, 57] Several animal models show evidence of waking HTN after induced apneas or hypoxia, but the applicability of these models to human OSAS remains uncertain.[58, 59]

HTN and OSAS are clearly linked by common risk factors, of which obesity is the strongest. Sixty to 80% of symptomatic OSAS patients appear to be at least 20%

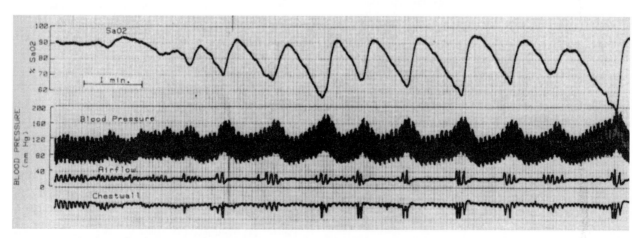

Figure 76–1. Segment of a sleep record demonstrating the changes in systemic blood pressure associated with apneas in a patient with obstructive sleep apnea. (From Shepard JW Jr. Gas exchange and hemodynamics during sleep. Med Clin North Am 69:1243–1264, 1985.)

overweight. Weight loss appears to reduce apnea frequency in patients with OSAS, but the mechanism by which obesity promotes sleep apnea has not been clarified.[60] Persons with OSAS tend to have predominantly upper body (i.e., central or "apple-type") obesity.[61, 62] An excess of neck fat has also been described in OSAS patients compared with weight-matched controls.[63] Mass loading studies suggest that large deposits of deep neck fat may predispose to the airway narrowing that occurs in OSAS.[64]

If, as noted previously, OSAS promotes the development of daytime HTN independently of known confounders, such as obesity and age, the causal mechanisms have yet to be defined. Increased directly measured neural activity has been described in awake, resting persons with OSAS,[65] and plasma and urinary catecholamines tend to be elevated in OSAS patients during waking hours.[66] Studies in rats have demonstrated that sympathetically mediated blood pressure increases can be produced by repetitive episodes of hypoxia.[59] Primary or secondary chemoreceptor abnormalities have also been proposed, with increased daytime sympathetic activity considered to be the final pathway responsible for the blood pressure increase.[67] Humoral and/or volume-related mechanisms have been postulated, but minimal supportive evidence is currently available.[68]

POTENTIAL CARDIOVASCULAR CONSEQUENCES

In theory, OSAS may increase cardiovascular morbidity and mortality by several mechanisms. Pulmonary artery pressures are increased in patients with OSAS, although repetitive changes in pulmonary artery pressures at night rarely lead to daytime pulmonary HTN and cor pulmonale in the absence of concomitant lung disease.[6]

The increase in nocturnal blood pressure may contribute to the typical cardiovascular complications of systemic HTN, including left ventricular hypertrophy, myocardial infarction, and stroke. Cardiovascular risk would be increased further if daytime HTN were a direct consequence of OSAS. The repetitive nocturnal blood pressure elevations and autonomic surges, as well as the hypoxemia, acidosis, and hypercapnea that accompany apneic episodes, have been postulated to produce endothelial and arteriolar wall damage, cardiac ischemia, and arrhythmias.[40] Whereas some retrospective studies have shown increased mortality associated with vascular complications in people with OSAS,[69, 70] others have not.[71]

TREATMENT OF HYPERTENSION IN PATIENTS WITH OSAS

Effective treatment of OSAS, e.g., with nCPAP, is likely to reduce nocturnal blood pressure but may or may not decrease daytime blood pressure. If daytime HTN persists after institution of OSAS therapy, treatment based on the standard guidelines for management of essential HTN is appropriate, and consideration should be given to potential coexisting conditions, such as obesity, diabetes mellitus, and cardiovascular disease. Medications that cause sedation

or increase daytime somnolence should be avoided. The 1997 sixth report of the Joint National Committee on Prevention, Detection, Evaluation, and Treatment of High Blood Pressure (JNC-VI) described OSAS as a "coexisting disease" with HTN, but did not provide specific recommendations for blood pressure management in patients with OSAS.[72]

Several small, controlled studies of antihypertensive drug therapy have been performed specifically in patients with HTN and OSAS, but evidence is insufficient to identify antihypertensive agents that either improve or exacerbate sleep apnea.[73–77]

CONCLUSIONS

1. Both OSAS and HTN are common medical conditions with similar, overlapping risk factors.
2. There is likely an association between OSAS and HTN, and although there is a suggestion from the current literature that OSAS may cause secondary daytime HTN, a clear causal association has not yet been established.
3. As there is evidence that patients with OSAS have increased sympathetic activity, it is likely, although unproved, that this is the mechanism by which patients with OSAS develop daytime HTN.
4. OSAS may contribute to cardiovascular morbidity and mortality, but this too requires further study.
5. Sleep testing is recommended for hypertensive patients with symptoms or conditions associated with OSAS, specifically excessive daytime sleepiness, loud snoring, and witnessed apneas.

References

1. Redline S, Strohl KP. Recognition and consequences of obstructive sleep apnea hypopnea syndrome. Clin Chest Med 19:1–19, 1998.
2. Strohl KP, Redline S. State of the art: Recognition of obstructive sleep apnea. Am J Respir Crit Care Med 154:279–289, 1996.
3. Schwab RJ. Upper airway imaging. Clin Chest Med 19:33–54, 1998.
4. Winakur SJ, Smith PL, Schwartz AR. Pathophysiology and risk factors for obstructive sleep apnea. Semin Respir Crit Care Med 19:99–112, 1998.
5. Strollo PJ, Rogers RM. Current concepts: Obstructive sleep apnea. N Engl J Med 334:99–104, 1996.
6. Epstein LJ, Weiss JW. Clinical consequences of obstructive sleep apnea. Semin Respir Crit Care Med 19:123–132, 1998.
7. American Thoracic Society Position Paper. Sleep apnea, sleepiness, and driving risk. Am J Respir Crit Care Med 150:1463–1473, 1994.
8. Young T, Palta M, Dempsey J, et al. The occurrence of sleep-disordered breathing among middle-aged adults. N Engl J Med 328:1230–1235, 1993.
9. Schwartz AR, Smith PL. Sleep apnea in the elderly. Clin Geriatr Med 5:315–329, 1989.
10. Hoch CC, Reynolds CF III, Monk TH, et al. Comparison of sleep-disordered breathing among healthy elderly in the seventh, eighth, and ninth decades of life. Sleep 13:502–511, 1990.
11. Kales A, Cadieux RJ, Shaw LC, et al. Sleep apnoea in a hypertensive population. Lancet 2:1005–1008, 1984.
12. Lavie P, Ben-Yosef R, Rubin AE. Prevalence of sleep apnea syndrome among patients with essential hypertension. Am Heart J 108:373–376, 1984.
13. Williams AJ, Houston D, Finberg S, et al: Sleep apnea syndrome and essential hypertension. Am J Cardiol 55:1019–1022, 1985.
14. Fletcher EC, DeBehnke RD, Lovoi MS, Gorin AB. Undiagnosed sleep apnea in patients with essential hypertension. Ann Intern Med 103:190–195, 1985.

15. Worsnop CJ, Naughton MT, Barter CE, et al. The prevalence of obstructive sleep apnea in hypertensives. Am J Respir Crit Care Med 157:111–115, 1998.

16. Oparil S. Arterial hypertension. *In* Bennett JC, Plum F (eds). Cecil Textbook of Medicine, 20th ed. Philadelphia, WB Saunders, 1996; pp 256–271.

17. Hypertension Detection Follow-up Program Cooperative Group. The Hypertension Detection and Follow-up Program: A progress report. Circ Res 40(suppl I):I-106–I-110, 1977.

18. Fletcher EC. The relationship between systemic hypertension and obstructive sleep apnea: Facts and theory. Am J Med 98:118–128, 1995.

19. Silverberg DS, Oksenberg A. Essential and secondary hypertension and sleep-disordered breathing: A unifying hypothesis. J Hum Hypertens 10:353–363, 1996.

20. Carlson J, Davies R, Ehlenz K, et al. Working Group on OSA and Hypertension: Obstructive sleep apnea and blood pressure elevation: What is the relationship? Blood Press 2:166–182, 1993.

21. Millman RP, Neumeyer D, Kramer NR. Diagnostic strategies. Semin Respir Crit Care Med 19:133–138, 1998.

22. Crocker BD, Olson LG, Sanders NA, et al. Estimation of the probability of disturbed breathing during sleep before a sleep study. Am Rev Respir Dis 142:14–18, 1990.

23. Moser NJ, Phillips BA, Berry DTR, et al. What is hypopnea anyway? Chest 105:426–428, 1994.

24. Redline S. Epidemiology of sleep-disordered breathing. Semin Respir Crit Care Med 19:113–122, 1998.

25. Browman CP, Sampson MG, Yolles SF, et al. Obstructive sleep apnea and body weight. Chest 85:435–436, 1984.

26. Smith PL, Gold AR, Meyers DA, et al. Weight loss in mildly to moderately obese patients with obstructive sleep apnea. Ann Intern Med 103:850–855, 1985.

27. Phillips BA, Anstead MI, Pinto SJ. Behavioral management of obstructive sleep apnea. Semin Respir Crit Care Med 19:139–146, 1998.

28. Pasquali R, Colella P, Cirignotta F, et al. Treatment of obese patients with obstructive sleep apnea syndrome (OSAS): Effect of weight loss and interference of otorhinolaryngoiatric pathology. Int J Obes 14:207–217, 1990.

29. Pevernagie DA, Stanson AW, Sheedy PF II, et al. Effects of body position on the upper airway of patients with obstructive sleep apnea. Am J Respir Crit Care Med 152:179–185, 1995.

30. Strollo PJ, Sanders MH, Atwood CW. Positive pressure therapy. Clin Chest Med; 19:55–68, 1998.

31. Schmidt-Nowara W, Lowe A, Wiegand L, et al. Oral appliances for the treatment of snoring and obstructive sleep apnea: A review. Sleep 18:501–510, 1995.

32. Millman RP, Rosenberg CL, Kramer NR. Oral appliances in the treatment of snoring and sleep apnea. Clin Chest Med; 19.1: 69–75, 1998.

33. Eveloff SE, Rosenberg CL, Carlisle C, Millman RP. Efficacy of a Herbst mandibular advancement device in obstructive sleep apnea. Am J Respir Crit Care Med 149:905–909, 1994.

34. Sher AE, Schechtman KB, Piccirillo JF. The efficacy of surgical modifications of the upper airway in adults with obstructive sleep apnea syndrome. Sleep 19:156–177, 1996.

35. Powell NB, Riley RW, Robinson A. Surgical management of obstructive sleep apnea syndrome. Clin Chest Med 19:77–86, 1998.

36. Stradling JR, Thomas G, Warley ARH, et al. Effect of adenotonsillectomy on nocturnal hypoxaemia, sleep disturbance, and symptoms in snoring children. Lancet 335:249–253, 1990.

37. Riley RW, Powell NB, Guilleminault C. Obstructive sleep apnea syndrome: A surgical protocol for dynamic upper airway reconstruction. J Oral Maxillofac Surg 51:742–747, 1993.

38. Levinson PD, Millman RP. Causes and consequences of blood pressure alterations in obstructive sleep apnea. Arch Intern Med 151:455–462, 1991.

39. Coccagna G, Mantovani M, Brignani F, et al. Arterial pressure changes during spontaneous sleep in man. Electroencephalogr Clin Neurophysiol 31:277–281, 1971.

40. Shepard JW Jr. Hypertension cardiac arrhythmias, myocardial infarction, and stroke in relation to obstructive sleep apnea. Clin Chest Med 13:437–458, 1992.

41. Coccagna G, Mantovani M, Brignani F, et al. Continuous recording of the pulmonary and systemic arterial pressure during sleep in syndromes of hypersomnia with periodic breathing. Bull Physiopathol 8:1159–1172, 1972.

42. Motta J, Guilleminault C, Schroeder JS, et al. Tracheostomy and hemodynamic changes in sleep-induced apnea. Ann Intern Med 89:454–458, 1978.

43. Lies A, Nabe B, Pankow W, et al. Hypertension and obstructive sleep apnea: Ambulatory blood pressure monitoring before and with nCPAP-therapy. Z Kardiol 85(suppl 3):140–142, 1996.

44. McGinty D, Beahm E, Stern N, et al. Nocturnal hypotension in older men with sleep-related breathing disorders. Chest 94:305–311, 1988.

45. Davies RJO, Crosby J, Vardi-Visy K, et al. Non-invasive beat to beat arterial blood pressure during non-REM sleep in obstructive apnoea and snoring. Thorax 49:335–339, 1994.

46. Noda A, Okada T, Hayashi H, et al. 24-Hour ambulatory blood pressure variability in obstructive sleep apnea syndrome. Chest 103:1343–1347, 1993.

47. Wilcox I, Grunstein RR, Collins FL, et al. Circadian rhythm of blood pressure in patients with obstructive sleep apnea. Blood Press 1:219–222, 1992.

48. Hla KM, Young TB, Bidwell T, et al. Sleep apnea and hypertension—A population-based study. Ann Intern Med 120:382–388, 1994.

49. Bonsignore MR, Marrone O, Insalaco G, et al. The cardiovascular effects of obstructive sleep apnoeas: Analysis of pathogenic mechanisms. Eur Resp J 7:786–805, 1994.

50. Weiss JW, Remsburg S, Garpestad E, et al. Hemodynamic consequences of obstructive sleep apnea. Sleep 19:388–397, 1996.

51. Ringler J, Basner RC, Shannon R, et al. Hypoxemia alone does not explain blood pressure elevations after obstructive apneas. J Appl Physiol 69:2143–2148, 1990.

52. Hedner JA, Wilcox I, Laks L, et al. A specific and potent pressor effect of hypoxia in patients with sleep apnea. Am Rev Respir Dis 146:1240–1245, 1992.

53. Baruzzi A, Riva R, Cirignotta F, et al. Atrial natriuretic peptide and catecholamines in obstructive sleep apnea syndrome. Sleep 14:83–86, 1991.

54. Young T, Peppard P, Palta M, et al. Population-based study of sleep-disordered breathing as a risk factor for hypertension. Arch Intern Med 157:1746–1752, 1997.

55. Warley ARH, Mitchell JH, Stradling JR. Prevalence of nocturnal hypoxaemia amongst men with mild to moderate hypertension. Q J Med 256:637–644, 1988.

56. Stradling J, Davies RJO. Sleep apnea and hypertension—What a mess! Sleep 20:789–793, 1997.

57. Silverberg DS, Oksenberg A. Essential hypertension and abnormal upper airway resistance during sleep. Sleep 20:794–806, 1997.

58. Brooks D, Horner RL, Kozar LF, et al. Obstructive sleep apnea as a cause of systemic hypertension: Evidence from a canine model. J Clin Invest 99:106–109, 1997.

59. Fletcher EC. Sympathetic activity and blood pressure in the sleep apnea syndrome. Respiration 64(suppl 1):22–28, 1997.

60. Strobel RJ, Rosen RC. Obesity and weight loss in obstructive sleep apnea: A critical review. Sleep 19:104–115, 1996.

61. Levinson PD, McGarvey ST, Carlisle CC, et al. Adiposity and cardiovascular risk factors in men with obstructive sleep apnea. Chest 103:1336–1342, 1993.

62. Millman RP, Carlisle CC, McGarvey ST, et al. Body fat distribution and sleep apnea severity in women. Chest 107:362–366, 1995.

63. Horner RL, Mohiaddin RH, Lowell DG, et al. Sites and sizes of fat deposits around the pharynx in obese patients with obstructive sleep apnoea and weight matched controls. Eur Respir J 2:613–622, 1989.

64. Koenig JE, Thach BT. Effects of mass loading on the upper airway. J Appl Physiol 64:2294–2299, 1988.

65. Carlson JT, Hedner J, Elam M, et al. Augmented resting sympathetic activity in awake patients with obstructive sleep apnea. Chest 103:1763–1768, 1993.

66. Dimsdale JE, Coy T, Ziegler MG, et al. The effect of sleep apnea on plasma and urinary catecholamines. Sleep 18:377–381, 1995.

67. Przybylski J, Sabbah HN, Stein PD. Why do patients with essential hypertension experience sleep apnea syndrome? Med Hypotheses 20:173–177, 1986.

68. Guilleminault C, Robinson A. Sleep-disordered breathing and hypertension: Past lessons, future directions. Sleep 20:806–811, 1997.

69. He J, Kryger MH, Zorick FJ, et al. Mortality and apnea index in obstructive sleep apnea—Experience in 385 male patients. Chest 94:9–14, 1988.

70. Partinen M, Jamieson A, Guilleminault C. Long-term outcome for

obstructive sleep apnea patients. Mortality. Chest 94:1200–1204, 1988.

71. Wright J, Johns R, Watt I, et al. Health effects of obstructive sleep apnoea and the effectiveness of continuous positive airways pressure: A systematic review of the research evidence. BMJ 314:851–860, 1997.
72. Joint National Committee on Prevention, Detection, Evaluation, and Treatment of High Blood Pressure. The sixth report. Arch Intern Med 157:2413–2446, 1997.
73. Tochikubo O, Minamisawa K, Miyakawa T, et al. Blood pressure during sleep: Antihypertensive medication. Am J Cardiol 67:18B–25B, 1991.
74. Weichler U, Herres-Mayer B, Mayer J, et al. Influence of antihyper-

tensive drug therapy on sleep pattern and sleep apnea activity. Cardiology 78:124–130, 1991.
75. Grote L, Heitmann J, Schneider H, et al. Twenty-four-hour blood pressure control: Effect of cilazapril on continuous arterial blood pressure during sleep, and physical and mental load in patients with arterial hypertension and sleep apnea. J Cardiovasc Pharmacol 24(suppl 3):S78–S82, 1994.
76. Pelttari L, Rauhala E, Kantola I. Effects of antihypertensive medication on hypertension in patients with sleep apnoea. Blood Press 3(suppl 2):88–91, 1994.
77. Kantola I, Rauhala E, Erkinjuntti M, Mansury L. Sleep disturbances in hypertension: A double blind study between isradipine and metoprolol. J Cardiovasc Pharmacol 18(suppl 3):S41–S45, 1991.

CHAPTER 77

Renovascular Hypertension: Diagnosis and Treatment

Samuel Spitalewitz and Ira W. Reiser

SIGNIFICANCE

Renovascular hypertension results from renal ischemia and is usually caused by a partially or completely occlusive lesion of one or both renal arteries. It may affect up to 5% of patients with hypertension and is the most common cause of correctable (secondary) hypertension. Renovascular hypertension may lead to ischemic nephropathy and even end-stage renal disease (ESRD) in a significant proportion of affected patients.[1, 2] It is therefore a major public health problem. We have recently reviewed the diagnosis and treatment of renovascular hypertension.[3]

INCIDENCE AND CAUSE

Most patients with renovascular disease present with moderate to severe hypertension, although blood pressure rarely may be normal or only mildly elevated. Renovascular disease is less common in African Americans than in Caucasians, in whom it may cause accelerated or malignant hypertension in as many as 10 to 45% of affected patients.[4, 5] However, in those African American patients with clinical features suggestive of renovascular disease (see later section), the incidence may be as high as 20%.[5]

Although hypertension may result from any form of ischemic renal disease (e.g., scleroderma, vasculitis of the kidney or renal artery, atheroembolic disease, aneurysms, or other extrinsic compression of the renal arteries), atherosclerotic renal artery disease accounts for more than two thirds of cases of renovascular hypertension; the remainder are caused by fibromuscular dysplasia.[1] Atherosclerotic renovascular disease typically presents in patients older than 40 years of age, most commonly involves the renal ostium (extending from an aortic atherosclerotic plaque) or the proximal third of the renal artery, and has a male:female ratio of 2:1.[1, 6] Fibromuscular dysplasia, of which there are four types (medial fibroplasia, perimedial fibroplasia, medial hyperplasia, and intimal hyperplasia), is more commonly seen in younger patients, usually Caucasian females. Although the exact incidence of each type of fibromuscular dysplasia is unknown, medial fibroplasia is the most common and accounts for approximately two thirds of cases. The lesions of fibromuscular dysplasia are generally bilateral and, unlike those seen with atherosclerotic renovascular disease, affect the more distal portion of the renal artery.[7]

CLINICAL SIGNS AND SYMPTOMS

Because of its low incidence, screening all hypertensive patients for renovascular disease is not cost-effective. However, the clinician should screen those hypertensive patients who present with one or more of the following signs or symptoms:[1, 8]

1. Severe or refractory hypertension, with evidence of grade 3 or 4 hypertensive retinopathy (particularly in Caucasian patients)
2. Abrupt onset of moderate to severe hypertension, particularly in a previously well-controlled hypertensive or normotensive patient
3. Onset of hypertension before age 20 (early onset) or after age 50 (late onset), particularly in the absence of a family history of hypertension
4. Unexplained deterioration in renal function with or without hypertension, or in association with the administration of angiotensin-converting enzyme (ACE) inhibitors or angiotensin II receptor blockers (ARBs), or reduction of blood pressure to "normal" with other antihypertensive agents
5. Paradoxical worsening of hypertension with diuretic therapy
6. Spontaneous hypokalemia
7. Recurrent "flash" pulmonary edema or otherwise unexplained episodes of congestive heart failure

8. Generalized vascular disease
9. The presence of a systolic-diastolic abdominal bruit that lateralizes to one or both flanks (a systolic bruit alone is more sensitive but less specific)
10. Stigmata of cholesterol emboli

SCREENING TESTS

There are several screening tests for renal artery disease, each with its own advantages and disadvantages, that will be described in detail below. The tests we find most useful are radioisotope scanning, magnetic resonance angiography (MRA), and spiral (helical) computed axial tomography (CT). Because a negative screening test does not entirely preclude the presence of a renal artery lesion, if our clinical suspicion is high and a radiological or a surgical intervention is deemed emergent, we proceed directly to angiography (Fig. 77–1).

Radioisotope Scanning

Renal scintigraphy, with and without ACE inhibition, is our most frequently used initial screening test in patients without renal insufficiency (Fig. 77–2).[1, 9] A scintigraphic study without ACE inhibition (nonstimulated), using either I^{131} orthoiodohippurate (OIH) or ^{99m}Tc diethylenetriamine-pentaacetic acid (DTPA) as the radioisotope, is only as

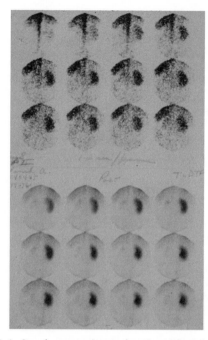

Figure 77–2. Renal scan, using technetium-99m–diethylenetri-aminepentaacetic acid as the radionuclide, demonstrates reduced and delayed blood flow to the left kidney due to renovascular disease of the left renal artery.

sensitive and specific as an intravenous pyelogram (see later) and is, therefore, of limited value as a screening test.[9–11] However, both the sensitivity and the specificity of the study can be greatly improved (to 90 to 95%) with a stimulated (captopril) scan.[12–15] When the pre- and postcaptopril (nonstimulated vs. stimulated) renograms are compared, a decrement in renal function may be seen in the involved kidney. This occurs because ACE inhibition attenuates the angiotensin-mediated vasoconstriction distal to the renovascular lesion, thereby reducing intraglomerular capillary pressure and, as a consequence, the glomerular filtration rate (GFR). Less often, an improvement in function may be demonstrated on the uninvolved side.[11, 16, 17] In addition to its high sensitivity and specificity, ACE-inhibition renography is easy to perform, does not require discontinuing antihypertensive medications (except ACE inhibitors and ARBs at least 48 hours prior to the study), and may predict the blood pressure response to revascularization.[12, 13, 15, 18–21] The following are consistent with a positive study:

1. Decreased relative uptake by the involved kidney, which in turn contributes less than 40% of the total renal function
2. Almost twice the usual time (5 min) to peak uptake of the isotope on the affected side
3. Delayed washout of the radioisotope of more than 5 minutes on the involved side compared with the contralateral kidney

The radionuclides of choice are DTPA, a marker of glomerular filtration, and OIH, a marker of renal plasma flow. No statistically significant difference in quantitative or qualitative accuracy has been demonstrated between the two markers in the absence of significant renal insuffi-

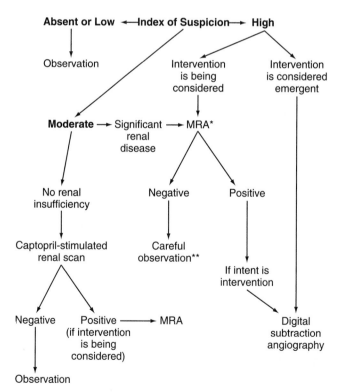

Figure 77–1. Schematic approach to the diagnostic investigation of renal artery stenosis. *A spiral computed tomography scan may be substituted for a magnetic resonance angiography (MRA) if there is no renal insufficiency or if an MRA is contraindicated or both. **If a patient's renal function significantly deteriorates or blood pressure cannot be controlled medically, proceed to angiography.

ciency.[22] However, in the presence of moderate renal insufficiency, OIH is more sensitive.[18] Mercaptoacetyltriglycine (Mag$_3$), a radionuclide with transport properties similar to those of hippuran, has also been utilized and is particularly useful when colabeled with ^{99}Tc, with which it better delineates renal anatomy and can estimate renal blood flow.[23]

Although stimulated renal scintigraphy is a practical screening test with high sensitivity and specificity, its use is limited in patients with advanced azotemia or bilateral renovascular disease. It has been suggested that stimulated renal scans not be used in patients with creatinine clearances of less than 20 ml/min because of diminished accuracy at this level of renal dysfunction.[10, 11, 15, 17, 24, 25] However, furosemide when combined with OIH in stimulated scintigraphy has recently been found to be both sensitive (96%) and specific (95%) in screening patients with varying degrees of renal insufficiency (serum creatinines 1.8 to 5.3 mg/dl). This study was done in only a small number of patients and must be confirmed by larger trials.[18]

We find radioisotope scanning most useful in patients with normal renal function and "resistant" or difficult-to-control hypertension. If the scan is negative, and the patient's moderate to severe hypertension is likely to be due to inadequate therapy or noncompliance, we will not proceed with any further screening tests. If the scan is positive, we usually proceed with a magnetic resonance angiogram.

Magnetic Resonance Angiography

Recent prospective studies indicate that three-dimensional MRA with gadolinium-based contrast agents (which are non-nephrotoxic) may be more sensitive than the screening tests described above (Fig. 77–3). A total of 80 patients were studied in two recent trials comparing MRA with

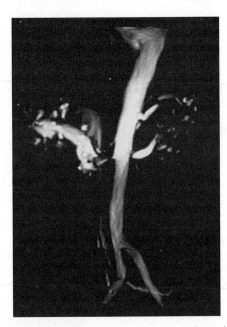

Figure 77–3. Time-of-flight magnetic resonance angiography demonstrates a small area of narrowing 6 mm from the origin of the right renal artery and a severe occlusion of the left renal artery at its origin with poststenotic dilatation.

digital subtraction angiography (DSA) (see later) or conventional renal angiography.[26, 27] A sensitivity approaching 100% and a specificity of 71 to 96% was found with MRA. When combined with cardiac synchronization, three-dimensional MRA can sharply delineate virtually the entire length of the major renal arteries. However, the visualization of distal, intrarenal, and accessory renal arteries that may have hemodynamically significant occlusive lesions remains suboptimal.[28–31] MRA can also noninvasively determine both the absolute renal blood flow and the GFR and thus assess the functional significance of renovascular lesions.[29]

This excellent screening modality remains limited by its expense, its availability, and its contraindication in patients with metallic clips and implants such as pacemakers and defibrillators. It is extremely valuable in providing us with a noninvasive method of visualizing the arterial anatomy and is often the decisive factor in determining whether nonmedical intervention is warranted.

Computed Axial Tomography

Spiral (helical) CT angiography with intravenous contrast administration has been used as a screening test for detecting renovascular lesions in patients with normal renal function. With this technique, the diagnostic accuracy in detecting renal artery lesions is quite good, with some investigators reporting a 98% sensitivity and a 94% specificity.[32] In a recent prospective study, spiral CT angiography and intra-arterial DSA were compared in patients with normal renal function suspected of having renal artery stenosis and in potential kidney donors. Spiral CT angiography demonstrated 27 of 28 accessory renal arteries and 100% of stenoses of 50% or more in the main renal arteries.[33] In another prospective study comparing it with Doppler ultrasound, spiral CT angiography was the more accurate screening technique.[34] If these initial observations are confirmed by larger studies in patients without renal insufficiency, spiral CT angiography may become the noninvasive screening technique of choice. However, both the sensitivity and the specificity of this test decline (to 93% and 81%, respectively) in the presence of renal insufficiency (serum creatinine concentration > 1.7 mg/dl).[32] Furthermore, the risk of radiocontrast-induced nephrotoxicity is significant because the volume of radiocontrast required is large (approximately 100 ml). These shortcomings have been the major limitations in its usefulness in our patient population, many of whom have significant renal insufficiency at presentation. We use spiral CT angiography if an MRA is contraindicated and there is no renal insufficiency or emergent need for nonmedical intervention.

Angiography

When they are negative, screening tests do not totally exclude the presence of a renal artery lesion, especially in the distal vessels. Therefore, the clinical index of suspicion should determine which screening tests, if any, should be done. The clinician may opt to proceed immediately with conventional renal angiography or an intra-arterial DSA, both of which remain the diagnostic gold standards (Fig. 77–4).[10, 11, 16] This is done when emergent radiological or surgical intervention is deemed appropriate. Because intra-arterial DSA requires the administration of less radiocontrast (25 to 50 ml) than conventional angiography (100 ml), it is preferred, especially in patients with compromised renal function.

Carbon dioxide digital angiography has been used as an effective alternative to iodinated contrast agents in patients with renal insufficiency. When used in combination with digital subtraction, intra-arterial carbon dioxide angiography provides diagnostic imaging similar to that achieved using standard contrast studies, while eliminating the potential nephrotoxicity of radiocontrast.[35] Despite these advantages, it does not always provide adequate visualization of the more distal vasculature and requires an experienced technician as well as sophisticated programming with electronic enhancement. In addition, the procedure may be complicated by air embolization, neurotoxicity, and renal ischemia due to "vapor lock." At present, it remains only an investigational tool.

Compared with intra-arterial injection, intravenous DSA is less invasive and does not pose a risk of cholesterol embolization. However, the renal vasculature is not as well delineated as with intra-arterial injection; the amount of radiocontrast required is greater (150 to 200 ml); and the sensitivity and specificity are 90% or less, compared with arterial studies.[36, 37] In addition, it requires more dye and is less reliable than a spiral CT scan. Therefore, we no longer use this test.

Duplex Doppler Ultrasonography

Similar to scintigraphy with Mag$_3$ colabeled with ^{99}Tc, ultrasonic duplex scanning of the renal arteries can provide both anatomical and functional information. This technique combines the direct visualization of the main renal arteries via B-mode ultrasound imaging with Doppler measurements of various hemodynamic parameters characteristic of renal artery lesions. Stenotic lesions are detected by comparing the acceleration time, the resistive indexes of each kidney and artery, and the systolic or end-diastolic flow in the involved renal artery to that in the aorta. Early experience with this technique demonstrated a significant false-negative rate of 8 to 20%. However, more recent studies have demonstrated greatly improved sensitivity and specificity when sonography was done prior to and then compared with the results of angiography.[38–42] As with radioisotope scanning, captopril (stimulated) Doppler ultrasound studies have further increased the sensitivity of the technique. The specific Doppler wave forms distal to the vascular lesion are enhanced by captopril and the sensitivity of the study may increase significantly and may approach 100% following captopril administration.[43]

A recent prospective study compared duplex Doppler scanning with captopril-stimulated renography in terms of ability to detect hemodynamically significant renovascular lesions and to predict the fall in blood pressure following percutaneous transluminal angioplasty. No significant difference between the two tests was found, and the positive predictive value of both for blood pressure cure or improvement approached 90%.[44] Intrarenal echo-Doppler velocimetric indexes (particularly the acceleration time and index) have also been used to assess the success of dilatation procedures, predict re-stenosis, and detect re-stenosis in arteries previously revascularized by angioplasty, stent placement, or surgery.[16, 40, 41]

Duplex Doppler scanning is noninvasive, does not require discontinuing any antihypertensive medications, and does not involve exposure to radiation or radiocontrast. Unlike the other screening tests described, it may be used with accuracy in patients with renal failure and it provides information regarding the presence of bilateral disease.

Despite these advantages, the usefulness of duplex Doppler ultrasonography as a screening tool is limited because it is very time-consuming, operator-dependent, and technically difficult to perform, and extensive training in the procedure is necessary in order to perform an accurate study. In addition, intrarenal vascular lesions and multiple (and even main) renal arteries may be missed, particularly in obese patients or in those with overlying intestinal gas.[16, 38, 42, 44] Its major use at present is to follow up lesions in patients in whom an MRA is contraindicated and who have significant renal insufficiency, precluding a spiral CT scan.

SCREENING TESTS OF LITTLE CLINICAL USEFULNESS

Intravascular Ultrasonography

This invasive sonographic procedure provides structural detail of the renal vascular lesion and, therefore, can distinguish between fibromuscular dysplasia and atherosclerotic renal artery lesions.[45] Compared with noninvasive sonography, it can more accurately assess the severity of occlusion and closely correlates with angiographic findings.[45, 46] Be-

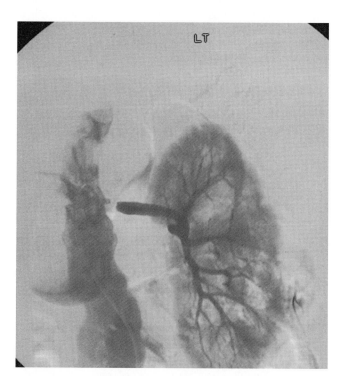

Figure 77–4. Selective renal angiography of the left renal artery demonstrates a 99% stenosis of the artery at its origin.

cause it estimates volumetric flow, it has also been used recently to assess the patency of renal arteries before and after angioplasty and stent placement.[47, 48] Intravascular ultrasonography is invasive and requires radiocontrast to guide the placement of the intra-arterial ultrasound probe. Therefore, its usefulness as a screening test is limited, especially in patients with impaired renal function.

Intravenous Pyelography

Decreased function of the kidney involved in renovascular disease may be detected by conventional intravenous pyelography (IVP), but greater sensitivity is achieved with a "hypertensive" IVP. With the latter technique, additional radiographs are taken at 1, 2, 3, 4, and 5 minutes. Thus, the hypertensive IVP is more likely to demonstrate a delay in the calyceal appearance or nephrogram of the affected kidney, which may be missed if only later films are viewed, as in a conventional IVP. Other IVP findings suggestive of renal artery disease include discrepancy in renal size or cortical thickness, hyperconcentration of the radiocontrast in the involved kidney, ureteral notching due to collateral circulation, and a prolonged nephrogram effect in the later films.[1] An IVP is now seldom used as a screening test for renovascular hypertension because of its low sensitivity and specificity (both approximately 75%), the risk of radiocontrast-induced nephrotoxicity, and its relatively high radiation dose.[16, 49] Furthermore, in the presence of bilateral renal artery disease, many of the above findings may be absent, especially if there is little difference in function between the two kidneys.[10]

Plasma Renin Activity

Elevated baseline plasma renin activity (PRA) is found in only 50 to 80% of patients with renovascular hypertension and may be observed in 16% of patients with essential hypertension. Thus, an elevated baseline PRA is of limited diagnostic significance, and its absence in no way excludes renovascular hypertension. The predictive value of PRA may be enhanced by measuring its increase 1 hour after the ingestion of 25 to 50 mg of captopril.[10, 16, 17] This "captopril test" improves the diagnostic accuracy of PRA, but the reported sensitivity and specificity of the procedure vary widely (63 to 100% and 72 to 100%, respectively), even when strict criteria for a positive result are met.[10, 17, 50] In addition, to perform this test accurately, antihypertensive agents affecting PRA must be discontinued, which may be dangerous in these patients, most of whom have moderate to severe hypertension. The usefulness of the captopril test is further limited because it is impractical and requires strict standardization; its accuracy is reduced in the presence of mild renal insufficiency (serum creatinine > 1.5 to 2.0 mg/dl), and its predictive value is less than that of a renogram obtained following ACE inhibition (see later).[9, 12-14, 51]

IS A RENAL ARTERY LESION CAUSING HYPERTENSION?

The presence of a renal artery lesion does not mean that it is the cause of hypertension. Therefore, prior to any intervention aimed at eliminating or controlling hypertension, the physiological significance of a lesion should be proven.[1] ACE-inhibitor scans, renal vein renin (RVR) measurements, and the pressure gradient across the renal artery lesion have been used to determine whether a stenosis is causing hypertension.[52] If a lesion is the cause of "renin-dependent" hypertension, renin secretion by the kidney distal to the renal vascular lesion should be increased, and secretion by the contralateral kidney should be suppressed, resulting in an RVR ratio of 1.5 or more (affected:nonaffected side). When the RVR ratio is used to predict reduction in blood pressure following intervention, a sensitivity of only 80% and a specificity of 62% have been reported.[36] However, the predictive accuracy of the RVR can be improved with the administration of ACE inhibitors prior to testing.[10] With unilateral renal artery disease and a captopril-stimulated lateralizing RVR, an improvement in blood pressure after revascularization is seen in up to 90% of patients.[11] However, the absence of lateralization does not necessarily mean that there will be no fall in blood pressure after intervention, for as much as 60% of these patients may still have an improvement in their blood pressures following revascularization.[11] Because of its low predictive value, the need for renal vein catheterization with radiocontrast injection, and the need to discontinue medications that may affect renin secretion, RVR measurements are no longer commonly used. More predictive than RVR measurements is the pressure gradient across the renal artery lesion as determined by intra-arterial renal angiography. The absence of a significant pressure gradient (10 to 15 mm Hg) suggests that the lesion is of little physiological significance and that revascularization in this setting will be of little benefit.

Because no single test is reliable enough to determine a causal relationship between a renal artery lesion and hypertension, the signs and symptoms previously described (items 1 through 7 under Clinical Signs and Symptoms), if present, should alert the clinician that it is highly likely that the lesion is causing hypertension. Once the diagnosis of renovascular hypertension is made, the clinician may attempt to control the patient's blood pressure with medical therapy alone and/or with percutaneous transluminal renal angioplasty (PTRA), placement of a vascular endoprosthesis (a stent), or surgery. The therapeutic approach is determined by the type of lesion causing the hypertension, the site and extent of renal artery involvement, the overall medical status of the patient, and the perceived risks which are, in part, based on the interventionist's skills in performing the procedures. The effectiveness of each approach in controlling hypertension as well as the role of revascularization in preserving renal function (many of these patients have associated ischemic nephropathy and renal insufficiency), are reviewed later.

MEDICAL THERAPY FOR HYPERTENSION

Medical therapy for renovascular hypertension is similar to that for essential hypertension, but because severe hypertension is more common in patients with renovascular disease, combination drug therapy is frequently necessary in that group. Nevertheless, blood pressure control is usually achieved in more than 90% of cases. Because the hypertension may be dependent on angiotensin II, antihypertensives that inhibit renin or angiotensin II production or block their actions are especially useful in renovascular hypertension. Therefore, β-blockers, ACE inhibitors, and ARBs have been extensively utilized, with ACE inhibitors being especially efficacious.[53–55] Studies have demonstrated control of blood pressure in 80% of patients when ACE inhibitors are used alone and in up to 90% when they are combined with diuretic therapy.[54, 55] However, ACE inhibitors should be used with caution, particularly in patients with bilateral renal artery stenosis (RAS) (see later). Although there is less clinical experience with the newer ARBs, in experimental models of renovascular hypertension, they are as potent as ACE inhibitors.[56]

Despite control of blood pressure with medical therapy, several studies have demonstrated that atherosclerotic renal artery lesions progress in 40 to 60% of patients within 7 years (with half of these lesions progressing within 2 years).[57–59] Patients with an initial stenosis of more than 75% have the fastest rate of progression, with total occlusion occurring in 40% of these lesions.[57] Renal function, however, may not necessarily decline concomitantly. In addition to the "natural" progression of the atherosclerotic vascular lesion, medical therapy, by reducing blood pressure, may result in chronic hypoperfusion distal to the lesion and may hasten tubular atrophy, interstitial fibrosis, and glomerulosclerosis in the affected kidney or kidneys.[60–62] Some investigators have demonstrated in animal models that at a given level of blood pressure, ACE inhibitors are more likely than other antihypertensive agents to induce these structural changes.[60, 61] However, to date, there are no clinical studies suggesting that ACE inhibitors or ARBs irreversibly hasten the loss of renal function when given on a long-term basis to patients with unilateral or bilateral atherosclerotic renovascular disease.[63] Nevertheless, when these drugs are used, especially when they are combined with diuretic therapy, patients' renal function should be frequently monitored. In addition to monitoring renal function with serum creatinine concentrations and 24-hour creatinine clearances, it has also been suggested that renal sizes and renal cortical blood flow velocity, using duplex scanning, be monitored too, as these parameters may provide earlier signs of irreversible renal function loss.[64] In this recent study of 122 patients, persistent stenosis increased the risk of long-term loss of renal mass, but this loss was more closely associated with the degree of renal artery stenosis and the level of systolic blood pressure than with the use of ACE inhibitors. In addition to a possible association with *chronic* hypoperfusion and nephron loss, ACE inhibitors, as well as the ARBs, may result in *acute* (usually reversible) renal failure in 10 to 20% of patients with bilateral RAS or with RAS affecting a solitary kidney. This is most likely to occur when patients are volume-contracted.

Compared with atherosclerotic RAS, the risk of progressive occlusion and renal ischemia with medial fibroplasia, the predominant form of fibrous renal artery disease, is low.[56, 57] In contrast, the lesions of perimedial fibroplasia, medial hyperplasia, and intimal fibroplasia frequently progress and may result in a deterioration of renal function similar to that seen with atherosclerotic RAS.[65, 66] There-

fore, renal function must be carefully monitored in these patients.[57]

ANGIOPLASTY AND STENTING FOR HYPERTENSION

PTRA is an angiographic technique by which stenotic renal arteries are dilated with a catheter containing a cylindrical inflatable balloon at its tip (Fig. 77–5). The success rate of PTRA is dependent on the site and type of the vascular lesion; it is most likely to be successful in lesions in which there is incomplete arterial occlusion, the length of the stenosis is less than 10 mm, and in lesions which do not involve the renal os.[67, 68]

Most studies of PTRA in patients with fibromuscular dysplasia report a high technical success rate (87 to 100%), an improvement in or cure of the hypertension in as many as 90% of patients, and a low incidence (10%) of re-stenosis.[66, 68–70, 72] In contrast to fibromuscular dysplasia, the technical success rate of PTRA when performed for unilateral atherosclerotic renovascular lesions may be as low as 70%, and long-term improvement in or cure rates of the hypertension vary widely.[66, 68–70, 72] The improvement in or cure of hypertension depends in large part on the location of the lesion. In a study of 100 patients, Canzanello and colleagues demonstrated an improvement in blood pressure of 86% in patients with nonostial unilateral lesions compared with 46% for patients with ostial unilateral lesions.[72] Acute reversible renal insufficiency complicated 21% of the procedures, and mechanical complications such as thrombosis, perforation, or dissection of renal arteries or diffuse atheroembolism occurred in 14% of the patients.

The preceding data were generated in uncontrolled trials. A recent randomized prospective trial comparing medical therapy (in 26 patients) with PTRA (in 23 patients) for unilateral RAS demonstrated that PTRA reduced the number of drugs necessary for blood pressure control at 6 months.[73] At baseline, 54% of the medically treated patients needed more than two antihypertensive medications, compared with 34% in the angioplasty group. With time, 88% of the medically treated group required two or more medications, compared with 35% of those who were postangioplasty. PTRA was complicated by one case of dissection with segmental renal infarction, and by re-stenosis in 18%. It should be noted, however, that more patients with ostial lesions at baseline (46% vs. 30%) were treated medically. Thus, the more favorable outcome observed with PTRA may reflect this selection bias. Of the medically managed patients, 27% were terminated from the study and subsequently underwent angioplasty because of refractory hypertension. It was not specified whether these "refractory" patients had ostial lesions and whether PTRA was successful. The results of this study are therefore difficult to interpret, and others are needed for a better comparison of these two approaches.

In contrast to this study, no improvement in blood pressure was observed in a group of 13 patients with unilateral RAS randomized to PTRA as compared with 14 treated with medical therapy and followed for up to 54 months (range, 3 to 54 months).[74] Major outcome events such as death, myocardial infarction, heart failure, stroke, and dial-

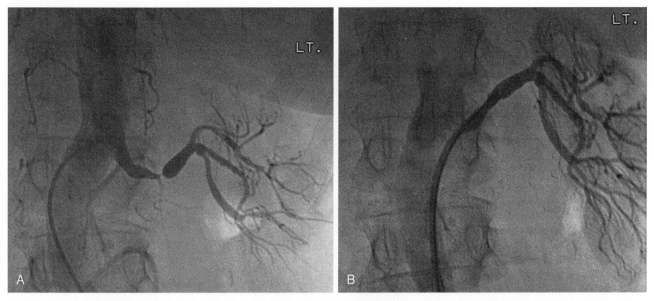

Figure 77–5. Nonostial renal artery lesion before **(A)** and after **(B)** percutaneous transluminal angioplasty.

ysis did not differ between the two groups. In addition, 28% of the patients who underwent angioplasty experienced complications attributable to the procedure, the most common of which was bleeding at the arterial puncture site (8 patients). Thus, it appears that when PTRA is used to control hypertension due to unilateral RAS, the potential gain, if any, is often outweighed by the risk and the discomfort of the procedure.

The results of PTRA in patients with bilateral RAS are equally unimpressive, due, at least in part, to the high incidence of ostial or completely occluding lesions, both of which are more difficult to dilate and are associated with a high complication rate.[67, 69, 72] Ramsay and Waller have recently reviewed 10 series of patients who underwent PTRA for treatment of atherosclerotic RAS.[69] In general, the selection criteria were ill-defined, and the patients chosen for the PTRA were carefully selected, which probably biased the findings in favor of angioplasty. The studies cited had significant variations in the technical failure rates and the estimates of cure or improvement in blood pressure. Further, the types of lesions treated were often not characterized. Despite the limitations of these studies, it appears that in bilateral atherosclerotic lesions, the technical failure rate may be as high as 60% and the cure rate for hypertension as low as 8%, with improvement in blood pressure in only 43%.[69] The results are especially disappointing when the bilateral disease is associated with an atrophic kidney, as total renal artery occlusion of the atrophic kidney is observed in half of the cases.[68] As demonstrated by Geyskes, PTRA in a patient with an atrophic kidney resulted in an improvement in blood pressure in only 8 of 57 (14%) and in a cure of the hypertension in only 5 patients (9%).[68]

In view of these data, it is reasonable to attempt PTRA only in the patients in whom medical therapy has failed and in whom an incomplete but high-grade ($\geq$75 to 90%) unilateral RAS distal to the os is present. Even with an initial successful therapeutic outcome, the incidence of re-stenosis following PTRA for RAS is significant (30% for nonostial lesions and 50% for ostial lesions) and may occur soon after the procedure (15 to 30% by 2 years). Reocclusion, however, does not preclude a repeat PTRA.[53]

To prevent re-stenosis and improve blood pressure control with PTRA for atheromatous ostial lesions, intravascular stents have been placed during angioplasty (Fig. 77–6).[75–77] One group of investigators has now performed this procedure without nephrotoxic radiocontrast by using a combination of intra-arterial carbon dioxide and gadepentetate dimeglumine, avoiding the risk of contrast-induced acute renal failure.[78] Initial studies of intravascular stenting reported a success rate of 65 to 70% and a risk of re-stenosis ranging from 13 to 39%.[75, 76] More encouraging results were recently demonstrated in 68 patients with ostial lesions after stent placement for unsuccessful PTRA.[77] The technical success rate was 100%; re-stenosis (defined as reocclusion of more than 50% of the vessel diameter) occurred in only 11% during a mean follow-up time of 27 months, and either cure or improvement of the hypertension was noted in 78%. No major complications were reported in this study. It is important to note that the majority of the patients (64%) were followed for only 12 months, with only 9% followed long-term (60 months). Furthermore, patients with a residual stenosis of up to 50% of the arterial lumen were classified as complete technical successes, even though they remain at a substantial risk for reocclusion. The study demonstrates the safety and short-term efficacy of the procedure but does not provide sufficient evidence to support long-term efficacy of endovascular stenting.[79] Nevertheless, it appears that renal arterial stenting may prove to be most useful in patients with ostial disease, re-stenosis after PTRA, or complications due to PTRA such as dissection.[66]

Primary renal artery stenting (i.e., without antecedent PTRA) has also been performed in atherosclerotic RAS.[80] The technical success rate is high and the rate of serious complications is low. Although the investigators do not specify what percentage of the patients had nonostial lesions, approximately 60% demonstrated cure or improvement of their blood pressure (regardless of whether there was unilateral or bilateral disease) at 6 months. At 1 and 4 years' follow-up, the improvement rate fell to 42%, and only 1% remained cured of their hypertension.[81, 82] At 6 months, 25% of the lesions were re-stenosed (proven angiographically), but longer-term patency rates of the stents are unknown because of lack of angiographic follow-up.[80–82]

Two other studies have been done in patients who have undergone primary and/or secondary stenting.[83, 84] In both studies, no clinically significant improvement in blood pressure was observed. In the study with the longest follow-up (5 years), despite an initial diminution in the number of antihypertensive medications required at 3 to 6 months, the number increased subsequently and was no different from before stent placement. Patency was angiographically determined at a mean of 8 months plus or minus 5 months (range 2 to 24 months). A re-stenosis rate of 50% or more occurred in 14%.[84]

Based on these data, stenting for control of blood pressure alone is not generally recommended. To date, no investigators have cited criteria that clearly define which patients with nonostial lesions should undergo primary renal artery stenting. We perform primary renal artery stenting in nonostial lesions in the patients in whom angiography demonstrates a very high-grade stenosis (≥90%) and/or a stenosis of 7 to 10 mm or longer, as the probability of success with PTRA alone is low.

Following successful PTRA, a reduction in blood pressure may be seen as early as 4 to 6 hours after the procedure, but the maximal antihypertensive effect is commonly achieved well after 48 hours.[53, 71] In some cases, the full antihypertensive benefit may not be observed until after several weeks. The absence of an early decline in

blood pressure suggests that significant long-term improvement of the hypertension is unlikely.[71]

Although PTRA and stenting are generally safe procedures, complication rates of approximately 5 to 15% have been reported. Most of these complications, such as hematoma formation at the puncture site and renal artery spasm, are of minor clinical significance. However, if it is severe, renal artery spasm can lead to local thrombosis and renal infarction. This can be prevented or reversed by the administration of intra-arterial nitroglycerin. Major complications frequently include reversible, contrast-induced acute tubular necrosis (approximately 20%) and, infrequently (<5%), renal artery perforation, dissection, or irreversible acute renal failure due to atheroembolization.

SURGERY FOR HYPERTENSION

Surgical revascularization for renovascular hypertension involves bypassing the site of the arterial lesion by grafting or anastomosing another vessel distal to the lesion and/or removing an atrophic kidney. Because PTRA is highly successful in patients with fibromuscular dysplasia, is less invasive, and is associated with lower morbidity and mortality rates than is surgical revascularization, surgery is not recommended as primary therapy for these patients. It is done, however, when PTRA is unsuccessful or is technically not feasible, as is the case when branch renal artery disease is present (30% of patients with fibrous renal artery disease).[85, 86] When surgery is done, 90 to 95% of patients with fibromuscular dysplasia are cured or see substantial improvement of their hypertension.[36, 66, 86–88]

Although surgical revascularization in patients with atherosclerotic RAS may result in cure or improvement of the

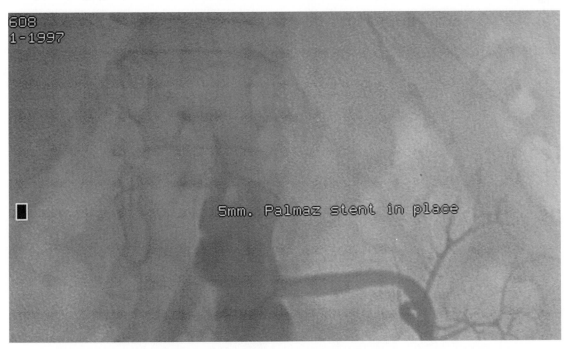

Figure 77–6. The renal ostial lesion depicted in Figure 77–4 is shown after placement of an intravascular stent.

hypertension in as many as 80 to 90% of patients, surgery other than a simple nephrectomy of an atrophic kidney is not recommended for blood pressure control alone in patients with unilateral or with bilateral atherosclerotic renal artery disease. These patients are generally older and commonly have extensive extrarenal vascular disease. Their long-term survival rate following surgery, particularly if they have bilateral RAS and diffuse atherosclerosis, is poor. Furthermore, their hypertension can usually be controlled with medical therapy. If surgery becomes the only option, the probability of successful control of blood pressure in unilateral RAS is inversely related to the duration of and vascular damage caused by preexisting essential hypertension, as well as to the degree that the renin angiotensin system is activated in the contralateral kidney (see later). In the presence of underlying contralateral RAS with renal ischemia, parenchymal small-vessel disease, or both, the antihypertensive response to surgery is significantly diminished.[66, 86-90]

The morbidity and mortality with surgical revascularization is significant. As with any major intra-abdominal vascular surgery, complications include those due to manipulation of the aorta (thrombosis, dissection, and atheroembolization), acute renal failure due to renal ischemia, pancreatitis, hemorrhage, splenic infarction, renal graft aneurysm formation, and postoperative RAS or renal artery thrombosis. Because of their younger age and absence of extrarenal vascular disease, mortality rates are very low in patients with fibromuscular disease. In contrast, mortality rates are significantly higher in patients with atherosclerotic disease unless they are carefully selected, in which case mortality rates may be as low as 3 to 5%. Mortality rates increase in patients older than 65 years of age, particularly if generalized atherosclerosis (coronary or cerebral vascular disease), congestive heart failure or significant renal disease is present. In order to decrease mortality, screening for and surgical correction of significant carotid or coronary artery disease should be attempted before revascularization.[85]

Hypertension may recur after surgery and is most often due to either recurrent atherosclerotic disease or anastomotic neointimal hyperplasia. Although recurrent lesions are generally clinically silent, in as many as 15%, either PTRA or another surgical procedure may be required. In approximately 10% of patients, bypass graft re-stenosis will occur and may be seen as late as 10 years after surgical revascularization.[53]

To date, no prospective randomized trials have been done comparing medical therapy, PTRA, and surgery in controlling atherosclerotic renovascular hypertension. However, the results of several nonrandomized studies have suggested that surgery is the most successful, whereas other studies have demonstrated no difference in control of blood pressure among the three approaches.[53, 91-93] Many of these studies were done prior to the widespread use of ACE inhibitors, and recent advances in surgical techniques make these earlier comparisons irrelevant to current management strategies.

In a more recent prospective randomized trial comparing PTRA and surgical revascularization in a group of patients with unilateral RAS, a higher success rate and a lower incidence of re-stenosis were found in the surgical group after 2 years. However, the effect on blood pressure was not different when both interventions were successful.[94]

In view of the current data, we manage hypertension in patients with RAS as follows:

1. Because of its low risk-to-benefit ratio, high success rate, and low rate of re-stenosis, PTRA is the treatment of choice for fibromuscular dysplasia uncomplicated by branch renal artery disease. If PTRA is unsuccessful, or if branch renal artery disease is present, surgical revascularization should be undertaken, as these patients are generally young and have excellent responses to surgery, obviating the need for long-term medical therapy.

2. Medical therapy should be the primary management in patients with atherosclerotic RAS with mild, controllable hypertension or with comorbid conditions such as diffuse atherosclerosis that place them at high operative risk. Because renal function may decline with progression of the underlying atherosclerotic lesions or with the medical therapy itself, we monitor renal function closely in these patients. If renal size diminishes significantly (due to renal ischemia) or if there is deterioration in renal function, PTRA or surgery should be performed to attempt to preserve or improve renal function. As discussed later, the modality chosen is highly individualized.

3. In the absence of diffuse vascular disease or other comorbid conditions that may increase operative risk, nonmedical intervention should be undertaken in those patients with atherosclerotic RAS and moderate to severe hypertension only if blood pressure is not well controlled by medical therapy or if deterioration of renal function occurs with blood pressure control. PTRA, with or without intravascular stenting, should then be done in the presence of a nonostial, partially occluding vascular lesion. In view of technically successful results with intravascular stenting, we attempt this procedure in patients with ostial lesions, with nonostial lesions that have re-stenosed after PTRA, and with lesions that have more than 90% stenosis or are 7 to 10 mm in length or longer, particularly in patients in whom the surgical risk is considerable. If the above approach is unsuccessful, surgical revascularization is performed, particularly in patients with unilateral RAS.

PRESERVATION OF RENAL FUNCTION

As previously discussed, atherosclerotic renal artery lesions narrow progressively. However, it is not known how many patients with bilateral renovascular disease develop ischemic nephropathy or ESRD, nor is it known over what time period this occurs. A recent retrospective study examined these issues.[95] The investigators studied the medical records of 51 patients with particularly severe bilateral RAS (total occlusion or stenosis of 90% or more in one renal artery, with at least 50% stenosis on the opposite side). Only medical therapy had been offered to these patients because of physician or patient preference, because the lesions were not amenable to angioplasty, because the kidneys were too small to salvage, or because the patient was not clinically suitable for surgical intervention. The overall mortality rate was high—38% within 2 years of renal angiography and 45% at 5 years. The incidence of ESRD was 12% at 5 years. The rate of decline of the GFR for all patients was 4 ml/min/year (range 1 to 16 ml/min/year). Those most likely to reach ESRD were those with more advanced renal failure (GFR < 25 ml/min) at the time of angiography and those whose renal function showed a decline in GFR of > 8 ml/min/year. It is impressive that in a large percentage of patients, little or no serial change in renal function was observed despite the presence of severe bilateral disease. Progressive renal dysfunction and narrowing of the arterial lumen does not inevitably occur, and the development of collateral circulation to the kidneys may offset the reduction in flow in the major renal arteries. Hence, even in the presence of severe RAS, collateral circulation may maintain renal viability and function.[96] This is not always the case, however, and it is clear that progressive but potentially reversible renal insufficiency results from bilateral renal artery disease. In the view of some investigators, this problem is becoming more common in older patients.[90]

It has been estimated that ischemic nephropathy is the cause of renal failure in 5 to 15% of patients over the age of 50 years, and it may account for 10 to 20% of all patients with ESRD. Despite dialytic therapy, mortality rates are high (>50% over 3 years), and 5- and 10-year survival rates are only 18% and 5%, respectively. In view of these grim statistics, restoration of renal function (either by surgery or by PTRA with or without stenting) is critically important and should be attempted whenever indicated.[59, 65, 97–99]

PTRA in patients with renal dysfunction due to ischemic nephropathy improves renal function in 40% of patients and stabilizes function in an additional 30 to 40%.[59, 72, 97, 100, 101] The majority of patients included in these studies had nonostial lesions. Because the success rate is reasonable and is comparable to that of surgical revascularization, which has a higher morbidity and mortality rate, PTRA should be the initial intervention in patients with nonostial atherosclerotic lesions who have deteriorating renal function.[102] Re-stenosis occurs in 10 to 30% of these patients, and many of them are amenable to repeat PTRA.[97]

Only 15 to 20% of atherosclerotic lesions are nonostial.[102] With ostial atherosclerotic lesions, PTRA without stenting has been largely ineffective because of the high technical failure rate due to elastic recoil of the artery and because of neointimal hyperplasia or recurrent atherosclerosis both of which commonly result in eventual failure.[102] As previously discussed, the placement of intravascular stents for ostial atherosclerotic lesions is a promising new technique to improve the safety and possibly the long-term patency rate and efficacy of PTRA.

Recent studies have examined the role of intravascular stenting in the preservation of renal function.[77, 81–83, 103] Following unsuccessful angioplasty, 68 patients with ostial lesions and normal renal function at baseline (serum creatinine < 1.4 mg/dl) underwent stenting. None had worsening of renal function at a mean follow-up of 27 months. Similarly, no deterioration of renal function was observed in the 30% of patients who had significant renal insufficiency at baseline.[77] In another study, 32 patients with a median serum creatinine of 2.9 mg/dl underwent renal artery stenting and were followed for a mean of 8 months (range 0 to 29 months). Of the 32, 11 patients (34%) showed significant improvement in renal function, 11 patients (34%) stabilized, and 9 patients (28%) worsened. In a subset of 23 patients, in whom the level of renal function prior to stenting was known for a sufficient time period that the reciprocal of the serum creatinine vs. time could be plotted, the rate of progression of renal failure was slowed in 18 (78%) following the procedure. Patients with baseline serum creatinine levels of less than 4.5 mg/dl were most likely to benefit from stenting.[83] In both studies, the re-stenosis rate was less than 15%.[77, 83]

Results of stenting for ischemic nephropathy in patients followed for longer periods have now been reported.[82, 84, 103] Of 163 patients who underwent primary stenting, Dorros and colleagues followed 145 for approximately 4 years.[82] The outcome of renal function was stratified according to whether the lesion was initially bilateral or unilateral. The baseline serum creatinine concentration in both groups was approximately 2.0 mg/dl. Of those with unilateral disease, 67% experienced improved or stable renal function, and the remainder progressed as reflected by an increase in the serum creatinine of more than 0.2 mg/dl above baseline. Of those with bilateral disease, 75% had stable or improved renal function, and 25% deteriorated. Overall survival, however, was worse for those with poorer renal function at baseline, regardless of whether stenting was successful. Survival at 4 years was good in patients with normal baseline renal function (92 ± 4%), fair (74 ± 7%) in those with mildly impaired renal function (serum creatinine 1.5 to 1.9 mg/dl), and poor (52 ± 7%) in patients with serum creatinine levels of 2.0 mg/dl or more. The rate of re-stenosis is not reported in this study.

Tuttle and colleagues followed 129 patients after primary or secondary stenting for a mean of 24 months. During this follow-up time, renal function, as assessed by creatinine clearances, remained stable, but no improvement in renal function was demonstrated regardless of baseline creatinine clearance (range 23 ± 3 to 53 ± 3 ml/min). However, of the 129 patients studied, 4 of the 8 who were initially dialysis-dependent recovered renal function after stenting. Their mean serum creatinine concentration was 2.3 ± 0.5 mg/dl at 15 ± 6 months (range 9 to 24 months). As demonstrated by angiography in 46 patients with a total of 49 stents, the re-stenosis rate was 14% at 8 ± 5 months.[84] Rundback and colleagues followed 45 patients with azotemia (serum creatinine > 1.5 mg/dl) and atheromatous RAS untreatable by, or recurrent after, PTRA for a mean of 54 months. Similar to the findings of Tuttle and colleagues, renal function remained stable (serum creatinine approximately 2.1 mg/dl).[103]

These reports are limited by the absence of a control group treated with medical therapy alone and by the fact that (except in a subset of patients in one study) no data are provided about whether intervention was performed because of on-going deterioration of renal function prior to stenting.[77] Nevertheless, PTRA with intravascular stenting may prove to be the best therapeutic option for patients with ostial atherosclerotic RAS who are deemed poor surgical risks or have refused surgery and are demonstrating worsening renal function or are on dialysis.

The results of surgical revascularization for the preservation of renal function in patients with atherosclerotic RAS have been similar to or slightly better than results with PTRA and, on occasion, have even reversed ESRD.[59, 65, 87, 97, 102, 104, 105] Improvement in renal function has been observed in approximately 50%, and stabilization of renal function has occurred in approximately 35%.[59, 65, 87, 97, 102, 104] Because the operative morbidity and mortality rates (11% and 3 to 6%, respectively) are significant, careful patient selection is imperative.[59, 88, 90, 104] If the disease is obviously progressing, if PTRA without stenting has failed, and if other patient-specific risk factors favor long-term survival, surgical revascularization should be undertaken before advanced renal failure is evident. Stenting precludes future surgical revascularization because the stent becomes endothelialized and is difficult to remove. Therefore, those patients who are younger and have lower operative risk should undergo surgery rather than stent placement. The best window of opportunity for renal survival achieved by surgical revascularization is when the serum creatinine concentration is between 1.5 mg/dl and 3.0 mg/dl.[90] Patients with diffuse atherosclerotic disease and congestive heart failure, or those undergoing simultaneous bilateral renal artery repair or revascularization in combination with another major vascular procedure, pose the greatest surgical risk.[102] As with surgical correction for renovascular hypertension, underlying coronary or cerebrovascular disease should, if possible, be corrected prior to surgery in order to reduce operative risk.

Successful surgical revascularization depends on the degree of renal insufficiency present, the rate at which renal function has deteriorated preoperatively, and the anatomy of the renal vasculature distal to the reno-occlusive lesion or lesions. In the presence of advanced renal failure (serum creatinine above 4.0 mg/dl), revascularization offers little benefit because significant irreversible renal parenchymal disease is invariably present.[85, 90] In addition to the absolute level of renal function, it appears that patients with the most rapid decline in renal function in the 6 months prior to surgery have the greatest recovery of renal function following revascularization.[106] Adequate collateral renal circulation is critical for surgical revascularization because it is necessary for the maintaining of viable glomeruli. Therefore, recovery or stabilization of renal function is more likely postoperatively when one or more of the following is present preoperatively:[85, 107–109]

1. Visualization of the collecting system on an IVP or during the pyelogram phase of the arteriogram
2. Renal length greater than 9.0 cm
3. Demonstration of retrograde filling of the distal renal vasculature from collateral circulation on the side of total renal artery occlusion during angiography
4. The presence of viable glomeruli on renal biopsy (done prior to or at the time of revascularization)

Because of the higher attendant risk of surgery, we adhere more strictly to these guidelines before attempting surgery but are much more flexible in attempting PTRA with or without stenting.

Renal artery disease is a major health problem that is the cause of high rates of morbidity and mortality. Appropriate management requires the combined expertise of nephrologists, interventional radiologists, and vascular surgeons.

The correct therapeutic approach, which is highly individualized, may lead to better management of blood pressure, stabilization or restoration of renal function and, perhaps, improved patient survival; it represents a continuing challenge to those caring for these patients.

References

1. Ploth DW. Renovascular Hypertension. *In* Jacobson HR, Striker GE, Klahr S, (eds). The Principles and Practice of Nephrology, 2nd ed. St. Louis, Mosby, 1995;379–386.
2. Kaplan NM, Rose BD. Who should be screened for renovascular or secondary hypertension? Uptodate Nephrol Hypertens 5:1–3, 1997.
3. Reiser IW, Spitalewitz S. Screening for renovascular hypertension: Which patients—what approach? J Crit Illness 13:301–308, 1998, and Reiser IW, Pallan TM, Spitalewitz S. How to treat renovascular hypertension: Medical therapy vs. revascularization. Ibid, pp 409–424
4. Davis BA, Crook JE, Vestal RE, et al. Prevalence of renovascular hypertension in patients with grade III or IV retinopathy. N Eng J Med 301:1273–1276, 1979.
5. Svetkey LP, Kadir S, Dunnick NR, et al. Similar prevalence of renovascular hypertension in selected blacks and whites. Hypertension 17:678–683, 1991.
6. Wollenweber J, Sheps SG, Davis GD. Clinical course of atherosclerotic renovascular disease. Am J Cardiol 21:60–71, 1968.
7. Pohl MA, Novick AC. Natural history of atherosclerotic and fibrous renal artery disease: Clinical implications. Am J Kidney Dis 5:120–130, 1985.
8. Rose BD. Pathophysiology of renal disease, 2nd ed. New York, McGraw-Hill, 1987; pp 512–515.
9. Nally JV. Provocative captopril testing in the diagnosis of renovascular hypertension. Urol Clin North Am 21:227–234, 1994.
10. Mann SJ, Pickering TG. Detection of renovascular hypertension. State of the art. Ann Intern Med 117:845–853, 1992.
11. Canzanello VJ, Textor SC. Noninvasive diagnosis of renovascular disease. Mayo Clin Proc 69:1172–1181, 1994.
12. Pederson EB. Angiotensin-converting enzyme inhibitor renography. Pathophysiological, diagnostic and therapeutic aspects in renal artery stenosis. Nephrol Dial Transplant 9:482–492, 1994.
13. Elliot WJ, Martin WB, Murphy MB. Comparison of two noninvasive screening tests for renovascular hypertension. Arch Int Med 153:755–764, 1993.
14. Wilcox CS. Ischemic nephropathy: Noninvasive testing. Semin Nephrol 16:43–52, 1996.
15. Setaro JF, Saddler MC, Chen CC, et al. Simplified captopril renography in diagnosis and treatment of renal artery stenosis. Hypertension 18:289–298, 1991.
16. Kaplan NM, Rose BD. Screening for renovascular hypertension. Uptodate Nephrol Hypertens 5:1–6, 1997.
17. Wilcox CS. Use of angiotensin-converting enzyme inhibitors for diagnosing renovascular hypertension. Kidney Int 44:1379–1390, 1993.
18. Erbsloh-Moller B, Dumas A, Roth D, et al. Furosemide-I^{131} hippuran renography after angiotensin-converting enzyme inhibition for the diagnosis of renovascular hypertension. Am J Med 90:23–29, 1991.
19. Mann SJ, Pickering TG, Sos TA, et al. Captopril renography in the diagnosis of renal artery stenosis: Accuracy and limitations. Am J Med 90:30–40, 1991.
20. Dondi M, Fanti S, De Fabritiis A, et al. Prognostic value of captopril renal scintigraphy in renovascular hypertension. J Nucl Med 33:2040–2044, 1992.
21. Chen CC, Hoffer PB, Vahjen G, et al. Patients at high risk for renal artery stenosis: A simple method of renal scintigraphic analysis with Tc-99m DTPA and captopril. Radiology 176:365–370, 1990.
22. Blaufox MD, Fine EJ, Heller S, et al. Prospective study of simultaneous orthoiodohippurate and diethylenetriaminepentaacetic acid and captopril renography. The Einstein/Cornell Collaborative Hypertension Group. J Nucl Med 39:522–528, 1998.
23. Dondi M, Monetti N, Fanti S, et al. Use of technetium-99m-MAG$_3$ for renal scintigraphy after angiotensin-converting enzyme inhibition. J Nucl Med 32:424–428, 1991.
24. Scoble JE, McClean A, Stansby G, et al. The use of captopril-DTPA scanning in the diagnosis of atherosclerotic renal artery stenosis in

patients with impaired renal function. Am J Hypertens 4(suppl):721S–723S, 1991.

25. Svetkey LP, Wilkinson R Jr, Dunnick NR, et al. Captopril renography in the diagnosis of renovascular disease. Am J Hypertens 4(suppl):711S–715S, 1991.

26. Postma CT, Joosten FB, Rosenbusch G, et al. Magnetic resonance angiography has a high reliability in the detection of renal artery stenosis. Am J Hypertens 10:957–963, 1997.

27. Rieumont MJ, Kaufman JA, Geller SC, et al. Evaluation of renal artery stenosis with dynamic gadolinium-enhanced MR angiography. Am J Roentgenol 169:39–44, 1997.

28. Schoenberg SO, Prince MR, Knopp MV, et al. Renal MR angiography. MRI Clin North Am 6:351–370, 1998.

29. Sommer G, Noorbehesht B, Pelc N, et al. Normal renal blood flow measurement using phase-contrast cine magnetic resonance imaging. Invest Radiol 27:465–470, 1992.

30. Klatzburg RW, Dumoulin CL, Buonocore MA, et al. Noninvasive measurement of renal hemodynamic functions using gadolinium-enhanced magnetic resonance imaging. Invest Radiol 29:5123–5126, 1994.

31. de Haan MW, Kouwenhoven M, Thelissen GRP, et al. Renovascular disease in patients with hypertension: Detection with systolic and diastolic gating in three-dimensional phase contrast MR angiography. Radiology 198:449–456, 1996.

32. Olbricht CJ, Paul K, Prokop M, et al. Minimally invasive diagnosis of renal artery stenosis by spiral computed tomography angiography. Kidney Int 48:1332–1337, 1995.

33. Kim TS, Chung JW, Park JH, et al. Renal artery evaluation: Comparison of spiral CT angiography to intra-arterial DSA. J Vasc Interv Radiol 9:553–559, 1998.

34. Halpern EJ, Rutter CM, Gardiner GA Jr, et al. Comparison of Doppler US and CT angiography for evaluation of renal artery stenosis. Acad Radiol 5:524–532, 1998.

35. Hawkins IF, Wilcox CS, Kerns SR, et al. CO_2 digital angiography: A safer contrast agent for renal vascular imaging. Am J Kidney Dis 24:685–694, 1994.

36. Working Group on Renovascular Hypertension. Detection, evaluation and treatment of renovascular hypertension. Final Report. Arch Int Med 147:820–829, 1987.

37. Dunnick NR, Svetkey LP, Cohan RH, et al. Intravenous digital subtraction renal angiography: Use in screening for renovascular hypertension. Radiology 171:219–222, 1989.

38. Olin JW, Piedmonte MR, Young JR, et al. The utility of duplex ultrasound scanning of the renal arteries for diagnosing renal artery stenosis. Ann Intern Med 122:833–838, 1995.

39. Kliewer MA, Tupler RH, Hertzberg BS, et al. Doppler evaluation of renal artery stenosis: Interobserver agreement in the interpretation of wave form morphology. AJR 162:1371–1376, 1994.

40. Starvos T, Harshfield D. Renal Doppler, renal artery stenosis, and renovascular hypertension: Direct and indirect duplex sonographic abnormalities in patients with renal artery stenosis. Ultrasound Q 12:217–263, 1994.

41. Marana I, Airoldi F, Burdick L, et al. Effects of balloon angioplasty and stent implantation on intrarenal echo-Doppler velocimetric indices. Kidney Int 53:1795–1800, 1998.

42. Hoffman U, Edwards JM, Carter S, et al. Role of duplex scanning for the detection of atherosclerotic renal artery disease. Kidney Int 39:1232–1239, 1991.

43. René PC, Oliva VL, Bui BT, et al. Renal artery stenosis: Evaluation of Doppler US after inhibition of angiotensin-converting enzyme with captopril. Radiology 196:675–679, 1995.

44. Kaplan-Pavlovcic S, Nadja C. Captopril renography and duplex Doppler sonography in the diagnosis of renovascular hypertension. Nephrol Dial Transplant 13:313–317, 1998.

45. Sheikh KH, Davidson CJ, Newman GE, et al. Intravascular ultrasound assessment of the renal artery. Ann Int Med 115:22–25, 1991.

46. Chavan A, Hausmann D, Brunkhorst R. Intravascular ultrasound to establish the indication for renal angioplasty. Nephrol Dial Transplant 13:1583–1584, 1998.

47. Savader SJ, Lund GB, Venbrux AC. Doppler flow wire evaluation of renal artery blood flow before and after PTA: Initial results. J Vasc Interv Radiol 9:451–460, 1998.

48. Carlier SG, Li W, Cespedes I, et al. Images in cardiovascular medicine. Simultaneous morphologic and functional assessment of a renal artery stent intervention with intravascular ultrasound. Circulation 97:2575–2576, 1998.

49. Nally JV, Olin JW, Lammert GK. Advances in non-invasive screening for renovascular disease. Cleve Clin J Med 61:328–336, 1994.

50. Frederickson ED, Wilcox CS, Bucci CM, et al. A prospective evaluation of a simplified captopril test for the detection of renovascular hypertension. Arch Intern Med 150:569–572, 1990.

51. Muller FB, Sealey JE, Case DB. The captopril test for identifying renovascular disease in hypertensive patients. Am J Med 80:633–644, 1986.

52. Derkx FH, Schalekamp MA. Renal artery stenosis and hypertension. Lancet 344:237–239, 1994.

53. Ram CVS, Clagett GP, Radford LR. Renovascular hypertension. Sem Nephrol 15:152–174, 1995.

54. Hollenberg NK. The treatment of renovascular hypertension: Surgery, angioplasty and medical therapy with converting enzyme inhibitors. Am J Kidney Dis 10(suppl 1):52–60, 1987.

55. Franklin SS, Smith RD. Comparison of the effects of enalapril plus hydrochlorothiazide versus standard triple therapy on renal function in renovascular hypertension. Am J Med 79:14–23, 1985.

56. Imamura A, Mackenzie HS, Lacy ER. Effects of chronic treatment with an angiotensin converting enzyme inhibitor or an angiotensin receptor antagonist in two-kidney, one-clip hypertensive rats. Kidney Int 47:1394–1402, 1995.

57. Pohl MA, Novick AC. Natural history of atherosclerotic and fibrous renal artery disease: Clinical implications. Am J Kidney Dis 5:120–130, 1985.

58. Schreiber MJ, Pohl MA, Novick AC. The natural history of atherosclerotic and fibrous renal artery disease. Urol Clin North Am 11:383–392, 1984.

59. Rimmer JM, Gennari FJ. Atherosclerotic renovascular disease and progressive renal failure. Ann Int Med 118:712–719, 1993.

60. Hricik DE, Dunn MJ. Angiotensin-converting-enzyme inhibitor–induced renal failure: Causes, consequences and diagnostic uses. J Am Soc Nephrol 1:845–858, 1990.

61. Michel JB, Dussaule JC, Choudat L. Effects of antihypertensive treatment in one-clip, two-kidney hypertension in rats. Kidney Int 29:1011–1020, 1986.

62. Veniant M, Heudes D, Clozel JP. Calcium blockade versus ACE inhibition in clipped and unclipped kidneys of 2K-1C rats. Kidney Int 46:421–429, 1994.

63. van de Ven P, Beutler JJ, Kaatee R, et al. Angiotensin converting enzyme inhibitor–induced renal dysfunction in atherosclerotic renovascular disease. Kidney Int 53:986–993, 1998.

64. Caps MT, Zierler ER, Polissar NL, et al. Risk of atrophy in kidneys with atherosclerotic renal artery stenosis. Kidney Int 53:735–742, 1998.

65. Jacobson HR. Ischemic renal disease: An overlooked clinical entity? Kidney Int 134:729–743, 1988.

66. Aurell M, Jensen G. Treatment of renovascular hypertension. Nephron 75:373–383, 1997.

67. Marshall FI, Hagen S, Mahaffy RG, et al. Percutaneous transluminal angioplasty for atheromatosis renal artery stenosis: Blood pressure response and discriminant analysis of outcome predictors. Q J Med 75:483–489, 1990.

68. Geyskes GG. Treatment of renovascular hypertension with percutaneous transluminal renal angioplasty. Am J Kidney Dis 12:253–265, 1988.

69. Ramsay LE, Waller PC. Blood pressure response to percutaneous angioplasty: An overview of published series. BMJ 300:569–572, 1990.

70. Libertino JA, Beckmann CF. Surgery and percutaneous angioplasty in the management of renovascular hypertension. Urol Clin North Am 21:235–243, 1994.

71. Bonelli FS, McKusick MA, Textor SC. Renal artery angioplasty: Technical results and clinical outcome in 320 patients. Mayo Clin Proc 70:1041–1052, 1995.

72. Canzanello VJ, Millan VG, Spiegel JE. Percutaneous transluminal angioplasty in management of atherosclerotic renovascular hypertension: Results in 100 patients. Hypertension 13:163–172, 1989.

73. Plouin PF, Chatellier BD, Raynaud A, for the ESSAI Multicentrique Medicaments vs. Angioplastie (EMMA) Study Group. Blood pressure outcome of angioplasty in atherosclerotic renal artery stenosis. A randomized trial. Hypertension 31:823–829, 1998.

74. Webster J, Marshall F, Abalalla M, et al. Randomized comparison of percutaneous angioplasty vs. continued medical therapy for hypertensive patients with atheromatous renal artery stenosis: Scottish

and Newcastle Renal Artery Stenosis Collaborative Group. J Hum Hypertension 12:329–335, 1998.

75. Rees CR, Palmaz JC, Becker GJ. Palmaz stent in atherosclerotic renal arteries involving the ostia of the renal arteries: Preliminary report of a multicenter study. Radiology 181:507–514, 1991.

76. van de Ven PJ, Beutler JJ, Kaatee R. Transluminal vascular stent for ostial atherosclerotic renal artery stenosis. Lancet 346:672–674, 1995.

77. Blum U, Krumme B, Flugel P. Treatment of ostial renal-artery stenoses with vascular endoprostheses after unsuccessful balloon angioplasty. N Engl J Med 336:459–465, 1997.

78. Spinosa DJ, Matsumoto AH, Angle JH, et al. Use of gadopentetate dimeglumine as a contrast agent for percutaneous transluminal renal angioplasty and stent placement. Kidney Int 53:503–507, 1998.

79. Novick AC. Treatment of ostial renal-artery stenoses with vascular endoprosthesis after unsuccessful balloon angioplasty. [Editorial comment] J Urol 158:983, 1997.

80. Dorros G, Jaff M, Jain A. Follow-up of primary Palmaz-Schatz stent placement for atherosclerotic renal artery stenosis. Am J Cardiol 75:1051–1055, 1995.

81. Dorros G, Jaff MR, Mathiak L, et al. Stent revascularization for atherosclerotic renal artery stenosis. One-year clinical follow-up. Tex Heart Inst J 25:40–43, 1998.

82. Dorros G, Jaff M, Mathiak L, et al. Four-year follow-up of Palmaz-Schatz stent revascularization as treatment for atherosclerotic renal artery stenosis. Circulation 98:642–647, 1998.

83. Harden PN, MacLeod MJ, Rodger RS, et al. Effect of renal-artery stenting on progression of renovascular renal failure. Lancet 349:1133–1136, 1997.

84. Tuttle KR, Chouinard RF, Webber JT, et al. Treatment of atherosclerotic ostial renal artery stenosis with the intravascular stent. Am J Kidney Dis 32:611–622, 1998.

85. Novick AC. Surgical correction of renovascular hypertension. Surg Clin North Am 68:1007–1025, 1988.

86. Novick AC. Current concepts in the management of renovascular hypertension and ischemic renal failure. Am J Kidney Dis 13(suppl 1):33–37, 1989.

87. Hansen KJ, Starr SM, Sands RE. Contemporary surgical management of renovascular disease. J Vasc Surg 16:319–331, 1992.

88. Stanley JC. The evolution of surgery for renovascular occlusive disease. Cardiovasc Surg 2:195–202, 1994.

89. Lawrie GM, Morris GC, Glaeser DH. Renovascular reconstruction: Factors affecting long-term prognosis in 919 patients followed up to 31 years. Am J Cardiol 63:1085–1092, 1989.

90. Textor SC. Revascularization in atherosclerotic renal artery disease. Kidney Int 53:799–811, 1998.

91. Olin JW, Vidt DG, Gifford RW Jr. Renovascular disease in the elderly: An analysis of 50 patients. J Am Coll Cardiol 5:1232–1238, 1985.

92. Greminger P, Luscher TF, Zuber J. Surgery, transluminal dilatation and medical therapy in the management of renovascular hypertension. Nephron 44(suppl 1):36–39, 1986.

93 Zech P, Finaz de Villaine J, Pozet N. Surgical versus medical treatment in renovascular hypertension. Restrospective study of 166 cases. Nephron 44(suppl 1):105–108, 1986.

94. Weibull H, Bergqvist D, Bergentz SE. Percutaneous transluminal angioplasty versus reconstruction of atherosclerotic renal artery stenosis. Prospective randomized study. J Vasc Surg 18:841–852, 1993.

95. Baboolal K, Evans C, Moore RH. Incidence of end-stage renal disease in medically treated patients with severe bilateral atherosclerotic renovascular disease. Am J Kidney Dis 31:971–977, 1998.

96. Meyrier A, Hill GS, Simon P. Ischemic renal diseases: New insights into old entities. Kidney Int 54:2–13, 1998.

97. Greco BA, Breyer JA. Atherosclerotic ischemic renal disease. Am J Kidney Dis 29:167–187, 1997.

98. Middleton JP. Ischemic disease of the kidney: How and why to consider revascularization. J Nephrol 3:123–136, 1998.

99. Mailloux LU, Napolitano B, Bellucci AG. Renal vascular disease causing end-stage renal disease, incidence, clinical correlates, and outcomes: A 20-year clinical experience. Am J Kidney Dis 24:622–629, 1994.

100. O'Donovan RM, Gutierrez OH, Izzo JL Jr. Preservation of renal function by percutaneous renal angioplasty in high-risk elderly patients: Short-term outcome. Nephron 60:187–192, 1992.

101. Sos TA. Angioplasty for the treatment of azotemia and renovascular hypertension in atherosclerotic renal artery disease. Circulation 83(suppl I):162–166, 1991.

102. Novick AC. Options for therapy of ischemic nephropathy: Role of angioplasty and surgery. Sem Nephrol 16:53–60, 1996.

103. Rundback JH, Gray RJ, Rozenblit G, et al. Renal artery stent placement for the management of ischemic nephropathy. J Vasc Interv Radiol 9:413–420, 1998.

104. Libertino JA, Bosco PJ, Ying CY. Renal vascularization to preserve and restore renal function. J Urol 147:1485–1487, 1992.

105. Kaylor WM, Novick AC, Ziegelbaum M. Reversal of end-stage renal failure in patients with atherosclerotic renal occlusion. J Urol 141:486–488, 1989.

106. Dean RH, Tribble RW, Hansen KJ. Evolution of renal insufficiency in ischemic nephropathy. Ann Surg 213:446–456, 1991.

107. Novick AC, Ziegelbaum M, Vidt DG. Trends in surgical revascularization for renal artery disease—Ten years' experience. JAMA 257:498–501, 1987.

108. Schefft P, Novick AC, Stewart BH. Renal revascularization in patients with total occlusion of the renal artery. J Urol 124:184–186, 1980.

109. Rose BD, Mailloux LU, Kaplan NM. Chronic renal failure due to ischemic renal disease. Uptodate Nephrol Hypertens 5:1–6, 1997.

CHAPTER

78 Adrenal Cortex

Emmanuel L. Bravo

GENERAL PRINCIPLES

Hypertension of adrenocortical origin is usually associated with symptoms and signs that raise clinical suspicion of the diagnosis and help the physician in planning a rational diagnostic and therapeutic approach. The diagnostic evaluation should start with a careful history and a thorough physical examination. Following this, a few basic laboratory tests are indicated (Table 78–1). The types of information thus obtained are categorized into groupings, each indicating either a diagnosis or a need for further testing. The adrenal cortex can cause hypertension through over-

production of deoxycorticosterone (DOC), aldosterone, or cortisol (Fig. 78–1). DOC and aldosterone are mineralocorticoids that produce hypertension through salt and water retention. Cortisol is a glucocorticoid that causes hypertension, in part, by exerting a mineralocorticoid effect because of incomplete metabolism at target tissues.

With rare exceptions, hypertension of adrenocortical origin is associated with hypokalemia, either spontaneous or diuretic-induced. Evaluation for adrenocortical hypertension is recommended under the following circumstances: (1) diuretic therapy results in serum potassium less than 3.0 mEq/L even if levels normalize after diuretics are

Table 78–1 Diagnostic Evaluation

CLINICAL HISTORY
Family history of primary aldosteronism
Age of onset of hypertension
Early death of affected family members resulting from cerebrovascular accidents
Development of secondary sexual characteristics

PHYSICAL EXAMINATION
Signs of chronic severe elevated blood pressure
 Fundoscopic eye changes
 Left ventricular hypertrophy
Absence of secondary sexual characteristics
Signs of androgen or cortisol excess

INITIAL LABORATORY EVALUATION
Serum electrolytes, blood urea nitrogen, creatinine
Plasma concentrations of aldosterone, cortisol, and plasma renin activity
24-hr urinary Na, K, Cr, aldosterone, and free cortisol

Table 78–2 Outpatient Oral Salt-Loading Protocol

PREPARATION
1. Discontinue all diuretic agents
2. Raise serum K if still <3.5 mEq/L after 1–2 weeks of diuretic abstinence
3. If elevated BP is a concern, use calcium antagonists, α-blockers, or β-blockers

PROCEDURE
1. At baseline, draw blood for Na, K, Cl, CO_2
2. On days 1 to 5 inclusive, add to usual dietary intake, 1 level full teaspoon of salt daily
3. On days 4 and 5 of increased salt intake, collect 24-hr urines for Na, K, Cr, and aldosterone
4. On day 6 (the morning after the last urine collection), draw blood for Na, K, Cl, CO_2, PA, and PRA

INTERPRETATION
Findings indicating inappropriate aldosterone production
 1. Renal K-wasting (serum K < 3.5 mEq/L with U_KV > 30 mEq/24 hr)
 2. PA > 22 ng/dl, urinary aldosterone > 14 μg/24 hr, PRA < 1.0 ng/ml, and $U_{Na}V$ ≥ 250 mEq/24 hr
Absence of hypokalemia and/or suppressed PRA does not preclude the diagnosis

Abbreviations: BP, blood pressure; PA, plasma aldosterone; PRA, plasma renin activity; U_KV, urinary potassium volume; $U_{Na}V$, urinary sodium volume.

withdrawn; (2) oral potassium supplementation and/or potassium-sparing agents fail to maintain serum potassium values of 3.5 mEq/L or greater in a patient on diuretics; or (3) serum potassium levels fail to normalize after 4 weeks off diuretics.

The initial assessment and subsequent studies should answer three questions: Is potassium loss renal or extrarenal? If renal, is it steroid- or nonsteroid-dependent? If steroid-dependent, what is its cause? A 24-hour urinary potassium excretion greater than 30 mEq when the serum potassium is less than 3.5 mEq/L usually reflects renal potassium wasting, whereas lower excretion rates suggest extrarenal loss caused by diarrhea, vomiting, or laxative

abuse. Renal potassium wasting should be investigated further after adequate repletion of total body potassium (serum potassium ≥3.8 mEq/L) with oral potassium chloride supplementation. The occurrence of hypokalemia (Table 78–2) accompanied by renal potassium wasting during oral salt loading suggests an exaggerated exchange of sodium for potassium at renal distal tubular sites. The re-

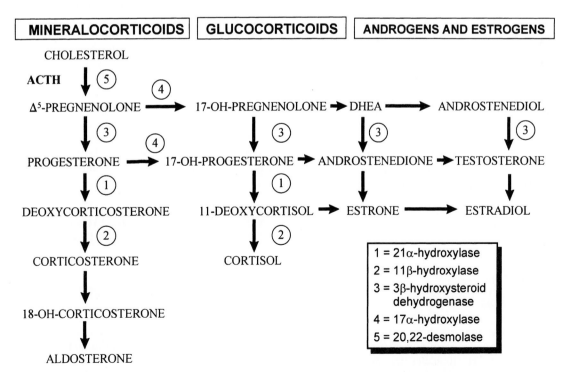

Figure 78–1. Pathways of adrenal hormone synthesis: 21α-hydroxylase; 11β-hydroxylase; 3β-hydroxysteroid dehydrogenase; 17α-hydroxylase; 20,22-desmolase. DHEA, dehydroepiandrosterone. (From Watts NB. Congenital adrenal hyperplasia. *In* Hurst JW [ed]. Medicine for the Practicing Physician, 4th ed. Stamford, CT, Appleton & Lange, 1996; p 566.)

sponse to spironolactone (50 mg four times daily for 3 to 5 days) can demonstrate conclusively whether renal potassium wasting is truly mineralocorticoid-dependent. If spironolactone produces an elevation in the serum potassium level with a concomitant reduction in urinary potassium excretion, potassium wasting is probably mediated by electrolyte-active steroids. The demonstration of true mineralocorticoid-dependent renal potassium wasting warrants further diagnostic studies to determine the most effective treatment. Liddle's syndrome, a familial, non–steroid-dependent renal potassium-wasting disorder associated with hypokalemia and hypertension, does not respond to spironolactone.[1]

HYPERTENSIVE SYNDROMES DUE TO EXCESS DEOXYCORTICOSTERONE PRODUCTION

Adrenocortical Enzyme Deficiency

The best-defined circumstance in which DOC plays a significant role in hypertension is in syndromes characterized by a deficiency of 11β- or 17α-hydroxylation of steroids (see Fig. 78–1).[2, 3] These disorders are usually congenital, but they may be induced by excessive production of estrogen[4] or androgens[5] from either a benign or a malignant tumor. In addition to these two hypertensive forms of congenital adrenal hyperplasia, excess DOC production occurs in a variety of disorders, including DOC-producing tumors[6] and primary glucocorticoid resistance.[7]

11β-Hydroxylase Deficiency

Findings on physical examination provide the most important clues to the presence of enzymatic deficiency. Virilization in females or precocious puberty with advanced masculinization in males (caused by increased androgen production) are prominent features of 11β-hydroxylase deficiency. Deficiency of 11β-hydroxylase results in reduced production of cortisol, corticosterone, and aldosterone. Subsequent overproduction of adrenocorticotropic hormone (ACTH) drives the zona fasciculata to increase production of DOC, which produces a type of mineralocorticoid hypertension. There is also increased formation of dehydroepiandrosterone (DHEA) and androstenedione, which produces hypergonadism. Deficiency of 11β-hydroxylase is confirmed by demonstrating increased levels of plasma 11-deoxycortisol (S) and urinary tetrahydro-S and 17-ketosteroids.

17α-Hydroxylase Deficiency

Abnormalities in steroid production in the 17α-hydroxylase deficiency syndrome result in reduced production of 17α-hydroxy progesterone and the distal steroids in the 17-hydroxy pathway, deoxycortisol and cortisol. Resultant overproduction of ACTH stimulates the uninvolved 17-deoxy pathway to increase the levels of progesterone, DOC, corticosterone (B), 18-OH DOC, and 18-hydroxycorticosterone. Because DOC causes salt and water retention, total suppression of renin synthesis and subsequent suppression of aldosterone result.

Deficiency of 17α-hydroxylase causes reduced production of all adrenal and gonadal androgens, including testosterone, DHEA, and androstenedione, resulting in a form of hypergonadotropic hypogonadism and abnormalities of sexual development. The hypogonadal consequences of the enzyme deficiency account for most of the clinical features of the disorder. Women with primary amenorrhea have disproportionately long limbs relative to the trunk, absent axillary and pubic hair, infantile breast and genital development, absent uterus, and an incomplete vagina. In men, the testes do not produce testosterone, causing decreased masculinization; male patients also have reduced axillary and pubic hair and ambiguous genitalia. Increased production of DOC and corticosterone as well as decreased androgen secretion establishes the diagnosis of 17α-hydroxylase deficiency.

In both 11β- and 17α-hydroxylase deficiency disorders, dexamethasone, by inhibiting ACTH release, decreases DOC production, resulting in normalization of arterial blood pressure and serum potassium concentration.

Glucocorticoid Resistance[8]

The control of cortisol synthesis is through a negative feedback loop in which cortisol feeds back on the pituitary to inhibit ACTH secretion. In generalized inherited glucocorticoid resistance, cortisol secretion remains ACTH-dependent, but is reset to a higher than normal level. Affected individuals do not develop features of Cushing's syndrome, since the peripheral tissues and pituitary are equally resistant. There is an ACTH-dependent increase in mineralocorticoids (primarily DOC) and adrenal androgens. Since there is no peripheral resistance to these hormones, they produce clinical effects. Therefore, the clinical presentation is caused by excess adrenal androgens (virilization, precocious puberty) and/or excess mineralocorticoids (hypertension, hypokalemia).

There are two strategies to treat generalized glucocorticoid resistance. The first employs an exogenous glucocorticoid, such as dexamethasone, to suppress adrenal stimulation by ACTH. Therapy is monitored by measuring the serum concentrations of cortisol, DOC, and androgen. Alternatively, mineralocorticoid or androgen antagonists can be used.

HYPERTENSIVE SYNDROMES DUE TO EXCESS ALDOSTERONE PRODUCTION

Primary Aldosteronism

Clinical Recognition and Diagnosis

The clinical manifestations of primary aldosteronism are not distinctive. The clinical decision to initiate a laboratory assessment is based on observing one of a number of clinical characteristics. Any of the following categories of hypertensive patients deserve strong consideration of additional studies to determine the presence of primary aldosteronism:

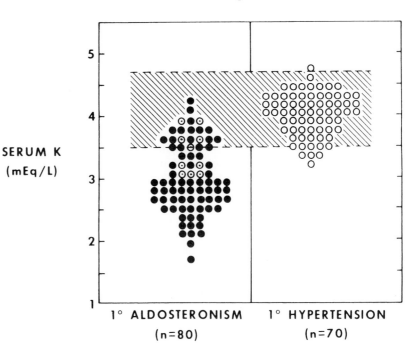

Figure 78–2. Serum potassium values during normal dietary sodium intake. Each point represents the mean of at least three determinations. For patients with primary aldosteronism, *solid circles* represent adenomas (*n* = 70) and *open circles with dotted centers* represent hyperplasia (*n* = 10). The *cross-hatched area* represents 95% confidence limits (3.5 to 4.6 mEq/L) of values obtained from 60 healthy subjects. (Reprinted from Am J Med, vol 74, Bravo EL, Tarazi RC, Dustan HP, et al. The changing clinical spectrum of primary aldosteronism. pp 641–651, copyright 1983 with permission from Excerpta Medica Inc.)

1. Patients who develop spontaneous hypokalemia (serum potassium concentration <3.5 mEq/L)
2. Patients who develop moderately severe hypokalemia (serum potassium concentration ≤3 mEqL), or patients who have difficulty maintaining normal serum potassium values despite concomitant use of oral potassium supplements or potassium-sparing agents during conventional doses of diuretics
3. Patients with serum potassium values that fail to normalize within 4 weeks off diuretic treatment
4. Patients with refractory hypertension with no evidence for a secondary cause.

For screening purposes, hypokalemia, whether spontaneous or provoked, provides an important clue to the presence of primary aldosteronism. A substantial number of patients with primary aldosteronism do not present with hypokalemia, however (Fig. 78–2); the serum potassium concentration is normal in 7 to 38% of reported cases.[9–12] In addition, 10 to 12% of patients with proven tumors may not have hypokalemia during short-term salt loading.[9] Plasma renin activity (PRA) less than 1 ng/ml/hr that fails to rise above 2 ng/ml/hr after salt and water depletion, and upright posture have been used as a screening test to exclude primary aldosteronism. However, a substantial number (about 35%) of patients have values that rise to greater than 2 ng/ml/hr when appropriately stimulated (Fig. 78–3). In addition, about 40% of subjects with essential hypertension have suppressed PRA, and 15 to 20% of these patients have values below 2 ng/ml/hr under conditions of stimulation.[9] The plasma aldosterone:renin ratio[13] and the captopril test[14, 15] are used to define the appropriateness of PRA for the circulating concentration of aldosterone. It is assumed that the volume expansion associated with the presence of an aldosterone-producing tumor suppresses the release of renin without affecting the autonomous production of aldosterone. Both tests are subject to the same

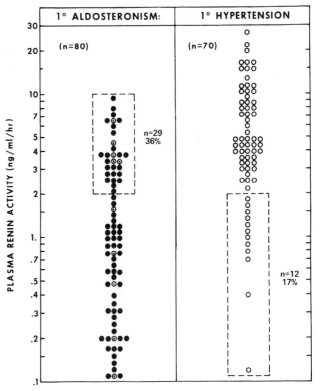

Figure 78–3. Stimulated plasma renin activity (PRA) in primary aldosteronism and primary hypertension. PRA was measured after 4 days of sodium deprivation. Blood was drawn between 8 and 9 AM after an overnight fast and at least 30 minutes of supine rest. For patients with primary aldosteronism, *solid circles* represent adenomas (*n* = 70) and *open circles with dotted centers* represent hyperplasia (*n* = 10). After sodium deprivation, 29 patients (36%) with primary aldosteronism had values greater than or equal to 2.0 ng/ml/hr, and 12 patients (17%) with primary hypertension had values less than 2.0 ng/ml/hr. The sensitivity and specificity of the test were 64% and 83%, respectively.

limitations. First, there is inherent variability in plasma levels of aldosterone even in the presence of a tumor,[16] which translates into variability in the absolute value of the ratio. Second, the use of drugs that result in prolonged stimulation of renin long after their discontinuation may alter the ratio.

The diagnosis of primary aldosteronism often can be established with relative ease. In the hypertensive patient receiving no treatment who demonstrates significant hypokalemia (≤3 mEq/L) with inappropriate kaliuresis (24-hour urinary potassium >30 mEq), PRA below 1 ng/ml/hr, and elevated plasma or urinary aldosterone values, the diagnosis is unequivocal. Often, however, the diagnosis is not obvious because of equivocal values. In such cases, multiple measurements are needed during salt loading. In the author's experience, the single best test for identifying patients with primary aldosteronism is the measurement of 24-hour urinary aldosterone excretion during salt loading.[9] An aldosterone excretion rate greater than 14 μg/24 hr following salt loading (see Table 78–2) distinguishes most patients with primary aldosteronism from those with essential hypertension; only 7% of patients with primary aldosteronism have aldosterone excretion values that fall within the range for essential hypertension (Fig. 78–4). In contrast, a substantial number (about 39%) of patients with primary aldosteronism have plasma aldosterone values that fall within the range for essential hypertension. The findings of hypokalemia and/or suppressed PRA provide corroborative evidence for the diagnosis of primary aldosteronism, but their absence does not preclude the diagnosis.

The most common cause (70 to 80% of all proven cases) of primary aldosteronism is an aldosterone-producing adenoma. Approximately 20 to 30% of cases are caused by hyperplasia of the zona glomerulosa layer of the adrenal cortex (idiopathic hyperaldosteronism). Some reports suggest the rare occurrence of a syndrome intermediate between adenoma and hyperplasia.[16] The distinction between these two processes is important because surgical intervention is much more likely to be effective in cases of adenoma than hyperplasia. An adenoma is likely in the presence of spontaneous hypokalemia of 3.0 mEq/L or below, plasma 18-hydroxycorticosterone values greater than 100 ng/dl,[17] and an anomalous postural decrease in plasma aldosterone concentration.[18] In addition, adenomas are largely unresponsive to changes in sodium balance[9] and appear to be exquisitely sensitive to ACTH, unlike hyperplasias, which are more sensitive to angiotensin II infusions.[19] A plasma 18-hydroxycorticosterone value below 100 ng/dl or a postural increase in plasma aldosterone, or both, are usually associated with adrenal hyperplasia, but do not completely rule out the presence of an adenoma.[9]

The adrenal computed tomography (CT) scan should be considered the initial step in localization. It is noninvasive, and all adenomas 1.5 cm in diameter or larger can be located accurately. Only 60% of nodules measuring 1.0 to 1.4 cm in diameter are detected by CT, however, and nodules smaller than 1.0 cm in diameter are very difficult, if not impossible, to detect. The overall sensitivity of localizing adenomas by high-resolution CT scanning exceeds 90%.[20–22] Adrenal venous aldosterone levels should be measured when the results of the adrenal CT scan are ambiguous and biochemical evidence for the presence of a tumor is overwhelming. Bilateral adrenal venous sampling for the measurement of aldosterone concentration is still the most accurate test for localizing aldosterone-producing tumors. When technically successful, and both adrenal veins are entered, the accuracy of comparative adrenal venous aldosterone levels in confirming either a tumor or hyperplasia exceeds 95%.[23] The ratio of ipsilateral:contralateral aldosterone usually is greater than 10:1. Correct placement of the catheter in the adrenal vein is essential and is best evaluated by obtaining simultaneous ACTH-stimulated selective adrenal venous cortisol levels. An aldosterone ratio of 10:1 or greater in the presence of a symmetric ACTH-induced cortisol response is diagnostic of an aldosterone-producing adenoma. Unfortunately, this procedure is invasive and technically demanding and requires considerable skill and experience. There is an appreciable incidence of complications, including adrenal and iliac venous thrombosis and extravasation of dye into the gland, which can lead to adrenal insufficiency.

A simplified approach to the diagnosis of primary aldosteronism is shown in Figure 78–5. In untreated patients who have spontaneous hypokalemia (serum potassium) ≤ 3 mEq/L), inappropriate kaliuresis (urinary potassium > 30 mEq/24 hr), PRA below 1 ng/ml/hr, plasma aldosterone greater than 22 ng/dl, and an aldosterone excretion rate greater than 14 μg/24 hr when the urinary sodium is 250 mEq/24 hr or greater, the diagnosis is incontrovertible. Under these conditions, additional biochemical studies to differentiate a tumor from hyperplasia can be performed, followed by an adrenal CT scan to determine which adrenal gland might be the site of an adenoma. Patients who are normokalemic but who have a history of becoming

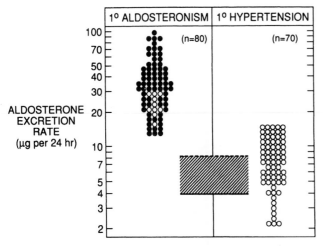

Figure 78–4. Aldosterone excretion rate after 3 days of high sodium intake. For patients with primary aldosteronism, *solid circles* represent adenomas (*n* = 70) and *open circles* represent hyperplasia (*n* = 10). The *cross-hatched area* represents the mean (4.0 μg/24 hr) and +2 standard deviations (8.0 μg/24 hr) of values obtained from 47 healthy subjects. No patient with primary aldosteronism had a value within the 95% normal range. Ten patients (14%) with primary hypertension had values that fell within the range obtained in patients with primary aldosteronism. Using a reference value of greater than 14 μg/24 hr after a high sodium intake for 3 days, the sensitivity and specificity of the test are 96% and 93%, respectively. (From Bravo EL, Tarazi RC, Dustan HP, et al. The changing clinical spectrum of primary aldosteronism. Am J Med 74:641, 1983.)

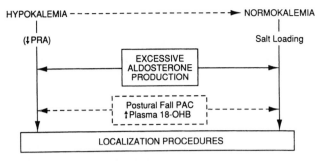

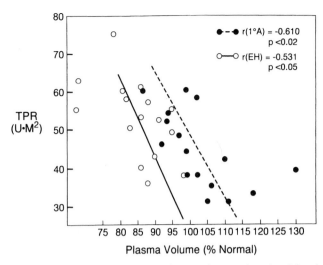

Figure 78-5. Algorithm for the diagnosis of primary aldosteronism. PRA, plasma renin activity; PAC, plasma aldosterone concentration; 18-OHB, 18-hydroxycorticosterone. (From Bravo EL. Primary aldosteronism. Urol Clin North Am 16:481, 1989.)

significantly hypokalemic on conventional diuretic therapy or who have persistent hypokalemia despite attempts at potassium repletion should have a salt-loading test. This can be accomplished in the outpatient setting (see Table 78–2). An aldosterone excretion rate greater than 14 μg/24 hr when the urinary sodium is at least 250 mEq/24 hr suggests excessive aldosterone production. Additional studies can then be performed to confirm and localize a tumor.

Rational Therapeutic Approaches Based on Understanding the Pathophysiology of Primary Aldosteronism

Mineralocorticoids lead to fluid retention and might be expected to increase intravascular volume. Early studies reported hypervolemia in primary aldosteronism, but this abnormality is not a universal finding. Many subjects with primary aldosteronism have either low or normal intravascular volume, and there is no correlation between arterial pressure and plasma or total blood volume in either men or women with untreated primary aldosteronism.[9] In contrast, there is a significant inverse correlation between volume and total peripheral resistance similar to that reported in essential hypertension, renal arterial disease, and normal subjects. These results might suggest that intravascular volume, as such, plays no role in the hypertension of primary aldosteronism. This conclusion, however, must be qualified by two observations: First, the correlation between volume and resistance in primary aldosterionism and in essential hypertension is similar only in its sign (negative) and slope; the two groups differ significantly in the levels of intravascular volume.[24] For any level of peripheral resistance, plasma volume is always greater in primary aldosteronism than in essential hypertension (Fig. 78–6). Second, with diuretic therapy, the arterial pressure response is directly and significantly related to the magnitude of intravascular volume alterations.[25]

Abnormalities in intravascular volume are associated with drug resistance in some patients with primary aldosteronism. Bravo and coworkers[26] studied 28 patients with primary aldosteronism (25 with a solitary adenoma) and resistant hypertension. All were on a combination of three to several drugs but were receiving small doses of diuretics. In 12 patients who underwent hemodynamic studies, plasma volume was either normal or elevated in most, despite marked elevations of total peripheral resistance

Figure 78-6. Correlation between plasma volume and total peripheral resistance (TPR) in patients with primary aldosteronism (1°A) and those with hypovolemic essential hypertension (EH). The slopes of the regression equations defining the two lines are not significantly different from each other, but the intercepts are. ●–●, primary aldosteronism ($n = 16$; $r = -0.531$; $p < .05$); ○–○, essential hypertension ($n = 16$; $r = -0.610$; $p < .02$). (From Tarazi RC, Ibrahim MM, Bravo EL, et al. Hemodynamic characteristics of primary aldosteronism. Reprinted, by permission. N Engl J Med 289:1330, 1973. Copyright 1973 Massachusetts Medical Society. All rights reserved.)

(Fig. 78–7). The addition of spironolactone (200 mg/day) and hydrochlorothiazide (50–100 mg/day) to previous multiple-drug therapy reduced blood pressure significantly in all 28 patients. The reduction in blood pressure was associated with decreases in intravascular volume (Fig. 78–8).

Therapeutic Choices

Medical therapy is indicated in patients with adrenal hyperplasia, in those with adenoma who are poor surgical risks, and in those with bilateral adrenal adenomas that may

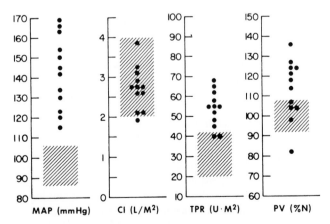

Figure 78-7. Hemodynamic characteristics of primary aldosteronism with refractory hypertension. At the time of the study, patients were on three to seven different drugs in combination. Despite marked increases in total peripheral resistance (TPR), patients were either normovolemic or hypervolemic. MAP, mean arterial pressure; CI, cardiac index; PV = plasma volume; %N, percent of normal; *cross-hatched areas* indicate ± 2 SD. (From Bravo EL. Primary aldosteronism. Endocrinol Metab Clin North Am 23:271, 1994.)

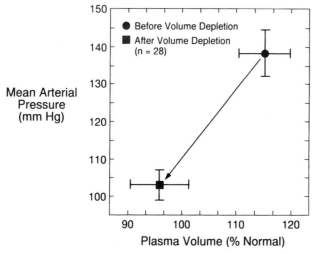

Figure 78–8. The effect of adequate volume depletion on the blood pressure of patients with primary aldosteronism and resistant hypertension. Spironolactone (200 mg/day) and hydrochlorothiazide (50 to 100 mg/day) were added to current therapy. Blood pressure and plasma volume values were those obtained after 8 to 12 weeks of continued therapy. Mean arterial pressure (MAP) was significantly reduced in all. For the group as a whole, it fell from 138 ± 2 to 103 ± 9 (SEM) mm Hg ($p < .01$). Associated with reductions in MAP were decreases in plasma volume (from 114 ± 3 to 97 ± 2 [SEM] % normal) ($p < .01$). (From Bravo EL. Primary aldosteronism. Endocrinol Metab Clin North Am 23:271, 1994.)

require bilateral adrenalectomy. Total bilateral adrenalectomy has no place in the management of primary aldosteronism because adrenal insufficiency may be more difficult to treat than hypertension caused by aldosteronism. The hypertension associated with primary aldosteronism is salt- and water-dependent and is best treated by sustained salt and water depletion.[26] The usual doses of diuretics are hydrochlorothiazide 25 to 50 mg/day or furosemide 80 to 180 mg/day in combination with either spironolactone 100 to 200 mg/day or amiloride 10 to 20 mg/day. These combinations usually result in prompt correction of hypokalemia and normalization of blood pressure within 2 to 4 weeks (Fig. 78–9). In some cases, the addition of either a β-adrenergic blocker or a vasodilator may be needed to normalize arterial pressure.

Spironolactone and amiloride are both capable of controlling blood pressure and normalizing serum potassium concentration in patients with primary aldosteronism. However, spironolactone may be more efficacious (Bravo EL, unpublished observations, 1998). In 11 of 24 patients who have taken both amiloride and spironolactone at different times in the course of long-term (≥ 5 years) medical therapy, the blood pressure was 123 ± 46 (SE) mm Hg systolic and 82 ± 18 (SE) diastolic on spironolactone and 134 ± 3.9 (SE) systolic and 80 ± 2.5 (SE) diastolic on amiloride. The serum potassium concentration on spironolactone was 4.6 ± 0.2 (SE) mEq/L and 4.1 ± 0.1 (SE) mEq/L on amiloride. None of the differences was statistically significant, perhaps because of the small number of patients. However, spironolactone was associated with more adverse effects. In 17 patients started on spironolactone, the most common complaints included breast tenderness in 13, breast engorgement in 8, muscle cramps in 7, and sexual dysfunction

in 5. These adverse events had no relationship to dose. The only adverse effect noted with amiloride was muscle cramping, which was usually related to dose.

Agents that block transmembrane calcium flux and inhibit in vitro aldosterone production induced by angiotensin II, ACTH, and potassium[27] are potent direct arteriolar vasodilators, and in some studies, are reported to have natriuretic properties.[28] For these reasons, calcium entry blocking agents should be ideally suited for treating the hypertension associated with excessive aldosterone production. In a study by Bravo and colleagues,[29] nifedipine (30 to 80 mg/day) was given to eight hypertensive patients with solitary adenomas for at least 4 weeks, followed by the addition of spironolactone (100 to 200 mg/day) for 4 weeks, after which nifedipine was discontinued and patients remained on spironolactone alone. The following factors were assessed in the 4th week of each phase of the study: weekly averages of supine home blood pressures, plasma volume, PRA, plasma aldosterone concentration, and serum electrolyte levels. Nifedipine decreased blood pressure but not to normal levels, and did not alter plasma volume, PRA, aldosterone, or serum potassium concentrations. Spironolactone normalized blood pressure and serum potassium concentration, reduced plasma volume, and increased PRA and plasma aldosterone concentration. Nifedipine plus spironolactone did not result in a greater antihypertensive effect than spironolactone alone (Table 78–3). These results suggest that nifedipine is not as efficacious as spironolactone in the treatment of primary aldosteronism.

In the majority of patients, surgical excision of an aldosterone-producing adenoma leads to normotension as well as reversal of the biochemical defects. At the very least, surgery renders arterial pressure easier to control with medications. Neither the duration (Fig. 78–10) and severity

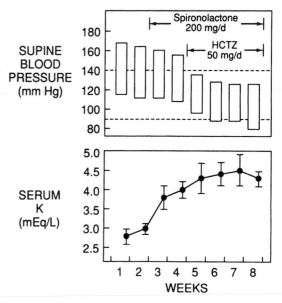

Figure 78–9. Diuretic therapy in primary aldosteronism. The effect of spironolactone combined with hydrochlorothiazide (HCTZ) on blood pressure and serum potassium concentrations in patients with aldosterone-producing tumors. (From Bravo EL, Dustan HP, Tarazi RC. Spironolactone as a nonspecific treatment for primary aldosteronism. Circulation 48:491, 1973. By permission of the American Heart Association, Inc.)

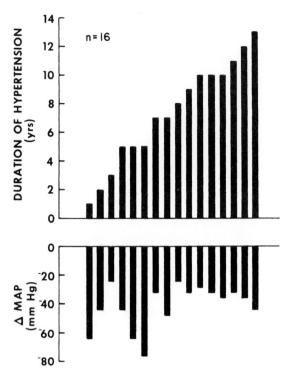

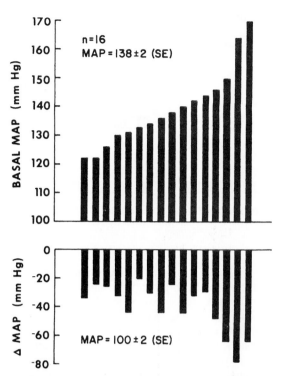

Figure 78–10. The relationship between duration of hypertension and blood pressure response after removal of an aldosterone-producing tumor. Postoperative blood pressure readings represent values obtained at 6 to 12 months after surgery. MAP, mean arterial pressure. (From Bravo EL. Pheochromocytoma and mineralocorticoid hypertension. *In* Glassock RJ [ed]. Current Therapy in Nephrology and Hypertension, 4th ed. St. Louis, Mosby–Year Book 1998; p 330.)

Figure 78–11. The relationship between severity of hypertension and blood pressure response after removal of an aldosterone-producing tumor. Postoperative blood pressure readings represent values obtained at 16 to 12 months after surgery. MAP, mean arterial pressure. (From Bravo EL. Pheochromocytoma and mineralocorticoid hypertension. *In* Glassock RJ [ed]. Current therapy in Nephrology and Hypertension, 4th ed. St. Louis, Mosby–Year Book, 1998; p 330.)

of hypertension (Fig. 78–11), nor the degree of target organ involvement has any relationship to the arterial pressure response after surgery. One year postoperatively, about 70% of patients are normotensive, but 5 years postoperatively, only 53% remain normotensive. The restoration of normal potassium homeostasis is permanent.

Patients undergoing surgery should receive drug treatment for at least 8 to 10 weeks, both to decrease blood

pressure and to correct metabolic abnormalities. These patients have significant potassium deficiency that must be corrected preoperatively because hypokalemia increases the risk of cardiac arrhythmias during anesthesia. Prolonged control of blood pressure (at least 3 months before surgery) permits the use of intravenous fluids during surgery without producing hypertension and decreases morbidity. Administration of antihypertensive medications usually is continued until surgery and glucocorticoid administration is not needed before surgery. After removal of an aldosterone-producing adenoma, selective hypoaldosteronism usually occurs, even in patients whose PRA had been stimulated with chronic diuretic therapy.[30] Potassium supplementation therefore should be given cautiously, and serum potassium values should be monitored closely. Residual mineralocorticoid activity is often sufficient to prevent excessive renal retention of potassium provided that sodium intake is adequate. If hyperkalemia does occur, furosemide in doses of 80 to 160 mg/day should be started. Treatment with fludrocortisone is not often necessary. If it is needed, 0.1 mg/day may be used as the initial dose and adequate salt intake continued. Abnormalities in aldosterone production can persist for as long as 3 months after tumor removal.

Table 78–3 Individual Blood Pressure Responses* to Calcium Entry Blocker (Nifedipine), Spironolactone, or Both in Patients With Primary Aldosteronism			
Patient No.	Nifedipine	Nifedipine + SPLT	SPLT
1	145/85	130/82	130/80
2	155/84	139/79	134/82
3	147/98	118/79	113/77
4	146/102	105/78	104/76
5	146/110	118/84	110/70
6	174/102	142/92	138/92
Mean	152/97	125/82†	122/80†
± SEM	4/4	5/2	5/3

From Bravo EL, Fouad FM, Tarazi RC. Calcium channel blockade with nifedipine in primary aldosteronism. Hypertension 8(suppl I):I-191, 1986.
Abbreviation: SPLT, spironolactone.
*Values are weekly averages of supine blood pressure taken twice daily during the 4th week of each treatment period.
†Values are significantly lower than nifedipine values only.

Glucocorticoid-Remediable Aldosteronism

Glucocorticoid-remediable aldosteronism (GRA) is an inherited autosomal dominant disorder that mimics an aldo-

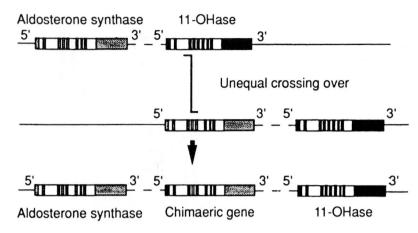

Figure 78–12. Diagram depicts unequal crossing over between aldosterone synthase and 11β-hydroxylase (11-OHase) genes. Each gene is represented by a *wide bar*, with the location of exons indicated by either *black* (11-OHase) or *stippled* (aldosterone synthase) *bands*. One of the two products of unequal crossing over will have a chimeric gene fusing sequences of the normal aldosterone synthase and 11-OHase genes. In this example, unequal crossing over is depicted as occurring in the intron between exons 3 and 4. (From Lifton RP, Dluhy RG, Powers M, et al. A chimaeric 11 beta-hydroxylase/aldosterone synthase gene causes glucocorticoid-remediable aldosteronism and human hypertension. Reprinted by permission from Nature 355:262, 1992. Copyright © 1992, Macmillan Magazines Ltd.)

sterone-producing adenoma.[31] GRA is caused by a genetic mutation that results in a hybrid or chimeric gene product fusing nucleotide sequences of the 11β-hydroxylase and aldosterone synthase genes.[32] This chimeric gene arose from unequal crossing between the 11β-hydroxylase and aldosterone synthase genes. These two genes are located in close proximity to human chromosome 8, are 95% homologous in nucleotide sequence, and have identical intron-exon structure. The structure of the duplicated gene contains 5′ regulatory sequences conferring the ACTH responsiveness of 11β-hydroxylase fused to more distal coding sequences of the aldosterone synthase gene (Fig. 78–12). This hybrid gene is expected to be regulated by ACTH and to have aldosterone synthase activity. It allows ectopic expression of aldosterone synthase activity in the ACTH-regulated zona fasciculata, which normally produces cortisol.[33] Aldosterone synthase oxidizes the C-18 carbon of a steroid precursor, such as corticosterone or cortisol, leading to the production of aldosterone and the hybrid steroids 18-hydroxy and 18-oxycortisol (Fig. 78–13). This abnormal gene duplication can direct genetic screening for this disorder with a small blood sample. An important clinical clue is the age of onset of hypertension. Patients with GRA typically are diagnosed with high blood pressure as children; conversely, patients with other mineralocorticoid excess disorders, such as aldosterone-producing adenomas and idiopathic hyperplasia, usually are diagnosed in their 30s to 60s. A strong family history of hypertension, often associated with early death of affected

family members from cerebrovascular accidents, is seen in some families with GRA.

No controlled studies of treatment of patients with GRA have been carried out. Theoretically, the suppression of ACTH with exogenous glucocorticoid should correct all GRA abnormalities. However, this therapy may be limited by complications of glucocorticoid administration. Another concern with glucocorticoid treatment is that patients may undergo a brief period of mineralocorticoid insufficiency when therapy is initiated before the renin-angiotensin axis recovers fully. Additional treatment modalities include mineralocorticoid receptor blockade with spironolactone or inhibition of the mineralocorticoid-sensitive distal tubule sodium channel with amiloride.

HYPERTENSIVE SYNDROMES DUE TO EXCESS CORTISOL PRODUCTION

11β-Hydroxysteroid Dehydrogenase Deficiency

11β-Hydroxysteroid dehydrogenase deficiency syndromes result in excessive activation of mineralocorticoid receptors by a steroid dependent on ACTH, rather than by the conventional mineralocorticoid agonist. This steroid appears to be cortisol. Mineralocorticoid receptors in the distal nephron have equal affinity for their two ligands—aldosterone and cortisol—but are protected from cortisol by the presence of 11β-dehydrogenase, which inactivates cortisol by

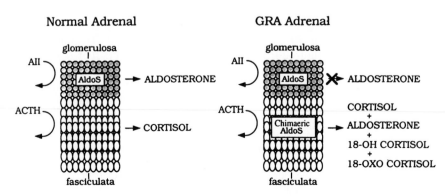

Figure 78–13. Regulation of aldosterone production in the zona glomerulosa and cortisol production in the zona fasciculata in the normal adrenal, and model of the physiologic abnormalities in the adrenal cortex in glucocorticoid-remediable aldosteronism (GRA). Ectopic expression of aldosterone synthase (AldoS) enzymatic activity in the adrenal fasciculata results in GRA. ACTH, adrenocorticotropic hormone. AII, angiotensin II. (From Lifton RP, Dluhy RG, Powers M, et al. Hereditary hypertension caused by chimaeric gene duplications and ectopic expression of aldosterone synthase. Reprinted by permission from Nat Genet 2:66, 1992. Copyright © 1992, Macmillan Magazines Ltd.)

converting it to cortisone.[34] The 11,18-hemiacetal structure of aldosterone protects it from the action of 11β-dehydrogenase so that aldosterone gains specific access to the receptors. When this mechanism is defective because of either congenital 11β-dehydrogenase deficiency or enzyme inhibition (by either licorice or carbenoxolone), intrarenal levels of cortisol increase, causing inappropriate activation of mineralocorticoid receptors (Fig. 78–14).[35] The resulting antinatriuresis and kaliuresis lead to hypertension and hypokalemia. Biochemically, there are elevations in urinary free cortisol excretion and the ratio of the urinary metabolites of cortisol to those of cortisone and prolongation of the half-life of titrated cortisol. Plasma cortisol concentrations usually are not elevated. The signs and symptoms are reversed by spironolactone or dexamethasone and are exacerbated by administration of physiological doses of cortisol.

Cushing's Syndrome (Ectopic ACTH Excess)

The recognizable causes of Cushing's syndrome include Cushing's disease (72%), ectopic ACTH excess (12%), adrenal adenoma (8%), carcinoma (6%), and hyperplasia (4%). The typical clinical presentation of Cushing's syndrome includes truncal obesity, moon facies, hypertension, plethora, muscle weakness and fatigue, hirsutism, emotional disturbances, and typical purple skin striae. Carbohydrate intolerance or diabetes, amenorrhea, loss of libido, easy bruising, and spontaneous fracture of ribs and vertebrae may also be encountered. Patients with ectopic ACTH excess may not have the typical manifestations of cortisol excess, but they may present with hyperpigmentation of the skin, severe hypertension, and marked hypokalemic alkalosis.

The incidence of hypokalemic alkalosis in the ectopic ACTH syndrome is greater than 90% compared with 10% in Cushing's syndrome of other causes.[36] It is widely supposed that corticosterone or 11-deoxycorticosterone is responsible for mineralocorticoid excess, but there is a poor correlation between the levels of these steroids and the degree of hypokalemia. A better predictor of hypokalemia is the level of cortisol.[37, 38] Several studies suggest that the ratio of cortisol:cortisone metabolites is increased in all forms of Cushing's syndrome.[39, 40] Ulick and associates[41] have advanced the hypothesis that excessive circulating cortisol overwhelms the enzyme, escaping conversion of cortisol to cortisone, thereby gaining inappropriate access to mineralocorticoid receptors. Walker and coworkers[42] demonstrated a negative correlation between the extent of impairment of 11β-dehydrogenase and plasma potassium concentration in 26 patients with Cushing's syndrome, 9 of whom had higher cortisol:cortisone ratios than the 15 with pituitary Cushing's and 2 with adrenal adenomas.

The determination of 24-hour urinary free cortisol is the best available test for documenting endogenous hypercortisolism.[43] A level above 100 μg/24 hr suggests excessive cortisol production. There are virtually no false-negative results. False-positive results may be obtained in non–Cushing's hypercortisolemic states (e.g., stress, chronic strenuous exercise, psychiatric states, glucocorticoid resistance, and malnutrition). If differentiation between pituitary and ectopic sources of ACTH cannot be made based on plasma levels alone, pharmacological manipulation of ACTH secretion should be performed. The overnight dexamethasone suppression test requires only a blood collection for serum cortisol the morning after the patient has taken a 1.0-mg dose of dexamethasone at 11 PM of the previous evening. In normal subjects, cortisol levels at 8 AM will be suppressed to 5.0 μg/dl or less.

When the syndrome has been diagnosed by appropriate biochemical testing, the cause must be identified. Radioimmunoassay of plasma ACTH is the procedure of choice for pinpointing the basis of hypercortisolism. In patients with ACTH-independent Cushing's syndrome, ACTH levels have usually been suppressed to below 5 pg/ml. In contrast, patients with the ACTH-dependent form tend to have either normal or elevated levels of ACTH, usually above 10 pg/ml. In patients with Cushing's disease, ACTH release can be inhibited only at much higher doses of dexamethasone

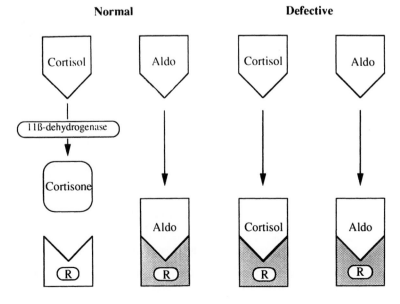

Figure 78–14. Enzyme-mediated receptor protection. Normal 11β-dehydrogenase converts cortisol to inactive cortisone, protecting mineralocorticoid receptors (R) from cortisol and allowing selective access for aldosterone (Aldo). When 11β-dehydrogenase is defective, e.g., in congenital deficiency or after licorice administration, cortisol gains inappropriate access to mineralocorticoid receptors, resulting in antinatriuresis and kaliuresis. (From Walker BR, Edwards CRW. Licorice-induced hypertension and syndromes of apparent mineralocorticoid excess. Endocrinol Metab Clin North Am 23:359, 1994.)

(2 mg every 6 hours for 2 days). The established criterion for the test is that suppression of the 24-hour urine and plasma steroids to less than 50% of baseline indicates pituitary Cushing's syndrome. Failure to suppress to less than 50% of baseline is considered consistent with an ectopic source of ACTH or ACTH-independent Cushing's syndrome. The best way to differentiate pituitary ACTH excess from the ectopic production of ACTH is with the inferior petrosal sinus procedure for ACTH concentration.[44] The test has been characterized in the literature as having 100% specificity and 100% sensitivity. The criterion currently used after corticotropin-releasing hormone administration is that the ACTH gradient between the inferior petrosal sinus and the peripheral site will be greater than 2 if the patient has Cushing's syndrome.

Surgical resection of a pituitary of ectopic source of ACTH or of a cortisol-producing adrenocortical tumor is the treatment of choice for Cushing's syndrome. For pituitary Cushing's syndrome, transsphenoidal pituitary adenomectomy is the treatment of choice,[45] but total hypophysectomy may be required in patients with diffuse hyperplasia or large pituitary tumors. Bilateral adrenalectomy for Cushing's disease is universally successful in alleviating the hypercortisolemic state; however, 10 to 38% of individuals may later develop pituitary tumors and hyperpigmentation (Nelson's syndrome).[46] Radiotherapy (i.e., external pituitary irradiation, seeding the pituitary bed with yttrium or gold) has also been used with occasionally good results.[47] The long-acting analogue SMS 201-995 (octreotide or sandostatin) has been used with varied success to treat ectopic ACTH syndromes;[48] some benefit has been reported in Cushing's disease and Nelson's syndrome. Cyproheptadine has had limited success in the treatment of Cushing's disease. Ketoconazole, an inhibitor of several steroid biosynthetic pathways, has been used for rapid correction of hypercortisolism awaiting definitive intervention.[49] Mitotane (o,p' DDD), an insecticide derivative, induces destruction of the zonae reticularis and fasciculata with relative sparing of the zona glomerulosa. Mitotane has been used to treat Cushing's syndrome associated with adrenal carcinoma or to suppress cortisol secretion in Cushing's disease.[50]

References

1. Liddle GW, Bledsoe T, Coppage WS. A familial renal disorder simulating primary aldosteronism but with negligible aldosterone secretion. Trans Assoc Am Physicians 76:199, 1963.
2. White PC, Speiser PW. Steroid 11 beta-hydroxylase deficiency and related disorders. Endocrin Metab Clin North Am 23:325, 1994.
3. Biglieri EG, Herron MA, Brust N. 17-Hydroxylation deficiency in man. J Clin Invest 45:1946, 1966.
4. Saadi HF, Bravo EL, Aron DC. Feminizing adrenocortical tumor: Steroid hormone response to ketoconazole. J. Clin Endocrinol Metab 70:540, 1990.
5. Azziz R, Boots LR, Parker CR Jr, et al. 11 Beta-hydroxylase deficiency in hyperandrogenism. Fertil Steril 55:733, 1991.
6. Biglieri EG, Kater CE, Brust N, et al. The regulation and diseases of deoxycorticosterone. In Mantero F, Takeda R, Scoggins BA, et al (eds). The Adrenal and Hypertension. From Cloning to Clinic. Serona Symposia Publication, vol 57. New York, Raven, 1989; p 355.
7. Lamberts SW, Poldermans D, Zweens M, et al. Familial cortisol resistance: Differential diagnostic and therapeutic aspects. J Clin Endocrinol Metab 63:1328, 1986.
8. Malchoff CD, Malchoff DM. Glucocorticoid resistance in humans. Trends Endocrinol Metab 6:89, 1995.
9. Bravo EL, Tarazi RC, Dustan HP, et al. The changing clinical spectrum of primary aldosteronism. Am J Med 74:641, 1983.
10. Conn JW. The evolution of primary aldosteronism: 1954–1967. Harvey Lect 62:257, 1966.
11. Ferriss JB, Beevers DG, Brown JJ, et al. Clinical, biochemical and pathological features of low-renin ("primary") hyperaldosteronism. Am Heart J 95:375, 1978.
12. George JM, Wright L, Bell NH, et al. The syndrome of primary aldosteronism. Am J Med 48:343, 1970.
13. Lins PE, Adamson U. Plasma aldosterone-plasma renin activity ratio. A simple test to identify patients with primary aldosteronism. Acta Endocrinol (Copenh) 113:564, 1986.
14. Hambling C, Jung RT, Gunn A, et al. Re-evaluation of the captopril test for the diagnosis of primary hyperaldosteronism. Clin Endocrinol (Oxf) 36:499, 1992.
15. Wambach G, Degenhardt S, Bonner G, et al. [Does the captopril test improve the diagnosis of primary hyperaldosteronism?] [German] Dtsch Med Wochenschr 117:1175, 1992.
16. Biglieri EG, Irony I, Kater CE. Identification and implications of new types of mineralocorticoid hypertension. J Steroid Biochem 32:199, 1989.
17. Biglieri EG, Schambelan M. The significance of elevated levels of plasma 18-hydroxycorticosterone in patients with primary aldosteronism. J Clin Endocrinol Metab 49:I-87, 1979.
18. Ganguly A, Melada GA, Luetscher JA, et al. Control of plasma aldosterone in primary aldosteronism: Distinction between adenoma and hyperplasia. J Clin Endocrinol Metab 37:765, 1973.
19. Fraser R, Beretta-Piccoli C, Brown JJ, et al. Response of aldosterone and 18-hydroxycorticosterone to angiotensin II in normal subjects and patients with essential hypertension, Conn's syndrome, and non-tumorous hyperaldosteronism. Hypertension 3:I87–I92, 1981.
20. Geisinger MA, Zelch MG, Bravo EL, et al. Primary hyperaldosteronism: Comparison of CT, adrenal venography, and venous sampling. AJR 141:299, 1983.
21. Linde R, Coulam C, Battino R, et al. Localization of aldosterone-producing adenoma by computed tomography. J Clin Endocrinol Metab 49:642, 1979.
22. White EA, Schambelan M, Rost CR, et al. Use of computed tomography in diagnosing the cause of primary aldosteronism. N Engl J Med 303:1503, 1980.
23. Melby JC, Spark RF, Dale SL, et al. Diagnosis and localization of aldosterone-producing adenomas by adrenal-vein catheterization. N Engl J Med 277:1050, 1967.
24. Tarazi RC, Ibrahim MM, Bravo EL, et al. Hemodynamic characteristics of primary aldosteronism. N Engl J Med 289:1330, 1973.
25. Bravo EL, Dustan HP, Tarazi RC. Spironolactone as a nonspecific treatment for primary aldosteronism. Circulation 48:491, 1973.
26. Bravo EL, Fouad-Tarazi FM, Tarazi RC, et al. Clinical implications of primary aldosteronism with resistant hypertension. Hypertension 11:I107–I111, 1988.
27. Schiffrin EL, Lis M, Gutkowska J, et al. Role of Ca^{2+} in response of adrenal glomerulosa cells to angiotensin II, ACTH, K^+, and ouabain. Am J Physiol 241:E42, 1981.
28. Kiowski W, Bertel O, Erne P, et al. Hemodynamic and reflex responses to acute and chronic antihypertensive therapy with the calcium entry blocker nifedipine. Hypertension 5:I70, 1983.
29. Bravo EL, Fouad FM, Tarazi RC. Calcium channel blockade with nifedipine in primary aldosteronism. Hypertension 8(suppl I):I-191, 1986.
30. Bravo EL, Dustan HP, Tarazi RC. Selective hypoaldosteronism despite prolonged pre- and postoperative hyperreninemia in primary aldosteronism. J Clin Endocrinol Metab 41:611, 1975.
31. Ganguly A, Grim CE, Weinberger MH. Anomalous postural aldosterone response in glucocorticoid-suppressible hyperaldosteronism. N Engl J Med 305:991, 1981.
32. Lifton RP, Dluhy RG, Powers M, et al. A chimaeric 11 beta-hydroxylase/aldosterone synthase gene causes glucocorticoid-remediable aldosteronism and human hypertension. Nature 355:262, 1992.
33. Lifton RP, Dluhy RG, Powers M, et al. Hereditary hypertension caused by chimaeric gene duplications and ectopic expression of aldosterone synthase. Nat Genet 2:66, 1992.
34. Edwards CR, Stewart PM, Burt D, et al. Localisation of 11 beta-hydroxysteroid dehydrogenase–tissue specific protector of the mineralocorticoid receptor. Lancet 2:986, 1988.
35. Funder JW, Pearce PT, Smith R, et al. Mineralocorticoid action:

Target tissue specificity is enzyme, not receptor, mediated. Science 242:583, 1988.

36. Howlett TA, Drury PL, Perry L, et al. Diagnosis and management of ACTH-dependent Cushing's syndrome: Comparison of the features in ectopic and pituitary ACTH production. Clin Endocrinol (Oxf) 24:699, 1986.

37. Christy NP, Laragh JH. Pathogenesis of hypokalemic alkalosis in Cushing's syndrome. N Engl J Med 265:1083, 1961.

38. Ritchie CM, Sheridan B, Fraser R, et al. Studies on the pathogenesis of hypertension in Cushing's disease and acromegaly. Q J Med 76:855, 1990.

39. Cost WS. Quantitative estimation of adrenocortical hormones and their alpha-ketotic metabolites in urine II: Pathological adrenocortical hyperfunction. Acta Endocrinol (Copenh) 42:39, 1963.

40. Phillipou G. Investigation of urinary steroid profiles as a diagnostic method in Cushing's syndrome. Clin Endocrinol (Oxf) 16:433, 1982.

41. Ulick S, Wang JZ, Blumenfeld JD, et al. Cortisol inactivation overload: A mechanism of mineralocorticoid hypertension in the ectopic adrenocorticotropin syndrome. J Clin Endocrinol Metab 74:963, 1992.

42. Walker BR, Campbell JC, Fraser R, et al. Mineralocorticoid excess and inhibition of 11 beta-hydroxysteroid dehydrogenase in patients with ectopic ACTH syndrome. Clin Endocrinol (Oxf) 37:483, 1992.

43. Tsigos C, Kamilaris TC, Chrousos GP. Adrenal diseases. In Moore WT, Eastman RC (eds). Diagnostic Endocrinology, Philadelphia, BC Decker, 1996; pp 125–156.

44. Oldfield EH, Chrousos GP, Schulte HM, et al. Preoperative lateralization of ACTH-secreting pituitary microadenomas by bilateral and simultaneous inferior petrosal venous sinus sampling. N Engl J Med 312:100, 1985.

45. Mampalam TJ, Tyrrell JB, Wilson CB. Transsphenoidal microsurgery for Cushing's disease. A report of 216 cases. Ann Intern Med 109:487, 1988.

46. Aron DC, Findling JW, Fitzgerald PA, et al. Cushing's syndrome: Problems in management. Endocr Rev 3:229, 1982.

47. Howlett TA, Plowman PN, Wass JA, et al. Megavoltage pituitary irradiation in the management of Cushing's disease and Nelson's syndrome: Long-term follow-up. Clin Endocrinol 31:309, 1989.

48. Lamberts SW, Krenning EP, Reubi JC. The role of somatostatin and its analogs in the diagnosis and treatment of tumors. Endocr Rev 12:450, 1991.

49. Tabarin A, Navarranne A, Guerin J, et al. Use of ketoconazole in the treatment of Cushing's disease and ectopic ACTH syndrome. Clin Endocrinol 34:63, 1991.

50. Luton JP, Mahoudeau JA, Bouchard P, et al. Treatment of Cushing's disease by o,p'DDD. Survey of 62 cases. N Engl J Med 300:459, 1979.

CHAPTER 79

Pheochromocytoma

William F. Young, Jr.

Catecholamine-producing tumors that arise from chromaffin cells of the adrenal medulla and the sympathetic ganglia are termed *pheochromocytomas* and *catecholamine-secreting paragangliomas (extra-adrenal pheochromocytomas),* respectively. Since the clinical presentation and therapeutic approach are similar, the term *pheochromocytoma* is used to refer to both adrenal pheochromocytomas and catecholamine-secreting paragangliomas.

CLINICAL PRESENTATION

Pheochromocytomas occur with equal frequency in men and women, primarily in the third, fourth, and fifth decades of life.[1] Patients harboring catecholamine-secreting tumors may be asymptomatic. However, symptoms usually are present and are due to the pharmacological effects of excessive levels of catecholamines or cosecreted peptide hormones. The hypertension may be sustained or paroxysmal. Episodic symptoms may occur in spells, or paroxysms, that can be extremely variable in presentation. Spells may be either spontaneous or precipitated by postural change, anxiety, medications (e.g., metoclopramide), exercise, or maneuvers that increase intraabdominal pressure. Although the interindividual variability in the types of spells is high, spells tend to be stereotypical for each patient.[2]

The familial autosomal neurocristopathic syndromes include familial pheochromocytoma, multiple endocrine neoplasia type IIA and IIB, neurofibromatosis,[3] and von Hippel-Lindau disease.[4-6] Advances in molecular genetics have uncovered many of the mutations responsible for these familial disorders. At least six germline mutations of the *RET* proto-oncogene on chromosome 10 (10q11.2) have been shown to be related to multiple endocrine neoplasia type IIA.[7] In addition, more than 300 von Hippel-Lindau germline mutations (von Hippel-Lindau tumor suppressor gene is on chromosome 3,3p25–26) have been identified and 32 of them are associated with pheochromocytoma.[8] A "founder effect" in the Black Forest region of Germany has been reported.[5, 6] Additional catecholamine-secreting tumor–related neurocutaneous syndromes include ataxia-telangiectasia, tuberous sclerosis, and Sturge-Weber syndrome. Other known associations that do not appear to have a familial basis are Carney's triad (gastric leiomyosarcoma, pulmonary chondroma, and extraadrenal pheochromocytoma),[9] cholelithiasis, and renal artery stenosis.

DIAGNOSTIC INVESTIGATION

Screening and Confirmatory Testing

Biochemical documentation of catecholamine hypersecretion should precede any form of imaging study. Refined laboratory techniques have overcome the problems associated with fluorometric analysis (e.g., false-positive results caused by α-methyldopa and other drugs with high native fluorescence). Catecholamines and their metabolites can be measured in the blood or the urine.

The 24-hour urinary excretion rates of catecholamines and their metabolites are the tests of choice to screen for catecholamine-secreting tumors.[10, 11] Catecholamine-secreting neoplasms are heterogeneous and have various qualitative and temporal secretory patterns. The *qualitative* pattern refers to the type or types of catecholamines or catecholamine metabolites that each patient with a pheochromocytoma secretes/excretes (e.g., norepinephrine, epinephrine, dopamine, metanephrine, normetanephrine, or vanillylmandelic acid). *Temporal* patterns refer to the unpredictable periodic hypersecretion of catecholamines and catecholamine metabolites that occur over time. Normal plasma or 24-hour urine catecholamine or metanephrine concentrations on one day may represent a trough between episodes of hypersecretion. Therefore, false-negative results may be obtained if patients are assessed at times when the catecholamine-secreting tumor is not hormonally active. The concept of periodic hormone excess is key to the appropriate evaluation of patients with possible catecholamine-secreting tumors.

Urine collections may be indexed to time (12 or 24 hours) or to creatinine levels.[11, 12] For a patient with episodic hypertension, the 24-hour urine collection should start with the onset of a spell. When it is collected in this manner, patients with pheochromocytoma have 24-hour urinary levels of catecholamines or metanephrines that are increased more than twofold above the upper limit of normal (Fig. 79–1). In 130 patients with benign sporadic adrenal pheochromocytomas operated on at Mayo Clinic from 1978 to 1995, we found that (1) 24-hour urinary metanephrines increased above the upper limit of normal in 94% of patients, (2) 24-hour urinary norepinephrine or epinephrine increased more than twofold above the upper limit of normal in 93% of patients, and (3) diagnostic increases occurred in either 24-hour urine metanephrines or catecholamines in 99% of patients.[13] Although it is best to evaluate patients who are not receiving any medication, treatment with most medications may be continued, with some exceptions (Table 79–1). Since the late 1970s, we have performed histamine and glucagon stimulation testing in 542 patients in whom pheochromocytoma was strongly suspected despite normal 24-hour urinary catecholamine or catecholamine-metabolite excretion; not one patient had positive results on the stimulation test in this setting.[11] Therefore, with current methodologies, there is no longer a role for provocative testing.

Many other approaches have been used to screen for and to confirm the presence of catecholamine-secreting tumors. Although plasma catecholamine measurements are convenient, they are not as sensitive as 24-hour urinary measurements and add little information.[14] Plasma concentrations of catecholamines are affected by diuretic treatment, smoking, and renal insufficiency. One report showed

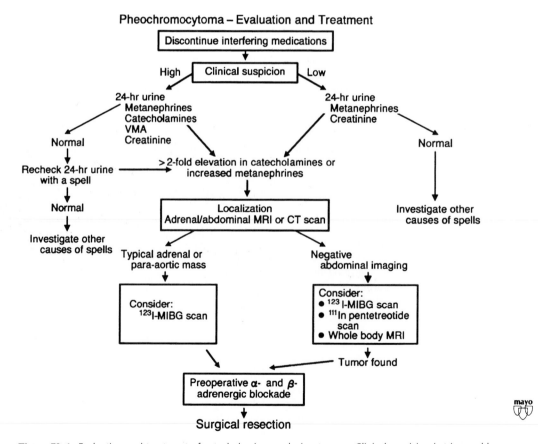

Figure 79–1. Evaluation and treatment of catecholamine-producing tumors. Clinical suspicion is triggered by: paroxysmal symptoms (especially hypertension); hypertension that is intermittent, unusually labile, or resistant to treatment; family history of pheochromocytoma or associated conditions; or incidentally discovered adrenal mass. The details are discussed in the text. VMA, vanillylmandelic acid; MRI, magnetic resonance imaging; CT, computed tomography; ^{123}I-MIBG, ^{123}I-metaiodobenzylguanidine. (Modified from Trends Endocrinol Metab, vol 4, Young WF Jr. Pheochromocytoma: 1926–1993, p 122, copyright 1993, with permission from Elsevier Science. By permission of Mayo Foundation.)

Table 79–1 Medications That May Alter Measured Levels of Catecholamines and Metabolites

INCREASE THE VALUES
Tricyclic antidepressants
Labetalol
Levodopa
Drugs containing catecholamines (e.g., decongestants)
Amphetamines, buspirone, and most psychoactive agents
Sotalol
Methyldopa
Withdrawal from clonidine hydrochloride (Catapres) and other drugs
Ethanol
Benzodiazepines

DECREASE THE VALUES
Metyrosine
Methylglucamine*

*A component of iodinated contrast media that may cause metanephrine values to be falsely normal for as long as 72 hours when measured with the Pisano spectrophotometric method.

that measurement of plasma concentrations of metanephrines is accurate for diagnosing pheochromocytoma.[14] If these data are confirmed, the plasma metanephrine assay will be another option for screening for catecholamine-secreting tumors. Plasma levels of chromogranin A and neuropeptide Y are increased in 80 to 90% of patients with catecholamine-secreting tumors.[15–17]

Localization

Localization studies should not be initiated until biochemical studies have confirmed the diagnosis of catecholamine-secreting tumor (see Fig. 79–1). Computer-assisted imaging of the adrenal glands and abdomen (magnetic resonance imaging or computed tomography) should be the first localization test (sensitivity > 95%; specificity > 65%).[18] Approximately 90% of these tumors are found in the adrenal glands and 98% in the abdomen.[10]

Catecholamine-secreting paragangliomas are found where chromaffin tissue is located (e.g., along the para-aortic sympathetic chain; within the organs of Zuckerkandl at the origin of the inferior mesenteric artery; wall of the urinary bladder; and the sympathetic chain in the neck or mediastinum).[19, 20] Tumor size is not correlated with the degree of increase in catecholamine levels.[21] If the results of abdominal imaging are negative, scintigraphic localization with ^{123}I-metaiodobenzylguanidine is indicated. This radiopharmaceutical agent accumulates preferentially in catecholamine-producing tumors; however, this procedure is not as sensitive as initially hoped (sensitivity 88%; specificity 99%).[22] Computer-assisted imaging of the chest, neck, and head and central venous sampling are localizing procedures that can also be used, but they are rarely required. Results of selective venous sampling for catecholamines are usually misleading because of periodic secretion; however, some medical centers have had positive results.[23, 24] Other localizing studies such as somatostatin-receptor imaging with ^{111}In-labeled pentetreotide may also be considered.[25, 26]

TREATMENT

Surgery

The treatment of choice for catecholamine-secreting tumors is surgical resection. Most pheochromocytomas are benign and can be excised totally. The details of preoperative preparation with combined α- and β-adrenergic blockade and the surgical approaches have been described elsewhere.[20, 27] Acute hypertensive crises should be treated with either nitroprusside or phentolamine. This is a high-risk surgical procedure and an experienced surgeon/anesthesiologist team is required.[28] Laparoscopy is being used more often for benign, sporadic, intraadrenal catecholamine-secreting tumors that are less than 8 cm in diameter.[29, 30] Blood pressure usually is normal by the time the patient is dismissed from the hospital; however, some patients remain hypertensive for up to 4 to 8 weeks postoperatively. Persistent hypertension may occur and may be related to accidental ligation of a polar renal artery, resetting of baroreceptors, established hemodynamic changes, structural changes in blood vessels, altered sensitivity of blood vessels to pressor substances, functional or structural changes in the kidney, or coincident essential hypertension.

Follow-Up Care

Approximately 2 weeks postoperatively, a 24-hour urine sample should be obtained for measurement of catecholamines and metanephrines. If the levels are normal, the resection of the catecholamine-secreting tumor can be considered to have been complete. Increased levels of catecholamines postoperatively indicate the presence of residual tumor, a second primary lesion, or occult metastases. The 24-hour urinary excretion of catecholamines should be checked annually for at least 5 years as surveillance for tumor recurrence in the adrenal bed, metastatic disease, or delayed appearance of multiple primary tumors.[31] Longer follow-up may be indicated if the DNA ploidy of the tumor is abnormal or if tumor telomerase activity is increased.[32–34]

The patient should undergo screening tests for multiple endocrine neoplasia type II, von Hippel-Lindau disease, and familial pheochromocytoma either preoperatively or at the first postoperative visit. Studies that should be considered include *RET* proto-oncogene or pentagastrin stimulation test,[7, 35] ophthalmology consultation, computerized imaging of the head, computerized imaging of the kidneys and pancreas (usually done preoperatively), and evaluation of 24-hour urine metanephrines in all immediate family members with hypertension.

References

1. Stenstrom G, Svardsudd K. Phaechromocytoma in Sweden, 1958–81. An analysis of the National Cancer Registry Data. Acta Med Scand 220:225, 1986.
2. Manger WM, Gifford RW Jr. Diagnosis. *In* Clinical and Experimental Pheochromocytoma. Cambridge, Blackwell Science, 1996.
3. Kalff V, Shapiro B, Lloyd R, et al. The spectrum of pheochromocytoma in hypertensive patients with neurofibromatosis. Arch Intern Med 142:2092, 1982.
4. Atuk NO, McDonald T, Wood T, et al. Familial pheochromocytoma,

hypercalcemia, and von Hippel-Lindau disease: A ten year study of a large family. Medicine 58:209, 1979.

5. Brauch H, Kishida T, Glavac D, et al. von Hippel-Lindau (VHL) disease with pheochromocytoma in the Black Forest region of Germany: Evidence for a founder effect. Hum Genet 95:551, 1995.

6. Gross DJ, Avishai N, Meiner V, et al. Familial pheochromocytoma associated with a novel mutation in the von Hippel-Lindau gene. J Clin Endocrinol Metab 81:147, 1996.

7. Eng C, Clayton D, Schuffenecker I, et al. The relationship between specific *RET* proto-oncogene mutations and disease phenotype in multiple endocrine neoplasia type 2: International *RET* mutation consortium analysis. JAMA 276:1575, 1996.

8. Atuk NO, Stolle C, Owen JA Jr, et al. Pheochromocytoma in von Hippel-Lindau disease: Clinical presentation and mutation analysis in a large multigenerational kindred. J Clin Endocrinol Metab 83:117, 1998.

9. Carney JA. The triad of gastric epithelioid leiomyosarcoma, pulmonary chondroma, and functioning extra-adrenal paraganglioma: A five-year review. Medicine 62:159, 1983.

10. van Gils APG, Falke THM, van Erkel AR, et al. MR imaging and MIBG scintigraphy of pheochromocytomas and extraadrenal functioning paragangliomas. Radiographics 11:37, 1991.

11. Young WF Jr. Phaeochromocytoma: How to catch a moonbeam in your hand. Eur J Endocrinol 136:28, 1997.

12. Heron E, Chatellier G, Billaud E, et al. The urinary metanephrine-to-creatinine ratio for the diagnosis of pheochromocytoma. Ann Intern Med 125:300, 1996.

13. Kudva YC, Young WF Jr. Sensitivity of 24-hour urine metanephrines and fractionated catecholamines in benign sporadic adrenal pheochromocytoma. [Abstract #OR28-5] *In* Programs and Abstracts of the 79th Annual Meeting of The Endocrine Society. Minneapolis, 1997; p 106.

14. Lenders JWM, Keiser HR, Goldstein DS, et al. Plasma metanephrines in the diagnosis of pheochromocytoma. Ann Intern Med 123:101, 1995.

15. Hsiao RJ, Parmer RJ, Takiyyuddin MA, et al. Chromogranin A storage and secretion: Sensitivity and specificity for the diagnosis of pheochromocytoma. Medicine 70:33, 1991.

16. Stridsberg M, Husebye ES. Chromogranin A and chromogranin B are sensitive circulating markers for phaeochromocytoma. Eur J Endocrinol 136:67, 1997.

17. Mouri T, Sone M, Takahashi K, et al. Neuropeptide Y as a plasma marker for phaeochromocytoma, ganglioneuroblastoma, and neuroblastoma. Clin Sci 83:205, 1992.

18. Jackson JA, Kleerekoper M, Mendlovic D. Endocrine grand rounds: A 51-year-old man with accelerated hypertension, hypercalcemia, and right adrenal and paratracheal masses. Endocrinologist 3:5, 1993.

19. Whalen RK, Althausen AF, Daniels GH. Extra-adrenal pheochromocytoma. J Urol 147:1, 1992.

20. O'Riordain DS, Young WF Jr, Grant CS, et al. Clinical spectrum and outcome of functional extraadrenal paraganglioma. World J Surg 20:916, 1996.

21. Ito Y, Fujimoto Y, Obara T. The role of epinephrine, norepinephrine, and dopamine in blood pressure disturbances in patients with pheochromocytomas. World J Surg 16:759, 1992.

22. Shapiro B, Gross MD, Fig L, et al. Localization of functioning sympathoadrenal lesions. *In* Biglieri EG, Melby JC (eds). Endocrine Hypertension. New York, Raven, 1990; p 235.

23. Newbould EC, Ross GA, Dacie JE, et al. The use of venous catheterization in the diagnosis and localization of bilateral phaeochromocytomas. Clin Endocrinol 35:55, 1991.

24. Walker IA. Selective venous catheterization and plasma catecholamine analysis in the diagnosis of phaeochromocytoma. J R Soc Med 89:216P, 1996.

25. Lamberts SWJ, Bakker WH, Reubi JC, et al. Somatostatin-receptor imaging in the localization of endocrine tumors. N Engl J Med 323:1246, 1990.

26. Tenenbaum F, Lumbroso J, Schlumberger M, et al. Comparison of radiolabeled octreotide and meta-iodobenzylguanidine (MIBG) scintigraphy in malignant pheochromocytoma. J Nucl Med 36:1, 1995.

27. Young WF Jr. Pheochromocytoma: 1926 to 1993. Trends Endocrinol Metab 4:122, 1993.

28. O'Riordain JA. Pheochromocytomas and anesthesia. Anesthesiol Clin 25:99, 1996.

29. Fernandez-Cruz L, Taura P, Saenz A, et al. Laparoscopic approach to pheochromocytoma: Hemodynamic changes and catecholamine secretion. World J Surg 20:762, 1996.

30. Thompson GB, Grant CS, van Heerden JA, et al. Laparoscopic versus open posterior adrenalectomy: A case-control study of 100 patients. Surgery 122:1132, 1997.

31. van Heerden JA, Roland CF, Carney JA, et al. Long-term evaluation following resection of apparently benign pheochromocytoma(s)/paraganglioma(s). World J Surg 14:325, 1990.

32. Cope C, Delbridge L, Philips J, et al. Prognostic significance of nuclear DNA content in phaeochromocytoma. Aust N Z J Surg 61:695, 1991.

33. Nativ O, Grant CS, Sheps SG, et al. The clinical significance of nuclear DNA ploidy pattern in 184 patients with pheochromocytoma. Cancer 69:2683, 1992.

34. Kubota Y, Nakada T, Sasagawa I, et al. Elevated levels of telomerase activity in malignant pheochromocytoma. Cancer 82:176, 1998.

35. Ledger GA, Khosla S, Lindor NM, et al. Genetic testing in the diagnosis and management of multiple endocrine neoplasia type II. Ann Intern Med 122:118, 1995.

CHAPTER

80 Hypertension in Pregnant Women

Marshall D. Lindheimer and Ayub Akbari

Hypertension during pregnancy, the most common medical complication of gestation, can be a challenging clinical problem, the approach to which differs considerably from that employed in nonpregnant populations. The practitioner must first consider additional entities in his or her differential diagnosis because of two pregnancy-specific disorders: preeclampsia—a complication associated with substantial maternal and fetal morbidity and mortality—and the relatively more benign disorder, gestational (transient) hypertension of pregnancy. In addition, there are two patients to deal with simultaneously, the hypertensive mother and her unborn child. This chapter, devoted to the hypertensive disorders of pregnancy, commences with a review of the striking alterations in hemodynamics that accompany normal gestation, then highlights problems related to classification and diagnosis. Its main focus, however, is preeclampsia because this disease is the most potentially ominous of the more common hypertensive disorders of

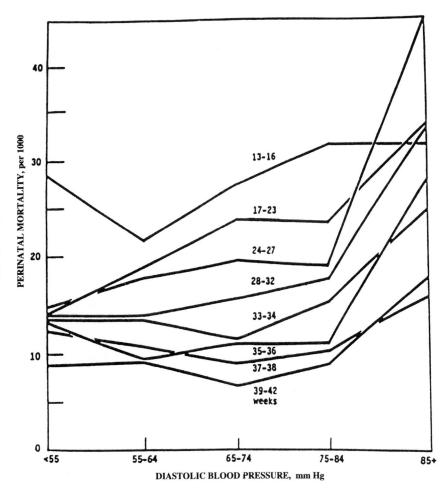

Figure 80–1. Prospective data from a collaborative trial involving 58,806 recruited subjects demonstrate trends in perinatal mortality rates as a function of diastolic pressure recordings analyzed from gestational week 13 through term. Note that perinatal mortality increases significantly once diastolic pressure exceeds 84 mm Hg. (From Friedman EA, Neff RK. Pregnancy and Hypertension. A Systematic Evaluation of Clinical Diagnostic Criteria. Littleton, MA, PSG Publishing, 1977.)

pregnancy. The chapter concludes with a discussion of the efficacy and safety of a number of antihypertensive drugs currently prescribed for pregnant women.

ALTERED HEMODYNAMICS AND VOLUME HOMEOSTASIS IN NORMAL PREGNANCY

Cognizance of the cardiovascular changes that occur during normal gestation should lead to earlier detection and management of the hypertensive complications. Blood pressure decreases during the luteal phase of the menstrual cycle and continues to decline after conception. Diastolic blood pressure levels average 10 mm Hg below nonpregnant values by midgestation.[1–6] Blood pressure then increases slowly, approaching nongravid levels near term, and may even exceed such levels transiently in the puerperium.[7] Cardiac output increases 30 to 50%, the increment also beginning soon after conception and peaking near gestational week 16, after which values are sustained until term.[8, 9] Given the magnitude of the increase in cardiac output, the fall in blood pressure levels must be due to a striking decrement in peripheral vascular resistance, and indeed, this is the case. Thus, normal pregnancy is a markedly vasodilated state. Finally, there are striking increments in total arterial compliance in pregnancy, as well as alter-

ations in pulsatile flow,[9] another adaptation that helps the gravida to accommodate greater intravascular volume (see Volume Homeostasis) without increasing her mean arterial pressure. Maladaptation, or reversal of such changes in compliance, could conceivably affect blood pressure control in pregnant women with hypertension.

The major implication of the cardiovascular changes in normal pregnancy described previously is the following: Although the definition of hypertension in gravidas remains diastolic and systolic blood pressure levels of greater than or equal to 90 and greater than or equal to 140 mm Hg, respectively, one should consider a diastolic value of 75 mm Hg in the second, and 85 mm Hg in the third trimester, and/or a systolic value of 120 mm Hg in midpregnancy and 130 mm Hg in late pregnancy as suspect. In this respect, two large epidemiological studies have demonstrated that fetal mortality rises significantly when diastolic pressure at any stage of gestation is 85 mm Hg,[2] and that perinatal mortality and growth retardation increase when mean blood pressure exceeds 90 and 95 mm Hg during the second and the third trimesters,[3] respectively (Fig. 80–1). One should also be aware that some women with undiagnosed mild essential hypertension experience a decrement in blood pressure to apparently normal levels early in pregnancy. They are then mislabeled when frankly elevated values occur at term. An astute clinician cognizant that a blood pressure of 124/78 mm Hg at gestational week 16 may be abnormal would avoid such errors.

Review of mechanisms that maintain blood pressure during pregnancy, including alterations in vasoconstricting and vasodilating hormones and autacoids, such as natriuretic peptides and endothelium-produced factors, is beyond the scope of this chapter, and is discussed elsewhere.[10–12] One notes, however, the marked increments in production and circulating levels of renin, angiotensin, and a host of corticoids, primarily aldosterone, desoxycorticosterone, and progesterone, during pregnancy. There is also a body of work suggesting that increments in production of vasodilating prostanoids and of nitric oxide synthase and the endothelium-derived relaxing factor nitric oxide are responsible for the marked decrease in peripheral vascular resistance characteristic of normal pregnancy.[13–15] Some of this is revisited when discussing the pathogenesis of hypertension in gestation.

Measuring Blood Pressure

There are controversies about the correct way to measure blood pressure during gestation, including the appropriate posture (e.g., lateral recumbency vs. sitting), and sound used to measure diastolic levels (Korotkoff four [K_4] muffling or Korotkoff five [K_5] disappearance). It is now apparent that the lower blood pressure levels observed when the subject is in lateral recumbency often reflect only the reduction in hydrostatic pressure observed when the cuff is positioned substantially above the left ventricle. Also, the view prominent in the literature that the hyperdynamic circulation of pregnant women often results in large differences between K_4 and K_5, the latter approaching zero, is incorrect. Work has affirmed that K_5 is the sound closest to true diastolic pressure,[16–19] and K_5 should be used to define diastolic pressure in gravidas. There is a growing literature on the role of ambulatory blood pressure monitoring in the detection of hypertensive disorders in pregnancy, but its efficacy and/or cost effectiveness remain to be established.[20–22]

Volume Homeostasis

Pregnant women gain approximately 12.5 kg of body weight, mainly because of fluid accumulation; total body water increases by 6 to 9 L, of which 4 to 7 L is extracellular.[11, 23] Plasma volume and red blood cell mass rise by approximately 50% and 20 to 30%, respectively, resulting in the "dilutional" anemia of pregnancy. Interstitial volume also increases, and edema is a normal feature of pregnancy. Finally, renal plasma flow and glomerular filtration rate (GFR) increase markedly, the rise in GFR being reflected by decreases in both creatinine and urea nitrogen levels, the upper limits of normal for these solutes being 0.8 mg/dl and 13 mg/dl, respectively. Thus, values considered normal in nonpregnant populations may be abnormal in pregnant women. Urinary protein excretion also rises in pregnancy, the upper limit of normal being 300 mg/24 hr (or twice that used for nonpregnant individuals in most institutions).

DETECTION AND CLASSIFICATION

The literature is filled with an assortment of terminologies used to describe high blood pressure in pregnancy. Terms such as *toxemia, pregnancy-induced or -associated hypertension, gestosis, preeclampsia,* and *preeclamptic toxaemia* present a source of confusion for many readers. The latter point is especially true when the same term (e.g., *pregnancy-induced hypertension*) is defined in different manners by various authors. Many of the classification schema are also complex and overdetailed. We use an approach developed by the American College of Obstetricians and Gynecologists Committee on Terminology in 1972 and endorsed most recently by the U.S. National High Blood Pressure Education Program (NHBPEP)[24] because it is concise and practical and accurately separates the more benign from the serious disorders. It divides high blood pressure in pregnancy into four categories: chronic hypertension (both essential and secondary); preeclampsia-eclampsia; preeclampsia superimposed on chronic hypertension; and gestational (transient) hypertension of pregnancy.

Chronic Hypertension

The incidence of high blood pressure in pregnant women ranges between 7 and 10%, about one quarter due to essential hypertension.[2, 24, 25] The latter diagnosis is most certain when history of the disease has been documented before pregnancy or when elevated blood pressure is detected before gestational week 20 or persists after the puerperium.[26, 27] Pregnancies in patients who fit this category are, for the most part, uneventful when pressure elevations are mild and target organ damage absent. However, as discussed later, these mothers experience increased incidences of superimposed preeclampsia, the cause of most of the morbidity in these gestations.[28]

Fortunately, "secondary" causes of hypertension in pregnant women are infrequent. In patients with scleroderma, periarteritis nodosa, and Cushing's syndrome, both mothers and fetuses do poorly. Pheochromocytoma, which has a propensity to present during pregnancy, is particularly ominous and was once associated with substantial lethality. Currently, the disorder is being detected and managed to successful outcomes, either surgically or pharmacologically (depending on the stage of gestation).[29, 30] Medical management involves α-blockade to control the blood pressure until delivery, after which the tumor, if operable, is resected[31] (see also Chap. 79, Pheochromocytoma). It is therefore prudent to screen for catecholamine excess at the slightest suspicion.

Both renal angioplasty and stent placement have been successfully performed in pregnant women with uncontrolled hypertension secondary to renal artery stenosis.[30–33] The course of pregnancy in women with aldosterone-producing tumors is variable. In some, the course appears similar to that in nongravid subjects with the disease. However, there are several well-documented instances in which patients have experienced amelioration of the kaliuresis, normalization of plasma potassium levels, and even spontaneous reductions in blood pressure, presumably due to the rise in progesterone production during pregnancy, as this hormone inhibits the effect of aldosterone on the renal tubule.[34]

Preeclampsia-Eclampsia

Preeclampsia, especially when superimposed on chronic hypertension or renal disease (category 3), is the hypertensive disorder most frequently associated with morbidity in pregnancy, jeopardizing the well-being of both mother and fetus.[2, 10–12, 26, 35, 36] For this reason, when uncertainty exists as to the underlying diagnosis, it is prudent to treat the patient as if she had preeclampsia.

Preeclampsia occurs primarily in nulliparas, after midpregnancy (although there are exceptions), most often near term. The cardinal features are hypertension and proteinuria, and many patients experience rapid weight gain and develop edema as well. The preeclamptic patient may also manifest liver function and/or coagulation abnormalities, especially thrombocytopenia.

Of considerable concern is the potential for this disease to progress rapidly to a life-threatening convulsive phase, termed *eclampsia*. The latter is frequently preceded by premonitory symptoms and signs including hyperreflexia, visual disturbances, severe headache, right upper quadrant or epigastric pain, and several laboratory changes (Table 80–1). Eclampsia can also occur suddenly, and without such warning signs and symptoms, in a patient whose blood pressure is only mildly elevated—one reason why preeclampsia, regardless of apparent severity, always presents a danger to mother and fetus.

There is a deceptively benign variant of preeclampsia characterized by minimal changes in blood pressure, borderline thrombocytopenia, modest increases in liver enzymes, and often, no renal dysfunction. This scenario leads to thoughts of temporization, especially when present before gestational week 34. However, this form of preeclampsia may rapidly become life-threatening, progressing within 24 to 48 hours into a florid syndrome characterized by hemolysis (of the microangiopathic hemolytic anemia variety with schistocytes present on the peripheral blood smear) and prominent changes in coagulation and liver function (platelet counts can decrease by $100,000/mm^3$ in a day, and transaminases and lactic dehydrogenase levels rise very quickly to exceed 1000 IU within 24 hours). This is the acronym, the HELLP syndrome (*h*emolysis, *e*levated *l*iver enzymes, *l*ow *p*latelet count). There can also be variants, such as HEL, EL, LP. This syndrome is associated with severe morbidity, unless the pregnancy is promptly terminated (see Controversy: "Aggressive" Versus "Conservative" Management When Preeclampsia Is Remote From Term, later in this chapter).

As noted, preeclampsia occurs primarily after midpregnancy or in the immediate puerperium, but exceptions exist. The disorder can occur before the 20th gestational week, in which case it is usually associated with one of the following conditions: hydatidiform disease, nonimmune fetal hydrops disorder (including α-thalassemia), abdominal pregnancy, and on rare occasions, chronic hypertension and renal disease. At the other end of the spectrum is a disorder termed *late postpartum eclampsia* that manifests more than 48 hours after delivery and within the first 2 weeks of the puerperium.

Gestational (Transient) Hypertension of Pregnancy

This entity is characterized by mild to moderate hypertension in late gestation or in the immediate puerperium, blood pressures normalizing rapidly postpartum, at which time the diagnosis of "transient" is confirmed. These events frequently recur in subsequent gestations, but pregnancies are otherwise benign. When such a scenario occurs late in the pregnancy of a nullipara, it may be difficult to distinguish transient hypertension of pregnancy from early preeclampsia, in which case it is prudent to manage the patient as if she had preeclampsia.[26] One author has suggested that transient hypertension in pregnancy is not benign, especially if hyperuricemia or decreasing platelet counts are noted.[37] Finally, there is evidence that some of the women manifesting transient hypertension of pregnancy are those destined to develop essential hypertension later in life. Thus, yearly follow-up blood pressure checks in such women should lead to earlier detection of frank hypertension.

There is an entity termed *late postpartum hypertension,* whose cause may be comparable to that of transient hypertension of pregnancy. This classification should be restricted to patients experiencing normotensive gestations, whose blood pressures first rise after the 2nd postpartum week and remain mildly elevated for up to 6 months, normalizing thereafter. The literature is sparse, there having been few studies of patients manifesting this strange chain of events. It is tempting to speculate that late postpartum

---

Table 80–1 Ominous Signs, Symptoms, and Laboratory Abnormalities in Women With Preeclampsia

Preeclampsia is always potentially dangerous, and the indicators listed here may be particularly ominous.

SIGNS AND SYMPTOMS

Blood pressure ≥ 160 mm Hg systolic or ≥ 110 mm Hg diastolic

Upper abdominal pain, especially epigastric and in the right upper quadrant

Headache, visual disturbances, and/or other cerebral signs

Cardiac decompensation (e.g., pulmonary edema), which usually is associated with underlying heart disease or chronic hypertension

Retinal hemorrhages, exudates, or papilledema (very rare without other indicators of severity; when present usually indicates underlying chronic hypertension)

LABORATORY ABNORMALITIES

Rapid increase in proteinuria, especially to ≥3 g/24 hr, combined with rapidly decreasing serum albumin levels

Increasing serum creatinine concentrations to ≥2 mg/dl (177 μmol/L) (unless known to be elevated previously)

Platelet count $10^5/mm^3$ or evidence of microangiopathic hemolytic anemia (e.g., schistocytes and/or increased lactate dehydrogenase or direct bilirubin levels)

In presence of intrauterine growth retardation and decreasing urine volumes, added vigilance is also required.

Modified from Akbari A, Lindheimer MD. Management of high blood pressure in pregnancy. *In* Epstein M (ed). Calcium Antagonists in Clinical Medicine, 2nd ed. Philadelphia, Hanley & Belfus, 1998; pp 321–344.

hypertension is another harbinger of essential hypertension later in life. Gravidas exposed to cocaine may present with syndromes that mimic both transient hypertension of pregnancy and preeclampsia.

In summary: The previously described classification schema should prove clinically useful. However, one must keep in mind that at times it may be very difficult to distinguish among preeclampsia, chronic, secondary, or transient hypertension, and combinations of these entities by clinical criteria alone. These dilemmas have been underscored in the older literature by the results of clinical correlation studies in which renal biopsy results were used to verify the diagnosis.[38] In one such study, in which a nephrologist and an obstetrician recorded their impressions before the biopsy, they were completely correct in only 58% of the patients (cited in ref. 38). This is why we approach the patient presenting with high blood pressure in pregnancy cautiously, managing her for the most ominous of possible disorders (Table 80–2).

PATHOPHYSIOLOGY AND MANAGEMENT OF PREECLAMPSIA

Preeclampsia is more than hypertension, it is a systemic disorder. This section summarizes its pathology and pathophysiology and discusses both management and preventive strategies.

Hypertension

Hypertension in preeclampsia represents a reversal of the vasodilatation characteristic of normal gestation, to a point where the striking increases in peripheral vascular resistance are so marked that blood pressure rises despite decreases in cardiac output. The vasoconstriction occurs because the vasculature in preeclamptic women becomes hyperresponsive to a variety of vasoactive peptides and amines, especially angiotensin II, whereas in normal pregnancy the vessels are resistant to these pressor hormones and/or autacoids.[11, 12, 26] Hypertension in preeclampsia is labile and may be accompanied by a reversal of the normal circadian blood pressure pattern.[11, 12]

The cause of the altered vascular reactivity remains obscure. Research has focused on changes in the ratio of vasodilating and vasoconstricting prostanoids, some suggesting increments in the production of thromboxane,[11, 12] as well as on the vasoconstricting potential of circulating pressor substances (e.g., angiotensin II and endothelin). Another focus of research is the question of whether increased vascular reactivity in preeclampsia is related to inhibition of the adaptive increments in the production of nitric oxide synthase as well as nitric oxide–dependent endothelium-derived relaxing factor. There is a search for mechanisms that would damage the endothelium (the site of prostanoid, endothelin, and endothelium-derived relaxing factor production) in preeclampsia, including a host of "bad" cytokines and insufficient antioxidant activity.[11, 12, 39, 40] Other investigators have focused on gestational aberrations in calciotropic hormone, insulin, and magnesium metabolism. As of 1999, however, all of their hypotheses remain to be proved.

Kidney and Volume Homeostasis

There is a characteristic renal lesion associated with preeclampsia. The glomerulus is enlarged and ischemic owing to hypertrophy and swelling of the intracapillary cells, termed *glomerular endotheliosis* (some regard this as further evidence of an abnormal endothelium in all the vessels

---

Table 80–2 Findings and Tests for Differentiating Preeclampsia (Pure or Superimposed) From Other Hypertensive Disorders

	Preeclampsia	Chronic Hypertension
Age	Extremes of age	Usually older (>30 yr)
Parity	Mainly in nulliparas	More often multiparas
Onset	Rare before gestational wk 20	Pressure may be elevated ≤20 wk
History	Negative	Positive; including hypertension in previous pregnancy
Physical examination	Funduscopic evidence of vasospasm, cardiac status usually normal, central nervous system irritability (visual signs, headaches, hyperreflexia), upper abdominal or epigastric pain	Target-organ findings with long-standing disease or uncontrolled pressure (i.e., arteriovenous nicking in fundi, cardiac hypertrophy), normal reflexes and abdominal examination
Complete blood count	Increased hematocrit suggesting hemoconcentration, decreasing platelet counts, schistocytes on smear	Normal (lupus erythematosus may mimic preeclamptic platelet changes)
Urinalysis and protein excretion	Often normal, but may contain red blood cells and even casts; proteinuria usually present	Normal in essential hypertension, "active" when glomerular diseases exacerbate; minimal or no proteinuria
Serum creatinine	Abnormal or increasing values, especially when oliguria present, suggest severe preeclampsia	Normal in essential hypertension, but may be increased in underlying glomerular disorders, which may exacerbate and mimic preeclampsia
Serum urate	Often increased out of proportion to changes in creatinine levels	Usually normal
Liver function	Abnormal enzymes (transaminases, lactic dehydrogenase), increased bilirubin	Normal

Modified from Akbari A, Lindheimer MD. Management of high blood pressure in pregnancy. *In* Epstein M (ed). Calcium Antagonists in Clinical Medicine, 2nd ed. Philadelphia, Hanley & Belfus, 1998; pp 321–344.

of preeclamptics). Both GFR and renal plasma flow are decreased, GFR decreasing 25% in mild cases. This may be due to a combination of renal vasoconstriction and structural changes that decrease the ultrafiltration coefficient at the nephron level.[41] Thus, despite morphological evidence of ischemia and obliteration of the urinary space, GFR in preeclamptics is still greater than that in nonpregnant women. This may not be appreciated if one is not aware of the upper limits of normal for serum creatinine in pregnancy (see later).

Uric acid clearances normally rise in gestation, but decrease, often early and before overt disease, in patients with developing preeclampsia. The decrement in uric acid clearance is generally greater than the decrement in GFR. In this respect, a circulating urate level of 5 mg/dl is abnormal in pregnancy. Renal calcium handling is also affected by preeclampsia. The normal hypercalciuria of pregnancy is replaced by hypocalciuria, which may relate to reductions in GFR that, at times, are too small to be detected by the measurement of endogenous creatinine clearance.[42]

Abnormal proteinuria usually accompanies preeclampsia, and the diagnosis should be suspect in its absence. Nevertheless, increased protein excretion can be a late feature of the disorder. The proteinuria may be minimal or severe and is nonselective.[38, 42, 43] Preeclampsia is the major cause of nephrotic range proteinuria in pregnancy.

Renal sodium handling may be impaired in preeclampsia and is the major cause of salt retention and sudden edema in these patients. However, the degree of impairment is variable, and some of the most severe forms of the disease occur in the absence of edema (the "dry" preeclamptic). This is underscored by a report where 26 of 67 eclamptics (women who convulsed) were edema free.[44] More importantly, even when edema is marked, plasma volume is below that of normal pregnancy, and hemoconcentration may be present. This decrease in intravascular volume represents, in part, extravasation of albumin into the interstitium (leaky vasculature secondary to endothelial damage or dysfunction), so that interstitial oncotic pressure rises.[12, 45] Hypoalbuminemia may be present when proteinuria and/or liver dysfunction are minimal. Central venous and pulmonary capillary wedge pressures tend to be low in preeclampsia because of the reduced intravascular volume. Because of the reduced intravascular volume, compromised placental perfusion, and decreased cardiac output, diuretics should be avoided in these patients.

The cause of the impaired renal sodium excretion in preeclampsia is not known. Filtered sodium, although decreased compared with levels in normal gestation, is still higher than in the nongravid state. More paradoxical is that the renin-angiotensin-aldosterone system is suppressed and circulating natriuretic factor(s) levels are increased, despite a decrease in intravascular volume. On the other hand, there is renal vasoconstriction and increased activity of the sympathetic nervous system in preeclampsia.[46]

Brain

Eclampsia (the convulsive phase) is still a leading cause of maternal death, while our knowledge of its cause remains fragmentary, leading to controversies about its treatment. Some suggest that eclampsia may relate to the coagulopathy associated with preeclampsia, noting fibrin deposition in the brain at autopsy.[47] Still others consider it a form of hypertensive encephalopathy,[48] a concept we find difficult to accept, as convulsions can occur suddenly in women with systolic blood pressure levels below 140 mm Hg. However, vasoconstriction in preeclampsia may at times be organ-selective, and investigations using ultrasonographic techniques suggest that severe cerebral vasospasm may occur even when peripheral vasoconstriction is less evident.[49] Studies utilizing techniques such as computed axial tomography and magnetic resonance imaging have produced varied results, but many describe abnormalities, usually transient, consistent with localized petechiae or edema. A problem with many of these studies is that they were performed in patients receiving considerable fluid administration, raising the specter that some of the findings may be iatrogenic. Most recently, Doppler ultrasonographic techniques have provided evidence that previous disagreements are due to the heterogeneity of the population studied. It appears that some patients may have normal cerebral vascular pressure indices and others high pressures and/or perfusion akin to hypertensive encephalopathy.[50, 51]

The best descriptions of gross and microscopic pathology in preeclampsia are contained in the large autopsy series published by Sheehan and Lynch in 1973.[52] Most of these necropsies were performed within an hour or two of death, eliminating most of the postmortem changes that might confound interpretation. There were varying degrees of hemorrhages and petechiae, some grossly visible, others at the microscopic level. These authors offer some of the most cogent arguments that the initiating events are vasoconstrictive and ischemic in nature and that edema is a late or postpartum feature of the process.

Uterus and Placenta

There is a decrease in uteroplacental blood flow in preeclampsia, reflecting both arterial lesions (termed *acute atherosis*) and a greater degree of placental infarction than is seen in normotensive gravidas. Decrements in flow may relate to changes in the vascular resistance indices, and evidence of reversal of blood flow is seen when the patient is examined using Doppler ultrasound technology.[12, 53] There is also evidence of abnormal placentation. Shortly after conception, a process begins whereby the uterine arteries are transformed from thick-walled muscular into saclike flaccid vessels that serve to accommodate a 10-fold increase intrauterine blood flow.[12, 54–58] This process, said to be due to endovascular trophoblastic invasion, is virtually complete by the end of the second trimester. In women who later develop preeclampsia, trophoblastic invasion of the spiral arteries is incomplete and the arteries remain thick-walled and muscular. There is evidence that in preeclampsia the cytotrophoblast cells fail to mimic a vascular adhesion phenotype and to express adhesion molecules believed crucial to the process of vascular invasion.[59] These changes add credence to the theory that relative placental hypoxemia is the proximate cause of the disease.[39]

Several other systemic manifestations of preeclampsia, including coagulation problems and liver dysfunction (including the ominous HELLP syndrome), have been discussed previously. The pathological changes in the liver, as well as rarer pathology in heart, lung, and pituitary and adrenal glands, are noted in the excellent monograph of Sheehan and Lynch.[52]

Preeclampsia Superimposed on Another Disorder

Superimposed preeclampsia, especially when it presents early in the latter half of pregnancy and/or in conjunction with preexisting hypertension, is associated with increased maternal and fetal risk. Such superimposition may be difficult to distinguish clinically from an exacerbation of either chronic hypertension or an underlying renal disorder.[28] Because preeclampsia can be explosive, and its course ominous, investigators continually search for tests to predict imminent disease, to distinguish preeclampsia from the more benign transient hypertension of pregnancy, or to decide whether superimposed preeclampsia has indeed occurred. They also search for markers that may help determine the cause of preeclampsia, as such markers could lead to strategies to prevent the disease or at least improve its management. In this respect, studies have focused on a host of autacoids, hormones, lipids, oxidant or antioxidant activity, markers of endothelial dysfunction, evidence of neutrophil activation, adhesion molecules, a multitude of cytokines, the isoelectric point of plasma albumin, urinary excretion of calcium, and other factors.[11, 12, 39] Both the sensitivity and the positive predictive value of virtually all of these tests are either unknown or appear modest, and as of 1999, none can be recommended. Table 80–2 suggests a clinical approach that may help in the differentiation of preeclampsia from chronic or transient hypertension in pregnancy.

Can Preeclampsia Be Prevented?

Interventions that succeed in preventing preeclampsia or that abort its development at an early or preclinical stage would revolutionize prenatal care. Sodium restriction and/or the administration of prophylactic diuretics, once a popular strategy but then discarded, was revived briefly in 1985 after a meta-analysis of approximately 7000 randomized patients suggested favorable results.[60] Analysis of the article, however, revealed no difference in the incidence of proteinuric hypertension; the seemingly positive effects were restricted to the ability of diuretics to reduce edema and/or provoke a modest decrement in blood pressure.

In the 1990s, two approaches were advocated, each based on plausible hypotheses. In the first, administration of low-dose aspirin (60 to 100 mg/day) commenced after the 12th gestational week, was based on the hypothesis that hypertension and coagulation abnormalities in preeclampsia were due to an imbalance in the production of vasodilating and vasoconstricting prostaglandins. Low-dose aspirin would inhibit platelet thromboxane synthesis, but spare prostacyclin production. Initially, extremely favorable meta-analyses, primarily of small series, led physicians to prescribe low-dose aspirin prophylactically, especially to "high-risk" patients, (e.g., pregnant women with chronic hypertension, renal disease, multiple gestations, and preeclampsia in a previous pregnancy—populations in which the incidence of preeclampsia may approach 20%). This optimism proved premature, as several large randomized, placebo-controlled multicenter trials that included more than 20,000 patients failed to reveal any effects of aspirin on the incidence of preeclampsia. More importantly, aspirin prophylaxis failed to affect a variety of adverse maternal and fetal outcomes.[23, 61]

The second approach—calcium supplementation starting early in gestation—was based on observations that preeclamptics are hypocalciuric and the hypothesis that calciotropic hormones play a role in the pathogenesis of the hypertension. In a manner similar to the aspirin study, initial reports were very encouraging, meta-analyses noting marked and significant reductions in preeclampsia. Again, a carefully conducted, large, blinded, randomized, and placebo-controlled multicenter trial comprising more than 4500 women failed to detect any effects of calcium supplementation on the incidence of preeclampsia.[62]

Are there other promising trials? Enthusiasm for fish oil or its ingredient eicosapentaenoic acid (surrogates for aspirin in their effects on prostaglandin metabolism) appears to have waned. Investigators are now contemplating new trials, again based on plausible hypotheses, including dietary supplementation of L-arginine, antioxidants, and magnesium. Such trials, when designed appropriately, are expensive. Hopefully, resources will focus on basic research designed to determine the cause of the disease first, before funds are committed to further trials that lack firm, statistically based hypotheses.

There are, however, certain populations where "prophylactic" strategies *may* improve outcomes. For instance, patients who have experienced early-onset preeclampsia (before or by gestational week 34) are said to harbor metabolic abnormalities or risk factors associated with vascular thrombosis. Screening such patients may reveal hyperhomocysteinemia, anticardiolipin antibodies, lupus anticoagulants, activated protein C resistance (factor V Leiden), or protein S deficiency.[63] The presence of any of these abnormalities increases the likelihood that a preeclampsia-like syndrome will recur in subsequent gestations and is an indication to consider prophylactic treatment with heparin and/or low-dose aspirin. In addition, women manifesting hyperhomocysteinemia may benefit from high-dose pyridoxine and folate.

MANAGEMENT

Because of its explosive nature, suspicion of preeclampsia is sufficient grounds to recommend hospitalization. There are exceptions in which, under carefully supervised circumstances, a well-informed patient may be managed by resting at home, and in this respect, the utility of home nurse visits, as well as electronic fetal monitoring services, is being evaluated. The aggressive approach, primarily early hospitalization, will diminish the incidence of convulsions, minimize diagnostic error, and improve fetal outcome. Near term, induction of labor is the treatment of choice, but earlier in pregnancy, one may carefully attempt temporization.[64] Delivery is indicated, regardless of gestational age, in the presence of uncontrolled severe hypertension for 24 to 48 hours or the appearance of "ominous signs" (see Table 80–1) or signs suggesting fetal jeopardy.

Controversy: "Aggressive" Versus "Conservative" Management When Preeclampsia Is Remote From Term

Contemporaneous texts stress that preeclampsia remote from term warrants termination of the pregnancy, citing a literature that attests to the low yield of successful fetal outcomes and, more importantly, substantial risk to the mother's well-being. However, several authors have questioned this practice, suggesting an expanded role for "conservative" management of severe disease.[65–69] Review of their reports reveals that the appeal for a conservative approach seems more apparent than real.

One group,[65–68] for instance, temporizes as long as blood pressure can be reasonably controlled and in the absence of ominous signs and symptoms such as headache, blurred vision, epigastric pain, laboratory evidence of coagulation or liver abnormalities, or indications of fetal jeopardy. This is precisely what we (see earlier) as well as others have recommended for decades when suggesting termination for severe disease. Of interest is a trial[65] in which the investigators assigned patients for pregnancy termination or conservative management after labeling their disease as *severe* based on a traditional classification pattern (e.g., level of blood pressure and degree of proteinuria), rather than by evolution of the clinical picture over a defined period of time. The positive results in the "conservative" arm are a cogent demonstration and a reminder that when managing women with hypertension in pregnancy, we treat not the diagnosis, but the evolving disease.

A second group stresses conservative management and makes therapeutic recommendations that we strongly question. Visser and Wallenburg[69] would temporize even when their patients develop early indications of the HELLP syndrome. Scrutiny of these authors' results suggests to us that their studies were inadequately controlled, that fetal loss was substantial even though pregnancies up to gestational week 34 were included, and that there was an increase in the number of maternal bleeding episodes. Such increments in maternal complications appear unacceptably risky to us. It is hoped that clinicians will continue to be vigilant in aggressively terminating gestations complicated by early-onset preeclampsia, using the clinical criteria noted by us previously and by Sibai and coworkers,[65] who paradoxically entitled their criteria *conservative management*. Finally, and of considerable importance, all the studies cited took place in tertiary care centers with maternal-fetal medicine intensive care units, facilities not readily available to most practitioners.

Management of Sudden Escalating Hypertension and of Imminent or Frank Eclampsia

When blood pressure rises rapidly near term or during delivery (usually with the presentation of pure or superim-posed preeclampsia), parenteral therapy may be required. There are debates concerning the level at which to commence therapy: We adhere to the 1999 NHBPEP Working Group recommendations (in press) that diastolic blood pressures above 105 mm Hg should be treated (although some current texts list this figure as 110 mm Hg). Certain circumstances may prompt treatment at lower levels, such as a teenage gravida whose recent diastolic pressures were 70 mm Hg or a patient demonstrating cerebral signs, such as an excruciating headache, confusion, or somnolence.[70]

There has been an acrimonious debate about the prevention and management of eclamptic convulsions. American obstetricians traditionally considered parenteral magnesium sulfate the drug of choice for both its preventative and its therapeutic value, whereas neurologists and many internists condemned the efficacy of this approach and, along with European consultants, prescribed diazepam or phenytoin. There were even some who questioned whether any therapy other than blood pressure control alone was necessary for prophylaxis.[48, 71] Two articles published in 1995 appear to have resolved these controversies. In a randomized trial of 1680 preeclamptic women, intravenous magnesium sulfate proved superior to both diazepam and phenytoin in preventing recurrent seizures.[72] A second study, scheduled to evaluate 4500 patients and compare magnesium sulfate with phenytoin as prophylaxis, had to be halted after only 2123 women had been randomized when it appeared that seizures were occurring only in the phenytoin arm.[73]

In summary, magnesium sulfate is the drug of choice once a convulsion appears, and it is superior to phenytoin in preventing preeclampsia. Neither trial answered the question of whether prophylactic therapy is necessary and whether blood pressure control alone will prevent preeclampsia. However, in the preventive trial, blood pressure was controlled similarly in each arm, but only the women receiving phenytoin convulsed. This suggests that phenytoin, the quintessential anticonvulsant, is a central nervous system irritant in preeclamptic women. Thus, parenteral magnesium sulfate is indicated both to treat and to prevent eclampsia.

CHRONIC HYPERTENSION[27]

Most pregnant women with chronic hypertension have the "essential" variety, often mild in nature and of recent origin. Over 85% of their gestations are uncomplicated, outcomes approaching or only slightly poorer than those of normotensive populations. A minority, however, manifest increased morbidity, which includes abruption, acute renal failure, cardiac decompensation, and cerebral accidents in the mother and growth retardation in the fetus. Most of these adverse outcomes are associated with the simultaneous presence of superimposed preeclampsia. Much of the morbidity occurs in gravidas over 30 years of age with poorly controlled blood pressure, sometimes of several years' duration, especially when there is evidence of target organ damage. Extremely obese women with chronic hypertension are also at special risk for cardiac decompensation near term, especially if volume overloading occurs in labor. Such patients warrant an echocardiac examination

Table 80–3 Drug Therapy for Acute and Severe Hypertension in Pregnancy*

Drug (FDA Category)†	Dose and Route	Onset of Action	Adverse Effects‡	Comments
Hydralazine (C)	5 mg IV or IM, then 5–10 mg every 20–40 min; or constant infusion of 0.5–10 mg/hr	IV: 10 min IM: 10–30 min	Headache, flushing, tachycardia, and possibly arrythmias, nausea, vomiting[86]	Drug of choice according to NHBPEP Working Group;[24] broad experience of safety and efficacy
Labetalol (C)	20 mg IV, then 20–80 mg every 20–30 min, up to 300 mg; or constant infusion of 1–2 mg/min to desired effect, then stop or reduce to 0.5 mg/min	5–10 min	Flushing, nausea, vomiting, tingling of scalp; older literature noted retroplacental bleeding	Experience in pregnancy considerably less than that of hydralazine
Nifedipine (C)	5–10 mg PO; repeat in 30 min if necessary, then 10–20 mg PO every 3–6 hr	10–15 min	Flushing, headache, tachycardia, nausea, inhibition of labor	May have synergistic interaction with magnesium sulfate; experience in pregnancy limited
Diazoxide (C)	30–50 mg IV every 5–15 min	2–5 min	Inhibition of labor; hyperglycemia, fluid retention with repeated doses; rarely used in 1990s	Doses of 150–300 mg may cause severe hypotension; may displace phenytoin from serum protein-binding sites
RELATIVELY CONTRAINDICATED Sodium nitroprusside (C)§	0.5–10 µg/kg/min by constant IV infusion	Instantaneous	Cyanide toxicity, nausea, vomiting	Use only in critical care unit at low doses for briefest time feasible; may cause fetal cyanide toxicity

Modified from Barron WM. Hypertension. *In* Barron WM, Lindheimer MD (eds). Medical Disorders During Pregnancy, 2nd ed. St. Louis, Mosby–Year Book, 1995.
Abbreviations: FDA, U.S. Food and Drug Administration; IV, intravenously; IM, intramuscularly; NHBPEP, National High Blood Pressure Education Program; PO, orally.
*Indicated for acute elevation of Korotkoff phase V blood pressure > 105 mm Hg; goal is gradual reduction to 90–100 mm Hg.
†For details on the FDA classification, see Table 80–5.
‡All agents may cause marked hypotension, especially in severe preeclampsia.
§We classify sodium nitroprusside in category D.

Table 80–4 Drug Therapy for Chronic Hypertension in Pregnancy*†

Drug (FDA Category)‡	Daily Dose	Adverse Effects and Comments
AGENT OF CHOICE Methyldopa (C)	500–300 mg preferably in 2 divided doses	Drug of choice according to the NHBPEP Working Group;[24] safety for mother and fetus (after 1st trimester) is well documented; good 7-year follow-up of neonates
SECOND-LINE AGENTS Hydralazine (C)	50–300 mg in 2–4 divided doses	Few controlled trials but extensive experience and few serious adverse effects documented; may cause neonatal thrombocytopenia
Labetalol (C)	200–1200 mg in 2–3 divided doses	Less experience than with methyldopa; efficacy and short-term safety appear equal to methyldopa
β-Adrenergic inhibitors (C)	Depends on specific agent used	May cause fetal bradycardia and impair fetal responses to hypoxia; risk of intrauterine growth retardation when begun in 1st or 2nd trimester[94]
Nifedipine (C)	30–120 mg of a slow-release preparation	Limited data; may inhibit labor; may have synergistic action with magnesium sulfate
Clonidine (C)	0.1–0.8 mg in 2 divided doses	Limited data
Prazosin (C)	1–30 mg in 2–3 divided doses	Very limited data
Thiazide diuretics (C by manufacturer, D assignation in reference 124)	Depends on agent used	Majority of controlled studies in normotensive pregnant women; few data in hypertensive gestation; can cause volume depletion, electrolyte imbalance, pancreatitis, and thrombocytopenia
CONTRAINDICATED ACE inhibitors (D)§	Depends on agent used	High rates of fetal loss in animals; in humans, *associated with oligohydramnios, fetopathy, intrauterine growth retardation, neonatal anuric renal failure in human pregnancies, occasionally fatal;* thus, use only when absolutely necessary to preserve maternal well-being and when other agents are unsuccessful

Modified from Barron WM. Hypertension. *In* Barron WM, Lindheimer MD (eds). Medical Disorders During Pregnancy, 2nd ed. St. Louis, Mosby–Year Book, 1995.
Abbreviations: FDA, U.S. Food and Drug Administration; NHBPEP, National High Blood Pressure Education Program; ACE, angiotensin-converting enzyme.
*Note that safety during the first trimester has not been established for any antihypertensive agent.
†Drug therapy indicated for uncomplicated chronic hypertension when phase V diastolic blood pressure ≥ 100 mm Hg. Treatment at lower levels may be indicated for patients with renal disease or diabetes mellitus.
‡For details on the FDA classification, see Table 80–5.
§We classify ACE inhibitors and angiotensin receptor blocking agents in category X.

during pregnancy to help evaluate ventricular compliance and performance.

The approach to treatment of chronic hypertension presented here follows the recommendations of the NHBPEP Working Group on Hypertension in Pregnancy, which have been incorporated into the fifth and sixth reports of the Joint National Committee for the Prevention, Detection, Evaluation, and Treatment of Hypertension.[74, 75] These recommendations are summarized in Table 80–3, and a review of antihypertensive medications prescribed for gravidas follows in the final section. One should be aware, however, that there have been few, if any, large randomized multicenter trials of the safety and efficacy of antihypertensive medications in pregnant women. Currently, antihypertensive treatment is indicated when diastolic blood pressure levels are 100 mm Hg or higher, or lower if other risk factors are present. Treatment of mild hypertension during pregnancy, advocated by some, is not recommended by us (see later), but we stress the need for further studies of this important question. Finally, an update of the NHBPEP report, scheduled to appear in 1999, should be compared with the previous documents and the recommendations noted here.

ANTIHYPERTENSIVE DRUG THERAPY IN PREGNANCY

When contemplating antihypertensive drug therapy in pregnancy, one must consider the following: There have been few, if any, large multicenter randomized trials conducted with the sophistication currently required by regulating agencies. Most studies have been limited in scope, often performed at the request of and with the support of industry. The vast majority of published data reflect studies in which therapy was started after midgestation, when virtually all of the risks of provoking congenital malformations have passed. Also, there are no rigorous animal testing requirements that must be met before trials in pregnant women are commenced, including standardized means of evaluating drug effects on the ability of the fetus to withstand hypoxic stress, as well as a more complete analysis of morphological and physiological variables in the newborn of these animal models. The latter issue is highlighted by reports that demonstrate that administration of aminoglycosides to pregnant rats has harmful tubular and glomerular effects on the fetal kidney, demonstrable only by sophisticated functional, histological, and biochemical evaluations.[76]

With the previous discussion in mind, we review the status of antihypertensive drug therapy in pregnancy in 1998. Table 80–4 summarizes current views on the major antihypertensive medications prescribed to pregnant women, and Table 80–5 explains the risk classification defined by the U.S. Food and Drug Administration (FDA), which is usually published in the *Physician's Desk Reference* (PDR). Very few drugs are listed as category A, highlighting the paucity of information in the field. Physicians tend to overutilize drugs listed in category C, interpreting this classification as evidence of safety. The danger of such an approach is exemplified by the history of the prescription of angiotensin-converting enzyme (ACE) in-

---

Table 80–5 U.S. Food and Drug Administration Classification of Risk in Pregnancy*

CATEGORY A
Controlled studies in women fail to demonstrate a risk to the fetus in the first trimester, and there is no evidence of a risk in later trimesters. The possibility of fetal harm appears remote.

CATEGORY B
Either animal reproduction studies have not demonstrated a fetal risk but no controlled studies have been performed in pregnant women, or animal-reproduction studies have shown an adverse effect (other than a decrease in fertility) that was not confirmed in controlled studies in women in the first trimester. There is no evidence of a risk in later trimesters.

CATEGORY C
Either studies in animals have revealed adverse effect on the fetus (teratogenic or embryocidal effects or other) and there are no controlled studies in women, or studies in women and animals are not available. Drugs should be given only if the potential benefit justifies the potential risk to the fetus.

CATEGORY D
There is positive evidence of human fetal risk, but the benefits of use in pregnant women may be acceptable despite the risk (e.g., if the drug is needed in a life-threatening situation or for a serious disease for which safer drugs cannot be used or are ineffective). There is an appropriate statement in the "warnings" section of the labeling.

CATEGORY X
Studies in animals or humans have demonstrated fetal abnormalities, or there is evidence of fetal risk based on human experience, or both, and the risk of the use of the drug in pregnant women clearly outweighs any possible benefit. The drug is contraindicated in women who are or may become pregnant. There is an appropriate statement in the "contraindications" section of the labeling.

*Plans have been made to modify this classification.

---

hibitors for pregnant women. Both captopril and enalapril were originally listed as category C in the PDR. Although reports of problems in animal models were cited in the early 1980s, these drugs remained as category C until 1992. By then, mounting evidence that ACE inhibitors were associated with renal failure and death in the neonate resulted in the manufacturers being required to cite a "black box" label warning and a change to category D in the PDR. (We had considered these drugs as X since 1985, and still do.[77]) Thus, we reiterate that drugs in FDA category C are not to be considered "safe." Rather, such a classification should be interpreted as a warning that unknown adverse fetal effects may be present. Finally, the FDA, aware of the inadequacies of its current classification schema, is contemplating new guidelines for 1999.

Central Adrenergic Inhibitors

Methyldopa is the drug of choice for initial therapy of hypertension during gestation. This view takes into account its long history of effective use in gravidas, as well as its having been prospectively evaluated in several randomized trials, one of which included periodic evaluation of the offspring for 7.5 years.[78–82] Hypertension experts frequently criticize obstetricians for using this drug, suggesting that methyldopa is less effective and more poorly tolerated than a host of newer medications, many of which can be prescribed once daily. However, all studies comparing this drug with others have failed to establish such superiority, and a well-documented side effect profile indicates that maternal side effects are generally mild and well tolerated.

Clonidine, another α-agonist, has been prescribed to pregnant women,[83, 84] but total experience with it is much less than with methyldopa. In one randomized trial, efficacy and safety of the two medications were said to be similar.[83] Another limited study in hospitalized patients found that clonidine, alone or in combination with a placebo or hydralazine, reduced the incidence of premature delivery.[84] Clonidine should be avoided in early gestation because it is suspected of causing embryopathy. In one small neonate follow-up study (22 patients), more sleep disturbances were noted in the clonidine group.[85]

Vasodilators

Parenteral hydralazine is the drug of choice to treat bouts of sudden severe hypertension in pregnancy. For management of chronic hypertension, however, its use is primarily as a second-line agent in conjunction with methyldopa or β-adrenergic blocking drugs (although some now use labetalol or calcium channel blockers in this role; see later). There are limited data on the use of hydralazine as monotherapy, although in one small study in which the drug was used alone, there were increased frequencies of palpitations, dizziness, and headache.[86]

β-Adrenergic Receptor Blockers

The safety of β-blocking agents in pregnant women and their therapeutic indications in these patients remain unclear, despite an extensive literature on the subject.[87–97] This is due to the heterogeneous nature of many of these studies and the fact that in many of them, drug was started late in gestation, making it hard to evaluate several concerns regarding its use, especially whether it causes fetal growth retardation. The major concern about β-adrenergic blocking agents in pregnancy relates to the fetus. Some worry that these drugs may alter the cardiovascular responses to hypoxia and cause bradycardia, respiratory depression, hypoglycemia, and growth retardation. Most of these concerns arose from animal studies and anecdotal reports from humans, and only growth retardation seems to have been documented adequately.[94] Most of the larger studies in humans have failed to detect adverse fetal effects.[88, 89, 91, 98–100] Nevertheless, these drugs are not preferred for long-term therapy of hypertension in pregnancy, unless methyldopa and hydralazine therapy (and even labetalol) have failed to control the blood pressure or cannot be administered for some other reason.

Combined α- and β-Adrenergic Receptor Blockers

Labetalol is the preparation in this class most commonly prescribed for pregnant women. The parenteral form is used to treat severe hypertension, some believing it controls pressure more efficiently and causes fewer side effects, including headaches, flushing, and cardiac arrhythmias, than parenteral hydralazine.[97–101] Other studies find the two drugs similar, and hydralazine remains the drug of choice, following the dictum that the medication with the longest uneventful history in pregnancy should prove the safest.

Data concerning the use of labetalol in chronic hypertension in pregnancy, limited to a few, albeit well-designed, randomized trials, have failed to establish any superiority of this drug over methyldopa.[102–104] Thorough follow-up studies of the infant are yet to appear. This drug may be explosively hepatotoxic in nonpregnant patients, and during pregnancy the liver may be more vulnerable. Thus, labetalol is currently recommended as a second-line agent.

α-Adrenergic Blockers

Data relating to the use of these drugs (primarily prazosin) in pregnancy are purely anecdotal and uncontrolled, and they should not be prescribed.[105–107] The single exceptions are the rare cases of pheochromocytoma, in which both prazosin and phenoxybenzamine have been used successfully.

Calcium Channel Blockers

These drugs have been used to treat both acute and chronic hypertension in pregnancy. Most studies are limited or anecdotal, and there is concern that when used to treat severe hypertension, the oral short-acting agent may provoke precipitous decreases in blood pressure. This is especially true when magnesium sulfate is infused, as the latter agent interferes with calcium-dependent excitation-contraction coupling. It is in this setting in which case reports of severe hypotension and neuromuscular blockade have appeared.[108, 109] Thus, calcium channel blockers are best avoided in the treatment of rapidly rising blood pressure late in gestation.

Data relating to calcium channel blockers and chronic hypertension in pregnancy are also limited.[97, 110–113] We hesitate to recommend these drugs, given the high incidence of superimposed preeclampsia in this population, which may result in the need to precipitously start magnesium sulfate in a patient receiving long-acting calcium channel blocking agents.[108, 109] Finally, one calcium channel blocker, nimodipine, utilized by neurologists when treating patients with cerebral bleeding, is under study as a therapeutic agent in women with eclampsia.[114]

Angiotensin-Converting Enzyme Inhibitors and Angiotensin II Receptor Antagonists

ACE inhibitors were discussed previously as an example of why drugs originally listed as FDA class C should be viewed with caution. These drugs have now been linked to fetopathy, and ACE inhibitors are associated with oliguria-anuria and fetal and neonatal death.[115–121] Since 1992, ACE inhibitors have been classified as category D (and here as X) with a warning on the label. The recommended approach to the newer angiotensin II receptor antagonists is similar. This is a prudent precaution, for there are few data relevant to use of this new drug class in pregnancy.

Diuretics

These drugs were once extensively prescribed "prophylactically" to prevent preeclampsia.[60] However, there are few data regarding use of these agents in pregnant women with hypertension. In one small study, diuretics prevented most of the physiological volume expansion associated with normal pregnancy.[122] Suboptimal plasma volume expansion in women with chronic hypertension has been associated with impaired fetal growth, but the data are far from persuasive.[11, 123]

Another problem with the use of diuretics is hyperuricemia, which may lead to a mistaken diagnosis of superimposed preeclampsia. Nevertheless, the NHBPEP Working Group, recognizing the role of diuretics in populations with "salt-sensitive" blood pressure, especially those who develop rapid refractoriness to vasodilator therapy alone, noted that diuretics could be continued during gestation if prescribed before conception. However, they discouraged the use of these agents in preeclampsia. Thiazide diuretics are the agents that seem to have the safest record in pregnancy.[60] The more potent "loop" diuretics should be avoided, and furosemide is embryotoxic.

Breast Feeding

Data are scarce, and this is unfortunate as many antihypertensive drugs can be detected in breast milk, sometimes in sufficient quantity to affect neonatal blood pressure. The reader is referred to the monograph by Briggs and colleagues,[124] recommendations of the Committee on Drugs of the American Academy of Pediatrics, and brief reviews by White[125] and Dillon and associates.[126] Many β-blocking agents concentrate in breast milk in quantities sufficient to cause symptoms in the neonate, but propranolol seems to be an exception.[127, 128] On the other hand, the concentrations of ACE inhibitors, calcium channel blockers, and diuretics are low, and mothers ingesting these agents can breast-feed without concern.

References

1. MacGillivray I, Rose GA, Rowe B. Blood pressure survey in pregnancy. Clin Sci 37:395–407, 1969.
2. Friedman EA, Neff RK. Pregnancy and Hypertension. A Systematic Evaluation of Clinical Diagnostic Criteria. Littleton, MA, PSG Publishing, 1977.
3. Page EW, Christianson R. The impact of mean arterial pressure in the middle trimester upon the outcome of pregnancy. Am J Obstet Gynecol 125:740–746, 1976.
4. Wilson M, Morganti AA, Zervoudakis I, et al. Blood pressure, the renin-aldosterone system and sex steroids throughout normal pregnancy. Am J Med 68:97–104, 1980.
5. Capeless EL, Clapp JF. Cardiovascular changes in early phase of pregnancy. Am J Obstet Gynecol 161:1449–1453, 1989.
6. Chapman AB, Zamudio S, Woodmansee W, et al. Systemic and renal hemodynamic changes in the luteal phase of the menstrual cycle mimic early pregnancy. Am J Physiol 273:F777–F782, 1997.
7. Walters BN, Thompson ME, Lee A, de Swiet M. Blood pressure in the puerperium. Clin Sci 71:589–594, 1986.
8. Robson SC, Hunter S, Boys RJ, Dunlop W. Serial study of factors influencing changes in cardiac output during human pregnancy. Am J Physiol 256:H1060–1065, 1989.
9. Poppas A, Shroff SG, Korcarz CE, et al. Serial assessment of the cardiovascular system in normal pregnancy. Circulation 95:2407–2415, 1997.
10. Lindheimer MD, Roberts J, Cunningham FGC (eds). Chesley's Hypertensive Disorders in Pregnancy, 2nd ed. Stamford, CT, Appleton & Lange, 1999.
11. Lindheimer MD, Katz AI. Renal physiology and disease in pregnancy. In Seldin DW, Giebisch G (eds). The Kidney: Physiology and Pathophysiology, 3rd ed. New York, Raven, 1999.
12. August P, Lindheimer MD. Pathophysiology of preeclampsia. In Laragh JH, Brenner BM (eds). Hypertension: Pathophysiology, Diagnosis, and Management, 2nd ed. New York, Raven, 1995; pp 2407–2426.
13. Fitzgerald DJ, Fitzgerald GA. Eicosanoids in the pathogenesis of preeclampsia. In Laragh J, Brenner BM (eds). Hypertension: Pathophysiology and Management. New York, Raven, 1990; pp 1789–1804.
14. McGiff JG, Carrol MA. Magnesium, platelets and the vasculature in preeclampsia-eclampsia. Hypertens Pregnancy 13:217–226, 1994.
15. Sladek SM, Magness RR, Conrad KP. Nitric oxide and pregnancy. Am J Physiol 272:R441–R463, 1997.
16. Johenning AR, Barron WM. Indirect blood pressure measurement in pregnancy: Kortokoff phase 4 vs phase 5. Am J Obstet Gynecol 167:573–580, 1992.
17. Blank SG, Helseth G, Pickering TG, et al. How should diastolic blood pressure be defined during pregnancy? Hypertension 24:234–240, 1994.
18. Shennan A, Gupta M, Halligan A, et al. Lack of reproducibility in pregnancy of Korotkoff phase 4 as measured by mercury sphygmomanometry. Lancet 347:139–142, 1996.
19. de Swiet M, Shennan A. Blood pressure measurement in pregnancy. Br J Obstet Gynaecol 103:862–863, 1996.
20. Halligan A, Shennan A, Thurston H, et al. Ambulatory blood pressure measurement in pregnancy: The current state of the art. Hypertens Pregnancy 14:1–16, 1995.
21. Penny JA, Halligan AW, Shennan AH, et al. Automated, ambulatory, or conventional blood pressure measurement in pregnancy: Which is the better predictor of severe hypertension? Am J Obstet Gynecol 178:521–526, 1998.
22. Hermida RC, Ayala DE. Diagnosing gestational hypertension and preeclampsia with the 24-hour mean of blood pressure. Hypertension 30:1531–1537, 1997.
23. Lindheimer MD, Katz AI. The normal and diseased kidney in pregnancy. In Schrier RW, Gottshalk CW (eds). Diseases of the Kidney, 6th ed. Boston, Little, Brown, 1977; pp 2063–2097.
24. National High Blood Pressure Education Program Working Group: Report on high blood pressure in pregnancy. Am J Obstet Gynecol 163:1689–1712, 1990.
25. Lindheimer MD. Preeclampsia-eclampsia 1996: Preventable? Have disputes on its treatment been resolved? Curr Opin Nephrol Hypertens 5:452–458, 1996.
26. Chesley LC. Hypertensive Disorders in Pregnancy. New York, Appleton-Century-Crofts, 1978.
27. August P, Lindheimer MD. Chronic hypertension and pregnancy. In Lindheimer MD, Roberts J, Cunningham FGC (eds). Chesley's Hypertensive Disorders in Pregnancy. Stamford, CT, Appleton & Lange, 1999.
28. Sibai BH, Lindheimer MD, Hauth J, et al. Risk factors for preeclampsia, abruptio placenta, and adverse neonatal outcomes in women with chronic hypertension. N Engl J Med 339:667–671, 1998.
29. Molitch ME. Pituitary, thyroid, adrenal, and parathyroid disorders. In Barron WM, Lindheimer MD (eds). Medical Disorders During Pregnancy, 2nd ed. St. Louis, Mosby–Year Book 1995; pp 89–127.
30. Lyons CW, Colmorgen GH. Medical management of pheochromocytoma in pregnancy. Obstet Gynecol 72:450–451, 1988.
31. Greenberg M, Moawad AH, Weties BM, et al. Extraadrenal pheochromocytoma: Detection during pregnancy using MR imaging. Radiology 161:475–476, 1986.

32. Easterling TR, Brateng D, Goldman ML, et al. Renal vascular hypertension during pregnancy. Obstet Gynecol 78:921–925, 1991.

33. Diego J, Guerra J, Pham C, Epstein M. Management of renovascular hypertension complicating pregnancy. [Abstract] J Am Soc Nephrol 7:1549, 1996.

34. Lindheimer MD, Richardson DA, Ehrlich EM, Katz AI. Potassium hemostasis in pregnancy. J Reprod Med 32:517–522, 1987.

35. Sibai BM. Eclampsia. *In* Rubin PC (ed). Hypertension in Pregnancy. Vol 10 of Birkenhäger WH, Reid JL (eds). Handbook of Hypertension. New York, Elsevier Science, 1988; pp 320–340.

36. Sibai BM, Justermann L, Velasco J. Current understanding of severe pre-eclampsia, pregnancy-associated haemolytic uremic syndrome, thrombotic thrombocytopenic purpura, haemolysis, elevated liver enzymes and low platelet syndrome, and postpartum acute renal failure: Different clinical syndromes or just different names? Curr Opin Nephrol Hypertens 3:436–445, 1994.

37. Brown MA, Buddle ML. What's in a name? Problems with the classification of hypertension in pregnancy. J Hypertens 15:1049–1054, 1997.

38. Fisher KA, Luger A, Spargo BH, Lindheimer MD. Hypertension in pregnancy: Clinical-pathological correlations and remote prognosis. Medicine 60:267–276, 1981.

39. Conrad KP, Benyo DF. Placental cytokines and pathogenesis of preeclampsia. Am J Reprod Immunol 37:240–249, 1997.

40. Ness RB, Roberts JM. Heterogenous causes constituting the single syndrome of preeclampsia. A hypothesis and its implications. Am J Obstet Gynecol 175:1365–1370, 1996.

41. Lafayette RA, Druzin M, Sibley R, et al. Nature of glomerular dysfunction in pre-eclampsia. (See also accompanying editorial by A. Chapman). Kidney Int 54:1240–1249, 1998.

42. Conrad K, Lindheimer MD. Renal and cardiovascular alterations. *In* Lindheimer MD, Roberts J, Cunningham FGC (eds). Chesley's Hypertensive Disorders in Pregnancy. Stamford, CT, Appleton & Lange, 1999.

43. Lindheimer MD, Katz AI. Renal Function and Disease in Pregnancy. Philadelphia, Lea & Febiger, 1977.

44. Sibai BM, McCubbin JH, Anderson GD, et al. Eclampsia: Observations from 67 recent cases. Obstet Gynecol 58:609–613, 1981.

45. Øian P, Maltau JM, Noddeland H, Fadnes HO. Transcapillary fluid balance in pre-eclampsia. Br J Obstet Gynaecol 93:235–239, 1986.

46. Schobel HP, Fischer T, Heuszer K, et al. Preeclampsia—A state of sympathetic overactivity. N Engl J Med 335:1480–1485, 1996.

47. Mckay DG, Merrill SJ, Weiner AE, et al. The pathologic anatomy of eclampsia, bilateral renal cortical necrosis, pituitary necrosis, and other acute fatal complications of pregnancy, and its possible relationship to the generalized Shwartzman phenomenon. Am J Obstet Gynecol 66:507–539, 1953.

48. Donaldson JO. Neurology of Pregnancy, 2nd ed. London, WB Saunders, 1989.

49. van den Veyver IB, Belfort MA, Rowe TF, Moise KJ. Cerebral vasospasm in eclampsia: Transcranial Doppler ultrasound findings. J Matern Fetal Med 3:9–13, 1994.

50. Williams K, Wilson S. Eclampsia occurs with a significant fall in cerebrovascular resistance. [Abstract] Am J Obstet Gynecol 178:S6, 1998.

51. Belfort M, Whiman I, Grunewald C, et al. Preeclamptic women with headache are much more likely to have abnormal cerebral perfusion than those without. Am J Obstet Gynecol 178:S3, 1998.

52. Sheehan H, Lynch JB. Pathology of Toxemia of Pregnancy, London, Churchill, 1973.

53. Cunningham FG, Macdonald PC, Gant NF, et al. Williams Obstetrics, 19th ed. Norwalk, CT, Appleton & Lange, 1993; pp 782–783.

54. Robertson WB, Brosens I, Dixon G. Maternal uterine vascular lesions in the hypertensive complications of pregnancy. *In* Lindheimer MD, Katz AI, Zuspan FP (eds). Hypertension in Pregnancy. New York, John Wiley & Sons, 1976; pp 115–129.

55. Fox H. The placenta in pregnancy hypertension. *In* Rubin PC (ed). Hypertension in Pregnancy. Vol 10 of Birkenhäger WH, Reid JL (eds). Handbook of Hypertension. New York, Elsevier Science, 1988; pp 16–37.

56. Khong TY, De Wolf F, Robertson WB, Brosens I. Inadequate maternal vascular response to placentation in pregnancies complicated by preeclampsia and by small for gestational age infants. Br J Obstet Gynaecol 93:1049–1059, 1986.

57. Pijnenborg R, Anthony J, Davey DA, et al. Placental bed spiral arteries in the hypertensive disorders of pregnancy. Br J Obstet Gynaecol 98:648–655, 1991.

58. Zhou Y, Damsky CH, Chiu K, et al. Preeclampsia is associated with abnormal expression of adhesion molecules by invasive cytotrophoblasts. J Clin Invest 91:950–960, 1993.

59. Zhou Y, Damsky CH, Fisher SJ. Preeclampsia is associated with failure of human cytotrophoblasts to mimic a vascular adhesion phenotype. One cause of defective endovascular invasion in this syndrome. J Clin Invest 99:2152–2164, 1997.

60. Collins R, Yusuf S, Peto R. Overview of randomised trials of diuretics in pregnancy. BMJ 290:17–23, 1985.

61. Caritis S, Sibai B, Hauth J, et al. Low dose aspirin to prevent preeclampsia in women at high risk. N Engl J Med 338:701–705, 1998.

62. Levine RJ, Hauth JC, Curet LB, et al. Trial of calcium for prevention of preeclampsia. N Engl J Med 337:69–76, 1997.

63. Kuperfermine MS, Eldor A, Steinman N, et al. Increased frequency of genetic thrombophilia in women with complications of pregnancy. N Engl J Med 340:9–13, 1999. (See also editorial by BH Sibai.)

64. Sibai BM, Akl S, Fairlie F, et al. A protocol for managing severe preeclampsia in the second trimester. Am J Obstet Gynecol 163:733–738, 1994.

65. Sibai BM, Mercer BM, Schiff E, Friedman SA. Aggressive versus expectant management of severe preeclampsia at 28–32 weeks gestation: A randomized controlled trial. Am J Obstet Gynecol 171:818–822, 1994.

66. Schiff E, Friedman SA, Sibai BM. Conservative management of severe preeclampsia remote from term. Obstet Gynecol 84:626–630, 1994.

67. Visser W, van Pampus MG, Treffers PE, Wallenburg HCS. Perinatal results of hemodynamic and conservative temporizing treatment in severe preeclampsia. Eur J Obstet Gynecol Reprod Biol 53:175–181, 1994.

68. Chari RS, Friedman SA, O'Brien JM, Sibai BM. Daily antenatal testing in women with severe preeclampsia. Am J Obstet Gynecol 173:1207–1210, 1995.

69. Visser W, Wallenburg HC. Temporarizing management of severe preeclampsia with and without the HELLP syndrome. Br J Obstet Gynaecol 102:111–117, 1995.

70. Hinchey J, Chaves C, Appignani B, et al. A reversible posterior leukoencephalopathy syndrome. N Engl J Med 334:494–500, 1996.

71. Chua S, Redman CW. Are prophylactic anticonvulsants required in severe preeclampsia? Lancet 337:250–251, 1991.

72. The Collaborative Eclampsia Group. Which anticonvulsant for women with eclampsia? Evidence from the Collaborative Eclampsia Trial. Lancet 345:1455–1463, 1995.

73. Lucas MJ, Leveno KJ, Cunningham FG. A comparison of magnesium sulfate with phenytoin for the prevention of eclampsia. N Engl J Med 333:201–205, 1995.

74. Joint National Committee on Detection, Evaluation, and Treatment of High Blood Pressure. The fifth report. Arch Intern Med 153:154–183, 1993.

75. Joint National Committee on Prevention, Detection, Evaluation, and Treatment of High Blood Pressure. The sixth report. Arch Intern Med 157:2413–2446, 1997.

76. Mallie JP, Coulon G, Billery C, et al. In utero aminoglycoside-induced nephrotoxicity in rat neonates. Kidney Int 33:36–44, 1988.

77. Lindheimer MD, Katz AI. Hypertension in pregnancy. N Engl J Med 313:675–680, 1985.

78. Redman CW. Fetal outcome in trial of antihypertensive treatment in pregnancy. Lancet 2:753–756, 1976.

79. Plouin PF, Breart G, Llado J, et al. A randomized comparison of early with conservative use of antihypertensive drugs in the management of pregnancy induced hypertension. Br J Obstet Gynaecol 97:134–141, 1990.

80. Kyle PM, Redman CW. Comparative risk-benefit assessment of drugs used in the management of hypertension in pregnancy. Drug Saf 7:223–234, 1992.

81. Leather HM, Baker P, Humphreys DM, Chadd MA. A controlled trial of hypotensive agents in hypertension in pregnancy. Lancet 2:488–490, 1968.

82. Cockburn J, Moar VA, Ounsted M, Redman CW. Final report of study on hypertension during pregnancy. The effects of specific treatment on the growth and development of the children. Lancet 1:647–649, 1982.

83. Horvath JS, Phippard A, Korda A, et al. Clonidine hydrochloride—A safe and effective antihypertensive agent in pregnancy. Obstet Gynecol 66:634–638, 1985.

84. Phippard AF, Fischer WE, Horvath JS, et al. Early blood pressure control improves pregnancy outcome in primigravid women with mild hypertension. Med J Aust 154:378–382, 1991.

85. Huisje HJ, Hadders-Algra M, Touwen BCL. Is clonidine a behavioral teratogen in the human? Early Hum Dev 14:43–48, 1986.

86. Rosenfeld J, Bott-Kanner G, Boner G, et al. Treatment of hypertension during pregnancy with hydralazine monotherapy or with combined therapy with hydralazine and pindolol. Eur J Obstet Gynecol Reprod Biol 22:197–204, 1986.

87. Fidler J, Smith V, Fayers P, de Swiet M. Randomised controlled comparative study of methyldopa and oxprenolol in treatment of hypertension in pregnancy. BMJ 286:1927–1930, 1983.

88. Rubin PC, Butters L, Clark DM, et al. Placebo-controlled trial of atenolol in treatment of pregnancy-associated hypertension. Lancet 1:431–434, 1983.

89. Bott-Kanner G, Hirsch M, Friedman S, et al. Antihypertensive therapy in the management of hypertension in pregnancy—A clinical double blind study of pindolol. Clin Exp Hypertens [B] 11:207–220, 1992.

90. Reynolds B, Butters L, Evans J, et al. First year of life after the use of atenolol in pregnancy associated hypertension. Arch Dis Child 59:1061–1063, 1984.

91. Pruyn SC, Phelan JP, Buchanan GC. Long-term propranolol therapy in pregnancy: Maternal and fetal outcome. Am J Obstet Gynecol 135:485–489, 1979.

92. Wichman K, Ryden G, Karlberg B. A placebo controlled trial of metoprolol in the treatment of hypertension in pregnancy. Scand J Clin Lab Invest 169:90–95, 1984.

93. Gallery EDM, Saunders DM, Hunyor SN, Gyory AZ. Randomised comparison of methyldopa and oxprenolol for treatment of hypertension in pregnancy. BMJ 1:1591–1594, 1979.

94. Butters L, Kennedy S, Rubin PC. Atenolol in essential hypertension during pregnancy. BMJ 301:587–589, 1990.

95. Montan S, Ingemarsson I, Marsal K, Stoberg NO. Randomised controlled trial of atenolol and pindolol in human pregnancy: Effects on fetal hemodynamics. BMJ 304:946–949, 1992.

96. Marlettini MG, Crippa S, Morselli-Labate AM, et al. Randomised comparison of calcium antagonists and beta-blockers in the treatment of pregnancy induced hypertension. Curr Ther Res 48:684–694, 1990.

97. Sibai BM. Treatment of hypertension in pregnant women. N Engl J Med 335:257–265, 1996.

98. Hogstedt S, Lindeberg S, Axelsson O, et al. A prospective controlled trial of metaprolol-hydralazine treatment in hypertension during pregnancy. Acta Obstet Gynecol Scand 64:505–510, 1985.

99. Rubin PC, Butters L, Clark D, et al. Obstetric aspects of the use in pregnancy-associated hypertension of the beta-adrenoreceptor antagonist atenolol. Am J Obstet Gynecol 150:389–392, 1984.

100. Wichman K. Metaprolol in the treatment of mild to moderate hypertension in pregnancy—Effects on fetal heart activity. Clin Exp Hypertens Pregnancy B5:195–202, 1986.

101. Bhorat IE, Naidoo DP, Rout CC, Moodley J. Malignant ventricular arrhythmias in eclampsia: A comparison of labetalol with hydralazine. Am J Obstet Gynecol 168:1292–1296, 1993.

102. Michael CA, Potter JM. A comparison of labetalol with other antihypertensive drugs in the treatment of hypertensive disease of pregnancy. In Riley A, Symonds EM (eds). The Investigation of Labetalol in the Management of Hypertension in Pregnancy. Amsterdam, Excerpta Medica, 1982; pp 101–110.

103. Plouin PF, Breart G, Maillard F, et al. Comparison of antihypertensive efficacy and perinatal safety of labetalol and methyldopa in the treatment of hypertension in pregnancy: A randomized controlled trial. Br J Obstet Gynaecol 95:868–876, 1988.

104. Sibai BM, Mabie WC, Shamsa F, et al. A comparison of no medica-

105. Lubbe WF, Hodge JV. Combined alpha- and beta-adrenoreceptor antagonism with prazosin and oxprenolol in control of severe hypertension in pregnancy. N Z Med J; 94:169–172, 1981.

106. Rubin PC, Butters L, Low RA, Reid JL. Clinical pharmacological studies with prazosin during pregnancy complicated by hypertension. Br J Clin Pharmacol 16:543–547, 1983.

107. Dommisse J, Davey DA, Roos PJ. Prazosin and oxprenolol therapy in pregnancy hypertension. S Afr Med J 64:231–233, 1983.

108. Snyder SW, Cardwell MS. Neuromuscular blockade with magnesium sulphate and nifedipine. Am J Obstet Gynecol 161:35–36, 1989.

109. Ben-Ami M, Giladi Y, Shalev E. The combination of magnesium sulphate and nifedipine: A cause of neuromuscular blockade. Br J Obstet Gynaecol 101:262–263, 1994.

110. Childress CH, Katz VL. Nifedipine and its indications in obstetrics and gynecology. Obstet Gynecol 83:616–624, 1994.

111. Levin AC, Doering PL, Hatton RC. Use of nifedipine in the hypertensive diseases of pregnancy. Ann Pharmacol Ther 28:1371–1378, 1994.

112. Lewis R, Sibai BM. The use of calcium-channel blockers in pregnancy. New Horiz 4:115–122, 1996.

113. Wide-Swensson DH, Ingemarsson I, Lunell NO, et al. Calcium channel blockade (isradipine) in treatment of hypertension in pregnancy: A randomised placebo-controlled study. Am J Obstet Gynecol 173:872–878, 1995.

114. Sibai BM. Diagnosis and management of chronic hypertension in pregnancy. Obstet Gynecol 78:451–461, 1991.

115. Magee LA, Schick B, Donnenfeld AE, et al. The safety of calcium channel blockers in human pregnancy: A prospective, multicenter cohort study. Am J Obstet Gynecol 174:823–828, 1996.

116. Belfort MA, Carpenter RJ Jr, Kirshon B, et al. The use of nimodipine in a patient with eclampsia: Color flow Doppler demonstration of retinal artery relaxation. Am J Obstet Gynecol 169:204–206, 1993.

117. Adverse drug reaction reporting systems. MMWR 46:240–242, 1997.

118. Rosa FW, Bosco LA, Graham CF, et al. Neonatal anuria with maternal angiotensin-converting enzyme inhibition. Obstet Gynecol 74:371–374, 1989.

119. Hanssens M, Keirse MJ, Vankelecom F, van Assche FA. Fetal and neonatal effects of treatment with angiotensin-converting enzyme inhibitors in pregnancy. Obstet Gynecol 78:128–135, 1991.

120. Piper JM, Ray WA, Rosa FW. Pregnancy outcome following exposure to angiotensin-converting enzyme inhibitors. Obstet Gynecol 80:429–432, 1992.

121. Barr M Jr, Cohen MM Jr. ACE inhibitor fetopathy and hypocalvaria: The kidney skull connection. Teratology 44:485–495, 1991.

122. Sibai BM, Grossman RA, Grossman HG. Effects of diuretics on plasma volume in pregnancies with long-term hypertension. Am J Obstet Gynecol 150:831–835, 1984.

123. Gallery EDM, Hunyor SN, Györy AZ. Plasma volume contraction. A significant factor in both pregnancy-associated hypertension (preeclampsia) and chronic hypertension in pregnancy. Q J Med 48:593–602, 1979.

124. Briggs GG, Freeman RK, Yaffe SJ. A Reference Guide to Fetal and Neonatal Risk: Drugs in Pregnancy and Lactation, 4th ed. Baltimore, Williams & Wilkins, 1994.

125. White WB. Management of hypertension during lactation. Hypertension 6:297–300, 1984.

126. Dillon AE, Wagner CL, Wiest D, Newman RB. Drug therapy in the nursing mother. Obstet Gynecol Clin North Am 24:675–696, 1998.

127. American Academy of Pediatrics, Committee on Drugs. The transfer of drugs and other chemicals into human breast milk. Pediatrics 84:924–936, 1989.

128. American Academy of Pediatrics, Committee on Drugs: The transfer of drugs and other chemicals into human milk. Pediatrics 93:137–150, 1994.

Anesthesia and Hypertension

CHAPTER **81**

James Gould, J. G. Reves, and Mark Phillips

The purpose of this chapter is to review the current knowledge of anesthesia and surgery in the hypertensive patient. It is hoped that internists, surgeons, and anesthesiologists will be able to use this information to better prepare patients for surgery by understanding how hypertension, its treatment, and anesthesia interact. Emphasis is placed on the cardiovascular pharmacology of anesthetic drugs, anesthetic techniques, the preoperative evaluation of the patient, and the implications of the operative procedure for management strategies. The risks of perioperative hypertension and the best way to minimize those risks are also discussed.

Elsewhere in this book the pathophysiology and treatment of hypertension and the therapy are discussed in detail. This chapter reviews the effects of anesthesia and surgery on the hypertensive patient from a physiological, pharmacological, and clinical outcome perspective. Hypertension (blood pressure [BP] > 140/90 mm Hg) and surgery are both very prevalent, particularly in the elderly.[1] It is important to have an understanding of the effect that hypertension has on anesthesia and surgery, as well as the effect that surgery and anesthesia have on hypertensive patients. It has been estimated that severe hypertension (180/110 mm Hg) is found in 11% of surgical patients.[2] The prevalence of hypertension depends on the surgical population; its incidence is increased in older patients and in those undergoing vascular and cardiovascular surgery.[3] Hypertension is common during surgery, occurring in 57% of patients undergoing abdominal aortic surgery, in 29% of those undergoing peripheral vascular surgery, and in 8% of those undergoing intraperitoneal procedures.[4] In patients having carotid artery or open heart surgery, the incidence of hypertension varies between 40 and 80%.[5, 6]

In the perioperative period, there are four classes of hypertensive patients (Table 81–1). The first class is the normotensive patient who experiences the many stresses of the perioperative period, such as anxiety, pain, and distended bladder, that evoke a catecholamine response and cause hypertension.[7] This form of hypertension is usually transient (self-limited) and can be successfully treated by removing the cause. The second class of patients includes those with a history of hypertension controlled (≤140/90 mm Hg) by pharmacological therapy. These patients are likely to respond to the multiple perioperative stressors of surgery with hypertension, but to a lesser degree than the third and fourth classes of patients. The third class of patients includes those with undiagnosed or uncontrolled hypertension (BP 160/90 to 180/110 mm Hg). These patients are likely to have recurrent hypertension in the perioperative period. The fourth class includes the hypertensive patients who may or may not be treated, but who present for anesthesia with uncontrolled hypertension (≥180/110 mm Hg). This class is at highest risk for perioperative hypertension, hypotension, and a labile hemodynamic course. These patients are at risk for possible morbid events and should generally have surgery delayed until the hypertension can be better controlled.[4, 8]

It is important to recognize that hypertensive patients often have comorbid diseases such as diabetes, renal disease, cerebrovascular disease, peripheral vascular disease, and cardiac disease, including coronary artery disease, left ventricular hypertrophy, and congestive heart failure (CHF). Hypertensive patients are at increased risk of hemodynamic fluctuations during the perioperative course,[9–12] which may result in myocardial ischemia,[9–11, 13] myocardial infarction,[4, 14] postoperative renal dysfunction,[15, 16] and an increased incidence of postoperative neurological deficits.[16–18] Hypertension generally confers added risk to anesthesia and surgery. This risk is further discussed later in the chapter.

The pathophysiology of hypertension is dealt with elsewhere in this book; however, from the anesthesia perspec-

Table 81–1 Perioperative Hypertensive Patients

Classification*	BP† (mm Hg)	Commentary‡	Disposition
1. Normotensive	<140/90	Controlled, resolves with removal of stressor	Treat q.s.
2. Controlled hypertensives	<140/90	Adequately controlled	Treat q.s.
3. Poorly controlled or undiagnosed hypertensives	140/90 ≤ 180/110	Poorly controlled	Dx and Rx, better Rx, arrange appropriate medical follow-up
4. Uncontrolled or undiagnosed hypertensives	≥110 diastolic	Uncontrolled	Dx and Rx, better Rx, arrange appropriate medical management, *delay elective surgery*

Abbreviations: BP, blood pressure; q.s., as needed during the perioperative period; Dx, diagnose; Rx, treat.
*Classification adapted from literature review and definitions of the Joint National Committee on Prevention, Detection, Evaluation, and Treatment of High Blood Pressure. The sixth report. Arch Intern Med 157:2413–2446, 1997.
†BP at preoperative evaluation or before anesthesia induction.
‡Hypertensive response (≥140/90) during the preoperative or perioperative period in patients who are diagnosed as hypertensive or not diagnosed as hypertensive, but who develop hypertension during the perioperative period.

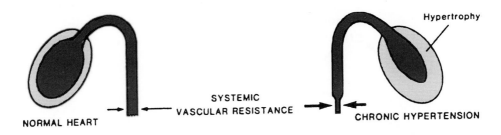

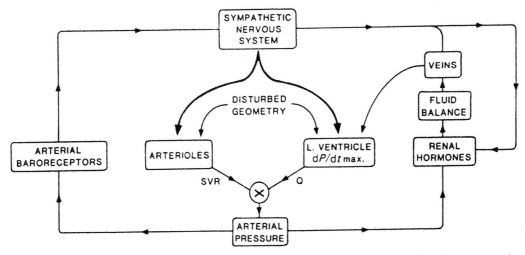

Figure 81–1. Schema of the hemodynamic perturbations induced in the hypertensive patient demonstrates the interactions of adaptive hypertrophy of the arteriolar media, and of the left ventricle, with sympathetic nervous activity. SVR, systemic vascular resistance. (From Prys-Roberts C. Anaesthesia and hypertension. Br J Anaesth 56:711–724, 1984.)

tive, general pathophysiological principles apply to most hypertensive patients. Figure 81–1 illustrates the effects of hypertension on the heart and identifies the important determinants of BP that are affected by anesthetic and antihypertensive drugs. The hypertensive patient is likely to have elevated systemic vascular resistance (SVR), reduced total blood volume, impaired cardiac contractility, and a hypertrophied myocardium. The hypertrophied left ventricle (which by its very pathology has higher oxygen requirements and potentially less oxygen supply) is vulnerable to subendocardial ischemia,[9, 19] particularly if there is tachycardia and/or if the perfusion pressure decreases during anesthesia. Almost all anesthetic drugs and most anesthetic techniques will produce vasodilatation (see the next section), and most inhalation anesthetics are direct negative inotropic drugs. Thus, hypertensive patients who may be volume depleted,[20] who have high SVR, and who may have depressed ventricular function are likely to experience hypotension with the induction of anesthesia. This hypotension can compromise myocardial oxygen delivery, which may lead to ischemic ventricular dysfunction.

The treatment of hypertension is particularly important for patients undergoing anesthesia and surgery for two reasons. It is well documented that patients under hypertensive control have fewer hemodynamic fluctuations in the perioperative period.[16, 19–21] The fewer the hemodynamic fluctuations (particularly tachycardia), the less likely patients are to have myocardial ischemia.[9, 22] Also, many of the drugs commonly used in the treatment of hypertension have pharmacological interactions with anesthetics. Anesthetic drugs and techniques (general, spinal, epidural) require a complex set of homeostatic reflexes to maintain cardiac output and BP, as illustrated in Figure 81–2.[23] Antihypertensive drugs that lower the plasma volume (e.g., diuretics),[24] the vasodilators, and the β-adrenergic antagonists accentuate the hypotensive effects of anesthesia and impair the autoregulatory responses of increased heart rate (HR), contractility, and vasoconstriction that occur in response to the primary effects of anesthesia.

Two classes of antihypertensive drugs that are especially helpful in the perioperative management of hypertensive patients are the β-adrenergic antagonists and the α$_2$-agonists. β-Blockers attenuate the hypertensive and tachycardic responses to perioperative stress and reduce myocardial ischemia.[9, 25, 26] α$_2$-Agonists such as clonidine reduce the incidence of hypertension and tachycardia as well as the need for additional anesthesia.[27] Patients whose hypertension is treated with these classes of drugs will likely have smoother perioperative courses. The failure of diuretics to provide smooth hemodynamics during anesthesia is attributed to the lower total blood volume, increased circulating vasoactive substances, and potassium depletion.[9] There is insufficient information on the many new antihypertensive drugs such as angiotensin II receptor, I1-imidazoline receptor, and serotonergic receptor antagonists to know how these agents affect the perioperative course.

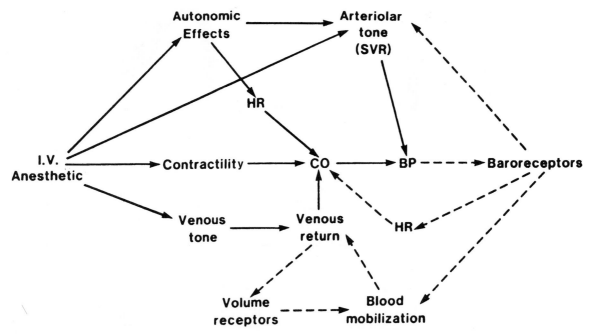

Figure 81–2. The multiple effects of anesthetic drugs on the cardiovascular system are shown. Direct *(solid arrows)* and indirect *(broken arrows)* effects of intravenous (I.V.) anesthetics on cardiovascular function. SVR, systemic vascular resistance; HR, heart rate; CO, cardiac output; BP, blood pressure. (From Reves JG, Gelman S. Cardiovascular effects of intravenous anesthetic drugs. *In* Covino F, Rehder K, Strichartz GR [eds]. Effects of Anesthesia. Bethesda, MD, American Physiological Society, 1985; pp 179–193.)

CARDIOVASCULAR PHARMACOLOGY OF SEDATIVE AND ANESTHETIC DRUGS

To better understand the hemodynamic effects of sedative, inhalation, and intravenous anesthetics, we review the major cardiovascular effects of drugs used in anesthesia as well as the cardiovascular effects of common anesthetic techniques. This section is a synopsis of material presented in earlier reviews of the pharmacology of anesthetic drugs.[23, 28–31] The cardiovascular effects of the various drugs and anesthetic techniques are summarized in Table 81–2.

Anesthetic Techniques

Anesthetic techniques can be divided into four categories. The first is general anesthesia, which is accomplished with a wide variety of intravenous and inhalation anesthetic drugs. The majority of general anesthetics are given with a hypnotic (usually a barbiturate or a benzodiazepine), an analgesic (an opioid and/or an inhalation drug) and a mus-

cle relaxant (neuromuscular blocking drugs). A second form of anesthesia is neuraxial block, which is accomplished by placing a local anesthetic in the spinal or epidural space. A third technique is a regional nerve block with a local anesthetic. The final anesthetic technique involves sedation of the patient and local anesthetic infiltration at the site of surgery. This is called *monitored anesthesia care* (MAC).

We have recently examined the effect of anesthetic technique on hypertensive patients.[32] General and neuraxial techniques result in the greatest hypotension because both techniques result in vasodilatation (Fig. 81–3). Loss of consciousness, as seen in normal sleep,[33] reduces HR, cardiac output, and BP. Most drugs used for general anesthesia have hemodynamic effects that, together with loss of consciousness, cause hypotension. Neuroaxial block produces hypotension by creating a complete sympathectomy to (or slightly above) the dermatome level of the anesthesia. This causes profound vasodilatation, reduced preload, lower cardiac output, and hypotension. The use of epidural anesthesia with general anesthesia significantly lowers the inci-

Table 81–2 Anesthetic Drugs/Techniques—Effects on Hemodynamic Variables				
Variable	Intravenous	Inhalation	Neuroaxial	Peripheral
Cardiac output	0 to −	−	− to 0	0
SVR	− to 0	−	−	0
Contractility	0	−	0	0
Heart rate	0	−	0	0
Stroke volume	0	−	0	0

Abbreviation: SVR, systemic vascular resistance.
Key: 0, no change; −, decrease.

dence of operative hypertension, but it is associated with greater hypotension and can evoke hypertension when it is withdrawn postoperatively.[34] Regional block and MAC have minimal hemodynamic effects and are less likely to cause hypotension in hypertensive patients. Hypertensive patients often have hypertensive responses during anesthesia, and all anesthetic techniques are associated with similar peak incidences of hypertension (Fig. 81–4; see also Fig. 81–3).

GENERAL ANESTHETIC CARDIOVASCULAR PHARMACOLOGY

General Anesthetic Induction Drugs

Thiopental (Pentothal) has survived the test of time as an intravenous anesthetic drug. Since Lundy introduced it in 1934, thiopental has become the most widely used induction agent because of the rapid hypnotic effect (one arm-brain circulation time), highly predictable effect, lack of vascular irritation, and general overall safety.[35] The principal hemodynamic change produced by thiopental is a decrease in myocardial contractility[36-38] due to reduced availability of calcium to the myofibrils.[39] There is also an increase in HR.[37, 40] The cardiac index (CI) is unchanged[41, 42]

or reduced,[37, 43] whereas the mean arterial pressure (MAP) is maintained[41, 44] or slightly reduced.[43] When thiopental is given to hypovolemic patients, which could include poorly controlled hypertensive patients, there is a significant reduction in cardiac output as well as an important decrease in BP. Thus, patients without adequate compensatory mechanisms may have serious hemodynamic depression with a thiopental induction.[45] This probably explains the disastrous results of thiopental administration at Pearl Harbor,[46] in which many wounded men who were hypovolemic experienced shock with the rapid administration of the newly released anesthetic thiopental.

Diazepam (Valium) is probably the most widely used 1,4-benzodiazepine in the world. It was introduced in the United States in 1963 and is used for sedation and anesthesia induction. The presumed mechanism of action of diazepam and other benzodiazepines in the central nervous system is by potentiation of the inhibitory effect of γ-aminobutyric acid on neuronal transmission.[47] All benzodiazepines have hypnotic, anticonvulsant, muscle relaxant, amnesic, and anxiolytic neuropharmacological properties. Induction with diazepam is characterized by hemodynamic stability. Filling pressures and CI remain unchanged,[48-53] with variable but modest changes in HR.[48-54] Although diazepam may be safely combined with other anesthetic drugs, there is some potential for hemodynamic depression.[55] The effect of the

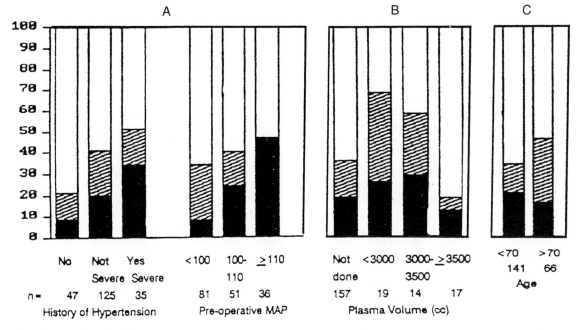

Figure 81–3. Percentage of patients with intraoperative hypotension *(black)*, hyper/hypotension *(cross-hatched)*, or neither high-risk pattern *(white)* according to preoperative characteristics. **A.** Patients are compared based on their history of hypertension and preoperative mean arterial pressure (MAP). A preoperative MAP greater than 110 mm Hg was a significant ($p < .0001$) predictor of intraoperative hypotension. **B.** Patients are compared based on their initial plasma volume as determined using Evans blue. Decreased plasma volume was a significant ($p = .03$) predictor of intraoperative hypotension and was associated with a higher incidence of intraoperative hyper/hypotension. **C.** Patients are compared based on age. Age greater than 70 years was a significant ($p < .006$) predictor of intraoperative hyper/hypotension. Age alone did not significantly increase the incidence of intraoperative hypotension. Preoperative hypertension was defined as a systolic blood pressure (BP) greater than 160 mm Hg or a diastolic BP greater than 95 mm Hg. Severe preoperative hypertension was defined as diastolic BP greater than or equal to 120 mm Hg. *Intraoperative hypotension* was defined as a decrease of greater than 20 mm Hg from preoperative MAP lasting 1 hour or longer. *Intraoperative hyper/hypotension* was defined as an increase of greater than or equal to 20 mm Hg above the usual MAP lasting more than 15 minutes combined with a decrease of greater than 20 mm Hg in MAP lasting less than 1 hour. (A–C. From Charlson ME, MacKenzie CR, Gold JP, et al. Preoperative characteristics predicting intraoperative hypotension and hypertension among hypertensives and diabetics undergoing noncardiac surgery. Ann Surg 212[1]:66–81, 1990.)

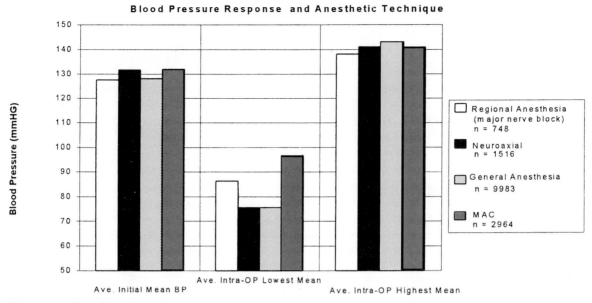

Figure 81–4. The effect of anesthetic technique on maximal changes in blood pressure (BP) is shown. BP drops (average intraoperative [intra-OP] lowest mean vs. average preoperative mean) are significantly ($p < .001$) greater with general and neuroaxial anesthetic techniques compared with regional (major nerve block) and monitored anesthetic care (MAC) techniques. The average intra-OP highest mean BP was similar among anesthetic techniques. *Regional anesthesia* refers to major peripheral nerve blocks such as brachial plexus blocks, lumbar plexus blocks, sciatic nerve blocks, and paravertebral blocks; *general anesthesia* refers to general anesthesia; neuroaxial anesthesia refers to spinal anesthesia, epidural anesthesia, and combined spinal/epidural anesthesia. See text for more details on anesthetic technique. (From Gould JD, Reves JG, D'Ercole FJ, et al. Effect of anesthetic technique on blood pressure response in hypertensive patients. Anesth Analg 88:SCA1–SCA126, 1999.)

combination of diazepam and morphine (indeed of any benzodiazepine and opioid) in patients who have ischemic heart disease[56, 57] and valvular heart disease[58] has been reported. The combination of diazepam (0.125 to 0.5 mg/kg) and fentanyl (50 mg/kg) used to induce anesthesia in patients for coronary artery bypass graft surgery[59] led to a supraadditive fall in BP that could be more pronounced in hypovolemic hypertensive patients. The authors concluded from this that diazepam ablates normal sympathetic tone.[59]

Midazolam (Versed, Dormicum) is a water-soluble benzodiazepine synthesized in the United States in 1975. It is unique among benzodiazepines with its rapid onset and short duration of action and relatively rapid plasma clearance.[60] It is the most commonly used benzodiazepine in anesthetic practice. The hemodynamic changes that result from the intravenous administration of midazolam (0.2 mg/kg) in premedicated patients who have coronary artery disease are usually minor.[53, 61] Changes of potential importance include a decrease in MAP of 20%[61] and an increase in HR of 15%.[61] The CI is maintained.[53, 61] Filling pressures are either unchanged or decreased in patients who have normal ventricular function,[53, 61] but are significantly decreased in patients who have an elevated pulmonary capillary wedge pressure (≥ 18 mm Hg).[62] Interactions between midazolam and other drugs are relatively mild and predictable. Premedication with both morphine and scopolamine decrease induction time. The combination of nitrous oxide (N_2O) (50%) with midazolam (0.2 mg/kg) does not cause increased cardiovascular depression.[53] The safe combination of N_2O and midazolam contrasts with the well-known additive depression of N_2O and narcotic agents.[63] Midazolam and halothane together are well tolerated,[64] and midazolam (0.15 mg/kg) and ketamine (1.5 mg/kg) have proved

to be a safe and useful combination for a rapid-sequence induction for emergency surgery.[44] If midazolam is given to patients who have received fentanyl, significant hypotension may occur, as seen with diazepam and fentanyl.[59] Midazolam is routinely combined with fentanyl for induction and maintenance of general anesthesia during cardiac surgery without adverse hemodynamic sequelae.[65, 66]

Although ketamine (Ketalar) produces rapid hypnosis and profound analgesia, respiratory and cardiovascular functions are not depressed as much as with most other induction agents. Disturbing psychotomimetic activity (described as vivid dreams, hallucinations, or other mental disturbances on emergence from ketamine anesthesia) as well as undesirable increases in myocardial oxygen consumption have limited the use of ketamine. One unique feature of ketamine is stimulation of the cardiovascular system. The most prominent hemodynamic changes are significant increases in HR, CI, SVR, and systemic and pulmonary artery pressures. Because of the hypertension after ketamine, this drug is seldom used in hypertensive patients.

Propofol (Diprivan; 2,6 di-isopropylphenol; ICI 35,868) is the most recent intravenous anesthetic to be introduced into clinical practice (in 1977).[67] It is an alkylphenol (substituted derivative of phenol) with hypnotic properties. The hemodynamic effects of propofol have been compared with the most commonly used induction drugs including the thiobarbiturates and etomidate.[68–72] Systolic pressure falls 15 to 40% after intravenous induction with ±2 mg/kg and maintenance infusion ±100 μg/kg/min propofol. Similar changes are seen in both diastolic pressure and MAP. The effect of propofol on HR is variable. Despite a significant decrease in MAP, some studies have shown no change in

HR,[73] a decrease in HR,[72] and an increase in HR.[74] The majority of studies have demonstrated significant reductions in SVR (9 to 30%), CI, stroke volume, and left ventricular stroke work index after propofol. In summary, propofol alone or in combination causes significant decreases in arterial pressure and CI secondary to increased venodilatation with decreased myocardial contractility. Its use in uncontrolled hypertensives could be problematic.

Drugs for Maintenance of Anesthesia

Contemporary inhalation anesthesia includes the use of six drugs—the volatile liquids halothane, enflurane, sevoflurane, desflurane, isoflurane and the inert gas N_2O. Each inhalation anesthetic has a specific cardiovascular profile, but all except N_2O are vasodilators and negative inotropes. As with the intravenous agents, their hemodynamic effects depend on several factors that include the drug per se, the cardiovascular status of the patient, and concurrent pharmacological therapy. Unlike the intravenous drugs, cardiovascular effects of the inhalation agents are more similar to one another than they are different. The inhalation anesthetics often reduce cardiac output. All of the inhalation agents exert a direct, dose-dependent negative inotropic effect on the myocardium in humans.[75–77] There are small differences among agents in the degree of myocardial depression and in the mechanism of myocardial suppression. In general, halothane and enflurane reduce cardiac output to a greater degree than isoflurane in healthy patients. The depressant effects of the volatile anesthetics on myocardial contractility in disease states such as ischemic heart disease are additive.[78] The influences of age, myocardial disease, premedication, and adjuvant drugs are also important additive depressant factors. Inhalation anesthetics must be used judiciously in hypertensive patients because of the propensity to cause hypotension.

Opioids are also used to provide analgesia during general anesthesia and postoperatively. The drugs commonly used are morphine, fentanyl, sufentanil, alfentanil, and remifentanil. Morphine causes more hemodynamic perturbations than the others. Morphine, because of release of histamine, causes vasodilatation that generally produces hypotension. The other synthetic opioids are devoid of this action, and their administration is marked by maintenance of SVR. All opioids tend to be vagomimetic, causing a decrease in HR. Opioids have little effect on cardiac output, stroke volume, cardiac filling, or baroreflex function. They are used in hypertensive patients to blunt sympathetic responses to painful stimuli. They are useful in hypertensive patients because they tend to minimize hemodynamic fluctuation, but they must be combined with other anesthetic drugs to accomplish total anesthesia. The hemodynamic interactions with these drugs can cause vasodilatation and hypotension.

EVALUATION AND PREPARATION OF THE HYPERTENSIVE SURGICAL PATIENT

There is no area in medicine where the collaborative team approach to patient care can be better employed than in evaluating and preparing the hypertensive patient for surgery. The internist (cardiologist, generalist), the surgeon, and the anesthesiologist all have important roles in the optimal care of these high-risk patients.[79] The objectives of the evaluation are listed in Table 81–3. Each specialist has a specific role: The surgeon must determine the appropriate operation; the internist must optimize the medical therapy; and the anesthesiologist must choose the appropriate monitoring, anesthetic technique, and postoperative pain strategy.

Table 81–1 lists the categories into which hypertensive patients fall when presenting for surgery. Patients who are optimally medically managed before, during, and after surgery have a smoother hemodynamic course. Patients in groups 3 and 4 of Table 81–1 have more labile courses than patients in groups 1 and 2.[2–4, 16, 20, 80] It is important in evaluating the hypertensive patient that comorbid conditions be detected (Table 81–4) and that antihypertensive therapy be optimized (BP ≤ 140/90).

The preoperative evaluation listed in Table 81–3, including relevant history and physical examination (see Table 81–4), can be made by the internist, the surgeon, or the anesthesiologist. It does not matter who has the initial responsibility. What is vital is that all of the objectives in Table 81–3 are successfully attained before surgery. The cause of hypertension should be determined, remembering that essential hypertension is most common. Knowing, wherever possible, the causes and pathophysiology of the hypertension (see Fig. 81–1) is critical to proper perioperative management. It is important to determine what antihypertensive medications the patient is taking, what the dosing regimen is, and whether this regimen should be continued or changed during the perioperative period. If the regimen cannot be continued, an alternative strategy must be developed. It is clear from multiple studies and reviews of this subject that it is best to continue the patient's antihypertensive medicines until the morning of surgery.[2–4, 9, 16, 19, 79, 80] The discontinuation of antihypertensive medication in anticipation of surgery can cause rebound hypertension, tachycardia, or myocardial ischemia,[19] which will be problematic in the perioperative management of the patient. Antihypertensive therapy should be continued after surgery and throughout the perioperative period as the patient's course indicates.

The single most important and most obvious preoperative assessment (see Table 81–4) is the adequacy of BP control. If the BP is greater than 110 mm Hg diastolic on the preoperative evaluation, it is generally recommended to delay elective surgery until the BP can be better controlled.[2, 3, 8, 16, 20] Unless the surgery is emergent or urgent, it is best to get the resting BP as close to the normal range

Table 81–3 Objectives of the Preoperative Evaluation of Hypertensive Patients

Diagnosis of hypertension (cause)
Ascertain antihypertensive medical therapy
Determine adequacy (optimization) of therapy
Identify comorbid diseases (see Table 81–4)
Obtain appropriate consultative services
Devise appropriate postoperative antihypertensive plan

Table 81–4 Identifying Comorbidity in the Hypertensive Patient

System	Effect of Hypertension	History	Physical	Tests*
Cardiovascular	CAD	Angina, MI		ECG,* ETT (other functional study), coronary angiography
	LVH (diastolic/systolic dysfn), pulmonary edema, ischemia	Dyspnea, orthopnea, PND, exercise tolerance, edema	S₃, S₄, rales, JVD, HJR, peripheral edema	CXR,* 2D-ECHO, ECG*
	Hypovolemia	Syncope, near syncope	Orthostatic BP	Orthostatic BP*
	PVD	Claudication	Peripheral pulses, ABI	Angiography HCT*
Renal	Renal impairment	Symptoms occur late in process		BUN,* Cr,* electrolytes,* UA*
Central nervous	Cerebrovascular disease	TIA, CVA, syncope	Carotid bruits, neurological deficits	Carotid Doppler, angiography, CT scan, MRI

Abbreviations: CAD, coronary artery disease; MI, myocardial infarction; ECG, electrocardiogram; ETT, exercise tolerance test; LVH, left ventricular hypertrophy; dysfn, dysfunction; PND, paroxysmal nocturnal dyspnea; S₃, S₄, third and fourth heart sounds; JVD, jugular venous distention; HJR, hepatojugular reflux; CXR, chest radiography; 2D-ECHO, two-dimensional echocardiography; BP, blood pressure; PVD, peripheral vascular disease; ABI, ankle/brachial index; HCT, hematocrit; BUN, blood urea nitrogen; Cr, creatinine; UA, urinalysis; TIA, transient ischemic attack; CVA, cerebrovascular accident; CT, computed tomography; MRI, magnetic resonance imaging.

as possible, or at least to below 110 mm Hg diastolic. It should be remembered that many patients who are faced with the prospect of surgery have conditions that may artifactually raise their BP, e.g., anxiety or pain. Therefore, a preoperative BP that is above the "normal" range, as defined for office readings in relaxed patients, is acceptable for the preoperative patient. It is also useful to obtain a supine and a standing BP as an assessment of the orthostatic component of BP control. This measurement can also indirectly gauge the blood volume. Routine perioperative evaluation of the hypertensive patient includes electrocardiogram and chest x-ray (looking for evidence of left ventricular hypertrophy), serum electrolytes (especially in patients treated with diuretics), blood urea nitrogen/creatinine to evaluate renal status, and a baseline hematocrit. Additional tests may be indicated based on the patient's history and physical examination to further evaluate the effects of hypertension on vital organs.

Preoperative evaluation of the surgical patient may reveal not only hypertension but also other important coexisting diseases (cardiac, renal, cerebrovascular). Each of these requires lifelong management, and one benefit of routine preoperative evaluation may be the discovery of these potentially life-threatening diseases.[79] Medical consultation should be obtained to be certain that the extent of the comorbid diseases is fully understood *and* that a long-term plan for management after surgery is put into place.

Consultations have an important role in the preoperative

evaluation of the hypertensive patient. To be most informative to the professionals involved, as well as to provide optimal patient care, consultations should include a number of important elements.[79, 81–83] Table 81–5 lists suggestions to make the consultative process most effective.[79] It is generally unproductive for professionals to stray from their own realm of expertise, no matter how great the temptation. Thus, medical consultants who "clear patients for surgery" encroach on the surgeon's ultimate decision. Likewise, internists' advice to anesthesiologists regarding monitoring or anesthetic techniques is noncontributory. The four key questions that surgeons and anesthesiologists have for their medical consultants are:

1. What diseases does the patient have?
2. Are the diseases being appropriately treated?
3. Is there any further medical therapy that should be instituted?
4. Who will be responsible for the postoperative treatment of the medical conditions that are identified?

HYPERTENSION, ANESTHESIA, AND SURGERY

After the preoperative evaluation, the anesthetic plan is made. It must include choice of anesthetic technique; monitoring strategy; method of anesthesia induction, maintenance, and emergence; and postoperative disposition. The patient's coexisting disease, the planned operative procedure, and the duration of the procedure all influence the anesthetic plan.

In general, anesthetic technique falls into one of four categories: centroneuraxial anesthesia, regional (major nerve block) anesthesia, MAC, and general anesthesia. *Centroneuraxial anesthesia* includes spinal and epidural anesthesia. *Major nerve block anesthesia* includes, but is not limited to, brachial plexus blocks (interscalene, supraclavicular, and axillary) for upper extremity surgery, lumbar plexus blocks and femoral-sciatic nerve blocks for lower extremity surgery, and paravertebral blocks for trunk sur-

Table 81–5 Essentials of Effective Perioperative Consultation

Establish clear communication
Ask specific questions in the realm of consultant's expertise
Avoid general statements on "clearance for surgery"
Avoid specific advice on matters for which another professional has ultimate decision
Specify whether anything can be done to improve patient status

A condensation of the authors' thoughts and those of Kleinman et al[79] and Goldman et al.[81]

gery. In simplest terms, *MAC* involves intravenous sedation, patient monitoring, and local anesthetic infiltration at the operative site. *Regional anesthesia* provides profound analgesia and muscle relaxation to a limited portion of the body, allowing the patient to maintain normal respiratory control, easy assessment of neurological status, and minimal physiological disturbance. *General anesthesia* involves inducing a state of unconsciousness with analgesia, amnesia, and immobility. Frequently, endotracheal intubation, mechanical ventilation, complete paralysis, and hemodynamic support are part of a general anesthetic.

Choice of Technique in Hypertensive Patients

With regard to anesthetic technique, two main questions need to be addressed:

1. How does the choice of anesthetic technique affect perioperative cardiovascular, neurological, and renal morbidity and mortality in the hypertensive patient?
2. What effect (consequence) does anesthetic technique have on the incidence of perioperative hypertension, hypotension, hemodynamic lability, and myocardial ischemia?

General Anesthesia

Most of the literature evaluating the cardiovascular responses of hypertensive patients to anesthetic techniques is with use of general anesthesia. The cardiovascular responses of hypertensive patients undergoing general anesthesia tend to be labile.[2, 9, 10, 13] Hypertensive patients become hypotensive with induction and have hypertensive responses to laryngoscopy, intubation, noxious stimuli, and emergence. Their response to rapid changes in anesthetic depth is also exaggerated. Intraoperative BP lability, hypertension, and hypotension place hypertensive patients at increased risk of myocardial ischemia,[9] myocardial reinfarction,[14] and perioperative renal dysfunction.[16, 20] Charlson and coworkers[20] have looked at the association between preoperative patient characteristics and intraoperative hemodynamics. Figure 81–3 shows these results. Patients older than 70 years (see Fig. 81–3C) with a preoperative MAP greater than 110 (see Fig. 81–3A) are at greatest risk for intraoperative hemodynamic lability (hypertensive/hypotensive episodes). Charlson and coworkers'[20] data also support a role for appropriate fluid management in decreasing hemodynamic lability; patients with a plasma volume greater than 3500 ml had a decreased incidence of intraoperative hypotension and hypertension episodes (see Fig. 81–3B).

Other than a few studies looking at spinal anesthesia in hypertensive patients,[16, 21] there have been no studies of the effects of anesthetic technique per se (comparing MAC, regional, centroneuraxial, and general) on the BP response in hypertensive patients. To help answer this question, we analyzed over 120,000 anesthetic records stored in the Duke Anesthesia Database compiled by an automated anesthesia information system used at Duke University.[32] From the database, 15,211 hypertensive patients where identified; their mean BP was recorded before initiating an anesthetic technique (MAC, centroneuraxial, major nerve block, or general) and then compared with their intraoperative highest and lowest mean BPs. Figure 81–4 shows the differences in change in MAP after induction of anesthesia among the anesthetic techniques. BP changes (drops) are significantly ($p < .001$) greater with general and centroneuraxial anesthetics compared with MAC and major nerve block. The maximal mean BP intraoperatively was similar with all techniques. We also found that patients with higher initial MAP regardless of techniques had larger intraoperative changes (drops) in BP after initiating anesthesia, confirming previous studies (see Fig. 81–3A).[20] These data support the notion that better BP control intraoperatively may be achieved with major nerve block anesthesia compared with general or centroneuraxial techniques. Of course, many operations cannot be performed with nerve block anesthesia.

Regional Anesthesia (Neuraxial and Major Nerve Blocks)

Some anesthesiologists believe that regional anesthesia has theoretical advantages in the high-risk patient.[84] Since regional techniques do not involve intubation, paralysis, or mechanical ventilation with positive pressure, one can make an argument that regional techniques are less physiologically intrusive and therefore may be better tolerated in patients predisposed to hemodynamic lability. Furthermore, the dense block provided by regional techniques almost eliminates the hypertensive response to surgical stimuli, and the excellent postoperative analgesia (with major nerve block or epidural) may prevent hypertensive or ischemic responses to postoperative pain.[34]

Epidural and spinal anesthesia involve the injection of local anesthetic in or around the spinal cord to interrupt afferent impulses. The result is usually a dense sensory and motor block to the lower half of the body (T4–T10 dermatomal level and below depending on dose and technique). This block also produces a profound sympathectomy to the lower extremities and part of the splanchnic circulation with resultant vasodilatation and venodilatation of these vascular beds. This reduction in preload, particularly in a hypertensive patient with mild hypovolemia, left ventricular hypertrophy, and diastolic dysfunction, can cause a marked drop in cardiac output and BP. Racle and colleagues[21] compared the cardiovascular responses of normotensive and hypertensive patients after spinal anesthesia and found that hypertensive patients, on average, had a significantly larger drop in systolic, diastolic, and mean BPs compared with normotensive patients. In general, patients with well-controlled hypertension tolerate lumbar and thoracic epidural block without unpredictable or profound decreases in arterial pressure. In contrast, a small group ($n = 5$) of patients with untreated hypertension showed an average decrease of 44% in systolic arterial pressure. Three of these patients required active intervention to correct the problem.[85] Finally, in a study by Garnett and associates,[34] looking at patients (42% hypertensive) undergoing elective aortic surgery, epidural anesthesia in combination with general anesthesia reduced the risk of intraoperative hypertension compared with general anesthesia alone. In the same study, epidural anesthesia did not prevent, and possibly intensified, hypotension during the procedure. This hypotension was associated with a higher incidence of electrocardiographic evidence of myocardial ischemia.

Hypertensive patients have perioperative hemodynamic characteristics that are associated with increased perioperative complications. Untreated and severe hypertensive patients are at higher risk. The hemodynamic patterns of the various anesthetic techniques in hypertensive patients are different, yet improved perioperative outcome has not been demonstrated unequivocally for any of them. Each anesthetic technique has certain benefits and risks as well as certain desirable and undesirable characteristics. For example, a technique that prevents hypertensive responses may make the patient prone to hypotension and ischemia. Rather than anesthetic technique, it is more likely that acute, aggressive treatment of perioperative hypotension, hypertension, and ischemia is the key to improving perioperative outcomes. Hypertension, hypotension, or ischemia, if treated appropriately and promptly, is unlikely to have negative sequelae, whereas prolonged periods place the patient at increased risk.[20] Thus, an anesthesiologist familiar with the consequences of the anesthetic technique, appropriate intraoperative monitoring to detect rapid hemodynamic changes and ischemia, and aggressive correction of the hemodynamic disturbances are more important than the choice of anesthetic technique alone.

Outcome Studies

The majority of studies evaluating anesthetic technique (centroneuraxial, regional, or general) on cardiac morbidity and mortality were carried out in patients undergoing peripheral vascular surgery[86–89] or carotid endarterectomy.[90–93] The studies in patients undergoing peripheral vascular surgery all compare a centroneuraxial technique with general anesthesia. The most recent and largest study by Bode and coworkers[86] randomly assigned 423 patients scheduled for elective femoral-distal vessel bypass surgery to one of three anesthetic techniques (spinal, epidural, or general). Using an intent-to-treat analysis, they reported no statistically significant differences between groups with regard to in-hospital mortality, nonfatal myocardial infarction, angina, or CHF. Other studies comparing general anesthesia with combined epidural-general anesthesia for abdominal aortic surgery found no differences in perioperative cardiovascular outcome.[94, 95] The carotid endarterectomy literature comparing regional anesthesia with general anesthesia has also failed to demonstrate a significant difference in cardiac outcome between techniques.

A study by Charlson and coworkers,[20] looking at patients at risk for postoperative renal dysfunction (hypertensives and diabetics), concluded that patients whose MAP fell below the preoperative baseline (<20 mm Hg) for greater than 60 minutes or rose above baseline (>20 mm Hg) for greater than 30 minutes and received less than 300 ml/hr of fluids had significantly increased postoperative renal dysfunction. It was also noted in this study that postoperative renal dysfunction varied with the anesthetic technique. The incidence of renal dysfunction was higher in patients receiving regional or centroneuraxial anesthesia than in those receiving general anesthesia. However, after further analysis, taking into account the occurrence of the

three significant predictors of renal dysfunction listed previously, the type of anesthesia was not an independent predictor of postoperative renal dysfunction in these patients.

The incidence of perioperative stroke in the general surgery population is low, and it is unlikely that a study comparing anesthetic technique with stroke rate in hypertensive patients would show a significant difference among techniques. In a prospective study by Larsen and colleagues,[18] looking at postoperative cerebrovascular accidents in general surgery, anesthetic technique was not found to be a significant predictor of postoperative cerebrovascular accidents. Furthermore, the carotid endarterectomy literature has failed to demonstrate a difference in neurological outcome between regional and general techniques. There are no particular anesthetic techniques or specific drug combinations that have been shown to be better than others for the hypertensive patient. The choice of general or regional anesthesia, or a combination of both, depends primarily on the skill and experience of the anesthesiologist rather than on the apparent suitability of any technique in the hands of others.[16]

Choice of Monitoring in Hypertensive Patients

Monitoring is a decision the anesthesiologist must make. A history of hypertension, by itself, is not an indication for additional hemodynamic monitoring. Rather, the patient's coexisting disease (coronary artery disease, CHF, renal insufficiency, cerebrovascular disease), the planned operative procedure, and the duration of the procedure weigh more heavily into monitoring decisions. Routine monitoring for anesthesia includes noninvasive BP cuff, pulse oximetry, capnography, continuous electrocardiographic monitoring, and temperature monitoring. Invasive hemodynamic monitors (arterial line, central venous pressure, or pulmonary artery catheter) should not be used without considering the risks. Five-lead electrocardiographic monitoring should be used in hypertensive patients, since it enhances ischemia detection with no additional patient risk. Bladder catheterization should be considered for longer procedures to monitor urine output.

Intracranial, intrathoracic, major vascular, and cardiac surgery require invasive monitoring based on the hemodynamic insults and hemodynamic requirements of the procedure alone. Whereas a patient with severe renal disease, hypertension, angina, and a history of CHF could undergo the creation of a primary arteriovenous fistula under MAC with routine monitors, the same patient would require invasive arterial and central venous monitoring for a total hip replacement. For major or prolonged operations, it is preferable to monitor BP through an arterial line. When an arterial line is planned, it should be inserted before induction, since induction is one of the phases when cardiovascular lability is greatest.[2] In extensive surgeries, procedures with large intravascular volume shifts, hypertensive emergencies, and in the presence of severe myocardial dysfunction, central monitoring with a central venous or pulmonary artery catheter should be undertaken.[2, 16, 19] When uncertainty exists regarding monitoring, it is probably safer to err in favor of the monitoring device. Increased monitoring of high-risk cardiac patients during the perioperative period has been shown to decrease postoperative morbidity.[96]

In summary, although various monitoring approaches can be recommended, we believe that there is no preponderant evidence to support any particular anesthetic approach over another in the hypertensive patient.

OPERATIVE COURSE

Before inducing anesthesia, the anesthesiologist must have a plan for managing intraoperative hemodynamics. This plan includes setting certain hemodynamic limits that will be tolerated intraoperatively. What are the safe levels for hypertension and hypotension? Some anesthesiologists attempt to maintain a patient's BP within 20% of the "preoperative baseline." Others review the medical record and pick a range of pressures at which the patient "normally lives" symptom free. For example, if a patient has a BP of 180/100 mm Hg during the daytime and 100/60 mm Hg at night, with neither causing physiological insult, the patient should be able to tolerate these extremes under anesthesia. A patient's coexisting disease(s), the effect of hypertension on cerebral autoregulation, and the operative procedure are all considered. Thresholds may be lowered to prevent rupture of vascular anastomoses and may be raised to prevent cerebral ischemia during carotid endarterectomy.

The goal of this section is not to define acceptable limits or give management strategies based on certain procedures, but rather to illustrate some of the issues involved in the decision-making process. After setting the physiological parameters, the pharmacological means to achieve these goals must be considered. Again, the operative procedure is a major factor. For example, aortic surgery and cardiac surgery demand precise hemodynamic control, and the use of a sodium nitroprusside infusion is routine. The management of cerebrovascular surgery also demands strict hemodynamic control. In this instance, the choice of pharmacological intervention must take into account the effects on cerebroautoregulation and intracranial pressure. Other procedures, such as resection of a carcinoid tumor or pheochromocytoma, have unique perioperative management strategies based on the pathophysiology of the hemodynamic derangement. For the majority of patients undergoing general surgical or orthopedic procedures, intermittent intravenous boluses of appropriate vasoactive drugs are used to control hemodynamics, whereas continuous infusion is used if the stimuli or causes of perturbation are judged to be persistent.

Induction and Intubation

Induction of anesthesia with rapidly acting intravenous drugs is acceptable, recognizing that an exaggerated decrease in BP may occur. The choice of induction agent is not as critical as the method of administration. A large initial bolus is more likely to cause hypotension than a slower, titrated induction. Using pharmacological agents that cause peripheral vasodilatation in a population with elevated SVR and mild hypovolemia explains the common occurrence of hypotension. Giving a small volume load

before induction may help attenuate this hypotensive response. Laryngoscopy and intubation of the trachea can result in a hypertensive and tachycardic response in normotensive patients. The response in hypertensive patients, even patients considered to be well treated, can be exaggerated. There are many ways of controlling the hemodynamic response to laryngoscopy and intubation:[97] Preoperative clonidine, topical treatment of the airway with lidocaine, intravenous lidocaine, intravenous nitroprusside, and intravenous esmolol before intubation are some of the reported methods.[25, 98–100] Using a modest dose of narcotic (fentanyl 5 to 8 μg/kg) before intubation and limiting laryngoscopy to 15 seconds or less are also very effective in reducing the hemodynamic response. After intubation, the patient is often placed on mechanical, positive-pressure ventilation. This can cause a reduction in preload with a resultant drop in cardiac output and BP. Usually, gentle volume expansion solves this problem.

Maintenance and Emergence

Maintenance of anesthesia can be accomplished with any of a number of techniques. Often, a "balanced" technique is used. The combination of N_2O, a narcotic, and a low-dose inhalation agent provides a technique that is rapidly titratable to operative stimuli and hemodynamic responses. The goal during maintenance of anesthesia is to anticipate surgical stimuli and adjust the anesthetic depth in order to minimize hemodynamic responses. Both inhalation and intravenous drugs should be given to maintain therapeutic levels; thus, continuous administration is the most rational method.[101] Appropriate fluid management to minimize direct and indirect intravascular volume change also limits hemodynamic lability during maintenance. Preoperative treatment with clonidine improves intraoperative hemodynamics in hypertensive patients,[102, 103] and perioperative β-blockers can blunt the hypertensive and tachycardic response to noxious stimuli.[12, 104] The benefits of perioperative β-blockers in reducing perioperative ischemia[9] and decreasing cardiovascular morbidity and mortality in high-risk patients[26] cannot be overemphasized.

Hypertension that occurs during maintenance of anesthesia can be treated by increasing anesthetic depth or by administering an intravenous antihypertensive agent. Drugs commonly used intraoperatively include labetalol, esmolol, metoprolol, and hydralazine. Intravenous calcium channel blockers and angiotensin-converting enzyme inhibitors are also available. Severe, resistant hypertension is usually managed with intravenous infusions of sodium nitroprusside or nitroglycerin, or a combination of both. Fenoldopam, a new selective dopamine D_1-agonist recently approved by the U.S. Food and Drug Administration, also shows promise in the management of resistant/emergent hypertensive episodes. Administered by a continuous infusion, fenoldopam has reported efficacy and titratability similar to those of nitroprusside. In addition to lowering BP, fenoldopam significantly increases urine flow, sodium excretion, and creatinine clearance.[105–107] Although further evaluation is needed, fenoldopam is an exciting new antihypertensive agent that may be the drug of choice in certain patient populations (i.e., those with renal insufficiency).

Table 81–6 Consequences of Perioperative Hypertension
Mortality
Myocardial ischemia
Myocarial infarction
Increased hemorrhage (surgical bleeding)
Intracranial hemorrhage
Disruption of vascular surgical incision sites
Congestive heart failure
Increased intracranial pressure
Hypertensive encephalopathy
Prolonged hospital stay
Added hospital costs

From Skarvan K. Perioperative hypertension: New strategies for management. Curr Opin Anaesthesiol 11:29–35, 1998.

Intraoperative hypotension can be treated by decreasing anesthetic depth, increasing intravenous fluids, or giving a sympathomimetic drug such as phenylephrine or ephedrine. Although phenylephrine and ephedrine usually resolve hypotension and help preserve vital organ perfusion, this treatment should be considered a temporizing measure until the underlying problem is sought and corrected.

Emergence from anesthesia involves turning off the anesthetic agents and allowing the patient to awaken. Tracheal stimulation from the endotracheal tube and operative pain can cause severe hypertension at this point secondary to catecholamine responses.[7] Extubation of the trachea under deep general anesthesia and using pharmacological means to blunt hemodynamics are options for managing emergence.

POSTOPERATIVE MANAGEMENT

Perioperative hypertension is associated with many adverse outcomes (Table 81–6). Therefore, when possible, it should be prevented. One of the most significant predictors of postoperative hypertension is a history of hypertension preoperatively.[108] Aggressive treatment to prevent myocardial ischemia, CHF, stroke, bleeding, and rupture of vascular suture lines is necessary. Although the hypertension may not have an identifiable cause, secondary etiologies should be considered. Excluding postoperative pain, hypoxia, and hypercarbia should be routine. Iatrogenic hypervolemia can cause hypertension, as can a distended bladder. Aggressive postoperative pain management may decrease the incidence of postoperative hypertension and cardiac morbidity.[109] Management of hypertension in the immediate postoperative period should be an extension of the intraoperative plan. Invasive monitoring should be continued until the patient becomes hemodynamically stable. The same intravenous agents used intraoperatively can be used postoperatively until the patient can return to his or her oral regimen, which should be restarted as soon as possible.[110] In some settings, it is appropriate to have an internist and/or cardiologist consultant assisting in the postoperative control of BP.

SUMMARY

Hypertension is the most prevalent circulatory disorder in the United States, affecting close to 60 million people.

Surgical patients with hypertension are at increased risk for perioperative hemodynamic lability, myocardial ischemia, myocardial infarction, CHF, renal failure, and stroke (see Table 81–6). Hypertensive patients often have significant coexisting diseases; appropriate preoperative evaluation and use of consultants are necessary to optimize these patients' medical management and minimize their perioperative risk. Patients with well-controlled hypertension have a lower risk for perioperative complications than patients with uncontrolled hypertension. Elective procedures should be postponed and appropriate medical management initiated when uncontrolled hypertension is evident (BP 110 mm Hg diastolic). No particular anesthetic technique (general, centroneuraxial, major nerve block, MAC) has been shown to improve morbidity and mortality in the hypertensive patient. However, familiarity with the hemodynamic consequences of the various anesthetic techniques, knowledge of the interactions between antihypertensive medications and anesthetic agents, appropriate hemodynamic monitoring, and early recognition and treatment of intraoperative hypertension, hypotension, and ischemia are necessary. The development of postoperative hypertension also requires swift detection and treatment to prevent perioperative complications (see Table 81–6). In short, the hypertensive surgical patient is at increased risk for perioperative morbidity and mortality. These risks can be minimized with optimal preoperative preparation and prompt assessment and treatment of adverse hemodynamic changes in the intraoperative and postoperative period.

References

1. Barker WH, Mullooly JP, Linton KLP. Trends in hypertension prevalence, treatment, and control in a well-defined older population. Hypertension 31:552–559, 1998.
2. Foex P. Anesthesia for the hypertensive patient. Cleve Clin Q 48:63–67, 1981.
3. Skarvan K. Perioperative hypertension: New strategies for management. Curr Opin Anaesthesiol 11:29–35, 1998.
4. Goldman L, Caldera DL. Risks of general anesthesia and elective operation in the hypertensive patient. Anesthesiology 50:285–292, 1979.
5. Estafanous FG, Tarazi RC, Viljonan JF, El Tawil MY. Systemic hypertension following myocardial revascularization. Am Heart J 85:732–738, 1973.
6. Hans SS, Glover JL. The relationship of cardiac and neurological complications to blood pressure changes following carotid endarterectomy. Am Surg 61:356–359, 1995.
7. Wallach R, Karp RB, Reves JG, et al. Pathogenesis of paroxysmal hypertension developing during and after coronary artery bypass surgery: A study of hemodynamic and humoral factors. Am J Cardiol 46:559–565, 1980.
8. Joint National Committee on Detection, Evaluation, and Treatment of High Blood Pressure. The fifth report. Arch Intern Med 153:154–183, 1993.
9. Stone JG, Foex P, Sear JW, et al. Risk of myocardial ischaemia during anaesthesia in treated and untreated hypertensive patients. Br J Anaesth 61:675–679, 1988.
10. Prys-Roberts C, Meloche R, Foex P, Ryder A. Studies of anaesthesia in relation to hypertension. I: Cardiovascular responses of treated and untreated patients. Br J Anaesth 43:122–137, 1971.
11. Bedford RF, Feinstein B. Hospital admission blood pressure: A predictor of hypertension following endotracheal intubation. Anesth Analg 59:367–370, 1980.
12. Prys-Roberts C, Foex P, Biro GP, Roberts JG. Studies of anaesthesia in relation to hypertension. Adrenergic beta-receptor blockade. Br J Anaesth 45:671–680, 1973.
13. Prys-Roberts C, Greene LT, Meloche R, Foex P. Studies of anaesthe-

sia in relation to hypertension. Haemodynamic consequences of induction and endotracheal intubation. Br J Anaesth 43:531–546, 1971.

14. Steen PA, Tinker JH, Tarhan S. Myocardial reinfarction after anesthesia and surgery. JAMA 239:2566–2570, 1978.

15. Charlson ME, MacKenzie CR, Gold JP, et al. Postoperative renal dysfunction can be predicted. Surg Gynecol Obstet 169:303–309, 1989.

16. Prys-Roberts C. Anaesthesia and hypertension. Br J Anaesth 56:711–724, 1984.

17. Asiddao CB, Donegan JH, Whitesell RC, Kalbfleisch JH. Factors associated with perioperative complications during carotid endarterectomy. Anesth Analg 61:631, 1982.

18. Larsen SF, Zaric D, Boysen G. Postoperative cerebrovascular accidents in general surgery. Acta Anaesthesiol Scand 32:698–701, 1988.

19. Estafanous F. Hypertension in the surgical patient: Management of blood pressure and anesthesia. Cleve Clin J Med 56:385–393, 1989.

20. Charlson ME, MacKenzie CR, Gold JP, et al. Preoperative characteristics predicting intraoperative hypotension and hypertension among hypertensives and diabetics undergoing noncardiac surgery. Ann Surg 212:66–81, 1990.

21. Racle JP, Poy JY, Haberer JP, Benkhadra A. A comparison of cardiovascular responses of normotensive and hypertensive elderly patients following bupivacaine spinal anesthesia. Reg Anesth 14:66–71, 1989.

22. Slogoff S, Keats AS. Does perioperative myocardial ischemia lead to postoperative myocardial infarction? Anesthesia 62:107–114, 1985.

23. Reves JG, Gelman S. Cardiovascular effects of intravenous anesthetic drugs. In Covino F, Rehder K, Strichartz GR (eds). Effects of Anesthesia. Bethesda, MD, American Physiological Society, 1985; pp 179–193.

24. Freis ED. Salt in hypertension and the effects of diuretics. Annu Rev Pharmacol Toxicol 19:13–23, 1979.

25. Sharma S, Mitra S, Grover VK, Kalra R. Esmolol blunts the haemodynamic responses to tracheal intubation in treated hypertensive patients. Can J Anaesth 43:778–782, 1996.

26. Mangano DT, Layug EL, Wallace A, Tateo I. Effect of atenolol on mortality and cardiovascular morbidity after noncardiac surgery. N Engl J Med 335:1713–1720, 1996.

27. Quintin L, Bouilloc X, Butin E, et al. Clonidine for major vascular surgery in hypertensive patients: A double-blind, controlled, randomized study. Anesth Analg 83:687–695, 1996.

28. Reves J, Sladen R, Newman M. Multicenter study of target-controlled infusion of propofol-sufentanil or sufentanil-midazolam for coronary artery bypass graft surgery. Anesthesiology 85:522–535, 1996.

29. Reves JG, Hill S, Berkowitz D. Pharmacology of intravenous anesthetic induction drugs. In Kaplan J, Reich DL, Konstadt SN (eds). Cardiac Anesthesia, 4th ed. Philadelphia, WB Saunders, 1999; pp 611–634.

30. Reves JG, Greeley WJ, Grichnik K, et al. Anesthesia and supportive care for cardiothoracic surgery. In Sabiston DC Jr, Spencer FC (eds). Surgery of the Chest, 6th ed. Philadelphia, WB Saunders, 1995; pp 117–152.

31. Dentz ME, Grichnik KP, Sibert KS, Reves JG. Anesthesia and postoperative analgesia. In Sabiston DC Jr (ed). Textbook of Surgery. Philadelphia, WB Saunders, 1996; pp 186–206.

32. Gould JD, Reves JG, D'Ercole FJ, et al. Effect of anesthetic technique on blood pressure response in hypertensive patients. Anesth Analg 88:SCA1–SCA126, 1999.

33. Khatri I, Freis E. Hemodynamic changes during sleep. J Appl Physiol 22:867, 1967.

34. Garnett RL, MacIntyre A, Lindsay P, et al. Perioperative ischaemia in aortic surgery: Combined epidural/general anesthesia and epidural analgesia vs. general anaesthesia and iv analgesia. Can J Anaesth 43:769–777, 1996.

35. Olesen A, Huttel M, Hole P. Venous sequelae following the injection of etomidate or thiopentone IV. Br J Anaesth 56:171, 1984.

36. Seltzer J, Gerson J, Allen F. Comparison of the cardiovascular effects of bolus v. incremental administration of thiopentone. Br J Anaesth 52:527, 1980.

37. Sonntag H, Hellberg K, Schenk H, et al. Effects of thiopental (Trapanal) on coronary blood flow and myocardial metabolism in man. Acta Anaesthesiol Scand 19:69, 1975.

38. Toner W, Howard P, McGowan W, et al. Another look at acute tolerance to thiopentone. Br J Anaesth 52:1005, 1980.

39. Frankl W, Poole-Wilson P. Effects of thiopental on tension develop-

ment, action potential, and exchange of calcium and potassium in rabbit ventricular myocardium. J Cardiovasc Pharmacol 3:554, 1981.

40. Christensen J, Andreasen F, Jansen J. Pharmacokinetics and pharmacodynamics of thiopentone. A comparison between young and elderly patients. Anaesthesia 37:398, 1982.

41. Filner B, Karliner J. Alterations of normal left ventricular performance by general anesthesia. Anesthesiology 45:610, 1976.

42. Reiz S, Balfors E, Friedman A, et al. Effects of thiopentone on cardiac performance, coronary hemodynamics and myocardial oxygen consumption in chronic ischemic heart disease. Acta Anaesthesiol Scand 25:103, 1981.

43. Flickinger H, Fraimow W, Cathcart R, et al. Effect of thiopental induction on cardiac output in man. Anesth Analg 40:694, 1961.

44. White P. Comparative evaluation of intravenous agents for rapid sequence induction—Thiopental, ketamine and midazolam. Anesthesiology 57:279, 1982.

45. Pedersen T, Engbaek J, Klausen N, et al. Effects of low-dose ketamine and thiopentone on cardiac performance and myocardial oxygen balance in high-risk patients. Acta Anaesthesiol Scand 26:235, 1982.

46. King E. The treatment of army casualties in Hawaii. Army Med Bull 61:18, 1942.

47. Richter J. Current theories about the mechanisms of benzodiazepines and neuroleptic drugs. Anesthesiology 54:66, 1981.

48. Rao S, Sherbanuik R, Prasad K, et al. Cardiopulmonary effects of diazepam. Clin Pharmacol Ther 14:182, 1973.

49. Prakash R, Thurer R, Vargas A, et al. Cardiovascular effects of diazepam induction in patients for aortocoronary saphenous vein bypass grafts. Abstracts of Scientific Papers, ASA Annual Meeting. San Francisco, October 1976.

50. Jackson A, Dhadphale P, Callaghan M, et al. Haemodynamic studies during induction of anaesthesia for open-heart surgery using diazepam and ketamine. Br J Anaesth 50:375, 1978.

51. McCammon R, Hilgenberg J, Stoelting R. Hemodynamic effects of diazepam and diazepam–nitrous oxide in patients with coronary artery disease. Anesth Analg 59:438, 1980.

52. Samuelson P, Lell W, Kouchoukos N, et al. Hemodynamics during diazepam induction of anesthesia for coronary artery bypass grafting. South Med J 73:332, 1980.

53. Samuelson P, Reves J, Kouchoukos N, et al. Hemodynamic responses to anesthetic induction with midazolam or diazepam in patients with ischemic heart disease. Anesth Analg 60:802, 1981.

54. D'Amelio G, Volta S, Stritoni P, et al. Acute cardiovascular effects of diazepam in patients with mitral valve disease. Eur J Clin Pharmacol 6:61, 1973.

55. Bailey P, Stanley T. Pharmacology of intravenous narcotic anesthetics. In Miller R (ed). Anesthesia. London, Churchill Livingstone, 1986; pp 745–798.

56. Hoar P, Nelson N, Mangano D, et al. Adrenergic response to morphine-diazepam anesthesia for myocardial revascularization. Anesth Analg 60:406, 1981.

57. Melsom M, Andreassen P, Melsom H, et al. Diazepam in acute myocardial infarction. Clinical effects and effects on catecholamines, free fatty acids and cortisol. Br Heart J 38:804, 1976.

58. Stanley T, Bennett G, Loeser E, et al. Cardiovascular effects of diazepam and droperidol during morphine anesthesia. Anesthesiology 44:255, 1976.

59. Tomichek R, Rosow C, Schneider R, et al. Cardiovascular effects of diazepam-fentanyl anesthesia in patients with coronary artery disease. Anesth Analg 61:217, 1982.

60. Reves J, Fragen R, Vinik H, et al. Midazolam: Pharmacology and uses. Anesthesiology 62:310, 1985.

61. Reves J, Samuelson P, Lewis S. Midazolam maleate induction in patients with ischemic heart disease. Haemodynamic observations. Can Anaesth Soc J 26:402, 1979.

62. Reves J, Samuelson P, Linnan M. Effects of midazolam maleate in patients with elevated pulmonary artery occluded pressure. In Aldrete J, Stanley T (eds). Trends in Intravenous Anesthesia. Chicago, Year Book Medical, 1980; pp 253–257.

63. Lunn J, Stanley T, Eisele J, et al. High-dose fentanyl anesthesia for coronary artery surgery. Plasma fentanyl concentrations and influence of nitrous oxide on cardiovascular responses. Anesth Analg 58:390, 1979.

64. Melvin M, Johnson B, Quasha A, et al. Induction of anesthesia with midazolam decreases halothane MAC in humans. Anesthesiology 57:238, 1982.

65. Newman M, Reves J. Pro: Midazolam is the sedative of choice to supplement narcotic anesthesia. [Review] J Cardiothorac Vasc Anesth 7:615–619, 1993.

66. Theil D, Stanley T, White W, et al. Midazolam and fentanyl continuous infusion anesthesia for cardiac surgery: A comparison of computer-assisted versus manual infusion systems. J Cardiothorac Vasc Anesth 7:300–306, 1993.

67. Kay B, Rolly G. ICI 35 868, a new intravenous induction agent. Acta Anaesth Belg 28:303, 1977.

68. Profeta J, Guffin A, Mikula S, et al. The hemodynamic effects of propofol and thiamylal sodium for induction in coronary artery surgery. Anesth Analg 66:S142, 1987.

69. De Hert S, Vermeyen K, Adriensen H. Influence of thiopental, etomidate and propofol on regional myocardial function in the normal and acute ischemic heart segments. Anesth Analg 70:600, 1990.

70. Mulier J, Wouters P, Van Aken H, et al. Cardiodynamic effects of propofol in comparison with thiopental: Assessment with a transesophageal echocardiographic approach. Anesth Analg 72:28, 1991.

71. Brussel T, Theissen J, Vigfusson G, et al. Hemodynamic and cardiodynamic effects of propofol and etomidate: Negative inotropic properties of propofol. Anesth Analg 69:35, 1989.

72. Patrick M, Blair I, Feneck R, Sebel P. Comparison of the hemodynamic effects of propofol (Diprivan) on thiopentone in patients with coronary artery disease. Postgrad Med J 61:23, 1985.

73. Vermeyen K, Erpels F, Janssen L, et al. Propofol-fentanyl anaesthesia for coronary bypass surgery in patients with good left ventricular function. Br J Anaesth 59:1115, 1987.

74. Stephan H, Sonntag H, Schenk H, et al. Effects of propofol on cardiovascular dynamics, myocardial blood flow and myocardial metabolism in patients with coronary artery disease. Br J Anaesth 58:969, 1986.

75. Brown B, Crout R. A comparative study of the effects of five general anesthetics on myocardial contractility. Anesthesiology 34:236, 1971.

76. Merin RG, Basch S. Are the myocardial functional and metabolic effects of isoflurane really different from those of halothane and enflurane? Anesthesiology 55:398–408, 1981.

77. Price ML, Price HL. Effect of general anesthetics on contractile response of rabbit aorta strips. Anesthesiology 23:16–20, 1962.

78. Mallow JE, White RD, Cucchiara RF. Hemodynamic effects of isoflurane and halothane in patients with coronary artery disease. Anesth Analg 55:135–138, 1976.

79. Kleinman B, Szinn E, Shah K, et al. The value to the anesthesia-surgical care team of the preoperative cardiac consultation. J Cardiothorac Anesth 3:682–687, 1989.

80. Wells PH, Kaplan JA. Optimal management of patients with ischemic heart disease for noncardiac surgery by complementary anesthesiologist and cardiologist interaction. Am Heart J 102:1029–1037, 1981.

81. Goldman L, Lee T, Rudd P. Ten commandments for effective consultations. Arch Intern Med 143:1753–1755, 1983.

82. Lee T, Pappius EM, Goldman L. Impact of inter-physician communication on the effectiveness of medical consultations. Am J Med 74:106–112, 1983.

83. Rudd P. Contrasts in academic consultation. Ann Intern Med 94:537–538, 1981.

84. Yaeger MP, Glass DD, Neff RK, Brinck-Johnsen T. Epidural anesthesia and analgesia in high-risk surgical patients. Anesthesiology 66:729–736, 1987.

85. Dagnino J, Prys-Roberts C. Evaluation of beta-adrenoceptor responsiveness during anesthesia in humans. Anesth Analg 62:255, 1983.

86. Bode RH, Lewis KP, Zarich SW, et al. Cardiac outcome after peripheral vascular surgery. Anesthesiology 84:3–13, 1996.

87. Cook PT, Davies MJ, Cronin KD, Moran P. A prospective randomized trial comparing spinal anaesthesia using hyperbaric cincocaine with general anaesthesia for lower limb vascular surgery. Anaesth Intensive Care 14:373–380, 1986.

88. Rivers SP, Scher LA, Sheehan E, Veith FJ. Epidural versus general anesthesia for infrainguinal arterial reconstruction. J Vasc Surg 14:764–770, 1991.

89. Christopherson R, Beattie C, Frank SM, et al. Perioperative morbidity in patients randomized to epidural or general anesthesia for lower extremity vascular surgery. Anesthesiology 79:422–434, 1993.

90. CASANOVA Study Group. Carotid surgery versus medical therapy in asymptomatic carotid stenosis. Stroke 22:1229–1235, 1991.

91. Executive Committee for the Asymptomatic Carotid Atherosclerosis Study. Endarterectomy for asymptomatic carotid artery stenosis. JAMA 273:1421–1428, 1995.

92. Godin MS, Bell WH, Schwedler M, et al. Cost effectiveness of regional anesthesia in carotid endarterectomy. Am Surg 55:656–659, 1989.

93. Shah DM, Darling RC, Chang BB, et al. Carotid endarterectomy in awake patients: Its safety, acceptability, and outcome. J Vasc Surg 19:1015–1020, 1994.

94. Haku E, Hayashi M, Kato H. Anesthetic management of abdominal aortic surgery: A retrospective review of perioperative complications. J Cardiothorac Anesth 3:587–591, 1989.

95. Baron JF, Bertrand M, Barre E, et al. Combined epidural and general anesthesia versus general anesthesia for abdominal aortic surgery. Anesthesiology 75:611–618, 1991.

96. Rao TLK, Jacobs KH, El-Etr AA. Reinfarction following anesthesia in patients with myocardial infarction. Anesthesiology 59:499–505, 1983.

97. Kovac AL. Controlling the hemodynamic response to laryngoscopy and endotracheal intubation. J Clin Anesth 8:63–79, 1996.

98. Stoelting RK. Circulatory response to laryngoscopy and tracheal intubation with or without prior oropharyngeal viscous lidocaine. Anesth Analg 56:618–621, 1977.

99. Stoelting RK. Circulatory changes during direct laryngoscopy and tracheal intubation: Influence of duration of laryngoscopy with or without prior lidocaine. Anesthesiology 47:381–384, 1977.

100. Stoelting RK. Attenuation of blood pressure response to laryngoscopy and tracheal intubation with sodium nitroprusside. Anesth Analg 58:116–119, 1979.

101. Smith BE, Reves JG. Computer-assisted continuous infusion of intravenous anesthesia drugs. Int Anesthesiol Clin, vol. 33, no. 3, 1995.

102. Ghignone M, Calvillo O, Quintin L. Anesthesia and hypertension: The effect of clonidine on perioperative hemodynamics and isoflurane requirements. Anesthesiology 67:3–10, 1987.

103. Flacke JW, Bloor BC, Flacke WE, et al. Reduced narcotic requirement by clonidine with improved hemodynamic and adrenergic stability in patients undergoing coronary bypass surgery. Anesthesiology 67:11–19, 1987.

104. Prys-Roberts C. Interactions of anaesthesia and high pre-operative doses of beta-receptor antagonists. Acta Anaesthesiol Scand 74:27, 1982.

105. Elliott WJ, Weber RR, Nelson KS, et al. Renal and hemodynamic effects of intravenous fenoldopam versus nitroprusside in severe hypertension. Circulation 81:970–977, 1990.

106. Murphy MB, McCoy CE, Weber RR, et al. Augmentation of renal blood flow and sodium excretion in hypertensive patients during blood pressure reduction by intravenous administration of the dopamine-1 agonist fenoldopam. Circulation 76:1312–1318, 1987.

107. Panacek EA, Bednarczyk EM, Dunbar LM, et al. Randomized, prospective trial of fenoldopam vs sodium nitroprusside in the treatment of acute severe hypertension. Acad Emerg Med 2:959–965, 1995.

108. Gal TJ, Cooperman LH Hypertension in the immediate postoperative period. Br J Anaesth 47:70–74, 1975.

109. Weiss SJ, Longnecker DE. Perioperative hypertension: An overview. Coron Artery Dis 4:401–406, 1993.

110. Joint National Committee on Prevention, Detection, Evaluation, and Treatment of High Blood Pressure. The sixth report. Arch Intern Med 157:2413–2446, 1997.

82 Hypertensive Crisis
David A. Calhoun

Hypertensive crisis is defined as a severe elevation in blood pressure, generally a systolic blood pressure greater than 220 mm Hg and/or a diastolic blood pressure greater than 120 to 130 mm Hg.[1] More important than the absolute blood pressure, however, is the rate of rise of the blood pressure in relation to previous levels of blood pressure. A person with chronic, poorly controlled blood pressure can tolerate a much higher blood pressure level than a previously normotensive person. Accordingly, in assessing the need for acute intervention, more important than the level of blood pressure is evidence of acute target organ deterioration. *Hypertensive emergencies* are severe elevations in blood pressure complicated by acute target organ dysfunction, such as coronary ischemia, stroke, intracerebral hemorrhage, pulmonary edema, or acute renal failure (Table 82–1). Hypertensive emergencies require immediate blood pressure reduction. This is most safely accomplished in the intensive care setting with use of an intravenous agent. *Hypertensive urgencies* are severe elevations in blood pressure without evidence of target organ deterioration. Immediate blood pressure reduction is not indicated, and instead, blood pressure should be reduced gradually in an outpatient setting. Acute blood pressure lowering with clonidine loading or short-acting nifedipine is not indicated and may be hazardous.

With the advent of better tolerated, long-acting antihypertensive agents, hypertensive crisis became less common, with an estimated prevalence rate of 1% among hypertensive patients.[2] This contrasts with a 7% incidence of accelerated hypertension with papilledema in patients with untreated primary hypertension before the availability of modern antihypertensive therapies.[3] There is concern, however, that the incidence of hypertensive crisis may be increasing. Between 1983 and 1992, hospital admissions for malignant hypertension increased from 16,000 to 35,000 in the United States.[4] This increase may be due in

part to differences in coding, but such differences likely would not account for the total increase. Hypertensive emergencies occur most frequently in patients previously diagnosed with primary hypertension but who are noncompliant. Men, African Americans, persons of lower socioeconomic status, and smokers are at increased risk.

The long-term prognosis of untreated severe or accelerated hypertension is abysmal. In 1939, Keith and colleagues[5] found that patients with hypertension and grade IV retinopathy had a mean survival of 10.5 months, with no survivors at 5 years. Most patients died of complications of uremia. With development of the first successful oral antihypertensive agents in the 1950s, survival improved dramatically. In 1958, Dustan and coworkers[6] found that among 84 patients being treated for malignant hypertension, 70% survived 1 year and 33% survived 5 years. The most common causes of death were renal failure, cerebral hemorrhage, and myocardial infarction. In the 1960s, with use of more effective and better tolerated antihypertensive agents, 5-year survival rates of patients treated for malignant hypertension were 50 to 60%.[7] With increased use of dialysis, 5-year survival rates continued to improve throughout the 1970s, reaching approximately 75%.[8] Current survival of patients with severe hypertension approaches that of patients with uncomplicated primary hypertension. Using life-table analysis, Webster and associates[9] estimated survival of patients with malignant hypertension at 18 years versus 21 years in patients with uncomplicated hypertension. The primary cause of death in patients with accelerated hypertension was myocardial infarction.

HYPERTENSIVE EMERGENCY

Pathophysiology

The cause of hypertensive crisis remains speculative. It is believed that an abrupt increase in systemic vascular resistance, such as occurs secondary to noncompliance, triggers an increase in circulating levels of vasoconstrictor substances, including norepinephrine, angiotensin II, and antinatriuretic hormone.[10] Arteriolar fibrinoid necrosis ensues as a consequence of the severely elevated blood pressure, precipitating endothelial damage, platelet and fibrin deposition, and loss of autoregulatory function, with resultant target organ ischemia. Ischemia, in turn, triggers the further release of vasoactive substances, thus initiating a vicious circle of further vasoconstriction and myointimal proliferation. If unchecked, target organ extravasation and/ or infarction ensues.

Treatment

The goal of therapy is to reduce systemic vascular resistance. Animal and human studies indicate that organ perfu-

---

Table 82–1 Types of Hypertensive Emergencies

Hypertensive encephalopathy
Intracerebral hemorrhage
Subarachnoid hemorrhage
Myocardial ischemia
Myocardial infarction
Acute pulmonary edema
Aortic dissection
Eclampsia
Acute renal insufficiency
Grade II or IV Keith-Wagner funduscopic changes
Microangiopathic hemolytic anemia
Catecholamine crisis (pheochromocytoma crisis, cocaine or "crack" overdose)
Acute withdrawal syndromes (β-blockers or centrally acting compounds, such as clonidine)

sion, particularly cerebral perfusion, is generally autoregulated within a fairly wide blood pressure range. However, abrupt changes greater than 25% may exceed the brain's ability to reliably maintain blood flow.[11] Based on these data, the approach in treating hypertensive emergency is to initially reduce mean arterial pressure by about 25%, with further reductions accomplished more gradually. The time course of the initial reduction varies from minutes to hours, according to concomitant target organ damage. In general, the initial reduction should be achieved over a period of 1 to 4 hours, with less rapid reduction over the ensuing 24 hours to a diastolic blood pressure of approximately 100 mm Hg. With the exception of patients with aortic dissection, the blood pressure should not be reduced to normotensive and especially hypotensive levels, as target organ hypoperfusion may result. Normalization of blood pressure should be accomplished later on an outpatient basis.

Drug Choice

The drug of choice for acutely reducing blood pressure, in most cases, is sodium nitroprusside (Table 82–2). It is very potent, with an almost instantaneous onset and withdrawal of action that allows for minute-by-minute titration. Be-

cause of its potency, use of an intraarterial line to monitor blood pressure is usually required to avoid overreduction in blood pressure. Cyanide and thiocyanate, potentially toxic metabolites of nitroprusside, can accumulate during prolonged or high-dose infusions, particularly in the setting of renal insufficiency.

Owing to its coronary vasodilator effect, nitroglycerin is the drug of choice for reducing blood pressure in the setting of myocardial ischemia or infarction. Nitroglycerin also dilates cerebral vessels such that headache, which is often severe, can be anticipated. The blood pressure response to nitroglycerin is not as predictable as with nitroprusside. In addition, tolerance will often occur with extended infusions.

Fenoldopam is a peripherally acting dopamine-1 agonist that was recently approved for use as a parenteral antihypertensive agent. Stimulation of the dopamine-1 receptor reduces blood pressure secondary to arterial vasodilatation. Fenoldopam is unique in that it maintains or even increases renal blood flow in the setting of reduced blood pressure.[12] In addition, fenoldopam has direct renal tubular–mediated natriuretic properties that may prove to be beneficial in certain subsets of patients, such as those with severe hypertension complicated by renal insufficiency.[13] Overall, in patients with and without renal insufficiency, fenoldopam

Table 82–2 Parenteral Agents for Treatment of Hypertensive Emergencies

Drug	Intravenous Dose	Onset of Action	Duration of Action	Adverse Effects/Comments	Indications/Comments
Nitroprusside	0.25–10 µg/kg/min	Immediate	1–2 min	Nausea, vomiting, tachycardia, fluid retention, fasciculations; risk of thiocyanate and cyanide toxicity increased with renal insufficiency, higher doses, and prolonged infusion; patient must be shielded from light	Most hypertensive emergencies
Nitroglycerin	5–100 µg/min	2–5 min	2–5 min	Headache, nausea; tolerance can occur with prolonged use; risk of methemoglobinemia increases with prolonged use	Angina, acute myocardial infarction
Labetalol	20–80 mg IV bolus q 5–10 min; 0.5–2.0 mg/min	5–10 min	3–6 hr	Heart block, bradycardia, heart failure, bronchospasm, nausea, scalp tingling, vomiting, paradoxical pressor response; may not be effective in patients receiving α- or β-antagonists	Most hypertensive emergencies, including aortic dissection and catecholamine crisis; avoid in heart failure
Fenoldopam	0.1–0.3 µg/kg/min	<5 min	30 min	Diuretic effects may exacerbate volume depletion	Most hypertensive emergencies
Hydralazine	5–10 mg q 20 min up to 20 mg	10–20 min	3–6 hr	Headache, nausea, tachycardia, flushing, worsening of angina, local thrombophlebitis (change infusion site after 12 hr)	Eclampsia
Enalaprilat	1.25–5 mg q 6 hr administered over a 5-min period	15–30 min	6–8 hr	Response variable; in high-renin states may see profound drop in blood pressure	Heart failure; pulmonary edema
Nicardipine	5 mg/hr, increase by 1–2.5 mg/hr q 15 min up to 15 mg/hr	5–10 min	1–4 hr	Tachycardia, worsening angina, headache	Most hypertensive emergencies except heart failure, angina, myocardial infarction
Esmolol	500 µg/kg/min for 1 min, then 50–300 µg/kg/min for 4 min; repeat sequence as needed	1–2 min	10–20 min	Nausea	Perioperative hypertension; aortic dissection when used in combination with a vasodilator such as nitroprusside
Phentolamine	5–10 mg q 5–15 min	1–2 min	3–10 min	Tachycardia, headache, angina, paradoxical pressor response	Catecholamine crisis

increases renal blood flow, urine output, creatinine clearance, and sodium and free water excretion with minimal effect on glomerular filtration rate.[14] Nitroprusside tends to have the opposite effects on these parameters.

Clinical studies have shown that fenoldopam is safe and as effective as nitroprusside in reducing blood pressure.[15–17] Its onset of action is less abrupt than nitroprusside such that use of an intraarterial line to monitor blood pressure can generally be avoided. It has other advantages over nitroprusside in that none of its metabolites are toxic, nor is it light sensitive. Fenoldopam is a pure arterial vasodilator and induces little, if any, reduction in right ventricular filling pressures or pulmonary capillary wedge pressure. Accordingly, it is not indicated for treatment of hypertension complicated by congestive heart failure.

Most patients who present with hypertensive crisis have volume depletion, presumably secondary to a pressure-related diuresis. In such cases, further diuresis may exacerbate the hypertension and cause further deterioration in renal function. Accordingly, the use of diuretic agents and/or fluid restriction should be reserved for patients who are clinically fluid-overloaded and should not be prescribed routinely.

SPECIFIC HYPERTENSIVE EMERGENCIES

Hypertensive Encephalopathy

Hypertensive encephalopathy, which had been common before the use of modern antihypertensive agents, is believed to be due to cerebral edema resulting from a failure of cerebral blood flow autoregulation. It occurs at a much higher blood pressure in patients with chronic hypertension than in previously normotensive persons. Symptoms of hypertensive encephalopathy include headache, nausea, vomiting, visual disturbances, confusion, and focal or generalized weakness. Clinical signs include disorientation, obtundation, focal neurological signs, generalized or focal seizures, and retinopathy (including papilledema). Hypertensive encephalopathy is a diagnosis of exclusion requiring that stroke, subarachnoid hemorrhage, mass lesions, seizure disorder, vasculitis, and encephalitis be ruled out.

Treatment goals are to reduce mean arterial pressure by approximately 25% within the first hour or to a diastolic blood pressure of 100 mm Hg, whichever value is higher. Reductions in blood pressure approaching 50% must be avoided, as cerebral hypoperfusion may result. If neurological function deteriorates during treatment, the blood pressure should be allowed to increase. Subsequent reductions in blood pressure should be effected more slowly.

Neurological Complications

Acute blood pressure lowering in the setting of stroke, intracerebral hemorrhage, or subarachnoid hemorrhage remains controversial.[18] In each of these cases, the increase in blood pressure may have contributed to or resulted from the neurological condition. In either event, systemic blood pressure regulation may be precarious, and even minimal intervention may produce precipitous drops in blood pres-

sure. Compounding the hazard is that autoregulation of cerebral blood flow may be compromised in the area of the infarction or bleed. Accordingly, it is generally recommended that acute blood pressure reduction not be attempted except in the case of extreme elevation.[1] If antihypertensive therapy is indicated, the blood pressure should be reduced gradually by approximately 25% or to a diastolic pressure less than 120 mm Hg over a 24-hour period.

Myocardial Ischemia or Infarction

Myocardial ischemia or infarction is a common complication of severe blood pressure elevation. Blood pressure should be reduced until the pain subsides or until a diastolic blood pressure of approximately 100 mm Hg is achieved. Intravenous nitrates, which reduce systemic resistance while improving coronary perfusion, are the antihypertensive treatment of choice. Labetalol can be used alternatively. Nitroprusside can induce a coronary steal–type syndrome and therefore should be reserved for refractory cases.

Congestive Heart Failure

Severe elevations in systemic vascular resistance may precipitate left ventricular failure. Sodium nitroprusside, administered in conjunction with oxygen, morphine, and a loop diuretic, is the treatment of choice, as it effectively reduces both preload and afterload. Nitroglycerin also reduces both preload and afterload and can be used in this setting.

Aortic Dissection

Aortic dissection must be excluded in any patient who presents with severe elevation in blood pressure and with pain in the chest, back, or abdomen. In the emergency department, the immediate reduction of blood pressure and shear stress is essential to halt extension of the dissection. The diastolic blood pressure should be quickly reduced to 100 mm Hg, or as low as can be tolerated without inducing target organ hypoperfusion. The treatment of choice for aortic dissection has classically been a vasodilator such as nitroprusside in combination with a β-blocker. Labetalol has also been effectively used in such cases.[19]

Renal Insufficiency

Acute renal insufficiency may both cause and/or result from severe elevations in blood pressure. In patients with kidney transplants, additional causes of hypertension include stenosis of the graft site, the use of cyclosporine and corticosteroids, and excessive secretion of renin by the native kidney. Therapy should aim to reduce systemic vascular resistance without compromising renal blood flow. Calcium antagonists, such as nicardipine, are used effectively in this setting. Fenoldopam, with its beneficial effects on renal blood flow, would seem to be a good choice, but experience is limited.

Eclampsia

Eclampsia is characterized by the onset of hypertension, edema, proteinuria, and seizures after gestational week 20. Definitive therapy is delivery of the fetus. Interim blood pressure reduction is generally accomplished with hydralazine, as it tends not to compromise uterine blood flow. A small number of studies suggest that labetalol is also effective and well tolerated.

Catecholamine Crisis

Catecholamine crisis is seen with pheochromocytoma and overdoses of cocaine or crack. In the latter case, the crisis is often complicated by drug-induced seizures, stroke, or myocardial infarction. Phentolamine is the classic drug of choice for catecholamine excess, although labetalol is also effective.

Withdrawal Syndromes

Abrupt cessation of centrally acting compounds, such as clonidine or β-blockers, may precipitate a withdrawal syndrome characterized by severe hypertension, nausea, diaphoresis, and/or angina. Treatment is to restart the discontinued agent after initially controlling the blood pressure with intravenous therapy.

HYPERTENSIVE URGENCY

Diagnosis and Treatment

If a patient presents with a severely elevated blood pressure but no evidence by history, physical examination, or laboratory analysis of acute target organ damage, the patient is said to be having a *hypertensive urgency*. Until recently, treatment recommendations were to acutely lower the blood pressure with oral agents, most often short-acting nifedipine or repeated doses of clonidine, on the assumption that the patient was at increased risk for an acute event. This approach was presumptive in that acute blood pressure lowering had never been shown to improve either short- or long-term outcome. In one of the few studies to actually evaluate treatment of hypertensive urgency, patients did equally well whether they received acute blood pressure reduction in the emergency room or were discharged home on standard outpatient therapy.[20] In contrast, there have been a number of anecdotal reports of catastrophic outcomes with sublingual administration of nifedipine.[21] In most cases, a precipitous drop in blood pressure induced a stroke or myocardial infarction. Accordingly, acute blood pressure reduction is not indicated for hypertensive urgency. If the patient had been on an antihyperten-

sive regimen but was noncompliant, the prior therapy should be resumed. If the patient had been compliant, her or his doses of medications should be increased or an additional agent begun. If the patient had not been previously treated, she or he should be started on long-acting monotherapy. In all cases, the patient should have follow-up within a week to ensure compliance and to make adjustments in medications as needed.

References

1. Calhoun DA, Oparil S. Treatment of hypertensive crisis. N Engl J Med 323:1177, 1990.
2. Gudbrandsson T. Malignant hypertension: A clinical follow-up study with special reference to renal and cardiovascular function and immunogenic factors. Acta Med Scand Suppl 650:1, 1981.
3. Calhoun DA, Oparil S. Hypertensive crisis since FDR: A partial victory. N Engl J Med 332:1029, 1995.
4. National Center for Health Statistics: Vital and Health Statistics. Detailed Diagnoses and Procedures for Patients Discharged from Short-Stay Hospitals: United States, 1983–1990. National Health Survey. Hyattsville, MD, U.S. Department of Health and Human Services, 1985–1993.
5. Keith NM, Wagener HP, Barker NW. Some different types of essential hypertension: Their course and prognosis. Am J Med Sci 196:332, 1939.
6. Dustan HP, Schnekloth RE, Corcoran AC, et al. The effectiveness of long-term treatment of malignant hypertension. Circulation 18:644, 1958.
7. Hood B, Orndahl G, Bjork S. Survival and mortality in malignant (grade IV) and grade III hypertension: Trends in consecutive, actively treated groups. Acta Med Scand 187:291, 1970.
8. Gudbrandsson T, Hansson L, Herlitz H, et al. Malignant hypertension—Improving prognosis in a rare disease. Acta Med Scand 206:495, 1979.
9. Webster J, Petrie JC, Jeffers TA, et al. Accelerated hypertension—Pattern of mortality and clinical factors affecting outcome in treated patients. Q J Med 865:485, 1993.
10. Kock-Weser J. Hypertensive emergencies. N Engl J Med 290:211, 1974.
11. Strandgaard S, Paulson OB. Cerebral autoregulation. Stroke 15:413, 1984.
12. Allison NL, Dubb JW, Ziemniak JA, et al. The effect of fenoldopam, a dopaminergic agonist, on renal hemodynamics. Clin Pharmacol Ther 41:282, 1987.
13. Hughes JM, Beck TR, Rose CE Jr, Carey RM. Selective dopamine-1 receptor stimulation produces natriuresis by a direct tubular action. J Hypertens 4(suppl 6):S106, 1986.
14. Calhoun D, Oparil S, Mathur V, et al. Fenoldopam: A novel, peripherally acting dopamine-1 agonist for parenteral treatment of hypertension. Drugs Today 33:729, 1997.
15. Holcslaw TL, Beck TR. Clinical experience with intravenous fenoldopam. Am J Hypertens 3:120S, 1990.
16. Panacek EA, Bednarczyk EM, Dunbar LM, et al, for the Fenoldopam Study Group. Randomized, prospective trial of fenoldopam vs sodium nitroprusside in the treatment of acute severe hypertension. Acad Emerg Med 2:959, 1995.
17. Tomlin JA, Dunbar LM, Oparil S, et al. Intravenous fenoldopam for the management of hypertensive emergency: A randomized, multicenter, double-blind, dose-comparison trial. (in press).
18. Tietjen CS, Hurn PD, Ulatowski JA, Kirsch JR. Treatment modalities for hypertensive patients with intracranial pathology: Options and risks. Crit Care Med 24:311, 1996.
19. Cumming AM, Davies DL. Intravenous labetalol in hypertensive emergency. Lancet 1:929, 1979.
20. Zeller KR, Kuhnert LV, Matthews C. Rapid reduction of severe asymptomatic hypertension: A prospective, controlled trial. Arch Intern Med 149:2186, 1989.
21. Grossman E, Messerli FH, Grodzicki T, Kowey P. Should a moratorium be placed on sublingual nifedipine capsules given for hypertensive emergencies and pseudoemergencies? JAMA 276:1328, 1996.

Appendix

Drug Tables

David A. Calhoun

Table A–1. Commonly Used Oral Antihypertensive Agents

Generic Name	Trade Name	Dosing Range (mg)	Frequency	Common Adverse Effects/Comments
DIURETICS				Hypokalemia; increased uric acid levels (may worsen gout); may increase cholesterol levels (less so of indapamide); hyponatremia (uncommon)
Chlorthalidone (g)	Hygroton	12.5–50	1	
Hydrochlorothiazide (g)	HydroDIURIL, Microzide, Esidrix	6.25–25	1	
Indapamide	Lozol	1.25–5	1	
Metolazone	Mykrox	0.5–1.0	1	
	Zaroxolyn	2.5–10	1	
LOOP DIURETICS				Hypokalemia; volume depletion
Bumetanide (g)	Bumex	0.5–4	2–3	
Ethacrynic acid	Edecrin	25–100	2–3	
Furosemide (g)	Lasix	40–240	2–3	
Torsemide	Demadex	5–100	1–2	
POTASSIUM-SPARING DIURETICS				Hyperkalemia—Use cautiously with potassium supplementation, ACE inhibitors, angiotensin II antagonists
Amiloride (g)	Midamor	5–10	1	
Spironolactone (g)	Aldactone	25–100	1	
Triamterene (g)	Dyrenium	25–100	1	
CALCIUM CHANNEL BLOCKERS				
Dihydropyridines				Ankle edema; flushing; headache; gingival hypertrophy (uncommon); increase in heart rate may occur
Amlodipine	Norvasc	2.5–10	1	
Felodipine	Plendil	2.5–20	1	
Isradipine	DynaCirc	5–20	2	
	DynaCirc CR	5–20	1	
Nicardipine	Cardene SR	60–90	2	
Nifedipine	Adalat CC	30–90	1	
	Procardia XL	30–90	1	
Nisoldipine	Sular	60–90	1	
Nondihydropyridines				AV node suppression; possible negative inotropic effect; constipation can occur with verapamil; Covera HS designed to be dosed at bedtime
Diltiazem	Cardizem CD, Dilacor XR, Tiazac	120–360	1	
Verapamil	Calan SR, Covera-HS, Isoptin SR, Verelan	120–480	1	
ACE INHIBITORS				Cough; much less common are angioedema, rash, hyperkalemia; contraindicated in pregnancy; use cautiously with renal artery stenosis
Benazepril	Lotensin	5–40	1–2	
Captopril (g)	Capoten	25–150	2–3	
Enalapril	Vasotec	5–40	1–2	
Fosinopril	Monopril	10–40	1–2	
Lisinopril	Prinivil, Zestril	5–40	1	
Moexipril	Univasc	7.5–15	1–2	
Quinapril	Accupril	5–80	1–2	
Ramipril	Altace	1.25–20	1–2	
Trandolapril	Mavik	1–4	1	

Table continued on following page

719

Table A–1. Commonly Used Oral Antihypertensive Agents *Continued*

Generic Name	Trade Name	Dosing Range (mg)	Frequency	Common Adverse Effects/Comments
ANGIOTENSIN II RECEPTOR BLOCKERS				Hyperkalamia; angioedema (rare); contraindicated in pregnancy; use cautiously with renal artery stenosis
Candesartan	Atacand	8–32	1–2	
Irbesartan	Avapro	150–300	1	
Losartan	Cozaar	25–100	1–2	
Telmisarten	Micardis	20–80	1	
Valsartan	Diovan	80–320	1	
β-BLOCKERS				Fatigue; sexual dysfunction; insomnia; bronchospasm; bradycardia; negative inotropic effect; may mask hypoglycemic symptoms; may worsen symptoms of peripheral vascular disease; may suppress exercise tolerance; may increase triglyceride levels (less true for agents with ISA); rebound syndrome (hypertension and/or angina) may occur with abrupt discontinuation; acebutolol both is cardioselective and has ISA
Nadolol	Corgard	40–320	1	
Propanolol (g)	Inderal	40–480	2–3	
Cardioselective Agents				
Acebutolol				
Atenolol (g)	Sectral	200–800	1	
Betaxolol	Tenormin	25–100	1	
Bisoprolol	Kerlone	5–20	1	
Metoprolol (g)	Zebeta	2.5–10	1	
	Lopressor (g)	50–300	1–2	
	Toprol XL	50–300	1	
Agents with ISA				
Carteolol	Cartrol	2.5–10	1	
Penbutolol	Levatol	10–20	1	
Pindolol (g)	Visken	10–60	1	
α-BLOCKERS				First-dose effect (can be minimized with gradual titration or taking first dose at bedtime)
Doxazosin	Cardura	1–16	1	
Prazosin	Minipress	2–30	2–3	
Terazosin	Hytrin	1–20	1	
COMBINED α- and β-BLOCKERS				With higher doses, similar to β-blockers
Labetalol	Normodyne, Trandate	200–1200	2	
CENTRAL α-AGONISTS				Dry mouth; fatigue; drowsiness; sexual dysfunction; symptoms minimized with patch, guanfacine; rebound syndrome can occur with abrupt discontinuation of clonidine and/or methyldopa pills
Clonidine (g)	Catapres	0.2–1.2	2–3	
	Catapres patch	TTS 1, 2, or 3	Weekly	
Guanfacine	Tenex	1–3	1	
Methyldopa (g)	Aldomet		2	
VASODILATORS				Fluid retention and tachycardic effects usually require concomitant use of a loop diuretic and a β-blocker; hydralazine is associated with a lupus-like syndrome, particularly with higher doses; minoxidil may induce pericardial effusion; hirsutism limits use of minoxidil in women
Hydralazine (g)	Apresoline	50–300	2	
Minoxidil (g)	Loniten	5–100	1	

Abbreviations: (g), available in generic formulation; ACE, angiotensin-converting enzyme; CR, controlled-release; SR, sustained-release; AV, atrioventricular; ISA, intrinsic sympathomimetic activity; TTS, through the skin.

Table A–2. Combination Antihypertensive Agents

Generic Name	Trade Name	Doses (mg/mg)
CALCIUM ANTAGONISTS AND ACE INHIBITORS		
Amlodipine/benazepril	Lotrel	2.5/10, 5/10, 5/20
Diltiazem/enalapril	Teczem	180/5
Felodipine/enalapril	Lexxel	5/5
Verapamil/trandolapril	Tarka	180/2, 240/1, 240/2, 240/4
ACE INHIBITORS AND DIURETICS		
Benazepril/hydrochlorothiazide	Lotensin HCT	5/6.25, 10/12.5, 20/12.5, 20/25
Captopril/hydrochlorothiazide	Capozide	25/15, 25/25, 50/15, 50/25
Enalapril/hydrochlorothiazide	Vaseretic	5/12.5, 10/25
Lisinopril/hydrochlorothiazide	Prinzide, Zestoretic	10/12.5, 20/12.5, 20/25
ANGIOTENSIN II RECEPTOR ANTAGONISTS AND DIURETICS		
Losartan/hydrochlorothiazide	Hyzaar	50/12.5
Valsartan/hydrochlorothiazide	Diovan HCT	80/12.5, 160/12.5
Irbesartan/hydrochlorothiazide	Avalide	150/12.5, 300/12.5

Table A–2. Combination Antihypertensive Agents *Continued*

Generic Name	Trade Name	Doses (mg/mg)
ß-BLOCKERS AND DIURETICS		
Atenolol/chlorthalidone	Tenoretic	50/25, 100/25
Bisoprolol/hydrochlorothiazide	Ziac	2.5/6.25, 5/6.25, 10/6.25
Metoprolol/hydrochlorothiazide	Lopressor HCT	50/25, 100/25, 100/50
Nadolol/bendroflumethiazide	Corzide	40/5, 80/5
Propranolol/hydrochlorothiazide	Inderide	40/25, 80/25
Propranolol/extended-release/hydrochlorothiazide	Inderide LA	80/50, 120/50, 160/50
Timolol/hydrochlorothiazide	Timolide	10/25
OTHER COMBINATIONS		
Amiloride/hydrochlorothiazide	Moduretic	5/50
Spirinolactone/hydrochlorothiazide	Aldactazide	25/25, 50/50
Triamterene/hydrochlorothiazide	Dyazide	37.5/25
	Maxzide, Maxzide-25	75/50, 37.5/25
Clonidine/chlorthalidone	Combipres	0.1/15, 0.2/15, 0.3/15
Hydralazine/hydrochlorothiazide	Apresazide	25/25, 50/50, 100/50
Methyldopa/chlorothiazide	Aldoclor	250/15, 250/25, 500/30, 500/50
Prazosin/polythiazide	Minizide	1/0.5, 2/0.5, 5/0.5

Abbreviations: ACE, angiotensin-converting enzyme; HCT, hydrochlorothiazide; LA, long-acting.

Index

Note: Page numbers in *italics* refer to illustrations;
page numbers followed by t refer to tables.

AASK (African-American Study of Kidney Disease), 346t, 356
ABCD (Appropriate Blood Pressure Control in Diabetes), 337, 344, 346, 346t–347t, 392
Acebutolol. See also β-*Adrenoreceptor antagonists.*
  elimination characteristics of, 594t
  pharmacodynamics of, 591t
  pharmacokinetics of, 592t
  in renal replacement therapy, 536t
Acetylcholine, endothelium-mediated response to, in resistance vessels, 130
Acidosis, metabolic, diuretic-induced, 588
ACTH syndrome, ectopic. See also *Cushing's syndrome.*
  diagnosis of, 683–684
  treatment of, 684
Adalat. See *Nifedipine.*
Adenoma, adrenal. See *Adrenal gland(s), adenoma of.*
Adipose tissue. See also *Obesity.*
  critical mass of, menarche triggered by, 26
  hypertension related to, in adolescents, 26
  increase of, after Westernization of lifestyle, 25
Adolescents. See also *Children.*
  blood pressure in, adult hypertension related to, 23
  rise of, synchronized with growth spurts, 25–26
Adrenal cortex–related hypertension. See *Adrenocortical hypertension.*
Adrenal gland(s), adenoma of, hyperaldosteronism due to, 678
  hypertension due to, 514
  localization of, 678
  surgical excision of, 680–681, *681*
  treatment of, 679–680
  angiotensin-converting enzyme distribution in, 93t, 94
  angiotensin-converting enzyme function in, 95t
  angiotensin II effects on, 621–622
  hormone synthesis in, 674, *675*
  in pathophysiology, of insulin resistance syndrome, *123,* 124

Adrenal vein, sampling of, for measurement of aldosterone, 678
Adrenalectomy, bilateral, for Cushing's disease, 684
Adrenergic inhibitors, combined with diuretics, 637
  ganglion blocking drugs as, 638–639
  in pregnancy, 697–698
  neurotransmitter synthesis and, 637–638, 638t
  postganglionic inhibitors as, 639–641
α-Adrenergic receptor(s), classification of, 596–597, 596t
  hyperresponsiveness of, hypertension related to, 50
  racial differences in, 50
  hypertensive role of, 595–596, *596*
α₂-Adrenergic receptor(s), functions of, 45
  modulation of neurotransmitters by, 44
  subtypes of, 45
β₂-Adrenergic receptor(s), functions of, 45
  modulation of neurotransmitters by, 44
  subtypes of, 45
Adrenocortical hypertension, 674–684
  diagnosis of, 674–676, 675t
  excess aldosterone production in. See *Hyperaldosteronism.*
  excess cortisol production in, 682–684
  excess deoxycorticosterone production in, 676
  management of, 514–515
α-Adrenoreceptor agonists, characteristics and dosage of, 720t
  in elderly, adverse effects of, 557
  in obese hypertensives, 209
  withdrawal from, hypertensive emergency due to, 718
α₂-Adrenoreceptor agonists, exercise interaction with, 474
  for orthostatic intolerance, 576
  in anesthesia, 703
  in chronic renal insufficiency, 288
α-Adrenoreceptor antagonists, 595–598.
    See also *Antihypertensive therapy;* specific agents, *e.g., Doxazosin.*
  cardiovascular risk factor improvement by, 597

α-Adrenoreceptor antagonists *(Continued)*
  characteristics and dosage of, 720t
  combined with other agents, ACE inhibitors, 604
    β-adrenoreceptor antagonists, in pheochromocytoma, 514–515
    in pregnancy, 698
    dihydropyridine calcium antagonists, 614
  effectiveness of, 597
  in benign prostatic hyperplasia and lower urinary tract symptoms, 597–598
  in chronic renal insufficiency, 288
  in obesity, 485
  in pregnancy, 515, 698
  in renal replacement therapy, 536t
  lipid-lowering effect of, 511
  mechanisms of action of, 597
  pharmacology of, 596, 596t
  quinazolines as, 596
α₁-Adrenoreceptor antagonists, in chronic renal insufficiency, 288
  in diabetes mellitus, 522
  in obese hypertensives, 209
    with diabetes, 485
  in renal replacement therapy, 534t, 535
β-Adrenoreceptor antagonists, 590–595.
    See also *Antihypertensive therapy;* specific agents, *e.g., Metoprolol.*
  α-adrenergic activity of, 593
  adverse effects of, 593, 595
  ALLHAT study of, 360–361
  as initial choice of therapy, clinical trials of, 342, 344
    in Australia, 386
    in Canada, 384, 384t, *385*
    in Germany, 386
    in left ventricular dysfunction, 485
    in Norway, 386
    in obesity, 484
    in Sweden, 386
    in United Kingdom, 385
    JNC VI recommendation for, 590
  ASCOT trial of, 346t, 351t, 355
  β₁-selectivity of, 591, 591t
  blood pressure effects of, 593
  breast feeding and, 699
  characteristics and dosage of, 720t

723

β-Adrenoreceptor antagonists *(Continued)*
  combined with other agents, α-adreno-
      receptor antagonists, 514–515
    in pregnancy, 698
    ACE inhibitors, 604
    adverse effects of, 595
    calcium antagonists, 570, 613, 614
    diltiazem, 613
    diuretics, 500, 501t, 570, 721t
    for resistant hypertension, 570
    nifedipine, for suppression of myo-
        cardial infarction, 612, 614
    verapamil, 595, 613
  contraindications to, in diabetes melli-
      tus, 485, 487, 510, 522, 593
    in specific disorders, 593
    when combined with other agents,
        595
  efficacy of, clinical trials of, 344, 345t
  elimination characteristics of, 594t
  exercise interaction with, 474–475
  in African Americans, 562
  in airways disease, 511
  in anesthesia, 703, 711
  in asymptomatic diastolic dysfunction,
      260
  in chronic renal insufficiency, 288
  in congestive heart failure, 512
    diastolic, 259
  in coronary artery disease, 512
  in elderly, 555, 557
  in ischemic heart disease, 542
  in obese hypertensives, 209
  in orthostatic intolerance, 576
  in peripheral vascular disease, 513
  in pregnancy, 515, 696t, 698
  in renal replacement therapy, 536t
  in renovascular hypertension, 667
  intrinsic sympathomimetic activity in,
      591, 591t
  lipoprotein levels affected by, 511
  membrane-stabilizing activity of, 591,
      591t
  partial agonist activity of, 591, 591t
  pharmacodynamic properties of, 591,
      591t, 592
  pharmacokinetics properties of, 592t,
      593, 594t
  protective effects of, clinical trials of,
      344, 345t
  resistance vessel remodeling and, 128,
      128, 128t
  ultra-short-acting, 593
  withdrawal from, hypertensive emer-
      gency due to, 718
β₁-Adrenoreceptor antagonists, in renal
    replacement therapy, 534t
Aerobic exercise. See *Exercise.*
Affect, angiotensin II receptor blocker
    effects on, 627
African Americans, absence of nocturnal
    lowering of blood pressure in, 506
  α-adrenergic responsiveness in, 50
  alcohol consumption by, blood pressure
      levels in, 211, *212,* 213, *214*
  angiotensinogen polymorphisms in, 81,
      84t
  antihypertensive therapy in, ACE inhibi-
      tors for, 562, 603

African Americans *(Continued)*
    with diuretics, 604
    general principles of, 561, 561t
    in diabetes mellitus, 522
      for protection against renal disease
          progression, 521t
      initial choice of, 483–484, 484t
      recommended agents in, 562
      threshold level for beginning, 561
  blood pressure level of, in chronic re-
      nal insufficiency, 288
  bradykinin hypersensitivity in, 196
  coronary disease in, mortality rate
      from, 532
  hypertension in, 558–562
    AASK study of, 346t, 356
    ALLHAT study of. See *Antihyperten-
        sive and Lipid-Lowering to Pre-
        vent Heart Attack Trial (ALL-
        HAT).*
    antecedents of, 558
    epidemiology of, 558
    in elderly, prevalence of, 551, 552
    isolated systolic, 558
    lifestyle modification for, 483, 561–
        562
    personality traits and, 63
    possible causes of, 7
    renal replacement therapy and, 532
    target organ damage in, mechanisms
        of, 559–561, *560*
      patterns of, 558–559, 559t
    therapeutic implications of, 561, 561t
  kallikrein excretion by, 196
  low potassium consumption by, hyper-
      tension related to, 450
  obesity in, 559–560, *560*
  renal failure in, genetic predisposition
      to, 519
  renal injury in, 560–561, *560*
  salt sensitivity of, 560
  sodium excretion abnormalities in,
      atrial natriuretic peptide and, 170
  stress response in, 59
  stroke risk in, 552
  ventricular hypertrophy in, genetics of,
      250
    wall thickness and mass in, 245–246
  women, antihypertensive therapy in,
      549
    lifestyle modifications for, 549
    obesity in, 559, 560
Africans, angiotensinogen polymorphisms
    in, 81, 84t
  blood pressure in, blood pressure in Af-
      rican Americans vs., 7
  low-to-normal, 8
Age and aging. See also *Elderly.*
  arterial stiffness in, hypertension re-
      lated to, 137
    pathophysiology of, 142–143, *145*
    pulse pressure elevation in, 228–229,
        229
  blood pressure changes related to, he-
      modynamic phases of, 229–230,
      229–230
  blood pressure rise associated with, 6,
      6, 229–230
  coronary blood flow alterations in,
      263–264

Age and aging *(Continued)*
  diastolic function affected by, 255–256
  dose-response variability due to, 494
  humoral changes in, 553, 553t
  increased levels of norepinephrine in,
      51
  physiological and pathological changes
      in, 552–553
  sympathetic nervous system hyperactiv-
      ity associated with, 51
  ventricular hypertrophy in, 250
AIPRI (Angiotensin-Converting Enzyme
    Inhibition in Progressive Renal
    Insufficiency), 291
Airway pressure, continuous positive
    nocturnal, for obstructive sleep
    apnea, 658
Airways disease, antihypertensive therapy
    and, 511
Aladotril (alatriopril), 652, *653*
Albumin, glycated, in diabetic renal
    disease, 520
Alcohol consumption, cardioprotective
    effects of, 468
  excessive, resistant hypertension due
      to, 567
  hypertension related to, 211–217
    alcohol restriction in, 217
    alcohol withdrawal and, 216
    epidemiologic studies of, 211–214
      cross-sectional studies in, 211–
          214, *212–214*
      in hospitalized alcoholics, 213–
          214
      problems in, 214
      prospective studies in, 213
    epidemiology of, 6–7, 466
    health outcomes in, 217
    historical background of, 211
    initial evaluation of, 299t, 300
    intervention studies in, 214–216
    pattern of drinking in, 466
    possible mechanisms in, 215–216,
        468
    proportion of hypertension attribut-
        able to alcohol in, 217
    recommendations regarding, 468–
        469
    resistance to antihypertensives in,
        466
  reduction of, blood pressure response
      to, randomized controlled trials of,
      466–468, *467,* 467t
  screening for, 469
  ventricular hypertrophy related to, 250–
      251
Aldactone. See *Spironolactone.*
Aldosterone, angiotensin II as
    secretagogue for, 622
  genetic mutation of, in glucocorticoid-
      remedial aldosteronism, 682, *682*
  secretion of, from adenoma, diagnosis
      of, 678
    hyperaldosteronism due to, 678
    in pregnancy, 690–691
  sodium restriction effects on, 438,
      439t, *440*

Aldosterone *(Continued)*
  synthesis of, by endothelin, 154
  24-hour urinary excretion of, in evalua-
      tion of hyperaldosteronism, 678,
      678
Aldosteronism. See *Hyperaldosteronism.*
Alfuzosin, 597
Alkalosis, metabolic, diuretic-induced,
    588
ALLHAT study. See *Antihypertensive and
    Lipid-Lowering to Prevent Heart
    Attack Trial (ALLHAT).*
Allopurinol, interaction of, with ACE
    inhibitors, 606
Alzheimer's disease, 11, 12. See also
    Dementia.
Ambulatory Blood Pressure Monitoring
    and Treatment of Hypertension Trial
    (APTH), 315
Ambulatory monitoring of blood pressure.
    See *Blood pressure, ambulatory
    monitoring of.*
American College of Obstetricians and
    Gynecologists, Committee on
    Terminology, 690
Amiloride, characteristics and dosage of,
    587t
  combined with hydrochlorothiazide,
      500
  for glucocorticoid-remedial aldosteron-
      ism, 682
  for hyperaldosteronism, 680
  with hydrochlorothiazide, resistance
      vessel remodeling and, 128
Amlodipine. See also *Calcium
    antagonists.*
  ALLHAT study of, 363
  ASCOT trial of, 346t, 351t, 355
  cilazapril vs., in chronic renal insuffi-
      ciency, 293
  combined with hydrochlorothiazide,
      dosage of, 501t
  exercise interaction with, 475
  fosinopril vs., FACET trial of, 392
  in ischemic heart disease, 542
  pharmacokinetics of, in renal replace-
      ment therapy, 536t
  PRAISE trial of, 542
  slow-onset and long-lasting preparation
      of, 617
  VALUE trial of, 338t, 346t, 351t, 355–
      356
Amphetamines, hypertension due to, 566
ANBP (Australian National Blood
    Pressure Study), 332t, 338t
ANBP2 (Australian National Blood
    Pressure Study–2), 346t, 351t, 354
Androgen(s), antagonists of, for
    glucocorticoid resistance, 676
  excess of, in women, metabolic abnor-
      malities due to, 114
  synthesis of, *675*
Anesthesia, 702–712
  cardiovascular pharmacology of, 704–
      707, *704*, 704t
  general, definition of, 709
    epidural anesthesia with, 704–705
    induction of, 705–707
    intraoperative hemodynamics in,
        705, 709

Anesthesia *(Continued)*
    maintenance of, 707
    response to, *706*, 709
    types of drugs in, 704
  hypotension due to, 703, 704, *705*,
      709–710
  in hypertension, anesthetic plan for,
      708–709
    antihypertensive therapy for, 703,
        704, 711
    choice of technique in, 709–710
    classification of hypertension in,
        702, 702t
    consultative process in, 708, 708t
    emergence from anesthesia and, 712
    general anesthesia in, 709
    induction and intubation in, 711
    intraoperative management of, 711–
        712
    maintenance of anesthesia in, 711–
        712
    monitoring in, 710–711
    outcome studies of, 709
    pathophysiology of, 702–703, *703*
    patient evaluation and preparation in,
        707–708, 707t–708t
    peak incidences of hypertension in,
        705, *706*
    postoperative management of, 712,
        712t
    regional anesthesia in, 709–710
  local (monitored anesthesia care), 704,
      705, 709
  major nerve block in, 708–710
  neuraxial block in, 704, 708, 709–710
  regional block in, 704, 705, 709–710
  techniques in, 704–705, *705–706*
Aneurysm(s), of abdominal aorta, as risk
    factor for hypertension, 301t
Anger, hypertension related to, 62
Angina, calcium antagonists for
    improving, 612, *612*
  Canadian Cardiovascular Society classi-
      fication of, 539
Angioedema, due to ACE inhibitor
    therapy, 606
Angiogenesis, defective, in hypertension,
    261
Angiography, carbon dioxide digital, in
    renovascular hypertension, 665
  coronary, in coronary artery disease,
      540
  digital subtraction (DSA), computed
      axial tomography vs., in reno-
      vascular hypertension, 664
    in renovascular hypertension, 665
    MRI vs., in renovascular hyperten-
        sion, 664
  in renovascular hypertension, 664–665,
      665
  radionuclide, of diastolic function, 256
Angioplasty, percutaneous transluminal,
    for coronary artery disease,
    540–542
  for renal artery stenosis, 667–669,
      668
    as initial therapy, 670
    renal function preservation with,
        671

Angioplasty *(Continued)*
    results of, 667–668
    stenting with, 668–669, *669*, 671,
        672
Angiotensin I, as substrate for
    angiotensin-converting enzyme, 92t,
    600
Angiotensin II, adrenal effects of, 622,
    623t
  cardiovascular effects of, 95–96, 449,
      622, 623t
  decreased levels of, in aging, 553
  elevation of, with increased tissue ACE
      activity, 94, 96
  endothelin interaction with, 154
  escape of, during ACE inhibition, 600
  fetal development and, 606
  functions of, 100
  glucose combined with, renal damage
      due to, 290
  in cardiovascular hypertrophy, 96
  in inflammation and tissue repair, 95
  interaction of, with ouabain, 45
    with sympathetic nervous system,
        44–45
  nervous system effects of, 622, 623t
  pathways for generation of, 621, *621*
  receptors for. See *Angiotensin II recep-
      tor(s).*
    dual, endothelin and, 155
  renal effects of, 622, 623t
  structural effects of, 622
  vascular effects of, 621–622, 623t
  ventricular hypertrophy related to, 251
Angiotensin II receptor(s), 100–108
  AT₁, 101–104
    binding requirements for, 103–104,
        103
    blockade of, consequences of, 106,
        108
    distribution of, 102
    functions of, 105–106, *105–107*
    gene for, 101–102
    signal transduction of, 102–103
    structure of, 101
    subtypes of, 101
  AT₂, 104–105
    distribution of, 104–105
    functions of, 105–106, *105–107*
    gene for, 104
    signal transduction of, 105
  discovery and classification of, 100–
      101, *101*
  distribution of, 622–623, 623t
Angiotensin II receptor antagonists. See
    also *Antihypertensive therapy;*
    specific agent, *e.g., Losartan.*
  adverse effects of, 630–631
  antihypertensive response to, 631
  behavior and affect effects of, 627
  cardiac effects of, 625–626
  characteristics and dosage of, 720t
  combined with other agents, ACE inhib-
      itors, 632
    diuretics, 501t, 720t
  development of, 623
  exercise interaction with, 475
  hemodynamic effects of, 625
  in cardiac disease, 631–632

Angiotensin II receptor antagonists
(*Continued*)
in cerebrovascular and neurological disorders, 633
in congestive heart failure, 512
in diabetes mellitus, 522
clinical trials of, 346, 346t–347t, 348
in elderly, 557
in left ventricular dysfunction, 485–486
in pregnancy, contraindications to, 483, 627, 698–699
in renal artery stenosis/renovascular hypertension, monitoring required with, 513, 515–516, 631, 667
renal failure due to, 513, 667
in renal failure, as initial choice of therapy, 486
physiologic effects of, 626–627
renoprotective effects of, 292, 513, 528, 632–633
with and without diabetes, 632–633
in renal replacement therapy, 534t, 536t
intraglomerular pressure reduction by, 510
nervous system effects of, 627
newer types of, 623–625, *625–626*
pharmacology of, 627–631
renal effects of, 626–627
renin inhibitors vs., 649, 650, 650t
safety of, 630–631
structure of, 624–625, *624–626*
Angiotensin-converting enzyme (ACE), 90–97
basic properties of, 90–93
catalytic sites for, 91–92
distribution and localization of, 93–94
in cardiovascular system, 93, 93t
in central nervous system, 93–94, 93t
in gastrointestinal tract, 93t, 94
in kidney and adrenal system, 93t, 94
in reproductive system, 93t, 94
functional role of, 94–96, 95t
genetic polymorphism of, cardiovascular and renal damage related to, 526
in predisposition to diabetic nephropathy, 519
renal effects of, 605
response to ACE inhibitors and, 605
response to antihypertensives and, 527–528
human gene for, 90–91, *92*
inhibitors of. See *Angiotensin-converting enzyme (ACE) inhibitors.*
isoforms of, plasma, 90, *91*
somatic, 90, *91*
testicular, 90, *91*
neutral endopeptidase inhibitor effects on, 652–654
pathophysiological role of, 96–97
in cardiovascular hypertrophy, 96
in hypertension, 96
in inflammation and tissue repair, 97
in myocardial infarction and cardiac remodeling, 96–97
structure of, 90, *91*
substrates of, 92t, 93

Angiotensin-converting enzyme (ACE) inhibitors, 599–606. See also *Antihypertensive therapy;* specific agent, *e.g., Enalapril.*
adverse effects of, 605–606
in women, 483
ALLHAT study of. See *Antihypertensive and Lipid-Lowering to Prevent Heart Attack Trial (ALLHAT).*
arterial stiffness reduced by, 148
as initial choice of therapy, in Canada, 384, 384t, *385*
in left ventricular dysfunction, 485
in New Zealand, 385
in obesity, 485
in renal failure, 486
in United States, 383
blood pressure response to, 602–603, 603t
breast feeding and, 699
calcium channel blockers vs., clinical trials of, 392
in chronic renal insufficiency, 291, 293
cardiovascular effects of, 605
characteristics and dosage of, 719t
class effect of, 601
combined with other agents, 603–604
α-antagonists, 604
angiotensin II receptor blockers, 632
β-blockers, 604
calcium channel blockers, common combinations in, 720t
efficacy of, 604, 614
in congestive heart failure, 512
pharmacology of, 501t, 502–503
diuretics, common combinations in, 720t
effectiveness of, 501–502, 501t–502t
for resistant hypertension, 570
in renal failure, 528, *529*
rationale for, 603–604
verapamil, 614
contraindications to, in pregnancy, 483, 515, 696t, 698–699
dosage of, 603t
drug interactions with, 600, 606
endothelial vasodilator function improvement with, 159–160
exercise interaction with, 475
for proteinuria reduction, in diabetic nephropathy, 510
in renal failure, 486
glomerular filtration rate decreased by, 510, 602, 605
reversal of, after cessation of therapy, 513
hemodynamic effects of, 602, 602t
in African Americans, 562, 603, 604
in airways disease, 511
in asymptomatic diastolic dysfunction, 260
in congestive heart failure, 511–512
clinical trials of, 339
diastolic, 259
in diabetes mellitus, AIPRI trial of, 291
clinical trials of, 337, 344, 346, 346t–347t, 348

Angiotensin-converting enzyme (ACE) inhibitors (*Continued*)
improvement of cardiovascular disease with, 114
insulin sensitivity and, 510
renoprotective effects of, 510, 521, 521t
with renal involvement, 604
in disorders associated with hypertension, 604
in elderly, 557
ANBP2 trial of, 354, 351t
in ischemic heart disease, 543
in isolated systolic hypertension, 604
in myocardial infarction, clinical trials of, 339
in obese hypertensives, 209
in radionuclide scanning, for renovascular hypertension, 663
in renal artery stenosis, monitoring required with, 288, 513, 667
renal failure due to, 513, 667
in renal failure, clinical trials of, 337
effectiveness of, 604–605
intraglomerular pressure reduction by, 510, 526
monitoring creatinine levels with, 487
proteinuria reduction by, 486, 527, 528, *529,* 605
renoprotective effects of, 290–292, 513, 604–605
in renal replacement therapy, anaphylactoid reaction to, 535
for comorbid conditions, 534t
pharmacokinetics of, 536t
in renovascular hypertension, 667
in elderly, 515–516
monitoring required with, 288, 513, 667
in stroke, PROGRESS trial of, 346t–347t, 349
indications for, 599, 600t
kininase interaction with, 193–194
lipophilicity of, 97
Losartan Intervention for Endpoint (LIFE) study of, 366–370
mechanisms of action of, 97, 599–600
nonsteroidal anti-inflammatory drug effects on, 600
pharmacology of, 600–601, 601t
renal hemodynamic effects of, 602, 602t
renin inhibitors vs., 647–650, *649,* 650t
resistance vessel remodeling reversed by, 129, *129,* 129t
Angiotensinogen, 77–87
blood pressure regulation by, 77–78
discovery of, 77
elevation of, due to estrogen, 77–78
gene for, diabetic nephropathy related to, 519
genetic studies of, 79–87
criteria for association studies in, 81, 87
initial reports of linkage and association in, 79–80, 79t, 82t–87t
linkage vs. association in, 79

Angiotensinogen *(Continued)*
  in tissues, 78
  polymorphisms of, in Africans and African Americans, 81, 84t
    in hypertensive subtypes, 81, 87t
    in Japanese, 81, 85t, 87t
    in whites, 80, 82t–83t, 87t
  renin interaction with, biochemical characteristics of, 77
  transgenic studies of, 78–79
Anglo-Scandinavian Cardiac Outcomes Trial (ASCOT), 338t, 346t, 351t, 355
Ankle edema, from calcium antagonists, 611–612
Anticoagulant therapy, for ischemic heart disease, 542–543
  for stroke prevention, 282–283
Antidepressants, tricyclic, hypertension due to, 566
Antihypertensive and Lipid-Lowering to Prevent Heart Attack Trial (ALLHAT), 360–365
  antihypertensive component of, comparison of drugs in, 360–361
    eligibility for, 362, 362t
    treatment program in, 362–363
  baseline characteristics of patients in, 364, 364t–365t
  cholesterol-lowering component of, eligibility for, 362, 363t
    Scandinavian Simvastatin Survival Study vs., 361–362
    treatment program in, 363
  endpoints for, 363–364, 363t
  hypotheses of, 360, 362, 362t
  objective and design of, 346t, 351t, 353–354, 360, 362, 362t
  rationale for conducting, 360–362
Antihypertensive therapy. *See also* specific class of agent, *e.g., Calcium antagonists.*
  adverse effects of, as measure of outcome, 325
    from excessive dosage, 495–496
    in elderly, 481
    in women, 549
    resistant hypertension due to, 565
  alcohol consumption and, 215, 466
  ALLHAT study of. *See Antihypertensive and Lipid-Lowering to Prevent Heart Attack Trial (ALLHAT).*
  approval process for, 579–583
    chemistry and biopharmaceutics in, 579
    clinical trials for, 580
    drug development after, 583
    review of application for, 580–583
      Action Letter in, 583
      Advisory Committee in, 583
      criteria of approvability in, 581–582
      filing requirements in, 581
      hard-endpoint trials and, 582
      primary review in, 582–583
      secondary reviews in, 583
      tertiary and quaternary reviews in, 583
    submission of application for, 580

Antihypertensive therapy *(Continued)*
    toxicological studies for, 579–580
  blood pressure goal in, clinical trials of, 336
    determination by HOT trial, 226–227, 381
    guideline recommendations for, 381–382, 382t
    in African Americans, 483–484
    in chronic renal failure, 513, 526, *526,* 528, 604
    in diabetes mellitus, 510, 518, 520–521, 521t
    in elderly, 481
    in isolated systolic hypertension, 481
    patient compliance and, 420–421, *421,* 421t
  blood pressure response to, in mild hypertension, 398, *398,* 400t
    in renal failure, genetic factors in, 527–528
  cardioprotective effects of. *See Cardioprotective effects.*
  changing approach to, 372–374
    for hypertensive urgencies, 374
    general guidelines in, 373–374
    initial choice of drug in, 372t, 373, *373*
    lifestyle modification in, 372–373, 372t
  chronotherapeutic methods in, 506–508, *507*
  clinical trials of. *See Clinical trial(s).*
  combined, 497–503. *See also* specific class of drug, e.g., *Calcium antagonists, combined with other agents.*
    advantages of, 497–499, 497t
    compliance with, 499
    disadvantages of, 499–500
    dose-dependent side effects of, pharmacology of, 498–499, *498*
    fixed-dose combinations in, 500–503, 501t, 720t–721t
    for resistant hypertension, 570
    for risk factor modification, 498
    general guidelines for, 374
    history of, 497
    in African Americans, 561
    in initial therapy, 487–488, 488t
    in renal replacement therapy, 535, 535t
    number of drugs in, as measure of outcome, 325–326
    objectives of, 497–498
    prescription strategy for, 499, 499t
    rationale for, 498, 498t
    tolerability of, 498
  commonly used agents in, 719t–720t
  community outreach for, 415
  compliance with, 419–429
    as measure of outcome, 325
    definition of, 420
    enlarged focus of, 423
    epidemiology of, 423–425
    goal blood pressure achievement and, categorization of patients for, 420–421, *421*

Antihypertensive therapy *(Continued)*
    distribution of adherence according to, 420, 421t
    implications of, 420, *421*
    historical perspectives in, 422–423
    in clinical trials, 339
    in combination therapy, 499
    initial choice of drug and, 387
    measures of, 422–423, 422t
    medication possession ratio as index of, 325
    patterns of medication-taking behavior in, 423–424, *424*
    predictors of, 424–425
    relative contributions of patient, physician, and pharmacist in, 419–420, *420*
    resistant hypertension and, 564t, 567
    strategies for improving, 425–429
      for clinicians, 425–427, 425t
      multifaceted, 427–428
      patient-physician collaboration in, 428–429
      pharmacokinetics as guide for, 428, *428*
    therapeutic implications of, 421–422, 421t
    therapeutic paradigm for, 420–421, *421*
  coronary blood flow effect of, 265–266
  cost effectiveness of. *See Cost effectiveness, of therapy.*
  decision to begin, blood pressure threshold for, 222–223, *223*
    risk assessment in, 221–222
  delayed-action agents in, calcium antagonists, lipophilic preparations of, 617, *617–618,* 618t
    slow-onset and long-lasting preparations of, 617, 618t
    slow-release (retarded) preparations of, 616–617, 618t
    verapamil, for control of early morning blood pressure surge, 507–508, *507*
  dose of, inappropriate, resistant hypertension due to, 564t, 565
    once-a-day, uneven blood pressure control with, 507
    patient compliance and, 427, *427*
  dose-response relationship of, 492–496
    adverse effects related to, 495–496
    clockwise hysteresis in, 493
    concentration-effect analysis of, 493, *494*
    counterclockwise hysteresis in, 492–493, *493*
    counterregulatory mechanisms in, 495
    group vs. individual variability in, 493, *494*
    in combination therapy, 498–499, *498*
    individualized therapy and, 496, *496*
    log-linear, 492, *492*
    temporal relationship in, 492, *493*
    variability in, 493–495, 495t
  drug interactions with, in elderly, 481

Antihypertensive therapy (Continued)
  resistant hypertension due to, 565
during anesthesia, 703, *704*, 711
efficacy of, acute hypotensive response
    as predictor of, 495
  definition of, 221
  published trials proving, 341, 342t–
    343t, 344
efficiency of, 221
endothelial vasodilator function improvement with, 160
exercise interaction with, 473–475
goal blood pressure in. See *Antihyper-*
  tensive therapy, blood pressure
  goal in.
guidelines for, adherence to, changes
    over time in, 384
  agreement in, 379–380, 379t
  calcium channel blocker recommen-
    dations in, 394
  cost of treatment and, 377–378
  critical assessment of, 375–382
  development of, 376–377
  differences in, 380–382, 380t–382t
  evidence-based vs. consensus-based,
    376–377
  implementation of, 378, *378*
  individualized therapy vs., 375
  initial choice of drugs and, 381–382,
    381t
  nonclinician use of, 376
  presentation of, 378–379
  reasons for using, 375–376
history of, 2–3
in African Americans. See *African*
  Americans, antihypertensive ther-
  apy in.
in asymptomatic diastolic dysfunction,
  260
in chronic hypertension, sympathetic
  nervous system activity and,
  50–51
in Cushing's syndrome, 514
in dementia, clinical trials of, 14
in diabetes mellitus. See *Diabetes melli-*
  tus, antihypertensive therapy in.
in elderly. See *Elderly, antihypertensive*
  therapy in.
in high-risk vs. low-risk patients, clinical trials of, 335–336, *335*
in hyperaldosteronism, 514, 679–681,
  679–681, 681t
in hypertensive encephalopathy, 279–
  280
in hypertensive stroke, choice of drugs
  in, 281
  controversies in, 280, *280*
  effects of, 280–281
  types of stroke prevented by, 278–
    279
in ischemic heart disease, 543–544
in migraine, 513
in mild hypertension, blood pressure response to, 398, *399,* 400t
  clinical trials of, 399, 400t, 401
    implications of, 401–403, *402*
in pheochromocytoma, 514–515
in pregnancy. See *Pregnancy, antihyper-*
  tensive therapy in.

Antihypertensive therapy (Continued)
  in renal failure. See *Renal failure,*
    chronic, antihypertensive therapy
    in.
in renal replacement therapy, 535–536,
  534t–536t
in renovascular hypertension. See *Reno-*
  vascular hypertension, antihyper-
  tensive therapy in.
in ventricular hypertrophy, regression
  of mass with, 242, 242t, 253
in women, 549
  adverse effects of, 483, 549
initial choice of, 383–387, 479–489
  aging and, 480–481, 480t
  algorithm for selection of, 373, *373*
  combined vs. single agent therapy in,
    487–488, 488t
  cost effectiveness of, 407
  demographic issues in, 480–487
  effect of drug choice in, 386–387
  for coexisting conditions, 372t, 373
  gender differences in, 482–483, 482t
  guideline recommendations for, 381–
    382, 382t
  in Australia, *383,* 385–386
  in Canada, *383,* 384–385, 384t, *385*
  in coronary disease, 485, 486t
  in diabetes mellitus, 487
  in Germany, *383,* 386
  in isolated systolic hypertension,
    481–482
  in left ventricular dysfunction, 485–
    486, 486t
  in New Zealand, *383,* 385
  in Norway, *383,* 386
  in obesity, 484–485, 484t
  in renal disease, 486–487, 486t
  in Sweden, *383,* 386
  in United Kingdom, *383,* 385
  in United States, 383–384, *383*
  lifestyle (hygienic) measures in,
    479–480, 479t
  planning for, 303–304
  racial issues in, 483–484, 484t
lifestyle modification vs. See *Lifestyle*
  modifications.
low-dose fixed combination. See *Antihy-*
  pertensive therapy, combined.
nursing clinics for, 409–414
outcome measurement with, 323–330
  intermediate measures in, 327–328,
    327t
  long-term measures in, 328–329,
    329t
  pros and cons of, 329–330, 330t
  short-term measures in, 324–327,
    325t
patient selection for, clinical trials of,
  335–336, *335*
rationale for, 323–324, *323*
regimen for, clinical trials of, 336–337,
  338t
  general guidelines for, 373–374
renoprotective effects of. See *Renopro-*
  tective effects, of antihypertensive
  therapy.
  clinical trials of, 337
  in chronic renal failure, 290–293

Antihypertensive therapy (Continued)
  resistance vessel remodeling reversed
    by, 128–129, *129,* 129t, 132
  risk stratification for, 224–227, *225–*
    226
  sequential monotherapy in, 407
  stepped care approach to, 495–496
  trough:peak variability in, drug compar-
    ison and, 428, *428*
  patient compliance and, 428
Antilipemic agents, ALLHAT study of,
  eligibility for, 362, 363t
  Scandinavian Simvastatin Survival
    Study vs., 361–362
  treatment program in, 354, 363
  ASCOT trial of, 338t, 346t, 351t, 355
  efficacy of, by compliance rate, 427,
    427
  endothelial vasodilator function im-
    provement with, 159
  for stroke prevention, 283
  goal of therapy with, 544
  in chronic renal insufficiency, 293
  in ischemic heart disease, 544
  reverse cholesterol transport in, 544
Antioxidants, for coronary artery disease,
  115, 545
Antiplatelet therapy, for ischemic heart
  disease, 542–543
  for stroke prevention, 282–283
Aorta, abdominal, aneurysm of, as risk
  factor for hypertension, 301t
  coarctation of, assessment of, in diagno-
    sis of hypertension, 303t
  disease of, as measure of outcome, 329
  dissection of, hypertensive emergency
    in, 717
  stiffness of. See *Artery(ies), stiffness*
    of.
Aortocarotid baroreceptors, 45–46
Apnea, definition of, 658
Apnea-hypopnea index (AHI), 658
Aprotinin, as tissue kallikrein inhibitor,
  192
APTH (Ambulatory Blood Pressure
  Monitoring and Treatment of
  Hypertension Trial), 315
Arachidonic acid, CYP-450–related
  metabolites of, conversion by
  cyclooxygenase, 177, *177*
  in preeclampsia, 180
  in spontaneously hypertensive rats,
    178–179
Area postrema, 42, 43, 622
L-Arginine, as substrate for nitric oxide,
  160–161
Arrhythmias, assessment of, as measure
  of outcome, 328
  calcium antagonists for, 612
Arterioles, as resistance vessels, 125
Arteriosclerosis, sympathetic nervous
  system effects of, 53
Artery(ies). See also *Resistance vessels.*
  compliance of, as index of stiffness,
    135t, 138
  as measure of outcome, 328
  elasticity of, 134–149
  historical concepts of, 135–137, *136*

Artery(ies) (Continued)
  in aging, 552–553
  properties of, 137–138, 138
  elastin of, fatigue and fracture of, with
    aging, 142–143, 230
  models of, 139–140
    distributed, 140, 141
    "lumped," 139–140, 140
  small, as resistance vessels, 125
  stiffness of, 134–139
    association of, with metabolic disor-
      ders, 146–147
    causes of, 230
    decreased diastolic pressure related
      to, 229, 230
    drug therapeutic effects in, 147–148,
      147–148
    gender differences in, 144, 145–146,
      230
    height and, 144, 146
    in aging, 552–553
    in hypertension, 137, 143–144
    indices of, 134, 135t, 138–139, 139
    pathophysiological implications of,
      141–142, 142–144
    pulse pressure elevation related to,
      228–229
    with aging, 137, 142–143, 145
Ascorbic acid, for coronary artery
  disease, 115
ASCOT (Anglo-Scandinavian Cardiac
  Outcomes Trial), 338t, 346t, 351t,
  355
Asian Americans, antihypertensive
  therapy in, 484
Asians. See also Japanese.
  alcohol consumption by, blood pressure
    levels in, 212
  calcium channel blocker therapy in,
    395
Aspartic proteinase, renin as, 647
Aspirin, ACE inhibitor interaction with,
  600
  for acute myocardial infarction, 542–
    543
  for coronary artery disease, 115, 544
  for stroke prevention, 282
  in preeclampsia, 694
  with streptokinase, for acute myocar-
    dial infarction, 542
Association for the Advancement of
  Medical Instrumentation (AAMI),
  validation of automatic blood
  pressure measurement devices by,
  310, 310t
Association studies. See also Linkage and
  association studies.
  criteria for, 81, 87
  purpose of, 79
Asthma, antihypertensive therapy and,
  511
  contraindications to β-blockers in, 591
AT₁ and AT₂ receptors. See Angiotensin
  II receptor(s).
Atenolol. See also β-Adrenoreceptor
  antagonists.
  combined with diuretics, 501t
  CONVINCE trial of, 337, 338t, 346t,
    351t, 354–355

Atenolol (Continued)
  elimination characteristics of, 594t
  exercise interaction with, 474–475
  pharmacodynamics of, 591t
  pharmacokinetics of, 592t, 593
    in renal replacement therapy, 536t
  resistance vessel remodeling and, 128,
    128, 128t
Atherosclerosis. See also Coronary artery
  disease; Lipoprotein abnormalities.
  accelerated, causes of, elevated factor
    VIII in, 112
    endothelial dysfunction in, 113,
      113t
  arterial stiffness related to, 147
  as measure of outcome, 328
  causes of, diabetes mellitus in, 544
    endothelial dysfunction in, 159
    hyperhomocysteinemia in, 283
    hyperinsulinemia in, 113, 113t
    hypertension associated with, genetic
      basis of, 111
    risk ratios in, 235, 236
  inflammation associated with, 301
  inhibition of, by calcium antagonists,
    513, 615
    QUIET trial of, 346t–347t, 348
    VHAS trial of, 613, 615
  nitric oxide inhibition of, 159
  of renal artery, hypertension due to,
    304, 662
    in elderly, 515
    progression of, 667
  plaque from, 506, 615
  pulse pressure and low DBP as indica-
    tors of, 230
Atrial fibrillation, calcium antagonists for,
  612
Atrial natriuretic peptide. See Natriuretic
  peptides.
Auscultatory method, of blood pressure
  measurement, 306–308
Australia, initial choice of
  antihypertensive treatment in, 383,
  385–386
Australian National Blood Pressure Study
  (ANBP), 332t, 338t
Australian National Blood Pressure
  Study–2 (ANBP2), 346t, 351t, 354
Australian Trial of Mild Hypertension
  (ATTMH), 342t–343t, 401, 402
Autacoids, kallikrein-kinin system
  interaction with, 195
Autonomic nervous system, in orthostatic
  hypotension. See Orthostatic
  hypotension.

Bandages, for external support, in
  orthostatic hypotension, 573
Baroreceptors, high-pressure
  (aortocarotid), 45–46
  low-pressure (cardiopulmonary), 45–46
Baroreflexes, failure of, orthostatic
  hypotension due to, 574–575
  causes of, 574
    clinical presentation of, 572t, 574
    diagnosis and treatment of, 574–
      575, 575

Baroreflexes (Continued)
  impairment of, by alcohol, 215
  resetting of, 46–47
Bartter's syndrome, genetic cause and
  phenotype of, 35t
  renin levels in, 74–75
  type III, genetic cause and phenotype
    of, 35t
Basic research, characteristics of, 389
  on cardiovascular risk of calcium chan-
    nel blockers, 389
Behavior, angiotensin II receptor blocker
  effects on, 627
Benazepril. See also Angiotensin-
  converting enzyme (ACE) inhibitors.
  combined with diuretics, 501t
  dosage of, 603t
  pharmacokinetics of, 601t
    in renal replacement therapy, 536t
  renoprotective effects of, 604
BENEDICT (Bergamo Nephrologic
  Diabetes Complication Trial),
  346t–347t, 348
Benign prostatic hypertrophy,
  α₁-adrenoreceptor antagonists
  for, 597–598
Bergamo Nephrologic Diabetes
  Complication Trial (BENEDICT),
  346t–347t, 348
Beta blockers. See β-Adrenoreceptor
  antagonists.
Betaxolol. See also β-Adrenoreceptor
  antagonists.
  combined with hydrochlorothiazide,
    500
  elimination characteristics of, 594t
  pharmacodynamics of, 591t
  pharmacokinetics of, 592t
    in renal replacement therapy, 536t
Biofeedback, for stress reduction, 66
Biological rhythms. See Blood pressure,
  circadian rhythm of.
Biometric analysis, of genetic vs.
  environmental causation, 31–32
Biopsy, gluteal, in resistance vessel
  studies, 127
Birth weight, hypertension associated
  with, 10–11, 11t, 24
  in African Americans, 558
Bisoprolol. See also β-Adrenoreceptor
  antagonists.
  combined with hydrochlorothiazide,
    501, 501t
  elimination characteristics of, 594t
  pharmacodynamics of, 591t
  pharmacokinetics of, 592t
    in renal replacement therapy, 536t
  with very-low-dose diuretic, for first-
    line therapy, 590
Blacks. See African Americans; Africans.
Bleeding risk, from calcium channel
  blockers, 394, 395–396
Blood pressure. See also Pulse pressure.
  adaptation of, to particular needs, in
    mammals, 21–22
  age-related changes in, 229–230, 229–
    230
  ambulatory monitoring of, advantages
    and disadvantages of, 310–311

Blood pressure *(Continued)*
APTH trial of, 315
automatic devices for, 310, 310t
combined with clinic and home monitoring, 311–312, *312*
for circadian rhythm of blood pressure, 504, *504*
for distinction of pseudohypertension, 565
HARVEST trial of, 317
in white-coat hypertension, prospective studies of, 319, *319*
birth weight effects on, 10–11, 11t, 24
circadian rhythm of, 504–506
ambulatory monitoring of, 504, *504*
cardiovascular events related to, 506
characteristic pattern of, 505, *505*
chronotherapeutics related to, 506–508, *507*
diurnal pattern of, 311, 504
in obesity, 207
nocturnal pattern of, absence of dip in, adverse effects of, 311, 325
conditions associated with, 311
in African Americans, 506, 558–559
in diabetes mellitus, 510
in elderly, 506
in obesity, 207
target organ damage in, 311
elevated blood pressure in, 505
in obstructive sleep apnea, 659, *659*
sympathetic nervous system and, 48, 505
classification of, 2, 5, 5t, 29
components of, 227
by age groups, 228, *229*
control of, as measure of outcome, 324–325
dementia associated with, 11–14
diastolic, J-curve relationship with cardiovascular events in, 231, 237, *237*, 265, 336
low, as predictor of cardiac events, 230–231, *231*
as supplementary risk, with high pulse pressure, 231
in coronary disease, 237, *237*
distribution of, in various populations, 5, *5*, 29, *29*
fall of, after alcohol consumption, 215
during sleep. See *Blood pressure, circadian rhythm of.*
gender differences in, 6, *6*, 546–547, *546*
goal for, in antihypertensive therapy. See *Antihypertensive therapy, blood pressure goal in.*
in industrialized populations, 6–8, *6–7*
factors affecting, 25
nonindustrialized populations vs., 8–9, 8t, *9*
in pregnancy, 689–690, *689*
level of. See also *Hypertension, threshold level of blood pressure in.*
in definition of hypertension, 5, 5t, 222, 298

Blood pressure *(Continued)*
in initial assessment of hypertension, 298, 298t
in renal replacement therapy, 532–533
myocardial reinfarction related to, 238, 238t
risk of coronary disease associated with, 235, 236t
mean arterial (MAP), in chronic renal insufficiency, 288–290
measurement of, 306–312
accuracy, errors, and bias in, 298, 307, 307t
ambulatory monitoring in. See *Blood pressure, ambulatory monitoring of.*
arm position and, 307, *307*
auscultatory gap in, 308
auscultatory method of, 306–308
automatic devices for, 310
basic techniques in, 306–308
combined methods in, 311–312, *312*
cuff inflation and deflation rate in, 308
cuff size and, 307, 307t
cuff-inflation hypertension in, 308, 565
during exercise, 312
finger cuff method of Penaz in, 309
finger monitors for, 310
history of, 1
home monitoring in, ambulatory monitoring combined with, 311–312, *312*
as predictor of future hypertension, 401
for comparison with office measurements, 371
in clinic situation, 309
in elderly, 312, 553–554
in infants and children, 312
in obesity, 312
in pregnancy, 312, 690
in reevaluation of hypertension, 304t
in white-coat hypertension, 315–316, *315*
oscillometric method of, 308–309
postural effects in, 309, *309*
regression dilution bias in, 311
self-monitoring in, 309–310
supplemental, away from clinic, 298
ultrasound techniques in, 309
variability in, 311
wrist monitors for, 310
migration effect in, 9–10
nocturnal fall of. See *Blood pressure, circadian rhythm of.*
psychosocial factors in, 10, *10*
regulation of, in acute stress response, 45, *56*
integrated cardiovascular-renal function in, 22–23
natriuretic peptides in, 168–169
pressure natriuresis mechanism in, 22
resistance vessel structure and, 130–132, *131*
rise of, cardiovascular events related to, 506

Blood pressure *(Continued)*
childhood antecedents in, 23
in aging, 6, *6*, 229–230
in nonindustrialized populations, 6, *6*
lack of, in nonindustrialized populations, 8–9
synchronization of, with growth spurts, 24, 25–26
sleep apnea effects on, during sleep, 658–659, *659*
in awake state, 659–660
systolic, age-related rise in, 230
augmentation of, from pulse-wave reflection, in elderly, 515
exercise effect on, 472
misconceptions about, 137
threshold level of, for hypertension. See *Hypertension, threshold level of blood pressure in.*
Blood vessels. See also *Artery(ies)*; specific type, *e.g., Coronary arteries.*
adaptive and maladaptive overload of, with increased peripheral resistance, 232
angiotensin II effects on, 621–622
angiotensin-converting enzyme distribution in, 93, 93t
clinical studies of, in white-coat hypertension, 318
compliance of, decreased, sympathetic nervous system effects in, 53
direct effects of diuretics on, 584
hypertrophy of, due to angiotensin II, 622
in mild hypertension, 403
sympathetic nervous system in, 52–53
obesity effects on, 207
remodeling of. See also *Resistance vessels, remodeling of.*
in pathophysiology of hypertension, 23
resistance in. See *Resistance; Resistance vessels.*
Body composition, hypertension related to, in obese adolescents, 26
Inuits as example of, 25
in elderly, 553
Body fluids. See *Fluid(s), body.*
Body mass index, association of, with blood pressure, 7, 11, 11t, 460
in definition of obesity, 460
in diagnosis of hypertension, 300
Body temperature. See *Temperature.*
Bosentan (endothelin receptor antagonist), 155t, 156, 644
BQ-123 and BQ-788 (endothelin receptor antagonists), 155, 155t
Brachial artery, rigid, pseudohypertension due to, 515
Bradbury-Eggleston syndrome, 572
Bradykinin(s). See also *Kinins.*
angiotensin-converting enzyme inhibitor interaction with, 600
as mediator of inflammation, 97
as substrate for angiotensin-converting enzyme, 92t, 97
beneficial effects of, 652
cardiovascular effects of, 95–96

Bradykinin(s) *(Continued)*
  hypersensitivity to, in African Americans, 196
  in coronary artery function, 262
  metabolism of, by angiotensin-converting enzyme, 95, 96
  protection of, by ACE and NEP inhibition, 652
Brain. See also *Central nervous system.*
  angiotensin-converting enzyme distribution in, 93–94, 93t
  angiotensin-converting enzyme function in, 95, 95t
  clinical studies of, in white-coat hypertension, 318
  hypertensive stroke distribution in, 278, *278–279*
  in preeclampsia/eclampsia, pathophysiology of, 693
Brain natriuretic peptide. See *Natriuretic peptides.*
Brain stem, in hypertensive models, 42–43
Brazilian Indians, low-to-normal blood pressure in, 8, 8t
Breast feeding, antihypertensive therapy with, 699
Bretylium, adverse effects of, 640
  hemodynamic effects of, 640
  pharmacology of, 639–640
British Heart Study, 8
British Medical Research Council. See *Medical Research Council.*
Bronchoconstriction, antihypertensive therapy and, 511
Bronchospasm, contraindications to β-blockers in, 591
Bumetanide (Bumex), characteristics and dosage of, 587t

Calcineurin, in ventricular hypertrophy, 248, *249,* 251
Calcitonin gene–related peptide, 182–188
  cardiovascular actions of, 183, *183*
  immunoreactive, distribution and localization of, 182–183
  in hypertension, CGRP$_{8-37}$ receptor antagonist effect in, 184–185, *185*
  counterregulatory effect of, 185
  deoxycorticosterone-salt–induced, 184–185, 184t, *185*
  during pregnancy, 186–187, *186*
  hypothesis for, 187–188, *188*
  in humans, 187
  in spontaneously hypertensive rats, 187
  substance P and, 187
  subtotal nephrectomy-salt–induced, 185, *185*
  modulation of neurotransmitters by, 45
  protection of, by NEP inhibition, 652
  receptors for, 183
  release of, from sensory nerve terminals, 183–184
Calcium, dietary, antihypertensive effect of, 202
  in preeclampsia, 694
  micronutrient interactions with, 203

Calcium *(Continued)*
  repletion of, 454–455
    interventional studies of, 454–455
    preclinical and observational studies of, 454, *454*
    recommendations for, 455
    sodium chloride interaction with, 202–203
  increased levels of, platelet abnormalities related to, 112, *112*
  intracellular, in ventricular hypertrophy, 248, *249,* 251
  urinary excretion of, in preeclampsia, 693
Calcium antagonists, 389–396, 609–619. See also *Antihypertensive therapy;* specific agent, *e.g., Verapamil.*
  adverse effects of, 611, 613
    in women, 483
  after acute coronary syndromes, for secondary prevention, 612
  ALLHAT study of, 353–354, 360–361
  angiotensin-converting enzyme inhibitors vs., in chronic renal insufficiency, 291, 293
  antianginal activity of, 612, *612*
  antiarrhythmic activity of, 612
  as initial choice of therapy, in African Americans, 483
    in New Zealand, 385
    in obesity, 485
    in renal failure, 486
    in United States, 383
  atherosclerosis inhibited by, 513
  bleeding risk related to, 394, 395–396
  blood pressure lowering by, 611–612, *611*
  breast feeding and, 699
  cancer risk related to, 392–394, 395
  cardiovascular disease risk related to, 390–392
    basic research in, 390–391
    clinical research in, 391
    flawed methodology in early studies of, 613
    observational epidemiological studies of, 391–392
    ongoing randomized studies of, 613
    randomized trials in, 392
    summary of evidence for, 395
  cellular action of, 609, *610,* 611
  classification of, 611
  combined with other agents, α$_1$-adrenoreceptor antagonists, 614
    ACE inhibitors, efficacy of, 604, 614
      in congestive heart failure, 512
      pharmacology of, 501t, 502
      types and dosage of, 720t
    β-adrenoreceptor antagonists, advantages and disadvantages of, 613
      for resistant hypertension, 570
    dihydropyridine, as initial therapy, for isolated systolic hypertension, 373, *373*
      characteristics and dosage of, 719t
      combined with other agents, 614
      for perioperative hypertension, 615
      structure of, *616*
  drug interactions with, 485, 614

Calcium antagonists *(Continued)*
  efficacy of, 614–615
    outcome studies of, 614–615
  exercise interaction with, 475
  hemodynamic actions of, 611–613, *611*
  historical background of, 609
  in African Americans, 562
  in asymptomatic diastolic dysfunction, 260
  in atherosclerosis, beneficial effects of, 615
  in chronic renal insufficiency, renoprotective effects of, 292–293
  in coronary artery disease, 512
  in cyclosporine-induced hypertension, 514
  in diabetes mellitus, renal effects of, 521–522, 521t
  in diastolic congestive heart failure, 259
  in hypertensive emergencies, in renal failure, 717
  in ischemic heart disease, 542
  in left ventricular hypertrophy, 615
  in obese hypertensive patients, 209
  in perioperative hypertension, 615
  in pregnancy, 515, 698
  in proteinuria reduction, in diabetic nephropathy, 510
  in pulmonary hypertension, 511
  in renal replacement therapy, 534t, 536t
  lipophilic preparations of, 617, *617–618,* 618t
  long-term safety of, 613
  new types of, 615–619, *616*
  nondihydropyridine, as initial choice of therapy, in left ventricular dysfunction, 485
    characteristics and dosage of, 719t
  nonsteroidal anti-inflammatory drug interaction with, 485
  pharmacokinetic improvements in, 616–618
  reduction of arterial stiffness by, 148
  reversal of resistance vessel remodeling with, 129
  safety of, clinical implications of, 394
    in elderly, 557
    summary of evidence and conclusions on, 395–396
    types of evidence in determination of, 389–390
  slow-onset and long-acting preparations of, 617, 618t
  slow-release (retarded) preparations of, 616–617, 618t
  spironolactone vs., for hyperaldosteronism, 680, 681t
  SYST-EUR trial of, 334, 613
  vascular selectivity of, 617–618, 618t
  vasodilator effects of, 611–612
Calcium channels, L-type, 609, 611
  blockade of, *610,* 611
  T-type, 611
Calciuresis, of hypertension, metabolic defect in, 202
Caloric intake. See also *Diet.*
  excess of, hypertension related to, 25
  sympathetic nervous system stimulation by, 47

Canada, initial choice of antihypertensive treatment in, *383*, 384–385, 384t, *385*

Canadian Cardiovascular Society, classification of anginal symptoms by, 539

Cancer, risk of, from calcium channel blockers, 392–394, 395

Candesartan cilexetil. See also *Angiotensin II receptor antagonists.*
  development of, 624
  drug interactions with, 629
  pharmacokinetics of, in renal replacement therapy, 536t
  pharmacology of, 629, *630*, 631t
  structure of, *626*

Capillary pressure, identification of peripheral resistance by, 125

Captopril. See also *Angiotensin-converting enzyme (ACE) inhibitors.*
  CAPPP trial of, 338t, 350, 1351t
  cardioprotective effects of, 605
  dosage of, 603t
    excess, adverse effects of, 495
  exercise interaction with, 475
  in diagnosis, of hyperaldosteronism, 677
  in radionuclide scanning, for renovascular hypertension, 663
  losartan vs., in ELITE trial, 632
  oral or sublingual, 604
  pharmacokinetics of, 601t
    in renal replacement therapy, 536t
  pharmacology of, 601
  renin inhibitors vs., 647–649, *649*
  renoprotective effects of, 604
  with clonidine, for congestive heart failure, 512
  with hydrochlorothiazide, dosage of, 501t
    mean blood pressure reduction with, 502t

Carbamazepine, amplification of, by calcium antagonists, 614

Cardiac output, aging effects on, 552
  in pregnancy, 689
  longitudinal study of, in hypertension, 471
  response to exercise, 472

Cardioprotective effects, of alcohol consumption, 468
  of antihypertensive therapy, ACE inhibitors and, 605
    after ten years of treatment, 224–225, *225*
    clinical trials of, 337, 339
  of captopril, 605
  of diltiazem, 612
  of diuretics, clinical trials of, 344, 345t
  of enalapril, 605
  of endothelin receptor antagonists, 155
  of estrogens, 114, *115*
    in hormone replacement therapy, 544–545
  of lisinopril, 605
  of trandolapril, 605
  of verapamil, 612

Cardiopulmonary baroreceptors, 45–46

Cardiovascular disease, anesthetic considerations in, 708, 708t

Cardiovascular disease *(Continued)*
  clinical trials of antihypertensive therapy for, ASCOT, 338t, 346t, 351t, 355
    HOPE, 346t–347t, 348–349
    PEACE, 346t–347t, 348
    QUIET, 346t–347t, 348
  endothelial dysfunction in, 159–160

Cardiovascular events, as measure of outcome, 329
  blood pressure rise as precipitating agent for, 506
  circadian pattern of blood pressure as factor in, 506
  coronary hypothesis of, 324, *324*
  in mild hypertension, increased risk of, 323, *323*
  in response to antihypertensive therapy, changing patterns of, 224–225, *225*
  J-curve relationship of, with diastolic pressure, 231, 237, *237*, 265, 336
  MRFIT study of mortality from, in ischemic heart disease, 539
    in mild hypertension, 399, 402, *402*
    in normotensive patients, 30, *30*
    with diuretic use, 584–585
  predictor of, carotid artery stenosis as, 230
    low diastolic pressure as, 230–231, *231*
    pulse pressure as, 225, *225*, 230–232
  renin level as risk factor for, 448–449, *449*
  risk stratification for, 224–227, *225–226*
  sodium restriction and, 447–448, *447–448*

Cardiovascular risk factor(s). See also *Risk.*
  antihypertensive therapy for, ACE inhibitors in, clinical trials of, 346t–347t, 348–349
    combination therapy in, 498
  assessment of, 371–372, 371t–372t
    guideline recommendations for, 380
  blood pressure as, continuous relationship in, 29, *30*
    genetics of, 29–31
    in normotensive patients, 30–31, *30*
    low diastolic pressure and, 230–231, *231*
    systolic vs. diastolic, 238
  calcium antagonists as. See *Calcium antagonists, cardiovascular disease risk related to.*
  chronic renal failure as, 525
  clustering of, 238–240, 239t
  coronary. See *Coronary artery disease, risk of.*
  heart rate as, 240, 240t
  hypertension as, arbitrary definition of hypertension and, 29, *29*
    coronary hypothesis of, 324, *324*
    in congestive heart failure, 248
    in coronary disease, 237–238, 236t–237t, *237*
    in elderly, 552, *552*
    in ischemic heart disease, 543–544

Cardiovascular risk factor(s) *(Continued)*
  in isolated systolic hypertension, 552, *552*
    level of blood pressure in, 14–15, *15*, 16t
    syndrome of abnormalities in, 323–324, 324t
  in elderly, risk stratification of antihypertensive therapy for, 555, 555t
  in renal replacement therapy, 532
  in white-coat hypertension, 318–319
  left ventricular hypertrophy as, 239–240, *240*, 244, *245*
  lipoprotein abnormalities as. See *Lipoprotein abnormalities.*
  pressure-related target organ damage as, 558, 559t
  renal failure risk factors in common with, 525–526, 525t
  renin level as, 239, 448–449, *449*

Cardiovascular Risk Reduction Dietary Intervention Trial, 203

Cardiovascular Study in the Elderly (CASTEL), 342t–343t

Cardiovascular system, ACE inhibitor effects on, 602, 602t
  alcohol effects on, 215
  anatomic/hemodynamic changes in, with aging, 552–553, 553t
  anesthetic interactions with, 703, 704, *704*, 704t
  angiotensin II receptor blocker effects on, 625
  angiotensin-converting enzyme distribution in, 93, 93t
  angiotensin-converting enzyme function in, 95t, 95–96
  calcitonin gene–related peptide effects on, 183, *183*
  hypertrophy of. See *Blood vessels, hypertrophy of; Heart, hypertrophy of.*
  obesity effects on, 206–207, *206*
  obstructive sleep apnea effects on, 660
  stress response of, as predictor of later hypertension, 64–65, *64*, 65t
  sympathetic nervous system regulation of, 45–47

Cardiovascular-renal homeostasis, in blood pressure regulation, 22–23

CARE (Cholesterol and Recurrent Events), 544

Carotid arteries, clinical studies of, in white-coat hypertension, 318
  endarterectomy of, for stroke prevention, 282, *282*, 282t
  stenosis of, as risk factor for cardiovascular events, 230
    assessment of, in diagnosis of hypertension, 301t
    pulse pressure and low diastolic pressure as indicators of, 230

Carteolol. See also β-*Adrenoreceptor antagonists.*
  elimination characteristics of, 594t
  pharmacodynamics of, 591t
  pharmacokinetics of, 592t
    in renal replacement therapy, 536t

Carvedilol. See also β-*Adrenoreceptor antagonists.*

Carvedilol *(Continued)*
α-adrenergic activity of, 593
elimination characteristics of, 594t
for congestive heart failure, 512, 593
pharmacodynamics of, 591t
pharmacokinetics of, 592t
in renal replacement therapy, 536t
Case-control studies, 390
CASTEL (Cardiovascular Study in the Elderly), 342t–343t
Catecholamine crisis, 718
Catecholamines. See also *Norepinephrine.*
circulating, "cardiovascular hormone" function of, 45
diastolic function affected by, 256
in chronic renal failure, 525
plasma, as marker of early hypertension, 49
in diagnosis of pheochromocytoma, 686–687
urinary excretion of, after alcohol consumption, 215–216
daily rate of, 638, 638t
in diagnosis of pheochromocytoma, 685–686, 687t
ventricular hypertrophy related to, 251
Catecholamine-secreting tumors. See also *Pheochromocytoma.*
location of, in chromaffin tissue, 687
qualitative vs. temporal patterns of, 686
Caucasian race. See *Whites.*
Celiprolol, elimination characteristics of, 594t
Central nervous system, angiotensin II effects on, 622
angiotensin-converting enzyme distribution in, 93–94, 93t
angiotensin-converting enzyme function in, 95t
Centrencephalon, vascular, distribution of strokes in, 278, *279*
Cerebral arteries, in hypertension, antihypertensive therapy effects in, 280–281, *280*
pathophysiology of, 278, *278*
middle (MCA), antihypertensive therapy effects in, 280
Cerebrovascular disorders. See also *Stroke.*
anesthetic considerations in, 708, 708t
assessment of, as measure of outcome, 329
in diagnosis of hypertension, 301t
hypertension in, ACE inhibitors for, 604
angiotensin II receptor blockers for, 633
angiotensinogen polymorphisms in, 81, 87t
gradual reduction of, 512
hypertensive emergency in, 717
CGS 30440 (vasopeptidase inhibitor), 653–654, *653*
Characteristic impedance. See *Impedance, characteristic.*
Chemotactic peptide, as substrate for angiotensin-converting enzyme, 92t, 97
inactivation of, by angiotensin-converting enzyme, 97

Children. See also *Adolescents.*
blood pressure measurement in, 312
hypertension in, definition of, 23
Chinese Lacidipine Event Reduction (CLEVER), 346t–347t, 349
Chinese Trial on Isolated Systolic Hypertension in Elderly (SYST-CHINA), 334, 338t, 342, 342t–343t
Chloride, plasma, renal hemodynamic effects of, 177
Chlorothiazide. See also *Hydrochlorothiazide.*
history of, 3
Chlorthalidone. See also *Diuretics.*
characteristics and dosage of, 586t
in ALLHAT study, 363
in obese hypertensive patients, 208
Cholesterol and Recurrent Events (CARE), 544
Chromaffin cells, cardiac, 45
location of catecholamine-secreting tumors in, 687
Chromogranin A, plasma, as marker of early hypertension, 49
Chronobiology, 504. See also *Blood pressure, circadian rhythm of.*
Cigarette smoking. See *Smoking.*
Cilazapril, amlodipine vs., in chronic renal insufficiency, 293
Circadian rhythm, of blood pressure. See *Blood pressure, circadian rhythm of.*
Cirrhosis, atrial natriuretic peptide in, 171
CLEVER (Chinese Lacidipine Event Reduction), 346t–347t, 349
Clinical trial(s), AASK (African-American Study of Kidney Disease), 346t, 356
ABCD (Appropriate Blood Pressure Control in Diabetes), 337, 344, 346, 346t–347t, 392
AIPRI (Angiotensin-Converting Enzyme Inhibition in Progressive Renal Insufficiency), 291
ALLHAT. See *Antihypertensive and Lipid-Lowering to Prevent Heart Attack Trial (ALLHAT).*
ANBP (Australian National Blood Pressure Study), 332t, 338t
ANBP2 (Australian National Blood Pressure Study–2), 346t, 351t, 354
APTH (Ambulatory Blood Pressure Monitoring and Treatment of Hypertension Trial), 315
ASCOT (Anglo-Scandinavian Cardiac Outcomes Trial), 338t, 346t, 351t, 355
ATTMH (Australian Trial of Mild Hypertension), 342t–343t, 401, 402
BENEDICT (Bergamo Nephrologic Diabetes Complication Trial), 346t–347t, 348
Bergen study, 402
CAPPP (Captopril Prevention Project), 338t, 350, 1351t
Cardiovascular Risk Reduction Dietary Intervention Trial, 203
CARE (Cholesterol and Recurrent Events), 544
CASTEL (Cardiovascular Study in the Elderly), 342t–343t

Clinical trial(s) *(Continued)*
CLEVER (Chinese Lacidipine Event Reduction), 346t–347t, 349
CONVINCE (Controlled Onset Verapamil Investigation of Cardiovascular Endpoints), 337, 338t, 346t, 351t, 354–355
CSGTEI (Collaborative Study Group Trial on Effect of Irbesartan), 346, 346t–347t, 348
DASH (Dietary Approaches to Stop Hypertension). See *Dietary Approaches to Stop Hypertension (DASH).*
DAVIT II (Second Danish Verapamil Infarction Trial), 612
DIAB-HYCAR (Diabetes Hypertension Cardiovascular Morbidity-Mortality and Ramipril), 346, 346t–347t
Diltiazem Multicenter Postinfarction Research Trial, 612
DISH (Dietary Intervention Study in Hypertension), 208
ELITE (Evaluation of Losartan in the Elderly), 339, 632
ELSA (European Lacidipine Study on Atherosclerosis), 613, 614, 615
European Working Party on High Blood Pressure in Elderly, 332t, 342t–343t, 554
FACET (Fosinopril vs. Amlodipine Cardiovascular Events Randomized Trial), 337, 392
GENEDIAB (Genetique de la Nephropathie Diabetique), 519
GISEN (Gruppo Italiano di Studi Epidemiologici in Nefrologia), 291
HAPPHY (Heart Attack Primary Prevention in Hypertension Trial), 342t, 344, 345t
HARVEST (Hypertension and Ambulatory Recording Venetia Study), 317
HCP (Hypertension Control Program), 461
HDFP. See *Hypertension Detection and Follow-up Program (HDFP).*
HDS (Hypertension in Diabetes Study), 346t, 356
Health Professionals Follow-Up Study, 450, 454, 456
HEP (Hypertension in the Elderly Prevention Trial), 342t–343t
HOPE (Heart Outcomes Prevention Evaluation), 346t–347t, 348–349
HOT. See *Hypertension Optimal Treatment Study (HOT).*
HPT (Hypertension Prevention Trial), 461
HSCSG (Hypertension-Stroke Cooperative Study Group), 342t–343t
HYVET (Hypertension in the Very Elderly Trial), 338t, 346t–347t, 349–350
in drug approval process, 580
INSIGHT (International Nifedipine GITS Study Intervention as a Goal in Hypertension Treatment), 338t, 346t, 350, 351t, 352

Clinical trial(s) *(Continued)*
INVEST (International Verapamil-Tran-
dolapril Study), 346t, 351t, 353
INWEST (Intravenous Nimodipine
West European Stroke Trial), 281
IPPPSH (International Prospective Pri-
mary Prevention Study in Hyper-
tension), 342t, 344, 345t
ISIS-2 (Second International Study of
Infarct Survival), 542
LIFE. See *Losartan Intervention for
Endpoint (LIFE) Reduction in Hy-
pertension Study.*
MACH-1 (Mibefradil in Patients with
Congestive Heart Failure), 542
MAPHY (Metoprolol Atherosclerosis
Prevention in Hypertensives),
342t, 344, 345t
MDRD. See *Modification of Diet in Re-
nal Disease (MDRD).*
Medical Research Council trials. See
Medical Research Council.
MIDAS (Multicenter Isradipine Di-
uretic Atherosclerosis Study), 392,
615
MRFIT (Multiple Risk Factor Intervention Trial). See *Multiple Risk Factor Intervention Trial (MRFIT).*
NASCET (North American Symptomatic Carotid Endarterectomy Trial),
282
NICS-EH (National Intervention Cooperative Study in Elderly Hypertensives), 338t, 346t, 350, 351t
NORDIL (Nordic Diltiazem Study),
346t, 351t, 355, 613, 614
Nurses Health Study II, 453, 454, 455
of blood pressure goal for therapy, 336
of calcium channel blockers, 391, 392
of diastolic hypertension therapy, 331,
332t–333t, 334
of isolated systolic hypertension therapy, 334–335
of lifestyle modification vs. medication,
335
of metabolic effects of antihypertensive
drugs, 337, 339
of patient selection for therapy, 335–
336, *335*
of treatment regimen, 336–337, 338t
ongoing or planned, 344–356
in special groups of patients, 344–
350, 346t–347t
African Americans and, 356
elderly and, 349–350
with previous cardiovascular disease, 346t–347t, 348–349
with type 2 diabetes, 344, 346,
346t–347t, 348, 356
of older vs. newer drugs, 350, 351t,
352–355
of second- and third-generation
drugs, 351t, 355–356
PATHS (Prevention and Treatment of
Hypertension Study), 466–468,
467, 467t
PATS (Post-Stroke Antihypertensive
Treatment Study), 342t–343t

Clinical trial(s) *(Continued)*
PEACE (Prevention of Events with Angiotensin-Converting Enzyme Inhibition), 346t–347t, 348
PEPI (Postmenopausal Estrogen/Proges-
tin Interventions), 548
PRAISE (Prospective Randomized Am-
lodipine Survival Evaluation), 542
PROGRESS (Perindopril Protection
Against Recurrent Stroke), 346t–
347t, 349
published results of, 341–344
of diuretics or β-blockers, 344, 345t
of treatment efficacy, 341–342, 342t–
343t, 344
QUIET (Quinapril Ischemic Event
Trial), 346t–347t, 348
REIN (Ramipril Efficacy in Nephropa-
thy), 291
RENAAL (Randomized Evaluation of
NIDDM with the Angiotensin II
Antagonist Losartan), 346t–347t,
348
Scandinavian Simvastatin Survival
Study (4S), 361
SCOPE (Study of Cognition and Prog-
nosis in Elderly Patients with Hy-
pertension), 346t–347t, 349
SHELL (Systolic Hypertension in El-
derly Long-Term Lacidipine
Trial), 338t, 346t, 351t, 352
SHEP. See *Systolic Hypertension in El-
derly Project (SHEP).*
SNAP (Sodium and Blood Pressure)
Study, 559
SOLVD (Studies of Left Ventricular
Dysfunction), 511–512
STAI (Studio della Ticlopidina nell' An-
gina Instabile), 543
STONE (Shanghai Trial of Nifedipine
in Elderly), 342, 342t–343t, 613,
614
STOP. See *Swedish Trial in Old Pa-
tients with Hypertension (STOP).*
SYST-CHINA (Chinese Trial on Iso-
lated Systolic Hypertension in El-
derly), 334, 338t, 342, 342t–343t
SYST-EUR. See *Systolic Hypertension
in Europe (SYST-EUR).*
TAIM (Trial of Antihypertensive Inter-
ventions and Management), 440,
442, *442*, 461–462, 461t
Tecumseh study, 402–403
TOHP. See *Trials of Hypertension Pre-
vention (TOHP).*
TOMHS. See *Treatment of Mild Hyper-
tension Study (TOMHS).*
TONE (Trial of Nonpharmacologic In-
terventions in Elderly), 445–446,
444–446
U.S. Public Health Service Trial, 332t
USPHS (United States Public Health
Service Hospitals Cooperative
Study Group), 342t–343t
VA-NHLBI Feasibility Study, 332t,
342t–343t
VALUE (Valsartan Amlodipine Long-
Term Utilization Evaluation), 338t,
346t, 351t, 355–356

Clinical trial(s) *(Continued)*
value of, 390
Vanguard studies as, 203
Veterans Administration trials as. See
Veterans Administration trials.
VHAS (Verapamil Hypertension Atherosclerosis Study), 613, 615
Walnut Creek Contraceptive Drug
Study, 548
WOSCOP (West of Scotland Coronary
Prevention) trial, 613
Clonidine. See also α-*Adrenoreceptor
agonists.*
combined with other agents, captopril
and, 512
hydrochlorothiazide and, 501t
exercise interaction with, 474
in acute stroke, 512
in diagnosis, of baroreflex failure, 575
in elderly, adverse effects of, 557
in migraine, 513
in obese hypertensive patients 209
in orthostatic intolerance, 576
in pregnancy, 515, 696t, 698
in resistant hypertension, 570
intraoperative use of, 711
pharmacology of, 640
preoperative, for induction, 711
withdrawal from, hypertensive emergency due to, 718
Clopidogrel, for prevention of myocardial
infarction, 543
for stroke prevention, 282
Coagulation disorders, associated with
hypertension, 111–112, 111t
in diabetes mellitus, 544
Coagulation factors, increased levels of,
in hypertension, 112
Coarctation of aorta, assessment of, in
diagnosis of hypertension, 303t
Cocaine, catecholamine crisis due to, 718
hypertension due to, 566
Cognitive decline. See *Dementia.*
Cohort studies, 390
Cold pressor (hand pain) test, in
baroreflex failure, 574–575, *575*
Collaborative Study Group Trial on
Effect of Irbesartan (CSGTEI), 346,
346t–347t, 348
Combination antihypertensive agents. See
Antihypertensive therapy, combined.
Community Hypertension Evaluation
Clinic (CHEC) Program, 546
Community outreach programs, 415–418
definition of, 415
for hypertension management, community health workers in, 417–418
community–health system partnership in, 417
ecological multidisciplinary model
in, 417
for gaps in care and control, 417
history of, 415–417
key principles of, 415
Comorbid conditions. See specific
disorder, *e.g., Renal failure, chronic.*
Compliance, as index of arterial stiffness,
135t, 138
capacitative, as index of arterial stiffness, 135t, 138–139

Compliance *(Continued)*
  cross-sectional, as index of arterial stiffness, 138
  oscillatory, as index of arterial stiffness, 135t, 138–139
  with antihypertensive therapy. See *Antihypertensive therapy, compliance with.*
Computed tomography (CT), for adrenal adenoma localization, 678
  of pheochromocytoma, 687
  spiral (helical), in renovascular hypertension, 664
  ultrafast, of coronary blood flow, 267
  of ventricular hypertrophy, 253
Congenital abnormalities, from ACE inhibitors, 483, 606
  from calcium antagonists, 614
Congestive heart failure. See *Heart failure, congestive.*
Conn's tumor, hypertension due to, 514
Continuous positive airway pressure, for nocturnal obstructive sleep apnea, 658
Contraceptives, oral, angiotensinogen elevation due to, 77–78
  estrogen and progestin dosage in, 548
  hypertension related to, pathophysiology of, 548
  resistant, 565–566
  risk of, 482–483
Contrast, genetic, 34–35
Controlled Onset Verapamil Investigation of Cardiovascular Endpoints (CONVINCE), 337, 338t, 346t, 351t, 354–355
Coping, active (John Henryism), 63
  defensive, 62
Coronary arteries, autoregulation of, alteration of, in left ventricular hypertrophy, 262–263
  blood pressure reduction effects on, 264–265, *264*
  blood flow in, arterial stiffening effects on, 142
  flow reserve abnormalities in, 260–267, *261*
    epicardial coronary disease and, 265
    in left ventricular hypertrophy, altered autoregulation and, 262–263
    antihypertensive therapy for, 265–266
    blood pressure reduction in, 264–265, *264*
    endothelial dysfunction in, 262
    hypertensive effects in, 263–264
    increased vascular water content in, 262
    medial wall thickening in, 261–262
    pathology of, 261–262
    perivascular and interstitial fibrosis in, 262
    rarefaction of arterioles in, 261
    in myocardial hypertrophy and wall stress, 262
    measurement of, confounding factors in, 263

Coronary arteries *(Continued)*
    noninvasive techniques in, 266–267, *267*
    radionuclide-labeled microspheres in, 266
Coronary artery disease. See also *Atherosclerosis; Heart disease, ischemic.*
  angiography of, 540
  antihypertensive therapy in, 512
    initial choice of, 485, 486t
  bypass graft surgery for, 542
  in hypertension, 235–243
    alcohol consumption and, 217
    atherosclerotic sequelae of, 235, *236*
    blood pressure components in, 238
    blood pressure threshold level in, 235, 236t
    coronary events related to, 237–238, *237*, 237t
    gender and metabolic issues in, 114–115, *115*
    in elderly, 240–241, 240t–241t, *241*
    initial assessment of, 301t
    myocardial infarction related to, reinfarction and death from, 238, 238t
      unrecognized, 237, 237t
    prevalence and incidence of, 235
    preventive strategies for, 241–242, 242t
  mortality from, 532
    in African Americans, 558
  percutaneous transluminal angioplasty for, 540–542
  risk of, blood pressure levels in, 15, *15*, 16t, *236*, 237–238, 237t
    from calcium channel blockers, observational studies of, 391–392
    randomized trials of, 392
    summary of evidence for, 395
    heart rate as factor in, 240, 240t, 242
    J-curve relationship with diastolic pressure and, 231, 237, *237*, 265, 336
    left ventricular hypertrophy as factor in, 239–240, *240*, 242
    ranking of, in Scottish Heart Health Study, 435, *436*
    reduction of, with antihypertensive therapy, 331
    relative, 221, *222*
    renin as factor in, 239
    risk factor clustering in, 238–240, 239t
    visceral obesity as risk factor for, 111
    wide pulse pressure as marker of, 232
Coronary heart disease. See *Coronary artery disease.*
Coronary hypothesis of hypertension, 324, *324*
Corticosteroids, fetal exposure to, hypertension related to, 24
  hypertension due to, 566
    sympathetic nervous system hyperactivity in, 51
Cortisol, excess production of, hypertension due to, 682–684

Cortisol *(Continued)*
  24-hour urinary excretion test of, 683
Cost effectiveness, of screening, for white-coat hypertension, 320
  of therapy, 405–408
    as measure of outcome, 326, 329
    drug costs in, 405
    estimation of costs in, 405–406
    guideline recommendations and, 377–378, 381
    hypertension specialists and, 408, 408t
    impact of managed care in, 407–408, 408t
    indirect costs in, 406
    outcome measurement and, 407
    secondary costs in, 406
    strategies in, 406–407, 406t
      optimization of drug use and, 407
      patient selection and, 406, 406t
      practical approaches to, 406–407
    variable costs in, 405, 405t
Cough, in ACE inhibitor therapy, 606
Counterpulsation, external enhanced, in coronary artery disease, 543
C-reactive protein, as risk factor, for hypertension, 301
Creatinine, evaluation of, in diagnosis of hypertension, 302, 304t
  rise of, with antihypertensive therapy, 528–529
CSGTEI (Collaborative Study Group Trial on Effect of Irbesartan), 346, 346t–347t, 348
C-type natriuretic peptide. See *Natriuretic peptides.*
Cuff, in blood pressure measurement, inflation of, hypertension due to, 308, 565
  rate of inflation and deflation of, 308
  size of, 307, 307t
    in infants and children, 312
    in obesity, 312
Cushing's syndrome, assessment of, in diagnosis of hypertension, 303t, 568t, 569–570
  causes of, 683
  hypertension in, 683–684
    antihypertensive therapy for, 514
    diagnosis of, 683–684
    treatment of, 684
Cyanide, from high-dose nitroprusside, 716
Cyclooxygenase (COX), conversion of CYP-450–derived arachidonate products by, 177, *177*
  vasoconstrictor derivatives of, nitric oxide dysfunction due to, 162
Cyclosporine, amplification of, by calcium antagonists, 614
  hypertension due to, 514, 566
Cyproheptadine, for Cushing's disease, 684
Cytochrome P450, arachidonate metabolites of, conversion of, by cyclooxygenase, 177, *177*
  in preeclampsia, 180
  in spontaneously hypertensive rats, 178–179

DASH. See *Dietary Approaches to Stop Hypertension (DASH)*.
DAVIT II (Second Danish Verapamil Infarction Trial), 612
Debrisoquin, for hypertension, in chronic renal insufficiency, 287
Defeat reaction, 59
Dehydroepiandrosterone sulfate, as risk factor, for hypertension and metabolic abnormalities, in women, 114
Delayed-action antihypertensives, calcium antagonists and, lipophilic preparations of, 617, *617–618*, 618t
  slow-onset and long-lasting preparations of, 617, 618t
  slow-release (retarded) preparations of, 616–617, 618t
  verapamil and, for control of early morning blood pressure surge, 507–508, *507*
Demadex. See *Torsemide*.
Dementia, 11–14
  antihypertensive therapy in, clinical trials of, 14
  changing concepts in, 11–12
  cognitive decline in, early, high blood pressure associated with, 12–13, *12–13*
  low blood pressure associated with, 13–14, *14*
  definition of, 11
  multi-infarct, 11
  risk factors for, 12
  vascular, 11–12
Deoxycorticosterone excess, hypertension due to, 676
Deoxycorticosterone-salt–induced hypertension, calcitonin gene–related peptide role in, 184–185, 184t, *185*
Depression, cardiovascular disorders related to, 63
  hypertension related to, 63
Deserpidine, combined with hydrochlorothiazide, dosage of, 501t
Development. See *Growth and development*.
Dexamethasone, for glucocorticoid resistance, 676
  suppression test with, for ACTH secretion, 683–684
Diabetes mellitus, 518–522
  antihypertensive therapy in, 520–522
    ACE inhibitors in, 337, 604
    β-adrenoreceptor blockers contraindicated in, 485, 487, 510, 522, 593
    benefits of, 331, 334
    blood pressure goal in, 510, 518, 520–521, 521t
    clinical trial(s) of, 344, 346, 346t–347t, 348
      ABCD, 337, 344, 346, 346t–347t, 348, 392
      BENEDICT, 346t–347t, 348
      CSGTEI, 346, 346t–347t, 348
      DIAB-HYCAR, 346, 346t–347t

Diabetes mellitus *(Continued)*
      FACET, 337, 392
      GENEDIAB, 519
      HDS, 346t, 356
      RENAAL, 346t–347t, 348
    comparison of agents in, 510, 521–522, 521t
    initial choice of, 487
      in obesity, 485
    optimal characteristics for, 510
  arterial stiffness related to, 147
  as risk factor, for hypertension, 299–300, 299t
  atherosclerotic process in, 544
  β-blockers contraindicated in, 485, 487, 510, 522, 593
  blood pressure in, absence of nocturnal dip in, 510
  coronary artery bypass graft surgery vs. percutaneous angioplasty in, 541
  coronary artery disease associated with, gender and metabolic issues in, 114–115, *115*
    treatment considerations in, 115–116
  hypertension associated with, angiotensinogen polymorphisms in, 81, 87t
    blood pressure control in, 518, *518*
    follow-up assessment of, 304t
    genetic predisposition to, 519
  incidence and prevalence of, 518
  intensive insulin therapy in, for prevention of complications, 544
  kallikrein excretion in, 195
  kallikrein-kinin system function in, 197–198
  nephropathy due to. See *Nephropathy, diabetic*.
  vascular disease in, 519–520
    elevated arterial pressure in, 519
    glycated albumin in, 520
    hyperglycemia/hyperinsulinemia in, 519–520, 520t
    predisposing factors in, 519, 519t
DIAB-HYCAR (Diabetes Hypertension Cardiovascular Morbidity-Mortality and Ramipril), 346, 346t–347t
Dialysis. See *Hemodialysis; Peritoneal dialysis; Renal replacement therapy*.
Diastolic blood pressure. See *Blood pressure, diastolic; Hypertension, diastolic*.
Diastolic function. See *Ventricle(s), diastolic function/dysfunction of*.
Diazepam, for induction of anesthesia, 705–706
  magnesium sulfate vs., in eclamptic convulsions, 695
Diazoxide, for preeclampsia/eclampsia, 696t
  intravenous, for hypertensive encephalopathy, 279
  pharmacology of, 641–642
Diet, 460–465
  calcium in. See *Calcium, dietary*.
  clinical trials of, 203–204. See also *Dietary Approaches to Stop Hypertension (DASH)*.
  excess caloric intake in, hypertension related to, 25

Diet *(Continued)*
  sympathetic nervous system stimulation by, 47
  fat in, 180, 462–463
  fruits and vegetables in, 463, *464*
  high-carbohydrate, blood pressure and insulin effects of, 462
  macronutrient alteration in, 457
  magnesium repletion in, 456–457
  micronutrients in, controversies and, 202, 204
  nutrient interactions and, 202–203
  nutrient patterns and, 203
  potassium repletion and, 450–454
  sodium in. See *Sodium, dietary*.
  sympathetic nervous system activity related to, 119–120
    insulin in, 119–120
    nutrient-specific effects in, 119
    thermogenesis and energy balance in, 120
  unsaturated fatty acids in, eicosanoid effects of, 180
  weight-reducing, clinical trials of, 461–462, 461t
    hypertension lowered by, 208
Diet Modification in Renal Disease. See *Modification of Diet in Renal Disease (MDRD)*.
Dietary Approaches to Stop Hypertension (DASH), blood pressure effect of, 433, *433*
  combination of nutrients in, 433–434
  ease of acceptance of, 465, 479
  food components in, 463, *464*, 556t
  low-fat dairy products in, 455
  nutrient patterns in, 203–204
Dietary Intervention Study in Hypertension (DISH), 208
Dietary thermogenesis, energy balance and, 120, *120*
99mTc Diethylenetriaminepentaacetic acid (DTPA), in radionuclide imaging, 663
Digoxin, for diastolic congestive heart failure, 260
  potentiation of, by telmisartan, 630
Diltiazem. See also *Calcium antagonists*.
  adverse effects of, 613
  cardioprotective effects of, 612
  combined with other agents, β-blockers and, 595, 613
    hydrochlorothiazide and, 501t
  Diltiazem Multicenter Postinfarction Research Trial of, 612
  drug interactions with, 614
  in arrhythmia, 612
  in chronic renal insufficiency, 292–293
  in diabetes mellitus, renoprotective effects of, 522
  in ischemic heart disease, 542
  NORDIL trial of, 346t, 351t, 355, 613, 614
  pharmacokinetics of, in renal replacement therapy, 536t
  slow-release (retarded) preparation of, 617
  structure of, *610*
Dipyridamole, echocardiography with, 540

Dipyridamole *(Continued)*
for stroke prevention, 282–283
DISH (Dietary Intervention Study in Hypertension), 208
Distensibility, arterial, as index of arterial stiffness, 135t, 138
Diulo (metolazone), 586t
Diuresis, due to natriuretic peptides, 168
Diuretics, 584–589
  ALLHAT study of, 353, 360–361
  as initial choice of treatment, clinical trials of, 342, 344
    in African Americans, 483
    in Australia, 386
    in elderly, 555
    in Norway, 386
    in obesity, 485
    in United Kingdom, 385
  breast feeding and, 699
  cardiovascular morbidity and mortality from, 584–585
  characteristics and dosage of, 585, 586t–587t
  combined with, ACE inhibitors, 528, 529, 603–604
    adrenergic inhibitors, 637
    β-blockers, 500–501, 501t, 721t
    common agents, 500, 720t–721t
      for resistant hypertension, 570
      low-dose, general guidelines for, 374
  complications of, 588–589, 588
  contraindications to, in hyperuricemia, 511
  currently available agents as, 585, 588
    dosage and features of, 586t–587t, 719t
  efficacy of, clinical trials of, 344, 345t
  exercise interaction with, 474
  in African Americans, 562
  in chronic renal failure, choice of agents in, 287–288
    combined with ACE inhibitors, 528, 529
    dosage of, 529
  in diabetes mellitus, 487, 510, 522
  in diastolic congestive heart failure, 259–260
  in elderly, 555
    ANBP2 trial of, 354, 351t
  in hyperaldosteronism, 680, 680
  in isolated systolic hypertension, 482
  in obese hypertensive patients, 208
  in pregnancy, 696t, 699
  in ventricular hypertrophy, regression of mass with, 253, 585
  inappropriate dose of, in resistant hypertension, 566
  loop of Henle agents as, characteristics and dosage of, 586t–587t, 719t
    long-acting, 585
  mechanisms of action of, 584–585, 585, 585t
  potassium-sparing, 500, 585, 588, 719t
  protective effects of, clinical trials of, 344, 345t
  resistance vessel remodeling and, 128
  sulfonamide-based, glucose metabolism and, 588–589
  therapeutic guidelines for, 589, 589t

Diuretics *(Continued)*
  with sodium restriction, in elderly, 516
Diurnal pattern of blood pressure. See *Blood pressure, circadian rhythm of.*
Dobutamine echocardiography, 540
DOC-salt–induced hypertension, calcitonin gene–related peptide role in, 184–185, 184t, 185
Dopamine, urinary excretion of, 638t
Doppler echocardiography. See *Echocardiography, Doppler.*
Dorsal root ganglia (DRG), calcitonin gene–related peptide synthesis in, 182
Doxazosin. See also α-*Adrenoreceptor antagonists.*
  effectiveness of, 596
  in ALLHAT study, 363
  lipid-lowering effects of, 597
  pharmacokinetics of, in renal replacement therapy, 536t
Drug abuse or overdose, assessment of, in diagnosis of hypertension, 303t
  catecholamine crisis due to, 718
Drug approval process. See *Antihypertensive therapy, approval process for.*
Dyrenium. See *Triamterene.*
Dyslipidemia. See *Lipoprotein abnormalities.*
Dysplasia, fibromuscular, progression of, 667
  renovascular hypertension due to, 662
    in women, 547–548

Echocardiography, contrast agents for, 253
  dobutamine, 540
  Doppler, of diastolic function, 256–257, 256–257
    Ar wave measurement in, 258
    emerging techniques in, 257–259
    pitfalls in interpretation of, 257
    tissue imaging in, 259
  in ischemic heart disease, 539–540
  M-mode, color, of diastolic function, 258–259
    of ventricular hypertrophy, 251–252, 252, 252t
  of ventricular hypertrophy, in white-coat hypertension, 317t
    specific methods in, 251–253
  three-dimensional, of ventricular hypertrophy, 253
  transesophageal, of coronary blood flow, 266
  transthoracic, of coronary blood flow, 266
  two-dimensional, of coronary blood flow, 266, 267
    of ventricular hypertrophy, 252–253
Eclampsia. See also *Preeclampsia.*
  as hypertensive emergency, 718
  cerebral pathophysiology in, 693
  convulsions in, magnesium sulfate vs. diazepam and phenytoin for, 695
  late postpartum, 691

Eclampsia *(Continued)*
  management of, 695, 696t
  signs and symptoms of, 691, 691t
Edecrin (ethacrynic acid), characteristics and dosage of, 587t
Edema, ankle, from calcium antagonists, 611–612
Eicosanoids, 176–181
  in hypertension, CYP-450–related arachidonic acid metabolites in, 178–179
    dietary unsaturated fatty acids and, 180
    prohypertensive prostanoids in, 178
  in preeclampsia, 179–180
  kinin synthesis related to, 195
  renal hemodynamic effects of, 176–178, 177–178
Elastic modulus, as index of arterial stiffness, 135t, 138
Elasticity, arterial. See *Artery(ies), elasticity of.*
Elastin, fatigue and fracture of, with aging, 142–143, 230
Elderly. See also *Age and aging.*
  antihypertensive therapy in, benefits of, 242
    drug metabolism and, 553
    efficacy of, 554–555, 555
    in isolated systolic hypertension, initial choice of therapy for, 481–482
    individualized, in comorbid conditions, 555, 557
    initial choice of, 480–481, 480t, 555, 557
    lifestyle modification in, 555, 556t
    management of, 515–516
    risk stratification in, 555, 556t
  blood pressure in, definition of, 551
    measurement of, 312
  blood pressure rise in, in nonindustrialized populations, 6, 6
    lack of, in nonindustrialized populations, 8–9
    physiology of, 229–230
  clinical trial(s) of hypertension in, ANBP2 (Australian National Blood Pressure Study–2), 346t, 351t, 354
    CASTEL (Cardiovascular Study in the Elderly), 342t–343t
    ELITE (Evaluation of Losartan in the Elderly), 339, 632
    European Working Party on High Blood Pressure in Elderly, 332t, 342t–343t, 554
    HEP (Hypertension in the Elderly Prevention Trial), 342t–343t
    HYVET (Hypertension in the Very Elderly Trial), 338t, 346t–347t, 349–350
    Medical Research Council Trial of Treatment of Hypertension in Older Adults, 333t, 342t–343t, 344, 345t, 554
    NICS-EH (National Intervention Cooperative Study in Elderly Hypertensives), 338t, 346t, 350, 351t

Elderly *(Continued)*
    ongoing or planned, 349–350
    SCOPE (Study of Cognition and
        Prognosis in Elderly Patients
        with Hypertension), 346t–347t,
        349
    SHELL (Systolic Hypertension in El-
        derly Long-Term Lacidipine
        Trial), 338t, 346t, 351t, 352
    SHEP. See *Systolic Hypertension in
        Elderly Project (SHEP)*.
    STONE (Shanghai Trial of Nifedi-
        pine in the Elderly), 342, 342t–
        343t, 613, 614
    STOP. See *Swedish Trial in Old Pa-
        tients with Hypertension
        (STOP)*.
    SYST-CHINA (Chinese Trial on Iso-
        lated Systolic Hypertension in
        Elderly), 334, 338t, 342, 342t–
        343t
    SYST-EUR (Systolic Hypertension
        in Europe), 554
    TONE (Trial of Nonpharmacologic
        Interventions in Elderly), 445–
        446, *444–446*
    distribution of blood pressure measure-
        ments in, 5, *5*
    hypertension in, 551–557
        cardiovascular risks in, 552, *552*
        coronary disease related to, 240–241,
            240t–241t, *241*
        diagnosis and clinical assessment of,
            553–554
        epidemiology of, 551–552
        prevalence of, 551–552, 552t
        pulse pressure as risk marker in, 232
        isolated systolic hypertension in. See
            Hypertension, isolated systolic.
    nocturnal lowering of blood pressure
        absent in, 506
    pseudohypertension in, 515, 554
    salt sensitivity of, in clinical trials, 437
    sodium restriction in, diuretics with,
        516
    TONE trial of, 445–446, *444–446*
    systolic pressure augmentation in, from
        pulse-wave reflection, 515
Electrocardiography, as screening method
    for hypertension, in LIFE study, 369
    during anesthesia, 710
    in diagnosis of hypertension, 302, 304t
    in ischemic heart disease, 539
Electrolytes, evaluation of, in diagnosis of
    hypertension, 302, 304t
ELITE (Evaluation of Losartan in the
    Elderly), 339, 632
ELSA (European Lacidipine Study on
    Atherosclerosis), 613, 614, *615*
Employment-related stress, 61–62
Enalapril. See also *Angiotensin-
    converting enzyme (ACE) inhibitors*.
    ABCD trial of, 344, 348
    cardioprotective effects of, 605
    dosage of, 603t
    exercise interaction with, 475
    in renal failure, *529*
    nisoldipine vs., ABCD trial of, 392
    pharmacokinetics of, 601t

Enalapril *(Continued)*
    in renal replacement therapy, 536t
    pharmacology of, 600–601
    renoprotective effects of, 604
    with hydrochlorothiazide, dosage of,
        501t
        mean blood pressure reduction with,
            502t
Enalaprilat, for hypertensive emergencies,
    604, 716t
    intravenous form of, 603
    renin inhibitors vs., 647–648
Enalkiren, 647, 649. See also *Renin,
    inhibitors of*.
Encephalopathy, hypertensive, 279–280,
    717
Endopeptidase, neutral (NEP), in
        metabolism of natriuretic peptides,
        167
    inhibition of, 172
        effects of, 651
    inhibitors of, advantages and disad-
        vantages of, 654
        rationale for development of, 651–
            652
        with affinity for ACE and NEP,
            652–654, *653*
Endothelial growth factors, in
    angiogenesis, 261
Endothelin(s), 152–156
    activation and role of, in hypertension,
        155–156, *156, 162*
    biological actions of, 152–154, 643
    eicosanoid effects on, 178
    humoral actions of, 154
    isoforms of, 152, *152*
    levels of, in chronic renal failure, 525
    medial wall thickening due to, 262
    myocardial actions of, 154
    natriuretic peptide interaction with,
        167, 170
    nitric oxide interaction with, 162
    receptor agonists of, 155, 155t
    receptor antagonists of, 643–645
        cardiopulmonary protective role of,
            155
        in experimental models of hyperten-
            sion, 644
        potential antihypertensive uses for,
            156, 644–645
        selective and nonselective types of,
            155t
        subtypes of, 643–644, 643t
    receptors for, 154–155, 155t
        blockade of, cardiopulmonary protec-
            tive effects of, 155
        in vascular tone regulation, 162
    renal actions of, 154
    vascular actions of, 152–154, *153*
Endotheliosis, glomerular, in
    preeclampsia, 692
Endothelium, agonists of, 158
    angiotensin-converting enzyme distribu-
        tion in, 93, 93t
    angiotensin-converting enzyme interac-
        tion with, 96
    dysfunction of, due to metabolic abnor-
        malities, 113, 113t, *114*
    in cardiovascular disease, 159–160

Endothelium *(Continued)*
    in chronic renal failure, cardiovascu-
        lar damage due to, 525
    in coronary artery disease, 262
    preeclampsia related to, 179
    estrogen effects on, 547
    mediation of acetylcholine response by,
        in resistance vessels, 130
    regulation of vascular tone by, 158–159
    vasodilation abnormalities in, in hyper-
        tension, 262
Endothelium-derived factor(s). See also
    Nitric oxide (NO).
    C-type natriuretic peptide as, 169
    interaction of, with nitric oxide, 162
    regulation of vascular tone by, 158–159
End-stage renal disease. See *Renal
    failure, chronic*.
Energy balance, dietary thermogenesis
    and, 120, *120*
Environment, blood pressure related to,
    31–33
    biometric analysis of, 31–32
    family environment in, 31–32
    family history studies in, 48–49
    gene–environment interaction in, 33,
        47–49
    genes vs. environment in, 32
    in individuals, 33, *34*
    polygenes in, 32–33, *33*
    population environment in, 32
    population genetics in, 32
    stress in, 61–62
    sympathetic nervous system activity
        and, 47–49
Ephedrine, combined with β-blockers,
    adverse effects of, 595
Epidemiology of hypertension, 4–16
    birth weight and, 10–11, 11t, 24
    dementia and, 11–14
    historical background of, 1–2
    in African Americans, 558
    in elderly, 551–552
    in industrialized populations, 6–8, *6–7*
    in nonindustrialized populations, 8–9,
        8t, *9*
    migration effect in, 9–10
    observational surveys in, 4–5, 4t, *5*
    on calcium channel blockers, 389–
        390, 391–392
    prevalence in, 4, 4t, *5*
    psychosocial factors in, 10, *10*
    risk factors in, 14–15, *15, 16t*
Epinephrine, circadian rhythm of, 505
    combined with β-blockers, adverse ef-
        fects of, 595
    dyslipidemia due to, in insulin-resis-
        tance syndrome, 121, *122, 124*
    urinary excretion of, 638, 638t
    in pheochromocytoma, 686
Epithelial cell(s), angiotensin-converting
    enzyme distribution in, 93, 93t
    angiotensin-converting enzyme function
        in, 95t
5,6-Epoxyicosatrienoic acid (EET),
    conversion to vasoconstrictor and
    vasodilator metabolites by, 177, *177*
    preeclampsia and, 180
Eprosartan, development of, 625

Eprosartan *(Continued)*
pharmacology of, 629–630
structure of, *625–626*
Erythropoietin therapy, in chronic renal insufficiency, hypertension related to, 287, 566
in orthostatic hypotension, 573
Esmolol, for hypertensive emergencies, 716t
for hypertensive stroke, 281
indications for, 593
intraoperative use of, 711
Estrogen(s). See also *Contraceptives, oral.*
angiotensinogen elevation due to, 77–78
blood pressure level related to, 547
endothelium-dependent vasodilation from, 547
PEPI trial of, 548
protective effects of, in coronary artery disease and hypertension, 114, *115*
replacement therapy with, arterial stiffness and, 146
cardioprotective effect of, 544–545
for stroke prevention, 284
hypertension in, 548–549
antihypertensive therapy for, 515
synthetic vs. natural estrogen for, 548
monitoring of blood pressure in, 482
stress response related to, 59
synthesis of, *675*
Ethacrynic acid (Edecrin), characteristics and dosage of, 587t
European Lacidipine Study on Atherosclerosis (ELSA), 613, 614, *615*
European Working Party on High Blood Pressure in Elderly, 332t, 342t–343t, 554
Evidence-based guidelines. See *Antihypertensive therapy, guidelines for.*
Exercise, 470–476
aerobic, as stress buffer, 66
antihypertensive therapy with, 473–475
arterial stiffness and, 146
blood pressure measurement during, 312
diastolic function affected by, in aging, 255–256
fitness related to, 472
health benefits of, 470–471, 471t
hemodynamic response during, 471–472, 472t
in African Americans, 562
in women, 549
isometric exercise/strength training in, 472
physiologic response to, 472
ambulatory blood pressure monitoring of, 473
blood pressure response in, 472
glucose/insulin effect of, 472
prescription for, 473
with weight loss, 509
Exercise stress testing, before beginning exercise program, 473

Exercise stress testing *(Continued)*
in ischemic heart disease, 539–540
Extracellular fluid volume, in chronic renal failure, 524, *524*
in renal replacement therapy, 535

FACET (Fosinopril vs. Amlodipine Cardiovascular Events Randomized Trial), 337, 392
Familial paraganglioma syndrome, 575
Family environment, blood pressure effects of, 31–32
Family studies, of sympathetic nervous system activity, 48–49
Fat. See also *Adipose tissue; Obesity.*
dietary, 180, 462–463
Felodipine. See also *Calcium antagonists.*
combined with hydrochlorothiazide, dosage of, 501t
in HOT trial, 392
pharmacokinetics of, in renal replacement therapy, 536t
slow-release (retarded) preparation of, 617
Fenoldopam, for hypertensive emergencies, 716–717, 716t
in renal failure, 717
intraoperative use of, 711
Fetus, abnormalities of, from ACE inhibitors, 483, 606
from calcium antagonists, 614
mortality in, with maternal diastolic hypertension, 689, *689*
Fibrillation, atrial, calcium antagonists for, 612
Fibrinoid necrosis, in pathophysiology of hypertensive emergency, 715
in resistance vessels, lacunar infarction due to, 278, *278*
Fibrinolytic disorders, associated with hypertension, 111–112, 111t
Fibroblasts, angiotensin-converting enzyme distribution in, 93t, 97
angiotensin-converting enzyme function in, 95t
Fibromuscular dysplasia, progression of, 667
renovascular hypertension due to, 662
in women, 547–548
Fight-or-flight response, hypothalamic control of, 43
integrated role of sympathetic nervous system in, 47
stress response vs., 59
Finger cuff method of Penaz, in blood pressure measurement, 309
Fish oils, 180, 462–463
Fludrocortisone, for orthostatic hypotension, 573
for orthostatic intolerance, 576
Fluid(s), body, angiotensin-converting enzyme distribution in, 93t
diuretic depletion of. See *Diuretics.*
extracellular volume of, in chronic renal failure, 524, *524*
in renal replacement therapy, 535
intraoperative management of, 711
intravascular volume of, in hyperaldosteronism, 679, *679*

Fluid(s) *(Continued)*
volume contraction of, from diuretics, 588
volume homeostasis of, in pregnancy, 690
volume overload with, in chronic renal failure, treatment of, 528
resistant hypertension due to, 566
Folate, for hyperhomocysteinemia prevention, 283
Food and Drug Administration, drug approval process of. See *Antihypertensive therapy, approval process for.*
Fosinopril. See also *Angiotensin-converting enzyme (ACE) inhibitors.*
dosage of, 603t
FACET trial of, 337, 392
pharmacokinetics of, 601t
in renal replacement therapy, 536t
phosphinyl group on, 601
Four Corners Approach, to genetic contrast, 35
Framingham Heart Study, of blood pressure, alcohol consumption and, 213
coronary disease risk in, *236*, 236t–237t, 237
gender differences in, 547
historical significance of, 2
rise of, with aging, 6, *6*
risk of coronary artery disease and, 15, 16t
of isolated systolic hypertension, 552, *552*
of stroke probability, 223, *223*
Furosemide, characteristics and dosage of, 586t
for hyperaldosteronism, 680
for hyperkalemia, after adenoma removal, 681
with orthoiodohippurate, in radionuclide imaging, 664

G protein, angiotensin AT_1 receptor binding with, 104
GABA, modulation of neurotransmitters by, 45
Ganglion blocking drugs, 638–639. See also *Postganglionic adrenergic inhibitors.*
adverse effects of, 639
clinical uses of, 639
hemodynamic effects of, 638–639
mechanism of action of, 638
Gastrointestinal system, angiotensin-converting enzyme distribution in, 93t, 94
circadian rhythm of, drug absorption and, 506
Gastrointestinal therapeutic system (GITS), for nifedipine, 616–617
Gender differences. See also *Women.*
in arterial stiffness, 144, *145,* 230
in blood pressure, 6, *6,* 546–547, *546*
in coronary artery disease, 114–115, *115*
in initial choice of therapy, 482–483, 482t

Gender differences *(Continued)*
  in left ventricular hypertrophy, 246
  in stress response, 59, 65, 65t
  in syndrome X, 146
  in ventricular hypertrophy, 250
Gene(s), expression of, in vascular
    growth and hypertrophy, 262
  in ventricular hypertrophy, 248, *249*
Gene therapy, 38–39
General adaptation syndrome, 47
General anesthesia. See *Anesthesia.*
Genetic homeostasis, impaired, syndrome
    of, 24
Genetic markers, of sympathetic nervous
    system activity, 48
Genetic mutation(s), in glucocorticoid-
    remediable aldosteronism, 682, *682*
  in pheochromocytoma, 685
  of lipoprotein lipase (LPL), lipoprotein
    abnormalities related to, 111
Genetic polymorphisms, in angiotensin-
    converting enzyme gene, 90–91
  in angiotensinogen gene, in Africans
    and African Americans, 81, 84t
  in hypertensive subtypes, 81, 87t
  in Japanese, 81, 85t, 87t
  in whites, 80, 82t–83t, 87t
  predisposition for renal and cardio-
    vascular damage related to, 526
  types of, 80
  ventricular hypertrophy related to, 250
Genetics, 29–39
  context-dependent effects of allelic vari-
    ations in, 26
  of angiotensinogen, 79–87
  of blood pressure, assumptions and
    models in, 29–31
    cardiovascular disease risk and, 29–
      31, *29–30*
    environment vs. genes in, 31–33
    testing for, 38
  of blood pressure disorders, 35–38, 35t
    molecular and genetic heterogeneity
      in, 35–36
    phenotypic clues in, 36
    phenotypic heterogeneity in, 36
  of diabetic nephropathy, 519
  of hypertension, 36–38
    candidate genes in, 36–37, 37t
    future therapies for, 38–39
    inconsistency of analysis in, 37–38
  of ventricular hypertrophy, 250
  research in, 33–35
    approaches to, 26–27
    avoiding extremes in, 35
    Baconian-Cartesian-Newtonian-
      Darwinian-Comtean paradigm
      in, 26
    future of, 38–39
    genetic contrast in, 34–35
    linkage and association studies in,
      33–35
    phenotypes and, 34
    sampling bias in, 34
Germany, initial choice of
    antihypertensive treatment in, *383,*
    386
Gestational (transient) hypertension,
    691–692, 692t

Giraffes, blood pressure adaptation in, 22
GISEN (Gruppo Italiano di Studi
    Epidemiologici in Nefrologia), 291
Gitelman's syndrome, genetic cause and
    phenotype of, 35t
Glomerular endotheliosis, in
    preeclampsia, 692
Glomerular filtration rate, decrease of, by
    angiotensin II receptor blockers,
    627
  in ACE inhibitor therapy, 510, 602,
    605
    reversal of, after cessation of ther-
      apy, 513
  in preeclampsia, 693
  in obesity, 208
  in pregnancy, 690
Glomerulus(i), angiotensin II effects on,
    622
  antihypertensive therapy for reduction
    of pressure in, ACE inhibitors in,
    510, 526
  renoprotective effect of, 510
  damage to, from hypertension, in
    chronic renal failure, 525
  in African Americans, 560
Glucocorticoid(s), resistance to, 676
  synthesis of, *675*
Glucocorticoid-remediable aldosteronism,
    681–682, *682*
Glucose. See also *Hyperglycemia.*
  exercise effect on, 472
  fasting test of, in diagnosis of hyperten-
    sion, 300, 302, 304t
  high normal levels of, as risk factor,
    for hypertension, 299–300, 299t
  homeostasis of, sympathetic nervous
    system regulation of, 47
  impaired fasting, 300
  increased metabolism of, sympathetic
    nervous system effects of, 119–
    120, *119*
  metabolism of, sulfonamide-based di-
    uretics and, 588–589
Glyburide, hypertension related to, in
    women, 115
Glycogen synthetase gene, diabetic
    nephropathy related to, 519
Glycoprotein IIb/IIIa inhibitors, for
    prevention of myocardial infarction,
    543
Gordon's syndrome
    (pseudohypoaldosteronism type II),
    genetic cause and phenotype of, 35t
  sodium retention due to, 514
Growth and development, acceleration of,
    hypertension related to, 25–26
  allometric dysfunction in, 24
  in pathophysiology of hypertension,
    23–24
  synchronicity of blood pressure rise
    with, 24
  vigorous, in modern children, 24
Growth factors, in angiogenesis, 261
  ventricular hypertrophy related to, 251
Gruppo Italiano di Studi Epidemiologici
    in Nefrologia (GISEN), 291
Guanabenz, exercise interaction with, 474
  pharmacology of, 640

Guanethidine, adverse effects of, 640
  combined with hydrochlorothiazide,
    dosage of, 501t
  hemodynamic effects of, 640
  pharmacology of, 639–640
Guanfacine. See also α-*Adrenoreceptor
    agonists.*
  for resistant hypertension, 570
  pharmacology of, 640
Guidelines. See *Antihypertensive therapy,
    guidelines for.*

Hand pain (cold pressor) test, in
    baroreflex failure, 574–575, *575*
HAPPHY (Heart Attack Primary
    Prevention in Hypertension Trial),
    342t, 344, 345t
HARVEST (Hypertension and
    Ambulatory Recording Venetia
    Study), 317
HCP (Hypertension Control Program),
    461
HDFP. See *Hypertension Detection and
    Follow-up Program (HDFP).*
Health aides, in community outreach
    programs, 417
Health Plan Employer Data and
    Information Set (HEDIS), 408
Health Professionals Follow-Up Study,
    450, 454, 456
Health resource utilization, as measure of
    outcome, 328
  frequency of physician visits in, 326
Heart, aging effects on, 552, 553t
  angiotensin II receptor blocker effects
    on, 625
  chromaffin cells of, 45
  composition of, in left ventricular hy-
    pertrophy, 246–247, *247*
  endocrine and paracrine functions of.
    See *Natriuretic peptides.*
  endothelin effects on, 154
  fibrosis of, left ventricular hypertrophy
    related to, 246–247
  hypertrophy of. See also *Ventricle(s),
    hypertrophy of.*
    angiotensin II in, 96, 622
    angiotensin-converting enzyme in,
      96
    in mild hypertension, 403
    in obesity, 207
    renin-angiotensin system in, 96
    sympathetic nervous system in,
      52–53
  obesity effects on, 207
    weight reduction and, 208
  remodeling of, after myocardial in-
    farction, angiotensin-converting
    enzyme in, 96–97
Heart Attack Primary Prevention in
    Hypertension Trial (HAPPHY), 342t,
    344, 345t
Heart disease, antihypertensive therapy in,
    511–512
  hypertension in, initial choice of ther-
    apy in, 485, 486t
  ischemic, 539–545. See also *Coronary
    artery disease.*

Heart disease *(Continued)*
 alternative therapy for, 543
 assessment of, as measure of outcome, 327–328
 clinical history in, 539
 coronary angiography in, 540
 echocardiography in, 539–540
 electrocardiography in, 539
 exercise stress testing in, 540
 incidence of, 539
 medical therapy for, 542–543
 noninvasive clinical evaluation of, 539–540
 revascularization for, 540–542, *541*
  coronary artery bypass graft surgery for, 542
  percutaneous transluminal angioplasty for, 540–542
 secondary prevention of, 543–545
 with blood pressure reduction, in left ventricular hypertrophy, 264, *264*
Heart failure, congestive. See also *Ventricle(s), hypertrophy of.*
 ACE inhibitors for, 339, 511–512, 605
 β-adrenoreceptor blockers in, 542
 angiotensin II receptor blockers in, 631–632
 atrial natriuretic peptide in, 170–171
 diastolic, antihypertensive agent effect in, 259–260
 hypertension as risk factor for, 248
 hypertensive emergency in, 717
 improvement of, by thiazide diuretics, 585
 low blood pressure as predictor of mortality in, 532
 prevention of, with antihypertensive therapy, 250, 331
 risk of, in elderly, 552
 sympathetic nervous system in, 52–53
Heart Outcomes Prevention Evaluation (HOPE), 346t–347t, 348–349
Heart rate, antihypertensive agents for lowering, 485, 486t
 as risk factor, for cardiovascular events, 507
  for coronary disease, 239–240, *240,* 242
  for future hypertension, 403
 in orthostatic hypotension, due to baroreflex failure, 575
 increase of, in response to antihypertensive therapy, 495
Heart rate–systolic blood pressure product, as index of myocardial oxygen demand, 508
Heart valve disease, antihypertensive therapy in, 511
Height, arterial stiffness and, 144, 146
HELLP syndrome, in preeclampsia, 691
Hematocrit, in mild hypertension, as indicator of coronary risk, 403
Hemodialysis, antihypertensive therapy in, anaphylactoid reaction to ACE inhibitors in, 535
 peritoneal dialysis vs., 533, 535
 pharmacokinetic properties of agents in, 536t

Hemodynamic system, ACE inhibitor effects on, 602, 602t
 angiotensin II receptor blocker effects on, 625
 calcitonin gene–related peptide effects on, 183, *183*
 calcium antagonist effects on, 611–613, *611*
 natriuretic peptide effects on, 168–169
 obesity effects on, 206–207
  weight reduction and, 208
 renal, obesity effects on, 207–208
 response to exercise in, 471–472, 472t
Hemorrhage, intracerebral, stroke due to, 278, *278*
 risk of, from calcium channel blockers, 394, 395–396
HEP (Hypertension in the Elderly Prevention Trial), 342t–343t
Heparin, low molecular weight, for prevention of myocardial infarction, 543
 renoprotective effect of, in chronic renal insufficiency, 293–294
Hepatocyte growth factor, in angiogenesis, 261
Heterogeneity, molecular and genetic, 35–36
 phenotypic, 36
HETEs. See *Hydroxyeicosatetraenoic acids (20-HETE).*
Hexamethonium, for hypertension, history of, 3
Hippel-Lindau tumor suppressor gene, mutations in, 685
Hispanic Americans, antihypertensive therapy in, 484
 coronary disease in, mortality rate from, 532
 prevalence of hypertension in, 552
Homeostasis, acute stress response vs., 45
 sympathetic nervous system function in, 45
Homocystinuria, 283. See also *Hyperhomocysteinemia.*
HOPE (Heart Outcomes Prevention Evaluation), 346t–347t, 348–349
Hopelessness, hypertension related to, 63
Hormone replacement therapy. See *Estrogen(s), replacement therapy with.*
Hostility, hypertension related to, 62, 66, *66*
HOT. See *Hypertension Optimal Treatment Study (HOT).*
HPT (Hypertension Prevention Trial), 461
HSCSG (Hypertension-Stroke Cooperative Study Group), 342t–343t
Hydralazine. See also *Vasodilator agent(s).*
 adverse effects of, 641
 combined with hydrochlorothiazide, 501t
 exercise interaction with, 475
 history of, 3
 in acute stroke, 512
 in hypertensive emergencies, 716t
 in preeclampsia/eclampsia, 696t

Hydralazine *(Continued)*
 in pregnancy, 515, 696t, 698
 intraoperative use of, 711
 pharmacokinetics of, in renal replacement therapy, 536t
 pharmacology of, 641
Hydrochlorothiazide. See also *Diuretics; Thiazide diuretics.*
 characteristics and dosage of, 586t
 combined with, ACE inhibitors or angiotensin II receptor blockers, 502, 502t
  amiloride, 128, 500
  β-blockers, 501, 501t
  common agents, 500
 CONVINCE trial of, 337, 338t, 346t, 351t, 354–355
 in hyperaldosteronism, 680
 in obese hypertensive patients, 208
 in ventricular hypertrophy, regression of mass with, 253
 lisinopril vs., in obese hypertensive patients, 209
HydroDIURIL. See *Hydrochlorothiazide.*
3-Hydroxy-3-methylglutaryl coenzyme A (HMG CoA) reductase inhibitors, in ALLHAT study, 354
 in chronic renal insufficiency, 293
Hydroxyeicosatetraenoic acids (20-HETE), conversion to vasoconstrictor vasodilator metabolites by, 177, *177*
 nitric oxide synthase inhibition by, 177, *178,* 179
 preeclampsia and, 180
11β-Hydroxylase, deficiency of, hypertension due to, 676
 genetic mutation of, in glucocorticoid-remediable aldosteronism, 682, *682*
17α-Hydroxylase deficiency, hypertension due to, 676
11β-Hydroxysteroid dehydrogenase, deficiency of, hypertension due to, 682–683, *683*
 placental, in pathophysiology of hypertension, 24
Hygroton. See *Chlorthalidone.*
Hyperaldosteronism, glucocorticoid-remediable, 681–682, *682*
 genetic cause and phenotype of, 35t
 hypertension in, 676–682
  aldosterone-secreting adenoma in, 678
  antihypertensive therapy for, choice of agents in, 514, 679–681, *680–681,* 681t
   rational approaches to, 679, *679–680*
  diagnosis of, initial assessment in, 303t
   simplified approach to, 678–679, *679*
   tests in, 677–679, *677–678*
  hemodynamic characteristics of, 679, *679*
 in pregnancy, 690–691
Hyperchloremia, renal hemodynamic effects of, 177

Hyperglycemia, angiotensin II in, renal damage due to, 290
   endothelial dysfunction due to, 113, 113t
   in diabetes mellitus, diabetic nephropathy related to, 519–520, 520t
      vascular disease related to, 519t, 544
   sympathetic nervous system stimulation by, 47
Hyperhomocysteinemia, as risk factor, for hypertension, 301
   causes of, 283
   treatment of, for stroke prevention, 283–284
Hyperinsulinemia, in diabetes mellitus, diabetic nephropathy related to, 519–520, 520t
   vascular disease related to, 519, 519t
   in hypertension, atherosclerosis due to, 113, 113t
   in obesity-related hypertension, 121, 460
   in sodium restriction, 449
   in women, coronary artery disease related to, 114–115
   resistant hypertension due to, 567
Hyperkalemia, after adenoma removal, treatment of, 681
   from ACE inhibitors, 606
      in renal failure, 513
   from potassium-sparing diuretics, 588
Hyperlipidemia. See *Lipoprotein abnormalities.*
Hyperparathyroidism, secondary, hypertension related to, 287
Hyperpiesia, 1
Hypertension, arterial stiffness in. See *Artery(ies), stiffness of.*
   classification of, 2, 5, 5t
   clinical trials of. See *Clinical trial(s).*
   combined systolic/diastolic, 228
   comorbid conditions in, 509–516. See also specific condition, *e.g., Hyperlipidemia.*
   control of, NHANES survey of, 398, 419, *420,* 479, 518, *518*
   coronary flow reserve abnormalities in, 260–267
   definitions of, by Joint National Committee on Prevention, Detection, Evaluation, and Treatment of Hypertension, 298, 551
      by National High Blood Pressure Education Program, 222
      by World Health Organization and International Society of Hypertension, 5, 5t
   dementia associated with, 11–14
   diagnosis of, 297–305
      blood pressure measurement in, 298, 371. See also *Blood pressure, measurement of.*
      changes in, 371–372
      initial assessment in, 302–303, *302,* 302t–303t
      reevaluation and follow-up in, 304–305, 304t
      risk factor assessment in, 298–301, 371–372, 371t–372t

Hypertension *(Continued)*
      target organ damage evaluation in, 301–302, 301t
   diastolic, fetal mortality related to, 689, *689*
      treatment of, clinical trials of, 331, 332t–333t, 334
   diastolic function in, 254–260
   diet in. See *Diet.*
   epidemiology of, 4–16
   exercise and, 470–476
   genetics of. See *Genetics.*
   historical aspects of, 1–3
   hyperkinetic borderline, 23–24
   in blacks. See *African Americans; Africans.*
   in coronary disease. See *Coronary artery disease, in hypertension.*
   in elderly. See *Elderly.*
   in pregnancy. See *Preeclampsia; Pregnancy.*
   in renal failure. See *Renal failure, chronic, hypertension in.*
   in renal replacement therapy, 531–537
   in women. See *Women.*
   isolated systolic, definition of, 228
      in elderly, as risk factor for cardiovascular mortality, 552, *552*
      in African Americans, 558
      prevalence of, 551
      resistance in, 564
      initial choice of therapy for, 481–482
      risk of cardiovascular disease with, 232
      treatment of, clinical trials of, 334–335
         with ACE inhibitors, 604
   lifestyle modifications for. See *Lifestyle modifications.*
   malignant, accelerated, peripheral resistance in, 232
      outcome of, 715
   metabolic abnormalities in. See *Metabolic abnormalities.*
   mild, 398–403
      approach to, 403
      cardiovascular events related to, 323, *323*
      clinical trials of antihypertensive therapy in, implications of, 401–403, *402*
         Medical Research Council Trial in Mild Hypertension and, *335,* 336, 342t–343t, 344, 345t, 400t, 401
         summary of results of major trials in, 399, 400t, 401
         Treatment of Mild Hypertension Study (TOMHS) and, 361, 400t, 401, 614
      incidence of, 398
      public health impact of, 399
      response to antihypertensive therapy in, 398, *399,* 400t
   natural history of, 2
   normotension vs., 5, *5,* 29
   obesity-related. See *Obesity.*
   pathophysiology of, 21–27
      cardiovascular-renal function in, 22–23

Hypertension *(Continued)*
      evolutionary needs and, 21–22
      genetics of, 26–27. See also *Genetics.*
      growth and development effects in, 23–24
      proximate and ultimate causation in, 24–26
   perioperative, calcium antagonists for, 615
   pulmonary, antihypertensive therapy and, 511
   renal failure related to. See *Renal failure, chronic.*
   renovascular. See *Renovascular hypertension.*
   resistance vessel remodeling in. See *Resistance vessels.*
   resistant, 564–570
      conditions associated with, 564t, 567
      counterregulatory systems vs., 495
      definition of, 564
      drug-related causes of, 564–566, 564t
      hemodynamic abnormalities in, 570, 570t
      modification of antihypertensive therapy in, 570, 570t
      prevalence of, 564, 564t
      pseudoresistance vs., 564–565, 564t
      secondary cause(s) of, 567–570, 568t
         Cushing's syndrome as, 568t, 569–570
         diagnosis and management of, 567–570, *568*
         hyperaldosteronism as, 568t, 569
         pheochromocytoma as, 568t, 569–570
         renal artery stenosis as, 568t, 569
         renal parenchymal disease as, 568t, 570
      volume overload in, 566
      with nonadherence to antihypertensive therapy, 564t, 567
   risk factor(s) for. See also *Cardiovascular risk factor(s); Risk.*
      alcohol consumption as, 299t, 300
      definition of, 298–299, 299t
      diabetes, glucose, and insulin resistance as, 299–300, 299t
      exercise and fitness in, 299t, 300
      lipid and lipoprotein levels as, 299, 299t
      potential factors in, 301
      renin as, 299t, 300–301
      smoking as, 299, 299t
      syndrome of abnormalities in, 323–324, 324t
      weight, build, and overweight as, 299t, 300
   secondary, adrenocortical, 674–684. See also specific disorders, *e.g., Hyperaldosteronism.*
      after prolonged antihypertensive therapy, 304
      circadian rhythm absent in, 505
      discovery of, 2
      from anesthesia, 702–712
      from obstructive sleep apnea, 657–660

Hypertension (Continued)
 from pheochromocytoma. See *Pheochromocytoma.*
 from renovascular hypertension, 662–672
 guidelines for diagnosis of, 302, 303t
 in pregnancy. See *Pregnancy.*
 in women, 547–548
 sympathetic nervous system hyperactivity in, 51–53
 stress in. See *Stress.*
 stroke related to. See *Stroke.*
 supine, in orthostatic hypotension, 573, 574
 threshold level of blood pressure in, for starting antihypertensive therapy, 222–223, *223*
  in African Americans, 561
  guideline recommendations for, 380–381, 380t
  in hypertensive crisis, 715
  in preeclampsia, 695
  in pregnancy, 689
 treatment of. See *Antihypertensive therapy.*
 untreated, mortality associated with, 15, *15*
 ventricular hypertrophy in. See *Ventricle(s), hypertrophy of.*
 white-coat, 314–320
  background and definition of, 315–316, *315*, 315t
  cardiovascular risk factors in, 318–319
  cost effectiveness of screening for, 320
  criteria for, 315, *315*
  cross-sectional target organ studies of, 316–318
   cardiac studies in, 316–317, *317*, 317t
   cerebral studies in, 318
   renal studies in, 318
   vascular studies in, 318
  evolution of, in untreated patients, 319–320
  implications of, 314
  pathophysiology of, 316
  prevalence of, 315, 315t
  prognostic studies of, with ambulatory monitoring, 319, *319*
Hypertension and Ambulatory Recording Venetia Study (HARVEST), 317
Hypertension Control Program (HCP), 461
Hypertension Detection and Follow-up Program (HDFP), community outreach programs and, 416
 mortality reporting in, 400t, 401, 552
 of antihypertensive therapy, in elderly, 554
 of pressure-related target organ damage, 558
 on antihypertensive therapy in women, 549
 on gender differences in blood pressure, 547
 published results of, 342t
Hypertension in the Elderly Prevention Trial (HEP), 342t–343t

Hypertension in the Very Elderly Trial (HYVET), 338t, 346t–347t, 349–350
Hypertension Optimal Treatment Study (HOT), goal blood pressure level determined by, 226–227, 336, 381
 of diabetes mellitus, 336
 of felodipine as initial therapy, 338t, 392, 614
 of safety of calcium antagonists, 613
 published results of, 342t–343t
Hypertension Prevention Trial (HPT), 461
Hypertension specialist, 408, 408t
Hypertension-Stroke Cooperative Study Group (HSCSG), 342t–343t
Hypertensive emergencies, blood pressure reduction in, 715–716
 blood pressure threshold for, 715
 definition of, 715
 drug choice for, 716–717, 716t
 from pheochromocytoma, treatment of, 687
 in baroreflex failure, 574
 pathophysiology of, 715
 types of, 715, 715t, 717–718
Hypertensive encephalopathy, 279–280, 717
Hypertensive urgencies, definition of, 715
 diagnosis and treatment of, 718
 short-acting calcium antagonists for, 374
Hypertonie, essentielle, 1
Hyperuricemia, diuretic-induced, 588
 diuretics contraindicated in, 511
Hypoalbuminemia, in preeclampsia, 693
Hypoaldosteronism, after adenoma removal, 681
Hypoglycemic agents, oral, amelioration of cardiovascular disease by, 114
Hypogonadism, hypergonadotropic, 676
Hypokalemia, diuretic-induced, exercise and, 474
 from high-dose therapy, 495
 mechanisms of, 588, *588*
 potassium infusions for, in diabetes mellitus, 487
 hypertension due to, renin levels in, 74
 in adrenocortical hypertension, evaluation of, 674–676, 97t
 in Cushing's syndrome, 683
 in hyperaldosteronism, correction of, before adenoma removal, 681
 evaluation of, 677, *677*
Hypomagnesemia, diuretic-induced, from high-dose therapy, 495
Hyponatremia, diuretic-induced, 589
Hypopnea, definition of, 658
Hypotension, in anesthesia, 703, 704, *705*, 709–710
 intraoperative, 712
 orthostatic. See *Orthostatic hypotension.*
Hypothalamus, in hypertensive models, 43
 sympathetic nervous system regulation by, 43
Hypothyroidism, secondary hypertension due to, diagnosis of, 304
HYVET (Hypertension in the Very Elderly Trial), 338t, 346t–347t, 349–350

Icatibant (HOE 140), renin-angiotensin system regulation by, 195
 reversal of ACE inhibitors by, 194
Idiopathic orthostatic hypotension, 572
Immunoradiometric assay (IRMA), for renin measurement, 75
Immunosuppressive agents, hypertension due to, 514
Impedance, characteristic, as index of arterial stiffness, 135t, 138
 doubling of, in arterial stiffness, 142, *142*
 elevation of, in hypertension, 143
Impedance modulus, aortic, arterial stiffening and, 141, *142*
Indomethacin, with ACE inhibitors, for reduction of proteinuria, 528
Industrialized populations, blood pressure in, 6–8, *6–7*
 factors affecting, 25
 nonindustrialized population blood pressure vs., 8–9, 8t, *9*
 environment stress exposure in, 61–62
Infants. See also *Children.*
 blood pressure measurement in, 312
Infarction(s), lacunar, 278, *278*
Inflammation, angiotensin-converting enzyme in, 97
Inotropic agents, for diastolic congestive heart failure, 260
INSIGHT (International Nifedipine GITS Study Intervention as a Goal in Hypertension Treatment), 338t, 346t, 350, 351t, 352
Insulin, levels of. See also *Hyperinsulinemia.*
 as risk factor, for hypertension, 118–119
 in response to high-carbohydrate diet, 462
 resistance to. See *Insulin resistance.*
 sensitivity to, α_1-adrenoreceptor antagonist effects on, 597
 antihypertensive effects on, 510
 sympathetic nervous system activity related to, 119–120, *119*
 obesity-related hypertension and, 120–121, *120–121*
 ventricular hypertrophy related to, 251
Insulin resistance, as risk factor, for hypertension, 299–300, 299t
 exercise effect on, 472
 in hypertension, endothelial dysfunction due to, 113, 113t
 in obesity, fat distribution and, 110, 118
  hypertension resulting from, 120–121, *121*
  metabolic abnormalities associated with, 110–111, 118
 microalbuminuria as marker for, 520
 sympathetic nervous system activity related to, 50
 syndrome of, components of, 119
 pathophysiology of, *123*, 124
 ventricular hypertrophy related to, 251
Insulin-like growth factor-1 (IGF-1), in hypertension, endothelial dysfunction due to, 113, *114*

International Nifedipine GITS Study Intervention as a Goal in Hypertension Treatment (INSIGHT), 338t, 346t, 350, 351t, 352
International Prospective Primary Prevention Study in Hypertension (IPPPSH), 342t, 344, 345t
International Society of Hypertension (ISH), definition of hypertension, 5, 5t
International Study of Infarct Survival, Second (ISIS-2), 542
International Union of Pharmacology, classification of angiotensin II receptors, 101
International Verapamil-Trandolapril Study (INVEST), 346t, 351t, 353
Intersalt study, hypotheses of, 434
    of nonindustrialized populations, 8–9, 8t, 9
    results of, 434, 435
Intervention studies, 390
Intrauterine environment, hypertension associated with, 11
Intravenous Nimodipine West European Stroke Trial (INWEST), 281
Intravenous pyelography (IVP), in renovascular hypertension, 666
Intubation, for anesthesia, 711
Inuit, body composition changes in, 25
INVEST (International Verapamil-Trandolapril Study), 346t, 351t, 353
INWEST (Intravenous Nimodipine West European Stroke Trial), 281
IPPPSH (International Prospective Primary Prevention Study in Hypertension), 342t, 344, 345t
Irbesartan. See also *Angiotensin II receptor antagonists.*
    CSGTEI trial of, 346, 346t–347t, 348
    development of, 624
    pharmacokinetics of, in renal replacement therapy, 536t
    pharmacology of, 628–629, 630, 631t
    structure of, 626
Ischemia, blood pressure increase as factor in, 506
    diastolic function affected by, 254–255
    early morning occurrence of, 506
Ischemic heart disease. See *Heart disease, ischemic.*
ISIS-2 (Second International Study of Infarct Survival), 542
Isolated systolic hypertension. See *Hypertension, isolated systolic.*
Isometric exercise, 472
Isradipine. See also *Calcium antagonists.*
    exercise interaction with, 475
    MIDAS study of, 392, 615
    pharmacokinetics of, in renal replacement therapy, 536t
    slow-release (retarded) preparation of, 617

Japanese, alcohol consumption by, blood pressure levels in, 213
    angiotensinogen polymorphisms in, 81, 85t, 87t

Japanese *(Continued)*
    calcium channel blocker therapy in, 395
    kallikrein and kinin excretion by, 196
JNC VI. See *Joint National Committee for the Prevention, Detection, Evaluation, and Treatment of High Blood Pressure (JNC VI).*
Job strain, as stress exposure factor, 61–62
"John Henryism," as coping style, 63
Joint National Committee for the Prevention, Detection, Evaluation, and Treatment of High Blood Pressure (JNC VI), classification of blood pressure, 5, 5t, 298, 551
    recommendations of, based on cardiovascular risk, 561
        on ACE inhibitors, 604
        on calcium channel blockers, 394
        on exercise, 471
        on initiation of therapy in mild hypertension, 403

Kallidin, 192
Kallikrein(s), tissue, atrial natriuretic peptide synthesis by, 195
    inhibitors of, 192
    regulation of, 194
    structure and functions of, 192
Kallikrein-kinin systems, 190–198
    angiotensin-converting enzyme inhibitor interaction with, 600
    in diabetes mellitus, 197–198
    in hemodynamic, excretory, and metabolic processes, 195–196
    in hypertension, 196–197, 198
    regulation of, 194, 194
    regulatory hormones and autacoid relationship with, 194–195
    renin-angiotensin system interaction with, 194–195
    structure and function of, 190–194
Kallistatin, as tissue kallikrein inhibitor, 192
Ketamine, for induction of anesthesia, 706
Ketoconazole, for hypercortisolism, 684
Kidney(s), ACE inhibitor effects on, 602, 602t, 604–605
    angiotensin II effects on, 622
    angiotensin II receptor blocker effects on, 626–627
    angiotensin-converting enzyme distribution in, 93t, 94
    angiotensin-converting enzyme function in, 95t
    damage of, obesity-related, in African Americans, 560, 560
        salt-induced, in African Americans, 560–561
    diabetic nephropathy of. See *Nephropathy, diabetic.*
    disease of. See *Renal disease.*
    failure of. See *Renal failure, chronic.*
    function of. See *Renal function.*
    medulla of, in pressure natriuresis mechanism, 22–23

Kidney(s) *(Continued)*
    obesity effects on, 206, 207–208
        weight reduction and, 208
    sensitivity to toxic exposures, in African Americans, 560
    transplantation of, hypertensive emergencies related to, 717
        immunosuppression for, hypertension due to, 514
Kinase(s), in angiotensin AT$_1$ receptor signal transduction, 102
    in ventricular hypertrophy, 248, 249
Kininases, 193–194
    angiotensin-converting enzyme inhibitor interaction with, 193–194
Kininogens, gene for, regulation of expression of, 190–191
    structure of, 190, 190
    structure and functions of, 191–192, 191
Kinins. See also *Bradykinin(s).*
    receptors for, functions of, 192–193
    renal hemodynamic function and, 196
Korotkoff sound method, of blood pressure measurement, 306

Labetalol, α-adrenergic activity of, 593
    characteristics and dosage of, 720t
    combined with diuretics, 500
    elimination characteristics of, 594t
    in hypertensive emergencies, 716t
        in aortic dissection, 717
        intravenous formulation for, 590, 593
    in myocardial infarction or ischemia, in hypertensive emergencies, 717
    in preeclampsia/eclampsia, 696t
    in pregnancy, 696t, 698
    intraoperative use of, 711
    pharmacodynamics of, 591t
    pharmacokinetics of, 592t
        in renal replacement therapy, 536t
Laboratory tests, frequency of, as measure of outcome, 326
Lacidipine, CLEVER trial of, 346t–347t, 349
    ELSA trial of, 613, 614, 615
    long duration of action of, 617, 617–618
    SHELL trial of, 338t, 346t, 351t, 352
Lacunar infarction(s), in white-coat hypertension, 318
    pathophysiology of, 278, 278
Lasix. See *Furosemide.*
Lay advisors, in community outreach programs, 417
Left ventricular hypertrophy. See *Ventricle(s), hypertrophy of.*
Licorice, overingestion of, sodium retention due to, 513–514
Liddle's syndrome, absence of spironolactone response in, 676
    genetic cause and phenotype of, 35t
    renin levels in, 74
    sodium retention due to, 514
Lifarizine, incidental antihypertensive effect of, in stroke patients, 281
LIFE. See *Losartan Intervention for Endpoint (LIFE) Reduction in Hypertension Study.*

Life insurance data on hypertension, 1, 4
Lifestyle modification(s). See also *Diet.*
  alcohol reduction as, randomized controlled trials of, 466–468, *467,* 467t
  antihypertensive therapy vs., TOMHS trial of, 335
  as initial choice of therapy, 479–480, 479t
  as measure of outcome, 325–326
  cost of, 406
  exercise as, 470–476
  in African Americans, 483, 561–562
  in elderly, 555, 556t
  in women, 549
  nursing clinics for management of, 411, 412t
  recommendations for, 372, 372t, 470t
  sodium restriction as. See *Sodium, dietary, restriction of.*
  weight reduction as. See *Weight, reduction of.*
Linkage, definition of, 79
Linkage and association studies, general principles of, 33–34
  of angiotensinogen, criteria for association studies in, 81, 87
  initial reports of, 79–80, 79t, 82t–87t
  linkage vs. association in, 79
Lipid profile, in diagnosis of hypertension, 302, 304t
Lipid-lowering agents. See *Antilipemic agents.*
Lipoprotein abnormalities. See also *Atherosclerosis.*
  antihypertensive therapy in, α-adrenoreceptor antagonists in, 597
  β-blockers in, 593
  choice of agents in, 510–511
  as risk factor, for cardiovascular damage, in chronic renal failure, 525
  for hypertension, 299, 299t
  for ischemic heart disease, 544
  dietary intervention for, in TOMHS trial, 461
  in chronic renal failure, 293, 527, *528*
  in diabetes mellitus, vascular disease related to, 519t
  in hypertension, genetic basis of, 111
  stroke related to, 283
  types of abnormalities in, 111, 111t
  in insulin-resistance syndrome, 121, *122,* 124
  in sodium restriction, 438, 439t
  lipid-lowering drugs for. See *Antilipemic agents.*
  platelet disorders related to, 113
Lipoprotein lipase (LPL), point mutation of, lipoprotein abnormalities related to, 111
  reduced activity of, in obesity, 111
12-Lipoxygenase, reversal of angiotensin-dependent hypertension by, 178
Lisinopril. See also *Angiotensin-converting enzyme (ACE) inhibitors.*
  cardioprotective effects of, 605
  combined with hydrochlorothiazide, dosage of, 501t
  mean blood pressure reduction with, 502t

Lisinopril *(Continued)*
  dosage of, 603t
  hydrochlorothiazide vs., in obese hypertensives, 209
  in ALLHAT study, 363
  pharmacokinetics of, 601t
  in renal replacement therapy, 536t
  renin inhibitors vs., 649, *649*
Lithium, interaction of, with ACE inhibitors, 606
Liver, cirrhosis of, 171
Local anesthesia (monitored anesthesia care), 704, 705, 709
Loop diuretics. See *Diuretics.*
Losartan. See also *Angiotensin II receptor antagonists.*
  combined with hydrochlorothiazide, blunting of hyperuricemia by, 502
  dosage of, 501t, 502
  development of, 623
  drug interactions with, 628
  ELITE trial of, 339, 632
  for congestive heart failure, 512
  in renal failure, *529*
  pharmacokinetics of, in renal replacement therapy, 536t
  pharmacology of, 627–628, 631t
  RENAAL trial of, 346t–347t, 348
  renin inhibitors vs., 649, *649*
  structure of, *625–626*
  uricosuric effect of, 631
Losartan Intervention for Endpoint (LIFE) Reduction in Hypertension Study, 366–370
  countries participating in, 367, *367*
  design of, 346t, 351t, 353, 366
  discussion of, 369–370
  eligibility for, 366
  methods in, 366–367
  patient characteristics in, 367–368, *368*
  protocol for, 366–367
  results of, 367–369, *367–369*
  statistical measures in, 367

Macronutrients, blood pressure effects of, 457
Macrophages, angiotensin-converting enzyme distribution in, 93t, 97
  angiotensin-converting enzyme function in, 95t
Magnesium, as predictor of hypertension, 456
  decreased levels of, with diuretic therapy, 495
  for eclampsia, eicosanoid augmentation by, 179–180
  for preeclampsia, 695
  repletion of, interventional studies in, 457
  preclinical and observational studies in, 456–457, *456*
  recommendations for, 457
Magnetic resonance imaging (MRI), in renovascular hypertension, 664, *664*
  of coronary blood flow, 267
  of pheochromocytoma, 687
  of ventricular hypertrophy, 253
Managed care, for management of hypertension, cost issues in, 407–408, 408t

Managed care *(Continued)*
  monitoring of performance of, 408
Manidipine, vascular selectivity of, 618
MAP kinase. See *Mitogen-activated protein (MAP) kinase.*
MDL 100,240 (vasopeptidase inhibitor), 652, *653*
Mean arterial pressure (MAP), in chronic renal failure, 288–290
Medical Research Council, Trial in Mild Hypertension, cardiovascular event reduction in, 400t, 401
  of diuretics and β-blockers, 344, 345t
  published results of, 342t–343t
  stroke reduction in, *335, 336*
  summary of, 332t
  Trial of Treatment of Hypertension in Older Adults, design of, 554
  of diuretics and β-blockers, 344, 345t
  published results of, 342t–343t
  summary of, 333t
Medulla, renal, in pressure natriuresis mechanism, 22–23
Menopause, blood pressure level related to, 547
Menstrual cycle, blood pressure level related to, 547
Mercaptoacetyltriglycine (Mag₃), in radionuclide imaging, 664
Metabolic abnormalities, 110–116. See also specific disorder, *e.g., Diabetes mellitus.*
  arterial stiffness related to, 146–147
  coagulation/fibrinolytic abnormalities in, 111–112, 111t
  endothelial. See *Endothelium, dysfunction of.*
  in mild hypertension, 402
  in outcome measurement, 327
  insulin resistance in. See *Insulin resistance.*
  lipoprotein abnormalities in. See *Lipoprotein abnormalities.*
  obesity in. See *Obesity.*
  platelet abnormalities in, 112–113, *112,* 113t
  syndrome of. See also *Syndrome X.*
  exercise effect on, 472
  in obesity, initial choice of therapy in, 485
  types of abnormalities in, 323–324, 324t
Metabolic acidosis, diuretic-induced, 588
Metabolic alkalosis, diuretic-induced, 588
[123]I-Metaiodobenzylguanidine scintigraphy, in pheochromocytoma, 687
Metalloendopeptidase. See *Endopeptidase, neutral (NEP).*
Metanephrine, plasma assay of, in pheochromocytoma, 687
  urinary excretion of, in pheochromocytoma, 686
Methyldopa. See also α-*Adrenoreceptor agonists.*
  adverse effects of, 640–641
  combined with hydrochlorothiazide, dosage of, 501t

Methyldopa *(Continued)*
  exercise interaction with, 474
  hemodynamic effects of, 640
  in pregnancy, 515, 696t, 697–698
  pharmacology of, 640
Metolazone, characteristics and dosage of, 586t
Metoprolol. See also β-*Adrenoreceptor antagonists.*
  combined with hydrochlorothiazide, dosage of, 501t
    mean blood pressure reduction with, 501t
  elimination characteristics of, 594t
  exercise interaction with, 474
  extended-release formulations of, 593
  intraoperative use of, 711
  MAPHY trial of, 344, 345t
  pharmacodynamics of, 591t
  pharmacokinetics of, 592t, 593
  in renal replacement therapy, 536t
Mibefradil, adverse effects of, 613, 618
  in ischemic heart disease, 542
  L-channel vs. T-channel blockade by, 611
  mode of action of, 618
  withdrawal of, from market, 618
Microalbuminuria, in diabetes mellitus, 520
Micronutrients. See *Diet.*
Midamor. See *Amiloride.*
MIDAS (Multicenter Isradipine Diuretic Atherosclerosis Study), 392, 615
Midazolam, for induction of anesthesia, 706
Migraine, hypertension in, antihypertensive therapy for, 513
Migration, blood pressure effect of, 9–10, 32
Mild hypertension. See *Hypertension, mild.*
Mineralocorticoid(s), apparent excess of (AME syndrome), genetic cause and phenotype of, 35t
    sodium retention due to, 513–514
  for glucocorticoid resistance, 676
  synthesis of, *675*
Mini-Mental State Examination (MMSE), 12
Minoxidil. See also *Vasodilator agent(s).*
  adverse effects of, 641
  for resistant hypertension, 570
  pharmacokinetics of, in renal replacement therapy, 536t
  pharmacology of, 641
Mitogen-activated protein (MAP) kinase, activation of, in vascular proliferation and hypertrophy, 262
  in angiotensin AT₁ receptor signal transduction, 102
  in ventricular hypertrophy, 248, *249*
Mitotane, for Cushing's disease, 684
Mitral valve prolapse syndrome, orthostatic intolerance in, 576
Mixanpril, 652–653, *653*
MMSE (Mini-Mental State Examination), 12
Modification of Diet in Renal Disease (MDRD), benefits of antihypertensive therapy in, 289

Modification of Diet in Renal Disease (MDRD) *(Continued)*
  blood pressure reduction goal in, 336, 486, 526, *526*
  progression of renal disease in, 289
Moexipril. See also *Angiotensin-converting enzyme (ACE) inhibitors.*
  dosage of, 603t
  pharmacokinetics of, 601t
    in renal replacement therapy, 536t
Monitored anesthesia care (local anesthesia), 704, 705, 709
Monitoring of Trends and Determinants of Cardiovascular Disease (MONICA), 4
Monitoring techniques, during anesthesia, 710–711
Monoamine oxidase inhibitors, adverse effects of, 641
  pharmacology of, 641
Mortality, as measure of outcome, 329
MRFIT (Multiple Risk Factor Intervention Trial). See *Multiple Risk Factor Intervention Trial (MRFIT).*
Multicenter Isradipine Diuretic Atherosclerosis Study (MIDAS), 392, 615
Multi-infarct dementia, 11
Multiple endocrine neoplasia type IIA, genetic cause and phenotype of, 35t
  pheochromocytoma related to, 685, 687
Multiple Risk Factor Intervention Trial (MRFIT), of blood pressure levels, in chronic renal insufficiency, 288, 334
  of cardiovascular mortality, from diuretics, 584–585
    in ischemic heart disease, 539
    in mild hypertension, 399, 402, *402*
    in normotensive patients, 30, *30*
Myocardial infarction. See also *Heart disease, ischemic.*
  adverse effects of nifedipine in, 485, 612
  ALLHAT study of. See *Antihypertensive and Lipid-Lowering to Prevent Heart Attack Trial (ALLHAT).*
  antihypertensive therapy with, ACE inhibitors in, 339, 605
    initial choice of agents in, 486t
  β-blocker benefits in, 595
  blood pressure rise as precipitating agent for, 506
  coronary blood flow reduction after, 265
  depression after, mortality related to, 63
  diltiazem after, cardioprotective effects of, 612
  hypertensive emergency in, 717
  inflammatory response in, angiotensin-converting enzyme in, 96
  reinfarction after, blood pressure increase and, 238, 238t
  renin as risk factor for, 449
  sodium restriction and, 447–448, *447*
  unrecognized, 237, 237t, 242
  verapamil after, cardioprotective effects of, 612

Myocardium. See also *Heart.*
  composition of, in left ventricular hypertrophy, 246–247, *247*
  membrane-stabilizing activity of β-blockers and, 591, 591t
  transmyocardial revascularization of, 543
Myographs, of resistance vessel remodeling, 129–130

NADH/NADPH oxidase, angiotensin AT₁ receptor and, 102
Nadolol. See also β-*Adrenoreceptor antagonists.*
  combined with diuretics, 501t
  pharmacodynamics of, 591t
  pharmacokinetics of, 592t, 593
  in renal replacement therapy, 536t
NASCET (North American Symptomatic Carotid Endarterectomy Trial), 282
National Cholesterol Education Program guidelines, 544
National Health and Nutrition Examination Survey (NHANES), of dietary calcium association with blood pressure, 454, *454*
  of gender differences in blood pressure, 546, *546*
  of sodium restriction and cardiovascular events, 448, *448*
  on poor control of hypertension, 398, 419, *420*, 479, 518, *518*
  prevalence data from, 4, 4t
    in elderly, 551–552
National Heart, Lung, and Blood Institute, 3
National High Blood Pressure Education Program, as form of community outreach, 416
  establishment of, 3
  recommendations of, on chronic hypertension of pregnancy, 697, 699
    on preeclampsia, 695, 696t
  threshold level of hypertension defined by, 222
National Intervention Cooperative Study in Elderly Hypertensives (NICS-EH), 338t, 346t, 350, 351t
Native Americans, antihypertensive therapy in, 484
Natriuretic effect, of angiotensin II receptor blockers, 627
Natriuretic peptides, 165–172
  antagonists of, 168
  atrial, chemistry and structure of, 165
    diuretic effect of, 168
    hemodynamic effects of, 168–169
    in chronic obstructive pulmonary disease, 171–172
    in cirrhosis, 171
    in congestive heart failure, 170–172
    in hypertension, 170
    in measurement of left ventricular filling, 258
    in nephrotic syndrome, 171
    in renal replacement therapy, 535
    metabolism of, 167
    natriuretic effect of, 168

Natriuretic peptides (Continued)
  regulation of secretion of, 167–168
  sympathetic nervous system activity
      modulation by, 169
  synthesis of, by tissue kallikrein, 195
  tissue distribution of, 166
  brain, chemistry and structure of, 165–
      166
    hemodynamic effects of, 168–169
    metabolism of, 167
    natriuretic effect of, 168
    regulation of secretion of, 167–168
    sympathetic nervous system activity
        modulation by, 169
    tissue distribution of, 166
  clinical applications of, 172
  C-type, chemistry and structure of, 166
    hemodynamic effects of, 169
    protection of, by NEP inhibition, 652
    sympathetic nervous system activity
        modulation by, 169–170
    tissue distribution of, 166
    vascular regulatory effects of, 170
  discovery of, 165
  guanylin and uroguanylin as, 172
  interaction among, 170
  physiological actions of, 168–170
  receptors of, 166–167
  urodilatin, chemistry and structure of,
      166
    natriuretic effect of, 168
    tissue distribution of, 166
  ventricular, 172
Nelson's syndrome, 684
NEP. See Endopeptidase, neutral (NEP).
Nephrectomy, subtotal (SN)-salt–induced
      hypertension and, calcitonin
      gene–related peptide in, 185, 185
Nephropathy, diabetic, angiotensin-
      converting enzyme inhibitors for,
      291, 292
  antihypertensive therapy in, choice
      of agents in, 510, 521–522,
      521t
    clinical trial(s) of. See Diabetes
        mellitus, antihypertensive
        therapy in, clinical trials of.
    renoprotective effect of, 290
  genetic predisposition in, 519
  hyperglycemia/hyperinsulinemia in,
      519–520, 520t
  prorenin as possible predictor of, 75
Nephrotic syndrome, atrial natriuretic
      peptide in, 171
Nephrotoxicity, in African Americans,
      560
Nerve block, major, 708–710
Nervous system. See Central nervous
      system; Sympathetic nervous system.
Neuraxial block, 704, 708, 709–710
Neurotransmitters. See also specific type,
      e.g., Norepinephrine.
  endothelin interaction with, 154
  in hypertensive models, 44
  intrasynaptic metabolism of, 44
  modulation of, by presynaptic receptors
      and cotransmitters, 44
Neutral endopeptidase (NEP). See
      Endopeptidase, neutral (NEP).

New Zealand, initial choice of
      antihypertensive treatment in, 383,
      385
NHANES. See National Health and
      Nutrition Examination Survey
      (NHANES).
Nicardipine. See also Calcium
      antagonists.
  for hypertensive emergencies, 716t
  NICS-EH trial of, 338t, 346t, 350, 351t
  pharmacokinetics of, in renal replace-
      ment therapy, 536t
  slow-release (retarded) preparation of,
      617
  vascular selectivity of, 617
NICS-EH (National Intervention
      Cooperative Study in Elderly
      Hypertensives), 338t, 346t, 350, 351t
Nifedipine. See also Calcium antagonists.
  adverse effects of, 613, 615–616
  combined with β-blockers, for suppres-
      sion of myocardial infarction, 612,
      614
  for preeclampsia/eclampsia, 696t
  gastrointestinal therapeutic system
      (GITS) for, 616–617
  in pregnancy, 696t
  INSIGHT trial of, 338t, 346t, 350,
      351t, 352
  myocardial infarction related to, 612
    favorable effect of β-blockers with,
        612
  oral or sublingual, adverse effects of,
      280, 374
    alternative short-acting agents vs.,
        374
    myocardial infarction related to, 485
  pharmacokinetics of, in renal replace-
      ment therapy, 536t
  short-acting, reflex tachycardia due to,
      613
  slow-release preparation of, 616
  spironolactone vs., for hyperaldosteron-
      ism, 680, 681t
  STONE trial of, 613
Nimodipine, for eclampsia, 698
  incidental antihypertensive effect of, in
      stroke patients, 281
Nisoldipine. See also Calcium
      antagonists.
  ABCD trial of, 344, 348
  coat core formulation of, 617
  enalapril vs., ABCD trial of, 392
  pharmacokinetics of, in renal replace-
      ment therapy, 536t
  vascular selectivity of, 617–618
Nitrates, for ischemic heart disease, 543
  for myocardial infarction or ischemia,
      in hypertensive emergencies, 717
Nitrendipine, in SYST-EUR trial, 392,
      394
Nitric oxide (NO), 158–163
  CYP-450–arachidonic acid metabolism
      inhibited by, 178–179
  decreased production of, in hyperten-
      sion, 160–161
  endothelin interaction with, 154
  in hypertension, 160–162
  increased destruction of, in hyperten-
      sion, 161–162

Nitric oxide (NO) (Continued)
  interaction with other endothelium-de-
      rived factors, 162
  modulation of neurotransmitters by, 45
  organ protective properties of, 262
  vascular biology of, 159
Nitric oxide synthase (NOS), forms of,
      159
  inhibition of, by 20-HETE, 177, 178,
      179
    in chronic renal failure, 525, 533
    preeclampsia related to, 179, 180,
        692
Nitroglycerin, for hypertensive
      emergencies, 716, 716t
  in aortic dissection, 717
  in congestive heart failure, 717
  intraoperative use of, 711
  reduction of arterial stiffness by, 147–
      148, 147–148
  transdermal, for supine hypertension,
      574
Nitroprusside, for hypertensive
      emergencies, 716, 716t
  in aortic dissection, 717
  in congestive heart failure, 717
  in pheochromocytoma, 687
  for hypertensive encephalopathy, 279
  for hypertensive stroke, 281, 512
  for preeclampsia/eclampsia, 696t
  intraoperative use of, 711
Nitrous oxide, for induction of anesthesia,
      706
Nocturnal pattern of blood pressure. See
      Blood pressure, circadian rhythm of.
Noise exposure, blood pressure levels
      associated with, 10
Nonindustrialized populations, blood
      pressure in, 8–9, 8t, 9
Nonsteroidal anti-inflammatory drugs
      (NSAIDs), antagonism of
      antihypertensives by, 565
  ACE inhibitors and, 600, 606
  in elderly, 481
  choice of antihypertensive agent with,
      485
  limitation of protein excretion by, in
      chronic renal insufficiency, 293
  renal functional response to, 176–178
Nordic Diltiazem Study (NORDIL),
      design and objectives of, 346t, 351t,
      355
  on diltiazem vs. β-blocker and/or di-
      uretic, 614
  on safety of calcium antagonists, 613
Norepinephrine, circadian rhythm of, 505
  circulating, "cardiovascular hormone"
      function of, 45
  "diabetogenic" properties of, 47
  increased levels of, after alcohol con-
      sumption, 216
  with aging, 51, 553
  metabolism of, 44, 638
  modulation of, by presynaptic receptors
      and cotransmitters, 44
  plasma levels of, as marker of early hy-
      pertension, 49
    in baroreflex failure, 575
  spillover of, as index of sympathetic
      nervous system activity, 44

Norepinephrine *(Continued)*
  microneurographic studies of, 49–50
  storage of, in granules, 44
  synthesis of, 637
  urinary excretion of, 638, 638t
    in pheochromocytoma, 686
  ventricular hypertrophy related to, 251
North American Symptomatic Carotid
    Endarterectomy Trial (NASCET),
    282
Norway, initial choice of antihypertensive
    treatment in, *383, 386*
Nucleus, rostral ventrolateral (RVL), 42,
    43, 45
Nucleus tractus solitarius (NTS), 42
Nurses Health Study II, of calcium
    intake, 454, 455
  of potassium supplementation, 453
Nursing clinics, 409–414
  caseload size in, 412–413
  cost effectiveness of, 407, 412
  equipment needs and setup for, 412,
    413t
  implementation of, 410–411
  reimbursement for services of, 413–
    414, 414t
  roles and responsibilities in, 411–412,
    412t
Nutrition. See *Diet.*

Obesity. See also *Adipose tissue; Diet;
    Weight.*
  as risk factor, for hypertension, 299t,
    300, 460
  blood pressure measurement in, 312
  body mass index in definition of, 460
  cardiovascular effects of, 206–207, *206*
  gastric restrictive surgery for, hyperten-
    sion reduction after, 462
  hypertension related to, 118–124
    antihypertensive therapy in, 208–209
    body fat distribution and, 118–119
    determination of, during in utero de-
      velopment, 26
    initial choice of therapy in, 483–484,
      484t
    insulin and sympathetic nervous sys-
      tem activity in, 120–121, *120–
      121*
    insulin resistance syndrome in, 119
    nature of association between, 118
    weight reduction effects on, 208
  in African Americans, renal injury due
    to, 560, *560*
    target organ damage related to, 559–
      560
  in pregnancy, cardiovascular risk re-
    lated to, 695
  in women, hypertension related to, 547
  insulin-resistance syndrome related to,
    abnormalities in, 119
  dyslipidemia in, 121, *122,* 124
  pathophysiology of, *123,* 124
  left ventricular abnormalities in, 246
  management of, 509
  obstructive sleep apnea related to, 657,
    660
  of upper body, as cardiovascular risk
    factor, 118

Obesity *(Continued)*
  insulin resistance and diabetes melli-
    tus related to, 118–119
  relative, in adolescents, hypertension re-
    lated to, 26
  renal effects of, 207–208
  resistant hypertension due to, 567
  sympathetic nervous system activity re-
    lated to, 50
  ventricular hypertrophy in, 250
  visceral, as risk factor for hypertension,
    111
    metabolic abnormalities associated
      with, 110–111, 111t
  waist:hip ratio of, as risk factor, for hy-
    pertension, 299t, 300
  weight reduction for. See *Weight, reduc-
    tion of.*
Observational studies, case-control vs.
    cohort types of, 390
  definition of, 390
  of blood pressure distribution, 4–5, 4t,
    5
  of calcium channel blockers, 389–390,
    391–392
Obstructive sleep apnea. See *Sleep apnea,
    obstructive.*
Octreotide, for ectopic ACTH syndrome,
    684
Omapatrilat, *653,* 654
Opioid analgesics, 707
Oral appliances, for obstructive sleep
    apnea, 658
Oral contraceptives. See *Contraceptives,
    oral.*
I^{131} Orthoiodohippurate, in radionuclide
    imaging, 663–664
Orthostatic hypotension, 572–576
  assessment of, in elderly, 554
  associated with dementia, 13
  features of autonomic disorders in,
    572, 572t
  from ganglion blocking drugs, 639
  in baroreflex failure, 574–575, *575*
  in pure autonomic failure, 572–574
    severity of, 572, *573*
    standing time as measure of, 572–
      573
    supine hypertension in, 573, 574
    treatment of, 573–574, *574*
Orthostatic intolerance, features of pure
    autonomic failure vs., 575, 575t
  nomenclature for, 575, 576t
  treatment of, 575
Oscillometric method, of blood pressure
    measurement, 308–309
Osler maneuver, for measuring
    pseudohypertension, 554, 565
Ouabain, angiotensin II interactions with,
    45
Outcome measurement, 323–330
  cost effectiveness of therapy related to,
    407
  intermediate measures in, 327–328,
    327t
  long-term measures in, 328–329, 329t
  pros and cons of, 329–330, 330t
  short-term measures in, 324–327, 325t
Outreach programs. See *Community
    outreach programs.*

Ovary, angiotensin-converting enzyme
    distribution in, 93t, 94
  angiotensin-converting enzyme function
    in, 95, 95t
Overweight. See *Obesity.*

Papilledema, as sign of hypertension, 1
Paraganglioma syndrome, familial, 574
Paragangliomas, catecholamine-secreting.
    See *Pheochromocytoma.*
PATHS (Prevention and Treatment of
    Hypertension Study), 466–468, *467,*
    467t
Patient compliance. See *Antihypertensive
    therapy, compliance with.*
Patient education, by nurses, 411, 412t
Patient satisfaction, as measure of
    outcome, 326–327
PATS (Post-Stroke Antihypertensive
    Treatment Study), 342t–343t
PEACE (Prevention of Events with
    Angiotensin-Converting Enzyme
    Inhibition), 346t–347t, 348
Penaz's finger cuff method of blood
    pressure measurement, 309
Penbutolol. See also β-*Adrenoreceptor
    antagonists.*
  elimination characteristics of, 594t
  pharmacodynamics of, 591t
  pharmacokinetics of, 592t
  in renal replacement therapy, 536t
Pentaquine, for hypertension, 3
Pentetreotide, ^{111}In-labeled, in
    pheochromocytoma, 687
PEPI (Postmenopausal Estrogen/Progestin
    Interventions), 548
Pepstatin, as renin inhibitor, 647
Perindopril, PROGRESS trial of,
    346t–347t, 349
  resistance vessel remodeling and, 128,
    128, 128t
Perioperative hypertension. See also
    Anesthesia, in hypertension.
  calcium antagonists for, 615
  classes of hypertensive patients in, 702,
    702t
  management of, 703, *704*
Peripheral blood vessels, disease of, ACE
    inhibitors in, 604
  antihypertensive therapy for, 513
  as measure of outcome, 329
  resistance in. See *Resistance, periph-
    eral.*
  stenosis of, as risk factor for hyperten-
    sion, 301t
Peripheral nerves, in hyperinnervated
    hypertensive models, 44
  modulation of sympathetic nervous sys-
    tem impulses in, 43–44
Peritoneal dialysis. See also *Renal
    replacement therapy.*
  drug clearance in, 536t
  management of hypertension in, 533,
    535, 536
Personality, alcohol consumption related
    to, 216
  hypertension related to, 48, 62–64
Phenotypes, as clues to blood pressure
    disorders, 36

Phenotypes *(Continued)*
  heterogeneity of, 36
  in genetic research, 34
  intermediate, 34
Phenoxybenzamine, 596
Phentolamine, 596
  for hypertensive crisis, due to pheochromocytoma, 687
  for hypertensive emergencies, 716t
Phenylpropanolamine, combined with β-blockers, adverse effects of, 595
Phenytoin, magnesium sulfate vs., in eclamptic convulsions, 695
Pheochromocytoma, 685–687
  antihypertensive therapy for, 514–515
  assessment of, 685–687, *686*
    clonidine in, 640
    in diagnosis of hypertension, 303t, 568t, 569–570
    localization studies in, 687
    plasma catecholamines in, 686–687
    urinary catecholamines in, 685–686, 687t
  baroreflex failure vs., 574
  clinical presentation of, 685
  follow-up care of, 687
  genetic mutations in, 685
  in pregnancy, 690
  in women, 548
  surgical treatment of, 687
  sympathetic nervous system hyperactivity in, 52
Physical fitness. See *Exercise.*
Physician visits, as measure of outcome, 326
Physicians, as hypertension specialists, 408, 408t
  satisfaction of, with antihypertensive therapy, as measure of outcome, 327
Pindolol. See also β-*Adrenoreceptor antagonists.*
  elimination characteristics of, 594t
  pharmacodynamic properties of, 591t
  pharmacokinetic properties of, 592t
  pharmacokinetics of, in renal replacement therapy, 536t
Pituitary gland, as ectopic source of ACTH, surgical resection of, 684
  tumors of, after bilateral adrenalectomy, 684
Placental abnormalities, in preeclampsia, 693–694
Plaque, atherosclerotic, calcium antagonist effect on, 615
  rupture of, from sudden blood pressure increase, 506
Plasminogen activator inhibitor-1 (PAI-1), increased levels of, in hypertension, 112
Platelets, abnormalities of, in diabetes mellitus, 544
  in hypertension, 112–113, *112,* 113t
Polycystic kidney disease, assessment of, in diagnosis of hypertension, 303
  genetic cause and phenotype of, 35t
Polygenic model of blood pressure, 32–33, *33*
Polymorphisms. See *Genetic polymorphisms.*

Polysomnography, for obstructive sleep apnea, 657, 658
Population environments, blood pressure effects of, 32
Population genetics, 32
Positron emission tomography (PET), of coronary blood flow, 266
Postganglionic adrenergic inhibitors, 639–641. See also *Ganglion blocking drugs.*
  guanethidine and bretylium, 639–640
  methyldopa, clonidine, guanabenz, and guanfacine, 640–641
  monoamine oxidase inhibitors, 641
  rauwolfia alkaloids, 639
  Veratrum alkaloids, 641
Postmenopausal Estrogen/Progestin Interventions (PEPI), 548
Postpartum hypertension, late, 691–692
Post-Stroke Antihypertensive Treatment Study (PATS), 342t–343t
Potassium. See also *Hyperkalemia; Hypokalemia.*
  evaluation of, in hyperaldosteronism, 677, *677*
  in salt substitutes, adverse effects of, with angiotensin II receptor blockers, 481
  infusions of, for diuretic-induced hypokalemia, in diabetes mellitus, 487
  protective effects of, 450–451
  repletion of, 450–454
    interventional studies of, 451–453, *452–453*
    observational studies of, 450–451, *451*
    recommendations for, 453–454
  sodium intake and, 450, 453
  supplementation with, interaction with ACE inhibitors, 606
Potassium-sparing diuretics, benefits of, 585
  characteristics and dosage of, 719t
  hyperkalemia due to, 588
  with thiazide diuretics, 500
Power motivation, hypertension related to, 62–63
PRAISE (Prospective Randomized Amlodipine Survival Evaluation), 542
Pravastatin, in ALLHAT study, 354, 363
Prazosin. See also α-*Adrenoreceptor antagonists.*
  combined with hydrochlorothiazide, dosage of, 501t
  effectiveness of, 596
  exercise interaction with, 475
  in pregnancy, 696t
  pharmacokinetics of, in renal replacement therapy, 536t
Prednisone, high-dose, hypertension due to, 514
Preeclampsia, differential diagnosis of, 692, 692t
  eicosanoid effects on, 179–180
  HELLP syndrome in, 691
  management of, 694–695. See also *Pregnancy, antihypertensive therapy in.*

Preeclampsia *(Continued)*
  aggressive vs. conservative, 695
  antihypertensive agents in, 696t
  magnesium sulfate in, 695
  with escalating blood pressure, 695
  pathophysiology of, 692–694
    cerebrovascular changes in, 693
    kidney and volume homeostasis in, 692–693
    ureteroplacental factors in, 693–694
    vascular changes in, 692
  pregnancy termination in, 695
  preventive measures in, 694
  signs and symptoms of, 691, 691t
  superimposition of, on preexisting hypertension, 694
  sympathetic nervous system hyperactivity in, 52
  variant of, 691
Pregnancy, 688–699
  antihypertensive therapy in, 697–699
    α-adrenoreceptor antagonists in, 698
    β-adrenoreceptor antagonists in, 698
    breast feeding and, 699
    calcium antagonists in, 698
    central adrenergic inhibitors in, 697–698
    choice of agents in, 515
    combined α- and β-adrenoreceptor antagonists in, 698
    contraindicated agents in, ACE inhibitors, 483, 606, 696t, 698–699
      angiotensin II receptor blockers, 483, 627, 698–699
      calcium antagonists, 614
    diuretics in, 699
    for chronic hypertension, 696t
    risk classification in, 697, 697t
    vasodilators in, 698
  blood pressure level in, 547
    measurement of, 312, 690
  hemodynamic changes in, 689–690, *689*
  hypertension in. See also *Eclampsia; Preeclampsia.*
    angiotensinogen polymorphisms in, 81, 87t
    calcitonin gene–related peptide in, 186–187, *186*
    chronic, causes of, 690–691
      treatment of, 695, 696t, 697
    classification of, 690–692
    gestational (transient), 691–692, 692t
    initial choice of therapy for, 483
    late postpartum, 691–692
  volume homeostasis in, 690
Prescribing practices. See *Antihypertensive therapy, initial choice of drug and.*
Pressure natriuresis, in blood pressure regulation, 22
Prevention and Treatment of Hypertension Study (PATHS), 466–468, *467,* 467t
Prevention of Events with Angiotensin-Converting Enzyme Inhibition (PEACE), 346t–347t, 348
Probucol, for coronary artery disease, 115
Progesterone, calcitonin gene–related peptide regulation by, 186

Progesterone (Continued)
  protective effects of, in coronary artery
      disease and hypertension, 114, 115
Progestin, in oral contraceptives,
      hypertension related to, 548
  PEPI trial of, 548
PROGRESS (Perindopril Protection
      Against Recurrent Stroke),
      346t–347t, 349
Propofol, for induction of anesthesia,
      706–707
Propranolol. See also β-Adrenoreceptor
      antagonists.
  breast feeding and, 699
  combined with diuretics, 501t
  elimination characteristics of, 594t
  exercise interaction with, 474–475
  extended-release formulations of, 593
  pharmacodynamics of, 591t
  pharmacokinetics of, 592t, 593
  in renal replacement therapy, 536t
Prorenin, 70–76. See also Renin.
  activation of, 72, 72
  as possible predictor of diabetic
      nephropathy, 75
  measurement of, in clinical hyperten-
      sion, 74–75
      methods for, 75
  regulation of, 72, 73t, 74, 74
  synthesis and biochemistry of, 71, 72
Prospective Randomized Amlodipine
      Survival Evaluation (PRAISE), 542
Prostacyclin, deficiency of, preeclampsia
      related to, 179
Prostaglandin(s), ACE inhibitor
      interaction with, 600
  in pregnancy, preeclampsia related to,
      179, 180
Prostaglandin E₂, preeclampsia related to,
      180
Prostaglandin H₂, hyperchloremia and,
      177
  hypertension related to, 178
Prostaglandin I₂, preeclampsia related to,
      179, 180
Prostanoids. See also Eicosanoids.
  endothelial dysfunction due to, 162
  preeclampsia related to, 692
Prostate, angiotensin-converting enzyme
      distribution in, 94
Prostatic hypertrophy, benign,
      α₁-adrenoreceptor antagonists for,
      597–598
Protein, dietary, restriction of, in chronic
      renal insufficiency, 293
  with ACE inhibitor therapy, 605
Protein tyrosine kinase, in angiotensin
      AT₁ receptor signal transduction, 102
Proteinuria, as cardiovascular risk factor,
      525
  in African Americans, 559
  in diabetic nephropathy, management
      of, 510
  in preeclampsia, 693
  in pregnancy, 690
  in renal failure, ACE inhibitors for re-
      ducing, 486–487, 486t, 526–527,
      527, 528, 605
      angiotensin II receptor blockers for
          reducing, 633

Proteinuria (Continued)
  as predictor of renal function loss,
      525
  blood pressure goal in, 526, 528
  calcium channel blockers for reduc-
      ing, 486, 486t
Pseudoephedrine, combined with
      β-blockers, adverse effects of, 595
Pseudohypertension, in elderly, due to
      rigid brachial artery, 515
  Osler maneuver for measuring, 554,
      565
  signs of, 565
Pseudohypoaldosteronism, type 1, mild,
      genetic cause and phenotype of,
      35t
  severe, genetic cause and phenotype
      of, 35t
  type II (Gordon's syndrome), genetic
      cause and phenotype of, 35t
Pseudoresistance, 564–565, 564t
Psychosocial factors, associated with
      blood pressure elevation, 10, 10,
      62–64
  in white-coat hypertension, 316
Pulmonary disease, chronic obstructive
      (COPD), antihypertensive therapy
      and, 511
  atrial natriuretic peptide in, 171–172
  contraindications to β-blockers in,
      591
Pulmonary hypertension, antihypertensive
      therapy and, 511
Pulmonary vein, inflow of, in
      measurement of diastolic function,
      258
Pulse pressure, 227–233. See also Blood
      pressure.
  age-related changes in, 229–230, 229–
      230
  as predictor of cardiac events, 225,
      225–226, 230
  definition of, 227
  elevated, clinical relevance of, 230
      due to arterial stiffness, 137, 142,
          143, 230
      low diastolic pressure as associated
          risk with, 231
  hemodynamic implications on, 228–
      229, 228
  historical perspective on, 227–228
  noninvasive pulse-wave analysis of,
      233
  resistance vessel media:lumen ratio cor-
      related with, 127
  wide, clinical correlates of, 232
      hemodynamic correlates of, 232
      in elderly, 553
      pathological correlates of, 231–232
      therapeutic correlates of, 232–233
Pulse-wave velocity (PWV), as index of
      arterial stiffness, 135t, 138, 139
  doubling of, with aging and arterial
      stiffness, 142, 145
  relationship of, with arterial elasticity,
      136
Pyelography, intravenous, in renovascular
      hypertension, 666

Quality of life, as measure of outcome,
      325
QUIET (Quinapril Ischemic Event Trial),
      346t–347t, 348
Quinapril. See also Angiotensin-
      converting enzyme (ACE) inhibitors.
  dosage of, 603t
  interaction with tetracycline, 606
  pharmacokinetics of, 601t
  in renal replacement therapy, 536t
  QUIET trial of, 346t–347t, 348

Race. See also specific racial group, e.g.,
      African Americans.
  α-adrenergic responsiveness and, 50
  alcohol consumption and, blood pres-
      sure levels in, 211, 212, 214
  angiotensinogen polymorphisms and,
      80, 82t–85t, 87t
  as determinant of blood pressure, 7, 7
  diabetes mellitus and, 518
  dose-response variability due to, 494
  hypertension and, initial choice of ther-
      apy and, 483–484, 484t
  stress response related to, 59
Radioimmunoassay, for plasma ACTH,
      683
  for renin measurement, 75
Radionuclide imaging, for renovascular
      disease, 663–664, 663
  of catecholamine-secreting tumors, 687
  of diastolic function, 256
  radiolabeled microspheres in, for coro-
      nary blood flow measurement, 266
Ramipril. See also Angiotensin-converting
      enzyme (ACE) inhibitors.
  dosage of, 603t
  HOPE trial of, 346t–347t, 348–349
  pharmacokinetics of, 601t
  in renal replacement therapy, 536t
  REIN trial of, 291
  renoprotective effects of, 604
Randomized Evaluation of NIDDM with
      the Angiotensin II Antagonist
      Losartan (RENAAL), 346t–347t, 348
Randomized trials. See Clinical trial(s).
Rauwolfia alkaloids, adverse effects of,
      639
  combined with hydrochlorothiazide,
      dosage of, 501t
  pharmacology of, 639
RB 106 (vasopeptidase inhibitor), 653,
      653
Regional anesthesia, 704, 705, 709–710
Regression dilution bias, in blood
      pressure measurement, 311
Reimbursement, for nursing clinic
      services, 413–414, 414t
REIN (Ramipril Efficacy in
      Nephropathy), 291
Relaxation therapy, for stress reduction,
      66
Remikiren, 647. See also Renin,
      inhibitors of.
RENAAL (Randomized Evaluation of
      NIDDM with the Angiotensin II
      Antagonist Losartan), 346t–347t, 348
Renal artery stenosis, angioplasty and
      stenting for, 513

Renal artery stenosis *(Continued)*
  assessment of, 303t, 666
  atherosclerosis in, 304
    progression of, 667
  hypertension due to. See *Renovascular hypertension.*
  in elderly, 515–516
  surgical revascularization for, 669–670
Renal disease. See also *Nephropathy, diabetic; Renal failure, chronic.*
  anesthetic considerations in, 708, 708t
  assessment of, in diagnosis of hypertension, 301t
  polycystic, assessment of, in diagnosis of hypertension, 303, 303t
  genetic cause and phenotype of, 35t
Renal failure. See also *Renal replacement therapy.*
  acute, due to ACE inhibitors or angiotensin II antagonists, in renal artery stenosis, 513, 667
  hypertensive emergency in, 717–718
  chronic, 524–529
    antihypertensive therapy in, 526–529. See also *Renoprotective effects.*
      ACE inhibitors in. See *Angiotensin-converting enzyme (ACE) inhibitors, in renal failure.*
      angiotensin II receptor blockers in, 292, 486, 513, 528, 626–627, 632–633
      benefits of, 331, 1334
      blood pressure goal in, 526, *526*
      genetic factors in response to, 527–528
      guidelines for, 528–529, *529*
      intraglomerular pressure reduction in, 526, *527*
      lipid profile improvement in, 527, *528*
      proteinuria reduction in, 526–527, *527*
      special considerations in, 528–529
      treatment schedule for, 528
    as measure of outcome, 329
    assessment of, in diagnosis of hypertension, 303t
    dietary protein excretion in, 293
    drug therapy of, hypertension due to, 514
    dyslipidemia in, 293
    heparin therapy for, 293–294
    hypertension in, 286–294
      assessment of, 568t, 570
      cardiovascular target organ damage in, 525
      goal blood pressure in, 288–290
      incidence of, 286
      initial choice of therapy in, 486–487, 486t
      management of, 513–514
      nonpharmacological therapy for, 287
      pathogenesis of, 286–287, 524–525, *524*
      pharmacological therapy for, 287–288
      prevalence of, 524

Renal failure *(Continued)*
    renal target organ damage in, 525–526, 525t
    renoprotective antihypertensive drugs for, 290–293
    sympathetic nervous system hyperactivity in, 52
    nonsteroidal anti-inflammatory drugs in, 293
    progressive function loss in, risk factors for, 525–526, 525t
    proteinuria in. See *Proteinuria.*
Renal function, abnormalities of, from anesthesia, 710
  in preeclampsia, 692–693
  ACE inhibitor effects on, 602, 602t, 667
  angiotensin II effects on, 622
  angiotensin II receptor blocker effects on, 626–627, 631, 632–633, 667
  assessment of, as measure of outcome, 327
    in diagnosis of hypertension, 302, 304t
  eicosanoid effects on, 176–178, *177–178*
  endothelin effects on, 154
  in African Americans, 560
  in blood pressure regulation, cardiovascular-renal homeostasis in, 22–23
  in white-coat hypertension, 318
  kallikrein-kinin system interaction with, 195–196
  obesity effects on, *206,* 207–208
    weight reduction and, 208
  renin inhibitor effects on, 649, *649*
Renal insufficiency. See *Renal failure, chronic.*
Renal medulla, in pressure natriuresis mechanism, 22–23
Renal replacement therapy,
  antihypertensive therapy in, management of, 514
  hypertension in, 531–537
    blood pressure level and, 532–533
    cardiovascular morbidity and mortality in, 532
    epidemiology of, 531–532
    management of, 533–536
      antihypertensive therapy in, 535–536, 534t–536t
      extracellular volume and, 535
      principles of, 533, 535
    pathogenesis of, 533
    prevalence of, 532
    renin-dependent, 533
    volume-dependent, 533
Renal salt wasting, renal sympathetic nerves and, 48
Renal sympathetic nerves, organ-protective effects of, 47
  renal salt wasting related to, 48
  stress effects on, hypertension related to, 48
Renal vein renin (RVR) measurement, 666
Renin, 70–76. See also *Prorenin.*
  angiotensinogen interaction with, biochemical characteristics of, 77

Renin *(Continued)*
    transgenic studies of, 78
  as risk factor, for cardiovascular events, 448–449, *449*
    for coronary disease, 239, 403
    for hypertension, 299t, 300–301
    for myocardial infarction, 449
  biochemistry of, 647
  circulating vs. local, 71–72, *72*
  discovery of, 70
  gene for, 70–71
  in renal vein (RVR), measurement of, 666
  increased levels of, after alcohol consumption, 216
  inhibitors of, 646–650
    ACE inhibitors and angiotensin II antagonists vs., 650, 650t
    advantages of, 75
    antihypertensive effects of, 647–649
    biochemistry of, 647, *648*
    discontinuation of development of, 650
    renal response to, 649–650, *649*
    specificity of, 646, *646*
    structure of, *648*
  low levels of, in African Americans, 559, *560*
  in orthostatic intolerance, 576
  measurement of, in clinical hypertension, 74–75
    in initial diagnosis of hypertension, 302
    methods for, 75, 300–301
  plasma levels of, conditions affecting, 73t
    in aging, 553
    in chronic renal failure, 525
    in evaluation, of hyperaldosteronism, 677–678, *677*
      of renovascular hypertension, 666
  regulation of, 72, 74, *74*
  sodium restriction effects on, 438, 439t, *440,* 448–449
  synthesis and biochemistry of, 70–71, *72*
  ventricular hypertrophy related to, 251
Renin-angiotensin system, activation of, by sodium restriction, 438, 440, 448
  aging effects on, 553
  circulating vs. local, concepts in, 72, *73*
  in cardiovascular hypertrophy, 96
  in chronic renal failure, 525, 533
  kallikrein-kinin system interaction with, 194–195
  physiology of, 70, *71*
  sympathetic nervous system interaction with, 44–45
  hypertension related to, 50
Renin inhibitors. See *Renin, inhibitors of.*
Renoprotective effects, of ACE inhibitors, in diabetes mellitus, 510, 521, 521t
  in renal failure, 290–292, 513, 604–605
  of angiotensin II receptor antagonists, 292, 513, 528, 632–633
  of antihypertensive therapy, clinical trials of, 337

Renoprotective effects (Continued)
    for reduction of glomerular pressure, 510, 526
    in chronic renal failure, 290–293
    of benazepril, 604
    of calcium antagonists, 292–293
    of captopril, 604
    of diltiazem, 522
    of enalapril, 604
    of heparin, 293–294
    of ramipril, 604
    of verapamil, 522
Renovascular hypertension, 662–672
    angioplasty and stenting for, 513, 667–669, 668–669, 670
    antihypertensive therapy in, ACE inhibitors in, in elderly, 515–516
        monitoring required with, 288, 513, 667
    angiotensin II receptor antagonists in, in elderly, 515–516
        monitoring required with, 513, 631, 667
    choice of agents in, 666–667
    causes of, 662
    clinical signs and symptoms of, 568t, 662–663
    from fibromuscular dysplasia, in women, 547–548
    in elderly, contraindications to ACE inhibitors and angiotensin II antagonists in, 515–516
    in pregnancy, 690
    incidence of, 662
    recommended management of, 670
    renal artery evaluation in, 666
    renal function preservation in, 670–672
    screening tests for, 569, 663–665
        angiography in, 664–665, 665
        computed axial tomography in, 664
        duplex Doppler ultrasonography in, 665
        intravascular ultrasonography in, 665–666
        intravenous pyelography in, 666
        magnetic resonance imaging in, 664, 664
        plasma renin activity in, 666
        radioisotope scanning in, 663–664, 663
    significance of, 662
    surgery for, 669–670
    sympathetic nervous system hyperactivity in, 51–52
Reproductive system, angiotensin-converting enzyme distribution in, 93t, 94
    angiotensin-converting enzyme function in, 95, 95t
Research. See also Clinical trial(s).
    basic, characteristics of, 389
    on cardiovascular risk, of calcium channel blockers, 390–391
Reserpine, combined with β-blockers, adverse effects of, 595
    combined with hydrochlorothiazide, dosage of, 501t
    for hypertension, history of, 3
    pharmacology of, 639

Resistance, peripheral, adaptive and maladaptive overload related to, 232
    in hyperaldosteronism, 679, 679
    location of, 125
    longitudinal study of, in hypertension, 471
    reduction of, by diuretics, 584, 585t
    systemic, in hypertension, 471
    vascular, in pathophysiology of hypertension, 24
        in renal failure, 533
        reduction of, by kinins, 196
Resistance vessels, 125–132
    definition of, 125
    endothelium-mediated responses of, 130
    fibrinoid necrosis in, lacunar infarction due to, 278, 278
    functional properties of, 130
    location of peripheral resistance and, 125
    rarefaction in, 125, 128
    remodeling of, definitions and classifications of, 126, 126
        eutrophic, 126, 126
        inward, 127, 127
        evidence for, 126–127
        hypertrophic, 126, 126
        inward, 126, 127
        hypotrophic, 126, 126
        in vitro demonstration of, 127–128, 127–128
        in vivo visualization of, 128
        measurement of, 129–130
        reversal of, with antihypertensive treatment, 128–129, 129, 129t, 132
    structure of, 125–126
        antihypertensive treatment and, 132
        blood pressure regulation and, 130–132, 131
Resistance/capacitance circuit, as model of arterial elasticity, 136
Resistant hypertension. See Hypertension, resistant.
RET proto-oncogene, mutations in, in pheochromocytoma, 685
Retina, assessment of, in diagnosis of hypertension, 301t
Revascularization, for coronary artery disease, 540–542, 541
    transmyocardial, 543
Risk, 221–227. See also Cardiovascular risk factor(s); Hypertension, risk factor(s) for.
    absolute, definition of, 221
        determination of, 297, 297
        in decision to treat, 223–224, 381
        in selection of blood pressure threshold, 223
    in hypertension, blood pressure threshold and, 222–223, 223
        decision to treat related to, 221–222
    relative, definition of, 221
        in decision to treat, 223–224
        in selection of blood pressure threshold, 222–223
    stratification of, in diagnosis of hypertension, 371–372, 371t–372t

Risk (Continued)
    in elderly hypertensives, 555, 555t
    in treated hypertensive patients, 224–227, 225–226
Rostral ventrolateral (RVL) nucleus, blood pressure regulation by, 42
    glutamate-sensitive neurons in, 45
    modification by hypothalamus, 43

Salt. See Sodium, dietary.
Sampatrilat, 653, 653
Sandostatin, for ectopic ACTH syndrome, 684
Sarafotoxin S6c (endothelin receptor agonist), 155, 155t
Saralasin, development of, 623
    exercise interaction with, 475
    limitations of, 623
Scandinavian Simvastatin Survival Study (4S), 361
SCOPE (Study of Cognition and Prognosis in Elderly Patients with Hypertension), 346t–347t, 349
Scottish Heart Health Study, 435, 436
Seasons, sympathetic nervous system effects of, 48
Secondary hypertension. See Hypertension, secondary.
Secular trends, in blood pressure, 32
Senile plethora, 1
Sensory nerves, calcitonin gene–related peptide release from, 183–184
Sex. See Gender differences.
Sexual development, abnormalities of, with 17α-hydroxylase deficiency, 676
Sexual function, antihypertensive effects on, in women, 549
Shanghai Trial of Nifedipine in Elderly (STONE), 342, 342t–343t, 613, 614
SHELL (Systolic Hypertension in Elderly Long-Term Lacidipine Trial), 338t, 346t, 351t, 352
SHEP. See Systolic Hypertension in Elderly Project (SHEP).
Signal transduction, of angiotensin AT$_1$ receptor, 102–103
    of angiotensin AT$_2$ receptor, 105
Simvastatin, Scandinavian Simvastatin Survival Study of, 361
Sleep, blood pressure fall during. See Blood pressure, circadian rhythm of, nocturnal pattern of.
Sleep apnea, obstructive, 657–660
    antihypertensive therapy in, 511, 660
    blood pressure changes in, in awake state, 659–660
        nocturnal, 658–659, 659
    cardiovascular consequences of, 660
    diagnosis of, 657–658, 658t
    mechanisms of, 657
    prevalence of, 657
    resistant hypertension due to, 567
    risk factors for, 657, 658t
    treatment of, 658
Slow-release antihypertensives. See Delayed-action antihypertensives.

Smoking, arterial stiffness related to, 147
  as risk factor, for cardiovascular death,
      in diabetes mellitus, 115–116
    for cardiovascular disease, 526
    for hypertension, 299, 299t
    for renal failure, 526
  blood pressure elevation from, 47
  in African Americans, 561
  resistant hypertension due to, 567
SNAP (Sodium and Blood Pressure)
    Study, 559
Social class, blood pressure rise
    associated with, 6–7
Social factors, in blood pressure levels,
    10, 10
Social support, as stress buffer, 65–66, 66
Socioeconomic status, blood pressure
    elevation related to, 61
Sodium, decreased level of, diuretic-
    induced, 589
  dietary, 433–450
    calcium interaction with, 202–203
    controversies in, 202
    extracellular fluid volume related to,
        524, 524
    Intersalt study of, 8–9, 8t, 9, 434–
        435, 435
    observational studies of, 434–450
    proteinuria related to, in chronic re-
        nal insufficiency, 287
    recommendations on, 449–450
    renal injury due to, in African Ameri-
        cans, 560–561
    restriction of, for volume overload
        prevention, 566
      gradual reduction in, 479–480
      historical background of, 2, 434
      in African Americans, 561–562
      in chronic renal failure, 287, 487,
          528
      in elderly, diuretics with, 516
      in renal replacement therapy, 535
      in women, 549
      interventional studies of, 435–447
        blood pressure changes in, 435,
            436, 437
        heterogeneity among, 437, 437
        meta-analyses of, 435–440, 436,
            438–440, 439t
        TAIM study in, 440, 442, 442
        TOHP Phase I in, 440, 441
        TOHP Phase II in, 442–445,
            443–444
        TONE study in, 445–446, 444–
            446
      lowering of hypertension by, 208
      neurohumoral effects of, 438,
          439t, 440
      with ACE inhibitor therapy, 605
    Scottish Heart Health Study of, 435,
        436
    SNAP study of, 559
  in diagnostic oral salt loading, for adre-
      nocortical hypertension, 675, 675t
    for hyperaldosteronism, 678
  renal wasting of, 48
  retention of, in African Americans, 59

Sodium (Continued)
  in chronic renal insufficiency, 286–
      287
  in preeclampsia, 693
  in response to antihypertensive ther-
      apy, 495
  nonmineralocorticoid, 513–514
  potential risks of, 447–448, 447–449
  sensitivity to, in African Americans,
      560
  in elderly, 437
Solomon Island societies, epidemiology
    of blood pressure in, 8
SOLVD (Studies of Left Ventricular
    Dysfunction), 511–512
Spinal cord, sympathetic nervous system
    and, 43–44
Spironolactone, characteristics and dosage
    of, 587t
  combined with hydrochlorothiazide,
      500
  for glucocorticoid-remediable aldoste-
      ronism, 682
  for primary aldosteronism, 514, 679,
      679, 680
  in Conn's syndrome, 514
  in evaluation of hypokalemia, 676
  nifedipine vs., for hyperaldosteronism,
      680, 681t
STAI (Studio della Ticlopidina nell'
    Angina Instabile), 543
Statine, as renin inhibitor, 647
Stenting, for renal artery stenosis, results
    of, 668–669, 669, 671
  surgical revascularization vs., 672
Steroids. See Corticosteroids.
Stiffness, arterial. See Artery(ies),
    stiffness of.
Stockings, counterpressure support, for
    orthostatic hypotension, 573
STONE (Shanghai Trial of Nifedipine in
    Elderly), 342, 342t–343t, 613, 614
STOP. See Swedish Trial in Old Patients
    with Hypertension (STOP).
Strength training exercise, 472
Streptokinase, with aspirin, for acute
    myocardial infarction, 542
Stress, 59–67
  acute, sympathetic nervous system and,
      47–48
  buffers and stress-reduction interven-
      tions for, 65–67, 66
  chronic, blood pressure effects of, 48
    socioeconomic status and, 61
  environmental, job-related vs. home-
      related, 61–62
  general adaptation syndrome and, 47
  hypertension due to, animal models of,
      59–61, 60
  oxidative, angiotensin AT_1 receptor in,
      102
  psychological, alcohol consumption re-
      lated to, 216
  renal sympathetic nerve tone and, 48
  response to, acute, blood pressure regu-
      lation in, 45, 46
    homeostasis vs., 45

Stress (Continued)
  cardiovascular response in, 64–65,
      64, 65t
  gender differences in, 59
  integrated role of sympathetic ner-
      vous system in, 47
Stroke, 277–284
  anesthesia-related, 710
  antihypertensive therapy in, angiotensin
      II receptor blockers in, 633
    choice of drugs in, 281, 512
    controversies in, 280, 280
    effects of, 280–281
    PROGRESS trial of, 346t–347t, 349
    stroke prevention by, clinical trials
        of, 335, 336
    types of stroke prevented by, 278–
        279
  as measure of outcome, 329
  hypertension-related, alcohol consump-
      tion and, 217
    pathophysiology of, 278, 278–279
  hypertensive emergency in, 717
  hypertensive encephalopathy in, 279–
      280
  PATS trial of, 342t–343t
  prevention of, 281–284
    antilipemic agents for, 283
    antiplatelet agents and anticoagulants
        for, 282–283
    carotid endarterectomy for, 282, 282,
        282t
    hyperhomocysteinemia prophylaxis
        in, 283–284
    postmenopausal hormone replace-
        ment therapy in, 284, 284
    primary and secondary methods of,
        277
  risk of, association of, with blood pres-
      sure, 15, 15
    based on Framingham study, 223,
        223
    in African Americans, 558
    in elderly, 552
    reduction of, with antihypertensive
        therapy, 331
    relative, 221, 222
  types of, 277, 277t
Studies of Left Ventricular Dysfunction
    (SOLVD), 511–512
Studio della Ticlopidina nell' Angina
    Instabile (STAI), 543
Study of Cognition and Prognosis in
    Elderly Patients with Hypertension
    (SCOPE), 346t–347t, 349
Substance P, as mediator of inflammation,
    97
  as substrate for angiotensin-converting
      enzyme, 92t, 97
  colocalization with calcitonin gene–
      related peptide, 183, 187
  in coronary artery function, 262
  in experimental hypertension, 187
  protection of, by ACE and NEP inhibi-
      tion, 652
  vasodilator activity of, 187
Superoxide anions, degradation of nitric
    oxide by, 161–162

Superoxide anions *(Continued)*
  sources of, 162
Superoxide dismutase, scavenging of
  superoxide anions by, 161
Surgery. See also *Anesthesia.*
  coronary artery bypass graft, 542
  for obstructive sleep apnea, 658
  for renal artery stenosis, 669–670
    angiography and stenting vs., 671–
      672
    perioperative hypertension in, calcium
      antagonists for, 615
    classes of hypertensive patients in,
      702, 702t
    management of, 703, *704*
Sweden, initial choice of antihypertensive
  treatment in, *383, 386*
Swedish Trial in Old Patients with
  Hypertension (STOP), evaluation of
  antihypertensive therapy in, 554
  long-term results of, 333t
  published results of, 342t–343t
  stroke reduction in, *335, 336*
Swedish Trial in Old Patients with
  Hypertension-2 (STOP-2),
  comparison of antihypertensive
  agents in, 346t, 351t, 352–353, 614
  on safety of calcium antagonists, 613
Sympathectomy, for hypertension, history
  of, 3
Sympathetic nervous system, ACE
  inhibitor interaction with, 600
  activation of, by sodium restriction,
    438, 440, 449
  aging effects on, 553
  angiotensin II receptor blocker effects
    on, 627
  "baroprotective role" of, 47
  benign prostatic hypertrophy and, 597–
    598
  central control of outflow from, 42, *43*
  circadian and seasonal effects on, 48,
    505, 506
  dietary influences on, 119–120
  in hypertension, 42–53
    chronic, 50–51
    circulating catecholamines and, 45
    early, 49–50
    genetic-environmental interaction in,
      47–49
    mild, 403
    neurotransmitters and, 44–45
    obesity-related, insulin and, 120–
      121, *120–121*
    peripheral hyperinnervation in, 44
    postsynaptic adrenergic receptors
      and, 45
    secondary, 51–53
  in insulin-resistance syndrome, *123,*
    124
  integrated cardiovascular and metabolic
    regulation by, 45–47
  natriuretic peptide modulation of, 169–
    170
  organization and function of, 42–45
  organ-protective effects of, 47
  renin-angiotensin system interaction
    with, 44–45

Sympathomimetic activity, intrinsic, of β-
  blockers, 591, 591t
Sympathomimetic amines, hypertension
  due to, 566
Syndrome X. See also *Insulin resistance;
  Metabolic abnormalities.*
  components of, diabetic vascular dis-
    ease related to, 519, 519t
  gender differences in, 146
  sympathetic nervous system activity re-
    lated to, 50
SYST-CHINA (Chinese Trial on Isolated
  Systolic Hypertension in Elderly),
  334, 338t
Systemic resistance, in hypertension, 471
SYST-EUR. See *Systolic Hypertension in
  Europe (SYST-EUR).*
Systolic blood pressure. See *Blood
  pressure, systolic.*
Systolic function. See *Ventricle(s),
  systolic function of.*
Systolic hypertension, isolated. See
  Hypertension, isolated systolic.
Systolic Hypertension in Elderly Long-
  Term Lacidipine Trial (SHELL),
  338t, 346t, 351t, 352
Systolic Hypertension in Elderly Project
  (SHEP), arterial stiffness and, 135
  goal blood pressure in, 481
  guidelines based on, 227–228
  long-term results of, 333t, 334
  on antihypertensive therapy, 554
  on heart failure improvement by thia-
    zide diuretics, 585
  on prevalence of isolated systolic hyper-
    tension, 551
  on risk of congestive heart failure, 250
  published results of, 342t–343t
Systolic Hypertension in Europe (SYST-
  EUR), goal blood pressure in, 481
  long-term results of, 333t, 334, 335
  on antihypertensive therapy, in elderly,
    554
    with short-acting calcium channel
      blockers, 554
  on cardiovascular effects of calcium an-
    tagonists, 334, 613
  published results of, 342, 342t–343t
  reduction of cardiovascular endpoints
    in, 392, 394
  stroke reduction in, *335, 336,* 614

Tachycardia, reflex, absence of, in
  lipophilic calcium antagonists, 617
  from nifedipine, 613, 616
  sinus, in prognosis of myocardial in-
    farction, 539
TAIM (Trial of Antihypertensive
  Interventions and Management), on
  sodium restriction effects, 440, 442,
  442
  on weight reduction, 461–462, 461t
Tamsulosin, 597
Target organ damage. See also specific
  organ, *e.g. Heart.*
  clinical studies of, in white-coat hyper-
    tension, 316–318

Target organ damage *(Continued)*
  evaluation of, in diagnosis of hyperten-
    sion, 301–302, 301t
  in chronic renal failure, 525–526
  in mild hypertension, 403
  pressure-related, as cardiovascular risk
    factor, 558
  in African Americans, mechanisms
    of, 559–561, *560*
  patterns of, 558–559, 559t
Tasosartan, development of, 624
  structure of, *626*
Tecumseh study, 402–403
Telecommunications, in management of
  hypertension, by nursing clinics,
  410–411
  in community outreach programs,
    416–417
Telmisartan. See also *Angiotensin II
  receptor antagonists.*
  development of, 624
  pharmacology of, 630, 631t
  structure of, *626*
Telomere(s), shortening of, hypertension
  related to, 24
Temperature, regulation of, by
  sympathetic nervous system, 47
Terazosin. See also α-*Adrenoreceptor
  antagonists.*
  effectiveness of, 596
  pharmacokinetics of, in renal replace-
    ment therapy, 536t
Testis, angiotensin-converting enzyme
  distribution in, 93t, 94
  angiotensin-converting enzyme function
    in, 95, 95t
Tetracycline, interaction with quinapril,
  606
Tetraethylammonium chloride, 638
Thallium-201 imaging, of coronary blood
  flow, 266–267
Thallium scintigraphy, with exercise
  electrocardiography, 540
Thermogenesis, dietary, energy balance
  and, 120, *120*
Thiazide diuretics. See also *Diuretics;
  Hydrochlorothiazide.*
  characteristics and dosage of, 586t
  combined with, ACE inhibitors, in left
    ventricular dysfunction, 485
    adrenergic inhibitors, 637
    benefits of, other agents, 487–488,
      488t
    loop-active diuretic, for chronic renal
      insufficiency, 287
    potassium-sparing diuretics, 500
  exercise interaction with, 474
  for calcium loss prevention, in women,
    483
  for isolated systolic hypertension, 482
  high-dose, adverse effects of, 495
  in elderly, 555
  in pregnancy, 696t, 699
  low-dose, in diabetes mellitus, 522
  recommendation for, 374
  reduction of left ventricular hypertro-
    phy by, 585

Thiazide diuretics *(Continued)*
   with sodium restriction, in elderly, 516
Thiazolidinedione(s), for diabetes
   mellitus, improvement of
   cardiovascular disease with, 114
Thiocyanate, early use of, 2
   from high-dose nitroprusside, 716
Thiopental, for induction of anesthesia,
   705
Thromboxane A$_2$, hyperchloremia and,
   177
   hypertension related to, 178
Ticlopidine, for prevention of myocardial
   infarction, 543
   for stroke prevention, 282
Time lost from work, as measure of
   outcome, 328
Timolol, combined with diuretics, 501t
   elimination characteristics of, 594t
   pharmacodynamics of, 591t
   pharmacokinetics of, 592t
   in renal replacement therapy, 536t
Tissue repair, angiotensin-converting
   enzyme in, 97
Tobacco use. See *Smoking.*
TOHP. See *Trials of Hypertension
   Prevention (TOHP).*
TOMHS. See *Treatment of Mild
   Hypertension Study (TOMHS).*
TONE (Trial of Nonpharmacologic
   Interventions in Elderly), 445–446,
   444–446
Torsemide, characteristics and dosage of,
   587t
   for hypertension, in chronic renal insufficiency, 287
Toxicology studies, in drug approval
   process, 579–580
Trandolapril. See also *Angiotensin-
   converting enzyme (ACE) inhibitors.*
   cardioprotective effects of, 605
   dosage of, 603t
   INVEST trial of, 346t, 351t, 353
   PEACE trial of, 346t–347t, 348
   pharmacokinetics of, 601t
   in renal replacement therapy, 536t
Transgenic studies, of angiotensinogen,
   78–79
Transplantation, immunosuppression for,
   hypertension due to, 514, 566
Treatment of Mild Hypertension Study
   (TOMHS), blood pressure response
   in, 400t, 401
   comparison of antihypertensive agents
   in, 361
   of calcium antagonists, 614
   of lifestyle modification, in women,
   549
   vs. antihypertensive therapy, 335
   with weight reduction, 461
Trial of Antihypertensive Interventions
   and Management (TAIM), on sodium
   restriction effects, 440, 442, *442*
   on weight reduction, 461–462, 461t
Trial of Nonpharmacologic Interventions
   in Elderly (TONE), 445–446,
   444–446

Trials of Hypertension Prevention
   (TOHP), of magnesium
   supplementation, 457
   of sodium restriction, in Phase I, 440,
   441
   in Phase II, 442–445, *443–444*
   of weight reduction, 461, 461t
Triamterene, characteristics and dosage
   of, 587t
   combined with hydrochlorothiazide,
   500
Trichlormethiazide, NICS-EH trial of,
   338t, 346t, 350, 351t
Tricyclic antidepressants, hypertension
   due to, 566
Trimethaphan camsylate, 638, 639
Troglitazone, for diabetes mellitus,
   improvement of cardiovascular
   disease with, 114

Ultrasonography. See also
   Echocardiography.
   duplex Doppler, in renovascular hypertension, 665
   in blood pressure measurement, 309
   intravascular, in renovascular hypertension, contraindications to, 665–666
United Kingdom, initial choice of
   antihypertensive treatment in, *383,*
   385
United States, initial choice of
   antihypertensive treatment in,
   383–384, *383*
United States Food and Drug
   Administration, drug approval
   process of. See *Antihypertensive
   therapy, approval process for.*
United States Public Health Service
   (USPHS), Hospitals Cooperative
   Study Group, 342t–343t
   Trial, 332t
Unsaturated fatty acids, eicosanoid effects
   of, 180
Urban areas, blood pressure rise
   associated with, 9–10
Uric acid clearance, decrement of, in
   preeclampsia, 693
Urinalysis, in diagnosis of hypertension,
   302, 304t
Urodilatin. See *Natriuretic peptides.*
Uterus, abnormalities of, in preeclampsia,
   179, 693
Uvulopalatopharyngoplasty, for
   obstructive sleep apnea, 658

Valsartan. See also *Angiotensin II
   receptor antagonists.*
   combined with hydrochlorothiazide,
   dosage of, 501t
   development of, 624
   drug interactions with, 628
   pharmacokinetics of, in renal replacement therapy, 536t
   pharmacology of, 628, 631t
   structure of, *626*

Valsartan *(Continued)*
   VALUE trial of, 338t, 346t, 351t, 355–
   356
Vanguard studies, 203
Vascular centrencephalon, distribution of
   strokes in, 278, *279*
Vascular dementia, 11–12. See also
   Dementia.
Vascular disease. See also *Cardiovascular
   disease.*
   hypertension in etiology of, historical
   background of, 3
   in diabetes mellitus, predisposing factors in, 519–520, 519t
Vascular endothelium. See *Endothelium.*
Vascular remodeling. See also *Resistance
   vessels, remodeling of.*
   in pathophysiology of hypertension, 23
Vascular resistance, in pathophysiology of
   hypertension, 24
   in renal failure, 533
   reduction of, by kinins, 196
Vascular system. See *Artery(ies); Blood
   vessels; Cardiovascular system.*
Vasoconstrictor agent(s), angiotensin II
   as, 621–622
   endothelin as, 152, 153
   endothelin receptors as, 154–155
   in preeclampsia, 692
   short-acting, for supine hypertension,
   574
Vasodilator agent(s), calcium antagonist
   as, 611, 612
   characteristics and dosage of, 720t
   direct-acting smooth muscle relaxants
   as, 641–642
   endogenous, decrease of, in chronic renal failure, 525
   exercise interaction with, 475
   for peripheral vascular disease, 513
   in pregnancy, 698
   in renal replacement therapy, 536t
Vasomotor control center, 42
Vasopeptidase inhibitors, 651–654
   advantages and disadvantages of, 654
   combined angiotensin-converting enzyme and neutral endopeptidase inhibitors with, 652–654, *653*
   rationale for, 651–652
Ventricle(s), aging effects on, 553t
   arterial stiffening effects on, 141–142,
   143
   diastolic function/dysfunction of, 254–
   260
   aging and, 255–256
   assessment of, in diagnosis of hypertension, 301t
   clinical presentation and etiology of,
   254, *254*
   factors affecting, 255–256, *255*
   hemodynamic load in, 255
   hormone and paracrine factors in,
   256
   in white-coat hypertension, 318
   initial choice of therapy in, 486, 486t
   ischemia in, 254–255
   noninvasive measurement of, 256–
   259, *256–258*

Ventricle(s) *(Continued)*
emerging techniques in, 257–259, *256*
pitfalls in interpretation of, 257
structural factors in, 254
systolic function affecting, 255
treatment effects in, in asymptomatic dysfunction, 260
in congestive heart failure, 259–260
hypertrophy of, 244–253. See also *Heart, hypertrophy of; Heart failure, congestive.*
antihypertensive therapy for, for risk reduction, 242, 242t
safest level of blood pressure reduction in, 265
as risk factor, for cardiovascular events, 244, *245*
for coronary disease, 239–240, *240*
assessment of, as measure of outcome, 328
for management of antihypertensive therapy, 512
in diagnosis of hypertension, 301t
causes of, 247–251
hemodynamic factors in, 247–248, 248t, *249, 250*
nonhemodynamic factors in, 248t, 250–251
concentric, 245, *245*
concentric remodeling in, 245, *245*
coronary flow reserve abnormalities in, 260–267
definition of, 244
eccentric, 245, *245*
geometric patterns of, 244–246, *245–246*, 246t
in mild hypertension, 403
in obesity, 207
LIFE study of, 366–370
measurement of, 251–253
M-mode echocardiography in, 251–252, *252*, 252t
MRI, CT, and three-dimensional echocardiography in, 252–253
two-dimensional echocardiography in, 252–253
myocardial composition in, 246–247, *247*
regression of, by ACE inhibitors, 604
by angiotensin II receptor blockers, 632
by calcium antagonists, 615
by thiazide diuretics, 585
clinical trials of antihypertensive agents in, 253
structure of, 244–247
mass of, in white-coat hypertension, 316–317, *317*, 317t
obesity effects on, 207
systolic function of, assessment of, in diagnosis of hypertension, 301t
diastolic function related to, 255

Ventricle(s) *(Continued)*
in white-coat hypertension, 317–318
initial choice of therapy in, 485–486, 486t
Verapamil. See also *Calcium antagonists.*
adverse effects of, 613
cardioprotective effects of, 612
combined with, angiotensin-converting enzyme inhibitors, 614
β-blockers, 595, 613
calcium channel blockers, 542
hydrochlorothiazide, 501t
controlled-release, for control of early morning blood pressure surge, 507–508, *507*
CONVINCE trial of, 337, 338t, 346t, 351t, 354–355
DAVIT II trial of, 612
drug interactions with, 614
exercise interaction with, 475
for arrhythmias, 612
in chronic renal insufficiency, 292–293
in diabetes mellitus, renoprotective effects of, 522
in migraine, 513
INVEST trial of, 346t, 351t, 353
pharmacokinetics of, in renal replacement therapy, 536t
slow-release (retarded) preparation of, 617
structure of, *610*
VHAS study of, 613, 615
Veratrum alkaloids, adverse effects of, 641
pharmacology of, 641
Veratrum viride, for hypertension, adverse effects of, 2–3
Veterans Administration trials,
VA-NHLBI Feasibility Study in, 332t, 342t–343t
Veterans Administration Cooperative Study on Antihypertensive Agents, comparison of antihypertensive agents in, 361, 554
combination therapy in, 487–488
history of, 3
long-term outcome of, 332t
published results of, 342t–343t
Veterans Administration Trial in Severe Hypertension, 332t
VHAS (Verapamil Hypertension Atherosclerosis Study), 613, 615
Vitamin B$_6$ and Vitamin B$_{12}$, for hyperhomocysteinemia prevention, 283
Vitamin C, for coronary artery disease, 115
Vitamin E, for coronary artery disease, 115
for ischemic heart disease, 545
HOPE trial of, 346t–347t, 348–349
Volume, of fluids. See *Fluid(s).*
von Hippel-Lindau tumor suppressor gene, mutations in, 685

Walnut Creek Contraceptive Drug Study, 548

Wave reflection, augmentation of, as index of arterial stiffness, 139, *139,* 228
in elderly, 515
early return of, in elderly, 228–229
in hypertension, 143
time for return of, as index of arterial stiffness, 139, *139*
Weight. See also *Obesity.*
hypertension associated with, birth weight and, 10–11, 11t, 24, 558
pathophysiology of, 460
weight distribution and, 300
reduction of, alcohol consumption and, 215
diet for, clinical trials of, 461–462, 461t
hypertension lowered by, 208
exercise in, 509
for obstructive sleep apnea, 658
hypertension lowered by, 460–462
additive effect of antihypertensive drugs with, 462
clinical studies of, 461–462, 461t
with or without salt restriction, 208
in African Americans, 562
in women, 549
Weight-lifting exercise, 472
West of Scotland Coronary Prevention (WOSCOP) trial, 613
Westernized societies. See *Industrialized populations.*
White-coat hypertension. See *Hypertension, white-coat.*
Whites, alcohol consumption by, blood pressure levels in, 211, *212,* 213, *214*
angiotensinogen polymorphisms in, 80, 82t–83t, 87t
Williams' trait, 190
Windkessel model of arterial elasticity, 136, *136,* 139, *140*
Women. See also *Estrogen(s); Gender differences; Pregnancy.*
African-American, antihypertensive therapy in, 549
lifestyle modifications for, 549
obesity in, 559, 560
alcohol consumption by, blood pressure levels in, 211, *212, 214*
ALLHAT study of. See *Antihypertensive and Lipid-Lowering to Prevent Heart Attack Trial (ALLHAT).*
arterial stiffness in, 144, *145*
blood pressure in, 546–547, *546*
coronary artery disease in, 114–115, *115*
hypertension in, 546–550
antihypertensive therapy in, 549
adverse effects of, 483, 549
from hormone replacement therapy. See *Estrogen(s), replacement therapy with.*
from oral contraceptives, 77–78, 482–483, 548
initial choice of therapy for, 482–483, 482t